Current Veterinary Therapy 3

Food Animal Practice

Consulting Editors

Jimmy L. Howard, D.V.M., M.S.
Special Therapy and Procedures
Dietary Management
Diseases of the Urinary System
Neurologic Diseases

William Braun, Jr., D.V.M.
Neonatal Diseases and Disease Management

Mark F. Spire, D.V.M.
Herd Health Management

Ivan W. Caple, B.V.Sc., Ph.D.
Metabolic Disorders

John C. Halliburton, V.M.D.
Physical and Chemical Disorders

A. Konrad Eugster, D.V.M., Ph.D.
Diseases Caused by Viruses, Chlamydiae, and Mycoplasma

Søren Rosendal, D.V.M., and John F. Prescott, Vet. M.B., Ph.D.
Bacterial and Fungal Diseases

Sarel R. Van Amstel, B.V.Sc., M.Med.Vet.(Med.)
Protozoal and Rickettsial Diseases

Jerome G. Vestweber, D.V.M., Ph.D.
Diseases of the Respiratory System

Donald R. Clark, D.V.M.
Diseases of the Cardiovascular and Hemolymphatic System

Glen Hoffsis, D.V.M.
Diseases of the Digestive System

Louis F. Archbald, D.V.M.
Diseases of the Reproductive System

Thomas C. Randolph, D.V.M.*
Diseases of the Urinary System

Cecil P. Moore, D.V.M.
Diseases of the Eye

Bruce L. Hull, D.V.M.
Diseases of the Musculoskeletal System

Danny W. Scott, D.V.M.
Dermatologic Diseases

---
*Deceased.

Jimmy L. Howard, D.V.M., M.S.
Diplomate, American Board of
Veterinary Practitioners
(Food Animal Practice)
Coordinator of Veterinary Technology
Amarillo College
Amarillo, Texas

Current Veterinary Therapy 3

Food Animal Practice

W.B. SAUNDERS COMPANY
A Division of Harcourt Brace & Company
Philadelphia   London   Toronto   Montreal   Sydney   Tokyo

W.B. SAUNDERS COMPANY
A Division of
Harcourt Brace & Company

The Curtis Center
Independence Square West
Philadelphia, Pennsylvania 19106

Library of Congress Cataloging-in-Publication Data

Main entry under title:

Current veterinary therapy.

Includes index.

1. Veterinary medicine.   I. Howard, Jimmy L.
   II. Title: Food animal practice 3.
SF745.C784 1986   636.089′55   85–2006
ISBN 0–7216–3633–0

CURRENT VETERINARY THERAPY 3: Food Animal Practice   ISBN 0–7216–3633–0

Copyright © 1993, 1986, 1981 by W. B. Saunders Company.

All rights reserved. No part of this publication may be reproduced or transmitted in any form or by any means, electronic or mechanical, including photocopy, recording, or any information storage and retrieval system, without permission in writing from the publisher.

Printed in the United States of America.

Last digit is the print number: 9   8   7   6   5   4   3   2

The editor would like to dedicate
this Third Edition of
CURRENT VETERINARY THERAPY:
Food Animal Practice
to a very special friend and colleague,
Dr. Thomas Clayton Randolph, Jr.,
who died suddenly in 1991 at a very young age.
Tom was our consulting editor
for the Urinary Disease Section.
Tom graduated from Sallisaw High School,
Sallisaw, Oklahoma.
He received his DVM, MS, and BS degrees
from Oklahoma State University.
At the time of his death,
Tom was associate professor,
Economic and Performance Medicine,
at Mississippi State University.
The profession has lost a very fine member,
and he will certainly be missed.

CONTRIBUTORS

I. D. AITKEN, BVMS, PhD, MRCVS
Professor and Director, Moredun Research Institute, Edinburgh, Scotland.
Q Fever

WILLIAM MAURICE ALLEN, DVSc, PhD, MSc, MRCVS
Senior Partner, Compton Paddock Laboratories, Newbury, Berkshire, United Kingdom.
Parturient Paresis (Milk Fever) and Hypocalcemia (Cows, Ewes, and Goats)

ARNOLD D. ALSTAD, DVM, PhD
Head, Equine-Ovine Section, Diagnostic Virology Laboratory, National Veterinary Services Laboratory, Ames, Iowa.
Sweet Clover Poisoning

N. KENT AMES, DVM, MS
Associate Professor, College of Veterinary Medicine, Michigan State University, East Lansing, Michigan.
Fractures; Tendon Injuries

NEIL ANDERSON, DVM, PhD
Professor and Small Ruminant Clinician, College of Veterinary Medicine, Kansas State University, Manhattan, Kansas.
Management of Respiratory Disease in Sheep

JOHN J. ANDREWS, DVM, PhD, MS
Professor of Veterinary Pathology, Veterinary Diagnostic Laboratory, Iowa State University, Ames, Iowa.
Diarrhea in Neonatal Swine

DONNA WALTON ANGARANO, DVM, Diplomate, ACVD
Associate Professor of Dermatology, Department of Small Animal Surgery and Medicine, College of Veterinary Medicine, Auburn University, Auburn, Alabama.
Congenital and Hereditary Skin Diseases

LOUIS F. ARCHBALD, DVM, PhD, MS, Diplomate, ACT
Professor of Reproduction, College of Veterinary Medicine, University of Florida, Gainesville, Florida.
Section 13, Diseases of the Reproductive Tract; Pyometra in Cattle; Dairy Herd Reproductive Efficiency

C. H. ARMSTRONG, DVM, PhD
Professor Emeritus, School of Veterinary Medicine, Purdue University, West Lafayette, Indiana.
Swine Mycoplasmosis

ROBERT ASSAF, Agr MScV
Adjunct Professor, Institut Armand-Frappier, Université du Quebec, Ville de Laval, Quebec, Canada.
Porcine Cytomegalovirus (Inclusion Body Rhinitis)

PAUL BÆKBO, DVM, PhD
District Veterinarian, Veterinary Department, The Federation of Danish Pig Producers and Slaughterhouses, Denmark.
Pasteurellosis in Swine

C. V. BAGLEY, DVM
Associate Professor and Extension Veterinarian, Utah State University, Logan, Utah.
Toxicants in Geothermal Waters, Cooling Waters, and Mine Tailings; Fluoride Toxicosis

KENNETH G. BATEMAN, DVM, MSc
Associate Professor, Department of Population Medicine, and Field Service Clinic Head, Veterinary Teaching Hospital, Ontario Veterinary College, University of Guelph, Guelph, Ontario, Canada.
Pasteurellosis in Cattle

VAL R. BEASLEY, DVM, PhD
Associate Professor of Toxicology, College of Veterinary Medicine, University of Illinois at Urbana, Champaign, Illinois.
Trichothecenes

H. NEIL BECKER, DVM, MS
Technical Services Veterinarian, Animal Health Research and Development, The Upjohn Company, Kalamazoo, Michigan.
Reproductive Management Problems in Swine

G. J. BENSON, DVM, MS, Diplomate, ACVA
Professor, Veterinary Clinical Medicine, Anesthesiology, University of Illinois, Urbana, Illinois.
Anesthesia in Ruminants and Swine; Regional Analgesia

DANIEL M. BETTS, DVM, MS, Diplomate, ACVO
Professor, Veterinary Clinical Sciences, Iowa State University, Ames, Iowa.
Ophthalmic Examination Techniques for Food and Fiber Animals

RUDOLPH D. BIGALKE, DVSc, BVSc, Diploma in Applied Parasitology, Diploma in Advanced Public Administration
Executive Director, Department of Agricultural Development, Pretoria, South Africa.
Besnoitiosis

DENNIS J. BLODGETT, DVM, PhD
Associate Professor, Virginia–Maryland Regional College of Veterinary Medicine, Blacksburg, Virginia.
Renal Toxicants

DAWN M. BOOTHE, DVM, PhD, Diplomate, ACVIM, ACVCP
Assistant Professor, Department of Veterinary Physiology and Pharmacology, College of Veterinary Medicine, Texas A&M University. Attending Clinician, Veterinary Teaching Hospital, The Texas Veterinary Medical Center, Texas A&M University, College Station, Texas.
Adverse Drug Reactions

ROBERT T. BRANDT, JR, PhD, MS
Associate Professor of Animal Science, Kansas State University, Manhattan, Kansas.
Use of Growth Stimulants and Feed Additives in Ruminant Animal Production

R. KENNETH BRAUN, DVM, MS
Professor and Department Chair, Department of Large Animal Clinical Sciences, and Chief of Staff, Large Animal Hospital, Veterinary Medical Teaching Hospital, College of Veterinary Medicine, University of Florida, Gainesville, Florida.
Dairy Replacement Rearing Programs

WILLIAM BRAUN, JR, DVM, Diplomate, ACT
Associate Professor, Department of Veterinary Medicine and Surgery, University of Missouri, Columbia, Missouri.
Section 2, Neonatal Diseases and Disease Management

ROGER BREEZE, BVMS, PhD, MRCVS
Director, U.S. Department of Agriculture, Agricultural Research Service, Plum Island Animal Disease Center, Greenport, New York.
Acute Bovine Pulmonary Edema and Emphysema; Vena Caval Thrombosis

KATHERINE BRETZLAFF, DVM, PhD
Associate Professor, Department of Large Animal Medicine and Surgery, Texas A&M University. Theriogenologist, Texas Veterinary Medical Center, College Station, Texas.
Production Medicine and Health Programs for Goats

JANICE C. BRIDGER, BSc, PhD
Principal Scientific Officer, Department of Microbiology, AFRC Institute for Animal Health, Compton, Berkshire, United Kingdom.
Bovine Astroviruses; Bovine Calici-like Viruses; Ovine Astroviruses

TALMAGE T. BROWN, JR, DVM, PhD
Professor of Veterinary Pathology and Pathologist, Veterinary Teaching Hospital, College of Veterinary Medicine, North Carolina State University, Raleigh, North Carolina.
Enteroviral Encephalomyelitis of Pigs (Teschen Disease)

GORDON W. BRUMBAUGH, DVM, PhD, Diplomate, ACVIM, ACVCP
Associate Professor, Department of Veterinary Physiology and Pharmacology, College of Veterinary Medicine, Texas A&M University. Staff, Department of Large Animal Medicine and Surgery, Texas A&M University, College Station, Texas.
Adverse Drug Reactions

CINDY J. BRUNNER, DVM, PhD
Assistant Professor, Department of Pathobiology, College of Veterinary Medicine, Auburn University, Auburn, Alabama.
Immunologic Disorders and Immunotherapy

WILLIAM B. BUCK, DVM, PhD, Diplomate ABVT
Professor of Toxicology, Department of Veterinary Biosciences, College of Veterinary Medicine, University of Illinois. Director, National Animal Poison Control Center, Urbana, Illinois
Copper-Molybdenum Toxicosis

MARIE S. BULGIN, DVM
Professor of Ovine Production Medicine, Caine Veterinary Teaching and Research Center, University of Idaho, Caldwell, Idaho.
Ovine Production Management and Preventive Medicine

ELIZABETH C. BURGESS, DVM, PhD
Assistant Professor, Department of Medical Sciences, School of Veterinary Medicine, University of Wisconsin, Madison, Wisconsin.
Borreliosis in Cattle

GEORGE E. BURROWS, DVM, PhD
Professor of Toxicology, College of Veterinary Medicine, Oklahoma State University, Stillwater, Oklahoma.
Principal Poisonous Plants in the Midwestern and Eastern United States

DANIEL G. BUTLER, DVM, MSc, PhD
Professor of Large Animal Medicine, Department of Clinical Studies, Ontario Veterinary College, and Veterinary Teaching Hospital, University of Guelph, Ontario, Canada.
Paratuberculosis (Johne's Disease)

JERRY CALLIS, DVM, DSc, MS
Formerly, Director of Plum Island Animal Disease Center, U.S. Department of Agriculture, Agricultural Research Service, Southold, New York.
Foot-and-Mouth Disease in Cattle; Foot-and-Mouth Disease in Sheep and Goats; Foot-and-Mouth Disease in Pigs

IVAN W. CAPLE, BVSc, PhD
Professor of Veterinary Medicine, School of Veterinary Science, University of Melbourne, Parkville, Australia.
Section 5, Metabolic Disorders; Acetonemia; Pregnancy Toxemia; Ruminant Hypomagnesemic Tetanies

JAMES R. CARLSON, PhD
Chair, Department of Animal Sciences, Washington State University, Pullman, Washington.
Acute Bovine Pulmonary Edema and Emphysema

WILLIAM W. CARLTON, DVM, PhD
Professor of Veterinary Pathobiology, Purdue University, West Lafayette, Indiana.
Ochratoxin; Citrinin; Stachybotryotoxicosis

R. L. CARSON, DVM, MS, Diplomate, ACT
Associate Professor and Chief of Theriogenology, School of Veterinary Medicine, Auburn University, Auburn, Alabama.
Diseases of the Male Internal Genitalia; Diseases of the Penis and Prepuce

T. L. CARSON, DVM, PhD, MS
Professor of Veterinary Pathology, College of Veterinary Medicine, Iowa State University. Veterinary Toxicologist, Veterinary Diagnostic Laboratory, Ames, Iowa.
Water Quality for Livestock; Organophosphorus and Carbamate Insecticides

ARTHUR A. CASE, DVM, MS*
Formerly, College of Veterinary Medicine, University of Missouri, Columbia, Missouri.
Principal Poisonous Plants in the Midwestern and Eastern United States

---
*Deceased.

HOWARD H. CASPER, PhD
Toxicology Section Supervisor, North Dakota Veterinary Diagnostic Laboratory, North Dakota State University, Fargo, North Dakota.
Sweet Clover Poisoning

ANTHONY E. CASTRO, DVM, PhD
Associate Adjunct Professor, School of Veterinary Medicine, University of California, Davis, California.
Malignant Catarrhal Fever

WILLIAM P. CHEEVERS, PhD
Professor, Department of Veterinary Microbiology and Pathology, Washington State University, Pullman, Washington
Caprine Arthritis-Encephalitis Virus

M. M. CHENGAPPA, BVSc, PhD
Professor of Microbiology, Department of Laboratory Medicine, College of Veterinary Medicine, and Director, Diagnostic Bacteriology and Mycology, Veterinary Medical Teaching Hospital, Kansas State University, Manhattan, Kansas.
Clostridial Enterotoxemia (Clostridium perfringens)

DONALD R. CLARK, DVM, PhD, Diplomate, ADVIM (Cardiology)
Professor, Department of Veterinary Physiology and Pharmacology, Texas A&M University, College Station, Texas
Section 11, Diseases of the Circulatory System; Cardiovascular Pathophysiology; Diseases of the General Circulation

BILLY R. CLAY, DVM, MS, Diplomate, ABVT
Adjunct Professor, College of Veterinary Medicine, Oklahoma State University, Stillwater, Oklahoma.
Oak Poisoning

N. ANDY COLE, PhD
Supervisory Research Animal Scientist, U.S. Department of Agriculture, Agriculture Research Service, Conservation and Production Research Laboratory, Bushland, Texas.
Nutritional Management of Stressed and Morbid Calves

B. KEITH COLLINS, DVM, MS, Diplomate, ACVD
Assistant Professor, Department of Veterinary Medicine and Surgery, College of Veterinary Medicine, University of Missouri, Columbia, Missouri.
Neuro-ophthalmology in Food Animals

JOSEPH F. CONNOR, DVM
Veterinarian, Carthage Veterinary Service, Ltd., Carthage, Illinois.
Swine Herd Health Management

ROBERT J. CONNOR, DVetMed, MVSc, MRCVS
Specialist in Regional Trypanosomiasis, Regional Tsetse and Trypanosomiasis Control Programme, Avondale, Harare, Zimbabwe, Central Africa.
Trypanosomiasis

PETER D. CONSTABLE, BVSc, MS, MRCVS, Diplomate, ACVIM
Clinical Instructor, College of Veterinary Medicine, The Ohio State University, Columbus, Ohio.
Introduction to the Ruminant Forestomach; Diseases of the Abomasum and Small Intestine; Diseases of the Large Intestine; Therapeutic Management of Cardiovascular and Hemolymphatic Diseases

LARRY R. CORAH, PhD
Professor, Animal Science Department, Kansas State University, Manhattan, Kansas.
Dietary Management of the Beef Breeding Herd

ROBERT M. CORWIN, DVM, PhD
Professor of Veterinary Medicine, University of Missouri, Columbia, Missouri.
Anthelmintic Therapy

ROSS P. COWART, DVM, MS, Diplomate, ABVP
Associate Professor, Food Animal Medicine and Surgery, College of Veterinary Medicine, University of Missouri, Columbia, Missouri.
Hypoglycemia and Hypothermia in Neonatal Pigs

ROBERT A. CRANDELL, DVM, BS, MPH
Formerly, Head, Diagnostic Microbiology, Texas Veterinary Medical Diagnostic Laboratory, Texas A&M University, College Station, Texas.
Diagnosis of Viral Diseases; Infectious Bovine Rhinotracheitis; Pseudorabies (Aujeszky's Disease, "Mad Itch"); Bovine Papular Stomatitis; Contagious Ecthyma; Arthrogryposis-Hydranencephaly in Sheep: Cache Valley Virus Infection; Porcine Pseudorabies (Aujeszky's Disease)

WILLIAM H. CRAWFORD, DVM, MVSc, Diplomate, ACVS
Staff Surgeon, Young-Crawford Veterinary Clinic, Mercer, Pennsylvania.
Stifle Injuries and Patellar Luxations

RANDALL C. CUTLIP, DVM, PhD
U. S. Department of Agriculture, Agricultural Research Service, National Animal Disease Center, Ames, Iowa.
Maedi-Visna (Ovine Progressive Pneumonia, Zwoegerziekte); Sheep Pulmonary Adenomatosis (Sheep Pulmonary Carcinoma; Jaagsiekte)

LLOYD E. DAVIS, DVM, PhD, Diplomate, ACVCP
Professor of Clinical Pharmacology, College of Veterinary Medicine, and Veterinary Medical Teaching Hospital, University of Illinois, Urbana, Illinois.
Drugs Affecting the Digestive System

SCOTT A. DEE, DVM, MS
Swine Practitioner, Swine Health Center, Morris, Minnesota.
Eubacterium suis

A. J. DELLA-PORTA, BSc, PhD
Deputy Head of Laboratory, CSIRO, Australian Animal Health Laboratory, Geelong, Victoria, Australia.
Akabane Disease in Cattle; Akabane Disease in Sheep and Goats

STANLEY M. DENNIS, BVSc, PhD, FRCVS, FRCPath
Professor of Pathology, College of Veterinary Medicine, Kansas State University, Manhattan, Kansas.
Congenital Defects of Cattle and Sheep; Listeriosis (Circling Disease, Silage Sickness)

LUC A. DEVRIESE, DVM
Werkleider (Chef de Travaux), Faculty of Veterinary Medicine, University of Ghent, Ghent, Belgium.
Staphylococcal Diseases

DANIËL THEODORUS DE WAAL, BVSc
Assistant Director, Protozoology Division, Veterinary Research Institute, Onderstepoort, South Africa.
Babesiosis

G. ARTHUR DONOVAN, DVM
Associate Professor, Department of Large Animal Clinical Sciences, College of Veterinary Medicine, University of Florida. Service Chief, Rural Animal Medicine Service, Veterinary Medical Teaching Hospital, Gainesville, Florida.
Dairy Cow Production Medicine; Dairy Replacement Rearing Programs

J. C. DOYLE, DVM, PhD
Staff, Nutrition Service Associates, Technical Services, Hereford, Texas.
Mineral Supplementation for Beef Cattle on Rangeland

J. P. DUBEY, MVSc, PhD
Senior Scientist, Zoonotic Diseases Laboratory, Livestock and Poultry Sciences Institute, U. S. Department of Agriculture, Beltsville, Maryland.
Toxoplasmosis; Sarcocytosis

JOHN DUFTY, BVSc, RDA
Principal Research Scientist, Commonwealth Scientific and Industrial Research Organization, Division of Animal Health,

Animal Health Research Laboratory, Parkville, Victoria, Australia.
Bovine Veneral Campylobacteriosis

B. C. EASTERDAY, DVM, PhD
Dean and Professor, School of Veterinary Medicine, University of Wisconsin, Madison, Wisconsin.
Swine Influenza

A. J. EDWARDS, DVM, PhD
Professor Emeritus, Feedlot Specialist, Kansas State University, Manhattan, Kansas.
Feedlot Health Management

WILLIAM C. EDWARDS, DVM
Interim Director, Oklahoma Animal Disease Diagnostic Laboratory, Oklahoma State University, Stillwater, Oklahoma.
Petroleum and Petroleum Products

TERRY J. ENGELKEN, DVM, MS
Assistant Professor, Diagnostic and Field Service Program, College of Veterinary Medicine, Mississippi State University, Mississippi State, Mississippi.
Management of Large-Producer Calf/Cow Herds

E. DENIS ERICKSON, DVM, PhD
Professor, Department of Veterinary Science, University of Nebraska, Lincoln, Nebraska.
Streptococcal Disease

A. KONRAD EUGSTER, DVM, PhD
Executive Director, Texas Veterinary Medical Diagnostic Laboratory, College Station, Texas.
Section 7, Viruses, Chlamidiae, and Mycoplasma; Bovine Chlamydiosis; Caprine and Ovine Herpesviruses

M. L. FAHNING, DVM, PhD
Professor and Head, Theriogenology Division, College of Veterinary Medicine, University of Minnesota, St. Paul, Minnesota.
Retained Fetal Membranes

JOHN M. FAIRBROTHER, BVSc, PhD
Associate Professor Faculté de Medecine Vétérinaire, Université de Montréal, St. Hyacinthe, Quebec.
Escherichia coli Infections in Farm Animals

JAMES G. FLOYD, Jr, DVM, MS, Diplomate, ACT
Extension Veterinarian and Associate Professor, Department of Animal and Dairy Sciences, and Adjunct Associate Professor, Department of Large Animal Surgery and Medicine, College of Veterinary Medicine, Auburn University, Auburn, Alabama.
Urolithiasis in Food Animals (Urinary Calculi, Waterbelly, Calculosis)

MURRAY E. FOWLER, DVM
Professor Emeritus, School of Veterinary Medicine, and Zoological Medicine Service, Veterinary Medical Teaching Hospital, University of California, Davis, California.
Poisonous Plants in Harvested or Prepared Foods; Cardiotoxic Plants; Hepatotoxic Plants; Zootoxins

GLYNN H. FRANK, DVM, PhD, MS
Veterinary Medical Officer, U. S. Department of Agriculture, Agricultural Research Service, National Animal Disease Center, Ames, Iowa.
Parainfluenza-3 Virus

MERWIN L. FREY, DVM, PhD
Head, Bovine-Porcine Viruses Section, Diagnostic Virology Laboratory, National Veterinary Services Laboratories, Ames, Iowa.
Bovine Mycoplasmosis

DEBORAH S. FRIEDMAN, DVM, Diplomate, ACVO
Clinical Ophthalmologist, Animal Emergency Center, Milwaukee, Wisconsin.
Ophthalmology of South American Camelids: Llamas, Alpacas, Guanacos, and Vicuñas

JOSEPH H. GAINER, DVM
Veterinary Medical Officer, Food and Drug Administration, Beltsville, Maryland.
Encephalomyocarditis Virus

FRANCIS D. GALEY, DVM, PhD, Diplomate, ABVT
Assistant Professor of Clinical Diagnostic Veterinary Toxicology, California Veterinary Diagnostic Laboratory System, University of California, Davis, California.
Arsenic Toxicosis

DONNA M. GATEWOOD, DVM, MS
Veterinary Medical Officer, National Veterinary Services Laboratories, U. S. Department of Agriculture, APHIS, Ames, Iowa.
Clostridial Enterotoxemia (Clostridium perfringens)

E. PAUL J. GIBBS, BVSc, PhD, FRCVS
Professor of Virology, College of Veterinary Medicine, and Chief, Microbiology and Parasitology Service, University of Florida, Gainesville, Florida.
Cowpox and Bovine Vaccinia Mammillitis; Pseudocowpox; Sheep and Goat Pox

JULIET RATHBONE GIONFRIDDO, DVM, MS, Diplomate, ACVO
Clinical Ophthalmologist, Eye Clinic for Animals, Overland Park, Kansas.
Ophthalmology of South American Camelids: Llamas, Alpacas, Guanacos, and Vicuñas

ROBERT D. GLOCK, DVM, PhD
Director, Veterinary Diagnostic Laboratories, Colorado State University, Fort Collins, Colorado.
Swine Dysentery

ROBERT A. GODKE, PhD
Professor of Animal Science, Department of Animal Science, and Adjunct Professor of Veterinary Physiology, Department of Physiology, Pharmacology and Toxicology, School of Veterinary Medicine, Louisiana State University, Baton Rouge, Louisiana.
Synchronization of Estrus

DAN E. GOODWIN, DVM, PhD
Formerly, Director, Oklahoma Animal Disease Diagnostic Laboratory, College of Veterinary Medicine, Oklahoma State University, Stillwater, Oklahoma.
Abortion—An Approach to Diagnosis

DOUGLAS GREGG, DVM, MEd, PhD
Veterinary Pathologist and Electron Microscopist, Foreign Animal Disease Diagnostic Laboratory, U. S. Department of Agriculture, NVSL, APHIS, Greenport, New York.
Foot-and-Mouth Disease in Cattle; Foot-and-Mouth Disease in Sheep and Goats; Foot-and-Mouth Disease in Pigs

DEENA G. GREGORY, DVM
Veterinary Toxicology Resident, Oklahoma Animal Disease Diagnostic Laboratory, College of Veterinary Medicine, Oklahoma State University, Stillwater, Oklahoma.
Oak Poisoning

JOHN C. HALLIBURTON, VMD
Texas A&M University, Amarillo, Texas.
Section 6, Physical and Chemical Disorders

FAROUK M. HAMDY, DVM, PhD
Co-Director, Mexico–U.S. Commission for Prevention of Foot and Mouth Disease and Other Exotic Animal Diseases, Laredo, Texas.
Rinderpest

MICHAEL S. HAND, DVM, PhD, Diplomate, ACVN
Research Veterinarian, Mark Morris Associates, Topeka, Kansas. Adjunct Professor, College of Veterinary Medicine, Kansas State University, Manhattan, Kansas. Adjunct Professor, College of Veterinary Medicine, North Carolina State University, Raleigh, North Carolina.
Field Calculations for Ration Formulation; Special Dietary Management in Lactation and Gestation; New Concepts for Measuring Proteins for Cattle

SEBASTIAN E. HEATH, Vet MB, MVSc, MRCVS, Diplomate, ACVIM
Assistant Professor and Section Chief, Large Animal Medicine, Purdue University, West Lafayette, Indiana.
Bovine Mastitis

R. P. HERD, MVSc, PhD
Professor, College of Veterinary Medicine, The Ohio State University, Columbus, Ohio.
Trematode Infections in Cattle, Sheep, and Goats; Cestode Infections in Cattle, Sheep, Goats, and Swine; Nematode Infections in Cattle, Sheep, Goats, and Swine

STAN HERR, BVSc, BVSc(HONS), MMedVet (Gyn), Diplomate, AgRIC
Assistant Director, Bacteriology/Reproduction (Head of Section), Onderstepoort Veterinary Institute, Onderstepoort, South Africa.
Trichomoniasis in Cattle

WERNER P. HEUSCHELE, DVM, PhD, Diplomate, ACVM
Adjunct Professor, Department of Pathology, School of Medicine, University of California, San Diego, California. Adjunct Professor, Department of Veterinary Science, University of Arizona, Tucson, Arizona.
Bovine Viral Diarrhea–Mucosal Disease

CLAIR M. HIBBS, DVM, MS, PhD
Pathologist, Kansas State University, Manhattan, Kansas.
Salmonellosis

CHARLES A. HJERPE, DVM
Professor of Veterinary Medicine, School of Veterinary Medicine, and Director, Veterinary Medical Teaching Hospital, University of California, Davis, California.
The Bovine Respiratory Disease Complex; Respiratory Therapeutics

WALTER E. HOFFMAN, DVM, PhD
Professor, Veterinary Pathobiology, University of Illinois, College of Veterinary Medicine, Veterinary Medical Teaching Hospital, Urbana, Illinois.
Appendix: A Partial List of Reference Ranges

GLEN F. HOFFSIS, DVM, MS, Diplomate, ACVIM
Professor, Food Animal Medicine and Surgery, and Director, Veterinary Teaching Hospital, The Ohio State University, Columbus, Ohio.
Section 12, Diseases of the Digestive System; Diseases of the Abomasum and Small Intestine

JIMMY L. HOWARD, DVM, MS, Diplomate, ABVP
Coordinator of Veterinary Technology, Amarillo College, Amarillo, Texas.
Section 1, Special Therapy and Procedures; Section 4, Dietary Management; Section 14, Diseases of the Urinary System; Section 16, Neurologic Diseases

J. T. HUBER, PhD
Professor of Ruminant Nutrition, Department of Animal Sciences, University of Arizona, Tucson, Arizona.
Dietary Management of Dairy Cattle

R. S. HUDSON, DVM, MS, Diplomate, ACT
Consultant in Veterinary Medicine in Japan.
Diseases of the Male Internal Genitalia; Diseases of the Penis and Prepuce

BRUCE L. HULL, DVM, MS, Diplomate, ACVS
Professor, Department of Veterinary Medicine, The Ohio State University, Columbus, Ohio.
Section 17, Diseases of the Musculoskeletal System; Introduction to the Musculoskeletal System; Sole Abscesses; Vertical Wall Cracks; Horizontal Wall Cracks; Rusterholz Ulcer; Verrucose Dermatitis; Spondylitis

ELAINE HUNT, DVM, Diplomate, ACVIM
Associate Professor, College of Veterinary Medicine, North Carolina State University, Raleigh, North Carolina.
Diarrheal Diseases of Neonatal Ruminants

J. E. HUSTON, PhD
Professor of Animal Science, Texas Agricultural Experimental Station, Texas A&M University, San Angelo, Texas.
Dietary Management in Goats; Mineral Supplementation for Beef Cattle on Rangeland

DAVID P. HUTCHESON, PhD
Professor of Animal Nutrition, Texas Agricultural Experiment Station, Texas A&M University, Amarillo, Texas.
Cattle Feeding

LYNN F. JAMES, PhD
Research Animal Scientist, U. S. Department of Agriculture, Agricultural Research Service, Poisonous Plant Research Laboratory, Logan, Utah.
Principal Poisonous Plants in the Western United States; Effects of Plant Toxins on the Central Nervous System; Oxalate Accumulators; Selenium Accumulators

A. EARL JOHNSON, MS
Formerly, U. S. Department of Agriculture, Poisonous Plant Research Laboratory, Logan, Utah.
Plants Producing Dermal Injury

LaRUE W. JOHNSON, DVM, PhD
Associate Professor, Department of Clinical Sciences, Colorado State University, Fort Collins, Colorado.
Llama Herd Health Management

ROBERT KAINER, DVM, MS
Professor Emeritus, Department of Anatomy, College of Veterinary Medicine and Biomedical Sciences, Colorado State University, Fort Collins, Colorado.
Food Animal Ocular Neoplasia

THOMAS R. KASARI, DVM, MVSc, Diplomate, ACVIM
Associate Professor, Food Animal Medicine, Department of Large Animal Medicine and Surgery, Texas A&M University, College Station, Texas.
Omphalitis and Its Sequelae in Ruminants

ARNOLD F. KAUFMANN, DVM, MS
Acting Chief, Mycotic Diseases Branch, Division of Bacterial and Mycotic Diseases, National Center for Infectious Diseases, Centers for Disease Control, Atlanta, Georgia.
Anthrax

RICHARD F. KEELER, PhD
Research Chemist, Poisonous Plant Research Laboratory, Logan, Utah.
Plants Teratogenic in Livestock

DAVID P. KELBERT, DVM
Private Practitioner, Jacksonville, Florida.
Dairy Cow Production Medicine

JOE D. KENDALL, DVM, MS
Research Associate, Department of Pathology, University of Missouri, Columbia, Missouri.
Taxus (Yew) Poisoning; Chlorinated Hydrocarbon Insecticides

GEORGE A. KENNEDY, DVM, PhD, Diplomate, ACVP
Professor, Diagnostic Laboratory, Kansas State University, Manhattan, Kansas.
Salmonellosis

LARRY A. KERR, DVM, MS
Associate Professor, University of Tennessee, College of Veterinary Medicine, Knoxville, Tennessee.
Perilla frutescens (Purple Mint) Toxicosis in Cattle; Fescue Toxicosis

KARL W. KERSTING, DVM, MS
Assistant Professor, Department of Veterinary Clinical Sciences, and Head, Food Animal Section, Veterinary Teaching Hospital, College of Veterinary Medicine, Iowa State University, Ames, Iowa.
Diseases of the Ruminant Forestomach

CLEON V. KIMBERLING, DVM, MPH
Extension Veterinarian, Colorado State University, Fort Collins, Colorado.
Sheep Feedlot Management

DONALD P. KNOWLES, Jr, DVM, PhD
Veterinary Medical Officer, U. S. Department of Agriculture, Agricultural Research Service, Department of Veterinary Mi-

crobiology-Pathology, Washington State University, Pullman, Washington.
Caprine Arthritis-Encephalitis Virus

GERARD J. KOENIG, DVM, MS
Veterinary Clinician, Veterinary Medical Teaching and Research Center, University of California at Davis, Tulare, California.
Choke; Fescue Foot

L. D. KONYHA, DVM, MS
Director, Southeast Region Veterinary Services, U. S. Department of Agriculture, APHIS, Tampa, Florida.
Tuberculosis

M. M. KOTHMANN, PhD, MS
Professor, Department of Range Science, Texas A&M University, College Station, Texas.
Nutrition for Livestock Grazing Rangelands and Pasturelands

PALLE KROGH, DVM, PhD*
Formerly, Professor, Veterinary Pathology and Toxicology, Purdue University, West Lafayette, Indiana.
Ochratoxin

JERRY P. KUNESH, DVM, PhD, MS
Professor of Veterinary Clinical Sciences, College of Veterinary Medicine, Iowa State University, Ames, Iowa.
Swine Erysipelas

VERNON C. LANGSTON, DVM, PhD, Diplomate, ACVCP
Assistant Professor, College of Veterinary Medicine, Department of Basic Sciences, Mississippi State University, Mississippi State, Mississippi.
Therapeutic Management of Inflammation; Therapeutic Management of Urinary Diseases

VAUGHN L. LARSON, DVM, PhD,
Professor, Clinical and Population Sciences Department, College of Veterinary Medicine, and Clinician, Veterinary Teaching Hospital, University of Minnesota, St. Paul, Minnesota.
Upper Respiratory System Diseases

J. A. LAWRENCE, BSc, DPhil, MRCVS, DTVM
Department of Veterinary Medicine, University of Malawi, Lilongue, Malawi, Africa.
Theileriosis

G. H. K. LAWSON, BVM & S, PhD, BSc, MRCVS
Reader, Faculty of Veterinary Medicine, Edinburgh University, Veterinary Field Station, Easter Bush, Roslin, Lothian, United Kingdom.
Campylobacter Proliferative Enteropathies of Pigs

---
*Deceased.

H. W. LEIPOLD, DVM, MS, PhD
Professor of Pathology, Kansas State University, Manhattan, Kansas.
Congenital Defects of Cattle and Sheep

THOMAS L. LESTER, DVM, PhD, ACVM
Veterinary Virologist, Texas Veterinary Medical Diagnostic Laboratory, College Station, Texas.
Bovine Rotavirus; Calf Coronavirus Diarrhea; Ovine Rotavirus

PETER B. LITTLE, DVM, PhD, MS, Diplomate, ACVP
Professor, Department of Pathology, and Head of Laboratory Services, Veterinary Teaching Hospital, University of Guelph, Guelph, Ontario, Canada.
The Haemophilus somnus Complex

D. H. LLOYD, BVetMed, PhD, FRCVS
Senior Lecturer in Dermatology, Royal Veterinary College, University of London, Herts, United Kingdom.
Dermatophilosis

R. K. LOVEDAY, BVSc, Diplomate, MedVet
Professor Emeritus, Faculty of Veterinary Science, University of Pretoria, Onderstepoort, South Africa. Staff, Department of National Health, Pretoria.
Porcine Eperythrozoonosis

S. K. LYLE, DVM, Diplomate, ACT
Veterinarian, Tampa Bay Veterinary Referral, Inc., Largo, Florida.
Lactation Failure

JOHN A. LYNCH, DVM, MSc, DVSc, Diplomate, ACVM
Adjunct Faculty, Ontario Veterinary College, Department of Veterinary Microbiology and Immunology, University of Guelph. Chief Microbiologist, Agricultural and Food Laboratory Services Branch, Ontario Ministry of Agriculture and Food, Guelph, Ontario, Canada.
Nocardioses

JAKOB MALMO, BVSc, FACVSc
Senior Academic Associate, Faculty of Veterinary Science, University of Melbourne, Melbourne, Australia. Director, Rural Veterinary Unit at Maffra, Victoria, Australia.
Downer Cow Syndrome

DEBORAH MARSH, BS
Research Associate, Colorado State University, Fort Collins, Colorado.
Sheep Feedlot Management

ROGER MARSHALL, BVSc, PhD, MS
Associate Professor, Department of Veterinary Pathology and Public Health, Faculty of Veterinary Science, Massey University, Palmerston North, New Zealand.
Nonvenereal Campylobacteriosis

W. B. MARTIN, DVSM, PhD, CIBiol, FIBiol, FRSE, MRCVS
Formerly, Scientific Director, Moredun Research Institute, Edinburgh, United Kingdom.
Bovine Mammillitis

DONALD MATTSON, DVM, PhD
Associate Professor, Veterinary Immunology Service, Veterinary Diagnostic Laboratory, College of Veterinary Medicine, Oregon State University, Corvallis, Oregon.
Bovine Adenoviruses; Ovine and Caprine Adenoviruses; Porcine Adenoviruses

DAVID McCLARY, DVM, MS, Diplomate, ACT
Research Scientist, Lilly Research Laboratories, Eli Lilly and Co., Greenfield, Indiana.
Bovine Somatotropin

C. PAT McCOY, DVM, MS
Professor of Veterinary Toxicology and Pathology, College of Veterinary Medicine, Mississippi State University, Mississippi State, Mississippi.
Ionophores: Monensin, Lasalocid, Salinomycin, and Narasin

CHRISTOPHER J. McCAUGHAN, BVSc, MACVSc
Senior Research Fellow, Faculty of Veterinary Science, University of Melbourne, Werribee, Australia.
Postparturient Hemoglobinuria

H. A. McDANIEL, DVM, PhD
Formerly, U. S. Department of Agriculture, APHIS, Hyattsville, Maryland.
African Swine Fever

SHEILA M. McGUIRK, DVM, PhD, Diplomate, ACVIM
Associate Professor, Department of Medical Sciences, and Head, Section on Large Animal Medicine, University of Wisconsin, Madison, Wisconsin.
Diseases of the Abomasum and Small Intestine

JAMES D. McKEAN, DVM, MS, JD
Extension Veterinarian, Iowa State University, Ames, Iowa.
Neonatal Polyarthritis in Swine

J. G. McLEAN, BVSc, PhD
Dean, Faculty of Applied Science, Swinburne Institute of Technology, Hawthorn, Australia.
Acetonemia; Pregnancy Toxemia

LINDA MEDLEAU, DVM, MS, Diplomate, ACVD
Associate Professor of Dermatology, Department of Small Animal Medicine, College of Veterinary Medicine, University of Georgia, Athens, Georgia.
Fungal Dematoses

WILLIAM L. MENGELING, DVM, PhD
Research Leader, U. S. Department of Agriculture, Agricultural Research Service, National Animal Disease Center, Ames, Iowa.
Porcine Parvovirus–Induced Reproductive Failure of Swine; Mystery Pig Disease; Encephatis–Vomiting and Wasting Disease Complex of Swine; SMEDI and Other Porcine Enteroviruses

PAULA I. MENZIES, DVM, MPVM
Assistant Professor, Ruminant Health Management Group, Department of Population Medicine, Ontario Veterinary College, University of Guelph, Guelph, Ontario, Canada.
Corynebacterium *Species Infections in Food Animals*

H. DWIGHT MERCER, DVM, PhD
Professor of Toxicology and Dean of the College of Veterinary Medicine, Mississippi State University, Mississippi State, Mississippi.
Prevention and Management of Drug and Chemical Residues in Meat and Milk

W. DUANE MICKELSEN, DVM, MS, Diplomate, ACT
Associate Professor, and Chief, Theriogenology, Department of Veterinary Clinical Medicine and Surgery, Washington State University, Pullman, Washington.
Evaluation of Reproductive Efficiency in Beef Cattle Herds

DUANE MIKSCH, DVM, MS
Extension Veterinarian, University of Kentucky, Princeton, Kentucky.
Management of Farm Cow/Calf Herds

JANICE M. MILLER, DVM, PhD, MS, BS
Veterinary Medical Officer, U. S. Department of Agriculture, Agricultural Research Service, National Animal Disease Center, Ames, Iowa.
Bovine Leukemia Virus

ROBERT B. MILLER, DVM, PhD
Associate Professor and Head, Food Animal Section, College of Veterinary Medicine, University of Missouri, Columbia, Missouri.
Infectious and Parasitic Eye Diseases of Cattle

WILLIAM H. MILLER, Jr, VMD
Associate Professor of Medicine, College of Veterinary Medicine, Cornell University, Ithaca, New York.
Nutritional, Endocrine, and Keratinization Abnormalities

SASHI B. MOHANTY, BVSc, PhD
Professor and Associate Dean, Virginia-Maryland Regional College of Veterinary Medicine, University of Maryland, College Park, Maryland.
Bovine Reoviruses; Ovine and Caprine Reoviruses; Porcine Reoviruses

CECIL P. MOORE, DVM, MS, Diplomate, ACVO
Associate Professor, Department of Veterinary Medicine, College of Veterinary Medicine, and Head, Ophthalmology Section, Veterinary Teaching Hospital, University of Missouri, Columbia, Missouri.
Section 15, Diseases of the Eye; Infectious and Parasitic Eye Diseases of Cattle; Selected Eye Diseases of Sheep and Goats

LARRY F. MOORE, DVM
Veterinarian, Senior Professional Services, Food Animal Products, Shawnee Mission, Kansas.
External Parasiticides

SANDRA E. MORGAN, DVM, MS
Assistant Professor and Ambulatory/Field Service Clinician, Food Animal Section, Department of Medicine and Surgery, Boren Veterinary Medical Teaching Hospital, Oklahoma State University, Stillwater, Oklahoma.
Ammoniated Feed Toxicosis; Gossypol Toxicosis

JOHN C. MORRILL, DVM, PhD
Chief, Clinical Immunology Department, U. S. Army Medical Research Institute of Infectious Diseases, Fort Detrick, Maryland.
Rift Valley Fever in Cattle; Rift Valley Fever in Sheep and Goats

C. ANNE MUCKLE, DVM, MSc, PhD
Veterinarian, New Hazards Laboratory and Health of Animals Laboratory, Guelph, Ontario, Canada.
Corynebacterium *Species Infections in Food Animals*

MICHAEL J. MURPHY, DVM, PhD, Diplomate, ABVT
Assistant Professor, Department of Veterinary Diagnostic Medicine, College of Veterinary Medicine, University of Minnesota, St. Paul, Minnesota.
Rodenticides

STEVEN S. NICHOLSON, DVM
Associate Professor, Department of Veterinary Pharmacology, Physiology, and Toxicology, Louisiana State University, Baton Rouge, Louisiana.
Cyanogenic Plants

PAUL NICOLETTI, DVM, MS
Professor, Department of Infectious Diseases, College of Veterinary Medicine, University of Florida, Gainesville, Florida.
Brucellosis

JENS PETER NIELSEN, DVM, PhD
Research Officer, National Veterinary Laboratory, Copenhagen, Denmark.
Pasteurellosis in Swine

CELESTINE O. NJOKU, DVM, PhD, FRVCS
Professor of Veterinary Pathology and Dean, Faculty of Veterinary Medicine, and Chief Consulting Pathologist, Veterinary Teaching Hospital, Ahmadu Bello University, Zaria. Visiting Professor, School of Veterinary Medicine, University of the West Indies, St. Augustine, Trinidad.
Lumpy Skin Disease

CHERYL F. NOCKELS, PhD
Professor, Department of Animal Sciences, Colorado State University, Fort Collins, Colorado.
Stress Impacts of Metablic-Hormonal Regulation and Immune Function

PETER T. OBEREM, BSc, BVSc(HONS)
Manager, Scientific Affairs, Hoechst Animal Health (Pty) Ltd., Kempton Park, South Africa.
Heartwater

FREDERICK W. OEHME, DVM, PhD
Professor of Toxicology, Medicine, and Physiology; and Director, Comparative Toxicology Laboratories, Department of Clinical Sciences, College of Veterinary Medicine, Kansas State University, Manhattan, Kansas.
Coal Tar and Phenols

OLIMPO OLIVER, DVM, MSc
Assistant Professor, Department of Animal Health, Facultad de Medicina Veterinaria Y Zootecnia, Universidad Nacional, Bogota, Colombia. DVSc Candidate at the Veterinary Teaching Hospital, Ontario Veterinary College, University of Guelph, Guelph, Ontario, Canada.
Diseases Caused by Clostridium *Species: Tetanus; Botulism; and Clostridial Myositis, Cellulitis, Hemoglobinuria, Abomastis, and Hepatitis*

A. E. OLSON, MS
Formerly, Research Associate Professor, Veterinary Science, Utah State University, Logan, Utah.
Toxicants in Geothermal Waters, Cooling Waters, and Mine Tailings; Fluoride Toxicosis

CARL OLSON, DVM, PhD
Professor Emeritus, Department of Veterinary Science, College of Agricultural and Life Sciences, School of Veterinary Medicine, University of Wisconsin, Madison, Wisconsin.
Papillomatosis in Cattle; Papillomatosis in Sheep and Goats

DAVID P. OLSON, DVM, PhD, MS
Head, Serology Section, Diagnostic Bacteriology Laboratories and National Veterinary Services Laboratories, Ames, Iowa.
Prevention of Cold Stress in Calves

WILLIAM G. OLSON, DVM, MS, PhD, Diplomate, ACVN
Associate Professor, Clinical Nutrition, College of Veterinary Medicine, University of Minnesota, St. Paul, Minnesota.
Evaluation of Heat- or Mold-Damaged Ensiled Feeds and Their Effects on Livestock

BENNIE I. OSBURN, DVM, PhD
Professor of Pathology, Department of Pathology, School of Veterinary Medicine, University of California, Davis, California. Acting Director, Veterinary Medical Teaching and Research Center, School of Veterinary Medicine, University of California, Tulare, California.
Border Disease

GARY D. OSWEILER, DVM, PhD, MS
Professor, Veterinary Diagnostic Laboratory, College of Veterinary Medicine, Iowa State University, Ames, Iowa.
Ergotism

RANDALL S. OTT, DVM, MS, Diplomate, ACT
Professor of Theriogenology, Department of Veterinary Clinical Medicine, College of Veterinary Medicine, University of Illinois, Urbana, Illinois.
Management of Reproduction of Sheep and Goats

DALE PACCAMONTI, DVM, MS, Diplomate, ACT
Assistant Professor of Theriogenology, Department of Veterinary Clinical Sciences, and Theriogenologist, Veterinary Teaching Hospital and Clinics, School of Veterinary Medicine, Louisiana State University, Baton Rouge, Louisiana.
Potential Problems with the Use of Artificial Insemination in Cattle

JOSEPH C. PAIGE, DVM, MPH
Special Assistant, Division of Voluntary Compliance and Hearings Development, Center for Veterinary Medicine, Food and Drug Administration, Rockville, Maryland.
Residues in Food Animals: Regulatory and Veterinary Responsibility

KIP E. PANTER, PhD
Adjunct Research Assistant Professor, College of Agriculture, Utah State University. Research Animal Scientist, U. S. Department of Agriculture, Agricultural Research Service, Poisonous Plant Research Laboratory, Logan, Utah.
Principal Poisonous Plants in the Western United States; Effects of Plant Toxins on the Central Nervous System; Plants Teratogenic in Livestock; Oxalate Accumulators; Selenium Accumulators

JAMES E. PEARSON, DVM, MS
Chief, Diagnostic Virology Laboratory, National Veterinary Services Laboratory, Ames, Iowa.
Hog Cholera; Japanese Encephalitis (Flavivirus)

B. L. PENZHORN, DSc, BVSc
Professor and Head, Department of Parasitology, Faculty of Veterinary Science, University of Pretoria, Onderstepoort, South Africa.
Coccidiosis

H. B. PETERSON, PhD
Professor Emeritus, Department of Agriculture and Irrigation Engineering, Utah State University, Logan, Utah.
Toxicants in Geothermal Waters, Cooling Waters, and Mine Tailings; Fluoride Toxicosis

ROBERT H. POPPENGA, DVM, PhD, Diplomate, ABVT
Assistant Professor of Veterinary Toxicology, Animal Health Diagnostic Laboratory, and the Department of Pathology, College of Veterinary Medicine, Michigan State University, East Lansing, Michigan.
Sodium Ion Toxicosis

JOHN F. PRESCOTT, Vet MB, PhD
Professor, Department of Veterinary Microbiology and Immunology, Ontario Veterinary College, University of Guelph, Guelph, Ontario, Canada.
Section 8, Bacterial and Fungal Diseases; Systemic Mycoses; Leptospirosis

MERL F. RAISBECK, DVM, PhD, MS
Associate Professor, Veterinary Toxicology, College of Agriculture, University of Wyoming, Laramie, Wyoming.
Taxus (Yew) Poisoning; Chlorinated Hydrocarbon Insecticides

RICHARD F. RANDLE, DVM, MS
Specialist, Veterinary Extension Ruminant Health, College of Veterinary Medicine, University of Missouri, Columbia, Missouri.
Urinary Disorders Associated with the Neonate; Infectious Pyelonephritis and Pyelonephritis in Cattle

THOMAS C. RANDOLPH, DVM*
Formerly, Assistant Professor, College of Veterinary Medicine, Mississippi State University, Mississippi State, Mississippi.
Section 14, Diseases of the Urinary System

HUGH W. REID
Head, Division of Immunobiology, Moredun Research Institute, Edinburgh, United Kingdom.
Nairobi Sheep Disease

IAN M. REID, BSc, MNS, PhD, MRCPath
Head, Animals Research Branch, Agricultural and Food Research Council, Swindon, United Kingdom.
Fat Cow Syndrome and Subclinical Fatty Liver

---
*Deceased.

GAVIN F. RICHARDSON, DVM, MVSc, BA, Diplomate, ACT
Associate Professor of Theriogenology, Department of Health Management and Veterinary Teaching Hospital, Atlantic Veterinary College, University of Prince Edward Island, Charlottetown, Canada.
Metritis and Endometritis; Bovine Vaginitis

ROBERT K. RIDLEY, DVM, PhD
Professor of Veterinary Parasitology, College of Veterinary Medicine, Kansas State University, Manhattan, Kansas.
Parasites of the Respiratory System

D. MICHAEL RINGS, DVM, MS
Associate Professor, Food Animal Medicine and Surgery, College of Veterinary Medicine, The Ohio State University, Columbus, Ohio.
Pharyngeal Lacerations and Retropharyngeal Abscesses in Cattle; Diseases of the Abomasum and Small Intestine; Contagious Foot Rot of Sheep

ZORANA RISTIC, DVM
Dermatology Resident, Department of Small Animal Medicine, College of Veterinary Medicine, University of Georgia, Athens, Georgia.
Fungal Dermatoses

C. JEREMY ROBERTS, BVSc, PhD, MRCVS
Superintending Inspector, Home Office, Shrewsbury, United Kingdom.
Fat Cow Syndrome and Subclinical Fatty Liver

STEVEN M. ROBERTS, DVM, MS, Diplomate, ACVO
Associate Professor, Department of Clinical Sciences, College of Veterinary Medicine and Biomedical Sciences, Colorado State University, Fort Collins, Colorado.
Food Animal Ocular Neoplasia

SØREN ROSENDAL, DVM, PhD
Professor, Department of Veterinary Microbiology and Immunology, Ontario Veterinary College, University of Guelph, Ontario, Canada.
Section 8, Bacterial and Fungal Diseases; Porcine Actinobacillus *Pleuropneumonia; Ovine and Caprine Mycoplasmoses*

BRUCE D. ROSENQUIST, DVM, PhD
Professor, Department of Veterinary Microbiology, College of Veterinary Medicine, University of Missouri, Columbia, Missouri.
Bovine Rhinoviruses

RICHARD F. ROSS, DVM, PhD
Professor, Veterinary Microbiology, College of Veterinary Medicine, Iowa State University, Ames, Iowa.
Swine Mycoplasmosis

EDMUND J. ROSSER, Jr, DVM, Diplomate, ACVD
Associate Professor of Dermatology, Department of Small Animal Clinical Sciences, Veterinary Medical Center, Michigan State University, East Lansing, Michigan.
Parasitic Dermatoses

ALLEN J. ROUSSEL, Jr, DVM, MS, Diplomate, ADVIM
Assistant Professor, Department of Large Animal Medicine and Surgery, College of Veterinary Medicine, Texas A&M University. Staff, Veterinary Teaching Hospital, Texas Veterinary Medical Center, College Station, Texas.
Fluid Therapy, Transfusion, and Shock Therapy; Colostrum and Passive Immunity

LOYD D. ROWE, DVM
Veterinary Toxicologist, U. S. Department of Agriculture, Agricultural Research Service, Food Animal Protection, Research Laboratory, College Station, Texas.
Plants Producing Dermal Injury; Organic Herbicides; Petroleum and Petroleum Products

A. C. ROWLAND, BSc, MRCVS
Senior Lecturer, Faculty of Veterinary Medicine, Edinburgh University, Veterinary Field Station, Easter Bush, Roslin, Lothian, United Kingdom.
Campylobacter *Proliferative Enteropathies of Pigs*

WILSON K. RUMBEIHA, BVM, PhD
Post-doctoral Fellow and Resident in Toxicology, Department of Clinical Sciences, College of Veterinary Medicine, Kansas State University, Manhattan, Kansas.
Coal Tar and Phenols

DANIEL P. RYAN, PhD
Research Scientist (Post-doctoral), Texas A&M University Research Station, Beeville, Texas.
Synchronization of Estrus

LINDA J. SAIF, PhD, MS
Professor, The Ohio State University, Columbus, Ohio. Research Assistant, Food Animal Health Research Program, Ohio Agricultural Research and Development Center, Wooster, Ohio.
Porcine Rotavirus; Transmissible Gastroenteritis Virus; Porcine Epidemic Diarrhea Virus

JULIE M. SANDERSON, MS
Formerly, Research Assistant, Department of Plant Pathology, University of Wisconsin, Madison, Wisconsin.
Slaframine (Slobber Factor)

BERNARD FREDERICK SANSOM, DPhil, MA
Compton Paddock Laboratories, Newburn, Berkshire, United Kingdom.
Parturient Paresis (Milk Fever) and Hypocalcemia (Cows, Ewes, and Goats)

DAVID SCHMITZ, DVM, MS
Associate Professor, Department of Medicine and Surgery, College of Veterinary Medicine, Texas A&M University, College Station, Texas.
Diagnostic Ultrasonography

DANNY W. SCOTT, DVM, Diplomate, ACVD
Professor of Medicine, Department of Clinical Science, College of Veterinary Medicine, Cornell University, Ithaca, New York.
Section 18, Dermatologic Diseases; Viral Skin Diseases; Protozoal Skin Diseases; Immunologic Skin Diseases; Environmental Skin Diseases; Disorders of Pigmentation and Epidermal Appendages; Miscellaneous Skin Diseases; Neoplastic Skin Diseases

GORDON R. SCOTT, BSc, PhD, MS, FRCVS
Honorary Fellow, Centre for Tropical Veterinary Medicine, Royal (Dick) School of Veterinary Studies, University of Edinburgh, Easter Bush, Roslin, Lothian, United Kingdom.
Bovine Ehrlichiosis and Nofel; Ovine Ehrlichiosis; Swine Ehrlichiosis; Bovine Petechial Fever; Tick-Borne Fever and Pasture Fever

PATRICIA E. SHEWEN, BSc, DVM, MS, PhD
Associate Professor, Ontario Veterinary College, University of Guelph, Guelph, Ontario, Canada.
Pasteurellosis in Cattle

JAMES A. SHMIDL, DVM, MS
Manager, Toxicology and Regulatory Affairs, Miles, Inc., Animal Health Division, Shawnee Mission, Kansas.
External Parasiticides

J. L. SHUPE, DVM
Formerly Professor, Veterinary Medicine, Utah State University, Logan, Utah.
Plants Teratogenic in Livestock; Toxicants in Geothermal Waters, Cooling Waters, and Mine Tailings; Fluoride Toxicosis

JOHN C. SIMONS, DVM
Formerly, Director of Science Division, Eastern Wyoming College, Torrington, Wyoming.
Field Calculations for Ration Formulation; Special Dietary Management in Lactation and Gestation; New Concepts for Measuring Proteins for Cattle

EUGENE B. SMALLEY, PhD
Professor of Plant Pathology, University of Wisconsin, Madison, Wisconsin.
Slaframine (Slobber Factor)

NONIE L. SMART
Veterinary Microbiologist, Ontario Ministry of Agriculture and Food, Nepean, Ontario, Canada.
Haemophilus parasuis (Glasser's Disease)

ALVIN W. SMITH, DVM, PhD
Professor of Veterinary Medicine, College of Veterinary Medicine, Oregon State University, Corvallis, Oregon.
Vesicular Stomatitis Virus in Cattle; Calicivirus (Vesicular Exanthema of Swine Virus); Swine Vesicular Disease; Vesicular Stomatitis Virus in Swine

MALCOLM H. SMITH, DVM, PhD
Professor and Chairman, Department of Veterinary and Microbiological Sciences, North Dakota State University, Fargo, North Dakota.
Bovine Respiratory Syncytial Virus

MARY C. SMITH, DVM
Associate Professor, Large Animal Medicine, New York State College of Veterinary Medicine, Cornell University. Staff, Ambulatory Clinic, Cornell University, Ithaca, New York.
Inflammatory Neurologic Diseases of Small Ruminants

ROBERT A. SMITH, DVM, MS, Diplomate, ABVP
McCasland Chair in Beef Health and Production, College of Veterinary Medicine, Oklahoma State University, Stillwater, Oklahoma.
Backgrounding and Stocker Calf Management

J. GLENN SONGER, PhD
Professor, Department of Veterinary Science, University of Arizona, Tucson, Arizona.
Swine Mycobacterial Disease

MARK F. SPIRE, DVM, MS, Diplomate, ACT
Head, Agricultural Practices Section, Kansas State University, Manhattan, Kansas.
Section 3, Herd Health Management; Management of Large-Producer Cow/Calf Herds

P. B. SPRADBROW, DVSc, BVSc, PhD
Professor, Veterinary School, University of Queensland, Brisbane, Australia.
Bovine Ephemeral Fever

HENRY STAEMPFLI, DVM, DrMedVet, Diplomate, ACVIM (Large Animals)
Assistant Professor, Large Animal Medicine, Department of Clinical Studies, and Section Head, Large Animal Medicine, Veterinary Teaching Hospital, Ontario Veterinary College, University of Guelph, Guelph, Ontario, Canada.
Diseases Caused by Clostridium *Species: Tetanus; Botulism; and Clostridial Myositis, Cellulitis, Hemoglobinuria, Abomastis, and Hepatitis*

ALBERTO STEPHANO, DVM, MC
Professor, Pig Production Department, Veterinary School, National Autonomous University of Mexico, Cuidad Universitaria, Mexico.
Paramyxovirus (Blue Eye Disease of Swine)

COLIN G. STEWART, BVMS, BVSc(Hons), MSc
Professor, Faculty of Veterinary Science, Medical University of Southern Africa, Medunsa, South Africa.
Cryptosporidiosis; Ovine Eperythrozoonosis

GUY ST. JEAN, DVM, MS, Diplomate, ACVS
Assistant Professor, Department of Veterinary Clinical Sciences, College of Veterinary Medicine, Kansas State University, Manhattan, Kansas.
Septic Arthritis

G. L. STOKKA, DVM
Resident, Production Medicine, Kansas State University, Manhattan, Kansas.
Feedlot Health Management

WILHELM HEINRICH STOLTSZ, BVSc
Research Veterinarian, Veterinary Research Institute, Onderstepoort, South Africa.
Bovine Anaplasmosis

J. STORZ, DVM, PhD, Diplomate, ACVM
Professor and Head, Department of Veterinary Microbiology and Parasitology, School of Veterinary Medicine, Louisiana State University, Baton Rouge, Louisiana.
Bovine Parvoviruses

BARBARA STRAW, DVM, PhD
Professor, Swine Veterinary Extension, University of Nebraska, Lincoln, Nebraska.
Causal Factors in Swine Pneumonia

ROBERT N. STREETER, DVM
Clinical Instructor, The Ohio State University, Columbus, Ohio.
Traumatic Reticuloperitonitis and Its Sequelae

DAVID A. STRINGFELLOW, DVM, MS
Associate Professor, Department of Pathobiology, College of Veterinary Medicine, Auburn University, Alabama.
Potential of Embryo Transfer for Infectious Disease Control

JOHN M. SULLIVAN, DVM, MS
Veterinary Toxicologist, Animal Disease Diagnostic Laboratory, Purdue University, West Lafayette, Indiana.
Ochratoxin; Citrinin; Stachybotryotoxicosis

STEPHEN F. SUNDLOF, DVM, PhD, Diplomate, ABVT
Associate Professor of Veterinary Toxicology, College of Veterinary Medicine, Department of Physiological Sciences, University of Florida, Gainesville, Florida.
Polybrominated Biphenyls (PBBs); Polychlorinated Biphenyl (PCB) Toxicosis

G. E. SWAN, BVSc, MMedVet(Pharm et Tox)
Coopers Professor in Pharmacology, Faculty of Veterinary Science, University of Pretoria, Onderstepoort, South Africa.
Coccidiosis

ROBERT C. THALER, PhD
Assistant Professor and Extension Swine Specialist, South Dakota State University, Brookings, South Dakota.
Dietary Management in Pigs

PHILIP G. A. THOMAS, BVSc, MACVSc, Diplomate, ACT
Graduate Assistant, Cornell University, Ithaca, New York.
Elective Termination of Pregnancy

JAMES R. THOMPSON, DVM, MS
Associate Professor, Department of Veterinary Clinical Sciences and Food Animal Section, Veterinary Teaching Hospital, College of Veterinary Medicine, Iowa State University, Ames, Iowa.
Diseases of the Ruminant Forestomach

LARRY J. THOMPSON, DVM, Diplomate, ABVT
Clinical Toxicologist, Diagnostic Laboratory, New York State College of Veterinary Medicine, Cornell University, Ithaca, New York.
Copper-Molybdenum Toxicosis

J. C. THURMON, DVM, MS, Diplomate, ACVA
Professor and Head Anesthesiology Section, Department of Veterinary Clinical Medicine, University of Illinois, Urbana, Illinois.
Anesthesia in Ruminants and Swine; Regional Analgesia

DEOKI N. TRIPATHY, BVSc&AH, PhD, MS
Professor, Department of Veterinary Pathobiology, College of Veterinary Medicine, University of Illinois, Urbana, Illinois.
Swine Pox

RODERICK C. TUBBS, DVM, MS, Diplomate, ACT
Clinical Assistant Professor, Department of Veterinary Medicine and Surgery, College of Veterinary Medicine, and Swine Veterinarian, Commercial Agriculture Program, University of Missouri, Columbia, Missouri.
Cystitis, Pyelonephritis, and Miscellaneous Diseases of Swine

ERIC TULLENERS, DVM, Diplomate, ACVS
Associate Professor of Surgery, University of Pennsylvania, Philadelphia, Pennsylvania. Chief, Section of Surgery, New

Bolton Center, University of Pennsylvania, Kennett Square, Pennsylvania.
Coxofemoral Luxations

JEFF W. TYLER, DVM, MPVM, PhD
Assistant Professor, Department of Large Animal Surgery and Medicine, College of Veterinary Medicine, Auburn University. Staff, Large Animal Clinic, Auburn University, Auburn, Alabama.
Immunologic Disorders and Immunotherapy

SAREL R. VAN AMSTEL, BVSc, MMedVet(Med)
Professor and Head, Department of Medicine, and Head, Production Animal Clinic, Onderstepoort Veterinary Academic Teaching Hospital, Faculty of Veterinary Science, Onderstepoort, South Africa.
Section 9, Protozoal and Rickettsial Diseases

MARTIN L. VAN DER LEEK, BVSc, MS, MRCVS
Research Assistant, Department of Infectious Diseases, College of Veterinary Medicine, University of Florida, Gainesville, Florida.
Dairy Cow Production Medicine; Dairy Replacement Rearing Programs; Reproductive Management Problems in Swine

H. H. VAN HORN, PhD
Professor, Dairy Nutrition and Management, Department of Dairy Science, University of Florida, Gainesville, Florida.
Protein Nutrition and Nonprotein Nitrogen

JILL VAUGHAN, BAppSci, FAIMLS, MASM
Research Microbiologist, Commonwealth Scientific and Industrial Research Organization, Division of Animal Health, Animal Health Research Laboratory, Parkville, Victoria, Australia.
Bovine Venereal Campylobacteriosis

JEROME G. VESTWEBER, DVM, PhD
Professor, Department of Surgery and Medicine, College of Veterinary Medicine, Kansas State University, Manhattan, Kansas.
Section 10, Diseases of the Respiratory System; Pathophysiology of the Respiratory Tract; Pneumonia in Cattle, Sheep, and Swine; Respiratory Tract Diagnostic Methods

R. D. WALKER, MS, PhD
Professor, Michigan State University, East Lansing, Michigan.
Actinobacillosis and Actinomycosis

LAURIE MILLS WALLACE, DVM, MVSc
Assistant Professor, Veterinary Medicine and Surgery, Large Animal Clinic, Veterinary Teaching Hospital, University of Missouri, Columbia, Missouri.
Selected Eye Diseases of Sheep and Goats

THOMAS E. WALTON, DVM, PhD
U. S. Department of Agriculture, Agricultural Research Service, Arthropod-Borne Animal Diseases Research, Laramie, Wyoming.
Bluetongue in Cattle; Bluetongue in Sheep

WALLACE M. WASS, DVM, PhD
Professor, Department of Veterinary Clinical Sciences and Food Animal Section, Veterinary Teaching Hospital, College of Veterinary Medicine, Iowa State University, Ames, Iowa.
Diseases of the Ruminant Forestomach

A. DAVID WEAVER, PhD, FRCVS
Professor of Veterinary Medicine and Surgery, College of Veterinary Medicine, University of Missouri, Columbia, Missouri.
Aseptic Laminitis of Cattle; Interdigital and Digital Dermatitis; Interdigital Phlegmon (Interdigital Necrobacillosis)

ERIC M. WEAVER, MS
Graduate Resident Assistant, South Dakota State University, Brookings, South Dakota.
Dietary Management in Pigs

JANICE WEBB, DVM
Deputy Director, Residue Evaluation and Planning Division, Food Safety and Inspection Service, U. S. Department of Agriculture, Washington, D.C.
Residues in Food Animals: Regulatory and Veterinary Responsibility

BIMBO WELKER, DVM, MS
Clinical Associate Professor and Director, Ohio State University, Ambulatory Services, Marysville, Ohio.
Diagnostic Methods in Food Animal Cardiology; Acquired Diseases of the Heart; Interdigital Fibroma; Osteomyelitis

DAVID M. WEST, BVSc, PhD, FACVSc
Senior Lecturer, Faculty of Veterinary Science, Massey University, Palmerston North, New Zealand.
Ruminant Hypomagnesemic Tetanies

MAURICE E. WHITE, DVM
Professor of Medicine, and Chief, Section of Medicine, College of Veterinary Medicine, Cornell University. Staff, Ambulatory Clinic, Cornell University, Ithaca, New York.
Cerebellar Disease in Cattle

S. D. WHITE, DVM, Diplomate, ACVD
Associate Professor, College of Veterinary Medicine and Biomedical Sciences, Colorado State University, Fort Collins, Colorado.
Bacterial Skin Diseases

NORMA E. WHITE-WEITHERS, DVM
Dermatology Resident, Department of Small Animal Medicine, College of Veterinary Medicine, University of Georgia, Athens, Georgia.
Fungal Dermatoses

HOWARD W. WHITFORD, DVM, PhD
Head, Diagnostic Microbiology, Texas Veterinary Medical Diagnostic Laboratory, College Station, Texas.
Bovine Spongiform Encephalopathy (Cow Madness, Raging Cow Disease, Mad Cow Disease); Scrapie

HOWARD L. WHITMORE, DVM, PhD, MS
Professor Emeritus, College of Veterinary Medicine, University of Illinois, Urbana, Illinois. Consultant in private practice.
Bovine Ovarian Cysts

MARLYN S. WHITNEY, DVM, PhD, Diplomate, ACVP
Assistant Professor, Department of Veterinary Pathobiology, College of Veterinary Medicine, and Clinical Pathologist, Veterinary Teaching Hospital, Texas A&M University, College Station, Texas.
Hematology of Food Animals

STEVEN E. WISKE, DVM, Diplomate, ACVP
Associate Professor of Food Animal Medicine, Department of Large Animal Medicine and Surgery, College of Veterinary Medicine, Texas A&M University, College Station, Texas.
Evaluation of Reproductive Efficiency in Beef Cattle Herds

DWIGHT F. WOLFE, DVM, MS
Associate Professor and Head, Food Animal Section, Department of Large Animal Surgery and Medicine, College of Veterinary Medicine, Auburn University, Auburn, Alabama.
Management of the Repeat Breeder Female; Diseases of the Testis and Epididymis

GERALD N. WOODE, DVetMed, BVetMed
Professor, Department of Pathobiology, College of Veterinary Medicine, College Station, Texas.
Bovine Breda Virus (Torovirus)

PHILIP R. WOODS, DVM, PhD, MRCVS
Resident, Large Animal Medicine, Department of Large Animal Medicine and Surgery, College of Veterinary Medicine, Texas A&M University, College Station, Texas.
Colostrum and Passive Immunity

R. S. YOUNGQUIST, DVM
Professor and Head, Theriogenology, and Veterinary Teaching Hospital, University of Missouri, Columbia, Missouri.
Therapeutic Management of Reproduction

PREFACE TO THE THIRD EDITION

Current Veterinary Therapy 3: Food Animal Practice presents a timely update in the field of food animal practice. More than 250 authors and 15 consulting editors have contributed to this edition. There are more than 100 new authors and nine new consulting editors, giving the book new dimensions. This edition features additional international contributors, particularly in the bacterial and protozoal sections, which provides a broader spectrum. The response to the first two editions has been excellent. Therefore, the format and style have not been drastically changed. However, in order to include in one volume as much as possible that which is current in food animal practice, references have been made to articles in previous editions when little or no change has taken place. This is especially true in the section on the nervous system. Please look for these references in the Table of Contents.

This edition continues to have the same purpose as originally intended, that is, a quick, concise resource book concerning prevention, therapy, and management of food animal diseases. It is not encyclopedic in scope; however, some sections, such as nutrition, toxicology, and infectious diseases, are miniature books within a book.

The responsibility for the scientific material contained in each article is solely that of the article's author. The consulting editors and I have attempted to standardize the manuscript form without affecting the scientific content. The authors have presented outstanding, up-to-date material in excellently prepared manuscripts. The word *current* in the title remains a true reflection of the contents.

It is impossible to thank everyone who had a part in producing this edition. However, I will take space to thank God, my wife, the consulting editors, and the authors for making this possible. A special thanks is due the outstanding editorial staff of W. B. Saunders Company for their excellent work. Those due personal recognition and thanks are Rosanne Hallowell, Linda Mills, Carol Robins, and Ray Kersey. Finally, I would like to thank those who ultimately make the whole thing possible, the purchasers and users of the book.

I hope that you will find this book to be a worthwhile addition to your library, and I recommend that you use it often.

JIMMY L. HOWARD

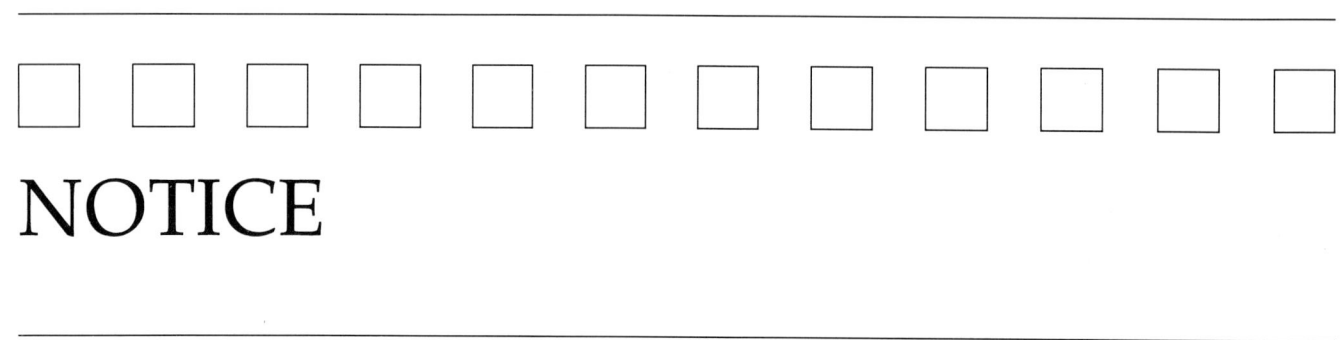

NOTICE

Food animal practice is an ever-changing field. But as new research and clinical experience grow, changes in treatment and drug therapy become necessary or appropriate. The authors and editors of this work have carefully checked and verified drug dosages to assure that dosage information is precise and in accord with standards accepted at the time of publication. Readers are advised, however, to check the product information currently provided by the manufacturer of each drug to be administered to be certain that changes have not been made in the recommended dose or in the contraindications for administration. This is of particular importance in regard to new or infrequently used drugs. Recommended dosages for animals are sometimes based on adjustments in the dosage that would be suitable for humans. Some of the drugs mentioned have been given experimentally by the authors. Others have been used in dosages greater than those recommended by the manufacturer. In these kinds of cases, the authors have reported on their own considerable experience. It is the responsibility of those administering a drug, relying on their professional skill and experience, to determine dosages, the best treatment for the patient, and whether the benefits of giving a drug justify the attendant risk. The editors cannot be responsible for misuse or misapplication of the material in this work.

THE PUBLISHER

CONTENTS

SECTION 1
Special Therapy and Procedures 1
JIMMY L. HOWARD, Consulting Editor

Fluid Therapy, Transfusion, and Shock
Therapy 1
ALLEN J. ROUSSEL, JR.

Therapeutic Management of Inflammation 8
VERNON C. LANGSTON

Immunologic Disorders and Immunotherapy 12
CINDY J. BRUNNER
JEFF W. TYLER

Stress Impacts of Metabolic-Hormonal
Regulation and Immune Function 16
CHERYL F. NOCKELS

Adverse Drug Reactions 20
DAWN M. BOOTHE
GORDON W. BRUMBAUGH

Diagnostic Ultrasonography 26
DAVID SCHMITZ

Residues in Food Animals: Regulatory and
Veterinary Responsibility 29
JANICE WEBB
JOSEPH C. PAIGE

Prevention and Management of Drug and
Chemical Residues in Meat and Milk 39
H. DWIGHT MERCER

Bovine Somatotropin 42
DAVID McCLARY

Anthelmintic Therapy 47
ROBERT M. CORWIN

External Parasiticides 51
LARRY F. MOORE
JAMES A. SHMIDL

Anesthesia in Ruminants and Swine 58
J. C. THURMON
G. J. BENSON

Regional Analgesia 77
G. J. BENSON
J. C. THURMON

See **Current Veterinary Therapy 2** for the following article:
Antimicrobial Therapy 8
WILLIAM L. JENKINS

SECTION 2
**Neonatal Disease and Disease
Management** 89
WILLIAM BRAUN, JR., Consulting Editor

Congenital Defects of Cattle and Sheep 89
H. W. LEIPOLD
STANLEY M. DENNIS

Colostrum and Passive Immunity 97
PHILIP R. WOODS
ALLEN J. ROUSSEL, JR.

Omphalitis and Its Sequelae in Ruminants 101
THOMAS R. KASARI

Diarrheal Diseases of Neonatal Ruminants 103
ELAINE HUNT

Diarrhea in Neonatal Swine 111
JOHN J. ANDREWS

Neonatal Polyarthritis in Swine 115
JAMES D. McKEAN

Prevention of Cold Stress in Calves 116
DAVID P. OLSON

Hypoglycemia and Hypothermia in
Neonatal Pigs 119
ROSS P. COWART

SECTION 3
Herd Health Management 121
MARK F. SPIRE, Consulting Editor

Management of Farm Cow/Calf Herds 121
DUANE MIKSCH

Management of Large-Producer Cow/Calf
Herds 124
TERRY J. ENGELKEN
MARK F. SPIRE

Backgrounding and Stocker Calf
Management 130
ROBERT A. SMITH

Feedlot Health Management 135
A. J. EDWARDS
G. L. STOKKA

Dairy Cow Production Medicine 142
MARTIN L. VAN DER LEEK
DAVID P. KELBERT
G. ARTHUR DONOVAN

Dairy Replacement Rearing Programs 147
MARTIN L. VAN DER LEEK
G. ARTHUR DONOVAN
R. KENNETH BRAUN

Ovine Production Management and Preventive
Medicine 153
MARIE S. BULGIN

Sheep Feedlot Management 159
CLEON V. KIMBERLING
DEBORAH MARSH

Production Medicine and Health Programs
for Goats 162
KATHERINE BRETZLAFF

Swine Herd Health Management 167
JOSEPH F. CONNOR

Llama Herd Health Management 172
LaRUE W. JOHNSON

SECTION 4
Dietary Management 178
JIMMY L. HOWARD, Consulting Editor

Nutritional Management of Stressed and
Morbid Calves 178
N. ANDY COLE

Use of Growth Stimulants and Feed Additives
in Ruminant Animal Production 180
ROBERT T. BRANDT, JR.

Field Calculations for Ration Formulation 188
JOHN C. SIMONS
MICHAEL S. HAND

Special Dietary Management in Lactation
and Gestation 204
JOHN C. SIMONS
MICHAEL S. HAND

Protein Nutrition and Nonprotein Nitrogen 224
H. H. VAN HORN

New Concepts for Measuring Proteins
for Cattle 232
JOHN C. SIMONS
MICHAEL S. HAND

Cattle Feeding 250
DAVID P. HUTCHESON

Dietary Management of the Beef Breeding
Herd 253
LARRY R. CORAH

Dietary Management of Dairy Cattle 260
J. T. HUBER

Dietary Management in Goats 272
J. E. HUSTON

Dietary Management in Pigs 278
ROBERT C. THALER
ERIC M. WEAVER

Nutrition for Livestock Grazing Rangelands
and Pasturelands 285
M. M. KOTHMANN

Mineral Supplementation for Beef Cattle on
Rangeland 293
J. C. DOYLE
J. E. HUSTON

See **Current Veterinary Therapy 2** for the following articles:

General Pediatric Feeding: Milk Replacers in Pediatric Feeding 239
  LAVERNE M. SCHUGEL

Dietary Management in Sheep 259
  F. C. HINDS

Deficiencies of Mineral Nutrients 278
   JAMES T. BAXTER

SECTION 5
Metabolic Disorders 304
IVAN W. CAPLE, Consulting Editor

Parturient Paresis (Milk Fever) and
Hypocalcemia (Cows, Ewes, and Goats) 304
   WILLIAM MAURICE ALLEN
   BERNARD FREDERICK SANSOM

Acetonemia 309
   IVAN W. CAPLE
   J. G. McLEAN

Pregnancy Toxemia 312
   IVAN W. CAPLE
   J. G. McLEAN

Fat Cow Syndrome and Subclinical Fatty
Liver 315
   C. JEREMY ROBERTS
   IAN M. REID

Ruminant Hypomagnesemic Tetanies 318
   IVAN W. CAPLE
   DAVID M. WEST

Downer Cow Syndrome 321
   JAKOB MALMO

Postparturient Hemoglobinuria 323
   CHRISTOPHER J. McCAUGHAN

SECTION 6
Physical and Chemical Disorders 327
JOHN C. HALLIBURTON, Consulting Editor

Feed-Related Toxicoses 327

Ammoniated Feed Toxicosis 327
   SANDRA E. MORGAN

Sodium Ion Toxicosis 328
   ROBERT H. POPPENGA

Ionophores: Monensin, Lasalocid,
Salinomycin, and Narasin 329
   C. PAT McCOY

Gossypol Toxicosis 331
   SANDRA E. MORGAN

Mycotoxicoses 332

Trichothecenes 332
   VAL R. BEASLEY

Ergotism 334
   GARY D. OSWEILER

Ochratoxin 336
   JOHN M. SULLIVAN
   WILLIAM W. CARLTON
   PALLE KROGH*

Citrinin 337
   JOHN M. SULLIVAN
   WILLIAM W. CARLTON

Slaframine (Slobber Factor) 338
   EUGENE B. SMALLEY
   JULIE M. SANDERSON

Stachybotryotoxicosis 340
   JOHN M. SULLIVAN
   WILLIAM W. CARLTON

Evaluation of Heat- or Mold-Damaged Ensiled
Feeds and Their Effects on Livestock 341
   WILLIAM G. OLSON

Plant Toxicoses 343

Poisonous Plants in Harvested or Prepared
Foods 343
   MURRAY E. FOWLER

Principal Poisonous Plants in the Western
United States 345
   LYNN F. JAMES
   KIP E. PANTER

Principal Poisonous Plants in the Midwestern
and Eastern United States 349
   GEORGE E. BURROWS
   ARTHUR A. CASE*

Cardiotoxic Plants 352
   MURRAY E. FOWLER

Hepatotoxic Plants 354
   MURRAY E. FOWLER

Effects of Plant Toxins on the Central
Nervous System 356
   LYNN F. JAMES
   KIP E. PANTER

Sweet Clover Poisoning 358
   HOWARD H. CASPER
   ARNOLD D. ALSTAD

---

*Deceased.

Plants Teratogenic in Livestock 359
RICHARD F. KEELER
KIP E. PANTER
J. L. SHUPE

Plants Producing Dermal Injury 361
LOYD D. ROWE
A. EARL JOHNSON

Oxalate Accumulators 364
LYNN F. JAMES
KIP E. PANTER

Selenium Accumulators 366
LYNN F. JAMES
KIP E. PANTER

Cyanogenic Plants 367
STEVEN S. NICHOLSON

Perilla frutescens (Purple Mint) Toxicosis
in Cattle 368
LARRY A. KERR

Fescue Toxicosis 370
LARRY A. KERR

Taxus (Yew) Poisoning 371
MERL F. RAISBECK
JOE D. KENDALL

Oak Poisoning 372
BILLY R. CLAY
DEENA G. GREGORY

Water Quality 375

Water Quality for Livestock 375
T. L. CARSON

Toxicants in Geothermal Waters, Cooling
Waters, and Mine Tailings 377
J. L. SHUPE
C. V. BAGLEY
H. B. PETERSON
A. E. OLSON

Pesticides, Rodenticides, and Herbicides 380

Chlorinated Hydrocarbon Insecticides 380
JOE D. KENDALL
MERL F. RAISBECK

Organophosphorus and Carbamate
Insecticides 381
T. L. CARSON

Rodenticides 383
MICHAEL J. MURPHY

Organic Herbicides 386
LOYD D. ROWE

Heavy Metals and Trace Elements 394

Arsenic Toxicosis 394
FRANCIS D. GALEY

Copper-Molybdenum Toxicosis 396
LARRY J. THOMPSON
WILLIAM B. BUCK

Fluoride Toxicosis 398
J. L. SHUPE
C. V. BAGLEY
A. E. OLSON
H. B. PETERSON

Miscellaneous Toxicoses 403

Polybrominated Biphenyls (PBBs) 403
STEPHEN F. SUNDLOF

Polychlorinated Biphenyl (PCB) Toxicosis 405
STEPHEN F. SUNDLOF

Petroleum and Petroleum Products 407
LOYD D. ROWE
WILLIAM C. EDWARDS

Coal Tar and Phenols 409
WILSON K. RUMBEIHA
FREDERICK W. OEHME

Zootoxins 411
MURRAY E. FOWLER

See **Current Veterinary Therapy 2** for the following articles:

*Management and Treatment of Toxicosis in
Cattle* 341
   E. MURL BAILEY, JR.

Urea and Other Nonprotein Nitrogen Sources 354
   W. EUGENE LLOYD

Iodine 357
   WILLIAM B. BUCK

Aflatoxins 363
   ROBERT W. COPPOCK

*Sporidesmins Facial Eczema and
Pithomycotoxicosis* 375
   C. V. BAGLEY
   J. L. SHUPE

Tremorgenic Toxins 378
   WILLIAM B. BUCK

Zearalenone (F-20) 380
   LAWRENCE P. RUHR

Nitrate Accumulators 392
   LAWRENCE P. RUHR
   GARY D. OSWEILER

Principal Poisonous Plants in the Southwestern
United States 412
   E. MURL BAILEY, JR.

Lead 439
   J. W. SEXTON
   WILLIAM B. BUCK

Mercury Toxicosis 440
   GARY D. OSWEILER
   BARBARA S. HOOK

Toxic Gases 456
   STANLEY E. CURTIS

Lightning Strike and Electrocution 458
   F. K. RAMSEY
   J. R. HOWARD

Heat Prostration 459
   E. MURL BAILEY, JR.

Cold Stress 461
   DAVID ROBERTSHAW

SECTION 7
Viruses, Chlamydiae, and Mycoplasma 414
A. KONRAD EUGSTER, Consulting Editor

Diagnosis of Viral Diseases 414
ROBERT A. CRANDELL

Viral Disease of Cattle 417

Infectious Bovine Rhinotracheitis 417
ROBERT A. CRANDELL

Bovine Mammillitis 419
W. B. MARTIN

Malignant Catarrhal Fever 421
ANTHONY E. CASTRO

Pseudorabies (Aujeszky's Disease,
"Mad Itch") 422
ROBERT A. CRANDELL

Cowpox and Bovine Vaccinia Mammillitis 423
E. PAUL J. GIBBS

Pseudocowpox 425
E. PAUL J. GIBBS

Bovine Papular Stomatitis 426
ROBERT A. CRANDELL

Lumpy Skin Disease 427
CELESTINE O. NJOKU

Bovine Adenoviruses 429
DONALD MATTSON

Papillomatosis in Cattle 430
CARL OLSON

Bovine Parvoviruses 431
J. STORZ

Bovine Viral Diarrhea–Mucosal Disease 432
WERNER P. HEUSCHELE

Bovine Reoviruses 434
SASHI B. MOHANTY

Bluetongue in Cattle 435
THOMAS E. WALTON

Bovine Rhinoviruses 437
BRUCE D. ROSENQUIST

Foot-and-Mouth Disease in Cattle 437
JERRY CALLIS
DOUGLAS GREGG

Bovine Rotavirus 439
THOMAS L. LESTER

Calf Coronavirus Diarrhea 440
THOMAS L. LESTER

Rift Valley Fever in Cattle 441
JOHN C. MORRILL

Akabane Disease in Cattle 442
A. J. DELLA-PORTA

Parainfluenza-3 Virus 443
GLYNN H. FRANK

Rinderpest 444
FAROUK M. HAMDY

Bovine Respiratory Syncytial Virus 447
MALCOLM H. SMITH

Vesicular Stomatitis Virus in Cattle 447
ALVIN W. SMITH

Bovine Ephemeral Fever 449
P. B. SPRADBROW

Bovine Leukemia Virus 450
JANICE M. MILLER

Bovine Breda Virus (Torovirus) 451
GERALD N. WOODE

Bovine Astroviruses 452
JANICE C. BRIDGER

Bovine Calici-like Viruses 453
JANICE C. BRIDGER

Bovine Spongiform Encephalopathy (Cow
Madness, Raging Cow Disease, Mad Cow
Disease) 454
HOWARD W. WHITFORD

Chlamydial Disease in Cattle 455

Bovine Chlamydiosis 455
A. KONRAD EUGSTER

Mycoplasmosis in Cattle 457

Bovine Mycoplasmosis 457
MERWIN L. FREY

Viral Diseases of Sheep and Goats 459

Caprine and Ovine Herpesviruses 459
A. KONRAD EUGSTER

Sheep and Goat Pox 459
E. PAUL J. GIBBS

Contagious Ecthyma 460
ROBERT A. CRANDELL

Ovine and Caprine Adenoviruses 461
DONALD MATTSON

Papillomatosis in Sheep and Goats 462
CARL OLSON

Border Disease 462
BENNIE I. OSBURN

Foot-and-Mouth Disease in Sheep and Goats 464
JERRY CALLIS
DOUGLAS GREGG

Ovine and Caprine Reoviruses 465
SASHI B. MOHANTY

Bluetongue in Sheep 465
THOMAS E. WALTON

Ovine Rotavirus 467
THOMAS L. LESTER

Nairobi Sheep Disease 468
HUGH W. REID

Rift Valley Fever in Sheep and Goats 469
JOHN C. MORRILL

Akabane Disease in Sheep and Goats 470
A. J. DELLA-PORTA

Maedi-Visna (Ovine Progressive Pneumonia,
Zwoegerziekte) 470
RANDALL C. CUTLIP

Caprine Arthritis-Encephalitis Virus 472
DONALD P. KNOWLES, JR.
WILLIAM P. CHEEVERS

Ovine Astroviruses 474
JANICE C. BRIDGER

Arthrogryposis-Hydranencephaly in Sheep:
Cache Valley Virus Infection 474
ROBERT A. CRANDELL

Scrapie 475
HOWARD W. WHITFORD

Sheep Pulmonary Adenomatosis (Sheep
Pulmonary Carcinoma, Jaagsiekte) 477
RANDALL C. CUTLIP

Ovine and Caprine Mycoplasmoses 478
SØREN ROSENDAL

Viral Disease of Swine 480

Porcine Pseudorabies (Aujesky's Disease) 480
ROBERT A. CRANDELL

Porcine Cytomegalovirus (Inclusion Body
Rhinitis) 481
ROBERT ASSAF

Swine Pox 482
DEOKI N. TRIPATHY

Porcine Adenoviruses 483
DONALD MATTSON

Porcine Parvovirus–Induced Reproductive
Failure of Swine 484
WILLIAM L. MENGELING

Mystery Pig Disease 485
WILLIAM L. MENGELING

African Swine Fever 486
H. A. McDANIEL

Calicivirus (Vesicular Exanthema of
Swine Virus) 488
ALVIN W. SMITH

Enteroviral Encephalomyelitis of Pigs (Teschen
Disease) 490
TALMAGE T. BROWN, JR.

Swine Vesicular Disease 491
ALVIN W. SMITH

Encephalitis–Vomiting and Wasting Disease
Complex of Swine 492
WILLIAM L. MENGELING

SMEDI and Other Porcine Enteroviruses 493
WILLIAM L. MENGELING

Encephalomyocarditis Virus 493
JOSEPH H. GAINER

Foot-and-Mouth Disease in Pigs 494
JERRY CALLIS
DOUGLAS GREGG

Hog Cholera 495
JAMES E. PEARSON

Japanese Encephalitis (Flavivirus) 496
JAMES E. PEARSON

Porcine Reoviruses 497
SASHI B. MOHANTY

Porcine Rotavirus 497
LINDA J. SAIF

Transmissible Gastroenteritis Virus 498
LINDA J. SAIF

Porcine Epidemic Diarrhea Virus 500
LINDA J. SAIF

Swine Influenza 501
B. C. EASTERDAY

Paramyxovirus (Blue Eye Disease of Swine) 502
ALBERTO STEPHANO

Vesicular Stomatitis Virus in Swine 504
ALVIN W. SMITH

Mycoplasmosis of Swine 504

Swine Mycoplasmosis 504
C. H. ARMSTRONG
RICHARD F. ROSS

See **Current Veterinary Therapy 2** for the following articles:

Rabies in Cattle *501*
GEORGE M. BAER

Rabies in Sheep and Goats *527*
GEORGE M. BAER

*Chlamydia-Induced Diseases of Sheep and
Goats* *532*
J. STORZ

Rabies in Pigs *555*
GEORGE M. BAER

Chlamydial Infections of Swine *555*
J. STORZ

SECTION 8
Bacterial and Fungal Diseases 506
JOHN F. PRESCOTT and SØREN ROSENDAL,
Consulting Editors

Haemophilus parasuis (Glasser's Disease) 506
NONIE L. SMART

Nonvenereal Campylobacteriosis 507
ROGER MARSHALL

Bovine Venereal Campylobacteriosis 510
JOHN DUFTY
JILL VAUGHAN

Campylobacter Proliferative Enteropathies
of Pigs 513
G. H. K. LAWSON
A. C. ROWLAND

Borreliosis in Cattle 515
ELIZABETH C. BURGESS

Escherichia coli Infections in Farm Animals 517
JOHN M. FAIRBROTHER

Eubacterium suis 519
SCOTT A. DEE

Nocardioses 521
JOHN A. LYNCH

Dermatophilosis 522
D. H. LLOYD

Systemic Mycoses 524
JOHN F. PRESCOTT

Swine Mycobacterial Disease 529
J. GLENN SONGER

Tuberculosis 531
L. D. KONYHA

Paratuberculosis (Johne's Disease) 533
DANIEL G. BUTLER

Actinobacillosis and Actinomycosis 534
R. D. WALKER

Corynebacterium Species Infections in
Food Animals 537
C. ANNE MUCKLE
PAULA I. MENZIES

Leptospirosis 541
JOHN F. PRESCOTT

The Haemophilus somnus Complex 546
PETER B. LITTLE

Porcine Actinobacillus Pleuropneumonia 549
SØREN ROSENDAL

Brucellosis 551
PAUL NICOLETTI

Pasteurellosis in Cattle 555
PATRICIA E. SHEWEN
KENNETH G. BATEMAN

Pasteurellosis in Swine 559
JENS PETER NIELSEN
PAUL BÆKBO

Swine Dysentery 560
ROBERT D. GLOCK

Salmonellosis 562
GEORGE A. KENNEDY
CLAIR M. HIBBS

Anthrax 565
ARNOLD F. KAUFMANN

Diseases Caused by Clostridium Species:
Tetanus; Botulism; and Clostridial Myositis,
Cellulitis, Hemoglobinuria, Abomasitis, and
Hepatitis 567
HENRY STAEMPFLI
OLIMPO OLIVER

Clostridial Enterotoxemia (Clostridium
perfringens) 573
DONNA M. GATEWOOD
M. M. CHENGAPPA

Streptococcal Disease 575
E. DENIS ERICKSON

Staphylococcal Diseases 578
LUC A. DEVRIESE

Swine Erysipelas 579
JERRY P. KUNESH

Listeriosis (Circling Disease, Silage Sickness) 580
STANLEY M. DENNIS

SECTION 9
Protozoal and Rickettsial Diseases 584
SAREL VAN AMSTEL, Consulting Editor

Babesiosis 584
DANIEL THEODORUS DE WAAL

Bovine Anaplasmosis 588
WILHELM HEINRICH STOLTSZ

Besnoitiosis (Elephant Skin Disease,
Olifantsvelsiekte [Afrikaans], Anasarque des
Bovidés) 596
RUDOLPH D. BIGALKE

Coccidiosis 599
B. L. PENZHORN
G. E. SWAN

Trypanosomiasis (Surra; Nagana, Samore, or
Tsetse Fly Disease) 604
ROBERT J. CONNOR

Trichomoniasis in Cattle 608
STAN HERR

Cryptosporidiosis 612
COLIN G. STEWART

Ovine Eperythrozoonosis 613
COLIN G. STEWART

Porcine Eperythrozoonosis 614
R. K. LOVEDAY

Bovine Ehrlichiosis and Nofel 616
GORDON R. SCOTT

Ovine Ehrlichiosis 617
GORDON R. SCOTT

Swine Ehrlichiosis 618
GORDON R. SCOTT

Bovine Petechial Fever 618
GORDON R. SCOTT

Tick-Borne Fever and Pasture Fever 620
GORDON R. SCOTT

Q Fever 622
I. D. AITKEN

Toxoplasmosis 623
J. P. DUBEY

Sarcocystosis 625
J. P. DUBEY

Theileriosis 627
J. A. LAWRENCE

Heartwater (Cowdriose, Kaboa, Daji, Enguruti, Khadar, Modikulogo) 628
PETER T. OBEREM

SECTION 10
Diseases of the Respiratory System 633
JEROME G. VESTWEBER, Consulting Editor

Pathophysiology of the Respiratory Tract 633
JEROME G. VESTWEBER

Upper Respiratory System Diseases 637
VAUGHN L. LARSON

Pneumonia in Cattle, Sheep, and Swine 640
JEROME G. VESTWEBER

Acute Bovine Pulmonary Edema and Emphysema 643
ROGER BREEZE
JAMES R. CARLSON

Venal Caval Thrombosis 647
ROGER BREEZE

The Bovine Respiratory Disease Complex 653
CHARLES A. HJERPE

Causal Factors in Swine Pneumonia 664
BARBARA STRAW

Management of Respiratory Disease in Sheep ... 670
NEIL ANDERSON

Parasites of the Respiratory System 673
ROBERT K. RIDLEY

Respiratory Tract Diagnostic Methods 675
JEROME G. VESTWEBER

Respiratory Therapeutics 678
CHARLES A. HJERPE

SECTION 11
Diseases of the Circulatory System 681
DONALD R. CLARK, Consulting Editor

Cardiovascular Pathophysiology 681
DONALD R. CLARK

Diseases of the General Circulation 682
DONALD R. CLARK

Diagnostic Methods in Food Animal Cardiology 684
BIMBO WELKER

Acquired Diseases of the Heart 686
BIMBO WELKER

Hematology of Food Animals 690
MARLYN S. WHITNEY

Therapeutic Management of Cardiovascular and Hemolymphatic Diseases 699
PETER D. CONSTABLE

SECTION 12
Diseases of the Digestive System 706
GLEN F. HOFFSIS, Consulting Editor

Introduction to the Ruminant Forestomach 706
PETER D. CONSTABLE

Choke 712
GERARD J. KOENIG

Pharyngeal Lacerations and Retropharyngeal Abscesses in Cattle 713
D. MICHAEL RINGS

Diseases of the Ruminant Forestomach 714
    Lactic Acidosis (Rumen Overload, Rumen Acidosis, Grain Overload, Engorgement Toxemia, Rumenitis) 714
      KARL W. KERSTING
      JAMES R. THOMPSON
      WALLACE M. WASS

    Rumenitis (Ruminal Parakeratosis, Chronic Rumen Acidosis) 716

    Ruminal Tympany (Bloat) 717

Traumatic Reticuloperitonitis and Its Sequelae 719
ROBERT N. STREETER

Diseases of the Abomasum and Small Intestine 723
GLEN F. HOFFSIS
SHEILA M. McGUIRK
PETER D. CONSTABLE
D. MICHAEL RINGS

    Left Displaced Abomasum 723
      GLEN F. HOFFSIS
      SHEILA A. McGUIRK

    Right Displaced Abomasum and Abomasal Volvulus (Torsion) 725
      GLEN HOFFSIS
      SHEILA M. McGUIRK

Vagus Indigestion 730
  GLEN F. HOFFSIS
  SHEILA M. McGUIRK

Abomasal Impaction 732
  GLEN F. HOFFSIS
  SHEILA M. McGUIRK

Intussusception 733
  GLEN F. HOFFSIS
  SHEILA M. McGUIRK

Volvulus of the Root of the Mesentery 734
  GLEN F. HOFFSIS
  SHEILA M. McGUIRK

Strangulated Inguinal Hernia 734
  GLEN F. HOFFSIS
  SHEILA M. McGUIRK

Abdominal Pain 735
  GLEN F. HOFFSIS
  SHEILA M. McGUIRK

Gastric Ulcers of Swine 735
  PETER D. CONSTABLE

Abomasal Emptying Defect of Sheep 736
  D. MICHAEL RINGS

Diseases of the Large Intestine 738
PETER D. CONSTABLE

  Cecal Dilation 738
  Cecocolic Volvulus (Cecal Volvulus) and Cecal
    Torsion 739
  Colonic Obstruction 740
  Atresia Coli 740
  Rectal Prolapse 741
  Rectal Stricture 742
  Atresia Ani and Recti 742

Nematode Infections in Cattle, Sheep,
Goats, and Swine 743
R. P. HERD

Trematode Infections in Cattle, Sheep,
and Goats 755
R. P. HERD

Cestode Infections in Cattle, Sheep, Goats,
and Swine 757
R. P. HERD

Drugs Affecting the Digestive System 758
LLOYD E. DAVIS

See **Current Veterinary Therapy 2** for the following articles:
  Abomasal Ulcers 740
    ROBERT H. WHITLOCK
  Liver Disease (Hepatitis) 741
    ROBERT H. WHITLOCK

SECTION 13
Diseases of the Reproductive Tract 762
LOUIS F. ARCHBALD, Consulting Editor

Bovine Mastitis 762
  SEBASTIAN E. HEATH

Lactation Failure 768
  S. K. LYLE

Retained Fetal Membranes 769
  M. L. FAHNING

Metritis and Endometritis 770
  GAVIN F. RICHARDSON

Pyometra in Cattle 772
  LOUIS F. ARCHBALD

Bovine Vaginitis 773
  GAVIN F. RICHARDSON

Bovine Ovarian Cysts 774
  HOWARD L. WHITMORE

Synchronization of Estrus 776
  ROBERT A. GODKE
  DANIEL P. RYAN

Potential Problems with the Use of Artificial
Insemination in Cattle 779
  DALE PACCAMONTI

Management of the Repeat Breeder Female 781
  DWIGHT F. WOLFE

Potential of Embryo Transfer for Infectious
Disease Control 785
  DAVID A. STRINGFELLOW

Abortion—An Approach to Diagnosis 787
  DAN E. GOODWIN

Elective Termination of Pregnancy 791
  PHILIP G. A. THOMAS

Diseases of the Male Internal Genitalia 793
  R. L. CARSON
  R. S. HUDSON

Diseases of the Testis and Epididymis 794
  DWIGHT F. WOLFE

Diseases of the Penis and Prepuce 796
  R. L. CARSON
  R. S. HUDSON

Dairy Herd Reproductive Efficiency 798
LOUIS F. ARCHBALD

Evaluation of Reproductive Efficiency in
Beef Cattle Herds 800
W. DUANE MICKELSEN
STEVEN E. WIKSE

Management of Reproduction of Sheep
and Goats 803
RANDALL S. OTT

Reproductive Management Problems
in Swine 805
MARTIN L. VAN DER LEEK
H. NEIL BECKER

Therapeutic Management of Reproduction 809
R. S. YOUNGQUIST

SECTION 14
Diseases of the Urinary System 817
JIMMY L. HOWARD and THOMAS C. RANDOLPH,*
Consulting Editor

Therapeutic Management of Urinary
Diseases 817
VERNON C. LANGSTON

Urolithiasis in Food Animals (Urinary, Calculi,
Waterbelly, Calculosis) 819
JAMES G. FLOYD, JR.

Urinary Disorders Associated with the
Neonate 821
RICHARD F. RANDLE

Renal Toxicants 822
DENNIS J. BLODGETT

Infectious Pyelonephritis and Pyelonephritis
in Cattle 826
RICHARD F. RANDLE

Cystitis, Pyelonephritis, and Miscellaneous
Diseases of Swine 827
RODERICK C. TUBBS

SECTION 15
Diseases of the Eye 829
CECIL P. MOORE, Consulting Editor

Ophthalmic Examination Techniques for
Food and Fiber Animals 829
DANIEL M. BETTS

*Deceased.

Infectious and Parasitic Eye Diseases of
Cattle 834
CECIL P. MOORE
ROBERT B. MILLER

Selected Eye Diseases of Sheep and Goats 839
CECIL P. MOORE
LAURIE MILLS WALLACE

Ophthalmology of South American Camelids:
Llamas, Alpacas, Guanacos, and Vicuñas 842
JULIET RATHBONE GIONFRIDDO
DEBORAH S. FRIEDMAN

Food Animal Ocular Neoplasia 846
STEVEN M. ROBERTS
ROBERT KAINER

Neuro-ophthalmology in Food Animals 851
B. KEITH COLLINS

SECTION 16
Neurologic Diseases of Food Animals ... 858
JIMMY L. HOWARD, Consulting Editor

Cerebellar Disease in Cattle 858
MAURICE E. WHITE

Inflammatory Neurologic Diseases of Small
Ruminants 860
MARY C. SMITH

See **Current Veterinary Therapy 2** for the following
articles:

Neurologic Examination of Cattle 848
THOMAS J. DIVERS

Infectious Causes of Meningitis and Encephalitis 852
THOMAS J. DIVERS

Toxic Encephalopathies in Cattle 855
JOHN A. SMITH

*Metabolic Diseases That Cause Neurologic
Syndromes* 866
RAYMOND W. SWEENEY

Polioencephalomalacia in Ruminants 868
STEPHEN G. DILL

Rabies 870
F. H. FOX

Spinal Cord Problems in Cattle 872
KAREN H. BAUM

Diseases of the Peripheral Nerves 874
WILLIAM C. REBHUN

Neurologic Disease in Swine 879
BARBARA STRAW

SECTION 17
Diseases of the Musculoskeletal System 864
BRUCE L. HULL, Consulting Editor

Introduction to the Musculoskeletal System 864
BRUCE L. HULL

Sole Abscesses 864
BRUCE L. HULL

Vertical Wall Cracks 865
BRUCE L. HULL

Horizontal Wall Cracks 865
BRUCE L. HULL

Rusterholz Ulcer 866
BRUCE L. HULL

Verrucose Dermatitis 867
BRUCE L. HULL

Aseptic Laminitis of Cattle 867
A. DAVID WEAVER

Interdigital and Digital Dermatitis 868
A. DAVID WEAVER

Interdigital Phlegmon (Interdigital Necrobacillosis) 869
A. DAVID WEAVER

Fescue Foot 870
GERARD J. KOENIG

Interdigital Fibroma 871
BIMBO WELKER

Contagious Foot Rot of Sheep 872
D. MICHAEL RINGS

Septic Arthritis 873
GUY ST. JEAN

Stifle Injuries and Patellar Luxations 874
WILLIAM H. CRAWFORD

Coxofemoral Luxations 876
ERIC TULLENERS

Spondylitis 877
BRUCE L. HULL

Fractures 878
N. KENT AMES

Tendon Injuries 880
N. KENT AMES

Osteomyelitis 881
BIMBO WELKER

SECTION 18
Dermatologic Diseases 882
DANNY W. SCOTT, Consulting Editor

Parasitic Dermatoses 882
EDMUND J. ROSSER, JR.

Fungal Dermatoses 890
LINDA MEDLEAU
ZORANA RISTIC
NORMA E. WHITE-WEITHERS

Bacterial Skin Diseases 894
S. D. WHITE

Viral Skin Diseases 898
DANNY W. SCOTT

Protozoal Skin Diseases 900
DANNY W. SCOTT

Immunologic Skin Diseases 900
DANNY W. SCOTT

Environmental Skin Diseases 901
DANNY W. SCOTT

Congenital and Hereditary Skin Diseases 907
DONNA WALTON ANGARANO

Nutritional, Endocrine, and Keratinization Abnormalities 911
WILLIAM H. MILLER, JR.

Disorders of Pigmentation and Epidermal Appendages 913
DANNY W. SCOTT

Miscellaneous Skin Diseases 915
DANNY W. SCOTT

Neoplastic Skin Diseases 915
DANNY W. SCOTT

APPENDIX 919

A Partial List of Reference Ranges 919
WALTER E. HOFFMAN

Availability of Some Common Products 921

Addresses of Some Companies Manufacturing Common Drugs 926

Table of Common Drugs: Approximate Doses ... 930

Conversion Tables 934

Index 935

SECTION 1
Special Therapy and Procedures

JIMMY L. HOWARD, DVM, MS, Consulting Editor

Fluid Therapy, Transfusion, and Shock Therapy

ALLEN J. ROUSSEL, JR., DVM, MS, DIPLOMATE, ACVIM

Water and salt, known for centuries to be elements essential for life, are as critical to survival today as ever. Because of the extreme importance of water and electrolytes to biologic processes, many organ systems are involved in their regulation and balance. The gastrointestinal tract, kidneys, skin, and several endocrine glands function to maintain body water and electrolyte concentration in delicate balance despite large changes in intake and loss. However, life-threatening imbalances can occur rapidly when these homeostatic mechanisms are overwhelmed.

WATER AND ELECTROLYTE BALANCE

Total body water comprises approximately 60 per cent of the mass of the adult ruminant and pig. Total body water is inversely related to body fat; therefore, fattened livestock have relatively less body water. On the other hand, neonates have relatively more body water, as much as 86 per cent of body mass. Total body water is divided into 2 major physiologic compartments that have imperfect anatomic corollaries. The largest compartment is the intracellular fluid compartment (ICF), which accounts for about two thirds of total body water. The extracellular fluid compartment (ECF) makes up the balance. Extracellular water can further be divided into the intravascular fluid compartment and the interstitial fluid compartment. Intravascular fluid or plasma volume makes up about 5 per cent of total body mass. Water and certain molecules, such as urea, move freely from one compartment to the next, but the movement of certain ions and molecules is restricted or controlled by membrane channels and pumps. The osmolality of body fluids is relatively constant in healthy animals, about 300 mOsm/kg in the ECF and 400 mOsm/kg in the ICF. Sodium, the most important extracellular cation, constitutes about 95 per cent of the total cation pool. Major ECF anions include chloride and bicarbonate. The most important intracellular cation is potassium. The inverse relation of sodium and potassium inside and outside of the cells is maintained by the Na^+-K^+-ATPase pump found in almost all mammalian cell membranes. Phosphate, proteins, and other anions balance the charge of K^+ and the other cations inside the cells.

When dehydration occurs, all fluid compartments are affected, but not uniformly. Rapid dehydration causes disproportionate reduction in the intravascular compartment, followed by contraction of the interstitial fluid compartment and then by contraction of the intracellular fluid compartment. In time equilibration occurs, and all compartments become dehydrated.

Depletion of body water and electrolytes usually occurs simultaneously, but the relative amount of water and electrolytes lost is not constant. If excess free water is lost owing to evaporative loss or water deprivation, electrolyte *content* of the ECF will not increase, but electrolyte *concentration* will increase. This can be most easily measured by analyzing plasma sodium, which will rise above normal concentration. If body water and electrolytes are lost in the same relative proportions as they are found in the ECF, volume contraction or dehydration will be isotonic. Measuring plasma electrolytes will reveal a normal sodium concentration. In some situations, sodium loss may exceed water loss, which results in hypotonic or at least hyponatremic dehydration. This is seen in ruminants with ruptured bladder when sodium ion moves into the peritoneal cavity, and in some calves with diarrhea when sodium is lost in the feces. Most clinically dehydrated ruminants and swine have isotonic or nearly isotonic fluid losses. Therefore it is essential to supply electrolytes, particularly sodium, in addition to water for rehydration and volume replacement. Failure to do so will result in relative water excess, which will be quickly corrected by the kidneys, subsequently returning the animal to a volume-depleted state again.

FLUID AND ELECTROLYTE REPLACEMENT THERAPY

Fluid therapy in food animals is both challenging and rewarding. Although it is often technically difficult, labor-intensive, and inconvenient, this basic therapeutic modality produces clinical results that no sophisticated surgical technique or expensive miracle drug can duplicate.

The principles of therapy are relatively simple; the physical, logistical, and economic restraints can be (and have been) overcome by creative, resourceful practitioners. Administration of effective and economical fluid and electrolyte replacement therapy is achievable by every large animal practitioner.

Many of the principles of fluid therapy are the same for all classes of livestock. However, there are enough differences between neonates and mature ruminants in terms of the abnormalities frequently encountered and by solutions subsequently required to correct them to warrant separate discussions. Most of the research and clinical experience has been derived from cattle, but the same principles apply to other ruminants as well.

Fluid Therapy for Calves

The most frequent indication for fluid therapy for calves is neonatal calf diarrhea. Regardless of the etiologic organism, the metabolic changes resulting from diarrhea in calves are similar. They include (1) dehydration, (2) acidosis, (3) electrolyte abnormalities, and (4) negative energy balance and/or hypoglycemia.

The major cause of dehydration of these calves is fecal fluid loss, which can be as much as 13 per cent of body weight in 24 hours. Compounding this problem is decreased intake from either anorexia or withdrawal of milk by the owner.

Acidosis results from bicarbonate and strong cation loss in the stool, lactic acid accumulation in tissues, decreased renal excretion of acid, and increased production of organic acid in the colon in malabsorptive diarrheas. Along with water and bicarbonate, sodium, chloride, and potassium are lost in the feces, which results in a total body deficit of these ions.

Negative energy balance occurs consistently in diarrheic calves owing to decreased milk intake, decreased digestion or absorption of nutrients, or replacement of milk with low-energy oral rehydration solutions. In some calves with malabsorptive disease, acute hypoglycemia may occur. Increased energy demand, such as that resulting from cold weather or fever, exacerbates these problems.

Patient Assessment

DEHYDRATION. Acute dehydration can most accurately be quantitated by monitoring body weight. This is seldom possible except during rehydration because accurate baseline weights are usually not available. Serial measurement of packed cell volume (PCV) and total plasma protein (TPP) provide assessment of the relative state of hydration, but without baseline data, these measurements can be misleading. The range for PCV in healthy neonatal calves is 22 to 43 per cent, much too variable to provide quantitative information on hydration status, at least with a single sampling. The TPP is even more variable, depending greatly on the degree of colostral immunoglobulin absorption that occurred, as well as hydration. The PCV aids in assessment of rehydration efforts and can be used to help prevent overhydration, but TPP may be less useful. Proteins are contained in other fluid compartments, which makes the volume of distribution of plasma proteins larger than the plasma volume. Therefore, PCV is a more reliable indicator of changes in blood volume than is TPP.

Without a reliable quantitative measure for hydration status, we must rely on estimates based on clinical signs. Table 1 provides a rough guideline for estimating the degree of dehydration in cattle. However, this table, like many others, is based on clinical experience and response to therapy, not on scientific evidence. Naylor found that calves assessed to be 8 to 10 per cent dehydrated by a clinical scoring system, and rehydrated accordingly, gained only about 5.2 per cent of their body weight in 24 hours, even though they were no longer clinically dehydrated. Perhaps the ICF compartment had not equilibrated; thus restoration of total body water was not accomplished, or perhaps our method of assessment overestimates dehydration. Regardless, rehydration based on estimated degree of dehydration is clinically successful. Veterinarians, however, should not become overly concerned with pinpointing the exact degree of dehydration. Rather, we should be concerned whether intravenous therapy is needed, or whether voluntary or forced oral supplementation will suffice.

Traditionally, 8 per cent dehydration is the severity beyond which it is considered that oral fluid therapy will not suffice. Clinical signs associated with severe dehydration include marked enophthalmos, prolonged skin tenting, dry mucous membranes, and moderate to severe depression. Calves displaying these signs will benefit the most from intravenous therapy. In general, calves that readily suckle quantities of rehydration solution sufficient to meet their replacement, maintenance, and ongoing loss needs will respond to oral solutions. Many more severely dehydrated calves will respond to forced oral solutions as well, but intravenous replacement is preferred.

ACIDOSIS. Acidemia can quickly and accurately be assessed when a blood gas analyzer is available, but access to such a unit is uncommon in private practice. It may be beneficial for practitioners to have several samples analyzed occasionally as a means of evaluating how effective their empirical treatment regimens are. A recent study showed that blood samples submerged in ice water can be held up to 24 hours before analysis for pH and blood gases. Therefore practitioners could have the samples analyzed after the fact as a self-education experience for help in future cases. Samples should be collected into a heparinized syringe anaerobically, and the needle should be capped with a rubber stopper immediately. Consult your laboratory for details.

Total carbon dioxide analyzers are an alternative at a reasonable cost. These are only valid in assessment of nonrespiratory acidosis or alkalosis, which is the type of acid-base disturbance most frequently encountered in conscious animals. In most cases in practice, the degree of acidosis will be estimated. Although some authors have published tables that suggest estimated base deficit based on the same criteria as dehydration, these estimates have not been evaluated experimentally. Kasari and Naylor attempted to use a depression score by evaluating a battery of clinical signs of diarrheic, acidemic calves. Unfortunately, the scoring system was inaccurate at predicting the degree of acidosis in calves. In fact, in another report, these same authors described several calves with moderate to severe metabolic acidosis without diarrhea or dehydration. Still another study determined that dehydrated calves greater than 1 week of age had more severe acidosis (mean base deficit of 19.5 mEq/L) than did those less than 1 week of age (mean base deficit of 14.4 mEq/L). As a rule of thumb, severely diarrheic calves less than 1 week of age can be assumed to have a base deficit of 10 to 15 mEq/L whereas those greater than 1 week of age can be assumed to have a base deficit of 15 to 20 mEq/L.

ELECTROLYTE IMBALANCE. Laboratory analysis of serum or plasma electrolytes is of limited benefit in evaluating the replacement needs of diarrheic calves and, if misinterpreted, could lead to inappropriate therapy. Plasma represents a very small portion of total body water, and the concentration of

Table 1. GUIDE TO ESTIMATION OF FLUID REPLACEMENT REQUIREMENT

Percentage of Body Weight Needed	Clinical Signs
6–7	Slight enophthalmos, skin turgor slightly increased, mucous membranes moist
8–9	Eyes obviously sunken, skin turgor obviously increased, mucous membranes tacky
10–12	Eyes deeply sunken in orbits, skin tents and does not return, mucous membranes dry, depression evident

electrolytes in a blood sample must be interpreted in light of that fact. If sodium and chloride are within normal limits and a calf has lost 10 per cent of ECF volume, then the calf has a total body sodium and chloride deficit of approximately 10 per cent. Because plasma sodium and chloride concentrations are usually within or below accepted norms in diarrheic calves, it is extremely important to provide these electrolytes in replacement solutions. Failure to do so will result in dilution of the already deficient ions.

Potentially more misleading than plasma sodium and chloride laboratory values is potassium. Many dehydrated, acidemic calves are hyperkalemic, yet they have a total body potassium deficit. This paradox is the result of a shift of potassium out of the ICF compartment into the ECF compartment during acidemia. The ECF, which normally contains only about 5 per cent of the body's total exchangeable potassium, has a greater than the normal concentration of potassium. Because of the fecal and urinary losses, however, ICF potassium concentration and total body potassium content are decreased.

BLOOD GLUCOSE. Blood glucose determination can be made by a serum analyzer or by a dipstick method. Hypoglycemia in calves results in weakness, lethargy, coma, convulsions, and opisthotonos. Negative energy balance is not easily quantitated because it can result from inadequate intake, malabsorption-maldigestion, or increased metabolic demand due to fever or low ambient temperature. If milk is withheld for more than 48 hours, especially in cold weather, serious energy deficits can occur. Weak or recumbent calves that do not appear to be dehydrated, but are emaciated, are usually suffering from malabsorption or malnutrition. Sometimes these calves respond, at least temporarily, to intravenous dextrose infusion.

Estimating Fluid and Electrolyte Replacement Requirements

The first priority in treatment of a dehydrated calf should be restoration of ECF volume. When estimating the volume of fluid needed by a patient, the veterinarian should consider not only the deficit, but also maintenance requirement and compensation for continuing loss. Daily maintenance fluid requirement for the neonatal calf is 50 to 100 ml/kg, whereas ongoing fluid loss can range from minimal amounts to as much as 4 L in 24 hours. One must avoid overemphasizing the estimate of the degree of dehydration and the calculation of volume *replacement* needed, while neglecting to include maintenance and ongoing loss into the calculations. In many cases, the actual deficit is less than half of the total 24-hour volume requirement.

Second in priority to correcting ECF volume depletion is correcting acidosis. It has been suggested that the restoration of ECF volume alone would allow the kidneys to eliminate acid in sufficient quantity to restore normal acid-base balance. This has been disproved in calves with moderate to severe acidemia. Two studies, one using intravenously administered solutions and one using orally administered solutions, have demonstrated the failure of nonalkalinizing solutions to resolve acidosis expeditiously even though ECF volume was restored.

Acidosis can be corrected by the administration of sodium bicarbonate ions or so-called bicarbonate precursors, salts of weak organic acids. Alternatives to bicarbonate include lactate, acetate, gluconate, and citrate. Studies in calves have demonstrated the superior alkalinizing efficiency of bicarbonate, compared with L-lactate and acetate.

Sodium bicarbonate is the most economical and readily available alkalinizing agent; however, it cannot be heat sterilized. It also should not be used in solutions containing calcium because an insoluble compound, calcium carbonate, will be formed.

Alternative alkalinizing agents offer advantages and disadvantages as well. Lactate is probably the most widely used alkalinizing agent in veterinary medicine, although it has several shortcomings. Hepatic perfusion and function are necessary for its metabolism, and endogenous lactate (lactic acid) that accumulates during hypovolemia and shock can reduce its metabolism. Also, commercial preparations of lactated Ringer's solution contain racemic mixtures of D- and L-lactate. Only the L-isomer is metabolized efficiently, whereas most of the D-isomer is excreted in the urine unchanged. Therefore, the alkalinizing potential of the racemic mixture is only about half of the alkalinizing potential of an equimolar amount of the L-isomer. Acetate has the advantage of being metabolized by peripheral tissues and of having no significant endogenous source and no unmetabolized isomer. Citrate can be used in oral rehydration solutions, but its calcium-chelating properties preclude its inclusion in solutions for intravenous administration. Gluconate, an alkalinizing agent used in combination with acetate in some commercially prepared solutions for intravenous administration to humans, dogs, and horses, has been shown to be ineffective as an alkalinizing agent in calves when administered intravenously, but it is effective when administered orally.

Rate of administration of alkalinizing agents, especially sodium bicarbonate, is a controversial subject. Some concern is warranted because rapid intravenous administration of 8.3 per cent sodium bicarbonate can cause serious side effects. Rapid injection of this solution can cause hypernatremia and hyperosmolality as well as rapid alkalinizing. Another complication reported to be associated with the use of sodium bicarbonate for alkalinization is cerebrospinal fluid (CSF) acidosis. This condition was reported in 1967 in 2 human patients who received sodium bicarbonate infusions; however, whereas numerous warnings about CSF acidosis can be found in veterinary literature, the author is not aware of a documented clinical case of CSF acidosis in domestic animals and therefore does not hesitate to replace the total calculated deficit of bicarbonate in the initial deficit replacement solution.

When blood gas analysis is available, the value for the base deficit (BD) can be used to calculate total base requirement by use of the formula

$$0.6 \times BD \times body\ weight = base\ requirement\ in\ mEq$$

We have found 0.6 to be an accurate estimate of the bicarbonate space in young calves, although other factors as small as 0.3 have been recommended for mature cattle. When the value for total carbon dioxide or bicarbonate is known, it can be subtracted from 25, and the difference can be used in place of BD in the formula. When it is not possible to quantitate acid-base status, an estimate of 10 to 20 mEq/L may be used to formulate fluids for intravenous use for diarrheic calves. Remember that calves greater than 1 week of age tend to become more severely acidotic.

The addition of glucose to rehydration solutions has 3 benefits. In orally administered solutions, glucose enhances sodium absorption in the small intestine via a transmembrane cotransport system. Once absorbed or injected, glucose also stimulates the release of insulin, which in turn enhances the movement of potassium from the ECF to the ICF. Last, glucose provides readily available energy. Glucose concentrations of 1 to 2 per cent in intravenously administered solutions have produced favorable clinical results and usually do not result in significant glucosuria or osmotic diuresis. Additional glucose may be provided in oral solutions. In selected cases, total or partial parenteral nutrition may be beneficial to calves with severe prolonged malabsorptive diarrhea. In one study, calves receiving parenteral nutrition gained more weight but did not have better survivability than those receiving traditional therapy.

The importance of replacing sodium and chloride should not be overlooked. Remember that total body sodium and chloride are deficient in dehydrated calves, even when plasma concentrations are normal.

The administration of potassium to a hyperkalemic patient seems absurd at first, but the objective is to replace the total body potassium deficit that exists despite hyperkalemia. Administration of potassium to hyperkalemic acidemic calves can be safely accomplished by concurrently administering bicarbonate and dextrose. As previously mentioned, dextrose and bicarbonate enhance the movement of potassium from the ECF to the ICF. Ideally, the initial liter or so of intravenously administered rehydration solution should contain less potassium than in subsequent volumes. However, practicality often dictates the use of a single solution for rehydration. There seems to be little danger in including up to 20 mEq of potassium per liter if bicarbonate and dextrose are included in the solution.

Formulating a Solution for Intravenous Administration

There are as many "correct" ways to formulate solutions for intravenous administration in calves as one can imagine. The following is a list of suggested criteria for intravenously administered solutions.

1. Osmolality between 300 and 450 mOsm/L.
2. Sodium and chloride concentrations near or slightly less than normal plasma concentrations.
3. Potassium concentration 10 to 20 mEq/L. (Because 1 g of potassium chloride contains 14 mEq potassium, inclusion of 1 g of potassium chloride per liter fulfills this criterion.)
4. Dextrose at 10 to 20 g/L of solution (1 to 2 per cent).
5. Sodium bicarbonate or a suitable metabolizable base calculated to meet the measured deficit (or an estimated base deficit of 10 to 20 mEq/L if laboratory values are not available).

Of course, commercial solutions like lactated Ringer's can be used. In most cases, sodium bicarbonate will be required in addition to correct acidosis. Dextrose and additional potassium should also be added. Remember that bicarbonate should not be mixed in the same container with calcium-containing solutions, such as lactated Ringer's.

Whereas it may be ideal to rehydrate a patient over 24 to 48 hours, bovine practitioners must often use the maximal safe infusion rate rather than the ideal. Overhydration and hypertension can be detected when central venous pressure is monitored, but this luxury is seldom available to the practitioner. A maximum of 80 ml/kg/hr has been suggested as a "safe" flow rate. A more conservative rate of 50 ml/kg/hr is probably a reasonable, relatively safe maximal infusion rate. With use of this infusion rate, most calves can be rehydrated in 2 to 3 hours. During rapid intravenous administration of fluids, the veterinarian or attendant should periodically monitor heart rate, respiratory rate and character, and attitude, adjusting the flow rate if necessary.

When possible, it is desirable to administer approximately 1 L of the solution rapidly to reverse hypovolemic shock, and then administer the balance over a period of hours. This will maximize the benefit of the therapy by minimizing the diuresis that is sometimes induced by rapid fluid administration. If it is impractical or impossible to administer the total 24-hour requirement, or even the total deficit by intravenous infusion, 1 or 2 L of fluid administered intravenously may be enough to improve the circulatory status of a calf so that the balance of the calf's requirement may be provided by the oral route. In other words, a relatively small volume of fluids administered intravenously may convert a calf from the "intravenous fluid required" to the "oral fluid satisfactory" category. Fluids for maintenance and continued loss may be administered orally or by slow intravenous infusion.

Oral Rehydration Therapy for Calves

The growth in popularity of oral rehydration solution (ORS) for calves is an accurate reflection of the success of this therapeutic modality. Veterinarians and stockmen alike have witnessed the results of oral rehydration and have promoted its use. There are many products commercially produced (Table 2), each with its own claim to superiority. The following discussion should help veterinarians make informed decisions concerning the use of these products.

ADVANTAGES OF ORS. There are several obvious advantages of oral fluid therapy over intravenous fluid therapy. Economy of materials, time, and equipment is the major advantage in treating food animals. The ORS can be carried and stored in dry form, mixed with tap water, administered by nursing bottle or by stomach tube, and administered as infrequently as every 12 hours. Whereas suckling delivers the solution more directly to the abomasum by inducing reticular groove closure, intubation is also an accepted means of delivery in neonatal calves. A slight delay in absorption may occur after intubation, which could be beneficial if a depot effect is desired rather than an immediate effect. Finally, the gradual absorption of the ORS allows more flexibility in the formulation of these solutions than of those for intravenous use. Greater concentrations of potassium, glucose, and total osmoles can be supplied in ORS than in intravenous solutions.

CHARACTERISTICS OF ORS. Several types and numerous individual formulations of ORS are available commercially. Although a significant difference in constituents exists, almost all of these solutions have been used successfully. Included in all ORS formulations are substantial amounts of sodium, chloride, potassium, and glucose. Most contain bicarbonate or another alkalinizing agent. Many contain glycine, acetate, or citrate to enhance sodium and water absorption. Calcium, magnesium, and phosphorus are present in some. Additives such as mucopolysaccharides and pregelatinized starch are now included as antidiarrheal agents.

The major differences between formulations occur in the following constituents: glucose, alkalinizing agents, and total osmolality. The variety of combinations of constituents in today's commercial ORS market allows the veterinarian to choose the type of solution that will perform best in a given situation. High-energy solutions approach the maintenance needs of the calf and reduce weight loss, compared with low-energy solutions. However, if a significant amount of glucose reaches the colon, it may exacerbate diarrhea. When milk intake is withdrawn or reduced for more than 24 hours, moderate- to high-energy solutions should probably be used.

Whenever acidosis is moderate to severe, ORS with alkalinizing agents must be used to restore normal acid-base status in a timely manner. According to Naylor's work, alkalinizing solutions are more likely to be needed for older calves. Nonalkalinizing solutions are indicated for clients who monitor calves closely and institute fluid therapy early in the course of disease before dehydration or acidosis becomes severe. Alkalinizing potential and alkalinity of solutions do not necessarily parallel each other. Solutions containing sodium bicarbonate as an alkalinizing agent are alkaline, whereas some solutions

Table 2. GUIDE TO ORAL ELECTROLYTE REPLACERS

Product (Manufacturer)	Na^+ (mEq/L)	K^+ (mEq/L)	Ca^{2+} (mEq/L)	Mg^{2+} (mEq/L)	Cl^- (mEq/L)	HCO_3^- (mEq/L)	Glycine (mEq/L)	Dextrose (g/L)	Osmolality (mOsm/L)	pH	How Supplied (ml)	Comments
Biolyte (Upjohn Company)	134	22.8	—	6.6	75.8	81.0	—	68	698	—	800-g bottle (80 g/L)	For re-establishment and maintenance of electrolyte balance and energy for neonatal calves with dehydration due to diarrhea
Life Guard H. E. (SmithKline Beecham)	100	24	11.5	3.1	49	76.0	2.4	76	—	—	178-g pkt (1 pkt/2 quarts)	For use as an electrolyte replacement and nutrient supplement after oral administration; refrigerate if not used immediately; discard unused solution after 24 hours
Resorb (SmithKline Beecham)	73.2	15.5	—	—	73.2	—	3.1	22.3	315	4.3	64-g pkt (1 pkt/2 quarts)	For use as an aid in replacing vital fluids, nutrients, and electrolytes in dehydrated calves; is not alkalinizing; contains citrate (2.8 mEq/L)
Revive (TechAmerica)	90	25	—	—	85	(60)	3.75	72	705	—	162.5-g pkt (1 pkt/2 quarts)	Aid in replacement of normal body fluids and electrolytes for energy-rich nutritional support in young diarrheic calves, lambs, and foals; may be mixed with milk replacers; HCO_3^- provided as acetate

Source: Modified from Frederick GS, Hannaway CD, Hunt E: Oral electrolyte replacement solutions. Vet Clin North Am [Food Anim Pract] 6(1):149–183, 1990.

containing a metabolizable base are actually acidic when consumed. Bicarbonate-containing solutions are therefore more likely to alkalinize the abomasum and allow the proliferation of bacteria and possibly the passage of pathogens to the intestines. The clinical significance of this is unproven, but experimentally it is easier to produce colibacillosis in calves if sodium bicarbonate is administered before bacterial challenge.

The high-energy solutions mentioned must also be hyperosmolar, because the energy source is glucose. Reasonable arguments can be made for both isosmolar and hyperosmolar solutions. Intuitively, it seems reasonable that consumption of hyperosmolar solutions would result in movement of free water into the gastrointestinal lumen along the osmotic gradient. Such a shift in water would exacerbate the pre-existing dehydration. There is evidence that a slight transient shift occurs, but no adverse effects have been shown. On the other hand, a villous countercurrent mechanism causes the interstitium of the villus tip to become hyperosmolar during absorption, which makes a hyperosmolar solution "isosmotic" relative to the interstitial fluid in closest proximity. However, the merit of creating a luminal osmolality equal to the interstitium is questionable, because one of the theories explaining the purpose of the countercurrent mechanism and resulting villous hyperosmolality is that the gradient established between the lumen and interstitium enhances water absorption from the lumen. If this gradient is reduced or negated by hypertonic solutions, water absorption could theoretically be reduced.

There is probably not one "ideal" ORS for all situations. In addition to the medical and physiologic considerations, other factors (such as cost, convenience, and palatability) must be considered when an ORS is chosen.

Using ORS for Optimal Results. In order to maximize the benefit of ORS, there are certain practices to adopt and others to avoid. The controversy over whether ORS should be used as a supplement to milk feeding or as a replacement is still unsettled, but a consensus is forming on a few points. There is evidence in people that removing all food from the diet results in rapid loss of digestive and absorptive capability of the intestines. In calves, weight loss is accelerated by withdrawing milk and replacing it with ORS, especially the lower-energy solutions. Therefore it is desirable to maintain calves on milk if the intestinal damage is not so great that a severe malabsorptive osmotic diarrhea results. However, recent studies show that consumption of bicarbonate-containing solutions interspersed between milk feedings results in poor digestibility of the milk. Also, if ORS is mixed 1:1 with milk, diarrhea results. From these studies, it can be concluded that ORS should not be mixed with milk or milk replacer and that non–bicarbonate-containing solutions may be preferred if calves are not taken off milk during the time that fluids are being administered. If milk is withdrawn from the diet, it should probably be reintroduced after 48 hours or less to avoid excessive weight loss.

FLUID THERAPY IN MATURE RUMINANTS

The sheer size of mature cattle and the great quantity of fluid required to rehydrate them has prevented many veterinarians from taking full advantage of intravenous rehydration therapy. We should not be any less willing to take the time and charge the appropriate fee to administer intravenous solutions to a cow in endotoxic shock due to coliform mastitis than we are to perform a cesarean section on a cow in dystocia. Both can be lifesaving procedures.

Although many of the principles of fluid therapy of mature ruminants are similar to those of calves and other species, many important exceptions exist. When assessing hydration status, one must remember that body weight and rumen fill can be misleading. Cattle with carbohydrate engorgement may not lose weight and may actually look full, but much of the fill is intraruminal water, which is unavailable to the animal. Also, skin tent and enophthalmos must be evaluated in light of the body condition. Emaciated cows may have sunken eyes and skin that tents, regardless of their hydration status. When deciding on route of administration, one should consider not only hydration status but cardiovascular status as well. For example, cattle with strangulating-obstructing gastrointestinal disease, especially those soon to undergo standing surgery, will benefit from intravenous fluid therapy even if they are not severely dehydrated because they may be in or near shock and cardiovascular collapse.

The volume required for complete rehydration of a large cow or bull is substantial and may dissuade practitioners from using this mode of therapy. It should be remembered that 10 to 20 L of fluid administered rather rapidly may be lifesaving, even though it represents less than half of the total fluid deficit. By use of at least some intravenous fluid, intravascular volume can be restored, an underlying problem can be remedied by surgical or medical means, and oral fluids can be supplied to replace the rest of the deficit. To reduce the cost of administering intravenous fluids, practitioners may consider formulating their own solutions. Dry ingredients can be preweighed and packaged and mixed with sterile distilled water immediately before administration. Another disadvantage of prepackaged solutions, besides the expense, is that there are relatively few solutions appropriate for most cattle.

Unlike neonates, adult ruminants do not usually require alkalinizing fluids when they are dehydrated. A few conditions (such as choke, carbohydrate engorgement, severe diarrhea, and diabetes mellitus) are consistently associated with acidosis. Renal failure, fatty liver–ketosis, and pregnancy toxemia are sometimes associated with acidosis. Abomasal volvulus, displacement and impaction, intussusception, and cecal torsion are causes of moderate to severe alkalosis. Many cattle with metritis, mastitis, pneumonia, and other conditions are alkalotic or have normal acid-base status. Therefore, nonalkalinizing solutions will be the fluid of choice for most dehydrated mature ruminants. Usually accompanying alkalosis is hypochloridemia. Sequestration of chloride in the proximal small intestine, abomasum, and rumen results in hypochloridemic alkalosis. Alkalosis and anorexia result in hypokalemia in many sick cattle. Lactating dairy cattle are often hypocalcemic as well. In order to address these metabolic problems, we have used the following formulation at our hospital:

160 g NaCl
20 g KCl
10 g $CaCl_2$
q.s. to 20 L

This solution may be administered intraruminally via tube or intravenously. If it is administered intravenously, 1 bottle of commercially prepared calcium borogluconate solution may be substituted for the calcium chloride, and up to a liter of 50 per cent dextrose may be added if ketosis is a concurrent problem.

When administering solutions intraruminally, the author prefers to pass a medium-sized nasogastric tube through the nasal cavity instead of using a Frick mouth speculum. The procedure is less stressful to the patient and allows the veterinarian to administer fluids unassisted. Be aware that on a relative weight basis, the nasal cavity of the cow is smaller than that of the horse, so a relatively smaller tube must be used. If nutritional supplementation is needed, pelleted feed (with no large pieces of grain) can be soaked in warm water, made into a slurry, and pumped in by use of a marine bilge pump or a commercially available cattle pump system.

Intravenous administration is usually accomplished through a jugular catheter. A 10- to 14-gauge catheter is sufficient to permit rapid fluid administration. Cyanocrylic glue is effective for affixing the catheter to the skin. The author prefers to use a 30-inch extension set connected to the catheter and held in place by elastic tape wrapped around the cow's neck. The extension set may be taped so that the end is positioned at the dorsum of the cow's neck to allow easy access for attachment to the intravenous administration set or for injections. An alternative to the jugular is the ear vein. It is easily accessible and is more convenient to use if cattle must be restrained in a head-catch during fluid administration. A 16- to 18-gauge 1- or 2-inch catheter is placed in the vein, glued and taped in place, with or without an extension set (Fig. 1). Because of the smaller size of the vein, speed of fluid administration is limited; however, the rate of administration is great enough to rehydrate even a severely dehydrated cow. An ear catheter can also be used as an access for repeated intravenous infusions. One must be aware that an artery is present and prominent on the dorsal surface of the pinna. It should be identified by palpation of a pulse and avoided.

USE OF BLOOD AND PLASMA

WHOLE BLOOD. Whole blood is indicated when the red cell mass is below that necessary to carry an adequate amount of oxygen to the tissues. The point at which transfusion is necessary is determined in large part by the time course over which the red cells were lost or destroyed. The slower the process, the more tolerant the animal is to a low PCV. Cattle that become anemic gradually can tolerate a PCV as low as 8 per cent if they are not stressed. Transfusion has been recommended at a PCV of 12 to 15 per cent if the anemia develops acutely. However, the most important indicator for determining if transfusion is indicated is the overall condition of the animal determined by respiratory rate and character, heart rate, and neurologic status. Another important fact to consider before deciding to transfuse is whether the stress of transfusion itself is likely to result in death.

Although plasma is more desirable, whole blood transfusion can be used to provide immunoglobulins to calves with failure of passive transfer. Achieving an adequate plasma immunoglobulin concentration in a calf with complete failure of passive transfer with the use of whole blood is difficult because the volume required may result in volume overload, polycythemia, and/or hemolytic icterus. Therefore whole blood is most useful in calves with partial failure of passive transfer. Up to 2 L of whole blood can be safely administered to a 45-kg calf.

Transfusion reactions are extremely rare in cattle that have not been transfused previously. A practical means of determining compatibility is to infuse a small quantity of blood, about 0.5 ml/kg body weight, and wait 10 minutes before proceeding with the transfusion. Blood should be administered slowly (10 ml/kg/hr or less) through a blood administration set with an appropriate filter. Usually, 10 to 15 ml/kg are administered. Reported signs of transfusion reaction include hiccoughing, dyspnea, muscle tremor, salivation, lacrimation, and fever. Epinephrine hydrochloride 1:1000 should be administered (at 4 to 5 ml intramuscularly to an adult cow) if signs of anaphylaxis occur.

Although many diseases are transmissible by transfusion, bovine leukosis and anaplasmosis are two of the most important. If a known uninfected donor is unavailable, the donor should probably be a herdmate of the recipient. This will at least prevent inadvertent introduction of a new pathogen into the herd.

It is safe to remove 10 to 15 ml/kg of blood from a healthy donor. Remember, however, that if this same dose is given to a recipient the rise in PCV will be small (3 to 4 per cent) and the duration short because exogenous red blood cells are rapidly destroyed by the recipient.

When blood is collected for immediate use, sodium citrate

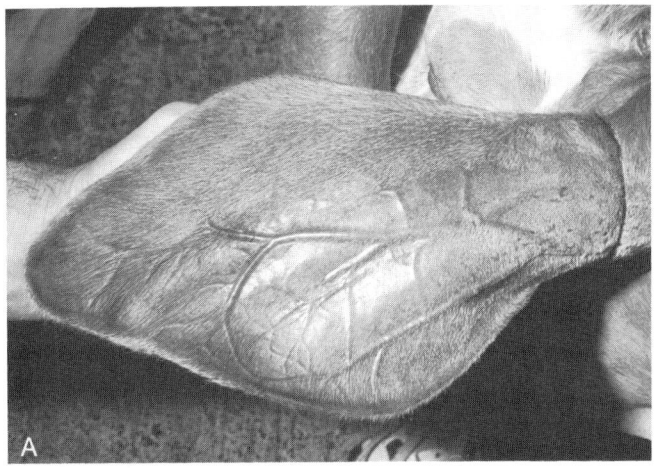
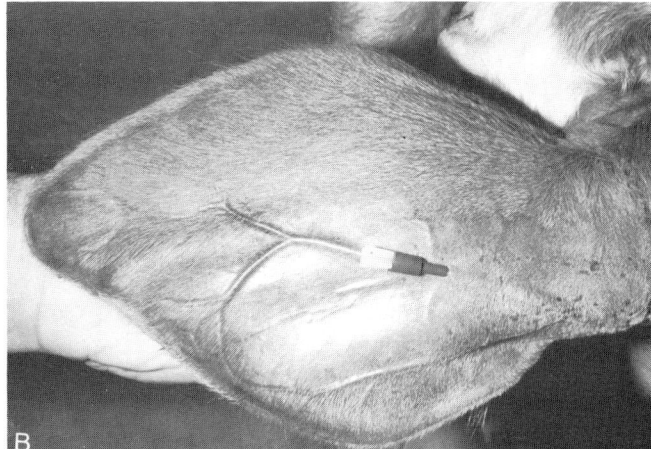
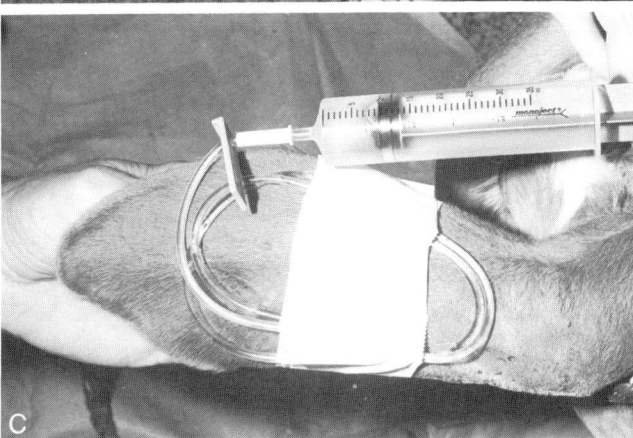

Figure 1. *A*, Distended veins on the dorsal surface of the bovine ear. Note the rubber band serving as a tourniquet. *B*, Catheter in place attached to the extension set and glued to the skin. *C*, Catheter and extension set taped to the ear, ready for attachment to the fluid administration set.

is an effective and inexpensive anticoagulant. It should be purchased or formulated to a 2.5 to 4 per cent solution and added as 1 part solution to 9 parts of blood. In our hospital, we stock gallon jugs with 400 ml of sterile sodium citrate solution ready for collection. If blood is to be stored for more than a few hours, acid citrate dextrose solution should be used.

PLASMA. Plasma is indicated in cases of hypoproteinemia and failure of passive transfer. Because ruminant red blood cells do not settle by gravity, centrifugation is required. The large volumes required to raise the recipient's plasma protein concentration significantly make plasma transfusion a relatively uncommon practice. In attempting to provide an acceptable immunoglobulin concentration to a calf with complete failure of passive transfer, 2 L of plasma should be administered.

SHOCK

Shock in its broadest sense is a condition in which there is decreased tissue perfusion, cellular hypoxia, and ultimately cell death.

There are three major types of shock: hypovolemic, cardiogenic, and vasculogenic. The type of shock most commonly encountered in cattle is vasculogenic, specifically endotoxic or septic shock. Endotoxin is a constituent of the cell wall of gram-negative bacteria. It is released when bacterial cells die. Causes of endotoxic shock in cattle include colisepticemia, coliform mastitis, septic metritis, and pasteurellosis.

Endotoxic shock is characterized by dyspnea, depression, congested mucous membranes, recumbency, and death. Cardiovascular effects include decreased mean arterial blood pressure and cardiac output, and increased pulmonary arterial pressure. The most important treatment for shock in food animals is rapid intravenous infusion of crystalloid solutions, usually a polyionic balanced solution. The rate of administration should be rapid, especially initially. In most cattle, 75 ml/kg/hr is probably safe for at least 30 to 60 minutes. In people, dogs, and horses, hypertonic saline (7 per cent NaCl solution) 4 ml/kg administered rapidly intravenously has been used successfully to treat shock. One study in calves failed to demonstrate superiority over conventional therapy. Hypertonic saline should not be used in dehydrated animals.

In endotoxic shock, corticosteroids and flunixin meglumine have been shown to be effective in reducing the cardiopulmonary effects. The "shock" dose of dexamethasone for horses is said to be 5 mg/kg, although many veterinarians use smaller doses. Flunixin meglumine may be approved for cattle by the time this book is published. The recommended dose will probably be 2.2 mg/kg, twice that recommended for horses (Table 3).

Table 3. DRUG REFERENCE LIST

Name of Drug	Company	Species	Dose
Dexamethasone	Many	Bovine	5 mg/kg for shock
Flunixin meglumine (Banamine)	Schering-Plough, Kenilworth, NJ	Bovine	2.2 mg/kg

BIBLIOGRAPHY

Naylor JM: Severity and nature of acidosis in diarrheic calves over and under one week of age. Can Vet J 28:168–173, 1987.

Roussel AJ: Fluid and electrolyte therapy. Vet Clin North Am [Food Anim Pract] 6:1, 1990.

Schotman AJH: The acid-base balance in clinically healthy and diseased cattle. Neth J Vet Sci 4:5–23, 1971.

Therapeutic Management of Inflammation

VERNON C. LANGSTON, DVM, PhD, Diplomate, ACVCP

Inflammation plays a prominent role in many afflictions. Indeed, the inflammatory process is a part of the normal defense mechanisms that first localize and then aid in the repair of damaged tissue. This is true most notably in the acute phases. However, widespread or chronic inflammation may become detrimental. In these cases, therapeutic interruption of the inflammatory process is required to avoid inadequate tissue perfusion, tissue fibrosis, and loss of function. Because pharmacologic intervention is usually performed at the inflammatory mediator level, a brief review of the inflammatory process is in order.

After an insult to tissue, a variety of mediators derived from cells, plasma, or tissues are released. Those mediators that can be manipulated pharmacologically include histamine and the eicosanoid mediators (prostaglandins, leukotrienes, and thromboxanes).

Histamine is found in mast cells and basophils. After its release, it causes prominent vasodilation and edema, which result in the well-known signs of inflammation: redness (erythema), warmth, swelling, pain, and loss of function. Histamine is the prominent mediator, however, for only the first 30 to 60 minutes after injury.

Whereas histamine is of obvious importance in such acute conditions as anaphylactoid shock, in most other instances it plays a secondary role to the eicosanoid mediators. As Figure 1 illustrates, after tissue injury, phospholipases convert the fatty acids of cell membranes (e.g., arachidonic acid) into intermediaries that are subsequently acted upon by either lipoxygenases or cyclo-oxygenases, which produce leukotrienes or prostaglandins, respectively.

The leukotrienes are responsible for a variety of actions on vascular and airway smooth muscle including pronounced bronchoconstriction. Additionally, many of them are strongly chemotactic to white blood cells, which move into an area to remove the offending organism or agent. If the white blood cells are overwhelmed and die in significant numbers, their lysosomal enzymes containing large amounts of free radicals will be released into the tissues, thereby aggravating the inflammation. At present, there are no clinically available drugs that can selectively inhibit the lipoxygenase pathway.

Prostaglandins are a group of autacoids with tremendously diverse and often opposite actions. The exact role of the prostaglandins (and related thromboxanes) in inflammation and disease is not totally understood. It is, however, well accepted that these agents are capable of sensitizing pain receptors, causing fever, and altering blood flow. Because prostaglandins regulate a number of normal body mechanisms including gastrointestinal mucus production and renal blood flow, it is not surprising that drugs that interfere with cyclo-oxygenase activity cause gastrointestinal ulceration and renal papillary necrosis as common side effects.

Table 1 presents an overview of the common anti-inflammatory drugs.

ANTIHISTAMINES

Antihistamines act by binding to the H_1-receptors of cells, thereby serving as a competitive antagonist to histamine. Although they have been suggested for treatment of a variety of illnesses including laminitis, mastitis, pneumonia, and others, their use in food animals has remained empiric. They are

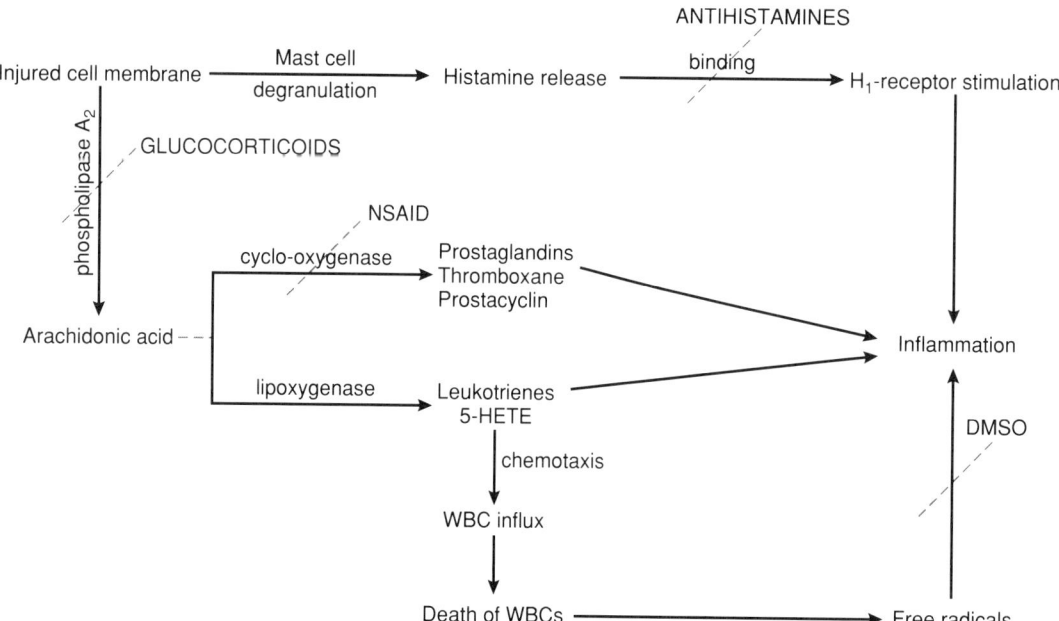

Figure 1. Site of action of common anti-inflammatory agents.

Table 1. COMMON ANTI-INFLAMMATORY DRUGS AND THEIR DOSAGES

Generic Name	Trade Name	Source	Species	Dosage
Antihistaminic Drugs				
Pyrilamine maleate	Histavet-P	Schering Corporation, Kenilworth, NJ	Cattle	1 mg/kg IM or IV q 6–12 hr
Tripelennamine	ReCovr Injection*	Solvay Veterinary Inc., Princeton, NJ	Cattle	1 mg/kg IM or IV q 6–12 hr
			Swine	1 mg/kg IM or IV q 6–12 hr
Diphenhydramine	Benadryl	Parke-Davis, Morris Plains, NJ	Cattle	0.5–1 mg/kg IM or IV q 8 hr
Nonsteroidal Anti-Inflammatory Drugs[1]				
Aspirin	Aspirin 60-gr tablets*	Veterinary Laboratories Inc., Lenexa, KS	Cattle	100 mg/kg po q 12 h
			Swine	10 mg/kg po q 6 h
Phenylbutazone	Butazolidin	Pitman-Moore, Inc., Washington Crossing, NJ	Cattle	10 mg/kg IV or po q 48 h
			Swine	4 mg/kg IV or po q 24 hr
Dipyrone	Novin Injection	Haver; Mobay Corporation, Shawnee, KS	Cattle	20 mg/kg IV, IM, SC q 8–12 hr
Flunixin	Banamine Injection	Schering Corporation, Kenilworth, NJ	Cattle and swine	1.1–2.2 mg/kg IV, IM[2]
Steroids[1]				
Dexamethasone				
Sodium phosphate	Azium SP	Schering Corporation, Kenilworth, NJ	Cattle and swine	Shock: 1 mg/kg IV
				Inflammation: 0.15 mg/kg IV or IM q 24–48 hr
Solution[3]	Azium**	Schering Corporation, Kenilworth, NJ	Cattle and swine	Same as sodium phosphate form
Prednisolone				
Sodium succinate	Solu-Delta-Cortef	Upjohn Company, Kalamazoo, MI	Cattle and swine	Shock[4]: 5–10 mg/kg IV
Sodium phosphate	Cortisate 20	Schering Corporation, Kenilworth, NJ	Cattle and swine	Shock[4]: 5–10 mg/kg IV
				Inflammation: 1 mg/kg IM s.i.d.
Prednisone suspension	Meticorten	Schering Corporation, Kenilworth, NJ	Cattle and swine	Inflammation: 1 mg/kg IM s.i.d.
Isoflupredone acetate	Predef 2X*	Upjohn Company, Kalamazoo, MI	Cattle	Ketosis: 0.04 mg/kg IM
Dimethyl Sulfoxide				
DMSO solution	Domoso	Syntex, West Des Moines, IA	Cattle and swine	CNS inflammation: 1 g/kg IV as a 10% solution s.i.d.

*Labeled for use in the United States in cattle at the stated dose.
**Labeled for use in the United States in cattle but dose quoted is higher than label recommendation (withdrawal times may be longer). No asterisk indicates use in the United States is extra-label.
1. Adjust to lowest effective dose if therapy exceeds 3 to 5 days.
2. Repeat flunixin as needed based on clinical response but not more often than every 8 to 12 hours in cattle or every 12 to 24 hours in pigs.
3. Product is in a solution with propylene glycol and alcohol. Although it may be given slowly intravenously, the sodium phosphate form is preferred for this route because of its quicker onset and minimal cardiovascular depression.
4. Doses 3 to 5 times that stated are commonly quoted.
IM = intramuscular; IV = intravenous; SC = subcutaneous; po = per os (by mouth); s.i.d. = once a day.

of doubtful efficacy in most food animal diseases with the exception of allergies. When they are used, the following points should be kept in mind.

1. Antihistamines do not reverse the effects of histamine; they only prevent its binding. In an acute allergic reaction (i.e., anaphylaxis), primary emphasis must be placed on physiologically reversing life-threatening hypotension, laryngeal edema, and so on. In such situations, epinephrine and fluid support are usually the preferred treatment with antihistamines used as ancillary agents to minimize the effects of subsequent histamine release.

2. Antihistamines commonly have anticholinergic properties and cause a drying effect on epithelial surfaces. This is of special importance in regard to the respiratory tract, in which secretions may become thick and tenacious. Their use in respiratory disease is probably best avoided unless an allergic component is suspected. If they are used, patient hydration should be well maintained.

3. All of the antihistamines used in veterinary medicine cross the blood-brain barrier and may cause sedation. Paradoxically, sudden high concentrations as seen with rapid intravenous administration may cause central nervous system (CNS) stimulation. Therefore, they should be dosed by intramuscular, subcutaneous, or slow intravenous administration to avoid excitation.

4. A rare use in humans is the control of drug-induced extrapyramidal signs such as after a phenothiazine overdose. Diphenhydramine is usually the preferred agent in this situation.

CYCLO-OXYGENASE INHIBITORS (NONSTEROIDAL ANTI-INFLAMMATORY DRUGS)

The cyclo-oxygenase–inhibiting drugs, also known as nonsteroidal anti-inflammatory drugs (NSAIDs), are one of the most commonly used classes of drugs in veterinary practice. Members of this family typically have a triad of effects, namely, anti-inflammatory, analgesic, and antipyretic. These agents have occasionally been referred to as antiprostaglandins; however, this nomenclature would seem to imply that the drugs work by either binding prostaglandins or blocking their effects. In actuality they do neither but rather work by inhibiting the cyclo-oxygenase (i.e., prostaglandin synthetase, prostaglandin H synthase) enzyme system, thereby reducing prostaglandin and thromboxane production.

Although classified as anti-inflammatory drugs, they are probably used more in veterinary medicine for their analgesic and antipyretic effects; the analgesic action occurs by virtue of decreasing the synthesis of prostaglandins that sensitize pain receptors (peripheral and central mechanisms may exist), and the antipyretic effects occur by resetting the temperature regulatory center of the hypothalamus toward normal. The NSAIDs possess rather limited anti-inflammatory capabilities by comparison to the glucocorticoids; however, they are occasionally used for this purpose because of the high incidence of side effects associated with glucocorticoid therapy. Typically, a larger dose is required for the purpose of combating inflammation as opposed to control of fever and pain. There is evidence that these agents are helpful in combating endotoxic shock.

As a group, the NSAIDs tend to behave as weak acids often highly bound to plasma proteins. They are metabolized extensively by the liver and removed by the kidney. As with most drugs that undergo extensive hepatic metabolism, interspecies pharmacokinetic variation is high, and extrapolation of doses between species is not recommended.

If all NSAIDs worked by the same mechanism, it might be presumed that they would all have the same clinical uses. This is not the case because there is tremendous variation between drugs, particularly when they are used as analgesics. An adequate explanation of why some drugs perform better for certain conditions than for others has not been established.

ASPIRIN. The first NSAID to be used in modern medicine was aspirin (acetylsalicylic acid). Aspirin is only given orally and, after its absorption, is quickly converted to salicylic acid, which serves as the active metabolite. Other salicylates exist but are seldom used in clinical medicine. Aspirin is unique from the other NSAIDs in that in all common domestic animals except cattle, it irreversibly binds to platelet cyclo-oxygenase, producing a mild anticoagulant effect. This irreversibility is not seen with the other salicylates or NSAIDs and occurs at a dose much smaller than that required for other effects. Cattle and horses rapidly excrete the drug and therefore require large doses for maintenance of therapeutic plasma concentrations. It is effective as an antipyretic and for the control of mild to moderate somatic pain (skin, muscle). Aspirin has little effect on visceral pain. It is the only NSAID labeled in the United States for use in food animals.

PHENYLBUTAZONE. Phenylbutazone is an NSAID classified as a pyrazolon derivative. It has the ability to block mild to moderate somatic and visceral pain, and its use is increasing in cattle. Like salicylates, phenylbutazone has large species differences in metabolism with an elimination half-life of 36 hours in the cow versus 4 hours in the horse. This long half-life makes it particularly attractive in treating fractious cattle because dosing can be done at 48-hour intervals rather than the 12-hour intervals needed with most other NSAIDs. The long half-life, coupled with the potential to cause aplastic anemia in humans, does warrant prudent use in animals destined for slaughter. Food animal veterinarians should realize that the use of this drug falls under the extra-label drug use policy of the Food and Drug Administration. Because of its long elimination half-life and extensive protein binding, a loading dose of 1.5 to 2 times the maintenance dose is commonly employed.

DIPYRONE. Dipyrone is closely related to phenylbutazone but has less anti-inflammatory action. It has developed a reputation primarily as an antipyretic but can also control mild to moderate somatic and visceral pain. Unlike aspirin (given orally) or phenylbutazone (given orally or intravenously), dipyrone can be given subcutaneously or intramuscularly. This versatility combined with its low cost makes it suitable in a number of situations. Like phenylbutazone, it has the potential to cause bone marrow suppression.

FLUNIXIN. Flunixin meglumine is an NSAID approved for use in the horse but is commonly used in the cow and pig. The drug has excellent analgesic activity especially for control of severe visceral pain. It also performs well as an antipyretic and anti-inflammatory agent. It has been shown to be effective in reducing signs and lesions associated with PI_3 viral pneumonia in cattle. Flunixin may be one of the few drugs effective in the treatment of 3-methylindole intoxication (atypical bovine pulmonary emphysema). It is reputed to be useful in the management of endotoxemia such as that associated with coliform mastitis and *Pasteurella* pneumonia in cattle and agalactia-hypogalactia in swine. Because it is relatively nonirritating, subcutaneous or intramuscular injections can be given.

KETOPROFEN. An NSAID approved for use in horses, ketoprofen may have some ability to inhibit lipoxygenase and cyclo-oxygenase pathways. At present, not enough data exist to recommend its use.

Contraindications and Side Effects

By far the most common side effect of the NSAIDs is gastrointestinal ulceration with associated gastrointestinal bleeding, which also represents the major contraindication to the use of these drugs. The reason is not totally known but appears to be due, in part, to an alteration of the normal mucus that protects the gastrointestinal system (PGE_1, PGE_2, and PGA are involved in normal mucus production). Although this effect has long been noted with aspirin and phenylbutazone, it is seen with all drugs of this category.

Nephrotoxic effects are occasionally reported. Most commonly a renal papillary necrosis is observed. Because PGE_2 is necessary for normal renal blood flow, blocking its production with resultant impaired circulation may be the underlying pathophysiologic mechanism of nephrotoxicity.

Thromboxane production by platelets is a major contributing factor to normal coagulation. Cyclo-oxygenase inhibition thus results in some degree of impaired platelet adhesion and may cause a tendency toward increased bleeding. (As mentioned previously, this effect is not seen in cattle.) This is normally a reversible process except when aspirin is used.

Other side effects sometimes seen include bronchoconstriction, delayed parturition, and hypersensitivities. Because of their ability to displace other highly protein-bound drugs, adverse drug interactions involving anesthetics or coumarin anticoagulants have been observed. Bone marrow suppression has been reported as a rare but serious complication of NSAID therapy. This occurs most commonly with the pyrazolon derivatives phenylbutazone and dipyrone.

GLUCOCORTICOIDS

Of all the anti-inflammatory agents, there is no doubt that the glucocorticoids are the most effective. A variety of mechanisms have been proposed to explain their actions, including stabilization of lysosomal membranes and decreased influx of white blood cells. It is now well accepted that their major anti-inflammatory effects occur by inhibition of phospholipase. As seen in Figure 1, this early interruption of the arachidonic acid cascade leads to decreased production of all the eicosanoids.

Although the glucocorticoids have many common physiologic effects, there are differences that make certain agents preferable for a given situation. Table 2 lists the common glucocorticoids and their potency, mineralocorticoid activity, and duration of hypothalamic-pituitary suppression (biologic half-life). Several points deserve mention here. First, regarding potency, note that this term is intended for comparison between agents in achieving a stated effect, not whether one agent is capable of achieving an effect that another cannot. For example, normal cortisol secretion is approximately 1 mg/kg/day. To have an anti-inflammatory effect, a good rule of thumb is that 5 times that amount is required. Thus a dose of 5 mg/kg/day of cortisol approximates 1 mg/kg/day prednisolone or 0.15 mg/kg/day dexamethasone. In selecting a glucocorticoid, potency is not an important concern as long as proper dosage adjustments are made. Primarily, one should consider (1) how rapid an onset is required, (2) the desired duration of effects, (3) the desirability of mineralocorticoid activity, and (4) whether abortifacient activity is an issue.

Table 2. CHARACTERISTICS OF SOME COMMON GLUCOCORTICOIDS

Glucocorticoid	Anti-inflammatory Potency[1]	Mineralocorticoid Potency[1]	Biologic Half-Life	Abortifacient Potential
Hydrocortisone	1	1.0	8–12 hr (short)	+
Prednisolone	4	0.8	12–36 hr (intermediate)	+
Triamcinolone	5	0.0	12–36 hr (intermediate)	+
Isoflupredone	17	0.0	—	+
Dexamethasone	29	0.0	36–54 hr (long)	+ + +
Betamethasone	30	0.0	36–54 hr (long)	+ + +
Flumethasone	30	0.0	36–54 hr (long)	+ + +

[1]Potency is relative to hydrocortisone.

In selecting an agent for administration in regard to onset and duration, it is important to realize that both the drug and its formulation must be considered. If a rapid onset is desired, it could be argued that prednisolone achieves intracellular penetration earlier than does dexamethasone, which makes it more desirable in acute situations. However, in large animal medicine, the longer biologic half-life (allowing less frequent dosing) and lower cost make dexamethasone a preferred glucocorticoid. Whereas these characteristics of the parent drug are of obvious importance, formulation of the glucocorticoid preparation is often more relevant. When an immediate effect is desired, the water-soluble form of the steroid is preferred (i.e., sodium phosphate or sodium succinate salts), whereas if a long duration is desired, the water-insoluble (repository) form would be used (i.e., acetate, acetonide, or dipropionate salts). For example, in treating endotoxic shock, because of its rapid onset the sodium phosphate form (Azium SP) is preferable over conventional dexamethasone base (in propylene glycol and water [Azium]). Dexamethasone acetate would be inappropriate in such a condition because of its delayed onset.

Differences also exist in the mineralocorticoid activity of the glucocorticoids. Usually this attribute is of limited clinical significance. A possible exception is cardiac disease, in which fluid retention may further decompensate the patient.

Of particular importance to food animal veterinarians is the abortifacient activity of the differing agents. Although all glucocorticoids have the potential to induce abortion, this phenomenon is seen most often in ruminants in the last half of gestation after administration of C-16–methylated agents such as dexamethasone. Steroid-induced abortion usually results in placental retention. When glucocorticoids must be administered to the pregnant animal, the nonmethylated compounds such as prednisolone or isoflupredone will decrease the risk of abortion.

Clinical Uses

The glucocorticoids have been used in a number of specific clinical conditions including shock, CNS edema, and ketosis. The benefit of glucocorticoids in shock has remained controversial; although seldom contraindicated, it now appears that they are of limited benefit in most forms of shock. An exception to this is in endotoxic (septic) shock in which early large doses of glucocorticoids may stabilize the condition of the animal, allowing correction of the underlying infection. (There is evidence from human clinical trials that steroids do not change the eventual mortality rate in septic shock; that is, the patient improves only to die later.)

Dexamethasone and methylprednisolone both have the ability to limit damage after CNS trauma provided large doses are given shortly after the injury. They are also effective in reducing cerebral edema associated with certain CNS neoplasms. Because of their immunosuppressive properties, care should be taken to rule out the presence of CNS infection before proceeding with glucocorticoid therapy.

The glucocorticoids are also used to treat bovine ketosis. Although these agents decrease the peripheral utilization of glucose, the gluconeogenic properties produce higher blood glucose concentrations, thereby ameliorating CNS signs. Actually, many of the beneficial effects seen in lactating dairy cattle may come from their ability to decrease milk production, thereby decreasing energy demands. It is probably wise to warn the dairyman of this side effect when lactating dairy cattle are treated.

Dexamethasone, betamethasone, and flumethasone have been shown to increase surfactant production in the fetus. In those instances in which completion of the full term of pregnancy is unlikely, treatment of the dam with small doses (i.e., 0.02 mg/kg intramuscularly) 24 to 48 hours before induction or cesarean section may reduce the incidence of neonatal respiratory distress syndrome.

The following "rules of thumb" apply to the clinical uses of glucocorticoids in the general treatment of inflammatory disease.

1. A single large dose of a glucocorticoid seldom causes harm.

2. If glucocorticoids are used in bacterial infections, bactericidal antimicrobials may be preferred to bacteriostatic agents because of glucocorticoid-induced dysfunction of phagocytes. Animals suffering from infectious diseases controlled primarily by cell-mediated immunity (i.e., systemic mycoses, mycobacterial infections) should not receive glucocorticoids (unless clinical judgment deems them absolutely necessary and if appropriate antifungal-antimycobacterial therapy is instituted).

3. If chronic therapy is required, the smallest possible dose that achieves the desired effect should be sought. Every-other-day therapy with a nonrepository intermediate-acting agent further decreases the incidence of adrenal insufficiency and immunosuppression. Because iatrogenic hypoadrenocorticism is a rare but serious consequence of chronic steroid administration, doses should be gradually rather than abruptly decreased.

4. Remember that glucocorticoids are primarily palliative therapy. Diagnosis and treatment of the underlying disease should be instituted.

Contraindications and Side Effects

Few drugs affect such a wide variety of tissues as do the glucocorticoids. Of the myriad effects that can occur after their use, clinically the contraindications against short-term administration of a glucocorticoid include gastrointestinal ulceration, systemic mycoses, and mycobacterial infections. Corneal ulceration prohibits ophthalmic use. All of the drugs in this class tend to delay healing and promote infection; therefore, their use in animals with bone fractures or after abdominal or thoracic surgery is discouraged. If they must be used in any of these conditions, an intermediate-acting water-soluble product such as prednisolone sodium succinate or prednisolone phosphate is preferred so that the duration of activity is minimized. If sepsis is suspected, bactericidal antimicrobials are preferred to bacteriostatic agents because phagocyte activity is inhibited by glucocorticoids. Less frequently encountered conditions that may be exacerbated by glucocorticoid administration include diabetes mellitus (due to anti-insulin effect), pancreatitis, osteoporosis (due to increased calcium excretion), and renal disease (due to catabolic effects). In addition to their abortifacient activity, these agents are teratogenic in the first trimester, which makes their use in pregnant animals undesirable. Prednisone (inactive prodrug) should not be used in patients with hepatic failure because a functioning liver is required for transformation to active prednisolone.

DIMETHYL SULFOXIDE (DMSO)

DMSO has a large number of characteristics that make it a useful agent in the treatment of inflammation. Although most of the anti-inflammatory effects have been attributed to its ability to scavenge free radicals, it also may potentiate endogenous glucocorticoid effects, decrease the influx of white blood cells into an area, and limit fibrous tissue formation after injury. Its ability to act as a percutaneous carrier for other drugs with molecular weights less than 3000 has also attracted a great deal of interest.

Topically, its approved route in the dog and horse, DMSO can be used to treat a variety of musculoskeletal conditions such as tendinitis or desmitis. It is also used in an extra-label manner intravenously to treat CNS edema-trauma or pneumonia.

When DMSO is used to treat CNS edema or trauma, a dose of 0.5 to 1.0 g/kg is usually given intravenously once daily as a 10 per cent solution. Higher concentrations (which can cause hemolysis) or rapid administration may cause nonspecific histamine release, with resultant collapse. Even the 10 per cent solution is still quite hypertonic, and a marked diuresis is common.

Surprisingly, no scientific data exist to document the efficacy of DMSO as an adjunct treatment in bovine pneumonia. It has been used empirically at intravenous doses of 0.02 to 1 g/kg.

In addition to the hemolysis and histamine release mentioned, DMSO is a potential teratogen and should ideally be avoided in pregnant animals. DMSO may potentiate the effects of cholinesterase-inhibiting agents such as organophosphate insecticides or phenothiazine tranquilizers. Although chronic large-dose administration has been reported to cause cataract formation in the dog, this is of doubtful clinical significance.

BIBLIOGRAPHY

Booth NH, McDonald LE (eds): Veterinary Pharmacology and Therapeutics, 6th ed. Ames, IA, Iowa State University Press, 1988.
Calvert CA, Cornelius LM: Symposium on the use and misuse of steroids (peer reviewed). Vet Med August: 810–865, 1990.
Ellis C (ed): International Symposium on Nonsteroidal Anti-inflammatory Agents. Orlando, FL, Veterinary Learning Systems, 1986.
Upson DW: Upson's Handbook of Veterinary Pharmacology, 2nd ed. Lenexa, KS, VM Publishing, 1985.

Immunologic Disorders and Immunotherapy

CINDY J. BRUNNER, DVM, PhD
JEFF W. TYLER, DVM, MPVM, PhD

The immune system, like other organ systems of the body, is susceptible to disease and responsive to therapy. Clinical laboratory assessment of immunologic competence in veterinary patients is now possible, as is modification of the immune response through immunotherapy. Thirty years ago, immunology in the veterinary curriculum typically consisted of discussion of serologic tests for the detection of bacterial and viral infections. Now, many veterinary schools devote an entire course to the study of the basic principles of immunology and a second course to the clinical problems associated with immune system dysfunction in veterinary patients. The importance of continuing education in the field of veterinary immunology cannot be overemphasized.

COMPONENTS AND FUNCTION OF THE IMMUNE SYSTEM

Resistance to infection in animals requires the participation of a variety of nonspecific and specific immunologic mechanisms. The nonspecific mechanisms of resistance include physical and chemical barriers at epithelial surfaces, phagocytic leukocytes (monocytes and neutrophils), natural killer cells, and the complement system. Immunologically specific resistance to infection occurs through the ability of B and T lymphocytes to recognize subtle differences among antigenic determinants on microorganisms and to undergo clonal expansion and differentiation when exposed to those antigens.

During a critical period in the primary lymphoid organs, T and B lymphocytes acquire receptors that will enable each cell to react with a unique antigen. These antigen receptors are the products of genes that have undergone random and nonrandom mutation, which results in an array of lymphocytes that will recognize virtually all the infectious agents in the animal's environment. Also during maturation in the primary lymphoid organs, immature lymphocytes undergo a selection process to eliminate those cells that would mistake the animal's own tissues as foreign. Upon release from the primary lymphoid organs, T and B lymphocytes are capable of distinguishing "self" from "nonself" and of responding appropriately when exposed to an antigen.

Lymphocytes that mature under the influence of hormones and epithelial cells of the thymus are called T lymphocytes. T lymphocytes participate in cell-mediated immune reactions, which result in the destruction of neoplastic cells, virus-infected cells, fungi, protozoan parasites, and microorganisms that replicate intracellularly. In addition, T lymphocytes produce soluble factors called lymphokines that are important in the initiation and regulation of an immune response. On the basis of their function and of characteristic cell-surface proteins, T lymphocytes can be classified as helper (CD4) or suppressor-cytotoxic (CD8) cells.

Lymphocytes that develop under the influence of hormones and epithelial cells of the fetal liver and the bone marrow are called B lymphocytes. B lymphocytes respond to antigens by proliferating and differentiating into plasma cells. Each clone of plasma cells secretes antibodies of unique antigenic specificity. Antibodies can be classified according to their biochemical structure into one of five isotypes (IgM, IgG, IgA, IgE,

IgD). The isotype influences the biologic activity of the antibody and its distribution in the body. Although each plasma cell clone produces antibodies of only one antigenic specificity, a B lymphocyte may change the isotype it produces during the course of an immune response. This isotype switch accounts for the change from IgM to IgG that occurs between primary and secondary immune responses.

Many endogenous factors determine whether an immune response takes place. The most critical are (1) possession of appropriate genetic information for recognizing and responding to an antigen, (2) development of all the necessary components of the immune system, (3) balanced participation of all components in an immune response, and (4) effective regulation of the response, once it is initiated. External factors such as drugs, nutritional status, age, hormone levels, and the unique characteristics of a pathogenic microorganism can have a significant influence on the outcome of an immune response.

IDENTIFICATION AND TREATMENT OF IMMUNOLOGIC DISORDERS

Illness can result from abnormalities in either the development or the function of components of the immune system. In some cases, these abnormalities can be detected with routine veterinary diagnostic procedures. However, definitive diagnosis of an immunologic disorder often requires the use of special techniques available only at veterinary teaching hospitals or commercial diagnostic laboratories. Three types of immunologic disorders occur in animals.

Immunodeficiencies

The most common form of immunodeficiency in veterinary medicine is hypogammaglobulinemia caused by failure of a newborn animal to absorb colostral immunoglobulins. Although most domestic animal species are able to respond to some antigens at birth, the response may be inadequate because of immaturity of the immune system and because of the prolonged lag phase that occurs in a primary immune response. As a result of these factors, the newborn animal is particularly susceptible to infectious diseases unless it receives passive immunization from its dam. Newborn calves, piglets, lambs, and kids are particularly susceptible to failure of passive transfer because they must obtain all their passive immunity through ingestion of colostrum, rather than receiving some through transplacental transfer of antibodies. Animals with failure of passive transfer commonly present with septicemia, omphalophlebitis, polyarthritis, meningitis, or panophthalmitis. The high frequency of life-threatening bacterial infections in these patients reflects the critical role of serum antibodies in opsonizing bacteria to facilitate their removal by phagocytic cells. A simple assay of serum gamma globulins by zinc sulfate or sodium sulfite turbidity analysis will indicate whether passively transferred immunoglobulin is present in the serum of the neonate; a concentration less than 800 mg/dl is indicative of inadequate passive transfer. Other tests to measure immunoglobulins include radial immunodiffusion, glutaraldehyde coagulation, nephelometry, and enzyme-linked immunosorbent assay (ELISA). Some of these assays are available in kits for use on the farm.

If the hypogammaglobulinemic patient is more than 24 to 48 hours old, immunoglobulins will no longer be absorbed across the intestinal mucosa, so treatment consisting of oral administration of colostrum will be ineffective. Instead, therapy must be provided parenterally, by intravenous or subcutaneous injection of serum or plasma (approximately 30 ml/kg body weight) or whole blood (40 to 50 ml/kg). Transfusion reactions after administration of blood or blood products are rarely reported in food animals, despite the complexity of blood group systems in those species. Nevertheless, care should be taken to monitor the patient for a transfusion reaction during and after administration of the blood or blood product. Donor animals should be free of common blood-borne infections, including anaplasmosis, retrovirus infections, and viral diarrhea.

After the disappearance of colostral antibodies from the circulation, the neonate normally begins to mount its own immune responses. During this transition period, congenital absence or dysfunction of components of the immune system (primary immunodeficiency) will become apparent as chronic, recurrent infectious disease. The congenitally immunodeficient animal will be susceptible to infections caused by opportunistic or mildly pathogenic agents such as coliform bacteria, *Cryptosporidium* spp., *Pneumocystis carinii*, *Aspergillus* spp., or *Candida* spp. or will suffer from generalized infections with herpesviruses or papillomaviruses. Some animals also develop generalized infections with microorganisms from attenuated live vaccines. Infections may be controlled temporarily with chemotherapy, but they usually recur once treatment is stopped.

Congenital immunodeficiencies may be hereditary or may be induced by viral infection in utero or ingestion of a toxic substance by the dam during pregnancy. Congenital immunodeficiencies are rarely diagnosed in food animals, although a few have been well characterized because of their value as animal models of human diseases. For example, Chédiak-Higashi syndrome is an autosomal recessive problem that results from structural and functional abnormalities in neutrophils and other cells with granules. Chédiak-Higashi syndrome has been reported in partial albino Hereford cattle as well as in other species of wild and domestic animals. Another metabolic defect of neutrophils called granulocytopathy syndrome occurs as an autosomal recessive trait in some Holstein cattle. Combined immunodeficiency, which is characterized by hypogammaglobulinemia and the complete absence of lymphocytes from blood and lymphoid organs, is familiar to most veterinarians as a problem in Arabian foals, but a case was recently reported in an Angus calf. Thymic aplasia and deficiency of T lymphocytes occurs in some lines of Black Pied Danish cattle as the result of an inherited zinc malabsorption syndrome. Selective deficiency of IgG_2 has been described in some Red Danish cattle. Single cases of other congenital disorders have also been reported.

Secondary, or acquired, immunodeficiencies are much more common than are primary immunodeficiencies in food-producing animals. In a secondary immunodeficiency, the immune system usually develops normally, but its function is depressed by an external factor such as nutritional imbalance, viral infection, pregnancy, exogenous glucocorticoid administration, or physiologic changes associated with the response to a stressor. An animal with a secondary immunodeficiency is susceptible to infection with many of the same microorganisms that are observed in primary immunodeficiency disorders. In a secondary immunodeficiency, the course of an infection may be longer or more severe than in normal animals, but the prognosis is seldom as grave as with a primary immunodeficiency.

Diagnostic tests that can be used to detect primary and secondary immunodeficiencies are listed in Table 1. As is noted in the table, routine laboratory procedures can sometimes be used to rule out immunodeficiency, but if a definitive diagnosis is desired, a veterinary clinical immunology laboratory should be contacted. Primary immunodeficiencies should be distinguished from secondary immunodeficiencies whenever

Table 1. DIAGNOSTIC TESTS FOR IMMUNODEFICIENCIES

Nonspecific Compartment—Neutrophils and Monocytes
  Differential leukocyte count*
  Phagocytosis of latex beads or bacteria
  Chemotaxis
  Bactericidal activity
  Iodination
  Nitroblue tetrazolium reduction
  Chemiluminescence

Specific Compartment—Lymphocytes
T lymphocytes
  Differential leukocyte count*
  Intradermal injection of phytohemagglutinin*
  Lymph node biopsy*
  Skin allo(iso)graft rejection*
  Post-mortem examination: lymphoid hypoplasia*
  T lymphocyte count (flow cytometry)
  Lymphocyte blastogenesis test (PHA, Con A)
  Lymphokine production (migration inhibition factor, interferon-γ, interleukin-2)
B lymphocytes
  Lymph node biopsy*
  Electrophoresis of serum proteins
  Radial immunodiffusion or ELISA for specific Ig isotype*
  Specific antibody response after vaccination*
  Immunoelectrophoresis
  B lymphocyte count (flow cytometry)

*The tests marked with an asterisk can be performed with standard equipment and technical skills in a clinical laboratory. Special tests (unmarked above) require submission of samples to a clinical immunology laboratory at a veterinary college, major veterinary hospital, or properly equipped and staffed commercial diagnostic facility.

Abbreviations: PHA = phytohemagglutinin; Con A = concanavalin; ELISA = enzyme-linked immunosorbent assay.

possible, because the treatment of primary immunodeficiencies is impractical in food animals, and the prognosis is usually poor. Features of primary immunodeficiencies that are helpful in distinguishing them from secondary immunodeficiencies are the age at onset, the severity of clinical illness, the presence of other congenital anomalies, a history of exposure to predisposing factors in utero (but not after birth), or evidence of a similar problem in a full sibling or closely related animal.

An animal with a congenital immunodeficiency can be restored to normal immunocompetence only by replacement of the missing component of the immune system through tissue transplantation or genetic manipulation. Long-term administration of leukocyte growth factors such as granulocyte colony–stimulating factor, interferon-γ, or interleukin-2 may provide partial relief. Neither of these approaches is likely to be successful or practical in food-producing animals, so therapy is rarely considered. Despite the impracticality of treating primary immunodeficiencies in food animals, veterinary teaching hospitals sometimes accept these patients as referrals because of their value in teaching and research.

With the exception of failure of passive transfer, the best therapy in secondary immunodeficiency is elimination of the underlying cause of the problem. One can also consider administration of hyperimmune serum or leukocyte growth factors to support the patient until immunocompetence is restored.

Hypersensitivity Reactions

A hypersensitivity reaction is inflammation and tissue damage resulting from an excessive or inappropriate immune response. Hypersensitivity reactions are classified into four types in order to distinguish the immunopathologic mechanisms causing the tissue damage. Some of the clinical manifestations of these four types are listed in Table 2.

Type 1 hypersensitivity reactions are also called immediate hypersensitivity reactions because of the short interval between exposure to the antigen and the appearance of clinical signs. This category includes atopy and anaphylaxis as well as most other allergic disorders. Type 1 reactions occur when multivalent antigen molecules bind to and cross-link IgE antibodies located on the surface of a mast cell. The binding of antigen molecules to IgE triggers degranulation of the mast cell, releasing potent inflammatory mediators that include histamine, serotonin, leukotrienes, prostaglandins, heparin, and leukocyte chemotactic factors. Resultant changes in the diameter and permeability of small blood vessels produce the familiar signs of inflammation, including edema, congestion, and leukocytic infiltration. Type 1 hypersensitivity is probably one mechanism responsible for the increased severity of pulmonary disease reported in cattle vaccinated with some bovine respiratory syncytial virus vaccines and *Pasteurella* bacterins. Although local type 1 hypersensitivity reactions are mild, intravenous absorption of the antigen can trigger massive release of inflammatory mediators, leading to a life-threatening systemic anaphylactic reaction. Type 1 hypersensitivity is suggested by a history of acute inflammation of the respiratory tract, skin, or gastrointestinal tract after exposure to an antigen. The diagnosis is confirmed by intradermal injection of the suspected antigen. Edema and erythema at the injection site after 10 to 15 minutes indicates immediate hypersensitivity. Antigen-specific IgE can also be measured in the serum with a radioallergosorbent test, but the clinical usefulness of this test in veterinary medicine is controversial.

Type 2 hypersensitivity reactions result from binding of antibodies (IgG or IgM) to antigenic structures on the animal's own cells. Damage to the cells can result if the complement system is activated, as occurs with immune-mediated hemolytic anemia. If the antibodies bind to a receptor for a hormone or other biologic ligand, the receptor may be blocked and the response to the hormone diminished. Alternatively, antibodies can bind to hormone receptors and mimic the biologic activity

Table 2. CLINICAL MANIFESTATIONS OF HYPERSENSITIVITY REACTIONS

Type 1	Eczema
	Allergic inhalant dermatitis
	Atopic rhinitis
	Milk allergy
	Hypersensitivity pneumonitis
	Drug allergy (also vaccine reactions)
	Insect bites and stings
	Urticaria
Type 2	Bullous skin disorders (pemphigus complex)
	Hemolytic anemia, thrombocytopenia
	Drug allergy
	Neonatal isoerythrolysis
	Blood transfusion incompatibility
	Myasthenia gravis
	Anemia due to hemoparasitism
Type 3	Glomerulonephritis
	Serum sickness
	Rheumatoid arthritis
	Vasculitis
	Hypersensitivity pneumonitis
	Drug allergy
Type 4	Allergic contact dermatitis (dyes, metals, plant resins)
	Encephalomyelitis
	Tuberculin skin reaction
	Hypersensitivity pneumonitis
	Orchitis, epididymitis
	Granulomatous inflammation (mycobacteria, actinobacilli)
	Insect bite hypersensitivity

of the hormones themselves. Myasthenia gravis, a neuromuscular disorder in animals and humans, and certain endocrinopathies, including some forms of thyroiditis and diabetes mellitus, are thought to be the result of binding of antibodies to receptors on cells. Antibodies on the surfaces of cells in tissues can be detected by immunofluorescence microscopy of biopsy specimens collected in Michel's transport medium. Antibodies on erythrocytes can be detected with the Coombs' direct antiglobulin test. Antibodies that participate in type 2 reactions can sometimes be detected in the serum, but this indirect approach is less reliable in animals than it is in humans.

Type 3 hypersensitivity reactions are also called immune complex–mediated reactions because they involve activation of complement by antigen-antibody complexes in the circulation or in tissues. Complement activation generates molecules that cause vasodilation, increased vascular permeability, and local influx of leukocytes (particularly neutrophils). In a futile attempt to eliminate the antigen-antibody complexes, the neutrophils release enzymes extracellularly; the result is neutrophil-mediated damage to adjacent normal tissue. When type 3 reactions occur locally, they are called Arthus reactions. Alternatively, if the antigen-antibody complexes form in the circulation, they are typically deposited in the kidneys and in blood vessel walls, causing glomerulonephritis and vasculitis. Immune complex–mediated glomerulonephritis and vasculitis are seen in hog cholera, African swine fever, bluetongue, and streptococcal infections and as an occasional sequela to passive immunotherapy. Diagnosis of type 3 hypersensitivity reactions is based on a history of chronic antigenic stimulation, the appearance of inflammatory lesions in the target organs, and the detection of immune complexes in the affected tissues with immunofluorescence microscopy.

Type 4 hypersensitivity reactions occur when T lymphocytes predominate in an immune response to an antigen. Type 4 reactions are also called delayed-type hypersensitivity reactions, because activated T lymphocytes release lymphokines that trigger the gradual accumulation of other lymphocytes and monocytes. Granulomatous inflammation seen in histoplasmosis, actinobacillosis, and mycobacterial infections represents a type 4 reaction. Delayed-type hypersensitivity is usually diagnosed by intradermal injection of antigen and examination of the injection site for induration and redness 48 to 72 hours later. The intradermal tuberculin test is a familiar example of a delayed-type hypersensitivity reaction. Delayed-type hypersensitivity can also be detected with a laboratory test called lymphocyte blastogenesis, in which lymphocytes from a blood sample are cultured with suspected antigens to see if the lymphocytes proliferate.

A peculiar form of type 4 reaction is cutaneous basophil hypersensitivity, also called a Jones-Mote reaction. Basophils predominate in these lesions, which are seen in dermatitis caused by fleas, ticks, and biting flies. Cutaneous basophil hypersensitivity contributes to the apparent resistance of some cattle to ectoparasites.

All four types of hypersensitivity reactions are initiated and sustained by antigen, so the most effective and permanent treatment is elimination of the antigen. The signs of inflammation that are seen can be diminished by administration of small-dose glucocorticoids, which act principally by blocking the increase in vascular permeability. Stronger immunosuppressive drugs may be necessary in some cases but are contraindicated if the suspected antigen is an infectious agent. Long-term remission can sometimes be maintained by hyposensitization, which involves repeated subcutaneous or intradermal injection of the offending antigen. Hyposensitization is effective in type 1 reactions and some type 4 reactions, but it can be harmful in hypersensitivity reactions whose immunologic mechanisms involve IgG antibodies.

Autoimmune Disorders

Autoimmune disease develops from bypass of the normal regulatory pathways of the immune system, with a resultant loss of immunologic tolerance to structures on the animal's own cells. In autoimmune disease, the relevant antigen is present constantly, and the subsequent tissue damage can be classified into one of the types of hypersensitivity reactions mentioned in the previous section.

Examples of autoimmune disorders in animals include cytolytic reactions against blood cells (hemolytic anemia or thrombocytopenia), reactions against antigens in solid tissues (polyneuritis, encephalitis, pemphigus-type bullous skin diseases), and generalized autoimmune reactions involving immune complexes (lupus erythematosus and rheumatoid arthritis). Potent immunosuppressive therapy is usually required to control autoimmune reactions. Autoimmune diseases are seldom encountered in food animal practice.

IMMUNOTHERAPY

Recent advances in understanding the regulation of immune responses have accelerated the development of products for treatment of immunologic disorders. Chemical and biologic immunostimulants should actually be called immunomodulators or biologic response modifiers because they do not always stimulate immunity. Most are capable of either enhancing or suppressing immunity, depending on the dose and timing of their administration and the patient's immunocompetence.

Adjuvants

The simplest and most common method of potentiating an immune response is addition of an adjuvant to increase immunogenicity of a vaccine. Many commercial vaccines are administered with aluminum-containing adjuvants such as aluminum hydroxide. Newer synthetic adjuvants may be useful with weakly immunogenic products such as inactivated viral vaccines, subunit vaccines, or vaccines produced with recombinant DNA technology. Most adjuvants enhance immunogenicity by improving the processing of antigens by macrophages. They may enhance specific immune responses in marginally immunocompetent as well as in normal animals.

Passive Immunization

Passive immunization by administration of antibodies is another common form of immunotherapy. Plasma and hyperimmune serum provide temporary immunologic protection against infection in animals that did not absorb colostral antibodies or that fail to produce their own immunoglobulins. Both polyclonal and monoclonal antibodies against specific structural components or virulence factors of microorganisms are available commercially (e.g., Genecol 99,[1] Pro-Immune 99,[2] snakebite antivenin, tetanus antitoxin). These specific antibodies may temporarily prevent colonization, replication, or clinical illness caused by specific microorganisms. One serious disadvantage of administration of passive antibodies is that they may block active immunization in the recipient and may limit the intensity and duration of an ongoing immune response.

---

[1]Available from Schering-Plough Animal Health, Kenilworth, NJ 07033.
[2]Available from SmithKline Beecham Animal Health, Exton, PA 19341.

Bacterial Products

Immunologic activity can be stimulated nonspecifically with bacterial cells or cell products from *Mycobacterium* spp. (Nomagen,[1] Ribigen-B,[2] bacillus Calmette-Guérin or BCG), *Propionibacterium acnes* (Immunoregulin[3]), and *Staphylococcus aureus* (Staphage Lysate SPL[4]). One clinical problem in which immunotherapy with mycobacterial cell wall products has been moderately successful is ocular squamous cell carcinoma of cattle. It should be noted that mycobacterial extracts may cause a false-positive reaction with the intradermal tuberculin test for *Mycobacterium bovis*. Regulatory agencies restrict the use of bacterial products to specific animal species and defined medical conditions. Veterinarians contemplating the use of these products in livestock should consult appropriate sources to determine whether such use is permitted.

Cytokines

Cytokines are specific leukopoietic hormones that regulate cell interactions and leukocyte maturation. Several cytokines have been identified in food animals and have been synthesized in vitro with use of recombinant DNA technology. Examples include interferon-α, interferon-γ, interleukin-2, and granulocyte–colony-stimulating factor. These hormones produce transient increases in numbers and activity of specific types of leukocytes. Recombinant cytokines may have prophylactic and therapeutic effects in high-risk patients and may enhance the efficacy of vaccines. The use of these products in animals is currently experimental, and the compounds are generally not available to practitioners.

Chemical Immunomodulators

The anthelmintic levamisole has seen widespread use as an immunostimulant in cattle. Despite anecdotal claims of its effectiveness, controlled studies have failed to demonstrate any clear benefits of small-dose levamisole immunotherapy in livestock.

Vitamin C (ascorbic acid) has also received much attention as a potential immunostimulant in animals as well as in humans. Administration of vitamin C to feeder calves has been claimed to reduce the incidence and severity of respiratory disease associated with shipping. Large farm animals produce adequate amounts of endogenous vitamin C, except during the early postnatal period and possibly during times of stress. Controlled trials in cattle have failed to demonstrate increased plasma ascorbate concentrations after administration of moderately large doses of vitamin C.

Recent studies have linked decreased blood selenium concentrations to increased incidence and severity of mastitis in dairy cattle. A more complete understanding of the role of diet in disease resistance in animals can be expected within the next decade.

BIBLIOGRAPHY

Archambault D, Morin G, Elazhary Y: Influence of immunomodulatory agents on bovine humoral and cellular immune responses to parenteral inoculation with bovine rotavirus vaccines. Vet Microbiol 17:323–334, 1988.

Bennett K (ed): Compendium of Veterinary Products. Port Huron, MI, North American Compendiums Inc., 1991.

Halliwell REW, Gorman NT: Veterinary Clinical Immunology. Philadelphia, WB Saunders, 1989.

Mulcahy G, Quinn PJ: A review of immunomodulators and their application in veterinary medicine. J Vet Pharmacol Therapeut 9:119–139, 1986.

Reddy PG, et al: Bovine recombinant interleukin-2 augments immunity and resistance to bovine herpesvirus infection. Vet Immunol Immunopathol 23:61–74, 1989.

Roth JA, Frank DE: Recombinant bovine interferon-gamma as an immunomodulator in dexamethasone-treated and nontreated cattle. J Interferon Res 9:143–151, 1989.

Tizard IR: Veterinary Immunology: An Introduction. Philadelphia, WB Saunders, 1987.

---

[1]Available from Fort Dodge Laboratories, Inc., Fort Dodge, IA 50501.
[2]Available from Ribi Immunochem Research, Inc., Hamilton, MT 59840.
[3]Available from ImmunoVet, Inc., Tampa, FL 33610.
[4]Available from Delmont Laboratories, Inc., Swarthmore, PA 19081.

Stress Impacts of Metabolic-Hormonal Regulation and Immune Function

CHERYL F. NOCKELS, PhD

Animals alter their metabolism in response to noxious stimuli or stress. This change in metabolism is primarily to provide the animal with a continuing source of energy and amino acids for protein synthesis derived from its own resources. Not only does the animal begin to use its own tissues for energy production, but it routes the energy sources to specific tissues while decreasing it to others. This coordination of energy production, distribution, and utilization is a tightly controlled process regulated by specific hormones. Whereas the metabolic control exerted by some hormones has been known for some time, newly recognized hormones and their functions are just now beginning to be discerned. With more sophisticated biochemical techniques, more hormones and their regulation of our life processes will be elucidated. Hormones orchestrate the activity of the metabolic pathways through which compounds pass by altering the activity of the rate-regulating enzymes of that pathway. In stress, although many metabolic pathways such as those involving fatty acids, glucose, and certain proteins may be catabolic in supplying a continued energy source, others such as acute-phase protein synthesis are anabolic as long as energy is sufficient. In this redistribution of metabolic effort, some processes, such as certain facets of the immune system, may be sharply curtailed. As we understand how metabolic changes incurred during stress impinge on the immune system, our ability to rectify or prevent some of them will aid animal recovery and health.

The following thesis attempts to integrate the metabolic changes in the Bovidae, when possible, as the animal goes from a fed to a fasted state while being subjected to increasing stress and trauma and discusses how some of these changes impact immune function. In order to illustrate the dynamic alterations in metabolism when stress and trauma intensify, data obtained from cattle arriving at the feedlot are presented.[4] Generally, as stress intensity and length increased, so did blood levels of cortisol, glucose, creatine phosphokinase, serum aspartate aminotransaminase, urea-nitrogen, creatinine, and fibrinogen; decreases in albumin (A) and increases in globulin (G) reduced the A:G ratio, although total protein remained constant.

STRESS HORMONES AND IMMUNE RESPONSE

In trying to determine the cause of these biochemical changes, the different noxious stimuli producing the stress response need to be identified. These stimuli are, at least in part, handling, transport, physical trauma, fasting, fatigue, and unfamiliar environment. Any one or all of these elicit the following hormonal changes.[56, 58] Increased adrenocorticotropic hormone (ACTH) release from the pituitary occurs, which augments adrenal cortex release of cortisol and aldosterone.[18] Additionally, through neural stimulation, the adrenal medulla releases to the circulation the catecholamines epinephrine and norepinephrine. Furthermore, β-endorphin is cosecreted with ACTH from the pituitary, and enkephalins are cosecreted with epinephrine from the adrenal medulla. Both of these peptide hormones are also produced by activated macrophages and lymphocytes. These hormones may in part regulate inflammation, immune function, and temperature control in infection.[7] Norepinephrine may also be released at most sympathetic postganglionic nerve endings. Additional blood hormonal changes result from alterations in blood glucose levels.[37]

The immunosuppressive effects of glucocorticoids in stress have been well documented.[20] "Shipping fever" or the bovine respiratory disease complex is a good example of stress-associated infectious disease.[56] Researchers have presented evidence that glucocorticoids reduced immunity in cattle by decreasing antibody production, lymphocyte blastogenesis, and neutrophil function.[56] Further adverse effects of stress on immune function such as lymphoid tissue atrophy and inhibition of synthesis of interleukin-1 (IL-1), interleukin-2 (IL-2), and the IL-2 receptor on lymphocytes have been reported.[27]

Epinephrine may also adversely affect immune function by increasing the eicosanoids, prostaglandins, thromboxanes, leukotrienes, and lipoxins.[24] This catecholamine activates phospholipase A_2 (PLA_2), which frees arachidonate from membrane phospholipids. IL-1 is also an enhancer of PLA_2 activity and stimulates arachidonate metabolism through the following pathways, the products of which regulate much of the immune response.[41] The arachidonate may be converted to leukotrienes and lipoxins via the lipoxygenase pathway or by cyclo-oxygenase to form prostaglandin and thromboxane.[35] Increased levels of prostaglandin have been shown to inhibit the production of lymphokines, induce nonspecific suppressor T-cell activity, and inhibit the response of T cells to mitogens.[63] Leukotrienes alter vascular permeability, attraction and activation of leukocytes, inflammation, and immediate hypersensitivity reactions; lipoxin inhibits natural killer cell cytotoxicity and causes chemotaxis.[59] Other products produced in these pathways are highly reactive oxygen-derived molecules (ROM), peroxides, and free radicals.[17] Hydroperoxide, hydrogen peroxide, and free radicals such as hydroxy, superoxide, and peroxy radicals may be increased in stress and may prove injurious to animal health and disease resistance. In tissue injury, the inflammatory response results from leukotriene and ROM effects. These ROM are produced in all cells within membranes and in the cytosol and in activated phagocytes. Cells may be destroyed if these ROM are not controlled by antioxidants or degraded by specific metalloenzymes.[17, 33, 47] In addition to ROM synthesis as part of eicosanoid metabolism during stress, they are also produced by the adrenal gland concomitantly with glucocorticoids and during enhanced oxidative metabolism.[36] Free radicals generated in active phagocytes as a means of destroying ingested particles may cause self-destruction and damage to adjacent tissues if antioxidant systems are inadequate.[64] Extracellular superoxide radical is also a chemotactic factor that increases migration of unactivated neutrophils to the site of activated ones.[7] Because stress may also increase loss of metals necessary to enzymes that deactivate ROM,[48] ROM levels may potentially remain higher in tissues for a longer time and produce more damage.

One of the means by which ROM may damage cells is through lipoperoxidation of its membranes.[33] When this occurs, cellular enzymes penetrate the membrane and enter the circulation, where their high level is diagnostic of tissue injury. Circulating levels of creatine phosphokinase and aspartate aminotransaminase were found to increase to very high levels in stressed cattle,[4] but it was not known whether this was due to ROM levels or tissue trauma.

HORMONES ALTER METABOLISM

When hormones respond to stress and affect the immune response, they concomitantly affect metabolism. Blood glucose levels are maintained at a fairly constant level by regulation of the amount entering the circulation from the liver and kidney or its uptake by glucose-utilizing tissues. These changes in entry and removal are hormonally regulated. Blood glucose rises rapidly when catecholamines initiate hepatic glycogenolysis. This increase in blood glucose in turn increases insulin secretion, which enhances the extrahepatic uptake of glucose. When blood glucose decreases during fasting, insulin declines, and glucagon and cortisol secretion are enhanced. Glucagon and cortisol are gluconeogenic and promote glucose production by the kidney and liver in order to maintain blood glucose levels. These hormones act to provide carbon compounds from body tissues from which glucose is ultimately synthesized. The metabolic pathways of glycogenolysis, proteolysis, and lipolysis are catabolic and are increased in activity by these hormones. Whereas all tissues can use glucose for energy synthesis, the red blood cells and portions of the central nervous system have an absolute requirement for it. In order to partition and protect the low level of glucose produced for the red blood cells and the central nervous system during fasting, cortisol prevents glucose entry into other tissues. Insulin, which is low at this time, is needed for glucose entry into all tissues except the liver, red blood cells, and central nervous system. When glucose is kept pooled in the blood, it may reach quite high levels, as found in chronically stressed cattle.[4] This high glucose level has been shown to impair ascorbic acid entry into the neutrophil[50] and decrease its function.[9, 55, 57] The source of carbon compounds from which glucose is synthesized is also ensured by cortisol. During stress and when energy is limited, protein synthesis in most tissues is largely curtailed; certain proteins are preferentially degraded in some tissues to furnish amino acids for glucose synthesis and energy and for the production of other proteins. These changes in protein metabolism are discussed later.

Energy Metabolism

The primary energy source for tissues other than the red blood cells and the central nervous system is fatty acids arising from fat stored in adipose tissue. Enzymes responsible for fat catabolism (lipolysis) so that the fatty acids may exit adipose tissue are responsive to ACTH, thyroid-stimulating hormone (TSH), epinephrine, norepinephrine, and glucagon. Most of these lipolytic events require the presence of glucocorticoids and thyroid hormone for an optimal effect. Fatty acids leaving the adipocyte combine with albumin for transport as free fatty acids, which rise in the circulation. Large quantities of free fatty acids are removed by the liver. Generally, in the fed animal, some of these fatty acids contribute to energy production of the liver via oxidative phosphorylation, with the majority converted into very-low-density lipoproteins (VLDL) and introduced back into the blood. However, both energy and VLDL production are greatly diminished in the fasted animal so that the free fatty acids remain in the liver. In an effort to reduce fatty livers and export an energy source elsewhere, the free fatty acids are converted to ketone bodies, which are returned to the circulation. The two primary ketone bodies are 3-hydroxybutyric acid and acetoacetic acid. These ketoacids may lead to a metabolic acidosis. Cattle arriving at the feedlot may have a metabolic acidosis from ketoacidosis and lactic acid production. These stressed cattle may suffer from serious mineral deficiencies as a result of acidosis, high aldosterone and cortisol production, and tissue catabolism.[48] Losses of elements such as zinc, copper, and magnesium, which are instrumental in developing immunocompetence,[10, 16, 38] may jeopardize the animals' defense mechanisms.

Furthermore, acidosis may suppress immunity by inhibiting the synthesis of the active form of vitamin D, 1,25-dihydroxycholecalciferol (1,25-D_3).[8] This hormone-vitamin is needed for several immunologic events including the differentiation of promonocytes and monocytes to macrophages, macrophage functions, phagocytic activity, and cytotoxicity.[28, 34, 53] Acidosis has been shown to reduce renal synthesis of 1,25-D_3. Within the promoter region of the osteocalcin gene, there is a binding site for 1,25-D_3 as well as a separate binding site for dexamethasone.[44] The osteocalcin promoter was repressed by dexamethasone, which slowed or inhibited transcription of the osteocalcin gene. Genes or gene products regulated by 1,25-D_3, such as immunoglobulins and growth factors needed in immunity,[40] might similarly be repressed by glucocorticoids.

Protein, Amino Acid Metabolism

In the initial stages of fasting, cellular proteins are degraded first in the liver, kidney, and intestine, whereas decreases in skeletal muscle occur much later.[45] Certain proteins within these tissues are marked for degradation and hydrolyzed to their amino acids.[12, 25] The freed amino acids may be catabolized to provide energy within the cell or released to be used elsewhere. When amino acids are catabolized in the cell, the amino group is captured by α-keto acids with a net production of alanine and glutamine. The relative proportion of these two released amino acids may be regulated by hormone levels. Glucagon increases the efflux from skeletal muscle of alanine relative to glutamine, which is a better substrate in the liver for gluconeogenesis.[62] Glutamine release relative to alanine was increased by ammonium chloride–induced metabolic acidosis, which would provide the better substrate for renal ammoniagenesis in reducing hydrogen ion excesses.[62] All forms of acidosis in rats, including ketoacidosis, produced significant increases in muscle glutamine synthetase in skeletal muscle; this increases glutamine synthesis and its efflux, which may result in muscle atrophy.[14] Smith[62] hypothesized that both the amount and pattern of amino acids released from skeletal muscle are regulated to match the requirements of other tissue. Glutamine released into the circulation may be an important nutrient for the immune system.[46]

Most of the circulating alanine and glutamine in neutral pH conditions as well as other amino acids arising from muscle proteolysis enter the liver, where they may have a variable fate. After removal of the amino group from amino acids by transaminases, whose activity is increased by cortisol, the carbon skeleton enters the glucose synthetic pathway as directed by the gluconeogenic hormones. The ammonia is combined with another waste product, carbon dioxide, in the urea cycle, whose enzyme activity is increased by glucagon and glucocorticoids.[2] When catabolism of protein is high, as in stressed cattle, blood urea levels rise. As muscle protein is degraded, creatinine levels also increase as creatinine is released from the tissue. Another important fate of amino acids arising from proteolysis is their resynthesis into different vital proteins, which may occur in the liver and other organs and tissues.

Interorgan transport of amino acids arising in stress or disease is very important in providing the substrate for synthesis of acute-phase proteins in the liver, clonal expansion of immune cells, immunoglobulins, and cytokines.[26] Induction of hepatic acute-phase protein synthesis occurs in response to interleukin-6 (IL-6), which is synergistically aided by IL-1[41] and induced in vitro by either IL-1 or tumor necrosis factor (TNF).[1] A few of the acute-phase proteins produced are C-reactive protein and serum amyloid A (both are immunosuppressive), haptoglobin, ceruloplasmin (increases serum copper, scavenges free radicals), α_1-acid glycoprotein (potentiates clotting), fibrinogen (fibrin precursor), and C3 (protective part of the complement pathway).[63] Increases in acute-phase proteins produce hypoferremia, hypozincemia, and hypercupremia in animals in response to cytokines.[22, 26, 43] Induction of procoagulant activity on endothelial cells by TNF and IL-1[31] may be one reason for the difficulty noted in obtaining blood from highly stressed cattle.[4] Proteins that are decreased in the acute-phase response are albumin, prealbumin (transthyretin), retinol-binding protein, and transferrin.[15]

Acute-phase response effects on plasma proteins are demonstrated after bacterial or parasitic infection, mechanical or thermal trauma, malignant growth, or ischemic necrosis.[15] Injury but not protein-energy depletion reduces albumin levels.[15] The decline in plasma albumin and increase in fibrinogen in highly stressed cattle[4] demonstrate that a functional acute-phase response is occurring. Part of the stress these cattle have received may be trauma that results in cell and tissue damage. Products from the damaged cells probably increase chemotaxis of macrophages and neutrophils to the injured site to begin recovery from the injury. Arriving leukocytes, macrophages, and mast cells then release IL-1, IL-2, IL-6, and TNFα. These cytokines initiate hormonal changes that activate proteolysis of destroyed proteins so that new tissue rebuilding may occur. Evidence that serum TNF is increased with severe tissue damage was reported by Reuter and colleagues.[54] Serum TNF values increased in patients suffering from burns or multiple injuries with and without sepsis relative to controls. Furthermore, the increase in TNF was directly correlated to the severity of the pathologic process. These polypeptide cytokines perform various functions, including alterations in acute-phase protein levels in plasma.[15] Because stressed cattle[4] evidence increased acute-phase protein changes that are augmented by cytokines, this is indirect evidence that cytokine levels may be increased in stressed, traumatized cattle. The interactions between immune cells and inflammatory cells are conducted largely by the seven interleukins and TNF. Their production, cell receptors, immune function, and toxic effects are beyond the scope of this paper and have been recently reviewed.[1, 29, 31, 41, 60, 61] Instead, the influence of IL and TNF on metabolism is described.

CYTOKINES AFFECT METABOLISM

Receptors to the cytokines are present in many or most tissues of the body so that they may have not only paracrine but also endocrine function. They are very much involved in enhancing immune function and recovery of injured tissue, which requires a source of energy and amino acids. Much of what is known regarding metabolic changes in infection, inflammation, and repair processes is directed by IL-1 and/or TNF.[51] IL-1 has been shown to stimulate ACTH secretion with consequent adrenal release of glucocorticoids; TNF directly causes adrenal catecholamine release. The secretion of ACTH in response to IL-1 increases glucocorticoid release, which acts by a feedback mechanism to control the immune response through immunosuppression by reducing further production of IL-1.[32] Besides causing anterior pituitary secretion of ACTH, IL-1 also promotes growth hormone, luteinizing hormone, and TSH secretion.[5] IL-1 was also reported to stimulate pancreatic secretion of insulin and glucagon.[51] Cytokine-induced production of these hormones would then initiate the metabolic strategies previously described. Metabolic rate would be expected to increase as a result of enhanced TSH secretion stimulating thyroid hormone release[21] as well as from the fever caused by the cytokines.[22] An initial hyperglycemia due to epinephrine-induced hepatic glycogenolysis and glucose release may be followed by hypoglycemia due to ensuing insulin-induced glucose entry into extrahepatic tissues. Hypertriglyceridemia may occur as free fatty acids from adipose tissue are converted by the liver to triglyceride-containing VLDL, followed by a mild ketoacidosis. Proteolysis may result in increases in blood urea and amino acids, which would provide the substrate for increased production of some of the acute-phase proteins and immune proteins. Evidence for these metabolic changes induced by the cytokines is increasing and is reported subsequently.

Differences in glucose metabolism occur after burns, trauma, and sepsis; nonseptic burn patients have increased glucose production, which is depressed with sepsis.[51] These findings suggest that different forms of injury produce different mediators that do not produce uniform changes in carbohydrate metabolism. Administration of IL-1 to mice was temporally associated with increased insulin, corticosterone, and glucagon and decreased glucose blood levels; the investigators indicated that cytokine-induced hypoglycemia was entirely due to the hyperinsulinemia.[11] TNF injections into mice did not elicit a change in blood glucose, insulin, or corticosterone. IL-1 administered to rats induced a febrile response, increased blood insulin levels, and increased glucose utilization in skeletal muscle and diaphragm and in macrophage-rich tissues, including the lung, spleen, liver, and skin.[30] However, these investigators believe that the increase in tissue glucose utilization occurred by insulin-dependent mechanisms. Dogs given TNF responded with a hypoglycemia associated with increased blood levels of ACTH, cortisol, glucagon, and epinephrine.[13] Glucagon production increased, as did increased blood glucose disappearance and clearance. As blood glucose declined, hindlimb glucose uptake and clearance increased markedly despite a 50 per cent fall in mean serum-insulin level. Hindlimb release of lactate and pyruvate rose 2- to 3-fold after TNF administration. The investigators state that the increased hindlimb glucose uptake was neither mediated by insulin nor due to the increased body temperature. IL-1 and TNF have both been implicated in producing lactic acidosis and reduced oxygen consumption by shifting glucose utilization to anaerobic metabolism.[26]

Lipid metabolism is also affected by cytokines. Lipoprotein lipase (LPL) is an enzyme that releases fatty acids in the blood from their lipoprotein carrier, such as chylomicrons and VLDL. This then allows entry of the fatty acids into the tissue. LPL is attached to the endothelial capillaries adjacent to most tissues, including heart, liver, and adipose and muscle tissue. TNF, IL-1, and IL-2 have been shown to reduce lipoprotein lipase activity in adipose tissue but not elsewhere.[51] This inhibition of LPL synthesis in adipose tissue results in a continual loss from this depot with no reentry of fatty acids. An increased concentration of VLDL in plasma has been observed after decreased LPL activity.[23, 52] This repartitioning of the fatty acids through LPL regulation is energetically feasible because the fatty acids are needed for energy production elsewhere.

Chronic TNF production causes cachexia, a potentially lethal syndrome, which involves lipid and protein wasting.[52] Earlier work reported that IL-1 produced skeletal muscle proteolysis similar to that caused by endotoxin.[51] However, more recent research has shown that purified IL-1 did not stimulate whole-body leucine flux, oxidation, and muscle breakdown although it induced fever, increased plasma acute-phase protein levels, and decreased serum iron and zinc.[51] TNF, a possible contaminant of early IL-1 preparations, has been shown to increase total leucine oxidation and muscle catabolism. Coadministration of both IL-1 and TNF had a synergistic effect on increasing skeletal muscle breakdown and reducing the percentage of protein in muscle.[51]

TNF administration in rats has profound effects on individual amino acid utilization.[3] This cytokine increases both the total hepatic amino acid uptake and the individual uptake of gluconeogenic amino acids while decreasing the uptake of leucine, isoleucine, and phenylalanine. Mealy and associates[39] sought to determine if effects exerted by TNF were mediated by glucocorticoids in rats. Whereas either TNF or corticosterone decreased nitrogen balance and carcass nitrogen content, only TNF induced increased liver DNA and protein content and diminished jejunal mucosal DNA and protein level, which suggested that TNF may have effects independent of glucocorticoid.

Cytokines, although promoting peripheral protein wasting and nitrogen excretion, are essential for supplying amino acids needed for acute protein synthesis, immune cell proliferation, and peptide modulators of the neural and endocrine systems. Another common manifestation of cytokine production is a decrease in food intake followed by a depression in body weight. TNF and IL-1 have both been found to produce anorexia,[42] another acute-phase response. TNF is instrumental in the pathogenesis of cachexia.[6] Continuous administration of TNF into rats or mice produced changes in nitrogen balance and a slight reduction in body weight followed by a gradual increase to normal levels associated with fluid retention.[26]

Many effects of administering recombinant bovine TNF to cattle were reported by Ohmann and colleagues.[49] Depending on the amount and length of TNF administration, some of the responses found were hyperthermia; leukopenia; decreased serum iron and zinc; increased serum copper and urea; depression; anorexia; cachexia; diarrhea; atrophy of the thymus, heart, and skeletal muscle; and loss of body fat.

Many of the changes precipitated by cytokine administration are classic signs observed in highly stressed cattle arriving at the feedlot. Cytokines are multifunctional in the regulation and integration of metabolism and immunity. Whereas energy repartitioning during acute stress may be advantageous to survival, prolonged endocrine-induced effects may prove pernicious. As our knowledge in this area expands, opportunities for preventing some of the deleterious effects of stress and trauma may be realized.

REFERENCES

1. Akira S, Hirano T, Taga T, Kishimoto T: Biology of multifunctional cytokines: IL6 and related molecules (IL-1 and TNF). FASEB J 4:2860–2867, 1990.
2. Anonymous: Regulation of urea cycle enzymes. Nutr Rev 46:326–327, 1988.
3. Argiles JM, Lopez-Soriano FJ: The effects of tumour necrosis factor-α (cachectin) and tumour growth on hepatic amino acid utilization in the rat. Biochem J 266:123–126, 1990.
4. Bennett BW, Kerschen RP, Nockels CF: Stress induced hematological changes in feedlot cattle. Agri-Practice 10:16–28, 1989.
5. Bernton EW, Beach JE, Holaday JW, et al: Release of multiple hormones by a direct action of interleukin-1 on pituitary cells. Science 238:519–521, 1987.

6. Beutler B, Cerami A: Tumor necrosis, cachexia, shock and inflammation: a common mediator. Ann Rev Biochem 57:505–518, 1988.
7. Braezile JE: The physiology of stress and its relationship to mechanisms of disease and therapeutics. Vet Clin North Am [Food Anim Pract] 4:441–480, 1988.
8. Ching SV, Fettman MJ, Hamar DW, et al: The effect of chronic dietary acidification using ammonium chloride on acid-base and mineral metabolism in the adult cat. J Nutr 119:902–915, 1989.
9. Crandon JH, Lennihan R, Mikal S: Ascorbic acid economy in surgical patients. Ann NY Acad Sci 92:246–267, 1961.
10. Davis GK, Mertz W: Copper. *In* Mertz W (ed): Trace Elements in Human and Animal Nutrition, 5th ed, vol 1. New York, Academic Press, 1987, pp 335–336.
11. Del Rey A, Besedovsky H: Interleukin-1 affects glucose homeostasis. Am J Physiol 253:R794–R798, 1987.
12. Dice JF: Molecular determinants of protein half-lives in eukaryotic cells. FASEB J 1:349–357, 1987.
13. Evans DA, Jacobs DO, Wilmore DW: Tumor necrosis factor enhances glucose uptake by peripheral tissues. Am J Physiol 257:R1182–R1189, 1989.
14. Falduto MT, Hickson RC, Young AP: Antagonism by glucocorticoids and exercise on expression of glutamine synthetase in skeletal muscle. FASEB J 3:2623–2628, 1989.
15. Fleck A: Clinical and nutritional aspects of changes in acute-phase proteins during inflammation. Proc Nutr Soc 48:347–354, 1989.
16. Fletcher MP, Gershwin ME, Keen CL, Hurley L: Trace element deficiencies and immune responsiveness in human and animal models. *In* Chandra RK (ed): Nutrition and Immunology. New York, Alan R. Liss, 1988, pp 215–239.
17. Freeman BA, Crapo JD: Biology of disease free radicals and tissue injury. Lab Invest 47:412–426, 1982.
18. Ganong WF: Hormonal control of calcium metabolism and the physiology of bone. *In* Review of Medical Physiology, 13th ed. Norwalk, CT, Appleton and Lange, 1987, p 331.
19. Goldstein L: Interorgan glutamine relationships. Fed Proc 45:2176–2179, 1986.
20. Golub MS, Gershwin ME: Stress-induced immunomodulation: What is it, if it is? *In* Moberg GP (ed): Animal Stress. Bethesda, MD, American Physiological Society, 1985, pp 177–192.
21. Granner DK: Thyroid hormones. *In* Murray RK, Granner DK, Mayes PA, Rodwell VW: Harper's Biochemistry, 21st ed. Norwalk, CT, Appleton and Lange, 1988, pp 496–501.
22. Grimble RF: Cytokines: their relevance to nutrition. Eur J Clin Nutr 43:217–230, 1989.
23. Grunfeld C, Gulli R, Moser AH, et al: Effect of tumor necrosis factor administration in vivo on lipoprotein lipase activity in various tissues of the rat. J Lipid Res 30:579–585, 1989.
24. Hadden JW: Neuroendocrine modulation of the thymus-dependent immune system. Ann NY Acad Sci 496:39–48, 1987.
25. Hershko A: Ubiquitin-mediated protein degradation. J Biol Chem 263:15237–15240, 1988.
26. Johnstone BJ, Klasing KC: Aspects nutritionnels des cytokines leucocytaines. Nutr Clin Metabol 4:7–27, 1990.
27. Kelley KW: Cross-talk between the immune and endocrine systems. J Anim Sci 66:2095–2108, 1988.
28. Koeffler HP, Reichel H, Tobler A, Norman AW: Macrophages and vitamin D_3. *In* Zembala M, Asherson GL (eds): Human Monocytes. New York, Academic Press, 1989, pp 345–351.
29. Kunkel SL, Remick DG, Strieter RM, Larrick JW: Mechanisms that regulate the production and effects of tumor necrosis factor-α. Crit Rev Immun 9;93–117, 1989.
30. Lang CH, Dobrescu C: Interleukin-1 induced increases in glucose utilization are insulin mediated. Life Sci 45:2127–2134, 1989.
31. Le J, Vilcek J: Biology of disease. Tumor necrosis factor and interleukin-1: cytokines with multiple overlapping biological activities. Lab Invest 56:234–248, 1987.
32. Lumpkin MD: The regulation of ACTH secretion by IL-1. Science 238:452–454, 1987.
33. Machlin LJ, Bendich A: Free radical tissue damage: protective role of antioxidant nutrients. FASEB J 1:444–445, 1987.
34. Manolagas SC, Hustmyer FG, Yu X: 1,25-Dihydroxyvitamin D_3 and the immune system. SEBM 192:238–245, 1989.
35. Mayes PA: Metabolism of unsaturated fatty acids and eicosanoids. *In* Murray RK, Granner DK, Mayes PA, Rodwell VW (eds): Harper's Biochemistry, 21st ed. San Mateo, CA, Appleton and Lange, 1988, pp 210–217.
36. Mayes PA: Biological oxidation. *In* Murray RK, Granner DK, Mayes PA, Rodwell VW (eds): Harper's Biochemistry, 21st ed. San Mateo, CA, Appleton and Lange, 1988, pp 100–107.
37. Mayes PA: Regulation of carbohydrate metabolism. *In* Murray RK, Granner DK, Mayes PA, Rodwell VW (eds): Harper's Biochemistry, 21st ed. San Mateo, CA, Appleton and Lange, 1988, pp 100–107.
38. McCoy JH, Kenney MA: Magnesium and immunocompetence. *In* Watson RR (ed): Nutrition, Disease Resistance and Immune Function. New York, Marcel Dekker, 1984, pp 223–247.
39. Mealy K, van Lanschot J, Robinson BG, et al: Are the catabolic effects of tumor necrosis factor mediated by glucocorticoids? Arch Surg 125:42–48, 1990.
40. Minghetti PP, Norman AW: 1,25-$(OH)_2$-Vitamin D_3 receptors: gene regulation and genetic circuitry. FASEB J 3:2043–3053, 1988.
41. Mizel SB: The interleukins. FASEB J 3:2379–2388, 1989.
42. Moldawer LL, Anderson C, Gelin J, Lundholm KG: Regulation of food intake and hepatic protein synthesis by recombinant-derived cytokines. Am J Physiol 254:G450–G456, 1988.
43. Moldawer LL, Marano MA, Wei H, et al: Cachectin/tumor necrosis factor-α alters red blood cell kinetics and induces anemia in vivo. FASEB J 3:1637–1643, 1989.
44. Morrison NA, Shine J, Fragonas J, et al: 1,25-Dihydroxyvitamin D–responsive element and glucocorticoid repression in the osteocalcin gene. Science 246:1158–1161, 1989.
45. Mortimore GE: Regulation of hepatic protein degradation by circulatory amino acids. Fed Proc 45:2169–2172, 1986.
46. Newsholme EA, Crabtree B, Ardawi MS: Glutamine metabolism in lymphocytes: its biochemical, physiological and clinical importance. Q J Exp Physiol 70:473–489, 1985.
47. Nockels CF: The role of vitamins in modulating disease resistance. Vet Clin North Am [Food Anim Pract] 4:531–542, 1988.
48. Nockels CF: Mineral alterations associated with stress, trauma, and infection and the effect on immunity. Compendium 12:1133–1139, 1990.
49. Ohmann HB, Campos M, Snider M, et al: Effect of chronic administration of recombinant bovine tumor necrosis factor to cattle. Vet Pathol 26:462–472, 1989.
50. Pecoraro RE, Chen MS: Ascorbic acid metabolism in diabetes mellitus. Ann NY Acad Sci 498:248–257, 1987.
51. Pomposelli JJ, Flores EA, Bistrain BR: Role of biochemical mediators in clinical nutrition and surgical metabolism. J Parenteral Enteral Nutr 12:212–217, 1988.
52. Porat O: The effect of tumor necrosis factor α on the activity of lipoprotein lipase in adipose tissue. Lymphokine Res 8:459–469, 1989.
53. Reinhart TA, Hustmyer FG: Role of vitamin D in the immune system. J Dairy Sci 70:952–962, 1987.
54. Reuter A, Benier J, Gysen P, et al: A RIA for tumor necrosis factor (TNFα) and interleukin 1β (IL-1β) and their direct determination in serum. *In* Powanda MC, Oppenheim JJ, Kluger MJ, Dinarello CA (eds): Monokines and Other Non-Lymphocytic Cytokines. New York, Alan R. Liss, 1988, pp 377–381.
55. Roth JA, Kaeberle ML: Effects of in vivo dexamethasone administration on in vitro bovine polymorphonuclear leukocyte function. Infect Immun 33:434–441, 1981.
56. Roth JA, Kaeberle ML: Effect of glucocorticoids on the bovine immune system. J Am Vet Med Assoc 18:894–901, 1982.
57. Roth JA, Kaeberle ML, Hsu WH: Effects of ACTH administration on bovine polymorphonuclear leukocyte function and lymphocyte blastogenesis. Am J Vet Res 43:412–416, 1982.
58. Rulofson FC, Brown DE, Bjur RA: Effect of blood sampling and shipment to slaughter on plasma catecholamine concentrations in bulls. J Anim Sci 66:1223–1229, 1988.
59. Samuelsson B, Dahlen SE, Lindgren JA, et al: Leukotrienes and lipoxins: structures, biosynthesis and biological effects. Science 237:1171–1176, 1987.
60. Sisson SD, Dinarello CA: Interleukin-1. *In* Zembala M (ed): Human Monocytes. New York, Academic Press, 1989, pp 183–215.
61. Smith KA: Interleukin-2. Inception, impact and implications. Science 240:1169–1176, 1988.
62. Smith RJ. Role of skeletal muscle in interorgan amino acid exchange. Fed Proc 45:2172–2176, 1986.
63. Tizard IR: Regulation of the immune response. *In* Immunology: An Introduction, 22nd ed. New York, Saunders College Publishing, 1988, pp 261–283.
64. Weiss SJ, Buglio AF: Biology of disease phagocyte-generated oxygen metabolites and cellular injury. Lab Invest 47:5–18, 1982.

Adverse Drug Reactions

DAWN M. BOOTHE, DVM, PhD, DIPLOMATE, ACVIM, ACVCP
GORDON W. BRUMBAUGH, DVM, PhD, DIPLOMATE, ACVIM, ACVCP

Adverse drug reactions are defined as any unintended and undesirable response to a drug and can be categorized as either type A or type B. Type B (idiosyncratic or "bizarre") drug reactions are unpredictable responses to a drug. Whereas they affect only a small percentage of the animal population, they occur regardless of the dose of drug administered. Drug hypersensitivities and genetic idiosyncrasies are examples of type B reactions. In contrast, type A (idiopathic or "augmented") drug reactions are not uncommon and may occur in most animals in a given population. Type A adverse reactions are usually dose-dependent and are more likely to occur when an improper dosing regimen is used. Normally, dosing regimens recommended for a species are designed to generate plasma drug concentrations within a therapeutic range. However, if plasma drug concentrations develop above the therapeutic range, a type A reaction may occur and will be manifested as either an exaggerated pharmacologic response or a toxic response (i.e., tissue damage). Alternatively, if plasma drug concentrations develop below the therapeutic range, therapeutic failure may result.

TYPE A ADVERSE REACTIONS

Type A adverse reactions are more likely to occur if plasma drug concentrations increase above the toxic concentration or fall below the minimum effective concentration. Although the dosing regimen is an important determinant of plasma concentrations of a drug, the disposition of that drug in the body is equally important. Events that determine drug disposition include the rate and extent of drug absorption from the site of administration, distribution of the drug from the circulation into tissues, and clearance of the drug by metabolism or excretion. The chemical structure of the drug largely determines the role each of these events has in the drug's disposition. However, these events can be altered in a patient by a variety of factors; thus the potential of type A adverse drug reactions is increased. These factors can be described as physiologic, pharmacologic, or pathologic.

Physiologic Factors

Many type A adverse reactions occur because a dosing regimen in one species has been inappropriately extrapolated to another. Generally, species that are physiologically similar tend to have the same pattern of drug disposition. Thus, whereas a similar dosing regimen might be used for ruminants, a different one is often needed for monogastrics (pigs). Species differences occur in all phases of drug disposition.

The major determinants of gastrointestinal absorption of a drug include gastrointestinal pH, which determines the percentage of diffusible drug available for absorption; surface area; motility; and blood flow. Each of these determinants may vary between species, with resultant differences in the rate and extent of absorption. For example, the gastrointestinal pH of pigs varies from 1 to 7. Although ruminal pH is less variable (pH 5.5 to 6.5), it can be markedly affected by diet. Ruminants present another unique challenge to orally administered drugs. Ruminal contents might dilute the drug and can destroy (or be destroyed by) the drug before the drug reaches the site of absorption (e.g., chloramphenicol, trimethoprim/sulfadiazine, and digoxin). Differences in reticular groove function have been cited as the reason that plasma drug concentrations are higher in adult sheep compared to other adult ruminants following oral administration. The site of parenteral administration may also lead to a different rate and extent of drug absorption. For example, studies in calves have shown that the most consistent parenteral drug absorption follows administration either intramuscularly in the middle gluteal muscles or subcutaneously over the ribs.

The major determinants of drug distribution include the extent of binding to plasma proteins (particularly albumin); the fat-to-lean body weight distribution; and the size of body compartments to which the drug might be distributed. The plasma concentration of a drug varies inversely with the amount of tissue to which the drug is distributed. For example, fat can represent a compartment to which a water-soluble drug may not distribute but a lipid-soluble drug might. Administration of a lipid-soluble drug to animals with a greater proportion of body fat, such as pigs, finished steers, and lambs, may decrease the amount of drug available to target tissues, resulting in therapeutic failure. Alternatively, if the drug does not penetrate fat, but the animal is dosed on the basis of total body weight, plasma drug concentrations may be higher, compared with lean animals (i.e., unfinished animals, steers, goats, or cows), and an exaggerated response may occur. Another potential difference in distribution among food animals results from large body compartments. The gastrointestinal tract of ruminants and the mammary glands of dairy cattle represent tissues to which drugs may or may not be distributed. Distribution into these tissues depends on the chemical structure of the drug, its degree of ionization in the tissue, and its lipid solubility. If the pH difference among tissues and plasma is appropriate, a drug can be ionized and thus nondiffusible or trapped in the tissue. Large amounts of a drug can accumulate in tissues in this manner. Two potential problems can occur: (1) less drug is available for distribution to target organs; and (2) the drug may be trapped in the milk of a lactating cow, where it serves as a source of drug exposure to nursing calves or human consumers of milk products. In the latter case, violative milk residues become a major concern.

Species differences in drug metabolism can be profound and clinically significant. Drug metabolism occurs primarily in the liver in two phases. Phase I metabolism chemically changes the drug so that it is more susceptible to phase II metabolism. Phase II reactions are synthetic: a large molecule (e.g., glucuronic acid or sulfate) is added to the drug or its phase I metabolite. With rare exception, phase II reactions inactivate the drug and increase its water solubility so that drug excretion is facilitated. Few differences in metabolism have been documented among food animals. Deficiencies in phase II sulfation, a reaction important to the elimination of a number of drugs (e.g., sulfonamides), have been reported in swine. Differences in the metabolism of some nonsteroidal anti-inflammatory drugs have also been reported. The elimination half-life of phenylbutazone is at least 36 hours in cows and 19 hours in goats but much less (i.e., 9 hours) in several other species. If cows are dosed by use of regimens recommended for other species, toxicity would probably occur. Drug metabolism by microbes in the gastrointestinal tract can also result in type A reactions, particularly therapeutic failure. For example, chloramphenicol is destroyed by ruminal microflora. Species differences in drug excretion are also likely to exist among food animals, although their role in the advent of type A adverse drug reactions has not been established.

Another physiologic difference between species that may lead to adverse reactions is pharmacodynamic response. Species differences in pharmacodynamic responses may reflect differences in receptor numbers, receptor sensitivity, or other unidentified differences in physiology. For example, cattle, and particularly Brahman, are more sensitive to the sedative effects of xylazine than are other animals. In contrast, inhibition of rumination by xylazine is more likely to cause bloat in sheep than in cattle. Other examples of pharmacodynamic differences between species include: (1) the likelihood of cattle to become excited rather than sedated following administration of morphine derivatives, and (2) the greater sensitivity of sheep to the adverse effects of the anthelmintic haloxone.

Age-induced differences in drug disposition can also play a significant role in the advent of adverse drug reactions, although these differences are not as important in food animals. Briefly, the pediatric patient is predisposed to changes in drug disposition because

1. The gastrointestinal tract is more permeable, particularly for the first 24 hours after birth. More drug is absorbed than in adult animals. This might be problematic if increased drug absorption in veal calves results in violative tissue drug residues.
2. Drug is distributed to a larger volume of tissue. Total body water is greater and the concentration of serum albumin is less in the pediatric patient, compared with adults.
3. Drug metabolism is generally less, particularly in neonates, because drug-metabolizing enzymes mature at different rates during the first 3 months of life.
4. Finally, renal elimination of drugs is less than that of adults for the first few weeks of life.

Predicting the effects of physiologic changes in drug disposition in neonatal or pediatric animals can be difficult. Differences in drug distribution, which tend to decrease plasma drug concentrations, may be offset by differences in absorption and elimination, which tend to increase plasma drug concentrations. A few studies have characterized differences in the disposition of a few drugs in pediatric animals. For example, several drugs, including chloramphenicol, apromycin, and trimethoprim/sulfadiazine, can reach therapeutic concentrations following oral administration in calves, but not adult ruminants.

Age-induced changes in drug disposition in the geriatric patient can be more dramatic than those in the pediatric patient. Total body and organ mass decline by approximately 25 per cent in older patients. The decline in mass is accompanied by a decline in the general function of remaining cells. In addition, the geriatric patient may be suffering from diseases that can adversely alter drug disposition. Therapy of these diseases may require multiple drugs, which may lead to drug interactions. In general, drug absorption is decreased in the geriatric patient because gastrointestinal motility, pH, and blood flow decrease. These changes are most likely to lead to therapeutic failure. Drug distribution in the geriatric patient varies. These patients are often overweight and have a higher proportion of body fat. Drugs may accumulate in fat, which would prevent drug distribution to target tissues. If the drug is not distributed to fat, plasma drug concentrations might be higher than anticipated. Drug metabolism in the geriatric patient is decreased, and the elimination of drugs is generally slower because both hepatic and renal mass and function decrease. Thus clearance of most drugs is impaired, and response to many drugs may be exaggerated.

Sex differences in drug disposition have not been documented in food animals. In those species in which they have been identified, the sequelae are usually minor and clinically insignificant. However, the female of all species is predisposed to selected type A adverse reactions because of her reproductive activity. Drugs may cause embryocidal or teratogenic effects, abortion, changes in parturition, or altered lactation. Occasionally, the male reproductive tract is selectively susceptible to some type A adverse reactions.

Type A adverse reactions may reflect inter- or intraspecies variations in the ratio of body mass to body weight. Whereas body surface area is the best estimate of body mass, drugs are usually dosed on a per unit body weight (i.e., pounds or kilograms). Unfortunately, conversion of weight to body surface area charts that have been validated for large animals are not available to the practitioner. Generally, large animals should receive a smaller dose per unit body weight, compared with a small animal, because the larger animal has a smaller body surface area per unit body weight. In addition, differences between body weight and "true lean body weight" can be important contributors to adverse reactions in selected populations of animals: the obese versus starved animal; animals with edema or ascites; dehydrated animals; animals with large tumors; and animals with filled gastrointestinal compartments. Body surface area should be used to calculate dosages of those drugs that are potentially toxic.

A final physiologic factor that can lead to type A adverse reactions is environmental temperature. Blood flow to sites of parenteral drug administration can be altered, which will change drug absorption. For example, hypothermia can cause peripheral vasoconstriction and subcutaneously administered drugs may be poorly absorbed. Alternatively, metabolic processes may be decreased. The newborn animal is particularly susceptible to the effects of hypothermia.

Pharmacologic Factors

Pharmacologic factors, or drug interactions, occur whenever the action or disposition of one drug is modified by another concurrently administered drug. The incidence of drug interactions increases proportionately with the number of drugs included in the preparation, with the number of drugs administered during a single dosing interval, and with the duration of drug therapy. Drug interactions can be pharmaceutic, pharmacokinetic, or pharmacodynamic, depending on the phase of drug action in which they occur.

Pharmaceutic Drug Interactions

Pharmaceutic drug interactions occur when two or more chemically incompatible drugs are combined (Tables 1 and 2). This may occur before (in vitro) or after (in vivo) administration. Interactions in preparations can occur among drugs or additives (e.g., base or salt forms, solubilizers, stabilizers). Pharmaceutic drug interactions are often accompanied by a

Table 1. EXAMPLES OF PHARMACEUTIC DRUG INTERACTIONS

Drug	In Vitro Interactions
Atropine sulfate and barbiturates	Diazepam
Chloramphenicol and hydrocortisone sodium succinate	Heparin sodium, chlorpromazine hydrochloride, gentamicin, penicillins, tetracyclines
Gentamicin sulfate	Carbenicillin, cephalosporins, chloramphenicol sodium succinate, heparin sodium quinolones
Tetracyclines	Di- and trivalent cations (calcium, aluminum, magnesium), cephalosporins, tylosin, chloramphenicol sodium succinate, hydrocortisone sodium succinate, sodium bicarbonate
Meperidine and barbiturates	Sodium bicarbonate, heparin sodium, methylprednisolone sodium succinate
Calcium gluconate and carbonate	Phosphate, sulfate salts, tetracyclines, others
Semisynthetic penicillins	Aminoglycosides, barbiturates, diazepam, phenothiazine neuroleptics, vitamin B complexes, and any drugs

Drug	In Vivo Interactions
Aminoglycosides	Penicillins
Tetracyclines	Di- or trivalent cations
Protamine	Heparin
Calcium gluconate and sodium sulfonamide	Can form gels in veins
Kaolin	Rifampin, lincomycin, and other drugs after oral administration

Table 2. EXAMPLES OF PHARMACEUTIC DRUG–FLUID INTERACTIONS

Drug	Fluid
Ampicillin	Glucose and dextran fluids
Oxytetracycline	Ca^{+2} or Mg^{+2}, glucose fluids
Gentamicin sulfate	Any (>1 g/L)
Diazepam	Any
Methylprednisolone	Sodium succinate and sodium lactate solutions
Sodium bicarbonate	Sodium lactate, Ringer's, any solution with Ca^{+2}

Table 4. DRUGS THAT AFFECT GASTRIC MOTILITY

Drug	Effect
Anticholinergics	Decreased
Adrenergics	Decreased
Neuroleptics	Decreased
Antihistamines	Decreased
Opioid analgesics	Decreased
Cholinergics	Increased
Metaclopramide	Increased

change in the physical or chemical nature of the drug. These changes usually alter the dissolution of the drug and its diffusion through tissues. Absorption and distribution can be affected. In some instances, one or more drugs are inactivated. The most common pharmaceutic interactions are those that occur when drugs intended for injection are mixed with fluids (Table 2) or with one another for convenience before administration. In the case of orally administered drugs, pharmaceutic incompatibilities can occur in the gastrointestinal tract after administration but before absorption. Occasionally, interactions between a drug and dietary constituent can lead to adverse drug reactions (Table 3).

Pharmacologic factors involving only one drug can also lead to adverse drug reactions. Drug preparations designed for slow delivery are an example. Slow-release preparations, such as benzathine penicillin, may be convenient, but drug release following intramuscular administration may be so slow that therapeutic plasma drug concentrations are never reached. Drugs or their carriers can cause tissue necrosis at the site of intramuscular injections. Necrosis can lead to lameness, abscessation, and financial loss at meat inspection.

Pharmacokinetic Drug Interactions

Pharmacokinetic drug interactions occur when one drug alters the disposition of a second, concurrently administered drug. They occur in vivo during any phase of disposition. These interactions can be profound and occasionally life-threatening. Pharmacokinetic drug interactions that alter drug absorption usually follow oral administration. For example, some drugs (H_2-receptor blockers) increase gastric pH, thus altering the disintegration and dissolution of weakly acidic drugs and delaying or decreasing their absorption. The effect of changes in gastric motility depend on the site of drug absorption (Table 4). Because most drugs are absorbed from the small intestine, drugs that slow gastric motility tend to delay gastric emptying and the rate of absorption. Whereas the total amount of drug absorbed might not be affected, peak plasma drug concentration may be decreased. Drugs that increase gastric motility may have the opposite effect. Drugs that alter small intestinal motility frequently do not change the absorption of an orally administered drug because the surface area of the intestines is too large. However, drugs that increase or decrease blood flow in the gastrointestinal tract may cause parallel changes in the absorption of some drugs. Finally, some drugs can cause malabsorption of other drugs or nutrients owing to their toxic effects on the gastrointestinal tract.

Absorption of parenterally administered drugs can also be altered by another drug. For example, absorption from intramuscular and subcutaneous sites can be decreased by drugs that decrease regional blood flow. Some topical drug preparations contain drugs that are included to increase the permeability of the skin (i.e., DMSO) and thus drug absorption.

Most clinically important pharmacokinetic drug interactions that alter drug distribution result from competition between highly (>85 per cent) protein-bound drugs for protein-binding sites. Examples of highly protein-bound drugs include most nonsteroidal anti-inflammatory drugs and some sulfonamides. Because protein-binding is reversible, the drug with the highest affinity for protein (usually albumin) will displace the drug with less affinity. Because the free (unbound) form of the drug is pharmacologically active, the potential for adverse reactions is increased. Competition for protein-binding can also occur in tissues. Drug distribution to organs may also be changed by drugs that alter regional blood flow.

Changes in drug metabolism induced by pharmacokinetic drug interactions can be profound and clinically significant. Phase I hepatic drug-metabolizing enzymes are susceptible to induction or inhibition by other compounds. Many drugs have been identified as potential inducers or inhibitors (Table 5); some drugs (i.e., phenylbutazone) are capable of either effect, depending on the enzyme involved. If induction of enzymes occurs, drug metabolism increases. Clearance of concurrently administered drugs that are also metabolized by the liver will increase, and therapeutic failure may follow. However, drug toxicity or a pharmacologic response may also occur if production of a toxic phase I metabolite or a pharmacologically active drug is increased. Drugs vary in their ability to induce enzymes, and several days to weeks of drug administration may be required for enzyme induction to occur. A similar period may be necessary for resolution of induction after the drug has been discontinued.

Drugs can also inhibit metabolizing enzymes, although these

Table 3. EXAMPLES OF INTERACTIONS BETWEEN DRUGS AND DIETARY CONSTITUENTS

Drug or Dietary Nutrient	Effect
Sulfafurazole	Impaired absorption
Ampicillin and other semisynthetic penicillins (except amoxicillin)	Impaired absorption
Cephalexin	Impaired absorption
Tetracyclines	Impaired absorption
Lincomycin	Impaired absorption
Rifampin	Impaired absorption
Griseofulvin	Enhanced absorption in presence of fat

Table 5. DRUGS THAT INDUCE OR INHIBIT DRUG METABOLISM ENZYMES

Inducers
Chlorinated hydrocarbons
Griseofulvin
Phenobarbital (and other barbiturates)
Phenylbutazone
Phenytoin
Theophylline
Inhibitors
Chloramphenicol
Cimetidine, ranitidine
Prednisolone
Phenylbutazone
Quinidine

effects are probably not as clinically significant as are those resulting from induction. Clearance of a concurrently administered drug that is metabolized by the liver is usually decreased. As the drug accumulates, the potential for toxicity effect or an exaggerated pharmacologic response increases. Generally, inhibition does not require long-term administration of the drug, and the effects of inhibition may resolve faster than do those of induction. Drug metabolism may also be decreased by drugs that decrease hepatic blood flow (e.g., theophylline and cimetidine). However, this interaction is significant only for drugs characterized by extensive and rapid hepatic clearance (e.g., propranolol, lidocaine). In such instances, the clearance of drug will decline in concert with decreased hepatic blood flow.

Pharmacokinetic drug interactions also alter the excretion of some drugs, although these changes are probably not as clinically important as are those that affect drug metabolism. Changes in biliary elimination are rare and usually result from competition for excretory proteins. Pharmacokinetic drug interactions during renal excretion often reflect drug-induced changes in renal blood flow and glomerular filtration. In addition, drugs, and particularly weak acids, compete for active tubular secretion. Finally, renal excretion of a drug may be changed by drugs (or diets) that alter urinary pH. As the drug becomes more ionized, less is resorbed from the tubules and more is excreted. If the pH increases the amount of un-ionized drug, more drug is resorbed from the tubules into the plasma. Clearance of the drug would then be decreased.

Pharmacodynamic Drug Interactions

Pharmacodynamic drug interactions occur when one drug directly alters the physiologic response to another drug (Table 6). They can enhance the response to a drug (i.e., agonistic), or they can inhibit the response (antagonistic). Agonistic interactions can be additive or synergistic. This may occur either at the same receptor site or at different sites but with the same physiologic reaction. Antagonistic interactions decrease the response to a drug owing to competition at the same receptor site (e.g., atropine and anticholinesterases) or at distant but physiologically related sites. Combination of a bactericidal and bacteriostatic might be considered an antagonistic pharmacodynamic response. Whereas antagonistic pharmacodynamic drug interactions often produce an undesirable side effect, they may also be of therapeutic benefit. Examples of some therapeutically beneficial antagonistic interactions include the combination of chemicals for restraint or anesthesia, the reversal of narcotics, or the combination of selected antimicrobials.

Pathologic Factors

The dosage regimens recommended for a pharmaceutic preparation generally are based on controlled studies in the normal, healthy animal. However, the target patient is usually diseased. Pathophysiologic changes that accompany disease can profoundly alter drug disposition, which predisposes the diseased patient to type A adverse drug reactions. Diseases of the liver and kidneys are probably most important because they are responsible for most drug clearance.

The effects of renal disease on drug disposition have been well documented in selected species. Disease-induced decreases in glomerular filtration and tubular secretion will markedly decrease clearance of drugs and metabolites. In general, the clearance of drugs eliminated by glomerular filtration will decline proportionally with decreased renal blood flow. These changes become important if the drug is toxic and particularly if the drug is nephrotoxic (i.e., aminoglycosides). The effects of renal disease on drug clearance can be estimated on the basis of changes in the patient's creatinine clearance. Likewise, dosing regimens of drugs that are excreted by glomerular filtration can be individualized to the patient on the basis of the patient's creatinine clearance (pt CrCl) or its serum creatinine concentrations, according to the formula

$$\text{New dose} = \text{normal dose} \times \frac{\text{pt CrCl}}{\text{normal CrCl}} \left[or \; \frac{\text{normal creatinine}}{\text{pt creatinine}} \right]$$

$$\text{New interval} = \text{normal interval} \times \frac{\text{normal CrCl}}{\text{pt CrCl}} \left[or \; \frac{\text{pt creatinine}}{\text{normal creatinine}} \right]$$

Physiologic changes that accompany renal disease may alter other determinants of drug disposition. Examples include changes in serum protein-binding (due to protein loss through the glomerulus or due to competition with accumulated endogenous substrates) and fluid, electrolyte, and acid-base imbalances.

The effects of hepatic disease on drug disposition are very complex. Both hepatic blood flow and metabolic enzyme activity decline with progressing hepatic disease. Hepatic clearance of drugs proportionately decreases. Changes in protein-binding also occur as a result of decreased synthesis of albumin or increased formation of globulins. These will affect the rate of hepatic clearance because unbound drugs are generally cleared faster by the liver than are protein-bound drugs. Changes in hepatic clearance are particularly important for orally administered drugs that undergo hepatic first-pass metabolism (i.e., most of the drug is removed from the blood by the liver the first time the drug passes through the liver). The

Table 6. EXAMPLES OF PHARMACODYNAMIC DRUG INTERACTIONS THAT INCREASE DRUG TOXICITY

Drug 1	Toxicity	Drug 2
Aminoglycosides	Ototoxicity and nephrotoxicosis	Furosemide
Aminoglycosides	Neuromuscular and cardiac	Most general anesthetics[1]
Pancuronium gallamine	Enhanced neuromuscular blockade	Lincomycin
		Clindamycin
		Polymyxins
Tetracyclines	Neuromuscular blockage	General anesthetics (or during hypocalcemia)
Halothane and methoxyflurane	Sensitized myocardium to arrhythmogenic effects of catecholamines	Thiobarbiturates potentiate the effect[2]
Diamidine antiprotozoals	Anticholinesterase inhibitors	Organophosphates
Succinylcholine	Prolonged flaccid paralysis	Cholinesterase inhibitors
Methoxyflurane	Renal failure	Tetracyclines

[1]Reversed with Ca^{+2} and anticholinesterase antagonist.
[2]Premedication with acepromazine, lidocaine, or propranolol reduce this effect.

bioavailability of such drugs increases as hepatic blood flow decreases. Plasma drug concentrations may develop in the toxic range if the normal oral dose is administered. Changes in protein concentration can also alter drug distribution, as can changes in fluid balance and electrolyte and acid-base balance. The effects of hepatic disease on drug disposition depend on the drug, its degree of protein-binding, how rapidly the drug is removed by the liver, the type of hepatic disease, and the species to which the drug is being administered. Unfortunately, the complexity of hepatic disease precludes making general recommendations regarding the alteration of dosing regimens in the patient with hepatic disease. Caution should be exercised when potentially toxic drugs and particularly drugs that are hepatotoxic are administered.

Because cardiac output is important to the normal function of all body organs, cardiovascular disease can affect all determinants of drug disposition. These effects can be profound in an animal suffering from hypotensive or endotoxic shock. In general, regional blood flow to body organs decreases in the presence of cardiac disease. Both oral and parenteral absorption can decrease. Regional distribution of drugs to target organs declines. Because blood flow to the heart and brain is maintained, these organs may receive a greater proportion of drug and are susceptible to drug-induced toxic effects. Blood flow to organs of excretion (i.e., kidney and liver) parallels cardiac output; consequently, drug excretion decreases.

Diseases of other body systems can also dramatically alter drug disposition. For example, gastrointestinal disease may alter drug absorption owing to changes in the gastrointestinal pH, epithelial permeability, or motility. Malnutrition can alter drug disposition as a result of hypoproteinemia and altered metabolism. Endocrine disorders can alter body metabolism as well as fluid and electrolyte homeostasis. Fever is known to change the disposition of several drugs. Finally, diseases of any organ will affect the response of the organ to a drug. If the organ is the target of drug therapy, therapeutic failure may occur owing to changes in receptors, intracellular messengers, or subcellular physiology. Alternatively, diseased organs are not as capable of repair after drug-induced toxic effects as are healthy organs. A final consideration to be made regarding disease-induced changes in drug disposition is the effects of successful therapy. As the pathologic effects of disease are reversed, disposition is apt to change again, which may predispose the patient to adverse drug reactions.

TYPE B ADVERSE REACTIONS

In contrast to type A reactions, type B reactions are bizarre reactions that are unrelated to the dose or the normal pharmacologic effect of the drug. Because they are unpredictable, occurring in a very small percentage of the population, they are hard to avoid. Type B reactions have been attributed to genetic or idiosyncratic reactions or drug hypersensitivities (allergic reactions). Some species reactions that reflect differences in receptor sensitivity may be considered type B. For example, cattle, and particularly Brahman, are more sensitive to the depressant effects of xylazine; sheep tend to react adversely to haloxon. Cattle react to morphine by exhibiting excitation rather than depression.

The most common type B adverse reactions probably result from drug hypersensitivity. The incidence of drug hypersensitivities is not great. Most drugs are too small to induce an immune response. Rather they (or their metabolites) must covalently bond with a larger endogenous macromolecule in order to induce an allergic response. The drug molecule is referred to as a "hapten" (as opposed to antigen), and the allergic reaction can be manifested against the drug, the macromolecule, or both. Drugs can cause any type of immune-mediated response (i.e., types 1 through 4), and any component of a drug preparation can cause the allergic reaction. For example, carriers and solubilizers may result in sudden release or activation of autacoids such as histamine, serotonin, kinins, prostaglandins, leukotrienes, and platelet-activating factors. Signs indicative of an anaphylactic response may occur. Microbiologic (contaminating) products may also stimulate an immune reaction. Cross-reactivity between closely related compounds (e.g., β-lactam antibiotics such as penicillins and cephalosporins, or any of the chemically related sulfonamides, including furosemide) may result in a similar response.

Drug allergies are characterized by the following conditions: (1) previous exposure to the drug must have occurred; (2) the reaction will recur every time the drug and, in some cases, similar drugs are administered; (3) the reaction is not correlated to the amount of drug administered; and (4) the response will recur regardless of the dose.

AVOIDANCE OF ADVERSE DRUG REACTIONS

The incidence of type A adverse drug reactions can be decreased by (1) limiting one's clinic pharmacy to selected, representative drugs; (2) becoming familiar with these drugs, particularly their therapeutic indications, disposition, interactions with other drugs, and adverse effects associated with their use; (3) being informed of the clinical status of the patient, particularly any species-, age-, and disease-related factors that may predispose the patient to adverse reactions; (4) collecting appropriate baseline data before initiating drug therapy, with emphasis on organs of drug elimination and organs that are targets for drug-induced toxic effects; (5) altering the dosing regimen (dose or interval) if indicated, based on clinical assessment, clinical laboratory tests, or therapeutic drug monitoring; (6) selecting the least toxic drug; (7) avoiding concurrent administration of drugs in order to reduce the incidence of drug interactions; (8) alternating the times at which multiple drugs are administered; (9) following the recommended dosing regimen for each species without modifying the drug preparations; and (10) monitoring the patient for response and discontinuing the drug if it is indicated by therapeutic success, failure, or toxic effect.

Clinical signs, biochemical monitoring, and therapeutic drug monitoring are important tools that can be used to guide drug therapy in the patient predisposed to drug-induced toxic effects. However, signs due to drug toxicity can be difficult to discern from signs due to the patient's illness. Whereas biochemical tests are more specific, some drugs induce changes in tests that are not necessarily indicative of drug-induced organ disease. Practitioners must be informed regarding the potential of a drug to alter tests before an assumption of drug toxicity is made. Therapeutic drug monitoring is the most specific means of guiding drug therapy. It is particularly applicable to therapy with selected antimicrobials (i.e., aminoglycosides), antiarrhythmics, and anticonvulsants. Measurement of plasma drug concentrations is important for drugs that are toxic, when therapeutic success is critical (i.e., when an organ or life is threatened), or when therapeutic response is difficult to assess (i.e., antimicrobials). Several laboratories throughout the United States offer therapeutic drug monitoring services. Clinical pharmacology consultation is offered at these and other locations to support efforts of practitioners in reducing the incidence of adverse drug reactions.

BIBLIOGRAPHY

Baggott J: Principles of Drug Disposition in Domestic Animals: The Basis of Veterinary Clinical Pharmacology. Philadelphia, WB Saunders, 1979, pp 73–112.

Brater DC, Chennavasin P: Effects of renal disease: altered pharmacokinetics. In Benet LZ, Massoud N, Grunbertoglio JU (eds): Pharmacokinetic Basis for Drug Treatment. New York, Raven Press, 1985, pp 149–172.

Green TP, Mirkin BL: Clinical Pharmacokinetics: Pediatric Considerations. Philadelphia, Lea and Febiger, 1976, pp 269–282.

Massoud N: Pharmacokinetic Considerations in Geriatric Patients. Philadelphia, Lea and Febiger, 1976, pp 283–310.

Pond SM: Pharmacokinetic drug interactions. In Benet LZ, Massoud N, Grunbertoglio JU (eds): Pharmacokinetic Basis for Drug Treatment. New York, Raven Press, 1985, pp 195–220.

Riviere JE: Veterinary clinical pharmacokinetics. Part I. Fundamental concepts. Compend Contin Educ Sm Anim Pract 10:24–30, 1988.

Wilkinson GR, Branch RA: Effects of hepatic disease on clinical pharmacokinetics. In Benet LZ, Massoud N, Grunbertoglio JU (eds): Pharmacokinetic Basis for Drug Treatment. New York, Raven Press, 1985, pp 49–62.

Diagnostic Ultrasonography
DAVID SCHMITZ, DVM, MS

GENERAL PRINCIPLES

Diagnostic ultrasonography is becoming established as the preferred and accepted means of evaluating soft tissues in all animal species. The tremendous use and application of this technology in recent years has largely resulted from the facts that this diagnostic modality is noninvasive and, as far as is currently known, does not induce or cause any biologic change in the imaged tissues. There is no known biologic hazard resulting from the use of diagnostic ultrasonography in domestic animals, nor is there any apparent hazard to the operator of sonographic equipment when the equipment is used in an appropriate manner. Other advantages of this technology are that size, shape, location, and consistency of soft tissues can be evaluated and changes in these parameters can be monitored over time. Also, function can be evaluated to a limited degree—for example, evaluation of the heart or some other moving structure in an awake animal.

For understanding the image that is generated by an ultrasound transducer, certain basic facts and principles must be kept in mind. First, air and bone act as very strong reflectors of the ultrasonographic beam. As a result of this, the sound wave does not "penetrate" beyond the air or bone surface, and therefore nothing beyond the interface can be imaged. Air and bone can be thought of as "stopping" the ultrasonographic beam. This principle applies to all mineralized tissue as well; thus certain types of pathologic processes, such as dystrophic mineralization within tissues or mineralized nephroliths or hepatoliths, can cause a very bright reflection and result in acoustic shadowing beyond the interface. An air interface likewise serves as a very strong reflector, and nothing can be visualized beyond the air interface. This principle comes into play when tissues that normally contain air (i.e., lung and portions of the intestinal tract) are examined. The air interface makes it impossible to visualize tissue deep to the interface. When air is present in an abnormal location within the body, this same principle applies and allows the sonographer to identify the bright reflection as a possible air interface.

Fat causes attenuation of the ultrasound beam and makes imaging tissues in an obese animal difficult. The presence of fat around any tissue results in poor resolution of the tissue and gives a generalized "hazy" appearance to the sonographic image. A higher-power setting on the ultrasound machine is required to scan an obese animal adequately, compared with a thin animal, and the sound wave will not penetrate as deep into tissue in an obese animal.

The white specks that cumulatively make up an ultrasonographic image are the result of the sound wave's passing through cells or tissues with different physical properties and characteristics. Because of this, every tissue has a sonographic appearance that is generally characteristic for that tissue. When sound passes through tissue that is homogeneous, however, no reflective "specks" are generated. This results in a black or anechoic area on the sonogram. This is most evident when sound passes through a fluid medium such as blood, serum, peritoneal or pleural fluid, and the like. Although an anechoic area is not pathognomonic for fluid, no other normal tissue has an anechoic appearance. As the particulate matter in a fluid medium increases, however, the sonographic appearance of the fluid may become more echogenic. This occurs if the particles suspended in the fluid are large enough to generate an echo rather than just scatter the sound wave.

Most tissues have an echo pattern that is somewhere between the anechoic appearance of fluid and the extremely echogenic appearance of bone or air. Organs that have a greater amount of fibrous connective tissue stroma typically demonstrate an increased echogenicity or brightness. In most animals, bone and air are most echogenic, followed in decreasing order by fibrous tissue, spleen, liver, kidney, and fluid or very homogeneous tissue.

The ability to evaluate a desired soft tissue structure adequately is also dependent on the frequency of the sound wave. General rules of thumb to be remembered are that the lower the frequency of the sound wave, the greater the depth of penetration into tissue but the poorer the resolution of the image. Conversely, a high-frequency sound wave allows very good resolution of a desired tissue, but high-frequency sound waves are rapidly attenuated by tissue and therefore do not penetrate very deep into tissue. For these reasons, a low-frequency transducer must be used to evaluate deeper structures within the body, whereas a high-frequency transducer is used to evaluate those structures for which good resolution is required and where the transducer can be placed very close to the desired tissue.

Most conventional ultrasound transducers are manufactured so that the sound wave is focused at a certain distance beyond the end of the transducer. For some distance on either side of this "focal point," the sound wave is relatively focused in a "focal zone." It is within this focal zone that imaged tissues have their greatest resolution. For most transducers, particularly sector transducers, this focal zone is established at manufacture for each transducer, and it is not something the operator can change. As a result, one must choose the appropriate frequency transducer with a suitable focal zone to obtain the optimal sonographic image of a desired tissue or organ. Most manufacturers of ultrasonographic equipment make a variety of transducers that can be used with a single machine. Relatively recent changes in technology, however, have made it possible for some linear and annular array systems to have variable focusing, whereby the focal zone can be selectively placed anywhere in the image's depth. This variable focusing technology is optional and is available only on certain models of ultrasonographic equipment.

Another aspect of sonographic imaging that is fundamental in understanding and interpreting the sonogram is knowing that the ultrasonographic image is a two-dimensional representation of a three-dimensional object. The operator must think in terms of the spatial relationship between the desired tissue and adjacent structures. One must become familiar with

Table 1. SCANNING LOCATIONS AND TECHNIQUES FOR VARIOUS ORGANS AND STRUCTURES

Organ	Location	Depth	Frequency (in MHz)
Heart	R 3–4 ICS in axillary space	10–30 cm	2.5–3.0
	L 3–4 ICS in axillary space	10–30 cm	2.5–3.0
Liver	R 8–12 ICS at level of shoulder joint and below	5–15 cm	3.0–5.0
Gallbladder	R 9–10 ICS ventral to costal arch	5–15 cm	2.5–5.0
Kidney	R kidney: 11–12 ICS below transverse vertebral processes	10–20 cm	2.5–5.0
	L kidney: caudal to R kidney in R flank		
Uterus, ovaries, cervix, rectum		2–10 cm	5.0–7.5
Testes, scrotal contents		1–15 cm	5.0–7.5
Penis		2–5 cm	5.0–7.5
Udder		1–20 cm	5.0–7.5
Teats		1–5 cm	5.0–7.5
Lymph nodes		1–10 cm	5.0–7.5
Subcutaneous veins		1–5 cm	7.5
Retrobulbar space		5–10 cm	5.0–7.5
Umbilical structures		2–15 cm	5.0–7.5
Back fat thickness and rib eye area		5–20 cm	2.5–3.0

ICS = intercostal space; MHz = megahertz; R = right; L = left.

the cross-sectional anatomy of the species being scanned in order to adequately interpret the sonographic image.

EQUIPMENT REQUIRED

Two types of ultrasound machines are available for use on domestic animals. Linear array machines have the advantages of being less expensive and having fewer moving parts, which makes them somewhat more durable. They allow good tissue resolution in all fields, including the tissue in the field of view immediately adjacent to the transducer. Their major disadvantage is that they generally require a relatively large contact area on the animal's skin, which makes them less desirable for scanning tissue in the intercostal spaces or in other areas in which a small contact surface is necessary.

Mechanical sector scanners have the major advantage of providing a very small contact surface, which makes them ideal for scanning most areas of the body. There are also certain technical advantages that the sector scanners possess, but both types of machines can be used to obtain diagnostic images of many body parts and organs. Both types of machines are also available in portable units that can be readily taken to the animal.

Some means of preserving the generated image should be employed, because this examination ought to be included in the animal's medical record. Images can be preserved by various means including Polaroid cameras, heat-sensitive thermal paper printers, video cassette recorders (VCR), and formatting cameras that transfer the image onto x-ray film. Which of these recording devices will be used depends on the type of examination being performed and the expense and usefulness of each recording device in any given situation.

THE EXAMINATION PROCEDURE

Minimal preparation of the animal is necessary to perform transcutaneous ultrasonography. Many times, little or no tranquilization is required, but the patient must be adequately restrained. Because air "stops" the propagation of the sound wave, all air must be removed from the space between the transducer and the skin. This is accomplished by thoroughly wetting the skin in the desired area with copious amounts of coupling gel, mineral oil, or, in some cases, water and scan gel. Clipping the hair and thoroughly cleansing the exposed skin to remove dirt, oil, and debris before applying coupling gel will result in the best possible image. However, when clipping the hair is not possible or is undesirable, copious amounts of coupling gel or other suitable material may allow an adequate image to be obtained.

When a transrectal examination is being performed, every effort should be made to remove all air and feces from the rectum before the examination is begun. A couplant should be used in this examination also. Suitable materials would include mineral oil, obstetric lubricants, and water-soluble jellies.

Once the desired organ or tissue to be scanned has been identified, the examination is not complete until the tissue has been examined in its entirety. This necessitates examining the area in more than one plane and also in as many intercostal spaces and as far dorsally and ventrally in each intercostal space as is necessary to define the limits of the tissue fully. In some instances, it may be necessary to scan both sides of the animal in order to complete a thorough examination. Table 1 gives the approximate location for initial identification of various organs in the bovine.

Examination of the Thorax

The Cardiac Examination

The heart is not as readily identified and scanned in the bovine as it is in the horse. However, for evaluation of the heart, the right third intercostal space is a good place to begin. The heart should be scanned in long-axis and short-axis (transverse) views and from the apex to the heart base. The heart should be evaluated for motion and thickness of the heart wall; motion and structure of the valves, especially the right atrioventricular (tricuspid) valve; and the size of the chambers and outflow tracts. The entire length of the interventricular septum can be examined to evaluate the integrity of this structure.

The left side of the heart can sometimes be evaluated from the right side; but in adult cattle, one must often examine the left side of the heart from the left third or fourth intercostal spaces, in the axillary space at the level of the olecranon and above. A 2.5 or 3 MHz transducer is required to obtain a satisfactory cardiac examination in most adult cattle. A 5 MHz transducer is sufficient for most animals weighing less than 400 to 500 pounds and is the transducer of choice for cardiac examinations in calves.

The pericardial space should be evaluated when a cardiac examination is performed. Normally there is little or no fluid in the pericardial space, and the pericardium is not readily distinguishable from the epicardium. However, in cases of pericarditis or pericardial effusion, the pericardial sac may be distended and separated from the epicardium by an increased distance. Depending on the cellularity of the fluid in the pericardial sac, fluid may appear anechoic or exhibit some degree of echogenicity. Echogenic fibrous tags might also be observed attached to either side of the pericardial membrane.

The pleural space is best visualized during real-time examination of the thorax. The very bright echogenic margin of normal aerated lung can be observed to glide past the chest wall while the animal breathes. Normally, a very small amount of fluid is present in the pleural space, and this is best visualized in the ventral thorax adjacent to the heart. Any increase in quantity of pleural fluid can be readily detected by examining the ventral thorax and observing the lung margin to be separated from the chest wall by an increased distance. With chronic pneumonia or pleural effusion, echogenic fibrous bands are often noted in the pleural space in addition to the fluid accumulation. Transudates within the pleural space appear anechoic, whereas more cellular fluids appear echogenic to varying degrees.

The normal lung margin appears as a very bright echogenic line adjacent to the chest wall (Fig. 1). There are concentric reverberation lines deep to this initial line, and no soft tissue mass or structure is seen in the field of view. This is important to remember because significant pulmonary disease can be present, but if aerated lung lies between the pathologic area and the chest wall, the sonogram will not detect the abnormal area. However, when pathologic lesions are in the lung periphery adjacent to the chest wall, they can readily be detected by the ultrasonographic beam. To be complete, the entire pulmonary area on both sides of the animal should be evaluated during the course of the examination.

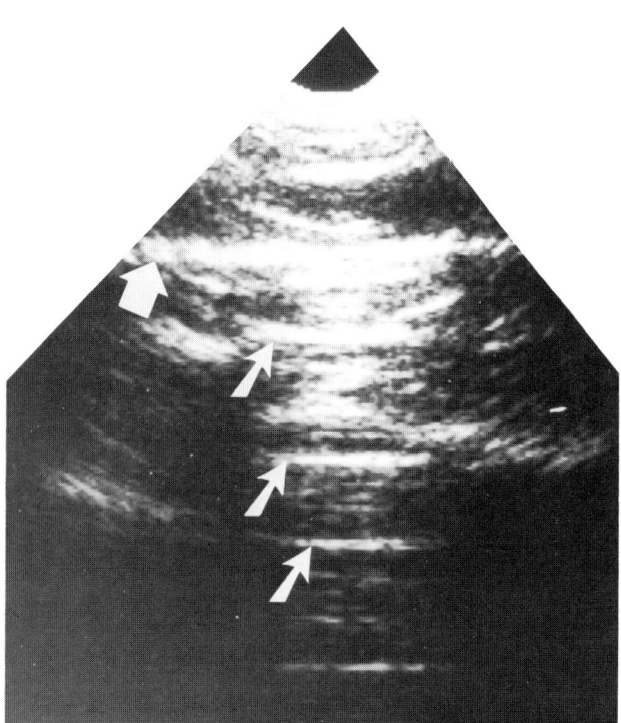

Figure 1. Ultrasonographic appearance of normal, aerated lung. Note the very echogenic lung surface (*large arrow*) and the concentric reverberation artifacts (*small arrows*).

Abdominal Examination

The presence of ascites is best determined by evaluating the right abdomen in the seventh to ninth intercostal spaces on the right side at about the level of the mid to lower third of the abdomen. Any excess peritoneal fluid is usually seen as an anechoic rim adjacent to the liver or other abdominal structure. Pure transudates have an anechoic appearance, whereas cellular fluids usually exhibit some degree of echogenicity.

The ruminoreticular area is best evaluated on the ventral abdomen, parasternally in the last few intercostal spaces and as far caudally as the xiphoid. The rumen normally lies adjacent to the ventral body wall, and ruminal contractions can be observed during real-time examination. Any suspected abnormal "mass" observed in the space between the rumen and reticulum must be differentiated from intraperitoneal adipose tissue. Ultrasonographic examination of this area can be useful in identifying abnormalities as well as in obtaining aspirates or biopsy specimens of suspicious lesions.

The liver is examined in the right eighth through twelfth intercostal spaces. The liver can be identified just ventral to the lung margin in these intercostal spaces, and the intrahepatic portal and hepatic veins are readily visualized. The caudal vena cava and the portal vein can often be seen on the medial border of the liver. The sonographic examination of the liver can be useful in determining changes in size, shape, location, and consistency of the liver parenchyma from normal. This information is not readily determined by other means excluding laparotomy. The gallbladder is usually visualized in the ninth or tenth intercostal spaces on the right side near the level of the costal arch. It is found on the medial, ventral border of the liver, has well-defined echogenic walls, varies in size, and has an oval to elliptical shape. The normal gallbladder should have a relatively echo-free lumen, but stones or sludge can cause acoustic shadowing.

The right kidney is readily evaluated transcutaneously in the right eleventh and twelfth intercostal spaces ventral to the transverse spinous processes. It is occasionally also seen at this level in the paralumbar fossa. The left kidney is not readily found on the left side but sometimes is seen caudal to the right kidney in the right flank. The kidney can also be scanned transrectally in appropriate situations. Bovine kidneys appear sonographically as lobulated structures with varying degrees of echo intensity. The cortical area is echogenic relative to the medulla, and a well-defined separation of these two regions is normally found. The renal pelvis has a very bright echogenic appearance owing to the presence of intrarenal fat. The kidney should always be examined in its entirety in two planes at right angles to each other. An attempt should be made to identify the renal artery and vein and the ureter. Renal diseases that generate abnormal scans include intrarenal cysts, pyelonephritis, nephroliths, hydronephrosis, and renal fibrosis.

The urinary bladder is best visualized via a transrectal approach. In order to thoroughly evaluate the bladder for patency or to examine the bladder wall, the lumen may be distended with fluid, or the animal may be examined when the bladder is full. Normal urine appears anechoic, but cellular debris and mucous within the bladder causes some degree of echo generation. In neonates, the bladder can be evaluated in the caudal ventral abdomen just cranial to the pelvis.

Reproductive System

For examination of the reproductive tract in the female, a 5 MHz transducer is employed with use of a transrectal approach. The ovaries, uterus, and cervix are readily identified, and abnormalities involving these structures can be detected if the abnormality causes morphologic change in the structure. Any of these organs or structures can be evaluated for change from normal in size, shape, or consistency.

The greatest use of diagnostic ultrasonography in females has been in early detection of pregnancy. For information concerning early pregnancy diagnosis, the reader is referred to other sources that cover this topic in detail. Diseases of the ovaries that can be diagnosed sonographically include ovarian cysts, tumors, and persistent corpora lutea. The uterus is readily evaluated for the presence of a fetus or some abnormal condition such as hydrometra or pyometra. With patience and some degree of acquired skill, one can also determine the sex of the fetus when the examination is performed around 75 days' gestation.

In the male, diagnostic ultrasonography is useful in evaluating the scrotum and its contents, the spermatic cords, and the penis. It also has application in evaluating the intrapelvic accessory sex glands.

Diagnostic ultrasonography is useful in evaluating the testes for change in size, shape, or consistency. When an abnormality is detected sonographically, it may be possible to obtain an aspirate or a biopsy specimen of the suspicious lesion while the organ is scanned. The scrotal contents can also be evaluated if enlargement or abnormal findings are discovered on physical examination. The presence of fluid or blood can be ascertained, as well as the presence of other abnormal contents such as portions of the intestinal tract (i.e., scrotal hernia). The epididymal structures can be examined, and the spermatic cords can be evaluated for change in size, shape, and position. The intrapelvic penis can be scanned transrectally, and the external penis can be examined beginning just cranioventral to the pelvis and continuing toward the glans penis.

SPECIAL EXAMINATIONS

Diagnostic ultrasonography can potentially be utilized in any situation in which soft tissue evaluation is desired. Some areas in which ultrasonography is just beginning to find application are in the examination of the udder and teats; examination of enlarged lymph nodes and various lumps and bumps; determination of the patency of large veins such as the jugular vein and subcutaneous milk vein; evaluation of the retrobulbar space; identification of the contents of umbilical swellings in calves; and as an aid in obtaining biopsy specimens of a suspected lesion. Diagnostic ultrasonography has also been used in carcass evaluation for measuring the amount of back fat present in market weight cattle and hogs and in determining the size of the rib eye muscle in live cattle. With so many potential applications for this diagnostic modality, the use of diagnostic ultrasonography in the future will increase dramatically.

BIBLIOGRAPHY

Baxter GM: Umbilical masses in calves: diagnosis, treatment, and complications. Compend Contin Educ Pract Vet 11:505–527, 1989.
Braun U: Ultrasonographic examination of the liver in cows. Am J Vet Res 51:1522–1526, 1990.
Cartee RE, Ibrahim AK, McLeary D: B-mode ultrasonography of the bovine udder and teat. J Am Vet Med Assoc 188:1284–1287, 1986.
Curran S, Pierson RA, Ginther OJ: Ultrasonographic appearance of the bovine conceptus from days 10 through 20. J Am Vet Med Assoc 189:1289–1294, 1986.
Curran S, Pierson RA, Ginther OJ: Ultrasonographic appearance of the bovine conceptus from days 20 through 60. J Am Vet Med Assoc 189:1295–1302, 1986.
Miles KG: Basic principles and clinical applications of diagnostic ultrasonography. Compend Contin Educ Pract Vet 11:609–624, 1989.
Yamaga Y, Too K: Diagnostic ultrasound imaging in domestic animals: fundamental studies on abdominal organs and fetuses. Jpn J Vet Sci 46:203–212, 1984.
Yamaga Y, Too K: Echocardiographic detection of bovine cardiac diseases. Jpn J Vet Res 34:251–267, 1986.
Yamaga Y, Too K: Diagnostic ultrasound imaging of vegetative valvular endocarditis in cattle. Jpn J Vet Res 35:49–63, 1987.

Residues in Food Animals:
Regulatory and Veterinary Responsibility

JANICE WEBB, DVM
JOSEPH C. PAIGE, DVM, MPH

Concerns over the adulterants found in our food supply have steadily increased during the 20th century. Pesticides, environmental contaminants, animal drug residues, compounds that leach from food packaging materials, and a myriad of other compounds are perceived by the public as unacceptable. Average consumers do not routinely consider factors such as concentration, tolerance, acceptable daily intake, assessed risk to health, hazard, exposure, and carcinogenicity. Drug residues in meat and poultry have not escaped the critical eyes of those who maintain vigilance over the safety of food. As a logical consequence, the veterinarian's role in ensuring accurate drug use, dose, withdrawal time before slaughter, and appropriate extra-label usage has received attention nationally and internationally.

Drugs and chemicals are essential to the efficient production of animals intended for food in the United States. They are used to treat animals for disease and to promote growth. Animals may be treated with drugs by injection, by implant, or orally in the form of boluses, pastes, premixes in feed or water, or drenching. Because of widespread use, it is a continuing concern of consumers that various drugs, chemicals, pesticides, therapeutic agents, and environmental contaminants will result in above-tolerance or illegal residues in the food supply.

Government regulations concerning veterinary drugs as presented by Baldwin[1] and drug surveillance information, drug usage patterns, and drug development presented by Mercer[2] provide excellent background material for this chapter. The objectives of this article are to provide (1) information on the regulatory agencies that are responsible for identifying and controlling drug and agricultural chemical residues in food animals; (2) references to the veterinary practitioner regarding regulatory requirements for approved drugs, including withdrawal times and extra-label use; (3) information on specific residues of concern, including problem areas by drugs and specific slaughter class; (4) veterinary ethics as a mechanism for affecting residue control; (5) a list of reference sources; and (6) agency contacts for answers to questions. In addition, a glossary of commonly used terms is provided.

HISTORICAL PERSPECTIVE

Responsible Agencies for Residue Control

Two books, the 1906 publication of Upton Sinclair's *The Jungle* and the 1962 publication of Rachael Carson's *Silent*

Spring, contributed significantly to the public's awareness of the need for measures that would help ensure the safety of meat and poultry in the United States. Regulatory authority was vested in three agencies within the federal government: the Environmental Protection Agency (EPA), the Food and Drug Administration (FDA) within the Department of Health and Human Services (HHS), and the Food Safety and Inspection Service (FSIS) within the United States Department of Agriculture (USDA). All three agencies work together in their various areas of expertise to help ensure an integrated approach to residue problems. In addition, residue control efforts are increasing at the state government level.

EPA Responsibility in Residue Identification and Control

The EPA is responsible for safety and efficacy evaluations and for establishing tolerances for pesticides. Legal authority comes from the Federal Insecticide, Fungicide, and Rodenticide Act (FIFRA) and also from several provisions of the Federal Food, Drug, and Cosmetic Act (FFDCA). EPA is notified by the FDA or the FSIS when pesticide residue violations occur. If pesticide violations occur as the result of failure to adhere to the label directions, EPA has authority to take regulatory action against the misuser of the compound. When a residue violation is present in a product as a result of actions other than misuse, FDA has legal authority to protect the consumer.

FDA Responsibility in Residue Identification and Control

FDA, through the Center for Veterinary Medicine (CVM), is responsible for ensuring that animal drugs are safe and effective for their intended use and that food from treated animals is safe for human consumption.

Hormones, antibiotics, and other chemical compounds for use in food-producing animals are "new animal drugs" within the meaning of the FFDCA. Whether something is a "new animal drug" is dependent on a *lack* of general recognition of safety and efficacy for the labeled conditions of use. For an expert to determine if something can be recognized as safe and effective, there must be published adequate and well-controlled studies demonstrating the safety and efficacy of the product under those labeled conditions.

The marketing of new animal drugs is controlled by the FFDCA. Premarket approval of "new animal drugs" and animal feeds containing "new animal drugs" (medicated feeds) is required. A major purpose in the requirement for premarket approval is to establish a proper use of the product that will result in either no residues in edible animal products or residues at a safe level for humans consuming this food. Therefore, for all new animal drugs approved by the agency for use in food-producing animals, the law requires, among other things, (1) a description of practicable methods for determining the quantity, if any, of the drug in or on food and (2) the proposed tolerance or withdrawal period or other use restrictions for the drug if tolerance, withdrawal period, or use restrictions are required in order to ensure that the proposed use of the drug will be safe.

Tolerances for residues of new animal drugs in food are specified in the Code of Federal Regulations. The tolerances are based on residues in edible products of food-producing animals and established as part of the approval process. The tolerances include a built-in safety factor for ensuring that the drug will have no harmful effects on consumers of the food. Appropriate tolerances consider the presence of finite residues, the carcinogenicity, and the drug metabolites and are dependent on the availability of practicable methods of determining the quantity of the residue.

The approval of an animal drug is based on toxicologic and clinical and chemical data submitted by the sponsor of the drug. One of the most important factors in determining the approval of a new animal drug is an evaluation of its carcinogenicity. A carcinogenic new animal drug cannot be approved under the FFDCA if scientific tests fail to show a dietary level at which the compound poses no significant risk of human carcinogenesis or if a regulatory method is not present that can reliably measure the derived safe level. If a product is a carcinogen, it must be demonstrated to be safe within this context, and a method of monitoring must be available.

Under the FFDCA, new animal drugs are "unsafe," among other things, when there is no approved New Animal Drug Application (NADA) on file or when labeling and use of the drug do not conform to the approved application. Animal feeds bearing or containing new animal drugs may also be deemed "unsafe" when there is no approved NADA on file, when there is no approved medicated feed application on file, or when the labeling and use do not conform to the approved, published conditions and indications for use.

These "unsafe" new animal drugs, medicated feeds, and edible animal products such as meat, milk, or eggs are considered adulterated under the FFDCA. The drugs and individuals responsible for causing the adulteration are subject to regulatory penalties. Such penalties may be seizure of the adulterated products, injunction, citation, and/or prosecution of the responsible firms and individuals.

The central focus of CVM's program on residues in meat and poultry is on public health. CVM is also concerned about the illegal distribution and misuse of veterinary drugs, the extra-label use of animal drugs, and the bulk drug issue. As a primary prevention factor, CVM encourages good husbandry practices.

The one action responsible for elevating tissue residues to the level of public health concern had its origin with FDA's regulatory action on the use of chloramphenicol in food animals (pigs and cattle). Chloramphenicol is not approved for use in food animals because it may cause aplastic anemia in sensitive people. Chloramphenicol was withdrawn from the market, and a potential public health problem was averted. However, as producers and veterinarians have moved away from using chloramphenicol, additional drugs have emerged (streptomycin, dimetridazole, gentamicin sulfate, neomycin, and others) as areas of concern.

The FDA/CVM Tissue Residue Program has both a preventive (public health) and a regulatory approach. One of the basic functions of public health is the collection and analysis of data. This approach is being utilized by FDA to understand the complexity and frequency of occurrence of residues and identify areas in which preventive strategies can be applied.

It is inconceivable that an effective Tissue Residue Reduction Program can be planned, implemented, monitored, and evaluated without a reasonable data base. Within FDA, the Tissue Residue Information Management System (TRIMS) has been developed to utilize data generated from FDA follow-up investigations. The TRIMS data will be utilized as follows:

1. To describe the frequency of occurrence and distribution of drug residues within an animal slaughter class by animal (species, slaughter class, sex, age), place (geographic distribution), and time (temporal sequence, i.e., seasonal).
2. To identify risk factors responsible for the development of residues in food animals, that is, drug carry-over, illegal drug use, improper mixing, improper withdrawal times, extra-label use, and so on.

3. To provide feedback to FDA district offices and all states under cooperative agreement with FDA for residue investigations.

4. To provide information essential to the planning, implementation, and evaluation of policies necessary for residue prevention and to establish priorities among these policies.

The regulatory function of the Tissue Residue Program is to enforce the FFDCA; these efforts are supported by FDA field operations personnel. FDA field operations are organized into 6 regions with 21 district offices throughout the United States and Puerto Rico and are managed from the commissioner's office of FDA.

When an illegal residue is detected, FSIS reports the violation to the appropriate FDA district office. The district office may then conduct an investigation. FDA investigators visit the farm or feedlot from which the animal was shipped to slaughter. They may additionally interview others who may be involved in the presentation of adulterated animals for slaughter for human food or the introduction of adulterated animals into interstate commerce, such as haulers, dealers, auction barns, slaughterhouses, and veterinarians. The investigation is aimed at determining the cause of the residue and identifying those responsible for it.

FDA will seek voluntary compliance from responsible individuals and encourage good husbandry practices for avoiding potential residues. If compliance is not forthcoming, regulatory actions as mentioned will be considered.

FSIS Responsibility in Residue Identification and Control

FSIS has responsibility for ensuring that USDA-inspected meat and poultry products are safe, wholesome, free of adulterating residues, and accurately labeled. FSIS conducts the National Residue Program (NRP) to identify, prevent, and control residue problems in food-producing animals. Legal authority for such actions is derived from the Federal Meat Inspection Act and Poultry Products Inspection Act. FSIS comprises two programs that are responsible for the NRP: Inspection Operations and Science and Technology. Inspection Operations is composed mostly of the field force of veterinarians and lay inspectors who serve as the primary "eyes and ears" of FSIS. It is these efforts toward residue awareness and control at this "grass roots" level that enhance the capability of the agency to perform most efficiently, for example, testing healthy animals (monitoring) or the suspect–obviously sick animal (surveillance).

The Residue Evaluation and Planning Division (REPD) within Science and Technology develops the National Residue Program Plan, which identifies species, slaughter class, target tissues, and compounds for which analyses are to be performed in relation to domestic animals and imported products. A yearly publication, the *Compound Evaluation and Analytical Capability National Residue Program Plan,* is produced for distribution to anyone interested in the residue program. Using the procedure set forth in *The Compound Evaluation System,* REPD evaluates old and new compounds for their ability to produce residues, toxicity, and potential use-misuse that could cause residues in meat and poultry. See Glossary that follows this article for a discussion of the contents of and the address for both publications.

The NRP contains three programs that serve to identify, control, and prevent residues in food-producing animals. Violators identified in either the Monitoring Program or the Surveillance Program will be asked to submit additional animals for residue testing. The purpose of additional animals for testing is to ensure that subsequent animals from a producer do not contain violative concentrations of drugs or other chemical compounds. Once this is accomplished, future animals submitted for slaughter will be subject to the routine inspection regulations.

MONITORING PROGRAM. The Monitoring Program is designed to test randomly selected, healthy-appearing animals (the carcass is not retained pending analysis). Results of monitoring provide information on residues in the national herd.

SURVEILLANCE PROGRAM. The Surveillance Program allows testing of animals that are retained on ante or post mortem inspection, suspected of having been treated with adulterating compounds, or that are from producers who have a history of presenting residue-adulterated animals for slaughter. FSIS inspectors may use one of several in-plant rapid screen tests for aid in the determination of the adulteration status of an animal (Table 1). Presumptive positive carcasses are retained, pending laboratory confirmation. The Swab Test on Premises (STOP) detects antibiotic residues and was developed primarily for use in cows. The Calf Antibiotic and Sulfonamide Test (CAST) detects both antibiotics and sulfonamides and is used only on bob veal calves. In response to the laboratory detection of sulfonamides in cull dairy cows, FSIS is currently developing an in-plant test, the Fast Antibiotic Screen Test (FAST), which can detect sulfonamides and can be used for all slaughter classes of cattle. The STOP, CAST, and FAST are microbial inhibition tests. The Sulfa-on-Site (SOS) is a thin-layer chromatography test that detects only sulfonamides in swine.

Producers and veterinarians can use a variety of tests before marketing animals. Table 2 contains a list of some of the widely used tests.[3] A more in-depth list of tests and manufacturers can be found in Veterinary Science Information published by the Cooperative Extension Service, Pennsylvania State University.[4] For in-depth discussion of regulatory and producer-veterinary–oriented tests, see the article by McKean on tools available for residue testing.[5] Neither FSIS nor FDA guarantees these tests; thus any false-negative screening test may subject users to regulatory action.

EXPLORATORY PROGRAMS. The third program in the NRP is generally reserved for compounds of special interest that have no established tolerance.

Laboratory Capabilities

Specimens requiring qualification or quantification of compounds are sent to one of three Technical Support Laboratories

Table 1. FSIS TESTS USED IN SLAUGHTER ESTABLISHMENTS FOR DETECTION OF ANTIMICROBIAL RESIDUES IN MEAT AND POULTRY

Test Name	Acronym	Type of Test	Species or Slaughter Class	Detects Antibiotics/Sulfonamides
Swab Test on Premises	STOP	Microbial zone of inhibition	Bovine (primarily cull cows), hogs, turkeys, chickens	Yes/No
Calf Antibiotic and Sulfonamide Test	CAST	Microbial zone of inhibition	Bob veal	Yes/Yes
Sulfa-On-Site	SOS	Thin-layer chromatography	Swine	No/Yes

Table 2. SPECIFIC SCREENING TESTS FOR ANTIBIOTIC RESIDUES[1]

Environmental Diagnostics, Inc.
P.O. Box 908
2990 Anthony Road
Burlington, NC 27215
800-334-1116

Tests Available	Detection Limit	Test Matrix	Approximate Price/Test	Time to Perform	Equipment Needed
Chloramphenicol	5 ppb	Urine, milk, feed, tissue	$ 7.50	15 min	None
Gentamicin	50 ppb	Same as above	$12.00	15 min	None
Sulfamethazine	10 ppb	Same as above	$ 7.50	15 min	None
Sulfadimethoxine	10 ppb	Same as above	$ 7.50	15 min	None
Tylosin	50 ppb	Same as above	$12.50	15 min	None
Sulfonamides:					
Sulfa-on-Site test	100–400 ppb	Swine urine	$ 1.50	30 min	Ultraviolet TLC reader

Idetek, Inc.
1057 Sneath Lane
San Bruno, CA 94066
800-433-8351

Tests Available	Detection Limit	Test Matrix	Approximate Price/Test	Time to Perform	Equipment Needed
β-lactam family	5–10 ppb	Urine, serum, milk	$ 1.40	30 min	Spectrophotometer
Gentamicin	15 ppb	Same as above	$ 3.25	30 min	None
Sulfamethazine	10 ppb	Same as above	$ 3.25	30 min	None

Idexx Corporation
100 Fore Street
Portland, ME 04101
800-548-6733

Tests Available	Detection Limit	Test Matrix	Approximate Price/Test	Time to Perform	Equipment Needed
β-lactam family	5–10 ppb	Milk	$ 2.20	15 min	None
Gentamicin	30 ppb	Milk	$ 3.20	5 min	None
Sulfa trio:					
Sulfamethazine	10 ppb	Milk	$ 3.20	15 min	None
Sulfathiazole					
Sulfadimethoxine					
Tetracycline	20–40 ppb	Milk	$ 3.20	5 min	None

Neogen Corporation
620 Lesher Place
Lansing, MI 48912–1509
517-372-9200

Tests Available	Detection Limit	Test Matrix	Approximate Price/Test	Time to Perform	Equipment Needed
Sulfamethazine	10 ppb	Milk	$ 3.50	30 min	Neogen reader
	100–400 ppb	Serum			
	1 ppb	Feed			

SmithKline Animal Health Products
1600 Paoli Pike
P.O. Box 2650
West Chester, PA 19380
800-877-7303

Tests Available	Detection Limit	Test Matrix	Approximate Price/Test	Time to Perform	Equipment Needed
Sulfamethazine	10 ppb	Urine, serum, milk, tissue	$ 2.50	30 min	None
Gentamicin	10 ppb	Same as above	$ 3.30	30 min	None
Neomycin	10 ppb	Same as above	$ 3.30	30 min	None

Some Precautions on These Rapid Tests
1. Most tests require refrigeration and must be brought to room temperature before use.
2. Each test has a limited shelf life; *be sure to check expiration dates.*
3. Most tests come in "kits," usually containing 50 to 100 tests/kit. Therefore prices quoted can be misleading. Call the manufacturer to find out minimum purchases.
4. These tests are only for screening purposes. Confirmation of the presence of antibiotics is suggested.

From Veterinary Service Information: Drug residue tests for use on milk, urine, serum, and tissues. VSE 0-3, Cooperative Extension Service, The Pennsylvania State University, University Park, Pa 16802.

located in Alameda, California; St. Louis, Missouri; or Athens, Georgia. All test results are sent to the respective Residue Officer in one of five FSIS regions and to REPD. If the specimen was determined to contain violative concentrations of residues (e.g., concentrations above the tolerance level), the appropriate Regional Residue Officer will write the producer of the animal and also notify FDA.

Additionally, violator case information is recorded in the Residue Violation Information System (RVIS), a computerized data base shared between FSIS and FDA. Its purpose is interagency communication and information on violator activities, the type and frequency of occurrence of violations, and slaughter establishment information.

First-time violators may be visited by a state representative responsible for investigating tissue residue violations, whereas a repeat violator is visited by FDA. A repeat violator is a producer who has had 2 violations (in any species) within a 12-month period.

The *Domestic Residue Data Book* is published annually by FSIS and contains the results (by species, slaughter class, and compound) of monitoring and surveillance testing from the FSIS NRP. It can be obtained from the address given for the *Compound Evaluation and Analytical Capability* (see Glossary).

SPECIFIC REGULATORY POLICIES AND PROCEDURES

Extra-Label Use

Veterinarians are afforded the extra-label use of drugs in treating food-producing animals in accordance with the CVM Compliance Policy Guide.[6] Extra-label use refers to the use of a new animal drug in a food-producing animal in a manner that is not in accordance with the drug labeling.

Under this policy, extra-label use of drugs in treating food-producing animals may therefore be considered only in special circumstances. The "exempting" criteria do not include drug use in treating food-producing animals by the layman. Lay persons cannot be expected to have sufficient knowledge and understanding concerning animal diseases, pharmacology, toxicology, drug interactions, and other scientific parameters to use drugs in treating food-producing animals in any way other than as labeled.[6]

Certain drugs may not be used in treating food-producing animals even under the cited criteria (e.g., diethylstilbestrol, dimetridazole, ipronidazole, and chloramphenicol). Extra-label uses of drugs in treating food-producing animals for improving rate of weight gain, feed efficiency, or other production purposes or for routine disease prevention are inappropriate, as is use for therapeutic purposes other than under the circumstances described. Also, the criteria cited do not sanction the sale and use, for any purpose, of new animal drugs that are not approved, such as diethylstilbestrol (DES). Furthermore, a drug (including a bulk drug) may not be mixed into feed for any use or at a potency level not specifically permitted by the regulations, even if it is prescribed or ordered by a veterinarian.[6]

The criteria for extra-label drug use in animals require strict adherence.[6]

1. A careful medical diagnosis is made by an attending veterinarian within the context of a valid veterinarian-client-patient relationship.
2. A determination is made that (a) there is no marketed drug specifically labeled for treatment of the condition diagnosed or (b) drug therapy at the dosage recommended by the labeling has been found clinically ineffective in the animals to be treated.
3. Procedures are instituted to ensure that identity of the treated animals is carefully maintained.
4. A significantly extended time period is assigned for drug withdrawal before marketing meat, milk, or eggs; steps are taken to ensure that the assigned timeframes are met, and no illegal residues occur.

The use of new animal drugs in treating food-producing animals in any manner other than in accordance with the approved labeling causes the drugs to be adulterated under the FFDCA and may cause edible tissues to be adulterated. FDA will consider regulatory action when use contrary to the extra-label policy is found, whether by a veterinarian, producer, or other person, or when a violative residue occurs. Regulatory action will also be considered against distributors and others who might cause the adulteration.

Additional information regarding the CVM Compliance Policy Guide for extra-label drug use can be obtained from the Office of the Director, FDA, Center for Veterinary Medicine, 7500 Standish Place, HEV–1, Rockville, MD 20855, (301) 295–8740.

Withdrawal Times and Tolerances

In addition to the basic scientific studies for drug approval, FDA requirements for drugs used in food animals include drug residue studies in target animals, metabolism studies, and toxicity studies for determination of safe levels of residues. The development of drug residue data is a very costly step in the drug approval process for food animals. The establishment of proper withdrawal times and setting of tolerances are important aspects of the approval process.

The withdrawal time is the time before marketing for slaughter during which the drug is not used in the animal. This allows the animal to deplete the drug in its system to a below-tolerance concentration (this concept also involves depletion from milk and eggs). This period is intended to ensure that edible tissue does not contain a harmful concentration of the compound. Because the withdrawal period is based on residue studies, drug residues in excess of tolerances should not be present in animal tissues if the drug is used in accordance with label instructions. Table 3 contains a list of drugs that have been associated with residues along with their withdrawal times and dosage form. Additional drugs that cause a significant number of residue violations are gentamicin and neomycin.[7] If further information is needed, contact FDA, CVM Industry Information Staff, HFV–12, 5600 Fishers Lane, Rockville, MD 20857.

Tolerances represent the maximal level of the active principle of a specific drug or a metabolite that can be permitted in the tissue of an animal. The tolerances are intended to ensure that residual drugs will have no harmful effects if they are ingested. The following drugs are currently of concern to CVM as posing enough risk to require FDA investigators to perform on-site investigations of initial violations: (1) banned or unapproved drugs such as diethylstibestrol, dimetridazole, ipronidazole, and chloramphenicol; and (2) drugs considered

Table 3. DRUG* WITHDRAWAL TIMES FOR FOOD ANIMALS

Species	Preslaughter Withdrawal Time in Days	Dosage Form
Swine		
Procaine penicillin G	6–7	Injectable
Sulfamethazine	15	Injectable
Sulfathiazole	10	Injectable
Chlortetracycline	1–5	Oral
Carbadox	70	Feed
Beef Cattle		
Procaine penicillin G and dihydrostreptomycin sulfate	30	Injectable
	15–28	Injectable
Oxytetracycline	18	Oral
Tetracycline (boluses)	12	Oral
Sulfamethazine	10	Oral
Streptomycin	2	Oral
Dairy Cattle (Nonlactating)		
Oxytetracycline	15–28	Injectable
Sulfamethazine	10	Injectable
Sulfamethazine (Rx)	16–28	Oral

*These drugs have been identified as frequently causing residue violations.

a toxicologic risk to human and animal safety, such as carbadox, fenbendazole, thiabendazole, ivermectin, penicillin, and sulfamethazine. Dibutyltin dilaurate is also of concern because it is considered a potential carcinogen.

How to Calculate Withdrawal Times[8]

In order to help avoid residues and in keeping with proper drug usage, the authors advise all veterinary practitioners and producers to adhere to the 10 drug use tips listed in the following.

Each withdrawal day is a full 24 hours starting with the last time an animal or bird receives the drug. Here is an example of the preslaughter withdrawal time:

A drug with a 5-day preslaughter time is withdrawn from the animals at 9 A.M. on Friday. At 9 A.M. on Saturday, the treated animals have completed their first withdrawal day. The fifth withdrawal day will end at 9 A.M. on Wednesday.

If the drug in use has a withdrawal time, it will be found on the label, the package insert, or the feed tag.

See clock chart below.*

Critical Elements for Proper Drug Usage

It has been shown by numerous FDA reports that failure to observe preslaughter withdrawal times for animal drugs is one of the major causes of violative drug residues in tissues of food animals in the United States. Failure to adhere to withdrawal periods accounted for 61 per cent (279 of 460) of the violations, and the use of unapproved drugs accounted for 10 per cent (48 of 460) of the violations. In cases in which the residue violation could be stratified according to route of administration, intramuscular injection accounted for 60 per cent of the residue violations. Oral administration accounted for 28 per cent, and intramammary infusion accounted for 9 per cent of the residue cases.[7]

Ten Drug Use Tips[8]

1. Read the label carefully; labeling directions may change.
2. Use drugs only in animal species listed on the label; drugs used in other species may cause adverse reactions or illegal residues, and possible animal deaths.
3. Use the proper dose for the species and size of animal to be treated; overdosing can cause illegal residues.
4. Calculate preslaughter drug withdrawal and milk discard times accurately; withdrawal and discard times begin with the last drug administration.
5. Use the correct route of administration; giving drugs incorrectly can lead to drug ineffectiveness, adverse reactions, illegal residues, and possible animal deaths.
6. Do not "double dose"; use of the same drug in the feed and by injection can cause illegal residues or adverse drug reactions.
7. Select needle size and injection sites carefully, if injections are necessary; misuse can lead to tissue damage, adverse drug reactions, reduced effectiveness, or illegal residues.
8. Allow proper withdrawal times for feed containing drugs; during the withdrawal time, storage bins and feeders must be completely free of medicated feed, and only drug-free feed should be used or illegal residues may result.
9. Keep accurate records of drugs used and animals dosed; poor records can be costly if drug residue violations occur.
10. Seek the advice of your veterinarian; your records will allow him or her to provide safer and more effective treatment and save you money by preventing illegal residues.

SPECIFIC RESIDUE PROBLEMS: SLAUGHTER CLASSES AND COMPOUNDS

In assessing the frequency of residue occurrence according to specific types of animals and drugs, patterns have emerged. Residues continue to occur predominantly in culled cows, veal calves, hogs, and "roaster" pigs. Sulfamethazine (SMZ) and gentamicin are antibacterials that cause regulatory concern because of the high frequency of residue violations they produce.

Culled Cows

As an annual estimate, 70 to 75 per cent of females are retained to maintain herd size. Others are culled for genetic or reproductive problems, management reasons, disease, or lameness. Culled animals have been grouped according to culling classification schemes as follows.

EMERGENCY CULLS. These include those likely to die and those with acute disease.

EXCESS TO REQUIREMENT CULLS. These are cows sold because the potential population increase by the herd exceeds the desired herd size.

FAILURE TO PERFORM CULLS. These are animals culled because of low production or failure to conceive.[9]

When animals in these groups are presented for slaughter, they represent a population with high risk for harboring drug residues because the proper withdrawal period has not been observed.

Residues in Bob and Formula-Fed Veal

The calf slaughter classes present opportunities for veterinarians and producers to dramatically affect the occurrence of residues. Calves are divided by weight and age into four groups: bob veal, formula-fed veal, non–formula-fed veal, and heavy calves (see Glossary for definition of terms). The first two categories, bob veal and formula-fed veal, are the most susceptible to stress from the environment and disease and thus are the most likely candidates for treatment with antimicrobials. Both bob veal and formula-fed veal are slaughtered at young ages: any medications administered to these animals provide enhanced residue potential because their drug clearance mechanisms may not be fully developed. Dry cow treatments that subsequently contaminate colostrum, milk from cows being treated, and milk replacers containing medication serve to adulterate bob veal, sometimes without owners even being aware that they are giving residue-causing substances to

* Friday 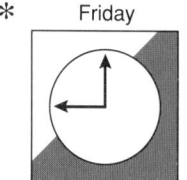 Saturday  Sunday 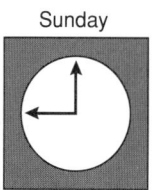 Monday 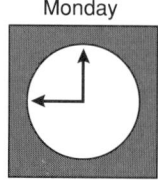 Tuesday 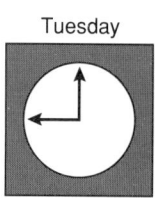 Wednesday

calves. Calves fed milk-colostrum from medicated cows account for 9 per cent (39 of 460) of the violations and represent one area in which FDA intends to focus on a prevention strategy.[7]

In non–formula-fed veal and heavy calves, the occurrence of antimicrobial residues is relatively infrequent.

Residues of zeranol have been identified in veal calves. The animals are being treated with zeranol by injection of three 12-mg pellets in the ear. The drug is not approved for use in veal calves; zeranol has a zero tolerance in the edible tissue of cattle. The presence of zeranol residues in veal calves constitutes a violation of the FFDCA.[10]

Residues in Swine

Market hogs, boars-stags, and sows slaughtered in the United States have historically been plagued with residues. The FSIS monitoring data before 1978 indicated that up to 13 per cent of slaughtered hogs had violative residues of sulfonamides in liver. Most were SMZ.[11] Monitoring data after 1978 indicate an oscillation of the percentage of sulfonamide residues. In 1989, sulfonamide residues detected were 1 per cent in market hogs, 3.6 per cent in boars-stags, 1.2 per cent in sows, with an overall slaughter class violation of 1.1 per cent.[12]

This dramatic reduction in residues can be attributed to widespread publicity concerning the potential carcinogenicity of SMZ. Industry effectuated a successful response by encouraging proper withdrawal times and implementing quality assurance programs. The need to maintain a viable market for pork products provided incentive to producers, drug manufacturers, veterinarians, feed companies, and other related industries to stress the importance of sulfonamide residue prevention. Regulatory agencies also promoted efforts made toward prevention. FSIS implemented the in-plant SOS test, and FDA gave priority to follow-up investigations of sulfonamide violations found in swine. The reduction to overall 1 per cent level in market hogs is a success story.

Residues in "Roaster" Pigs

"Roaster" pigs have recently received attention by FSIS and FDA as being a subslaughter class with residues. "Roaster" pigs are defined as being 2 to 4 months of age and 40 to 125 pounds in weight. They are unusual because although they are sold as feeder pigs, they are slaughtered as "roaster" pigs. Some medications that are commonly fed to this age pig have long withdrawal times (e.g., carbadox and SMZ). Producers and veterinarians can legally medicate feeder pigs. Once they are offered for slaughter, they are no longer feeder pigs, and the withdrawal period for the drugs has not been met. Because most "roaster" pigs are slaughtered for consumption by ethnic groups (Asian Americans) and for use as whole-hog barbecue in some areas of the United States, concern has arisen for consumption of high levels of SMZ and carbadox. The concentration consumed would most likely be higher than if the edible tissues were consumed as a comminuted product (e.g., sausage).

Sulfamethazine (SMZ) in Tissues and Milk

Sulfonamides are widely used drugs in food-producing animals. FDA has reported that approximately 70 to 80 per cent of all swine marketed in the United States receive some form of sulfonamide medication, of which SMZ is the drug most often used.[13]

During 1989, FSIS conducted additional tests on specimens that were determined to be positive on in-plant STOP tests. In FSIS Technical Support Laboratories, specimens were also analyzed for chloramphenicol, tylosin, gentamicin, sulfamethazine, and sulfadimethoxine.

Approximately 90 per cent of the specimens came from cows. FSIS cannot specifically state that these cows were cull dairy cows; however, it can be stated that specimens came from slaughter establishments that slaughter primarily cull dairy cows. Although most of the carcasses were negative for sulfonamides, those that were positive contained concentrations well above tolerance. In fact, the concentrations were high enough to indicate recent and intense therapeutic treatment, as opposed to lower concentrations, which would lead one to believe inadequate withdrawal from the sulfa therapy.

CVM is concerned about possible contamination of the public's milk supply with animal drugs. Although SMZ is not approved for use in lactating dairy cattle, it was found in most milk samples collected in 1988 from local stores in 10 geographic locations within the United States. A nationwide survey of milk by FDA approximately a year later found no violative residues of any antibiotic, but trace levels of SMZ were found at a detection limit of 10 ppb.[14] Several residues were reported and confirmed at 2 to 3 ppb. To further ensure the wholesomeness and safety of the nation's milk, the FDA has to (1) implement the National Residue Milk Monitoring Program, which will regularly monitor raw milk for the presence of drug residues; this will supplement the testing carried out by the states under the National Conference of Interstate Milk Shippers (NCIMS); and (2) work through the NCIMS for adoption by the states of appropriate new procedures and analytic methods. FDA encourages the continuation of programs that educate the dairy farmer about proper drug use and residue prevention.

In addition, FDA will continue research, development, and validation of new analytic methods for detection of residues in milk.

Because of public health concern, FDA is proposing to withdraw approval of SMZ (see discussion of unsafe new animal drugs). This proposal is based on the studies at the National Center for Toxicological Research (NCTR), which found that sulfamethazine was a carcinogen in mice and rats. NCTR concluded that the drug produced tumors (follicular cell adenoma) in the thyroid gland of male and female mice at moderate to large doses.

SMZ is, therefore, no longer shown to be safe by adequate tests by all methods reasonably applicable. Often, label directions have not been followed in practice. CVM has concluded that this new evidence provides a reasonable basis from which serious questions about the ultimate safety of the drug and its residues can be raised.

Gentamicin Sulfate

Gentamicin is one of the more prevalent antibiotics used in large animal veterinary practice. It is a broad-spectrum aminoglycoside that is effective against many gram-positive and gram-negative pathogens. It is not approved for therapeutic purposes in dairy or beef cattle in the United States; thus there is no tolerance for residues of this drug in edible tissues from cattle.

Gentamicin sulfate residues showed a sharp increase in frequency of occurrence over fiscal year 1987. Intramammary infusion accounted for 9 per cent of the residue cases, all of which occurred in culled dairy cows. In addition to the administration of gentamicin to culled dairy cows by intramammary infusion, violations resulting from intramuscular injection have increased in both culled dairy cows and calves.[7]

Given the increased numbers of gentamicin residues detected in cattle, regulatory concern has increased. Gentamicin has not been approved for oral or injectable use in cattle. Regulatory letters have been sent to producers charging them as being in violation of the FFDCA because residues were found in cows offered for slaughter. FDA is currently conducting a regulatory review of gentamicin to reassess its potential to cause a threat to public health.

ETHICAL ISSUES AND STRATEGIES FOR CONTROL OF DRUG RESIDUES

The ethical issues pertaining to residues in meat and poultry are intense for veterinarians in private practice, the food animal industry, the drug companies, academia, and regulatory agencies.

They need to know about the difference between virtues, obligations, and ideals; about competing analyses of "rights" and "welfare"; about the differences between descriptive, official, administrative, and normative veterinary ethics; about how the law affects and is affected by ethical judgments; about how empirical investigations of animal mentality and behavior relate to animal welfare. [They] need to know about controversies relating to merchandizing and marketing, to the extra-label use of drugs, to farm or sport animal welfare, and to the use of animals in research.[15]

In short, veterinarians in any phase of veterinary medicine need to understand not only the ethics of their chosen veterinary arena but also the ethics of other veterinary arenas. Simplistic as it may sound, if the basic premise for *anyone* involved in the issue of residues were "I'm producing food for my family and friends," and if ethical issues were thoroughly understood and appreciated, one could anticipate a dramatic reduction in residues in food animals.

Veterinary responsibilities are prominent in each piece of the residue puzzle. Those in academia should stress the importance to all veterinary students. Those in industry, drug companies, research, and regulatory areas should make efforts to grasp the total picture. Those in private practice should take the time to educate technicians, producers, local farming organizations, feed mills and stores, and others. Perhaps it is timely here to push for an approach similar to that used by the United Kingdom. In 1987, the Code of Practice for the Safe Use of Veterinary Medicines on Farms was distributed to all farms with livestock.[16] Success of the approach is yet undetermined, but it certainly provides the beginning premise of everyone "starting off on the same foot together." We all have a role in residue prevention and control. It is the responsibility of each member of the agricultural marketing chain to use livestock drugs safely and effectively by following label directions and using products for their approved purpose. It is only through concerted efforts that the issue will be placed in proper perspective; for example, food residues receive considerable attention and publicity, but microbial contamination is the most significant risk to the public's health. Once the issue of residues is conquered, veterinarians, producers, and the consuming public will all benefit.

Multiple Strategies for Residue Control

As with most large-scale undertakings, time will be needed to accomplish the goal of residue reduction. Several prominent publications and efforts stand out.

Food Animal Residue Avoidance Databank Trade Name File, A Comprehensive Compendium of Food Animal Drugs (FARAD)[17]

This publication by Sundlof, Riviere, and Craigmill provides quick reference to product trade names by the company that markets the product and an alphabetical index of all product trade names. Active ingredients, classification, formulation, product type, approved species, withdrawal times, indications and directions for use, references, and additional information are also given for each compound.

Copies of FARAD are available at a reasonable price; it is highly recommended for any veterinarian or producer or for those interested in residues, regardless of special interests. FARAD can be purchased from Publications, Institute of Food and Agricultural Sciences, Building 644, University of Florida, Gainesville, FL 32611.

Memorandum of Understanding (MOU) Between FSIS and Industry

MOUs are prevention programs that identify critical sources of exposure, such as drugs, feed, fat, and others. They establish effective means of control, such as drug and feed inventories, protocols on drug usage, and adequate record systems. In some instances, MOUs have served as models that stimulated industry to develop its own prevention programs.

The Residue Avoidance Program

As a result of knowledge gained from tracking residue problems to their source, FSIS and the Cooperative Extension Service (ES) concluded that production losses associated with violative residues can be prevented. Therefore, in 1984, FSIS contracted with ES to produce pamphlets and other educational material on residues in food animals. This material is directed toward the producer and can be obtained from most local ES offices. It is excellent information for introducing the idea of residue control to producers.

Cooperative Residue Program

FDA-CVM is actively pursuing a Cooperative Residue Program in which USDA-FSIS, Animal and Plant Health Inspection Service (APHIS), Packers and Stockyard Administration, states, and industry can explore regulatory approaches, voluntary control programs, and other prevention strategies for preventing the marketing of products with potentially harmful drug residues.

During the late 1980s, programmatic activities by FDA-CVM included cooperative work with the states of Colorado, Washington, Arkansas, and Ohio to conduct a pilot program to consider state control of the distribution and use of veterinary drugs. These and other activities resulted in the interest of the American Association of Veterinary State Boards and the National Association of Boards of Pharmacy in the regulation of animal drug distribution and use at the state level.

Currently, CVM is experiencing tremendous cooperation among leaders in the meat and milk industries, veterinary schools, and private practitioners in initiating quality control procedures for reducing residues. This cooperation exists largely because of a desire to provide the consumer with meat, milk, and eggs that are wholesome and free of drug residues.

The current move in residue reduction is toward improved quality control in drug use and animal production. Much of this has gained momentum since the 1987 Symposium on Animal Drug Use . . . Dollars and Sense. The Symposium was sponsored by FDA-CVM, USDA-FSIS, and ES.

FDA-CVM has worked closely with the Association of Food and Drug Officials in the development and adoption of a model veterinary drug code. The intent of the code is to support the legal apparatus of the states for a more exacting enforcement of the existing laws and regulations and to serve as a template for new laws and regulations. For additional information on the Model Veterinary Drug Code, contact Association of Food and Drug Officials, P.O. Box 3425, York, PA 17402.

Other examples of commitment toward improved quality control and food safety include the following:

- The National Pork Producers Council position on swine identification and its effort toward reducing the SMZ violations in swine. For more information, contact Director of Industry Information, P.O. Box 10383, Des Moines, IA 50306.
- The National Cattlemen's Association Task Force Report on Beef Safety Assurance (1987). For more information, contact Vice President, Communications, 5420 S. Quebec Street, Englewood, CO 80155.
- The National Broiler Council's publication "Good Manufacturing Practices for Fresh Broiler Products." For more information, contact National Broiler Council, Director of Economic Research, 1155 15th Street, NW, Washington, DC 20005.
- The Quality Assurance Program of the American Veal Association. For more information, contact President, American Veal Association, Naperville Plaza, 1804 Naper Boulevard, Suite 241, Naperville, IL 60563.
- The Dairy Quality Assurance Program (currently being developed by the National Milk Producers Federation and the American Veterinary Medical Association). For more information, contact National Milk Producers Federation, Director, Public Relations, 1840 Wilson Boulevard, Arlington, VA 22201.
- The American Veterinary Medical Association's Guidelines for Supervising Use and Distribution of Veterinary Prescription Drugs.[18] The guidelines were designed to heighten the practitioner's level of awareness on the subject and to promote appropriate animal drug use by practitioners as well as by animal owners. FDA-CVM believes that these guidelines should be consulted and followed.

CONCLUSIONS

Drugs and chemicals play a major role in the production of our meat and poultry supply. The course of residue awareness, prevention, and control has evolved to an intricate pattern of veterinary and nonveterinary involvement. Consumer concerns have never been greater and less justified. Three federal agencies strive to manage the situation, and substantial federal money is spent to ensure a safe meat and poultry supply. Overall, the story is one of success. More pointedly, some problems still persist; for example, cull dairy cows, bob and formula-fed veal, "roaster" pigs, and specific residues of compounds—SMZ, carbadox, gentamicin, neomycin, penicillin, (dihydro-) streptomycin—still persist. Ethical issues are confounded when approaches to residue control are not understood. Educational efforts have been sporadic and not coordinated. However, one definite conclusion can be made: veterinary medicine is at the very heart of residue control. The veterinary profession is the logical group to assume the leadership role in ensuring that the supply of meat, poultry, milk, and eggs is free of residues. It is from veterinary medical ethics, prominent professional projection of stories on "what we have done right," and the never-ending education of our profession, as well as of the producing and consuming public, that we will influence the occurrence of residues in food-producing animals. By assuming this leadership role, we will continue to ensure that safe meat, poultry, milk, and eggs will be available to the American consumer.

Note: The views represented in this paper are those of the authors and do not necessarily reflect agency policy.

CONTACTS IN THE FEDERAL AGENCIES

Each agency handles information sharing in different ways. EPA and FSIS prefer a single contact point through which responses to inquiries will be made. FDA prefers multiple contact points that can address general or specific questions. Titles, addresses, and telephone numbers for the various agency contacts are listed.

EPA Contact

United States Environmental Protection Agency
Office of Pesticides Programs
Field Operations Division
Public Information Branch
401 M Street, NW
Washington, DC 20460
(703) 557-7410 or (703) 557-2805

FDA Contacts

Director, Center for Veterinary Medicine
Food and Drug Administration
7500 Standish Place
Rockville, MD 20855
(301) 295-8740

Director, Office of New Animal Drug Evaluation
Center for Veterinary Medicine
Food and Drug Administration
7500 Standish Place
Rockville, MD 20855
(301) 295-8620

Director, Office of Surveillance and Compliance
Center for Veterinary Medicine
Food and Drug Administration
7500 Standish Place
Rockville, MD 20855
(301) 443-3400

Director, Office of Science
Center for Veterinary Medicine
Food and Drug Administration
7500 Standish Place
Rockville, MD 20855
(301) 443-6510

The FDA encourages anyone to contact these offices. Questions relating to the safety and effectiveness of new animal drugs, the safety for human consumption of drug residues in food derived from treated animals, monitoring of marketed veterinary drugs, food additives to ensure their continued safety and effectiveness, and adverse drug experience are welcomed.

FSIS Contact

United States Department of Agriculture
Food Safety and Inspection Service
Information and Legislative Affairs
14th & Independence Avenue, Room 1160
Washington, DC 20250
(202) 720-9113

GLOSSARY

In order for the reader to better understand the terminology used in this article or in dealing with residue-related issues, the authors felt that it would be beneficial to include a glossary of terms commonly used in the residue arena.

Adverse Drug Reaction (ADR). Any unexpected side effect, injury, toxicity, or sensitivity reaction (or any unexpected incidence or severity thereof) associated with clinical uses, studies, investigations, or tests, whether or not determined to be attributable to the new animal drug.

New Animal Drug (NAD). Any drug intended for use in animals that is not generally recognized by qualified experts as safe and effective for use under the condition prescribed, recommended, or suggested in the labeling thereof.

Calves. This slaughter class is divided into 4 groups:

1. Bob veal—up to 3 weeks of age or 150 pounds in weight.
2. Formula-fed or fancy veal—between 150 and 400 pounds; maintained on a liquid diet (milk or milk replacer).
3. Non–formula-fed veal—between 150 and 400 pounds; maintained on a solid diet (grain, silage, forage, and so on).
4. Heavy calves—over 400 pounds.

Code of Federal Regulations (CFRs). The codification (systematic classification) of the general and permanent rules published in the *Federal Register*. Title 40 pertains to EPA. Title 21 pertains to FDA, and Title 9 pertains to USDA.

Compound Evaluation and Analytical Capability National Residue Program Plan. (Commonly called the Blue Book.) This publication contains (1) references to *Code of Federal Regulations;* (2) tolerances for compounds of interest; (3) list of compounds considered; (4) cross-reference of compounds; and (5) FSIS residue analytical capability. It can be obtained by request from the United States Department of Agriculture, Food Safety and Inspection Service, Science and Technology, Residue Evaluation and Planning Division, 300 C Street, SW, Cotton Annex Bldg., Room 602, Washington, DC 20250.

Compound Evaluation System. Used by FSIS to determine the potential impact of a compound on public health. In this system, if the first evaluation element indicates that a residue can be formed, then the potential impact on public health is expressed as a function of two other elements: hazard (adverse effects that may be produced by a given compound) and exposure (residue concentration and factors affecting concentration, such as use patterns, withdrawal times, duration or frequency of exposure of product containing the residues of concern).

Domestic Residue Data Book National Residue Program. (Commonly called the Red Book.) Contains results (by individual years, slaughter class, and compound) of the National Residue Program and can be obtained from the same source given for the Blue Book.

Extra-label. Refers to the use that occurs when the user of a drug product does not follow the directions on the label.

Federal Register. A document that contains Notices and Proposed Final Rules formulated by the "executive" departments and agencies of the Federal Government.

Illegal Drug. This term refers to drugs that are illegal to use because they are unapproved new animal drugs, prohibited for use in show and performing animals, or otherwise do not meet the legal requirements for distribution or use, that is, diethylstilbestrol in food animals, chloramphenicol in food animals, extra-label use of drugs for production purposes, and dimetridazole in all species. *Note:* These examples relate only to illegal drugs used in food animals.

Over-the-Counter (OTC) Drugs. Those drugs that are not under a veterinary prescription. They can be purchased and used by laymen without the supervision of a veterinarian. *Note:* As a rule, OTC drugs cannot be used legally (by livestock producers, truckers, buyers, and others) for any purpose or dosage not stated on the drug's label.

Residue Violation. The occurrence of a drug or chemical residue above the tolerance level in edible tissue, fat, kidney, liver, muscle, meat by-products, or skin of a food producing animal.

Residue Violator. An individual producer, hauler, or trucker who has been identified by FDA or FSIS as having 2 or more violations within a 12-month period. The 12-month period begins with the initial date of notification to the violator. *Note:* In some instances, owners of sales barns have been issued regulatory letters for residue violations.

"Roaster" Pigs. Pigs usually 2 to 4 months of age and weighing 40 to 125 pounds. "Roasters" traditionally are consumed by ethnic populations, used for whole-hog barbecues, or served as baby-back ribs.

Safe Level. The amount of substance resulting in adulteration. A "safe level" is not a tolerance level or other binding rule of law. Safe levels do not limit FDA's enforcement discretion, and they do not protect producers, veterinarians, or other users from enforcement action.

Tolerance Level. The maximal level or concentration of a drug or chemical that is permitted in or on animal feed ingredients or animal tissues at the time of slaughter.

Unapproved Drugs. An unapproved drug is a product that is not the subject of an approved new animal drug application (NADA). *Note:* A drug approved in a foreign country but not approved in the United States is an unapproved drug.

Withdrawal Period. The interval from the time an animal is removed from medication until the permitted time of slaughter. This interval is established to prevent violative levels of drug residues in edible tissues for human consumption.

Zero Residue. FDA-CVM interprets zero residue to mean below the detection limit of the approved method.

REFERENCES

1. Baldwin RA: Government regulations concerning veterinary drugs. *In* Howard JL (ed): Current Veterinary Therapy: Food Animal Practice, 1st ed. Philadelphia, WB Saunders, 1981.
2. Mercer HD: Prevention management of drug and chemical residues in meat and milk. *In* Howard JL (ed): Current Veterinary Therapy: Food Animal Practice. Philadelphia, WB Saunders, 1986.
3. Bright SA, et al: Rapid tests for the detection of antibiotic residues. Proceedings of the International Symposium on Bovine Mastitis: National Mastitis Council and American Association of Bovine Practitioners, Indianapolis, 1990, pp 271–275.
4. Veterinary Service Information: Drug residue tests for use on milk, urine, serum, and tissues. VSE 0–3, Cooperative Extension Service, The Pennsylvania State University, University Park, PA 16802.
5. McKean JD: A veterinary approach to residue testing. Large Anim Vet Sept-Oct:38–42, 1987.
6. Food and Drug Administration, Center for Veterinary Medicine Compliance Policy Guide No. 7125.06: Extra-label use of new animal drugs in food-producing animals. Rockville, MD, Office of Surveillance and Compliance, Center for Veterinary Medicine, Food and Drug Administration, November 1986.
7. Center for Veterinary Medicine: Tissue Residue Program. Annual Report—Fiscal Year 1988. Rockville, MD, Center for Veterinary Medicine, Office of Surveillance and Compliance, Food and Drug Administration, 1990.
8. CVM Memo, Drug Use Guide: Beef cattle and calves. H.H.S. Publ. No. (FDA) 89–6015. Rockville, MD, United States Department of Health and Human Services, Public Health Service, Food and Drug Administration, 1989.
9. Radostits OM, Blood DC: Herd Health Management. Philadelphia, WB Saunders, 1985.
10. Federal Food, Drug, and Cosmetic Act, as Amended, and Related Laws. Washington, DC, Superintendent of Documents, U.S. Government Printing Office, 1985.
11. Cordle MK: USDA regulation of residues in meat and poultry products. J Anim Sci 66:413–433, 1988.

12. United States Department of Agriculture, Food Safety and Inspection Service, National Residue Program. Unpublished data, 1989.
13. Guest G: Keeping our food safe from animal drugs. FDA Consumer. Rockville, MD, Consumer Affairs Office, Food and Drug Administration, 1986.
14. HHS News. Rockville, MD, United States Department of Health and Human Services, Food and Drug Administration, P90–10, 1990.
15. Tannenbaum J: Recognizing professional ethics as a useful discipline. J Am Vet Med Assoc 197:168–169, 1990.
16. Knowles ME: Surveillance of the veterinary residues in meat. Food Sci Technol Today 2:193–196, 1988.
17. Sundlof SF, et al: Food Animal Residue Avoidance Databank Trade Name File, A Comprehensive Compendium of Food Animal Drugs. Gainesville, University of Florida, 1988.
18. AVMA guidelines for supervising use and distribution of veterinary prescription drugs. J Am Vet Med Assoc 193:1–8, 1988.

Prevention and Management of Drug and Chemical Residues in Meat and Milk

H. DWIGHT MERCER, DVM, PhD

The use of drugs in food-producing animals is an established and well-recognized requirement in the production of essential foodstuffs for a growing world population. Inherent in this widespread use of drugs are the problems associated with the fact that most chemical substances administered to animals will produce residual levels in various tissues and body fluids. Thus drug withdrawal periods must be established and also become a criterion for usage.

ATTITUDES CONCERNING DRUG RESIDUES

Most food animal producers are aware of the concerns related to drug residues. Educational efforts by drug manufacturers, the Animal Health Institute, the United States Department of Agriculture (USDA), and the United States Food and Drug Administration (FDA) have been effective in increasing awareness of the importance of drug residues.

Awareness, however, has not always been accompanied by complete understanding. For example, a producer may be aware of label instructions that define a drug withdrawal requirement but have difficulty in understanding how residues of a few parts per billion could possibly affect human health. Veterinarians may also view such small residues, which are comparable to a single drop in a railway tank car, with skepticism.

There is some justification in these viewpoints and attitudes; an association of residues of a few parts per billion with human health hazards is difficult to document. Molecular particles that cannot be detected by sight, touch, or smell have been associated with potential causes of cancer; the presence of these molecules in food is one of the most complex of current scientific and regulatory issues.

Regulatory issues are not the only concern; in an affluent society, consumer acceptance influences the profitability of food products. Avoidance of drug residues is most effectively implemented by producers and practicing veterinarians. Therefore producers and veterinarians should be aware of the beliefs and concerns of consumers.

There have been several recent circumstances that have escalated the power posture of consumers in the food demand equation. The media (newspapers and television) have become more aware of and willing to report residue problems vis-à-vis a recent New York milk supply study that was paid for and conducted by the media. Another vivid example is the current posture of 5 major food chains with regard to the pending marketing of a new biotechnology product, bovine somatotropin, in which milk from treated cows will not be sold through their respective chains. This trend is likely to continue and perhaps escalate. Food safety is now assuming a much broader base of support through consumer communication, and the responses can have devastating effects on the marketplace (*Salmonella* in and on chicken pieces and parts). Valuable drugs with 30- to 40-year histories of use (sulfonamides) are now under the scrutiny of both the regulatory agencies (FDA) and respected scientific organizations National Institutes of Health (NIH) and National Science Foundation (NSF).

CIRCUMSTANCES ASSOCIATED WITH VIOLATIVE DRUG RESIDUES

In advising practitioners on how to avoid drug residues, the recommendation to use only approved drugs, the recommended route of administration, and the dose recommended on the label and to follow label withdrawal times is overly simplistic. No doubt, the multimillion-dollar research expenditures that enable the FDA and drug manufacturers to make the label recommendations provide adequate assurance that drug residues will be avoided if the recommendations are followed. In practice, however, many difficult and often conflicting circumstances enhance the possibilities of producing animals with violative drug residues.

The most common example is that some disease conditions require drug doses in excess of label recommendations. Also, intratracheal, intrauterine, and other nontraditional routes of administration of approved and nonapproved antibiotics and other drugs are often associated with violative drug residues; it is commonly believed that little of the drug is absorbed via these routes.

The following drugs, use combinations, and conditions are often associated with violative drug residues:

- Oral neomycin given intravenously or intramuscularly.
- Administration of dimethyl sulfoxide (DMSO) cocktails (which enhance the absorption of drugs) for calf pneumonia.
- Intramuscular or intravenous administration of lincomycin-spectinomycin combinations that are labeled for poultry use (such administration is often used to prevent shipping fever in cattle).
- Acute septicemia if the microbial isolates are found to be sensitive only to gentamicin, kanamycin, chloramphenicol, or other nonapproved drugs.
- Nonapproved drugs that are required to treat diseases in minor food animal species, such as fish, goats, sheep, quail, ducks, and rabbits.
- New drugs that are approved for a single animal species but that are reported in the literature to be effective against a broad spectrum of organisms in many species.
- Minor diseases, such as fascioliasis in sheep, for which no drugs have been approved.
- Anesthetics and analgesics that have been used for years in food animals but yet have no established withdrawal times (e.g., barbiturates and xylazine hydrochloride).
- New drugs that have been approved for use in humans but that have demonstrated unique activity against common and difficult animal pathogens (e.g., carbenicillin and such related synthetics as carfecillin and ticarcillin for *Pseudomonas* infections).

- Homemade mixtures of antibiotics used for convenience and economic reasons and because they are believed to provide broad-spectrum coverage.

Whenever these or similar circumstances occur in a food animal practice, the veterinarian is placed in the precarious position of responding simultaneously to the needs of the animal, the concerns of the producer, the veterinarian's own legal liability, and the protection of the consumer. The conflicts among these concerns are troublesome to food animal veterinarians.

Veterinarians often must make extra-label use of drugs and consequently come into potential conflict with federal regulations. In such situations, clinical judgments are critical and must be balanced with desirable outcomes.

NEW DRUG DEVELOPMENT

The search for new drugs and their subsequent development follows a long and intense scientific pathway. Development of manufacturing methods, analytic procedures, formulations, stability, posology, toxicology, packaging, and marketing are only a few of the major scientific endeavors required for new drugs. The FDA adds several additional requirements for use in food animals, including drug residue studies in target animals, metabolism studies, and data relating potential toxicity in humans. The development of drug residue data is one of the most costly steps in drug development for food animals. The establishment of drug withdrawal requirements and setting of tolerances to ensure that the intended drug usage will not pose a threat to public health is the single most important aspect of the FDA's responsibilities in approving new drugs for use in food animals. Pharmacokinetics is the quantitative study of absorption, distribution, metabolism, and excretion of drugs and their pharmacologic, therapeutic, or toxic responses in animals and humans. In order to understand the problems of drug residues, it is necessary to have an appreciation of drug kinetics.

Conventional methods used to determine the residual nature of a drug in food animals may involve the following sequence of events.

1. Develop an analytic method for quantitative determination of the parent drug in biologic fluids and tissues.
2. Dose a series of animals via the intended route with the proposed formulation. Radiolabeled compounds are often used for this purpose.
3. At various intervals after dosing (i.e., at 0, 1, 3, 5, 7, 9, 12 days), slaughter at least 3 animals, collect a variety of tissues, including liver, muscle, fat, and kidney, and conduct assays to establish the necessary withdrawal interval.
4. Provide supporting toxicology data for establishing tolerances.
5. Refinement and modifications of the analytic procedure to the desired sensitivity level (parent drug and/or metabolites) may be necessary.
6. Establish withdrawal requirements. In many instances, the duration and extent of drug dosage for efficacy purposes may provide considerable concern from a residue standpoint. In striving to develop a drug that maintains concentrations in serum and tissues for a lengthy time interval, it is often found that this desired characteristic is incompatible with a short withdrawal interval. In fact, this is the paradox of the drug residue problem for the practitioner.

Figure 1 represents a conceptual model for drug kinetics as it relates to the problem of drug residues. On the basis of this

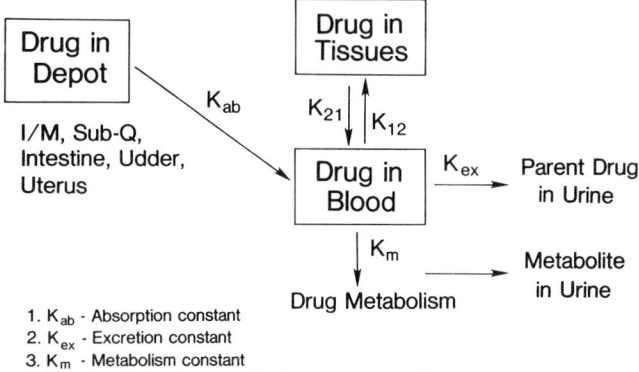

1. K_{ab} - Absorption constant
2. K_{ex} - Excretion constant
3. K_m - Metabolism constant
4. K_{12}/K_{21} - Rate of drug distribution into and out of tissue (Relates to volume of distribution)

Figure 1. Conceptual model of drug kinetics as it relates to the problem of drug residues.

model, it becomes apparent that the majority of drug residue problems can be associated with the drug either in depot phase or in tissue phase. A group of characteristics has been developed that often explains why certain drugs cause residue problems. These characteristics have been grouped into 3 major types of drugs. These criteria provide the most realistic basis for understanding the drug residue problem.

Criteria for Type I Drugs

1. Rapid absorption rate constant (k_{ab}).
2. High degree of absorption (>90 per cent). Absorption of drugs from aqueous solutions is rapid and almost complete.
3. Low volume of distribution (V_d) [organic acids] <0.2 to 0.25 L/kg.
4. Short biologic half-life ($t_{1/2} \leq 1$ hour); for example, penicillins and cephalosporins.
5. One- and two-compartment model drugs; for example, the drug generally remains in the central blood compartment.
6. Low affinity for tissues.

Most drugs that meet these criteria will provide relatively high blood concentrations that are diminished at a rapid rate. The use of this type of drug requires repetitive dosing on a daily basis for maintenance of therapeutic concentrations in the blood.

These properties are highly desirable from the standpoint of drug residue with use in food animals. Classic examples include most of the penicillins, cephalosporins, sulfisoxazole, and sulfadiazine. It is often the objective with this class of drugs to lengthen the dosage interval. The formulation (e.g., less soluble salts and oil bases) required to lengthen the dosage interval often leads to type II drugs in this classification scheme.

Criteria for Type II Drugs

1. Moderate to rapid absorption rate constants.
2. Moderate degree of absorption (>70 per cent): vehicle effects; for example, propylene glycol, polyvinylpyrrolidone, and certain oil-type bases.
3. High volume of distribution (>1 L/kg) (often true for organic bases).
4. Median biologic half-life (3 to 8 hours); for example, sulfamethazine, oxytetracycline, and erythromycin.
5. Two-compartment model drugs.
6. Indications of drug depot problems; for example, injection site problems with oxytetracycline and sulfonamides.

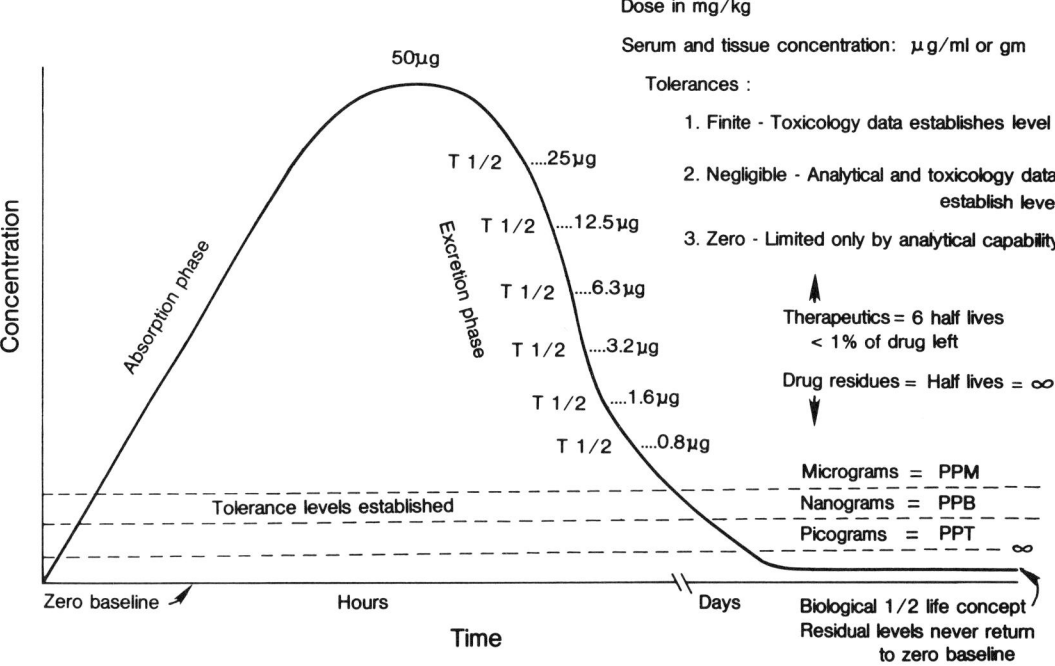

Figure 2. Biologic half-life concept.

7. Drugs such as erythromycin lactobionate and procaine penicillin G are examples of conversion from a type I drug to a type II drug.

A more extensive effort is required in the development of a drug residue profile for type II drugs. Subcutaneous or intravenous routes of administration might be chosen if intramuscular sites contain residues for long periods. The oral route may be the only acceptable route. Depot problems may be solved by route or vehicle modifications. This type of drug is considered a greater residue-producing risk, and its use may be more closely monitored and controlled. Also, it is more costly to develop this type of drug because of the greater increase in residue studies required. Classic examples include intramuscularly administered oxytetracycline, benzathine penicillin, and certain of the sulfonamides.

Criteria for Type III Drugs

1. Slow absorption rate constant.
2. Incomplete absorption (<50 per cent).
3. High volume of distribution.
4. Long half-life (<12 hours).
5. Two or more compartment drugs.
6. Strong affinity for tissue depots and binding; for example, chlorinated hydrocarbons accumulate in fat and kidneys, the aminoglycosides bind to kidney tissue.

Extreme caution and extensive residue data are required for the development of this type of drug. Usage patterns should be strictly limited to therapeutic purposes, with stringent restrictions recommended to the practitioner. Marketing channels should be limited to professional use only. Several classic examples are parenteral streptomycin and neomycin, long-acting sulfonamides (sulfadimethoxine), and chlorinated hydrocarbons. Whereas the goal of restricted use for this type of drug has not been realized, it is reasonable to expect that the practicing veterinarian will ultimately be given this responsibility. This should be particularly true if drug residue problems continue to occur and other means fail to control the incidence of drug residues in food animals. Alternatively, it is likely that these type drugs will be removed from the marketplace or restricted to non–food animal use.

Figure 2 is used to illustrate the biologic half-life concept of a drug in the animal body. The absorption phase is a rate-limiting phase. As indicated earlier, problems with absorption often translate to drug residue problems. It generally requires about 6 half-lives for a drug to be depleted below its therapeutic usefulness. This generally occurs within a matter of hours. After this point in time, the depletion pattern becomes reflective of the residual nature of the drug. Once depletion reaches the ppm, ppb, or ppt levels, it is at these concentrations for which tolerances are established. Theoretically, once a drug has entered the system, it will require an infinite time for the last molecule to be eliminated. Thus, establishment of tolerances becomes a necessity. There are several types of tolerances as illustrated in Figure 2. A discussion of tolerances is prohibited here, but a thorough discussion is available.[1]

CLINICAL APPROACH

As a consultant to food animal practitioners and producers, the author believes that a systematic and reasonable approach must be devised to deal with these issues. It is difficult to fulfill the responsibilities of the food animal veterinarian while

---

[1] A thorough and detailed presentation on the problems of drug residues along with tabulated withdrawal times for a variety of commonly used drugs is included in Chapter 66 of the fifth edition of Booth and MacDonald's *Veterinary Pharmacology and Therapeutics*. Every effort to avoid duplication of this material has been exercised in preparing this chapter.

maintaining total compliance with federal requirements and label restrictions of currently available veterinary drugs. An approach that has met with good success has involved implementation of risk assessment and the application of the drug's pharmacologic profile.

Risk Assessment

An important consideration is whether the food animal patient is likely to be slaughtered while the drug residues are violative. Valuable breeding stock, high-producing dairy cattle, show stock, and lightweight feeder-stocker calves destined for winter grazing and then for the feedlot are considered low-risk animals. Animals in these classes either are not immediately intended for slaughter or are not intended to be slaughtered for at least 100 to 150 days.

Surveillance data by the United States Department of Agriculture, Food Safety and Inspection Service (FSIS) indicate that the following high-risk classes of food animals must receive special and conservative treatment:

- Low-producing dairy cows with chronic mastitis or other metabolic disorders.
- Animals already in the feedlot.
- Animals with short finishing periods (e.g., 175-lb pigs in feedlots).
- Bob veal calves.
- Minor food animal species (e.g., quail and rabbit) for which little is known about drug residues.

The assignment of animals to low- and high-risk categories often enables the veterinarian to recommend special handling and written instructions regarding residue avoidance.

Pharmacokinetic Drug Profile

Many drugs that are indicated for use in food animals have pharmacokinetic characteristics that have been described in the literature. Drugs may be classified according to such properties as absorption constants, biologic half-life, rate of elimination, volume of distribution, extent of compartmentalization, and binding qualities of the drug. These characteristics enable reasonable estimates of the potential for prolonged residues and can be used to make a clinical judgment before the drug is used in a food animal.

Pharmacokinetic data can also be used to project withdrawal times for drugs and chemicals that accidentally contaminate food animals. Serum, urine, or tissue specimens from contaminated animals are required for estimates of the pharmacokinetics of the substance in the affected population. These analytic and mathematical calculations usually require expertise beyond the immediate resources of the practitioner, but practitioners should be aware of the availability and utility of such pharmacokinetic analysis. Such analyses have now become a reality and a ready resource to veterinary practitioners. This service is called the Food Animal Residue Avoidance Databank (FARAD); regional telephone access numbers have been published and are available through the *Journal of the American Veterinary Medical Association*.

REGULATORY AND CONSUMER CONCERNS

In recent years, several congressional subcommittees have examined the FDA's policies relating to the regulation of veterinary drugs. One of the subcommittee's findings was that more than 70 per cent of the animal drugs and animal drug metabolites that leave residues in meat, milk, and eggs are not being monitored. This finding, along with the rest of the subcommittee's report, signals an increasing effort to monitor food animal products for illegal drug residues. Food animal veterinarians as well as producers and middlemen in the drug marketing chain (cooperatives, feedstores, and door-to-door drug salesmen) play a major role in controlling drug residues. The current consumer attitudes, which are clearly escalating, along with more stringent testing by regulatory agencies will continue to focus attention on drug residues. The regulatory mechanisms for detection of violative residues are in place, and funds for increased testing have been appropriated. The ultimate outcome of less drug availability is likely if the incidence and occurrence of violative residues are not controlled.

The practicing food animal veterinarian, although not always directly involved in the drug usage pattern, represents the individual in the community who has the training and experience to educate and advise on the problems of drug residues. As drugs become more potent and their potential uses become more sophisticated, the role of the veterinarian will become more essential as an advisor.

BIBLIOGRAPHY

Baggot JD, Gingerich DA: Pharmacokinetic interpretation of erythromycin and tylosin activity in serum after intravenous administration of a single dose to cows. Res Vet Sci 21:318–323, 1976.
Booth NH, McDonald LE: Veterinary Pharmacology and Therapeutics, 5th ed. Ames, IA, Iowa State University Press, 1982, pp 1065–1113.
Koritz GD: Practical aspects of pharmacokinetics for the large animal practitioner. Compend Contin Educ Pract Vet 11:201–204, 1989.
Mercer HD: Antimicrobial drugs in food producing animals. Control mechanisms of government agencies. Vet Clin North Am 5:3–33, 1975.
Mercer HD: Residue avoidance: withdrawal times for drugs not labelled for food animals. *In* Proceedings of the 10th Annual Food Animal Medicine Conference on the Use of Drugs in Food Animals. Columbus, OH, Ohio State University Press, 1985, pp 7–24.
Mercer H: How to avoid the drug residue problem in cattle. Compend Contin Educ Pract Vet 12:124–126, 1990.
Mercer HD, Baggot JD, Sams RA: Applications of pharmacokinetic methods to the drug residue profile. J Toxicol Environ Health 2:787–801, 1977.
Nouws JFM, Ziv G: A kinetic study of β-lactam antibiotic residues in normal dairy cows. Zentralbl Veterinarmed [A] 25:312–326, 1978.
Nouws JFM, Ziv G, Van Ginneken CAM, Vree TB: Clinical pharmacokinetics of carbenicillin, carfecillin, ticarcillin, and BL-P 1654 in dairy cows. J Vet Pharmacol Ther 7:35–43, 1984.
Pilloud M: Pharmacokinetics, plasma protein binding and dosage of oxytetracycline in cattle and horses. Res Vet Sci 15:224–230, 1973.
Rasmussen F, Svendsen O: Tissue damage and concentration at the injection site after intramuscular injection of chemotherapeutics and vehicles in pigs. Res Vet Sci 20:55–60, 1976.
Talbot RB, Menning EL: Safe meat and poultry from farm to table and the National Animal Disease Surveillance Program. Proc AAVMC 11:84–118, 1985.
Ziv G, Shani J, Sulman FG: Pharmacokinetic evaluation of penicillin and cephalosporin derivatives in serum and milk of lactating cows and ewes. Am J Vet Res 34:1561–1565, 1973.

Bovine Somatotropin

DAVID McCLARY, DVM, MS, DIPLOMATE, ACT

Bovine somatotropin (bST) is a high-molecular-weight protein hormone (approximately 191 amino acids) produced by the anterior pituitary gland in the cow. Somatotropin is directly involved in numerous physiologic processes, including promotion of growth in young animals, deposition of muscle protein in growing animals, and regulation of milk production in lactating cows. The first evidence of the galactopoietic

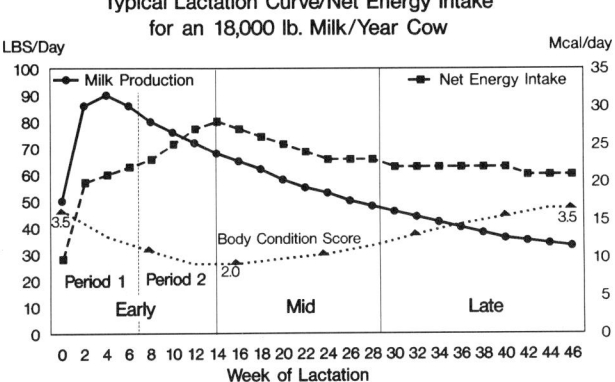

Figure 1. Milk production and nutrient intake during lactation.

activity of somatotropin was discovered in the 1930s when Russian scientists found injection of pituitary extracts into lactating cows increased milk yield.[1] During the 1940s, somatotropin was identified as the pituitary product responsible for enhancing milk production.[2] Although the potential for increasing milk production with pituitary bST has been recognized for years, commercial utilization was not considered feasible because of the large number of cadaver pituitary glands (approximately 200) required for a single treatment. In 1982, the first experiment using recombinant bST (r-bST) was reported.[3] Today, large-scale production of r-bST makes long-term research trials and eventual commercial utilization possible.

MECHANISM OF ACTION

Lactogenesis requires the interaction of a number of hormones including somatotropin. Somatotropin release is regulated by a balance between growth hormone–releasing factor (GRF) and growth hormone–inhibiting factor (somatostatin). Somatostatin usually provides the prime control of bST release, but episodic release of GRF produces variations in circulating somatotropin concentrations.

Early in lactation, serum concentrations of pituitary bST decline from an initial high level, mirroring the lactation curve. Serum insulin concentrations, however, are generally low in early lactation and increase as days-in-milk progress.[4] Studies[5,6] have shown that cows with higher milk production potential tend to have higher mean serum concentrations of bST.

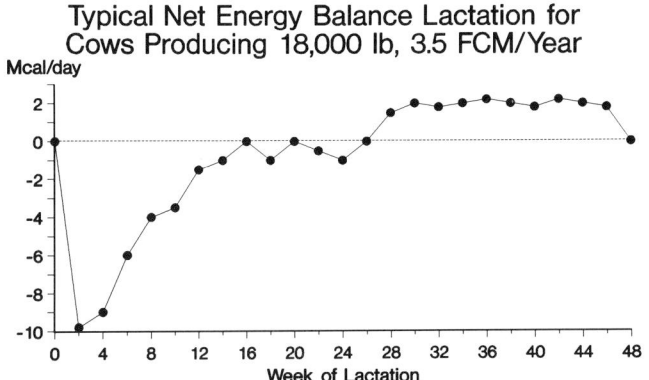

Figure 2. Energy balance during lactation.

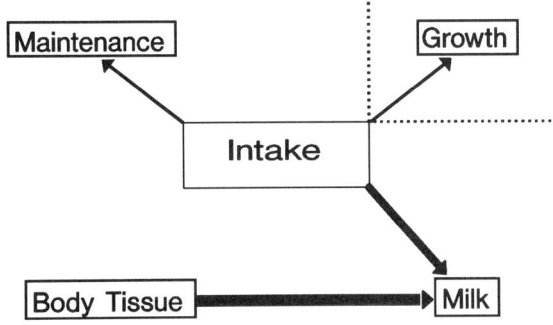

Figure 3. Nutrient partitioning, early lactation (1 to 40 days-in-milk).

The biologic action of bST can be manifested only in those tissues with somatotropin receptors. Receptors for bST have been isolated from a number of body cells, including liver, kidney, skeletal and cardiac muscle, ovary, lymphocytes, and fibroblasts. No somatotropin receptors have been identified in mammary gland secretory cells. Somatotropin action on the mammary gland is apparently mediated through related peptides called somatomedins. The specific somatomedins associated with the mammary tissue are insulin-like growth factors 1 and 2 (IGF-1 and IGF-2). Somatotropin appears to enhance the production and secretion of IGF-1, which in turn increases the metabolic activity of mammary secretory cells.[7]

Increased metabolic activity by secretory cells increases the rate of protein, fat, and lactose synthesis, which in turn increases the demand for nutrients supplied to the mammary gland. Somatotropin apparently increases milk production by increasing mammary gland secretory activity and by diverting nutrients away from nonmammary tissues and to the mammary gland.

NUTRIENT PARTITIONING

The dairy cow normally reaches peak milk production 4 to 8 weeks into lactation; maximum dry matter intake does not occur until 4 to 10 weeks later[8] (Fig. 1). During early lactation, the high-producing cow must mobilize body fat to supply the energy requirements for additional milk yield. This places her in a net negative energy balance (Fig. 2). After the nutritional

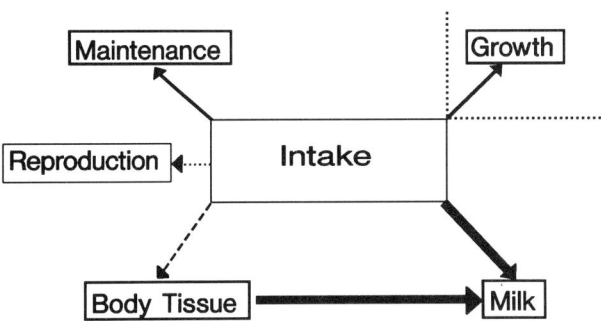

Figure 4. Nutrient partitioning, early lactation (40 to 100 days-in-milk).

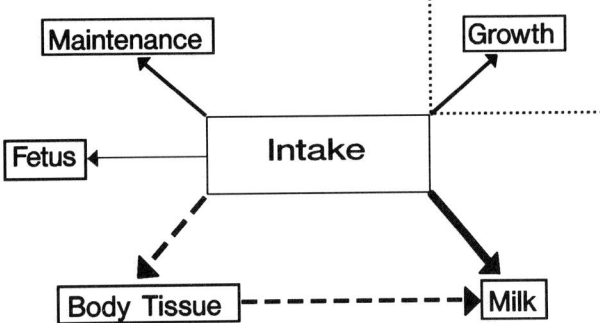

Figure 5. Nutrient partitioning, mid lactation (100 to 200 days-in-milk).

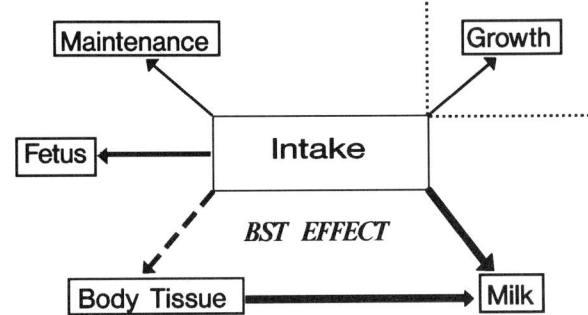

Figure 7. Nutrient partitioning, bST (BST) effect early in treatment (first 8 to 12 weeks).

requirements for maintenance and growth have been met, nutrients are partitioned away from body tissue reserves and toward the mammary gland (Fig. 3). As the cow proceeds in lactation, feed intake gradually increases. After peak lactation, daily milk production starts to decline (Fig. 4). Eventually nutrient intake equals and later exceeds nutrient loss to milk, and the cow gradually starts to replenish body tissue reserves (Figs. 5 and 6).

Bovine somatotropin also has a nutrient partitioning effect on the cow. During the first few weeks of bST supplementation, nutrients are diverted from body reserves and toward the mammary gland. Initial increases in milk production are supported primarily by increased mobilization of body fat reserves just as in early lactation (Fig. 7). After 8 to 12 weeks of bST supplementation, nutrient intake increases to compensate for increased milk production[9] (Fig. 8).

BODY CONDITION

Because bST mobilizes body fat reserves to support milk production, it would be expected to accelerate the normal rate of body condition loss. Some long-term studies have demonstrated a significant reduction in body condition score (BCS) when bST supplementation was initiated early in lactation.[10,11] Body composition studies have measured significant reduction in body fat content in bST-supplemented cows.[10,12,13]

Body condition score should be closely monitored throughout lactation regardless of bST usage. Ideally, cows should be examined for body condition score at 5 or 6 times during lactation: calving; early lactation (breeding); mid lactation (pregnancy examination); late lactation; drying-off; and mid-dry period. The cow's body condition score at calving should be at least 3.5 to ensure adequate fat reserve to maximize peak milk yield and maintain persistency throughout lactation. Over-conditioning (BCS >4.0) in late lactation and dry period should be avoided because it leads to depressed appetite and results in exaggerated losses in body condition during the early stages of the subsequent lactation. Body condition loss should not exceed 1 condition score in early lactation. Excessive loss may significantly depress first-service conception rate and increase days-open. Body condition score at drying off should have returned to 3.5 so that adequate reserve for the subsequent lactation is ensured.

Cows with poor condition scores (BCS <2.0) or cows rapidly losing condition should not be given supplemental bST. These cows should be maintained on energy-dense rations for help in meeting the demands of high milk production. Careful monitoring of body condition score will be useful in designing bST treatment programs tailored to the individual cow.

MILK PRODUCTION RESPONSE TO bST

Bovine somatotropin administered in a variety of dosage forms—including daily subcutaneous and intramuscular injections, and 14- and 28-day sustained-release subcutaneous injections—has consistently demonstrated increases in 3.5 per

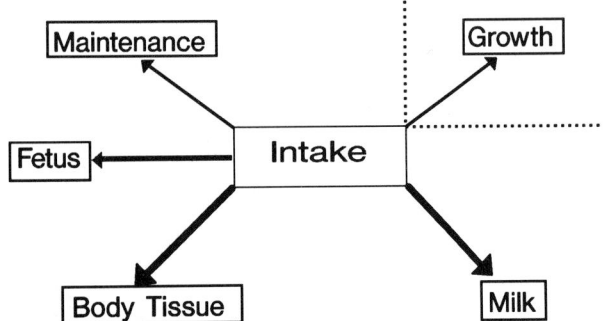

Figure 6. Nutrient partitioning, late lactation (200 to 300 days-in-milk).

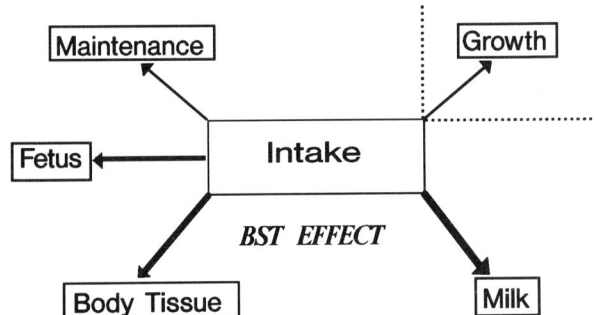

Figure 8. Nutrient partitioning, bST (BST) effect later in treatment (after week 12).

cent fat-corrected milk (FCM) yield of 8 to 10 pounds per day.[14] The level of milk production response varies among individual trials and individual cows. The response ranges from no significant increase in one trial[15] to greater than 20 pounds FCM per day in others.[16, 17] Some studies[18, 19] have shown a lesser response in primiparous compared with multiparous cows, whereas others[20, 21] have shown the response to be similar between parity groups. Variations in bST response by heifers, compared with multiparous cows, appear to be related to the size, body condition, and feed intake of the heifer at the start of bST treatment.

ANIMAL SAFETY AND HEALTH

Numerous studies have been conducted to determine the safety of bST and its impact on animal health. Safety studies have included trials with cows receiving bST over 2 lactations (the dose was at least 5 times the anticipated recommended dose); acute toxicity trials in which cows received 25 times the anticipated recommended dose; and long-term, multiple lactation studies.[11, 22] Some studies include serum clinical chemistry and hematology profiles during the trial with complete necropsy and histopathologic examinations at the completion of the study. Cows involved in bST research are closely monitored for evidence of abnormalities and diseases considered common to dairy cattle. Almost all studies have shown no significant increase in the incidence or severity of these conditions.[23-32] When an increase in the incidence of digestive problems or lameness has been reported, the increase has been associated with the highest (5 times) dose level.[22]

Although bST increases the mobilization of body fat reserves in the cow during the early treatment period, the incidence of clinical ketosis is not increased.[33, 34] Studies monitoring the incidence of subclinical ketosis by measurement of serum concentrations of β-hydroxybutyrate have shown no increase in the incidence of subclinical ketosis in r-bST–supplemented cows, compared with controls.[35-37] Apparently the increased lipolysis associated with bST supplementation is accompanied by increased utilization of free fatty acids.

Data from most bST trials have shown no significant increase in udder health problems. This includes incidence of clinical mastitis,[24, 28, 29] percentage of quarters infected,[38] and somatic cell counts.[23, 37-43] Reports indicating increases in the incidence of clinical mastitis or somatic cell counts in bST-treated animals involved animals receiving greater than the anticipated approved level of bST.[22, 44]

REPRODUCTION

Studies of bST's effect in reproduction have shown conflicting results. Some studies have indicated no effect on reproductive indices,[18, 32, 35, 39, 46, 47] whereas others indicated slight increases in days to first service, days-open, calving interval, and/or services per conception when bST supplementation was initiated before breeding.[21, 22, 28, 40, 48-50] Two factors must be considered when the effect of bST on reproductive efficiency in the dairy cow is evaluated: (1) number of days postcalving when BST supplementation was initiated and (2) effect of increased milk production on reproductive efficiency.

Numerous studies over the past 35 years have demonstrated an inverse relationship in milk yield and reproductive efficiency in dairy cows under similar management systems.[51-57] For each 100 pounds in milk production in the first 120 days of lactation, days-open will increase 0.3 days, and the number of services per conception will increase by 0.005 services.[56] The inverse relationship between milk production and reproductive efficiency appears to be related to the level of negative energy balance.

Maximal negative energy balance usually occurs at approximately 14 days-in-milk. The first postpartum ovulation usually occurs 20 to 30 days postcalving or approximately 10 days after maximal negative energy balance. Whereas nutrient requirements for ovarian function are likely not large, priority for nutrient partitioning to reproductive functions is low at this time. If the cumulative negative energy balance is increased owing to either increased milk yield or reduced nutrient intake, the return to cyclic ovarian activity will be delayed,[58] and a corresponding increase in days to first service and days-open can be expected.

Increased negative energy balance contributes to reduced luteal function and depressed serum progesterone concentrations subsequent to early postpartum ovulation.[59] Inadequate luteal function may contribute to the reduced first-service conception rates often seen with early postpartum breeding of high-producing cows in negative energy balance.

If bST supplementation is initiated early post partum (i.e., 30 to 40 days-in-milk), cumulative negative energy balance can be increased, bringing a corresponding increase in days to first service and days-open. However, much of the negative impact on reproduction can be negated by increasing nutrient intake by the early postpartum cow. If bST supplementation is initiated after the period of maximal negative energy balance (i.e., 80 to 100 days-in-milk), the negative impact of bST supplementation on reproductive efficiency will be minimal.

Studies in superovulated embryo transfer cows indicate a significant increase in the number of transferable embryos in bST-supplemented cows.[60] Apparently increased bST concentrations affect the development and recruitment of large ovarian follicles.[61] This explains the significant increase in the multiple birth rate demonstrated in some trials when cows were bred during bST supplementation.[62]

MANAGEMENT CONSIDERATIONS FOR bST SUPPLEMENTATION

Supplemental bST will not be recommended for all dairy operations. Within operations using bST, it will not be indicated for all cows or for the same stages of lactation on all cows. Maximal return from a bST supplementation program requires use programs tailored to individual cows. Parity, level of milk production, body condition score, nutrient intake, reproductive status, and overall health will need to be considered before the initiation of bST supplementation. Bovine somatotropin will not likely be indicated for high-producing cows in early lactation, cows rapidly losing body condition, poorly managed or under-conditioned first-lactation heifers, or cows with health problems. In these animals, bST usage should be delayed until after peak milk production and the animals have started to regain body condition. If a slight increase in calving interval or the increased possibility of twinning is considered undesirable in certain cows, bST supplementation should be delayed until after breeding.

Recommendations by herd health consultants will be extremely valuable in making management decisions regarding bST supplementation. Correlating reproductive information, body condition score, feed intake, and milk production records will be important for efficient usage of bST on individual cows.

Cows supplemented with bST are similar to genetically superior cows in that they produce higher levels of milk. Production medicine programs for bST-supplemented herds will be similar to programs designed for high-producing herds.

Bovine somatotropin–supplemented cows will differ from high-producing cows in the rate of accumulation of total milk production during lactation. Genetically superior cows reach a higher peak milk production level than do average cows, then start a typical decline in production of 8 to 9 per cent per month during the last two thirds of the lactation. The bST-supplemented cow will be more persistent in milk production and produce a higher percentage of her total milk production in the later part of lactation. The shift in the rate of milk production and profit accumulation toward the end of lactation may somewhat reduce the need for maintaining a minimum calving interval and reduce the pressure for early postpartum breeding.

REFERENCES

1. Asimov GJ, Krouze NK: The lactogenic preparations from the anterior pituitary and the increase of milk yield in cows. J Dairy Sci 20:289, 1937.
2. Young FG: Experimental stimulation (galactopoiesis) of lactation. Br Med Bull 5:155, 1947.
3. Bauman DE, DeGeeter MJ, Peel CJ, et al: Effect of recominantly derived bovine growth hormone (bGH) on lactational performance of high-yielding dairy cows. J Dairy Sci 65(Suppl 1):121 (abstract), 1982.
4. Koprowski JA, Tucker HA: Bovine serum growth hormone, corticoids and insulin during lactation. Endocrinology 93:645, 1973.
5. Flux DS, MacKenzie DDS, Wilson GF: Plasma metabolite and hormone concentrations in Friesian cows of differing genetic merit measured at two feeding levels. Anim Prod 38:377, 1984.
6. Barnes MA, Kazmer GW, Akers RM, et al: Influence of selection for milk yield on exogenous hormones and metabolites in Holstein heifers and cows. J Anim Sci 60:271, 1985.
7. Glimm DR, Baracos VE, Kennelly JJ: Effect of bovine somatotropin on the distribution of immunoreactive insulin-like growth factor-1 in lactating bovine mammary tissue. J Dairy Sci 71:2923, 1988.
8. National Research Council: Nutrient Requirements of Dairy Cattle, 6th ed. Washington, DC, National Academy Press, 1989, pp 2–52.
9. Bauman DE, Hard DL, Crooker BA, et al: Long-term evaluation of a prolonged-release formulation of n-methionyl bovine somatotropin in lactating dairy cows. J Dairy Sci 72:642, 1989.
10. Soderholm CG, Otterby DE, Linn JG, et al: Effects of recombinant bovine somatotropin on milk production, body composition, and physiological parameters. J Dairy Sci 71:355, 1988.
11. McClary DG: The impact of bST on animal health and reproduction. In Bovine Somatotropin: Proceedings of Symposia. Elanco Products Company and Lilly Research Laboratories. Columbus, OH, October 16, 1989; St. Paul MN, October 26, 1989, pp 5–11.
12. McGuffey RK, Spike TE, Basson RP: Partitioning of energy in the lactating dairy cow receiving bST. J Daily Sci 72(Suppl 1):535 (abstract), 1989.
13. Brown RH, Taylor SJ, dePeters EJ, et al: Influence of sometribove USAN recombinant methionyl bovine somatotropin on the body composition of lactating cattle. J Nutr 119:633, 1989.
14. Chilliard Y: Long-term effects of recombinant bovine somatotropin on daily cow performances. Ann Zootech 37:159, 1989.
15. Mollett TA, DeGeeter MJ, Belyea RL, et al.: Biosynthetic or pituitary extracted bovine growth hormone–induced galactopoiesis in dairy cows. J Dairy Sci 69(Suppl 1):118 (abstract), 1986.
16. Bauman DE, Eppard PJ, DeGeeter MJ, et al: Responses of high-producing dairy cows to long-term treatment with pituitary somatotropin and recombinant somatotropin. J Dairy Sci 68:1352, 1985.
17. Annexstad RJ, Otterby DE, Linn JG, et al: Responses of cows to daily injections of recombinant bovine somatotropin (bST) during a second consecutive lactation. J Dairy Sci 70(Suppl 1):176 (abstract), 1987.
18. Hansen WP, Otterby DE, Linn JG, et al: Multi-farm use of bovine somatotropin (bST) and its effects on lactation, health, and reproduction. J Dairy Sci 72(Suppl 1):429 (abstract), 1989.
19. Tessman NJ, Radloff HD, Dhiman TR, et al: Effect of dietary forage:grain ratio on reponse of lactating dairy cows to recombinant bovine somatotropin. J Dairy Sci 71(Suppl 1):121 (abstract), 1988.
20. Peel CJ, Hard DL, Madsen KS, et al: Bovine somatotropin: mechanism of action and experimental results from different world areas. In Meeting the Challenges of New Technology, Syracuse, NY, Monsanto Technical Symposium, Oct 24, 1989, p 6.
21. Cleale RM, Rehman JD, Robb EJ, et al: On-farm lactational and reproductive responses to daily injections of recombinant bovine somatotropin. J Dairy Sci 72(Suppl 1):429 (abstract), 1989.
22. Cole WJ, Eppard PJ, Lanza GM, et al: Response of lactating dairy cows to multiple injections of sometribove, USAN (recombinant methionyl bovine somatotropin) in a prolonged release system. Part II. Health and reproduction. J Dairy Sci 71(Suppl 1):184 (abstract), 1988.
23. Aguilar AA, Jordan DC, Olsen JD, et al: A short-term study evaluating the galactopoietic effects of the administration of sometribove (recombinant methionyl bovine somatotropin) in high-producing dairy cows milked three times per day. J Dairy Sci 71(Suppl 1):208 (abstract), 1988.
24. Chalupa W, Kutches A, Swager T, et al: Responses of cows in a commercial dairy to somatotropin. J Dairy Sci 71(Suppl 1):210 (abstract), 1988.
25. Cole WJ, Franson SE, Hoffman RG, et al: Response of cows throughout lactation to sometribove, recombinant methionyl bovine somatotropin, in a prolonged release system—a dose titration study. Part II. Health and reproduction. J Dairy Sci 72(Suppl 1):451 (abstract), 1989.
26. deBoer G, Kennelly JJ: Sustained-release bovine somatotropin for dairy cows. J Dairy Sci 71(Suppl 1):432 (abstract), 1989.
27. Galton DM, Samuels WA: Evaluation of sometribove, USAN (recombinant methionyl) bovine somatotropin on milk production and health. J Dairy Sci 72(Suppl 1):450 (abstract), 1989.
28. Huber JT, Willman S, Marcus K, et al: Effect of sometribove (SB), USAN (recombinant methionyl bovine somatotropin) injected in lactating cows at 14-day intervals on milk yields, milk composition, and health. J Dairy Sci 71(Suppl 1):207 (abstract), 1988.
29. Lamb RC, Anderson MJ, Henderson SL, et al: Production response of Holstein cows to sometribove USAN (recombinant methionyl bovine somatotropin) in a prolonged release system for one lactation. J Dairy Sci 71(Suppl 1):208 (abstract), 1988.
30. Larson RA, Otterby DE, Linn JG, et al: Responses of dairy cows to recombinant bovine somatotropin in a sustained-release vehicle. J Dairy Sci 72(Suppl 1):329 (abstract), 1989.
31. McDaniel BT, Gallant DM, Fetrow J, et al: Lactational, reproductive, and health responses to recombinant bovine somatotropin under field conditions. J Dairy Sci 72(Suppl 1):429 (abstract), 1989.
32. Samuels WA, Hard DL, Hintz RL, et al: Long-term evaluation of sometribove, USAN (recombinant methionyl bovine somatotropin) treatment in a prolonged release system for lactating dairy cows. J Dairy Sci 71(Suppl 1):209 (abstract), 1988.
33. Peel CJ, Bauman DE: Somatotropin and lactation. J Dairy Sci 70:474, 1987.
34. Bauman DE: National Workshop on Bovine Somatotropin. St. Louis, MO, October 24, 1987, pp 46–65.
35. Eppard PJ, Bauman DE, Curtis CR, et al: Effects of 188-day treatment with somatotropin on health and reproductive performance of lactating dairy cows. J Dairy Sci 70:582, 1987.
36. Hutchinson CF, Tomlinson JE, McGee WH: The effects of endogenous recombinant or pituitary-extracted bovine growth hormone on performance on dairy cows. J Dairy Sci 69(Suppl 1):152 (abstract), 1986.
37. Lanza GM, Eppard PJ, Miller MA, et al: Response of lactating dairy cows to multiple injections of sometribove, USAN (recombinant methionyl bovine somatotropin) in a prolonged release system. Part III. Changes in circulating analytes. J Dairy Sci 71(Suppl 1):184 (abstract), 1988.
38. Rowe-Bechtel CL, Muller LD, Deaver DR, et al: Administration of recombinant somatotropin (rbST) to lactating cows beginning at 35 and 70 days postpartum. I. Production responses. J Dairy Sci 71(Suppl 1):166 (abstract), 1988.
39. Bunn KB, Jenny BF, Pardue FE, et al: Effect of sustained-release bovine somatotropin (bST) on reproduction and mammary health of dairy cows. J Dairy Sci 72(Suppl 1):325 (abstract), 1989.
40. Elvinger F, Head HH, Wilcox CJ, et al: Effects of administration of bovine somatotropin on lactation milk yield and composition. J Dairy Sci 70(Suppl 1):121 (abstract), 1987.
41. Hemken RW, Harmon RJ, Silvia WJ, et al: Response of lactating dairy cows to a second year of recombinant bovine somatotropin (bST) when fed two energy concentrations. J Dairy Sci 71(Suppl 1):122 (abstract), 1988.
42. McGuffey RK, Green HB, Ferguson TH: Lactation performance of dairy cows receiving recombinant bovine somatotropin by daily injection or in sustained release vehicle. J Dairy Sci 70(Suppl 1):176 (abstract), 1987.
43. Rock DW, Patterson DL: Lactation performance of dairy cows given a sustained release form of recombinant bovine somatotropin. J Dairy Sci 72(Suppl 1):431 (abstract), 1989.
44. Crist WL: Oral presentation. Teaching and Extension Dealing with the Use of Somatotropin: bST and Health Aspects in the Dairy Cow. Lexington, KY, ADSA/ASAS Conference, August 4, 1989.
45. Samuels WA, Hard DL, Hintz RL, et al: Long-term evaluation of sometribove, USAN (recombinant methionyl bovine somatotropin) treatment in a prolonged release system for lactating dairy cows. J Dairy Sci 71(Suppl 1):209 (abstract), 1988.
46. Chalupa W, Baird L, Soderholm C, et al: Responses of dairy cows to somatotropin. J Dairy Sci 70(Suppl 1):176 (abstract), 1987.
47. Rajmahendran R, Desbottes S, Shelford JA, et al: Effect of recombinant bovine somatotropin (rbST) on milk production and reproductive performance of dairy cows. J Dairy Sci 72(Suppl 1):444 (abstract), 1989.
48. Palmquist DL: Response of high-producing cows given daily injections of recombinant bovine somatotropin from D 30-296 of lactation. J Dairy Sci 71(Suppl 1):206 (abstract), 1988.
49. Burton JH, McBride BW, Bateman K, et al: Recombinant bovine somatotropin: effects on production and reproduction in lactating cows. J Dairy Sci 70(Suppl 1):175 (abstract), 1987.
50. Hard DL, Cole WJ, Franson SE, et al: Effect of long-term sometribove,

USAN (recombinant methionyl bovine somatotropin), treatment in a prolonged release system on milk yield, animal health, and reproductive performance—pooled across four sites. J Dairy Sci 71(Suppl 1):210 (abstract), 1988.
51. Boyd LJ, Seath DM, Olds D: Relationship between level of milk production and breeding efficiency in dairy cattle. J Anim Sci 13:89, 1954.
52. Spalding RW, Everett RW, Foote RH: Fertility in New York artificially inseminated Holstein herds in dairy herd improvement. J Dairy Sci 58:718, 1975.
53. Olds D, Cooper T, Thrift FA: Relationship between milk yield and fertility in dairy cattle. J Dairy Sci 62:1140, 1979.
54. Burger PJ, Shanks RD, Freeman AE, et al: Genetic aspects of milk yield and reproductive performance. J Dairy Sci 64:114, 1981.
55. Laben RL, Shanks RD, Burger PJ, et al: Factors affecting milk yield and reproductive performance. J Dairy Sci 65:1004, 1982.
56. Hamudikuwanda H, Erb HN: Effects of 60-day milk yield on postpartum breeding performance in Holstein cows. J Dairy Sci 70:2355, 1987.
57. Lean IJ, Galland JC, Scott JL: Relationship between fertility, peak milk yields and lactational persistency in diary cows. Theriogenology 31:1093, 1989.
58. Butler WR, Smith RD: Interrelationships between energy and postpartum reproductive function in dairy cattle. J Dairy Sci 72:767, 1989.
59. Villa-Godoy A, Hughes TL, Emery RS, et al: Association between energy balance and luteal function in lactating dairy cows. J Dairy Sci 71:1063, 1988.
60. Herrler A, Farries E, Neimann H: A trial to stimulate insulin-like growth factor 1 levels to improve superovulatory responses in dairy cows. Theriogenology 33:248, 1990.
61. Spicer LJ, Enright WJ: Concentrations of insulin-like growth factor I (IGF-I) in follicular fluid (FFL) of preovulatory bovine ovarian follicles: effect of daily injections of potent growth hormone (GH)–releasing factor (GRF) analog and/or thyrotropin-releasing hormone (TRH). J Dairy Sci 72(Suppl 1):346 (abstract), 1989.
62. Wilkinson JID, McGuffey RK: Recent developments in somatotropin research. Fourth International Symposium on Modern Cattle Production, German Cattle Breeders Association (DGL), Giessen, FRG, November 24–26, 1989.

Anthelmintic Therapy

ROBERT M. CORWIN, DVM, PhD

Effectiveness or efficacy of an anthelmintic drug against target species of helminth parasites to relieve the host animal of that burden is the apparent rationale for its delivery. Usually the target parasite species is one of a complex deemed most important from a clinical, subclinical (economic), or pathophysiologic appraisal, such as the cattle abomasal worm *Ostertagia ostertagi*, which is part of the parasitic gastroenteric complex of worm species. *Ostertagia* is considered to be the most important worm parasite of cattle on a worldwide basis and was selected as a target species for testing the efficacy of the newer generation of anthelmintic drugs. This efficacy is determined by controlled-critical studies in which necropsy of experimental cattle is performed at a specific time after drug treatment; the *O. ostertagi* parasites remaining in abomasa from treated versus nontreated animals are then compared. A less precise measurement is qualitative and quantitative fecal examination for parasite eggs before and after treatment. Variability in egg production occurs per parasite species during the different parasitic phases in the host and with changes in host physiologic conditions, which thus makes this observation less reliable.

In addition to specific efficacy, spectrum of activity must be established in terms of the number of parasite species affected, the degree of removal of each (such as ≥90 per cent), and the stages eliminated (e.g., larval vs. adult). With the cattle parasitic gastroenteric complex, there are a number of trichostrongylid species, which include *Haemonchus, Ostertagia, Trichostrongylus, Cooperia,* and *Nematodirus;* the strongylid *Oesophagostomum;* perhaps the whipworm *Trichuris;* the tapeworm *Moniezia;* and, extending outside this environment, the lungworm *Dictyocaulus*. In the past 30 years, drugs developed and marketed have shown exceptional activity against many if not all these worm species, especially against their adult stages. Some have larvicidal activity as well, which is so important with *O. ostertagi* infections in which the inhibited fourth-stage larva (L_4) and the emergent fifth stage (L_5) or immature stage can be devastating in a sequela of pathophysiologic changes. Thus, anthelmintic drugs with a broad spectrum of activity including larvicidal are desirable, have been developed, and are marketed.

Safety as determined by therapeutic index is of paramount importance. This is monitored by changes in feed consumption; loss of weight or depressed weight gain and scouring; aberrant nervous behavior; chronic debilitation; reproductive abnormalities such as fetal anomalies, abortion, and stillbirths; and acute to chronic death. If there has been evidence of teratogenicity, mutagenicity, and the like, then avoidance of a certain period during gestation is stated. Most of the newer generations of anthelmintic drugs are quite safe as indicated by a factor greater than 3 to greater than 100 times the recommended dose; these are mandated to list any potential toxic problems at higher than recommended dose levels, for administration during times of stress (especially during breeding and pregnancy or physical debilitation), or for a given breed such as *Bos indicus*. Tissue residue as a food safety factor has received much attention recently. This includes retention of the drug and its metabolites in meat, milk, and excreta. Withdrawal times are given for each of these more recently approved drugs, whereas this might not be stated for older compounds.

Response of individuals and herds or flocks to administration of an anthelmintic drug should be monitored by overall appearance and conditioning, presence or absence of adverse reactions, and efficacy as determined by decrease of parasite eggs per gram in a 3- to 5-week period after treatment. Variability in response might be due to the following factors.

1. Stage of parasite development at time of treatment. Newer drugs are more likely to have larvicidal as well as adulticidal effects, including activity against inhibited or dormant and migrating larvae. Post-treatment examination of fecal samples is necessary to determine this effect. Be aware that under natural field conditions, reinfection does occur; but also consider prepatent periods of 2 to 4 weeks dependent on parasite species and dormancy of larvae, namely, *O. ostertagi* of 14 to 18 weeks.

2. Climate conditions or seasonality. Seasonality of treatment has been tested in the field from 1980 to 1990; this varies per geographic region, by husbandry, and by climatic conditions with each year. Precipitation, temperature, forage and soil type, conventional versus intensive rotational grazing, and stocking rate per given season are major influences in maintenance of pasture contamination and possible infection rate. Strategic deworming programs for livestock have been recommended on the basis of target parasite species, climatic conditions, and herd management. For beef cow and calf production, cows should be dewormed after the calving season, that is, just before turnout onto summer pasture, spring calves by midsummer, and all stock at weaning in late fall. If this is a fall calving operation, then cows should be dewormed before overwintering and all stock in the spring before summer pasturing. Yearling spring calves and fall calves, grazed as stockers, should be dewormed in the late spring and, if on intensively grazed summer pasture, again in the summer. All backgrounded stock brought into the feedlot should be dewormed (including a flukicide) when they are received. These programs should greatly reduce *Ostertagia* populations, including inhibited larvae.

For sheep, deworming is necessary before breeding and lambing. All sheep in the flock need to be dewormed at 3- to 4-week intervals when forage is lush, the temperature warm, and precipitation adequate for forage growth. *Haemonchus contortus* is the target species.

3. Drug metabolism and kinetics. Pharmacokinetics of a given drug varies per host species, breed, and individual. Some drugs are more effective at repeated small doses, whereas others are quite effective with one administration.

4. Physical and immunologic condition of the host. Certainly the best-conditioned animal will respond best to a well-designed drug and well-conceived program. If the animal metabolizes poorly or is immunodeficient, poor response will be observed regardless of these efforts. Observe others in the herd to appreciate overall effect.

5. Nutritional status of the host. Those animals with nutritional deficiencies due to metabolic abnormalities or inexperience with a given ration will not utilize the best of drugs.

6. Genetics of the host and of the parasite. Selective breeding of cattle, sheep, and goats has been and is under way to establish breeds and lineage within a breed for response to parasite infection. There have also been demonstrated differences in genetic response for drug metabolism; for example, some breeds are more susceptible to organophosphates or to larger than recommended dose levels of a given drug.

Strains of parasite respond differently to their environment, including outside and within the host, and to given drug classes. Physical factors such as degrees of ensheathment, response to sudden environmental changes such as cold stress, escaping immune response, and ability to metabolically avoid otherwise effective drugs are described for given species and strains.

7. Parasite resistance to drugs. Resistance of parasites to anthelmintic drugs has been documented and is being monitored. This has occurred in countries such as Australia and New Zealand where stock are dewormed more intensively but has appeared in the United States in the late 1980s. Sheep are involved most frequently, but goats have been also. When eggs per gram are made from fecal samples of treated animals, those with resistant parasite species will show a lessened response or increasing number of eggs over time in spite of continuing drug use. For avoiding development of drug resistance in a parasite population, classes of compounds should be alternated each year and their activity monitored. Do not alternate within a given class, such as with albendazole and fenbendazole in the benzimidazole group.

A number of factors confuse this issue, namely, poor or inadequate administration, poor scheduling, and use of a drug not targeted for a given species of parasite. Another consideration is identification of the species involved; for example, there are a number of trichostrongylid species, but with the exception of *Nematodirus* spp., larvated eggs need to be cultured to the infective L_3 stage for specific identification. *Cooperia* spp. are more numerous in population size and seemingly more drug tolerant, and therefore eggs per gram alone do not substantiate resistance.

The following description of anthelmintic drugs is presented alphabetically by class of compounds, that is, avermectins, benzimidazoles, and so on. A brief chemical description, mode and spectrum of activity, dose level and mode of administration, possible adverse effects, therapeutic index, and approved host use are included. Compounds not readily available or no longer marketed are mentioned at the end of this article.

AVERMECTINS

The avermectins are derived from fermentation products of the soil microorganism *Streptomyces avermitilis* and as such are antibiotics, although their antimicrobial activity is insignificant but some do possess anthelmintic and ectoparasiticide properties.

Ivermectin

Currently, ivermectin (Ivomec[1]) is the only avermectin approved and marketed as an anthelmintic for livestock including cattle, sheep, and swine. Its mechanism of action is to stimulate release of γ-aminobutyric acid (GABA), an inhibitory neurotransmitter that causes paralysis and slow death of target parasitic nematodes and certain arthropods. Because tapeworms, flukes, and protozoans such as coccidia do not possess GABA, ivermectin is not effective against them. In the mammalian host, GABA is present only in the central nervous system and would be unaffected by ivermectin in the normal healthy animal because of the blood-brain barrier.

The recommended dose level for cattle is 200 µg/kg. This is effective for the treatment and control of *Haemonchus placei, Ostertagia ostertagi* (adults; fourth-stage larvae including inhibited), *O. lyrata, Trichostrongylus axei, T. colubriformis, Cooperia oncophora, C. punctata, C. pectinata, Oesophagostomum radiatum, Nematodirus helvetianus* (adults only), *N. spathiger* (adults only), the lungworm *Dictyocaulus viviparus,* ectoparasites such as cattle grubs *Hypoderma bovis* and *H. lineatum,* the sucking lice *Linognathus vituli* and *Haematopinus eurysternus,* and the scabies mites *Psoroptes ovis* and *Sarcoptes scabiei* var. *bovis.*

Ivermectin is available as a 1 per cent solution for subcutaneous injection in cattle only and is *not* to be administered by intramuscular or intravenous injection. Doses greater than 10 ml should be divided between 2 injection sites in the neck region. Each milliliter of ivermectin per 110 pounds or 50 kg body weight will provide the recommended dose of 200 µg/kg. Observation should be made of treated cattle for injection site reactions, which would be swelling and discomfort that may progress to clostridial infection. As with any grubicide, proper timing of treatment by geographic region is necessary to avoid bloat, paralysis, and possible death due to disintegration of grubs in esophageal and spinal cord sites. In safety studies, toxic signs appeared only with doses exceeding 30 times the recommended dose. The recommended dose does not affect breeding performance of bulls or cows. Cattle must not be treated within 35 days of slaughter. Because a withdrawal time has not been established for milk, ivermectin should not be used in dairy cows of breeding age.

Ivermectin binds to the soil and is inactivated over time, but free ivermectin may affect fish and water-borne organisms adversely so that contamination of lakes, streams, and ponds must be avoided, including run-off from feedlots.

In 1990, ivermectin (Ivomec Sheep Drench 0.08 per cent solution with 3 per cent benzyl alcohol) was approved and marketed for sheep *only.* It is available in 4.8 L containers, ready to use as a free-flowing solution with any standard drenching equipment. Administration is 0.2 mg/kg orally or 3 ml/26 lb; this appears to be much more than the cattle dose, but note the percentage solution of each preparation. In sheep, ivermectin is effective against the adult and L_4 stages of gastrointestinal worms *Haemonchus contortus, Ostertagia circumcincta, Trichostrongylus axei, T. colubriformis, Cooperia curticei, Nematodirus spathiger, N. battus,* and *Oesophagostomum columbianum* and the lungworm *Dictyocaulus filaria;* adults only of *Haemonchus placei, Cooperia oncophora, Strongyloides papillosus, Oesophagostomum viviparus, Trichuris ovis,* and *Chabertia ovina;* and all larval stages of the nasal

---

[1]MSD AGVET, Division of Merck & Co., Inc., Rahway, NJ 07065.

bot *Oestrus ovis*. Do not administer within 11 days of slaughter, and as with dairy cows, do not administer to milking ewes. Other animal species should not be given Ivomec Sheep Drench.

Ivermectin (Ivomec Swine Injectable) is available for swine in 2 formulations, a 0.27 per cent solution for grower-feeder pigs at 1 ml/20 lb body weight and a 1 per cent solution for adult pigs at 1 ml/75 lb body weight, both given by subcutaneous injection in the neck region. This delivers 300 µg/kg body weight and is effective in the removal of *Ascaris suum* (adults, L_4), *Oesophagostomum* spp. (adults, L_4), *Metastrongylus* spp. (adults), *Hyostrongylus rubidus* (adults, L_4), *Strongyloides ransomi* (adults), *Haematopinus suis*, and *Sarcoptes scabiei* var *suis*. Withdrawal is 18 days before slaughter.

Warning: do *not* give this to other animal species not approved as cited in the preceding. Fatalities have occurred with livestock formulations given to dogs.

Precaution: do *not* expose containers of ivermectin to ultraviolet light because this breaks down the drug; heat and freezing do *not* affect the product.

BENZIMIDAZOLES

There are 3 benzimidazole carbamate anthelmintic drugs now approved and marketed for livestock. Thiabendazole is the progenitor of this group with later analogues collectively called substituted benzimidazole carbamates. All inhibit fumarate reductase blocking mitochondrial function in the parasite which depletes glycogen reserves. Each may have specific but different activities as well.

Albendazole

Albendazole (Valbazen[1]) is the most recently approved of this group for cattle only in the United States, where it is not approved for use in sheep, goats, or swine. It differs from the other benzimidazoles in being effective in killing adult liver flukes, *Fasciola hepatica*, at 8 weeks after infection. It is also effective for all parasitic stages of *Ostertagia ostertagi* (including inhibited L_4); adult and L_4 stages of *Haemonchus contortus* and *H. placei*, *Trichostrongylus axei*, *Nematodirus spathiger* and *N. helvetianus*, and *Cooperia punctata* and *C. oncophora*; *Bunostomum phlebotomum* (adults); *Trichostrongylus colubriformis* (adults); *Oesophagostomum radiatum* (adults); *Dictyocaulus viviparus* (adults, L_4); and *Moniezia* spp. (scolices and segments). Albendazole is administered as an 11.36 per cent suspension in an oral drench at 10 mg/kg or 4.54 mg/lb. It has no overt toxic effects at 4.5 times the highest recommended therapeutic dose level, and it is tolerated at 7.5 times the recommended therapeutic dose. At 2.5 times the highest recommended therapeutic dose, it had no significant effect on pregnancy, incidence of stillborn calves, or condition of calves at birth. However, because an adequate margin of safety for administration during breeding or early gestation has not been established, albendazole should not be administered during the first 45 days of pregnancy.

Fenbendazole

Fenbendazole (Panacur[2]) was approved for use in cattle in the United States in 1983. The dosage approved was 5 mg/kg, which is effective in the removal of adult *Haemonchus contortus*, *Ostertagia ostertagi*, *Trichostrongylus axei*, *T. colubriformis*, *Bunostomum phlebotomum*, *Nematodirus helvetianus*, *Cooperia* spp., *Oesophagostomum radiatum*, and the lungworm *Dictyocaulus viviparus*. Subsequent approvals provide label indication for removal of immature stages of most gastrointestinal nematodes at 5 mg/kg and removal of inhibited L_4 of *O. ostertagi* and the tapeworm *Moniezia* spp. at 10 mg/kg. Fenbendazole is available as a 10 per cent suspension and in a multidose 10 per cent paste cartridge. Withdrawal is 8 days before slaughter. Feed grade formulations of fenbendazole are also available. The Enproal/Safe-Guard Deworming Supplement Block provides fenbendazole in a dose of 5 mg/kg over a 3-day consumption period. Cattle must not be slaughtered within 11 days after the last treatment. A 20 per cent type A fenbendazole premix is also available to be mixed in the complete feed for a 1-day treatment providing 5 mg/kg. The premix can also be used to manufacture medicated crumbles, pellets, and cubes. Most recently, a fenbendazole free-choice mineral mix has become available to deworm cattle. The total dose of 5 mg/kg can be consumed over a 3- to 6-day period. Cattle must not be slaughtered within 13 days after the last treatment. Because a withdrawal time has not been established, do not use any of the fenbendazole formulations in dairy cattle of breeding age.

For swine, fenbendazole was introduced in the United States in 1984. At a total dose of 9 mg/kg over a consecutive 3- to 12-day period, it is effective in removal of the large roundworm *Ascaris suum* (adults and larvae in the liver, lung, and intestine), the nodular worms *Oesophagostomum dentatum* and *O. quadrispinulatum*, the small stomach worm *Hyostrongylus rubidus*, the whipworm *Trichuris suis* (adults and larvae in the intestinal mucosa), the kidney worm *Stephanurus dentatus* (adults and larvae), and the lungworm *Metastrongylus apri* and *M. pudendotectus*. Fenbendazole is available as an 8 per cent premix. There is no slaughter withdrawal time in pigs for use as labeled.

Fenbendazole has a broad margin of safety; 100 times the recommended dose for cattle is not toxic. It can be used safely in all breeding animals and concurrently with vaccines, growth implants, and organophosphate treatments in cattle and with feed additive antibiotics in swine without adverse effects.

Thiabendazole

Thiabendazole (TBZ[1]) was approved for use in cattle, sheep, goats, and swine in the early 1960s. In cattle, the recommended dosage is 66 mg/kg in a 43 per cent cattle paste, 2 g or 15 g boluses, 3.3 per cent cubes, and a suspension for *Haemonchus* spp., *Ostertagia* spp., *Trichostrongylus* spp., and *Oesophagostomum radiatum*. A dose of 110 mg/kg is recommended for severe infections of these parasites and for *Cooperia* spp. Treatment may be repeated within 2 to 3 weeks if indicated. Cattle should not be treated within 3 days of slaughter, and milk from treated cows must be withheld from market for 96 hours after treatment (8 milkings).

For sheep and goats, a dosage of 44 mg/kg (6.6 per cent pellets) is recommended for control of *Haemonchus* spp., *Ostertagia* spp., *Trichostrongylus* spp., *Cooperia* spp., *Nematodirus* spp., *Bunostomum* spp., *Strongyloides* spp., *Chabertia* spp., and *Oesophagostomum* spp. In goats with severe infections, 66 mg/kg is recommended. Milk from dairy goats must be withheld from market for 96 hours; sheep and goats must be withheld from slaughter for 30 days after treatment.

Thiabendazole is approved for baby pigs infected with *Strongyloides ransomi* as a paste at 62 to 83 mg/kg with

---
[1]Norden Laboratories, Inc., 601 W Cornhusker Hwy., P.O. Box 80809, Lincoln, NE 68501.
[2]Hoechst-Roussel Agri-Vet Co., Rt. 202–206 North, Somerville, NJ 08876.

[1]MSD AGVET, Division of Merck & Co., Inc., Rahway, NJ 07065.

retreatment in 5 to 7 days if necessary. For *Ascaris suum* prevention, thiabendazole is added to the feed at 0.05 to 0.1 per cent per ton of feed for 2 weeks and then at 0.005 to 0.02 per cent per ton for 8 to 14 weeks. A withdrawal time of 30 days before slaughter is necessary.

Thiabendazole has been shown to be safe at 20 times the therapeutic level even for debilitated and very young animals and is safe for pregnant animals.

CLORSULON

Clorsulon (Curatrem[1]) is a flukicidal drug commercially available for control of *Fasciola hepatica* in cattle. It is a 4-amino-6-trichloroethenyl-1,3-benzenedisulfonamide that inhibits glycolytic pathways of flukes. It has greater than 99 per cent efficacy against adult *F. hepatica* and 94 per cent against stages over 8 weeks of age in the bile ducts. It is administered as an oral drench (1-qt container) at 7 mg/kg body weight with an 8-day withdrawal period and can be used in conjunction with other anthelmintics. Commercial recommendations are that cattle should be treated in the northern United States in the fall after freezing and again in late winter–early spring and in the southern United States in late fall and in late spring to reduce adult *F. hepatica* populations and consequently egg production and pasture contamination.

IMIDAZOTHIAZOLES

Levamisole

Levamisole (Tramisol,[2] Levasole[3]) is the L-isomer of DL-tetramisole and was approved for use in cattle, sheep, and swine in the United States in the late 1960s and early 1970s. It is available as a phosphate salt for subcutaneous injection in cattle, as a hydrochloride salt in an oral gel for cattle, as oral boluses for cattle and sheep and as a soluble powder for drenching cattle and sheep, as a pour-on for cattle, and for drinking water for pigs.

In cattle, levamisole is indicated for the removal of the gastrointestinal nematodes *Haemonchus* spp., *Ostertagia* spp., *Trichostrongylus* spp., *Cooperia* spp., *Nematodirus* spp., *Bunostomum* spp., and *Oesophagostomum* spp., and the lungworm *Dictyocaulus viviparus*. At 8 mg/kg, it is highly effective against adult forms of these parasites and less so against immature stages. Withdrawal of treatment before slaughter is 2 days for oral administration, 7 days for injection, and 9 days for the pour-on. It is not to be used in dairy cows of breeding age.

The approved dose for sheep formulations is 8 mg/kg for removal of *Haemonchus* spp., *Ostertagia* spp., *Trichostrongylus* spp., *Nematodirus* spp., *Bunostomum* spp., *Oesophagostomum* spp., *Chabertia* spp., and *Dictyocaulus viviparus*. Withdrawal of treatment for sheep is 3 days.

For swine, levamisole is recommended at 8 mg/kg for removal of *Ascaris suum*, *Oesophagostomum* spp., *Strongyloides*, *Stephanurus*, and *Metastrongylus*. A withdrawal time of 3 days must be observed.

Levamisole has a narrow margin of safety; slight muzzle foaming occurs in cattle given 2 times the subcutaneous injection dose recommended with occasional swelling at the site of injection. Usually, reactions disappear in a short time. It is not contraindicated in pregnant animals.

---

[1]MSD AGVET, Division of Merck & Co., Inc., Rahway, NJ 07065.
[2]American Cyanamid Co., P.O. Box 400, Princeton, NJ 08540.
[3]Pitman-Moore, P.O. Box 344, Washington Crossing, NJ 08560.

ORGANOPHOSPHATES

Dichlorvos

Dichlorvos (Atgard[1]) is formulated in a polyvinyl chloride resin that adds stability to and delays release of the drug, thus reducing its toxicity and enhancing overall delivery to the gastrointestinal tract. It is approved for use in swine only of the food-producing group. Formulations include Atgard as resin pellets in a litter-pack to be added to the ration at time of use and Atgard-C and XLP-30 for bulk feeds. Dichlorvos is indicated for the removal of adult and immature *Ascaris suum*, *Oesophagostomum* spp., *Trichuris suis*, and *Ascarops strongylina*. Atgard added to the feed and administered shortly after mixing is approximately 17 mg/kg as a single treatment and may be repeated in 4 to 5 weeks. Atgard-C given for a single treatment is 479 g/ton of feed or 348 g/ton for 2 consecutive days. For pregnant sows, XLP-30 is fed at 334 to 500 g/ton for the last 30 days' gestation, providing 1 g/head/day.

Dichlorvos is generally safe in swine, although softening of stools may occur occasionally; at a too-large dose, organophosphate toxicosis may be seen. This drug should not be used with other cholinesterase inhibitors. When it is mixed with complete feeds, feeds must not be pelleted and must remain dry. There are no withholding requirements for slaughter of treated pigs.

PIPERAZINE

Generic piperazine salts have been available since the 1930s. Salts include adipate, citrate, hydrochloride, phosphate, sulfate, and tartrate. Efficacy of these is similar. Piperazine is available in powder for drinking water and premix for feed. It is primarily a swine anthelmintic with moderate efficacy for removal of *Ascaris suum* and *Oesophagostomum* at a single dose of 110 mg/kg. Herd treatment is accomplished with 0.2 to 0.4 per cent piperazine in feed or 0.1 to 0.2 per cent in water. All medicated feed or water should be consumed in 8 to 12 hours; therefore fasting or withholding of water overnight may be useful before treatment. Retreatment is recommended after 2 months. Drug withdrawal times have not been established for swine. It has a wide margin of safety and can be used during pregnancy.

TETRAHYDROPYRIMIDINES

Morantel

In the United States, morantel tartrate (Rumatel,[2] Nematel[2]) is commercially available for cattle as an oral bolus or as a medicated premix. The premix is added to complete feeds to provide 0.968 mg/100 kg of morantel tartrate. Do not mix in feeds containing bentonite. At 9.68 mg/kg (4.4 mg/lb), mature *Haemonchus* spp., *Ostertagia* spp., *Trichostrongylus* spp., *Cooperia* spp., *Nematodirus* spp., and *Oesophagostomum radiatum* are removed. Do not use with severely debilitated cattle or in dairy cows of breeding age. Withdrawal time before slaughter is 14 days.

Pyrantel

Pyrantel tartrate (Banminth[2]) is approved for use as a swine premix. It is recommended for addition to the ration at 800

---

[1]SDS Biotech Corp., Animal Health Business, Painesville, OH 44077.
[2]Pfizer, Inc., Agricultural Division, 235 E 42nd St., NY, NY 10017.

mg/ton (22 mg/kg) for a single treatment in removal of *Ascaris suum* and *Oesophagostomum* spp. or at 96 g/ton (2.6 mg/kg) for a 3-day treatment for removal and prevention of *A. suum* and prevention of *Oesophagostomum* spp. Pyrantel is also supplied as a fixed combination product with carbadox for swine up to 34 kg. Withdrawal before slaughter is 24 hours with pyrantel only, and 10 weeks with carbadox.

Pyrantel does have some cholinergic activity, but there is no evidence against its use with other cholinergic drugs. It is safe to use during the growth phase and pregnancy.

MISCELLANEOUS

Anthelmintics once used often but now infrequently or not at all include organophosphates such as coumaphos and haloxon, phenothiazine, and hygromycin. For information about these, please refer to Current Veterinary Therapy: Food Animal Practice 2.

External Parasiticides

LARRY F. MOORE, DVM
JAMES A. SHMIDL, DVM, MS

External parasiticides are compounds used in the control of insects and arachnids (mites, ticks, and so on). They are more commonly referred to as animal insecticides. External parasiticides are normally used on food-producing animals (1) to treat severe infestations that result in clinical disease, (2) to increase production of meat and other products of animal origin, and (3) to stop or prevent the spread of insect or arachnid-borne disease.

BOTANICAL AND CHLORINATED HYDROCARBON COMPOUNDS

The first products used for the control of external parasites of food-producing animals were botanicals. Examples are rotenone, nicotine, and natural pyrethrin. These compounds had limited application and usefulness. The first highly effective compounds were the chlorinated hydrocarbons, such as DDT and toxaphene. Their development coincided with the beginning of the modern era of agriculture, at which time there occurred a great increase in agricultural productivity. Humanity was no longer at the mercy of parasitic pests that affected its domesticized plants or animals.

The chlorinated hydrocarbon insecticides, although highly effective, had some serious shortcomings. They were quite persistent, being chemically stable and slow to degrade in the environment. In addition, a stable body residue developed in exposed organisms. With some compounds, an interesting phenomenon developed, termed biologic magnification. Biologic magnification, which led to harmful consequences in the environment, began as a residue in the lowest or the first organism in the food chain. An aquatic insect with a residue was eaten by a fish, which in turn was consumed by a larger fish, which was eaten by a bird. Each succeeding species accumulated a greater body residue than did the organism it consumed. In some cases, this process extended toxic manifestation to the species at the top of the food chain. Even after years of extensive study, these compounds' toxic mode of action was poorly understood, and there were no antidotes. Most chlorinated hydrocarbons have been removed from the market owing to environmental issues with the re-registration process required by the Environmental Protection Agency (EPA).

ORGANOPHOSPHATE COMPOUNDS

The subsequent development of organophosphate compounds gave the agriculturist and the veterinarian effective tools to control pests on plants or animals. These compounds are systemic in action, that is, they are translocated in the body of the plant or animal. Dermal application of a systemic organophosphate compound controls parasites in remote anatomic locations. The most important indicator of the presence of organophosphate compounds is cholinesterase depression. This class of compounds is in general more acutely toxic than are the chlorinated hydrocarbon compounds. Atropine is the most effective antidote for organophosphate parasiticides, but with the bovine an elevated dose is required; thus, the label should be consulted for dosage directions. The oxime compound 2-PAM, in combination with atropine, is effective for treating intoxication by organophosphate compounds. Organophosphate compounds are rather unstable after application and do not magnify in the environment. They are rapidly metabolized and eliminated from the body. The re-registration process by EPA has caused elimination of many products because of environmental issues and/or economics.

PYRETHROIDS

Some of the more recently developed external parasiticide compounds are synthetic pyrethrin or pyrethroid compounds. They are more effective and economical than are the natural pyrethrins. The advent of insecticide ear tags was followed by a wide variety of usages and formulations containing these pyrethroids.

AVERMECTINS

The newest animal parasiticides developed are the avermectins. Avermectins have a broad spectrum of activity against both internal and external parasites. These compounds were isolated from fermentation of the soil organism *Streptomyces avermitilis* and have a neurotoxic action on the parasite.

External parasites controlled by avermectins include grubs, mites, and sucking lice. Formulations for food animals include an injectable for cattle and swine, a combination injectable avermectin and flukicide for cattle, and an oral drench for sheep. A pour-on formulation is approved in other countries but has not yet been approved in the United States.

PARASITICIDE USE

Modern chemistry provided the veterinarian highly effective external parasiticides, but it is important that they be used according to label recommendations. Every product should be used solely on the animal species for which it is labeled, and only the label-prescribed dose should be applied for that specific parasitic infestation. The misuse of animal medications has brought unfavorable publicity because of illegal residues in human food. When examining a label, one must pay strict attention to the duration after treatment in which milk must be discarded or animals held from slaughter for food. To adhere to all label recommendations is the professional responsibility of every veterinarian who uses or recommends the use of an animal medication. Veterinarians must resist the thought that a product labeled for the control of a parasite in one species of animal may be used in another species without residue or toxic problems. The product should not be used on a host species for which there is no label recommendation. There could be several reasons for lack of label recommendations, including a lack of residue data, excessive residue of the compound or its metabolites in the host, and insufficient margin between safe and harmful doses. Products vary in safety factors. In any occurrence of toxicity associated with an external parasiticide, there is usually a history of accidental exposure or use contrary to label directions. Veterinarians are often required to make difficult clinical decisions when they encounter a severe infestation that is causing a pathologic condition in host animals that may be complicated by adverse climatic conditions. A product and method of application must be selected that will control the parasite without causing undue stress to the host animal. The products that are available as external parasiticides for use on food animals have all been reviewed and approved by a government agency for ensuring that the product is effective as labeled, is safe to the host species, and will not result in an unacceptable residue.

Treatment

Active ingredients have been formulated into a number of products for application by several treatment methods. These include the following approaches.

Pour-on products are formulated in a dilute solution so that they may be poured down the back of the animal. They are easy to use and have become a popular method for treating cattle for grubs (*Hypoderma* spp.). Some of these products are also approved for the control of cattle and swine lice.

The low-volume products such as Spotton (fenthion) and Dursban (chlorpyrifos) are formulated with a higher concentration of active compound than are the pour-on products. They are also applied to the backs of cattle. They are easy to apply, and their spectrum of activity is similar to that of pour-on products.

Solutions for dip vat use and whole body spray (applied with a high-pressure sprayer) have similar uses, advantages, and disadvantages. These treatment methods are effectively used for ticks, flies, grubs, lice, and mange control. The dip vat is an effective application method and is used in cattle feedlot operations and tick control programs. Whole-body sprays, although still used, are not as popular as they were in earlier times. The main disadvantage of both treatment methods is their use during severe cold weather.

The backrubber is one of the oldest "self-treatment" methods used for applying parasiticides to cattle or swines. There are several types on the market. This application method has several advantages, one of which is ease of application, because infested animals tend to seek out and use a rubber. The disadvantage of the backrubber is that it must be serviced regularly so that proper dispensing of the parasiticide is ensured.

Dust bags have generally the same advantages as the backrubber has but are usually more effective because they require less servicing and dispense the parasiticide more consistently when used by cattle. The dust bags are especially effective for horn fly and lice control, and their use has grown in recent years. They may be hung where cattle are forced to dust themselves, such as in gateways to pastures, or they may be located where cattle congregate and use them at will.

The insecticide ear tag containing pyrethroids was widely used in the early 1980s. It proved to be a useful method for horn fly control, especially when continuous control was important. Approved insecticidal ear tags gave season-long control in some areas. The pyrethroid-resistant fly became a problem in the mid 1980s; therefore insecticide ear tags were developed containing organophosphate compounds. In the late 1980s, second-generation pyrethroids (i.e., λ-cyhalothrin and cyfluthrin) were introduced in an ear tag formulation.

Other methods of application, such as mist sprayers, foggers, and treadle sprayers, do not have wide application. They may be of use in special situations.

The introduction of avermectins in injectable formulation represented an alternative to the dip vat and pour-on products. Market figures show wide acceptance because of spectrum and/or dosage form.

In determining what product or treatment method to use, several considerations need to be made. It is obvious that the treatment of choice should be effective in the control of the parasite, cause no untoward reaction in the host, and be easy to apply and economical to use. These several considerations are the reasons that so many products and methods of application have been developed.

Tables 1 to 4 list common products used for external parasite control on cattle, sheep, goats, and swine. The products are listed by common (generic) name and trade name when possible. These tables are not intended to be an all-inclusive listing of products for the noted indications but are only representative. The current label must be studied thoroughly

Text continued on page 58

Table 1. SOME COMMON PRODUCTS USED FOR EXTERNAL PARASITE CONTROL ON CATTLE

Product	Company and Address	Marketed Formulation	Pest	Method of Application	Withdrawal Period Before Slaughter (days)	Comments
Chlorpyrifos CPF44 Dursban	Fort Dodge Laboratories Fort Dodge, IA 50501	Low-volume pour-on	Lice and horn flies	Backline treatment	14 (after initial treatment)	Read precautions statement (discontinued as of 12/90)
Coumaphos All formulations	Mobay Corporation Animal Health Division Box 390 Shawnee Mission, KS 66201	Wettable powder	Horn flies, lice, ticks, grubs, screwworms, and mites	Spray or dip	0	Treat lactating dairy cattle only at lower dilution
		Flowable	Horn flies, lice, ticks, screwworms, and mites	Spray or dip	0	Treat lactating dairy cattle only at lower dilution

Table 1. SOME COMMON PRODUCTS USED FOR EXTERNAL PARASITE CONTROL ON CATTLE Continued

Product	Company and Address	Marketed Formulation	Pest	Method of Application	Withdrawal Period Before Slaughter (days)	Comments
		Liquid (ELI)	Horn flies, face flies, lice, ticks, and grubs	Spray or backrubber	0	Treat lactating dairy cattle only at lower dilution
		Dust (1%)	Horn flies and lice	Dust bag or shaker can	0	Apply no more than 2 oz per animal per day
		Dust (5%)	Screwworms and ear ticks	Spot treatment	0	Treat wounds with light, but thorough coverage
		K.R.S. spray foam	Screwworms, fly maggots, and ear ticks	Aerosol spray	0	Spray wound until complete coverage is obtained
Dichlorvos Vapona	Fermenta Animal Health 10150 N Executive Hills Blvd. Box 901350 Kansas City, MO 64190–1350	Liquid	Horn flies, face flies, stable flies, and house flies	Spray	0	Do not exceed 2 oz per animal daily as a fine-mist spray
Dichlorvos-tetrachlorvinphos Ravap	Fermenta Animal Health Kansas City, MO 64190–1350	Liquid	Horn flies, face flies, lice, and ticks	Spray or backrubber	0	Approved for lactating dairy and beef cattle; do not spray more often than every 10 days
Famphur Warbex	American Cyanamid Co. P.O. Box 400 Princeton, NJ 08540	Pour-on	Grubs and lice	Backline treatment	35	Do not treat lactating dairy cattle or within 21 days of freshening; do not treat Brahman bulls
Fenthion Lysoff	Mobay Corporation Shawnee Mission, KS 66201	Pour-on	Lice and horn flies	Backline treatment	21 (single treatment)	Dilute with water before use; do not use in female dairy cattle of breeding age
Spotton	Mobay Corporation Shawnee Mission, KS 66201	Low-volume pour-on	Grubs and lice	Spot treatment on the backline	45	Do not treat dairy cattle of breeding age
Tiguvon	Mobay Corporation Shawnee Mission, KS 66201	Pour-on	Grubs and lice	Backline treatment	35 (single treatment)	Do not treat lactating dairy cattle
Ivermectin Ivomec	MSD AGVET Div. of Merck & Co., Inc. Rahway, NJ 07065–0912	Injectable	Grubs, mites, and sucking lice	Inject subcutaneously	35	Do not use in female dairy cattle of breeding age
Ivomec F	MSD AGVET Rahway, NJ 07065–0912	Injectable	Grubs, mites, and sucking lice	Inject subcutaneously	49	Do not use in female dairy cattle of breeding age
Lindane Screwworm and Ear Tick Killer	Pitman-Moore 421 E Hawley St. Mundelein, IL 60060	Pressurized spray	Screwworm larvae, fleeceworms, and Spinose ear ticks	Direct application	0	Use sparingly on calves under 3 months of age; do not treat lactating dairy cattle

Table continued on following page

Table 1. SOME COMMON PRODUCTS USED FOR EXTERNAL PARASITE CONTROL ON CATTLE *Continued*

Product	Company and Address	Marketed Formulation	Pest	Method of Application	Withdrawal Period Before Slaughter (days)	Comments
Permethrin						
Atroban or Expar	Pitman-Moore Mundelein, IL 60060	Liquid	Horn and face flies, mites, ticks, lice, and various other flies	Spray	0	Repeat application as needed but not more often than every 14 days
Atroban Delice or Expar	Pitman-Moore Mundelein, IL 60060	Pour-on	Lice, horn flies, and face flies	Backline treatment	0	Repeat application as needed but not more often than every 14 days
Ectiban	Numerous suppliers	Liquid	Horn and face flies, mites, ticks, lice, and various other flies	Spray	0	Repeat application as needed but not more often than every 14 days
Liquid Duster	Pitman-Moore Mundelein, IL 60060	Self-application device	Horn and face flies	Topical dust	0	Repeat application as needed but not more often than every 14 days
Permectrin II	Boehringer-Ingelheim Animal Health 2621 N Belt Hwy. St. Joseph, MO 64502	Liquid	Horn flies, face flies, stable flies, horse flies, lice, ticks, and mites	Spray	0	Retreat not more than once every 2 weeks
		Wettable powder	Horn flies, face flies, stable flies, horse flies, lice, ticks, and mites	Spray	0	Retreat not more than once every 2 weeks
		Dust	Horn flies, face flies, stable flies, horse flies, lice, ticks, and mites	Direct application	0	Retreat not more than once every 2 weeks
Phosmet						
GX118	Zoecon Corporation 12200 Denton Drive Dallas, TX 75234	Liquid	Grubs, lice, horn flies, ticks, and mites	Spray, dip, or pour-on	21	For use on beef cattle only
Lintox HD–Prolate	Zoecon Corporation Dallas, TX 75234	Liquid	Horn flies, lice, mites, and ticks	Spray or (L intox HD) backrubber	3	Do not use on nonlactating cattle within 28 days of freshening
Tetrachlorvinphos						
Rabon	Fermenta Animal Health Kansas City, MO 64190–1350	Wettable powder	Horn flies, lice, and ticks	Spray	0	Do not treat dairy cattle
		Dust	Horn flies and lice; aids in control of face flies	Dust bag or shaker can	0	Apply 2 oz per animal per treatment
Trichlorfon						
Neguvon	Mobay Corporation Shawnee Mission, KS 66201	Pour-on	Grubs and lice	Backline treatment	21	Do not treat dairy cattle of breeding age
Pour-On	Kaw Valley 1801 S 2nd Street Leavenworth, KS 66248	Pour-on	Grubs and lice	Backline treatment	21	Do not treat dairy cattle of breeding age

Table 2. INSECTICIDE EAR TAG AND LARVICIDE PRODUCTS USED FOR EXTERNAL PARASITE CONTROL ON CATTLE

Product	Company and Address	Marketed Formulation	Pest	Method of Application	Withdrawal Period Before Slaughter (days)	Comments
Insecticide Ear Tags						
Pyrethroids						
Cyfluthrin						
Cutter Gold	Mobay Corporation Shawnee Mission, KS 66201	Ear tag	Horn flies	Two tags per animal, one in each ear	0 Remove tags at the end of the fly season or before slaughter	Approved for lactating dairy cattle
Fenvalerate						
Ectrin	Fermenta Animal Health Kansas City, MO 64190–1350	Ear tag	Horn and face flies, Gulf Coast and Spinose ear ticks	Two tags per animal, one in each ear	0 Remove tags before slaughter	Approved for lactating dairy cattle
λ-Cyhalothrin						
Saber	Pitman-Moore Mundelein, IL 60060	Ear tag	Horn flies (including the pyrethroid-resistant population) and face flies	Two tags per animal, one in each ear	0 Remove tags before slaughter	Do not use in lactating dairy cattle
Permethrins						
Atroban or Expar	Pitman-Moore Mundelein, IL 60060	Ear tag	Horn and face flies, Gulf Coast and Spinose ear ticks	Two tags per animal, one in each ear	0 Remove tags before slaughter	Approved for lactating dairy cattle
Ear Force	Boehringer-Ingelheim St. Joseph, MO 64502	Ear tag	Horn and face flies, Gulf Coast and Spinose ear ticks	One tag per animal for horn flies; two tags for face flies	0	Approved for lactating dairy cattle
Gard Star Plus	Y-Tex Corporation 1825 Big Horn Avenue Cody, WY 82414	Ear tag	Face flies, susceptible horn flies and Gulf Coast ticks	One tag per animal for horn flies; two tags for face flies	0 Remove tags before slaughter	Approved for lactating dairy cattle
Pyrethroid-Organophosphate						
Permethrin, chlorpyrifos, and piperonyl butoxide						
Ear Force Ranger	Boehringer-Ingelheim St. Joseph, MO 64502	Ear tag	Horn and face flies, Gulf Coast and Spinose ear ticks	One tag per animal for horn flies; two tags for face flies	0	Do not use in lactating dairy cattle
Cypermethrin, chlorpyrifos, and piperonyl butoxide						
Max-Con	Y-Tex Corporation Cody, WY 82414	Ear tag	Horn and face flies, Gulf Coast and Spinose ear ticks	Two tags per animal, one in each ear	0	Approved for lactating dairy cattle
Organophosphatases						
Diazinon						
Optimizer	Y-Tex Corporation Cody, WY 82414	Ear tag	Horn flies (including pyrethroid-resistant population), Gulf Coast and Spinose ear ticks	Two tags per animal, one in each ear	0	Do not use in lactating dairy cattle
Terminator	Fermenta Animal Health Kansas City, MO 64190–1350	Ear tag	Horn flies (including pyrethroid-resistant population)	Two tags per animal, one in each ear	0	Do not use in lactating dairy cattle
Pirimiphos-methyl						
Tomahawk	Pitman-Moore Mundelein, IL 60060	Ear tag	Horn flies (including pyrethroid-resistant population)	Two tags per animal, one in each ear	0 Remove tags before slaughter	Do not use in lactating dairy cattle

Table continued on following page

Table 2. INSECTICIDE EAR TAG AND LARVICIDE PRODUCTS USED FOR EXTERNAL PARASITE CONTROL ON CATTLE *Continued*

Product	Company and Address	Marketed Formulation	Pest	Method of Application	Withdrawal Period Before Slaughter (days)	Comments
Larvicide-Type Products						
Diflubenzuron Vigilante	American Cyanamid Princeton, NJ 08540	Standard release bolus	Horn flies, face flies, house flies, and stable flies	½–2 boluses	0	Approved for lactating dairy cattle; do not administer to cattle weighing less than 300 lb, and no more than two boluses to any single animal
Methoprene (IGR) Inhibitor	Zoecon Corporation Dallas, TX 75234	Standard release bolus	Horn flies	½–1 bolus	0	Approved for lactating dairy cattle; do not administer to cattle too small to swallow boluses
Stirofos Rabon	Fermenta Animal Health Kansas City, MO 64190–1350	Oral larvicide premix	Horn flies, face flies, house flies, and stable flies	Mixed in feed	0	Mix uniformly into cattle feed ration

TABLE 3. SOME COMMON PRODUCTS USED FOR EXTERNAL PARASITE CONTROL ON SHEEP AND GOATS

Product	Company and Address	Marketed Formulation	Pest	Method of Application	Withdrawal Period Before Slaughter (days)	Comments
Coumaphos All formulations	Mobay Corporation Shawnee Mission, KS 66201	Wettable powder	Lice, ticks, horn flies, screwworms, fleeceworms, and keds; mites in sheep only	Spray or dip	15	Do not treat lactating dairy goats
		Dust	Screwworms and ear ticks	Spot treatment	0	Dust into the infested wound or ear
		K.R.S. spray foam	Screwworms and fly maggots	Aerosol spray	0	Spray wounds until complete coverage is obtained
Fenvalerate Ectrin WDL	Fermenta Animal Health Kansas City, MO 64190–1350	Liquid	Lice and keds	Spray and pour-on	2	Repeat at 30-day intervals on sheep and nonlactating goats
Ivermectin Ivomec Drench	MSD-AGVET Rahway, NJ 07065–0912	Drench	Nasal bots	Oral drench	11	No label directions for goats
Methoxychlor-malathion	Boehringer-Ingelheim St. Joseph, MO 64502	Dust	Lice and keds	Dust or powder duster	0	Do not apply to lactating goats
Permethrin Atroban or Expar	Pitman-Moore Mundelein, IL 60060	Liquid	Keds, lice, ticks, and various flies	Spray	0	Repeat applications as needed but not more often than every 14 days; no label directions for goats
Atroban Delice or Expar	Pitman-Moore Mundelein, IL 60060	Pour-on	Lice and keds	Pour-on	0	Repeat applications as needed but not more often than every 14 days
Ectiban	Various suppliers	Liquid	Lice and keds	Spray	0	Repeat applications as needed but not more often than every 14 days; no label directions for goats
Permectrin II	Boehringer-Ingelheim St. Joseph, MO 64502	Liquid	Lice, ticks, and blowflies	Spray	0	No label directions for goats
		Wettable powder	Lice, ticks, and blowflies	Spray	0	No label directions for goats

TABLE 4. SOME COMMON PRODUCTS USED FOR EXTERNAL PARASITE CONTROL ON SWINE

Product	Company and Address	Marketed Formulation	Pest	Method of Application	Withdrawal Period Before Slaughter (days)	Comments
Coumaphos All formulations	Mobay Corporation Shawnee Mission, KS 66201	Wettable powder	Lice, ticks, horn flies, and screwworms	Spray	0	Repeat as necessary
		Liquid (ELI)	Lice	Spray	0	Apply to complete wetting
		Dust	Lice	Shaker can	0	Repeat as necessary, but not more than once every 10 days; bedding may be treated
		K.R.S. spray foam	Screwworms and fly maggots	Aerosol spray	0	Spray wounds until complete coverage is obtained
Fenthion Tiguvon	Mobay Corporation Shawnee Mission, KS 66201	Ready-to-use pour-on	Lice	Pour-on	14	Pour uniformly along the animal's back
Fenvalerate Ectrin WDL	Fermenta Animal Health Kansas City, MO 64190–1350	Liquid	Lice and mites	Spray and pour-on (lice only)	1	Repeat in 14 days if necessary
Ivermectin Ivomec	MSD AGVET Rahway, NJ 07065–0912	Injectable	Lice and mites	Inject subcutaneously	18	Severe lice infestations may require repeat treatments
Methoxychlor-malathion	Boehringer-Ingelheim St. Joseph, MO 64502	Dust	Lice	Direct application	0	Repeat in 10 days or thereafter as needed
Permethrin Atroban or Expar	Pitman-Moore Mundelein, IL 60060	Liquid	Lice and mites	Spray	5	Repeat application as needed but not more often than every 14 days
Ectiban	Various suppliers	Dust	Lice	Direct application	0	A second treatment in 14 days is recommended
Permectrin II	Boehringer-Ingelheim St. Joseph, MO 64502	Liquid	Lice, ticks, horn flies, and mites	Spray, paint, or dip	5	Retreat after 4–6 weeks
		Wettable powder	Lice, ticks, horn flies, and mites	Spray, paint, or dip	5	Retreat after 4–6 weeks
		Dust	Lice, ticks, horn flies, and mites	Direct application	5	Retreat after 4–6 weeks
Phosmet Prolate	Zoecon Corporation Dallas, TX 75234	Liquid	Lice and mites	Spray	1	Repeat in 14 days if needed
Tetrachlorvinphos Rabon	Fermenta Animal Health Kansas City, MO 64190–1350	Wettable powder	Lice	Spray	0	Repeat in 2 weeks if necessary
		Dust	Lice	Direct application and bedding	0	Repeat in 2 weeks if necessary
		Oral larvicide premix	House flies	Mixed into feed	0	Mix uniformly into daily feed

Anesthesia in Ruminants and Swine

J. C. THURMON, DVM, MS, Diplomate, ACVA
G. J. BENSON, DVM, MS, Diplomate, ACVA

before the use of any external parasiticide for specific use directions, safety considerations, and proper meat or milk withdrawal periods.

Progress in the development of anesthetic drugs, equipment, and techniques for food animals has not kept pace with that for companion animals or humans, especially in the United States. The animal welfare movement has drawn attention to the importance of humane treatment of all animals. Humane treatment demands that anesthetics and analgesics be used when appropriate in all animal species. However, acute awareness of this problem has done nothing to increase the availability of approved drugs for use in our food-producing animals. It should be clearly understood that animals perceive pain no differently than people do. The requirement of analgesia for prevention of pain in food-producing animals is just as important as in companion animals and in people. This is indeed a major and legitimate problem for the conscientious food animal practitioner.

Over the years, researchers have used food-producing animals (e.g., calves) to develop surgical techniques for eventual use in humans. These studies have contributed significantly to our understanding of safe anesthesia in the food animal species. With the advent of cardiopulmonary bypass and the subsequent use of ruminants for development of surgical techniques and equipment, safe general anesthetic techniques for ruminants and swine have evolved.[1-6] Studies of the influence of selected drugs on maternal-fetal circulation[7-10] and of anesthetic requirements during pregnancy[11] have also contributed a great deal to our understanding of maternal-fetal responses to anesthetic and other related drugs.

Although these methods offer relatively safe and reliable anesthesia for major surgical intervention, it must be emphasized that they are expensive, are time-consuming, and require a large investment in equipment and are therefore not readily adaptable to field use. Nonetheless, it would be naive to imply that procedures requiring major surgical intervention (e.g., thoracic surgery, orthopedic surgery, and the like) can be performed safely without appropriate anesthetic drugs and equipment.

It is not unreasonable to suspect that most general anesthesia in food animals is performed with use of unapproved drugs. The overtones of this speculation hint of anesthetic tissue residues, but yet this is absolutely not the case. The drugs most commonly used in anesthesia have extremely short halflives. Thus the probability of an animal's carrying anesthetic residues within its edible tissues after the surgical incision has healed (i.e., at least 14 days after surgery) is nearly unthinkable. Further, the majority of anesthetic drugs employed today have been previously approved for use in humans.

Owing to economic influences, most surgical procedures in food-producing animals are performed under field conditions, where local or regional analgesia or a brief period of general anesthesia is satisfactory. Because ruminants are docile by nature, they are rather easily handled and restrained with proper equipment. Unlike horses, cattle will accept mechanical restraint (e.g., cattle chute, head catch, nose tongs) without inflicting severe injury on themselves or their handlers. It is partly for this reason that local analgesic and mechanical restraint techniques have achieved a high degree of development and are widely employed in cattle. Large numbers of field operations are completed with use of regional analgesia in cattle.[12] Local and regional techniques are described in the following chapter. Local analgesics are economical, and many surgical manipulations can be performed best with the animal in a standing position. Another factor contributing to the refinement of local analgesic techniques is the untoward physiologic alterations of respiratory and cardiovascular function occurring during the course of general anesthesia when large ruminants are placed in an unnatural postural position. Performing surgery in the standing position helps eliminate these potential problems. However, valuable breeding or production animals requiring major surgery are generally transported to large animal hospitals, where appropriate facilities, equipment, and drugs are available.

The objective of this chapter is to review anesthetic techniques that have proved safe and effective in ruminants and swine. As has already been mentioned, a large number of the drugs discussed in this chapter are not approved for use in food-producing animals. Thus it is the responsibility of the veterinarian to ensure that animals receiving these drugs be kept from the human food chain until such time as the drugs have been cleared from their body tissues (generally 2 to 4 weeks). Because of limited space, major emphasis will not be placed on physiologic and pharmacologic responses to drugs. A number of well-written textbooks are readily available for those wishing greater detail on these two subjects.[13-16]

As previously stated, relatively few anesthetics and anesthetic adjuncts are currently approved for use in ruminants and swine in the United States, but techniques employing unapproved as well as approved drugs are reviewed because, as veterinarians, it is our responsibility to prevent pain and suffering in all animal species. Perhaps in the future some of the unapproved drugs will be approved for use in food animals.

PHYSICAL CHARACTERISTICS OF RUMINANTS

When ruminants are restrained in either dorsal or lateral recumbency, the massive weight of the abdominal viscera is shifted downward and anteriorly. This places massive pressure on the diaphragm. The diaphragm is forced further into the thoracic cavity, which decreases lung functional residual capacity.[17] In addition, in dorsal recumbency, the viscera rest on the major abdominal vessels in addition to the diaphragm. This pressure may impede venous blood flow returning to the heart with resultant decreases in cardiac output, arterial blood pressure, and ultimately tissue perfusion. This situation can be further aggravated by advanced pregnancy. In spite of these physiologic alterations, blood pressure is reasonably well maintained in cattle anesthetized with halothane in oxygen.

Clinical observations suggest that lateral or dorsal recumbency is more detrimental to pulmonary function than is sternal recumbency. Abnormal positioning (lateral or dorsal recumbency) leads to mismatching of pulmonary ventilation and perfusion. Alterations in ventilation-perfusion are progressive, leading ultimately to hypoxemia as a result of right-to-left shunting of blood. In addition, hypoventilation and hypercapnia can result because diaphragmatic excursion is limited by the weight of the abdominal contents. Deep sedation or general anesthesia enhances the insults to pulmonary function induced by abnormal body position through depression of the central nervous system and function of the muscles of respiration. Anesthetic-induced depression of the cardiovascular system decreases tissue perfusion.[1] Large quantities of ruminal gas are produced by the unfasted animal. Normally, these gases cannot be eructated when the animal is in lateral or dorsal recumbency. Thus intraruminal pressure can become extremely high, further limiting diaphragmatic excursion and the animal's ability to breathe. Hypoxemia and hypercapnia (causing respiratory acidemia) can become life-threatening in ruminants that are not properly prepared before long-term general anesthesia.

To a degree, these untoward cardiopulmonary alterations can be avoided by preanesthetic patient preparation, supplemental administration of oxygen, and mechanical ventilation. Availability and cost of equipment often precludes use of these measures. In cows breathing room air, given xylazine (0.22 mg/kg intramuscularly), and restrained in dorsal recumbency, the authors found arterial oxygen partial pressure to be dangerously low (45 to 60 torr). Supplemental oxygen given by nasal tube (flow rate, 10 to 15 L/min) helped relieve hypoxemia. However, placing the animals in sternal position or returning them to a standing position was ultimately found to be the most effective means of correcting hypercapnia and hypoxemia.

ANESTHETIC HAZARDS

Regurgitation

In the anesthetized ruminant, regurgitation is common and of major concern.[18] It may be classified as either active or passive ("silent regurgitation"). Active regurgitation is more likely to occur in light planes of anesthesia, whereas passive regurgitation is associated with deep surgical anesthesia. Active regurgitation, as the term implies, is characterized by explosive discharge of large quantities of ruminal contents. During regurgitation, ruminal contents are frequently aspirated deep into the respiratory tract. Massive amounts reaching the smaller airways often initiate acute bronchial constriction, hypoxia, and finally asphyxiation. If the animal does not succumb to asphyxia, the subsequent development of progressive foreign body pneumonia (in spite of all therapeutic measures) is a real possibility. The successful outcome of aspiration pneumonia probably depends more on the amount and pH of foreign material aspirated than on methods or drugs employed as treatment. Bronchospasm occurring at the time of aspiration may be treated with bronchodilators. Aminophylline (2 to 4 mg/kg intravenously) injected over a 5-minute period may be helpful. A more rapid rate of administration causes myocardial stimulation, accompanied by increased oxygen requirements[19] at a time when hypoxemia is of major concern. Suction may be employed for aspirate removal, but because of particulate size and aspiration into the deep recesses of the respiratory passages, suction has not proved to be of much value. Oxygen should be administered by mask or nasal tube. If the animal does not succumb to asphyxia, corticosteroid and broad-spectrum antibiotic therapy may be helpful. For decreasing the likelihood of regurgitation, the following measures are indicated.

1. Withhold food and water for 24 hours before induction of anesthesia in adult animals. Young calves (i.e., before full rumen development) should be starved of food and water for no more than 12 hours.
2. Position the animal in left lateral or sternal recumbency during intubation.
3. Avoid vigorous manipulation of the rumen and other internal abdominal organs during surgery.
4. Place a sandbag or some other device beneath the animal's neck to elevate the occiput.[13] This measure will tend to prevent passive regurgitation and allow saliva to flow out of the animal's mouth so that its aspiration is avoided.

Because regurgitation cannot be totally prevented, either a cuffed endotracheal tube or a correctly fitting Cole's tube should be placed into the trachea of all anesthetized ruminants. Regurgitation occurring in animals in which the trachea has been properly intubated does not pose a major hazard, if upon recovery the tube is removed with the cuff inflated. This extubation technique allows removal of massive amounts of regurgitant that may have accumulated in the trachea cephalad to the tube cuff. Before the tube is removed, the mouth, nares, and pharynx may be flushed safely with water to remove regurgitant and decrease the likelihood of its aspiration. A hose connected to a water hydrant can be used effectively and safely for this purpose.

Regurgitation may occur during intubation; often it is precipitated by poor induction and intubation techniques. Some have sought to avoid this problem by intubating before induction. This requires good patient restraint (i.e., cattle chute or strapping the patient to the surgical table) and the use of a mouth wedge held securely in place to prevent the animal from chewing the tube and one's hand and fingers during intubation. Such procedures are highly stressful. Generally, the hazards of regurgitation before intubation are avoided by not attempting intubation until surgical anesthesia has been attained. At this point, the tube is quickly and accurately placed in the trachea and the cuff quickly inflated. In the lightly anesthetized animal, accidental insertion of the endotracheal tube into the esophagus with to-and-fro movement for ascertaining its location is sure to initiate active regurgitation. In the event that the onset of regurgitation is recognized before intubation can be completed, the endotracheal tube can be quickly passed into the esophagus and the cuff inflated, allowing ruminal contents to flow out of the mouth while another tube is being placed in the trachea.

Ruminal Tympany (Bloat)

Bloat commonly occurs in anesthetized ruminants,[13, 20] but it is not always serious. In a series of 99 cattle in which general anesthesia was maintained with halothane in oxygen, Weaver[21] considered bloat not to be a serious problem. The use of a stomach tube to relieve bloat was required in 1 animal only. However, in this study, duration of anesthesia averaged only 80 minutes, and 11 of the animals were starved of food for 1 to 5 days and denied water for 4 hours.

Although bloat cannot be totally prevented, its incidence and severity can be decreased by starving ruminants of food and water for 24 hours before anesthesia. Fasting does not cause a major decrease in ruminal contents, but it decreases the rate of fermentation and thus the rate of ruminal gas production.

Should acute bloat occur, provided that it is not of a "frothy" type, pressure can be relieved by passing a stomach tube; trocarization of the rumen is discouraged except under the severest of circumstances, for fear of gross contamination of the peritoneal cavity and subsequent peritonitis. Some veterinarians routinely pass a stomach tube into the rumen before or shortly after induction of anesthesia. This precaution may lead ultimately to a more acute problem, because the tube, acting as a foreign body in the esophagus, may initiate regurgitation. For this reason, the authors employ a stomach tube for bloat relief only when it is absolutely necessary and when the animal has an endotracheal tube in place. An alternative method is to position the animal in sternal recumbency. In this position, ruminal decompression occurs naturally. Positional relief of bloat is usually unacceptable during an operation, but it is the most acceptable means once the procedure has been completed. Moderate external pressure applied to the abdominal wall over the rumen will aid initiation of eructation.

Salivation

Ruminants normally produce copious quantities of saliva (cattle 50 L/day and sheep 6 to 16 L/day), which continues to flow during anesthesia. The amount seems to increase with some anesthetics (e.g., ether), whereas it may decrease with others (e.g., halothane).[22]

Hall[13] suggests that using atropine as an antisialagogue is of little value because it does not decrease the amount of saliva secreted and because atropine causes an increase in saliva viscosity, which makes it more difficult to remove from the respiratory passages if it is inhaled. Inhalation does not occur if the trachea has been properly intubated. Clinical observations suggest, however, that the oropharynx is drier in cattle given atropine, although the period of decreased saliva flow is indeed brief. Weaver[21] found that atropine, given at a dose of 30 mg to adult cattle, decreased saliva production from 5 and 10 ml/100 kg/min to 1 and 5 ml/100 kg/min.

When inhalation anesthesia is to be employed, atropine may be given 10 to 20 minutes before induction. Once the trachea has been intubated, the amount and consistency of saliva produced is of minor importance. However, in animals with decreased respiratory passage secretions (e.g., bronchitis, tracheitis), the drying effect of atropine will inhibit the effectiveness of ciliated cell activity.

PREANESTHETIC MEDICATION

Table 1 summarizes the tranquilizers and sedatives used as preanesthetic medications in ruminants and swine.

Parasympatholytic Agents

Atropine sulfate, a parasympatholytic, is given to decrease saliva production and prevent bradycardia but is contraindicated in animals with tachycardia. The following doses of atropine have been found to be helpful in decreasing salivation for short periods of time in ruminants and swine:

Cattle, sheep, and goats: 0.06 to 0.12 mg/kg intramuscularly.
Swine: 0.04 mg/kg intramuscularly.

Ataractics-Tranquilizers

Phenothiazine tranquilizers have been used to decrease apprehension in nervous animals, which makes them easier to handle. Because of their limited effectiveness (i.e., minimal sedation without analgesia) and adverse side effects (hypotension, hypothermia), this group of tranquilizers has only limited use in ruminants and swine. Hypotension and hypothermia are more likely to occur in ill animals or when an actual or relative overdose of the tranquilizer has been given. Tranquilizers given to cattle before induction of general anesthesia will decrease the amount of anesthetic required, but recovery will generally be delayed. Because a rapid return of protective mechanisms (i.e., cough and swallowing reflex) and righting reflexes in ruminants recovering from anesthesia is highly desirable, tranquilizers should be given only to unruly animals that cannot otherwise be handled safely. Further, these drugs may induce relaxation of the esophagus and cardia, thus fostering regurgitation.[27] Tranquilizers may be given to cattle undergoing surgery in a standing position with use of regional or field analgesia. Under these circumstances, the dose of tranquilizer must be greatly decreased; otherwise, the animal is likely to lie down during the operation.

Phenothiazine tranquilizers should be avoided in the ill or debilitated animal because of their tendency to complicate such existing conditions as hypovolemia, anemia, hypothermia, shock, and hepatic dysfunction. Patients suffering from hypotension after receiving a tranquilizer should be treated first by rapid fluid loading. In the event that vigorous fluid therapy is ineffective, a catecholamine having strong $alpha_1$ action is indicated (e.g., phenylephrine 0.004 to 0.008 mg/kg, methoxamine 0.04 to 0.08 mg/kg intravenously). Finally, all tranquilizers cross the placenta, causing fetal depression.

Administration of Tranquilizers

These drugs may be given intramuscularly or intravenously. For intramuscular administration, a small-bore needle of sufficient length (i.e., 3.8 to 5.1 cm) to allow drug deposition in muscle tissue should be used. Depositing the drug in fat, which has low blood flow, will result in slow absorption and in delayed and often decreased animal response. The amount should be decreased to the smallest recommended dose when the drug is given intravenously, and the injection should be given slowly. Rapid administration can cause severe reactions. Jones[27] suggests the intravenous route for phenothiazine tranquilizers should be avoided because a number of deaths in cattle have been reported after intravenous injection.

Tranquilizers should be given under circumstances that cause the least possible distress to the patient. The animal should be in a quiet place and left undisturbed until the desired effect occurs. Repeated stimulation of the animal for assessment of tranquilization before full onset of action will be accompanied by excitement, often resulting in a less than desirable response. If phenothiazine tranquilizers are to be used, they must be used judiciously in order to ensure a desirable response.

Sedatives

Xylazine (Rompun, AnaSed)

Xylazine is the most useful sedative in ruminants.[32] However, it is not approved for use in food-producing animals in the United States. Xylazine is generally classified as a sedative[13, 33] with strong analgesic, hypnotic, muscle relaxant, and autonomic properties.[34] Because xylazine is in broad use in European and other western countries, a great deal of clinical information on its use has been published. As with most anesthetic and anesthetic-related drugs, some undesirable side effects accompany the use of xylazine. It abolishes ruminal motility at large doses,[35] and bloat often occurs in unfasted animals. The respiratory and pulse rates are decreased, as is myocardial contractility. These responses are most severe after rapid intravenous injection. The profuse salivation and bradycardia that accompany its administration can be counteracted to a large degree by atropine. However, the increase in heart rate after atropine in the face of an increased peripheral vascular resistance may be detrimental. Postadministration diarrhea is common, but it is generally self-limiting, clearing in approximately 36 hours.[36] Xylazine has been used as a preanesthetic and as a sedative combined with local analgesia for a wide variety of surgical procedures. For example, 5 to 10 mg of xylazine alone or combined with 5 to 10 mg of

Table 1. PREANESTHETIC MEDICATION: TRANQUILIZERS AND SEDATIVES (mg/kg)[1]

Generic Name	Trade Name (Manufacturer)	Cattle[2]		Sheep and Goats[2]		Swine[2]		Comments
		IV	IM	IV	IM	IV	IM	
Chlorpromazine hydrochloride	Thorazine (Pitman-Moore Washington Crossing, NJ 08560)	0.22–1.0[4]	1.0–4.4[14]	0.55[14]	2.2	0.55–3.3[23, 24]	2.0–4.0[25]	Use IV route with caution; give lowest effective dose
Promazine hydrochloride	Sparine (Wyeth Laboratories Division of American Home Products Corp. Philadelphia, PA 19101)	0.44–1.0	0.4–1.0	0.44–1.0	0.44–1.0	0.44–1.0	0.44–1.0	Intravenous route in cattle may nullify sedative effect[17, 18]
Triflupromazine hydrochloride	Vetame (E. R. Squibb & Sons Princeton, NJ 08540)	0.1 (maximum: 40 mg)	0.2 (maximum: 150 mg)	0.1 (maximum: 40 mg)	1.0 (maximum: 40 mg)	0.88	1.3	Not as effective as chlorpromazine in cattle[26]
Acepromazine maleate	Acepromazine maleate injectable (Ayerst Laboratories Division of American Home Products Corp. New York, NY 10017)	—	0.03–0.1[13]	—	0.03–0.1[13]	—	0.03–0.1	Use of IV route questionable in cattle[27]; injections require approximately 35 minutes for full onset of tranquilization[28]
Propiopromazine hydrochloride	Tranvet (Diamond Laboratories Des Moines, IA 50304)	0.22–1.0[14]	0.22–1.0[14]	0.5[14]	—	0.55–1.0[14]	0.55–1.0[14]	Do not give to young calves
Ethylisobutrazine	Diquel (Jensen-Salsbery Laboratories, Division of Richardson-Merell Kansas City, MO 64141)	0.55[14]	0.55–1.10[14]	—	—	1.25	2.2–4.4[14]	
Xylazine hydrochloride	Rompun (Haver-Lockhart Laboratories Shawnee, KS 66201)	0.05–0.15	0.1–0.33	0.05–0.11	0.1–0.22[29]	—	—	IV route can be hazardous; dosage should be decreased to ½ of that given IM; xylazine is not an effective sedative when used alone in swine; usually combined with ketamine
Azaperone	Stresnil (Pitman-Moore Washington Crossing, NJ 08560)	—	—	—	—	—	4.0–8.0 small swine[30] 2.0 large swine[31]	When given at 2.5 mg/kg, azaperone will prevent fighting in newly mixed animals[31]
Diazepam	Valium (Hoffman-LaRoche Nutley, NJ 07110)	—	—	0.4–1.0	0.8–2.0	—	5.5–8.5	In miniature swine, maximal sedation occurs in approximately 30 mins[25]; the use of diazepam at this dose will decrease the anesthetic dose of pentobarbital about 50%
Chlorprothixene	Taractan (Hoffman-LaRoche Nutley, NJ 07110)	—	—	—	—	0.3–1.0[27]	—	Optimal effect 5–10 minutes after injection
Fentanyl citrate and droperidol	Innovar-Vet (Pitman-Moore Washington Crossing, NJ 08560)	—	—	—	—	—	1 ml/12–25 kg body weight	Atropine premedication is required to prevent severe bradycardia; droperidol alone may be just as effective as the combination

[1]Read package insert for approval of use in food-producing animals and for milk discard and slaughter withdrawal times.
[2]Superscript numbers in dosage columns indicate references.
IV = intravenous; IM = intramuscular.

butorphanol intravenously provides effective sedation and enhances regional analgesia in the standing adult cow. Xylazine has also been used to immobilize bulls for electroejaculation and semen collection.[37]

PRECAUTIONS. Xylazine given to cows in the last trimester of pregnancy may cause premature parturition and retention of fetal membranes.[36] The use of xylazine should be avoided in ruminants with pronounced debilitating disease. More specifically, it should not be given to animals suffering from hypovolemia or with urinary tract blockade. In healthy cows, xylazine (0.22 mg/kg intramuscularly) caused urine output to increase 6-fold 2 hours after administration.[38] If given intravenously, particularly in young or small ruminants and when used at 10 per cent (100 mg/ml) concentration, xylazine should be diluted in 3 to 5 ml saline and given over 2 to 3 minutes. The dose probably should not exceed 0.11 to 0.22 mg/kg.

After being given xylazine, ruminants should be observed closely for 30 minutes to 2 hours. Some animals may remain recumbent for more than 2 hours if undisturbed. Bloat is of greater concern in animals that have not been properly fasted of food and water and when the larger dose of xylazine has been given. Ruminants recovering from xylazine sedation may appear to be in a general state of wakefulness but later may lie down in lateral recumbency and die from acute bloat. It is advisable to observe them closely for a time and to encourage them to move about until they have fully recovered or to administer an antagonist that will be discussed later.

ADMINISTRATION. Xylazine may be given intravenously[39] or intramuscularly. The onset of action by the intravenous route is immediate. The intravenous route is more acutely stressful on cardiovascular function than is the intramuscular route and therefore should be used with caution in unhealthy patients.

When xylazine is given intramuscularly, a small-bore needle (i.e., 18- to 20-gauge) sufficient in length to penetrate muscle tissue (3.8 to 5.1 cm) must be used, or drug deposition will occur in fatty tissue. When a large-bore needle is used, drug may leak from the needle puncture site; however, when the high concentration (100 mg/ml) is used, the needle used to withdraw the dose of xylazine should not be removed from the syringe before intramuscular needle placement, because the xylazine filling the dead space of the needle will be lost, decreasing the total dose injected. Even though it is known that the degree of sedation induced by xylazine is variable among animals, drug loss at the needle puncture site, deposition in fat, or perhaps a decrease in potency after prolonged storage may, in part, account for some of the variability of animal response.[33]

Because xylazine is available in 2 per cent (20 mg/ml) and 10 per cent (100 mg/ml) concentrations, the dose should always be calculated on the basis of milligrams per kilogram of body weight. Inadvertent substitution of the 10 per cent concentration (large animal) for the 2 per cent concentration (small animal) will result in a dose 5 times that intended if it is calculated on the basis of milliliters per given amount of weight (e.g., 5 ml [10 per cent]/1000 lb, a gross overdose).

Xylazine alone is not an effective sedative in swine even when given in a large dose. It is, however, an extremely useful drug when given in combination with one of the dissociatives, ketamine or Telazol. Combining xylazine with ketamine enhances muscle relaxation and analgesia. Effective doses of xylazine in ruminants are as follows:

Cattle: 0.05 to 0.22 mg/kg intravenously; 0.1 to 0.44 mg/kg intramuscularly; standing surgery, 0.025 to 0.05 mg/kg intramuscularly, when used to supplement regional analgesia. An alternative in the average 450-kg cow is 5 to 10 mg xylazine combined in the same syringe with 5 to 10 mg of butorphanol (total dose) given intravenously.

Sheep and goats: 0.05 to 0.10 mg/kg intravenously; 0.1 to 0.33 mg/kg intramuscularly.

Because the sedative response to xylazine is due primarily to its agonistic effect on α_2-receptors located in the central nervous system, drugs that block these receptor sites may be used effectively to antagonize xylazine sedation. Yohimbine* and doxapram† given in combination intravenously at dosages of 0.25 mg/kg and 0.3 to 0.5 mg/kg, respectively, have proved to be effective for this purpose, but neither drug is very effective when used alone. Tolazoline‡ 0.4 to 4.0 mg/kg intravenously is an effective antagonist for xylazine sedation in ruminants. Perhaps the most effective xylazine antagonist is atipamezole, which is currently undergoing clinical testing.§ These antagonists have proved to be very useful when animals have been accidentally overdosed or when rapid recovery from xylazine sedation is desirable.

Capture of Free-Ranging Cattle

Before capture of an escaped or feral ruminant is attempted, all efforts should be made to lure the animal into a corral or physically trap it before chemical immobilization is utilized. Chemical immobilization is much more dangerous to both the animal and people involved and more often unsuccessful than is live trapping. One must be fully aware that all of the drugs used to capture or immobilize ruminants are potent and toxic to people. The potential for a serious accident is ever present. It is incumbent upon the veterinarian to be fully knowledgeable of the chosen drug's pharmacology. In the event of accidental self-administration, the veterinarian must know the appropriate actions to take. A number of drugs and drug combinations have been used to capture wild cattle.[28] Xylazine, although not ideal, has been used extensively for this purpose.[40] Free-ranging wild cattle do not respond to xylazine with the same degree of sedation and immobilization as do more docile animals. Therefore, after the free-ranging animal has become recumbent, it should be approached quietly from its blind side and physically restrained.

For capture purposes, xylazine may be administered with a Cap-Chur-type gun.‖ However, in large animals, the gun may be incapable of delivering an immobilizing volume of 2 per cent xylazine. Use of the 10 per cent concentration helps to overcome this problem. When large doses are administered, the sedated animal should be observed closely for several hours so that side effects such as bloat and prolonged recumbency can be effectively treated. Wild cattle captured by Stewart were given an estimated dose of xylazine ranging from 0.66 to 0.88 mg/kg.[40] Recumbency occurred in 3 to 7 minutes, but the cattle were not always sufficiently sedated to prevent fleeing when they were approached. Subsequently, a second dose was given, estimated to be 0.52 to 0.53 mg/kg. The interval between first and second dose ranged from 2 to 70 minutes. Total doses of this magnitude should be used with extreme caution. Further, a specific antagonist (e.g., yohimbine-doxapram) should be readily available and administered when it is required to antagonize excessive sedation and other responses that could prove to be life-threatening (e.g., bloat).

Ketamine may be used in combination with xylazine, but total volume then becomes a concern. This problem can be overcome to a limited extent by freeze-dried ketamine¶ and reconstituting it to a higher concentration (i.e., 200 to 300 mg/

---

*Yobine, Lloyd Laboratories, Shenandoah, IA.
†A. H. Robins, Richmond, VA 23220.
‡Sigma Chemical Co., St. Louis, MO 63178.
§Farmos Group Ltd., Turku, Finland.
‖Palmer Chemical and Equipment Co., Douglasville, GA 30134.
¶Telazol, A. H. Robins, Richmond, VA 23220.

ml). Ketamine powder may be reconstituted in 100 mg/ml xylazine, thus providing a highly concentrated solution of both drugs.

Recently a 1:1 combination of tiletamine-zolazepam* in a lyophilized form became available in 500-mg vials. This amount can easily be reconstituted in 1 ml of liquid (e.g., saline or even xylazine). Studies have shown that calves administered Telazol 4 mg/kg and xylazine 0.1 to 0.2 mg/kg intramuscularly became recumbent in 2 to 3 minutes. Calves were able to stand unassisted in approximately 2 hours. Whereas respiratory depression occurred with the large dose of xylazine, this would not be expected in free-ranging adult cattle.[41] In England, a neuroleptanalgesic combination of acepromazine and etorphine† is used to immobilize cattle. The concentration ratio is 10 mg/ml of acepromazine to 2.45 mg/ml of etorphine. It is supplied along with an etorphine antagonist, diprenorphine (Revivon). The dose in cattle is as follows: acepromazine, 100 μg/kg; etorphine, 22.5 μg/kg; and the antagonist diprenorphine, 30 μg/kg. This drug combination may cause a moderate degree of excitement when it is given in a dose insufficient to induce rapid immobilization. In addition, excitement may appear some hours after the antagonist has been given. Postrecovery excitement is thought to be due to enterohepatic cycling of etorphine. Because of this possibility, animals should be kept under surveillance in a well-secured enclosure for 12 hours after reversal.[42] In the authors' experimental studies with etorphine in ponies, postrecovery excitement was observed in one animal. Excitement was adequately controlled by intravenous acepromazine. A more rational approach to the problem would have been administration of diprenorphine.

Etorphine is available in the United States; however, it is approved for use in zoo animals only. Because etorphine is a very potent opioid, it must be handled with extreme caution. The antagonist should be drawn into a syringe and immediately available in case of accidental self-administration. Diprenorphine[42] is given intravenously at approximately 1.5 to 2 times the dosage of etorphine.

Chloral Hydrate

Chloral hydrate has been used effectively to sedate confined animals that could not otherwise be approached or handled. Denying animals water for 24 to 36 hours makes them thirsty enough to consume water containing chloral hydrate. The dose is as follows:

Adult cattle: 100 to 150 g in 8 to 10 L of drinking water.
Light to medium narcosis: 5 to 7 g/100 kg intravenously.

Choral hydrate has been given to pigs for general anesthesia at a dose of 4 to 6 ml of a 5 per cent solution per kilogram of body weight intraperitoneally. The high incidence of peritonitis induced precludes the use of chloral hydrate by this route of administration.

Pentobarbital

Clinical experience has shown that pentobarbital is a useful sedative in cattle. The concentration that can be given intramuscularly without causing severe tissue necrosis (approximately 3 per cent) requires too large a volume for practical use; therefore it is generally given intravenously. By this route, pentobarbital is given slowly until noticeable unsteadiness and rear limb weakness occur. This response generally occurs after

---
*Immobilon, Reckitt and Colman, Hull, England.
†Available from American Cyanamid.

1 to 2 g have been given to an adult cow. Usually 3 g will induce recumbency.

Since the introduction of xylazine, sedation with pentobarbital has been less commonly used. For profound sedation, a combination of xylazine and pentobarbital can be given to effect.

INJECTABLE ANESTHETIC DRUGS FOR RUMINANTS AND SWINE

Barbiturates

The period of surgical anesthesia induced by the short-acting and ultrashort-acting barbiturates is brief, but complete recovery may be exceedingly prolonged in young calves, particularly if subsequent doses are given, lasting up to 24 hours.[26] When used for induction of anesthesia and followed by maintenance with an inhalation agent, the barbiturates are nearly ideal and are widely used for this purpose, both alone and in combination with other drugs (e.g., guaifenesin). It is not advisable to use barbiturates alone for anything other than the briefest of surgical procedures.[22] Although anesthesia can be prolonged by supplemental injections, regurgitation with aspiration, apnea, and death are likely to occur unless the trachea has been intubated.

Once a barbiturate has been injected, control of anesthetic depth and rate of recovery is clearly out of the hands of the veterinarian and depends on redistribution to non-nervous tissues and metabolism of the drug. In cattle, rate of barbiturate metabolism may have a greater influence on recovery time than does tissue redistribution. The reverse appears to be true for sheep, goats, and swine.[43] In either case, anesthetic depth cannot be as precisely controlled with barbiturates as it can with the inhalation anesthetics.

Barbiturates rapidly cross the placenta. Severity of fetal depression is directly related to total dose administered to the dam. Barbiturates are not recommended for cesarean section when given in large dose. An ultrashort-acting drug (e.g., thiopental) may be used safely as an induction agent in animals destined for cesarean section when an inhalation agent (e.g., halothane or isoflurane) is to be used as the maintenance anesthetic.

Specific antagonists are not available for barbiturates. Analeptics such as doxapram* will stimulate the respiratory centers, increasing respiration rate and tidal volume in barbiturate-depressed animals. Subsequently, the animal may revert to a deep state of depression because of decreased arterial carbon dioxide content. Apnea is more appropriately treated with mechanically controlled ventilation until adequate spontaneous breathing resumes. Barbiturate overdose may be treated by administering sodium bicarbonate (to increase blood pH) and balanced electrolyte solutions in conjunction with a diuretic. Peritoneal dialysis could be considered as well as administration of fresh whole blood to increase the availability of albumin for barbiturate binding. Although hemodialysis is used in human medicine, its practicality in large animals is doubtful. Aside from therapeutic measures, the patient should be kept warm and should not be allowed to remain in one position for a prolonged period. Adequate ventilation and oxygen supplementation are important. Prophylactically, antibiotics will help avoid secondary bacterial infection.

Endotracheal intubation is essential. A properly placed endotracheal tube with inflated cuff will provide protection from aspiration of saliva and regurgitated ruminal contents.

---
*Dopram-V, A. H. Robins, Richmond, VA 23220.

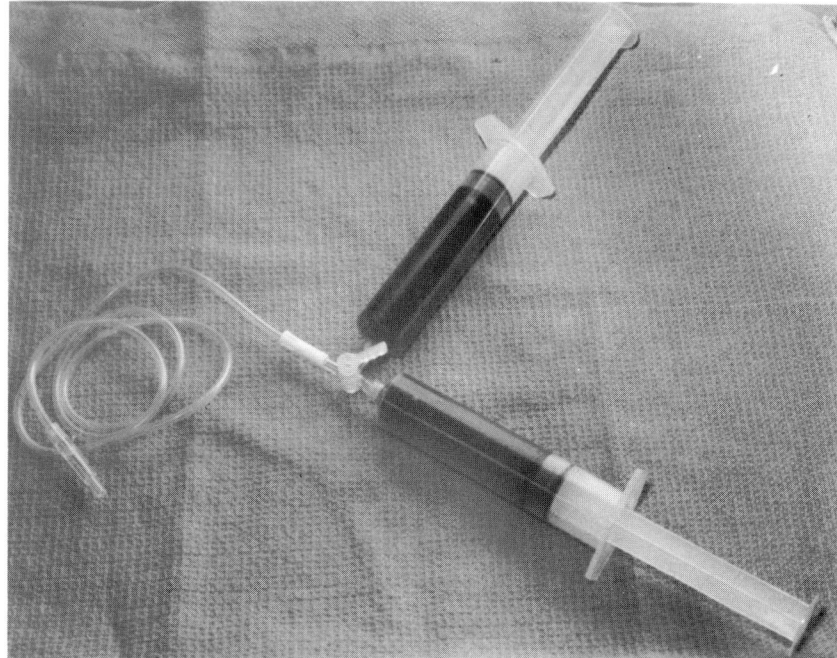

Figure 1. Syringes, stop-cock, and plastic tube extension used for rapid intravenous administration of a large volume of anesthetic.

In addition, apnea, which is common with barbiturate anesthesia, can be dealt with effectively.

Pentobarbital

Pentobarbital is not suitable for general anesthesia in adult cattle but may be used in calves over 1 month of age.[13] A prolonged recovery time is to be expected in animals younger than 1 month.[14] In adult sheep and goats (that have been properly fasted) and in swine, pentobarbital will provide 20 to 30 minutes of relatively safe anesthesia. Supplemental injections for prolonging anesthesia are not recommended unless they are given under ideal hospital conditions with appropriate respiratory support equipment available. Analgesia and muscle relaxation are poor, except in deep planes of anesthesia, and recovery is prolonged, which requires close patient surveillance if satisfactory results are to be achieved. Recommended doses are as follows:

Calves: 15 to 30 mg/kg intravenously (over 1 month of age).
Sheep and goats: 20 to 30 mg/kg intravenously.
Swine: 15 to 30 mg/kg intravenously.

Thiobarbiturates

With the increasing popularity of inhalation anesthesia, thiobarbiturates are used more extensively for induction in cattle, sheep, goats, and swine than is pentobarbital. When surgical anesthesia is to be maintained with inhalation anesthesia, thiopental* or thiamylal† is given by rapid intravenous injection. This method of administration is often referred to as a "crash induction" and is generally preferred in large, thrifty animals because uncontrollable excitement is seldom encountered. If a thiobarbiturate is given slowly, a much larger dose will be required, and recovery will be prolonged. A 10 per cent concentration is desirable to allow the required volume to be contained in a single large syringe. This high concentration is caustic and will likely cause varying degrees of phlebitis. Phlebitis is seldom recognized unless one has occasion to examine the vessel 24 to 48 hours later. Accidental perivascular injection (occurring in inappropriately restrained animals and with faulty vessel cannulation) can cause tissue necrosis and slough. For these reasons, it is probably safer to use a 5 per cent solution.

For induction of anesthesia, a precalculated dose of either thiopental or thiamylal is drawn into a syringe and injected rapidly into the jugular vein. In cows, the milk vein has been used, although it should be realized that phlebitis would be potentially more harmful in this vessel. The vein employed should be well cannulated. A 7.5- to 10-cm needle of 16 to 18 gauge should be used in order to ensure ease of injection and decrease the possibility of perivascular injection.

When a lower concentration (e.g., 5 per cent) is to be used, one end of a short (25 to 30 cm) length of plastic tubing is attached to the intravenous needle or catheter, and a 3-way stop-cock is connected at the other end. Two syringes containing the calculated dose of barbiturate are attached, one at each of the open stop-cock ports (Fig. 1). The contents of one syringe are injected rapidly, the stop-cock valve is rotated, and contents of the second syringe are injected rapidly. The entire injection procedure should be completed in 5 to 10 seconds. Fifteen to 20 seconds after completion of the injection, the animal will develop posterior limb weakness followed by rapid collapse to its sternum. Apnea lasting 15 to 30 seconds is not uncommon and should give rise to little concern in the physically fit animal. Intubation should be completed at once. Inadequate jaw relaxation, chewing, and the likelihood of regurgitation can occur if intubation is delayed or prolonged.

Because the potency of thiamylal is greater than that of thiopental, a slightly smaller dose of thiamylal should be given. Recommended dosages vary among reports, but in the authors' experience, the following dosage schedule has proved safe for induction in thrifty animals unpremedicated with tranquilizers:

Cattle: thiopental, 6 to 12 mg/kg intravenously; thiamylal, 4 to 8 mg/kg intravenously.
Sheep and goats: thiopental, 10 to 16 mg/kg intravenously; thiamylal, 8 to 14 mg/kg intravenously.

The larger dose is used in vigorous lightweight animals and the smaller dose in older heavy animals. The dose of thiobar-

---
*Pentothal, Abbott Laboratories, North Chicago, IL 60064.
†Surital, Parke-Davis, Detroit, MI 48232.

biturate should be decreased by approximately 1/4 to 1/3 in patients premedicated with a tranquilizer or sedative, such as xylazine. "Crash induction" is contraindicated in animals with circulatory shock or uncompensated cardiovascular disease. A safer method is to administer guaifenesin containing a barbiturate to effect.

In swine, anesthesia is induced by injecting a barbiturate into an ear vein. The anterior vena cava has been used but cannot be recommended because of the likelihood of perivascular injection or possibly direct intracardiac injection. "Crash induction" is not generally employed in this species because of the lack of a vein large enough for rapid injection. A lesser concentration of barbiturate (5 per cent or less) should be used in order to avoid phlebitis and necrosis of the ear. Swine are difficult to restrain for venipuncture unless they have been properly premedicated with a tranquilizer or sedative. They frequently shake their heads and ears, causing needle dislodgment and perivascular injection.

For injection into a pig's ear vein, a small-bore needle or catheter (18- to 22-gauge, 2.5 to 3.8 cm in length) is suitable. It is helpful to use a short length of plastic tubing* between the needle and syringe to avoid dislodging the needle if the pig struggles during the injection procedure. For intravenous injection, the vein is raised by placing a tight-fitting rubber band at the base of an ear. When the vessel has been suitably cannulated, the rubber band is cut free. Aspiration of a small quantity of blood into the syringe will ensure that the needle has not been dislodged and injection can begin. One third to 1/2 of the calculated dose is given rapidly. Swine restrained with a nose snare will sink down on their rear quarters 15 to 20 seconds after the initial injection. Close observation at this time is important to ensure that the pig is breathing. The injection is continued, with anesthesia slowly increased to the desired depth. Surgical anesthesia from the initial injection will last for 10 to 15 minutes, with complete recovery requiring approximately 1 hour. If inhalation anesthesia is to be used, there will be adequate time for tracheal intubation. Extending anesthesia time with supplemental injections of barbiturates will greatly prolong the recovery period and increase the likelihood of apnea.

Induction doses for swine are thiopental, 10 to 20 mg/kg intravenously; thiamylal, 6 to 18 mg/kg intravenously.

Thiobarbiturate and Guaifenesin Combination

Guaifenesin (GG) is a muscle relaxant acting at the level of the internuncial neurons of polysynaptic fibers arising within the spinal cord. Respiratory function is little affected by GG beyond the changes associated with abnormal postural position. Cardiovascular function remains stable in the healthy animal.

It should be clearly understood that GG induces little if any analgesia. When combined with a low level of barbiturate for maintenance of surgical anesthesia, it should be supplemented with local analgesia. Thiopental and thiamylal may be combined with GG and used as an induction agent for cattle.[44, 45] For sheep and goats, this combination probably does not offer any great advantages over thiobarbiturates alone when it is used specifically for induction. In cattle, it has the advantage of being effective when administered more slowly than thiobarbiturates alone, thus allowing titering of anesthesia to the desired depth. This combination has proved to be safe for immobilization of mature cattle for procedures that require only a minimal degree of analgesia. For example, the application of a plaster of Paris cast can be safely performed with a barbiturate and GG drip. Light anesthesia with adequate muscle relaxation is easily and safely achieved if painful manipulations are not required.

Administration. Guaifenesin solution is prepared by adding 50 g to 1 L of 5 per cent dextrose in water to make a 5 per cent solution. The mixture is heated in a water bath to dissolve the GG. Thiopental or thiamylal is generally added at the rate of 2 g/L. Greater amounts of barbiturate (3 to 4 g/L) may be added if immobilization is to be continued for longer than 45 minutes to 1 hour. Another alternative is to continue with a second liter of the standard solution. In either event, the greater the total dose of barbiturate, the more prolonged the recovery. Recovery to the point at which an animal will regain its righting and protective reflexes usually does not extend beyond 45 minutes to 1 hour once administration is discontinued.

For induction, the GG-barbiturate combination must be administered rapidly by gravitational flow or by pressurizing the administration vial. A 12-gauge needle or catheter is required for rapid administration in adult cattle. Once immobilization, muscle relaxation, and light general anesthesia have been achieved, the flow rate is decreased to a slow drip just sufficient to sustain immobilization. At this point, the animal's trachea should be intubated, a prerequisite to general anesthesia in ruminants. The GG-barbiturate combination can be continued as an infusion for short minor procedures, or the animal can be connected to an inhalation machine for induction and maintenance of deep surgical anesthesia.

For safety's sake, the dose of GG-barbiturate combination should not exceed 2 ml/kg of a 5 per cent solution for induction purposes. The total dose should not exceed 4 ml/kg when it is used as a continuous infusion for maintaining anesthesia. For a 5 per cent solution of GG with 2 g of thiobarbiturate per liter, the total dose for specific purposes is as follows:

Induction: 1.5 to 2 ml/kg given rapidly intravenously.

Maintenance: should not exceed 4 ml/kg over the entire course of administration, usually 45 minutes to 1 hour and 45 minutes.

Guaifenesin-Ketamine-Xylazine ("Triple Drip")

Extensive clinical experience with a solution of 5 per cent GG in 5 per cent dextrose containing 1 to 2 mg/ml of ketamine and 0.1 mg/ml of xylazine has shown that this combination of drugs, when given intravenously, induces safe and reliable general anesthesia in cattle, sheep, and goats. Initially, 0.55 ml/kg of this solution is given rapidly intravenously. Thereafter, "Triple Drip" is given at a rate of 2.2 ml/kg/hr. This infusion rate is calculated as follows.

When infusion rates are calculated on the basis of body weight in pounds:

$$\frac{(\text{body wt in kg}) \times (2.2 \text{ ml/kg/hr}) \times 15 \text{ drops/ml}}{60 \text{ min/hr}}$$
$$= \text{drops/min of "Triple Drip"}$$

$$\frac{(\text{body wt in lb}) \times (1 \text{ ml/lb/hr}) \times 15 \text{ drops/ml}}{60 \text{ min/hr}}$$
$$= \text{drops/min of "Triple Drip"}$$

For example, the infusion rate for a 500-lb heifer would be as follows:

$$\frac{(500 \text{ lb}) \times (1 \text{ ml/lb/hr}) \times 15 \text{ drops/ml}}{60 \text{ min}}$$
$$= 125 \text{ drops/min of "Triple Drip"}$$

The authors have maintained satisfactory general anesthesia

---

*Butterfly, Abbott Laboratories, North Chicago, IL 60064.

for up to 2.5 hours in calves and mature cattle with this drug combination. Surgical procedures, including femoral fracture plating and pinning, umbilical hernia repair, and cesarean section, were performed. The trachea was intubated, and supplemental oxygen (5 to 10 L/min) was given during the course of anesthesia. Increased inspired oxygen concentration is necessary only for prolonged procedures (i.e., longer than 1 hour) or in debilitated patients. "Triple Drip" is equally effective in sheep and goats when they are dosed at the same rate as cattle.

"Triple Drip" has proved to be nearly ideal as an injectable anesthetic in swine. For use in swine, the concentration of xylazine must be increased to 1 mg/ml. This is 10 times the concentration of xylazine used in "Triple Drip" for ruminants. Inadvertent use of "Triple Drip" prepared for swine in ruminants will result in a massive xylazine overdose and, if not promptly recognized and treated, can result in a lethal outcome. "Triple Drip" for swine consists of a 5 per cent solution of guaifenesin in 5 per cent dextrose and water containing 2 mg/ml of ketamine and 1 mg/ml of xylazine. This combination of drugs is initially given rapidly in a central ear vein at a dose of 0.5 to 1 ml/kg to induce anesthesia. Thereafter, the infusion is continued at a rate of 2 ml/kg/hr (see calculations for ruminants). This combination of drugs has been used to safely maintain surgical anesthesia for up to 2.5 hours in large numbers of swine of all ages. Muscle relaxation and analgesia are quite profound. Recovery is rapid (30 to 40 minutes) once infusion is discontinued and can be hastened by administration of yohimbine or tolazoline 10 to 15 minutes after the infusion is discontinued.

Dissociative Anesthetics

These drugs induce a peculiar state of unconsciousness often referred to as "cataleptoid" or dissociative anesthesia. This anesthetic state differs markedly from that induced by barbiturates. Generally, the patient's eyelids remain open, front limbs are extended, rear limbs are flexed, and pupils are dilated; nystagmus is not uncommon; and muscle tone is increased, particularly in light planes of anesthesia. Protective reflexes (i.e., cough, swallowing), to a degree, remain intact. The myotactic reflexes are hyperexcitable; thus, the usefulness of these agents for operations on or about tendinous structures is decreased. These reflexes can be obtunded by the addition of guaifenesin and/or xylazine. Somatic analgesia is profound, but visceral analgesia is poor. Patient movement during anesthesia is rather common and does not necessarily indicate pain perception unless the reaction corresponds directly with surgical manipulation.

With ketamine alone, postanesthetic excitement has been observed in mature cattle and in swine.[46] It is most likely to occur when the drug is given intramuscularly and when the patient is not permitted to recover in a quiet, darkened environment. A sedative dose of barbiturate (e.g., 2 to 4 mg/kg pentobarbital) will adequately control excitement.[46]

Ketamine

Cattle

Ketamine, although not approved by the United States Food and Drug Administration (FDA), has been investigated more than any of the dissociatives for use in food-producing animals. Fuentes and Tellez[47] reported on the use of ketamine in 10 cows undergoing minor and major surgeries ranging from toe amputation to laparotomy. Subsequently, the use of ketamine and xylazine for cesarean section was reported by the same authors.[48] The neonate had tachycardia and tachypnea that disappeared shortly after delivery. In their study, cows for elective surgery were starved of food and water for 24 hours. Atropine was not given. They reported that regurgitation, bloat, and salivation were "absent." Anesthesia was induced by rapid intravenous injection of ketamine, 2 mg/kg, followed by constant intravenous infusion. The solution was prepared by adding ketamine to normal saline (2 mg/ml). The ketamine-saline solution was infused intravenously at a rate of 10 ml/min in these cows.

Our clinical experience suggests that in cattle premedicated with xylazine (0.1 to 0.2 mg/kg IV), anesthesia can be induced safely with ketamine, 2 mg/kg administered as a bolus intravenously. The smaller dose of xylazine is suggested in cattle larger than 700 kg. Although jaw muscle relaxation is not as profound as that induced by GG-barbiturates, tracheal intubation can be accomplished by the use of a mouth wedge. The authors have used this technique extensively for induction of anesthesia in large bulls and cows under field conditions for foot trims and other surgeries about the feet.

Sheep and Goats

Numerous reports have appeared on the use of ketamine in sheep.[49-55] Although the results are generally good, two major limiting factors remain: lack of FDA approval for use in food-producing animals and a relatively high cost.

Taylor and colleagues[53] reported on the successful use of ketamine in pregnant ewes. Initially, 2 mg/kg of ketamine was given intravenously for induction; anesthesia was maintained by continuous infusion with 5 per cent dextrose in water containing 2 mg/ml of ketamine infusion at a rate of 4 ml/min. Length of the surgical procedures ranged from 1 to 2 hours. In their study, the sheep were not starved or given premedication. Bloat, regurgitation, and salivation were not reported to be a problem. Thurmon and coworkers[54] found that ketamine, 22 mg/kg given intramuscularly, will induce satisfactory anesthesia in sheep premedicated with atropine 0.22 mg/kg and acepromazine 0.55 mg/kg. The duration of analgesia was brief, but muscle relaxation was good. In this study, duration of surgical anesthesia was extended to 1 to 1.5 hours by intermittent intravenous injection of ketamine at a rate of 2 to 4 mg/kg. Total dose required was 33 to 44 mg/kg. Clinical experience has shown that anesthesia can be safely induced in sheep and goats by combining xylazine 0.11 mg/kg and ketamine 2.2 mg/kg in the same syringe and injecting this combination intravenously. Anesthesia may be extended by repeat injection of half the original dose of both drugs. An alternative way to extend anesthesia would be to infuse "Triple Drip" as described earlier.

In goats, a combination of atropine, xylazine, and ketamine has been used to induce and maintain surgical anesthesia for a wide variety of surgical procedures (laparotomy, eyeball enucleation, amputation of claws, abomasotomy, and enterotomy).[29] Atropine 0.4 mg/kg was given initially, followed in 20 to 25 minutes by xylazine 0.22 mg/kg intramuscularly. Ketamine (11 mg/kg intramuscularly) was administered after the onset of sedation. Surgical anesthesia was maintained for 2.25 to 2.75 hours by supplemental increments of ketamine (6 mg/kg intramuscularly) or a mixture of xylazine and ketamine (0.045 mg/kg and 2.45 mg/kg, respectively, intramuscularly). For extending surgical anesthesia, ketamine supplementation was preferred over the xylazine-ketamine mixture. Clinical experience suggests that ketamine 2 to 4 mg/kg should be given intravenously to extend surgical anesthesia for brief periods, whereas the intramuscular route should be used if a longer duration is required.

Even though regurgitation has not been reported to be a

serious problem with ketamine anesthesia, tracheal intubation complements sound judgment in the wise use of all general anesthetics in ruminants.

A combination of steroids, alfaxalone and alfadolone (Saffan*), has been used in sheep and goats to induce and maintain surgical anesthesia. Saffan is generally given at 2 to 4 mg/kg intravenously. It will provide 10 to 20 minutes of anesthesia. Anesthesia time may be extended by continuous intravenous infusion, 0.24 mg/kg/min. Recovery occurs in approximately 30 minutes once the infusion is discontinued.

Swine

Ketamine has been used rather extensively in swine for minor surgical and diagnostic procedures.[46] Atropine (0.04 mg/kg intramuscularly) may be given to suppress salivation. Immobilization after intramuscular injection (11 mg/kg) occurs in 3 to 5 minutes. Muscle relaxation is poor, and analgesia is brief. Xylazine 2 to 3 mg/kg intramuscularly will enhance both muscle relaxation and analgesia. For prolonging the duration of surgical anesthesia, ketamine (2 to 4 mg/kg) may be given intravenously. Injection of 2 per cent lidocaine at the surgical site can also be safely used to enhance analgesia.

Clinical trials suggest that the intravenous route is safe and recovery is less likely to be accompanied by excitement than when ketamine is given intramuscularly, particularly in mature swine. The authors have used ketamine (3 to 5 mg/kg) and xylazine (1 to 2 mg/kg) injected intratesticularly to immobilize large boars for castration. For best results, half the calculated dose should be injected into each testicle. Barbiturates have also been used in this manner (pentobarbital 18 to 20 mg/kg) but are less effective. Surgical removal of the testicle also removes a significant amount of the anesthetic, which hastens recovery. The testicles should not be discarded where they may be consumed by other animals, lest they may become anesthetized.

Physical restraint sufficient for intravenous injection is often difficult to achieve in swine. A combination of ketamine 2 mg/kg, xylazine 2 mg/kg, and oxymorphone 0.075 mg/kg mixed in the same syringe and given intravenously has been used to induce and maintain surgical anesthesia. When the intramuscular route was chosen, each of the drug doses was doubled.[56] In our limited experience with this combination, the authors have found it to induce relatively good analgesia and muscle relaxation. Recovery was smooth and could be hastened by administration of naloxone. Major drawbacks to use of this combination center on hypoventilation, cost, and lack of FDA approval.

Saffan (alfaxalone and alfadolone) given intravenously or intramuscularly has been used to induce general anesthesia in swine. Unlike barbiturates, this product does not cause pronounced respiratory depression. Intravenous injection induces only a brief period of anesthesia; thus frequent supplemental doses are required to prolong anesthesia. Even with repeated injections, recovery is reported to be smooth and brisk. Premedicating pigs with xylazine (2 to 3 mg/kg) will decrease the initial dose of Saffan required to induce anesthesia by approximately half. The initial intravenous dose is 4 to 6 mg/kg. The intravenous route is generally used because intramuscular administration requires a larger dose, which necessitates a large volume of Saffan.

Telazol

Telazol† is a proprietary combination of tiletamine and zolazepam in a 1:1 ratio. Tiletamine is a dissociative similar to ketamine but considerably more potent. Likewise, zolazepam is a benzodiazepine similar to diazepam. Zolazepam is a central muscle relaxant and anticonvulsant. Telazol is approved for use in dogs and cats only but has been used effectively in a wide variety of species. Telazol is supplied as a sterile powder in glass vials containing 500 mg (tiletamine 250 mg, and zolazepam 250 mg). It is normally reconstituted to 100 mg/ml by adding 5 ml of sterile water but can be reconstituted in a much greater concentration (e.g., 500 mg/ml). When Telazol is used alone, immobilization is rapid but analgesia does not appear to be adequate for painful procedures. This shortcoming can be easily corrected by the concomitant administration of xylazine. When Telazol was combined with xylazine and given intramuscularly in calves, recumbency occurred in approximately 2.5 minutes and lasted approximately 2.5 hours. Muscle relaxation and analgesia were excellent.[57] Telazol-xylazine can also be used in place of a barbiturate for intravenous induction before inhalation anesthesia:

Cattle: Telazol, 1 mg/kg intravenously; xylazine, 0.05 mg/kg intravenously.

Intramuscular injection (calves, sheep, and goats): Telazol, 4 mg/kg intramuscularly; xylazine, 0.1 mg/kg intramuscularly.

As in calves, Telazol-xylazine is an excellent drug combination for use in swine. In our laboratory and clinics, the authors have used Telazol-xylazine extensively.[57] When it was given intramuscularly in pigs weighing 20 to 30 kg, anesthesia occurred in 1 to 2 minutes and lasted approximately 1 hour. If desired, tracheal intubation can be easily accomplished. The effective intramuscular dose in pigs is Telazol, 6.6 mg/kg; xylazine, 2.2 mg/kg. The drugs may be combined in the same syringe. In large boars and sows, intramuscular administration of Telazol alone or with xylazine may result in prolonged recoveries. Because of this problem, the intravenous route seems to be preferable. In adults, the intravenous dose should not exceed 1 mg/kg Telazol and 1 mg/kg xylazine. When intended for intravenous use in swine, Telazol may be dissolved in 5 ml of xylazine (100 mg/ml). The resulting solution contains 100 mg/ml of both Telazol and xylazine. This solution can be safely administered intravenously at the rate of 1 ml/50 kg to 100 kg body weight. As previously stated and as with all anesthetics, larger animals require proportionately less drug per kilogram of body weight, and further, the drug should always be given to effect.

Prolonged recovery in swine appears to be related to the zolazepam fraction of Telazol. In order to decrease the amount of zolazepam administered, the authors have dissolved Telazol by adding 2.5 ml of ketamine (100 mg/ml) and 2.5 ml of xylazine (100 mg/ml). Each milliliter of the resulting mixture contains tiletamine (50 mg), ketamine (50 mg), zolazepam (50 mg), and xylazine (50 mg). This mixture has proved to be safe and effective when administered intravenously at the rate of 1 ml/75 kg. Anesthesia can be safely extended by supplemental doses of 0.5 ml/75 kg intravenously. Supplemental injections should be given over 60 seconds for avoidance of pronounced respiratory depression.

INHALATION ANESTHESIA

Without question, inhalation anesthesia is the safest and most satisfactory means of maintaining surgical anesthesia in ruminants and swine. Until recently, inhalation anesthesia was used primarily in research laboratories and hospitals dealing with valuable animals requiring major surgical intervention. Presently, the reasonable cost of halothane has stimulated a renewed interest in inhalation anesthesia for food-producing

---
*Glaxo Laboratories, Triangle Park, NC.
†A. H. Robins, Richmond, VA 23220.

animals as well as in the progressive development of advanced surgical techniques being employed in valuable animals. At this time, equipment cost, the economic value of the average animal, and the inconvenience of transporting equipment to the field are major disadvantages to the use of inhalation anesthesia in general food animal practice. However, it should be emphasized that there is no satisfactory substitute for inhalation anesthesia in valuable animals requiring general anesthesia for major surgical procedures.

Surgical Table Padding

Cattle do not appear to be as susceptible as are horses to generalized myositis. This does not mean that padding is unnecessary, because partial radial nerve paralysis may occur in heavy cattle kept deeply anesthetized for prolonged periods. The usual 5 to 7.5 cm of foam rubber padding or air mattress is not adequate in all cases. Clinical experience has shown in both horses and cattle that an automobile tire inner tube strategically placed beneath the animal's shoulder, combined with a moderate amount of table-top padding, will prevent radial nerve paralysis. For proper placement of the inner tube, the animal is rolled to its back, and the tube is fitted over the dependent leg. The animal is turned back to its side, and the tube is inflated. Inflation of the tube tends to raise the animal's front quarters, taking body weight off the brachial plexus where body contact is made with the table-top padding. In this position, the scapula is allowed to fall away from the thoracic wall, thus relieving pressure on and around the brachial plexus.

Inhalation Anesthetics

Ether, chloroform, and cyclopropane were the first inhalation agents used in ruminants and swine. They have, for the most part, been replaced by halothane and isoflurane.

Halothane and Isoflurane

These compounds are potent, volatile anesthetics with a rather broad safety margin. The physical and pharmacologic characteristics of halothane and isoflurane make them highly desirable anesthetics for use in large species. Owing to halothane's and isoflurane's high volatility, high potency, and low solubility, depth of anesthesia can be regulated quickly and precisely. Recovery is relatively rapid. Ruminants in light surgical anesthesia are generally able to assume sternal recumbency 10 to 15 minutes after administration is discontinued. Excitement during the recovery period is rarely observed.

Halothane and isoflurane cross the placental barrier and induce fetal depression. However, once breathing is initiated after birth, blood concentrations of these anesthetics decrease rapidly, and central nervous depression disappears, being most rapid for isoflurane. Because of high vapor pressure, it is unsafe to use halothane or isoflurane as an open drip. Safety can be ensured only when these anesthetics are administered with a precision vaporizer, using a circle or to-and-fro rebreathing system.

Carbon Dioxide–Oxygen Anesthesia for Processing Piglets

Concerns for humane treatment and prevention of pain in baby pigs subjected to surgical procedures such as castration, tail docking, and ear notching are increasing in frequency. In order for these procedures to be accomplished painlessly and, therefore, humanely, general anesthesia is required. Anesthesia for such a purpose must be safe, simple, effective, and economical with rapid onset and recovery without leaving tissue residues. In an attempt to meet these criteria, the authors have developed a system for anesthetizing piglets with carbon dioxide and oxygen. This method uses 50 per cent carbon dioxide and 50 per cent oxygen administered by nose cone, which induces unconsciousness in approximately 30 seconds. Recovery also occurs in approximately 30 seconds when administration is discontinued. A 50/50 per cent concentration of carbon dioxide and oxygen (flow rate of 2 L/min of each) administered by nose cone was used to anesthetize 34 male piglets for castration. Mean time for loss of consciousness was 31 seconds. Castration required 33 seconds. Recovery to standing required 28 seconds. Total time required for induction, castration, and recovery to walking required 92 seconds. There were no deaths. The total cost per pig was less than 4 cents. This technique can easily be used in any neonatal animal (e.g., lambs and kids).[58] The device for administering carbon dioxide and oxygen is illustrated in Figure 2.

Inhalation Anesthetic Equipment

Today, several companies manufacture anesthesia machines designed for use in large animals. These machines are well constructed and durable but extremely expensive. Although originally designed for horses, they are ideal for adult cattle. Machines designed for use in people or veterinary small animal practice are large enough for calves, sheep, goats, and swine. Details of these machines have been described in numerous texts.[13-16]

Rebreathing Systems

The machine shown in Figure 3 is equipped with calibrated vaporizers for halothane located out of the breathing circuit. With this arrangement, a precise volume percentage of anesthetic vapor can be delivered to the breathing circuit. The out-of-circuit vaporizer is preferred with halothane and isoflurane. This machine uses a circle rebreathing system that routes exhaled gases through a carbon dioxide absorbent for removal of carbon dioxide. The rebreathing systems are used as semiclosed or closed. Generally, the semiclosed method is pre-

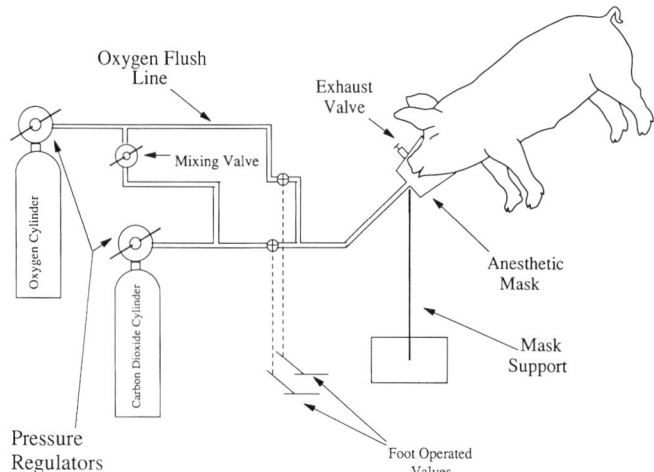

Figure 2. Schematic drawing of a device used to administer 50/50 carbon dioxide–oxygen to anesthetize pigs for castration. This device utilizes combination regulator/flowmeters to meter gas flows to the anesthetic mask. Line pressures at 50 psi and gas flow rates of 2 L/min are maintained. (Patent applied for.)

vaporizer is available, a to-fro canister can be used to administer inhalation anesthesia economically in large animals. To use a to-fro system with a small animal machine, the fresh gas delivery line is disconnected from the circle rebreathing stem and attached to the fresh gas inflow port of the to-fro canister. Oxygen flow rate and concentration of anesthetic vapor delivered to the to-fro canister are determined by flowmeter and vaporizer setting, respectively, on the small animal machine.

Nonrebreathing systems (e.g., Ayres "T" piece, Norman elbow) can be used in small food-producing animals. However, owing to the high fresh gas flow rates required, they are uneconomical in all but the smallest of patients (e.g., piglet, newborn lamb) and cause excessive environmental contamination unless properly scavenged.

Oxygen Flow Rates and Anesthetic Vapor Concentration

Because the concentration of nitrogen in the lungs is approximately 80 per cent in animals breathing ambient air, high oxygen flow rates are necessary for rapid denitrogenation during the induction period. An alternative method is to flush the rebreathing system and the animal's lungs several times with oxygen as soon as the endotracheal tube is connected to the anesthetic machine. Denitrogenation will ensure against early hypoxia and promote rapid induction of anesthesia. After induction with an injectable anesthetic (e.g., barbiturate, GG-barbiturate), the oxygen flow should be set at 5 to 8 L/min in mature cattle and 2 to 4 L/min in small ruminants and swine. The out-of-circuit vaporizer is adjusted to deliver 3 to 5 per cent halothane or isoflurane, depending on the rate of induction desired. When a 5 per cent setting is used, particularly in small animals (i.e., sheep, goats, pigs, and calves), the patient should be observed closely in order to prevent overdose. The oxygen flows and vaporizer settings are gradually decreased as the animal approaches surgical anesthesia, which will usually require 15 to 20 minutes. When surgical anesthesia has been

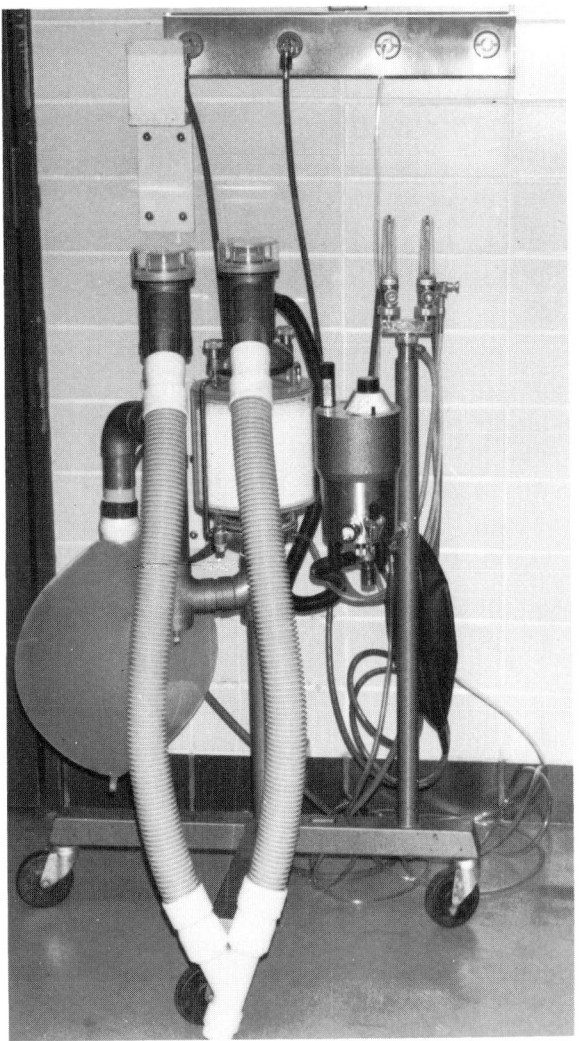

Figure 3. Inhalation anesthetic machine designed for use in large animals (i.e., adult cattle and horses). North American Drager, Telford, PA 18969.

ferred in large patients. Semiclosed indicates that the volume of fresh gas delivered to the rebreathing system (i.e., oxygen-anesthetic vapor) is greater than that required for the patient's metabolic needs. For prevention of overfilling of the breathing circuit and production of excessive airway pressure, the exhaust valve remains open for escape of the excess inflow of gases.

With the closed system, fresh gas inflow into the breathing system just meets the patient's metabolic requirement. This method is more economical but requires closer monitoring to ensure safe and stable anesthesia. Hypercapnia will not occur so long as the carbon dioxide absorbent is active. Neither will hypoxia occur so long as the rebreathing bag contains an amount of gas that exceeds the patient's tidal volume.

The original rebreathing system employed with inhalation agents was the to-fro canister (Fig. 4). The term "to-fro" means that inhaled and exhaled gases travel back and forth through the carbon dioxide absorbent, instead of in a circular pattern as in the circle system. Although not as satisfactory as a circle system, it is an economical substitute that can easily be "home made." Details for construction of a large to-fro canister have been published.[59]

When a small animal machine equipped with a precision

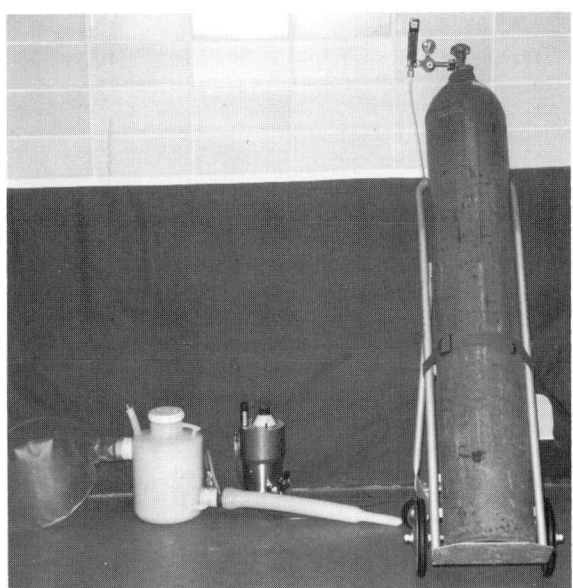

Figure 4. Home-constructed to-fro rebreathing canister is shown here with reservoir bag and Cole's endotracheal tube attached. A precision vaporizer is employed to supply anesthetic vapor to the breathing system. An oxygen tank with pressure regulator–flowmeter combination makes this a simple but complete anesthetic delivery system for large animals.

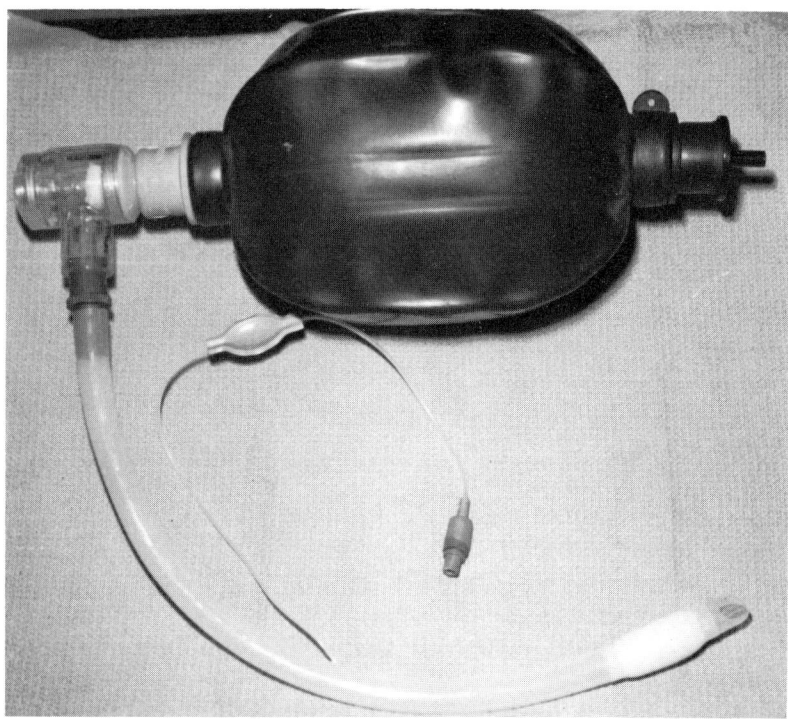

Figure 5. Hand-operated resuscitator with cuffed endotracheal tube attached. When desirable, oxygen can be metered into the resuscitator at a port located on the end opposite the endotracheal tube connection.

attained, the oxygen flow rate should be decreased to 3 to 5 L/min in adult cattle and 1 to 2 L/min in smaller animals. Vaporizer settings of 1.5 to 3 per cent will be required to maintain surgical anesthesia in most animals. In a mature cow, the higher vaporizer setting will be required with low oxygen flow rates. It is more appropriate to rely on patient response than on specific oxygen flow and vaporizer settings to determine induction rate and anesthetic depth.

Termination of Anesthesia

Shortly before completion of the surgical procedure, the anesthetic vapor concentration is decreased to approximately half of that required for maintenance. Just before completion of surgery, the anesthetic vaporizer is turned off, and the rebreathing system is flushed with oxygen. The animal should remain connected to the anesthetic machine and breathe oxygen until signs of recovery—active palpebral reflex, limb movement, chewing, and swallowing—are readily apparent, at which time it should be moved to a quiet, darkened recovery area. The patient should be observed closely for character and rate of respiration and color of mucous membranes until it is able to support itself in sternal recumbency. The endotracheal tube should not be removed until strong protective reflexes—chewing and swallowing—are present. If a cuffed endotracheal tube has been used, it should be removed with the cuff inflated in order to remove foreign material (e.g., saliva, regurgitant) that may have accumulated in the trachea proximal to the cuff. Animals are usually able to stand within 30 to 40 minutes after being moved to the recovery area.

Endotracheal Intubation

Whenever general anesthesia is induced, the importance of tracheal intubation cannot be overemphasized. Tracheal intubation ensures a patent airway (preventing aspiration of saliva or regurgitant), provides a rapid and safe means for controlling ventilation if apnea occurs, and establishes a route for delivery of oxygen or inhalation anesthetics. Assisted or controlled ventilation is effective only when the trachea is intubated. Even with the best-fitting face mask, there will be leaks, and positive-pressure ventilation with a mask will force gas into the rumen or stomach, particularly in swine, increasing intra-abdominal pressure and decreasing the effectiveness of positive-pressure ventilation or normal breathing. Death during general anesthesia occurs most often from respiratory arrest. When the trachea is intubated and the patient connected to an anesthetic machine, ventilation can be controlled by squeezing the reservoir bag. When injectable anesthesia is used in small ruminants and swine, one has only to blow into the endotracheal tube until breathing is resumed. A hand-operated resuscitator is economical and effective and can be used to support ventilation with room air (Fig. 5). Oxygen supplementation by connecting an oxygen line to the resuscitator may be used when necessary.

Types of Endotracheal Tubes

Two types of tubes are used in adult cattle: the cuffed tube and the Cole's tube (Fig. 6). The cuffed tube provides a complete seal between the tube and tracheal wall when the cuff is properly inflated. The cuff should be inflated to a pressure that will just prevent escape of gas between cuff and tracheal wall when 25 to 30 cm water positive pressure is applied. Most foreign material (i.e., saliva, regurgitant) accumulating in the trachea anterior to the cuff will be extracted to the oropharynx when the tube is removed with the cuff inflated; it is for this reason that cuffed tubes are generally used. However, the Cole's tube has been used satisfactorily in large numbers of cattle. Instead of a cuff, it has an air seal, which is adequate for positive-pressure ventilation, that is achieved between tube and airway wall in a rather unique way. In adult cattle, the large diameter of the tube extends through the larynx, where the shoulder presses upon the first tracheal ring. The smaller diameter of the tube extends into the trachea. A snug fit inside the larynx and shoulder contact with the first tracheal ring create an effective air seal. If foreign material should proceed distal to the tube's contact with the

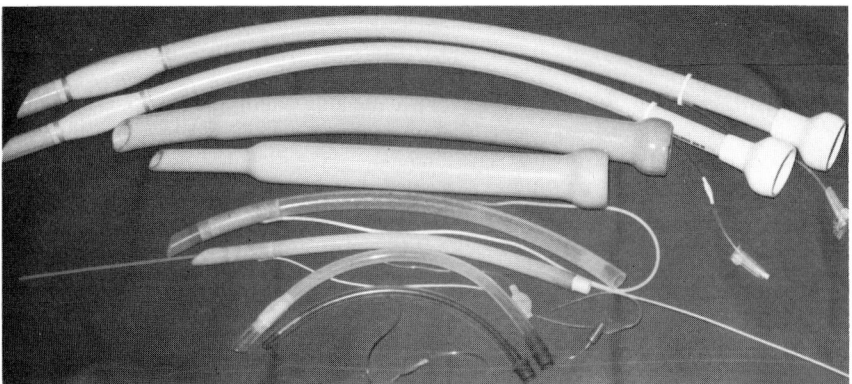

Figure 6. An assortment of endotracheal tubes. The two large tubes with tapered end are Cole's tubes. The plastic stylet (in the tube third from the bottom) is used as an aid to tracheal intubation.

tracheal rings, it would not be extracted with tube removal. On the other hand, tracheal contamination has not been identified as a problem when the Cole's tube is properly placed and anchored to the lower or upper jaw with adhesive tape or gauze. Regurgitant accumulating in the oropharynx may be safely rinsed from the mouth with a water hose before extubation.

Sizes of Endotracheal Tubes

The largest tube that can be placed into the trachea without injury to the delicate airway tissues should be used. It is the internal diameter that determines the amount of resistance to breathing created by a given size tube. Thin-walled tubes are desirable, but if the wall is too thin, the tube can become kinked easily if the animal's neck is flexed. Overinflation of the cuff can cause tubes with thin walls to collapse, creating airway obstruction.

Endotracheal tube sizes for cattle are listed in Table 2.[22] Although the diameters listed in the table have been found to be appropriate, the lengths are a bit excessive in some animals. The portion of endotracheal tube extending out of the animal's mouth constitutes mechanical dead space and should be removed in order to promote effective ventilation. Connecting the Y-piece of the rebreathing system as closely to the animal's mouth as possible eliminates most of the unnecessary dead space. Large sheep and goats will require a tube having an internal diameter of 10 to 16 mm. Tubes with internal diameters of 6 to 10 mm will be adequate for smaller ruminants; for this group, the disposable tubes used in people and dogs are quite satisfactory. In general, tubes required for goats will be one to two sizes smaller than those required for sheep of the same weight.

Proportionately, swine will require considerably smaller tubes than will goats or sheep. For example, a 50-kg pig will require a 9-mm tube.[22] A 10- to 14-mm internal diameter tube is satisfactory for adult sows, whereas smaller swine will require tubes of 6 to 10 mm.

Before induction of anesthesia, tube size for ruminants can be approximated by external palpation of the trachea. It is wise to have 3 tubes at hand: one the size judged to be appropriate by tracheal palpation, one a size larger, and one a size smaller.

Technique

Intubation of Cattle

Two basic techniques are employed for tracheal intubation in cattle. With either method, a dental wedge* is essential for preventing injury to the anesthetist's hand and damage to the endotracheal tube by the animal's teeth (Fig. 7). The mouth wedge should be left in place during anesthesia and until extubation. Adhesive tape or gauze placed around the animal's muzzle in front of the mouth wedge will prevent its dislodgment if the animal becomes lightly anesthetized and begins chewing.

The first method for tracheal intubation has been well described.[13] A mouth wedge is inserted and held in place by an assistant who also extends the head, decreasing the orotracheal angle and creating a straight pathway from mouth to trachea. The tongue is drawn out of the mouth, and the anesthetist's hand is passed between the dental arcades until contact is made with the epiglottis and arytenoid cartilages. The tube is then passed alongside or beneath the anesthetist's

---
*Jorgensen Laboratories, Loveland, CO 80538.

Table 2. ENDOTRACHEAL TUBE SIZES FOR USE IN CATTLE

	Internal Diameter (mm)	Approximate External Diameter (mm)	Length (cm)
Large bulls	30	38	100
Mature cows	25	31	80
Yearlings	20	26	80
Calves			
6 months	18	22.5	60
3 months	16	19.5	60

Adapted from Soma LR (ed): Textbook of Veterinary Anesthesia. Baltimore, Williams & Wilkins, 1971.

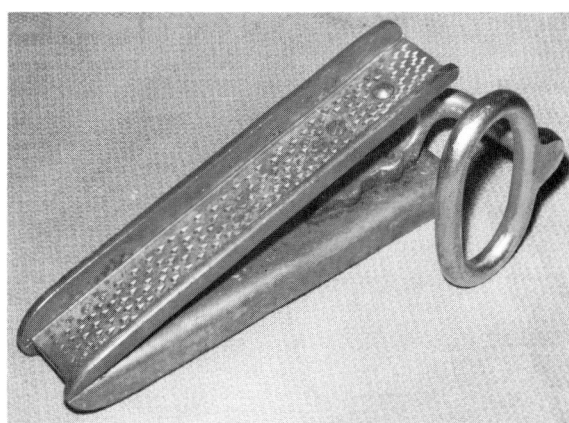

Figure 7. Dental wedge used to hold the mouth of adult cattle open for tracheal intubation.

arm and is gently guided with the fingertips through the laryngeal opening and into the trachea. The cuff is quickly inflated.

The procedure for the second method is the same as that for the first, up to the point of passing the endotracheal tube. At this point, a small stiff tube (horse stomach tube 3 times longer than the endotracheal tube) is passed into the trachea. The anesthetist's hand is withdrawn from the animal's mouth, and the endotracheal tube is passed over the small tube into the trachea (Fig. 8).[20] The small tube is removed. This method is preferred in medium-sized cattle and in all animals in which the Cole's tube is used.

Intubation of Calves, Sheep, and Goats

In animals with a small oral cavity, a laryngoscope with a long illuminated blade (Rawson or extension on human blade) (Fig. 9) can be used to visualize the laryngeal opening directly for tracheal intubation. Because the mouth of herbivores cannot be opened widely, the combination of laryngoscope blade and large endotracheal tube may occlude one's view of the laryngeal opening. In such cases, a plastic catheter can be passed into the trachea to act as a stylet over which the endotracheal tube is passed (see Fig. 6). When the endotracheal tube is in place, the stylet is removed and the cuff is quickly inflated.

Fetal Tracheal Intubation

Apnea may be encountered when a fetus is delivered by cesarean section. Tracheal intubation before delivery provides a means of dealing with this problem. When the fetal head is delivered through the incision in the uterine wall, the laryngoscope is used to visualize the laryngeal opening for tracheal intubation. With the tube in place, fluids can be aspirated from the upper airways. Mechanical ventilation with use of a hand-operated resuscitator (see Fig. 5) is commenced and may be continued until spontaneous breathing is initiated. Oxygen may be delivered to the fetus via the resuscitator when it is available and required. These maneuvers can all be completed before disruption of the placental-umbilical circulation, if so desired.

When apnea persists in the presence of a strong fetal heartbeat, a small dose of doxapram (0.2 to 0.4 mg/kg intravenously) or some other analeptic may aid in the establishment of spontaneous breathing.

Intubation of Swine

Pigs are more difficult to intubate than are small ruminants because of several physical features, including a relatively small larynx, inability to open the mouth widely, blending of cricoid cartilage into the laryngeal orifice, and a ventral slope from larynx to trachea. With light basal anesthesia, laryngeal spasms often occur when endotracheal intubation is attempted. Spraying the laryngeal mucosa with 2 to 4 per cent lidocaine shortly before proceeding with intubation will usually prevent laryngeal spasms, making the procedure less hazardous.

The technique for tracheal intubation in swine is essentially the same as that for small ruminants. A mouth wedge can be used to keep the mouth open. An alternative is to place loops of small-diameter rope around the upper and lower jaws immediately behind the canine teeth. An assistant applies traction on each loop, opening the mouth widely. A laryngoscope is nearly essential for intubation unless one has had a great deal of experience. With the laryngoscope, the laryngeal opening can be directly visualized and the tube passed into the trachea. As in sheep and goats, a small-gauge plastic catheter, 3 times the length of the endotracheal tube, can be passed into the trachea, serving as a stylet over which the endotracheal tube may be passed (see Fig. 6).

A technique whereby a small cuffed tube is placed into each nostril and connected to a Y-piece, which in turn is connected to the Y-piece of the anesthetic machine, has been used as a substitute for endotracheal intubation. Tape or gauze is placed around the pig's snout to prevent open-mouth breathing. Although anesthesia can be effectively maintained, this technique does not provide protection against aspiration of foreign materials or prevent inflation of the stomach when positive-pressure ventilation is used. It is, therefore, no less hazardous than a well-fitted nose cone and is not acceptable as a substitute for tracheal intubation.

STAGES AND PLANES OF ANESTHESIA

Traditionally, general anesthesia has been divided into stages and then into planes.[60] The signs associated with each stage are empiric at best, but nonetheless, they do serve as a useful noninvasive method for rough assessment of patient anesthetic response.

Monitoring methods, including blood pressure measurement, electrocardiogram, alveolar or blood anesthetic concentration, blood gas tensions, and acid-base status, will provide accurate information for assessment of anesthetic depth and physiologic response; however, equipment for these measurements is expensive, and the techniques are time-consuming and generally unavailable to the practicing veterinarian. As a result, the traditional signs as originally described for ether anesthesia in humans (Guedel) and since described in animals by several authors[13, 14, 44, 45] are generally used. From stage III to stage IV, the signs are based on vital system function, degree of muscle relaxation, eye reflexes, and progressive eyeball movement, which appears to be most informative in the bovine species.[45] Preanesthetic medications (tranquilizers, sedatives, and the like) modify the signs associated with each stage of anesthesia.

Stage I

This is the stage in which an animal is capable of resisting restraint in order to avoid induction of anesthesia. Rapid breathing or breath-holding may be encountered. Excitement may be associated with voiding of urine and feces. These are signs of apprehension and fear and are more prevalent in unpremedicated patients.

Stage II

This is often referred to as the involuntary excitement stage. Consciousness is lost abruptly, but reflex responses to stimuli are exaggerated. The respiratory pattern is irregular, and struggling is associated with breath-holding. The jaw muscles are unrelaxed, and attempts to intubate will initiate chewing and coughing. Reflex responses, including chewing movements, coughing, and likelihood of active regurgitation in ruminants, are common in stage II.

When surgical anesthesia is attained by rapid intravenous injection of a precalculated dose of barbiturate, this stage of anesthesia is passed through so quickly that it generally goes unidentified. Progressing rapidly from consciousness to surgical anesthesia usually avoids problems occurring in stage II. However, in the debilitated animal, "crash induction" should be avoided.

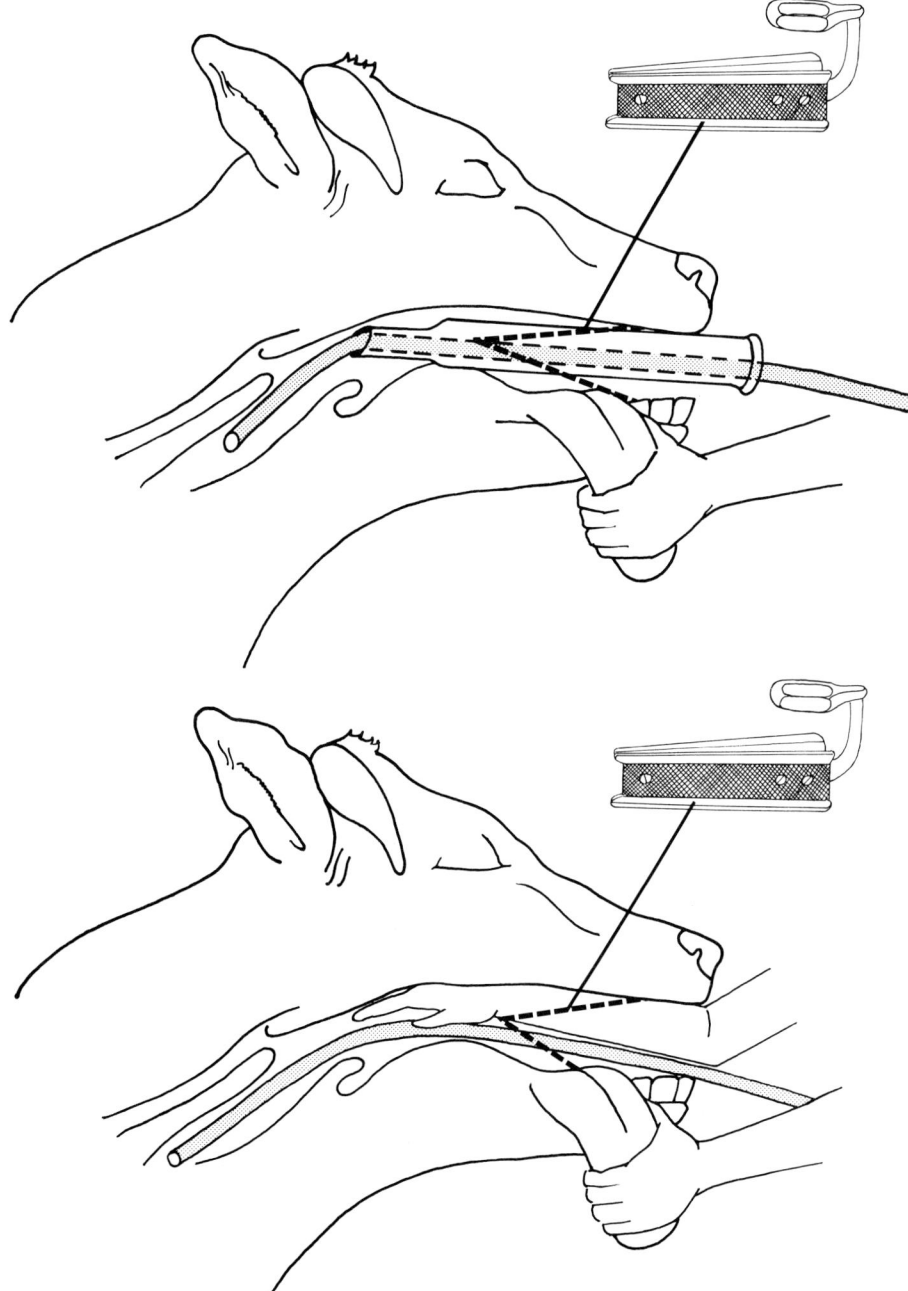

Figure 8. These drawings illustrate a method for passing an endotracheal tube in the cow. A dental wedge is used to prevent injury of hand and arm, and a small tube three times the length of the endotracheal tube is inserted into the trachea. This tube serves as a guide for directing the endotracheal tube into the trachea.

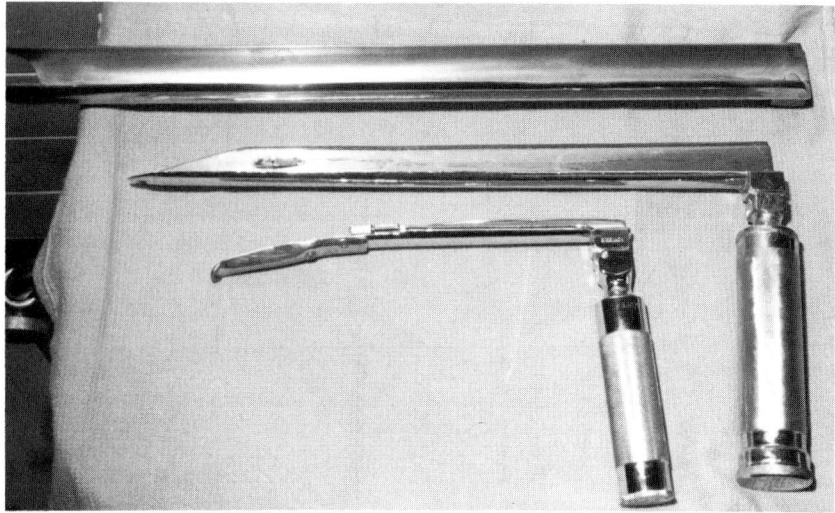

Figure 9. *Top,* Large animal laryngoscope with two types of blades. *Bottom,* The human laryngoscope has been modified by adding an extension to the blade. It is ideal for visualizing the laryngeal opening in small ruminants and swine.

Stage III

Surgical Anesthesia

PLANE 1. It is at this level of anesthesia that breathing becomes regular and analgesia is present. Nystagmus may be evident but rapidly disappears as anesthesia progressively deepens; this sign is not as common in cows as in horses. In ruminants, esophageal stimulation may evoke regurgitation, which extends to the early part of plane 2. Minor surgical procedures can be performed at this plane, but the degree of muscle relaxation is poor. Palpebral and corneal reflexes are strong.

PLANE 2. Respiration remains stable. Laryngeal reflexes progressively weaken and are eventually lost as plane 3 is achieved. Palpebral reflexes are sluggish or inactive. The corneal reflex is active, but the degree of muscle relaxation is sufficient for most surgical procedures to be accomplished without initiating reflex responses. Intercostal muscle activity is diminished.

PLANE 3. This plane is characterized by loss of intercostal muscle activity and depressed diaphragmatic function, which result in an uneven respiratory pattern. Respiration rate is generally increased, but tidal volume is decreased. Muscle relaxation is profound; the corneal reflex is weak or absent, with the eye being fixed centrally between the palpebrae.

Stage IV

The pupil is widely dilated, and all other eye reflexes have waned. Respiration is purely diaphragmatic in character, with excessive abdominal movement occurring with each agonal breath. Cardiac function is rapidly failing, the anus is dilated, and feces and urine may be passively voided. At this point in time, if respiration is not mechanically supported, anesthetic concentration is not decreased, and fluids are not administered rapidly to support the failing cardiovascular system, death is inevitable.

ANESTHESIA AND EYEBALL ROTATION IN CATTLE

Rotation of the eyeball in cattle has been described in detail[45] and has proved to be reliable for monitoring anesthetic depth as well as progression of recovery from anesthesia.

The eyeball is normally centered between the palpebrae in the unanesthetized cow in lateral recumbency (Fig. 10 A). As anesthesia is induced, the eyeball rotates ventrally, with the cornea being partially obscured by the lower eyelid (Fig. 10B and C). As depth of anesthesia increases, the cornea becomes completely hidden by the lower eyelid (Fig. 10D); this sign indicates stage III, plane 2 anesthesia. A further increase in the depth of anesthesia is accompanied by dorsal rotation of the eyeball. Dorsal movement is complete when the cornea is centered between the palpebrae (Fig. 10E); this sign indicates deep surgical (stage III, plane 3 or greater) anesthesia with profound muscle relaxation. With this depth of anesthesia, the patient's vital signs must be monitored closely and the anesthetic percentage must be decreased to a maintenance level. Otherwise, anesthesia may progress rather quickly to stage IV. During recovery, eyeball rotation occurs in reverse order to that observed during induction.

MALIGNANT HYPERTHERMIA IN SWINE

Malignant hyperthermia (MH) is a condition occurring in some strains of swine subjected to stress. The predisposition to MH appears to be inherited as an autosomal dominant gene with incomplete penetrance.[61] It is encountered most often in animals with a high proportion of muscle to body mass. The incidence of MH is higher in confined swine of Pietrain, Landrace, Spotted Swine, Large White, and Hampshire breeds. Other breeds are not immune, but the incidence does appear to be less in Durocs.[62] MH is characterized by rapid onset of tachycardia, muscle rigidity, hyperthermia, tachypnea that progresses to dyspnea, and finally apnea, cardiac dysrhythmias, bradycardia, and death. In susceptible animals, MH usually occurs shortly after exposure to halothane, although the authors have observed MH with all halogenated anesthetics. When anesthesia is induced with a thiobarbiturate, the onset of MH seems to be slower. In susceptible swine, the syndrome can be induced by any stressful condition (e.g., castration or even restraint for vaccination). Thus it is important to understand that the MH syndrome is not peculiar to stress associated with induction of halothane anesthesia.

Succinylcholine has been shown to induce MH in susceptible swine, but dantrolene,* a muscle relaxant, 1 to 2 mg/kg, has been shown to prevent the syndrome.[63] A rapid rise in body

---

*Dantrium, Norwich-Eaton Pharmaceutical, Norwich, NY 13815.

temperature and the rapid onset of muscle rigidity are the first characteristic signs of the onset of MH.

The rectal or body core temperature of swine subjected to general anesthesia should be monitored closely. Any sudden increase indicates the likelihood of MH onset. Treatment after the condition is clinically evident is generally unsuccessful. If MH is detected in the earliest stage, elimination of halothane, ventilation with oxygen, administration of sodium bicarbonate, and rapid body cooling with ice packs may be beneficial.

Swine known to harbor genes specific for the MH syndrome should not be anesthetized unless it is absolutely necessary. In special situations, pretreatment of swine with dantrolene (1 to 2 mg/kg) is effective in preventing the onset of MH; if given early, dantrolene may be used successfully to treat the condition after its initiation.

SUPPORTIVE FLUID THERAPY DURING ANESTHESIA

In the healthy patient subjected to short-term, light surgical anesthesia, administration of supportive fluids is not absolutely necessary unless the animal has been starved of food and water for 24 hours or more. Prolonged deep surgical anesthesia, on the other hand, is best managed with intravenous fluid support.

Catheterization of the jugular vein with a large-bore cannula (i.e., 10- to 13-gauge) will allow rapid delivery of large amounts of fluid in large adult ruminants when required. In addition, a route is established for administration of emergency drugs (e.g., cardiotonic or antidysrhythmics). Through the large catheter, maintenance fluids can be delivered continuously. Fluids best suited for this purpose are balanced electrolyte solutions (e.g., lactated Ringer's, Normosol solutions) unless laboratory results indicate a specific electrolyte deficiency, in which case fluids fortified with the deficient electrolyte will be required. If serum electrolyte analysis is unavailable, balanced electrolyte solutions should be selected because they tend to return either low or high electrolyte concentrations toward normal.

For maintenance purposes, fluids are generally given at a rate of 4 to 8 ml/kg/hr. In emergency situations (e.g., shock, acute blood loss, hypotension), rapid administration is required. With a large catheter (10- to 13-gauge) in place, gravity flow should allow a rapid enough expansion of circulating fluid volume. With a smaller catheter (e.g., 16-gauge), it will be necessary to pressurize the fluid vial with a rubber bulb hand pump or large syringe in order to attain a rapid fluid delivery rate. Volumes of 4 to 8 L are usually necessary to arrest falling blood pressure in adult cattle. Larger amounts will be required in adult patients in shock. For example, it is not improper to administer 25 to 30 L of a balanced electrolyte solution to a large bull or cow suffering from septic shock. Continuous monitoring of cardiopulmonary function is vital when large amounts of fluids are given. Hematocrit and serum protein

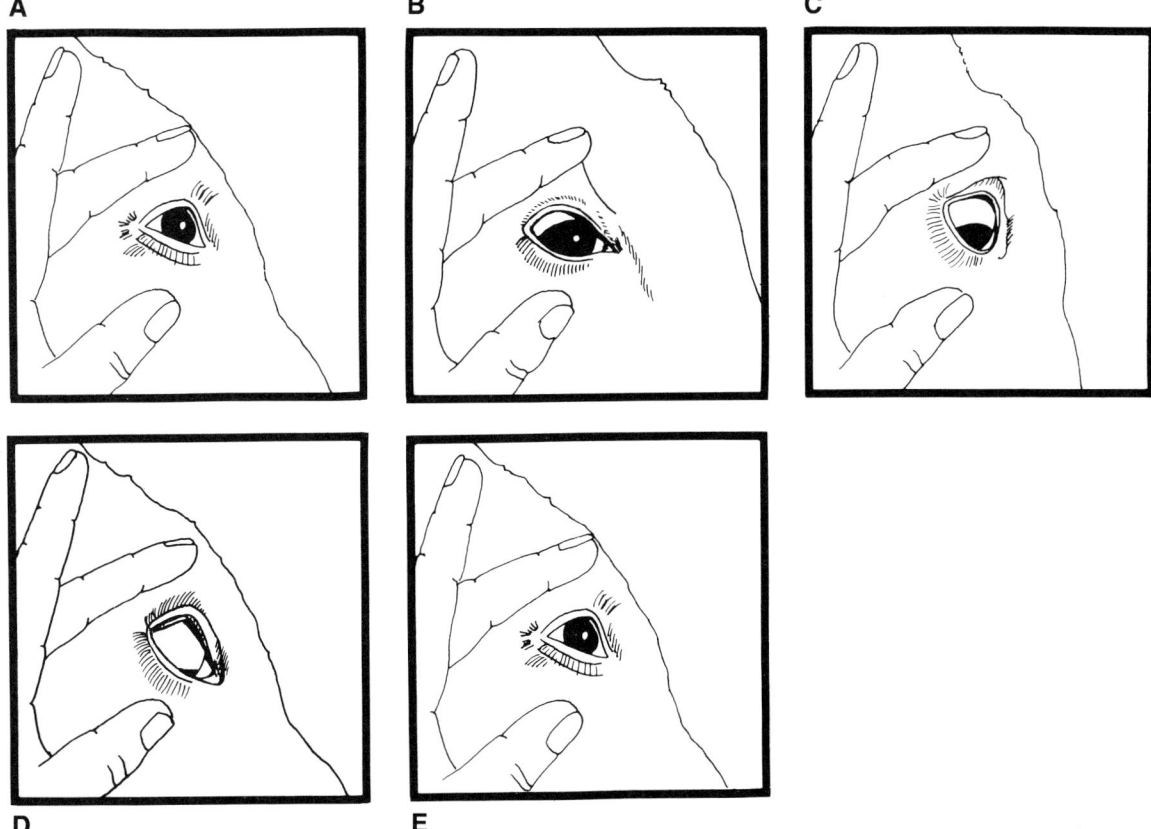

Figure 10. Eyeball position during induction and maintenance of general anesthesia of cattle. *A*, Position of eye when cow is unanesthetized and positioned in lateral recumbency. *B* and *C*, With induction of anesthesia, the eye rotates ventrally, the cornea being partially obscured by the lower eyelid. *D*, As depth of anesthesia is increased (stage III, plane 2–3), the cornea is completely hidden by the lower eyelid. *E*, Further increases in the depth of anesthesia cause the eye to rotate dorsally to a central position between the palpebrae. At this point, deep surgical anesthesia has been attained, and muscle relaxation is profound. Decreasing the depth of anesthesia is accompanied by eye movements occurring in a reverse order.

values should be used to evaluate response to fluid volume expansion. When the hematocrit values decrease to 20 per cent or less, blood transfusion would seem necessary. Serum protein concentrations less than 4.5 g/100 ml indicate excessive blood dilution. Under such circumstances, continued administration of crystalloid solutions can easily result in pulmonary edema.

Of major importance is fluid loading in sows presented for cesarean section that are hypotensive or demonstrate other signs of shock. With a 16-gauge, over-the-needle catheter placed in a large central ear vein, 2 to 3 L of fluid can be given rather rapidly by pressurizing the fluid vial. This procedure is often the single most important measure that can be taken to promote safe anesthesia in a sow presented for cesarean section. This is particularly true if the sow is toxic from dead piglets in utero and when epidural anesthesia is to be used.

REFERENCES

1. Donawick WJ, Hirmath I, Baue AE: Anesthesia, ventilation, and experimental thoracotomy in the calf. Am J Vet Res 30:533–541, 1969.
2. Gerring EL, Scarth SC: Anesthesia for open heart surgery in the calf. Br J Anaesth 46:455–460, 1974.
3. McFarlane JK, Robillard FA, Blundell PE: Anesthesia for cardiopulmonary bypass in calves. Can Anaesth Soc J 14:240–245, 1967.
4. Mishzawa T, Morris DT, Couves CM: Surgical techniques for total artificial heart replacement in calves. Can J Surg 17:261–265, 1974.
5. Short CE, Keats AS, Liotta D, Hall W: Anesthesia for cardiac surgery in calves. Am J Vet Res 29:2287–2294, 1968.
6. Steffey EP, Holland D: Halothane anesthesia in calves. Am J Vet Res 40:372–376, 1979.
7. Kumar A: Physiologic, biochemical and clinical effects of ketamine hydrochloride in goats (Capra hircus) with and without premedication. PhD Thesis, University of Illinois, 1973.
8. Palahniuk RJ, Shnider SM: Maternal and fetal cardiovascular and acid-base changes during halothane and isoflurane anesthesia in the pregnant ewe. Anesthesiology 41:462–472, 1974.
9. Smith JB, Manning FA, Palahniuk RJ: Maternal and fetal effects of methoxyflurane anaesthesia in the pregnant ewe. Can Anaesth Soc J 22:449–459, 1975.
10. Wallis KL, Shnider SM, Hicks JS, Spivey HT: Epidural anesthesia in the normotensive pregnant ewe. Anesthesiology 4:481–487, 1976.
11. Palahniuk RJ, Shnider SM, Eger EI: Pregnancy decreases the requirement for inhaled anesthetic agents. Anesthesiology 41:82–83, 1974.
12. Pearson H: The treatment of surgical disorders of the bovine abdomen. Vet Rec 92:245–254, 1973.
13. Hall LW, Clark KW: Veterinary Anaesthesia, 8th ed. London, Bailliere Tindall, 1983.
14. Lumb WV, Jones EW: Veterinary Anesthesia. Philadelphia, Lea & Febiger, 1984.
15. Short CE: Principles and Practice of Veterinary Anesthesia. Baltimore, Williams & Wilkins, 1987.
16. Soma LR: Textbook of Veterinary Anesthesia. Baltimore, Williams & Wilkins, 1971.
17. Steffey EP: Some characteristics of ruminants and swine that complicate management of general anesthesia. Vet Clin North Am [Food Anim Pract] 2:507–516, 1986.
18. Horney FD: Anesthesia in the bovine. Can Vet J 7:224–230, 1960.
19. Collins VJ: Principles of Anesthesiology, 2nd ed. Philadelphia, Lea & Febiger, 1976.
20. Massery A, Jones EW: Endotracheal intubation in cattle. Vet Rec 68:32–33, 1956.
21. Weaver AD: Complications in halothane anaesthesia of cattle. Zentralbl Vet Med [A] 8:409–416, 1971.
22. Jennings S: General anesthesia of ruminants and swine. In Soma LR (ed): Textbook of Veterinary Anesthesia. Baltimore, Williams & Wilkins, 1971.
23. Ritchie HE: Chlorpromazine sedation in pigs. Vet Rec 69:895–900, 1957.
24. Vaughn LC: Anesthesia in the pig. Br Vet J 117:383–391, 1961.
25. Regan HA, Gillis MF: Restraint, venipuncture, endotracheal intubation and anesthesia of miniature swine. Lab Anim Sci 23:409–419, 1975.
26. Jennings S: Anesthesia in cattle. Br Vet J 117:377–382, 1961.
27. Jones RS: A review of tranquilizers and sedation of large animals. Vet Rec 90:613–617, 1972.
28. Kidd ARM, Boughton E, Done JT: Sedation and immobilization of cattle in the field. Vet Rec 88:679–687, 1971.
29. Kumar A, Thurmon JC, Hardenbrook HJ: Clinical studies of ketamine HCl and xylazine HCl in domestic goats. Vet Med Small Anim Clin 71:1707–1713, 1976.
30. Ferguson AR: The use of azaperone in pig practice. Ir Vet J 25:61–64, 1971.
31. Callear JFF, Van Gestel JFE: An analysis of the results of field experiments in pigs in the United Kingdom and Ireland with the sedative neuroleptic azaperone. Vet Rec 89:453–458, 1971.
32. Reynolds WT: Anesthesia in cattle. Aust Vet J 51:270–272, 1975.
33. Clarke KW, Hall LW: "Xylazine": a new sedative for horses and cattle. Vet Rec 85:512–517, 1969.
34. Hopkins TJ: The clinical pharmacology of xylazine in cattle. Aust Vet J 48:109–112, 1972.
35. Seifelnasr E, Salch M, Soliman FA: In vivo investigations on the effect of Rompun on the rumen motility in sheep. Vet Med Rev 2:158–165, 1974.
36. Rosenberger G, Hempel E, Baumeister M: Contributions to the effect and applicability of Rompun in cattle. Vet Med Rev 2:137–142, 1969.
37. Rickard LJ, Thurmon JC, Lingard DR: Preliminary report on xylazine hydrochloride as a sedative agent in bulls for electroejaculation and semen collection. Vet Med Small Anim Clin 69:1029–1031, 1974.
38. Thurmon JC, Nelson DR, Hartsfield SM, Rumore CA: Effects of xylazine hydrochloride on urine in cattle. Aust Vet J 54:178–180, 1978.
39. Lane DR: The sedation of cattle. Vet Rec 86:358, 1970.
40. Stewart JM: Observations on the restraint and immobilization of uncontrollable cattle with Rompun. Vet Med Rev 3:197–204, 1972.
41. Thurmon JC, Lin HC, Benson GJ, et al: Combining Telazol and xylazine for anesthesia in calves. Vet Med August:824–830, 1989.
42. Dobbs HE, Ling CM: Reversible immobilization and analgesia in the bullock. Vet Med Rev 91:11–15, 1973.
43. Sharma RP, Stowe CM, Good AL: Studies on the distribution and metabolism of thiopental in cattle, sheep, goats, and swine. J Pharmacol Exp Ther 172:128–137, 1970.
44. Garner HE, Mather EC, Hoover TR, et al: Anesthesia of bulls undergoing surgical manipulation of the vas deferentia. Can J Comp Med Vet Sci 39:250–255, 1975.
45. Thurmon JC, Romack FE, Garner HE: Excursions of the bovine eyeball during gaseous anesthesia. Vet Med 63:967–970, 1968.
46. Thurmon JC, Nelson DR, Christie GJ: Ketamine anesthesia in swine. J Am Vet Med Assoc 160:1325–1330, 1972.
47. Fuentes VO, Tellez E: Ketamine dissociative analgesia in cattle. Vet Rec 94:482, 1974.
48. Fuentes VO, Tellez E: Mid-line caesarean section in a cow using ketamine anesthesia. Vet Rec 99:338, 1976.
49. Ivankovich AD, Miletich DJ, Reimann C, et al: Cardiovascular effects of centrally administered ketamine in goats. Anesth Analg 53:924–931, 1974.
50. Kumar A, Thurmon JC, Dorner JL: Hematologic and biochemical findings in sheep given ketamine hydrochloride. J Am Vet Med Assoc 165:284–287, 1974.
51. Kumar A, Thurmon JC, Nelson DR, Link RP: Effects of ketamine hydrochloride on maternal and fetal arterial blood pressure and acid-base status in goats. Vet Anesth 5:28–33, 1978.
52. Levinson G, Shnider SM, Gildea JE, DeLorimier AA: Maternal and foetal cardiovascular and acid-base changes during ketamine anesthesia in pregnant ewes. Br J Anaesth 45:1111–1115, 1973.
53. Taylor P, Hopkins L, Young M, McFadyen IR: Ketamine anesthesia in the pregnant sheep. Vet Rec 90:35–36, 1972.
54. Thurmon JC, Kumar A, Link RP: Evaluation of ketamine hydrochloride as an anesthetic in sheep. J Am Vet Med Assoc 162:293–297, 1973.
55. Thurmon JC, Kumar A, Cawley AJ: Changes in the acid-base status of sheep anesthetized with a combination of atropine sulphate, acepromazine and ketamine hydrochloride. Aust Vet J 51:484–487, 1975.
56. Breese CE, Dodman NH: Xylazine-ketamine-oxymorphone: an injectable anesthetic combination in swine. J Am Vet Med Assoc 184:182–183, 1984.
57. Thurmon JC, Benson GJ, Tranquilli WJ, et al: The anesthetic and analgesic effects of Telazol and xylazine in pigs: evaluating clinical trials. Vet Med August:841–845, 1988.
58. Thurmon JC, Lin HC, Curtis SE: Carbon dioxide and oxygen anesthesia for castration of baby piglets (abstract). 71st Conference of Research Workers in Animal Disease, Chicago, IL, November 5–6, 1990, p. 34.
59. Thurmon JC, Benson GJ: Inhalation anesthetic delivery equipment and its maintenance. Vet Clin North Am [Large Anim Pract] 3:73–96, 1981.
60. Jones LM: Veterinary Pharmacology and Therapeutics, 3rd ed. Ames, IA, Iowa State University Press, 1965.
61. Nelson TE, Jones EW, Hendrickson RL, et al: Porcine malignant hyperthermia. Observation on the occurrence of pale, soft, exudative musculature among susceptible pigs. Am J Vet Res 35:349–350, 1972.
62. Wagner AJ: The porcine stress syndrome. Vet Med Rev 1:68–77, 1972.
63. Gronert GA, Milde JH, Theye RA: Dantrolene in porcine malignant hyperthermia. Anesthesiology 44:488–495, 1976.

Regional Analgesia

G. J. BENSON, DVM, MS, DIPLOMATE, ACVA
J. C. THURMON, DVM, MS, DIPLOMATE, ACVA

Regional analgesia is a pharmacologically induced, temporary loss of sensation in a defined body area without loss of consciousness. Local analgesics act on nerve endings or nerve trunks to induce analgesia and loss of muscle function. Economically, regional analgesia is well suited for use in food-producing animals. Postoperative sequelae are few because physiologic alterations due to the analgesic are minimal. Major procedures can be done with the animal standing; therefore, casting and prolonged recumbency are avoided. The techniques, although requiring skill, are easily learned. Finally, regional analgesia may be induced with a minimal amount of help and equipment.

The major disadvantage of regional analgesia is that the patient is not immobilized. The judicious use of sedatives and physical restraint may be used to control the patient. Regional techniques are contraindicated in patients with pathologic processes involving the site of injection, such as infection, fibrosis, and deficient blood supply.

The major objectives of this article are to review the pertinent anatomy, physiology, and pharmacology associated with regional analgesia and to describe common regional analgesic techniques.

CLASSIFICATION OF REGIONAL ANALGESIA

Regional analgesia is classified by the site of analgesic contact with the nerve.

Terminal analgesia occurs when an analgesic acts directly on the nerve ending as a result of

1. Absorption from surface application with subsequent diffusion to the nerve endings. Examples of such surfaces are the mucous membranes, the cornea, and the synovial membranes of joints and tendon sheaths.
2. Infiltration of the operative field, placing the drug in contact with the nerve endings. An example is a line block for abdominal incision, in which the analgesic is injected beneath the skin and onto the peritoneum.
3. Intravenous injection of the drug into a limb around which a tourniquet has been applied proximal to the site of injection. Whereas this technique induces profound analgesia, it does not immobilize the limb.

Field analgesia results from injection of an analgesic around the periphery of the operative site, which blocks conductance of nerve impulses arising from within. An example is the "backwards 7" block for left paralumbar laparotomy.

Conduction analgesia occurs when the analgesic contacts major nerve trunks innervating large regions of tissue. Examples are

1. Epidural-spinal analgesia: deposition of the drug within the spinal canal.
2. Paravertebral analgesia: infiltration of spinal nerves where they emerge from intervertebral foramina.
3. Infiltration of peripheral nerves (e.g., pudendal, digital).

ANATOMY

Successful induction of regional analgesia is in large part dependent on an understanding of the spinal cord, the meninges, and the spinal and peripheral nerves. The central nervous system comprises the brain and spinal cord. The spinal cord is encased within the vertebral canal and extends from the foramen magnum to approximately the midsacrum in food animal species. Spinal nerves leave the cord at each spinal segment and exit the canal at the intervertebral foramen. The spinal nerves are composed of an efferent ventral motor branch and an afferent dorsal branch. The caudal portion of the vertebral canal contains the cauda equina, which contains descending spinal nerves. In the fetus, all spinal nerves exit at right angles to the spinal cord. In the adult, however, owing to differential growth rates between the spinal cord and the bony vertebral canal, the nerves must run posteriorly to reach their respective intervertebral foramina. This feature is significant and affects the level of analgesia induced by the deposition of analgesic within the spinal canal. Variations of innervation occur among and within species. Table 1 gives a summary of the areas of motor and sensory innervation supplied by the spinal nerves.

The meninges (dura mater, arachnoidea, and pia mater), which surround the spinal cord, are important in uptake and distribution of analgesic injected into perivertebral areas. Various spaces are associated with the meninges and are important to understanding spinal anesthetic techniques and nomenclature (Fig. 1). The dura mater has 2 layers within the cranial vault, an inner or visceral layer and an outer layer adherent to the cranial periosteum. The inner or visceral layer invests the spinal cord and dorsal and ventral nerve roots; the outer layer is absent in the vertebral canal of some species. The epidural space is the space within the spinal canal outside the visceral layer of dura mater. It has also been referred to as the extradural space, and in those species having both layers of dura, it is called the intradural space. The dura adheres to the periosteum of the foramen magnum, thereby preventing communication of the spinal epidural space with the cranial epidural space. The epidural space contains blood vessels, lymphatics, and fat, and it communicates with the paravertebral tissues via the intervertebral foramina. This communication may be interrupted in older animals by fibrous connective tissue, bony malformation, or arthritis and in obese patients by fat.

The subarachnoid space is located between the arachnoidea and pia mater. The subarachnoid space contains cerebrospinal fluid and is continuous with the cranial subarachnoid space. Because no direct communication occurs between the subarachnoid and epidural spaces, drugs cannot pass directly from the epidural space to the cerebrospinal fluid. However, analgesics can diffuse through the dura and arachnoidea to reach the cerebrospinal fluid. Arachnoid granulations protrude through the dura into the epidural space at the dural root sleeve and may afford a preferential pathway for passage of drugs between the epidural space and the cerebrospinal fluid.

The pia mater is 1 cell layer thick and lies directly on the spinal cord. Diffusion of agents from the cerebrospinal fluid to the spinal cord itself is relatively unimpaired.

At each segment, dorsal and ventral nerve roots emerge from the cord to form the bilateral spinal nerves. The spinal nerves contain sympathetic nerve fibers that regulate vascular tone. As the nerve roots leave the spinal cord, they pierce the meninges and carry a layer of each with them. These nerve roots with their meningeal covers join to form the spinal nerves. The meningeal covers fuse at their junction and extend no farther peripherally. Either spinal or epidural injection may be given at the lumbosacral junction in ruminants and in swine.

In nonmyelinated nerve fibers, conduction of impulses is relatively slow but increases as the fiber's diameter increases. Fibers in which frequent rapid transmission occurs are enclosed

Table 1. SENSORY AND MOTOR INNERVATION RELATED TO SPINAL CORD SEGMENTS

Spinal Segment	Nerves	Sensory Innervation	Motor Innervation
Coccygeal	All	Tail	Coccygeal muscles
Sacral	5, 4	Tail base and croup Anal region and sphincter Vulva Perineum	Anus Terminal rectum Vagina Penis, bladder, and urethra
Lumbar	3, 2, 1 6, 5, 4	Croup	Parts of lumbosacral plexus
Lumbosacral plexus	Posterior gluteal Greater sciatic	Lateral-posterior aspect of hip-thigh Midtibia to digits	Extensors of hip Flexors of stifle Flexors-extensors of hock and digit
	Anterior gluteal Obturator Femoral	Lateral thigh Medial aspect of thigh Anterior aspects of limbs as low as hock	Flexors-abductors of hip Abductors of hip Flexors of hip Extensors of stifle
Lumbar	3	Loins Croup Anterior stifle Scrotum, prepuce Inguinal region of mammary gland	Sublumbar muscle group Posterior parts of abdominal muscles
	2	Loins, flank Anterior-lateral thigh Prepuce Mammary gland	Sublumbar muscle group Posterior parts of abdominal muscles
	1	Loins Posterior abdomen Lateral thigh	Posterior parts of abdominal muscles
Thoracic	Last two	Abdominal wall and flank posterior to umbilicus	Abdominal muscles
	Mid to last	Anterior-ventral abdominal wall	Intercostal muscles Anterior abdominal muscles

in a myelin sheath that insulates the fiber. This myelin sheath is broken at intervals (i.e., the nodes of Ranvier) to allow direct contact of the cell membrane with the extracellular fluid. Depolarization can occur only at the nodes of Ranvier, so the impulse "jumps" from node to node along the course of the fiber, increasing rate of conduction.

Onset and duration of blockade of peripheral nerves is a function of fiber type and number within the nerve. Myelin limits the area of immediate contact between cell membrane and local analgesic to the nodes of Ranvier. Therefore, a higher concentration of analgesic is needed to block myelinated fibers than to block nonmyelinated fibers. Large-diameter fibers present less surface area per unit of volume for absorption of analgesic agent than do small-diameter fibers, which have a large surface area per unit volume. Therefore, small-diameter fibers are blocked more readily than are large-diameter fibers. Onset of blockade depends on diffusion of the local analgesic into the nerve trunk and fixation or stabilization of the cell membrane in individual fibers. Conduction of impulses is prevented by stabilization of the membrane potential, precluding depolarization. Thus, in a large mixed nerve, the fibers will be blocked in order of their susceptibility (i.e., size and thickness of myelin covering) (Table 2). Autonomic paralysis and vasomotor tone are lost first, followed by analgesia and finally by muscle paralysis. Not uncommonly, pain sensation will be lost while motor function and touch perception are retained, a phenomenon known as differential blockade. This occurrence may be confusing when the veterinarian attempts to assess the degree of analgesia. Recovery from blockade occurs in reverse order, so that muscle control

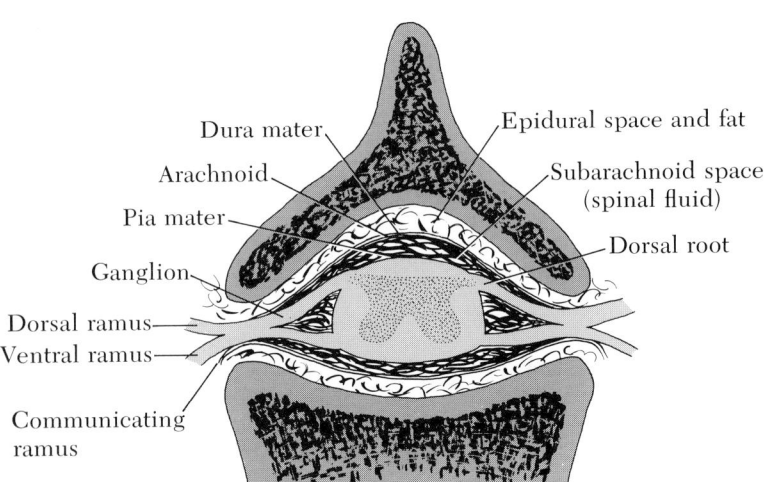

Figure 1. Anatomic detail of cross-section of spinal canal at level of intervertebral foramen.

Table 2. SEQUENCE OF NERVE MODALITY BLOCK

Vasomotor
Temperature
Pain (slow, then fast)
Tactile sensation
Paralysis of motor function
Joint sensation, proprioception
Deep pressure

is regained first, followed by pain sensation and finally vasomotor tone. Because vasomotor tone returns slowly, the patient may be intolerant of positional changes, loss of body fluid, and systemic drug effects associated with hypotension after apparent recovery from spinal analgesia. Reversal or recovery from nerve blockade depends on diffusion of the drug from a high concentration in the nerve fiber into the vascular system, where it will subsequently be redistributed, metabolized, and excreted.

ANALGESIC DRUGS

Local analgesics are drugs that, applied to a nerve, temporarily block conduction without producing permanent damage. The rates of diffusion and absorption may be altered by the addition of epinephrine or hyaluronidase. By delaying absorption, epinephrine prolongs the duration of action and decreases systemic toxicity of local analgesic. Conversely, hyaluronidase, by promoting diffusion and absorption, increases the area of infiltration affected by the drug. Because hyaluronidase is of little benefit in conduction-type techniques and because of its cost, it is seldom used in veterinary practice. Table 3 compares some commonly used analgesic drugs.

The commonly used local analgesics are weak bases. They are generally marketed as acid solutions of the water-soluble salts. Their acidity increases the stability of the solution and of the vasoconstrictor when present. In tissue, the acid salt is neutralized, liberating the base. Because it is the basic form that can penetrate cell membranes, causing blockade, it is readily apparent that a local analgesic will be less effective in inflamed tissue, where pH is decreased, because less of the basic form is liberated.

Local analgesics can cause adverse side effects. Hyperimmune reactions may occur with use of ester-type compounds (e.g., procaine hydrochloride), particularly on repeated use. These reactions may manifest as allergic-type dermatitis, asthma-like attacks (in humans), and anaphylaxis. Pretreatment with an antihistamine decreases systemic reaction in sensitized patients. Epinephrine and aminophylline are used to treat anaphylaxis and bronchospasm (asthmatic syndrome). Hypersensitivity reactions are rarely seen with use of the amide analgesics (e.g., lidocaine).

Overdosing causes central nervous system stimulation followed by depression. In the most severe cases, muscle twitching and opisthotonos rapidly progress to convulsions. Subsequently, death is due to asphyxia. Because respiratory muscle function is ineffective during convulsions, treatment is directed at seizure control and ventilatory support. Patients suffering from convulsive seizures should receive an anticonvulsant. Diazepam or a barbiturate will effectively control convulsions. The trachea should be intubated, and oxygen administered.

If the dose of a local analgesic is sufficiently large, depression will follow stimulation. Cortical centers are affected first, followed by medullary depression. Clinical signs include deep sedation, generalized analgesia, loss of consciousness, muscle flaccidity, hypotension, tachycardia, and a weak, thready pulse. Death ensues owing to cardiovascular collapse and respiratory arrest. Treatment consists of cardiovascular and respiratory support. This entails the establishment of a patent airway, administration of oxygen, and the rapid intravenous administration of balanced electrolyte solutions and a vasopressor (e.g., ephedrine or mephentermine). In general, the theapy is commensurate with that for any form of central cardiovascular collapse.

Regardless of the route of administration, the toxicity of local analgesic is the direct result of excessive blood concentrations. Plasma concentrations are a function of site of administration, total dose of the drug (volume × concentration), concurrent use of vasoconstrictor, rate of injection, rate of tissue redistribution, degree of protein binding, and rate of metabolism. Depending on local blood flow, infiltration of tissues with lidocaine hydrochloride results in maximal blood levels within 30 minutes. The toxic dose of infiltrated lidocaine is approximately 6 g in the adult horse or cow.

Biotransformation and detoxification of local analgesics vary with the drug and the species. Amides (e.g., lidocaine) are primarily metabolized by the liver, with the rate of metabolism being increased by enzyme induction. Lidocaine is slowly metabolized, but because of its high lipid solubility, it is 90 per cent redistributed within 1 hour of administration. Ester (e.g., procaine) metabolism is species-dependent, being by pseudocholinesterase in some species and by the hepatic enzymes in others.

SPINAL ANALGESIA

The nomenclature of various types of spinal analgesia in human and veterinary literature is confusing. For purposes of

Table 3. SOME COMMONLY USED ANALGESIC AGENTS

	Esters		Amides		
	Procaine (Novocain)	*Tetracaine (Pontocaine)*	*Lidocaine (Xylocaine)*	*Bupivacaine (Marcaine)*	*Mepivacaine (Carbocaine)*
Potency[1]	1:1	10:1	1.5–2:1	3–4:1	3:1
Toxicity[1]	1:1	10:1	1.0–1.5:1	3:1	0.75:1
Recommended concentration (%)					
Spinal	2	0.2–0.5	2–5	0.5–0.75	2
Epidural	1–2	0.2	2–4	0.5–0.75	1.5–2
Large nerve	2	0.2	2	0.5	2
Infiltration	0.5	0.1	0.5	0.25	0.5–1
Onset (minutes)[2]	1–3	5–10	1–3	5–25	3–10
Duration (hours)[2]	1–1.5	2–3	0.75–1	3.5–6	2.5–4

[1]Procaine = 1.
[2]Of spinal analgesia.

this discussion, spinal analgesia refers to all types of analgesia resulting from deposition of a local analgesic within the spinal canal. There are two types of spinal analgesia: (1) subarachnoid or "true" spinal analgesia, in which the drug is deposited in the subarachnoid space and, therefore, into the cerebrospinal fluid; and (2) epidural analgesia, the technique more commonly utilized in veterinary medicine, in which the drug is deposited within the epidural space. The epidural technique is further described by the site of injection; thus, caudal epidural describes the epidural injection of an agent at the sacrococcygeal or intercoccygeal spaces. Caudal epidural analgesia is said to be either high or low, being differentiated by the total dose of local analgesic administered. High caudal epidural analgesia results when the drug is injected at the tail head in a dose sufficient to cause paralysis of the rear limbs. In low caudal epidural analgesia, the dose is small and results in analgesia of the perineal region only, without affecting motor function to the rear limbs. Lumbosacral subarachnoid and lumbosacral epidural analgesia result from injection at the lumbosacral junction. Either technique causes paralysis of the rear limbs. Segmental epidural analgesia from the epidural injection of a drug in the lumbar or thoracic region results in a band of analgesia encircling the body. Motor function anterior and posterior to the area contacted by the drug within the epidural space is generally not affected, so the patient remains standing. Although this technique was first reported in cattle, it is not commonly used because alternative methods of producing analgesia of the same regions (e.g., paralumbar block) are easier to perform.

Because the epidural space usually communicates with the paralumbar space, and arachnoid villi in the spinal meninges allow diffusion of drugs from the epidural space into the cerebrospinal fluid, local analgesics injected into any one of the three spaces may be found in the other two. Probably there are multiple sites of action for local analgesics around the spinal cord, including the cord itself, the dorsal and ventral nerve roots, and the spinal nerves. Analgesia induced by epidural injection of procaine coincides with procaine concentration in cerebrospinal fluid. Diffusion of the drug through the dural root sleeve may allow the subperineural (submeningeal) blockade of the nerve roots. After repeated injections in the cow, procaine may be recovered from the cerebrospinal fluid, this finding would indicate that the meninges are not an effective barrier to drug diffusion. Analgesia induced by epidural injection depends on complex diffusion processes but is principally due to the agent's effects on nerves and nerve roots within the epidural and paravertebral spaces.

The effect of analgesics in the epidural space is influenced by (1) the size of the epidural space, that is, condition, age, pregnancy, and length; (2) the volume of solution; (3) the concentration of solution; (4) the speed of injection; (5) gravity; and (6) technique.

The epidural space contains blood vessels, lymphatics, and fat. Engorgement of vessels, which occurs in pregnancy, or increased quantities of fat, as in obesity, will decrease the volume of epidural space available for the analgesic. Therefore, a given volume of drug migrates farther from the site of injection in the pregnant or obese animal. For this reason, the dose of analgesic should be decreased by ⅓ during late pregnancy and in obese patients. Anterior migration of epidural drugs is also enhanced by transfer of negative pleural pressure to the epidural space.

The larger the epidural space, the larger the dose of drug required for a given level of blockade. Thus patients with longer "crown to rump" measurements will require larger doses of epidural drugs than will those having short "crown to rump" measurements. The epidural space attains maximal size in the young adult. It is smallest in young (immature) and old patients.

Extent of blockade is a function of total mass (volume × concentration) of drug. Increasing either volume or concentration without changing the other parameter will increase the extent of blockade, but concentration has a more profound effect than does volume on extent of blockade. Increasing the speed or force with which injection is made increases migration of the drug but may result in uneven distribution of drug within the epidural space and a "patchy" block. In subarachnoid injections, intermittent injection and withdrawal ("barbotage") of the agent with cerebrospinal fluid increases the spread of blockade. Migration of drugs in the epidural space is influenced by gravity, whereas that of drugs placed in the cerebrospinal fluid occurs according to their specific gravity relative to that of cerebrospinal fluid. Drugs with a lower specific gravity than cerebrospinal fluid (hypobaric, e.g., lidocaine) will "float" like oil on water and migrate anteriorly if the head or forequarters are elevated. Mixing of local analgesics with 50 per cent dextrose renders them hyperbaric. Thus they sink in cerebrospinal fluid, migrating to the dependent portions of the subarachnoid space.

In general, arterial blood pressure is decreased in proportion to the areas of the blockade during subarachnoid or epidural analgesia. The exact mechanism has not been conclusively identified, but it appears to be related to blockade of autonomic nerve fibers. If blockade does not extend anterior to the fifth thoracic segment, compensation occurs to maintain normal arterial blood pressures. Skarda and Muir[1] reported no effects on arterial blood pressure, blood gases, or pH in healthy unsedated cows after segmental subarachnoid analgesia extending from T9 to L4 on both sides of the spine. Concurrent use of sympatholytic drugs such as the phenothiazine derivative tranquilizers will prevent compensation. Decreased venous return due to α-receptor blockade will promote venous pooling of blood in relaxed skeletal muscle and will result in reduced cardiac output. Opening the peritoneal cavity, hypoxemia, hemorrhage, and surgical packing or traction on the viscera may further exacerbate this problem. In all likelihood, the decrease in arterial blood pressure is caused primarily by preganglionic sympathetic blockade and secondarily by decreased cardiac output. Patient positioning influences the alterations in blood pressure, with horizontal and head-down positions causing the least hypotension. In unsedated patients, centrally mediated and adrenal-mediated effects play a role in pressure regulation. Circulatory effects are more pronounced in patients experiencing stress of late pregnancy, parturition, and hypotension, for example.

Subarachnoid or epidural analgesia compromises respiratory function as the level of blockade progresses anteriorly. There is progressive depression of the intercostal muscles and depression of the diaphragm as phrenic nerve roots are blocked. Medullary depression and respiratory arrest can occur with excessive subarachnoid injections. When correct analgesic doses and techniques are employed, such complications are unlikely. Other effects of subarachnoid or epidural techniques are bowel contraction, splenic engorgement, and gastrointestinal sphincter relaxation.

Circulatory and respiratory changes should be treated if they endanger the patient. Respiratory failure necessitates establishment of a patent airway by endotracheal intubation and mechanical control of ventilation. Analeptics (e.g., doxapram) are of no use in respiratory failure induced by subarachnoid or epidural analgesia. Increased intra-abdominal pressure caused by abdominal packs, large abdominal tumors, a gravid uterus, or severe retraction may further increase respiratory embarrassment. Decreased arterial blood pressure and cardiac output are best treated by enhancing venous return. Rapid administration of balanced electrolyte solutions via a large venous catheter may be used to prevent or treat hypotension. Should hypotension occur, vasopressors and a head-down tilt are helpful.

The inadvertent subarachnoid injection of large doses of local analgesic, which may occur when epidural technique and dose are intended, results in "total spine." Controlled ventilation and cardiovascular support with fluids and vasopressors are indicated until the analgesic is eliminated. The patient should be positioned so that anterior migration of the drug is restricted or prevented. If a hypobaric drug (e.g., lidocaine) is injected subarachnoidally, the patient is placed in a head-down position so that the drug will be concentrated caudally. If a hyperbaric drug (e.g., lidocaine-dextrose) is administered in excess into the cerebrospinal fluid, the head is elevated above the rest of the body to prevent the drug from reaching the brain and upper spinal cord.

Other untoward sequelae of subarachnoid or spinal techniques include emesis due to unobtunded vagal reflexes arising from visceral manipulation; damage to spinal veins, arteries, or nerves; meningitis; and transient neurologic sequelae. In people, headaches, urine retention, fecal incontinence, loss of peripheral sensation, and loss of sexual functions have been reported. Spinal cord and meningeal injury or infection may result from improper technique or the analgesic itself. Paraplegia has been reported in people and animals, possibly as a result of exacerbations of pre-existing spinal disease. Inadvertent intravascular injection of a drug may result in cardiovascular collapse. Although the reported incidence of severe complications is relatively low, care should be taken to avoid intravascular injection.

In patients that are toxic or are experiencing cardiovascular collapse or shock, subarachnoid or epidural techniques should be viewed in light of their cardiovascular effects. Indiscriminate use of these techniques may result in cardiac decompensation and death. In such patients, subarachnoid or epidural techniques must be used judiciously, with particular attention given to cardiopulmonary function. Circulatory support should begin before spinal analgesic injection.

Extreme obesity with excessive epidural fat or venous engorgement favors greater anterior migration of the analgesic in the epidural or subarachnoid spaces. Orthopedic spinal disease may result in partial closure of the paravertebral foramina, causing increased retention and anterior movement of the analgesic within the epidural space.

Specific Technique for Subarachnoid and Epidural Analgesia

Local and regional analgesic techniques should be preceded by aseptic preparation of the site for needle introduction. Because drugs used for subarachnoid or epidural analgesia come into direct contact with the spinal cord, spinal nerves, and meninges, meticulous care must be taken to ensure that chemical or bacterial contamination does not occur. The cleanest possible technique should be used in order to avoid contamination and sequelae such as meningitis (Fig. 2). The injection site should be clipped free of hair and scrubbed as for a surgical incision. The veterinarian should scrub his or her hands and should wear sterile gloves. Syringes, needles, and drugs should be sterile. The smallest amount of detergent left on a needle entering the cerebrospinal fluid can cause permanent neurologic damage. Therefore, needles and syringes should be steam-autoclaved with stylets and plungers removed. The injection site may be draped with an eye drape.

A spinal needle should be used. It has a stylet to prevent clogging with tissue plugs, a short bevel to enhance tactile

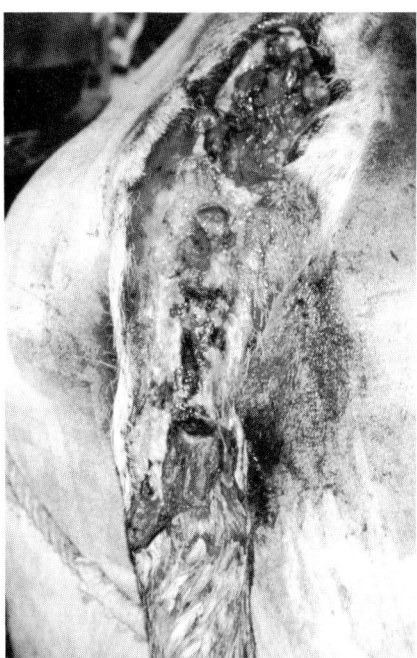

Figure 2. Osteomyelitis, meningitis, and necrosis of the tail subsequent to caudal epidural injection in the cow resulting from septic contamination of the epidural space.

sensation as various tissues are penetrated, and a notch on the hub to indicate the bevel direction. The bevel should be directed toward the area to be rendered analgesic, usually anteriorly. Needle size and length vary with the species and size of the patient. The technique for continuous epidural analgesia requires a special type of needle. The Tuohy needle opens at an angle to the shaft for introduction of a catheter into the epidural space. The analgesic can be repeatedly injected through this fine-gauge catheter.

Epidural and Subarachnoid Techniques in the Cow

In principle, any surgical procedure caudal to the diaphragm may be completed under epidural or subarachnoid analgesia. These techniques are commonly used for laparotomy and operations on the hindquarters of cattle, swine, and small ruminants. Epidural and subarachnoid analgesia may be indicated when general anesthesia is impractical. Contraindications for epidural and subarachnoid techniques include

1. Pathologic conditions of the lumbar or sacral vertebrae.
2. Pathologic conditions of the spinal cord or meninges.
3. Stenotic orthopedic processes of the vertebral canal.
4. Infection at the site of injection or within the spinal canal.
5. Congenital or acquired deformities of the spinal canal.
6. Paresis or lameness of nervous origin of the hindquarters.
7. Hypotension or circulatory collapse.
8. Cardiovascular disease.

Epidural analgesia in cattle is most commonly induced at the caudal region, either at the sacrococcygeal junction or between the first and second coccygeal vertebrae (Fig. 3). Raising and lowering the tail enables the veterinarian to locate the space between the vertebrae. The needle is inserted on the midline in the center of the space. If insertion is between the first two coccygeal vertebrae, the needle is directed ante-

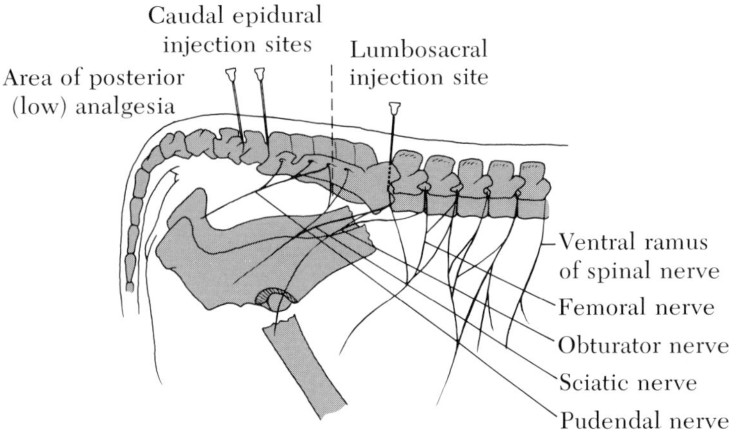

Figure 3. Anatomic relationships and injection sites for epidural analgesia in cattle.

riorly at a 45° angle. At the sacrococcygeal junction, the angle should be steeper, about 60° to the skin. Penetration of the interarcuate ligament can be felt at a depth of 2 to 4 cm in the adult. If the needle strikes bone, insertion is too deep, and the needle should be withdrawn about 0.5 cm. With the tip of the needle in the epidural space, there should be no blood in the needle or resistance to air injection. Low caudal epidural analgesia suitable for operations of the tail, anus, rectum, vulva, and perianal skin in the standing patient may be induced by injecting 8 to 15 ml of 2 per cent procaine or 5 to 8 ml of 2 per cent lidocaine in adult cows. High caudal epidural analgesia resulting in hindlimb paralysis and recumbency is suitable for most procedures caudal to the diaphragm. Dose depends on the surgical site and patient size; 60 to 100 ml of 2 per cent lidocaine is sufficient for laparotomy incisions caudal to the umbilicus in adult cows.

Lumbosacral epidural analgesia can be readily induced in the cow. The site for injection is the lumbosacral space, which is located between the dorsal iliac spines and between the lumbar spinous process anteriorly and the sacral spines caudally (Fig. 3). The patient is restrained in the standing position. The skin and underlying tissues over the lumbosacral space are infiltrated with a small amount of analgesic. The needle is inserted on the midline perpendicular to the skin. Resistance will be noted as the needle pierces the ligamentum flavum at a depth of 11 to 13 cm. At that point, the needle will be in the epidural space. Neither blood nor cerebrospinal fluid will be observed on withdrawal of the stylet or by aspiration. There will be no resistance to the injection of air or analgesic agent. If the needle is advanced farther, the meninges may be penetrated. Removal of the stylet allows the escape of cerebrospinal fluid from the needle. If the position of the needle is in doubt, the veterinarian should attempt to aspirate cerebrospinal fluid. Aspiration of cerebrospinal fluid confirms penetration of the dura and arachnoidea, and "true" spinal analgesia may be induced. In mature cows, 35 to 50 ml of 2 per cent lidocaine is sufficient to induce lumbosacral epidural analgesia extending anteriorly to the umbilicus. For subarachnoid analgesia, the dose is decreased by 35 to 50 per cent. Injection is made with the bevel of the needle facing anteriorly.

Epidural and Subarachnoid Analgesia in the Goat, Sheep, and Pig

Lumbosacral subarachnoid and epidural analgesia may be readily induced in the goat, sheep, and pig (Fig. 4). The landmarks for injection are the same as for the cow. In the goat and sheep, the dose is 1 ml/5 kg body weight of 2 per cent lidocaine for epidural analgesia caudal to the umbilicus.

Total dose should not exceed 15 ml of 2 per cent lidocaine in any size sheep or goat.

In the pig, the landmarks for location of the lumbosacral space are more difficult to identify. However, with practice, the technique is readily mastered. Depth of spinal needle insertion depends on the size and condition of the patient, with ranges from 2 to 3.5 cm in 10- to 20-kg pigs to 9 cm in 100-kg pigs. In heavy boars and sows, depth of penetration may be 10 to 13 cm. The dose for lumbosacral epidural analgesia with 2 per cent lidocaine is 1 ml/10 kg body weight to a maximum of 25 ml in the adult. This will provide analgesia caudal to the umbilicus suitable for laparotomy and cesarean section.

Xylazine has been used effectively to induce epidural analgesia in horses, cattle, and swine. In cattle, 0.05 mg/kg of xylazine, diluted to 5 ml with saline administered at C1–C2,

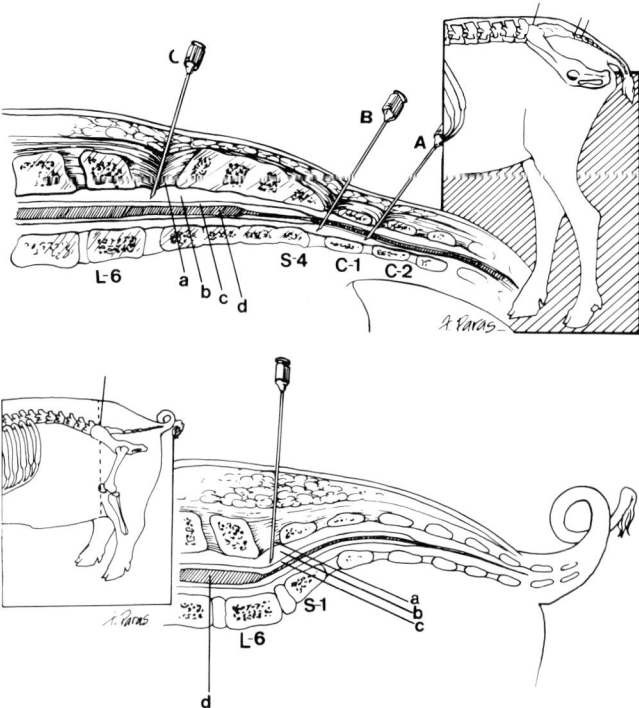

Figure 4. Sites for injection of local analgesic to induce epidural analgesia in the goat and pig: *a*, interarcuate ligament; *b*, epidural space; *c*, subarachnoid space; *d*, spinal cord. (From Skarda RT: Techniques of local analgesia in ruminants and swine. Vet Clin North Am [Food Anim Pract] 2:621–663, 1986.)

induced low caudal analgesia and sedation. Analgesia persisted for approximately 2 hours. In cows with cardiopulmonary disease, this technique may be contraindicated.[3] In a separate study comparing xylazine with lidocaine, 0.06 mg/kg xylazine in 5 ml of saline, when injected into the epidural space at the sacrococcygeal junction, induced a higher degree and longer duration of perianal analgesia than did 5 ml of 2 per cent lidocaine. Xylazine induced signs of sedation, salivation, vocalization, bradycardia, and ataxia. In addition, uterine motility was significantly increased from 20 to 50 minutes after administration.[4]

Preliminary studies in our hospital have shown that xylazine may be safely combined with lidocaine for induction of lumbosacral epidural analgesia in cattle and swine. Used in sows for cesarean section, 0.05 to 0.10 mg/kg xylazine added to 1 ml/15 kg of 2 per cent lidocaine induced excellent analgesia to the level of the umbilicus with mild sedation. In large sows or boars, the total dose of 2 per cent lidocaine should not exceed 15 ml when it is combined with xylazine. In the mature cow, injection of 30 ml of 2 per cent lidocaine containing 0.05 mg/kg xylazine at the lumbosacral junction induces strong analgesia caudal to the umbilicus and sedation.

Paravertebral Analgesia

Paravertebral analgesia is regional analgesia of the spinal nerves induced either proximally, as they emerge from the intervertebral foramina, or distally, as they cross the tips of the transverse processes of the lumbar vertebrae. The primary indication for paravertebral analgesia is laparotomy in the standing patient. The advantages of paravertebral over infiltration techniques include a lower total dose of analgesic inducing a wide area of analgesia; better muscle relaxation, which allows easier manipulation of viscera and decreases intra-abdominal pressure; no interference by the drug with healing; and the procedure is simple, safe, and yet elegant enough to discourage the use of feedstore drugs by the owner.

The paralumbar fossa is innervated principally by the thirteenth thoracic and first and second lumbar spinal nerves. Occasionally, fibers of the twelfth thoracic nerve supply cutaneous innervation to the cranial portion of the fossa. Infrequently, the third lumbar nerve supplies fibers to the caudal portion of the fossa, but blockade of the third lumbar nerve should be avoided because it supplies motor fibers to the rear limb. The nerves routinely blocked to provide paralumbar analgesia are T13, L1, and L2.

As the spinal nerves emerge from the intervertebral foramen, they divide into dorsal and ventral branches. The dorsal branch further divides into medial and lateral branches. The medial-dorsal branch innervates the dorsal lumbar muscles (loins). The lateral-dorsal branch provides cutaneous innervation to the dorsal half of the paralumbar fossa. The ventral branch of the spinal nerves innervates the skin of the ventral half of the paralumbar fossa to the ventral midline and innervates the muscles and peritoneum of the abdominal wall. As the spinal nerves run laterally, they sweep posteriorly to pass above and below the tips of the lumbar transverse processes. Thus the lateral-dorsal branch passes above and the ventral branch of T13 passes below the tip of the transverse process of the first lumbar vertebra. The branches of the first lumbar nerve are located in a like manner at the tip of the transverse process of the second lumbar vertebra, and the branches of the second lumbar nerve are located at the tip of the transverse process of the fourth lumbar vertebra (Figs. 5 and 6).

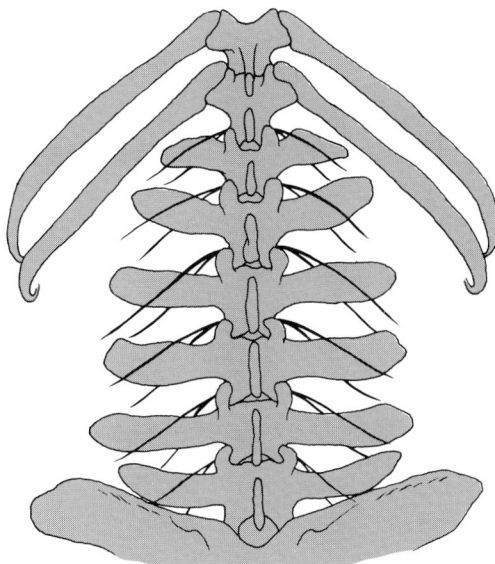

Figure 5. Anatomic relationships of spinal nerves and lumbar vertebrae for paravertebral analgesia in cattle.

The proximal technique has been described by several authors. The tips of the transverse processes of L1 and L2 are palpated. The skin is infiltrated above the anterior and posterior border of the transverse process of L1 and the posterior border of L2, 2 to 5 cm off the midline, depending on patient size. After an analgesic skin bleb, a 14-gauge, 1-cm needle is inserted through the skin to act as a cannula. An 18-gauge, 15-cm needle is used for injection. This needle is inserted through the cannula needle perpendicular to the skin. The authors have found it best to "walk" the needle off the transverse process by repeated insertion in order to ascertain the depth and location of the nerves. The thirteenth thoracic nerve is located just anterior to the edge of the transverse process of L1. As the needle is advanced, the intertransverse ligament can be felt as it is penetrated at the depth of the transverse process. The injection is made above and below the ligament over an area of 2 to 4 cm from top to bottom (Fig. 6). This process is repeated over the posterior border of the transverse process of L1 and L2 to block their corresponding nerves. If necessary, T12 may be blocked by injecting just anterior to the edge of the thirteenth rib at the level of the tips of the transverse processes of L1. Ten to 30 ml of 2 per cent lidocaine is injected at each site. As the veterinarian becomes more adept at locating the spinal nerves, less analgesic will be required. Analgesia develops within 5 to 10 minutes of injection. Induction time is a function of dose and accuracy in placement of the drug on the spinal nerves. Because the dorsal branch of the spinal nerve is blocked, scoliosis is induced as the muscles of the back relax on the affected side.

The distal block (Cakala block) is performed at the tips of the transverse processes of L1, L2, and L4. In this technique, an 18-gauge, 6-cm needle is inserted horizontally, and 15 ml of 2 per cent lidocaine is infiltrated directly above and below the tips of the transverse process. Because only the ventral and lateral-dorsal branches are affected, scoliosis does not occur; this is an advantage in the very sick or debilitated individual, who might not be able to stand after relaxation of the dorsal lumbar muscles.

Either the proximal or distal paralumbar technique can be utilized in goats or sheep.

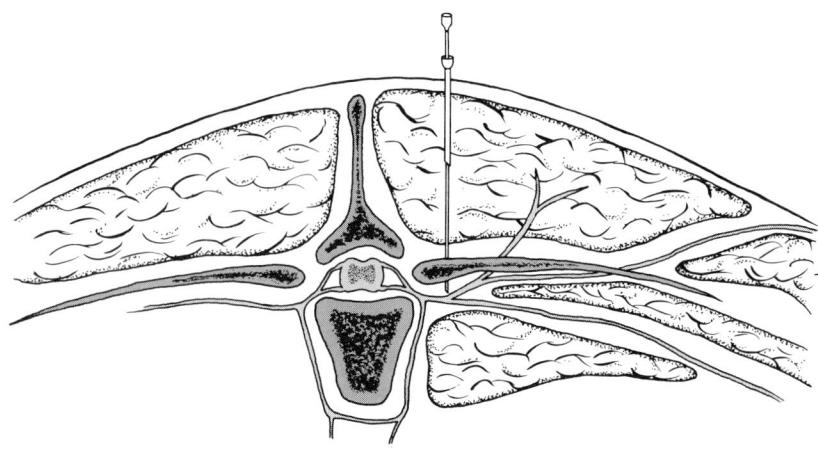

Figure 6. Anatomic relationships of spinal nerves and lumbar vertebrae for paravertebral analgesia in cattle.

ANESTHESIA OF THE PENIS

Pudendal Nerve Block

The pudendal nerve may be blocked in ruminants for exposure and analgesia of the penis, relaxation of the retractor penis muscle, and analgesia to at least a portion of the prepuce. This block has also been recommended for relief of straining induced by vaginitis or prolapse of the uterus; however, in these situations, low caudal epidural analgesia works equally well. Caudal epidural techniques have been used for exposure and analgesia of the penis but have the disadvantage of causing hindlimb paresis or paralysis at an effective dose. Therefore the pudendal block is preferred for examination and treatment of the penis in the standing patient.

The pudendal nerve is located by rectal palpation at the lesser sciatic notch and foramen medial to the sacrosciatic ligament. The nerve lies caudal and dorsal to the internal pudendal artery at the cranial angle of the notch and is the size of a wheat straw. The site for injection is the ischiorectal fossa, which is bounded laterally by the sacrosciatic ligament (sacrotuberous ligament), ventrally by the ischial tuberosity (pin bone), and medially by the anus-rectum and tail head. The area should be clipped and prepared as for surgery. A skin bleb is made at the deepest part of the fossa. In the bull, a 14-gauge, 1-cm cannula needle is inserted through the skin. With one hand in the rectum, an 18-gauge, 15- to 20-cm needle is passed through the cannula and directed cranially and somewhat ventrally to the pudendal nerve. Correct placement of the tip of the needle is determined by palpation; 25 ml of 2 per cent lidocaine is deposited on the pudendal nerve, and 5 to 10 ml is deposited 2 to 3 cm caudal and dorsal on the middle hemorrhoidal nerve. The process is repeated on the opposite side. Care must be taken to avoid intravascular injections or laceration of the pudendal artery or nerve. Maximal analgesia and relaxation occur in 30 to 40 minutes and last approximately 2 hours.

Pudendal nerve block can also be performed in the sheep and goat. The nerve is located by digital palpation per rectum. The injection site is the same as for the bull, and 7 ml of 2 per cent lidocaine is sufficient at each side. Analgesia and relaxation occur within 5 to 10 minutes of injection.

Dorsal Penile Nerve Block

Alternatively, blockade of the dorsal nerve of the penis may be used to induce analgesia and relaxation of the penis. This technique is somewhat easier than the pudendal nerve block to perform and is equally effective. The nerve is blocked as it crosses the ischial arch and gives rise to branches innervating the retractor penis muscle. The injection site is approximately 10 cm below the anus at the level of the ischial tuberosities (pin bones) and about 2.5 cm off the midline, just lateral to the penis on each side. The skin is infiltrated. The needle is inserted and is directed cranially and somewhat medially to contact the pelvic floor at the ischial arch near the midline. The needle is withdrawn 1 cm, and 20 to 30 ml of 2 per cent lidocaine is injected. The procedure is repeated from the opposite side. Care must be taken to avoid intravascular injection of the analgesic, because the nerve is accompanied by the dorsal artery of the penis. Onset of analgesia and relaxation occurs in 20 to 30 minutes and lasts 1 to 2 hours. This procedure is also applicable to the sheep and goat.

ANESTHESIA OF THE HORN

The cornual nerve supplying sensory innervation to the cow's horn is blocked for dehorning. The nerve is located just off the edge of the frontal crest, beneath the skin and fascia. It is best blocked in the upper third to half of the frontal crest. The needle is inserted off the lateral edge of the crest and directed medially, being kept ventral and as close to the crest as possible; 5 ml of 2 per cent lidocaine is injected at a depth of 0.5 to 1 cm. The cornual artery and vein run just lateral to the nerve; intravascular injection will prevent nerve blockade. In exotic breeds, especially the Simmental, it is also necessary to block the infratrochlear nerve, which innervates the medial aspect of the horn. This nerve is best blocked by infiltrating a line of analgesic subcutaneously from the midline to the facial crest dorsal to the eye across the forehead. The infratrochlear nerve in cattle divides into several branches that pass around the supraorbital process and then across the forehead; a line block, as illustrated in Figure 7, provides effective blockade of this nerve.

The horn of the goat is made analgesic by blocking the cornual and infratrochlear nerves (Fig. 8). The cornual nerve is located just posterior to the root of the supraorbital process beneath the skin, fascia, and frontalis muscle. The infratrochlear nerve may be palpated beneath the skin above the dorsomedial margin of the orbit. In the adult, 1 to 2 ml of 2 per cent lidocaine is used at each site. Care must be taken to avoid overdosing young kids, particularly during infiltration of nerves about the head; 1 to 2 ml of 2 per cent lidocaine is sufficient to block all four sites in a young kid. Volume could be increased by diluting with saline in order to keep the dose to a minimum. In addition to blockade of the nerve supply to the horn, it is helpful to sedate goats (e.g., 0.025 to 0.05 mg/kg xylazine intravenously) to be dehorned or disbudded.

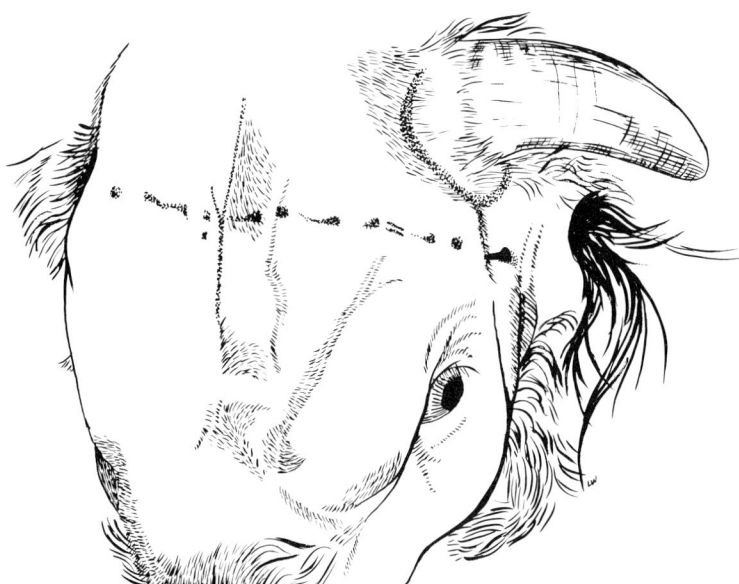

Figure 7. Injection sites for induction of analgesia of the horn in cattle. Cornual and infratrochlear nerves.

Sedation renders them more tractable and also prevents vocalization, which may be distressing to the owner.

ANESTHESIA OF THE EXTREMITIES AND DIGITS

The digital nerve supply in the ruminant is complex and variable, which makes regional analgesia of the digits difficult. Precise location of the nerves by palpation is not easy, because the skin is tense distal to the carpus, and the subcutaneous tissues are fibrous. Therefore, many believe that simple ring block, in which local analgesic agent is infiltrated through a transverse plane around the limb, is the most reliable method of inducing analgesia of the digits. Nevertheless, precise blockade of the digital nerves may be accomplished below the fetlock joint. There are 4 sites for injection to induce analgesia of 1 digit, or 6 sites to induce analgesia of the entire foot (Fig. 9). Injection sites are located on the midline of the anterior and posterior aspects of the pastern at the middle of the first phalanx. Injection at these two points will induce analgesia of the interdigital tissues and the medial aspect of the digits that is suitable for removal of corns or other interdigital procedures. For induction of analgesia of the entire digit, a line is drawn between the anterior and posterior injection sites around the digit. The line is divided into thirds, and injection is made at ⅓ and ⅔ of the distance between the initial injection sites. This will induce analgesia to the entire digit for amputation or extensive procedures involving the sole and third phalanx. Injection is made with the needle perpendicular to the skin beneath the deep fascia; 5 ml of 2 per cent lidocaine at each site is sufficient.

Intravenous injection of lidocaine effectively induces analgesia of the digits and extremities. This technique provides good cutaneous analgesia of the limbs and digits, but in the authors' experience it does not consistently induce adequate interdigital analgesia for such procedures as amputation of the digit. Increasing the dose to 50 to 60 ml will often overcome this problem. A tourniquet is placed around the limb proximal to the tarsus or carpus. For analgesia of the rear limbs, a roll of gauze should be placed in the depression between the tibia and the tendocalcaneus for improving the efficacy of the tourniquet (Fig. 10). The hair is clipped, and the skin is scrubbed over the radial or metatarsal vein; 30 ml of 2 per cent lidocaine is administered intravenously as close to the surgical site as possible. Analgesia occurs within 10 minutes. The tourniquet is left in place until the operation is completed.

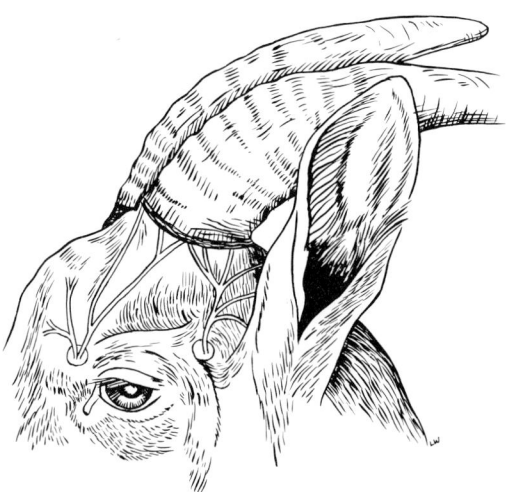

Figure 8. Injection sites for induction of analgesia of the horn in the goat. Cornual and infratrochlear nerves.

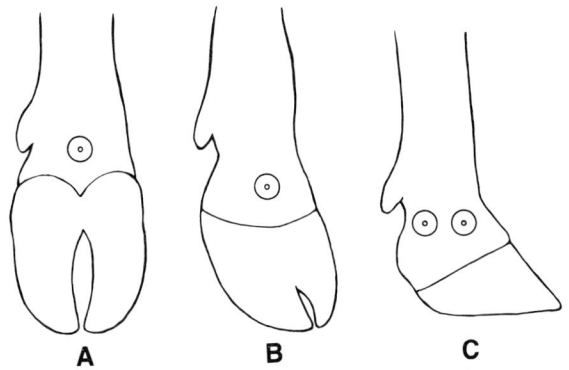

Figure 9. Injection site for induction of analgesia of the bovine foot by blockade of the digital nerves. *A*, Volar (plantar); *B*, dorsal; *C*, lateral and medial.

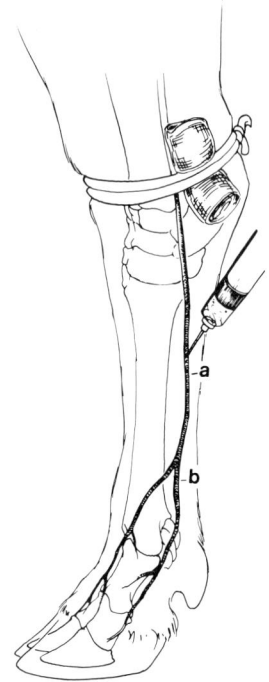

Figure 10. Technique for intravenous regional analgesia of the left rear limb of the cow; *a* is the cranial branch of the lateral saphenous vein, *b* the lateral plantar digital vein. (From Skarda RT: Techniques of local analgesia in ruminants and swine. Vet Clin North Am [Food Anim Pract] 2:621–663, 1986.)

The tourniquet may be left in place up to 75 minutes with no ill effects; lameness and edema may occur if the tourniquet is left in place for 2 hours or more. Upon completion of the operation, the tourniquet should be slowly released over a period of 15 seconds, then reapplied for 2 minutes. This sequence should be repeated several times so that the lidocaine is prevented from being released too rapidly into the systemic circulation.

Analgesia and paralysis of the forelimb distal to the elbow may be induced by blockade of the brachial plexus. This procedure is ideal for closed reduction and external fixation of fractures in the distal limb. The site for injection is 12 to 14 cm in front and at the level of the acromion. The needle is advanced horizontally and posteriorly to the lateral aspect of the first rib. Care should be taken to avoid intravascular injection. The needle is serially withdrawn and redirected ventrally so that an area 6 to 8 cm long is infiltrated along the lateral aspect of the first rib with 10 to 15 ml of 2 per cent lidocaine in calves, sheep, and goats. A total of 40 to 60 ml is required in a mature cow.

ANALGESIA OF THE UDDER

In ruminants, operations involving the udder may be performed with high caudal or lumbosacral epidural or subarachnoid analgesia. However, if the procedure is to be done in the standing patient, regional analgesia must be used. Principal innervation of the udder is derived from the second and third lumbar nerves and the perineal nerve. Occasionally, the skin of the anterior aspect of the udder receives fibers from the first lumbar nerve. Therefore, the first three lumbar nerves and the perineal nerves are blocked to render the udder analgesic (Fig. 11). Blockade of the lumbar nerves has been discussed previously. The perineal nerve is blocked at the ischial arch just beneath the skin and fascia about 2 cm lateral to the midline, with 5 ml of 2 per cent lidocaine. If analgesia of the entire udder is desired, the nerves should be blocked bilaterally. In this situation, it is best to use a distal paravertebral technique for preserving tone in the dorsal lumbar musculature.

Surgery of the teats may be accomplished with subcutaneous infiltration around the base of the teat. Procedures involving the teat orifice and canal will also require analgesia of the mucous membrane. The quarter is drained, and 10 ml of 2 per cent lidocaine is infused via the teat canal. In goats, the dose is 2.5 ml of 2 per cent lidocaine. Analgesia extends to the milk cistern.

ANALGESIA AND AKINESIS OF THE EYE AND EYELIDS OF THE RUMINANT

The eyelids receive motor innervation from the auriculopalpebral branch of the facial nerve. Blockade of the auriculopalpebral nerve results in paralysis of the upper and lower eyelids without analgesia. This nerve block is useful for allowing full examination of the eyeball and topical application of medications. The nerve runs from the base of the ear rostrally along the dorsal border of the facial crest. It may be blocked in the cow with 10 ml of 2 per cent lidocaine injected at the base of the ear, just dorsal to the zygomatic arch beneath the fascia (Fig. 12). An alternative method is to infiltrate around the orbital rim. With either method, the third eyelid is unaffected.

Analgesia of the eyelids is induced by infiltrating along the dorsal and ventral rims of the orbit to block the fibers of the ophthalmic and maxillary nerves (Fig. 12). The needle is inserted dorsal to the medial canthus and directed laterally to deposit 5 ml of 2 per cent lidocaine. The procedure is repeated ventral to the medial canthus. Innervation of the eye is complex. The lids and conjunctiva receive sensory innervation from the ophthalmic nerve and the maxillary branch of the

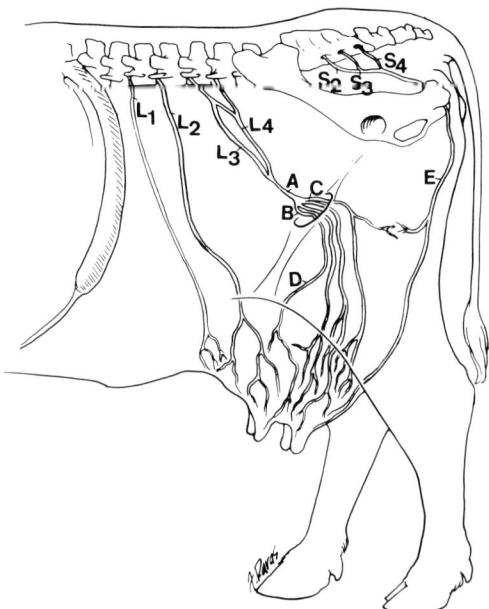

Figure 11. Nerve supply to the cow's udder. *A*, Inguinal nerve; *B*, internal anterior inguinal nerve; *C*, posterior inguinal nerve; *D*, external inguinal nerve; *E*, perineal nerve. (From Skarda RT: Techniques of local analgesia in ruminants and swine. Vet Clin North Am [Food Anim Pract] 2:621–663, 1986.)

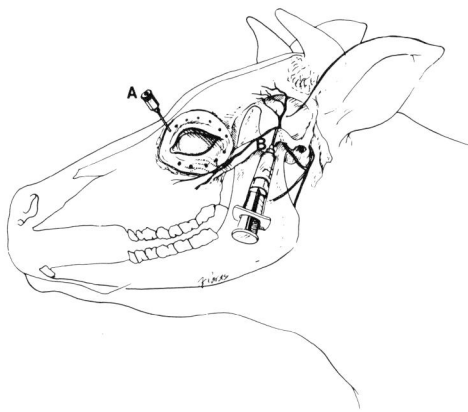

Figure 12. Technique for sensory (A) and motor (B) blockade of the eyelids of the cow. (From Skarda RT: Techniques of local analgesia in ruminants and swine. Vet Clin North Am [Food Anim Pract] 2:621–663, 1986.)

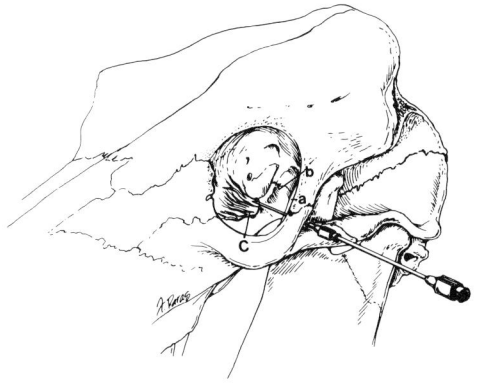

Figure 13. A technique for the Peterson eye block of the cow. *a*, coronoid process; *b*, pterygoid crest; *c*, foramen rotundum orbitale. (From Skarda RT: Techniques of local analgesia in ruminants and swine. Vet Clin North Am [Food Anim Pract] 2:621–663, 1986.)

trigeminal nerve. The straight and oblique muscles of the eyeball receive motor fibers from the oculomotor, abducens, and trochlear nerves. The eyeball itself receives sensory innervation from the ciliary branch of the ophthalmic nerve. The oculomotor, trochlear, ophthalmic, and maxillary branches of the trigeminal and abducens nerves may be blocked as they emerge from the foramen rotundum orbitale. Injection at this point results in analgesia of the eyeball, conjunctiva, eyelids, and skin of the forehead and paralysis of the ocular muscles. The auriculopalpebral nerve must be blocked as previously described for inducing motor paralysis of the eyelids and because it occasionally gives rise to some sensory fibers as well. Clinical experience suggests that subcutaneous infiltration completely around the orbital rim will eliminate patient response when the eyelids are incised for complete eye enucleation. It is extremely important to deposit 5 ml of lidocaine as a separate injection into the base of the third eyelid.

There are several techniques for approaching the nerves as they emerge from the foramen rotundum orbitale. An approach made 1.5 cm lateral to the medial canthus has been described. Topical analgesia of the conjunctiva is induced with either lidocaine or proparacaine. The needle is inserted through the conjunctiva below the eyeball and directed toward the base of the horn of the opposite side. After crossing the floor of the bony orbit, the needle is directed 10° to 15° more ventrally to a depth of 10 to 11 cm. Deeper penetration may result in the needle's entering the foramen rotundum orbitale and reaching the brain. In the adult cow, 20 ml of 2 per cent lidocaine will induce analgesia.

An alternative method is the Peterson technique (Fig. 13). A curved needle 12 cm long with a 25-cm radius of curvature is used. The needle is inserted at the angle between the supraorbital process and the zygomatic arch, with the concave surface posterior and the hub slightly above the point of insertion. The needle is pushed ventrally to strike the coronoid process and then past it until the needle contacts the bony floor of the pterygopalatine fossa.

A third method is insertion through the trochlear notch on the mediodorsal aspect of the orbit (Fig. 14). The needle is inserted at the notch and directed medially and ventrally to a depth of 10 to 12 cm, where it contacts the floor of the pterygopalatine fossa. Deeper insertion may result in the needle's entering the foramen. In the adult cow, 20 ml of 2 per cent lidocaine will induce analgesia suitable for enucleation or for surgical procedures of the eyeball and conjunctiva.

Retrobulbar injections may be used to induce proptosis of the eyeball for exposure and immobilization as well as to induce global analgesia. Topical analgesia of the conjunctiva is also required. An 18-gauge, 6-cm needle is inserted through the conjunctiva at either the medial or lateral canthus to its full depth. The needle is inserted tangential to the eyeball so that the tip penetrates the periorbital tissue, giving the sensa-

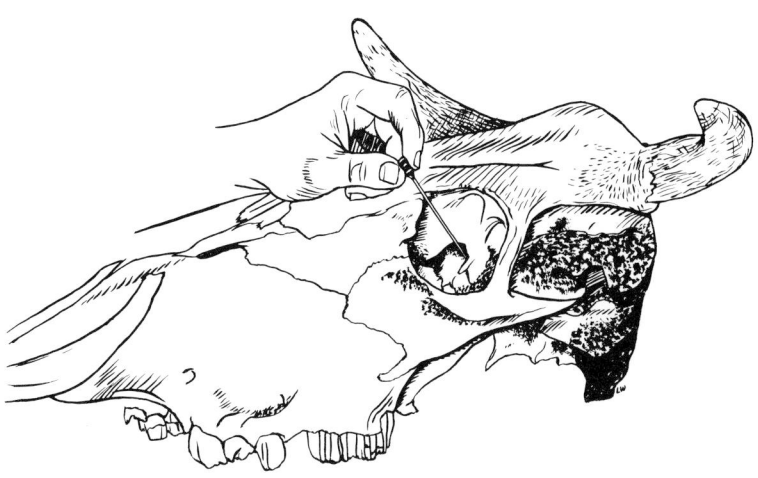

Figure 14. Insertion of needle at the trochlear notch for injection of agent in the foramen rotundum orbitale.

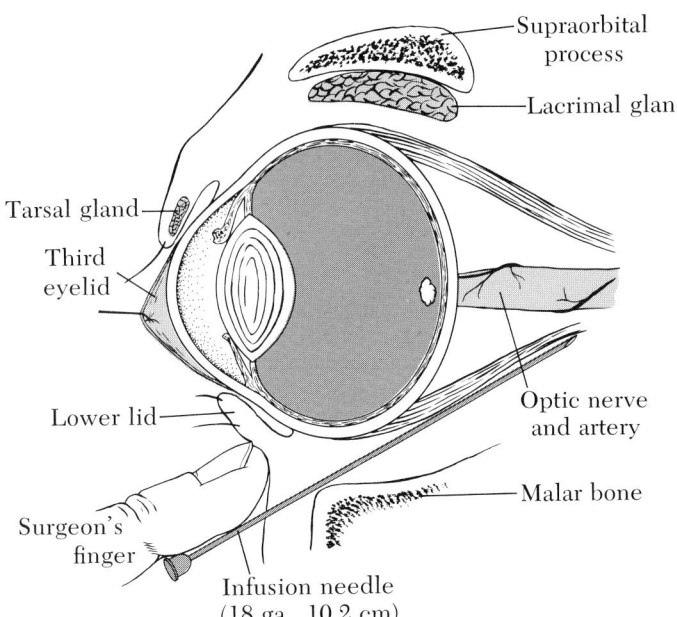

Figure 15. Retrobulbar injection of the bovine eye.

tion of penetrating a drum head (Fig. 15); 10 ml of 2 per cent lidocaine and 5 to 15 ml of sterile saline are deposited behind the eyeball. Analgesia of the eyeball and cycloplegia (paralysis and dilation of the iris) are induced. Exophthalmos is induced, and retraction of the eyelids results in proptosis. The procedure is satisfactory for removal of small tumors of the cornea or sclera but should be avoided if there are corneal ulcers or lacerations that would predispose to rupture of the globe. After completion of the surgical procedure, the eyeball can be returned to its normal position. An antibiotic ophthalmic ointment should be applied to prevent drying. Suturing the eyelids closed for 24 hours will ensure eyeball protection while the anesthetic-saline mixture is being absorbed.

REFERENCES

1. Skarda RT, Muir WW: Effects of segmental subarachnoid analgesia on arterial blood pressure, gas tensions, and pH in adult conscious cows. Am J Vet Res 42:1747–1750, 1982.
2. Schreiber J: Die anatomische Grundlagen der Leitungsanasthesie beim Hund. I. Die Leitungsanasthesie der Kopfnerven. Wien Tierarztl Fortschrift 42:129, 1955.
3. St. Jean G, Skarda RT, Muir WW, Hoffsis GF: Caudal epidural analgesia induced by xylazine administration in cows. Am J Vet Res 51:1232–1236, 1990.
4. Ko JCH, Althouse GC, Hopkins SM, et al: Effects of epidural administration of xylazine or lidocaine on bovine uterine motility and perineal analgesia (abstract). Theriogenology 32:779, 1989.

BIBLIOGRAPHY

Branson KR, Thurmon JC: Performing epidural anesthesia in swine. Vet Med 85:1345–1350, 1990.
Hall LW, Clark KW: Anaesthesia of the ox. Veterinary Anaesthesia, 8th ed. London, Bailliere Tindall, 1983, pp 245–272.
Lumb WV, Jones EW: Local anesthesia and nerve blocks. In Veterinary Anesthesia, 2nd ed. Philadelphia, Lea & Febiger, 1984, pp 371–391.
Skarda RT: Techniques of local analgesia in ruminants and swine. Vet Clin North Am [Food Anim Pract] 2:621–663, 1986.
Skarda RT: Local and regional analgesia. In Short CE (ed): Principles of Veterinary Anesthesia. Baltimore, Williams & Wilkins, 1987, pp 91–133.
Skarda RT, Muir WW: Segmental thoracolumbar subarachnoid analgesia in cows. Am J Vet Res 42:632–638, 1981.
Westhues W, Fritsch R: Spinal anesthesia. In Westhues W, Fritsch R (eds): Animal Anesthesia. Edinburgh, Oliver & Boyd, 1961, pp 153–170.

SECTION 2

Neonatal Disease and Disease Management

WILLIAM BRAUN, Jr., DVM, MS, Consulting Editor

Congenital Defects of Cattle and Sheep

H. W. LEIPOLD, DVM, PhD, MS
STANLEY M. DENNIS, BVSc, PhD, FRCVS, FRCPath

Congenital defects may be caused by genetic or environmental factors, by their interaction or by unknown factors. Many different types of defects have been described, ranging from minor variations compatible with life to semilethal defects to lethal monstrosities. Many more defects, particularly those involving formation and function, will undoubtedly be described as our knowledge expands. Veterinarians and livestock breeders are the prime sources for identifying and controlling genetic disease. Genetic defects may spread insidiously through a breed or species until they are difficult to control. It is necessary, therefore, to recognize genetic problems early in order to prevent their spread.

VETERINARIAN'S ROLE

Since recorded time, congenitally defective animals have evoked curiosity and fear. To veterinarians they pose a diagnostic challenge and also warn of dangers in the human environment.

Many malformed animals are stillborn or die soon after birth, whereas other defects are linked with embryonic and fetal deaths, abortions, and resorptions. Many defective animals are not reported; thus the various monitoring systems are bypassed.

Identifying the cause may be difficult, but failure to do so results in diagnostic and control problems. Veterinarians advise on control that may include adjusting breeding programs if the defect is genetic or altering herd management practices if it is environmentally induced.

DEFINITIONS

Congenital defects are abnormalities of structure or function present at birth. This definition excludes causes. *Congenital* means present at birth and is not synonymous with *hereditary*.

Many, but not all, congenital defects are caused by genetic factors; most are the result of simple autosomal recessive factors. A *teratogen* is any agent causing abnormal development. *Teratology* is that division of embryology and pathology dealing with abnormal development and congenital defects.

CAUSES

Many congenital defects are of unknown cause, others are caused by environmental or genetic factors or their interaction.

Environmental factors in general include toxic plants, viruses, drugs, trace elements, and physical causes such as undue pressure during rectal examination. Environmental factors do not follow familial patterns but rather seasonal factors, stressful conditions, or maternal disease.

Plants

Crooked calf disease, characterized by permanent joint contractures; axial skeletal defects such as various degrees of torticollis, scoliosis, or kyphoscoliosis; and various degrees of cleft palate may be due to ingestion of *Lupinus caudatus, L. sericeus,* or *L. nootkatensis* during the first trimester of pregnancy. Fetuses are at greatest risk if the plants are eaten between days 40 and 70 gestation. The teratogenic agent is an alkaloid, anagyrine. Other plants causing similar deformities have been described such as *Conium* sp., *Senecio* sp., *Indigofera spicata* sp., and others.

Veratrum californium (skunk cabbage) has caused epizootics of craniofacial malformations and gigantism in lambs. The defects are caused by pregnant ewes ingesting *V. californium* on day 14 gestation.

Locoweed poisoning in range cattle and sheep may cause emaciation, visual deficits, neurologic signs, habituation, abortion, and congenital defects of musculoskeletal and reproductive systems. It is also an effective and specific inhibitor of the enzyme α-mannosidase.

Physical Factors

Rectal palpation and pressure on the amnion during bovine organogenesis between day 33 and 40 gestation may cause atresia of the colon and sometimes the jejunum. Micrencephaly, brain cavitation, and retarded growth have been observed in lambs exposed to hyperthermia in vivo.

Intrauterine Viral Infections

Akabane virus in cattle and sheep has produced abortions, premature births, and congenital defects such as hydranencephaly and arthrogryposis.

Bovine viral diarrhea (BVD) has different effects on developing bovine fetuses, depending on stage of pregnancy of susceptible cows and the strain of virus. Impaired immunologic defenses, cerebellar dysplasia, ocular defects, brachygnathia, dysmyelinogenesis, and dysmaturity.

Hairy shaker (hypomyelinogenesis) lambs, abortion, stillbirths, birth of abnormally small lambs, and dysmorphogenesis of brain and skeleton have been associated with intrauterine border disease (BD) virus infection. It has been shown that intrauterine inoculation of ewes with Cache Valley virus between day 27 to 54 gestation may cause arthrogryposis, hydranencephaly, mummification, and resorption.

The effects of intrauterine bluetongue virus infection are similar to those of BVD and BD virus infections.

Genetic Defects

Hereditary defects are pathologic or pathophysiologic and are caused by mutant genes or chromosomal aberrations regardless of environment. Several chromosomal aberrations in cattle and sheep cause infertility or reduced fertility. One of the most common chromosomal defects in cattle is 1/29 robertsonian translocation. Worldwide, it has been reported with widely varying frequencies in 50 breeds of cattle and in sheep.

There is no visible effect on carriers of such chromosomal translocations, and the only reported consequence is reduced fertility from increased embryonic mortality resulting from karyotypically unbalanced embryos. Several countries have eradication policies for this chromosomal defect.

Many defects may be either monogenic or polygenic. Most genetic diseases result from mutation of a single autosomal recessive gene. Therefore genetic diseases run in families and are encountered in typical intergenerational transmission patterns and intragenerational frequencies. Modes of transmission include (1) recessive, (2) dominant, (3) incompletely dominant, (4) overdominant, (5) sex-linked, and (6) polygenic, with or without a threshold. Diagnosis of genetic diseases requires enumerating normal and abnormal offspring and identifying the familial relationship. Statistical methods are used to analyze such data. However, breeding trials with conventional methods or by employing superovulation, embryo transfer, and early gestation cesarean section may be necessary to confirm inheritance patterns. Biochemical tests may be developed to detect genetic deficiencies. Such tests would be useful for selecting breeding animals. Polygenic disorders are caused by mutant genes at various loci. These liability genes may increase the risk of faulty development owing to environmental factors.

All genetic defects have their counterparts in environmentally induced phenocopies. The problem is to recognize which are genetic and which, environmental.

Genetic analysis proceeds on the basis that genetic diseases run in families and that closely related animals have a greater chance of receiving the same copy of mutant and normal genes. Genetic diseases may be caused by a pair of mutant genes (simple autosomal recessive), a single mutant gene (dominant), or by multiple genes with or without a threshold.

The simple autosomal recessive genetic pattern involves only two types of calves, normal and defective. However, among normal cattle there are a few that can transmit the disease. Defective calves are born to normal parents; each normal parent producing an abnormal calf transmits one of the two abnormal genes. Most normal animals, however, cannot transmit the disease. When noncarriers of disease are mated with other noncarriers, or even with normal carriers, they produce only normal calves.

When normal animals that have produced a defective calf are mated repeatedly, 25 per cent of their calves will be defective and 75 per cent will be phenotypically normal. However, two of every three normal calves from such parents are heterozygous for the abnormal gene that can be transmitted to the offspring. Thus recessive defects are "carried" in a breed for generation after generation by normal-appearing heterozygous animals (carriers). Genetic defects of autosomal recessive nature are exposed only when such animals are mated to others like themselves (heterozygotes) and produce a defective calf (homozygote).

Eliminating defective calves usually keeps simple autosomal recessive defects at low frequencies, but breeds in which only a few animals produce most of the breeding bulls or in which many animals, particularly herd bulls, are closely related to a single outstanding animal are vulnerable to outbreaks of genetic defects (founder effect). Defects are exposed when descendants of such animals are mated.

A dominant inheritance pattern is the reverse of a recessive pattern; normal animals breed true, and abnormals mated to each other produce both normal and abnormal calves. Dominant diseases are easily recognized and can be controlled by eliminating all defective animals. Incomplete dominance is characterized by the birth of normal, slightly abnormal, and severely abnormal animals. The normal and severely abnormal cattle breed true. Matings of slightly abnormal animals produce one fourth normal, one half slightly abnormal, and one fourth severely abnormal calves. That pattern is easily controlled by eliminating all abnormal calves.

Overdominance is similar to incomplete dominance. Three kinds of animals are observed: normal, superior, and abnormal. The normal and abnormal animals breed true. Superior animals mated together, however, produce one fourth normal, one half superior, and one fourth defective calves. Replacements are selected from superior animals in preference to normals, with a resultant loss of up to 25 per cent of their calves when mated to other superior animals. Therefore, overdominant traits are difficult to control because superior animals carry the undesirable gene, and there is reluctance to choose inferior animals for breeding.

Congenital defects may also be inherited in a polygenic manner, with or without a threshold. Multiple gene defects may be inherited as dominant characteristics, but most are recessive. The control measures are the same; one needs to find families with little or no defects of the kind to be controlled. There are a few reports describing diseases in cattle that are linked with sex.

RESULTS OF CONGENITAL DEFECTS

Congenital defects have the following effects:

1. Reduced value of affected animals
2. Increased neonatal mortality
3. May be part of an embryonic and fetal mortality syndrome
4. Lowered productivity because of longer calving intervals

5. Common maternal sequelae of dystocia and infertility
6. Reduction of herd improvement through loss of replacements and consequent decrease in culling potential
7. Requires changing breeding programs as control measures
8. Differential diagnosis

CONTROL

Control of congenital diseases is difficult. Environmentally induced defects may be eliminated by adjusting management practices. Control of genetically caused defects requires accurate diagnosis of the defects and identification of the genetic transmission patterns. Once a sire has been identified as a carrier of a recessive defect, it is the breeder's responsibility to notify his customers of the presence of such a defective gene in the bull. Further control should be attempted by test matings.

CHARACTERISTICS OF CONGENITAL DEFECTS

A defective neonate is an adapted survivor from a disruptive event at one or more stages in the complexly integrated sequences of embryonic or fetal development. If the disruptive event is not immediately lethal, it is followed by the remaining normal developmental sequences that accommodate the event and its sequelae in succession. Often this is not possible, and the affected embryo or fetus dies before completing development and is resorbed or aborted, frequently without detection.

Susceptibility to injurious agents varies with the stage of development and decreases with age. Before day 14 in cattle (period of preattachment), the zygote or embryo is resistant to teratogens but susceptible to genetic mutations and chromosomal aberrations. During the embryonic period (days 14 to 42), the embryo is highly vulnerable to teratogens, but this decreases with embryonic age as critical development periods for the various organs are passed. The fetus (day 42 plus) becomes increasingly resistant to teratogenic agents with age except for later differentiating structures such as the cerebellum, palate, and urogenital system.

Defects may affect a single structure or a single function, may involve several body systems, or may combine functional and structural alterations. All body structures and functions may be affected. Defects may be obvious grossly, but some are not recognized without careful clinicopathologic and postmortem examinations. The frequency with which various parts of the body are affected varies according to breed, geographic location, season, sex, age of parent, and level of nutrition.

Developmental defects may be lethal, semilethal, or compatible with life. Other congenital defects may have little effect, may impair viability, or may affect esthetic quality only.

Although economic losses due to congenital defects are less than those from infectious, chemical, and nutritional agents, they may be economically important to individual animal breeders. With the increasing use of artificial insemination in cattle, no congenital defect can be considered rare, and all are important. Collectively, congenital defects cause economic losses by increasing perinatal calf mortality, decreasing maternal productivity, decreasing the value of viable defective calves, and decreasing the value of relatives of affected calves.

Classification. Congenital defects are usually classified by the body system primarily affected. Other methods include etiologic factors and the affected embryonic tissue. The principal body system classification is usually followed since it is also clinically useful.

Frequency of Congenital Defects. The frequency of congenital defects in animals is not known. The frequency of individual defects or defects of each body system and the total number of defects likely in a species varies among breeds, geographic areas, and years and seasons. Estimates of frequency of congenital defects are not easily obtained, because many go unreported.

It has been estimated that 0.5 to 1 per cent of calves and 0.2 to 2.0 per cent of lambs are born with congenital defects. The incidence reported ranges from 1/500 to 1/100 births; 40 to 50 per cent of these are born dead, and only small fraction of the defects are not visible externally. For comparison, congenital defects in humans are estimated at 1 to 3 per cent. The relative frequency of the various body systems involved in 2293 congenitally defective calves collected over a 9-year period was as follows: central nervous system, 21.6 per cent; musculature, 13.7 per cent; anomalous twins, 10 per cent; congenital systemic disturbances such as hydrops, 9.7 per cent; defects of large body cavities such as schistosomus reflexus, 6.9 per cent; digestive system, 4.3 per cent; urinary and reproductive systems, 4.3 per cent; bone and cartilage, 2.8 per cent; heart and vessels, 2.7 per cent; skin, 2.0 per cent; and other, 1.7 per cent.

Types of Malformation

Arrested development, absence (agenesis or aplasia), or incomplete development (hypoplasia) of organs or structures may be seen. There may be failure of an embryonal or fetal structure to disappear when it normally should—e.g., persistence of the ductus arteriosus or thyroglossal duct; failure of overlying skin to disappear from the anal opening (atresia ani); or certain openings, grooves, and fissures may fail to close properly. Many of these defects occur in the midline—e.g., cranioschisis and rachischisis from lack of neural groove closure; palatoschisis, or cleft palate; patent foramen ovale or ventricular septal defect in the heart; persistent cloaca owing to rectal and external genital openings not separating; and defects of the ventral abdominal wall. Closure defects such as hernias are common. Aberrant (ectopic or heterotopic) structures resulting from displacement of tissue to a location where it is not normally found, such as accessory organs (adrenals and thyroid gland) and islands or foci of pancreatic tissue in the wall of the stomach or adrenal tissue in the kidney or pelvic tissue. Displacement of cutaneous and mucosal tissue is considered to be the cause of dermoid cysts. Embryonic remnants of developmental vestiges are useless structures for adult animals and are of phylogenic importance only; embryogenically, the organs are formed but regress later. Duplication may involve many parts of the body—diprosopus, dicephalus, cranial or caudal duplication, or incomplete twinning. Duplicated organs such as penis and prepuce or toes (polydactyly) may be seen. Hypertrophy and hyperplasia are other mechanisms that can cause defects such as double muscling in cattle. Disturbances of cartilage and bone formation may lead to chondrodystrophy fetalis or dwarfism. Inborn errors of carbohydrate, lipid, and amino acid metabolism are of major importance in humans; however, little is known about these defects in domestic animals.

Blood defects in humans are well documented but are little understood in domestic animals.

SPECIFIC DEFECTS

Selected specific defects and their economic significance in cattle and sheep breeding are discussed here.

The most frequently encountered congenital defects involve the skeletal, central nervous, and muscular systems. Common bovine defects include arthrogryposis, cleft palate, hydrocephalus, and syndactyly; common defects in sheep are craniofacial, atresia ani, skeletal, hypospadias, cryptorchidism, and heart defects.

Central Nervous System

Congenital defects of the central nervous system (CNS) are common, and structural change may involve both skeletal structures and the central nervous system or only the latter. Functional defects also occur. CNS defects are of economic significance and of comparative interest.

Anencephaly is of unknown cause, involving nonclosure of the cranial portion of the neural tube and failure of the cranium to develop. Arhinencephaly, rare in cattle, is characterized by unilateral or bilateral absence of the corpus callosum or absence of all or part of the corpus callosum; the cause is unknown.

Hydranencephaly is complete or almost complete absence of cerebral hemispheres in a cranium of normal conformation; the space is filled with cerebrospinal fluid surrounded by thin membranous cerebral tissue. It occurs sporadically or in epizootics in calves. Associated changes include cerebellar hypoplasia, muscular atrophy, cleft palate, scoliosis, spina bifida, abortion, stillbirths, and premature births. Seasonal occurrence in unrelated herds of different breeds and epidemiologic, serologic, and pathologic changes have incriminated Akabane virus as a causative agent.

Hydrocephalus, an accumulation of excessive fluid within the ventricular system, is common and appears to be inherited in many breeds as a simple autosomal recessive trait. Calves affected with internal hydrocephalus are born dead or die within a few days. Congenital hydrocephalus in Hereford and Shorthorn calves is accompanied by stenotic aqueduct, cerebellar hypoplasia, myopathy, and multiple ocular anomalies (retinal detachment and dysplasia, cataract, microphthalmia, and persistent pupillary membranes).

Meningoencephalocele, or protrusion of meninges and brain tissue through a cranial cleft, usually with a liquid-filled sac, commonly occurs in the frontal region, but is sometimes found in the midfrontal, parietal, or occipital region. The cause in cattle is unknown.

The Arnold-Chiari malformation consists of herniation of tongue-like processes of cerebellar tissue through the foramen magnum into the anterior cervical spinal canal, with caudal displacement and elongation of the medulla oblongata, pons, and the fourth ventricle. It is rare, and the cause is unknown. Associated defects are spina bifida, hydrocephalus, and meningomyelocele.

Dandy-Walker syndrome, a rare defect of unknown cause, consists of hydrocephalus; aplasia or hypoplasia of the cerebellar vermis; cystic enlargement of the fourth ventricle, which is covered by a markedly thinned medullary velum, and associated tela choroidea; and an inner ependymal layer, which represents the roof of the expanded fourth ventricle.

Neuraxial edema (maple syrup urine disease) in Polled Hereford calves is characterized by extensor spasms and inability to stand. Histopathologic examination reveals edema of the terminal portions of myelinated bundles and gray substance containing heavily myelinated fibers. Genetic analysis indicates autosomal recessive transmission.

Shaker calves in newborn horned Hereford in Canada had tremulous shaking of the head, body and tail, difficulty in rising, a wobbly spastic gait, and atonia. This condition is considered to be transmitted as a simple autosomal recessive disease.

Spastic and Paralytic Diseases

Spastic paresis is characterized by spastic contracture of muscles and extension of the stifle and tarsal joints of one or both hindlimbs. Spasticity characteristically affects the gastrocnemius and superficial flexor muscles and tendons, and in some cases, the biceps femoris, semitendinosus, semimembranosus, quadriceps, and abductor muscles. Many breeds are affected.

Radiographic changes are fairly consistent and are characterized by increased angle of joints, osteoporosis and exostosis around the distal epiphyseal line of the tibia, curvature and exostoses of the dorsal side of the calcaneus, and widening of the epiphyseal line of the calcaneus. Central nervous system lesions have not been verified. Recent breeding experiments have indicated that transmission of spastic paresis is not by the simple recessive mode. Polygenic influences and environmental factors may interact to express spastic paresis.

Spastic syndrome, a chronic, progressive disease of cattle, is characterized by sudden spastic muscular contraction of both hind legs and, often, the back, neck, and front legs. Between attacks, muscle function is normal; however, complete recovery never occurs. Inheritance is thought to be by an autosomal dominant gene with incomplete penetrance.

Bovine progressive degenerative myeloencephalopathy ("weaver"), a genetic disease in Brown Swiss cattle, is diagnosed by four criteria: (1) onset of bilateral hindleg weakness and ataxia between 5 and 8 months of age, (2) deficient proprioceptive reflexes and normal motor and sensory reflexes with no other clinically detectable neurologic abnormality, (3) absence of clinically significant skeletal or muscular abnormality, and (4) adherence to familial relationship. Axonal degeneration is most severe in the thoracic spinal cord, with selective degeneration of Purkinje cells. It is transmitted by the simple autosomal recessive mode.

Spinal muscular atrophy in Brown Swiss calves causes weakness of the rear legs at 3 to 4 weeks of age. Further stages are characterized by severe muscular atrophy, quadriparesis, and sternal recumbency. Degeneration and loss of motor neurons in the ventral horns of the spinal cord and neurogenic atrophy of muscles are consistent histopathologic findings. Electron microscopy reveals accumulation of neurofilaments and mitochondria in affected neurons. It is most likely transmitted as a simple autosomal recessive trait.

The most significant storage diseases involving the CNS of cattle are GM_1 gangliosidosis, glyconeogenesis and α- and β-mannosidosis. α-Mannosidosis is due to deficiency of α-mannosidase transmitted as a simple autosomal recessive trait in Angus, Galloway, Simmental, and Murray Grey cattle. Clinically, it is characterized by ataxia, incoordination, head tremor, aggression, and failure to thrive. Occasionally, calves may be affected at birth. Clinical signs usually appear at several weeks or months of age, and affected cattle die within the first 12 months of life. Neuronal vacuolation is typical. Cytoplasmic vacuolation also occurs in lymph node macrophages, exocrine pancreatic cells, and kidney cells. It is controlled by testing of α-mannosidase levels. Affected calves have zero activity whereas carrier cattle have levels one half that of normal.

β-Mannosidosis was identified recently in neonatal Salers calves. Affected calves have short and round faces, nystagmus, marked intention tremor, and are unable to rise. They are deficient in lymphocyte and brain β-mannosidase. Cytoplasmic vacuolation of neurons and other tissues is widespread. On gross pathologic examination, the calves have internal hydrocephalus and swollen, green kidneys. The disease is inherited as a simple autosomal recessive trait.

Protoporphyria, a photosensitizing disease in Limousin cattle, is due to homozygosity of a simple autosomal recessive gene. Affected cattle may exhibit ataxia and convulsions.

Spinal cord defects have rarely been described in calves. Spinal dysraphism, characterized by a synchronized hopping gait and ataxia, is of unknown cause. Lesions are segmental; usually hydromyelia (dilation of central canal) and syringomyelia (cavitation of the spinal cord) occur in the lumbar area. Short spine lethal, perosomus elumbis, and occipital-atlantalaxial malformations have rarely been reported in calves.

Internal hydrocephalus has been observed in lambs, and other brain defects have occurred sporadically. Spina bifida, for example, has occurred in lambs. Among other defects, holoprosencephaly has been described. Holoprosencephaly, characterized by fusion of the cerebral hemispheres, presence of one single ventricle, and facial defects, has occurred in Border Leicester sheep. It is inherited as a simple autosomal recessive trait.

Daft lamb disease, or cerebellar cortical atrophy, has been reported in various sheep breeds as an autosomal recessive trait. Clinical signs vary in degree between breeds, and Purkinje cell development is deficient. Locomotor deficiency is expressed as inability to stand or walk. In Dorset sheep the onset of clinical signs of globoid cell leukodystrophy is between 3 and 4 months of age. These signs are hindleg ataxia, incoordination, and head tremor, progressing to tetraplegia. There is destruction of myelin with occurrence of PAS–positive laden globoid cells in perivascular spaces. This is a simple autosomal recessive disease, and lysosomal enzyme β-galactosidase is almost completely lacking in homozygous, affected lambs. The heterozygous carrier has about one half the normal activity of this enzyme. A glycogen storage disease in Corriedales has been described as a simple autosomal recessive trait. The glycogen is stored in neurons of brain stem and spinal cord and in cardiac, skeletal, and smooth muscles. Neuraxial dystrophy in various breeds of sheep has been suggested to be inherited in a simple autosomal recessive mode. Signs of neuraxial dystrophy vary from "weaving" to progressive ataxia, collapse of the hindquarters and legs, and finally death. Histopathologic changes were bilateral spheroid formation in brain stem nuclei and spinal cord.

Congenital Eye Defects

Relatively few ocular defects have been described in cattle as either single or multiple defects restricted to the eye, observed in conjunction with defects in other organs, or associated with pigment deficiencies. Ocular defects in cattle frequently include abnormalities in other body organs, especially in the central nervous system. Anophthalmia may be associated with taillessness. Hereditary encephalomyopathy and internal hydrocephalus in Hereford calves are combined with retinal dysplasia. In grade Shorthorn calves, multiple ocular defects such as retinal detachment, cataract, microphthalmia, persistent pupillary membrane, and retinal dysplasia have been associated with internal hydrocephalus. Congenital defects of the caudal segments of the vertebral column and high ventricular septal defects occur together with anophthalmia and microphthalmia. The frequency of anophthalmia and microphthalmia has been estimated in six United States breeds to range from one in 7500 to one in 50,000 births. Prenatal infection with bovine virus diarrhea virus causes cerebellar hypoplasia combined with ocular defects (retinal atrophy, acute and chronic neuritis, cataract, and microphthalmia with retinal dysplasia).

Ocular dermoids in Hereford cattle are characterized by skin with hair on the cornea. Visual impairment ranges from slight to severe. It is transmitted as a polygenic trait.

Oculocutaneous hypopigmentation in Angus cattle is due to homozygosity of a simple autosomal recessive gene. The hair is brown and skin surface a grayish-brown. The iris is light blue and white, which gives it a double-ring appearance.

Romney sheep have an autosomal dominant congenital cataract, which is expressed between 2 and 4 months of age and progresses to total lens opacity by 1 year of age. Other breeds of sheep also have cataracts.

Muscular System

Congenital defects of muscle are common in cattle and are economically important. Congenital flexure of the pasterns occurs in Jersey and other breeds owing to homozygosity of a simple autosomal recessive gene. Calves knuckle over in the front pasterns; the hind legs are only occasionally affected. The condition is reversible, and affected calves usually recover in 1 to 8 weeks.

Arthrogryposis, permanent abnormal joint fixation present at birth, is one of the most frequent congenital defects observed in calves. The arthrogryptic syndrome includes more than one etiologic or pathologic entity, is worldwide in distribution, and has been described in all major breeds of cattle.

Arthrogryposis and associated defects in Charolais calves consist of tetramelic arthrogryposis and cleft palate. The leg contractures are symmetric. Metacarpophalangeal and metatarsophalangeal joint surfaces are incongruent, and the distal trochlea of the femur and the patella are hypoplastic. Some calves also have kyphoscoliotic deformities of the vertebral column. The muscular system is affected by wasting and replacement of muscle fibers by fat cells. Arthrogryposis in Charolais calves is inherited as a simple autosomal recessive trait with incomplete penetrance.

Muscular hypertrophy (doppellender, double muscling, and muscular hyperplasia) is encountered in most major beef breeds; the degree of hypertrophy varies widely. Characteristic is the rounded outline of the hindquarters frequently referred to as "ham-like." The tail is attached more anteriorly than normal. The muscles of the shoulders, back, rump, and hindquarters are separated by distinct deep creases, with those between the semitendinosus and biceps femoris and between the longissimus dorsi muscles of either side being particularly noticeable. Necks of double-muscled cattle are shorter and thicker and the heads smaller and lighter. Many double-muscled cattle stand in a stretched stance. The diaphyses of the long bones tend to be shorter. Variable degrees of macroglossia may be present. Additional signs are infantile genital tracts, slower sexual maturity, impaired reproduction, lengthened gestation, and increased birth weight combined with dystocia. The double-muscled calves are less viable and are particularly susceptible to rickets and joint problems.

Muscular hypertrophy also occurs in lambs, but it seems to be rare. Arthrogryposis and hydranencephaly occur as a result of intrauterine exposure to Cache Valley fever virus. Bent-limb defect in different breeds of sheep is characterized by bent forelegs with rigid joints. Torticollis may cause dystocia. It is inherited as a simple autosomal recessive trait. Bent-limb defect is associated with blood group locus I and certain histocompatibility antigens.

Muscular dystrophy in Merino sheep has been attributed to a simple autosomal recessive trait. Clinical signs commencing at 1 month of age are a stiff gait that worsens with exercise.

Affected lambs starve under field conditions. Histopathologic lesions of a bilateral symmetric nature have been described in the quadriceps muscles.

Skeletal System

The entire skeletal system is affected, which results in dwarfism and osteopetrosis, or single regional defects may be encountered. Dwarfism is a universal problem in all cattle breeds and was an economic problem to the American beef cattle industry. It is a defect of interstitial growth of epiphyseal, articular, and basicranial cartilages, resulting in variable shortness of legs, cranial base, and vertebral column. Various types of dwarfism are distinguished such as short-headed, long-headed, and Telemark, all considered to result from recessive genes. In addition, the Dexter, compressed, and compact mutants (generally considered to be dominants) are part of a complex of conditions from more than one locus and seem to be related to the recessive types.

Osteopetrosis in black and red Angus, Hereford, and Simmental calves is a simple autosomal recessive trait characterized by small size and birth weight, inferior brachygnathia with impacted molar teeth, misshapen coronoid and condyloid processes, open fontanelle, thickened cranial bones, agenesis or hypoplasia of major foramina of the skull, and complete lack of bone marrow cavities. Radiographically, the bones have a "bone-within-bone" appearance. There is lack of remodeling of the primary spongiosa that persists throughout the metaphyseal and diaphyseal areas. Osteopetrotic calves are born prematurely at 251 to 272 days (mean 262) gestation and may be clinically misdiagnosed as abortion.

Acroteriasis congenitale (amputated) is a simple recessive syndrome consisting of low birthweight, amputation of all four legs, facial skeletal defects, cleft palate, inferior brachygnathia, microtia, and hydrocephalus.

Osteogenesis imperfecta, reported in Charolais and Holstein calves is inherited as either a simple autosomal recessive or incomplete dominant trait. The main feature is reduction in bone mass leading to spontaneous fractures.

Arachnomelia, described in German Simmental calves, is characterized by dolichosteomelia with extreme fragility of long bones, deviation of vertebral axis, tetramelic arthrogryposis, inferior brachygnathia, and cardiac defects. It is due to homozygosity of a simple autosomal recessive gene.

A number of regional skeletal defects are of concern in cattle. Cleft palate frequently occurs and is associated with other defects, particularly arthrogryposis. Cheilognathoschisis in Shorthorn calves has been reported as a simple autosomal recessive trait.

The jaws may be affected with campylognathia or lateral deviation of the face with normal development of the mandible. Abnormal length of the upper or lower jaw is referred to as superior or inferior prognathia, respectively. Short upper and lower jaw are termed superior and inferior brachygnathia. Inferior brachygnathia (short lower jaw, parrot beak, parrot mouth) may be a single, isolated congenital defect in cattle that varies considerably in degree of involvement. In Angus calves, it may be accompanied by cerebellar hypoplasia, a lethal condition believed to be due to homozygosity of a simple autosomal recessive gene. In calves inferior brachygnathia combined with other defects may result from an autosomal trisomy chromosomal defect. Austrian Simmental calves affected with short lower jaw are considered to have homozygosity of a simple autosomal recessive gene. Craniofacial dysplasia ("sheep head") described in the Limousin breed of France reveals deficient ossification of the frontal sutures, convex profile of the nose, inferior brachygnathia, bilateral xerophthalmia, scoliosis of the upper jaw, macroglossia, and defects of omasum and heart. Short-spine lethal recessive trait in several breeds is characterized by fusion of spine and ribs and reduction of ribs from the normal 13 to 6 or 7. Fusion of the occipital area with the atlas is seen in horses and calves.

Perosomus elumbis or agenesis of the caudal segments of the vertebral column is relatively rare. Other defects of the spinal column include kyphosis (dorsal deviation), lordosis (ventral deviation), scoliosis (lateral deviation), and their combinations. Kyphoscoliotic deformities are commonly associated with arthrogryposis. Lateral deviation of the neck is referred to as torticollis or wryneck. In cattle total agenesis (anury) and partial agenesis (brachyury) of the caudal part of the spinal column are commonly found associated with defects in other organs such as the eye and heart. Taillessness is most likely not an inherited condition.

Tibial hemimelia, a recessive lethal trait, is common in Galloway cattle. Adactyly, also a recessive lethal trait, has been described in Shorthorn calves. Development of additional digits (polydactyly) has occasionally been described and is genetically caused.

One of the commonest skeletal defects in Holstein-Friesian cattle in the United States is syndactyly; other breeds affected are Angus, Chianina crossbred cattle, and Simmental cattle in Austria. It is defined as fusion or nondivision of functional digits.

Syndactyly in Holstein-Friesian cattle is a recessive trait with incomplete penetrance and varying degrees of expressivity. The right front foot is more frequently affected, followed in order of frequency by the left front, right rear, and left rear feet. The degree of fusion or nondivision is always more advanced in the right front foot when more than one foot is affected. Osteologic defects in syndactylous feet have followed certain sequences; the second phalanges are frequently horizontally fused, followed by the third and then the first phalanges. Osteologic anomalies parallel the asymmetric external pattern. Muscles, blood vessels, and nerves accommodate the syndactylous deformities. Hereditary bovine syndactyly is accompanied by a functional defect expressed as hyperthermia that is triggered by higher outside temperatures. When syndactylous cattle and control cattle were subjected to controlled conditions in a climatic chamber, all five syndactylous Holstein-Friesian cattle developed signs of malignant hyperthermia. This complemented experience with syndactylous cattle (kept at Kansas State University) that had succumbed to environmental stresses such as higher ambient temperatures and calving. The use of preterminal cesarean section and recovery of fetuses can accelerate breeding trials considerably.

Mandibular hypoplasia to aplasia or agnathia is commonly observed in lambs. It is inherited as a simple recessive trait. Vertebral malformations reported in sheep mostly were tail defects. However, kyphoscoliosis, spina bifida, and perosomus elumbis do occur. Tailless lambs have been reported in various breeds of sheep. The defect is inherited as a dominant trait causing death of the tailless homozygous lamb in utero. Spider Suffolk and Hampshire lambs (chondrodysplasia) have been described. The affected lambs have long, bent and deformed legs, kyphoscoliosis of the thoracolumbar area, and twisted and deformed sternum and ribs. In addition, there is an abnormal profile of the facial bones, abnormal cartilage islands in the epiphyses, and erosion of articular cartilage. Most studies implicate simple autosomal recessive inheritance.

Joint Defects

Congenital disorders of joints may be generalized or localized. Bilateral osteoarthritis of the stifle joint in Holstein-

Friesian and Jersey cattle has been described as an autosomal recessive trait. Hip dysplasia in Hereford and Charolais cattle seems to be hereditary. Joint diseases are of considerable importance, but hereditary components and pathologic and other etiologic factors remain largely unstudied.

Skin

Developmental defects of the skin and adnexa may be generalized or localized. Epitheliogenesis imperfecta due to homozygosity of a simple autosomal recessive gene affects skin distal to the carpal and tarsal joints, and calves also have one or more defective claws. Epithelial defects usually involve the muzzle, nostrils, tongue, hard palate, and cheeks. Calves affected with epitheliogenesis imperfecta die shortly after birth from septicemia.

Fragility of skin similar to the Ehlers-Danlos syndrome in humans has been identified in cattle. Affected calves have hyperelasticity of skin and articular ligaments, cutaneous fragility, and delayed healing of skin wounds.

Lethal keratogenesis imperfecta appears a few months after birth. This is a recessively inherited disease causing exudative dermatitis of the legs and intestinal tract erosions (oral cavity, esophagus, and forestomachs) described in black-pied Danish, Pinzgauer, and Holstein-Friesian calves. Some affected calves develop diarrhea, whereas others develop conjunctivitis, rhinitis, bronchopneumonia, or central nervous system signs. This is a hereditary zinc deficiency syndrome associated with immunodeficiency, skin disease, and other signs.

Collagen dysplasia, a simple autosomal recessive trait, in sheep has been described in various breeds. Excessive fragility of skin leads to severe lacerations. Ewes heterozygous for this condition have hemoglobin phenotype AB. Homozygous affected lambs are characterized by absence of a 34-kd collagen-binding protein. Suffolk and Southdown-Dorset, Down lambs affected with epidermolysis bullosa exhibit bullae on skin and in the oral cavity as well as partial sloughing of the hooves. The genetic transmission pattern has not been studied, but the occurrence of the defect is familial in sheep.

Defects of Hair

Congenital hypertrichosis has been described in European cattle. Polypnea occurs during hot weather. Abnormal curliness of hair transmitted as an autosomal dominant has been reported in Ayrshire calves.

Six different types of hypotrichosis are distinguished in cattle:

1. Hairless lethal hypotrichosis is encountered in exotic breeds. Affected calves die shortly after birth owing to this simple autosomal recessive trait.

2. Semihairlessness has been reported only in Polled Herefords and is characterized by thin coat at birth. Later, the hair coat is sparse and patchy, and the skin is wrinkled and scaly. It is inherited as a recessive trait.

3. Hypotrichosis associated with anodontia has been described in Maine-Anjou calves as a recessive trait.

4. Viable hypotrichosis, encountered in Guernseys and exotic breeds and characterized by partial to complete absence of hair at birth, is due to homozygosity of a simple autosomal recessive gene.

5. Hypotrichosis with missing incisor teeth has been reported in Holstein-Friesian calves. The trait possibly is dominant.

6. Streaked hairlessness in Holstein-Friesians, characterized by vertical hairless streaks over hip joints and sometimes over the body and legs, is a dominant sex-linked gene.

Hypotrichosis in horned and Polled Hereford cattle ranges from slight to severe, resulting in skin infections and problems from the environment. The skin of affected calves is thin, with only a few hairs per unit area. In addition, hair over the eyelids, preputial, and umbilical areas, and the switch of the tail is thin, wavy, and silky. Histopathologic examination of skin biopsies easily identifies hypotrichosis by the degenerative changes in Huxley's layer characterized by trichohyalin macrodroplets. The condition is inherited as a simple autosomal recessive trait.

Cross-related hypotrichosis in Simmental-Angus and other crossbreeds is recognized by a short, curly, malformed, sparse hair coat. Affected cattle appear to grow less than their contemporaries. The cause may be due to color-dilution mutants present in European breeds such as Simmental, Gelbvieh, and Charolais.

A new syndrome in Polled Hereford calves, consisting of anemia, alopecia, and dyskeratosis, has been described. The skin changes were hyperkeratosis and generalized hair loss. The anemia was reported as nonprogressive, normochromic and normocytic to macrocytic. The syndrome appears to be transmitted as a simple autosomal recessive.

Gray coat color in Karakul sheep is inherited as a dominant trait. However, the homozygous gray Karakuls reveal a digestive disorder that usually leads to death.

Albinism

Partial albinism is characterized by a blue and white iris, and the coat color is usually either characteristic or a dilute color of the breed. A form of partial albinism, which includes abnormally large, membrane-bound organelles in various cell types and increased susceptibility to infection, is recessively inherited in the Chédiak-Higashi syndrome. Incomplete albinos, having inherited the trait as autosomal dominant, usually have pure white hair, and a few cattle may have small pigmented body areas. Iris color varies from blue to gray to white and may contain brown segments. Incomplete albinos have colobomas of the nontapetal fundus and tapetal fibrosum hypoplasia. Complete albinism is a simple autosomal recessive trait and is characterized by pure white coat, white to pink irises, but a normal tapetum lucidum.

Chédiak-Higashi syndrome, an inherited disease in Hereford and Brangus cattle, is characterized by photophobia, partial albinism, a tendency to bleed, recurrent pyogenic infections, and, finally, death. Peripheral blood leukocytes and other tissues have enlarged, pleomorphic, cytoplasmic granules, morphologically compatible with lysosomes. Hair is irregularly distributed, and there is clumping of melanin granules.

Albinism has occurred in lambs and is characterized by white coat, pink iris, and photophobia. This mutation at the color locus is an autosomal recessive inheritance.

Cardiovascular System

Most congenital cardiac defects have been reported as single cases. In a 14-year study of defective calves, 36 were affected with 78 congenital cardiac defects: ectopia cordis cervicalis, 10; common aortic trunk, 3; dextroposed aorta, 8; duplicated major trunk, 1; hypoplastic aorta, 2; interventricular septal defect, 11; interatrial septal defect, 2; left ventricular hypoplasia, 10; patent ductus arteriosus, 5; patent foramen ovale, 5; right ventricular hypoplasia, 10; cor triloculare biatriatum, 1; endocardial fibroelastosis with calcification, 3; and valvular hematomas, 7. The septal defects were high in location and ranged from 5 to 35 mm in diameter. The major clinical signs of congenital heart defects were poor appetite, reduced growth rate, dyspnea, tachycardia, and cyanosis. Studies of congestive cardiomyopathy in cattle have indicated a genetic predisposition.

Ectopia cordis is a common cardiac malformation, but its cause is unknown. The heart may be located in the cervical region, outside the thoracic cavity through a sternal fissure, or within the abdominal cavity. Ventricular septal defects, considered common in cattle, may be single isolated defects or may be combined with abnormalities of the large vessels, which are referred to by the nomenclature of their human counterparts.

A lethal autosomal recessive trait in Australian Polled Hereford cattle is characterized by cardiomyopathy and a woolly haircoat.

Ventricular septal defects, observed in 44 lambs, included 9 cases of tetralogy of Fallot and one lamb with 2 septal defects; these septal defects were high in location (73.3%) and less than 1 cm in diameter. Twenty of the 44 lambs had congenital defects of the skeletal system. Septal defects in Southdown sheep were reported as simple autosomal recessive traits.

Blood and Other Organs

Erythrocyte glutathione deficiency is expressed by causing anemia due to ingestion of kale. In Finnish Landrace it causes a shorter than normal life span of the red blood cell.

A glomerular nephritis of a dominant trait with a variable degree of expression in heterozygous lambs has been studied in Finnish Landrace. The basic defect is postulated to be the inability to synthesize the complement fraction C3, thus leading to deposition of immune complexes in glomeruli. Onset of clinical disease varies from 6 to 8 weeks and from 16 to 18 weeks and is characterized by anorexia, enlargement of the kidneys, central nervous system signs, and, finally, death.

Neonatal death and hypothyroidism characterized by silky coat, swollen joints, and sensitivity to cold has been described in sheep with congenital goiter. This is a simple autosomal recessive trait constituting a defect in thyroglobulin synthesis.

A hepatic transport defect as a simple autosomal recessive trait has been described in Southdown and Corriedale sheep. The affected lambs have jaundice, testicular atrophy, hydrothorax and ascites, and renal radial fibrosis.

Lymphatic System

Dysplasia of the lymphatics in Ayrshire calves and other breeds is due to an autosomal recessive defect of the lymphatic system that results in generalized edema.

Digestive System

Smooth tongue in Dutch Friesians is characterized by diminution of filiform papillae, fragility of the mucosa, velvety hair coat, soft horns, and microcytic hypochromic anemia. Smooth tongue in American Brown Swiss is considered to be due to an incompletely penetrant dominant gene. Defects of the intestine such as atresia of the ileum, colon, and other regions are usually localized and disrupt patency. The cause of intestinal tract defects may be polygenic in nature.

Studies in Germany indicated that colonic atresia may be caused by rectal palpation. A recent study postulated a genetic cause for atresia of the colon in Holstein calves. Atresia ani is common in lambs and claimed to be inherited.

Large Body Cavity

Hernias such as scrotal, inguinal, and in particular umbilical, are common in cattle. Outbreaks of umbilical hernia in cattle have variously been attributed to an incomplete dominant gene, homozygosity of a simple autosomal recessive gene, and polygenic inheritance.

Schistosomia (schistosomus reflexus), an extreme closure defect of the abdominal cavity, is a common lethal defect in cattle. Studies concerning its cause are scarce. Schistosomia is considered to be a polygenically caused defect that is part of a complex of umbilical hernia-abdominal fissures. Of 329,961 cases submitted to 12 United States and Canadian veterinary college hospital clinics, 1,315 were diagnosed with congenital umbilical hernia, 705 with congenital inguinal hernia, and 57 with congenital scrotal hernia. Several breeds of cattle were at risk for one or both types of hernia. Introduction of American Holsteins into northern Germany has led to increased frequency of umbilical hernia in that breed.

Congenital hernias that are not uncommon in sheep include diaphragmatic, umbilical, scrotal, abdominal, inguinal, perineal, and schistosomus reflexus. Inguinal hernia in lambs is inherited as an autosomal recessive trait.

Enzyme System

Deficiency of uridine-5-monophosphate synthase (DUMPS) causes embryonic mortality in Holstein cattle. It is inherited as a simple autosomal recessive trait. To maintain reproductive fitness, matings between heterozygotes should be avoided.

Urinary System

There are few reports of urinary defects in animals, and they are usually associated with defects of other body systems. Renal oxalosis has been observed in calves, and gross and histologic evidence of various developmental abnormalities were also seen in these calves. The events that precede or initiate catabolic degradation of glycine and its intermediary products are not currently known.

Urinary defects in lambs include hydronephrosis, cystic and polycystic kidneys, renal agenesis, megaloureters, renal dysgenesis, lobulated kidneys, hypospadias, and patent urachus.

Reproductive System

Various deviations of the penis and prepuce are not common and frequently are of unknown causes. Duplication of the penis has been reported in cattle and sheep. Persistent penile frenulum, interfering with copulation, common in Shorthorn and Angus, is claimed to be inherited. Hypospadias, a defect of the extrapelvic urethra resulting from partial or complete lack of fusion of the urethral folds, has been reported in sheep and occasionally in cattle. The most common opening in lambs is perineal, and associated defects are common.

Since the study in Swedish Highland cattle, numerous other reports have described testicular hypoplasia (bilateral or unilateral, partial or complete). Chromosomal changes in testicular hypoplasia included inversions, translocations, and sticky chromosomes.

Testicular hypoplasia and aspermatogenesis in two rams had an XXY sex chromosome complement.

Cryptorchidism, defined as incompletely descended testicle, unilateral or bilateral, is the most common defect in animals. Few studies in cattle suggest the cause. Four cases of unilateral left cryptorchidism in purebred Hereford bulls indicated possible genetic transmission.

Segmental aplasia, characterized by lack of isolated portions derived from the wolffian duct, mostly in the epididymal head, is usually unilateral.

Multiple defects of the male genital tract, including segmental aplasia of the wolffian duct, gonadal hypoplasia, and intermittent cryptorchidism, were found to have a karyotype XXX.

An intersex is an animal with congenital anatomic variations that confuse diagnosis of sex; it may have some reproductive organs of both sexes or may be genetically one sex and phenotypically the other.

Hermaphrodites have anatomic features of both sexes. By definition, a true hermaphrodite has gonads of both sexes, either an ovary and a testis or both, combined into an ovotestis. Hermaphroditism occurs occasionally in cattle and sheep.

A pseudohermaphrodite is an animal with the gonads of one sex and the reproductive organs, together with some characteristics, of the opposite sex; it is classified as a male or female by the presence of testes or ovaries. Pseudohermaphroditism is more common than hermaphroditism. Testicular feminization characterized by a male karyotype and female external genitalia has been reported in cattle, sheep, goats and pigs.

Female

Freemartinism in heifers born co-twin to a male is characterized in 93 per cent of cases by variable hypoplasia or agenesis of organs developing from the müllerian ducts and stimulated development of the wolffian duct system. Freemartins have male characteristics and are usually sterile. This defect may be a function of sex chromosome chimerism.

Freemartinism has rarely been reported in sheep.

Ovarian hypoplasia, with or without associated defects of the tubular reproductive system, may be total or partial and unilateral or bilateral. The clinical incidence in cattle has been estimated at around 2 per cent.

Defects of oviducts, uterus, cervix, and vagina have been described in several cattle breeds, with fusion of the müllerian ducts either lacking or exaggerated. Slaughterhouse specimens have been classified into three groups: partial or complete duplication of the uterine body and cervix, partial or complete duplication of cervix, and vaginal septa. A high incidence of duplication of the cervix was reported in two closely related Hereford herds.

White heifer disease falls into two distinct classes of morphologic aberrations, both with partial or total hymen persistence and one with additional defects cranial to the hymen. Common to both are functional ovaries and localized accumulation of secretory products. Although the defect is most common in white Shorthorn cattle, occurrence in other breeds and colors occurs.

Rectovaginal constriction (RVC), affecting the anus and vulvovestibular area, is due to simple autosomal recessive inheritance and is a common defect of Jersey cattle. The defect is characterized by inelastic constrictions at the junction of the anus, rectum, vestibule, and vulva. The male is affected with anal stenosis. Affected cows have dystocia, and calves are delivered following episiotomy or cesarean section. Rectal examination and artificial breeding are difficult to perform in affected cattle. In addition, Jersey cows affected with RVC are prone to develop peripartum udder edema, frequently followed by severe mastitis.

Studies have identified differences between RVC-affected carrier and normal Jersey cattle and have suggested possible ways to identify heterozygotes. Electromyograms from the external anal sphincter muscle of age-matched normal, carrier, and affected Jersey cows revealed highly significant differences among the three types. In addition, immunohistochemical studies utilizing purified antibodies to various collagen types revealed type II collagen within the connective tissue of the external anal sphincter of RVC-affected and RVC carrier animals.

In most dairy breeds and sheep, prolonged gestation has been recorded as hereditary, and two distinct pathologic conditions have been distinguished in cattle. In the first, due to a single autosomal recessive gene, the calf continues to grow in utero and is carried up to 100 days past normal term. Calves born or taken by cesarean section are weak and die in hypoglycemic crisis. In the second type, also caused by homozygosity of a recessive gene, the fetus ceases to grow beyond 7 months and may have craniofacial defects.

BIBLIOGRAPHY

Baird JD, Wojcinski W, Wise AP, Godkin, MA: Maple syrup urine disease in five Hereford calves in Ontario. Can Vet J 28:505–511, 1987.
Bryan L, Schmutz S, Hodges SD, Snyder, FF: Bovine β-mannosidase deficiency. Biochem Biophys Res Com 173:491–495, 1990.
Dennis SM, Leipold HW: Ovine congenital defects. Vet Bull 233–239, 1979.
El-Hamidi M, Leipold HW, Vestweber JGE, Saperstein G: Spinal muscular atrophy in Brown Swiss calves. J Vet Med 36A:731–738, 1989.
Leipold HW, Huston K, Dennis SM: Bovine congenital defects. Adv Vet Sci Comp Med 27:197–271, 1983.
Long SE: Chromosomes of sheep and goat. Adv Vet Sci Comp Med 34:105–129, 1990.
Popescu PC: Chromosomes of the cow and bull. Adv Vet Sci Comp Med 34:41–71, 1990.
Steffen DJ, Leipold HW, Gibb J, Smith JE: Congenital syndrome with alopecia and anemia in polled Hereford calves. Vet Path 28:234–240, 1991.

Colostrum and Passive Immunity

PHILIP R. WOODS, DVM, PhD, MRCVS
ALLEN J. ROUSSEL, Jr, DVM, MS, Diplomate, ACVIM

Lack of neonatal disease resistance in the immediate postparturient period is a significant cause of reduced livestock productivity and consequent economic loss. The ability to manage the food animal neonate so that it does not succumb to disease is of paramount importance.

NEONATAL IMMUNITY

Protective immunity in the neonate is achieved primarily by passive immunity in the form of colostrum ingested shortly after birth. Food animal species do not have the luxury of in utero–derived passive immunity because of syndesmochorial-epitheliochorial placentation, which does not permit the transplacental transfer of antibody.

The developing fetus is able to respond immunologically to a variety of infectious challenges. Antibody to parainfluenza-3 virus is detected in the fetal calf at approximately 120 days of gestation and to infectious bovine rhinotracheitis virus at approximately 170 days of gestation. These observations reflect maturation of the immune system and development of the capacity to respond immunologically to a specific disease challenge.

Although there is a capacity to respond immunologically to disease, the neonate is incapable of protecting itself against the massive infectious challenge it faces as soon as it is born. This is primarily due to a combination of hypogammaglobulinemia and immunologic naiveté. Correlation between high rates of neonatal mortality and lack of passive immunity emphasizes the importance of colostrum administration in reducing neonatal losses.

CONTENTS OF COLOSTRUM

Colostrum has both nutritional and disease-preventing functions. Bovine colostrum has 20 to 25 per cent total solids, being relatively rich (compared with milk) in immunoglobulins, casein, fats, and vitamins.

Colostral immunoglobulin (Ig) provides specific immunity against infection, IgG being the predominant antibody class in all farm animal species. IgA and IgM are present in colostrum in smaller but significant amounts. In pigs, as lactation progresses, IgA becomes the major antibody class in mammary secretions. Lactoperoxidase, lactoferrin, and lysozyme activity provides nonspecific protection against infection. Colostral immunoglobulins are protected from enzymatic digestion by the presence of a trypsin inhibitor. A prolene-rich colostral protein has lymphocyte mitogen activity that may be important for the development of neonatal immunity.

The cellular component of colostrum consists of a significant population of macrophages and lymphocytes. In the mammary gland these cells are an integral part of the secretory immune system.

ALTERNATIVES TO FRESH COLOSTRUM

A variety of colostrum substitutes are available. Many of these commercial products are named to suggest that their content is similar to that of colostrum. Unfortunately, most do not as yet appear to have the protective qualities of fresh colostrum in establishing adequate passive immunity, particularly in regard to immunoglobulin (Ig) content. One product, an ultrafiltrate of cheese whey, is interesting because there is some attempt to prove therapeutic efficacy. Encouraging clinical trials have been reported by the manufacturer. The product has relatively low concentrations of Ig but appears to have some protective effect on calves challenged with a pathogenic *Escherichia coli* bolus. (Whether such a challenge regime reflects what happens on the farm is a matter of debate.)

Other alternatives to fresh colostrum include frozen, fermented, acid-treated, pasteurized, and formaldehyde-treated colostrum. Levels of antibody activity in these forms of colostrum are considerably reduced compared with fresh colostrum. These fresh colostrum substitutes are of significant economic value as an alternative nutritional source.

FORMATION OF COLOSTRUM

Colostrum is primarily a product of the mammary gland. The elevated protein concentrations found in colostrum, compared with milk, are in part accounted for by elevated levels of Ig. Accumulation of Ig in colostrum in the final few weeks of gestation is mediated by a variety of gestational hormone influences. In the cow, increasing estrogen concentrations during the last 5 weeks of gestation are associated with accumulation of IgG in the mammary gland.

In farm animals, colostral IgG is produced systemically and is selectively transferred into the mammary gland; as IgG accumulates in the mammary gland, systemic concentrations of IgG can fall by 50 per cent. IgA and IgM in colostrum appear to be produced both systemically and locally. The cellular components of colostral immunity are derived systemically (intramuscular vaccination of the dam results in the appearance of sensitized lymphocytes in colostrum) and from the secretory immune system of the mammary gland.

A variety of factors are associated with the quality and quantity of colostrum produced, including the following:

1. Breed. Dairy cows produce more colostrum than do beef cows. Jersey and Holstein cows are reported to have a higher quality colostrum. Guernsey cows are reported to have lower concentrations of colostral IgA and IgM. Considerable variations in colostral IgG have been noted among breeds of sheep, and among rams within a breed.

2. Parity. First-calf heifers produce less and poorer quality colostrum than cows. Sows in their third or later lactation produce more lacteal IgA.

3. Season. Calving in the summer is associated with better quality colostrum than with calving at other times of the year.

4. Nutrition. An energy-deficient diet reduces the quantity of colostrum produced. In sheep, underfeeding during the third trimester of pregnancy results in a significantly reduced colostral yield in the first 18 hours after lambing. This is due to reduced prenatal accumulation of colostrum and a reduced rate of mammary gland secretion.

5. Loss of colostrum. Leakage of colostrum and periparturient milking reduce the total amount of colostrum available. Epidemiologic studies have shown leakage to be the major cause of low colostral Ig levels. Immunoglobulin concentrations between the first two milkings after calving can drop by at least 50 per cent.

6. Vaccination status of dam. High titers of specific Ig in the dam's colostrum are associated with a lower prevalence of neonatal disease and reduced shedding of infectious agents by the neonate, compared with nonvaccinated cohorts. Vaccinating sows against *Haemophilus somnus* 5 weeks and 2 weeks prior to farrowing results in a significantly reduced prevalence of associated disease in their offspring. Vaccination of pregnant cows with an experimental bovine rotavirus vaccine confers protective immunity in their offspring to rotavirus infection.

ABSORPTION OF COLOSTRUM BY THE NEONATE

Colostrum ingested by the food animal neonate is nonselectively absorbed from the gastrointestinal lumen by pinocytosis. After about 24 hours of age, the ability to absorb colostral Ig is dramatically reduced to the point at which further administration of colostrum does not enhance serum Ig concentrations further. However, colostrum administered after Ig absorption has stopped has significant effects in neutralizing enteric pathogens.

Cellular immunity associated with lymphocytes and macrophages in colostrum appears to be functional in the neonate. Lymphocytes migrate across the neonatal gastrointestinal wall and are functional for a time. The presence of rotavirus-sensitized colostral lymphocytes in neonatal calves is associated with reduced virus shedding by such calves.

Many parameters affect the eventual passive immune status of the neonate. Environment and behavior of both dam and neonate play significant roles in the quality and total amount of colostrum absorbed. Factors affecting absorption include the following:

1. Some "slow-acting" corticosteroids used to induce parturition are reported to reduce absorption of colostral Ig in the neonate.

2. Temperature stress reduces colostrum absorption by the neonate.

3. Calves that are delivered by induced parturition or by cesarean section or that are dysmature/premature have a slower uptake of colostrum.

4. Mothering and cow-calf bonding affect uptake of colostrum. Calves taken from their dam at birth absorb less colostral IgG compared with calves left with their dams for the first 24 hours, despite ingesting the same amounts of colostrum. Piglets weaned at 24 hours of age have reduced immunity compared with piglets weaned at 6 weeks of age.

5. Calves born in a stall may orient toward a dark corner instead of the udder, whereas at pasture the neonate has no such confusing and time-wasting options.

6. Poor udder and teat conformation (e.g., poorly developed teats on first-calf heifers and pendulous udders on old milkers) may result in the neonate's inability to find the teat.

In more general terms, the later the neonate starts to suckle, the less chance it has to achieve its theoretically maximum absorption of colostrum.

FAILURE OF PASSIVE TRANSFER

Failure of passive transfer (FPT) is the absence of adequate concentrations of plasma IgG with the potential consequence of a diseased neonate. This does not imply that the neonate will automatically become sick but is a statistically significant indicator of higher risk. It also identifies the need to monitor the identified neonate if not to provide prophylactic measures. Septicemia and diarrhea are the most common diseases to which susceptible neonates succumb; these topics are considered elsewhere. In the calf and lamb, 1600 mg of IgG/dl of plasma is considered adequate, 800 to 1600 mg/dl is considered partial FPT, and less than 800 mg/dl is considered complete FPT.

Continuing research is beginning to identify other dependent variables associated with neonatal mortality. Results suggest that reliance on the single parameter of neonatal serum Ig concentrations as an indicator of neonatal well-being is inappropriate because (1) protection against infectious agents is conferred by specific antibody titers, not total Ig levels, and (2) other factors such as management and infectious challenge contribute to the risk of disease. The protective effect of a particular Ig concentration in the neonate is modified by environment; elevated levels of ammonia in a piggery cause an increased prevalence of *Bordetella bronchiseptica* rhinitis in piglets. At least two well-controlled studies have failed to show any significant association between passive transfer and neonatal health. It has been shown that nonspecific serum factors such as complement may be of much greater significance in the neonatal pig. Obviously, we still have much to learn.

ASSESSMENT OF PASSIVE IMMUNITY

Evaluation of immune status in the neonate is of considerable economic and practical significance. A number of tests that can be relatively inexpensive in relation to the information obtained and the subsequent savings realized are available. Adequacy of colostral transfer is most specifically assessed by measurement of serum Ig concentrations in the neonate. This value appears to correlate well with survival. In one study it was noted that a neonatal serum IgG concentration of less than 1000 mg per dl in calves at 36 hours of age was associated with a significantly greater likelihood of dying before weaning.

The single radial immunodiffusion test (SRID) is a simple, specific quantitative test, but 24 to 48 hours is required to obtain a result, limiting its value as a field test upon which to base immediate management decisions.

Refractometry is a simple, nonspecific test that measures total plasma protein. The test assumes that the presuckle neonate has a relative hypoproteinemia that is corrected by adequate intake of colostrum. The test shows a good correlation with quantitative Ig assays in normal animals. A plasma protein concentration of greater than 6 g/dl indicates adequate passive immunity in a normally hydrated animal, less than 5 g/dl constitutes failure of passive transfer.

The zinc sulfate precipitation test is a quantitative assay but is time-consuming and requires sophisticated instrumentation. It is possible to get a rough estimate of Ig concentrations by visual inspection of degree of turbidity. However, comparison of visual inspection results with SRID does not show a worthwhile correlation, and visual inspection of zinc sulfate turbidity alone cannot be relied on.

The sodium sulfite precipitation test is a simple, semiquantitative test that requires a minimal amount of equipment. Three solutions of sodium sulfite, one each at 14, 16, and 18 per cent are used, and turbidity is noted in each one after addition of test serum. Turbidity is noted in all three tubes at >1500 mg/dl IgG; in the 16 and 18 per cent tubes at 500 to 1500 mg/dl IgG (Fig. 1) and in only the 18 per cent tube at <500 mg/dl.

A latex agglutination test has been described for use in the calf. It is a semiquantitative test that comes as a kit and requires no additional equipment. The kit is easy to use and is reported to give a quick and accurate result. The kit is marketed in the United Kingdom.

A variety of other techniques involving ELISA and similar solid-phase methods are potentially applicable to field evaluation of the food animal neonate, but as yet they are not available commercially.

Evaluation of colostrum before it is administered to the neonate is of value. There is a good correlation between

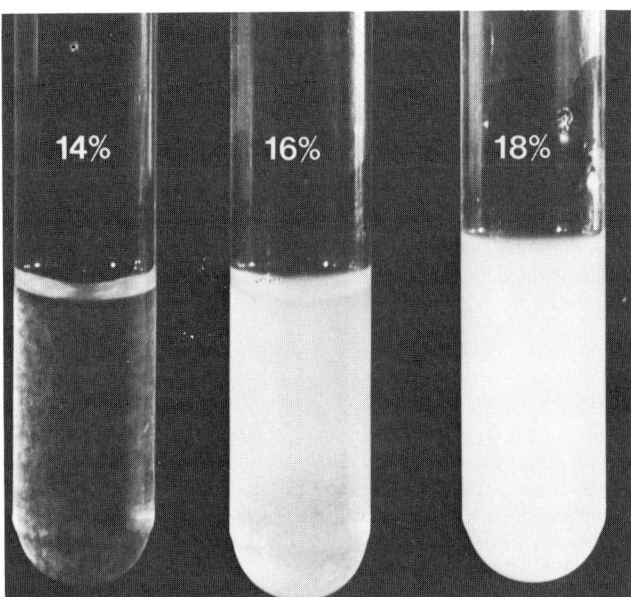

Figure 1. Partial failure of passive transfer detected by the sodium sulfite precipitation test: 0.1 ml serum was added to 1.9 ml of sodium sulfite solution, which was allowed to stand at room temperature for 30 minutes. Note the relative lack of turbidity in the 14% sodium sulfite solution.

colostral Ig concentration and neonatal serum Ig concentration. Refractometry has been reported as a simple and reliable method of estimating the quantity of Ig in colostral whey. In dairy calves it has been shown that reduced fecal shedding of rotavirus and *Cryptosporidium* is associated with more than 9 g/dl total protein of ingested colostrum.

The colostrometer has been shown to be of considerable value in estimating the quantity of Ig in colostrum. There is a positive correlation between colostral specific gravity and colostral Ig concentration. A specific gravity of more than 1.050 implies a colostral Ig concentration of 6 g/dl. Ideally, colostrum with an Ig concentration of 6 g/dl should be used for administration to the newborn neonate. Colostrum with a specific gravity below 1.050 is probably best saved and used in later feedings after gastrointestinal absorption of colostral Ig has stopped.

Although quantification of Ig concentrations appears to be useful in managing herd health, it must be recognized that this is not an infallible tool. It is becoming more apparent that a sick neonate metabolizes Ig faster and thus requires higher concentrations of antibody for protection. It is also recognized that Ig with appropriate activity against relevant pathogens is required for protective immunity.

From a practical point of view, the astute veterinarian or owner will be able to make some basic estimates of the probability that adequate transfer of colostral immunity will occur. A checklist based on the following questions can be developed to evaluate the risk of FPT: Does the dam have a history of poor nursing ability? Is the conformation of the teats and udder adequate? What is the physical nature of the first postpartum mammary fluids? Did the dam have any significant leakage of colostrum prior to parturition? Is the neonate premature or dysmature, and did the dam have any illness during the last trimester of pregnancy?

CORRECTION OF FPT

Several strategies can be employed in correcting FPT. The initial decision to be made is whether the neonate still has the capacity to absorb ingested colostrum. If the neonate is a potential FPT candidate and is less than 12 hours old, it is probably of value to administer an adequate amount of good quality colostrum per os, preferably by a bottle and nipple: for example, a Holstein calf requires 3 to 5 liters of first colostrum over a 4 to 6 hour period. Further colostrum feeds should be administered so that the neonate receives approximately 10 to 15 per cent of its body weight in colostrum by 24 hours of age. Similarly, lambs should be bottle fed to attain approximately 10 to 15 per cent of body weight in colostrum at 24 hours of age.

Once the gastrointestinal tract no longer has the ability to absorb colostrum, the only way to achieve protective levels of passive systemic immunity is a plasma or serum transfusion. Ideally, cells should be separated, but when necessary, whole-blood transfusions can be used. Consideration must be given to the increased risk of disease transmission (e.g., leukosis, anaplasmosis) when using whole blood for transfusion. Plasma or serum at 20 to 40 ml/kg should be administered slowly, intravenously or intraperitoneally. Ideally, the plasma or serum should be from the dam or animals in the same herd, ensuring that the plasma has immune reactivity to local environmental pathogens. This system is equally effective in calves, lambs, and kids. There is little information on use in piglets, but given the current popularity for Vietnamese potbellied pigs, work needs to be done. At Texas A and M the authors have had success with ear vein and intraosseous techniques of fluid administration in pigs.

MANAGEMENT TO OPTIMIZE PROTECTIVE IMMUNITY

Good maternal nutrition is important for allowing optimal intrauterine growth and adequate maternal immunity. A dairy cow body score condition of 3 in the last 2 months of pregnancy is recommended.

The dam should be kept in her normal environment during the last trimester to minimize stress and to allow development of good environmental immunity. Vaccination of the dam at 7 and 9 months of gestation will produce a colostrum rich in vaccinal IgG. Vaccines used depend on the diseases affecting neonates in the locality. Cows may be vaccinated or boosted with vaccines against infectious bovine rhinotracheitis, bovine virus diarrhea, bovine respiratory syncytial virus, parainfluenza-3 (PI-3), *Leptospira pomona*, *E. coli* pili, rotavirus, and coronavirus. Care should be taken not to use abortigenic forms of the vaccine during gestation.

Cows need a dry period of 5 to 8 weeks before parturition in which to produce and accumulate adequate amounts of colostrum. It is best not to foremilk, since the titer of colostral IgG can fall dramatically as it is removed from the udder and presumably reflects changing hormonal influences on the udder in the postparturient period.

Monitoring colostral Ig concentrations, especially when pooled, allows for strategic use of both high- and low-quality colostrum.

It is important to have access to a colostrum bank to supplement any neonate that is a potential FPT candidate. Ideally, colostrum from such a bank should be fresh, should contain 6 g/dl IgG, and should be from healthy cows that have a known relevant vaccination status. Care should be taken not to use colostrum from bovine leukemia virus–positive cows or from caprine arthritis–encephalitis–positive goats. In the case of small ruminants, bovine colostrum is a good substitute if no other colostrum is available.

It has been shown that giving early assistance in suckling to satiation optimizes colostral absorption; in the calf, 3 to 5 liters colostrum providing 80 to 100 g of Ig in the first 4 hours should be the goal.

With valuable livestock, it is best to assume that any neonate of a sick dam (dystocia, milk fever, mastitis, etc) is in need of colostrum supplementation. Evaluation of all neonates within 12 hours of birth and assessment of passive transfer at 12 to 24 hours allows management decisions about the need to treat, monitor, or cull individuals.

Environmental control is a major consideration and can significantly reduce the prevalence of neonatal problems regardless of plasma Ig concentration. Particular attention should be paid to cleaning, disinfection, ventilation, air-filtering, and feeding regimes with the goal of reducing stress and infectious challenge. Parturition in an outdoor, nonstressful environment is probably the most ideal situation for ruminants. Calves taken from their dam at 24 hours of age should be placed in individual pens; calf hutches outside are probably best.

In conclusion, it is important to recognize that although Ig measurements may be useful in evaluating the neonate, many factors can modify the usefulness of the information. Placing emphasis on neonatal Ig concentrations alone may be inappropriate but is of value when assessed in association with other variables that contribute to neonatal health.

Omphalitis and Its Sequelae in Ruminants

THOMAS R. KASARI, DVM, MVSc, DIPLOMATE, ACVIM

The umbilical cord (umbilicus) of bovine, ovine, and caprine fetuses in utero consists of an outer amniotic membrane surrounding (1) two veins that fuse intra-abdominally to a single vein that returns blood from the placenta to the liver of the fetus, (2) two arteries that communicate with internal iliac arteries and carry blood from the fetus to the placenta, and (3) the urachus, a tubular structure connecting the urinary bladder with the allantoic cavity. Normally, at parturition, as the fetus is expelled from the pelvic canal of the dam, the umbilicus is torn a few inches from the body wall. In response to this tearing action, umbilical arteries usually constrict and retract into the abdomen to the level of the bladder, with only remnants of amniotic membrane left surrounding the externally exposed umbilical veins and urachus. The umbilical veins and urachus gradually close, and the remnants of amniotic membrane dry up and fall from the neonate within 1 week after birth.

Localized inflammation or infection of the contents of the umbilical cord external to the body wall is referred to as omphalitis (navel ill). Omphalophlebitis, omphaloarteritis, and urachitis are terms used to further describe the extension of inflammation or infection from the external umbilicus to the intra-abdominal segments of the umbilical vein, umbilical arteries, and urachus, respectively. More than one of these structures may be infected in the same animal.

Delineation of the extent of inflammation or infection to the external or intra-abdominal segments of the umbilicus is dependent on thorough palpation and other aids such as ultrasonography. Presenting clinical signs are ordinarily different, depending on the location of infection within umbilical structures. Furthermore, resolution of an umbilical mass via either surgery or a medical treatment and overall prognosis are predicated on whether external or intra-abdominal involvement of these structures is present.

OCCURRENCE

Although surveys on the incidence of omphalitis in domestic ruminants is lacking, it is perceived by veterinarians to be a commonly encountered problem. Most health problems and deaths in lambs and kids from birth to 1 to 2 days of age are the result of dystocia, starvation, exposure, and predation. Pathologic and microbiologic conditions causing death are relatively minor in importance during this time. Postnatal infections become more important near the end of the first week of life when either diarrhea and pneumonia or omphalitis and septicemia occur.

Whereas most cases of navel ill in lambs and kids will be presented for examination by 3 months of age, enlargement of the umbilicus and clinical signs referable to navel ill in calves can be seen as early as 2 to 5 days after birth. Owners are more apt to present the bovine neonate at this time for examination of an observable swelling of the umbilicus. However, if the umbilicus appears relatively normal and intra-abdominal segments of the umbilicus are involved, cases may be up to 3 months of age or older before presentation.

ETIOLOGY AND PATHOGENESIS

Infection of the umbilicus is presumed to occur soon after birth, often as a consequence of poor hygiene, hypogammaglobulinemia, and neonatal weakness. The lumen of umbilical veins, arteries, and urachus do not close immediately after birth, which leaves a portal of entry for pathogenic bacteria. Provided the infection remains restricted to the external umbilicus, either localized cellulitis or an abscess with a thick fibrous capsule forms. The urachus is overwhelmingly the most frequently involved intra-abdominal umbilical remnant, followed by umbilical vein and, rarely, umbilical arteries.

Urachal involvement may remain localized to the urachal stalk, or infection may migrate retrograde to the bladder mucosa. Cystitis and signs of pollakiuria, stranguria, and dysuria in an animal of any age, particularly those individuals without any enlargement of the umbilicus, can be the first indication that a urachal stalk abnormality exists. The changes in frequency and nature of urination are thought to be the result of mechanical interference with normal filling and emptying of the bladder. The urachus fixes the apex of the bladder to the ventral abdomen which, in effect, stretches the bladder longitudinally and reduces the functional volume. The reduced holding capacity of the bladder allows smaller volumes of urine to stretch the detrusor muscles and stimulates frequent voiding of small amounts of urine. If a patent urachus accompanies umbilical swelling, the end of the umbilicus may remain moist, persistent dribbling of urine from this structure may occur, or fluid may dribble from the umbilicus concomitant with the act of urination.

Extensive omphalophlebitis often results in abscessation of the liver. Omphaloarteritis may promote the development of septicemia if bacteria gain entrance to the system's arterial circulation through the umbilical arteries.

Bacteria isolated from umbilical masses and deeper structures are generally confined to those genera that have the capability to grow under anaerobic conditions. *Actinomyces pyogenes* (formerly *Corynebacterium pyogenes*) is probably the most frequently isolated pathogen. This bacterial organism has a propensity for abscess formation with a thick fibrous capsule. *A. pyogenes* may also be isolated as part of a mixed infection with coliforms, particularly *Escherichia coli*, or *Staphylococcus* spp., *Proteus* spp., *Streptococcus* spp., and *Enterococcus*. Less frequently reported bacterial isolates include *Salmonella dublin* and *Mycoplasma alkalescens*. Many of these bacteria cause toxemia.

CLINICAL SIGNS

Neonates with omphalitis can show signs of disease as early as 2 to 5 days after birth. The umbilicus is enlarged, warmer than surrounding skin, and painful when palpated. The mass can be firm with pitting edema, if cellulitis is present, whereas fluctuance may exist if an abscess has developed. There should not be any intra-abdominal cylindric structures coursing anteriorly or posteriorly from the body wall directly above the umbilicus. The umbilical stump may be dry, moist, or, less frequently, draining purulent debris. Tachycardia and tachypnea may be present owing to pain. Variable degrees of depression usually exist, resulting in a loss of appetite. Fever may be evident.

Calves appear to be more sensitive than are lambs and kids to the effects of infection to the umbilical vessels and urachus. Calves with omphalophlebitis usually present at 1 to 3 months of age, most often for unthriftiness. The umbilicus may not be noticeably enlarged. The key diagnostic feature of this form of navel ill is that deep abdominal palpation detects a cylindric structure 3 to 5 cm in diameter coursing from the umbilicus in the direction of the anterior abdomen. The animal may need to be restrained in lateral or dorsal recumbency to facilitate thorough abdominal palpation. Palpation usually elicits a painful reaction from the animal. Inappetence and a low-grade fever usually accompany omphalophlebitis along with variable degrees of depression. Dehydration and tachycardia may exist as a consequence of low-grade toxemia.

Animals with omphaloarteritis will present a clinical picture very similar to that of omphalophlebitis with the exception that abdominal palpation reveals a space-occupying mass above the umbilicus that courses in a dorsocaudal direction.

Animals with urachitis will exhibit abdominal palpation findings identical with those of animals with omphaloarteritis. However, clinical signs of pollakiuria, dysuria, and stranguria as well as changes in urine parameters consistent with cystitis (if a communicating urachal abscess is present) frequently accompany the palpatory findings. Unlike other umbilical remnant diseases that occur characteristically during the suckling period, urachal abnormalities can escape detection in cattle until after they are weaned or are yearlings. A urachal stalk abnormality that mechanically impedes urination normally has no untoward effects on body condition, appetite, and demeanor.

Various reported sequelae to omphalitis, omphalophlebitis, omphaloarteritis, and urachitis include diffuse gangrene of the limbs, peritonitis, intestinal strangulation, hepatic abscessation, and septicemia (signs of pneumonia, panophthalmitis, meningitis, septic arthritis, osteomyelitis, and endocarditis).

CLINICOPATHOLOGIC ABNORMALITIES

Clinicopathologic abnormalities that are specific or pathognomonic for navel ill do not exist. Neutrophilic leukocytosis with or without immature bands and hyperfibrinogenemia may be found and reflect the infectious nature of this disease. Mild anemia may coexist. If septicemia is present and the causative bacterial organism is gram-negative, particularly *E. coli*, disseminated intravascular coagulation may develop (thrombocytopenia, hypofibrinogenemia, prolonged prothrombin and partial thromboplastin times, and increased fibrin degradation products). Many calves, lambs, and kids will also exhibit hypoproteinemia from hypogammaglobulinemia due to failure of passive transfer of maternal immunoglobulins. Those animals with cystitis will show hematuria, pyuria, proteinuria, and bacteriuria. Serum concentrations of aspartate transaminase, alkaline phosphatase, and γ-glutamyl transferase may be elevated in instances in which extensive liver abscessation is present as a sequela to omphalophlebitis.

DIAGNOSIS

Diagnosis of omphalitis, omphalophlebitis, omphaloarteritis, and urachitis is dependent on thorough abdominal palpation. The umbilical vein and arteries and the urachus are not palpable intra-abdominally in the normal animal. Consequently, palpable intra-abdominal structures emanating from the umbilicus should be viewed as abnormalities. A diagnosis of omphalitis or other umbilical remnant disease is warranted provided appropriate signalment and characteristic presenting signs accompany the palpatory findings.

The primary differential diagnosis for a simple umbilical hernia is complicated by other pathologic processes, including omphalitis. An uncomplicated umbilical hernia will be reducible, that is, the contents of the mass can be manipulated back into the abdomen through the abdominal wall defect, whereas omphalitis will not respond in a similar manner. In the case of an umbilical hernia involving any or all of the remnants of the umbilical cord, manipulation of the contents allows partial reduction of the mass adjacent to the body wall through a distinct and uniformly smooth hernial ring except for the firm nonreducible portion of the mass associated with the umbilicus. Skin overlying the nonreducible portion is firmly attached to the mass. Depending on the direction in which the ventral component of the mass courses intra-abdominally, omphalophlebitis, omphaloarteritis, or urachitis should be considered.

Diagnosis of an umbilical abscess can be made by aspiration of purulent material from the mass with a large-bore needle. Ultrasonography should be considered if confusion exists over the composition of an umbilical mass or if the significance of an intra-abdominal structure originating from the umbilicus is unclear. A 7.5-MHz transducer is preferred for this procedure because of its improved resolution. Positive contrast cystography or intravenous contrast urography provides meaningful information if a urachal stalk abnormality is suspected. Normally, the urinary bladder is well within the pelvis; however, with urachal involvement, the bladder shows filling well out of the pelvis and in a cranioventral direction. In older animals that are amenable to rectal palpation, immobility of the bladder may be detected with digital manipulation. If the umbilicus has a fistulous opening, radiopaque contrast material can be injected retrograde in an attempt to outline the affected structures.

TREATMENT

Antimicrobial therapy can be quite beneficial in those cases in which cellulitis is present in the external umbilicus. Examples of suitable antimicrobial drugs for *A. pyogenes* and *E. coli*, the two most common bacterial isolates, are listed in Table 1. When abscessation of the umbilicus has occurred, surgical drainage should be instituted. A stab incision is made in the most ventral aspect of the abscess; the cavity is drained and lavaged with a 7 per cent iodine solution. Several days of this treatment may be necessary to achieve satisfactory resolution of the abscess. For cases that show signs of systemic toxemia associated with umbilical abscessation, antimicrobial therapy in addition to surgical drainage is recommended.

Infected intra-abdominal segments of the umbilicus are best

Table 1. ANTIMICROBIAL AGENTS WITH ACTIVITY AGAINST *ESCHERICHIA COLI* AND *ACTINOMYCES PYOGENES*

Drug	Route	Dosage
E. coli		
Potentiated sulfonamides	IV,PO	15.0 mg/kg, bid
Ampicillin trihydrate	IM,SC	22.0 mg/kg, bid
Amoxicillin trihydrate	IM	5.0 mg/kg, bid
Ceftiofur	IM	2.2 mg/kg, bid
Gentamicin sulfate	IM,IV	2.0 mg/kg, bid
Amikacin	IM,SC	6.6 mg/kg, bid
A. pyogenes		
Penicillin G		
Sodium salt	IV	50,000 IU/kg, qid
Potassium salt	IV	50,000 IU/kg, qid
Procaine	IM,SC	20,000 IU/kg, sid
Erythromycin	IM	44.0 mg/kg, sid
Ampicillin trihydrate	IM,SC	22.0 mg/kg, bid
Amoxicillin trihydrate	IM	5.0 mg/kg, bid

IM = intramuscular; IV = intravenous; PO = per os; SC = subcutaneous.

managed by surgical correction. Urachal infections extending to the bladder require excision of the apex of the bladder and ligation of the umbilical arteries along with any external umbilical structures. Infection of the umbilical vein can be localized anywhere along its length or become diffuse and involve the liver with sequelae of abscessation. Localized omphalophlebitis that does not involve the liver can be managed by ligation and removal of the affected umbilical vein. Liver abscessation is best handled by marsupialization of the infected umbilical vein. This procedure entails securing the wall of the abscessed umbilical vein to the ventral body wall in the right paramedia area approximately 5 cm caudal to the xiphoid. Contents of the abscess are allowed to drain externally from the now patent umbilical vein stalk. The tract should be flushed daily with a 10 per cent povidone-iodine solution until drainage ceases. When the umbilical arteries are involved, the treatment of choice is ligation and resection of the involved arteries along with any external umbilical tissue.

PREVENTION

Infection of the umbilicus is presumed to occur soon after birth owing to the interaction of poor hygiene, neonatal weakness, and hypogammaglobulinemia. Consequently, improving hygiene in the maternity area, providing prompt attention and intervention to females experiencing dystocia, and ensuring adequate early ingestion of colostrum will decrease the potential for umbilical infection. Although dipping the umbilical cord in tincture of iodine at birth is a time-honored procedure, there is not good supportive information that this antiseptic is effective in prevention of subsequent bacterial infection of the umbilicus.

BIBLIOGRAPHY

Trent AM, Smith DF: Surgical management of umbilical masses with associated umbilical cord remnant infections in calves. J Am Vet Med Assoc 185:1531–1534, 1984.

Diarrheal Diseases of Neonatal Ruminants

ELAINE HUNT, DVM, Diplomate, ACVIM

Calf mortality causes a net loss per year of $50 million to $120 million from the American agricultural economy. Diarrheal disease is the number one killer of the neonatal bovine. Diagnosis of the etiologic agents causing neonatal diarrhea is enhanced by new diagnostic tests that have evolved through the recent advances in biotechnology. New knowledge has also been developed in the field of oral and intravenous fluid therapy for calves. Chapters in prior editions of this book and other recent publications have been devoted to this subject, so actual principles of fluid therapy will not be covered in this section. The second edition of this book also provides an excellent section on prevention and control of neonatal diarrhea in ruminants. For avoidance of repetition, the reader is referred to those book sections.

FACTORS PREDISPOSING TO ENTERIC DISEASE

The calf is born immunoincompetent, requiring large quantities of passively acquired colostral immunoglobulin to provide antibodies necessary for protection against disease. These antibodies function systemically (when absorbed) and locally within the gut. Colostral IgA, IgG_1, and IgG_2 function particularly to protect the calf against proliferation of enteropathogens. Calves rely on colostrum and whole milk for daily replenishment of local immunoglobulin (especially IgA) in the gut. Because the half-life of this immunoglobulin is short, calves fed milk replacers rapidly become IgA-depleted and may be more likely to develop enteric infections. Early ingestion of colostrum is important; calves fed within 1 hour of birth were found to experience significantly less diarrhea than did calves receiving delayed feedings. This may be because specific IgG_1 antibody ingested the first day of life persists for at least 5 days within the gut, apparently protected from the normal proteolytic activity of the gut. This same antibody does not persist in the bowel lumen when calves are fed colostrum on day 2. Absorbed antibody also appears to be released slowly from the systemic circulation into the bowel, providing low-level immunity against rotavirus infection. Obviously, any compromise in early ingestion of quality colostrum rich in both specific and nonspecific immune factors may predispose the calf to enteric disease.

Overwhelming pathogen exposure will predispose the calf to enteric disease. One calf with diarrhea is capable of infecting its environment, leaving 10^{10} pathogenic organisms per milliliter of diarrhea in a lethal aerosol, or directly contaminating ground, stalls, or bedding. A seasonal effect on incidence of scours has been demonstrated in calves less than 14 days of age in the northeastern United States. Because dairymen also alter breeding schedules to encourage calving during the late fall and early winter, large calf populations coincide with the onset of inclement weather. In the northern United States and Canada, cattle are often housed during the winter months. Large populations of neonates may be confined to small spaces in close contact with older calves that are actively shedding organisms. Small calves may have to compete with others for food, warmth, dry bedding, and space. All these stress factors can be expected to contribute to an increased incidence of infectious enteritis during winter months.

PATHOGENIC MECHANISMS IN DIARRHEAL DISEASE

Four mechanisms through which diarrhea occurs in the calf have been demonstrated to be important. Hypersecretion of ions (and water) into the bowel lumen occurs with enterotoxigenic *Escherichia coli* (ETEC). Increased osmotic pressure from maldigestive-malabsorptive disease is caused by damage to the enterocytes in *Cryptosporidium parvum* infection and viral diarrheas. Increased intestinal mucosal permeability is characteristic of the inflammatory bowel disease of salmonellosis or cryptosporidiosis. The least important mechanism is alteration in intestinal motility. With each of these mechanisms, net loss of bicarbonate, chloride, sodium, potassium, and water may result in mild to overwhelming dehydration, acidosis, serum potassium aberrations, and cardiovascular collapse. In-depth discussions of these mechanisms are available but are beyond the scope of this text.

ROTAVIRUS INFECTION

This disease is caused by a virus of the family Reoviridae. The primary clinical sign of these viral infections is diarrheal disease of the young. Calf rotavirus is ubiquitous throughout the world and may be the most common infectious cause of calf diarrhea.

Clinical Signs

Diarrhea can be noted in calves as young as 12 hours of age; susceptibility persists until the virus is encountered. Clinical disease is most common in calves less than 8 weeks of age and most severe in calves less than 3 weeks of age. Systemic viremia does not occur, so calves appear bright until onset of weight loss, dehydration, and acidosis. The stool may be yellow, voluminous, or pudding-like at first; with time, the stool may become watery.

Pathophysiology

The primary site of infection is the absorptive cells of the tips of the small intestinal villi. Infected enterocytes die and are replaced by immature epithelial cells with squamous to cuboidal morphologic features. Collapse of the villus does not occur, but the dysmature cells lack the enzymes necessary for nutrient digestion, so bowel absorptive and digestive processes are compromised, resulting in osmotic diarrhea of a few days' duration. Infection progresses from the proximal small intestine to the posterior bowel. Severity of disease is influenced by the age of the calf when it is exposed, the strain of rotavirus involved, specific and nonspecific colostral immunity, stress, environmental conditions, and concurrent infection with other enteropathogens (*E. coli,* coronavirus, or *C. parvum*). Fatalities are not uncommon in some herds. Rotavirus generally produces a more transient and self-limiting diarrhea than does coronavirus or *Cryptosporidium*.

In addition to the damage done by the virus, the damaged villi provide a more suitable environment for secondary coliform adherence and proliferation. Subsequent enterotoxin elaboration may result in hypersecretory diarrhea in addition to maldigestive disease. Calves contracting the virus at an early age with concurrent exposure to enterotoxigenic *E. coli* (ETEC) are especially threatened because these calves experience significantly greater rotavirus colonization and more severe villous atrophy than do mono-infected calves; a synergic interaction appears to develop between the two infections.

Infection occurs through ingestion of the rotavirus from objects in the environment contaminated with feces (e.g., teats, calf hutches, calf pens, feeding equipment). The virus may be transported into the enterocyte via pinocytosis during the period of macromolecular gut permeability immediately after birth. The virus remains viable in feces or water for a prolonged period of time (at least 7 months at room temperature), and large numbers of virus particles are shed in the environment from affected calves. Aerosol exposure has been speculated upon but not documented in the calf. Most adult cattle are seropositive, but there is little correlation between serum antibodies and viral infection.

Diagnosis

Diagnostic techniques include virus identification through fecal electron microscopy (EM), tissue or fecal fluorescent antibody (FA), fecal enzyme-linked immunosorbent assay (ELISA), and fecal latex agglutination. It is advisable to determine what method is utilized by your diagnostic laboratory, because sample handling and sensitivity are variable among the different techniques.

The fecal ELISA test is a more sensitive technique than is EM for diagnosis of infection, but neither test lends itself well to field diagnosis. This author prefers the latex agglutination kits (for human rotavirus), which accurately detect bovine rotavirus on fresh or frozen calf feces. Tests can be performed on the farm with vigorous hand rotation of the sample for 5 minutes. Thirty fecal samples or controls can be performed for about $120. When fecal ELISA test or latex agglutination is not possible, fecal EM or FA (on feces or tissue) may be necessary; 2 g of fresh, chilled feces from early clinical cases can be submitted for FA or EM. Tissue FA is a more accurate technique than is fecal FA. Several small bowel segments must be obtained within an hour of death. Mailed samples should not be frozen, except at $-70°$ F, because conventionally frozen tissues (20° F) suffer disruption of intestinal cells, which makes interpretation impossible.

Therapy

The most important therapy for a calf with acute, severe rotavirus infection is properly maintained hydration and electrolyte and acid-base status. Depending on the severity of dehydration, intravenous, oral, or subcutaneous fluids can be administered. In the past, calves experiencing diarrhea were generally taken off milk feedings and maintained with oral or intravenous electrolyte solutions. This is dangerous because calves kept off feed or primarily on electrolyte solutions for several days will emaciate very rapidly! Calves with multiple enteropathogen infections actually maintain body weight better and experience better regeneration of gut mucosa when milk feedings are continued throughout the diarrheic phase as long as supplemental electrolyte solutions are bicarbonate-free.

Oral antibiotics will not be useful against rotavirus, although secondary ETEC may be responsive to antimicrobials in some instances. Feeding small quantities of milk frequently may be particularly important in dual infections because enzyme activity increases in unaffected portions of the bowel as a compensatory mechanism to enhance the digestive process.

Prophylaxis

Efficacy of the modified live combination (rotavirus-coronavirus) vaccines for pregnant cows or newborn calves has been questioned. The attenuated vaccine for oral inoculation of the newborn calf is dependent on viral replication of the virus in the intestine for stimulation of local immunity. The oral vaccine has been reported to decrease mortality and morbidity, compared with infection rates reported by farms during previous calving seasons. Vaccine failures can be expected because the attenuated virus is neutralized by ingested colostrum. Because oral administration should occur at least an hour before colostrum ingestion, this product is prone to failure unless suckling can consistently be delayed. Usefulness of the product was not substantiated when it was evaluated in double-blind trials, possibly because of colostral antibody neutralization of the product.

The modified live virus vaccine intended to stimulate lactogenic immunity has also been controversial. The vaccine commonly available in the United States in the early 1980s was incapable of increasing specific antibody titers (primarily IgG_1) in the serum or colostrum of the dam. A Canadian study found no prophylactic benefit from using the vaccine in calves or in their dams. Yet, the European literature continues to document greater success with rotavirus combination vaccines than has been described in North America. This may be due to variations in vaccine production (times and routes of administration, use of adjuvant, or differing doses of virus), variation in virulence (which has been demonstrated in at least four of nine cytopathic strains of rotavirus), failure of vaccine virus to confer reciprocal protection against some field virus strains, or type of virus manipulation (virulent, attenuated, or inactivated).

Recently, a killed vaccine (for rotavirus, coronavirus, and ETEC) for use in pregnant cows was released in North America. Using a different adjuvant, this vaccine is reported to result in 4-fold increase in antibody titers above those achieved by the previous vaccine. Strict guidelines must be adhered to in order to avoid vaccine failure. Boosters must be administered within 40 days of calving; if the vaccination-to-calving interval exceeds 40 days, revaccination is necessary. This author is presently unaware of any scientific studies documenting or challenging the ability of this product to stimulate adequate lactogenic immunity.

A factor of unknown significance in the pathophysiology and prophylaxis of rotavirus is cross-species immunity and susceptibility. Calves may potentially be infected from rotavirus that originated in other species. Cross-species protection has been implied among ruminants. Lambs experiencing severe rotavirus diarrhea within hours of birth responded well when they received bovine colostrum from cows vaccinated against rotavirus and *E. coli* (50 ml/lamb by stomach tube). Simian and porcine rotavirus strains are related antigenically to the bovine strain and have been reported to prevent rotavirus in vaccinated calves. Future vaccine development may take these factors into account. Additionally, rotavirus-specific milk antibody preparations for oral therapy or prophylaxis may become available in the future. This would be useful since the half-life of colostral antibody within the gut is so short.

ENTEROTOXIGENIC *Escherichia coli* (ETEC)

Although colibacillosis can manifest in several forms (colisepticemia in the colostrum-deprived calf, enteroinvasive colibacillosis, and the common diarrheal form of enterotoxigenic *E. coli*), this discussion is limited to the enterotoxigenic form. ETEC is caused by encapsulated *E. coli*, a hardy organism that can persist for months in a dirty environment. About 90 per cent of bovine ETEC is caused by strains that are positive for the K99 pilus adherence antigen; strains carrying the F41 and FY adhesins are also capable of causing ETEC but are not as widespread. Differing serotypes are responsible for neonatal septicemia and coliform mastitis. The original source of the infection may be the environment or the dam (pathogenic serotypes will colonize the adult gut briefly, but frequently). The infected calf then contaminates the environment by producing up to 10^{13} infectious bacteria per 12-hour period.

Clinical Signs

Variable degrees of diarrhea and dehydration are manifest in neonatal enterotoxigenic colibacillosis. Onset of "pineapple juice" diarrhea may be so acute and severe that dehydration with collapse occurs in 7 to 12 hours, and the calf is simply found dead. Calves are rarely febrile and most frequently suffer hypothermia, particularly as dehydration, acidosis, and cardiovascular collapse progress. Blood is rarely present in the stool. Acute uncomplicated ETEC occurs in calves less than 5 days old because K99 binding sites are lost by 72 hours of age. Mild cases may recover spontaneously. Dairy calves are affected earlier and more frequently than are beef calves owing to intensive husbandry (crowding and feeding) practices.

Pathophysiology

Bovine ETEC is caused by encapsulated coliforms capable of secreting enterotoxin. The capsule is important for colonization because it inhibits phagocytosis, prevents intestinal effluent "wash off," and blocks immunoglobulin attachment. Pathogenic strains also contain the plasmid necessary for adherence to the villus, the $K99^+$ pilus antigen, which is common to most pathogenic bovine coliform strains. The $K99^+$ antigen is important to coliform colonization because it allows the bacteria to attach to epithelial cell-receptor sites and to colonize the small intestine, overcoming the cleansing effects of peristalsis. The bacteria must also be capable of secreting enterotoxin, which causes hypersecretory diarrhea. Enterotoxin also disrupts the normal motility of the bowel, depressing the rhythmic mixing contractions. The bowel will become dilated and flaccid and experience periods of quiescence followed by single abnormally long peristaltic rushes that forcefully propel the luminal fluid into the colon.

Coliforms rapidly colonize the gut of the newborn; this is not difficult because there is no competitive microflora present, and the abomasum is too alkaline to destroy gram-negative bacteria until the calf is 24 to 36 hours of age. Early ingestion and absorption of colostrum is necessary to provide the calf with local specific and nonspecific immunity against colonization of the small intestine by ETEC.

If a $K99^+$ coliform capable of enterotoxin production is an early and successful colonizer, the calf is at a high risk of developing clinical colibacillosis. The bacteria bind to mature enterocytes and elaborate toxin that affects the crypt cells; the cells begin to secrete an isotonic solution, which becomes rich in bicarbonate, sodium, and chloride. Extreme depletion of the extracellular fluid may occur from rapidly developing diarrhea. Minimal destruction occurs to the enterocytes, unless concurrent viral infection is present. Because enterocyte damage is minimal, oral electrolyte solutions are often successful in maintaining the hydration status of the animal if dehydration is not too severe.

Acutely dehydrated calves, particularly those with ETEC, suffer extreme metabolic acidosis. Hyperkalemia develops because severe acidosis results in whole-body intracellular hydrogen-potassium exchange in an attempt to buffer the increasing quantities of free hydrogen ion. Cardiotoxic hyperkalemia, manifest by bradycardia, may ultimately cause cardiac arrest in these acidotic calves. This hyperkalemia is paradoxical because a whole-body cellular hypokalemia exists from potassium loss into the diarrheal effluent.

Diagnosis

Diagnostic techniques are not foolproof because coliforms are normally an inhabitant of the lower intestinal tract of the neonatal calf. Histologic examination of intestinal segments collected immediately after death should show minimal small intestinal mucosal lesions without evidence of invasion of the organisms into the underlying tissues. The identification of specific $K99^+$ serotypes is necessary in order to confirm that ETEC is a significant pathogen in a particular outbreak of diarrhea. Two tests utilized to identify $K99^+$ coliforms are available. One is a modified ELISA, the other a latex agglutination kit; both tests are quickly performed on fresh feces. The ELISA test utilizes monoclonal antibody to cause a visible color change if $K99^+$ antigen is in the feces. It is also semiquantitative. Either test should be performed only on calves with diarrhea that are less than 5 days of age and that have not received an oral $K99^+$ vaccine. The cost for these diagnostic tests is $4 to $8 per sample.

Therapy

The administration of oral antimicrobial agents is not advisable in these calves; binding sites quickly disappear, and the $K99^+$ coliform can no longer adhere in the gut. Antibiotics should be relied on only when evidence of systemic complications (bacteremia, navel infections, or infectious arthritis) is noted.

Advancements in biotechnology may provide natural means for therapy of ETEC in the future. An example of this is the experimental use of bacteriophages to control multiplication of particular strains of enteropathogenic *E. coli*. Spraying contaminated litter with phage suspensions or administration of phage organisms into the small intestine of the calf can prevent disease of the neonate. This type of biotherapy is unlikely to be utilized at the present; postprandial acidity of the abomasal–proximal duodenal chyme and the core body temperature of calves adversely influence the virulence and survivability of many of these phage types.

Prophylaxis

A successful coliform vaccine has been developed using the $K99^+$ antigen; significantly elevated titers to $K99^+$ *E. coli* can be demonstrated in vaccinated cows. This vaccine is most useful when it is administered to the pregnant cow twice in a short period before calving. Yearly boosters are then required before calving. If the calf ingests colostrum immediately after birth, it is provided with antibody specific for the $K99^+$ antigen. Protection is not guaranteed and should still be accompanied by proper hygienic precautions. The $K99^+$ vaccine is effective and will prevent deaths in calves, although transient diarrhea may still occur in exposed animals. Oral $K99^+$ monoclonal or antisera antibody preparations are similarly successful in preventing mortalities. These are more expensive than the $K99^+$ vaccine and require careful management because the preparations must be administered shortly after birth. Nonimmunized cow's colostrum provides some protection (usually nonspecific) against ETEC, but it is not comprehensive and can fail to protect calves exposed to ETEC. Milk replacers and colostral supplements are now available that contain some $K99^+$ passive antibody.

CORONAVIRUS INFECTION

Coronavirus causes a severe and long-lasting disease with high morbidity and moderate mortality in neonatal calves. Coronavirus infection is said to be less widespread than rotavirus infection.

Clinical Signs

Calves are commonly affected between 5 and 21 days of age. Severe depression is noted; diarrhea and dehydration progress through a course of 4 to 5 days, by which time the calf is often moribund. Dysentery is not a feature of this infection, but mild respiratory disease can occur when aerosolized virus is inhaled.

Pathophysiology

The cells destroyed by the virus are the mature enterocytes on the tip and along the sides of the villus. These tall columnar cells are replaced by immature cuboidal epithelium lacking in digestive enzymes, which gives the villus a blunted appearance and impairs the normal absorptive processes of the villus. Hypersecretion of sodium and water also occurs. The unabsorbed nutrients within the bowel lumen also exert an osmotic effect that contributes to the diarrheal process. The undigested carbohydrates are hydrolyzed to organic acids by the intestinal bacteria, and colonic pH may decrease.

Respiratory infection may be important in the transmission of the enteric disease and may be followed by typical enteric disease with fecal shedding.

Diagnosis

In the necropsy specimen, immunofluorescent examination of the intestinal tissues (particularly the spiral colon) is necessary for diagnosis. Histologic or gross examination of colonic tissues under a dissection microscope may support the diagnosis if blunted villi are detected. If a laboratory equipped for this test is not immediately available, fresh tissues should be submitted chilled and shipped on ice directly to a laboratory. If the tissues are frozen before submission, cell disruption makes fluorescent antibody detection more difficult. Feces (fresh or frozen) collected from a live calf immediately after onset of diarrhea may also show typical coronavirus with electron microscopic examination.

Prophylaxis

Supportive therapy is not as effective in decreasing mortality rates in this diarrheal disease as in those previously mentioned, partially owing to the duration of the infection. Certainly, antimicrobials will have a very limited usefulness. Killed vaccine for colostral antibody is available that combines the coronavirus and rotavirus. A discussion of the problems associated with vaccination is included in the segment on rotavirus. No coronavirus antibody has been detected in milk, colostrum, or serum as a result of administration of the vaccine available before 1989, but studies have not yet been reported on the newer vaccine product.

ENTEROTOXEMIA (*Clostridium perfringens* type C)

Several manifestations of *Clostridium perfringens* infection are lumped together under the name of enterotoxemia. This is an acute, noncontagious disease that often affects the healthiest, fastest growing calves yet is easily and inexpensively prevented.

Clinical Signs

Type C enterotoxemia results in development of an acute, fatal hemorrhagic enteritis in calves less than 2 weeks of age. Frequently, those affected are offspring of cows producing large quantities of milk. Death may occur so rapidly that signs of abdominal pain or depression are never witnessed. If survival is prolonged, neurologic signs may prevail. Salivation and moderate increase in body temperature may occur.

Diagnosis

Diagnosis is generally made on the basis of necropsy. Necropsy may demonstrate extensive hemorrhage in the small intestine and mesenteric lymph nodes; jejunum and ileum can be expected to give evidence of extensive hemorrhage. Petechiae may be noted in abdominal organs, and edema and neuronal degeneration may occur in the brain. Mouse toxin inoculation is necessary to verify presence of clostridial toxin.

Therapy

Treatment of clinical cases with hyperimmune serum, extra-label dosages of penicillin, fluid therapy, and nonsteroidal anti-inflammatory drugs for endotoxic shock may be successful if they are administered early. Prevention of deaths in newborns can be ensured through vaccination of the dam twice before parturition, followed by yearly boosters. Passive immunity will last for about 3 weeks. Calves should be vaccinated with toxoid for preventing problems when they begin ingesting grain and become susceptible to type D enterotoxemia.

CRYPTOSPORIDIOSIS (*Cryptosporidium parvum*)

The pathogenic significance of this coccidian was not recognized for several years because it was assumed that this organism did not invade host tissues. Significance of the organism was also missed because it could be identified in calves, humans, and many mammalian species suffering from acute, chronic, or no diarrhea. Prevalence rates in 1- to 3-week-old calves on infected farms are often greater than 50 per cent. *C. parvum* has been transmitted from calves to healthy humans and is associated with persistent and fatal diarrhea in the immunologically compromised human with acquired immune deficiency syndrome (AIDS) and in Arabian foals with severe combined immune deficiency (SCID). Generally, a lower incidence occurs in arid regions.

Clinical Signs

Clinical signs of this disease are nonspecific and vary from anorexia and mild diarrhea to protracted, watery, nonresponsive diarrhea and debilitation that is not affected by conventional antimicrobial therapy. In experimental studies, feces often contain blood, bile, mucus, and undigested milk, but dysentery is not frequently noted in field cases. Dehydration is not necessarily present, but emaciation is the most common gross necropsy finding. Duration of disease appears to be 6 to 10 days; it can occur as early as 5 days of age but often is noticed during the second week of life.

Pathophysiology

At the point where the organism attaches to the microvillus border, a host-plasma membrane surrounds the organism, allowing it to develop as an intracellular but extracytoplasmic parasite. This environment is probably responsible for the protection *Cryptosporidium* enjoys from the various antimicrobial and antimalarial drugs used unsuccessfully against infections. Infection is associated with atrophic villi, degenerate villous epithelial cells, and/or villous hyperplasia; maldigestive-malabsorptive diarrhea results.

Immunologic studies suggest that cell-mediated immunity is not the mechanism by which epithelial destruction occurs, but functional T cells are necessary for infection resolution. *Cryptosporidium* has been shown to be susceptible to certain immune modulators (e.g., surface protein-specific monoclonal antibodies). Deprivation of normal colostrum has not influenced infection rates, but administration of hyperimmune bovine colostrum has significantly reduced parasite infections in calves. Colostral IgA and IgG_1 appear to confer more immunity than does IgG_2 or IgM. Calves are susceptible to infection until a functional rumen develops. Immunity develops after clinical disease. Colostrum deprivation does not influence infection rates. Diarrhea presumably occurs as a result of brush border destruction and subsequent maldigestion.

The oocysts are resistant to disinfectants (including phenols, chloroform, perchlorethylene, perchloracetic acid), even remaining viable after 30-minute acid immersion. Early reports suggesting coccidiostats are efficacious against cryptosporidia were incorrect. Lasalocid (a monensin-like drug) did help prevent infection when it was administered at a dosage that caused calf mortality. The organism is resistant to all other conventional drugs.

Xylose tolerance tests are abnormal in affected calves. If affected calves do not become too debilitated, most will recover. Although contribution of the infection to overall mortality rates or economic significance is as yet unknown, virtually 100 per cent of all calves in an area may become infected and shed oocysts for more than 3 weeks.

Diagnosis

Day 12 of life is the optimal sampling time, because a large percentage of naturally infected calves are shedding oocysts on this day. Fecal diagnosis in the live calf can be made through many techniques. Fecal flotation is commonly used (do not use sugar solutions for flotation), and slides are stained with Giemsa or acid-fast stains. Oocysts are identified by microscopic examination of Giemsa or acid-fast stains by the magenta granules in their cytoplasm. Direct fecal smears can be evaluated with use of a modified carbolfuchsin stain technique. A drop of feces, a drop of oil, and the carbolfuchsin stain are combined; a dark background is seen in which the cryptosporidia oocyst is highlighted because it does not take up the stain. Large numbers of calves can be sampled and assessed in a short period of time by use of air-dried rectal swabs that are stained with auramine-O and interpreted under an epifluorescent microscope. Experimental ELISA tests have also been developed for diagnosis in the live animal but are not widely available.

Diagnosis in the dead calf is not enhanced by gross necropsy alone because gut lesions are relatively nonspecific: moderate enteritis with adherent mucofibrinous exudate present in the lower small intestinal mucosa and sometimes involving cecal and colonic mucosa. Microscopic examination of ileal mucosal scrapings or fixed tissue sections is a useful means of identifying infection in the recently dead calf.

Fixation of tissues must occur soon after the death of the animal; it is difficult to identify the organism after degeneration of the gut epithelium occurs. Careful histologic examination of the intestine of infected calves will demonstrate organisms present on the microvillus border in the small intestine; the microvilli are destroyed in advanced infection. Villus atrophy is most notable in the ileum, with cuboidal and squamous epithelium replacing the columnar epithelium upon the villus. In the large intestine, *C. parvum* is present in the crypts in addition to the mucosal surface. An inflammatory infiltration of the lamina propria is noted, and a mixed cellular exudate is present within the gut.

Proper techniques should be utilized to identify other enteric pathogens even when the suspicion of *Cryptosporidium* infection is very great; multiple pathogen infections are common and contribute to the severity of disease. *Cryptosporidium* infection coupled with coronavirus infection is particularly severe.

Therapy

Maintenance of hydration, electrolyte, and acid-base status is necessary and requires protracted intensive care. Because emaciation is so prevalent in this disease process, milk must continually be offered. Besides maintaining electrolyte and fluid balance, small quantities of whole milk administered frequently is the only means of therapy this author currently utilizes.

Prophylaxis

Although immunologic prophylaxis does not presently exist for *C. parvum* infection, administration of hyperimmune bovine colostrum suppresses parasite development. Production of this hyperimmune colostrum includes multiple infusions of inactivated oocysts into each teat, a procedure limiting practical application of this prophylaxis.

Without adequate therapeutic or immunologic prevention available, management techniques become critical for farms experiencing significant *C. parvum* infections. Control is made more difficult by the resistance of the organisms to conventional disinfectants. Strict cleanliness is helpful in minimizing severity of infection, but prior environmental contamination is difficult to overcome. Raising calves in hutches that are moved frequently is helpful. Because oocyst "drying" is a means of natural destruction, hutches placed on sand or pea gravel may be more beneficial than are those located on grassy areas. Hutches must be cleaned between calves and turned upside down to facilitate access of sunlight to the oocysts. Prolonged moist heat treatments also result in loss of infectivity of the oocysts.

This organism is infectious to humans, so be careful when handling infected calves. Veterinary students are at a particularly high risk of developing the disease, and hospitalization is occasionally required. Physicians need to be apprised that opiate therapy is contraindicated owing to the immediate infectivity of oocysts and potential for superinfections when gut motility is disrupted.

SALMONELLOSIS

Salmonellosis is an enteric disease of cattle capable of high morbidity and high mortality in neonates and adults alike. It is the second most economically significant bacterial disease of the bovine gastrointestinal tract ($53 million annually, as per 1978 estimates). The effects of salmonellosis are particularly severe in the neonate. The disease may cause peracute septicemia, acute or chronic enteritis, or infectious osteomyelitis or arthritis.

Clinical Signs

Salmonella typhimurium

Calves are almost always over 10 days of age when diarrhea first develops. Veal calves are most susceptible shortly after introduction to the veal barn. The diarrhea is intractable, resulting in metabolic acidosis (with or without dehydration) and is characterized by a "septic tank odor" and by dysentery with chunks and flakes of fibrin (or even putrid fibrin casts) present in the stool. Although some calves develop only enteric disease, meningitis, polyarthritis, pneumonia, leukopenia, degenerative left shift, and vascular thrombosis are all sequelae to septicemia. If the calf survives the initial dehydration, diarrhea may not resolve for over 3 weeks. Survivors are often poor doers or chronic carriers.

Salmonella dublin

Often no diarrhea is noted, but the calf is severely depressed and shows signs of ill thrift, septicemia, meningitis, polyarthritis, osteomyelitis, fatal peracute pneumonia, or vasculitis-thrombosis and gangrene of the skin of the extremities.

Pathophysiology

Salmonella typhimurium is the bacterium most commonly affecting cattle in the eastern United States; *S. dublin* is a major problem in the western states but has been found occasionally as far east as North Carolina. This gram-negative organism secretes a potent endotoxin that is responsible for hypersecretory diarrhea within the gut. The organism penetrates the submucosa, causing superficial necrosis and sloughing of the mucosa. Infection is introduced per os, and the organism probably penetrates pharyngeal tissues and small intestine to gain access to the lymphatic system. It probably localizes in the lymph nodes of the mediastinum, then spreads to the gut through migrating phagocytic cells. By becoming intracellular parasites, the bacteria are protected from antimicrobials and are capable of dissemination throughout the body. If the infection is confined to the gut, only signs referable to the alimentary tract will be recognized. Appearance and severity of clinical disease is stress-related and is also affected by virulence of strain, dose, age, and immune status (especially cell-mediated immunity). If septicemia occurs, fatal meningitis or endotoxic shock is a common cause of death. Size of challenge dose, colostrum ingestion, and concurrent stress are factors that may influence morbidity and mortality rates. Death losses may approach 100 per cent in neonatal calves. *S. typhimurium* is less of a long-term problem than is *S. dublin*, which persists in carriers that intermittently shed *S. dublin* in feces and milk. *S. typhimurium* is not host-specific, and infected calves pose a health risk to all species, particularly the horse and human. *S. dublin* is host-adapted to the bovine but is associated with higher mortality rates in humans than are most salmonellae.

There is no breed predisposition, but dairy calves are most commonly affected as a result of intensive rearing techniques. Housed veal calves and calves purchased from sale barns, where exposure rate is high, are particularly frequently involved. Infected animals may become clinical or subclinical carriers. The organism may persist in the lymph nodes or tonsils and not be shed in the feces. Any type of environmental stress can cause a subclinical carrier to develop clinical disease. Injudicious use of antimicrobial drugs can also lead to explosive outbreaks of salmonellosis, because destruction of the more antimicrobial-sensitive indigenous microflora eliminates one of the major means of controlling pathogen overgrowth. What little efficacy antimicrobial agents may have against *Salmonella* infection is rapidly lost because organisms are capable of sexual conjugation with drug-resistant coliforms.

Diagnosis

Diagnosis is achieved in the living animal by submitting at least 6 1-g fecal samples for enrichment culture (selenite tetrathionate broth) over a 2- or 3-day period to the local bacteriology laboratory. If a group is cultured one time only, at least 6 affected animals should be sampled. Culture from rectal biopsies is an effective means of reaching a definitive diagnosis in the equine.

Leukocyte anomalies occur in enteric and septicemic salmonellosis. Calves often develop a marked leukopenia and neutropenia with enteric salmonellosis. Neutrophil cytology may also be affected; toxic granulation may be abundant. The presence of fecal leukocytes on the fibrin tags in the stool is supportive of *Salmonella* infection. Calves that survive several days and continue to drink water often are moderately hyponatremic and hypoalbuminemic.

If necropsy is possible, submit gut and mesenteric lymph nodes for enrichment culture. Gross necropsy often shows a pseudodiphtheritic membrane lining the distal small bowel and large colon; an inflammatory response is noted with histopathologic examination. In the ruminant, the gallbladder should always be cultured because few organisms but *Salmonella* survive there.

An experimental ELISA test has been developed for *S. dublin*–infected cows that successfully differentiates between uninfected cows, recently infected but recovered cows, and *S. dublin* mammary gland carrier animals. Adoption of this test for identification of the last group may make it possible to detect and eliminate those animals that pose a significant threat to human and calf health.

Therapy

Oral antimicrobials rapidly become ineffective against enteric disease; systemic antimicrobials prolong recovery and prolong the carrier state by inhibiting indigenous and beneficial coliforms. Antibiotics should be reserved only for those animals that are individually valuable and show signs of septicemia (tachycardia, scleral injection, and so on). In these cases, drug sensitivity should be evaluated; many resistance factors (plasmids) exist that are frequently exchanged by sexual conjugation with other gram-negative organisms. For this reason, susceptibility patterns are constantly evolving. Some aminoglycosides have a useful in vitro spectrum against many strains of *Salmonella;* clinical efficacy is often disappointing because aminoglycosides are unable to penetrate the phagocytic cell where the live organisms remain. Ampicillin, amoxicillin, and nitrofurans are only occasionally useful. Trimethoprim-sulfamethoxazole may be useful if organisms are not resistant, because it readily penetrates the phagocyte.

Valuable septicemic animals should receive intravenous flunixin meglumine, intensive fluid therapy, and other appropriate shock therapy. Prolonged administration of oral electrolyte solutions is necessary in enteric infections, and intravenous fluids are often necessary as well. It is inadvisable to restrict milk intake in affected neonates because they rapidly become emaciated with this disease process anyway. Frequent feeding with small quantities of milk is certainly advisable in these instances.

Prophylaxis

Because large doses of the organism are necessary to cause infection, measures to eliminate stress and environmental contamination are imperative in the neonate, particularly considering that morbidity and mortality rates are so high. Wherever possible, calves should be purchased directly from a dairy that has no history of calf losses due to *Salmonella*, rather than dealing with a buyer or purchasing directly from a sale barn. Appropriate colostrum ingestion is a must. If a buyer is necessary to supply the number of calves needed, then similarly aged calves should be purchased at one time, and no younger susceptible calves should be brought into the barn at a later date (all-in, all-out premise). Because a buyer acquires calves from many different dairies at the same time, it is inevitable that mixed groups of calves will harbor *Salmonella* infections.

A live, mutant vaccine has been of some use against *S. dublin* infections in England, but this vaccine may never be released in the United States. Although many mutant strain vaccines of *S. typhimurium* have been explored, these have been largely unsuccessful or too dangerous to release. Commercial killed bacterins are available that may be partially beneficial in certain situations, but some vaccinates may die from what appears to be acute endotoxic shock. Because of this potential, commercial bacterins should be administered by a veterinarian on a cool day, when an adequate supply of epinephrine, furosemide, and nonsteroidal anti-inflammatory drugs are available. Bacterins made from local isolates for severely affected farms have had mixed results and require 10^9 formalin-killed adjuvanted bacteria per milliliter of proper serotype administered to the calf at birth. Some of the failure associated with the bacterins is due to the inability of a bacterin to stimulate effective, prolonged cell-mediated immunity. Bacterin administration to pregnant cows has not resulted in demonstrable passive antibody production.

Salmonella sp. affects the young, old, and debilitated of many mammalian species. Be careful when handling carrier animals, because this organism is a potent zoonotic.

OTHER UNCOMMON PATHOGENS

In many cases of neonatal bovine diarrhea, the causative agents are never discovered. Certainly in the future we will learn more about uncommon pathogens and those that we have yet to discover.

Giardia is probably the most important newly recognized organism capable of causing calf diarrhea. Signs associated with this disease include chronic, pasty diarrhea, weight loss, and failure to thrive. Diarrhea can be intermittent or continuous, lasting up to 6 weeks; giardiasis should be considered when persistent, nonresponsive diarrhea is noted in calves up to 5 months of age. Fecal flotation (do not use sugar solutions) can be used to concentrate the cysts. A fresh fecal sample is required for trophozoite identification. A direct smear suspended in a little saline on the slide and stained with Lugol's iodine will make the trophozoites visible. Cysts are found most commonly in formed or semiformed stools; trophozoites predominate in unformed feces. Negative samples on 3 successive days are necessary before this disease can be eliminated as a cause of diarrhea. If fecal samples are to be mailed to a diagnostic laboratory for analysis, preserve them in equal volumes of 5 per cent formalin in saline (19 parts normal saline added to 1 part 40 per cent formaldehyde solution). Dimetridazole therapy (50 mg/kg for 5 days) will cause resolution of the diarrhea by elimination of the parasite.

Another new pathogen that is evolving in importance is enteropathogenic *E. coli* (EPEC). This type of coliform is capable of attaching to and effacing the gut microvilli. The EPEC is thought to excrete a Shiga-like cytotoxin also called Verotoxin. Bloody diarrhea lasts 4 to 8 days in these calves.

Campylobacter jejuni/coli has been identified as an enteropathogen in Ontario causing over 10 per cent of infectious diarrhea in dairy calves, particularly in calves raised in group pens. Mortality rates could not be correlated with infections with this organism. "Small round viruses" that have been detected in the stool of calves with diarrhea include enterovirus, parvovirus, Norwalk agent–like viruses, and astroviruses. *Bacteroides fragilis* has been associated with diarrheal disease in calves in Montana and Idaho.

BIBLIOGRAPHY

GENERAL INFORMATION

Argenzio RA: Pathophysiology of neonatal calf diarrhea. Vet Clin North Am [Food Anim Pract] 1:461–470, 1985.

Bolton JR, Pass DA: The alimentary tract. *In* Robinson WF, Huxtable CRR (eds): Clinicopathologic Principles for Veterinary Medicine, New York, Cambridge University Press, 1988, pp 163–193.

Curtis CR, Erb HN, White ME: Descriptive epidemiology of calfhood morbidity and mortality in New York Holstein herds. Prevent Vet Med 5:293–307, 1988.

Howard JL (ed): Current Veterinary Therapy: Food Animal Practice 2. Philadelphia, WB Saunders, 1986.

Roussell AJ (ed): The Veterinary Clinics of North America: Food Animal Practice. Philadelphia, WB Saunders, 1990.

ROTAVIRUS INFECTION

Acres SD, Radostits OM: The efficacy of a modified live reo-like virus vaccine and an *E. coli* bacterin for prevention of acute undifferentiated neonatal diarrhea of beef calves. Can Vet J: 17:197–212, 1976.

Archambault D, Morin G, Elazhary Y, et al: Immune response of pregnant heifers and cows to bovine rotavirus inoculation and passive protection to rotavirus infection in newborn calves fed colostral antibodies or colostral lymphocytes. Am J Vet Res 49:1084–1091, 1988.

Besser TE, Gay CC, McGuire TC, Evermann JF: Passive immunity to bovine rotavirus infection associated with transfer of serum antibody into the intestinal lumen. J Virol 62:2238–2242, 1988.

Burki F, Mostl K, Spiegl E, et al: Reduction of rotavirus-, coronavirus- and E. coli–associated calf-diarrheas in a large-size dairy herd by means of dam vaccination with a triple-vaccine. J Vet Med [B] 33:241–252, 1986.

Castrucci G, Ferrari M, Frigeri F, et al: Experimental infection and cross protection tests in calves with cytopathic strains of bovine rotavirus. Comp Immunol Microbiol Infect Dis 6:321–332, 1983.

Castrucci G, Frigeri F, Ferrari M, et al: Neonatal calf diarrhea induced by rotavirus. Comp Immunol Microbiol Infect Dis 11:71–84, 1988.

DeLeeuw PW, Ellens DJ, Talmon FP, Zimmer GN: Rotavirus infections in calves: efficacy of oral vaccination in endemically infected herds. Res Vet Sci 29:142–147, 1980.

Ellis GR, Daniels E: Comparison of direct electron microscopy and enzyme immunoassay for the detection of rotavirus in calves, lambs, piglets and foals. Aust Vet J 65:133–135, 1988.

Haralambiev H, Georgiev G, Mitov B, Tsvetkov P: Application of an attenuated vaccine, RoCo-81, against viral enteritis of calves. Acta Vet Hung 35:469–473, 1987.

Heath SE, Naylor JM, Guedo BL, et al: The effects of feeding milk to diarrheic calves supplemented with oral electrolytes. Can J Vet Res 53:477–485, 1989.

Killen JR, Hugill MC, Jones HL: Treatment of scour in lambs [correspondence]. Vet Rec 122:494, 1988.

Mebus CA, Newman LE: Scanning electron, light and immunofluorescent microscopy of intestine of gnotobiotic calf infected with reovirus-like agent. Am J Vet Res 38:553–558, 1977.

Reynolds DJ, Morgan JH, Chanter N, et al: Microbiology of calf diarrhea in southern Britain. Vet Rec 119:34–39, 1986.

Runnels PL, Moon HW, Matthews PJ, et al: Effects of microbial and host variables on the interaction of rotavirus and *Escherichia coli* infections in gnotobiotic calves. Am J Vet Res 47:1542–1550, 1986.

Saif LJ, Smith KL, Landmeier BJ, et al: Immune response of pregnant cows to bovine rotavirus immunization. Am J Vet Res 45:49–58, 1984.

Schroeder BA, Sproule R, Saywell D: Prevalence of rotavirus in dairy calves as diagnosed by ELISA. Surveillance 12:2–3, 1985.

Snodgrass DR: Evaluation of a combined rotavirus and enterotoxigenic *Escherichia coli* vaccine in cattle. Vet Rec 119:39–42, 1986.

Snodgrass DR, Terzolo HR, Sherwood D, et al: Aetiology of diarrhoea in young calves. Vet Rec 119:31–34, 1986.

Stiglmair-herb MT, Pospischil A, Hess RG, et al: Enzyme histochemistry of the small intestinal mucosa in experimental infections of calves with rotavirus and enterotoxigenic *Escherichia coli*. Vet Pathol 23:125–131, 1986.

Thurber ET, Bass EP, Beckenahuer WH: Field trial evaluation of a reo-coronavirus calf diarrhea vaccine. Can J Comp Med 41:131–136, 1977.

Twiehaus MJ, Mebus CA: Licensing and use of the calf scour vaccine. Proc Annu Meet US Anim Health Assoc 77:55–58, 1974.

Waltner-Toews D, Martin SW, Meek AH, et al: A field trial to evaluate the efficacy of a combined rotavirus-coronavirus/*Escherichia coli* vaccine on dairy farms in south-western Ontario. Can J Comp Med 49:1–9, 1985.

Waltner-Toews DV: Dairy calf management, morbidity, mortality and calf-related drug use in Ontario Holstein herds. Dissertation Abstr Interna B 46:2589, 1986.

ENTEROTOXIGENIC *Escherichia coli* (ETEC)

Contrepois MG, Girardeau JP: Additive protective effects of colostral antipili antibodies in calves experimentally infected with enterotoxigenic *Escherichia coli*. Infect Immun 50:947–949, 1985.

Okerman L: Enteric infections caused by non-enterotoxigenic *Escherichia coli* in animals: occurrence and pathogenicity mechanisms. A review. Vet Microbiol 14:33–46, 1987.

Williams Smith H, Huggins MB, Shaw KM: The control of experimental *Escherichia coli* diarrhoea in calves by means of bacteriophages. J Gen Microbiol 133:1111–1126, 1987.

Williams Smith H, Huggins MB, Shaw KM: Factors influencing the survival and multiplication of bacteriophages in calves and in their environment. J Gen Microbiol 133:1127–1135, 1987.

CORONAVIRUS INFECTION

Heckert RA, Saif LJ, Hoblet KH, Agnes AG: A longitudinal study of bovine coronavirus enteric and respiratory infections in dairy calves in two herds in Ohio. Vet Microbiol 22:187–201, 1990.

Rodak L, Babiuk LA, Acres SD: Detection by radioimmunoassay and enzyme-linked immunosorbent assay of coronavirus antibodies in bovine serum and lacteal secretions. J Clin Microbiol 16:34–40, 1982.

Wieda J, Bengelsdorff HJ, Bernhardt D, Hungerer KD: Antibody levels in milk of vaccinated and unvaccinated cows against organisms of neonatal diarrhoea. J Vet Med [B] 34:495–503, 1987.

ENTEROTOXEMIA (*Clostridium perfringens* type C)

Fleming S: Enterotoxemia in neonatal calves. Vet Clin North Am [Food Anim Pract] 1:509–514, 1985.

Cryptosporidium parvum

Anderson BC: Cryptosporidiosis in calves: epidemiologic questions, diagnosis and management. Proc 14th Convention AABP 14:92–94, 1982.

Anderson BC: Moist heat inactivation of *Cryptosporidium* sp. Am J Public Health 75:1433–1434, 1985.

Campbell I, Tzipori S, Hutchinson G, Angus KW: Effect of disinfectants on cryptosporidium oocysts. Vet Rec 111:414–415, 1983.

Gobel E: Diagnose und Therapie der akuten Cryptosporidiose beim Kalb. [Diagnosis and treatment of acute cryptosporidiosis in the calf.] Tierarztl Umschau 42:863–869, 1987.

Lazo A, Barriga OO, Redman DR, Bech-Nielson S: Identification by transfer blot of antigens reactive in the enzyme-linked immunosorbent assay (ELISA) in rabbits immunized and a calf infected with *Cryptosporidium* sp. Vet Parasitol 21:151–163, 1986.

Moon HW, Woode GN, Ahrens FA: Attempted chemoprophylaxis of cryptosporidiosis in calves. Vet Rec 110:181–182, 1982.

Ongerth JE, Stibbs HH: Prevalence of *Cryptosporidium* infection in dairy calves in western Washington. Am J Vet Res 50:1069–1070, 1989.

Robert B, Ginter A, Antoine H, et al: Diagnosis of bovine cryptosporidiosis by an enzyme-linked immunosorbent assay. Vet Parasitol 37:9–19, 1990.

Sobieh M, Tacal J, Wilcke BW, et al: Investigation of cryptosporidial infection in calves in San Bernardino County, California. J Am Vet Med Assoc 191:816–818, 1987.

Tilley M, Fayer R, Guidry A, et al: *Cryptosporidium parvum* (Apicocomplexa: Cryptosporidiidae) oocyst and sporozoite antigens recognized by bovine colostral antibodies. Infect Immun 58:2966–2971, 1990.

Tzipori S, Campbell R, Angus KW: The therapeutic effect of 16 antimicrobial agents on *Cryptosporidium* infection in mice. Aust J Exp Biol Med Sci 60:187–190, 1982.

Tzipori S, Smith M, Halpin C, et al: Experimental cryptosporidiosis in calves: clinical manifestations and pathological findings. Vet Rec 112:116–120, 1983.

SALMONELLOSIS

Butler DG: Bovine salmonellosis. Bov Proc 18:14–19, 1986.

Clarke RC, Gyles CL: Galactose epimeraseless mutants of *Salmonella typhimurium* as live vaccines for calves. Can J Vet Res 50:165–173, 1986.

Smith BP, Oliver DG, Singh P, et al: Detection of *Salmonella dublin* mammary gland infection in carrier cows, using an enzyme-linked immunosorbent assay for antibody in milk or serum. Am J Vet Res 50:1352–1360, 1989.

OTHER PATHOGENS

Changer N, Hall GA, Bland AP, et al: Dysentery in calves caused by an atypical strain of *Escherichia coli* (S102-9). Vet Microbiol 11:241–253, 1986.

Kirkpatrick CE: Giardiasis in large animals. Compend Contin Educ 11:80–84, 1989.

Myers LL, Shoop DS, Firehammer BD, Border MM: Association of enterotoxigenic *Bacteroides fragilis* with diarrheal disease in calves. J Infect Dis 152:1344–1347, 1985.

Okerman L: Enteric infections caused by non-enterotoxigenic *Escherichia coli* in animals: occurrence and pathogenicity mechanisms. A review. Vet Microbiol 14:33–46, 1987.

Reckling KF: Electron microscopic observations on small round viruses in intestinal and faecal samples from healthy and diarrhoeic calves. Monatsschr Veterinarmed 42:272–275, 1987.

St. Jean G, Couture Y, Dubreuil P, Frechette JL: Diagnosis of *Giardia* infection in 14 calves. J Am Vet Med Assoc 191:831–832, 1987.

Waltner-Toews D, Martin SW, Meek AH: An epidemiological study of selected calf pathogens on Holstein dairy farms in southwestern Ontario. Can J Vet Res 50:307–313, 1986.

Diarrhea in Neonatal Swine

JOHN J. ANDREWS, DVM, PhD, MS

Diarrhea in baby pigs is a common and important economic problem in rearing of swine. In spite of improvements in management and veterinary care, diarrhea is still the most frequent clinical disease observed. The attending veterinarian needs to be able to determine the exact cause or causes of neonatal enteritis, treat effectively when possible, and recommend management changes or other preventive measures that will allow the producer to minimize the economic impact of neonatal diarrhea.

ETIOLOGY

A variety of infectious agents contribute to the production of diarrhea in preweaned pigs. The most frequent of these include various enteropathogenic strains of *Escherichia coli*, *Clostridium perfringens* type C, transmissible gastroenteritis (TGE) virus, rotaviruses, and coccidia (*Isospora suis*). Occasionally, other infectious agents such as *Salmonella* spp., *Clostridium perfringens* type A, *Pasteurella haemolytica*–like organisms, cryptosporidia, and adenoviruses have been associated with enteritis in preweaned pigs; however, these agents are not currently recognized as common pathogens.

Frequently, more than one of these agents contribute to diarrhea problems in a given herd. It is not uncommon to find an endemic TGE virus and rotavirus infection in a herd that also has enteropathogenic *E. coli* and *I. suis* producing clinical diarrhea.

The diet (or lack of diet, i.e., partial starvation), a lack of adequate colostral transfer, the environmental temperature and humidity, concurrent infections with agents that may be immunosuppressive (i.e., encephalomyocarditis virus, parvovirus, eperythrozoonosis, and others), and many other factors also play important roles in the pig's resistance to the infectious agents that produce diarrhea.

Understanding the multifactorial etiology of diarrhea, the pathogenesis of the various diarrhea-producing agents, and the means available to confirm the presence of the various agents in a herd is needed to develop an effective treatment and control program.

PATHOGENESIS: MECHANISMS OF DIARRHEA PRODUCTION

The mechanisms that protect the intestines and those by which an agent may produce diarrhea are important in determining therapeutics and control as well as in determining an etiologic diagnosis. Whereas exact mechanisms may be complex, there are some general features of these mechanisms.

Mechanisms of Gut Protection. The pig has a number of protective mechanisms by which diarrhea can be either prevented or controlled. Soon after birth, the sterile intestine is rapidly populated with usually nonpathogenic bacterial organisms. These nonpathogens compete for attachment sites and nutrients and thus block the colonization of pathogenic bacteria. *Lactobacillus* sp. generally colonize the stomach; α-hemolytic streptococci (frequently referred to as fecal streptococci) and lower numbers of lactobacilli colonize the small intestines; and *Clostridium* sp., *E. coli*, and lactobacilli heavily colonize the colon. These organisms also stimulate local immune responses. Heavy plasmacyte infiltration of the lamina propria and submucosa of the duodenum, the upper jejunum, and the colon is evidence of this immune stimulation. The acidic environment of the stomach and upper duodenum also plays a role in determining the types of bacteria that colonize these areas.

Ingested immunoglobulins in the colostral and lactation milk play a major role in preventing the attachment, penetration, and toxin production of many of the infectious agents. The plasmacytes located in the lamina propria of the duodenum and jejunum secrete locally active immunoglobulins (mainly IgA and IgM) and contribute to the immunologic protection of the gut as early as 5 to 10 days after birth.

The ability of the small intestine to replace lost epithelium is sluggish at birth but becomes more rapid in response to colonization of the small intestine by pathogenic and nonpathogenic bacteria and viruses.

The colon has a remarkable ability to absorb excessive fluid presented to it. Diarrhea occurs when the large intestine is not able to absorb the fluid presented to it from the small intestines. Whereas this may seem like a simplistic principle, the capacity of the colon to absorb fluid increases with age and is a major reason that diarrheal diseases are devastating in the young but are uncommon in adults. Infectious agents producing diarrheal diseases in growing and finishing swine often have direct effects on the colon (i.e., swine dysentery and enteric salmonellosis).

General Mechanisms of Diarrhea Production. In the neonatal pig, the most important and common of these include the following:

1. The destruction and loss of absorptive intestinal epithelial cells.
2. The presence of high osmolarity gut contents exerting a negative influence on absorption.
3. Toxic effects on the intestinal epithelial cells resulting in fluid loss into the gut lumen.
4. Toxic effects on the epithelium, lamina propria, and underlying tissues producing changes from epithelial effacement to necrosis and ulceration.
5. Invasion of organisms into the underlying tissues inciting an inflammatory response.

Specific Mechanisms of Diarrhea Production

Escherichia coli

Most *Escherichia coli* organisms that produce enteritis in neonatal piglets attach to the villous epithelium of the small and large intestines by means of structures called pili. The coliforms then colonize the epithelium and produce the classic heat-labile (LT) or heat-stable (ST) enterotoxins. The enterotoxins stimulate the mucosal epithelium to secrete excess alkaline fluid, which results in diarrhea. The 3 major pilus antigens that mediate this attachment have been identified as K88, K99, and 987P. Most coliform diarrheas in the near-weaning to postweaning time period are caused by K88–pilus containing *E. coli*, whereas coliform enteritis occurring during the first 2 weeks of life is caused by a mixture of K88, K99, and 987P organisms. Vaccines containing pilus antigens are now marketed to provide colostral and lactation antibodies to block this attachment. Coliforms without identifiable K88 or other pilus antigens may also colonize the small intestines and produce diarrhea. Non-K88 coliforms usually colonize the lower portions of the small intestines; pilus-containing *E. coli* frequently colonize the entire small intestine with the exception of the acidic portions of the upper duodenum.

E. coli organisms may also produce a cytotoxin called Shiga-like toxin, which is absorbed systemically and produces the vascular lesions of edema disease (gut edema). This toxin has also been associated with coliforms contributing to postweaning diarrheas. The Shiga-like toxin is probably not, however, the only toxin that contributes to these syndromes. Shiga-like toxin may also play a role in the 10-day to 2-week diarrheas of pigs that are associated with systemic effects such as purplish discoloration of the ears, snouts, and feet. The strains of *E. coli* responsible for this syndrome are often hemolytic on blood agar. A large amount of endotoxin is also released by the hemolytic *E. coli* organisms and may be responsible for most of the systemic effects seen in this syndrome.

Recently recognized strains of *E. coli* may also attach to the apical portions of the enterocytes and produce microvillus damage, thus effacing the gut surface. Loss of microvilli associated with cupping of the epithelial surface at the sites of bacterial attachment is the most common ultrastructural change. These strains are called attaching-effacing *E. coli* (AEEC). This attaching-effacing ability may exist in organisms that also possess the ability to produce the classic enterotoxins. Whereas AEEC strains of *E. coli* isolated from human diarrheas have produced diarrhea in gnotobiotic piglets, attaching-effacing coliforms have been infrequently isolated from naturally occurring diarrheas of neonatal swine.

Gut stasis also mediates the attachment and colonization of the small intestines with *E. coli*. It has long been recognized that chilling of neonatal pigs increases their susceptibility to coliform enteritis. It has been experimentally confirmed that the normal peristaltic movement of the gut is slowed at temperatures below 25° C.

Clostridium perfringens *Type C*

Clostridium perfringens type C produces a severe hemorrhagic necrotizing enteritis in neonatal pigs. The organisms attach to the surface of the small intestinal epithelium and produce powerful locally active necrotizing toxins. This results in coagulative necrosis of the adjacent epithelium, the lamina propria, and often the submucosa. A distinct line of necrosis can be seen microscopically, which reflects the concentration of the diffusing toxin into the lamina propria. An intense line of inflammatory cells infiltrates the margin of the necrotic mucosa. Gas produced by the bacteria distends the lymphatics in the gut wall. Because the disease is difficult to reproduce experimentally, very little is known about the exact pathogenesis. The production of the necrotizing β-toxin is a major pathogenic factor.

If piglets survive the acute stages of *C. perfringens* type C enteritis, the necrotic intestines are quickly colonized with other bacteria, and the numbers of *C. perfringens* type C drop. These animals are often unthrifty and may die several days after the initial infection. The necrosis and loss of the intestinal mucosa, with little chance of complete healing, leaves pigs unthrifty for several weeks after the initial infection.

Viral Enteritis (TGE Virus and Rotavirus)

The intestinal lesions produced by the TGE virus and porcine rotavirus occur as a result of the replication of the virus in enterocytes with subsequent destruction of the epithelial cells. The extent of the damage and the severity of the disease may result in part from a number of factors including the virulence of the virus, the viral exposure, and the immunity of the host. Environmental factors such as chilling may also increase the severity of the clinical disease. Once damaged epithelium has been sloughed, the lamina propria contracts, thus reducing the surface area of the intestines available for absorption of nutrients. This so-called villous atrophy causes a malabsorption syndrome that manifests clinically as diarrhea if the amount of fluid reaching the large intestines exceeds the ability of that organ to absorb it. The lactose (milk sugar) present in the intestines is converted to lactic acid, which exerts a negative osmotic effect on attempts to absorb the excess fluid.

Diarrhea may also be observed in piglets infected with either TGE or rotavirus before there is appreciable epithelial loss and villus damage. This suggests that virus replicating in epithelium may reduce the cells' ability to function before structural damage can be seen.

Coccidia (Isospora suis)

Piglets infected with the coccidium *Isospora suis* develop lesions that may resemble both viral and bacterial enteritides. The coccidia replicate in the enterocytes and rupture the cells during the organism's life cycle. In the early stages of coccidiosis, the lesions may resemble a viral enteritis with marked villous blunting. After the coccidial rupture of the epithelium, the denuded basement membrane of the intestines is rapidly colonized with bacteria, and a fibrinonecrotic membrane composed of necrotic debris, bacteria, and inflammatory exudates may form. This lesion closely resembles that produced by subacute infections with *C. perfringens* type C.

CLINICAL SIGNS

Age of Occurrence

The age of the neonatal pig with diarrhea may offer some clues as to the possible cause or causes of the enteritis.

In the immediate perinatal period, *E. coli*, *C. perfringens* type C, and TGE virus may and often do produce disease. Rotavirus rarely produces enteritis in the immediate neonatal period because of the endemic nature of the disease and the presence of colostral antibodies. The severe hemorrhagic lesions of *C. perfringens* type C are rarely seen in pigs over 2 to 3 days old. Pigs from 3 to 20 days of age may, however, have the more chronic fibrinonecrotic lesions associated with subacute to chronic *C. perfringens* type C enteritis.

Both rotavirus and TGE virus may produce disease in the immediate postnatal period; the devastating losses due to TGE virus are usually limited to pigs under 2 to 3 weeks of age. The endemic nature of rotaviruses usually means that neonatal piglets will receive colostrum containing antibody to rotavirus. Thus severe rotavirus infections are not common unless colostrum has been lacking or inadequate in anti-rotavirus antibodies. Experimental rotavirus infections in colostrum-deprived neonatal pigs produce lesions closely resembling TGE. Both TGE virus and rotaviruses may produce lesions and clinical disease in pigs as the colostral immunity begins to fade at 2 to 4 weeks. The cessation of lactation antibodies in the diet (weaning) also allows viral agents to produce clinical disease in the immediate postweaning period. Although viral infections of the intestines are often regarded as predisposing to bacterial colonization of the intestines, the mechanism by which this occurs has not been clearly identified.

Because of the time required for the life cycle of *I. suis*, clinical signs of coccidiosis are not commonly recognized in pigs younger than 5 days of age, with the most severe clinical signs generally occurring at 10 days to 2 weeks of life. Clinical coccidiosis in pigs older than 2 weeks is rarely reported.

Lesions and Diagnostic Implications

So-called villous atrophy is produced by the loss of the small intestinal epithelium with a resultant contraction of the underlying lamina propria. This can be recognized grossly by the thin-walled appearance of the intestine and by the sub-gross observation of the shortening of the intestinal villi. The gut wall may appear translucent, and intestinal contents can be seen through the thin-walled intestine.

Three diarrhea-producing agents in piglets are capable of producing villous atrophy. TGE produces the most consistent and extensive villous damage, but both coccidiosis and rotavirus infections are also capable of producing both gross and microscopic evidence of villous damage. It is not uncommon to have all 3 agents present and active in the same herd.

Thin-walled intestines can also result from post-mortem autolysis and by overdistention of the intestines with gas or fluid. It is, therefore, important to use only freshly euthanatized pigs for the determination of villous atrophy. Piglets that have been nursing agalactic sows will swallow excessive amounts of air, and this will also distend the upper small intestines, giving them a thin-walled appearance.

Sub-gross observation of the villus length can be accomplished by several techniques. Perhaps the simplest is to invert several sections of small intestines in a test tube of water. The hypotonic water will cause the villi to swell slightly and become more visible. The convex curvature of the test tube will produce a slight magnification and will allow the visualization of the villi without the aid of magnifying equipment.

Because mature villous epithelium is needed to absorb fat from the small intestine, the presence or absence of chyle in the lacteals and mesenteric lymphatics may be used as an indirect method for determining the presence of villous damage. In piglets ingesting protective antibodies to TGE virus and rotavirus, villous atrophy may be regional, primarily located in the lower small intestines. Likewise, *I. suis* replicates primarily in the lower half of the small intestines, and thus villous damage in that infection is most severe in this location. This can be recognized at necropsy by the cessation of chyle absorption from the proximal to distal small intestines. In the normal piglet with limited fat in the diet, fat may not be seen in the lymphatics of the upper or lower intestines, or it may be present only in the upper regions. Therefore, the lack of chyle in the lacteals is not, by itself, evidence of villous loss. Sub-gross examination of the intestines for villous atrophy should be done primarily in gut regions with evidence of reduced chyle in the lacteals and lymphatics.

Normal length villi are present in most acute to subacute *E. coli* infections and may be seen regionally in the small intestine in rotavirus, coccidia, and endemic TGE infections.

The presence of fibrinonecrotic membranes in the small intestines of neonatal pigs indicates the presence of either coccidiosis or *C. perfringens* type C in the subacute to chronic stages.

Acute *C. perfringens* type C enteritis may be recognized by the hemorrhagic necrosis of the small intestinal mucosa and the frequent presence of gas bubbles in the lymphatics of the gut wall. Lesions of subacute *C. perfringens* type C are seen as thickened intestines with diffuse fibrinonecrotic membranes on the mucosal surface. This may be confused with the lesions of subacute to chronic coccidiosis. *C. perfringens* type C enteritis lesions have a tendency to localize in the upper ½ to ¾ of the small intestines, and the necrotic membrane is usually a grayish color. This is contrasted by a golden-yellow to yellowish-gray fibrinonecrotic membrane in the lower half of the small intestines with coccidiosis.

DIAGNOSIS

Pig-Side Tests

Several pig-side tests may be used to establish an etiologic diagnosis of neonatal enteritis.

Determining the pH of the colon contents in baby pigs with diarrhea by use of strips of pH paper may be of diagnostic value in the very early stages of the diarrhea. Acidic colonic contents (pH 5 to 6) occur in the early stages of TGE. As TGE progresses, the pH of the colon returns to a more normal neutral pH. The colonic pH in the acute stages of *E. coli* enteritis tends to be neutral to slightly alkaline (pH 7 to 8). If the colon contents have become semisolid or solid, the colonic pH is of little diagnostic value.

Sub-gross examination of the intestines for villous atrophy has been mentioned earlier and will offer clues to the presence of agents associated with villous blunting (TGE virus, rotavirus, coccidia).

When coccidiosis is suspected, impression smears of the intestinal mucosa should be examined for the immature forms of coccidia. To make the impression smears, open the intestines and gently blot the mucosal surface with a paper towel. Then lightly touch a clean glass slide to the mucosal surfaces. Touch the same area of mucosa several times while moving down the glass slide to obtain adequate numbers of epithelial cells, bacterial organisms, and coccidia in the smear. Make smears from at least 4 to 6 different areas of the intestine because the lesions and organisms of coccidiosis and colibacillosis may be regional. If fibrinonecrotic mucosal lesions exist, make smears from the necrotic areas as well as from the transitional regions at the proximal and distal ends of the necrotic areas. Immature coccidial forms are crescent-shaped, staining light blue with a distinct reddish nucleus when stained with blood smear stains such as Wright's or Wright's Giemsa.

Intestinal mucosal impression smears made as described in the preceding can also be stained with Gram's stain for bacteria to evaluate the numbers of gram-positive and gram-negative organisms. In enteric colibacillosis with organisms attaching to the villous surfaces, numerous gram-negative rod-shaped bacteria (usually over 100 per $1000\times$ field) can be seen in these smears. In the acute hemorrhagic form of *C. perfringens* type C enteritis, high numbers of gram-positive rods can be found. In the subacute stages of *C. perfringens* type C enteritis, impression smears may be misleading because numerous other organisms replace the clostridia in the necrotic surface exudates.

Laboratory Diagnosis

Probably the most critical procedure in establishing a specific diagnosis in neonatal diarrheas of pigs is the selection of the animal or animals to be necropsied and examined. If only animals that have died from the diarrhea are available for examination, the chances of obtaining a specific and correct diagnosis are very poor. The most valuable specimen to examine is the live, acutely affected, untreated piglet. Several end-stage chronically affected animals might also be examined; however, examining only end-stage animals is a serious mistake. A reference diagnostic laboratory is often necessary for confirming the presence of certain lesions and organisms and should be frequently utilized in attempting to define the infectious etiologic agents affecting specific problem herds.

Multiple live pigs delivered to a laboratory are probably the best samples to submit, but it is not always possible or practical to send entire pigs to a laboratory. Dead pigs submitted to the laboratory are probably the worst possible sample. There are few diagnostic clues left 20 to 30 minutes after the death of a piglet because of the relatively rapid post-mortem decomposition of the gastrointestinal tract. Likewise, rapid invasion and overgrowth by post-mortem contaminants can greatly alter the results of bacterial examinations.

If live pigs cannot be submitted, then specimens collected by the veterinarian from recently euthanatized, acutely affected, untreated pigs with diarrhea can be used.

Specimens from these pigs should include:

1. Multiple chilled 3- to 6-inch segments of small intestines for bacteriologic culturing. The segments should be packaged separately in multiple sterile bags. At least 1 segment of high jejunum (or duodenum), 1 segment of mid–small intestine, and 1 segment of terminal ileum should be submitted from each pig. In most cases of neonatal enteritis in neonatal pigs, bacteriologic culturing of other organs will not add to the diagnostic information generated.

2. A minimum of 2 1-inch segments of fresh, chilled (4° C, not frozen) jejunum and ileum for TGE fluorescent antibody (FA) examination. Examinations of autolyzed intestines for TGE virus by FA techniques are of little value.

3. Chilled, frozen, or fixed (with a little 10 per cent formalin) feces or gut contents taken from the colon or lower ileum for ELISA and electron microscopic examinations for rotavirus. The most commonly used ELISA test for rotavirus will detect only group A rotaviruses. From 60 to 95 per cent of the rotavirus infections in midwestern swineherds are due to group A rotaviruses.

4. Multiple ½-inch segments of small intestine and colon in 10 per cent neutral buffered formalin for histopathologic examinations. The short length is very important for obtaining adequate fixation. Gently hold the gut segments open with a pair of scissors as the sections are immersed in the formalin so that immediate contact with the fixative is ensured. In most neonatal enteritides, the upper half of the intestinal villous epithelium is affected. Unfortunately, this is the portion of the small intestines that first sloughs during autolysis. Virtually nothing can be gained from histologic examination of autolyzed small intestines.

5. Impression smears taken from multiple locations in the lower jejunum and ileum. Air dry these smears before mailing. The smears can be stained and examined for such organisms as coccidia or bacteria.

PREVENTION AND TREATMENT

In diarrheal diseases of any species, maintaining body fluid is critical to minimizing death losses. In swine, it is often difficult to justify the administration of fluids to piglets with diarrhea because of the cost of the labor to accomplish this task. Dehydrated pigs will frequently consume fluid from pans placed in the pens even while nursing the sow. Pan-fed solutions can be useful in providing needed fluid and electrolytes to diarrheal pigs but may also act as a source of infectious agents if they are not changed frequently. Force feeding electrolyte solutions to calves has proved valuable at a rate of 3 to 4 per cent of body weight every 6 to 8 hours. Comparable treatment is of value if the economics justify the approach. Flexible plastic tubes mounted on the end of large syringes have been used to facilitate quick and relatively easy administration of electrolytes. Occasional aspiration pneumonia or esophageal and pharyngeal tears can result if the handlers are not careful.

Intravenous electrolytes are not usually economically justified and are difficult to administer to young pigs. Intraperitoneal injections have been attempted; however, peritonitis from organisms carried in from the skin can cause serious problems.

Early weaning in the face of diarrheal outbreaks in neonatal pigs can produce inconsistent results and is generally not recommended. Lactogenic immunity in the form of IgA is still present in the sow's milk for many days after parturition, and this may be beneficial in controlling infectious agents in the gut.

Stopping the spread of the agent becomes an important consideration in controlling neonatal diarrhea in a farrowing house. Antibiotic therapy given to affected litters as well as to adjacent litters can slow the spread of *E. coli*.

Frequent cleaning of pens after outbreaks of diarrhea reduces the number of infectious organisms; however, this must be done in such a way as to ensure a dry, warm environment for the pigs. Both warmth and dryness will kill many infectious agents. Viruses such as TGE, for example, do not survive long in dry, warm environments. Thorough cleaning and disinfection of pens between litters is a must for all facilities.

Competitive colonization of the intestines with high numbers of nonpathogenic organisms such as *Lactobacillus* sp., enterococci, and nonpathogenic *E. coli* has met with variable clinical success in preventing *E. coli* enteritis. The feeding of small amounts of soil collected from swine-free fields has been used by confinement farrowing facilities to populate neonatal guts or to repopulate intestines after intensive antibiotic therapy.

Orally administered or injectable antibiotics are useful in preventing and treating bacterial enteritis such as that produced by *E. coli* and *C. perfringens* type C. Numerous antibiotic products are available for use in the treatment of neonatal enteritis caused by *E. coli* in pigs. The choice of antibiotics is usually dictated by the cost and the antibiotic sensitivity patterns of the bacterial isolates. The *Clostridium* spp. are ordinarily sensitive in vitro to penicillin and penicillin derivatives. Sustained-release antibiotics may provide preventive levels of antibiotic for several days and help control diarrhea in problem herds.

The common coccidiostats, such as amprolium and decoquinate, have not been approved for use in swine. The use of various sulfonamide products has had some success in preventing and treating coccidiosis in swine. Physical removal of manure and oocysts from the pens and maintaining clean, dry pens constitute one of the most effective means for control of coccidiosis.

Antitoxins containing the anti–β-toxin of *C. perfringens* are available commercially and are beneficial in controlling and preventing *C. perfringens* type C enteritis. These antisera are usually given subcutaneously to pigs shortly after birth at dosages recommended by the manufacturer. Dosages may be increased if sufficient protection is not obtained. Additional administration of antitoxin orally has been suggested as an adjunct to parenteral administration. The goal of oral administration is to block the attachment of the clostridial organism to the gut mucosa. The effectiveness of this procedure has not been substantiated experimentally.

Vaccines administered to the dams at various times during gestation are marketed for TGE virus, rotavirus, *E. coli,* and *C. perfringens* type C. *C. perfringens* vaccines are marketed as both bacterins and as toxoids. Blocking the attachment of TGE virus or *E. coli* organisms to the gut epithelial cells requires the presence of immunoglobulins in the lumen of the intestinal tract. This has been accomplished by vaccinating sows so that colostrum and lactational milk contain specific anti–*E. coli* or anti-TGE virus immunoglobulins. Especially effective have been the vaccines containing the attachment pili of *E. coli*. Before the advent of *E. coli* pili vaccines, many veterinarians used milk-grown cultures of *E. coli,* fed to sows, for providing this colostral immunity. This procedure is still used but with much less frequency.

With any prevention program that relies on adequate colostral transfer of immunity, farrowing management is extremely important. Prolonged parturition, for example, may delay the ingestion of colostrum by the last-born pigs so that these animals do not receive adequate protection even in a well vaccinated herd. The prevention or rapid treatment of mastitis and agalactia is of obvious importance in effective colostral transfer.

In spite of the presence of adequate immunoglobulins in the gut lumen, non-IgA classes (IgM and IgG) of immunoglobulins may be digested, particularly in pigs over 1 week of age. This then frees the infectious agent (i.e., TGE virus) to attach to and infect the cells of the lower portion of the small intestines. This may partially explain the localization of the lesions of endemic TGE to the lower half of the small intestines.

Vaccination against the hemolytic *E. coli* infections in 10-day-old to 2-week-old pigs may produce variable results. These organisms are potent toxin producers, much of which is probably endotoxin. Vaccine reactions, probably due to the presence of endotoxins, are frequent after the administration of autogenous bacterins prepared from these organisms.

The effective prevention, treatment, and control of infectious enteritis in neonatal swine can be accomplished if specific etiologic diagnoses are established and there is an understanding of the mechanisms by which these diseases are produced.

BIBLIOGRAPHY

Andrews JJ, Holter JA, Daniels GN, et al: Diagnostic necropsy of suckling swine. Vet Clin North Am [Food Anim Pract] 2:159–172, 1986.
Collins JE, Benfield DA, Duimstra BS: Comparative virulence of two porcine group-A rotavirus isolates in gnotobiotic pigs. Am J Vet Res 50:827–835, 1989.
Garwes DJ: Transmissible gastroenteritis (review). Vet Rec 122:462–463, 1988.
Moxley RA, Olson LR: Clinical evaluation of transmissible gastroenteritis virus vaccines and vaccination procedures for inducing lactogenic immunity in sows. Am J Vet Res 50:111–118, 1989.
Niilo L: Toxigenic characteristics of *Clostridium perfringens* type C in enterotoxemia of domestic animals. Can J Vet Res 51:224–228, 1987.
Okerman L: Enteric infections caused by non-enterotoxigenic *Escherichia coli* in animals: occurrence and pathogenicity mechanisms. A review. Vet Microbiol 14:33–46, 1987.
Prestwood AK: Coccidiosis in swine (review). Vet Hum Toxicol 29(Suppl 1):65–67, 1987.
Stuart BP, Lindsay DS: Coccidiosis in swine. Vet Clin North Am [Food Anim Pract] 2:455–468, 1986.

Neonatal Polyarthritis in Swine

JAMES D. McKEAN, DVM, MS, JD

Polyarthritis is the concurrent inflammation of multiple articular joints in an animal. The joints most commonly affected and most easily observed in swine are the knees, elbows, and hock joints. The stifle, shoulder, hip, and vertebral column are less frequently infected. A wide variety of organisms including *Streptococcus* sp., *Staphylococcus* sp., and *Escherichia coli* in suckling pigs and *Erysipelothrix insidiosa*, *Mycoplasma hyorhinis*, *Mycoplasma hyosynoviae*, *Haemophilus parasuis*, and, occasionally, *E. coli* in older pigs have been identified as primary causes of polyarthritic lesions. In suckling pigs, *Streptococcus* sp. of the groups C and L are the most commonly isolated bacteria. A systemic distribution of these organisms may be coexistent or act as a precursor for meningitis, polyserositis, or endocarditis lesions.

CLINICAL SIGNS

Swelling of periarticular tissues with accompanying pain and lameness is generally the first sign noted. The knee and hock joints are the most commonly observed sites. Resultant locomotor dysfunction causes increased preweaning mortality. In some cases, preweaning mortality may be double that expected in a noninfected group. Clinical signs may appear from 1 to 8 weeks of age but most commonly occur from 8 to 21 days of age. Individual pigs or entire litters may be affected. Litters from females in their first parities are most likely to be affected. Purulent extra-articular exudates are observed with streptococcal, staphylococcal, and actinomycial infections; *E. coli* produces a fibrinous to fibrinopurulent exudate. Chronic joint lesions, common sequelae in perinatal infections, demonstrate organization and induration of the exudate; often, permanently reduced joint function results.

EPIDEMIOLOGY AND PATHOGENESIS

Incidence of polyarthritis is sporadic under normal conditions. Variability is influenced by the presence of pathogenic organisms, herd and individual female immunity levels, environmental conditions, and trauma. Although seasonal incidence has not been reported, adverse environmental or sanitary conditions may predispose to clinical disease. Gilt litters have a slightly higher infection frequency than do litters from older sows. Large numbers of pigs within a litter are exposed to pathogens, but clinical disease is apparent in those lacking adequate antibody protection or under stressful conditions, or both. Skin abrasions of the knees and of the face caused by struggling for nursing position, improper needle teeth clipping or tail docking, and rough floors may open pathways for infection.

Hemolytic streptococcal invasions are the most commonly observed infections in suckling pigs. *Streptococcus equisimilis* is most frequently observed, but other group C and groups D and L species have been reported. Exposure occurs during the early perinatal period, primarily from dam to litter. Aerosol transmission and vaginal contamination during birth are the primary sources of infection, with the tonsil and intestinal tract, umbilicus, and abraded skin areas the primary entry sites. Infectious organisms spread via blood from these primary sites and are filtered by periarticular capillaries. Rarely, these infections result in sudden death with no premonitory signs. Lesions observed are those associated with acute septicemia. Initially, synovial fluid in affected joints increases in volume and develops a creamy or white appearance. Subacute and chronic infections result in a more organized fibrinopurulent synovitis, pericarditis, or meningitis, or a combination of these signs. Generally, in an outbreak of streptococcal meningitis, meninges become opaque and hyperemic, but on a few occasions, gross lesions are not notable. Pericarditis characterized by a fibrinopurulent exudate on the pericardial surfaces can be observed.

Streptococcus suis II infections may cause meningitis and polyarthritis. Pigs between 4 and 8 weeks of age that have recently undergone the stress of mixing and moving are most susceptible, although suckling pigs are also commonly affected. Morbidity in a group is low to moderate, but mortality among meningitis-affected pigs is high. Aerosol transmission from carrier swine, either from dam to litter or within a group, is the most common contamination method. Organisms localize on the tonsil and await appropriate entry conditions. Incubation periods are variable but may be as short as 24 hours to as long as several months. Sudden death and signs of general septicemia are observed when circulating *S. suis II* organisms reach the meninges. Affected pigs will have acute symptoms associated with localization of the organisms on the meninges. Death occurs within 24 to 36 hours after signs develop. Early symptoms include dull attitude, fever, reluctance to move, and separation from the group. Neurologic signs of incoordination, paralysis, and tetanic spasms follow rapidly and terminate in death. In younger pigs, these organisms may localize in the joints and develop polyarthritis rather than meningitis.

Coliform invasions from the intestinal tract may cause meningitis, polyarthritis, and polyserositis. Suckling pigs are most commonly affected. Clinical signs consist of depression, fever, rough hair coat, labored breathing, and death within several days of onset. Diarrhea in affected pigs is not a consistent sign. Strains of *E. coli* most prominently isolated are O strains and are not enteropathogenic. Post-mortem examination reveals large volumes of fibrinous pericardial, pleural, and peritoneal exudates. Fibrinonecrotic pneumonia may be seen with this systemic disease. Meningitis and polyarthritis are less often observed. Morbidity is generally low, although sporadic outbreaks characterized by high morbidity and mortality have been reported.

Staphylococcus spp. produce polyarthritis symptoms and lesions similar in appearance to those caused by *Streptococcus* spp., but the relative incidence is quite low.

Septicemias caused by any of the aforementioned bacteria may result from invasion of the umbilical cord, of castration sites, of other skin or mucous membrane wounds, or of the small intestine.

DIAGNOSIS

Differential diagnosis may be obtained from presence of clinical signs and by isolation of causative organisms from affected joints, meninges, and pleural, peritoneal, or pericardial cavities. Blood cultures are generally unrewarding because the number of organisms decrease rapidly after the initial septicemia. Gram-stained smears of exudates may be helpful in determining the causative organism. Small abscesses at the umbilicus or at the castration or tail docking site, skin abrasions on knees or hocks, or the presence of gingivitis may be helpful in determining the bacteria's portal of entry. However, in many affected pigs, an external portal of entry is not easily identified, and the tonsil or intestinal tract is presumed to be the entry site.

TREATMENT AND PREVENTION

Because of the sporadic nature of neonatal polyarthritis, prevention can be difficult and frustrating. Introduction of new breeding females may result in an increased incidence in disease within their litters. As herd immunity develops, incidence will fall to previous levels. Therefore, gilt or new herd additions may be treated more aggressively. Each herd should be evaluated for the costs of disease at basal levels and the costs of proposed preventive programs. Sensitivity patterns of isolates will indicate which medications may be effective for parenteral treatment and for prevention. Prophylactic treatment of each pig at initial processing with 22,000 IU/kg penicillin, 11 mg/kg lincomycin, 8.8 mg/kg tylosin, or 11 mg/kg tiamulin has proved effective. Treatment of existing infections may be successful when these same medications are administered parenterally for 2 or 3 days at an early stage of infection. For severe streptococcal infections, use of large doses of tetracyclines (200 to 400 g/ton) or penicillin (100 to 250 g/ton) in feed for 2 to 4 weeks before farrowing may be justified to reduce the carrier state within the sow population. Commercial and autogenous vaccines against *Streptococcus suis II* infections have been more effective control measures than have been experienced with other streptococcal infections. Many practitioners believe that autogenous vaccines are more effective, but the data are generally anecdotal. Morbidity and mortality can be expected to be significantly reduced, but mortality after appearance of clinical signs is unaffected. Autogenous vaccines from *E. coli* isolates have been usefully administered to prefarrow females and in suckling pigs to reduce clinical disease. Other bacterial infections rarely are of sufficient economic magnitude to warrant institution of a prophylactic vaccination program.

Good nursing care and strict adherence to sanitary practices are important measures for reducing economic impact. Management practices that may reduce problems are sanitizing of the farrowing area and nursing facilities between groups; dipping of the umbilical cord into strong tincture solutions of iodine (7 per cent) immediately after birth; farrowing in dry, comfortable conditions; minimization of sharp or rough surfaces on farrowing pen floors; and placing of mats or rug material in the suckling area for 1 to 3 days after farrowing. Farrowing house personnel should be cautioned about opening new routes of infection or of transferring infection by improper or unsanitary tail docking and castration or by careless clipping of needle teeth.

Prevention of Cold Stress in Calves

DAVID P. OLSON, DVM, PhD, MS

Beef calves are often born under range conditions in the northern and western regions of the United States during late winter and early spring. As a result, they may be exposed to adverse climatic conditions such as cold, fluctuating air temperature, and excessive wind and moisture. Because of common cow/calf herd management practices, beef calves often have no access to natural or manmade protection and are especially susceptible to weather-related stress. Field observations indicate that dairy calves, born during the winter and reared under unfavorable management conditions, may also suffer from environmental stress.

TEMPERATURE REGULATION IN ANIMALS

Calves and many other warm-blooded species are classified as homeothermic animals, which means they are able to maintain their core body temperature (CBT; approximately 100° F for calves) within narrow limits despite variation in environmental temperature. Core body temperature refers to tissue temperatures within the body core, such as the major visceral organs and cardiac blood. Homeothermic animals readily maintain a balance between production and loss of body heat when air temperatures are within the thermoneutral zone (range between 50° and 95° F, depending on animal species). Body heat is normally lost by conduction, convection, and radiation; from exhaled air and voided urine and feces; and by evaporation of water from the body surface. Exposure to ambient temperatures slightly below the thermoneutral zone results in behavioral (crowding and periods of inactivity) and physiologic responses (peripheral vasoconstriction) that minimize heat loss and conserve body heat. Young calves normally have the capacity to generate adequate amounts of body heat from perirenal, abdominal, and pericardial deposits of thermogenic brown fat and by shivering thermogenesis. Exposure to colder ambient temperatures triggers maximal heat conservation and an increase in body heat production in order to maintain homeothermy. However, the CBT of these animals will decrease and they will become hypothermic when maximal heat production fails to equal or exceed the amount of body heat loss due to severe cold stress.

COLD STRESS IN CALVES

Clinical and Physiologic Changes

Calves from 1 to 4 days of age are most susceptible to severe cold exposure, although animals as old as 7 days may also be affected in a similar manner provided the environmental stress is sufficiently severe. Clinical signs seen in cold-stressed calves are often directly related to the severity and duration of the environmental conditions. For example, cold-stressed calves are frequently exposed to excessive wind and moisture and to air temperatures that are near or below freezing. Under these severe weather conditions, young calves may develop rapid and progressive hypothermia despite intensive shivering thermogenesis and efforts to conserve body heat. Shivering thermogenesis is usually diminished or ceases when the CBT has decreased by 10° to 14° F. As body cooling proceeds, calves become depressed and less responsive to their immediate surroundings, and they are reluctant to walk or stand and nurse owing to progressive physical weakness. In addition, breathing becomes shallow and irregular and heart sounds are indistinct in these animals. Death in comatose, recumbent cold-stressed calves occurs from respiratory arrest if their CBT has decreased by more than 17° F. The time required to induce hypothermia and eventual death of cold-stressed calves under field conditions will vary between 6 and 24 hours depending on ambient temperature, wind velocity, and moisture content of the environment.

The CBT is a reliable indicator of the ability of homeothermic animals to regulate body temperature. During severe cold stress and development of hypothermia, various tissues cool at different rates, depending on their location. As expected, the CBT is least affected by cold exposure and decreases more slowly than do temperatures of other body regions. Rectal and oral temperatures decrease linearly with time and closely approximate (within 1° F) the changes in CBT. Temperatures within skeletal muscle of the pelvic and pectoral limbs decrease in a curvilinear fashion despite the fact that these tissues are directly involved in heat production by shivering thermogenesis. Temperatures of subcutaneous tissues decrease most rapidly and approximate environmental temperatures as a result of conductive, convective, radiative, and evaporative heat losses and peripheral vasoconstriction.

Severe cold stress evokes important changes in cardiovascular function. Initially, there is a significant increase in heart rate and slight increase in aortic blood pressure. After the CBT has decreased by about 5° F, there is a rapid and significant decrease in both heart rate and blood pressure. In addition, hypothermia produces major changes in electrocardiographic waveforms characterized by extraneous and erratic peaks.

Laboratory Findings

Numerous clinical pathologic changes have been noted in cold-stressed calves. Increases in hematocrit and hemoglobin concentration reflect a state of dehydration in these animals. Leukopenia, due primarily to neutropenia, has also been noted. Cold-induced changes in blood chemistry include consistent and significant increases in plasma concentrations of glucose, cortisol, and catecholamines. Large increases in concentrations of several other plasma constituents may also be seen in cold-stressed calves.

The passive immune status of severely cold-stressed calves may be adversely affected. Studies have shown a delay in onset and a significant decrease in the rate of absorption of colostral immunoglobulins for the first 15 hours of age of hypothermic calves. Thus, during this early period of life, the cold-induced hypogammaglobulinemia represents a serious compromise of the nonspecific immune status of these animals. It is unclear whether the cell-mediated host defense status of cold-stressed young calves is adversely affected.

Lesions consistently seen in calves that have died from the effects of severe cold stress include extensive subcutaneous edema and hemorrhages in the pelvic and pectoral limbs, beneath the sternum, and occasionally in the head region. Moderate to severe hemorrhages may also be seen in one or both hock joint cavities. Internal deposits of brown adipose tissue are also diminished in severely cold-stressed calves.

In addition to the clinical and physiologic changes in calves, exposure to adverse winter weather may also produce other conditions that are potentially harmful to calves. Many pathogenic microorganisms are transmitted by the aerosol route and by direct contact between animals. In general, cold temperatures are less harmful to certain viral and bacterial pathogens than are high temperatures. Cold stress–induced increases in concentrations of catecholamines and glucocorticoids may increase the viscosity of mucus and decrease the mucociliary clearance of pathogens from the lungs. Lung hypoxia, due to the reduced rate and depth of respiration during cold stress, also decreases mucociliary action and alveolar macrophage activity. Increased levels of cold stress–induced glucocorticoids also suppress host defense mechanisms in general by decreasing the normal activities of phagocytic and lymphocytic cells.

REDUCING STRESS OF YOUNG CALVES

Evidence from field observations and controlled laboratory experiments indicates that severe cold stress produces a variety of adverse changes that may threaten the survival of young calves. In addition, calf losses at birth and during the first few weeks of life are also caused by diseases, poor growth performance, and death. Following is a summary of clinical and herd health management practices, identified by field observations and the cooperation of cow/calf producers, that may help prevent these losses in beef calves.

Protective Shelters

The task of providing protective shelter for beef calves is often difficult because these animals usually commingle with their dams on range and are normally not kept under confinement. Despite these circumstances, a system has been developed to provide temporary, protective shelter for beef calves. The idea of protecting beef calves from environmental stress was borrowed from a calf management practice commonly used by many dairymen in which single calves are reared in shelters called "calf hutches." The shelters currently in use by many beef cow/calf producers are made of exterior plywood, have no flooring, and are 8′ (width) × 8′ (depth) × 4′ (height in the front; 3′6″ height in the rear). Each shelter is open on one side and designed to house a maximum of 10 calves at one time. The shelters are placed in rows on higher ground within the calving yard and bedded with clean, dry straw; avoid use of wood shavings for bedding material. A plank is placed across the open side to prevent access by adult animals. Shelters are positioned so that the open side faces away from the usual source of prevailing winds and storms. Further, shelters must be relocated and rebedded regularly to avoid concentration of pathogenic microorganisms. Beef calves should have access to protective shelters for the first 3 weeks of life. An alternative, V-shaped protective shelter that is simpler in design consists of 2 corral panels, 41″ × 6″ boards, 4 rubber cords, and a solid plastic tarp.

Excellent results have been obtained by producers from use of protective shelters for beef calves. Most calves spontaneously seek cover within the shelters during inclement weather and at night. During the day, calves routinely leave the shelters to suckle and exercise. Field data also suggest that morbidity and mortality are reduced in sheltered compared with nonsheltered animals.

Cow Management at Calving

Calving Facilities. Calving facilities often consist of a pole barn–type structure with a sand or gravel floor covered with straw bedding, full-sized entry and exit doors on each end, a center alley, and individual pens on both sides. These buildings are unheated except for a calving/equipment room and a warming area for cold-stressed calves. Calving facilities allow close supervision of the cows during calving and the calves during the first 12 to 24 hours of life. Pens are cleaned, sanitized, and rebedded before occupancy by succeeding cow/calf pairs.

Calving Ease. Calving ease refers to the ease or difficulty encountered by cows during parturition. A numerical score indicating calving ease should be recorded for each animal at parturition. Except for first calf heifers, most beef calves are born by unassisted delivery. Calves born after assisted or prolonged unassisted delivery may lack normal vigor and stamina and should be given individual attention if required.

Lactation and Mothering Score. Cows should be observed daily for evidence of a healthy udder and sufficient milk to properly nourish their calves. In addition, they should be evaluated daily for mothering ability and willingness to groom and care for their calves. A numerical scoring system can be used to evaluate lactation and mothering activities. Special attention should be given to calves whose dams have an inadequate amount of milk or exhibit passive behavior or rejection of the calf.

Quality of Colostrum. Regardless of age or breed, the total immunoglobulin concentration of colostrum from beef cows is generally superior and ranges between 96.5 and 99 mg/ml. This is almost twice the concentration of total immunoglobulin normally found in colostrum from dairy cows. A useful method for estimating the quality of colostrum is with a colostrometer. A colostrometer measures the specific gravity and thus the approximate total immunoglobulin concentration of a colostrum sample. Information gained from routine sampling and testing of colostrum quality in beef cows is useful in assessing the passive immune status of their calves.

Early Calf Management

Birth Date, Breed, Sex, and Identification. A complete cow/calf herd record system should include information about the birth date, breed, sex, and ear tag numbers identifying all calves. These data are important as a basis for short- and long-term health, breeding, and feeding management decisions for the herd.

Weighing Calves. Body weights should be obtained for all calves at birth, at 1 month of age, and at weaning. Hanging or portable platform scales are commercially available and can be conveniently located close to where the calves are confined. Weight data for calves provide important information on the breeding and feeding management of the herd. In addition, weight data help identify calves that are unthrifty because of poor nutrition or disease.

Body Temperature. Rectal temperatures should be obtained and recorded on all calves at birth and on a representative number of calves for the first 3 days of life. Mercury or electronic digital thermometers are commercially available and are rapid and convenient to use. Normal rectal temperatures of beef calves range between 99.8° and 102° F and are not affected by breed, sex, or age of the respective dams. Elevation of rectal temperature often occurs before other clinical signs of disease become apparent and provides an opportunity for early detection and treatment.

Vigor and Suckling Activities. Calves should be observed one or more times a day for the first 3 weeks of life for evaluation of their vigor, behavior, responses to surroundings, and interest in maintaining a close physical relationship with their dams. Attention should also be given to the aggressiveness and frequency of suckling. A numerical scoring system can be developed to record the information for individual calves. Vigor and suckling scores are generally high for healthy beef calves, regardless of their age, sex, or age of the respective dams. In contrast, vigor and suckling scores of sick calves are usually low, indicating a direct effect of disease on these behavioral characteristics.

Age at First Suckling. Close attention must be given to the age when newborn beef calves first suckle. This information is important because they must consume adequate amounts of high-quality colostrum before gut closure at 24 to 36 hours of age. Approximately 50 per cent of normal beef calves suckle unassisted for the first time by 2 hours of age, whereas 90 per cent suckle unassisted for the first time by 5 hours of age. There are no differences in age at first suckling between beef bull and heifer calves. Calves from middle-aged dams (3 to 5 years old) tend to suckle at an earlier age than do calves from older-aged dams (6 to 13 years old). It is recommended that first suckling by newborn beef calves occur within the first hour after birth for ensuring maximal passive immune protection. This may require that a person be available to assist calves unable to suckle by this early age.

Pocket Field Book

A pocket field book has been developed for beef cow/calf producers as part of the National Integrated Resource Management (IRM) Program. This book is designed so producers can easily record important health and management information about their herds during the calving and postcalving periods as well as other events during the yearlong production cycle. Data summarized from these production record books can be used by the producer, veterinarian, feed and equipment suppliers, and lending agencies to identify areas in which management practices can be changed for improvement in production efficiency of the herd.

BIBLIOGRAPHY

Olson DP: Field studies of protective shelters for beef calves. Bovine Pract 21:19–22, 1986.

Olson DP, Duren EP, Bramwell KA, et al: Clinical observations and laboratory analysis of factors that affect the survival and performance of beef cattle. Bovine Pract 24:4–11, 1989.

Hypoglycemia and Hypothermia in Neonatal Pigs

ROSS P. COWART, DVM, MS, Diplomate, ABVP

The neonatal piglet is highly dependent on a steady flow of nutrition in the form of colostrum or milk from the dam and on a warm, draft-free environment. Interruption of a regular suckling routine, for whatever reason, is often associated with severe and potentially life-threatening metabolic derangements. Chilling is also directly or indirectly responsible for a large percentage of preweaning deaths in pigs. The majority of preweaning deaths, including those resulting from crushing by the dam, can be related to chilling, inadequate nutritional intake, or both.

During the first few days of life, the normal piglet will suckle from the dam every 1 to 2 hours and will consume approximately 10 per cent of its body weight in a 24-hour period. Abnormalities of the dam or piglet may interrupt the normal suckling routine. Lactation failure in the dam is commonly responsible for inadequate nutritional intake by the neonate. Piglets with physical defects such as splay-leg or congenital tremors may be unable to get to the udder to suckle. Small and weak piglets often have difficulty competing with their littermates for space at the udder. Unfortunately, the weakness of these piglets is perpetuated by the lack of adequate nutrition, and they often succumb to hypoglycemia, hypothermia, or crushing by the dam.

Because of its small size (i.e., the ratio of body surface area to body mass is relatively high), relatively sparse hair coat, and meager subcutaneous fat deposits, the neonatal piglet is highly susceptible to chilling. The piglet also lacks brown fat, which is associated with nonshivering thermogenesis in some other species. Drafts, moisture, and cool surfaces such as concrete or wire mesh floors can intensify heat losses to the environment. The lower critical temperature is the effective environmental temperature below which heat losses are so great that the piglet must increase its metabolic rate to maintain normal body temperature. The neonatal piglet's lower critical temperature is estimated at 34° C; therefore, at temperatures below 34° C, the piglet is stressed from chilling.

PATHOGENESIS

Hypoglycemia

Carbohydrate, lipid, and protein may all be metabolized for energy. Some organs, such as muscle, may utilize lipid (in the form of fatty acids) directly for energy. However, other organs such as the brain are absolutely dependent on glucose as an energy source. Thus the maintenance of normal levels of glucose in the blood is a high metabolic priority. Pigs greater than 10 days of age are readily able to maintain blood glucose within normal limits, even during a prolonged (up to 21-day) period of fasting. However, the neonatal pig faces special metabolic problems during fasting. Two mechanisms for maintaining blood glucose that are of special importance to the neonate are presented.

Utilization of Stored Carbohydrate. The neonatal pig is born with stores of carbohydrate in the form of liver and muscle glycogen. However, these glycogen stores are rapidly utilized regardless of nutritional intake. Within 12 hours of birth, the suckling pig has already utilized 75 per cent of its liver glycogen and 41 per cent of its muscle glycogen. Liver glycogen is effectively depleted after 18 to 24 hours of fasting.

Synthesis of Glucose from Noncarbohydrate Precursors. The metabolic process of synthesizing glucose from noncarbohydrate precursors (primarily lipid or protein) is known as gluconeogenesis. The primary site for gluconeogenesis is the liver. Gluconeogenesis appears to be relatively effective in suckling piglets but not in fasting piglets. The enzymes and hormones necessary to support hepatic gluconeogenesis appear to be functional in both the suckling and fasting piglet. The most likely cause for defective gluconeogenesis in the fasting neonatal piglet is the lack of metabolizable precursors. The normal response of an older pig to fasting is to increase the mobilization of fat and to increase the circulating levels of free fatty acids. The fasting neonate is unable to mobilize fat and sustain circulating levels of free fatty acids primarily because of limited body reserves. The piglet is born with only 1 to 2 per cent body fat, and some of this may not be readily available for mobilization. Adequate consumption of colostrum and milk provides the neonatal piglet with the necessary metabolic precursors of gluconeogenesis. Although sow's milk does contain carbohydrate (in the form of lactose), the amount of carbohydrate present is not sufficient to sustain the pig's glucose and energy requirements. Sow's milk is relatively high in fat. Digestion and absorption of milk fat provides free fatty acids to feed hepatic gluconeogenesis.

Hypothermia

As the effective environmental temperature drops below the lower critical temperature, the piglet begins to increase its metabolic rate to produce heat for maintenance of body temperature. This is usually manifested by shivering and by heat-conserving behavior such as huddling with littermates. If the piglet is able, it will increase its energy intake by consuming more milk to meet the increased energy demands. However, the smaller or weaker piglets in a litter will often not be able to increase their intake because of competition from the rest of the litter. As cold stress increases, a point is reached at which the piglet will not be able to produce enough heat, and body temperature will decline. The piglet may also become hypoglycemic owing to the negative energy balance.

CLINICAL SIGNS

Hypoglycemia and hypothermia often occur together and therefore share many of the same clinical signs. However, not all hypothermic pigs (especially those greater than a week of age) are hypoglycemic; therefore laboratory data are needed to confirm a diagnosis. Mildly hypothermic pigs will often huddle together in a corner of a pen and shiver. More severely hypothermic and hypoglycemic pigs will become lethargic and anorectic. These pigs will often have a weak, crying squeal when disturbed. The skin will appear pale and feel cold to the touch as the circulatory system fails. Profound hypoglycemia may be associated with central nervous system disturbances such as ataxia and convulsions. Coma and death often occur 24 to 36 hours after the onset of clinical signs.

DIAGNOSIS

A tentative diagnosis can be based on the typical clinical signs. Hypoglycemia can be confirmed via clinical pathology. Blood glucose levels of 50 mg/dl or lower are considered diagnostic of hypoglycemia. Coma usually occurs when blood glucose levels drop below 40 mg/dl. Blood glucose levels of less than 10 mg/dl have been reported. Hypothermia is confirmed by a rectal temperature of less than 37° C. Post-mortem findings are not specific, although the lack of milk curd in the stomach can support a diagnosis of hypoglycemia.

The clinician should rule out other causes of depression and death in baby piglets. Infectious enteritis (e.g., colibacillosis, transmissible gastroenteritis, rotaviral enteritis, clostridial enteritis, and coccidiosis) is usually characterized by diarrhea and dehydration. However, hypoglycemia may be a sequel to infection with transmissible gastroenteritis. Neonatal septicemias caused by agents such as *Escherichia coli* or *Streptococcus* may closely mimic hypoglycemia or hypothermia in clinical presentation. The ataxia and convulsions occasionally seen with hypoglycemia cannot be distinguished clinically from those seen with pseudorabies or bacterial meningitis.

TREATMENT

Treatment of neonatal pigs in an acute hypoglycemic-hypothermic crisis can be dramatic and lifesaving. Unfortunately, in many commercial swine units, these pigs are written off as "starve-outs," and little if any effort is made to save them. Treatment need not be excessively expensive or impractical to accomplish on the farm. The principles of therapy are simple: the pig must be provided a source of metabolizable energy and a warm environment.

Piglets that are severely depressed or comatose from hypoglycemia should receive parenteral glucose injections. Recommended dosages vary from 1 to 2 g of glucose per kilogram of body weight. The most convenient route of administration for the neonatal pig is intraperitoneal injection. A 1 g/kg dose can be achieved with 20 ml/kg of a 5 per cent glucose solution, 10 ml/kg of a 10 per cent solution, or 5 ml/kg of a 20 per cent solution. Although the piglet appears to tolerate the injection of a 20 per cent glucose solution into the peritoneal cavity, this may cause transient hemoconcentration. This is likely due to the hyperosmolarity of the 20 per cent glucose solution; water is drawn from the circulation into the peritoneal cavity. Glucose solutions with concentrations greater than 20 per cent should not be injected into the peritoneal cavity. The objective of parenteral glucose therapy is simply to restore the blood glucose to a normal level and thereby restore normal central nervous system function. With this accomplished, energy intake should be sustained via oral nutritional supplementation.

After the administration of glucose, the pig should be gradually warmed to a normal body temperature of 39° C. Although a hospital incubator is nice, a cardboard box with straw bedding and a heat lamp will suffice. In either case, caution is advised to avoid getting the pig too hot and to avoid creating a fire hazard. The temperature in the box should be monitored periodically by laying a thermometer beside the pig. The pig should be removed from the box when its body temperature returns to normal.

Many pigs will show a remarkable improvement in attitude and appetite within 2 or 3 hours after glucose therapy and rewarming. Occasionally, a pig will be refractory to therapy. This is usually a pig in the advanced stages of hypoglycemic coma that might have responded had therapy begun earlier.

Once a pig has recovered from the acute hypoglycemic-hypothermic crisis, it must begin a regular routine of nutrient intake to avoid relapse. There is no better food for the neonatal piglet than sow's milk. If the piglet's dam is lactating adequately, then the piglet should be returned to its dam. If the sow is not lactating properly or if she is already nursing too many piglets, then pigs should be cross-fostered onto other lactating sows so that the opportunities for the piglets to suckle are equalized.

A number of sow's milk and colostrum replacers are available from commercial vendors. A homemade sow's milk replacer can be formulated by mixing together 1 quart of whole cow's milk with 1 ounce of white syrup or honey and 1 ounce of cream or corn oil. In the author's opinion, all milk replacers are best utilized as a supplement to rather than a replacement for actual sow's milk. These solutions can be placed in a shallow container (e.g., a muffin tin) in the creep area of the farrowing pen. Most piglets will learn to drink out of the container fairly rapidly.

A nutritional supplement containing a high concentration of fatty acids and vitamins in a readily available form may be administered orally to individual baby pigs.[1] The fatty acids should provide the necessary precursors to activate hepatic gluconeogenesis.

PREVENTION AND CONTROL

Adequate dietary intake and a warm, comfortable environment should effectively prevent hypoglycemia and hypothermia. The effective environmental temperature for the baby pig should be maintained at 34° to 36° C. Some of the treatments mentioned (e.g., cross-fostering pigs to equalize litter size, routine supplementation with fatty acid preparations,[1] providing supplemental milk replacer) may also be useful as preventive therapy. Preventive therapy would be especially useful for the smaller or weaker pigs in a litter.

BIBLIOGRAPHY

Blood DC, Radostits OM: Veterinary Medicine, 7th ed. London, Baillière Tindall, 1989, pp 1144–1146.
Curtis SE: Responses of the piglet to perinatal stressors. J Anim Sci 38:1031–1036, 1974.
Elmore RG, Martin CE: Mammary glands. In Leman AD, Straw B, Glock RD, et al. (eds): Diseases of Swine, 6th ed. Ames, IA, Iowa State University Press, 1986, pp 168–183.
Mersmann HJ: Metabolic patterns in the neonatal swine. J Anim Sci 38:1022–1030, 1974.
Pégorier JP, Duée PH, Nunes CS, et al: Glucose turnover and recycling in unrestrained and unanesthetized 48-h-old fasting or post-absorptive newborn pigs. Br J Nutr 52:277–287, 1984.
Stanton HC, Mueller RL: Performance of swine chilled during artificial rearing. Am J Vet Res 38:1003–1006, 1977.
Swiatek KR, Kipnis DM, Mason G, et al: Starvation hypoglycemia in newborn pigs. Am J Physiol 214:400–405, 1968.
van Lith PM, Niewold TA, Vandenbooren CJMA, et al: A longitudinal study of starvation in piglets and the introduction of a modified liver biopsy technique. Vet Q 10:145–150, 1988.

---

[1]Available as Survival Plus from NOBL Laboratories, Inc., Sioux Center, IA 51250.

SECTION 3
Herd Health Management

MARK F. SPIRE, DVM, MS, Diplomate, ACT, Consulting Editor

Management of Farm Cow/Calf Herds

DUANE MIKSCH, DVM, MS

A large proportion of beef produced in the United States originates in small (farm) cow herds. Over half of all beef cows are in herds of fewer than 100; 93 per cent of all herds consist of fewer than 100 cows. Most states, including Kentucky and even Texas, have fewer than 20 cows in the average herd. In contrast, 4 per cent of feedyards (1650) marketed 84 per cent of "finished" cattle in 1989.

CHALLENGES

Where beef cattle are part of an agronomic farming operation, they seldom command a majority of the farmer's attention. Cows are usually kept to utilize existing forage, rather than forage being produced to feed the cows. As important as records are, records on cattle will be kept only to the extent that the farmer enjoys record-keeping.

This does not suggest that cow/calf operations are not important to anyone. It shows, really, that a lot of people like to own cattle. People who own cattle usually care about their health and appearance. Cattle are produced even when a profit is very unlikely. The situation creates a challenge for veterinarians to provide acceptable and affordable preventive health programs in sometimes difficult or improbable circumstances. Health programs will necessarily vary somewhat, depending on locale, inherent disease or health problems, and management preferences.

The smaller the herd, the greater will be the cost per animal for health maintenance. Adequate handling facilities can be especially expensive in small herds. Yet having "adequate" facilities is often the key to implementing or continuing a viable health maintenance program. Challenge No. 1 for the veterinarian may be to design adequate and affordable handling facilities for clients with small beef enterprises of varied description. Handling facilities, like health maintenance programs themselves, must be tailored to individual needs.

The smaller the herd, the less opportunity there is for the cattleman to gain needed experience in distinguishing between normal and abnormal animal behavior, castrating and dehorning calves, giving injections, and handling calving. Frequency of repetition may be insufficient to reinforce learning adequately. Likewise, most veterinary practices serving farmers are less than 50 per cent food animal medicine. Beef cattle are often a rather small part of the practice of the veterinarian supplying their health services. The veterinarian may be given little opportunity to become proficient in rectal palpation. Special equipment needed, such as an electroejaculator, may be hard to justify.

OPPORTUNITIES

Despite the difficulties of delivering adequate veterinary service at an affordable cost, preventive health programs are very important to the productivity of small beef herds. The death of one or a few animals before the cause is identified is relatively more costly in a small herd. Herd replacements are more apt to be bought than raised in a small herd; thereby, the risk of introducing disease is increased. A one-bull herd is in the greatest jeopardy of delayed calving if the bull is not sound at breeding time.

Owners of a small herd can benefit greatly from the use of artificial insemination. They cannot afford to keep a variety of bulls to breed cows and to breed heifers and to produce the best breed combinations. They can afford to use better bulls through artificial insemination than they can afford to own.

The operator of a small herd will probably not personally become a proficient inseminator. Once-a-year breeding of a few cows is not sufficient for most people to develop and retain adequate proficiency. Professional inseminators are usually only available in areas with considerable dairying. More often, a dairyman who inseminates his own cows inseminates for a neighbor with beef cows. Superior health management is essential for artificial insemination to be successful. The veterinarian may be the appropriate supplier of artificial insemination service. It brings the practitioner and producer together on the positive note of improved production rather than the less positive concept of disease prevention. As provider of both herd health and artificial insemination services, the veterinarian will become better acquainted with the herd and its management. The availability of products to synchronize breeding, some of which are prescription drugs, has made veterinarian-provided artificial insemination service more practical and appropriate.

In some regards, a group practice may be better able to provide programmed preventive health service than will a veterinarian practicing alone. One veterinarian in the group may be able to specialize in cattle or, at least, in food animals. In a group practice, there is less interference with appointments by emergencies. This can be very important in keeping

121

a client on a preventive health program. A producer should, however, be the client of one veterinarian. Rotating veterinarians on herd work, or sending whoever is available, negates much of the advantage of a herd health program.

Veterinarians providing health care to beef herds should be active members of local and state cattle-producer organizations and participate in planning sessions of the County Extension Council beef commodity group. Veterinarians within a geographic area should strive to give uniform recommendations to producers. They should also actively work toward uniform recommendations with other professionals giving advice in disciplines that overlap. Credibility and effect are diminished when producers receive conflicting advice. Conversely, repetition and replication reinforce good advice.

Products used in herd health maintenance are available to the cattle producer from a variety of suppliers. Veterinarians providing health care must directly address discrepancies in prices between sources. They must (1) convince clients that the advice provided with the product warrants a higher charge, (2) write prescriptions and direct clients to a least-cost source, or (3) find a way to be cost-competitive with other sources. Disguising products or suggesting that one label is superior to another label of the same product is generally counterproductive. All nonprescription products widely used by veterinarians in herd health work are also available with over-the-counter labels.

CLIENT EDUCATION

One of the greatest challenges to veterinarians serving farm beef herds is to be adequately compensated for producer education and consultation in a way acceptable to the producer. Client education is a necessary and desirable part of an effective herd health program. The better producers understand their problems and the proper solutions to those problems, the more they will realize the benefits of good veterinary service. Client education will be rewarded by better results from the veterinarian's efforts, and in most cases it will lead to more demand for veterinary services.

It is important for the veterinarian to understand and to emphasize to clients the relative merit of each health management practice. For example, proper feeding is relatively more important than is vaccination. Stress load should be considered when herd work is scheduled. Age and condition of animals, weather, and harshness of each intended procedure are all important considerations. Weaning results in considerable stress on calves and should not be combined with several other stressful procedures. Weaning should follow or precede major processing of calves by a minimum of 3 weeks.

The veterinarian providing health recommendations and services must remain acutely aware of the need to constantly caution against animals being slaughtered with potential drug residues. For example, cows are quite often treated with pour-on for grub control at the same time they are examined for pregnancy and physical soundness. Treated cull cows may be immediately sent to slaughter if the owner is not reminded of withdrawal requirements of all drugs used. Proper injection techniques and choice of products are necessary for ensuring that muscle is not scarred or abscesses are not produced.

Raising herd replacements should be encouraged for disease prevention and genetic improvement. Buying replacements increases the risk of introducing disease into the herd and makes genetic progress difficult. The necessity for adequate quarantine and retesting of animals being introduced to a herd must be emphasized.

The cattleman should be trained in calving management: (1) he needs to know the importance of frequent observation; (2) he must be able to distinguish between normal parturition and dystocia; (3) he should develop competence and confidence within his capabilities; and (4) he should be taught to seek professional help at the proper time.

Calf scours during calving season should be anticipated and the cattleman taught the principles of calf scours prevention. The importance of prompt and adequate treatment should be learned. Timely treatment should seldom require parenteral administration or a visit by the veterinarian. The relatively greater importance of combating dehydration and acidosis compared with controlling the causative organism must be emphasized.

Castrating and implanting with a growth stimulant may best be done by the educated herdsman on an as-born basis. Dehorning and castration should not be put off until weaning or fall roundup. The earlier they can be done, the easier it is on the calf. Dehorning can be done without attracting flies, and using implants favors early castration. Calves need blackleg protection early. The importance of revaccination for long-term protection must be stressed.

NUTRITION

A short calving season is prerequisite to a workable preventive health program. Nutritional management is the most important single factor in maintaining a short calving season. Heifers must be fed adequately from weaning to breeding if they are to calve at 2 years of age. Puberty is a function of both age and weight. Failing to feed heifers adequately before breeding results in delayed skeletal development and calving difficulty in addition to a low pregnancy rate. If feed levels are excessive, heifers will become overly fat, dystocia will increase, milk production may be lowered, productive life span may be shortened, and feed costs will be prohibitive.

The limiting nutrient related to reproduction is usually energy. Feed requirements of cows vary during the reproductive cycle. The greatest demand occurs from calving to breeding. Protein is also an important consideration in feeding. Young growing animals are often underfed protein, whereas mature dry cows are often overfed protein. Lactating cows require twice as much protein as dry cows do. Other nutrients that are frequently deficient and require supplementation include phosphorus and selenium. The beef cow's reproductive cycle and her varying nutrient requirements are illustrated in Tables 1 and 2.

HERD HEALTH CALENDAR

A preventive health program is most easily understood and communicated on a calendar. Practices can be adjusted on the calendar for geographic area, for calving season, and so on. The calendar concept emphasizes the need for a concise calving season. It provides a framework for integrating the recommendations from persons in the various disciplines serving beef herd enterprises. It is a starting place for veterinarians

Table 1. BEEF COW YEAR BY NUTRIENT REQUIREMENT PERIODS

Period 1 (82 days)	Period 2 (123 days)	Period 3 (110 days)	Period 4 (50 days)
Calving to breeding	Breeding to weaning of calf	Weaning of calf to 50 days before calving	Last 50 days of pregnancy

Table 2. NUTRIENT REQUIREMENTS FOR BEEF COWS OF VARIOUS WEIGHTS BY PERIOD

Body Weight (lb)	Daily Requirements						
	TDN	NE_m	Crude Protein (lb)	Digestible Protein (lb)	Ca (g)	P (g)	Vitamin A (Units × 1000)
Period 1: Calving to Breeding[1]							
900	11–14	10.7–13.6	1.8–2.6	1.1–1.6	25–45	25–41	21–34
1100	12–15	11.6–14.6	2.0–2.8	1.2–1.7	27–46	27–43	24–38
1300	13–16	12.6–15.5	2.2–3.0	1.3–1.8	28–46	28–44	27–43
Period 2: Breeding to Weaning Calf[1]							
900	9–11	8.7–10.7	1.5–2.1	0.9–1.3	22–41	22–37	21
1100	10–12	9.7–11.6	1.6–2.3	1.0–1.4	24–42	24–39	24
1300	11–13	10.7–12.6	1.7–2.4	1.1–1.5	25–42	25–39	27
Period 3: Weaning Calf to 50 Days Before Calving							
900	8.0	7.8	0.82	0.43	13	13	21
1100	8.5	8.2	0.90	0.45	13	13	24
1300	9.0	8.7	0.99	0.49	14	14	27
Period 4: Last 50 Days of Pregnancy							
900	8.8	8.5	1.0	0.48	14	14	21
1100	10.0	9.7	1.1	0.53	15	15	24
1300	11.1	10.8	1.2	0.58	17	17	27

[1]Requirements depend on milking ability, age, and condition.
TDN = total digestible nutrients; NE_m = net energy for maintenance.

within a geographic area to work toward uniformity in their recommendations.

Example Health Calendar *(March-April Calving)*

January

Vaccinate fall-weaned calves against BVD, IBR, and PI_3 with a replicating virus vaccine. This revaccination should be scheduled sometime between 30 days postweaning and 30 days prebreeding for replacement heifers that were vaccinated before weaning: (1) they will be over the stress of weaning; (2) they will be old enough to develop a solid, lasting immunity; (3) they should be away from the cows, so there will be no danger of exposing pregnant cows to vaccine virus; and (4) there will be no danger of interference with conception or pregnancy in the vaccinates.

Feed supplemental magnesium to cows from 60 days before calving until start of breeding in areas where grass tetany is a problem.

Treat for lice twice within 21 days to break the louse life cycle, if lice were not adequately controlled in the fall.

Inject vitamin A if feed is deficient and dietary supplementation is impractical. Booster calf scours vaccine 2 weeks before calving.

February

Begin calving heifers about 3 weeks ahead of calving cows: (1) they can be given the extra attention they need and (2) they will have the extra time they need to be cycling at start of breeding.

First colostrum from older cows should be available for heifers' calves that require it. This may necessitate keeping frozen colostrum from the previous year.

March-April

See that calves get colostrum immediately for maximal absorption of immunoglobulins. Calve cows and remainder of heifers.

Identify calves and record calving events for use in selection and culling.

Evaluate bulls for breeding soundness. This should include fertility determination, physical examination, and mating behavior observation.

Evaluate replacement heifers for breeding soundness. Determine pelvic size, and cull those that do not measure up.

Assess body condition and make feeding recommendations for the postcalving period.

Dehorn and castrate calves early, before they reach 4 months of age.

Implant steer calves with a growth promotant at the time they are castrated.

Vaccinate breeding herd against leptospirosis and vibriosis.

April-May

Deworm yearlings 3 weeks and 6 weeks after they are turned on pasture.

Deworm cows in areas where a "periparturient rise" is a problem. Worms do survive winter, both on pasture and in the cattle.

Initiate horn fly and face fly control. Apply insecticide ear tags at full label recommendation. Rotate products and take every precaution available to delay insecticide resistance in the fly population.

May-June-July

Breed replacement heifers 45 days only. Begin breeding heifers 3 to 4 weeks before starting to breed cows. Expose 50 per cent more heifers than needed as replacements.

Breed cows for 65 days only.

Vaccinate calves for blackleg and malignant edema soon after all calves are born.

Complete castrating, implanting, and dehorning calves.

Deworm in July with an anthelmintic effective against inhibited *Ostertagia* if location and environment indicate a need.

August

Examine heifers for pregnancy. Select replacements from heifers pregnant after 45 days of breeding. Cull open heifers from the breeding herd.

Table 3. LIVESTOCK WEATHER SAFETY INDEX

Temperature °F \ Relative Humidity (%)	5	10	15	20	25	30	35	40	45	50	55	60	65	70	75	80	85	90	95	100
75									70	70	71	71	72	72	73	73	74	74	75	75
76							70	70	70	71	72	72	72	73	74	74	74	75	76	76
77						70	70	71	71	72	72	73	73	74	74	75	75	76	76	77
78					70	70	71	71	72	72	73	74	74	75	75	76	76	77	78	78
79				70	70	71	72	72	73	73	74	74		76	77	77	78	78	79	79
80			70	70	71	72	72	73	73	74	74	75	Alert 76	77	78	78	79	79	80
81		70	70	71	71	72	73	73	74	75	75	76	77	77	78	78	79	80	80	81
82		70	71	71	72	73	73	74	75	75	76	77	77	78	79	79	80	81	81	82
83	70	71	71	72	73	73	74	75	75	76	77	78	78	79	Danger	81	82	82	83
84	70	71	72	72	73	74	75	75	76	77	78	78	79	80	80	81	82	83	83	84
85	71	72	72	73	74	75	75	76	77	78	78	79	80	81	81	82	83	84	84	85
86	71	72	73	74	74	75	76	77	78	78	79	80	81	81	82	83	84	84	85	86
87	72	73	73	74	75	76	77	77	78	79	80	81	81	82	83	84	85	Emergency	87
88	72	73	74	75	76	76	77	78	79	80	80	81	82	83	84	85	86	86	87	88
89	73	74	74	75	76	77	78	79	80	80	81	82	83	84	85	86	86	87	88	89
90	73	74	75	76	77	78	79	79	80	81	82	83	84	85	86	87	87	88	89	90
91	74	75	76	76	77	78	79	80	81	82	83	84	85	86	86	87	88	89	90	91
92	74	75	76	77	78	79	80	81	82	83	84	84	85	86	87	88	89	90		
93	75	76	77	78	79	80	80	81	82	83	84	85	87	87	88	89	90			
94	75	76	77	78	79	80	81	82	83	84	85	86	87	88	89	90				
95	76	77	78	79	80	81	82	83	84	85	86	87	88	89	90					
96	76	77	78	79	80	81	82	84	84	86	87	88	89	90	91					
97	77	78	79	80	81	82	83	84	85	86	87	88	90	91						
98	77	78	79	80	82	83	84	85	86	87	88	89	90							
99	78	79	80	81	82	83	84	86	87	88	88	90								
100	78	79	80	82	83	84	85	86	87	88	90	91								
105	80	82	83	84	86	87	88	90	91											

Halter and tie all replacement animals. This should include pregnant yearlings and heifer calves that are prospective replacements.

Observe Livestock Weather Safety Index (Table 3) when working with cattle in hot weather.

Deworm suckling calves if location and environment indicate a need.

Re-implant steer calves according to schedule recommended for the product used.

September-October

Examine cows for pregnancy and physical soundness. Record body condition scores. Mark for culling those that are open, old, or impaired.

Collect blood samples from the breeding herd. Achieve and maintain a "brucellosis certified free herd." Request blood samples be screened for anaplasmosis, leptospirosis, and other diseases of concern for which tests are reliable.

Vaccinate calves for leptospirosis, IBR-PI$_3$, BVD, BRSV, blackleg-malignant edema, *Hemophilus somnus*, and pasteurellosis.

Certify calves as "preconditioned" where a program is available. This will enhance the value of feeder calves. It will encourage extended ownership of stockers and development of replacements for the breeding herd.

Halter and tie all bred heifers and heifer calves that are prospective replacements.

Treat all cattle for grubs and lice. Retreat within 21 days to preclude necessity of treating during the winter.

Vaccinate heifer calves against brucellosis. Age at vaccination will depend on other management practices and current regulations. Do not combine brucellosis vaccination with weaning or other severe stresses.

A veterinarian-directed health program for farm herds should evolve from on-site services twice a year. One visit should center around pregnancy determination, collecting blood samples, and vaccinating calves for brucellosis. Body condition scoring, additional vaccinations, and other services can be provided. A second key visit should center around evaluating bulls and replacement heifers for breeding soundness. Providing and monitoring a records system can help maintain contact with the client.

Emphasize quality assurance with judicious use of drugs, proper injection techniques, and adequate withdrawal periods.

November-December

Wean and deworm calves.
Plan winter feeding program completely and carefully.
Initiate calf scours program by vaccinating heifers.

Management of Large-Producer Cow/Calf Herds

TERRY J. ENGELKEN, DVM, MS
MARK F. SPIRE, DVM, MS, Diplomate, ACT

Because of high operating costs, high interest rates, and fluctuating calf prices, many cattle producers must operate within a narrow profit margin. The reasons for the difference between calf prices and operating costs are numerous and complex. With many items competing for the food dollar, consideration of increased prices for calves sold as the primary means of increasing profitability in a herd is unrewarding. The most viable alternative is to improve herd efficiency through increasing the number and weight of calves sold and decreasing the cost of production.

Efficiency in the cow/calf operation can be defined in terms of both biologic and economic efficiency. Biologic efficiency describes the amount of marketable product available for the producer to sell. Measures such as percentage calf crop, calf weaning weight, calves weaned per cow exposed, and calving distribution describe biologic efficiency. These impact the total pounds of calf produced per cow each year. Economic efficiency can be measured by net return per cow/calf pair, cost of production per calf marketed, and income less variable costs per cow. The relationship between biologic and economic efficiency will vary from operation to operation. Oftentimes these efficiencies are closely related, but depending on the economic costs associated with a particular level of production, they may not be. The challenge has become one of maximizing production while keeping production costs as low as possible.

The specific components of a production medicine program will vary depending on problem identification, client confidence and acceptance, management changes recommended, and the operator's economic constraints. A strategy for meeting a reasonable set of production goals should be mapped out by the producer and veterinarian. A critical level of production within these goals should be identified as one requiring intervention by the veterinarian. The lower end of the normal range of production could serve as the "action" level for the herd (Table 1). Production goals should be set high enough to offer a challenge, but not so excessive as to risk client discouragement with the program.

A program such as this will require the veterinarian to be active in many different areas of the client's beef enterprise. These basic areas will include (1) chuteside management, (2) record analysis, (3) interpretation and management recommendations, (4) nutritional consultation, (5) replacement heifer development, and (6) program evaluation and documentation. A herd preventive medicine program, based on the concept of "risk-level management," is incorporated into the chuteside management and heifer development areas. This concept enables the veterinarian to identify herds at risk of a disease outbreak and to customize a preventive program. It is particularly useful in assessing the probability of viral agent introduction into a particular herd setting, based on animal flow patterns. This allows the delivery of needed vaccinations and treatments at times when animals are normally handled. This type of total package will enable the veterinarian to play an expanding role in the management of a client's herds. By being in a position to identify a producer's strengths and weaknesses, the practitioner can help optimize production efficiency in the cow/calf enterprise.

CHUTESIDE MANAGEMENT

This component of the production medicine program is the particular area in which the information gathering begins. At the time of pregnancy evaluation, basic information such as cow age, breed, identification number, body condition score, and estimated days pregnant should be recorded. Additional information concerning the bull battery is also noted. The day the bulls entered and left the pastures, bull breed, identification, and pasture assignment can be helpful in data analysis. All this information is recorded chuteside on the day a particular group of breeding females is processed.

Cull animals can represent a large part of the yearly income for an individual herd. It is essential that a criterion be established to identify these animals consistently. Obviously, open and late-calving cows should be marked for culling. Other candidates would include "smooth-mouthed" cows, poor producers, cows exhibiting lameness or ocular lesions, and those animals with an undesirable disposition. The producer should be given a listing of these cows and the reason that they are being eliminated from the herd. This list can easily be produced as these cows are run through the chute.

Methods of chuteside data recording can vary from simple to complex. The use of "lap top" computers with specifically designed software can facilitate rapid data entry and generation of reports. However, the cost of the equipment can be high, and the success of this option is dependent on the user's expertise. Another option for data collection is to simply use NCR paper. The information is recorded by hand, and a copy of the raw data is given to the producer. The data are then taken with the veterinarian for further analysis and report generation. Regardless of the collection method, the data are useful only if they are analyzed and reported back to the client.

If the veterinarian has the computer capability, he or she may want to function as a processing center for herd record maintenance and analysis. There are also commercial processing centers that will generate herd reports on the basis of data sent in by the veterinarian. These commercial operations usually charge on a per head basis and return computer printouts to the practitioner. Factors impacting on the chosen option include available computer space, level of computer literacy, available technical support staff, and time constraints imposed by other practice endeavors.

RECORD ANALYSIS

Previously, the criterion used in analyzing the success of the breeding season was total breeding percentage. This factor measured the percentage of females that became pregnant during the breeding season. This is a useful measure, but it does not give any indication as to when individual cows became pregnant or the percentages by heat cycle. A more contemporary and complete analytical tool is the Breeding Season Evaluation. This type of analysis allows the veterinarian and

Table 1. COW/CALF PRODUCTION EVALUATORS

	Goal	Monitor	Action
Reproduction			
Calf crop (%)	>90	85–90	<85
60-day pregnancy rates (%)	>95	90–95	<90
First 20-day pregnancy rates (%)	>65	55–60	<50
Median calving date	<17	18–25	>25
Herd			
Average cow age	5–6	4–5, 6–7	<4, >7
Body condition score (1 = thin, 9 = fat)			
Mid-gestation	4.5–6	4–4.5	<4
Calving	5–6	4.5–5	<4.5
Dystocia			
Adult (%)	<5	6–7	>8
Heifer (%)	<15	20–25	>25
Gestational losses (%)	<2	2–3	>3
Perinatal mortality (%)	<5	5–9	>10
Cow death loss (%)	<2	3–4	>5
Culling rate (%)	15–20	10–14, 20–25	<10, >25

Information compiled from the 1989 Summary of the North Dakota Beef Cow Herd Analysis Program, 1989 Iowa CHAPS Herd Summary, Kansas Cow Herd Surveys of 1984 and 1985, and Summary Data from Kansas State University Commodity Program Herds, 1986 through 1990.

Table 2. REPRODUCTIVE PROFILE OF A COW HERD

Cow Age (yrs)	H	2	3	4–8	9–10	>10
Average Group BCS	6.3	4.0	4.4	6.2	5.6	5.0
21-Day Breeding Interval	Percentage Pregnant					
1	65	30	40	78	59	50
2	19	35	30	13	25	20
3	7	18	16	6	11	15
% Open	9	17	14	3	5	15
% Culling	9	13	8	3	7	18

This format compares the interaction of age, body condition score (BCS), and 21-day interval to pregnancy status. This facilitates problem identification and client communication.

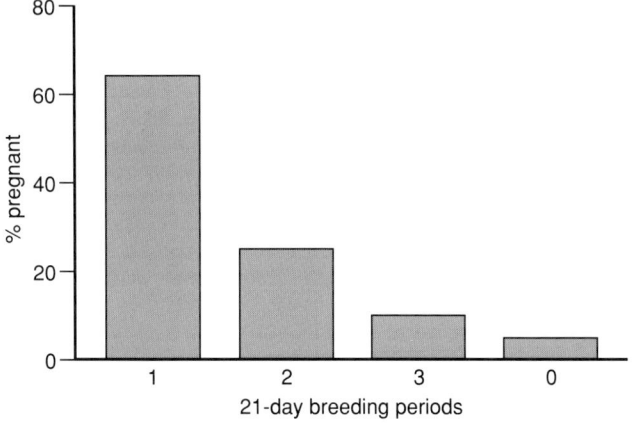

Figure 1. Breeding season evaluation graph showing percentage pregnant by 21-day breeding periods.

producer to track individual cow reproductive profiles, bull battery performance, replacement heifer development, and nutritional status of the herd. From the information collected at chuteside, variations in female reproductive performance based on age, breed, and body condition score can be assessed (Table 2). A histogram can be constructed to predict the herd's conception and calving pattern. This is based on 21-day intervals and shows the percentage of females bred in each estrus cycle (Fig. 1). This may be done for the whole group, or it may be broken down by breed, age, body condition score, pasture location, or other factors. This type of analysis facilitates both problem identification and program modification.

An important indicator of herd reproductive efficiency is median pregnancy date (MPD). By using the pregnancy data and calving histogram, the veterinarian can determine when 50 per cent of the females in the group became pregnant. The percentage pregnant in the first 21-day period is divided by 21 to give the percentage pregnant per day. This quotient is then divided into 50 to give the MPD. In herds that are able to get 60 to 65 per cent of the females bred in the first cycle, the MPD will occur approximately 17 days after the onset of the breeding season. Obviously, the more females that become pregnant during the first 21-day period, the lower the MPD, and the tighter the calving season.

When the MPD is known and the gestation length is estimated, one can now predict median calving date (MCD). This gives the day of the calving season by which 50 per cent of the calves are born. MCD can also be determined in retrospect, provided that calving dates have been recorded. By knowing the MCD, the producer can manipulate the beginning of the breeding season to produce a tighter calving season. This avoids the economic consequences of a high culling rate and subsequent replacement with heifers. Open cows are not included in the MCD calculation, explaining why this measure will be slightly lower than the MPD. If available, these data are particularly useful in herds with a prolonged breeding season, poor conception rates in the first 21-day period, and a high number of late calving cows. Mossman has determined that in herds such as these, the breeding season should begin 280 days from 17 to 18 days before the MCD of the previous year. This can also be expressed as beginning the breeding season 297 days from the previous year's MCD.

An economic analysis can be used to determine program costs and returns. The accuracy of this analysis is dependent on being able to select and monitor repeatable input and output parameters. Information concerning only the costs and returns of the cow herd is considered. Fixed inputs, such as machinery and buildings, used in more than one enterprise are charged to the cow herd, based on the percentage of their use. In midwestern operations, the largest variable cost is associated with the feeding program. Much of this is incurred during the winter supplementation period. This emphasizes the need for forage analysis and proper feeding practices so that feed costs are kept within reasonable limits.

On the output side, pounds of calf produced per exposed breeding female is a good indicator of overall production. Factors such as percentage calf crop, weaning rate, and weaning weight all impact heavily on this measurement. By tracking the number of calves weaned, their average weaning weight, and the breeding female inventory, one can calculate this value. It is essential that this type of information be recorded to enable both the practitioner and client to monitor changes in conception rates, calf mortality, and weaning weights.

Once the various inputs and outputs of the operation are known, an enterprise budget for the cow herd can be constructed. The purpose of this budget is to assist the producer in identifying the level of profitability and to facilitate both short- and long-term planning. This budget will need to deal with the level of production and the associated gross sales (cows and calves sold), variable inputs and costs, and fixed or ownership costs (Table 3). This information is organized yearly for tax purposes by the producer, and a finished budget may be already available. By tracking the changes in yearly profitability shown by this budget, the practitioner and client can monitor the economic impact of the production medicine program.

Table 3. USE OF AN ENTERPRISE BUDGET TO COMPARE COW HERD PROFITABILITY

	Lower 1/3	Middle 1/3	Upper 1/3
Gross returns	$370.00	$369.00	$409.00
Operating costs	236.00	209.00	148.00
Fixed costs	134.00	44.00	32.00
Net returns	−0.74	116.00	228.00
Number of cows	96.00	102.00	146.00
Average weaning weight (lb)	521.00	503.00	550.00
Calf crop (%)	85.00	87.00	92.00
Pounds of calf/cow exposed	442.00	437.00	505.00
Principal, interest/cow	112.00	38.00	22.00
Operator investment/cow	1497.00	1465.00	1817.00
Total investment/cow	2677.00	2379.00	2007.00
Building/equipment/cow	107.00	98.00	88.00
Feed costs (cash)/cow	162.00	164.00	104.00

Source: Simms DD, Marston TT: Cow/calf profitability: case studies of Kansas cattle producers. KAES Report of Progress #592. Manhattan, KS, Kansas State University Extension Service, 1990.

INTERPRETATION

Once information has been collected chuteside and analyzed, the task becomes one of recognizing trends, identifying problems, and recommending the proper management procedures. Trends associated with reproductive efficiency, calf performance, and production costs must be identified. Identifying the cause of these trends may be more difficult. In some instances, the effects of a disease process are not readily separated from environmental effects. In this situation, the practitioner is the one who is best suited to evaluate the conditions to which the herd is subjected, to form a diagnostic plan, collect the proper specimens, and decide which resource people to consult. Once the problem is identified, management procedures are instituted for correction of the situation.

In established herd programs, a reduction in reproductive efficiency from the previous year could indicate poor bull fertility; inadequate group nutrition; a disease process due to *Campylobacter*, IBR, BVD, or *Trichomonas*; or any combination of these. In this situation, open cows can be of great value in providing clues to problem identification. Reproductive tracts should be carefully palpated, and diagnostic samples, such as cervical mucus, should be taken to identify reproductive diseases. In herds not on a routine program, poor reproductive efficiency often accompanies a prolonged breeding season. In these herds, emphasis should be placed on factors that influence the first 21-day breeding interval, especially the percentage of cows cycling at the start of the breeding season. Cow age, postpartum interval, and body condition score will affect this percentage. By comparing the number of females found pregnant with the calving percentage, one can determine when reproductive losses are occurring. Disease organisms normally associated with early, middle, or late gestation, should be targeted once the timing of the reproductive losses is determined. Once the cause of the problem is identified, management decisions involving bull battery evaluation, initiation of herd vaccination programs, or nutritional consultation can be instituted.

Calf performance is measured primarily in terms of weaning weight and total pounds of beef produced. This measure can be negatively affected by improper genetic selection, inadequate cow herd nutrition, and poor milking ability of the cows. Calf age at weaning plays a central role in determining weaning weight. Improper genetic selection can lead to mismatches between the cow and her environment. This results in poor cow condition, decreased milk production, and a longer postpartum interval. Inadequacies in the herd nutrition program can prevent cows from producing at their genetic potential, in terms of both reproduction and milking ability. The grouping of cows to breed early and thus calve early has a great impact on weaning weight, because older calves are usually heavier. By using the calving histogram and determining the effects of age, precalving body condition, and breed on the first 21-day conception rate, the practitioner can evaluate the impact of these various factors on calf performance and recommend the appropriate management changes (Fig. 2).

NUTRITIONAL CONSULTATION

The nutritional status of the herd has a major impact on its reproductive efficiency and, hence, profitability. This is especially true for the last 100 days before calving, because the plane of nutrition will affect dystocia level, colostral quality, milk production, postpartum interval, and conception rate. Oftentimes, too little emphasis is placed on this particular area of the cow/calf operation, unless a major problem develops.

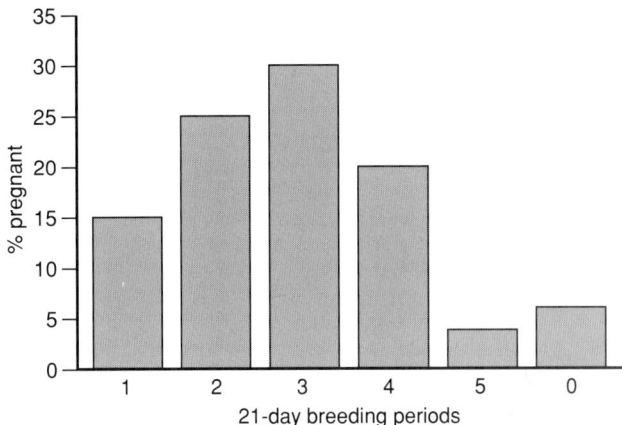

Figure 2. Breeding histogram depicting the results of an inadequate nutritional program resulting in a prolonged breeding season and poor conception rates per 21-day interval.

Usually by the time a problem is recognized, it is too late to prevent an economic loss. In order to properly evaluate a herd's nutritional needs and feeding program, the veterinarian must take into consideration the current body condition of the breeding herd (heifers and cows), their expected level of production, the quantity and quality of the client's feedstuffs, and the veterinarian's own ability to balance rations and make nutritional recommendations. This particular phase of the total program can begin chuteside at the time of herd pregnancy diagnosis when the females are in mid- to late-gestation, precalving, or before the start of the breeding season.

The evaluation of the herd's nutritional status begins with body condition scoring. The scoring system assigns a numerical value to each female, based on the amount of fat cover over the ribs, loin, and tailhead (Table 4). It is preferred to have the females in a moderate condition (5 or 6), because this will tend to optimize reproductive efficiency. This system is easily learned and can even be performed by the client while the veterinarian is pregnancy checking. Once all the cows have been scored, they can then be placed into different management groups, depending on their intended use and nutritional requirements. Cows in moderate body condition need only to gain the weight of the developing fetus. These cows can be fed a maintenance type of ration until they calve. If not provided with adequate energy supplementation, females that are thin at pregnancy examination tend to remain in poor body condition throughout the winter feeding period. If these cows are allowed to calve in poor condition, they become an economic liability as a result of prolonged postpartum intervals and reduced conception rates.

Once these thin cows are identified and grouped separately, a reconditioning program is constructed to bring pregnant cows into a moderate body condition before calving. In order to prepare such a program, one must know the needed weight gain, the number of days available, and the nutrient analysis of the available feedstuffs. On the basis of pregnancy information collected chuteside, the veterinarian can predict the beginning of the calving season. Since a target weight can be determined from the desired change in body condition score, the average daily gain can then be calculated. Animal requirements, based on body weight and stage of pregnancy, are available from National Research Council (NRC) publications. Invariably, the use of cereal grains such as corn or milo as an energy source is needed to feed these females adequately.

Forage samples from different sources, crops, and cuttings can be collected for analysis from baled hay with the use of a

Table 4. SYSTEM OF BODY CONDITION SCORING (BCS) FOR BEEF CATTLE

Group	BCS	Description
Thin condition	1	*Emaciated:* Cow is extremely thin with no palpable fat detected over spinous processes, transverse processes, hip bones, or ribs; tail head and ribs project quite prominently; needs to gain 350 lb
	2	*Poor:* Cow still appears somewhat emaciated, but tail head and ribs are less prominent; individual spinous processes are still rather sharp to the touch, but some tissue cover exists along the spine; needs to gain 300–350 lb
	3	*Thin:* Ribs are still individually identifiable, but not quite as sharp to the touch; there is obvious palpable fat along the spine and over tail head with some tissue cover along dorsal portion of the ribs; gain of 200–300 lb needed
Borderline condition	4	*Borderline:* Individual ribs are no longer visually obvious; the spinous processes can be identified individually on palpation but feel rounded rather than sharp; some fat cover over ribs, transverse processes, and hip bones; needs to gain 150–200 lb
Optimal moderate condition	5	*Moderate:* Cow has generally good overall appearance; upon palpation, fat cover over ribs feels spongy, and areas on either side of tail head now have palpable fat cover; needs to gain 100 lb (weight of fetus)
	6	*High moderate:* Firm pressure now needs to be applied to feel spinous processes; a high degree of fat is palpable over ribs and tail head; gain needed is weight of fetus
	7	*Good:* Cow appears fleshy and obviously carries considerable fat; very spongy fat over ribs and around tail head; some fat around vulva and in crotch; no weight gain needed
Excessive condition	8	*Fat:* Cow very fleshy and overconditioned; spinous processes almost impossible to palpate; cow has large fat deposits over ribs, around tail head, and below vulva; could lose 50–150 lb
	9	*Extremely fat:* Cow obviously extremely wasty and patchy and looks blocky; tail head and hips buried in fatty tissue; bone structure no longer visible and barely palpable; animal's motility may be impaired; could lose 100–200 lb

core sampler. Several random samples of each source are pooled and sent in for a separate analysis. Silage samples may be collected by the client as they are being harvested or unloaded. In obtaining samples from bunker or pit silos, the crust is removed before sampling. These samples should be taken at a level of 10 to 12 inches deep. A post hole auger makes a handy tool for collecting samples from these types of silos. Be sure to replace and repack the top crust in the area of sample collection to prevent any excess spoilage. These samples must be representative and random in order to be of value. The laboratory that performs the analysis should be contacted so that proper sample packaging and timely shipping are ensured. Once the analysis is obtained, least cost ration formulation for thin cows and those cows in proper body condition can be performed. Retention of open cows of poor body condition as possible replacements or to take advantage of seasonal cull cow price upswings will present a different set of requirements. In this case, it is imperative to take advantage of any available crop residue. Program economics will dictate which feedstuffs are used and for how long, because any increase in cull animal value must be greater than the added feed costs. When set up properly, these programs will ensure appropriate allocation of feed resources and prevent costly feeding errors.

Nutritional management of the replacement heifer involves many of the same principles as for a reconditioning program. However, in this case, the veterinarian has the opportunity to take a more proactive approach. By being able to track the growth of these heifers from weaning, the practitioner can prevent many of the pitfalls associated with improper feeding. Because heifer weight has such a large impact on the onset of puberty, the goal of any heifer nutritional program becomes one of maximizing the number of females that cycle before the beginning of the breeding season (Table 5). After the postweaning adjustment period, potential replacement heifers need to be placed on a growing ration that will enable them to develop structurally, but will not allow them to become too fat. Determination of the average daily gain needed to reach puberty, forage analysis, proper ration formulation, and periodic weighing of the heifers are some of the tools needed for ensuring adequate development. As these heifers enter the breeding season, those that are pasture-bred should maintain adequate growth on the available forage. Heifers that are managed in dry lot, for the purpose of being artificially inseminated, should be fed to gain 1.25 to 2 pounds per day. In either case, heifer body condition scores are then evaluated at the time of pregnancy examination, and any needed changes in their nutritional management are instituted.

HEIFER DEVELOPMENT

With an average annual cow turnover rate in midwestern herds of 15 to 25 per cent, proper heifer development becomes an essential part of any production medicine program. Emphasis needs to be placed on the production of highly fertile females that will achieve a high conception rate during a limited breeding season. These heifers must then be managed during gestation and calving to minimize dystocia, decrease the postpartum interval, and maximize successful rebreeding. The nutritional management of these heifers has been discussed previously and represents a major component of any development program. Other aspects include the selection process, estrus synchronization, bull selection, a gestational program, and calving management.

Table 5. ESTIMATES FOR HEIFERS REACHING PUBERTY AT VARIOUS WEIGHTS (LB) AT 13 TO 16 MONTHS OF AGE

	Percentage Reaching Puberty		
	50%	*70%*	*90%*
Angus	550	600	650
Brahman	700	750	800
Brangus	600	650	700
Charolais	700	750	775
Hereford	600	650	700
Limousin	650	700	750
Santa Gertrudis	700	750	800
Shorthorn	500	550	600
Simmental	625	675	750
Braham × British	675	725	750
British × British	575	625	675
Charolais × British	675	725	775
Limousin × British	650	700	775
Simmental × British	625	675	750

Source: Beverly JR: Management of replacement heifers for a higher reproductive and calving rate. Texas Agricultural Extension Service, Texas A&M University, College Station, TX, No. B/1213, 1980.

The initial selection process begins at weaning. Heifers with obvious conformational defects, ocular lesions, and poor overall development are immediately eliminated from the replacement pool. Individual heifer weights can be taken at this time to facilitate the selection process. If calving dates are available and if the heifers have been individually identified at birth, selection of heifers from the early part of the calving season should be emphasized. These heifers will be older and have a better chance of cycling before the beginning of the breeding season. Delivery of the needed vaccines to protect against respiratory and clostridial disease should be performed at this time and booster injections given 10 to 14 days later. By identifying cull heifers early, the client is afforded more in the way of marketing options. Depending on the feed supply and expected economic return, the producer has the option of marketing cull animals immediately or retaining ownership for feeding.

The next phase of the selection process occurs when the heifers are 12 to 14 months of age. At this time, heifers are processed for the delivery of vaccines against reproductive diseases and for pelvic measurement. Additional boosters for respiratory disease can be given as well. Regardless of which pelvimeter is used, a vertical and horizontal measurement is taken to determine the pelvic area. The shape of the pelvis is also ascertained and the level of group cyclicity estimated via reproductive tract palpation. Pelvic information is then indexed for individual heifers by dividing their measurement by the group average. Heifers indexing below 92 should be culled because of the likelihood of calving difficulty. Additionally, those heifers with infantile tracts, abnormally shaped or small pelvises, and obvious physical defects are eliminated as potential replacements. Ideally, heifers would be weighed again to monitor their growth rate and permit timely modification of the feeding program.

Because birth weight still has the largest impact on dystocia, proper bull selection is a necessity. Matching a bull's expected progeny difference (EPD) for birth weight to a particular set of heifers enables the producer to minimize calving problems. The EPDs simply predict how future progeny of a sire will perform for a particular trait. The values given for birth weight are usually expressed in pounds, but there may be breed to breed variation in how these are reported. In herds utilizing artificial insemination, bulls with higher EPDs for birth weight can be mated to heifers with larger pelvises. This will enable the producer to take advantage of the increased performance of these bulls' offspring. There is an increasing interest in the pelvic area of bulls, and it is becoming more important as a selection criterion. This trait tends to be highly heritable, but industrywide minimal values for bull pelvises have not been established. All bulls used in natural mating situations should have a breeding soundness examination at least 30 days before the start of the breeding season.

In order to maintain lifetime reproductive performance, heifers must calve early and over a short period of time. By breeding heifers to calve 2 to 3 weeks before the rest of the cow herd, special attention can be given to them during the subsequent calving season. This also allows the heifers additional time to undergo uterine involution and prepare to rebreed. Estrus synchronization programs offer the client the means to have replacement heifers calve early, decrease bull requirements, and, in some cases, increase conception rates. The programs currently offering the most predictable results are the melengestrol acetate–prostaglandin combination, 2 injections of a prostaglandin 11 days apart, and the combination of a norgestomet implant with an estradiol valerate injection. The particular program used must be matched with the producer's availability of labor, facilities, and time. Response to any synchronization program is dependent on the level of cyclicity within the group. Therefore, the physical development, the genetic base, and the reproductive status of the heifers must be evaluated before synchronization recommendations are made.

The gestational program is similar to that of the cow herd. After the breeding season, the pregnancy and nutritional status of the heifers is determined. Vaccines to prevent reproductive losses and products to control internal and external parasites are delivered at this time. Antigens against calf enteric disease are also given during gestation. The reproductive performance of the heifers is evaluated in the same way as for the cow herd, and a nutritional program is instituted. This program should enable the heifers to continue growing at a constant rate and allow them to enter the calving season in moderate body condition. The nutritional management of these heifers is critical to their longevity within the herd, the amount and quality of colostrum production (Table 6), and their ability to rebreed.

Once a replacement heifer has survived the selection process, been bred to calve early, and been maintained in a moderate body condition, calving season management becomes an exercise in client education. The producer must be able to recognize the signs of dystocia and provide the appropriate intervention. When the decision to intervene is made, cleanliness and the proper use of obstetric equipment should be emphasized to the client. The producer must also recognize when veterinary assistance is needed. Within 12 hours of birth, these calves should receive high-quality colostrum. If stored colostrum is given, calves need 5 to 10 per cent of their body weight. Colostral quality can be determined by use of a colostrometer or even with an antifreeze tester. A record system should be in place to keep track of when calves are born, cow and calf identification, and dystocia score (0 = unassisted through 5 = cesarian). Records of birth dates serve to evaluate the accuracy of pregnancy palpation and will aid in future heifer selection. Calf identification will enable the producer to determine the level of heifer production at weaning time. The dystocia scoring system will give the veterinarian and client an indication as to how well heifer development was matched to bull selection. This type of record system can also be used for the cow herd and should be kept as simple as possible.

PROGRAM EVALUATION AND DOCUMENTATION

The evaluation process begins with the identification of selected performance indices that are economically important to the operation. Parameters such as percentage calf crop, weaning weight, pounds of calf produced per breeding female,

Table 6. EFFECT OF CONDITION SCORE AT CALVING ON INTERVAL FROM CALVING TO STANDING, COLOSTRUM PRODUCTION, AND IMMUNOGLOBULIN CONCENTRATION

	Condition Score			
	3	4	5	6
Calving to standing (min)	59.9	63.6	43.3	35.0
Colostrum production (ml)	1525.0	1111.5	1410.9	—
Calf serum IgG (mg/dl)	1988.1	2178.8	2309.8	2348.9
Calf serum IgM (mg/dl)	145.9	157.2	193.1	304.1

Source: Odde KG, et al: Effect of body condition and calving difficulty on calf vigor and calf serum immunoglobulin concentrations in two-year old beef heifers. Ft. Collins, CO, Proceedings of the Colorado State University Beef Program Report, 1986.

and income over variable costs are all factors that have an impact on profitability. The ability to evaluate the impact of management recommendations depends on the completeness of production records, both before and after changes are initiated. Increases in production and decreases in production costs need to be identified. If possible, each phase of the production medicine program should be assessed independently in order to identify those parts that had the greatest impact on the operation. This evaluation is done at the end of each year, with the results being documented for the client.

Depending on how the program is set up, client communication and documentation may take several forms. If time and expertise are available, a complete written report can be generated for the client. This report will need to detail the practitioner's analysis of the herd's reproductive performance, nutritional status, and health delivery program. Needed management changes should also be outlined and the framework for program evaluation detailed. Consultation on an as-needed basis and periodic meetings with individual producers enable the client and veterinarian to keep in synchrony. Preseasonal reports enable the veterinarian to outline weaning programs, calving management, and cow herd processing before the occurrence of these events. This gives the producer time to obtain needed products and equipment and have any remaining questions answered. An organized and rational approach to the documentation process will enable the practitioner to track the progress of the production medicine program. This process will serve as the backbone of the yearly comparison and enable the client to appreciate the benefits of the program.

SUMMARY

The basic areas of a cow/calf production medicine program have been outlined. This type of veterinary service should enable the practitioner to expand his or her role in the management of the client's herds. With the evolution of today's cow/calf units into larger, more cost-conscious entities, the veterinarian will be increasingly called on to act as a production analyst. Production parameters will be evaluated and compared with herd indices. Animal health will be evaluated as part of the whole in its relationship to herd performance and economic return. Economic justification and impact, data management, documentation, and long-range planning will be phrases stressed in this type of practice setting. This will require increased awareness on the part of the practitioner in the areas of economics, computerized records, and reproductive management. These are the basics of production medicine, and this represents the next generation of veterinary service.

BIBLIOGRAPHY

Engelken TJ, Spire MF, Simms DD, et al.: Management practices that increase beef herd profitability. Vet Med 86:851–857, 1991.
Mossman DH: Analysis of calving. In Proceedings, J. D. Stewart Memorial Refresher Course on Beef Cattle Production, 68:201–222, 1984. University of Sydney, Australia.
Odde KG, Field TG: Economic efficiency in cow-calf production. Agri-Practice 8:28–32, 1987.
Osburn DD, Schneeberger KC: Using enterprise budgets. In Modern Agricultural Management, 2nd ed. Reston, VA, Reston Publishing Company, 1983, pp 202–217.
Rice LE: Development of replacement beef heifers. Compend Contin Educ Pract Vet 10:543–551, 1988.
Spire MF: Breeding season evaluation of beef herds. In Howard JL (ed): Current Veterinary Therapy: Food Animal Practice 2, 2nd ed. Philadelphia, WB Saunders, 1986, pp 808–811.
Spire MF: Immunization of the beef breeding herd. Compend Contin Educ Pract Vet 10:1111–1118, 1988.
Spire MF: Cow/calf production records: justification, gathering, and interpretation. Proceedings, American Association of Bovine Practitioners, 23rd Annual Convention, 1991, pp 93–95.

Backgrounding and Stocker Calf Management

ROBERT A. SMITH, DVM, MS, Diplomate, ABVP*

Backgrounding describes a management system by which cattle, generally recently weaned calves, are assembled from many sources with little or no knowledge of their history and are kept for a period of time before they are placed in a feedlot. Stocker calves of similar ages are assembled and placed on forage, generally grass or small grain pastures. When they are grown to a suitable size, they will be sold to the feedlot. Heifers intended for future breeding can also be handled in stocker operations.

Health management of calves in backgrounding or stocker programs can be among the greatest challenges facing the food animal practitioner. Calves in these programs have often been extremely stressed under the current management and marketing systems. Most are recently weaned, moved through auction markets where they are exposed to many pathogens for the first time, commingled, and then transported long distances. At the backgrounding or stocker operation, the calves must establish a new social order, adapt to different feedstuffs, and frequently must acclimate to new weather conditions. The result is that the calves suffer from fatigue, dehydration, hunger, and psychological stress, which makes them quite susceptible to bovine respiratory disease and other stress-related diseases. Many calves have been given antibiotics before arrival. Often these are given at incorrect dosages, for too short a time, and often in combination with corticosteroids. Morbidity in newly received calves is frequently 40 to 50 per cent, and mortality is often 5 per cent or more.

MANAGEMENT ON ARRIVAL

Calves should be inspected as they are unloaded for determination of health status and shipping injuries. If they are unacceptable, the seller should be contacted immediately for determining their disposition. Calves that have been trampled or seriously injured during transit should not be accepted and are the responsibility of the trucker. Calves should be weighed upon arrival for determining shrinkage. Shrinkage of 7 to 8 per cent or more is often associated with greater health problems, and affected calves will require more intensive management during the receiving period. Occasionally, newly received calves will have unusually low shrinkage or even weigh more on arrival than their purchase weight, which suggests nutritional mismanagement and possibly increased management problems during the receiving period.

Once the calves are accepted, they should be placed in drylots with free access to good-quality grass hay and fresh water and allowed to rest overnight. Drylots offer several advantages over grass traps. Calves kept in drylots have lower morbidity and mortality rates, improved gains, and lower labor costs. Traps allow calves too much room to walk fences,

---

*American Board of Veterinary Practitioners—Food Animal.

causing more physical stress, and allow them to stray too far from feedbunks and water sources. Confining calves for up to 3 weeks before turning them out to pasture is often necessary for allowing recovery from stress-related diseases that occurred during the receiving period. Water tanks with water running from a hydrant will often encourage calves to drink, because many are not accustomed to drinking from automatic waterers. Calves are not usually very competitive at the feedbunk, so a minimum of 1.5 feet of bunk space per animal should be provided. One to 2 pounds per head of a palatable protein pellet should be offered in the feedbunk on arrival.

NUTRITION

Newly received stressed calves have special nutritional problems. Inadequate or stress-inducing nutrition practices compound health problems. Such animals often eat too little for nutrient levels that aid in recovery to be achieved. With many feeds, animals initially eat too little and later eat too much, which can lead to digestive upset and other health problems.

As seen in Table 1, the percentage of calves eating daily is less than satisfactory during the first 10 days after arrival. Feed intake is also low, ranging from 0.5 to 1.5 per cent of their body weight on a dry matter basis during the first week. Feed intake increases through the third week and follows a plateau during the fourth week, indicating that normal feed intake is achieved during the third week. It is essential that a palatable ration be offered, and nutrient densities must be raised when feed intake is low. Pounds of nutrients consumed during the receiving period are of greater importance than are percentages of nutrients in rations. The use of silage in receiving rations is generally associated with higher morbidity and mortality rates. Silage should not be included in receiving rations during the first 2 weeks after arrival. Silage is generally low in protein; therefore calves should be supplemented with natural protein for meeting daily requirements. Alfalfa hay, although palatable and of good nutrient value, often causes bloat and contributes to loose stools. Moldy or poor-quality hay decreases consumption and should be avoided.

Concentrate levels above 55 per cent during the receiving period are often accompanied by higher morbidity and higher medication costs; however, average daily gain and feed efficiency will be improved. Feeding good-quality, long-stem hay, such as prairie or oat hay, results in the lowest morbidity and mortality rates. A good balance of health, average daily gain, and feed efficiency is obtained when a ration approximating 72 per cent concentrate is fed (Tables 2 and 3). Limit-feeding a concentrate ration for obtaining a calculated average daily gain and cost of gain offers advantages of controlling weight gains to achieve desired weights for future grazing or to take advantage of more favorable markets. Feeding long-stem grass hay free-choice, such as prairie hay, with up to 2 pounds/day of a palatable 38 to 40 per cent natural protein pellet (Table 4) results in excellent health performance, and gains of 1 to 2 pounds/day can be expected during a 28-day receiving period.

Coccidiostats in receiving rations provide effective control of both clinical and subclinical coccidiosis. Clinical coccidiosis in newly received calves is quite common and results in noticeable losses in production as well as in higher medication costs and deaths. Subclinical infections cause more subtle losses but can be costly owing to reduced performance and increased incidence of other stress-related diseases. Decoquinate (Deccox[1]) for 28 days as a feed additive at a dosage of 22.7 mg/45 kg body weight and amprolium (Corid[2]) crumbles at 5.06 mg/kg body weight for 21 days are effective preventive agents. Amprolium is also available as a liquid for use in drinking water. Improved average daily gain and feed efficiency result from the use of a coccidiostat during the receiving period. Rumensin[1] or Bovatec[2] can be placed in the ration after the calves have begun consuming normal quantities of feed, generally at about 3 weeks after arrival. These compounds aid in the control of coccidiosis, but their use during the early receiving period may reduce feed intake.

Calves from some origins may be selenium or copper deficient. Appropriate laboratory testing should be done so that trace mineral deficiencies can be documented. A nutritionist should be consulted to develop a premix suitable for calves from particular origins. Oversupplementation can be as detrimental as a deficiency. Vitamin E supplementation in the receiving ration at 400 IU per head per day generally improves health and performance of newly received stressed calves.

PROCESSING

Proper handling and management of cattle during processing is essential to minimize stress, to reduce the risk of injury, and to detect sick cattle as soon as possible. The veterinarian plays a vital role in the success of this phase of the receiving program by providing detailed instructions to employees of the backgrounding yard or stocker operation on proper techniques to be used in processing calves, on the procedures to be performed, and on sanitation and the proper use and handling of vaccines and other drugs. The consulting veterinarian should provide a written processing protocol to both managers and their employees.

Processing should not be delayed for more than 24 to 36 hours after arrival. Longer delays result in higher rates of morbidity and do not take full advantage of the protection offered by vaccines or preventive medications. Each day that processing is delayed results in a 1 per cent increase in morbidity. In many veterinary practices, facilities are available to process cattle before they are delivered to local backgrounding or stocker operations. This reduces the labor and facility requirements of the producer.

The following guidelines for procedures to be accomplished during processing may be modified to fulfill specific needs to meet local conditions.

1. Body temperature: Body temperature can reliably indicate sickness if a few simple rules are followed:
    a. Newly arrived cattle are rested overnight before processing. Body temperatures of cattle just unloaded from the truck are not reliable indicators of illness.
    b. Process small groups, so no animal is out of its pen or waiting to be processed for more than 30 minutes.
    c. Process early in the morning; temperature readings taken in the afternoon are seldom meaningful.
    d. Take extra care to move cattle through processing with a minimum of excitement or stress.
    e. Take body temperature as soon as the animal enters the chute.
    f. An electronic thermometer is essential. Calves with a body temperature of 104° F (40° C) or greater or showing other signs of illness should be separated from the group, placed in a treatment program, and kept in a hospital pen until they recover.
    g. Too much reliance can be placed on observed rectal temperatures. The appearance and history of the calves should be considered in deciding whether the calf is actually ill.

---

[1]Rhône-Poulenc Inc., Atlanta, GA 30342.
[2]MSD AGVET, Rahway, NJ 07065.

[1]Elanco Products Co., Indianapolis, IN 46285.
[2]Hoffmann-LaRoche Inc., Nutley, NJ 07110.

Table 1. THE PERCENTAGE OF CALVES EATING DURING THE FIRST 10 DAYS AFTER ARRIVAL

Day	Calves Eating (%)	Range
1	21.7	0–50
2	36.7	10–60
3	56.7	30–90
4	61.7	30–90
5	66.7	40–90
6	68.3	40–90
7	70.0	60–90
8	71.7	60–80
9	73.3	60–90
10	85.0	60–100

Source: Hutcheson DP: Observations on receiving new cattle. Amarillo, TX, Eighth Annual Texas Beef Conference Proceedings, 1980.

Table 3. SUPPLEMENT INCLUDED IN 72 PER CENT CONCENTRATE RATION

Ingredient	% Formula
Soy meal 44	89.347
Calcium carbonate	6.646
Potassium chloride	0.461
Salt	1.719
Trace mineral	0.075
Vitamin A 30	0.136
Vitamin E 50	0.109
Deccox	0.136
Dicalcium phosphate	1.372

Source: Gill DR: Extension Animal Scientist, Oklahoma State University, Stillwater, OK.

2. Vaccinations: It is tempting to use all available vaccines and bacterins to minimize disease. Many calves entering backgrounding or stocker operations are highly stressed; therefore they may be able to respond to only a limited number of antigens. The presence of colostrum-derived antibodies may also limit immunization against some diseases. Therefore the veterinarian must consider the following when outlining a vaccination program: risk of disease; stress; age of calf and the presence of colostral antibodies; stress induced by vaccine; efficacy of the vaccine; previous vaccination history; and the time of onset of disease after arrival. Vaccination programs should be tailored to meet the needs of calves of various ages, levels of stress, and origins.
    a. IBR and PI_3. The intranasal vaccine (MLV) should be used in calves less than 4 to 6 months of age and having colostral antibodies present. The intramuscular (MLV) vaccines are suitable for calves over 6 months of age and produce rapid immunity.
    b. BVD vaccine should be considered. The MLV vaccine is suitable for fresh, minimally stressed calves. Because the MLV vaccine is mildly immunosuppressive, it should be avoided in highly stressed, stale calves. Colostral antibodies may persist for 6 to 8 months and can interfere with immunization. Because killed vaccines require 2 injections, 14 days apart, protection is not afforded for about 21 days after the initial injection.
    c. BRSV vaccine. Both MLV and killed vaccines are available. Both types require 2 injections, 14 days apart. Maternal antibodies persist for up to 7 months and, although not protective, will interfere with immunization. The risk of clinical BRSV infection is greatest in the fall and winter with large temperature differentials between day and night and when wet feedstuffs are offered, such as high-moisture corn or silage.
    d. *Pasteurella* bacterins have shown no value in controlled trials and are not recommended in receiving programs.
    Inactivated subunit or modified live *Pasteurella* vaccines should be considered.
    e. Four-way *Clostridium* (*C. chauvoei, C. septicum, C. sordellii, C. novyi*) bacterin.
    f. *Leptospira pomona* bacterin in endemic areas.
3. Deworm: Products for internal parasite control are Ivomec injectable,[1] and pour-on Safe-Guard suspension,[2] TBZ paste,[3] Tramisol injectable or gel,[4] Levasole,[5] Valbazen,[6] or Synanthic.[7]
    Type II ostertagiosis is most prevalent in cattle originating in the southeast, particularly after long dry periods or in winter. Plasma pepsinogen levels can be determined by the state's diagnostic laboratories for ascertaining the incidence of type II ostertagiosis. Affected cattle should be dewormed with Ivomec, Valbazen, Synanthic, or Safe-Guard at twice the usual dosage.
4. External parasites: Systemic organophosphates should be avoided during the first 3 weeks after arrival. Lice can be treated with products such as Lysoff[8] or Ivomec pour-on. Ivomec injectable is also an effective grubicide. Grubicides should not be used after the regional cut-off dates because host-parasite reactions may occur, although they are not common in younger calves.
5. Vitamin A injection (1 million units) only if the calves originate from a vitamin A–deficient area.
6. Implant with growth stimulant: Products include Compudose,[9] Ralgro,[10] and Synovex-S[11] for steers, and Compu-

[1]MSD AGVET, Rahway, NJ 07065.
[2]Hoechst-Roussel Agri-Vet Co., Somerville, NJ 08876.
[3]MSD AGVET, Rahway, NJ 07065.
[4]American Cyanamid Co., Wayne, NJ 07470.
[5]Pitman-Moore, Inc., Mundelein, IL 60060.
[6]SmithKline Beecham Animal Health, Exton, PA 19341.
[7]Syntex Animal Health Inc., W Des Moines, IA 50265.
[8]Cutter Animal Health, Shawnee, KS 66201
[9]Elanco Products Co., Indianapolis, IN 46285.
[10]Pitman-Moore, Inc., Mundelein, IL 60060.
[11]Syntex Animal Health Inc., W Des Moines, IA 50265.

Table 2. A 72 PER CENT CONCENTRATE RECEIVING DIET

Ingredient	Amount (% as fed)
Rolled corn	53.030
Alfalfa pellets	7.850
Cottonseed hulls	19.200
Supplement	15.542
Molasses	4.378
Total	100.000

Source: Gill DR: Extension Animal Scientist, Oklahoma State University, Stillwater, OK.

Table 4. PERCENTAGE COMPOSITION OF PROTEIN PELLETS[1] USED IN RECEIVING PROGRAM

Ingredient	%
Soybean-oil meal	90.87
Limestone	1.50
Cottonseed hulls	1.75
Salt	3.00
Dicalcium phosphate	2.75
Vitamin mineral premix	0.12

[1]3/16 inch pellet.
Source: Gill DR, Armbruster S, Richey EJ: The nutrition of newly received stressed stocker cattle. Stillwater, OK, Proceedings of 1980 Oklahoma Beef Symposium.

dose, Synovex-H,[1] or Ralgro for heifers. Synovex-C[1] and Calf-oid[2] are approved for use in steers or heifers weighing less than 400 pounds. Synovex-S and Synovex-H should not be used in calves weighing less than 400 pounds. Periodically, observe implanting procedures to ensure that they are done properly because improper technique will not result in maximal benefit. Bulls intended for breeding should not be implanted. Synovex-C is approved for suckling heifers intended for breeding.

7. Tip horns.
8. Castrate.
9. Mass medication: If fresh cattle are received, and if there is sufficient skilled labor available, this practice may not be cost-effective. When there is a shortage of labor or when employees are not highly skilled at detecting sick cattle early, mass medication may be a useful management tool. It is of greatest benefit when it is used on sale-barn cattle assembled from several sources or on extremely stressed calves. In many instances, one mass medication treatment will be as effective as a 3-day program. Timing is important because mass medicating too far in advance of the onset of illness or too late will be ineffective. The selection of antimicrobials should be based on previous culture and sensitivity data or on clinical response.
10. Revaccination: When the morbidity within a pen suddenly increases or when feed intake drops, revaccination with an MLV IBR/PI$_3$ vaccine will generally reduce morbidity. An antibiotic administered concurrently aids in reducing morbidity.

After processing, all cattle, except those taken to the hospital pen, are moved to their home pen and offered a receiving ration. Sick cattle are placed on an appropriate treatment program.

DIAGNOSIS AND TREATMENT

The veterinarian should train the pen riders and doctoring crews to recognize the more common diseases affecting calves, especially respiratory diseases, in backgrounding or stocker operations. All cattle should be inspected daily, and pens of problem calves should be checked twice daily. Cattle with signs of illness should be removed from the pens to the hospital pen as quietly as possible for minimizing stress. They should remain in the hospital pen until they recover and are able to compete with penmates for feed and water. Sick cattle left in the pens another day or two in hope of spontaneous recovery often are less responsive to treatment than are those removed early and treated.

Once the cattle are in the hospital pen, the doctoring crews should take the body temperature, assign a degree of illness (severe, moderate, or slight), and begin a hospital treatment card (Figs. 1 and 2). Treatment should be based on written guidelines provided by the veterinarian, including duration of treatment, dosage, and route of administration. Drug selection should be based on culture results, sensitivity tests, and clinical response to treatment.

Sick cattle should be examined and evaluated daily for determining response to treatment. The degree of illness (severe, moderate, or slight) and body temperature should be evaluated in order to judge response. Depression, appetite, respiratory difficulties, and stool consistency are important factors to consider in assigning a degree to the illness. Useful criteria to consider in deciding to continue with the same medication or to change are as follows:

1. Ideally, a calf with a temperature of 104° F (40° C) or greater on the first day it was pulled will show a 2° F (1° C) reduction in fever or drop to less than 104° F (40° C) within 24 hours of treatment. The comparative severity of illness scores should also be considered. If the calf has improved markedly, as evidenced by improved appetite and reduced signs of illness, continue with the same drug.
2. Calves showing worsening severity of illness scores and a continued elevated body temperature should be changed to an alternative treatment and program outlined by the veterinarian.
3. A calf with a temperature of less than 104° F (40° C) on the first day must improve physically to be designated as

[1]Syntex Animal Health Inc., W Des Moines, IA 50265.
[2]The Upjohn Co., Kalamazoo, MI 49001.

Pen ________
Tag ________

Date	Temp	Severity of Illness	LA 200	Albon SR	Oxyject 100	Sulfa bolus	Erythro	Amoxicillin	Penicillin	Tylan	Naxcel	Thiamine	Corid	Neomycin			

Figure 1. Hospital card (side 1).

| Pen _____ Tag _____ Date First Pulled _____ Time of Day _____ |
| Body Temperature _____ Weight _____ |

Symptoms on date first pulled as sick:

Nose	Dry _____	Crusted _____	Discharge _____	Clear _____
Eyes	Clear _____	Cloudy _____	Ulcer _____	Watery _____
Breathing	Heavy _____	Labored _____	Rapid _____	Cough _____
Diarrhea (feces)	Blood _____	Watery _____	Black _____	
Abdomen	Bloated _____	Drawn _____	Full _____	
Foot Rot	Yes _____	No _____		
Nervous System	Staggering _____	Convulsions _____	Muscle Twitch _____	
Depression	Slight _____	Moderate _____	Severe _____	
Other				

Diagnosis: _____

Severity of Illness: _____

Remarks: _____

Figure 2. Hospital card (side 2).

responding to therapy. If it is not improving, the alternative treatment program should be utilized.

4. Once a calf is responding to a drug, it should be treated for at least 2 more days while fever, inappetence, depression, and other clinical signs are absent. It is often wise to extend the treatment of severely ill cattle for 2 to 3 additional days.

About 75 per cent of the calves suffering with respiratory disease require 3 days of therapy with an effective antimicrobial. Recent research (Smith and Gill, unpublished data) has shown that most of the calves not responding after 3 days of treatment will respond if they are given the same drug 2 additional days.

A rectal temperature of 103° F (39.5° C) may be normal for a calf that has been injected with antimicrobials for several days, especially when drugs such as erythromycin or tylosin are used. These drugs can cause severe muscle irritation when they are injected in large quantities for several days.

Calves sick on arrival or detected as sick too late are often nonresponsive or poorly responsive to therapy. A careful evaluation of pen surveillance and buying programs is necessary for differentiation between true "drug failures" and other management problems.

Treated calves should remain in a convalescent pen until they eat well enough to compete with penmates. A fortified, highly palatable hospital ration is often indicated for calves undergoing treatment. If the cattle in the home pen are on a high-concentrate ration, one must allow the treated calf to adjust to the higher concentrate ration before being returned to the home pen in order to avoid serious digestive upsets.

All dead cattle should undergo necropsy for determination of the type and extent of lesions present and the cause of death. Samples should be submitted to the laboratory for culturing, sensitivity testing, histopathologic examination, and virus isolation. The necropsy can be a useful instructional tool to show health crews why the animal failed to respond to therapy, the reason for the clinical signs, and the need for early detection of sick cattle before lesions advance.

RECORDS

Complete, accurate health records are essential. They provide documentation of charges, processing procedures, therapeutic regimens, and dispositions of cattle. They are necessary for the veterinarian to evaluate the overall health program effectiveness periodically and to determine the type and incidence of various health problems. Although an accurate, detailed, handwritten system is adequate, computerized health records allow the veterinarian and manager more flexibility in retrieving and evaluating data.

CONCLUSION

Consultation with backgrounders and stocker operators is still in its infancy; however, opportunities for increasing productivity and profits abound. Data regarding economic benefits of veterinary consultation input are lacking and are sorely needed. Producers are inundated with information, but the information received is often biased or not based on good factual research.

The veterinarian should provide written guidelines for preventive medicine and treatment programs. Records should be analyzed frequently to determine if production goals are realized. A thorough, systematic herd health program should be financially rewarding for the producer and the veterinarian alike.

BIBLIOGRAPHY

Hjerpe CA: Bovine vaccines and herd vaccination programs. Vet Clin North Am 6:169–260, 1990.
Hutcheson DP: Nutrient requirements of diseased, stressed calves. Vet Clin North Am 4:523–530, 1988.
Lofgren GP: Nutrition and management of stressed beef calves. Vet Clin North Am 5:87–101, 1983.
Lofgren GP: Nutrition and management of stressed beef calves. Vet Clin North Am 4:509–522, 1988.
Smith RA, Hays VS, Gill DR: Management of stockers. Agri-Practice 9:8–14, 1988.

Feedlot Health Management

A. J. EDWARDS, DVM, PHD
G. L. STOKKA, DVM

Livestock represent a vital link in the human food chain in America. Photosynthetic energy captured by agricultural areas must be cycled through livestock before becoming available for human consumption. The utilized agricultural area in the United States is about 1.06 billion acres, of which 64 per cent is range land (including government-owned and privately owned land). The only method of harvesting any return from this land is to utilize the grazing ability of cattle and sheep.

Feeder cattle are generally 10 to 18 months old when they are ready to be placed on feed in a feedlot; therefore they will have spent about 80 per cent of their lifetime on a roughage diet. They will spend the final 20 per cent of their life in the feedlot, where they will gain about 33 per cent of their total weight. The finishing phase is a very economical method of utilizing our grain resources as well as of aiding in producing the fine quality of meat protein that is such a vital part of our nutritious diet.

Feeding cattle in the feedlot represents a very intense period in beef production that utilizes solar energy for human food production. This involves some drastic changes for these animals: change from a high-roughage to a high-concentrate diet; change from range conditions to confined conditions; and change from minimal exposure to infectious agents to great exposure.

This brief period of time in the feedlot in which the animal makes such rapid body gains, and the changes in environment, nutrition, and exposure to infectious agents bring out the importance of a good feedlot management plan that includes a sound health program. Any depression of gain, whether it is due to disease or any other management factors, can contribute dramatically to decreased efficiency in production. A good health program can be very cost-effective in minimizing losses and therefore increasing the efficiency of cattle during the feeding period.

The role of the veterinarian in feedlot medicine has changed during the past decade from one who provides primary therapeutic care to one who is able to serve in an advisory capacity. This change has been brought about by the concentration that has taken place in the United States cattle feeding industry, in which over 80 per cent of the cattle are fed in about 250 feedlots. This concentration has made cattle feeding a very specialized industry that demands specialization from the veterinarians to service their industry needs.

DEVELOPING A FEEDLOT HEALTH PROGRAM

A feedlot health program should be considered a very important part of the operating procedure and overall production plan of a feedlot. Veterinarians are generally looked to for advice and assistance in treating sick cattle with the emphasis on treatment. This concept has been changing over the years as new demands are placed on veterinarians to provide plans on how to prevent or minimize losses due to disease. Many different plans or programs are now available to feedlot managers, but there are still a number of feedlots that use veterinarians for emergency services only and have not accepted the concept of veterinarians as providers of preventive medicine service. Perhaps part of the reason that these managers are not using a veterinarian in this role is that a health program has never been presented to them with the objectives and procedures spelled out and the program explained so they might better understand what they would be receiving for their money.

There are at least 3 factors contributing to the lack of feedlot health programs being presented to feedlot managers: the veterinarian does not have the time necessary to spend researching, designing, and then carrying out a preventive medicine program; feedlot managers are independent and prefer to run their own businesses and use veterinarians in the traditional role as emergency doctors; and veterinarians have a very difficult time charging for their advice and have not done a good job of marketing their expertise.

There is a real need for all of us in the veterinary profession to consider possible ways to better market our services. There are many programs already in use in some feedlots, swine units, and poultry operations that could be reviewed and at least some ideas utilized in developing new plans that might better meet the needs of the feedlot clients.

There are some feedlot managers or owners who simply have not been convinced that veterinarians are able to contribute on the management level. These feedlots might need a different plan, a different approach, or possibly a different veterinarian. Just as managers choose nutritional consultants, not on the basis of their geographic location, they are also free to choose their veterinarian as one who meets their particular needs and with whom they feel comfortable working.

Charging for advice is a relatively new concept in veterinary medicine. Collecting fees for client consultation and health care planning continues to be a controversial topic still criticized by some in the profession of veterinary medicine. The main solution to this problem will come from the innovative veterinarians who are able to professionally develop and market their plans without professional service fees being hidden in product mark-up costs.

There is no "health program" that will be equally effective for all feedlots. Health programs represent a disciplined set of instructions and directives for the implementation of a professional service.

A proper feedlot health program should include (1) a set of goals and objectives; (2) a health record system; (3) receiving schedules; (4) guidelines for detection of sick animals; (5) treatment schedules; and (6) recovery pen management.

GOALS AND OBJECTIVES

The primary goals of a feedlot health program are to reduce losses due to disease (both death losses and treatment costs); to minimize disease outbreaks through proper vaccination, early detection, and diagnosis; and to provide professional assistance in health management.

A set of objectives can be used to plot the course of action and to measure the accomplishments of the health program. This can be achieved by establishing and maintaining a health record system; providing schedules for processing and treatments; providing positive training for cattle crews in observation and handling of cattle, administration of vaccines and treatments, review of animal systems through post-mortem examination, use and action of drugs, sick pen management and nursing care, and sanitation and cleanliness; provision of critical evaluation of the overall feedlot operation to management in a written report to include a review of records, specific pen problems, treatment responses, general cattle health, progress of cattle crew in accomplishing assigned responsibilities, general feedlot conditions (pens, alleys, bunks, fences, and waterers), and cleanliness of processing and treatment areas; and communication with management relative to new developments, products, or techniques.

HEALTH RECORD SYSTEM

In order for any health program to be effective, it is essential to have a record system that maps the progress and can be expected to determine the success or failure of the program.

There are a number of individual treatment cards in use that are made up for each animal as it is removed from its pen for reasons of health. The treatment information is recorded, progress is noted, and the card is retained until that pen is closed out. There are a number of disadvantages to this system: it is necessary to complete a card for each animal pulled; location of individual cards can be difficult if the animal is brought back for retreatment; and accessible storage of the individual cards can be a problem.

1. The *pen treatment card* (Fig. 1) gives information on the health status of an entire pen or group of cattle without requiring a new card for each sick animal. It also lists drugs used, their effectiveness, withdrawal dates, the number of animals treated, and number and reason for deads.

The 6 × 9 pen treatment cards are kept in a file box in the treatment room at the feedlot where the procedures are carried out. Smaller operators find it convenient to keep them in a small, 3-ring notebook; for the farmer feeder who keeps only a few cattle around, keeping these in a zip-lock plastic bag with medical supplies works out very well.

Identifying the animal being treated with a numbered ear tag is most effective for positively identifying that individual animal. If that particular animal needs treatment later in the feeding period, the previous treatments will have been recorded. This aspect is so very important for ensuring that animals will not be marketed before the proper drug withdrawal time.

2. The *daily health reports* (Fig. 2) provide a means of accumulating the information for the monthly report as well as of informing the office or bookkeeper of the daily charges made to a particular pen. These forms can also be used to report cattle movements and processing procedures.

3. The *health summary sheet* (Fig. 3) has been developed to collect the data for the morbidity-mortality report.

4. The *morbidity-mortality report* (Fig. 4) should be used as a monthly summary and can be very valuable in identifying problems as well as in evaluating performance. This same form can be used to make quarterly and annual reports. This report not only summarizes the number of animals being treated for the various reasons, but also identifies the stage of the feeding period in which this occurs as well as the number of animals requiring retreatment. This information is important in evaluating the treatment response and is used to support the clinical impressions observed in the treatment hospital pens.

In larger feedlots, all of these records can be adapted to the computer. The treatment and diagnostic data can be entered either chuteside or from the office. Reports can be generated that will provide the same information as the pen treatment card and the health summary sheet.

The veterinarian should direct and monitor the health record system to ensure that it is accurate and current. The veterinarian should also make sure that the information from these reports is put to use in the health management program.

PEN TREATMENT RECORD

Vaccine Ser. No.

Pen No.______ Lot No.______ Date Rec'd.______ Date Processed______ ______ ______

No. Head______ In Wt.______ Implant______ ______ ______

______ Dip/Pour-on ______ ______ ______

Date Pulled	Hosp. Tag No.	Diagnosis	Day 1		Day 2		Day 3		Day 4		Pen C
			Temp	Treatment	Temp	Treatment	Temp	Treatment	Temp	Treatment	

Printed, Courtesy of Elanco Products Company, Manufacturers of Tylan* 200 Injection AJE

Figure 1. Example of the pen treatment card (6 × 9 file card).

DATE: _____

PEN NO.	HOSP. TAG NO.	DIAGNOSIS (Day 1 Only)		TREATMENT		DAYS ON FEED
		Resp.	Other	Code	Other	

Figure 2. Daily health report.

CLASSIFICATION OF FEEDLOT DISEASES

Classifying feedlot diseases by the systems affected seems to be the most logical method for grouping the diseases both from a diagnostic and from a treatment standpoint. Code numbers are assigned to each different disease. This simplifies and standardizes the record-keeping and aids in assigning treatments to the specific diagnosis.

This diagnostic "list" is made available to the cowboys and cattle crews on a small card that can be carried in the pocket and referred to so that the proper code numbers will be recorded on the pull sheets and daily health record (Fig. 2). Table 1 summarizes the incidence of feedlot diseases by system. Refer to the bibliography for more detailed disease descriptions.

Respiratory System

Code No. 1: Respiratory (Pneumonia)

This is the most common disease in feedlot cattle, accounting for up to 80 per cent of the morbidity and 50 to 60 per cent of the mortality. The symptoms include all of the signs associated with shipping fever, such as depression, nasal discharge, rapid breathing, and a gaunt appearance.

CODE	DIAGNOSIS	CODE	DIAGNOSIS	CODE	DIAGNOSIS
1	Respiratory	9	Overeating	17	Uterine Infection
2	Respiratory chronic	10	Coccidiosis	18	Waterbelly
3	Diphtheria	11	Foot Rot	19	Brainer
4	Allergic Pneumonia	12	Lameness	20	Buller Injury
5	Honker	13	Injury	21	Heat Stroke
6	Bloat	14	Downer	22	Unknown
7	Noneater	15	OB (Calving)	23	Misc
8	Scours	16	Prolapse		

DATE	FIRST TREATMENTS			DEADS (D) or BULLERS (B)			TRTMNT COST	NEW CATTLE RECEIVED	FIRST TRTMNT TOTAL
	Less than 45	45 - 90	Over 90	Less than 45	45 - 90	Over 90			
1/16									
2/17									
3/18									
4/19									
5/20									
6/21									
7/22									
8/23									
9/24									
10/25									
11/26									
12/27									
13/28									
14/29									
15/30									
31									

Figure 3. Health summary sheet.

Code No. 2: Respiratory (Chronic)

Animals with more advanced signs of respiratory infection or animals that have been treated and have failed to respond would fit into this classification. The signs observed would include severe depression, a dry crusty nose, rough hair coat, and a gaunt appearance.

Code No. 3: Diphtheria

This disease generally occurs after the cattle have been in the feedlot for at least 45 days. It is usually an acute infection manifested by difficult, noisy breathing. The incidence is generally less than 5 per cent of the morbidity. Differentiating this disease from the other two "hard-breathing" conditions, allergic pneumonia and honker, may seem academic because the treatments can be very similar. The importance of an accurate diagnosis becomes obvious when one considers the different etiologic agents and the different recommendations for prevention.

Code No. 4: Allergic Pneumonia

This disease is probably diagnosed more often on the basis of necropsy findings than from the clinical signs. The cause is not well understood, but the majority of evidence points to a

Feedlot _____ No. _____

Reporting Period _____

No. on feed end of period _____

No. received _____ Strs _____ Av wt _____

Hfrs _____ Av wt _____

	Diagnosis	Less than 45 days		45–90 days		Over 90 days	
		Trmts	Deads	Trmts	Deads	Trmts	Deads
Resp	[1]Respiratory	11	12	13	14	15	16
Resp	[2]Respiratory chronic	21	22	23	24	25	26
Resp	[3]Diphtheria	31	32	33	34	35	36
Resp	[4]Allergic pneumonia	41	42	43	44	45	46
Resp	[5]Honker	51	52	53	54	55	56
Diges	[6]Bloat	61	62	63	64	65	66
Diges	[7]Noneater	71	72	73	74	75	76
Diges	[8]Scours	81	82	83	84	85	86
Diges	[9]Overeating	91	92	93	94	95	96
Diges	[10]Coccidiosis	101	102	103	104	105	106
Skel	[11]Foot Rot	111	112	113	114	115	116
Skel	[12]Lameness	121	122	123	124	125	126
Skel	[13]Injury	131	132	133	134	135	136
Skel	[14]Downer	141	142	143	144	145	146
U/G	[15]OB (Calving)	151	152	153	154	155	156
U/G	[16]Prolapse	161	162	163	164	165	166
U/G	[17]Uterine infection	171	172	173	174	175	176
U/G	[18]Waterbelly	181	182	183	184	185	186
CNS	[19]Brainer	191	192	193	194	195	196
CNS	[20]Buller injury	201	202	203	204	205	206
Misc	[21]Heat Stroke	211	212	213	214	215	216
Misc	[22]Unknown	221	222	223	224	225	226
Misc	[23]Misc	231	232	233	234	235	236
	TOTALS						

Total hosp pulls [237] _____

Total repeats [238] _____

Cost/pull [239] _____

Total deads [240] _____

% of Inv. [241] _____

Dead in pen [242] _____

Bullers total [243] _____ [244] _____ [245] _____ [246] _____

No. Realizers Sold [247] _____ No. condemned [248] _____

Figure 4. Morbidity-mortality report.

Table 1. 5-YEAR SUMMARY OF 10 MIDWESTERN FEEDLOTS: MORBIDITY/MORTALITY REPORTS CLASSIFIED BY SYSTEM

				Morbidity					
		No. of				Percentage			
Year	No. Rec'd	Pulls	% of Rec'd	RESP	DIG	SKLT	U/G	CNS	Misc
1985	372,175	26,674	7	65	6	19	4	0	5
1986	377,634	27,769	7	71	4	17	4	0	3
1987	439,324	41,042	9	79	4	8	3	0	5
1988	486,899	33,469	7	67	5	6	5	0	17
1989	718,756	39,164	5	79	5	7	3	0	4
				Mortality					
						Percentage			
Year	No. Rec'd	No. Dead	% of Rec'd	RESP	DIG	SKLT	U/G	CNS	Misc
1985	372,175	2,420	.65	65	11	5	5	2	12
1986	377,634	2,157	.57	56	22	4	4	1	13
1987	439,324	3,382	.77	67	14	4	4	2	10
1988	486,899	3,259	.67	65	18	4	3	2	7
1989	718,756	5,202	.72	56	29	4	4	2	6

RESP = respiratory system, codes 1–5; DIG = digestive system, codes 6–10; SKLT = skeletal system, codes 11–14; U/G = Urogenital System, codes 15–18; CNS = central nervous system, code 19; Misc = miscellaneous diseases, codes 20–23;

gut-related condition probably triggered by a mold. The signs, if observed, are quite similar to diphtheria, except for more open-mouth breathing and increased respiratory grunting sounds common in animals suffering from emphysema. Examination of the bunks may reveal some build-up of caked feed and mold, and this evidence plus the typical heavy, wet lung devoid of pneumonia lesions at necropsy can be very helpful in arriving at a diagnosis.

Code No. 5: Honker

This syndrome has been recognized for the past several years in feedlot cattle. It is more prevalent during hot weather and can be triggered by increased exercise, such as when fat cattle are moved or handled and during bulling activity in a pen. The loud barking sounds made at expiration are a result of the severe edema of the lower tracheal mucosa-submucosa, which causes obstructive dyspnea.

Digestive System

Code No. 6: Bloat (Ruminal Tympany)

The incidence of feedlot bloat has been somewhat reduced since the development of the ionophores but still is No. 2 in cause of death, behind respiratory diseases.

Code No. 7: Noneater

A number of animals entering the feedlot do not readily accept the rations presented to them, are timid and refuse to go to the bunk, or simply do not consume an adequate amount of feed; therefore they seem to have a gaunt appearance, compared with other animals in their pens. These signs can be very similar to those associated with an early infection. They are generally differentiated from disease symptoms by a normal respiratory rate and a normal temperature. Animals can be removed from their pens because they are not competing and then can be held in a hospital environment for closer observation.

Code No. 8: Scours

Many digestive disorders are manifested by some type of scours or diarrhea. They may be caused by an infectious agent or simply be the result of a gastrointestinal upset due to a change in feed. The signs of scours include the presence of loose stools in the pen and also the feces-smeared hindquarters and generally gaunt appearance of the animal.

Code No. 9: Overeating (Enterotoxemia)

Enterotoxemia is usually diagnosed at necropsy on an animal that has been on feed for a time and then found dead in the pen. The symptoms observed of typical overeating would include a full appearance with possible drooling, a staggering gait, and usually a foamy diarrhea.

Code No. 10: Coccidiosis

Bloody or a black tarry diarrhea is generally quite diagnostic of coccidiosis. This disease is seen much less frequently since the ionophores and other prophylactic agents have been developed.

Musculoskeletal System

Code No. 11: Foot Rot (Infectious Pododermatitis)

The most obvious sign of foot rot in feedlot cattle is lameness in one limb. There is usually swelling between the toes of the affected foot from the invasion of this soft tissue with the invading soil organism. Differentiating this disease from BVD, founder (laminitis), or injury can be done by close observation of the type of lameness the animal exhibits and from an examination of the foot involved. Because this is caused by a soil organism, the history of the incidence of foot rot in the particular feedlot or area is important. Heavy soil seems to provide a better environment for the agent, and new pens, or pens that have been recently cleaned, are more likely to have a higher incidence of this disease.

Code No. 12: Lameness

This classification refers to animals that are obviously lame but not as a result of pododermatitis or injury (i.e., a swollen joint or reluctance of the animal to place weight on the limb). These symptoms need considerably more work-up for accurate diagnosis of the cause of the lameness.

Code No. 13: Injury

Not all feedlot cattle that are non–weight-bearing and have a foot lesion necessarily have infectious pododermatitis (foot rot). Injuries to the feet are not uncommon in cattle, and in many instances the evidence of some sort of trauma to differentiate it from pododermitis (foot rot) is detected only after a close inspection of the foot. The importance of differentiating becomes quite obvious when you consider the treatment for these diseases but even more important when preventive measures are considered.

Code No. 14: Downer

This is quite a general classification but has seemed appropriate for identifying those animals that are unable to rise because of injury, such as heifers might receive from being ridden when in heat, or animals that thaw out a depression in the frozen pen during severe cold and then traumatize themselves while trying to get up.

Urogenital System

Code No. 15: OB (Calving)

The early signs of parturition in fat heifers can be very similar to those of early respiratory infection, a noneater, or even bloat. If heifers are not examined for pregnancy at arrival and an abortion program is not followed, abortions may occur any time during the feeding period.

Code 16: Prolapse

The signs of prolapse are quite obvious and can occur at any time during the feeding period. The vaginal prolapses generally occur late in the feeding period and tend to be more breed-associated, with Hereford heifers being the most susceptible.

Code 17: Uterine Infection

A vaginal discharge after calving or an abortion is usually the sign of a uterine infection. Heifers that have been aborted with use of a prostaglandin and then determined to be sick should be rectally examined for determining whether a uterine infection is present.

Code No. 18: Waterbelly

Urinary calculi are not common in feedlot steers because the cause has become better understood and nutritionists are doing a much better job of keeping track of proper calcium and phosphorus balance.

Central Nervous System

Code No. 19: Brainer

All of the central nervous system diseases are grouped under one general heading and include diseases such as polioencephalomalacia, thromboembolic meningoencephalitis, nervous coccidiosis, and brain abscesses. The symptoms are so similar that it is very difficult to determine a diagnosis from the clinical signs alone. Generally, therapy is quite unrewarding. A differential diagnosis from gross and microscopic lesions is important so that prophylactic procedures might be initiated to prevent further losses.

Miscellaneous Diseases

Code No. 20: Buller Injury

Code No. 21: Heat Stroke

Code No. 22: Unknown

Code No. 23: Miscellaneous

SCHEDULES

Processing Schedule

Proper processing procedures should be considered very important. Properly trained workers can be one of the most effective ways of reducing the common problems associated with processing (i.e., crippled cattle and injection abscesses). Responsible people should be assigned to these tasks for ensuring that the proper dosages of all materials, the proper route of administration, and cleanliness in administering these products are closely adhered to.

A processing schedule should be developed by the veterinarian for each feedlot. An example of such a schedule follows:

PROCESSING SCHEDULE	
	_____ FEEDLOT
DATE:	VETERINARIAN:
VACCINATIONS	Multiple Clostridial Bacterin Multiple Polyvalent MLV Vaccine (IBR, BVD, PI$_3$, BRSV)
PARASITE CONTROL	
IMPLANT	
EAR TAG	
OTHER PROCEDURES:	Tip Horns Bob Tails Pregnancy Examine Heifers

Revaccination

Research has shown that *revaccinating* certain classes of feeder cattle at 7 days with a multiple polyvalent MLV vaccine (IBR, BVD PI$_3$, BRSV) is beneficial. The criteria used to determine which incoming cattle will be revaccinated include

1. Age. Newly weaned calves or cattle weighing under 500 pounds.
2. Source. Cattle direct from the farm or ranch.
3. Stress. Highly stressed cattle, when it is suspected that at least 10 per cent will need treatment during the first few weeks after receipt.
4. Special cases. Cattle that have a high morbidity rate in particular pens due to respiratory disease.

As soon as the processing procedures are completed, the cattle should be placed in a pen with feed and water available and adequate bunk space for the cattle to get to the feed. Some cattle may refuse to drink from the automatic waterers, and it may be necessary to place a large tank in the pen. Keeping new cattle separate from cattle that have already started on feed will give the new ones a better chance to compete as well as aid in reducing the spread of disease.

Treatment Schedule

Treatment schedules should be established by the veterinarian for the major diseases to be treated in the feedlot. Well-defined treatment schedules tend to put emphasis on the *time* of treatment rather than on the drug required to "save" the severely sick animal. The schedule serves as an accurate set of directions that includes the disease to be treated, the drug and dosage to be used, the route of administration of the drug, and the days withdrawal before slaughter. It is important that these schedules be closely followed and accurate records of the treatments be maintained. This allows proper evaluations to be made of the results (i.e., response of animals and drug selection). Any change in therapy must be based on results that do not meet the expectations of the veterinarian and hospital. Changes in therapy are applied to new pulls and should not be expected to succeed on cattle already treated for 3 days. Proper evaluations also ensure that animals will not be sent to slaughter until proper withdrawal time has elapsed.

TRAINING FEEDLOT PERSONNEL

The veterinarian should be actively involved in training of all employees associated with cattle at the feedlot. There are specific areas of training that should be given special attention for ensuring that the health program is being properly carried out.

The duties of the pen riders should be clearly spelled out. Regular training sessions can be very helpful for teaching riders to observe and detect critical signs in problem animals. Hospital crews need special training so that proper technique in administering prescribed treatments is ensured.

HOSPITAL PEN MANAGEMENT

Managing the hospital pens is an area that is often severely neglected in the feedlot health program. Good nursing care may be the best medicine that an animal can receive, and if this is neglected, it is usually of little value to waste expensive medicine on the animal. Hospital pens should be as the term implies, conducive to recovery. Having at least 4 hospital pens so that each day's hospital pulls can be kept separate is ideal. Not only does this provide a better environment for the sick animal, but it does not impose the added stress of sorting the animals daily. It is much easier for the personnel doing the treating to make evaluations on their treatments because they do not have to compare the recently pulled animal with one that has been treated for a number of days.

After the third day, the animal should be returned to its pen, retreated and placed back in a hospital pen, or placed in a separate chronic or realizer pen. It is very important that hospital pens be managed properly. Because animals are brought to the hospital pens every day, the same schedule should be followed for returning the recovered animals to their home pen on a daily basis.

The veterinarian should place a great deal of emphasis on proper hospital pen management and be very critical of the care that these animals receive. The ration should be kept fresh and should be very palatable. The animals should have clean water available, and good sanitation should be maintained for these recuperating animals.

SUMMARY

The veterinarian should assume a positive role in managing feedlot health. The health program should include a set of goals and objectives, a health record system, receiving schedules, guidelines for detecting sick animals, treatment schedules, and hospital pen management.

Implementation of any successful program involves effective communication and cooperation between the veterinarian and feedlot personnel.

BIBLIOGRAPHY

Blood DC, Radostits OM, Henderson JA, with contributions by Arundel JH, Gay CC: Veterinary Medicine: A Textbook of the Diseases of Cattle, Sheep, Pigs, Goats, and Horses, 7th ed. London, Bailliere Tindall, 1989.

Church DC: The Ruminant Animal: Digestive Physiology and Nutrition. Engelwood Cliffs, NJ, Prentice Hall, 1988.

Current Veterinary Therapy: Food Animal Practice 2. Howard JL (ed). Philadelphia, WB Saunders, 1986.

Jensen R, Mackey DR: Diseases of Feedlot Cattle, 3rd ed. Philadelphia, Lea & Febiger, 1979.

Jones TC, Hunt RD: Veterinary Pathology, 5th ed. Philadelphia, Lea & Febiger, 1983.

Jubb KVF, Kennedy PC, Palmer N: Pathology of Domestic Animals, 3rd ed. Orlando, Academic Press, 1985.

Kahrs RF: Viral Diseases of Cattle, 1st ed. Ames, Iowa State University Press, 1981.

Radostits OM, Blood DC: Herd Health: A Textbook of Health and Production Management of Agricultural Animals. Philadelphia, WB Saunders, 1985.

Slauson DO, Cooper BJ: Mechanisms of Disease: A Textbook of Comparative General Pathology. Baltimore, Williams & Wilkins, 1990.

Smith BP: Large Animal Internal Medicine: Diseases of Horses, Cattle, Sheep, and Goats. St. Louis, CV Mosby, 1990.

Veterinary Pharmacology and Therapeutics, 6th ed. Booth NH, McDonald LE (eds). Ames, Iowa State University Press, 1988.

Dairy Cow Production Medicine

MARTIN L. VAN DER LEEK, BVSc, MRCVS
DAVID P. KELBERT, DVM
G. ARTHUR DONOVAN, DVM

Veterinary involvement in dairy operations has evolved dramatically over the last 20 years. Today, the treatment and prevention of disease forms a vital but only minor part of what is more aptly referred to as production medicine. The components of a production medicine program are listed in Table 1. The ultimate goal of such a program is to maximize herd income by *optimizing* milk production within the unique constraints presented by each dairy operation. These include not only the physical constraints imposed by factors such as the available facilities and feedstuffs but, more important, those constraints imposed by the attitude and aspirations of the herd owner-manager and personnel. The successful dairy

Table 1. COMPONENTS OF A PRODUCTION MEDICINE PROGRAM

Record-keeping
Nutrition and feedbunk management
Reproduction
Milking management, udder health, and milk quality
Dry cows
Replacement rearing
Disease treatment, prevention, and control (health program)
Culling practices
Producer education and personnel training
Residue avoidance

practitioner is one who recognizes and works within these constraints, setting attainable goals with the producer and making realistic recommendations. Although many of the components making up a production medicine program may be in need of revision, the veterinarian needs to prioritize them and address them one at a time so as not to overwhelm the producer.

When a production medicine program is initiated, rapid results are important. The veterinarian should attempt to target those components that respond rapidly to changes. Herd nutrition is potentially most responsive, followed by udder health and then reproduction. The elimination, replacement, or reduced use of an expensive feed ingredient may boost profits almost immediately, whereas changes made in the replacement rearing program will impact the herd only 2 years later.

Regular farm visits and an appreciation of the dairy cows' needs afford the veterinarian an opportunity to become a vital part of the dairy production team, which may include computer experts, nutritionists, geneticists, milking machine specialists, agricultural economists, allied health professionals, and more.

This chapter, by no means exhaustive, attempts to provide some practical recommendations concerning each component of the production medicine program, particularly for the inexperienced practitioner initiating a dairy production medicine program. Numerous references are available detailing all aspects of herd health and production medicine programs (see bibliography), and several aspects are discussed elsewhere in this text.

RECORD-KEEPING AND DATA ANALYSIS

Individual animal identification and record-keeping are essential for determining the status of the operation. Once the

Table 2. RECORD-KEEPING SYSTEMS AND SELECTED COMPUTERIZED SYSTEMS AVAILABLE IN NORTH AMERICA*

No records	Programs of regional DHIAs
"Memorized" records	DairyChamp
Manual record-keeping	Dairy Comp 305
Card system	Dairy Herd Health Monitor
Cow wheel/clock	DairyTrak
Computerized record-keeping	VetCheck
On-farm system	VAMPP
Subscription service	

*This is not intended as a complete listing of programs available, nor does it imply an endorsement of these programs by the authors.

herd status is known, selected parameters can be monitored and trends can be analyzed. Although computers facilitate record-keeping and analysis, especially in large dairy herds, manual record-keeping systems can be used as effectively (Table 2). Key aspects to be considered when one is utilizing any record-keeping system include (1) the validity of the data, (2) the correct analysis of appropriate parameters, (3) the formulation of realistic recommendations, and (4) the need for continual re-evaluation to monitor trends.

In addition to the data and computer services offered by the Dairy Herd Improvement Associations (DHIAs), several software programs are available to assist in the management of dairy operations (Table 2). The computer hardware required might be prohibitively expensive for smaller dairy operations, which would provide the interested practitioner an opportunity to establish a subscription service using one of the available software packages. Many of these programs are compatible with DHIA programs, allowing the easy transfer of data by modem. Few of the computer programs are all-encompassing, and a combination of programs may have to be used to best serve the producer. The computer services of the DHIAs,

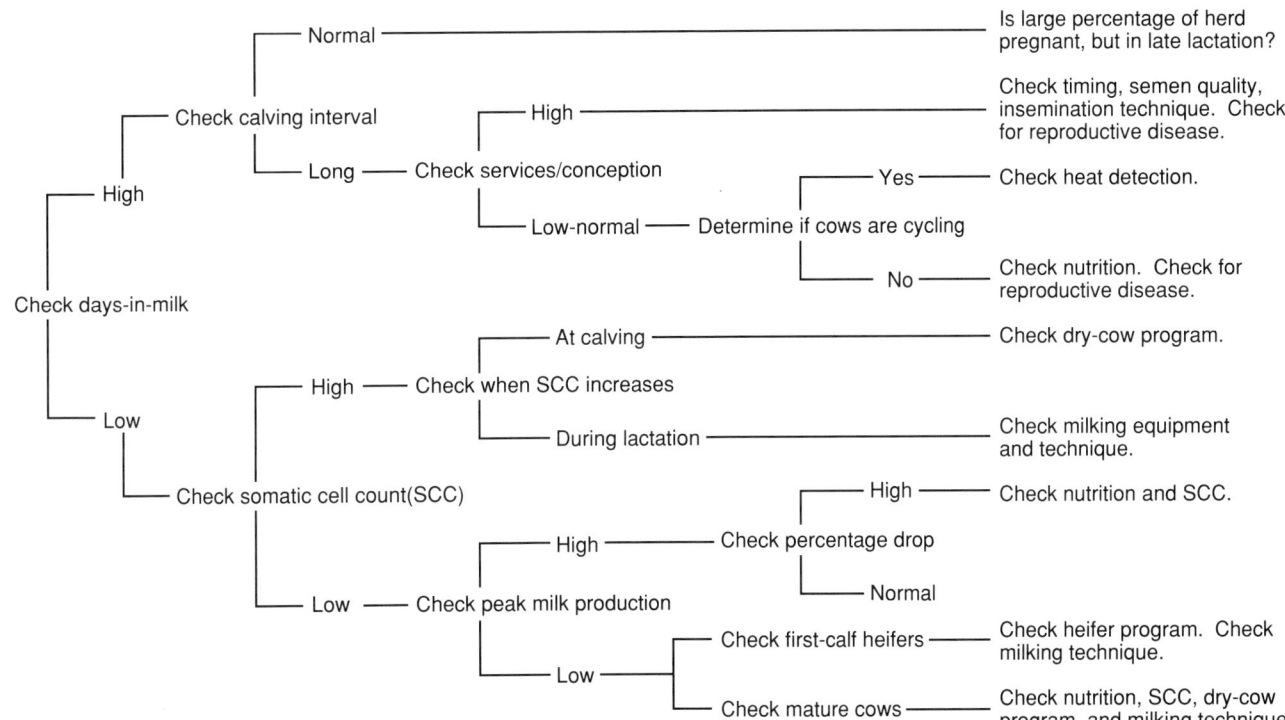

Figure 1. Flow diagram for investigating poor milk production. (Adapted from Gardner CE: Compend Contin Educ Pract Vet 8:F143–148, 1986.)

which concentrate on and provide good production and reproduction data, can be augmented by programs capable of handling disease data, body condition scores, and other factors. Alternatively, much of this data can be gleaned readily from individual cow cards or the daily log kept on most farms. When analyzed, such accumulated data can become a powerful tool for convincing a producer of shortcomings.

Because optimal herd milk production is the ultimate goal, a flow diagram useful for investigating poor milk production is illustrated in Figure 1.

NUTRITION

Ration analysis and formulation may not be the primary interest of every veterinarian, and many may prefer to consult with a nutritionist concerning these aspects. Dietary management of the dairy cow is discussed in Section 4. Without getting very involved in these aspects, however, the veterinarian can still play a valuable role in the nutrition program by monitoring (1) milk production trends, (2) feedbunk management, (3) cow body condition scores, and (4) the prevalence and incidence of nutrition-related diseases and conditions.

The primary objective of the nutritional program is to maximize dry matter intake during early to mid lactation because maximizing the intake above maintenance requirements will improve milk production and increase profits. Several factors that influence feed intake are listed in Table 3. Feedbunk management should be evaluated during every farm visit. Accurate records are essential for determining feed intake and should include the amounts of all feeds provided daily to each group, estimates of free-choice hays and parlor feed consumed, the amount of feed removed from the bunks ("weighback" feed), and the number of animals per production groups, where applicable. This information should be summarized weekly to monthly to allow comparisons with production data.

Body condition scoring should ideally be done 5 times (100 to 60 days before drying off, at drying off, at calving, 15 to 30 days post partum, and at pregnancy examination). A body condition score (BCS) of 3.5 ± 0.5 is recommended at drying off, which should be maintained through the dry period. During lactation, the BCS should never drop below 2.5. Nutrition-related diseases and conditions are outlined in Table 4.

REPRODUCTION

Rectal pregnancy and infertility examinations have traditionally formed the nucleus of herd health programs. The cows that should be presented routinely for palpation are listed in Table 5. The flow diagram illustrated in Figure 2 is useful in palpating a cow presented for pregnancy or as a problem breeder.

Numerous indices exist for evaluating herd reproductive performance. The American Association of Bovine Practitioners recently recommended those indices regarded as most useful and practical in an attempt to standardize their method of calculation (Table 6). Two useful indices of overall herd reproductive status are average days open (or calving-to-conception interval) and calving interval. These indices are a function of heat detection and conception rate. Heat detection is usually the weak link in most breeding programs, with 50 per cent of the cows in heat being missed on the average artificial insemination–bred herd (poor efficiency). In addition, up to 30 per cent of cows may be incorrectly identified as being in heat (poor accuracy).

Heat detection aids should be used as such but cannot replace adequate time set aside specifically for heat detection at least twice a day. Prostaglandin $F_{2\alpha}$ ($PGF_{2\alpha}$) can be used very successfully to synchronize cows, allowing the personnel to concentrate their heat detection efforts (Table 7). Best results are achieved when cows are subsequently bred when they are observed in heat, compared with timed inseminations. Dairy herd reproductive efficiency is discussed in Section 13.

Table 3. SEVERAL FACTORS TO CONSIDER IN EVALUATION OF FEED INTAKE

Ration Factors	Comments
Energy density	High-density rations require less dry matter intake per unit of milk produced
Forages and quality	Rations with <30–35% forage (dry matter basis) ↓ intake; ensure quality of forages
Rumen fill	Avoid rations containing high levels of poor-quality fiber
Rumen pH	Intake ↓ when rumen pH drops below 5.5
Palatability	Ensure that ingredients are fresh; consider palatability of ingredients (may have to limit-feed)
Moisture levels	Moisture levels >50% may ↓ intake, especially in rations containing fermented feed products
Ration changes	Minimize ration changes; avoid sudden changes
Feedbunk Management	**Comments**
Feed freshness	Check for stale or spoiled feed; bunks should be cleaned out daily; weighback should range from 5–6% of total feed fed daily
Bunk space	Recommended linear bunk space is 2.5–3 feet/cow
Parlor speed	Rapid parlor output requires more feedbunk space because more cows are consuming feed at the same time
Feeding frequency and timing	Feed should be available after each milking; multiple feedings improve intake and stabilize rumen pH (recommend at least 4 times); cows should be fed at the same times each day
Environment	Heat stress management vital in hot climates; fresh water should be available and accessible at all times; feeding areas should remain clean and accessible at all times
Grouping	Frequent regrouping ↓ feed intake (recommend no more than 3 times per lactation); inadvertent mixing of cows ↓ feed intake

Table 4. COMMON NUTRITION-RELATED DISEASES AND CONDITIONS

Disease/Condition	Cause
Anestrus	Energy deficiency and mineral imbalances
Bloat	Excessive grain or protein (especially from legumes)
Displaced abomasum	Low fiber, excessive grain before calving; abrupt changes in level of grain feeding
Fat cow syndrome	Energy excess during late lactation and dry period
Hypomagnesemia	Lush pasture (↓ magnesium, ↑ potassium and nitrogen); excessive protein, low fiber
Milk fever	Calcium imbalance and dietary cation-anion difference
Milk fat depression	Low fiber; glucogenic-lipogenic imbalance
Poor peak production	Low energy or protein level
Poor persistence	Low energy or protein level
Primary ketosis	Excessive protein (excessive butyrate); inadequate energy; overconditioned cows
Retained placenta	Selenium, vitamin E deficiency
Rumen acidosis Indigestion Laminitis	Excessive, pulsatile grain feeding; inadequate alkalinity or buffering of diet
Secondary ketosis	Low energy intake during late dry period

Source: Adapted from Ferguson JD, et al: Veterinary nutritional advisory services to dairy farms. Compend Contin Educ Pract Vet 9:F192–F200, 1987.

Table 5. COWS THAT SHOULD BE PRESENTED FOR RECTAL REPRODUCTIVE EXAMINATIONS

Group	Time	Action
Pregnancy	35 to 50 days after breeding	Follow flow diagram as in Figure 2
Prebreeding	15 to 30 days postcalving	Determine status of uterine involution
Problem breeders	Cows ≥ 50 days after calving and not showing heat; cows requiring repeated breedings; cows with abnormal heat cycles	Determine cause and treat accordingly (Fig. 2)
Dry-off rechecks	At dry-off	Confirm pregnant
Miscellaneous	Cows with discharge; cows confirmed pregnant but in heat; cows past due; cows that have aborted	Determined by reason for examination

Table 6. REPRODUCTIVE INDICES FOR WHICH THE AMERICAN ASSOCIATION OF BOVINE PRACTITIONERS HAS RECOMMENDED METHODS OF CALCULATION

Overall reproductive performance
  Projected minimum average days-open
  Past years days-open
  Projected calving interval
  Past calving interval
Estrus detection efficiency
  Percentage of possible breedings that were serviced
Conception efficiency
  Services per pregnancy (all cows)
  Services per pregnancy (pregnant cows)
  Service-specific conception rates
Pregnancy losses
  Abortions per known pregnancy (%)
Cows leaving the herd due to reproductive failure
  Reproductive cull rate (%)
Reproductive efficiency in herds using a bull
  Percentage pregnant by the bull
  Average days-open with the bull
  Average days-in-milk when turned to the bull
  Bull services per pregnancy
  Bull conception rate
  Bull usage rate

Additional aspects of the reproductive program that should be evaluated and monitored include calving area management and reasons for reproductive inefficiency. Calving area management evaluation should include the monitoring of dry cow BCS and the incidence and reasons for dystocia and calf mortality. The veterinarian should also help ensure that an adequate calving environment is provided. Reasons for reproductive inefficiency should be determined by monitoring the prevalence and incidence of retained fetal membranes, metritis and other urogenital infectious diseases (especially if bulls are used), cystic ovarian disease, abortions, fetal wastage, and retained placenta.

MILKING MANAGEMENT, UDDER HEALTH, AND MILK QUALITY

Occasional farm visits should be planned such that the veterinarian can specifically evaluate the parlor procedures during milking time. Several aspects of the parlor procedures that are easy to evaluate are outlined in Table 8.

A valuable tool for monitoring overall herd udder health and milk quality is bulk tank milk sampling. A bulk tank milk sample can be collected on every herd visit and submitted for analysis (Table 9). Bulk tank sampling should be augmented by herd somatic cell count profiles and the sampling of individual cows for culture and sensitivity to confirm the presence of udder pathogens or environmental pathogens and to determine appropriate control measures and antibiotic therapy. Mastitis is discussed in Section 13.

Of increasing importance is the veterinarian's role in milk quality by ensuring that milk is residue-free. Drug labeling of prescription drugs is the responsibility of the veterinarian and is particularly important when there is a need for extra-label drug usage. Before recommending the extra-label usage of drugs, the veterinarian should feel comfortable that a valid client-patient producer relationship exists. This relationship requires, among others, that the veterinarian is familiar with the operation. The veterinarian can also assist in ensuring that drugs are properly stored (to comply with the Pasteurized Milk Ordinance) and used appropriately and by recommending the use of on-farm milk residue tests or providing this service in his or her practice.

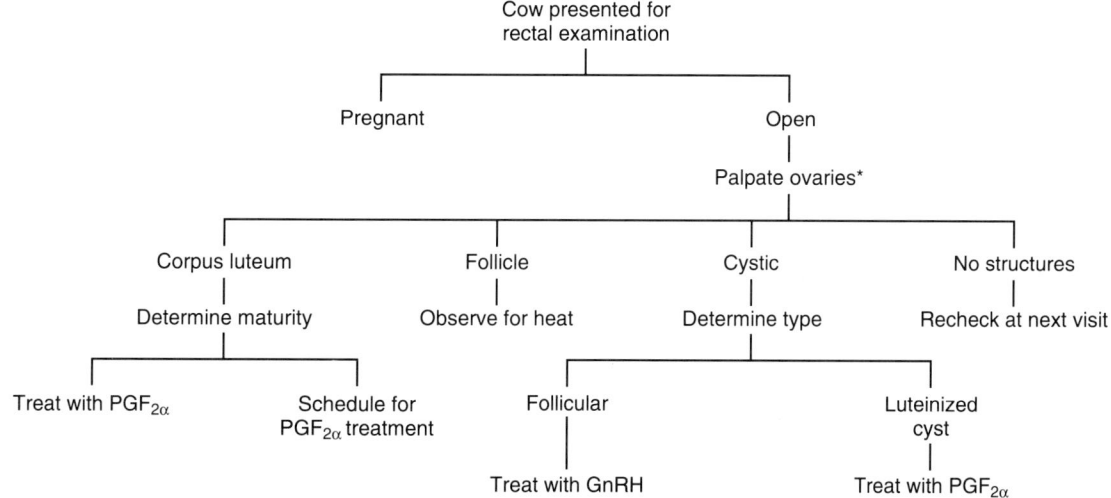

*Also evaluate uterine wall tone and thickness as well as the presence or absence of fluid

Figure 2. Flow diagram for use in performing rectal fertility examinations.

Table 7. UTILIZATION OF PROSTAGLANDIN $F_{2\alpha}$ ($PGF_{2\alpha}$) IN BREEDING PROGRAMS

Option	Comments
1. Cows are assigned for treatment after rectal palpation	2-week visits: cows with a corpus luteum are treated; monthly visits: cows with a corpus luteum are treated, other cows are assigned for later treatment depending on stage of cycle
2. All cows are treated at a fixed time postcalving, e.g., 45 days	Palpation not required; treatments are given on Mondays, allowing heat detection efforts to be concentrated on Wednesday through Friday
3. Progesterone assays are used to identify cows with a corpus luteum	Palpation not required; less $PGF_{2\alpha}$ is used; consider cost and accuracy of tests

Other considerations:
1. In options 2 and 3, cows are retreated a predetermined number of times. If they do not respond, they are presented for rectal palpation.
2. Good identification is essential for ensuring that pregnant cows are not treated with $PGF_{2\alpha}$ and for facilitating heat detection in treated cows.
3. Postpartum rectal examinations should be done as usual.
4. Too many cows should not be treated at once.

DRY COWS

Because most attention is usually focused on the milking herd, dry cow management (and replacement rearing) is often neglected. By routinely visiting the dry cows, the veterinarian can help ensure success by monitoring BCSs and by making certain that sufficient high-quality forage is available. The primary goals of dry cow management include (1) minimizing metabolic disease conditions during early lactation and (2) ensuring optimal body condition for maximal milk production and to prevent dystocia. During the last 2 to 3 weeks of the dry period, special consideration must be given to adapting the rumen environment to the components of the lactating cow ration.

REPLACEMENT REARING

Dairy replacement rearing programs are discussed in the preceding article.

HEALTH PROGRAMS

A single, all-encompassing health program is inappropriate, and the program should be tailored to each situation. The important components of a health program for adult cows are

Table 8. SELECTED ASPECTS OF MILKING PROCEDURES THAT SHOULD BE EVALUATED

Cow flow	Cow flow into the parlor should be quiet and voluntary
Udder preparation	Ensure that the udders are clean and dry
Milking technique	Monitor machine attachment, parlor and milker hygiene, milk letdown, and occurrence of liner slip
Teat dipping	Ensure that entire teat surface is covered
Milking routine	Promote establishment of a consistent milking routine within and between shifts
Equipment check	Examine the milking equipment for general condition and maintenance (inflations, short air tubes, pulsator hoses, milk hoses, pulsator function, vacuum level and fluctuation)

Table 9. APPROPRIATE ANALYSIS OF A BULK TANK MILK SAMPLE

Test	Indicative of
Somatic cell count	Level of mastitis (particularly subclinical cases)
Standard plate count	Milking hygiene, sanitation and refrigeration
Coliform count	Dirty udders, milking hygiene (fecal contamination)
Laboratory pasteurized count	Equipment washing and sanitation
Microbial identification	Contagious pathogens (*Streptococcus agalactiae*, *Staphylococcus aureus*, *Mycoplasma* spp.)
	Environmental pathogens (coliforms, other *Streptococcus* and *Staphylococcus* spp.)

listed in Table 10. Before recommendations are made, considerations should include the health status of the herd, whether the herd is managed as a closed herd, and the benefit-cost ratio of the procedures envisioned.

Even though a production medicine program concentrates on the herd as such, the individual animal must not be neglected. The regular examination of sick and poor-producing cows may provide valuable clues, particularly the presence and incidence of subclinical diseases.

The development of appropriate treatment protocols helps ensure that animals receive adequate treatment, but more important, such standardized protocols help ensure the absence of drug residues in milk and meat.

CULLING PRACTICES

The veterinarian can assist the producer in making culling decisions by providing accurate prognoses concerning cows with digestive disorders, infertility, mastitis, and feet and leg problems. By monitoring the reasons for which cows are culled and the number of culls per category (reproduction, production, feet and legs, disease, and so on), the veterinarian is better able to determine the health status of the herd. Residue avoidance again is a major issue, and careful consideration should be given before an animal is treated if there is a possibility that she will be culled.

PERSONNEL TRAINING AND PRODUCER EDUCATION

On-farm employee training sessions can be very valuable and may need to be repeated regularly if the employee turnover is high. Areas that should be addressed include disease recognition and treatment, milking technique and sanitation, feedbunk management, heat detection and artificial insemination, replacement rearing, and obstetrics.

Many dairy practices also sponsor regional producer meetings to discuss pertinent topics and to share new developments.

Table 10. COMPONENTS OF AN ADULT COW HEALTH PROGRAM

Vaccination program (particularly for reproductive and respiratory diseases)
External parasite control (flies, tail lice)
Internal parasite control
Strategic treatments (particularly dry cow treatment, but also the use of injectable vitamins such as vitamin E–selenium)
Hoof trimming
Disease monitoring
Disease seroprofiling
Establishment of treatment protocols

SUMMARY

It should be evident from this article that there are a wealth of areas in which the practitioner interested in dairy production medicine can get involved. By starting off in those areas in which he or she has some expertise, the opportunity will arise naturally to extend the program to other areas. The numerous trade journals currently available (often complimentary to veterinarians) are a valuable source of information. For those practitioners interested in a particular area (such as ration formulation, computer usage), regular seminars are presented by universities and extension services and also by the American Association of Bovine Practitioners.

Finally, it is very important that a report be written following each farm visit. Essentially this report should contain a section summarizing the activities of the visit and a section for comments and recommendations. At the end of the year, or even more frequently, a report should be prepared outlining the progress made, re-establishing goals, and identifying areas in need of improvement. The graphic representation of data enhances such reports.

BIBLIOGRAPHY

American Association of Bovine Practitioners: Practitioner's Guide to Drug Labelling and Storage on Dairy Farms. West Lafayette, American Association of Bovine Practitioners, 1990.
Braun RK, et al: Body condition scoring dairy cows as a herd management tool. Compend Contin Educ Pract Vet 8:F62–F67, 1986.
Ferguson JD, et al: Veterinary nutritional advisory services to dairy farms. Compend Contin Educ Pract Vet 9:F192–F200, 1987.
Fetrow J, et al: Dairy herd health monitoring. Part I. Description of monitoring systems and sources of data. Compend Contin Educ Pract Vet 9:F390–F398, 1987.
Fetrow J, et al: Dairy herd health monitoring. Part II. A computer spreadsheet for dairy herd monitoring. Compend Contin Educ Pract Vet 10:75–80, 1988.
Fetrow J, et al: Dairy herd health monitoring. Part III. Implementation and goal setting. Compend Contin Educ Pract Vet 10:373–378, 1988.
Fetrow J, et al: Calculating reproductive indices (recommendations of the American Association of Bovine Practitioners), Calgary, Proceedings, 21st Annual Convention of the American Association of Bovine Practitioners, 1988, pp 198–203.
Gardner CE: Using DHI reports in dairy production medicine. Compend Contin Educ Pract Vet 8:F143–F148, 1986.
Gardner CE (ed): Dairy practice management. Vet Clin North Am [Food Anim Pract] 5, 1989.
Gardner CE: An introduction to creation and analysis of lactation curves. Compend Contin Educ Pract Vet 12:277–283, 1990.
Hjerpe CA (ed): Bovine herd vaccination programs. Vet Clin North Am [Food Anim Pract] 6, 1990.
Jarrett JA: Maximizing feed intake for dairy cows. Compend Contin Educ Pract Vet 8:F23–F29, 1986.
Lesch TE (ed): Herd health management: dairy cow. Vet Clin North Am [Food Anim Pract] 3, 1981.
Mueller M: Computer aided dairy herd management. Agri-Practice 10:3–11, 1989.
Nordlund K: Using adjusted milk calculations. Agri-Practice 10:3–7, 1989.
Radostits OM, Blood DC: Herd Health. Philadelphia, WB Saunders, 1985.
Redlus HW: Interrelating dairy production and self-image psychology. Compend Contin Educ Pract Vet 10:1321–1327, 1988.
Redlus HW: Integrating motivational psychology and DHIA records into the dairy veterinary management program. Compend Contin Educ Pract Vet 9:F207–F211, 1987.

Dairy Replacement Rearing Programs

MARTIN L. VAN DER LEEK, BVSc, MS, MRCVS
G. ARTHUR DONOVAN, DVM
R. KENNETH BRAUN, DVM, MS

With an annual average herd turnover of 25 to 35 per cent, there is a constant need for replacement animals to maintain or increase herd production. Ideally, these replacements should calve for the first time at an age and body weight that would optimize their lifetime production and should be genetically superior. They should also represent a sound investment. Because the return on the investment in a replacement rearing program is delayed, the impact on future herd profitability is not always fully appreciated. As a result, many replacement rearing programs do not receive the attention they deserve.

In smaller herds, the existing facilities may suffice, and labor is more readily spared for raising the heifers needed. In contrast, the timely raising of sufficient heifers for a large dairy operation requires that a distinct replacement rearing program become recognized. Such a program needs dedicated management, sufficient skilled labor, adequate facilities, and priorities and goals. Individual animal identification and record-keeping are essential for determining the status of the operation and ensuring that attainable goals are set. Computers, though not essential, facilitate data-keeping and analyses, making monitoring easy. In addition to the computer services offered by the Dairy Herd Improvement Associations, several software programs are available that are capable of managing replacement herd data.

The goals of a replacement rearing program are to (1) raise more than 80 per cent of the heifer calves born; (2) have them calve at 24 months of age, with a precalving weight of 550 kg (~1200 lb) and a withers height of 140 cm (~55 inches); and (3) have them outproduce first calf heifers of the previous year by at least 90 kg (~200 lb) on a lactational basis.

Irrespective of the milking herd size, a producer should consider raising replacements only if the herd milk production exceeds the regional or state average. If not, resources are best utilized for improving milk production. This article outlines the important considerations for establishing and maintaining a sound replacement rearing program. Together with the input from others in the dairy field (such as animal scientists, nutritionists, allied health professionals, and economists), the veterinarian can help ensure the success of a replacement rearing enterprise, being uniquely qualified to appreciate the relationship between animal health, animal well-being, and herd profitability.

ECONOMIC CONSIDERATIONS

Determined by the herd turnover rate and the calf survival rate, the replacement herd size generally reflects 50 to 75 per cent of the milking herd size. The maintenance costs associated with these replacements account for 15 to 20 per cent of total milk production costs, ranking second only to feed costs. This significant financial input warrants that close attention be paid to the replacement rearing program so that optimal results are ensured. Recent studies show the cost of raising a heifer, from birth to 24 months, ranging from $1080 to $1353.

Other than raising their own, producers have the option of buying replacements or contracting with a calf-raising specialist. Producers raising their own replacements retain control over genetic progress and can ensure optimal growth and health. When contracting, the producer relinquishes control over growth and health while still retaining control over genetic progress. Buying replacements allows rapid returns, provided the animals remain healthy and produce as expected. An experienced eye is necessary to ensure success when heifers are bought, and the statement that "the most expensive diseases are the ones you buy" is especially true. Regional differences in the availability, quality, and price of pregnant heifers need to be taken into consideration. Market price changes make this difficult, and producers may ultimately decide on an option providing peace of mind, even if a more profitable alternative exists. The availability of sufficient space

Table 1. FACTORS TO BE CONSIDERED BEFORE INITIATING A REPLACEMENT REARING PROGRAM

Variable Costs	Fixed Costs	Other
Feed	Depreciation	Mortality
Labor	Interest	Morbidity
Semen	Repairs	Culling rate
Veterinary services	Taxes	Space
Drugs	Insurance	
Supplies		

may ultimately dictate the final decision, especially if herd expansion is being considered.

Partial budgeting is a useful technique for determining the expected net profit (or loss) associated with a replacement rearing program. Factors that should be considered include those listed in Table 1. Because assumptions may have to be made concerning various aspects of the enterprise, for example, calf mortality rate, feed costs, and the projected need for replacements, the analysis should be repeated under different sets of assumptions. Several spreadsheet programs have been developed for estimating the cost of raising dairy replacements.[1] A sensitivity or "what if?" analysis is done simply by replacing pertinent values and allowing the program to recalculate the cost. Finally, before a replacement rearing program is decided on, alternative investment opportunities should be investigated. Investment in a feed mill, for example, may prove to be more profitable.

THE DRY COW

In order to ensure the birth of a live, healthy calf, the dry cow should receive appropriate care. Environmental stress should be minimized and nutrition carefully monitored. Excessive summer temperatures can reduce birth weights owing to adverse effects on the vasculature supplying the fetus, especially during the third trimester when 2/3 of fetal growth occurs.

Cows should have a body condition score (BCS) of 3.5 ± 0.5 at dry-off that should be maintained throughout the dry period. This is achieved by appropriate feeding management throughout the lactation, but particularly during early lactation. Attempts to compensate for a poor BCS during the dry period may cause excessive fetal growth and result in dystocia.

The immunoglobulin content of colostrum can be enhanced by vaccination of the dry cow, although vaccines differ greatly in their ability to improve colostrum quality. Thus far, only vaccination with *Escherichia coli*, for the control of neonatal colibacillosis, has proved to be particularly efficacious.

CALVING AND COLOSTRUM MANAGEMENT

The future health of a calf is greatly influenced by the management actions employed around the time of calving. A clean calving environment, prompt and appropriate assistance during delivery if needed, disinfection of the umbilicus, and the early administration of colostrum are all important considerations. On large dairies, care should be taken to identify calves correctly.

The calving environment might range from an indoor calving pen to a pasture set aside only for calving. Irrespective of the nature of the calving facility, the primary goal should be to provide an environment minimizing exposure to potential pathogens. The importance of cleanliness and gentleness in providing calving assistance is also readily appreciated. Prompt disinfection of the umbilicus with an iodine-containing solution should prevent or decrease umbilical infections, preventing septicemia and arthritis. This is an opportune time to check for congenital abnormalities and to provide adequate, high-quality colostrum.

Because many calves fail to suckle adequately (up to 40 per cent), the administration of a sufficient volume of high-quality colostrum before gut closure is vital. Colostrum is easily collected, tested for immunoglobulin concentration using a colostrometer,[1] and stored for future use by refrigerating, souring, freezing, or adding formaldehyde (1 ml/gallon). Freezing colostrum in plastic milk jugs, coded for quality by the use of colored caps, allows long-term storage (6 months or less) and avoids the potential problems of abnormal fermentation with souring or poor palatability with use of formaldehyde. Irrespective of the method chosen, a sincere commitment from management and calf personnel is needed to ensure success. Calves should be fed colostrum containing greater than 50 mg/dl immunoglobulin and a volume equivalent to 8 to 10 per cent of their birthweight within a few hours after birth. If a colostrometer is not available, only colostrum from the first milking of long-standing, vaccinated herdmates should be stored for use as a first feeding. A practical recommendation is to force-feed 4 L (~1 gallon) colostrum as soon as possible after birth, repeating colostrum feeding at least once more within 12 hours (use an esophageal feeder if necessary). Poorer quality colostrum can be used at later feedings.

The success of a colostrum feeding program can be easily evaluated by means of a refractometer[2] for measurement of serum total protein (TP) concentration in calves from 2 to 10 days of age. The appropriate interpretation of serum TP values for Holstein calves is shown in Table 2. Calves with serum TP values in the gray zone will perform as well as calves with adequate serum TP levels, provided all aspects of management are superior. Other tests, some more difficult to perform and interpret, include radial immunodiffusion, zinc sulfate turbidity, sodium sulfite precipitation, and glutaraldehyde determination. Colostrum absorption is adversely affected by a number of factors, particularly temperature extremes and dystocia. The morbidity, mortality, and growth rate associated with different levels of serum TP are illustrated in Table 3.

HOUSING

Individual housing, designed to prevent contact between calves and the spread of pathogens, is preferred from birth until weaning. Calves can be raised successfully in groups, however, if careful attention is paid to sanitation and ventilation, and if different age groups are kept separated. Besides minimizing disease transmission, individual, separately housed calves are less likely to develop bad suckling habits.

---

[1]A computer spreadsheet program for estimating the cost of raising dairy replacements (for use with Lotus 1-2-3) is available from Dr. J. Fetrow, North Carolina State University, 4700 Hillsborough Street, Raleigh, NC 27601.

Costs to raise dairy heifers (for use with Lotus 1-2-3 or with Microsoft Excel) are available from Dr. A. J. Heinrichs, The Pennsylvania State University, 8 Borland Laboratory, University Park, PA 16802.

[1]Colostrometer, available from NASCO, PO Box 901, Fort Atkinson, WI 53538.

[2]Reichert-Jung Model Refractometer, available from Fisher Scientific, 145 Delta Drive, Pittsburgh, PA 15238.

Universal Hand Refractometer, available from NASCO, PO Box 901, Fort Atkinson, WI 53538.

Table 2. INTERPRETATION OF SERUM TOTAL PROTEIN VALUES (HOLSTEIN CALVES)

Total Protein (mg/dl)	Category
<5.0	Colostrum-deprived
5.0–5.5	Gray zone
5.5–7.5	Colostrum-satisfied
>7.5	Suspect dehydration

Equally as important as providing an environment minimizing exposure to pathogens is the need to keep calves dry and to provide adequate ventilation. This will help ensure optimal growth and will reduce the incidence of pneumonia. Enclosed, environmentally controlled calf barns are not recommended, and even naturally ventilated barns can become a liability because they are difficult to clean and disinfect. The excessive use of water to keep such facilities clean while occupied commonly predisposes calves to pneumonia. The portable hutch remains the superior housing choice under all weather conditions if it is managed correctly. Sufficient hutches should be available to allow them to be left vacant for at least 2 weeks after use, and adequate space is required to allow the hutches to be moved regularly.

Calves are grouped for the first time postweaning at 6 to 12 weeks of age with 10 to 12 calves per pen. They are later regrouped as needed after 6 months of age (up to 60 to 90 per pen). Although grouping is often done by age, it is essential to group calves in the same size and weight range together, which ensures that all calves have an equal opportunity to get to the feed trough. No special housing requirements exist for calves after 7 to 8 months of age, except for protection from weather extremes to help ensure optimal growth.

NUTRITION AND GROWTH

Calves can be fed whole milk, a high-quality milk replacer, or mastitic milk. Milk replacers should contain at least 20 per cent fat and 20 per cent protein if calves are to maintain good health and grow according to targets, especially in cold weather. The first 5 ingredients on the milk replacer label should preferably be of milk origin. Some controversy exists over the healthfulness and safety of feeding mastitic milk to calves. Although most data show no adverse effects on growth or health, it has been suggested that calves fed mastitic milk containing *Staphylococcus aureus* may subsequently develop mastitis. A general recommendation is to feed mastitic milk only if it looks like milk, that is, is not serum-like or grossly contaminated with pus, clots, or blood. The proper washing and sanitation of milk feeding equipment is important, and washing (soap and hot water) should always precede sanitation. Mixing milk replacers in a disposable plastic bag placed inside the mixing drum eliminates the need for cleaning and avoids fat build-up. Whole and mastitic milk should be properly handled and stored (kept cooled).

A starter grain ration, containing 18 to 20 per cent crude protein, should be offered from 3 days of age. This stimulates early rumen development and facilitates weaning. Calves should gain 0.5 kg/day (~1 lb/day) and be ready to wean at 4 to 6 weeks of age or when consuming more than 1 kg (~2 lb) grain per day.

After weaning, calves should be maintained on the starter ration and should be gaining 0.7 to 0.8 kg/day (~1.5 to 1.8 lb/day). At 5 to 6 months of age, calves can be turned out to pasture. Grain feeding (a grower ration, containing 14 to 15 per cent crude protein) and mineral supplementation should continue, and a good-quality hay should be provided to maintain normal rumen function. Nutrient requirements for heifers are presented in Table 4. It is helpful to convert all values to kilograms (pounds) of protein/energy required per head per day because such values are more tangible. This also underscores the need for suitable and accurate feed-weighing equipment to ensure that heifers are fed appropriately.

The desired growth rate of large-breed calves from 6 months of age to calving is 0.7 to 0.75 kg/day (~1.5 to 1.7 lb/day). Gains less than 0.7 kg/day may result in delayed first calving, or the producer may be tempted to breed underweight heifers, whereas gains in excess of 0.75 kg/day may result in the excessive deposition of fatty tissue in the developing mammary gland. The efficiency of weight gain (feed-to-gain ratio) decreases with age owing to increased body maintenance requirements (Fig. 1). As a result, attempts to make up for earlier poor gains are costly. The optimal growth rate may ultimately be determined by the feedstuffs and forage available. Approximate gains for various periods from birth to calving for large-breed calves are listed in Table 5.

Growth monitoring is important to ensure optimal calving age, height, and weight. Ideally, calves should be weighed, and their height measured (at the withers), five times as outlined in Table 6. Periods of poor growth can be identified, the nutritional value of pasture can be monitored, and grain feeding can be adjusted accordingly. Stragglers can be identified and sold to minimize losses or kept apart to receive special attention. Figures 2 and 3 illustrate growth curves (weight and withers height) for Holstein heifers. Similar graphs are available for other breeds.

Good feed trough management is essential. Each calf requires 15 to 18 inches of linear bunk space. Fence-line feeders, although management intensive compared with self-feeders, ensure the availability of fresh feed and allow the daily observation of heifers for growth and health. The addition of a coccidiostat is recommended for both its preventive and growth-promoting effects. Reasons for poor postweaning weight gains are listed in Table 7.

HEALTH

The most common preweaning health problem is diarrhea, caused by improper milk feeding management (poor-quality milk replacer, wrong mixing temperature) or several pathogens (*E. coli*, rotavirus, coronavirus, *Salmonella*, coccidia, and *Cryptosporidium*). Septicemia, caused by *E. coli* and other environmental bacteria and usually seen during the first 2 weeks of life, reflects poor sanitation *and* poor colostrum

Table 3. CALF MORBIDITY, MORTALITY, AND AVERAGE DAILY GAIN ASSOCIATED WITH DIFFERENT LEVELS OF SERUM TOTAL PROTEIN[1]

	Serum Total Protein (mg/dl)			
	<5.0	5.0–5.4	≥5.5	All
Number (%)	75 (14)	169 (33)	275 (53)	519
Morbidity				
Diarrhea	34.6%[a]	27.2%[a]	27.6%[a]	28.5%
Septicemia	9.3%[a]	4.7%[b]	3.6%[b]	4.8%
Mortality	6.7%[a]	0.6%[b]	1.1%[b]	1.7%
Average daily gain (kg/day) 0–150 days	0.71[a]	0.76[b]	0.76[b]	0.75

[1] Data from Holstein calves raised in Florida. (From Donovan GA, et al: Colostrum management in dairy calves. Calgary, Proceedings, Seminar 12, Annual Meeting of the American Association of Bovine Practitioners, 1988.)

[a], [b] Values in the same row with different superscripts are significantly different (p < .05).

Table 4. DAILY NUTRIENT REQUIREMENTS FOR HEIFERS[1]

Body Weight (lb)	Estimated Age (wk)	Daily Gain (lb)	NE (Mcal)	TDN (lb)	Crude Protein (lb)
Large Breeds					
Fed only milk or milk replacer					
90		0.60	1.76	1.32	0.24
110		0.80	2.13	1.70	0.29
Fed milk plus starter					
100		1.00	2.14	2.24	0.44
150		1.80	3.33	3.92	0.77
200	13	1.70	4.07	4.33	0.99
300	20	1.70	5.24	5.56	1.29
400	29	1.70	6.31	6.75	1.60
500	37	1.70	7.33	7.92	1.58
600	45	1.70	8.28	9.09	1.68
700	54	1.70	9.21	10.27	1.94
800	63	1.70	10.10	11.49	2.22
900	71	1.70	10.96	12.75	2.52
1000	80	1.70	11.79	14.07	2.84
1100	90	1.70	12.61	15.48	3.20
1200	100	1.50	12.93	16.09	3.41
1300	110	1.30	13.20	16.65	3.61
Small Breeds					
Fed only milk or milk replacer					
60		0.40	1.25	1.03	0.18
75		0.50	1.57	1.55	0.26
Fed milk plus starter mix					
100		1.10	2.30	2.24	0.44
150		1.30	2.96	3.92	0.77
200	26	1.10	3.64	3.76	0.87
300	37	1.30	5.01	5.32	1.26
400	48	1.30	6.07	6.56	1.34
500	59	1.30	7.08	7.80	1.46
600	70	1.30	8.02	9.07	1.75
700	81	1.30	8.93	10.41	2.07
800	92	1.30	9.81	11.85	2.43
900	105	1.10	10.19	12.52	2.65

[1] National Research Council, 1989 (revised edition).
NE = net energy for maintenance plus net energy for growth; TDN = total digestible nutrients.

Table 5. APPROXIMATE WEIGHT GAINS FOR LARGE-BREED HEIFERS FROM BIRTH TO CALVING

Age (months)	Average Daily Gain (kg)	Gain for the Period (kg)
0–2	0.5	40–70
2–6	0.8	70–165
6–15	0.7	165–355
15–24	0.7	355–550

create a sufficient fly-worry to affect weight gains. In addition, flies can spread the bacterium that causes pink eye and can traumatize teat ends. Respiratory diseases caused by IBR, PI$_3$, *Pasteurella*, and bovine respiratory syncytial virus (BRSV) remain a threat throughout the life of a heifer.

Recommendations applicable to all preventive medicine programs apply to replacement rearing. These include providing a stress-free environment, boosting immunity through vaccination when possible, using strategic treatments where possible, and ensuring that diseases are detected early and treated aggressively. Vaccination recommendations should be made after considering (1) the potential postvaccination sequelae (e.g., injection site abscesses when wet calves are vaccinated, and poor fertility when live viral vaccines are used immediately prebreeding); (2) the potential interference with acquired (colostral) immunity; (3) the potential impact on later serologic testing; (4) the timing of first and subsequent administrations (boosters); (5) the existence of a valid client-patient-veterinarian relationship; and (6) the benefit-cost ratio. Strategic treatments should include the use of injectable vitamins, the feeding of a coccidiostat, and the regular and timely use of dewormers.

Dehorning should be done at 4 to 8 weeks of age, preferably by use of a hot iron, but other methods are available (caustic paste, core dehorner). Extra teats can be removed when dehorning or when vaccinating at 5 to 6 months of age. Besides flies, several other factors may affect udder health. These include exposure to excessively abrasive weeds, mud, and contaminated water holes and the presence of a chronic suckler calf. This problem can be reduced significantly by training calves to drink out of open-faced pails. Blind and mastitic quarters should be monitored regularly and appropriate corrective action taken if needed.

An example health program is outlined in Table 8. A single, all-encompassing health program is inappropriate. The resources and limitations of each program need to be considered before final recommendations are made.

GENETICS–SEMEN SELECTION

Heifers represent all the genetic gains made in the herd over time. For ensuring continued improvement in herd milk production, artificial insemination with use of semen from bulls in the upper 30th percentile of their breed should be used. An increase of 80 to 100 kg milk per year (~200 lb) is

management. Colostrum absorption/management should always be evaluated when excessive losses are investigated in calves under 2 weeks of age. Immediately postweaning and associated with the feed change, calves are susceptible to intestinal clostridial infections. Growth in the older heifer is often stunted by the presence of gastrointestinal nematodes and external parasites. As few as 100 horn flies per animal

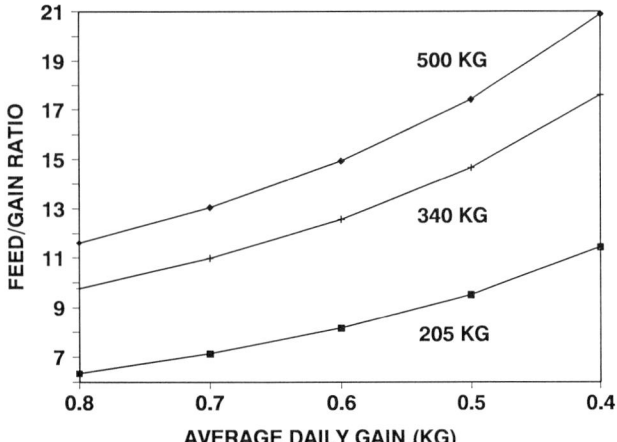

Figure 1. The efficiency of weight gain at various weights and average gains.

Table 6. MONITORING THE GROWTH RATE OF LARGE-BREED HEIFERS

Management Activity	Age (months)	Weight (kg)	Height (cm)
Move to group pens	2	70	85
Brucella vaccination	6	170	105
Regrouping	10	255	125
Prebreeding	14	340	130
Precalving	24	550	140

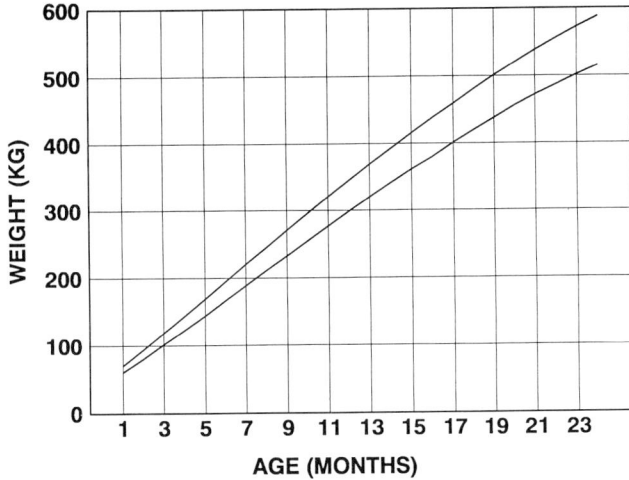

Figure 2. Range of recommended weights for Holstein heifers. (Produced from values recommended by The Pennsylvania State University, College of Agriculture, Cooperative Extension, and developed from data by Heinrichs AJ, Hargrove GL: Standards of weight and height for Holstein heifers. J Dairy Sci 70:653–660, 1987.)

attainable through artificial insemination alone. Because the genetic value of bulls used for natural mating rarely matches that of commercially available bull semen, the use of natural mating should be discouraged. If costs are an important consideration, semen from unproven sires should be used. Sires should have a calving ease of less than 10 per cent for improvement of calf livability and reduction of calving trauma. Care must be taken to ensure that undesirable body conformation traits do not undermine a breeding program. Breeding exclusively for milk production traits can have dire consequences in the long term. Traits affecting cow longevity and health, such as leg and udder conformation, deserve attention.

Genetic improvement is easily undermined by poor growth, chronic disease, and other factors such as a high calf mortality rate and poor breeding management. As calf mortality increases and the heifer pool decreases, the producer loses the ability to select only the superior animals. Poor breeding

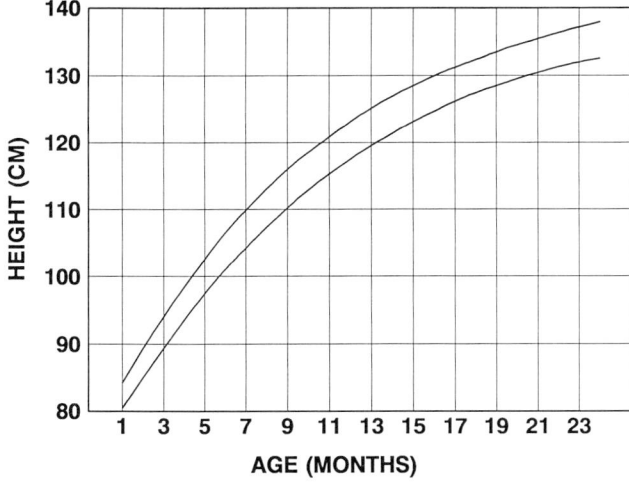

Figure 3. Range of recommended heights for Holstein heifers. (Produced from values recommended by The Pennsylvania State University, College of Agriculture, Cooperative Extension, and developed from data by Heinrichs AJ, Hargrove GL: Standards of weight and height for Holstein heifers. J Dairy Sci 70:653–660, 1987.)

Table 7. REASONS FOR POOR WEIGHT GAIN

Inadequate level of nutrition	Poor grouping
Poor feedbunk management	Disease
Poor pasture management	Environment
Parasitism	Genetics

management, in turn, requires multiple inseminations and forces the producer to use cheaper semen or to consider natural mating.

BREEDING AND THE PREGNANT HEIFER

Although a heifer will have a maximum first lactation milk yield if she calves at 30 to 32 months of age, her lifetime milk yield will be maximized if she calves at 22 to 24 months. A Holstein heifer is ready for breeding when she is 14 to 15

Table 8. EXAMPLE HEALTH PROGRAM FROM BIRTH TO CALVING

The Newborn (1 to 10 days of age)
Inject with 2 ml vitamin E and selenium for prevention of white muscle disease
Inject with 2 ml vitamin A and D (calves are born with small A and D reserves)
Vaccinate with intranasal IBR/PI$_3$, unless the dry cows have been vaccinated
Bleed to determine serum total protein (colostrum absorption)

The Month-old Calf
Dehorn with an electric dehorner
Tattoo with ID in left ear
Vaccinate with 7-way *Clostridium* toxoid/bacterin to prevent overeating disease and bloat
Suggest that hutches be moved regularly to prevent the excessive build-up of pathogens

From 2 to 5 Months of Age
Start an internal parasite control program
Start an external parasite control program, particularly for flies
Use a coccidiostat for control of coccidiosis and for its positive effect on weight gain
Monitor weight and height

At 5 to 6 Months of Age
Vaccinate with *Brucella abortus* strain 19
Vaccinate with IBR/PI$_3$ live virus vaccine; consider including BVD and BRSV vaccination
Booster with 7-way *Clostridium* bacterin
Remove extra teats and check udder
Deworm
Monitor weight, height, and body condition score to determine growth performance

From 6 to 13 Months of Age
Deworm and maintain external parasite control
Monitor growth and regroup as necessary
Observe daily for disease (easily done at feeding time)

Prebreeding
Vaccinate with IBR/PI$_3$; consider including BVD
Vaccinate with 5-way leptospirosis bacterin; consider including *Vibrio* bacterin if clean-up bulls are to be used
Deworm and pour with insecticide to control grubs
Check udders for abnormalities (mastitis, trauma, abscesses)
Monitor weight, height, and body condition score to determine if ready for breeding

At Pregnancy Check
Check body score
Deworm
Booster with 5-way leptospirosis bacterin

Pregnant Heifers
Monitor condition score
Deworm if necessary
Consider the use of injectable vitamin E and selenium 60 days before calving to promote udder health and fertility
Observe close-up heifers for udder edema and treat if necessary

152 □ DAIRY REPLACEMENT REARING PROGRAMS

Table 9. RECOMMENDED BREEDING WEIGHT AND AGE

Breed	Weight (kg)	Age (months)
Holstein	340–385	15
Brown Swiss	340–385	15
Milking Shorthorn	320–365	15
Guernsey	275–320	14
Ayrshire	275–320	14
Jersey	250–295	13

months of age, weighs 340 kg (~750 lb), measures 140 cm (~55 inches) at the withers, and has a BCS of ± 3.0. The suggested breeding weights and ages for heifers of various breeds are listed in Table 9. Besides the impact on future milk production, the additional financial burden of maintaining an open heifer should be considered. This cost, estimated at $3.00 per head per day, must be added to the costs for the additional space required for a larger heifer herd.

Synchronization of estrus is recommended, and various synchronization programs can be used. Estrus detection aids, such as tail paint, Kamar patches, or a teaser bull with a chin ball marker, are useful because heat detection is usually the weak link in the breeding program.

Growth and body condition should be monitored throughout pregnancy, aiming for a BCS of 3.0 at calving and a precalving body weight of 550 kg (~1200 lb). Excessive feeding late in gestation can result in excessive fat deposition in the pelvic canal, which, combined with increased fetal growth, may contribute to dystocia.

PERSONNEL TRAINING

Although a veterinarian may be directly involved, most of the aspects discussed are performed by the personnel on the farm. The veterinarian can play a valuable role by providing resource materials or by arranging personnel training sessions. Areas that benefit from such efforts include colostrum and feedbunk management, disease recognition and treatment, vaccination-deworming-processing procedures, and breeding programs. Something as simple as the correct placement of an ear tag may contribute positively to neonatal health and weight gains and prevent the need for retagging.

MARKETING A REPLACEMENT REARING PROGRAM

There are several easy procedures that could be used to promote a sound replacement rearing program. Traditionally, veterinary involvement in a replacement rearing program has meant dealing with disease outbreaks, dehorning calves, vaccinating calves for brucellosis, and checking heifers for pregnancy.

Table 10. EQUATION AND COEFFICIENTS FOR COMPUTING WEIGHT (LB) FROM GIRTH (INCHES)

	Weight = A * Girth$^{(B)}$	
Breed	A	B
Holstein	.0082	2.75
Jersey	.0058	2.83
Guernsey	.0041	2.91
Ayrshire	.0046	2.88

Data from Brody S: Bioenergetics and Growth. New York, Hafner Publishing Company, 1945.

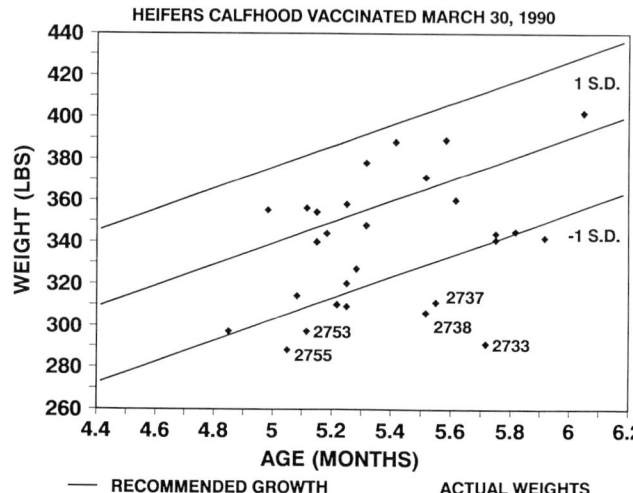

Figure 4. Example of the graphic output from a spreadsheet program for monitoring heifer growth. (Growth chart generator for Holstein heifers developed by Donovan GA. Output has been edited to improve print quality.)

Participation can be extended to include monitoring of the colostral absorption efficiency (bleed a few newborn calves and determine serum TP by refractometry) and growth monitoring (estimate weights with a tape, using the equation and coefficients provided in Table 10, and record body condition scores when the heifers are handled for any reason). Data accumulated in this way, relatively cost-free, can then be presented to the producer in an appropriate manner. Figure 4 illustrates a graph of heifer weights by age that was generated with available spreadsheet software. Several programs for generating such graphs are available.[1] The comparison of

[1]Growth chart generator for Holstein heifers (for use with Lotus 1-2-3) is available from Dr. G. A. Donovan, University of Florida, Box J-136, Gainesville, FL 32610.
Heifer growth analysis and economics (for use with Lotus 1-2-3) are available from Dr. K. Nordlund, 616 E. Lakeside Drive, Fergus Falls MN 56537.
Dairy heifer graphing worksheet (for use with Lotus 1-2-3) is available from Dr. A. J. Heinrichs, The Pennsylvania State University, 8 Borland Laboratory, University Park, PA 16802.

Table 11. TARGETS FOR A DAIRY REPLACEMENT REARING PROGRAM

Parameter	Target		
ME 305d improvement	>100 kg		
PTA of sire	Upper 30th percentile		
Calving ease index of sire	<10%		
Length of dry period of cow	50–60 days		
Body condition score at calving	3.5 ± 0.5 (3.0 – 3.5)[1]		
Calves born dead or alive for <24 hr	<6% (8%)		
Incidence of dystocia	<10% (20%)		
Incidence of mastitis at calving	<3% (7%)		
Incidence of blind quarters at calving	<0.5%		
First-service conception rate	>65%		
Heat detection rate	>80%		
Culling for reproduction	<5%		
Culling for disease/poor growth	<2%		
Calves with enlarged umbilical stumps	<10%		
	0–60 days	2–6 months	6–24 months
Mortality	<5%	<2%	<1%
Diarrhea	<20%	<5%	<1%
Pneumonia	<5%	<5%	<2%
Pinkeye	<1%	<5%	<5%

[1]Values for heifers in parentheses.
ME = Mature equivalent; PTA = predicted transmitting ability.

replacement herd data with established targets (Table 11) is valuable if farm data are available and accessible; however, a comparison with regional data may be more appropriate.

Although many areas of a replacement rearing program may be in need of help, it is important to prioritize problems on an economic basis and address them one at a time so as not to overwhelm the producer. Also, some areas may show dramatic improvement after relatively minor changes. It is important to consider the short- and long-term effects of such recommended changes. For example, an increase in calf survival may overburden the available labor and facilities and eventually become a financial burden because of the additional feed required as the heifers age.

BIBLIOGRAPHY

Braun RK, Donovan GA: Rearing herd replacements for optimum reproductive performance. Reproductive Herd Health Manual (Dairy Section). J Soc Theriog 16:51–64, 1990.
Brody S: Bioenergetics and Growth. New York, Hafner Publishing Company, 1945.
Clapp HJ: What height and weight should your heifers be? Hoards Dairyman 126:1250–1251, 1981.
Dairy Herd Workshop: Your Guide to Healthy, Profitable Calves. Minnetonka, MN, The Miller Publishing Company, March 15, 1990.
Donovan GA: Assessing herd performance in relation to replacement rearing. Buffalo, NY, Proceedings, 18th Annual Convention of the American Association of Bovine Practitioners, 1985, pp 50–51.
Donovan GA, Braun RK: Evaluation of dairy heifer replacement-rearing programs. Compend Contin Educ Pract Vet 9:F133–F139, 1987.
Donovan GA, Braun RK: Economics of rearing dairy replacements. Calgary, Proceedings, Seminar 12, Annual Meeting of the American Association of Bovine Practitioners, 1988.
Donovan GA, et al: Health considerations in rearing dairy replacement heifers. Calgary, Proceedings, Seminar 12, Annual Meeting of the American Association of Bovine Practitioners, 1988.
Donovan GA, et al: Colostrum management in dairy calves. Calgary, Proceedings, Seminar 12, Annual Meeting of the American Association of Bovine Practitioners, 1988.
Fetrow J, et al: Dairy herd health monitoring. Part II. A computer spreadsheet for dairy herd monitoring. Compend Contin Educ Pract Vet 10:75–80, 1988.
Harris B Jr, Shearer JK: Raising dairy replacement heifers. Circular 770, Florida Cooperative Extension Service, Institute of Food and Agricultural Sciences, University of Florida, Gainesville, FL, 1988.
Heinrichs AJ, Hargrove GL: Standards of weight and height for Holstein heifers. J Dairy Sci 70:653–660, 1987.
Heinrichs AJ, et al: Management of dairy heifers. Circular 385, Cooperative Extension, College of Agriculture, The Pennsylvania State University, University Park, PA, 1989.
Hoard's Dairyman, A supplement to: Raising Dairy Heifers. Fort Atkinson, WI, WD Hoard & Sons, 1990.
McGuirk SM: Practical colostrum evaluation. Calgary, Proceedings, 21st Annual Convention of the American Association of Bovine Practitioners, 1989, pp 108–111.
Radostits OM, Blood DC: Health management of dairy calves. In Radostits OM, Blood DC (eds): Herd Health. Philadelphia, WB Saunders, 1985.
Roberson JR, et al: *Staphylococcus aureus* intramammary infections (IMI): prevalence, sources and modes of transmission in dairy heifers. Proceedings, International Symposium Bovine Mastitis, 1990, pp 112–117.
White D: Feeding colostrum to calves. In Practice July 1987, pp 131–132.

Ovine Production Management and Preventive Medicine

MARIE S. BULGIN, DVM

The goal of production medicine is to optimize the profitability of a livestock enterprise. This is accomplished by the measuring of critical production parameters and identifying areas in which improvements can be made. By combining all facets of veterinary medicine with some concepts of animal science and business principles, production medicine attempts to maximize profits within the constraints of the particular management system. In most instances, this will be the maximization of pounds of lamb sold per production unit (ewe) at least cost.

Sheep producers make up a very diverse group. Many of these producers call veterinarians in only the direst of emergencies, whereas others expect the same medical treatment for their sheep as for their pets. However, the production medicine–oriented veterinarian knowledgeable about sheep production and management is usually able to offer some level of production medicine to meet most clients' goals. Maximizing pounds of lamb sold per ewe while minimizing the cost, the goal of production medicine, should also be the goal of most clients.

MARKETING PRODUCTION MEDICINE

Marketing is the process of making skills and services known so that they are understood and desired by potential clients. This involves establishing a relationship of trust with a client, usually by the practice of traditional veterinary medicine. Producers must feel that your primary interest is to help them and that your knowledge is broad enough to qualify you to advise on animal breeding, management, nutrition, marketing, environmental impact, and record-keeping. This involves keeping up with and being aware of the markets, new products, governmental regulations, and technologies affecting the industry. Taking the time to talk to your client, knowing your clients' problems, and informed discussions about markets and the sheep business all set the stage for clients' willingness to accept and pay for suggestions and recommendations affecting their whole enterprise.

One factor that often keeps us from the practice of production medicine is the perception of the low value producers place on the services we render and the difficulty quantifying our worth to a client. To rectify this problem, work out on paper the saving or increase in profit to the client by involvement in a production medicine program. Not only will this help sell the program when it is shown to the producer, but it will also give you, the practitioner, a clear sense of the program's real worth.

In setting fees, know that a certain percentage of time will be spent doing things for which the client cannot be billed. Charging by the procedure is most effective in a traditional veterinarian practice in which definite tasks are being carried out, but it does not fit well in production medicine. Remember, clients are accustomed to paying by the hour for other professionals (attorneys, accountants, servicemen), and billing for time spent in consultation as well as for definite tasks enables one to take the time to "talk" to the producer. It also allows compensation for working off the farm, that is, solving nutritional problems or reviewing rations. Some veterinarians use different rates for different types of work. Certain services should be defined that will be provided on a scheduled basis for a set fee, and extra services (such as necropsies, laboratory tests) can be additional charges as they occur. A written contract should be used to make clear exactly what is being provided and what payment is expected. A 1-year contract works well when certain goals of herd performance have been identified and the function of the veterinarian is to help reach these goals. At the end of the year, herd performance gains are reviewed, and the contract is renewed, modified, or forgotten.

GOALS

The ewe has the most untapped potential of any of the food animals. Not only can she commonly produce more than 1 lamb per gestation, but she has the potential of having 2 gestations and 4-plus lambs per year. Furthermore, sheep are more efficient converters of agricultural waste and poor-quality forage than are cattle. However, most alternative feeds require some kind of supplementation, and the nutritional knowledge of the production medicine–oriented veterinarian can make these feeds work for most producers.

Table 1 suggests some minimal goals as a guide. Five parameters to consider for trying to increase lambs marketed per production unit are conception rate, embryonic and fetal losses, lamb losses, pounds of lamb/ewe sold, and number of gestations per year. For documentation of the areas in which change could improve production, a record-keeping system must be in place that monitors those areas. In attempting to effect a change, special attention must be paid to management of prebreeding and breeding periods, pregnant ewes, lambing, control of lamb disease and nutrition, and choice of replacement breeding animals. Lambing more than once a year does not fit well into most management situations but can be very profitable when it does.

PREBREEDING AND BREEDING MANAGEMENT

Ideally, 90 per cent of the lambing should be completed within 45 days. The most desirable (or profitable) time to have lambs born must be selected. Winter lambing makes use of idle time for crop farmers and allows selling of lambs during the traditional period of peak lamb prices (May and June) and before hot, summer weather. Spring lambing, on the other hand, allows maximal use of grass and pasture and requires less labor and less elaborate lambing facilities. Ewes and rams tend to be more fertile later in the fall; thus lambing percentages tend to be higher and lamb losses from inclement weather are less likely. The decision as to when to lamb should be based on breed of sheep, feed costs, lamb prices, weather, labor availability, and lambing facilities.

An appointment should be set up for the client 180 days before the first day chosen for lambing (see Table 2). This farm visit should encompass a casual look at the ewes and breeding soundness examinations for the rams. The ewes should be checked for individual ear tag identification because no efficient production program can be instituted without keeping individual records. The veterinarian may need to assist the client in condition scoring both the ewe and ram flock. Condition scoring (CS) must be done by actual hands-on palpation of ribs, vertebral processes, and tuber coxae. The animals are rated 1 to 5 according to the following criteria:

1. extremely thin, emaciated
2. thin, but not emaciated; tuber coxae are prominent, vertebral processes and ribs are easily felt
3. tuber coxae, vertebral processes, and last 3 ribs can be felt but are not prominent; not fat, not thin
4. last 3 ribs can be felt with some difficulty; tuber coxae and vertebral processes are difficult to feel; the dorsum or back of the sheep is flat
5. no bones can be palpated; there is an obvious trough down the middle of the back; the brisket is filled with fat and does not hang loose; obese

Ovulation rate appears to respond to short-term increased energy intake within a specific intermediate range of body condition (i.e., CS 2–3). Condition scores above and below this range show no additional positive or negative effect.[1] For optimal ovulation and conception, ewes should be CS 2.5 approaching 3, that is, in a gaining mode during breeding time. That means that in 4 weeks' time when breeding begins, the ewes need to be CS approximating 2.5 and must be fed appropriately in the interim. When the rams are turned in, the ewes should then be fed for a weight gain of 10 to 15 pounds in 2 to 3 weeks' time. This procedure is called flushing.

It is not uncommon to find the ewes too fat (CS 5), in which case they need to have weight taken off before breeding. Implantation failures and early embryonic deaths are more common in obese ewes early in pregnancy, and fat ewes are more prone to dystocia and prolapses later in pregnancy. Furthermore, depending on the feed source, having and keeping ewes in this condition may be an unnecessary expense.

The selenium status of the flock could be determined at this time. Previous history of white muscle disease or known selenium status of the area may indicate that selenium supplementation is needed. Otherwise, 3 to 5 ewes should be bled into heparin or ethylenediaminetetraacetic acid (EDTA) tubes for either glutathione level determination or selenium analysis. If blood selenium levels are under 0.1 ppm or glutathione levels are below 2 mmol/L, supplementation at 90 ppm in loose salt will give positive results in weight gain, fetal and newborn health, and general herd health. Many so-called selenium salts are not supplemented with the maximal selenium concentration by law (90 ppm). The veterinarian should make it a point to check mineral concentrations in trace mineral salt mixes, with special attention not only to selenium but copper concentrations as well. Sheep require less copper than do most other animals and usually get more than enough in their diets. Never recommend trace mineral formulas with copper concentrations over 30 ppm for sheep.

Prebreeding is the time to cull all ewes that are not fully productive. The owner should examine teeth and udders of all ewes and remove those ewes that have problems. In farm flocks, front teeth (or even the lack of them) are not usually indicative of problems, but hard masses that can be palpated on the mandibles through the skin indicate tooth abscesses and osteomyelitis. Chronic health problems such as footrot, ovine progressive pneumonia, or caseous lymphadenitis, if present, should be recognized and taken care of or the ewe culled. The cause of an excessive number of culls (5 to 7 per cent over those culled for age) at this time should be identified

Table 1. PRODUCTION PARAMETERS

Culling	
Ewe culling due to problems other than age	<5–7%
Ram culling due to breeding soundness examination	<5–7%
Conception Rate (During September–December, Northern Latitudes)	
Number of mature ewes bred in 45 days	>90%
Number of mature ewes bred in 60 days	>95%
Ewes not lambing	<6–7%
Fetal Losses	
Abortion rate	<1%[1]
Stillbirths	<2%[1]
Lamb Losses	
Neonatal lamb losses	<12%[1]
Total lamb losses	<15%[1]
Weight Gains 0–60 Days	
Single lambs	>0.5 lb/day
Twin lambs (added together)	>0.8 lb/day

Number of lambs per ewe is dependent on breed, season bred, and nutrition. However, at least 150% should be a goal to strive for.

[1]Percentage of the total lambs.

and steps taken to rectify the problem in the upcoming year. Ewes that are kept and replacement ewe lambs should be vaccinated, dewormed, and treated for lice and keds, if necessary (Table 2).

The breeding soundness examination often reveals 5 to 10 per cent of the "normal rams" to be infertile or sterile owing to problems other than infections. Some of these are probably genetic. These rams go undetected in multisire operations without a breeding soundness examination. One good ram can cover for several less-than-adequate rams, because a fertile ram with good libido is able to adequately service at least 100 ewes in 45 days under natural breeding systems. However, keeping unnecessary ram power or rams that are not doing an optimal job is an expensive situation. Kimberling has estimated an annual maintenance cost of $175 and $225, excluding purchase price, for $200 and $300 rams, respectively.[2] In single-sire flocks, the importance of identifying an infertile ram before breeding season is obvious.

The breeding soundness examination should begin with a good general physical examination. Rams should be in CS 3 to 3.5. Feet should be trimmed if needed, and teeth, eyes, and prepuce should be checked. Ulceration of the prepuce (pizzle rot) should be treated at this time, and the scrotal contents should be palpated and measured. Any rams with hernias, epididymitis, or extremely soft or atrophied testicles should be culled. Although rams with testicles that are abnormally small (Table 3) but normal to palpation are generally fertile, productivity is limited. Daughters of early-maturing ram lambs with large scrotal circumference (>30 cm) at 9 months of age are more early-maturing and productive than are daughters of later-maturing rams with small testicle size (<28 cm). If epididymitis is discovered in any ram, all rams passing the semen examination should be bled for the *Brucella ovis* serum enzyme-linked immunosorbent assay (ELISA). Rams with epididymitis and rams testing positive on the ELISA test must be culled. For more detailed control methods for epididymitis and *B. ovis*, see other references.[3, 4]

A vasectomized or epidiymectomized ram introduced into the flock 2 to 3 weeks before breeding season is scheduled to start will stimulate the onset of estrus and advance the breeding season by a couple of weeks. A silent heat generally occurs within 6 days of the introduction of the ram, and a peak number of ewes will simultaneously come into estrus some 18 to 20 days later. Rams with epididymitis should not be chosen for vasectomies or epididymectomies. The causative agents of epididymitis reside also in the bulbourethral and secondary sex glands and can be transmitted to the ewes via mounting.

MANAGEMENT OF THE PREGNANT EWE

The most common causes of fetal wastage are infectious agents. A number of diseases may have early and midgestational impact. *Brucella ovis* transmitted by rams and bluetongue, common in areas of night temperatures over 45°F during breeding and early gestational periods, can cause early abortion and implantation failures. Late abortions and weak lambs may be caused by *Campylobacter* spp., *Chlamydia* spp., and border disease virus. *Campylobacter* spp., although usually associated with late abortion, also cause early abortions. A history of abortions, stillbirths, mummies, or nonpregnant ewes usually indicates an infectious disease in the flock. However, diagnosis after the fact is difficult, and proceeding with a good disease control program is probably the best way to attack the problem. Use of *B. ovis* ELISA-negative rams for breeding and vaccination of ewes against *Campylobacter* spp. will control losses due to those 2 organisms. Vaccine against bluetongue serotype 10 is commercially available*; however, it offers no protection against other serotypes. Vaccines against other serotypes of bluetongue are available in some states but, as of this writing, cannot be taken across state lines. Use of insect repellent sprays and fly tags and elimination of muddy areas in which *Culicoides*, the no-see-um gnat vector, breeds seem to help. The use of cattle vaccines against border disease has not been shown to be effective.

Pregnancy testing of ewes 30 to 45 days after the breeding season, with use of real-time ultrasonography, is now an accurate, practical, and economical practice and can be utilized to discover whether "dud" stud rams or early embryonic death is a problem in a flock. Used routinely, it identifies dry ewes early, allowing culling of noneconomical production units in the flock. It is not uncommon in a well-managed flock to have 3 to 4 per cent open ewes at lambing; however, more would indicate the presence of a problem. Because the average cost of feeding and maintaining a farm flock ewe ranges between $65 and $85 per year, it has been calculated by Kimberling that the cost of keeping a nonproducing ewe versus a producing ewe is $80 over the cost of feeding her.[5] Ewes carrying twins and triplets may also be identified, if desired, for special care or feeding or to allow a producer to sell off ewes having only

---

Table 2. VACCINATION AND WORMING SCHEDULE

30 Days Before Breeding
Condition score and separate culls
Vaccinate ewes and ewe lambs for *Campylobacter* spp. and chlamydial abortion
Deworm, pour-on if necessary
Perform breeding soundness examinations on rams
Adjust nutrition
Ear tag

21 Days Before Breeding
Turn in vasectomized ram

Breeding Time
Remove vasectomized rams
Turn in breeding rams

30 Days Before Lambing
Crutch or shear ewes
Vaccinate for enterotoxemia types C and D
Vaccinate for *Escherischia coli*, tetanus, *Clostridium septicum* if desired
Give selenium injections if necessary
Adjust nutrition
Worm
Begin use of coccidiostats in salt
Treat individuals for nasal discharge

Birth
Iodine navels
Check udders and milk of dam
Isolate dam and lamb(s)
Make sure lamb nurses
Record birth statistics
Weigh lamb (optional)

First Week of Life
Dock and castrate
Ear tag

3–4 Weeks of Life
Vaccinate for enterotoxemia types C and D
Supply coccidiostat in feed or salt for lambs
Supplement selenium if necessary, salt or injections

6–8 Weeks
Vaccinate for enterotoxemia types C and D
Weigh lambs if possible

Weaning
Choose replacement ewe lambs
Vaccinate replacement ewe lambs with abortion vaccine

---

*Colorado Serum Company, 4950 York St., Denver, CO 80216 (303-295-7527).

Table 3. BREEDING SOUNDNESS CRITERIA FOR RAMS

	Scrotal Circumference[1] Score								
	8	7	6	5	4	3	2	1	0
<12 months	>32 cm		30 cm		29 cm		28 cm		<25 cm
12–18 months	>36 cm		34 cm		32 cm		31 cm		<30 cm
>18 months	>39 cm		37 cm		35 cm		33 cm		<32 cm
Motility	—		—	>80	>60	>50	>30	>20	>20
Normal morphology	>90	>80	>70	>60	>50	>40	>30		>20

[1]Scrotal circumference normally decreases by 1 to 2 cm during anestrus periods.

Excellent >16 score; satisfactory 8–16 score; unsatisfactory <8 score or >5 white cells per high-power field or epididymitis in 1 or both testicles.

single fetuses. Under farm flock conditions, the current cost of maintaining a ewe requires a 130 to 160 per cent marketed lamb crop to pay for the ewe's maintenance. Thus pregnancy testing can help ensure that the lamb crop is adequate to pay the bills.

PRELAMBING MANAGEMENT

Twenty to 30 days before the beginning of lambing season, 3 necessary activities should be scheduled: shearing or crutching, veterinary care (vaccinating, worming, and control of coccidia and *Pasteurella* spp.), and adjustment of nutrition (see Table 2). This is an excellent time to schedule an examination of the ewe flock and lambing facilities, particularly if the owner is a novice.

Shearing or Crutching

Winter shearing is practiced by a limited number of producers with great success; however, shelter will need to be available in case of sudden winter storms immediately after shearing. Crutching, or the removal of wool from around the vulva and udder, is an important disease management practice for the control of both *Escherichia coli* scours and coccidia. Furthermore, it allows the producer to observe both the swelling of the vulva and enlargement of the udder, signs that lambing will occur within 1 or 2 weeks. These ewes can then be separated from the others for increased feed and attention.

Veterinary Activities

Some form of coccidial control should be instituted at this time. Coccidiostats such as lasalocid* or decoquinate† can be mixed into salt (2 lb 15 per cent lasalocid premix per 50 lb of salt or 2 lb 6 per cent decoquinate premix per 50 lb salt) and fed until lambing. Coccidial numbers are reduced in carrier ewes, thus reducing the dose to the newborn lamb.

Vaccination of the ewe flock at this time ensures having maximal levels of specific antibodies in the colostrum. Protection of the young lambs against *Clostridium perfringens* is important in any flock; other diseases, such as *E. coli* scours and tetanus, can be of importance in individual flocks with previous histories of those diseases. Vitamin ADE could be given as well if a poor-quality feed warrants it.

Ewes with heavy nasal discharge generally signify sinus infections with *Ovis estrus*, the nasal bot larvae, and *Pasteurella* spp. The discharge is a source of early *Pasteurella* infection of neonatal lambs transmitted as the dam licks them off. Individual treatment of these ewes with ivermectin* and long-acting tetracycline† usually alleviates the problem.

---

*Cleared for use in sheep in the United States.
†Not cleared for use in sheep in the United States.

Nutritional Adjustment

The ewes in their third trimester of pregnancy, the time of 75 per cent of the fetal growth, require dietary adjustment. The veterinarian can be of great help in planning and balancing diets. The utilization of least-cost nutritional computer programs makes this job exceptionally easy, but it can also be done by use of the tables found in *Nutrient Requirements of Sheep*.[7] The previous flock production history usually dictates current flock nutrition management unless multiparous ewes have been identified with real-time sonography. If so, they can be fed exactly what they need for the number of fetuses. Proper nutrition at this time will ensure vigorous newborn lambs and ewes coming into their milk at the proper time.

LAMBING MANAGEMENT

Lambing management is well covered in Norman Gate's book *A Practical Guide to Sheep Disease Management*,[8] which should be recommended reading for the producer. A barn sheet for record-keeping is a must. Lambs need to be identified, weighed (optional), and recorded. Birth weights are called for in most computer programs designed to evaluate ewe productivity. Neonatal lamb deaths should not exceed 10 to 12 per cent, but there are many management and disease problems that will quickly cause neonatal losses to soar.

The newborn lamb is not able to maintain its body temperature in the face of extreme environmental temperatures for the first 36 hours of life. Exposure to adverse weather for more than 1/2 hour can lead to hypothermia with resultant hypoglycemia, weakness, and death from starvation. Lambs with temperatures below 100°F should be tubed with colostrum and warmed. The use of hair dryers is probably the best method of warming hypothermic lambs. Warm water baths are effective, but then the warmed lamb is wet and tends to cool off again while drying, and often the odor of the ewe is washed off. Many ewes then reject the lamb upon its return. Use of 2 to 4 ounces of thawed or fresh cow, goat, or ewe colostrum for lambs inadequately supplied from their mothers increases survival rates.

Udders of the periparturient ewe should always be checked and stripped, making sure that a full-appearing udder is not actually "hard bag," the mastitic form of ovine progressive pneumonia virus. Ewes with abnormal milk should be treated immediately with an intramammary bovine mastitis product. *Staphylococcus aureus* is the most common agent causing subclinical infection and is also commonly implicated in gangrenous mastitis. *Streptococcus agalactiae* and *S. uberis*, *E. coli*, *P. multocida*, and *P. haemolytica* are also found in subclinical, acute, and generalized mastitis. Effective, practical control methods have not been worked out for mastitis in sheep.

Although starvation is the number-one cause of neonatal lamb death on most farms, exposure, trauma (being laid upon), and in utero disease may cause weak lambs and be the reason for the starvation. Diarrhea, occurring during the first 3 days after birth, is generally caused by enterotoxic *E. coli. Clostridium perfringens* type C, *E. coli*, and *Pasteurella* septicemia can also cause death this early but less commonly. *Pasteurella* septicemia and pneumonia are generally spread by the ewes, especially those with nasal discharges.

Diagnoses of most neonatal lamb problems can be made on gross necropsy, and the producer should be encouraged either to bring them in or to save them and have necropsy performed on a biweekly visit to the farm. Dead lambs under 60 days of age cool out rapidly, and the weather during lambing is usually cold. If carcasses are kept cool and where predators cannot reach them, they will usually remain in good enough condition for necropsy. Older sheep with functional rumens, particularly those with heavy fleeces, deteriorate rapidly. Six hours is usually the maximal allowable time between death and necropsy for them.

In the case of *E. coli* scours, or very-early-age pneumonia, antibiotics can be used prophylactically. One dose of an antibiotic, such as tribrissen,* gentamicin,* or spectinomycin,* given within the first 12 hours after birth is extremely effective but must be given orally for enterotoxic *E. coli*. Aminoglycosides are not excreted into the digestive tract. The same dose is used as for injection.

Docking and castration should be done early; 2 or 3 days of age is probably best, particularly when elastrators are used. The use of elastrators is very popular with producers because of ease, reduction of secondary infections and weight loss, lack of bloodshed, and elimination of fly strike in warmer weather. Tetanus, which has been associated with their use, can easily be prevented by the use of tetanus toxoid in the ewes before parturition. However, colostral antibodies last for only 3 weeks or so; thus elastrators should not be used after this time unless tetanus antitoxin is given before elastrating. Lambs need to be vaccinated for enterotoxemia, both type C and type D, at 3 to 4 weeks if dams have been vaccinated in the month before parturition. Otherwise, they should be vaccinated earlier, at 1 or 2 weeks of age.

Lambs should be weighed sometime before weaning for evaluation of both the milking ability of the ewe and the growth potential of the lambs. Average daily gain is a simple parameter used to compare ewe productivity for culling purposes and for choosing replacement breeding stock. It can also indicate the presence of a flock problem. Single lambs should gain at least 0.5 lb/day and twin lambs together should average at least 0.8 lb/day, and fast-growing and early-maturing breeds should do much better. If a large number of lambs are gaining less, energy and protein nutrition, mineral supplementation, and disease may all be implicated.

MAXIMIZING POUNDS OF LAMBS FOR SALE

In many farm flock situations, marketing lambs as early as possible has been economically advantageous. Generally, the earlier in the year the lambs go to market, the higher the price. Other advantages are that the producers have more free time and the lambs have less time for problems to develop. In this case, lambs should be started on concentrates as soon as possible. Subclinical coccidial infections, probably present in all lambs, interfere with optimal weight gains and should be controlled in any lamb feeding situation. Lasalocid† may have a further advantage over other coccidiostats because of improvement in feed efficiency. Sulfa drugs, the most effective agents for treatment and the most expensive, should be reserved for treatment of clinical cases.

Weaning

Weaning of lambs may be early, 3 to 4 weeks of age, done when ewes are to be bred back for twice-a-year lambing; late, 6 to 9 months, practiced in range or pasture management systems; or 60 to 90 days for early marketing. Lambs weaned at 6 to 9 months usually go straight to market weighing 110 to 120 pounds, depending on breed and feed. Lambs weaned at 60 days or 60 pounds can be grown out and fattened on pasture, in the feedlot, or on such things as turnips, onions, ensilage, and aftermaths of grass seed, alfalfa, sugar beet, or other crops. On a high-concentrate diet, lambs this age are able to gain an average of 1 lb/day, particularly when they are started on a high-concentrate creep feed at 3 weeks of age. Gains of creep-fed lambs will slump, however, if they are placed on high-roughage feeds after weaning because of the immaturity of the rumen at this age. Internal parasites, specifically helminths, can reduce gains or even cause clinical problems if lambs are placed on pasture or have been pastured before weaning with their dams.

Management of the early-weaned lambs is a little trickier because they cannot utilize roughages at 3 to 4 weeks of age, and a highly digestible protein substitute for the dam's milk must be fed if the lambs are going to do well. Soybean meal is very palatable to lambs and is probably the protein supplement of choice. Milk pellets are excellent but expensive; however, they may be cost-effective in small amounts. Because the immature rumen cannot handle fiber well, barley and oats are probably the least suitable of the grains for this age lamb. Rolled corn is usually chosen because of palatability and digestibility.

Most diseases of the feedlot lamb are diet- and management-related. Urolithiasis, for example, is related to the calcium-phosphorus ratio (Ca:P) in the diet; optimally 2:1 to 3:1 for prevention. In high-concentrate diets, it will be necessary to add calcium, usually in the form of limestone. Ammonium salts for acidifying urine may also be added in the form of ammonium chloride or ammonium sulfate as 1 per cent of the diet. Sodium chloride may be added as 1 to 2 per cent of the diet, as well, to increase water intake and decrease crystal formation in the bladder. Availability of water is of utmost importance particularly when salt is added to the feed.

Polioencephalomalacia may be caused by a thiamine deficiency exacerbated by the high demand for thiamine in the metabolism of carbohydrates, low amounts of thiamine in mixed feeds, or thiaminase-producing bacteria residing in the rumen. Addition of thiamine in the total diet at a concentration of 0.05 pound of thiamine per ton will usually eliminate cases of polio. However, high sulfates in feed or water have also been shown to cause a non–thiamine-responsive polioencephalomalacia in lambs and steers.

Rectal prolapses are most often seen in females of breeds that are more prone to internalize fat late in the feeding period. Coughing due to upper respiratory disease, dusty conditions that exacerbate coughing, and straining caused by enteritis (coccidia, *Salmonella* spp.) are also associated with prolapses. Prevention is difficult and is usually directed at the control of coughing or enteric problems.

Pneumonia is most often caused by *Pasteurella haemolytica* and is very similar to the shipping fever complex seen in cattle. It is most commonly seen in commercial feedlots in young lambs that have been recently weaned and transported. Many

---
*Not cleared for use in sheep in the United States.
†Cleared for use in sheep in the United States.

sheep carry the organisms in either their nose or tonsils. Stress appears to reduce the animal's normal defense mechanisms that keep these opportunists from causing disease. Antibiotics in the feed or water are helpful, if the organism is susceptible. However, lambs in new surroundings sometimes will not eat and drink the first few days. Availability of running water and familiar feeds or any innovative enticements to eat or drink reduces stress and disease. *Pasteurella* spp. are well known for becoming resistant to antibiotics, so necropsies and cultures are warranted when treatments do not work.

Enterotoxemia is prevented by vaccination against *C. perfringens* type C and type D. However, sporadic, sudden deaths are seen in vaccinated lambs on high-concentrate diets. Many producers attribute these to enterotoxemia vaccine breaks, but they are most likely due to acidosis. Diagnosis is relatively simple in the dead lambs by checking rumen pH with pH paper. Normally, rumen pH in lambs on high-concentrate diets is found to be around 6.5, whereas those dead of acidosis will be found to be around 4.5 to 5.5. Although acidosis may be due to sudden changes in feed, it often occurs apparently unrelated to any form of management change or error. Addition of buffers to the diet, such as sodium or calcium bicarbonate, can often reduce these losses.

OTHER CONSIDERATIONS OF PRODUCTION MEDICINE

Production medicine relies on good dependable records for identifying the areas of management that require changing for optimization of production. In smaller flocks, hand-kept records are adequate. However, in large flocks of over 100 ewes, record analysis may be made easier by use of a computerized system. Many producers have their own program or are subscribing to computerized records, and several of the breed associations are encouraging their members to subscribe. Data from computerized records indicate how many pounds of lamb and wool each ewe in the flock has produced, compare the production of young ewes with older ewes, keep track of health problems or other variables determined to be important, and compare performance of various sires. They also rank lambs on rate of gain, adjusted for sex, and type of birth (single, twin). Productivity of the ewes and rams is ranked, which allows the poorer producers and their offspring in the flock to be culled and the offspring of the higher producers to be chosen for replacements. Most extension agents have information about computerized production programs for sheep.

Replacement Ewe Lambs

Ewe replacements, preferably those from the outstanding production ewes, need to be identified at weaning or soon after and removed from the feeder lambs. Although high-concentrate diets with adequate protein contribute to fast growth rate, it is not beneficial to fatten replacement ewe lambs. Not only will losses from rectal prolapses be more likely, but as the udder fills with fat, milk-producing tissue is reduced and the ewe is never able to realize her full genetic milk-producing potential.

Ewes that breed and conceive as ewe lambs have been found to be more productive throughout their entire lifetime even when the first pregnancy is not counted. Ewe lambs selected on the basis of the dams' production should be the best ewes in the flock, and their offspring from production-selected sires should prove to be the best lambs in the flock. Breeding ewe lambs speeds up the genetic improvement of a flock.

Because ewe lambs continue to grow for another year, they have additional nutritional needs to those of older ewes. The duration of estrus is also shorter in ewe lambs than in the older females, and rams tend to show a preference for the more mature females. Thus ewe lambs need to be kept separately from the ewes for both breeding and feeding. Ewe lambs in heat tend to make little or no attempt to approach the ram but will accept service.

Lambing More Than Once a Year

For flocks that are *not* composed of Dorsets, Polypays, Finnsheep, Merinos, Rambouillets, or crosses thereof, lambing in the fall becomes a matter of artificially inducing estrus. In most cases, this is not practical. However, there are special cases in which producers enlist the aid of the veterinarian to fool nature. Intravaginal pessaries (sponges) utilizing a synthetic progesterone are available and are used extensively outside the United States, and producers in the United States often obtain them. They are extremely useful for inducing early mating of 9- to 11-month-old female lambs after they have reached an adequate body weight; increasing the number of lambings a year by mating ewes in the spring; facilitating the practice of artificial insemination or synchronizing lambing; and increasing the number of lambs, in which case pregnant mare serum gonadotropin (PMSG) is used in conjunction with the sponges.

There are some adverse effects of the synthetic progestogens on the survival of spermatozoa in the female genital tract, which makes it necessary to mate during the second half of heat (36 to 48 hours after initiation). Sponges are placed in the vagina for 10 to 12 days; longer reduces fertility. This treatment does not work well on lactating ewes; only 15 to 20 per cent will become pregnant.

Subcutaneous implants have also been used. Norgestomet* is used outside the United States, but Syncro-Mate B,† available in the United States for synchronizing cows, has been used with moderately good results. The 6-mg Syncro-Mate implant must be cut in half for use in sheep and implanted over the cartilage of the ear where it can be easily removed. The injectable norgestomet–estradiol valerate that is included is not required. Removal of the implant at the end of 10 to 12 days results in an onset of estrus in 24 hours. Cattle show a decrease in fertility if they are bred on the first heat; breeding on the second results in an increased pregnancy rate. It may be similar in ewes. The conception rate with use of the implants appears to be reduced 10 per cent compared with use of the sponges, but the prolificacy is about the same in adult ewes. However, the implants are not as effective in lambs unless PMSG injections are given when implants are removed.

The prostaglandin products (Lutalyse,‡ fenprostalene‡) used for synchronizing heat cycles of cattle have been used for synchronizing estrus in the cycling ewe. They will not initiate estrus during anestrus. As in the cow, for best results, 2 injections are required 11 days apart. Breeding on the first heat (which occurs 12 to 48 hours later) often causes a decrease in lambing percentage. For optimal lamb numbers, it may be better to breed the ewes on the second heat 17 to 18 days after the second injection. The dose is usually 1/3 to 1/4 that used in cows.

Light is the primary environmental factor controlling the natural onset of estrus. Estrus is triggered by decreasing light exposure to 10 hours. Cycling for most breeds will usually

---

*Available from Searle, Box 5110, Chicago, IL.
†Available from Ceva Laboratories, Inc., Overland Park, KS.
‡Not cleared for use in sheep in the United States.

begin 8 to 10 weeks after the longest day of the year, and this, too, can be very variable depending on the breed. Polypays, Finnsheep, Dorsets, Merinos, and Rambouillets have the longest breeding season, and individuals of those breeds may show a great deal of flexibility for breeding during the anestrus period. However, fertility generally is greatest during the middle of the breeding season for both rams and ewes.

Artificial alteration of illumination can alter the breeding season. For initiating estrus, fluorescent lights are recommended, 1 foot of bulb per 10 square feet of floor space. The ewes are exposed to 18 to 20 hours of light for 60 days, after which the light is reduced to 10 to 12 hours, and estrus should occur within several days. The rams require the treatment as well. Fifty to sixty per cent of the ewes should conceive. Outdoor exposure using mercury vapor lamps has also been reported to work.

The STAR sheep accelerated management system was developed at Cornell University for taking advantage of the sheep's potential 2 gestations a year without use of hormones.[9] It requires the use of a breed that is predominantly Merino, Rambouillet, Dorset, Finnsheep, or Polypay. By exposure of the dry flock to a ram or rams for 5 equally spaced 30-day periods, 5 back-to-back lambing-lactation cycles are produced annually. The shortest interval between lambing for each ewe is 7.2 months, with a second chance at 9.6 months and a third at a 12-month interval. In addition to increasing ewe productivity and improving feed utilization, the STAR system can maximize use of lambing and feeder lamb facilities, reduce risk, even out cash flow and labor requirements, and, most important, allow a year-round supply of young, efficiently grown lamb. Veterinarians and producers interested in this system should contact the Animal Science Department at Cornell University, Ithaca, NY.

REFERENCES

1. Gunn RG: The influence of nutrition on the reproductive performance of ewes. *In* Haresign W (ed): Sheep Production. Kent, England, Butterworth, 1983, pp 103–104.
2. Kimberling CV: The cost associated with maintaining a *Brucella ovis* (ram epididymitis) infected ram flock. Reno, Nevada, Proceedings, WRCC 46 (Ram Epididymitis and Footrot), 1987, pp 14–18.
3. Bulgin MS: Epididymitis in rams. Vet Clin North Am [Food Anim Pract] Vol 6, 1990.
4. Kimberling CV, Schweitzer D, Butler J, et al: A new way to eradicate ram epididymitis. Vet Med 82:424–429, 1987.
5. Kimberling CV: Just one more chance: does it make cents? Corvallis, Oregon, Proceedings, American Association of Small Ruminant Practice and WRCC 46 Conference 1990, pp 87–89.
6. Kott RW, Padula RF: Pregnancy diagnosis and fetal number determination in sheep. Boise, Idaho, Proceedings, American Association of Small Ruminant Practice and WRCC 46 Meeting, 1989, pp 29–37.
7. Subcommittee on Sheep Nutrition, Committee on Animal Nutrition, Agriculture National Research Council: Nutrient Requirements of Sheep, 6th ed. Washington, DC, National Academy Press, 1985.
8. Gates N: A Practical Guide to Sheep Disease Management. Moscow, Idaho, News-Review Publishing Company, 1985, pp 9–22.
9. Magee B: Star accelerated lambing system. Corvallis, Oregon, Proceedings, American Association of Small Ruminant Practice and WRCC 46 Meeting, 1990, p 47.

Sheep Feedlot Management

CLEON V. KIMBERLING, DVM, MPH
DEBORAH MARSH, BS

Throughout recorded history, sheep have played an important role in the welfare of mankind. The sheep is the most versatile domestic animal. From the conversion of forages alone, it has the ability to produce the finest quality meat, fiber, and milk. The feeding of concentrates to sheep has evolved primarily in the United States during the 20th century. Although the United States ranks 21st in total sheep population, it leads the world in lambs being fattened on concentrates. Sheep are extremely adaptable and can be incorporated into any type of farming or ranching enterprise.

The 1990 United States Department of Agriculture census estimates 7,650,000 breeding ewes in the United States. These sheep are distributed throughout 111,040 farms and ranches. Seventy-one per cent of the sheep in the United States are located in the western 10 states and are owned by 40 per cent of the producers. Fifty-four per cent of the sheep in the United States are in flocks of greater than 1000 head. Although Iowa has 10,500 farm operations with sheep, 92 per cent of these operations have less than 100 head. The current level of United States sheep production is a 95 per cent lamb crop with 10 to 11 pounds of grease wool per ewe. These figures clearly show the tremendous potential for improvement in production.

Depending on the practice location, there is an extreme variation in the flock size, the potential health problems, and the approach to these problems. Many of the smaller flocks will utilize the forage and feeds produced on the farm to conduct their own fattening program. These lambs may start on a creep at a few days of age, be weaned at 40 to 60 days, and be ready for market at 100 to 120 days. These programs are ideal because the veterinarian can monitor the health status on a continual basis.

In the case of the western states, very few lambs are fed or fattened on the ranch of origin. Some producers in the Mountain States produce a 100- to 120-pound fat lamb in 4 to 5 months directly from the high mountain forages. The majority of western lambs, however, will be weaned at 4 to 5 months, weighing from 65 to 85 pounds. The lighter-weight lambs may be shipped to areas where there are aftermath feeds (i.e., winter wheat, alfalfa, beet tops) to put on cheap gains and delay their finishing date. The heavier lambs may go directly to a custom feedlot for fattening. There are custom feedlots throughout the United States as shown in Table 1. These lots range in capacity from 600 to 150,000 head, with Colorado feeding 27 per cent of all lambs fed in the United States.

Custom lots provide a variety of services. A well-managed lot will have the computer capability to project break-even price and estimate rate of gain, slaughter date, least-cost rations, cost per pound of gain, and other projections the lamb producer may need.

A progressive custom lot will provide clients with a weekly progress report, exemplified in Table 2, showing the activities for that period. This is followed at the end of the month with a summary statement (Table 3). Finally, a closeout (Table 4) is provided at the end of the feeding period.

Each lot will have a different approach to health and

Table 1. DISTRIBUTION OF UNITED STATES CUSTOM SHEEP FEEDLOTS IN 1990

State	Number of Lots	State	Number of Lots	State	Number of Lots
CA	4	MT	1	TX	6
CO	12	NE	7	UT	1
ID	2	ND	2	WV	1
IA	11	OH	4	WI	3
KS	5	OK	1	WY	5
MI	1	OR	2		
MN	6	SD	13		

Data from American Lamb Industry Feedlot Directory.

Table 2. EXAMPLE OF A WEEKLY PROGRESS REPORT

Macho Feeders of Colorado

Lot: IOU
Date: July 15–21, 1990

Date Received	Shipper	Where Loaded	Truck Line	Off-Weight	Off-Count
07/15	El Borrego	Billings, MT	Cannon Ball Express	43,780	498 live/0 dead
07/19		San Fernando, CA	Cannon Ball Express	1,020	12 live/0 dead
07/20	B. Long	Mule Shoe, TX	Jack Sprat Express	44,800	558 live/0 dead

	Received	Shipped	Dead	Starting Balance	$2456
				Balance	Yardage
Sunday	498	0	1	2953	59.06
Monday	0	0	3	2950	59.00
Tuesday	0	0	2	2948	58.96
Wednesday	0	0	1	2947	58.94
Thursday	12	0	3	2956	59.12
Friday	558	0	1	3513	70.26
Saturday	0	0	1	3512	70.24
Totals	1068	0	12	21,779	$435.58
Handling	No. of hd.	0	0.25	0.00	
Hay	Bales	50	3.00	150.00	
Salt	Sacks	7	2.00	14.00	
3-way	No. of hd.	1068	0.38	405.84	
Re-vac	No. of hd.	567	0.10	56.70	
Shearing	No. of hd.	0	1.10	0.00	
Wool bags	No.	0	2.80	0.00	
Meds/SM	Lb	7	15.00	105.00	
			Subtotal	$731.54	
		TOTAL		$1167.12	

nutritional management. Because transportation stress is a major factor for most custom feedlots, an electrolyte program for the first 2 weeks is beneficial in preventing transport tetany. The entering lambs should be provided with long-stem hay and a starter ration (85 per cent roughage) and allowed 1 or 2 days of rest before processing (worming and vaccination). Processing should include *Clostridium perfringens* types C and D toxoid (some lots may use vaccines with additional clostridia strains). Worming is usually standard procedure unless the history of the lambs dictates otherwise. At this processing, any sick lambs or those not starting on feed can be sorted and treated separately. A clostridia booster should be administered in 2 weeks. Chlortetracycline can be added to the starter ration for the first 2 weeks at a 50 to 100 mg/head/day level. This procedure helps reduce pneumonia problems. If the incidence of a particular condition reaches 5 to 10 per cent of the lot, it may be best to mass treat the entire group.

As the lambs approach finish weight, the lot managers will assist with marketing. Unfortunately, there are only 9 packing plants operating in the United States (Colorado/2, California/2, Iowa/1, Kansas/1, New Mexico/1, Texas/1, and Washington/1), which limits marketing options.

Climatic and environmental conditions, origin of the lambs, rations (high-concentrate versus high-roughage diets), and general management practices will greatly influence the health management approach by the attending veterinarian. Conditions encountered in an enclosed barn operation, as seen in the upper Midwest, will vary greatly from the outside pen confinement system seen in Colorado. The veterinarian in the upper Midwest may need a basic knowledge of ventilation principles and humidity control for help in preventing pneumonia. On the other hand, for prevention of pneumonia in arid climates, the veterinarian will be concerned about population density per pen in controlling dust.

In lots in which lambs are received from distant locations, transportation tetany is a constant problem. Eliminating as many stresses as possible before and during shipping will likely reduce this problem. Stress and starvation deplete calcium and other ions that are involved with transport tetany. Some lambs are bought with an overnight drylot shrink, placed on trucks, and hauled for 24 to 36 hours. Eliminating these types of conditions will greatly improve the well-being of the lambs. When it is impossible to control these stress conditions, the veterinarian will need to establish a protocol of electrolyte therapy for incoming lambs. The veterinarian must be knowledgeable of the problems particular to his or her locality and be able to anticipate when these problems will arise in order to establish a viable health program.

The following paragraph describes the origin of lambs, inventory, feeding, and management practices of a typical Colorado commercial lamb feedlot for the period of February 1, 1985, to January 31, 1986. In this lot, the average inventory

Table 3. EXAMPLE OF AN END-OF-THE-MONTH STATEMENT

Macho Feeders of Colorado

El Borrego Land and Livestock
Bore Hole, MT

Lot: IOU   Date: 07/31/90

88,184 day	YARDAGE	0.02	1763.68
439 head	HANDLING	0.25	109.75
157 bales	HAY	3.00	471.00
21 sacks	SALT	2.00	42.00
2207 head	3-WAY	0.38	838.66
2724 head	RE-VAC	0.10	272.40
0 head	SHEARING	1.10	0.00
0 head	WOOL BAGS	2.80	0.00
15 lb	MEDS/SM	15.00	225.00
SUBTOTAL			$3,722.49
FEED (381,260 lb)			$23,087.62
TOTAL			$26,810.11
50% DUE			$13,405.06

THANK YOU!

Table 4. EXAMPLE OF A CUSTOM FEEDING CLOSEOUT STATEMENT

LOT: IOU	DATE:	11/13/90
	In	Out
Number of head	4,296	4,155
Payweight	378,240	559,070
Average weight	88.04	134.55
Price	$208,671.98	$312,013.63
Price/cwt	$55.17	$55.81
Off-truck weight	347,200	ADD WOOL
Shrink	8.21%	Head Sheared
Death loss	3.28%	Pounds Sheared

	Average weight	$0.00
	Price/lb	0.00
	Amount	0.00
	Total lambs and wool:	$312,013.63

Lamb days	316,837	
Average days	73.75	
Gain	$180,830	

Average daily gain	0.57	Lambs	$208,671.98
Lb/head/day	4.20	Feed cost	79,745.88
Lb/feed/lb gain	7.3	Interest	11,041.75
Feed cost/cwt gain	$44.10		
Total cost/cwt gain	$52.96	Total:	$311,748.21

	Sales		$312,013.63
	Purchases	$208,671.98	
	Expenses	$95,773.96	$304,445.94
	Net		$7,567.69
	Net per head		$1.76

Table 5. PREVALENCE OF DISEASE CATEGORIES FOR TWO COLORADO SHEEP FEEDLOTS (1985–1986)

	Cases		Prevalence (%)	
Disease	Feedlot 1	Feedlot 2[1]	Feedlot 1[2]	Feedlot 2[3]
Pneumonia	722	1243	4.90	13.00
Acidosis	491	734	3.33	7.68
Enterotoxemia	463	142	3.14	1.49
Transport tetany	71	229	0.48	2.40
Urolithiasis	74	33	0.50	0.35
Rectal prolapse	52	30	0.35	0.31
Salmonellosis	1	0	0.01	0.00
Enteritis	17	2	0.10	0.02
Polioencephalomalacia	5	0	0.04	0.00
Tetanus	0	1	0.00	0.01
Other	85	57	0.57	0.60
Total	1981	2471		

[1]Feedlot 2 reported a case-fatality rate of less than 100 per cent for pneumonia and transport tetany. All reported cases are included.
[2]The median monthly average population for feedlot 1 was 14,736.
[3]The median monthly average population for feedlot 2 was 9559.

of lambs on feed was 15,000 with a range of 4000 to 25,000. These lambs originated primarily from Texas, Colorado, Wyoming, Montana, Idaho, California, and Arizona. The ration consisted of whole corn, sun-cured alfalfa pellets, medicated starter for 2 weeks (chlortetracycline 70 mg/head/day for the first 2 days and 50 mg/head/day for the balance of the 2 weeks), and lamb finisher. During the adjustment period of 21 to 28 days, the ration changed from 85 per cent roughage–15 per cent concentrate to 15 per cent roughage–85 per cent concentrate. The ration was provided ad libitum via self-feeders, plus long-stem hay. The lambs were on feed 45 to 60 days and marketed at 110 to 140 pounds, depending on frame size and finish. During the 12-month study, all lambs received electrolytes via the water for the first 12 days. They were vaccinated with *Clostridium perfringens* types C and D toxoid, with a booster administered in 2 weeks. All lambs were wormed with levamisole or fenbendazole.

The lot increased its capacity in 1988 to 50,000 head with half of the lot designed for bunkline feeding to accommodate longer periods of higher-roughage feeding. This recent feeding change is in response to an industry shift toward evening out the marketing period. However, the most economical and efficient gains are still achieved with high-concentrate diets. This description plus a review of Figures 1 through 4 and Tables 5 and 6 will give the veterinarian an understanding of the complexity and economic impact of disease problems in the sheep feedlot.

Although there is an extreme fluctuation in the availability of feeder lambs throughout the year, many lots feed on a 12-month basis. With the majority of lambs being born in the spring, the peak numbers are in the feedlots in the fall and winter as shown in Figure 1.

The financial impact of these conditions as shown in Table 6 indicates where the practicing veterinarian should place the major preventive health emphasis. Death loss added $1.41 to the cost of every lamb entering the feeding program. This figure was the value of the animal at time of death based on

Table 6. FINANCIAL IMPACT OF DISEASES IN A COLORADO SHEEP FEEDLOT (1985–1986)

Annual Average Death Loss/Disease	Deaths	Loss ($)	100 Lambs Fed[1]
Pneumonia	722	49,077	0.79
Acidosis	491	33,241	0.54
Enterotoxemia	463	31,017	0.51
Transport tetany	71	4,798	0.08
Urolithiasis	74	4,555	0.08
Rectal prolapse	52	3,609	0.06
Salmonellosis	1	65	0.001
Enteritis	17	1,194	0.02
Polioencephalomalacia	5	396	0.01
Tetanus	0	0	0.00
Other	85	3,204	0.09
Total	1981	131,156	2.18

[1]The number of deaths was divided by the average of the number of lambs that arrived in the lot and the number of lambs that were sold from the lot. This was 91,683.

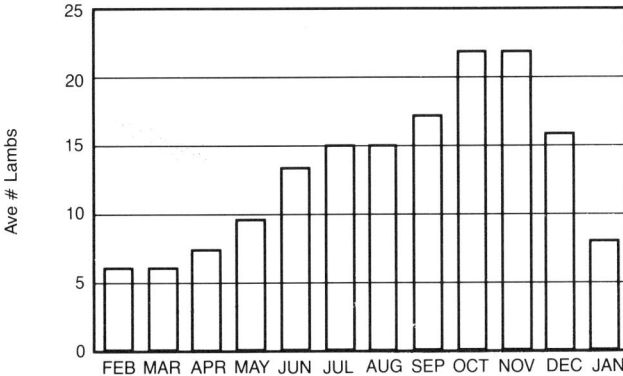

(thousands)
Figure 1. Monthly inventory for a Colorado sheep feedlot.

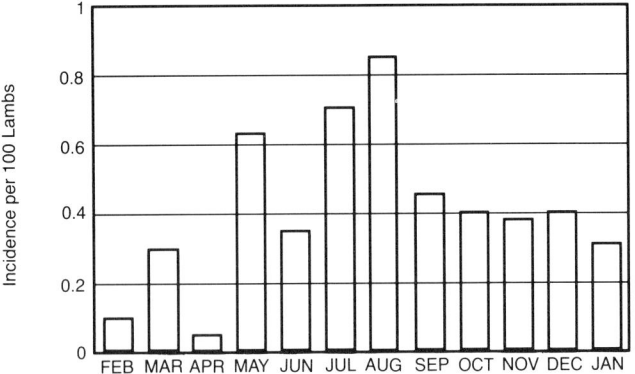

Figure 2. Incidence of pneumonia in a Colorado sheep feedlot.

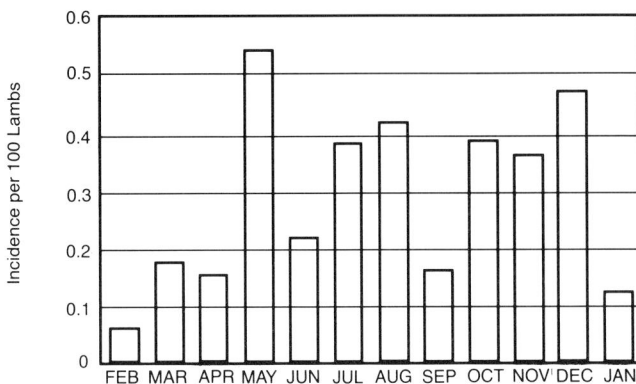

Figure 4. Monthly incidence of acidosis in a Colorado sheep feedlot.

its weight and that day's market price and did not include feed, labor, vaccinations, and the like. Pneumonia, enterotoxemia, and acidosis occur throughout the year, but the incidence is highest during the summer and fall (Figs. 2 to 4), as is also true for rectal prolapse and transport tetany. Urolithiasis is most common in the winter.

In a study of 2 Colorado feedlots, pneumonia, acidosis, and enterotoxemia were the major disease problems irrespective of differences in feeding and management practices (Table 5). This is consistent with other studies in which sheep are fed throughout the temperate climate.

After reviewing the most prevalent conditions affecting feedlot lambs (pneumonia, acidosis, enterotoxemia, transport tetany, urolithiasis), the veterinarian needs to direct his or her efforts toward prevention of these conditions.

If the lamb producer has used veterinary services on a limited basis, there is an excellent opportunity for the veterinarian to improve production and profitability. The economists refer to this as biologic and economic efficiency of the sheep enterprise. Measures of biologic efficiency include pregnancy rate, lambing rate, percentage lamb crop weaned, weaning weight, and pounds of lamb weaned per ewe exposed. Measures of economic efficiency include cost of production per weight of live animal marketed, net return per ewe, net return to the ewe enterprise, and return on investment. The large commercial feedlot may utilize a computer program that can estimate break-even price, project total cost of production, and estimate the economic impact of various decision alternatives, such as the return on investment of preventive health measures for pneumonia. However, for the majority of producers not on such a computer program, the veterinarian can play a major role.

A computer program, SHEEPMKT, was developed for the producer by Sharp, Gutierrez, and Holman at Colorado State University. This program is a Lotus 1-2-3 template that provides a format and procedure to evaluate the price and profit potential associated with alternative production and marketing strategies for a sheep operation. The program includes enterprise budgeting, break-even price by sales category, price and profit goals, and sensitivity analysis. Through this or similar programs, the veterinarian can assist the producer in making preventive health decisions by evaluating the potential economic impact these decisions will have on profitability.

To serve the lamb feeding industry and the sheep industry in general, the practicing veterinarian must have a thorough understanding of business, nutrition, and health. Problem-solving for total health management may necessitate the integration of assistance from a variety of disciplines. The veterinarian is the logical individual to determine the necessary expertise and coordinate a team to develop a total health and production program.

BIBLIOGRAPHY

Botkin MP, Field RA, Johnson CL: Sheep and Wool. Englewood Cliffs, NJ, Prentice Hall, 1988.
Kimberling CV: Diseases of Sheep, 3rd ed. Philadelphia, Lea & Febiger, 1988.
Salman MD, et al: Rates of diseases and their associated costs in two Colorado sheep feedlots (1985–86). J Am Vet Med Assoc 12:1518–1523, 1988.
Sharp R, Gutierrez P, Holman K: Sheep Integrated Resource Management: SHEEPMKT. Fort Collins, CO, Colorado State University Cooperative Extension, XCM–9016, April 1990.
Sheep Production Handbook. American Sheep Industries Development Program, Inc., 1988.

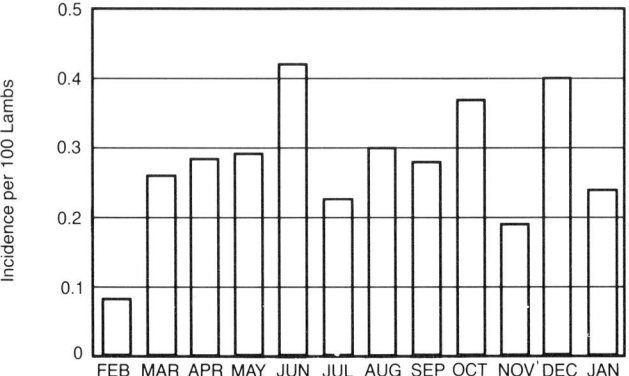

Figure 3. Monthly incidence of enterotoxemia in a Colorado sheep feedlot.

Production Medicine and Health Programs for Goats

KATHERINE BRETZLAFF, DVM, PhD

Goats can be generally classified by the commodity produced, that is, milk, meat, or fiber. Health programs vary with management schemes and the perceived value of animals.

Veterinary practitioners need to reflect on their role in small ruminant production medicine. Producers have access to most vaccines and dewormers at competitive prices and receive free advice from a variety of sources on health concepts. Application of economic resources to predator control, weed control, and pasture improvement may be a higher priority than are health programs in some rangeland areas. In regions with relatively small populations of goats, goat producers frequently voice disappointment in the lack of knowledge of or interest from their local practitioner. However, veterinarians may not be motivated to educate themselves about small ruminant medicine when producers are reluctant to pay for the value of the service rendered.

Ideally, a veterinarian who hopes to participate in a goat operation would be able to assist the producer in making an economic assessment of the operation. The veterinarian would then offer suggestions concerning management techniques that would increase productivity. This would almost certainly include, but not be limited to, health considerations. Unfortunately, many goat producers seek veterinary assistance only for sporadic health problems.

ECONOMIC ASSESSMENT OF GOAT OPERATIONS

Dairy Goats

Dairy goats and other types of pet or exotic goats are kept intensively, have individual animal identification, and frequently have sentimental value for the owner. Animals are observed frequently and are readily accessible for data collection or treatments. Producers perform most routine procedures such as disbudding, vaccinating, and castrating. Contagious diseases have the most impact on intensively reared goats.

Dairy goat producers can participate in the Dairy Herd Improvement Association programs available for cattle. Through the American Dairy Goat Association (ADGA),[1] breeders can arrange to have their goats classified according to conformation. In addition, ADGA-sanctioned dairy goat shows are held throughout the United States each year. Through the use of these records and artificial insemination, a buck sire summary has been compiled and is available through ADGA. By these means, some genetic gain has been realized in the dairy goat industry, and a basis for valuation of registered animals has been provided. However, the economic viability of dairy goat operations, aside from sale of breeding stock, is usually tenuous. Other than in a few major metropolitan markets, the sale of dairy goat products is inconsistent at best. Most dairy goat producers are in the business for the enjoyment or because they have a specific need or desire for goat milk products. Their desire or ability to pay for health care for their animals is often based on considerations beyond the dollar value of the individual goats and their products.

Fiber Goats

The majority of fiber produced by goats in the United States is mohair from Angoras. Most Angora goats are kept on rangeland in Texas. Under these conditions, contagious diseases are minimized, and nutrition, parasites, and predators become the limiting factors for health and production. Information on individual animals is frequently not available. The willingness of the producer to seek veterinary care to some extent parallels the value of the animals. This, in turn, is dependent on the price of mohair, which has varied 5-fold over the past decade (average market price in 1990 being $0.93 per pound). Most routine procedures are performed by the producer.

Approximately 85 per cent of the income from Angora flocks comes from sale of mohair. The rest comes from sale of replacement or breeding stock and sale of cull animals for meat. Determination of income from Angora flocks primarily involves the identification of the quality and quantity of hair produced. This is affected by an interaction of genetics and environment. Average mohair production is 7 to 8 pounds per year per animal obtained in 2 shearings. Selected goats under good management systems can produce twice this amount. Kids produce less hair, but the value of the fleece may be as great as or greater than that from adults because the quality of kid hair is higher. Average fiber diameter ranges from 24 to 40 μ. Reproductive efficiency affects mohair production because young animals produce the most valuable (smallest diameter) hair.

From gross income must be subtracted expenses including feed costs, insurance, taxes, depreciation, drugs and chemicals, equipment, labor, and predator control costs. This information alone allows a break-even price for mohair to be determined.

Computer software for Angora goats is commercially available.[1] Spreadsheet packages have also been devised by extension agents in areas of large Angora populations for financial analysis of Angora goat enterprises. Once herd productivity has been established, goals can be set to improve mohair production through animal selection and improved nutrition (including parasite control). If reproductive efficiency is a problem (weaned kid crops of 50 to 80 per cent are common, which leaves much room for improvement), management techniques for reducing stress abortions and neonatal losses can be discussed.

Movement of Angoras into nontraditional environments such as those in Oklahoma (improved pastures) or Michigan (feeding of harvested feeds) has led to the emergence of problems in Angoras that are similar to those seen with other intensively reared goats.

The cashmere goat industry in its present form is new to the United States. It includes imported breeding stock as well as native Spanish and dairy-type goats that are being bred to cashmere bucks to begin an upgrading process. A good-quality cashmere goat will produce 1 pound of cashmere per year. Many goats produce much less than this. Prices for cashmere in the United States vary with the international market. Producers received $45 per clean pound of cashmere fleece that averaged less than 16.5 μ in diameter or $35 for 16.5 to 19 μ fleeces in 1990. The prices for 1991 were $33 and $26, respectively. This meant that a number of first-generation half-Spanish ("bred-on") goats provided income of only $5 to $15 in 1991. It is difficult to predict for the long term whether cashmere goats will be able to support themselves on the production of fiber alone. However, by upgrading meat-type animals to cashmere production, an additional income could be realized from a meat goat operation. Presently, cashmere goats are rather scarce and in demand, and their value as breeding stock is considerably greater than the income they generate through production of cashmere. Computer software from Australia for evaluation of cashmere enterprises is commercially available.[2]

Meat Goats

The so-called Spanish goats found primarily in Texas and woodland areas of the Southeast are kept under extensive

---

[1] P.O. Box 865, Spindale, NC 28160.

[1] Roland Trees, P.O. Box 70, Mountain Home, TX 78058.
[2] CASHSTUD, Ann R. Dooling, P.O. Box 1339, Dillon, MT 59725.

management conditions. Management inputs are minimal in most cases. However, there has been an increasing interest in meat goats owing to (1) increasing ethnic populations that favor goat meat; (2) increasing interest in cashmere production, which is being investigated as an alternative income from meat-type goats; (3) increasing interest in environmentally sound methods of brush control; and (4) recognition of improved utilization of many rangeland areas by incorporation of goats into mixed-species grazing schemes.

Evaluation of meat goats should involve some parameter concerning meat produced per animal unit or acreage unit. In reality, this information is available from very few producers because of the lack of individual animal identification. In addition, the fact that the animals are handled on rare occasions makes meaningful data collection difficult. Another factor is the nature of the goat meat market. Although there are regional differences, many kid goats are sold on a per head basis rather than on a per pound basis. This reduces producer incentive to select animals for growth rates and shifts focus to selection for prolificacy and mothering ability. This is also difficult because many kids are lost at birth owing to predation and poor mothering ability. By the time kids are marked or weaned, the producer may have little idea which females produced twins or triplets. Improvements in reproductive efficiency and neonatal survivability can profoundly affect income to the meat goat producer.

Computer spreadsheet packages have been adapted by some extension agents for evaluation of meat goat enterprises on the basis of numbers of kids and nannies sold. Variable costs to be considered include feed, health costs, fuel, sales commissions, repairs, labor, and interest on credit; fixed costs include depreciation and land costs.

Assessment of fiber-producing or meat goat–producing operations may be severely limited by lack of individual animal identification. Ear tags have problems with retention, but they can be used with reasonable success. In the Angora industry, ear notching is sometimes used for identification. An alternative to permanent identification is to sort animals as they are worked into groups on the basis of some criterion of performance and keep them in separate pastures.

HERD HEALTH PROGRAMS FOR GOATS

Vaccinations

Clostridial spp.

A basic vaccination program for goats includes vaccinations against *Clostridium perfringens* type D (enterotoxemia) and tetanus. Some rangeland producers do not vaccinate for clostridial diseases because they feel the few animals they may lose to these diseases are not worth the expense of vaccinating the whole herd. Nevertheless, if animals are to be moved (sold), stressed, or subjected to changes in feed, or if animals are raised in confinement on processed feeds, vaccination for enterotoxemia should be strongly encouraged. Kids are generally vaccinated first at 4 weeks of age with boosters administered according to label directions for sheep. Administration of boosters should be emphasized; a second booster at the time of weaning is desirable if kids are put into a feedlot situation. Annual boosters of pregnant females 1 month before parturition will boost colostral immunity; other adults should receive annual boosters when it works into the ranch routine. Animals that are fed high amounts of processed feeds may need to receive boosters every 6 months for full efficacy. Vaccination with 7-way clostridial vaccines for cattle are acceptable in goats and may be desirable if clostridial diseases other than overeating are prevalent in livestock in the area or if they are more economical. Combination vaccines with tetanus are acceptable. Some of the combination products can cause significant local reactions in goats and should be administered in sites where a swelling would not be obvious in show animals. Occasionally, more severe reactions are observed after use of the combination vaccines including generalized stiffness, anorexia, bloating, and, rarely, sudden death.

Contagious Ecthyma

Contagious ecthyma or soremouth is common in goat enterprises and should be vaccinated for once it has been identified in a herd. Vaccination is not recommended in a closed herd in which the disease is not present because the vaccine will introduce the virus to the premises. Producers with closed herds who plan to begin showing their animals should seriously consider beginning a soremouth vaccination program in all their goats if animals from the show circuit will be reintroduced to the main herd. Initial vaccinations should be done in the whole herd; after that, only each year's new kid crop and unvaccinated purchased animals need be vaccinated. The site of vaccine administration should be chosen so that direct exposure of the udder of adult does to the vaccine virus is avoided.

Other

Vaccines for some other diseases that affect goats are available for sheep or cattle and can be used on an as-needed basis. Chlamydial vaccines for sheep can be used in goats just before the breeding season if chlamydial abortion is a problem. These can cause severe local reactions in goats, especially if they are not administered properly in the subcutaneous tissue. Vaccines for leptospirosis are not usually administered to goats unless they are kept near cattle in areas in which leptospiral abortions in cattle are a problem. An approved vaccine for caseous lymphadenitis is not available for goats. A newly released vaccine for sheep undoubtedly will be tried in goats, although the author has no experience with this product in goats.[1] Infectious keratoconjunctivitis (pinkeye) in goats is rarely caused by *Moraxella bovis*, so the cattle bacterin should not be used. Pinkeye in goats is usually caused by *Mycoplasma*, for which a vaccine is not available. Conjunctivitis can also be caused by *Chlamydia* but is due to a different strain from that which is contained in the abortion vaccine. No vaccine is available for control of caprine arthritis-encephalitis.

Although it is not a "vaccine," vitamin E–selenium injection is considered a "vaccination" by many owners because of the routine administration typically used in deficient areas. Treatments are given to pregnant does 30 days before parturition if indicated. If white muscle disease is still a problem, kids may also be injected soon after birth. If possible, it is advisable to supplement selenium in the feed.

Parasite Control Programs

Control of parasites is one of the most important facets of a goat herd health program. The degree of infestation varies with the goat-keeping system. Goats kept in drylots, such as dairy goats, may have minimal problems with nematodes. Kids on rangeland pastures have minimal problems with coccidiosis but in confined quarters are very susceptible to this disease. Goats kept on land with plenty of brush and tall weeds will

---

[1]Caseous D-T, Colorado Serum Company, P.O. Box 16428, Denver, CO 80216.

suffer little exposure to infective nematode larvae because of their preference for browsing over grazing. They also will develop little immunity and will be highly susceptible to infection if they are moved to a situation in which they are forced to graze infected pastures. Internal parasite infection may be of little significance in dry years in certain rangeland areas whereas it is a continual problem in moist, temperate areas. The degree of parasitic infection is a dynamic situation and one that needs to be continually monitored.

Nematodes

In fiber and meat goats, *Haemonchus contortus* is the most significant gastrointestinal nematode. In dairy goats, several other nematodes in addition to *H. contortus* may be of significance in certain geographic areas. Resistance of nematodes to many of the available dewormers has developed to varying degrees in different regions, largely owing to overuse or improper use of available drugs. Few dewormers are approved for use in goats, but many of the available cattle anthelmintics have been used on an extra-label basis. A number of the benzimidazoles, levamisole, and ivermectin have all been used safely in goats.

The dosages used for goats are frequently the same as those used in sheep. There is growing evidence that goats metabolize at least some of these compounds differently from sheep so that use of sheep dosages results in underdosing of goats. This may in turn contribute to development of resistant strains of parasites in goats. Clinical impressions from some practitioners indicate that twice the label dose of ivermectin is necessary for adequate control of *H. contortus* in Angora and dairy goats. Australian literature suggests that goats require larger doses of levamisole than do sheep. Scientific studies in this area are needed. Goats also have the reputation for not developing immunity to nematodes to the extent that sheep do. Whether this is due to an inherent difference in their immune system, a reduced exposure because of their preference to browse above the level of larval contamination, or both has not been resolved.

In order to determine whether a given anthelmintic is effective on a particular farm, pre- and post-treatment fecal egg per gram counts are recommended as in other species. The anthelmintics used should not be changed more often than once per year. The use of anthelmintics should be in conjunction with other methods of parasite control, such as strategic deworming and movement of goats to "safe" pastures after drenching. Safe pastures are those in which goats are not forced to graze close to the ground or that have not been grazed by goats or infected sheep for 3 months in warm weather or 6 months in cool weather. Treatments should be devised to prevent rather than treat clinical disease. Herd treatment should be considered when the average fecal egg count per individual exceeds 500 eggs per gram of feces. Strategic deworming times are similar to those in other species, that is, before parturition, before release onto spring pastures, as needed in late summer, and so on.

Coccidia

Coccidiosis can be a severe problem in kids. Management is similar to that in lambs and includes feeding of a creep feed with a coccidiostat whenever kids are brought or kept together on infected premises. Monensin at the level of 20 g per ton of feed or decoquinate fed at the rate of 0.5 mg/kg body weight per day during periods of exposure is approved for use in goats. Monensin may also improve feed efficiency in growing kids.

Parelaphostrongylus tenuis

The meningeal worm of white-tailed deer has been reported as a significant cause of paralysis and death of Angora goats in eastern Oklahoma and southwestern Missouri. The parasite is acquired by ingestion of the intermediate host (a snail). Prevention may be possible by timely deworming with ivermectin, but this may be cost-prohibitive for some producers. Treatment regimens still need to be worked out.

External Parasites

Sucking lice can cause anemia and biting lice can result in significant hair damage because of biting and rubbing by the goats to relieve itching. Hair goats can be treated for lice as they come out of the shearing pens if necessary, but it is best to wait 4 to 8 weeks to allow some regrowth of hair. Hair retains some of the pesticide, which improves control of the lice. Goats can be sprayed with a coarse high-pressure (300 to 350 psi) spray of malathion, permethrin (Ectiban or Atroban), fenvalerate (Ectrin), or other approved insecticide. Treatments with malathion or permethrin should be repeated in 2 weeks. Fenvalerate may give adequate control with just 1 application, although goats should be checked monthly to monitor the parasite load. Fenvalerate can also be applied as a pour-on. One quart of fenvalerate WDL and 1.25 ounces of liquid detergent can be mixed with 3 gallons of water and applied to goats at the rate of 1 ounce of mix per 50- to 100-pound animal. Care should be taken to use only approved products in lactating dairy goats.

Management Techniques

Reproduction and Neonatal Survival

DAIRY GOATS. Dairy goats are almost always subjected to controlled breeding programs in which does are hand-mated or artificially inseminated to selected bucks. Dairy goats are generally not expected to kid more than once per year because of selection for 10-month lactations; however, breeding some individuals during the nonbreeding season is desirable in order to maintain a uniform milk supply. This involves the use of a progestin such as one half of a Syncro-Mate B cattle ear implant for 9 to 11 days and the administration of 400 to 600 IU of PMSG (pregnant mare serum gonadotropin) 48 hours before removal of the progestin. Unfortunately, PMSG is not approved for use in the United States and so is not widely available. A new product (PG600[1]) that contains 400 IU PMSG and 200 IU HCG (human chorionic gonadotropin) in each dose has recently been approved for swine in the United States and no doubt will be tried in small ruminants. These hormones are not approved for use in goats, and should not be used in animals producing food for human consumption. An alternative to the use of hormones is manipulation of the photoperiod. Extra lights are used to expose does and bucks to 19- to 20-hour days from January 1 to March 1, at which time the extra lighting is shut off. Does will begin a short breeding season of approximately 60 days 7 to 10 weeks later.

With the advent of real-time ultrasonography, early pregnancy diagnosis is feasible. Dairy goats should be checked 45 days postbreeding for pregnancy. If fluid is seen in the uterus without placentomes or fetuses, the animal can be considered pseudopregnant and can be treated with prostaglandin and rebred.

Dairy goats frequently have multiple offspring and low neonatal mortality because of the intensive rearing practices

---
[1] Intervet America, Inc., P. O. Box 318, Millsboro, DE 19966.

under which they are kept. When high neonatal morbidity and mortality rates occur on dairy goat operations, they are usually due to contagious diseases associated with overcrowding, poor hygiene and failure of passive transfer. Management techniques recognized as important in other species, such as dipping navels and ensuring adequate intake of quality colostrum, are equally important in goats. Control programs for caprine arthritis-encephalitis that involve feeding of heat-treated colostrum (131°F for 1 hour) and pasteurized milk or milk replacer will also reduce the spread of other infectious agents such as *Mycoplasma* spp.

FIBER GOATS. Angora goats are generally managed under a controlled breeding season in the fall. Billies are kept separate from the nannies for 10 months of the year.

One of the most important target areas for improvement on fiber goat ranches is the number of kids born and weaned. Angora goat herds may have weaning rates of 50 to 80 per cent or even less in bad years. This is usually due to several factors. Angora goats have increased nutritional needs for mohair growth and are under relatively more nutritional stress than are other goats on rangeland. Low growth rates in nanny kids result in failure to breed the first breeding season after the animals are born. Poor body condition in adults results in failure of multiple ovulations. Angoras, especially young nannies, are sometimes subject to abortion because of chronic undernutrition and stress. High neonatal mortality due to birth of underweight kids, poor mothering ability especially in young nannies, and high predation rates on young Angora kids also contribute to a poor reproductive rate. Most Angora nannies breed exclusively during the autumn months.

Some producers feel single kids are desirable because they are larger and have a higher survival rate. They also feel more than one kid crop per year is not feasible owing to the limited nutrition available at certain times of the year and the physiologic stress already placed on the Angora for hair growth. They do not turn billies in with nanny kids the first autumn after they are born because they are too small to breed successfully and carry kids to term. However, in areas outside of west Texas where Angora goats are raised more intensively, Angoras have been shown to reproduce successfully by 1 year of age, to have a high percentage of twins, and to wean well over 100 per cent kid crops. Most of this can be accomplished by improved nutrition and supervised kidding.

The desire to invest money in extra feed, labor, and facilities will be determined to some extent by the market price for mohair. During times of depressed mohair markets, producers are less interested in increasing cost inputs to maximize reproductive efficiency.

Because of the more intensive management under which cashmere goats are currently kept, they will probably have fewer problems than Angoras will with poor reproductive efficiency. As the quantity of hair produced increases through selection, and as the goats are treated more as rangeland meat goats as the industry matures, more problems associated with nutrition may arise.

MEAT GOATS. Spanish nannies are more successful than are Angora goats in rearing kids but would be more productive if their tendency to breed almost year-round could be exploited. When billies are left with the nannies year-round, as is the case in many herds, some females will be seen kidding during 10 months of the year. Breeding is greatly reduced during April and May. This has led to the erroneous conclusion by some producers that Spanish goats can kid twice per year. Very few females can continually produce offspring every 6 months. Compared with a controlled breeding situation, this type of unsupervised reproduction is inefficient. When billies are not removed, the male effect is much reduced, and transitional nannies cannot be "shocked" into cycling all at one time. This type of management also makes health management of the herd difficult because animals are in different stages of the reproductive cycle at any given time. Controlled accelerated breeding programs (3 kid crops every 2 years) for meat goats can be successful by keeping billies separate from nannies except for defined breeding periods every 8 months. Progressive Spanish goat producers have shown that through selection alone, a herd of nannies that will breed at 6 to 8 months of age, continue to breed every 8 months with conception rates of 92 to 98 per cent depending on the time of year, and consistently have 2 or more kids can be maintained on rangeland if it is properly managed. This would lead to a goal of a 300 per cent kid crop weaned each year. A more realistic goal for most producers should be 200 per cent. For this to be successful, nutrition must be adequate to ensure that female kids are well grown by the time of first breeding and that kids born will not be too weak and small to survive. If neonatal losses prevent identification of females that had multiple offspring at marking time, those females can be identified by ultrasonography during gestation. Accelerated kidding requires early weaning and therefore attention to feeding of young kids if they do not go to market off the nannies. It also may predispose heavily milking females to mastitis so that females must be rigorously culled for udder conformation.

In dual-purpose meat and cashmere goats, the tendency of parturient nannies to shed their fleece and for lactation to inhibit the growth of new hair must be considered. Accelerated kidding programs may need to be devised that avoid fall kidding seasons when cashmere hair growth is at its maximum.

The male effect, by which billies are maintained separately from the nannies until their sudden introduction at the onset of a breeding season, contributes greatly to an accelerated kidding program. The use of teasers to get the nannies through the first, less prolific ovulations before turning in of fertile males should be considered. Although it is not clear whether the goat meat market will ever be on a per pound basis, it is probably advisable to select breeding billies from the largest, fastest-growing kids.

Rangeland goats should not be disturbed during kidding because they may become frightened and abandon their newborn kids. Nannies having multiple kids are more productive than are nannies having singles only if their kids survive, and because multiples are born smaller and weaker, they are more likely to die. If the producer will identify multiple-bearing nannies and manage them separately, many twins can be saved. Increased feeding during the last 6 weeks of gestation when the fetuses undergo 80 per cent of their growth will increase birth weight. Kidding the nannies in small pastures or in sheds will reduce abandonment of kids. In sheds, producers can assist newborn kids with colostral intake and see that they are bonded to their dams before they are turned out to pasture.

Whether any of these schemes is feasible will depend on the available facilities, labor, and motivation of the producer. Accurate record-keeping will be the only way by which to document the benefits of new management procedures.

Freeze Loss

High mortality rates can be seen in freshly shorn Angora or cashmere goats that are not provided shelter from inclement weather. Freeze loss can occur as readily in August in Texas as in February if wind and rain combine to produce a significant chill factor. Poor nutrition aggravates the freeze loss problem. Well-fed Angoras that have access to a windbreak will usually not succumb.

Testing for Caprine Arthritis-Encephalitis

Caprine arthritis-encephalitis (CAE) is an insidious disease that is highly prevalent in dairy goats. Over 80 per cent of dairy goats surveyed in some studies have been seropositive for the CAE virus. Although the incidence of clinical disease is much less than this, the disease is of great economic significance to the dairy goat industry through morbidity, labor required for eradication programs, and lost opportunity to export seropositive animals. The incidence of CAE in other populations of goats appears to be much less; large herds of Angoras or Spanish goats may be totally CAE-seronegative. However, with cross-breeding programs and use of dairy does as recipients for cashmere embryos, the potential for spread of the virus into other goat industries is great. *Every precaution to prevent the spread of the virus to uninfected flocks should be taken*. People purchasing goats for the first time or making additions to existing herds should insist on negative CAE tests in these animals. If animals are of dairy breeding, they ideally should be segregated from the rest of the herd until follow-up tests are found to be negative. Most goats become seropositive 4 to 16 weeks after they are infected. Segregation of animals for that period of time may seem difficult, but it would be a small price to pay to keep CAE out of a clean herd.

Dairy Goats

For dairy goat operations that milk goats for profit, monitoring of milk quality and udder health may be an important aspect of overall management. General approaches to diagnosis, treatment, and prevention of mastitis are similar to those in dairy cattle. Coagulase-negative staphylococci are a common and significant isolate from dairy goats. Somatic cell counts are useful for monitoring udder health, but care should be taken in interpretation. Healthy goats will frequently give higher readings than will cattle, with counts of 1.5 million being not uncommon in late lactation goats.

SUMMARY

Goat production medicine varies with the type of goat (dairy, hair, meat) being considered and the type of management system involved (intensive versus extensive). Economic assessment of the various goat production systems can be done with available computer software, being limited primarily by lack of identification of individual animals or the infrequent handling of animals. Basic vaccination programs include immunization against *Clostridium perfringens* type D, tetanus, and contagious ecthyma where it is endemic in the herd. Parasite control may be the most important aspect of goat production medicine. Although not approved for goats, many of the cattle dewormers have been used safely in goats. Monensin and decoquinate have been approved for control of coccidiosis in goats. Fenvalerate is widely used for control of external parasites in hair goats. Circumvention of seasonal limitations on reproduction in goats is an important aspect of improving production. Accelerated kidding programs are possible through good nutrition, genetic selection, and use of the male effect. Hormonal manipulations are also effective, but the necessary drugs are not approved for use in goats. Reduction of neonatal losses through good nutrition and supervised kidding can be a major factor in improving the production from a goat operation.

BIBLIOGRAPHY

Caprine Supply Catalogue (dairy goat supplies and sources of information). P.O. Box Y, 33001 West 83rd St., DeSoto, KS 66018.

Cashmere Producers of America Newsletter: Concerning Cashmere. P.O. Box 2F, Virginia Dale, CO 80548.

Proceedings of the Annual Conferences of the Cashmere Producers of America; contact the CaPrA office, currently P.O. Box 91106, Austin, TX 78709–1106.

Sheep and goat medicine. Vet Clin North Am [Large Anim Pract] 5, 1983.

Spanish meat goats: an alternative enterprise in South Texas. Texas Agricultural Extension Service, Corpus Christi, TX. A conference proceedings.

Texas Sheep and Goat Raisers publication: Ranch Magazine. P.O. Box 2678, San Angelo, TX 76902.

Swine Herd Health Management

JOSEPH F. CONNOR, DVM

Pork production is changing rapidly, and it behooves veterinary service to respond to and direct some of these changes. Although the surveys of the midwestern states show that the average sow herd size is 25 head, intensification of pork production has evolved over the last 10 years. Recent surveys indicate that 9.6 per cent of the production units in the United States produce 62.5 per cent of our total annual production.[1]

This change will not be slowed by veterinary service but, in actuality, presents a unique opportunity for members of our profession.

The Iowa State Enterprise Records show tremendous variation in profitability of the units, with as much as $34 per head difference in total costs between intensively managed units and low-profit units.[2]

One must expect that this trend will continue and that the low- and marginal-profit units will vanish. Owners and managers are now requesting professional consultation in the areas of health, reproduction, genetics, nutrition, environment, economics, personnel training, and quality assurance. All of these areas are interrelated, and our ability to address and tailor the needs of each individual herd will be of foremost importance. Because of their broad-based education, credibility, and continual desire to improve their skills, veterinarians can be intimately involved in the pork production system. Veterinarians are in the best position to coordinate production, health, and management schemes on an individual unit. They can utilize their knowledge and access to appropriate specialists to drive the swine enterprise to reach its goal, profit maximization. Recommendations can no longer be based on individual animal diagnosis and past experience but must be medically, scientifically, and, most important, financially correct. The cost of preventive treatment should not exceed the expected yield in return.

Opportunities exist not only in traditional roles but also in areas such as quality assurance programs, personnel training, marketing alternatives, and genetic programs. When a herd health program is initiated, communication is the key. The veterinarian, manager, and staff must be aware of each other's expectations. It is helpful for the veterinarian and the owner to discuss these expectations and to prioritize them. Producers who desire only consultation must be handled differently from those who wish to incorporate consultation with dispensing. It is imperative that the veterinary consultant determine the desires of herd management at the outset. Frequency of visits, amount of time spent per visit, phone consultation, fax charges, diagnostic work, and cost of total service are some points that should be discussed.

Fees should be based on return for time and structured according to service, competency, and client type. As production units grow, there is a tendency toward hourly compensation. This is probably most fair to both owner and veterinarian. Because of the necessary inputs for a successful unit, the owner should expect hourly charges that include phone consultation, record evaluation and interpretation, previsit preparation, and follow-up. Other methods of compensation include retainers, predetermined amount per pig weaned or marketed, and hourly fee plus mark-up on drugs. Whatever the type of fee scheduling chosen, it is important that the veterinarian review it with the owner annually and that the veterinarian be flexible enough to alter the fee schedule depending on the reasonable needs of the producer. Fee schedules must involve a mutual trust between owner, manager, and veterinarian if the program is to be successful. The most important ingredient in a herd production program is communication between veterinarian, owner, manager, and staff. The routes of communication should be established initially. For information to reach the employee who will carry out the task, the communication route and mode must address that employee's needs and education.

The owners or managers must realize that their job is to see that recommendations agreed on for the unit are accomplished by the staff.

Staff meetings on a regular basis are very helpful for reviewing routine procedures, schedules, goals, and progress. The owner, manager, and veterinarian must realize that the ultimate success of the unit is driven by their ability to provide information that will trigger the appropriate action by the staff. This motivation can be effected by establishing production goals and holding positive discussions with the various employees to clarify these goals and allow all parties to provide input toward achieving performance targets.

Some units or owners use financial incentives. These programs should be based on reasonable production targets and attainable goals. The best program splits the incentive package among all employees who are instrumental in achieving the production targets (see Production Targets section).

The incentive must be large enough to stimulate achievement of the goals yet still be fair to the owners as the targets are met. The package should also allow viewing of necessary long-term changes so the manager is not put in the position of being concerned with only short-term influences and effects.

Veterinarians should continue to strive to improve record-keeping on swine units. Success or failure of a program will be based on bottom-line economics. Unfortunately, in many units, financial records are the last ones to be established. Thus, decision-making is difficult to implement, and success in decision-making is difficult to evaluate. Decisions on the farm should be based on actual farm records rather than on published data bases. Intermingling of financial and production records allows evaluation of financial progress and decision-making. Partial budgeting and cash flows facilitate direct production decisions on the farm.

The first step in record-keeping is to establish production targets for an individual unit. After this, accurate records are mandatory in meeting the production targets. These records should be simple, practical, and usable. They can be hand-kept or computer-based.

Data should be collected and used for decision-making. Analysis of valid data allows the veterinarian to pinpoint problem areas of production and initiate remedial action. Unfortunately, many producers and veterinarians have not yet acquired the discipline to keep or interpret records. The best approach on the farm is initially to keep broad-based records. As the unit progresses, continue to narrow the record focus into individual areas. For many enterprises with no experience in keeping records, it is easiest to start with farrowing and sow production records because pigs and sows can be counted.

In the nursery through finishing phases, it is easier to examine the production areas as a whole and then to break them into the indiviudal phases of nursery-grower-finisher as the discipline of record-keeping and pig movement is established or as facilities change to allow records to be kept on a group basis. Veterinarians are frequently called on to evaluate and provide input for units with no records. In these instances, physical inventory can frequently provide aid in making decisions. Walking through the unit, the veterinarian can count sow inventory, number of available farrowing spaces, number of pigs weaned, and number of pigs in nursery, grower, and finisher categories. If the producer can provide the number of litters farrowed and pigs weaned over a particular time period, these parameters can be calculated: (1) litters per sow per year, (2) pigs weaned per sow per year, (3) farrowing crate utilization, (4) average farrowing rate, (5) pigs sold per sow per year, (6) pounds sold per sow per year, and (7) average age to market.

Record-keeping is required for the following production areas: (1) reproduction, (2) farrowing, (3) nursery, (4) grower, (5) finisher, (6) sales, and (7) feed usage. The other major requirements for record systems to be effectively implemented are sow identification and feed and animal weights.

Reproduction records should include inputs such as gilt source, selection age, sow herd death loss, matings, and pregnancy results. Information derived from this input will include conception rates, weaning to estrus interval, pregnancy rates, abortions, farrowing rates, culling reasons, and boar usage and performance.

Sow and litter records in the farrowing area should include farrowing date, number of pigs born alive, stillbirths, mummies, litter birth weight, number weaned, weaning weight, days to weaning, piglet deaths, and piglet death location. From this input, total number of pigs born alive, average stillbirths, average mummies, average born alive, average litter weights, average number weaned, average weaning weights, preweaning mortality, and death reasons can be derived. These will lead to an individual sow history and farm history for a given time period.

Nursery and growing-finishing records should indicate mortality, reasons for death, weights in, weights out, feed in, and feed out. Output includes percentage mortality, death loss reasons, average daily gain, feed per gain, facility turnover, and cost of gain. Records at the feed processing facility should include input ingredients, diet composition, production schedule, delivery location, and feed medication.

GUIDELINES FOR BREEDING STOCK REPLACEMENT

Most swine enterprises add new genetic material to the herd at some time. Data continue to accumulate showing the cost benefit of correct genetic programs on both maternal and terminal performance.

This new animal introduction has benefits but also carries the risk of disease introduction. This is an excellent opportunity for the recipient herd veterinarian to become involved in the production unit by being the individual who contacts the source herd veterinarian. From this communication, decisions can be made as to the compatibility of the source herd with the customer herd.

Proper isolation and acclimatization procedures should be established. It is important that veterinarians and producers be concerned only about economically important disease agents. Both the breeding stock supplier and producer monitor for the agents in question. Monitoring of the source herd should include (1) routine veterinary herd inspections; (2) quarterly or monthly slaughter checks; (3) routine necropsies; (4) feed, injectable, and water medication usage recording; and (5) serologic tests (for agents for which a reliable test exists).

If a producer's herd is currently infected with *Mycoplasma* or *Haemophilus parasuis*, for example, it is not necessary to demand a source herd free of these. The best criterion in addition to monitoring is the history of other herds supplied from the breeder's herd.

HERD HEALTH PROGRAM

No single herd health program can be written to cover all herds adequately. In fact, the unique opportunity that veterinarians have is the chance to customize a herd health program to an individual herd. Veterinarians must make reasonable immunization, parasite control, and therapeutic programs based on the (1) current health status of the herd; (2) efficacy of vaccines, pharmaceuticals, feed additives, pesticides, and the like; (3) cost benefit of vaccines, pharmaceuticals, feed additives, and pesticides; (4) comfort or insurance level; and (5) probability of infection or exposure to disease agents (including proximity to other swine herds).

A general herd health program is provided as a basis on which to establish more comprehensive programs as needed by the producer. Veterinarians should routinely review herd health programs and continue only procedures that are deemed cost-effective.

Herd health programs should revolve around quality assurance of pork products. Consumers are the final evaluators of pork quality. Veterinarians should direct and monitor correct product usage. This includes (1) withdrawal times; (2) mixing procedures, (3) proper administration or application, and (4) residue testing.

FACILITIES MANAGEMENT

Facility evaluation and correction of production bottlenecks are frequently requested. Problems abound in units, and because of the nature of the beast, solutions must be approached on an individual production unit basis. Anticipated economic return drives many units to crowd facilities, and unavailable production records cannot document that change will be cost-effective. The first step in optimizing pig flow is to identify the bottlenecks that restrict flow or do not maximize facility usage. For accomplishing this, animal flow must be based on some facility increment. The number of available farrowing crates has been and probably remains the best identifier on which to base population flow. In units with too much pig density in the grower-finisher, population should be based on usable square footage in this area. If one uses farrowing crates to establish population, the following rules apply:

Sow inventory	3-week weaning: Number of crates × 5.5
	4-week weaning: Number of crates × 6.0
Gilt pool	Number of crates × 6 weeks × 0.10
Boar inventory	Number of crates × 0.33
Hot-cold nursery	Number of crates × weaning average × 0.25 × weeks in nursery (7)
Grower-finisher	Number of crates × weaning average × 0.25 × weeks in grower-finisher (16)

If square footage is used to establish population, calculations are as follows:

Hot-cold nursery Weekly production × 3.0 sq ft/pig
Grower-finisher   Weekly production × 7.5–8 sq ft/pig

Environmental Quality

Drafts, waste gases, and dust aggravate the respiratory system and depress performance. Environmental analysis is frequently necessary to provide the correct environment for both pigs and people. The following maximal levels are recommended:[3]

Ammonia (ppm)	Carbon dioxide (ppm)	Hydrogen sulfide (ppm)	Carbon monoxide (ppm)	Methane	Dust	
					Total (mg/m^3)	Respirable (mg/m^3)
10	2000	3	20	1%	1.5	0.1

With the proper instruments, a veterinarian can effectively measure conditions within a building and direct the producer in making appropriate adjustments. This equipment necessary to evaluate air quality and ventilation performance includes (1) insect fogger or smoke sticks; (2) gas tubes for hydrogen sulfide, ammonia, carbon dioxide, carbon monoxide, and methane; (3) humidity meter; and (4) temperature meter.

In summary, the opportunities to work with swine production units are excellent. The unique training of veterinarians can be utilized in designing cost-effective production and health programs that maximize production and minimize cost to produce a residue-free consumer product.

GENERAL HERD HEALTH PROGRAM

I. Pregestation Period
   A. Gilt selection
      1. Select gilts 5 to 6 months old weighing 220 to 240 lb (100 to 110 kg)
      2. Select gilts with at least 12 well-spaced, prominent nipples from sows that
         a. have the highest breeding value sow productivity of their contemporary groups
         b. are conformationally sound
         c. have maternal genetics
   B. Boar selection
      1. Select boars 5 to 6 months old weighing 240 to 260 lb (109 to 118 kg)
      2. Select on the basis of
         a. Average daily gain
         b. Feed/Gain ratio (F/G)
         c. Conformation
         d. Lean gain
   C. Isolation/acclimatization of new breeding stock
      1. Isolation
         a. All purchased animals should be isolated for a minimum of 21 to 30 days
         b. Retest for brucellosis, pseudorabies virus (PRV), and other agents, depending on herd
         c. Medicate for ileitis prevention
      2. Acclimatization
         a. Begin after animals have been retested during isolation
         b. Feed back manure, mummies, and placentas from sow herd
         c. Expose boars and gilts to cull gilts or sows
         d. Test mate boars to one or more gilts

e. Vaccinate for disease agents that are present in the main herd or from which protection is desired
f. Treat for external and internal parasites
D. Immunizations
1. Vaccinate for parvovirus, leptospirosis (5- or 6-way), and erysipelas
2. Other vaccinations depend on history of recipient herd
E. Nutrition
1. Boars, developing gilts
a. Protein: 15 to 16 per cent
b. Calcium: 0.9 per cent
c. Phosphorus: 0.8 per cent
d. Feed intake: 4 to 6 lb (2 to 3 kg)

II. Breeding Period
A. Move gilts to a new location and provide boar contact to stimulate estrus or use a vasectomized boar
B. Flush gilts by increasing energy intake to 6 to 9 lb/day (3 to 4 kg/day)
C. Breed during second or third estrus or after 42-day isolation/acclimatization
D. Boars should be 8 to 9 months old
E. Use 1 boar for each 5 females to be bred in a 3-week period
F. Double-mate at 12 and 24 hours after onset of estrus using different boars
G. For hand-mating, provide 1 boar to 17.5 females
H. Reduce daily feed intake of gilt or sow immediately after breeding

III. Gestation Period
A. Nutrition
1. Maintain reduced feed intake until last trimester of pregnancy; gilts should gain between 70 and 100 lb (35 to 50 kg), sows between 50 and 60 lb (22.7 and 27 kg) during gestation; feed sows to condition during first trimester
2. Ration
a. Gilt
(1) Protein: 14 per cent, 250 g/day
(2) Calcium: 0.84 per cent, 16.0 g/day
(3) Phosphorus: 0.70 per cent, 13 g/day
(4) Feed intake: 4 lb (1.8 kg)/day
b. Sow
(1) Protein: 12 to 14 per cent, 250 g/day
(2) Calcium: 0.80 per cent, 15 g/day
(3) Phosphorus: 0.65 per cent, 13 g/day
(4) Feed intake: 4.5 lb (2 to 3 kg)/day
3. Increase feed to 3 kg in last trimester of pregancy
4. Heavy-milking white sows may require more feed
5. Increase energy intake during winter and outside housing
B. Immunization
1. *Clostridium perfringens* type C toxoid, when necessary, 5 weeks and 3 weeks before farrowing
2. *Escherichia coli* bacterin, when necessary, 5 weeks and 3 weeks before farrowing, or live oral milk vaccine
3. Transmissible gastroenteritis (TGE) vaccine if necessary
a. Injectable, 5 weeks and 3 weeks before farrowing
b. Oral, 5 weeks, 3 weeks, and 1 week before farrowing
4. Atrophic rhinitis bacterin, when necessary, 5 weeks and 3 weeks before farrowing
5. Erysipelas vaccine 3 weeks before farrowing, if not done before breeding
C. Retreat for mange 1 week before farrowing (unless mange free)
D. Deworm 7 to 10 days before farrowing if needed. (Biannual fecal examinations of breeding herd will determine need and anthelmintic.) Do not deworm with dichlorvos and treat with insecticide for mange simultaneously
E. Antibiotics are usually not added to gestation ration unless for attempting to control a specific disease, such as atrophic rhinitis or colibacillosis
F. House animals on a clean, dry surface to prevent MMA (mastitis, metritis, agalactia syndrome)

IV. Farrowing Period: Gilts or Sows
A. Thoroughly clean and disinfect the farrowing house
B. Wash and use mild disinfectant on gilts and sows to rid them of parasite eggs and dirt before placement in farrowing crate or stall
C. Feed a diet that will reduce constipation; use 7 lb (3.2 kg) potassium chloride or 20 lb (9 kg) DynaMate per ton of feed or top dress laxative for individual animals
D. Be present at farrowing to increase the number of pigs saved
E. Induce farrowing if breeding date is known
F. Treat sows early that show evidence of agalactia
G. Observe feed intake of sows closely; keeping farrowing room temperature below 80°F will help increase intake
H. Do not allow manure build-up in pen or behind sows in the crate

V. Farrowing to Weaning: Pig
A. Environment
1. Supply adequate heat with lamp or mats to avoid chilling at birth
2. Farrowing boxes or hovers provide direct heat for the pig and allow a lower farrowing house temperature for the sow
3. Split suckle pigs
4. Temperature for pig sleeping area should be 90° to 95°F
B. Administer a fat supplement to reduce weak pig death loss
C. Process pigs 12 to 24 hours after birth
1. Clip needle teeth
2. Dock tails
3. Notch ear to identify litter and week
4. Castrate
5. Inject 200 mg iron into the neck muscle
6. Treat with antibiotic if necessary to control diarrhea or navel ill; use sensitivity results to determine best antibiotic
7. Identify litters with genetic defects
D. If several sows are farrowing simultaneously, cross-foster to equalize piglet and litter size
E. Immunizations
1. Base on herd disease history
2. Administer atrophic rhinitis bacterin if needed
F. Nutrition
1. Provide water as a creep from day 1
2. Palatable creep feed provided at 14 days; feed small amounts daily
G. Wean pigs at 3 to 4 weeks

VI. Weaning Period
A. Environment
1. Place pigs in clean, warm (85°F) nursery, preferably with woven wire flooring or impervious perforated flooring
2. All-in/all-out farrowing and nursery will aid considerably in controlling disease
B. Nutrition

1. Recommendations: mixed-sex feeding
   a. 10 to 15 lb (5 to 7 kg)
      (1) Protein: 2.2 per cent
      (2) Lysine: 1.4 per cent
      (3) Calcium: 0.90 per cent
      (4) Phosphorus: 0.80 per cent
   b. 15 to 25 lb (7 to 11 kg)
      (1) Protein: 22 per cent
      (2) Lysine: 1.25 per cent
      (3) Calcium: 0.90 per cent
      (4) Phosphorus: 0.80 per cent
   c. 25 to 50 lb (11 to 24 kg)
      (1) Protein: 20 per cent
      (2) Lysine: 1.10 per cent
      (3) Calcium: 0.90 per cent
      (4) Phosphorus: 0.80 per cent
2. Diets need to be kept fresh, and pigs should be fed once or twice a day
3. Add antibiotics to the ration
C. Immunization (herd-specific)
   1. Atrophic rhinitis bacterin, when needed; second injection at 28 days
   2. Erysipelas vaccination if necessary at 8 weeks
   3. *Haemophilus pleuropneumoniae* bacterin, when necessary, at 8 to 12 weeks
   4. *Streptococcus suis* vaccination if necessary
D. Parasites
   1. Treat for lice and mange if needed
   2. Fecal samples should be collected at 16 weeks of age from a group of untreated pigs for determination of infections
      Deworm at 8 to 12 weeks when needed
E. Monitor for postweaning diarrhea
   1. Make definitive diagnosis and treat accordingly
   2. Medicate water if needed
F. Postmortem examination of pigs if disease outbreak occurs
VII. Growing-Finishing Period
A. Nutrition
   1. Recommendations: mixed-sex feeding
      a. 50 to 75 lb (23 to 34 kg)
         (1) Protein: 18 per cent
         (2) Lysine: 0.90 per cent
         (3) Calcium: 0.85 per cent
         (4) Phosphorus: 0.75 per cent
      b. 75 to 125 lb (34 to 57 kg)
         (1) Protein: 16 per cent
         (2) Lysine: 0.80 per cent
         (3) Calcium: 0.80 per cent
         (4) Phosphorus: 0.70 per cent
      c. 125 to 240 lb (57 to 109 kg)
         (1) Protein: 14 per cent
         (2) Lysine: 0.65 per cent
         (3) Calcium: 0.70 per cent
         (4) Phosphorus: 0.60 per cent
   2. Provide adequate feeder and waterer space
   3. Observe feed intake and adjust feeders to control waste
   4. Remove therapeutic antibiotics from diet at 50 to 75 lb (23 to 34 kg) of body weight; use growth promotant from 75 to 240 lb (34 to 109 kg)
B. Immunization (herd-specific)
   1. Second *Haemophilus pleuropneumoniae* bacterin, if needed, at 10 weeks and 14 weeks of age
   2. Other vaccinations as needed
C. Parasites
   1. Monitor fecal examination results twice a year and treat accordingly
   2. Inject or spray for lice and mange if needed
D. Check 30 pigs at slaughter at least twice a year for monitoring incidence of respiratory, enteric, skin, and joint problems
E. Conduct post-mortem examinations of pigs

The herd health program outlined here is only a reference, and each farm should develop its own set of specific guidelines. Many of the vaccinations will not be used on all farms because they are not necessary in all herds. The present trend is to eliminate as many vaccinations as possible from the program and to rely on strict isolation and sanitation for disease prevention.

PRODUCTION TARGETS

Reproductive Performance[4]

Gilt age at first mating	210 days
Gilt weight at first mating	260 lb
Total services	Herd-specific
Weaning to service interval	≤7 days
Percentage bred by 7 days	≥85 per cent
Breeding to first conception	
Gilts	85 per cent
Sows	90 per cent
Abortions	<1 per cent
Sows not in pig	<2 per cent
Entry to first service interval	28–49 days
Average nonproductive sow days	
Enter gilts at first service	≤35 days
Enter gilts at arrival	42–55 days
Sow mortality/year	3 per cent
Sow culling rate (disease)	<2 per cent

Farrowing Performance

Number of sows farrowed	Herd-specific
Average parity of farrowed sows	± (3.4–4.2)
Total pigs born alive	Herd-specific
Average total pigs born alive	≥11.2
Average total pigs born alive/litter	≥10.5
Average stillborn pigs/litter	≤0.5
Percentage stillborn pigs	≤5 per cent
Average mummies/litter	≤0.2
Percentage mummies	≤1.5 per cent
Average litter birth weight	≥32 lb
Farrowing rate	≥85 per cent
Farrowing interval	
± 3-week weaning	≤145 days
± 4-week weaning	≤149 days
Pigs weaned/sow farrowed	≥9.2
Litters/mated female/year	≥2.3
Litters/female/year	≥2.2

Weaning Performance

Number of litters weaned	Herd-specific
Total pigs weaned	Herd-specific
Pigs weaned/litter	≥9.2
Preweaning mortality	≤12.0 per cent
Average weaning weight	
± 3-week weaning	≥13.5 lb
± 4-week weaning	≥16.5 lb

Average age at weaning	
± 3-week weaning	21 ± 2 days
± 4-week weaning	28 ± 3 days
Adjusted 21-day litter weight	
± 3-week weaning	≥125 lb
± 4-week weaning	≥152 lb
Pigs weaned/mated female/year	≥21
Pigs weaned/female/year	≥20

Population

Percentage of herd:[5]	
P0	17%
P1	16%
P2	15%
P3	13%
P4	12%
P5	10%
P6	7%
P7	5%
P8	3%
P9	2%
Ending female inventory	Herd-specific
Average parity	± (2.6–3.4)
Average gilt pool inventory	Herd-specific
Ending boar inventory	Herd-specific
Female-boar ratio	17.5:1
Replacement rate	40 per cent ± 5 per cent
Culling rate	36 per cent ± 5 per cent
Death rate	4 per cent ± 1 per cent

Growth Performance

Mortality rate (standard rate method = percentage of inventory for the period interval)	
Hot nursery	≤1.0 per cent
Cold nursery	≤0.5 per cent
Standard nursery	≤1.5 per cent
Grower	≤0.5 per cent
Finisher	≤1.0 per cent
Grower-finisher	≤1.5 per cent
Average feeder pig weight	
8 weeks of age	44 lb
9 weeks of age	52 lb
10 weeks of age	59 lb
11 weeks of age	66 lb
12 weeks of age	77 lb
Percentage facility utilization	95 per cent
Turnover ratio (allows 2 days empty and clean-out time)	
3 weeks	15.9/year
4 weeks	12.2/year
5 weeks	9.9/year
6 weeks	8.3/year
7 weeks	7.2/year
8 weeks	6.3/year
9 weeks	5.6/year
10 weeks	5.1/year
11 weeks	4.6/year
12 weeks	4.2/year
13 weeks	4.0/year
14 weeks	3.7/year
15 weeks	3.4/year
16 weeks	3.2/year
17 weeks	3.0/year
18 weeks	2.9/year
19 weeks	2.7/year
20 weeks	2.4/year
21 weeks	2.4/year
Days to market	
200 lb	165 days
210 lb	170 days
220 lb	175 days
230 lb	180 days
240 lb	185 days
250 lb	190 days
260 lb	195 days
Rate of gain (varies with season, sale weight, age)	
Hot nursery	0.5 lb/day
Cold nursery	1.0 lb/day
Standard nursery	0.8 lb/day
Grower	1.5 lb/day
Finisher	1.7 lb/day
Grower-finisher	1.6 lb/day
Feed consumed/head/day (varies with season, sale weight, age)	
Hot nursery	0.75 lb/day
Cold nursery	1.90 lb/day
Standard nursery	1.40 lb/day
Grower	3.75 lb/day
Finisher	6.00 lb/day
Grower-finisher	5.30 lb/day
Feed conversion ratio	
Hot nursery	1.5 lb F/G
Cold nursery	1.9 lb F/G
Standard nursery	1.7 lb F/G
Grower	2.5 lb F/G
Finisher	3.5 lb F/G
Grower-finisher	3.3 lb F/G
Pounds sold/sow/year	
Farrow to finish	≥4500 lb
Farrow to feeder pig	≥800 lb

REFERENCES

1. Hogs and Pigs. National Agricultural Statistics Service for USDA, January 3, 1990.
2. Iowa State University College of Agriculture Swine Task Force. Ames, IA, December 1988.
3. Donham KJ. University of Iowa Institute of Agricultural Medicine, Iowa City, IA, 1982.
4. Pig CHAMP. University of Iowa Institute of Agricultural Medicine, University of Minnesota Department of Large Animal Clinical Science, College of Veterinary Medicine, St. Paul, MN, 1985.
5. DeKalb Swine Breeders, Inc., 1990.

Llama Herd Health Management

LaRue W. Johnson, DVM, PhD

The nature of a llama/alpaca herd health program has been markedly influenced by variables including owner's background, numbers of animals, purpose of animals, geographic location, economics, and, quite understandably, the background and species orientation of the veterinarian involved. In the following, a herd health program is discussed that includes some firm recommendations based on research and medical and management observations of the author. In addition, some theoretical options are discussed that have been shared with the author by professional colleagues and llama owners. The reader should not assume that this is *the* llama/alpaca herd health program; rather, it is a basic model by which to develop a custom-made program for the client and herd under consideration. For the client whose goals include breeding and subsequent sales, a reproductive herd health program will emerge as the launching pad for other aspects including neonatal care, nutrition, records, immunizations, parasite control, grooming–foot care, and facilities design. For the backyard companion animal owner and back country packer, only a portion of a complete herd health program may be applicable. In general, one should be prepared to encounter 2 extremes of clientele type. On the one hand is the novice livestock owner, having little previous experience with any pets or farm animals, whereas on the other is the extremely well informed llama owner who is probably qualified to advise you on many aspects of llama management. It is assumed that the reader has access to other reference books for background information about anatomic and physiologic uniqueness of the New World camelids.[1,2]

REPRODUCTION

Whereas the New World camelids are capable of breeding successfully at any time of the year, a tendency has emerged to avoid extremely hot and frigid seasons. The 11.5-month gestation period allows breedings to be easily spaced for avoidance of these compromising periods. This also creates 2 windows a year in northern climates, during which time problem breeders can be aggressively pursued, and creates options as to when to introduce young females into the breeding program. If a female of potentially breedable age (i.e., greater than 12 months and weighing two thirds of anticipated adult weight) is successfully bred in the spring, she obviously stays with the spring birthing group of females. If, however, she does not breed successfully with 2 mating attempts, do not assume she has a problem, but rather move her to the fall breeding group. The point is that there is a wide range of age for puberty expression. The wise breeder should be encouraged to detect and pursue early puberty in both the female and male for improving reproductive performance overall. The recently birthed female llama with no complications will have extremely rapid uterine involution and will be capable of successful rebreeding as early as 10 to 21 days post partum. Breeding at the earliest date to produce a pregnancy may increase the incidence of resorption, so generally it would be recommended to wait until 14 days post partum to breed.

Breeding programs vary widely from the extremes of pasture breeding to strictly managed hand breeding. Bearing in mind the follicular wave pattern[3,4] influencing female receptivity, hand breeding subjects female llamas to some unnecessary breedings. Without male exposure, most female llamas will have maximal male receptivity on an approximately 12-day cycle, during which time the ovulatable follicle reaches maximal size (10 to 14 mm). Without breeding, the follicle becomes atretic and is replaced by another follicle. Periods of minimal male receptivity are also observed on a 12-day cycle; however, many females will still be bred by an aggressive male in hand breeding programs. A challenge for the breeder as well as for the veterinarian is to detect the female llama that is the most receptive and to minimize the numbers of services necessary for a successful induced ovulation breeding. A veteran male in a pasture-breeding program will detect these receptive females by their proximity to him as well as by their excretion of estrogen conjugates in the urine. As such, there will tend to be 1 or 2 services per breeding. For hand-breeding programs, teasing of females is beneficial but requires individual interpretation of behavior of the female and male. Professional involvement can be beneficial, particularly for the problem breeder. Rectal palpation alone, but ideally in conjunction with ultrasonography, will enable monitoring of follicular development for prediction of the correct time for matings.

The approach to rectal palpation is basically no different from that in the mare or cow; however, size disparity of the operator's hand and rectal sphincter as well as pelvic cavity contents may preclude any other factors. In addition, however, consideration must be given to restraint, lubrication, behavior of the animal, and client acceptance of the procedure. The rectum of the llama is comparable to that of a mare, requiring gentle, well-lubricated examination procedures.

After a breeding resulting in an induced ovulation and beginning corpus luteum development, a female llama will behaviorly refuse any further matings. The combination of reduced estrogen and rising progesterone levels in her blood apparently accounts for this behavior change. Confirmation of pregnancy can be accomplished at virtually all stages of established gestation via various techniques, and depending somewhat on management as to applicability and interpretation. Persistent behavioral refusal on the part of the female from 14 days after breeding is very encouraging and should preclude other approaches. Transrectal ultrasonographic detection of pregnancy has been observed as early as 12 days of gestation; however, a practical time for the determination should occur at 21 to 28 days. An advantage of early ultrasonographic determination includes accurate estimation of gestation stage, in spite of unobserved pasture-breeding activity. Blood progesterone determination to date requires a commercial laboratory because no test kit has proved to be reliable in llamas. In addition, for accurate interpretation of results, the female subject must not be in contact with a breeding male for 14 to 21 days since the previous breeding or refusal because she may have been rebred and be already into a second luteal stage that would be indistinguishable from a pregnancy. The necessary turnaround time and possibility of a retained corpus luteum are additional disadvantages of progesterone analysis.

Transabdominal pregnancy diagnosis can be successfully accomplished in some females as early as the 35th day of gestation from the left flank fiberless area of the body. As the pregnant uterus becomes more gravid, it will shift positions such that by 90 days of gestation it will reside toward the right side. Although the fetus will not always be readily detected, healthy-appearing fluid and membranes will generally confirm a sustained pregnancy.

Rectal palpation alone can be used to confidently diagnose pregnancy in maiden females as early as the 30th day of gestation; however, many will be difficult to enter because of size disparity. Because of residual asymmetry of uterine horn size from the previous pregnancy, a veteran female will be somewhat difficult to confidently deem pregnant until 45 days of gestation. After 90 days of gestation, the gravid uterus becomes difficult to palpate, and pregnancy is suspected on the basis of cervical position and tone as well as inability to locate a nonpregnant uterus. Reconfirmation of pregnancy status sometime after 60 to 70 days is recommended because within the period from 30 to 60 days appears to be the prime time for pregnancy resorption.

Fertility and infertility work-ups for male and female llamas involve techniques that have been adapted from other species. Detailed descriptions of semen analysis and vaginoscopic, uterine biopsy, and uterine culture techniques are to be found elsewhere.[2]

NEONATAL CARE

A minimum of professional attention to the llama neonate includes a thorough physical examination with emphasis on cardiac auscultation, evaluation of umbilicus for hernia and adequacy of disinfection, determination of freedom from congenital defects, assessment of vigor, and determination of maturity status. A more aggressive approach will include determination of a hematocrit and total protein for establishment of normalcy before assessment of adequacy of colostral passive transfer at greater than 24 hours of age. On premises known to have had a problem with type C enterotoxemia, camelid neonates at birth have been administered up to 20 ml of C/D antitoxin subcutaneously with no deleterious effects. As a follow-up evaluation for neonates that are deemed suspect of passive transfer failure, a repeat of the hematocrit and total protein determination is to be made. Normal neonates at 24 hours of age will show a slight reduction of hematocrit from birth and a rise of total protein from generally less than 5 g/dl per cent to greater than 6 g/dl; whereas the total protein determination is not as accurate as are electrophoresis and llama-specific radial immunodiffusion techniques for estimating globulin content, the practicality of it makes it worthwhile as a rapid screening method. Although various other tests for globulins including Foal Check* and zinc sulfate turbidity have been used, we will be accurate in our estimates only when a llama globulin–specific test is available. Neonates falling into the obvious or suspicious category of failure of passive transfer should receive transfusion of plasma from a healthy donor or frozen plasma bank. As a practical guide, normally hydrated neonates having a 24- to 36-hour total plasma protein of less than 5.0 should receive 8 to 10 per cent of their body weight in plasma either intravenously or intraperitoneally. A veterinary practice is an ideal pivotal point for establishment of a plasma bank as well as a colostral bank. Client education on quality first-milking colostrum of ideally caprine species origin is often necessary because only in the case of stillbirth is there any llama colostrum to be spared for future neonates. Goat owners should be instructed to vaccinate their does before kidding with *Clostridium perfringens* C/D toxoid as well as tetanus toxoid and provide only first-milking colostrum to the colostrum bank.

IMMUNIZATIONS

Particularly in the area of immunizations do we currently observe the influence of a consulting veterinarian's background and other species orientation. No vaccines are officially approved for use in camelids. Without vaccination studies followed by serologic study and challenge procedures, little can be said with confidence about efficacy, duration of immunity, and frequency of vaccine administration. At best, vaccination decisions are currently made on the basis of theoretical indications and minimal observed complication risks and vaccines are administered with use of dosages, routes, and schedules derived from other species.

An effort should be made to coordinate the herd immunization program with one of the herd deworming schedules. Solid immunity to *Clostridium perfringens* C/D and tetanus should be a minimal goal in all llama herds. Thereafter, local and herd health problems based on opinion of the attending veterinarian should be considered. As such, the following recommendations and options are offered as guidelines:

- Annual C/D/tetanus toxoid for all juveniles and adults (3 ml of toxoid subcutaneously)
- C/D/tetanus booster to pregnant females 1 month before anticipated birthing

Note: Whereas there are 7-way and 8-way clostridial vaccines, they are observed to cause significant injection site reactions in llamas, and some correlation with postinjection abortions is emerging.

Neonates

- On enterotoxemia-endemic premises, 20 ml of C/D antitoxin (10 ml, 2 sites subcutaneously) at birth independent of dam's vaccination status and colostrum intake.

It appears that camelid neonates are immunocompetent at birth.[5] Independent of antitoxin administration and colostral intake, active immunization efforts have been initiated during the first week of life followed by 2 monthly boosters. Thereafter, they are annually boostered with the herd.

Immunization Options

- In leptospirosis-endemic areas, biannual vaccination of brood females should be considered with use of multivalent products available for other domestic species, once before breeding, once midgestation.
- In rabies-endemic areas, annual vaccination with a killed product should be considered.
- If risk of snake bite is real, annual vaccination for malignant edema may be justified.
- If close association with genus *Equus* is likely (especially zebras), vaccination with EHV-I killed vaccine quarterly should be considered.
- If theoretical indications arise for use of vaccines against any viral infections known to be a problem in other species, it would seem wise to avoid any modified live products until experimental work dictates otherwise. The only exception to that recommendation would be use of parainfluenza-3 (PI_3) vaccine intranasally as an attempt to alleviate chronic nasal discharge in young llamas.
- As an effort to provide colostral protection to the neonate, ScourGuard-III* has been administered to pregnant llamas without deleterious effects to the dam.
- CalfGuard* has been administered to newborn llamas on premises having significant diarrhea incidence with subjective assessed benefit.

NUTRITION

Knowledge of solid nutritional recommendations is sorely lacking for maintenance, growth, gestation, lactation, and work considerations. However, a veterinary practitioner can provide valuable guidance for most llama owners using general nutritional knowledge of quality forages and careful scrutiny of supplements. It is important to bear in mind that llamas, like their progenitors the wild guanacos, are adaptive animals, being able to build body stores during high caloric and protein intake that are utilized during the less nutritionally favorable times. In the North American management scene, most llamas are being offered a year-round high plane of nutrition, which makes many considerably overweight and unlikely to take advantage of their outstanding ability to reutilize urea for protein synthesis. The point of this information as it relates to a herd health program is, first, a veterinarian can aid in selection of quality grass hay of 8 to 10 per cent protein that will serve as the basis of herd nutrition. Core sampling and submission for nutrient analysis including selenium are en-

---

*These adapted for equine use.

*Available from SmithKline & Beecham, 812 Springdale Drive, Exton, PA 19341.

Table 1. BASIC FORAGE DIET ANALYSIS FOR MAINTENANCE FEEDING OF LLAMAS (DRY MATTER BASIS)

Nutrient	%	Nutrient	ppm
Protein	10	Mn	50
Fat	2	Cu	7.5
Fiber	30	Co	0.65
Total digestible nutrients	55	Zn	35
Ca	0.65	Fe	100
P	0.35	Mb	2.5
Mg	0.25	Se	0.35
K	2.0		
Na	0.25	Vitamin A: 20,000 units/kg	
S	0.21	Vitamin E: 25 units/kg	

couraged. Thereafter, protein supplementation with use of quality alfalfa hay for select groups including weanlings, late-gestation animals, and lactating mothers could be considered. Provision of a salt and mineral supplement is all that is additionally necessary. Table 1 indicates the nutrient contents of a basic maintenance forage diet for a mature llama and a mineral supplement (Table 2) that could be offered free-choice. An option for the mineral supplement involves the inclusion of additional selenium (90 ppm) and vitamin E (8000 units/lb) for use in areas that are considered deficient. This mineral mix could be bulk mixed, packaged, and made available to llama clients. Periodic blood sampling of the herd or peer groups for routine blood biochemical profiles including selenium, copper, zinc, and iron is recommended. Major alterations from published normal values[1, 2] would deserve consideration of mineral supplementation.

Consultation with owners on the subject of a growing number of llama supplement options can be both frustrating and rewarding. If one embraces the concept that these animals are adaptive to seasonal nutrition changes and that they are basically browsers and grazers, then significant levels of supplementation via pellets or cereal grains are likely unnecessary. Only nutritionally debilitated animals and animals subjected to extremely cold climates likely need caloric supplementation. As mentioned previously, protein supplementation can be provided by quality alfalfa hay. Therefore, the only consistent justification for supplements may be in the area of micronutrients, especially selenium. If a palatable low-energy, low-protein, high-fiber pellet can provide 2 mg of selenium per 100 kg of body weight, and if the amount consumed is no greater than 10 per cent of anticipated dry matter consumption, it can perhaps be justified. As such, a 150-kg (330-lb) llama should not be consuming any more than 300 g (2/3 lb) of pelleted supplement per day. A free-choice salt mineral mix remains a viable option.

It appears that there is rising skepticism concerning the use of injectable vitamin E–selenium preparations. Concerns over safety for use in pregnant females as well as in the neonate are foremost. In addition, the relatively short duration of elevated blood levels of selenium achieved after parenteral injections indicates this procedure alone is not adequate.

Table 2. COMPOSITION OF MINERAL SUPPLEMENT TO BE OFFERED FREE-CHOICE FOR ALL AGES OF LLAMAS

Bone meal	25 lb
Dry molasses	50 lb
Monosodium phosphate	25 lb
Trace mineralized salt	50 lb
ZinPro 100*	10 lb

*Zinpro Corp., 7825 Washington Ave. S., Edina, MN 55439-2441.

Consequently, oral supplementation via free-choice mineral mixes or palatable pellets would seem to be a better alternative.

Another area for veterinary involvement in nutrition is establishment of feeding groups. During any procedure, an attempt should be made to offer a subjective evaluation of body condition. This can be done by use of a 1 to 10 scoring system whereby 1 designates very thin and 10 designates very fat, with a score of 5 being ideal. Once body scores are established, animals of similar body condition in similar peer groups are fed together. The fact that this can perhaps be done without bias by an attending veterinarian makes it quite owner acceptable and is appreciated.

PROCEDURES

Consistent with the variation of backgrounds of llama owners will be the variation of their involvement with techniques including injection and deworming procedures as well as removal of fighting teeth. Consequently, a veterinarian should attempt to evaluate the need to be totally involved or serve strictly as a consultant. Except for occasions when a rapid attainment of drug blood levels is required, the subcutaneous route for parenteral administration has proved to be minimally invasive but effective in llamas. Preferred sites are more ventral locations in front or back of the shoulder where up to 15 ml/site have been administered without problems. Oral paste dewormers and drenches are readily used; paste dewormers are preferred. When ivermectin is deemed the desirable dewormer, the parenteral product (subcutaneously) is preferred.

Male llamas will generally need to have their fighting teeth cut by 2 to 2.5 years of age. Whereas numerous procedural options exist, cutting the teeth at the gum line with obstetric wire has emerged as the simplest, least invasive one and is accompanied by minimal complications. Ideally this should be done when all 6 teeth have erupted. Because many clients would prefer that this procedure be performed under anesthesia, it could well be combined with the gelding surgery. Without anesthesia, the procedure is best accomplished in a restraining chute,[6] where the animal is cross-tied and an assistant props the mouth open. A spray gun or water-filled syringe is used to cool the wire. So that the spread of disease is reduced, a new piece of wire should be used for each animal.

Under normal circumstances, it appears the ideal age to geld a llama is after 2 years of age. As with other species, this age decision is debatable. An anesthesia period of 20 to 30 minutes can be achieved by administering a ketamine-xylazine (10:1) mixture intramuscularly at 4.0 mg/kg ketamine and 0.44 mg/kg xylazine. The castration procedure is analogous to that performed in the horse, with minimal observed complications of swelling or infection.

PARASITE CONTROL

New World camelids are subject to infestations of both internal and external parasites. As regards internal parasites, it would appear that virtually all nematode parasites known to affect cattle, sheep, and goats are capable of infesting llamas; the protozoa coccidia remain species-specific. The migration of larval forms of the meningeal worm *Parelaphostrongylus tenuis* is a constant threat to llamas living in areas inhabited by white-tailed deer. Liver flukes are a problem in the same geographic areas as for traditional ruminant species. Tapeworm segments are occasionally passed in feces, which causes principally esthetic concerns. Toxoplasmosis does account for occasional abortions, and many llamas appear to be seropositive. Over the past 2 years, a significant incidence of blood parasite *Eperythrozoon* spp. has been demonstrated in llamas, most often affecting immunocompromised individuals. With the common usage of ivermectin, the incidence of mange in llamas is extremely low; however, considering their habits of using a community dusting area, it remains a constant possibility. There is in addition a need to regularly monitor the presence of both biting and sucking lice in these long-fibered species. In certain geographic locations, ticks will seasonally be a problem, causing the occasional case of tick paralysis.

Depending on many management factors, including geographic area, numbers of animals, groupings of animals, and pasture rotation and degree of confinement, a parasite control program should be tailor-made. Many llama owners have been led to believe that llamas are virtually parasite-free owing to their tendency to use a communal dunging pile. Fecal examinations of individual or composite samples from llama groups will generally allow interpretation of current parasite concerns. All animals in the groups should be wormed at the same time. Most nematode parasites have been controlled with use of fenbendazole preparations (paste or drench). When *Nematodirus* spp. or *Trichuris* spp. are diagnosed, up to 3 times the normal dose is used with effectiveness and safety. Tapeworms are also markedly reduced by these larger doses; however, albendazole appears to be more effective. Demonstration of fluke eggs will necessitate use of clorsulon for control. As with other species, demonstration of coccidia oocysts is common and elicits variable responses from owners and veterinarians. Unless an animal is stressed by other factors, clinical manifestations associated with coccidiosis are rarely observed. Consequently, most control measures are aimed at minimizing the problem in recently weaned youngsters with either decoquinate or amprolium and allowing them to develop immunity. Clinical cases are generally responsive to parenteral sulfadimethoxine.

Intervals between deworming procedures will vary principally with age of the group involved, degree of confinement, annual rainfall of environs, and parasite problems at hand. Locales having to deal with the meningeal worm problem are often found to be administering the parenteral ivermectin preparation at 21- to 30-day intervals. Under this scheme, most other nematodes should be controlled. Periodic fecal examinations would be indicated, however, for monitoring any development of resistance. In dry environments, a minimum of 2 deworming procedures per year is recommended. A springtime deworming should take place before the animals go on pasture with use of a product directed at nematode control. A fall deworming, 1 month after a killing frost with use of injectable ivermectin, would have an impact on nematodes as well as have a theoretical benefit of reducing nasal bots. If nasal bots are strongly suspected, a double dose of injectable ivermectin has been observed to be more effective. Traditional heavy parasite load locales (e.g., Pacific Northwest and southern states) should consider 2 or more additional dewormings per year, ideally coordinated with pasture rotations. With concerns for parasite resistance as well as available anthelmintics, rotation of products is a consideration. Table 3 lists various anthelmintic and coccidial drug options.

Recommendations for the prevention and control of eperythrozoonosis in llamas remain empirical and untested. At this point, it appears there may well be significant numbers of potential carrier animals in the camelid population, such that emphasis in prevention should be aimed at minimizing vector possibilities. Lice, mites, biting flies, gnats, midges, mosquitoes, and ticks should be controlled as best possible. In addition, emphasis should be placed on good hygiene practices for handling of any needles, syringes, tattoo pliers, or other equipment that could potentially transfer infected blood.

Table 3. ANTHELMINTICS AND COCCIDIAL DRUGS

Drug	Company	Dosage
Anthelmintic Drugs		
Fenbendazole		11–15 mg/kg (O) 1–3 days
Panacur	Hoechst-Roussel	
Safeguard	American Hoechst	
Ivermectin	Merck & Co.	2 mg/kg (SC) 1 day
Ivomec		
Thiabendazole	Merck & Co.	55–110 mg/kg (O) 1–3 days
Omnizole		
Levamisole		5.5–8.5 mg/kg (O or SC) 1 day
Ripercol	American Cyanamid Co.	
Levasol	Pitman-Moore	
Mebendazole	Pitman-Moore	22 mg/kg (O) 3 days
Telmin		
Albendazole	Norden Labs	6.5 mg/kg (O) 1 day
Valbazen		
Clorsulon	Smith Kline & Beecham	6.5 mg/kg (O) 1 day
Curatrem		
Praziquantel	Pfizer	2.2–3.3 mg/kg (O or SC) 1 day
Droncit		
Pyrantel pamoate		8.5 mg/kg (O) 1 day
Strongid-T	Pfizer	
Coccidial Drugs		
Prevention		
Amprolium	Merck & Co.	5 mg/kg, (1.25% crumbles in feed or 9.6% solution in drinking water) 21 days
Corid		
Decoquinate	Rhodia, Inc.	0.5 mg/kg, 28 days
Decox		
Therapy		
Sulfadimethoxine	Hoffman-LaRoche	Day 1: 55 mg/kg (SC)
Albon		Day 2–5: 22.5 mg/kg (SC)

O = orally; SC = subcutaneously.
Many of these preparations are sold under a variety of tradenames. Consult publications such as Veterinary Pharmaceuticals and Biologicals, 6th ed. Lenexa, KS, Veterinary Medicine Publishing Co, 1989/1990.

Blood donor animals for plasma or whole blood should ideally be free of the parasite. The problem as of this writing is to be absolutely sure of which animal is negative. Careful study of freshly made blood smears from animals that are borderline to severely anemic is recommended. In addition, serologic testing by use of an enzyme-linked immunosorbent assay (ELISA) test would appear to be the most rewarding procedure. Clinical cases have improved with oxytetracycline therapy (Table 4); however, recrudescence 2 to 3 weeks after treatment is predictable. Arsenilic acid therapy as ingested pellets is currently under evaluation for elimination of the carrier state.

Ectoparasites of principal concern in llamas include mange mites, and biting or sucking lice. Monitoring new additions to a herd, including visiting breeding animals, will minimize chances of introducing the problems. Lice can generally be demonstrated by parting fiber over the dorsal midline from shoulder to rump and using close inspection with the naked eye or a hand lens. It is important to determine whether the lice are biting or sucking varieties. Ivermectin will generally be effective against sucking lice (*Microthorcis cameli*) but only minimally effective for biting lice (*Damalinea breviceps*). Both

Table 4. *EPERYTHROZOON* THERAPY

Day 1	11 mg/kg oxytetracycline (IV)
	20 mg/kg oxytetracycline (LA-200 SC)
Days 3, 6, 9, 12	Repeat LA-200 above
Days 15–50	Aureomycin pellets, 22 mg/kg

IV = intravenously; SC = subcutaneously.

biting and sucking lice will be effectively treated with use of a 3 per cent fenthion (Tiguvon*) product as a pour-on administered at 31 ml/100 kg in direct contact with the skin through parted fiber on the dorsum of the back. Permectrin (Ectrin†) is another pour-on option that has been reported to be safe and effective.

Whereas llamas seem to have unlimited possibilities for dermatologic problems, mange remains a differential diagnostic consideration for any hyperkeratotic-parakeratotic lesion. Conventional skin scraping techniques will usually demonstrate the mites. Sarcoptic, chorioptic, and psoroptic mange have all been diagnosed. Generally one can anticipate a favorable response from parenteral ivermectin therapy (0.2 mg/kg subcutaneously); however, in the case of chorioptic mange, increased dosages appear to be indicated (0.4 mg/kg subcutaneously). Repeating the administered doses 21 days later is also recommended.

Tick control is as frustrating in llamas as in any other species. Use of parenteral ivermectin during the peak tick season should minimize chances of tick paralysis. Ectrin spray has been observed to be of value when it is repeated as a total body application on a 5- to 7-day basis. Avoiding heavily tick-infested areas in the spring of the year is probably the most effective recommendation.

---

*Available from Bayvet Division of Cutter Laboratories, Shawnee, KS 66201.
†Fermenta Animal Health Co., 10150 N. Executive Blvd., Kansas City, MO 64153.

Measures to prevent, control, and treat toxoplasmosis in llamas are essentially no different from any other species. Prevention is aimed at minimizing exposure to infective oocysts on the premises. This is best accomplished by maintaining a minimal cat population and at least keeping only mature cats that will shed minimal numbers of oocysts. Reminding llama owners of this relationship and encouraging good hygiene, including attention to cat litter boxes, should be part of a llama herd health program. There is essentially no economical effective treatment for animals infected with toxoplasmosis.

State-of-the-art record systems modeled after other species are slowly being developed but with emphasis on reproductive parameters, vaccinations, and deworming schedules. These can also be tailor-made to suit the client's goals and needs.

REFERENCES

1. Fowler ME: Medicine and Surgery of South American Camelids. Ames, IA, Iowa State University Press, 1979.
2. Johnson LW: Llama medicine. Vet Clin North Am [Food Anim Pract] 5:1, 1989.
3. Bravo W, Fowler ME: Basic physiology of reproduction in female llamas. Llamas 4:35–37, 1990.
4. Bravo W, et al: Ovarian follicular dynamics in female llamas. Biol Reprod 43:579–585, 1990.
5. Paul-Murphy J, et al: Immune response of the llama (Lama glama) to tetanus toxoid vaccination. Am J Vet Res 50:1279–1281, 1989.
6. Johnson LW: Restraining chutes. Llamas 5:30–32, 1987.

SECTION 4 ☐ ☐ ☐ ☐ ☐ ☐
Dietary Management

JIMMY L. HOWARD, DVM, MS, Consulting Editor

Nutritional Management of Stressed and Morbid Calves*

N. ANDY COLE, PhD

Feeder calves encounter physiologic and psychologic stresses during movement from one production point to another. Typically calves are both weaned and transported to a local auction market on the same day. The calf may then spend from 1 to 10 days in an order-buyer facility until transport to a stocker or feedyard operation. These calves are tired, dehydrated, anoretic, and highly susceptible to infectious diseases as a result of suppressed immune response. They present cattle producers and consultants with special nutritional, management, and health problems. Bovine respiratory disease (BRD) complex, as well as many other diseases, is caused by a combination of infectious agents and stress. The incidence of BRD can be reduced by immunization of calves against the major viral and bacterial organisms involved or by reducing stress encountered during movement from one production point to another, or both.

Stressors encountered by calves during movement from the farm to the stocker or feedyard operation include feed and water deprivation, weaning, inclement weather, antagonistic encounters, infectious agents, and transport. The physiologic effects of these stressors often appear to be additive. For example, a 24-hour fasting transport period is equivalent to about a 48- to 72-hour fasting nontransport period. During transport, calves held in individual crates lose only about 50 per cent as much weight as commingled calves.

Feeder calves lose appreciable quantities of nutrients during a fast, and these losses are accentuated by other stressors such as transport and infection. Nutrient deficiencies and excesses can have adverse effects on animal immunity. Because of increased research in this area, a new term, NAIDS (nutritionally acquired immune deficiency syndrome), has been coined.

Proper nutrition will generally not prevent stress or infection. Nonetheless, proper nutrition can help prepare for, reduce the adverse effects of, and enhance recovery from stressful periods.

PRESTRESS AND STRESS NUTRITION

Ruminants have a potentially large reserve of nutrients and water within the digestive tract. Improved performance and reduced morbidity and mortality can be realized if maximum use is made of this reserve. Hence the diet fed to calves before or during a stress period, or both, is as important as the diet fed upon arrival at the stocker or feedyard operation.

The diet of feeder calves at the farm of origin most often consists of grass and some milk, although calves receive less than 15 per cent of their nutrition from milk during the last 140 to 210 days after birth. As a result, the diet that calves receive before leaving the farm or ranch can be highly variable depending on the quality and quantity of grass available. Other factors—toxins such as the fescue endophyte (*Acremonium coenophialum*)—may have adverse effects on the nutrient status of calves when they leave the farm of origin.

One potential method to ensure that calves are properly nourished upon leaving the farm is to prewean the calf 4 weeks before sale and feed it a balanced ration. Practically, however, this procedure requires extra time, labor, investment, risk, and skills on the part of the cow-calf producer. Except when grass conditions are very poor, preweaning does not substantially help the cow herd. Research also indicates that preweaned calves do not have sufficient improvement in either health or performance at the feedyard for the cattle feeder to pay a premium for preweaning and feeding. On average, calves preweaned and fed for 30 days will gain 30 to 60 lb and consume 200 to 500 lb of a 50 per cent concentrate diet. Calves left with the cow will gain 10 to 50 lb during the same period. At the feedyard, preweaned calves will have about 20 per cent less sickness and death loss but 2 to 7 per cent poorer feed conversions than calves not preweaned.

A second method of providing proper nutrition that requires less investment and time is to feed calves limited creep rations during the last 60 to 90 days on the farm. Providing calves with 1 to 3 lb/head daily of a creep ration formulated to balance for grass conditions can yield a 0.2 to 0.5 lb/day increase in calf weight gain at a very reasonable cost. Once calves have learned to eat the creep ration, intakes can be limited via the use of salt. Limited creep rations have ranged from a simple 90 per cent cottonseed meal/10 per cent salt mixture to very complex formulations. Best results are obtained when the forage available is sampled and analyzed and the creep ration is formulated to balance for specific grass composition and availability. Data indicate that calves limit fed with creep feed have about 20 to 25 per cent less sickness and death loss and 0 to 3 per cent better feed conversions at the feedyard. Thus from a practical standpoint, limited creep feeding offers advantages over a preweaning program under most circumstances.

Because of costs and logistics, most auction and order-buyer facilities provide calves with a diet of only poor quality hay; properly formulated diets and supplements are usually not provided. Compared with calves fed poor quality hay, calves fed a 50 per cent concentrate pretransport diet will lose about

---

*All material in this article is in the public domain, with the exception of any borrowed figures or tables.

30 per cent less weight, 25 per cent less water, and 30 per cent less protein during a 24-hour transport period. However, because some calves will not eat a 50 per cent concentrate diet at the auction and order-buyer barns, calves should preferably be fed a 50 per cent concentrate diet plus good quality hay at these facilities. When offered both concentrate and hay, calves will normally consume 0.5 to 1 per cent of their body weight of the concentrate portion and 1 to 1.5 per cent of their weight of the hay. Hay intake will increase relative to concentrate intake as hay quality increases. If calves are accustomed to eating a concentrate diet, either because of previous creep feeding or preweaning, intakes of the concentrate portion will be greater. Most newly weaned calves will eat only enough hay or concentrate, or both, to meet their maintenance energy requirements during the short stay in the auction or order-buyer barn. Therefore the diet, should be formulated so that requirements for other nutrients (protein, vitamins, and minerals) are met with a limited intake (about 1 per cent of body weight). Calves fed a concentrate plus hay diet at the order-buyer facility will have 10 to 20 per cent less sickness and death loss at the feedyard compared with calves fed only poor quality hay.

By providing a nutritionally balanced diet before an extended transport period, the calf will have an increased capacity to tolerate transit stress, will start on feed faster, and will have fewer health problems at the feedyard.

POSTSTRESS NUTRITION

The diet fed during the first 2 to 4 weeks after arrival at the stocker or feedyard operation can significantly affect morbidity, mortality, performance, and cost of gain. There is probably no single best receiving program for the newly arrived stressed calf. The optimum program for each load of calves depends on their background, the amount of stress encountered during marketing and transport, and feed and cattle costs.

In general, as the energy concentration of the receiving diet increases, morbidity and mortality increase, performance improves, and costs of gain decline. The adverse health effects of feeding higher-energy diets to stressed calves can be overcome by providing free-choice good-quality hay along with the concentrate diet for the first 3 to 7 days after arrival. If alfalfa is used in the receiving program, it should be of average to good (not excellent) quality. If native hay or oat hay is fed, it should be of good to excellent quality.

Feeding 2 lb/head daily of a pelleted (3/16 inch) 40 per cent crude protein supplement along with good-quality hay has worked well in stocker operations with limited capacity to mix or feed complete rations. Under typical feedyard operations, however, the preferred method is feeding a 50 to 70 per cent concentrate complete diet plus hay because calves fed the supplement plus hay program during the first 4 weeks in the feedyard do not compensate for their early poor performance later in the feeding period.

The suggested nutrient concentrations in a receiving ration for stressed feeder calves are presented in Table 1. Actual nutrient requirements of stressed feeder calves (MCal, g, or mg/day) are not appreciably increased compared with those of normal calves; however, feeder calves usually have depressed feed intakes (less than 2 per cent of body weight) for 1 to 3 weeks after entering the feedyard. Thus to meet protein, mineral, and vitamin requirements, concentrations of these nutrients must be increased in the diet. As a general rule of thumb, receiving rations should be formulated so that the calf receives at least maintenance requirements for protein, vitamins, and minerals when feed consumption is 1 per cent of body weight.

Table 1. RECOMMENDED NUTRIENT CONTENT OF A FEEDYARD RECEIVING RATION FOR MARKET- AND TRANSPORT-STRESSED FEEDER CALVES

Nutrient	Suggested Range	Comments
Dry matter, %	82–90	Avoid high moisture feeds
NEm, Mcal/cwt	60–85[a]	Limit added fat to less than 4% of the ration dry matter
NEg, Mcal/cwt	36–51[a]	
Concentrate, %	50–70[a]	
Crude protein, %	13.0–14.5	Limit urea and other NPN
Calcium, %	0.5–0.7	
Phosphorus, %	0.4–0.5	
Potassium, %	1.0–1.3	Avoid high chlorine levels
Sodium, %	0.2–0.3	
Magnesium, %	0.2–0.3	
Sulfur, %	0.15–0.25	
Manganese, ppm	40–70	
Copper, ppm	10–15	
Iron, ppm	100–150	
Zinc, ppm	75–100	
Selenium, ppm	0.1–0.2	
Cobalt, ppm	0.1–0.2	
Vitamin A, IU/lb	1000–2000	If supplement is pelleted, double value to compensate for pelleting loss
Vitamin E, IU/lb	20–50	

[a]For calves weighing 400 lb or less use the greater value, for 500-lb calves use an intermediate value, and for 600-lb calves and yearlings use the lesser value. Ration should be fed with free-choice hay for the first 3 to 7 days.
NPN = nonprotein nitrogen; cwt = hundredweight.

Some additional guidelines for feeding stressed feeder calves include the following:

1. Limit use of high-moisture feeds like silage during the first 1 to 2 weeks after arrival.
2. Limit intake of urea to less than 1 oz (28 g) per head daily during the first 1 to 2 weeks after arrival.
3. Addition of B vitamins, especially niacin (100 to 200 ppm) and thiamine (1 g/head/day), is sometimes beneficial.
4. Addition of a coccidiostat, antibiotic, *Lactobacillus* culture, buffer, and/or yeast culture is sometimes beneficial.
5. Watch for calves that have been pulled late for treatment or were treated for an extended period of time because they may be more prone to acidosis, etc., when returned to their home pen from the hospital pen.

The cause(s) for depressed feed intake in marketing- and transport-stressed calves is still unclear, but a combination of reduced ruminal fermentative capacity, hormonal shifts, and altered sensitivity of the hypothalamus to satiety and hunger signals seems to be involved. Attempts to improve ruminal fermentation (and thus feed intake) via oral infusions of nutrient solutions or ruminal fluid from a donor animal, or both, have normally failed, except in severe cases, because the stress of infusion is often greater than potential benefits. During infection, reduced feed intake appears to be caused by increased secretion of interleukin-1 as well as fever.

SUPPORTIVE NUTRITION

Many stressed and morbid calves refuse to eat any diet offered to them. Under these circumstances and in cases of severe diarrhea it may become appropriate or necessary to provide supportive nutrition along with pharmaceutical treatment to keep the calf alive. In the morbid calf, simply reducing body temperature may be adequate to start the animal eating. Use of some microbial culture products containing *Lactobacillus acidophilus,* fungi, or yeast cultures may stimulate feed consumption in some animals. When other methods do not succeed, more strenuous measures such as intravenous, oral, intraruminal, or intraperitoneal infusions may be warranted.

Many oral and parenteral electrolyte and nutrient solutions are currently available. Advantages, disadvantages, and proper use of these solutions have been extensively reviewed in the article on fluid and electrolyte therapy.

MANAGEMENT PRACTICES

Many management factors can affect the health and performance of stressed feeder calves. The following is a list of general information and guidelines that may be beneficial:

1. Upon arrival (or sooner), calves should be classified into either low-risk or high-risk categories; this can be determined by their source (state of origin, marketing channels, etc.), appearance, and rectal temperature.
2. Castration and/or dehorning
   a. Castration and dehorning have adverse effects on animal health and performance; however, these adverse effects do not appear to be additive.
   b. Castrating and/or dehorning calves 30 days before sale will result in a net loss in weaning weight of about 3 per cent. For each month earlier, this effect on weaning weight will be reduced about 0.5 per cent (e.g., castration at 3 months before sale will reduce weaning weight 2 per cent).
   c. Calves that are castrated and/or dehorned upon arrival at the feedlot will have about 30 per cent more sickness and death loss, 3 per cent poorer daily gain, 3 per cent poorer feed conversion, and lower-quality grades compared with polled steers.
3. Vaccination
   a. Vaccinating calves against viral and bacterial agents usually associated with the BRD complex 30 days before sale will reduce weaning weight about 2 per cent. Earlier vaccination will reduce this loss but may also reduce immunity because of interference by maternal antibody.
   b. Compared with unvaccinated calves, calves vaccinated against the microbial agents associated with the BRD complex at the farm of origin will have about 20 to 30 per cent less sickness, 40 per cent less death loss, and similar feedyard performance.
4. Shrink
   a. Even in short-haul cattle, about 50 per cent of shrink is gut contents and about 50 per cent is tissue shrink.
   b. Calves can shrink too much but can also shrink too little. Concern about shrink should be based on deviation from "typical" shrink for cattle hauled similar distances. For example, calves hauled 24 hours normally shrink 6 to 9 per cent. Loads with shrinks of less than 6 per cent or more than 9 per cent may have more health problems.
5. During the stress of marketing and transport, subclinical infections such as *Salmonella* and coccidiosis may become clinical and add additional stress on calves.
6. Rectal Temperature
   a. During sunny and/or warm days, calf rectal temperature will increase about 0.27° C for each hour that calves are waiting for processing.
   b. During cold and/or rainy weather, rectal temperatures may decrease about 0.5° F for each hour that calves are waiting for processing.
   c. Off-truck rectal temperatures can be misleading. Best temperatures are obtained in rested calves, early in the morning before the sun warms them.
   d. Rectal temperatures must be evaluated considering other factors such as ambient temperature, sunlight, temperament of the animals, excitement, etc.
7. Highly stressed calves may benefit from a 12- to 24-hour rest period upon arrival at the feedyard. Generally processing should not be delayed for more than 48 hours. Sick calves should be treated as soon as possible.
8. Calves that have a gaunt or overfilled appearance at the auction generally have more health problems than "normal" calves.
9. Calves from fescue pastures infected with endophyte (as evidenced by origin in Missouri, Arkansas, or the northern parts of the southeastern United States and muddy, rough, long-hair coats) are prone to heat stress during the first 2 to 3 weeks after arrival but can have excellent performance if the heat stress is controlled.
10. Have several alternate plans and be ready for the unexpected.

SUPPLEMENTAL READING

Cole NA: Nutrition-health interactions of newly arrived feeder cattle. Proceedings, Symposium on Management of Food Producing Animals. Purdue University. May 1982, pp 683–701.
Cole NA: Preconditioning calves for the feedlot. Vet Clin North Am: Food Anim Pract 1:401–412, 1985.
Hutcheson DP: Nutrient requirements of diseased, stressed cattle. Vet Clin North Am: Food Anim Pract 4:523–530, 1988.
Lofgreen GP: Nutrition and management of stressed beef calves. Vet Clin North Am: Large Anim Pract 5:87–101, 1983.
Lusby KS: Limit fed creep feeds for nursing calves. The Bovine Proceedings. No. 21. April 1989, pp 92–95.

Use of Growth Stimulants and Feed Additives in Ruminant Animal Production

ROBERT T. BRANDT, JR, PHD, MS

The use of growth stimulants and feed additives to promote rate and efficiency of growth and animal health is prevalent in food animal production today and likely will be a key production component in the future. Most products on the market fall into two general categories: (1) anabolic agents (implants) and (2) feed additives. A third class of growth stimulants, known generically as nutrient partitioning agents (primarily growth hormone and β-adrenergic agonists), may be available for use in food animals in the future. It is the purpose of this article to describe briefly the compounds and products currently available for use, their modes of action, and recommendations for their use in field applications.

EFFICACY AND SAFETY

Products used to enhance animal production and health generally fall into one of two categories from a regulatory standpoint. Compounds that are "generally recognized as safe" (GRAS) are naturally occurring (e.g., buffers, some fermentation and plant extracts, yeasts) and are not regulated by the US Food and Drug Administration (FDA) unless therapeutic claims for the product are made. Compounds that do not fall into the GRAS category are regulated by the FDA and have undergone extensive research to prove that they are efficacious and nontoxic when used at approved levels and will not result in residues that pose any potential human health hazard. Thus when used properly, products available for food animal production are efficacious and safe. Problems arise when products are administered improperly or not used at approved levels, or when withdrawal times are not observed. Thus it is the responsibility of every professional involved in the livestock production industry to make knowledgeable, prudent recommendations to producers with respect to animal health and growth promotion products. Recent changes have been made in administration sites and withdrawal periods, and there are new uses for some products, which will all be addressed.

ANABOLIC GROWTH PROMOTANTS

An anabolic compound, by definition, is one whose use results in constructive metabolism, that is, lean tissue growth. It is important to remember that protein accretion (muscle growth) is an extremely dynamic process that is in a constant state of flux. Two metabolic processes occur continuously and simultaneously—namely, protein anabolism and protein catabolism. Thus net protein growth per unit of time is the difference between the amount of protein formed and that broken down. It follows that net protein growth rate can be increased by processes or compounds that increase protein anabolism or decrease protein catabolism. Estrogenic compounds apparently increase growth rate by increasing anabolic rate.

Mode of Action

For purposes of this discussion, anabolic compounds are classified as those having estrogenic activity or those having androgenic activity. Estrogens are phenolic steroids synthesized primarily by the ovary but also by the testes and the adrenal cortex. The primary role of estrogen is in female reproductive function and development of secondary sex characteristics, but research has shown that estrogens and compounds with estrogenic activity improve growth rate and feed efficiency when administered to beef cattle. The precise mode of action of estrogens and compounds exhibiting estrogen-like activity is unclear, although growth rate and efficiency responses are likely due at least in part to secondary effects of estrogen endocrine function. It has been shown that growing-finishing cattle treated with low levels of estrogen or estrogen-like compounds exhibit heavier pituitary weights and higher blood plasma concentrations of growth hormone (GH) when compared with nontreated control animals. Increased GH production with estrogenic implants is apparently directly related to increased pituitary weight. GH (as well as insulin) increases nitrogen retention and muscle growth rate, apparently by increasing amino acid uptake or protein synthesis by muscle cells, or both. The result is increased lean growth rate (daily gain). Also, because lean tissue is less expensive energetically to deposit in the carcass than fat (lean tissue contains approximately 85 per cent water), improvements in feed efficiency are a common result in animals treated with estrogenic substances. Zeranol (Ralgro*), originally isolated from mold growth, is not an estrogen but exhibits some estrogenic properties when administered to animals. As with estrogens, zeranol increases pituitary weight and plasma GH concentration.

Available Anabolic Products

Diethylstilbestrol (DES) was one of the first compounds identified to possess estrogen-like, anabolic properties. However, concern by FDA over the potential carcinogenicity of DES resulted in a total ban on its sale and use in 1979. Since the introduction of DES, several anabolic compounds have been introduced into the marketplace. Currently available implants, their active ingredients, and approved uses are summarized in Table 1.

*Available from Pitman-Moore, Inc., Mundelein, IL.

Table 1. ACTIVE INGREDIENTS AND APPROVED USES FOR CURRENTLY AVAILABLE ANABOLIC IMPLANTS

Trade Name	Active Ingredient(s)	Sex[a]	Growth Phase[b]
Ralgro[1]	36 mg zeranol	S,H	S,G,F
Synovex-C[2]	10 mg estradiol benzoate 100 mg progesterone	S,H	S
Compudose[3]	24 mg estradiol 17-β	S,H[c]	S,G,F
Synovex-S[2]	20 mg estradiol benzoate 200 mg progesterone	S	G,H[d]
Steer-oid[4]	20 mg estradiol benzoate 200 mg progesterone	S	G,F[d]
Synovex-H[2]	20 mg estradiol benzoate 200 mg testosterone propionate	H	G,F[d]
Heifer-oid[4]	20 mg estradiol benzoate 200 mg testosterone propionate	H	G,F[d]
Finaplix-S[5]	140 mg trenbolone acetate	S	G,F[e]
Finaplix-H[5]	200 mg trenbolone acetate	H	G,F[e]

[a]S = steer, H = heifer.
[b]S = suckling, G = growing, F = finishing.
[c]Heifer approval is for growing-finishing feedlot heifers only.
[d]For use in animals weighing 400 lb or more.
[e]For use in feedlot animals.
[1]Pitman-Moore.
[2]Syntex Animal Health.
[3]Elanco Products.
[4]The Upjohn Co.
[5]Hoechst-Roussel Agri-Vet. Co.

The effective payout time for enhanced growth promotion for the implants in Table 1 is approximately 70 to 100 days, with the exception of estradiol (Compudose*), whose life is 150 to 200 days. All implants listed in Table 1 have a zero-day withdrawal. Until July 1989, zeranol had a 65-day withdrawal period between final implantation and slaughter of the animals.

Proper Implant Location and Technique

All implants currently available should be administered subcutaneously in the *middle one third* of the back of the ear. Previously it was recommended that zeranol be implanted close to the base of the ear. It is critical that implants be administered in the proper location (middle of the ear) to achieve maximum response and to eliminate the potential for residues in meat removed from the head and neck regions of the carcass.

Proper implanting technique requires skill, patience, and common sense. Implants in Table 1 made by different companies have an applicator (implant gun) or applicators unique to that particular line of products. Thus familiarity with the applicator is needed. For most applicators the needle should be inserted between the skin and cartilage between major veins so that when inserted to the hub, the needle is in the middle one third of the ear. The needle should then be withdrawn approximately 1 cm to create a cavity in which to deposit the implant. The implant should then be deposited carefully, the needle withdrawn, and the wound gently pinched shut to prevent excessive bleeding as well as potential loss of a portion of the pellets composing the implant. Between uses the needle of the applicator should be wiped clean with an antiseptic solution to minimize the risk of infection and walling off of the implant. It cannot be overemphasized that proper technique and sanitation, not the speed with which animals are processed, are critical to realizing the profit potential afforded by implants. Net returns to implants range from $10 to $20 in suckling and growing situations and up to $25 to $40 in the feedlot. Improperly placed, walled off or missing implants result in the loss of this profit plus the cost of the implant.

Response to Implants

In this section response to implants over a range of beef cattle production segments is discussed. It is important to understand that the magnitude of improvement in rate and efficiency of gain is dictated by protein and energy adequacy of the diet. This point is illustrated in a summary of grazing studies evaluating estradiol efficacy in Table 2. Therefore, up to a point, implant response increases with increased plane of nutrition. Generally, implant responses are negligible in situations in which diet quantity or quality limits rate of gain to 1.0 lb/day or less.

SUCKLING CALVES. Implants cleared for use in suckling calves are Ralgro, Synovex-C,† and Compudose (steers only). Simms presented an excellent review on calf response to suckling implants.[8] In a summary of nine trials involving 1343 suckling steer calves, average weaning weights were improved 19.2 lb (range of 8.2 to 34 lb) by a single implant and 32.9 lb (range of 19.7 to 46 lb) for steers that were reimplanted later in the suckling phase. The wide range in response to suckling implants is probably the result of a number of interacting

Table 2. IMPLANT RESPONSE AS AFFECTED BY AVERAGE DAILY GAIN OF GRAZING CATTLE

No. Trials	Rate of Gain (lb/day)		Improvement over Control (%)
	Control	Implanted	
9	1.16	1.26	8.6
5	1.22	1.39	13.9
10	1.33	1.54	15.8
5	1.45	1.72	18.6

Source: Data adapted from Compudose Technical Manual, Elanco Products, Inc., Indianapolis, IN.

factors, including calf growth potential, dam milk production, and quantity and quality of available forage.

Considerable debate exists concerning the merit and risk of implanting heifer calves that may be used as replacements in the breeding herd. Kansas[8] and Missouri[6] data clearly indicate that implanting heifers at birth but *not* at 2 to 5 months of age dramatically reduces fertility as yearlings. Heifers implanted at birth cycled but did not conceive. Implanting *once* during the suckling phase, at 2 to 5 months of age, has generally had little or no effect on fertility. Although some studies (D. D. Simms, personal communication) have demonstrated increased pelvic size at weaning for implanted heifers, there is little or no difference in pelvic size at first calving between implanted and nonimplanted heifers. Therefore a single implant of Ralgro, Synovex C, or Calf-oid* at 2 to 5 months of age, while perhaps not counterproductive to fertility, may have little if any benefit for heifer reproductive performance.

GROWING CATTLE. Stocker cattle grown on high roughage diets in drylot or grazed on pastures will generally display increased weight gain in response to implants. A summary of four pasture studies comparing three implants with a negative control is presented in Table 3. Percentage responses by implanted cattle are similar to those reported in a summary by Ward, where daily gain was improved by an average of 15.1 per cent over nonimplanted control cattle (range of 8 to 28 per cent).[10]

It is often asked whether cattle implanted during suckling or initial growth phases will respond to subsequent growing phase implants. The research data are conflicting in this area, particularly when later growing phase rate of gain is low (less than 1.5 lb/day). There is enough positive data to make a general recommendation that previously implanted cattle should be reimplanted to maximize average daily gain (ADG) in later growing phases in pasture or drylot backgrounding programs. An exception would be if the client is going to retain ownership through the finishing phase, in which case implanting during the latter growth phase can be deferred to the finishing phase.

FINISHING CATTLE. Finishing cattle respond dramatically to implants, regardless of whether they have been implanted in previous growth phases. Implanting improves ADG and feed/gain by an average of 8 to 10 per cent. The value of reimplanting finishing cattle midway through the finishing period is demonstrated in Table 4. Implanting once at processing with estradiol has produced similar performance results to reimplant programs, with the added benefit of not having to work the cattle midway through the feeding period. There does not seem to be much if any benefit from reimplanting with an implant different from that used initially.

Trenbolone Acetate for Feedlot Cattle

Trenbolone acetate (TBA), an androgenic steroid that has been used in Europe for over 10 years as an anabolic agent,

---
*Available from Elanco Products, Indianapolis, IN.
†Available from Syntex Animal Health, West Des Moines, IA.

*Available from The Upjohn Co., Kalamazoo, MI.

Table 3. AVERAGE DAILY GAIN RESPONSE TO IMPLANTS BY GRAZING STEERS

Site	No. Steers	Trial Length (day)	Treatment[a]			
			Control	Synovex	Ralgro	Compudose
Kansas	442	145	1.45	1.71	1.67	1.70
California	120	193	1.70	1.91	1.79	1.89
New Mexico	114	149	1.10	1.22	1.20	1.24
Texas	236	160	2.05	2.39	2.26	2.32
ADG, lb			1.58	1.81	1.73	1.79
Increase over control, %				14.6	9.5	13.3

[a]ADG response in lb.
ADG = average daily gain.

has just recently been cleared for use in beef cattle in the United States. Marketed under the name of Finaplix* (Table 1), TBA apparently has a different mode of action than do estrogens in promoting protein growth. Estrogens and estrogen-like compounds exert their anabolic effects indirectly through the endocrine system, the net result being an increase in protein synthesis. Conversely, TBA apparently exerts its anabolic effect by reducing protein turnover. Although the mode of action is unclear, there is experimental evidence to suggest that TBA suppresses adrenocortical function, resulting in lowered cortisol production. Cortisol decreases protein deposition and muscle growth. Thus concomitant use of estrogen and TBA would theoretically have an additive effect on muscle growth by increasing protein synthesis and reducing protein breakdown.

Table 5 illustrates a summary of five trials conducted in the United States to evaluate the efficacy of TBA, alone or in combination with estradiol on animal performance. Estradiol was administered on day 1, and TBA (200 mg) was administered on either day 1 or days 1 and 63 (trials lasted 126 to 131 days). It is shown that the combination of estradiol and TBA was more efficacious for improving rate and efficiency of gain than either anabolic administered separately. Subsequent research has shown similar results with concomitant use of TBA with other estrogenic compounds (estradiol benzoate and zeranol).

The legality of TBA use in combination with estrogenic implants has been a highly controversial subject. In 1987, the FDA's Center for Veterinary Medicine (CVM) issued the statement, "Any individual or firms promoting the concomi-

*Available from Hoechst-Roussel Agri-Vet Co., Somerville, NJ.

tant use of Finaplix with other implanted growth promotants or the implant of the product in other than the approved site are violating the Federal Food, Drug and Cosmetic Act and are subject to regulatory action." This was interpreted to refer primarily to manufacturers, suppliers, and distributors. Further, CVM personnel stated that as long as a well-established patient-client relationship exists between the professional (nutritionist, veterinarian) recommending concomitant usage and the user, it is perfectly legal. However, if the "professional" functions both as a practitioner and distributor and calls on producers who are not established clients, then that person is considered a supplier, making it illegal for him or her to suggest such use. At this writing a new implant containing both TBA and estradiol is expected to be cleared for use in the near future.

Another concern with use of TBA with estrogen is its effect on carcass quality grade. A summary of several university studies indicates that grade reduction may be 8 to 10 per cent. Whether the observed reduction in quality grade can be overcome with additional days on feed, without losing the advantage of faster and more efficient gains, is unclear at this point.

Following is a list of important points regarding the use of TBA implants:

1. TBA is most effective when used in combination with estrogenic implants.
2. TBA should be administered when cattle have 70 to 100 days on feed remaining. There is no benefit from multiple implanting with TBA.
3. Quality grade can be reduced 8 to 10 per cent or more. A contributing factor seems to be reimplantation with less than 70 days on feed remaining.
4. TBA increases carcass weight and therefore should not be used when heavy-weight carcasses pose potential marketing problems. Conversely, TBA should be considered for light cattle to increase carcass weight.
5. TBA can be used to improve rate and efficiency of growth of Holsteins.

FEED ADDITIVES

Feed additives are essential to livestock production to enhance animal health, accelerate growth, and reduce the cost of production. Each additive offers specific benefits. In addition to improving rate or efficiency of gain, or both, some additives aid in the reduction of bovine respiratory disease (BRD) complex, coccidiosis, and incidence and severity of bloat, acidosis, liver abscesses, and foot rot.

Feed additives can generally be divided into six categories: (1) ionophore antibiotics, (2) nonionophore antibiotics, (3) coccidiostats, (4) estrus suppressants, (5) buffers, and (6) others. Each additive has its own characteristics and feeding

Table 4. EFFECT OF REIMPLANTING FINISHING STEERS AND HEIFERS IN KANSAS STUDIES

	Treatment		
	Control	One Implant[d]	Reimplant[e]
Steers[a]			
ADG, lb		2.69	2.84
Improvement, %			+5.6
Feed/gain		7.13	6.83
Improvement, %			+4.2
Heifers[b]			2.94
ADG, lb	2.58	2.86	+14.0
Improvement, %[c]		+10.9	7.60
Feed/gain	8.21	7.76	+7.4
Improvement, %[c]		+5.5	

[a]Nine-trial summary.
[b]Two-trial summary with 517 heifers fed 112 to 119 days.
[c]Relative to control heifers.
[d]Implanted at processing.
[e]Reimplanted after 60 to 75 days on feed.
ADG = average daily gain.

Table 5. FIVE-TRIAL SUMMARY OF THE EFFECTS OF TRENBOLONE ACETATE AND ESTRADIOL ON PERFORMANCE OF FINISHING STEERS

Treatment	ADG (lb)	Response (%)	Feed/Gain	Response (%)
Control	3.06[a]		6.79[a]	
Estradiol	3.41[b]	11.4	6.29[b]	7.4
TBA (days 1 and 63)	3.27[a,b]	6.9	6.29[b]	7.4
Estradiol + TBA (day 1)	3.67[c]	19.9	5.97[c]	12.1
Estradiol + TBA (days 1 and 63)	3.56[c]	16.3	5.95[c]	12.4

Source: Data adapted from Trenkle A: Combining trenbolone acetate and estrogen implants results in additive growth promoting effects in feedlot steers. Feedstuffs 59:43, 1987.

[a-c]Means in a column with different superscripts differ (P < .05).
TBA = trenbolone acetate.

limitations. Some are approved to be fed in combination with others. In this section we review feed additives currently available and make some recommendations for their use in field applications.

Ionophores

Ionophores are carboxylic polyether antibiotics that depress or inhibit the growth of specific ruminal microorganisms. The precise mode of action of ionophores on altering ruminal microflora is unknown, although it is probably related to their facilitation of passage of numerous monovalent and divalent actions through hydrophobic lipid membranes. However, the net results of ionophore additions to ruminant diets are well known. These include

1. Improvement in ruminal and whole animal energetic efficiency. This is accomplished mainly by an alteration in ratio of ruminal volatile fatty acids (VFA), resulting in a greater production of propionate, the only glucogenic VFA from rumen fermentation. Methane production is lowered, resulting in increased fermentation efficiency. Research also shows that ionophores may reduce the maintenance energy requirement of cattle.
2. Reduction in ruminal degradation of protein. This effect is most important from a practical standpoint for growing cattle fed a high-roughage, marginally deficient protein diet.
3. Increased lipid content of rumen microorganisms. Whether this is the result of microbial lipid synthesis acting as a hydrogen sink in response to an ionophore insult or the result of ionophores promoting ruminal microbial populations that synthesize greater proportions of lipid is unknown. However, increased lipid flow to the small intestine may in part help explain increased weight gains (grazing cattle) and increased feed efficiency (feedlot cattle) in animals fed ionophores.
4. Enhancement of animal health. Ionophores aid in the reduction of acidosis, bloat, and coccidiosis. Reduction of the incidence and severity of digestive disorders results in improved animal performance. Ionophores have also been shown to reduce the incidence of tryptophan-induced pulmonary edema and enphysema, probably by reducing ruminal conversion of tryptophan to the toxic 3-methyl-indole.

The two ionophores cleared for use in ruminant animal production are lasalocid sodium (Bovate*) and monensin sodium (Rumensin†). The following discussion outlines FDA-approved use levels, indications for use, and combination clearances with other feed additives. Lasalocid sodium and monensin sodium are available for application in liquid and dry supplements.

---
*Available from Hoffman-LaRoche, Inc., Nutley, NJ.
†Available from Elanco Products, Indianapolis, IN.

Lasalocid—Finishing Cattle

LABEL CLEARANCE. For improved feed efficiency, 10 to 30 g/ton in complete feed. Feed continuously to provide not less than 100 nor more than 360 mg/head daily. For improved rate of gain and feed efficiency use 25 to 30 g/ton of complete feed (250 to 360 mg/head daily).

COMBINATIONS ALLOWED. (1) Lasalocid (25 to 30 g/ton) plus oxytetracycline (OTC) (7.5 g/ton, to provide 75 mg OTC/head daily). For improved feed efficiency and increased rate of weight gain and reduction of the incidence and severity of liver abscesses. (2) Lasalocid (25 to 30 g/ton) plus melengestrol acetate (MGA; 0.25 to 0.50 mg/head daily) fed continuously for increased weight gain, improved feed efficiency, and suppression of estrus in beef heifers fed in confinement for slaughter. Discontinue MGA feeding 48 hours prior to slaughter.

Lasalocid—Growing Cattle

LABEL CLEARANCE. Feed continuously at a rate of no less than 60 mg nor more than 200 mg daily for increased weight gain of pasture cattle (stockers, feeders, slaughter cattle, and beef and dairy replacement heifers).

FORMULATION. If hand fed, the drug must be contained in at least 1 lb of feed. Free-choice loose salt and block formulations are available. Contact the sponsor (Hoffman-LaRoche, Nutley, NJ) for approved diet formulations.

Lasalocid—Coccidiosis

CATTLE. Feed continuously at a rate of 1 mg/2.2 lb body weight, up to a maximum of 360 mg/head daily (800 lb body weight) for the control of coccidiosis caused by *Eimeria bovis* and *E. zuernii*. Feed only to cattle weighing up to 800 lb.

SHEEP. Feed continuously to provide not less than 15 mg nor more than 70 mg/head daily (20 to 30g/ton) for the prevention of coccidiosis caused by *E. ovina, E. crandallis, E. ovinoidalis, E. parva,* and *E. intricata* in sheep maintained in confinement.

Monensin—Finishing Cattle

LABEL CLEARANCE. For improved feed efficiency, 5 to 30 g/ton in complete feed. Feed continuously to provide not less than 50 nor more than 360 mg/head daily.

COMBINATIONS ALLOWED. (1) Monensin (5 to 30 g/ton) plus tylosin (8 to 10 g/ton) for improved feed efficiency and the reduction of incidence of liver abscesses. (2) Monensin (5 to 30 g/ton) plus MGA (0.25 to 0.40 mg/head daily) for increased rate of weight gain, improved feed efficiency, and suppression of estrus in heifers fed for slaughter.

Monensin—Growing Cattle

LABEL CLEARANCE. For increased rate of weight gain in stocker cattle and dairy and beef replacement heifers weighing more than 400 lb on pasture. Feed continuously at a rate of 40 to 200 mg/head daily in not less than 1 lb of feed. After the fifth day, 400 mg can be offered every other day in not less than 2 lb of feed.

Monensin—Cows

LABEL CLEARANCE. Feed 50 to 200 mg/head daily in a minimum of 1 lb feed for improved feed efficiency. Feed can be restricted to 95 per cent of normal requirements when 50 g monensin is fed, and to 90 per cent at 200 mg. Clearance is for mature, reproducing beef cows in drylot or on pasture.

Ionophores—Field Applications

For livestock (nonpoultry) feeding, monensin has clearances for beef cattle only, while lasalocid has approved uses in cattle and sheep. These ionophores are toxic in varying degrees to other farm and pet species, and precautions should be taken to prevent other livestock from accessing ionophore-medicated feeds. Monensin is generally more toxic than lasalocid in cattle, sheep, and horses, although both can be lethal. Consistent signs of acute ionophore toxicity are anorexia, hyperactivity, skeletal muscle weakness, ataxia, decreased weight gains, and delayed deaths. Similar to other medicated feeds, following label directions is critical.

GROWING CATTLE. Table 6 shows pooled average daily gain responses to monensin by pasture cattle (200 mg/head daily) and by cattle fed harvested forages in confinement (150 to 200 mg/head daily). Monensin increased weight gains 14 to 16 per cent in growing cattle and improved feed efficiency an average of 15.3 per cent for cattle grown on harvested forages, where feed efficiency could be accurately measured. Optimal responses to both ionophores appear to differ as a function of energy level of the basal diet. For low-quality forages, 100 to 150 mg of lasalocid or monensin/head daily is recommended, compared with 150 to 200 and 200 mg/head daily for cattle on pasture and corn silage rations, respectively.

FINISHING CATTLE. Goodrich and colleagues reviewed the response to monensin by over 11,000 head of feedlot cattle in 228 trials.[4] Results are presented in Table 7. The response to monensin in feedlot rations is characterized by equal weight gains on lower dry matter consumption. Responses to lasalocid are similar, although lasalocid does not appear to reduce intake to the same degree as monensin.

This last point has important ramifications with respect to management of feedlot cattle. When starting cattle on feed, monensin step-up programs have proven useful. Feeding 10 g/ton during the step-up period and switching to 25 to 27 g/ton when cattle are placed on the finisher ration improves initial weight gain, intake, and feed efficiency compared with starting cattle on the higher level. However, this performance difference is lost over the entire feeding period. Conversely, cattle fed lasalocid require no adaptation period, thus precluding the need for an ionophore step-up period. One of the primary benefits of monensin in high-grain diets for beef cattle is maintenance of a less erratic, lower level of intake than for nonmedicated cattle. This aids in bunk management and lowers the risk of certain digestive upsets such as grain bloat and acidosis.

Much research effort has recently been expended on evaluation of daily or weekly ionophore rotation programs (IRP) in finishing cattle. This approach, which has proven beneficial in the poultry industry, is based on the hypothesis that microorganisms adapt to continuous feeding of one drug. Alternatively, it has been proposed that IRP may promote synergistic effects on animal performance because of different biologic modes of action. Hubbert and associates reviewed eight feedlot trials evaluating daily or weekly rotation of monensin and lasalocid in cattle finishing rations.[5] Tylosin (10 g/ton) was fed with monensin (25 g/ton), while lasalocid was included at 30 g/ton in the appropriate rations. The results (Table 8) showed that cattle fed lasalocid and monensin/tylosin in a daily rotation scheme gained 3.8 per cent faster and 2.2 per cent more efficiently than cattle fed monensin/tylosin alone. Subsequent research has failed to show improvement from IRP in rumen fermentation pattern or ration utilization. Therefore the small improvement seen in controlled studies may be offset by more erratic feed consumption patterns and increased bunk management problems. Further, implementation of the IRP requires additional supplement storage space or an on-site microingredient machine to medicate the feed with alternate drugs daily.

Table 7. EFFECT OF MONENSIN ON PERFORMANCE OF FEEDLOT CATTLE

Item	Control	Monensin	Change (%)
No. head	5696	5578	
Monensin, mg/head/day	0	246	
Daily gain, lb	2.4	2.42	0.8
Daily feed, lb DM	18.19	17.01	−6.4
Feed/gain	8.09	7.43	−8.2

Source: Data adapted from Goodrich RD, et al: Influence of monensin on the performance of cattle. J Anim Sci 58:1484, 1984.

Table 6. EFFECT OF MONENSIN ON CATTLE GROWN ON PASTURE OR HARVESTED FORAGES

	Pasture[a]		Harvested Forages	
Item	Control	Monensin	Control	Monensin
No. trials		24		12
Daily gain, lb	1.23	1.43[b]	1.35	1.54[b]
Improvement, %		+16.3		+14.1
Feed intake, lb DM			16.26	15.80[b]
Feed/gain			12.39	10.50[b]
Improvement, %				+15.3

Source: Adapted from Potter EL, et al: Effect of monensin on the performance of cattle on pasture or fed harvested forages in confinement. J Anim Sci 62:583, 1986.

[a]Control cattle received same amount of supplement as those fed monensin.
[b]Monensin differs from control within a forage system (P < .01).

Table 8. EIGHT-TRIAL SUMMARY OF THE EFFECT OF LASALOCID OR MONENSIN PLUS TYLOSIN FED ALONE OR IN DAILY OR WEEKLY ROTATION TO FINISHING CATTLE

	Treatment			
Item	L	MT	D	W
No. pens	32	32	25	32
Intake, lb DM	22.2[a]	21.7[b]	21.6[a-c]	21.8[b,c]
Daily gain, lb	3.66[a]	3.66[a]	3.80[b]	3.66[a]
Feed/gain	6.11[a]	6.01[b]	5.88[c]	5.97[b,c]

Source: Adapted from Hubbert ME, et al: Effect of short duration ionophore rotations on feedlot cattle performance (abstract 78). Proc 20th Biennial Conf on Rumen Function, Chicago, IL, 1989.

[a-c]Means with unlike superscripts differ (P < .05).
L = lasalocid; MT = monensin plus tylosin; D = daily; W = weekly.

Antibiotics

In ruminant animal production, antibiotics are most commonly fed (1) to finishing cattle fed high-grain diets, (2) in receiving rations, or (3) to aid in the control of specific disease states. There are a number of products available with a number of approved uses. The intent of the following discussion is to provide insight and recommendations for use in general ruminant livestock management. For a complete listing of FDA-approved feed-grade antibiotics and their approved uses and withdrawal times, the reader is referred to the Feed Additive Compendium (1991).[3]

FINISHING RATIONS. Antibiotics are fed to finishing cattle primarily to control liver abscesses. Data in Table 9 show the effect of liver abscess severity on cattle performance. Severe abscesses may reduce gain and increase feed requirements 10 per cent. These data, in agreement with other studies, indicate that a moderate degree of abscessation (A^-, A) does not negatively influence feedlot performance. Antibiotics have been shown to improve rate and efficiency of gain in feedlot cattle. This is probably primarily accomplished through a reduction in the incidence of severe liver abscesses, but beneficial alterations in gut microflora may also be involved. Antibiotics may also reduce the incidence of grain bloat, although the data are limited.

Tylosin fed at 10 g/ton is effective in reducing liver abscess incidence and severity and has the added advantage that it may be fed in combination with monensin. Recently, oxytetracycline (7.5 g/ton) has been cleared for use with lasalocid for the same purpose. Alternatively, tetracyclines can be fed intermittently with other feed additives to avoid nonapproved combination uses. Cattle fed 1 g/head daily for 3 out of 28 days or 400 mg/head daily for 7 out of 28 days have shown similar performance to those fed antibiotics continuously. It is important not to feed other medicated feeds during the periods of tetracycline feeding.

For sheep, chlortetracycline (20 to 50 g/ton) or oxytetracycline (20 g/ton) improves rate and efficiency of gain and reduces losses resulting from enterotoxemia.

RECEIVING RATIONS. Antibiotics are often included in receiving rations for prevention of bacterial pneumonia and shipping fever complex. Table 10 outlines approved uses for antibiotics commonly fed to cattle.

Combination clearances with ionophores have been previously discussed. For sheep, oxytetracycline can be fed at 50 to 100 g/ton as an aid in prevention of bacterial diarrhea, lamb dysentery, and white scours of lambs. Guidelines for choosing feed additives for receiving diets are presented in a subsequent section.

OTHER DISEASES. In addition to previously mentioned applications, feeding oxytetracycline is approved for anaplasmosis prevention in cattle. Feeding rates are 350, 500, and 750 mg/head daily for cattle weighing less than 700, 700 to 1000, and 1000 to 1500 lb, respectively. For cattle weighing over 1500 lb the approved rate is 0.5 mg/lb body weight daily. For all levels a 48-hour withdrawal period is required prior to slaughter of any animals.

Coccidiostats

Coccidiostats are primarily used in receiving rations to aid in the prevention or treatment of coccidiosis. Survey data indicate that approximately 75 per cent of all cattle in the United States harbor pathogenic coccidia. Clinical outbreaks can be caused by environmental and management stressors such as weather changes, auction barn commingling, trucking, processing, ration changes and others. Readily detectable clinical signs of coccidiosis include diarrhea, hemorrhaging, and dehydration. Subclinical cases may also cause performance losses as a result of damage to intestinal linings, which can decrease nutrient absorption.

PREVENTION. Amprolium, marketed under several trade names, is approved for use in beef and dairy calves at 227 mg/100 lb for a 21-day period to aid coccidiosis prevention. Use of amprolium requires a 24-hour withdrawal before slaughter of any animals. Decoquinate (Deccox), a product of Rhone-Poulenc), is approved for use at 22.7 mg/100 lb body weight. Decoquinate should be fed for 28 days in a preventive program. As previously discussed, the ionophore lasalocid is approved as a coccidiostat in cattle (1 mg/2.2 lb body weight) and sheep (20 to 30 g/ton) rations.

TREATMENT. Amprolium is approved for treatment of coccidiosis at 454 mg/100 lb daily, with a treatment period of 5 days.

Estrus Suppressants

The only estrus suppressant currently available commercially is MGA (melengestrol acetate) (marketed by TUCO, a division of Upjohn). MGA is a progestational steroid similar in structure and function to progesterone. Unlike progesterone, MGA is orally active in suppressing estrus and promoting growth. There is no evidence that progestins directly stimulate growth. Rather, it is thought that the stimulatory response is a function of an elevated baseline level of estrogen production in the animal resulting from maintenance of mature follicles on the ovaries. Long-acting implants containing progestins are in various stages of development. The main advantage of such an implant over oral administration is that implants would allow males and females to be fed together in backgrounding and growing-finishing situations.

FEEDLOT HEIFERS. Suppression of estrus in feedlot heifers is desirable (1) to prevent losses from injury resulting from riding and (2) because riding and chasing increases energy requirements and may reduce performance. Generally, feeding MGA increases rate and efficiency of gain 3 to 7 per cent. The response is additive to that from ionophores, and MGA is cleared to be fed at a level of 0.25 to 0.40 mg/head daily in combination with monensin, or at a level of 0.25 to 0.50 mg/head daily in combination with lasalocid. MGA must be withdrawn 48 hours before slaughter, which may increase the incidence of dark-cutting carcasses. Growth response to MGA in feedlot situations is variable and may depend on (1) the age of the heifers being fed, (2) the number of sources of heifers fed together, (3) the amount of feeding space per heifer, and (4) whether heifers have been implanted with other growth-promoting compounds.

ESTRUS SYNCHRONIZATION. Synchronization of estrus in

Table 9. EFFECT OF LIVER ABSCESS SEVERITY ON FINISHING CATTLE PERFORMANCE

Item	Liver Score			
	0	A^-	A	A^+
No. cattle	362	50	35	60
Daily gain, lb	2.63	2.73	2.59	2.32
Daily feed, lb DM	18.55	18.60	18.22	17.88
Feed/gain	6.94	6.71	6.94	7.63

Source: Brink D et al: How should efficiency of food utilization be evaluated. Nebraska Beef Cattle Report. MP 48, Agr Exp Sta, University of Nebraska, Lincoln, pp 19–20, 1985.

0 = no abscesses; A^- = one or two small abscesses or abscess scars; A = two to four well-organized abscesses, generally <1 inch in diameter; A^+ = one or more large, active abscesses and inflammation of liver tissue.

Table 10. APPROVED USES OF ANTIBIOTICS FOR APPLICATION IN CATTLE RECEIVING AND GROWING RATIONS

Indication	Drug and Level		
	Chlortetracycline	Oxytetracycline	Chlortetracycline + Sulfamethazine
Shipping fever	350 mg*[a]	0.5–2 g*[b]	350 + 350 mg*[c]
Bacterial diarrhea	70–100 mg*[d]	0.5–5 mg**	
Foot rot	70–100 mg*[d]		

*Values expressed as g or mg/head daily.
**Values expressed as mg/lb body weight daily.
[a]Discontinue use 48 hours before slaughter.
[b]If 2-g level is used, withdraw 5 days before slaughter.
[c]Feed in a 28-day program. Withdraw 7 days before slaughter.
[d]Use 70 and 100 mg/head daily for cattle weighing less than and more than 700 lb, respectively.

beef heifers can be very desirable. In addition to shortening the breeding season and allowing concentration of labor during breeding and calving, successful synchronization increases the practicality of artificial insemination. Kansas State University studies (L. L. Corah, personal communication) showed that feeding MGA at 0.5 mg/head daily for 14 days followed by injection of prostaglandin $F_{2\alpha}$ ($PGF_{2\alpha}$) 17 days later resulted in 908 out of 1451 (62.6 per cent) heifers responding to synchronization. Response rates ranged from 33 to 95 per cent at 11 locations. Locations with low response rates were also those with a high number of prepuberal heifers.

Buffers

Buffers resist change in ruminal pH and theoretically should be beneficial in maintaining health and high levels of performance in ruminants fed finishing diets. Feed additives that have been used as buffers include sodium bicarbonate, sodium sesquicarbonate, limestone, sodium bentonite, and magnesium oxide. Response in animal performance to buffers, however, has been extremely variable. This is in contrast to dairy cattle, where buffers have proven extremely useful in maintaining animal health and high levels of milk production. The routine use of buffers in beef cattle diets does not appear to be cost-effective.

Other Feed Additives

Other feed additives are available that claim enhanced performance of ruminant animals. Most are composed of naturally occurring GRAS compounds that are not FDA-regulated unless therapeutic label claims are made.

SARSAPONIN. Marketed as Sevarin,* sarsaponin is an extract of the yucca plant. The active ingredient(s) and mode of action have not been identified. Since it is not regulated, it can be included in any feeding program. The manufacturer recommends a rate of 0.5 g/head daily to be fed in conjunction with monensin or lasalocid. Controlled research studies have shown little or no performance benefit from sarsaponin-ionophore combinations.

YEASTS. Several products are commercially available that contain yeasts or fermentation extract, or both. Studies have shown that these products sometimes increase fiber digestion. Large improvements in cow milk production have also been reported. Performance responses in growing animals have generally been variable and small, although they may be beneficial in very high roughage diets. It is doubtful whether these products would be beneficial for animals fed high-grain diets, since few or no fungi normally exist in the rumen under these conditions.

PROBIOTICS. Probiotic is a term used for products containing "beneficial" microorganisms. A number of products are available for oral administration (pastes and gels), for intraruminal injection, or as feed additive preparations. Most contain either *Lactobacillus* spp. (primarily *L. acidophilus*) or *Streptococcus faecium*. In addition, many contain vitamins, trace minerals, and various "growth factors."

The conceptual basis for use of probiotics stems from the fact that beneficial strains of bacteria naturally inhabit the gastrointestinal tract of mammals and are believed to play an important role in regulating the growth of *Escherichia coli* and other pathogens along the digestive tract. Further, it has been observed that restriction of feed and water to laboratory animals resulted in reductions in lactobacilli and yeast, with a concomitant increase in coliforms and salmonella. Thus there has been great interest in the therapeutic value of lactobacilli and *S. faecium* for stressed animals.

Studies with poultry, swine, and preruminant calves have shown significant declines in fecal excretion of coliforms and corresponding improvements in health and performance with lactobacilli supplementation. However, a review of the available literature shows generally no response in functioning ruminants. In the few studies that have shown a response, it is difficult or impossible to ascertain whether the response was the result of the probiotic or the nutritional supplement (vitamins or trace minerals, or both) included in the particular preparation.

Lack of response in ruminants may be the result of (1) lack of sufficient viable microbial counts in the preparation, (2) low ruminal survivability, or (3) host species specificity for colonization (e.g., it has been observed that only lactobacilli indigenous to rats will attach to rat gastrointestinal epithelium). Until research is conducted to demonstrate site and mode of action of the various probiotic preparations, there can be no firm basis from which to recommend their routine use.

Use of Feed Additives in Receiving Rations

Determining the most beneficial feed additive to use in receiving diets for stressed animals can be confusing because of the number of compounds available and the approved uses for each. Therefore decisions should be based on (1) previous health history of the client's operation or animals being received, or both, (2) age and previous management of animals being received (e.g., calves versus yearlings; preconditioned versus freshly weaned calves), and (3) management capabilities of personnel at the particular operation where animals are received.

PREVIOUS HEALTH HISTORY. Previous experience can be extremely beneficial in developing a program for feed additive use. If a particular operation has a known history of problems

---
*Available from Distributers Processing, Inc., Porterville, CA.

with coccidiosis or purchases animals with which coccidiosis has been a problem in the past, inclusion of a coccidiostat in the receiving ration can be extremely beneficial. Conversely, where shipping fever complex, foot rot, or other bacterial-related disease problems have existed, an antibiotic program is indicated.

ANIMAL AGE AND PREVIOUS MANAGEMENT. Calves are more susceptible to stress and diseases incurred in marketing and transportation channels than are yearlings. As a result, feed consumption may be as low as 0.5 to 1 per cent of body weight for as long as 2 to 3 weeks after arrival, further compromising the ability of the animals to withstand a disease challenge. This situation can be exacerbated in freshly weaned calves, who have no prior experience with feed bunks and water tanks. Because ionophores reduce intake, they should not be included in stressed-calf receiving rations. Research has shown that feeding the coccidiostat decoquinate stimulates feed intake by stressed calves. This may be the result of controlling ruminal protozoal numbers, allowing bacterial species to proliferate and stimulate rumen digestive kinetics. Antibiotic feeding may help reduce the incidence of shipping fever complex, with no apparent detrimental effect on feed consumption. Thus both practices are beneficial, and decisions on which to use should be based largely on previous health history and experience.

MANAGEMENT. Another factor to consider in prescribing any animal health program is the day-to-day management capability of a given operation. Typically commercial feeding operations employ personnel to provide full-time animal health care. Some smaller operations with fewer employees may not be able to provide the same amount of constant care, particularly if other areas of the enterprise (e.g., harvesting, planting, mechanical breakdowns) require immediate attention. Although by no means a replacement for good management, antibiotic feeding to newly received calves will probably aid health management in smaller, diversified operations.

GROWTH PROMOTION—A FUTURISTIC LOOK

In the future, compounds that provide dramatic increases in lean tissue growth and production efficiency are expected to be available for use in domestic livestock production. One class of compounds, the beta agonists, are similar in chemical structure and pharmacologic function to the catecholamines. Their precise mode of action is unclear at this point because the interplay of several endocrine and physiologic factors is probably involved. However, increased protein accretion (via reduction in protein turnover) and increased rates of lipolysis have been observed. Thus these compounds have been termed "nutrient partitioning" agents. One compound expected to be available soon for use in swine and beef cattle is ractopamine. Table 11 demonstrates the potency of ractopamine for improving rate and efficiency of gain and carcass lean deposition in steers when administered during the last 38 to 45 days of the finishing period. Note that the 30-ppm level increased gain and feed efficiency 18.5 and 15.7 per cent, respectively. This level also had dramatic effects on carcass traits. Repartitioning agents have also been shown to have a very dramatic effect on increasing lean meat production from cull cows.

Somatotropins also enhance lean tissue deposition. However, as a protein hormone it must be injected to maintain biologic activity. Beta agonists, on the other hand, may be administered orally. Further, while beta-agonists are effective across different species, somatotropins are highly species specific. If somatotropins or beta-agonists are cleared for use in ruminant animal production, work will be needed to evaluate their impact on animal nutritional requirements.

Table 11. SIX-TRIAL SUMMARY OF THE EFFECTS OF RACTOPAMINE ON FEEDLOT PERFORMANCE AND CARCASS TRAITS OF FINISHING STEERS FED LAST 38 TO 45 DAYS OF FINISHING PERIOD

Item	Ractopamine (ppm)			
	0	10	20	30
Daily gain, lb	2.75[a]	2.95[b]	3.06[b]	3.26[c]
Daily feed, lb	20.7	20.5	20.7	20.5
Feed/gain	7.69[a]	7.14[b]	6.90[b]	6.48[c]
Carcass traits				
Hot weight, lb	714[a]	719[b]	724[c]	730[d]
Dress, %	60.71[a]	60.75[a]	61.02[b]	61.03[b]
Ribeye area, in^2	12.29[a]	12.37[a,b]	12.48[b]	12.75[c]
Marbling score	557[a]	550[a]	548[a,b]	535[b]
Yield grade	2.96[a]	3.01[a]	2.98[a]	2.89[b]
Conformation score	20.18[a]	20.45[a]	20.74[b]	20.99[c]

[a–d]Means in a row with different superscripts differ (P < .05).
Source: From Carroll LH et al: Ractopamine HCl dose titration in feedlot steers: performance and carcass traits. J Anim Sci 68(Suppl 1):294, 1990.

REFERENCES

1. Brink D, Lowry S: How should efficiency of feed utilization be evaluated. Nebraska Beef Cattle Report. MP 48, Agr Exp Stat, University of Nebraska, Lincoln. pp 19–20, 1985.
2. Carroll LH, Laudert SB, Parrott JC, et al: Ractopamine HCl dose titration in feedlot steers: performance and carcass traits. J Anim Sci 68(Suppl 1):294, 1990.
3. Feed Additive Compendium. Minnetonka, MN, Miller Publishing, 1991.
4. Goodrich RD, Garrett JE, Gast DR, et al: Influence of monensin on the performance of cattle. J Anim Sci 58:1484, 1984.
5. Hubbert ME, Johnson AB, Peterson LA: Effect of short duration ionophore rotations on feedlot cattle performance (abstract 78). Proc 20th Biennial Conf on Rumen Function, Chicago, IL, 1989.
6. Morrow RA, Brooks A, Fairbrother T, et al: Effects of implanting with Ralgro® on growth and reproductive performance of beef heifers. Animal Science Report 103, MO Agr Exp Sta, University of Missouri, Columbia. p 52, 1983.
7. Potter EL, Muller RD, Wray MI, et al: Effect of monensin on the performance of cattle on pasture or fed harvested forages in confinement. J Anim Sci 62:583, 1986.
8. Simms DD: Ralgro® implants in suckling calves and growing cattle. Proc Management for Growth Conf, Orlando, FL, sponsored by IMC, Inc, Terre Haute, IN. p 177, 1985.
9. Trenkle A: Combining trenbolone acetate and estrogen implants results in additive growth promoting effects in feedlot steers. Feedstuffs 59:43, 1987.
10. Ward JK: Growth stimulants for beef cattle. Proc Range Beef Cow Symp V. p 69, 1977.

Field Calculations for Ration Formulation

JOHN C. SIMONS, DVM
MICHAEL S. HAND, DVM, PHD, DIPLOMATE, ACVN

Any practical approach to food animal nutrition involves mathematical computation. Current methods and instruments enable us to calculate these nutrition formulae rapidly. In many cases, equations and tables have been derived and formulated that enable the computation of significantly accurate requirements for maintenance, weight change, gestation, lactation, and work.

A balanced ration has acceptable palatability and contains

within the limits of daily consumption all of the nutrients necessary for daily maintenance and production. The entities commonly measured include various categories of energy, protein, minerals, and vitamins. Water needs are expected to be met by offering potable water in unlimited quantities.

To balance rations we need to know (1) the daily nutrient requirement according to species, body weight, and physiologic state and (2) the nutrient concentrations in the specific available feeds. The primary sources of information about requirements and nutrient concentrations are the publications of the National Research Council (NRC) of the National Academy of Sciences.* Current NRC publications concerning food animals include the following:

- Nutrient Requirements of Dairy Cattle, 6th rev. ed., update 1989, 0-309-03826-X
- Nutrient Requirements of Swine, 9th rev. ed., 1988, 0-309-03779-4
- Nutrient Requirements of Sheep, 6th rev. ed., 1985, 0-309-03596-1
- Nutrient Requirements of Poultry, 8th rev. ed., 1984, 0-309-03486-8
- Nutrient Requirements of Beef Cattle, 6th rev. ed., 1984.
- Nutrient Requirements of Warm-Water Fishes and Shellfishes, rev. ed., 1983, 0-309-03482-8
- Nutrient Requirements of Cold-Water Fishes, 1981, 0-309-03187-7
- Nutrient Requirements of Rabbits, 2nd rev. ed., 1977, 0-309-02607-5

Related publications include the following:

- Predicting Feed Intake of Food Producing Animals, 1987, 0-309-03695-X
- Vitamin Tolerance of Animals, 1987, 0-309-03728-X

Nutrient requirements are expressed in heat units, weight units, or international units per animal per day. Nutrient concentrations are expressed as heat units, weight units, or international units per weight unit of feed. Table 1 demonstrates the mode of expression in the metric system.

The nutrient requirements for a given species are not strictly linear according to body weight for all physiologic states. Energy and protein requirements for maintenance and gain vary according to body weight to the 0.75 power (as weight doubles, the requirements increase about 75 per cent).

The formulation of balanced rations requires considerable computation involving arithmetic and algebraic functions. Practical application requires electronic calculation. Calculators having exponential, logarithmic, and storage capability modes in addition to ordinary arithmetic functions are essential. Within the last 10 years, computer hardware has become economically feasible and convenient to use. Usable software programs have been produced by universities, commercial agricultural enterprises, computer manufacturers, and private enterprises interested in selling information. Access to microcomputers and to networks using centrally located mini and mainframe computers is available to all.

This article is not concerned with computer literacy or programming, but the material presented is essential to such programming, and the understanding of this material should be valuable in evaluating computer hardware and related software.

ENERGY REQUIREMENTS (GENERAL)

Energy is the most important item to be considered in animal nutrition. It has no measurable dimensions or mass and is measured as heat in kilocalories (kcal) or megacalories (Mcal).

Energy is the capacity to do work, and work is accomplished by matter in motion. When matter is organized, it contains potential energy. When organized matter becomes disorganized, it releases kinetic energy and work may be accomplished. The energy involved in nutrition is chemical energy, that is, energy stored or released by chemical reactions. Endergonic reactions absorb and store energy. Examples include photosynthesis, growth, fat deposition, gestation, and lactation. Exergonic reactions release kinetic energy. Examples include glycolysis, the Krebs cycle, and electron transport. Kinetic energy released by exergonic reactions may be used to make muscles contract or glands secrete, or both. This kinetic energy may also be stored by endergonic reactions.

The kinetic energy released by exergonic reactions of energy nutrient metabolism contains free energy available for work and energy dissipated as heat. Some of the potential energy contained in feeds is lost in feces, combustible gases, and urine. Thus it is necessary to define a number of energy categories and understand their interrelationships.

1. Gross energy (GE), or heat of combustion, is the quantity of heat resulting from complete oxidation of a unit of feed.
2. Fecal energy (FE) is the quantity of heat resulting from complete oxidation of the fecal matter resulting from the digestion of a unit of feed. It includes energy contained in
   a. undigested feed,
   b. enteric microbes and their products,
   c. excretions from the gastrointestinal tract, and
   d. cellular debris from the gastrointestinal tract.
3. Energy from combustible gases (CGE) is the quantity of heat resulting from the complete oxidation of nonabsorbable gases, which result from the digestion of a unit of feed (primarily methane).
4. Digestible energy (DE) is GE minus FE.
5. Urinary energy (UE) is the heat resulting from the complete oxidation of the urine produced by the metabolism of a unit of feed.
6. Metabolizable energy (ME) is DE minus (UE + CGE).
7. Net energy (NE) is ME minus the heat increment (H_i) that results from the utilization of a unit of feed: $NE = ME - H_i$. Net energy is divided into two categories:
   a. net energy for maintenance (NE_m), which includes the heat produced by basal metabolism (H_b) plus the heat produced by normal activity (H_a) and
   b. net energy for production (NE_p), which includes the energy deposited in the products of gestation (NE_r), energy deposited in milk (NE_l), and energy used to perform work (NE_w).

---
*Further information and additional titles of Board of Agriculture publications and prices are available from the National Academy Press, 2101 Constitution Avenue NW, Washington, DC 20418.

Table 1. METRIC EXPRESSIONS OF NUTRIENT REQUIREMENTS OF ANIMALS AND NUTRIENT CONCENTRATIONS IN DM FEEDS

Nutrient	Daily Requirement Expressed As	Nutrient Concentration Expressed As
Energy	kcal or Mcal/animal day	kcal or Mcal/kg of feed
Protein	g or kg/animal day or % DM	g/kg feed or % DM
Urea potential	Not applicable	g urea equivalent/kg DM (+ or −)
Bulk minerals	g/animal day or % ration	g/kg of feed
Trace minerals	mg/animal/day	mg/kg of DM feed or ppm
Vitamin A	IU/animal/day	mg β carotene/kg of feed
Vitamins (general)	IU/animal/day	IU/kg of feed

The interrelationships among the energy categories are demonstrated schematically in Figure 1.

One of the implications of the second law of thermodynamics is that the total energy of any system is divided into two portions: (1) "bound energy" unavailable for work, called entropy, and (2) "free energy" available for work:

$$\Delta H = \Delta F + \Delta S$$

where ΔH is total energy in the system, ΔF is the free energy, and ΔS is the bound energy, or entropy. In nutrition ME corresponds to the total energy change in a system, H_i corresponds to the bound energy, or entropy, and NE corresponds to the free energy available for work. Thus

$$\Delta H = \Delta F + \Delta S \text{ (thermodynamics)}$$

and

$$ME = NE + H_i \text{ (nutrition)}$$

For most species the energy requirements and concentrations in feeds are measured as DE or ME. It is generally accepted that each gram of total digestible nutrients (TDN) contains 4.409 kcal of DE. The mathematical relationships between DE and ME vary according to species and type of diet as follows:

For swine: $ME = DE \times 0.96$
For sheep: $ME = DE \times 0.82$
For beef cattle: $ME = DE \times 0.82$
For dairy cattle: ME (Mcal/kg dry matter [DM]) = $-0.45 + 1.01$ DE (Mcal/kg DM)

For swine, sheep, and beef cattle ME is computed as a direct linear function of DE and TDN. In these cases any of the categories may be used without loss of accuracy. In the dairy cattle equation, ME as a percentage of DE varies linearly from 80 per cent at 50 per cent digestibility to 88 per cent at 80 per cent digestibility. In this case the use of ME as a standard should give a more accurate prediction than will DE or TDN.

For ruminant animals, metabolizable energy is still not a satisfactory measurement. The heat increment (H_i) that results from the metabolism of roughages is significantly greater than that of concentrates, and the ME system tends to overrate roughages as an energy source, especially in the production area. For this reason, Lofgreen and Garrett, in the late 1960s, developed what is now known as the "California Net Energy System."[24] This work was published in 1968 and has been accepted by the feeding industry. The NRC publications for beef cattle have used this system in their requirement and feed concentration tables since 1972. The development of the system is of more than passing interest. To tabulate energy requirements there must be a way to measure heat production. The pioneers in the field used respiration calorimeters, but only three of these were ever built. It is obvious then why there was so little available information about net energy. Lofgreen and Garrett used a different system based on simple algebra. It has been stated that in nutrition

$$ME = NE + H_i$$

If $ME = NE + H_i$, then

$$NE = ME - H_i$$

and

$$NE = NE_m + NE_p$$

Therefore

$$NE_m + NE_p = ME - H_i$$

and

$$NE_m + H_i = ME - NE_p$$

Since NE_m = heat of basal metabolism (H_b) + heat of necessary activity (H_a), then

$$H_b + H_a + H_i = ME - NE_p$$

or

$$\text{Total heat } (H_b + H_a + H_i) = ME - NE_p$$

Therefore if we can measure ME and the energy deposited in a product, we can measure total heat production resulting from the use of a unit of feed without a respiration calorimeter. ME is obtained by subtracting FE, CGE, and UE from GE. Lofgreen and Garrett[24] measured NE by the "comparative slaughter technique" as follows:

1. A large number of animals are selected for uniformity.
2. A portion of these animals are weighed, slaughtered, and measured for carcass specific gravity (CSG).
   a. The dead carcass is weighed in air.
   b. The dead carcass is reweighed in water.
   c. The CSG is measured mathematically and used to calculate body composition.
3. The remaining animals are fed for a prescribed period.
   a. A valid sample of the fed animals is chosen and slaughtered.
   b. CSG for these animals is measured.
   c. Carcass composition is calculated from CSG.
   d. Energy in the final sampling minus energy in the initial sampling equals NE_p (in this case NE_g).

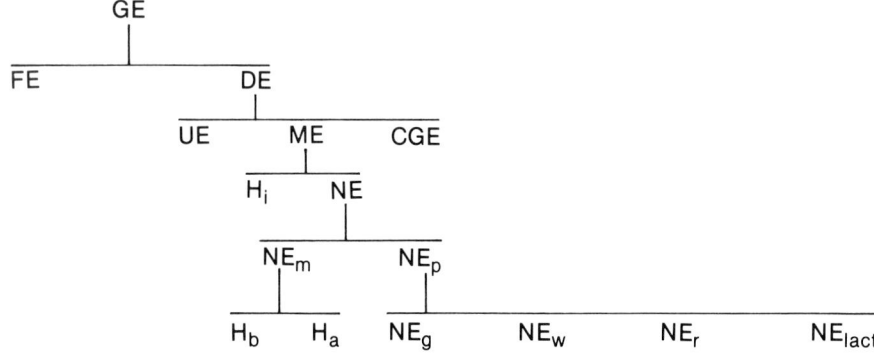

Figure 1. Schematic representation of the interrelationships among the energy categories (see text).

Validity of the specific gravity technique has been established by comparative quantitative and qualitative chemical analysis.

Modern nutritionists have access to combustion (bomb) calorimeters. These are standardized by the use of specifically purified benzoic acid. The caloric value of the benzoic acid has been determined by electrical units and computed in terms of joules/gram mole. The calorie has been standardized to equal 4.184 joules.[27]

Net Energy for Maintenance and Gain in Cattle

The big problem in predicting gain from ME is the discrepancy in heat production between roughage and concentrate feed components. An experiment performed in California demonstrated that a ration consisting of 19.45 lb of alfalfa DM provided an ME intake of 20.714 Mcal and an NE_g intake of 2.810 Mcal. A second ration containing 98 per cent concentrate produced 2.810 Mcal of NE_g from a total ME intake of 13.919 Mcal. These results show that ME does not provide a good prediction of the production energy produced by a specific unit of feed. This is particularly true in ruminant rations where mixtures of roughages and concentrates are used to provide the energy requirement. The same is true of TDN or DE. If a valid prediction is to be made, NE must be the unit of measurement. This principle is of less importance for monogastric animals, whose production rations are largely composed of concentrates.

The California Net Energy System provides a method of determining heat production in a large number of animals. It is now possible to measure heat production at different levels of intake and, by extrapolation, the NE required for maintenance. Such measurements tell us that at thermoneutral temperatures (15 to 25°C), the NE_m requirement in feedlot conditions is 77 kcal/ × (both weight [BW in kg])$^{0.75}$. Thus

$$NE_m \text{ (in Mcal)} = 0.077 \times (BW_{kg})^{0.75}$$

The NE_m requirement is modified by weather. High temperatures and humidity may depress feed intake up to 30 per cent. Low humidity and cool nighttime conditions tend to moderate the effect. Relatively high roughage diets are affected more severely than are high-concentrate diets. Conversely, feed intakes may be increased up to 30 per cent by low temperatures, particularly if the cattle remain dry. Extensive precipitation and muddy conditions can depress feed intake both in the thermoneutral zone and at lower temperatures. Rain and mud can also depress feed intake for beef cows on winter range. Forage intake may be depressed up to 50 per cent during and following storms that produce low temperatures and snow cover.

The availability of nutrients from roughages may be altered by environmental temperature. DE, ME, and NE values may be adjusted by the following formula:

$$A = B + B(0.001[T-20])$$

where A is the nutrient concentration adjusted for environmental temperature, B is the unadjusted value, and T is the effective ambient temperature (0). Thus if the listed NE_m value of a feed is 1.6 Mcal/kg and the ambient temperature is 10° below the thermoneutral zone (5°C), the adjusted NE_m concentration for the feed is

$$1.6 = 1.6(0.001[5-20]) = 1.585 \text{ Mcal/kg DM}$$

The NE_m requirement should be adjusted for exposure to temperature outside the thermoneutral zone. Requirements for adapted animals should be modified to allow for changes in the basal metabolic rate and possibly for acute exposure to heat or cold. Requirements for unadapted animals should be modified for acute exposure to heat or cold only. For adapted animals, energy expenditure is inversely proportional to temperature unless normal respiration is affected by high temperature. The following equation expresses the NE_m requirement:

$$\text{Mcal } NE_m = (a) \text{ W/kg}^{0.75}$$

For animals acclimated to the thermoneutral zone, the factor (a) is taken to be 0.077. For each degree Celsius above or below the thermoneutral zone, 0.0007 should be subtracted or added to (a) in the equation. Thus for cattle exposed to a temperature of 30°C, (a) = 0.077 − (10 × 0.0007) = 0.070. For cattle exposed to a temperature of 0°C, (a) = 0.077 + (20 × 0.0007) = 0.091. For acute heat stress, where the animals are showing rapid shallow breathing, add 7 per cent to (a). If the animals are showing open-mouthed panting, add 11 to 25 per cent to (a).

For acute cold stress, NE_m expenditures are increased according to exposures to temperatures below the lower critical temperature (LCT). The LCT for a specific animal depends on the animal's insulation and heat production. Wind velocity influences insulation and is an important environmental factor. Handley at Colorado State University proposed the use of the term temperature wind index (TWI), in which a wind velocity of 1 mph is equal to a decrease in temperature of 1°F. This would especially apply at temperatures below the thermoneutral zone. It also seems reasonable to use a figure of 0.6°C for each degree Celsius below the thermoneutral zone. Thus if the temperature was 5°C and the wind velocity was 10 mph, the TWI would equal 5°C − (10°C × 0.6) = −1°C. The (a) value in the formula $NE_m = (a) W/kg^{0.75}$ would be 0.077 + (0.0007 × 21) = 0.092.

The LCT value varies widely among different species and classes of animals. For a 1-week-old calf exposed to a low dry wind, the LCT is estimated to be 7.7°C. For a yearling steer gaining 1.1 kg/day and exposed to a low dry wind, the LCT is estimated to be −34.1°C. The increase in ME required per degree Celsius below the LCT is from 1 to 3 per cent. For details on calculation of the energy requirements of acute cold exposure see NRC.[29]

The energy concentrations in specific feeds have been determined by difference trials and by equations derived from data acquired from difference trials. Table 2 illustrates the results of a difference trial used to determine the NE_m concentration in alfalfa. In this trial 64 g of feed yields 77 kcal retention. Therefore

Table 2. DETERMINATION OF NE_m CONCENTRATION IN ALFALFA HAY*

Feed Level	Feed Eaten g(BW)$^{0.75}$†	ME Intake kcal (BW)$^{0.75}$	Heat Production kcal (BW)$^{0.75}$	Energy Gain kcal (BW)$^{0.75}$
1. Fasting	0	0	77	−77
2. Maintenance‡	64	131	131	0
3. Difference	64	131	54	77

*Level in fasting.
†Birth weight (BW) in kilograms.
‡Level 2 is at equilibrium.

$$NE_m \text{ conc.} = \frac{77}{64} = 1.2 \text{ kcal/g of feed}$$

or

$$NE_m = 1.2 \text{ Mcal/g}$$

Some NE_g values in feed have been established by difference trials. Such values must be evaluated on a sample of feed used above the maintenance level, as shown in Table 3. 82 g of feed yields 42 kcal NE_g. Therefore

$$NE_g \text{ conc.} = \frac{42}{82} = 0.51 \text{ kcal/g}$$

or

$$NE_g = 0.51 \text{ Mcal/kg}$$

Interconversions between DE, ME, and NE values of feedstuffs are possible. The following relationships have been estimated (all units are Mcal/kg DM):

$$ME = 0.82 \text{ DE (NRC, 1976; ARC, 1965)}$$
$$NE_m = 1.37 \text{ ME} - 0.138 \text{ ME}^2 + 0.0105 \text{ ME}^3 - 1.12$$
$$(\text{Garret}[18])$$
$$NE_g = 1.43 \text{ ME} - 0.174 \text{ ME}^3 + 0.0122 \text{ ME}^3 - 1.65$$
$$(\text{Garret}[18])$$

The NE requirements for growth are estimated as the amount of energy deposited as nonfat organic matter (mostly protein) plus the energy deposited as fat. Relative caloric values include 9.4 kcal/g of fat and 5.6 kcal/g of nonfat organic matter. The relative quantities of fat and protein being deposited are dependent on two factors: (1) the intake of energy above the maintenance requirement (assuming all other nutrient requirements are satisfied) and (2) the phase of growth. For most conditions the energy content of a unit of weight gain will be between 1.2 (energy content of fat-free body) and 8 Mcal/kg gain (energy content of adipose tissue). All relationships to estimate the caloric value of weight gain have been determined for some particular breeds and sex classes. These relationships may have to be adjusted for more precise use for other breeds and conditions.[1] The observed weight gain is also influenced by the contents of the digestive tract. The weight of these contents can vary from less than 5 to 21 per cent of the shrunk weight of cattle depending on the diet and the weighing conditions.

The primary relationships used in the 1984 NRC manual for beef cattle[30] to calculate the net energy values of empty body weight gains are taken from data furnished by Garrett.[18] In these equations, RE (retained energy) is equivalent to NE_g. RE requirements for medium-frame British breed steers and heifers receiving hormonal adjuvants include:

For steers: $RE = (0.0635 \text{ W}^{0.75})(\text{EBG}^{1.097})$
For heifers: $RE = (0.0783 \text{ W}^{0.75})(\text{EBG}^{1.119})$

In these equations EBG (empty body weight gain) and W (body weight) are in kilograms. RE is in Mcal/day and is equal to NE_g.

These basic relationships are easily modified for application to specific practical conditions. Examples include the following:

1. Data summarized by Garrett[18] indicate that cattle not receiving hormonal adjuvants require a 5 per cent increase in energy per unit of gain. Thus the equation for steers not implanted becomes

$$RE = 1.05(0.0635 \text{ W}^{0.75})(\text{EBG}^{1.097})$$

or

$$(0.0667 \text{ W}^{0.75})(\text{EBG}^{1.097})$$

2. Other modifications can be used to estimate RE or NE_g requirements for cattle with different frame sizes or sex classes.
   a. It is assumed that energy retention in a large-frame steer or medium-frame bull will be 15 per cent lower per unit of gain relative to that of a medium-frame steer. In this case the steer equation becomes

$$RE = (0.0635[0.85 \text{ W}]^{0.75})(\text{EBG}^{1.097})$$

or

$$RE = (0.0562 \text{ W}^{0.75})(\text{EBG}^{1.097})$$

   b. Other modifications of the primary equations have been made to estimate the energy requirements of large-frame bulls and heifers (see NRC,[30] pp. 38–39).

The primary equations are based on empty body weight (EBW) and EBG. Under practical conditions these do not exist. The NRC equations in Table 4 are based on shrunk body weights (overnight without feed or water) and shrunk weight gains.[30] The approach is simple and is based on a number of general assumptions:

1. Shrunk weight and shrunk weight gains are called live weight (LW) and live weight gains (LWG), respectively.
2. The assumed relationships include
   a. EBW = 0.891 LW, and
   b. EBG = 0.956 LWG.

For further information see ARC[1] and/or NRC,[30] p. 4.

For an example we will calculate the RE needs for a 450-kg LW, medium-frame steer being fed in a thermoneutral environment to gain 1.2 kg/day:

$$RE = 0.0635([450 \times 0.891]^{0.75})([0.0956 \times 1.2]^{1.097})$$
$$= 6.61 \text{ Mcal/day}$$

The relationship used to estimate NE_m requirements (0.77 Mcal/$W^{0.75}$) is not adjusted for EBW. Thus in this example the NE_m requirement is assumed to be $450^{0.75} \times 0.077 = 7.52$ Mcal.

Current information is inadequate to modify the general system describing the energy values of feeds and the energy requirements of all cattle in all production situations. Users are encouraged to adjust the primary equations if a consistent over- or underestimation of animal performance appears.

Other procedures for adjusting generally determined energy requirements to specific conditions have been suggested.[1, 13, 17a, 49]

The primary equations used to predict energy requirements have been rearranged to estimate daily gain when animal weight and feed consumption are known. Table 4 lists prediction equations for estimating nutrient requirements and feed intake of beef cattle. These equations are extracted from NRC,[30] section 6. The energy equations in Table 4 are limited to those pertaining to LWG.

In the basic energy ration formulation it is probably practical to decrease the estimated DMI by about 2 per cent. This allows for the addition of nonenergy nutrient supplements (minerals, vitamins) without extending the dry matter intake (DMI) beyond the capacity of the animal.

Net Energy for Gestation and Lactation

Energy deposition in the products of conception of female beef cattle has been determined by Ferrell and colleagues[12] and can be calculated from the data of Prior and Laster. The gross efficiency of ME use for the products of conception has been estimated as 11 to 15 per cent for cattle[12] and 12 to 13 per cent for sheep.[39] The average figure (13 per cent) is used

Table 3. DETERMINATION OF NE_g CONCENTRATION IN ALFALFA HAY*

Feeding Level	Feed Eaten $g(BW)^{0.75}$†	ME Intake $kcal(BW)^{0.75}$	Heat Production $kcal(BW)^{0.75}$	Energy Gain $kcal(BW)^{0.75}$
1. Maintenance	64	131	131	01
2. >Maintenance‡	146	298	256	42
3. Difference	82	167	125	42

*Level 1 is at maintenance.
†Birth weight (BW) in kilograms.
‡Level 2 is ad libitum.

Table 4. PREDICTION EQUATIONS FOR ESTIMATING NUTRIENT REQUIREMENTS AND FEED INTAKE OF BEEF CATTLE*

Energy

A. Maintenance requirements (Mcal/day) of steers, heifers, bulls, and cows:

$$NE_m = 0.077\ W^{0.75}$$

B. NE_g required for live weight gain (LWG):

Medium-frame steer calves:

$$NE_g = 0.0557\ W^{0.75}\ (LWG)^{1.097}$$

Large-frame steer calves, compensating medium-frame yearling steers, and medium-frame bull calves:

$$NE_g = 0.0493\ W^{0.75}\ (LWG)^{1.097}$$

Large-frame bull calves and compensating large-frame yearling steers:

$$NE_g = 0.0437\ W^{0.75}\ (LWG)^{1.097}$$

Medium-frame heifer calves:

$$NE_g = 0.0686\ W^{0.75}\ (LWG)^{1.119}$$

Large-frame heifer calves and compensating yearling heifers:

$$NE_g = 0.0608\ W^{0.75}\ (LWG)^{1.119}$$

Mature thin cows:

$$6.2\ Mcal/kg\ gain$$

C. Energy required for pregnancy (expressed as kcal NE_m/day):

$$NE_m = \text{calf birth weight}\ (0.0149 - 0.0000407t)e^{0.05883t - 0.0000804t^2}$$

Using the previous formula, we have calculated NE_m for gestation requirements for cows carrying small (70 lb), medium (88 lb), and large (110 lb) birthweight calves in the seventh, eighth, and ninth months of gestation expressed as Mcal/day as follows:

Month	Small Calf	Medium Calf	Large Calf
7	1.24	1.55	1.94
8	2.05	2.56	3.20
9	2.76	3.45	4.31

D. Energy required for lactation (expressed as NE_m, Mcal/kg milk):

$$NE_m = 0.1\ (\%\ fat) + 0.35$$

E. Estimation of live weight gain (LWG) from NE_g available for gain:

Medium-frame steer calves:

$$LWG = 13.91\ NE_g^{0.9116}\ W^{-0.6837}$$

Large-frame steer calves, compensating medium-frame yearling steers, and medium frame bulls:

$$LWG = 15.54\ NE_g^{0.9116}\ W^{-0.6837}$$

Large-frame bull calves and compensating large-frame yearling steers:

$$LWG = 17.35\ NE_g^{0.9116}\ W^{-0.6837}$$

Medium-frame heifer calves:

$$LWG = 10.96\ NE_g^{0.8936}\ W^{-0.6702}$$

Large-frame heifer calves and compensating yearling heifers:

$$LWG = 12.21\ NE_g^{0.8936}\ W^{-0.6702}$$

Protein

Factorialized Protein Requirement:

$$CP = \frac{F + U + S + G + C + M}{D \times BV \times CE}$$

CP = Crude protein in g/day
F = Metabolic fecal protein loss = 3.34% DMI
U = Endogenous urinary protein loss = $2.75W^{0.5}$
S = Scurf protein loss = $0.2W^{0.6}$
G = Tissue protein deposition (in g) = $(268 - 29.4 \times$ energy content of gain, Mcal/kg) daily gain in kg
C = Conceptus, 55 g/day, last third of pregnancy
M = Milk protein production (in g) = $33.5 \times$ milk production in kg
D = True protein digestibility = 0.90
BV = Biologic value = 0.66
CE = Conversion of dietary to postruminal protein = 1

Urea Potential

g/kg dry feed = $11.78NE_m + 6.85 - 0.0357\ CP \times DEG$† or
g/kg dry feed = $31.64 - 3.558\ CP + ([945\ NE_m - 887 - 179\ NE_m^2])^{0.5}$‡

CP = Crude protein (%)
NE = Net energy maintenance (Mcal/kg)
DEG = Ruminal degradation of protein (%)

Calcium and Phosphorus

Calcium, g/day = $((0.0154\ W_{kg}) + 0.071$ (protein gain in g/day) + 1.23 (milk/day in kg + 0.0137 (fetal growth, g/day))/0.5

Phosphorus, g/day = $((0.0280\ (W_{kg}) + 0.039$ (protein gain g/day) + 0.95 (milk/day in kg) + 0.0076 (fetal growth, g/day))/0.85

Feed Intake

Breeding Females:
Daily feed intake (kg DM) = $W^{0.75}\ (0.1462\ NE_m - 0.0517\ NE_m^2 - 0.0074)$

Growing and Finishing Cattle:
Daily feed intake (kg DM) = $W^{0.75}\ (0.1493\ NE_m - 0.0460\ NE_m^2 - 0.0196)$.
NE_m = net energy maintenance (Mcal/kg DM diet)

Adjustments for Size:
None for medium-frame steer calf, large-frame heifer, and medium-frame bull.

+10% for large-frame steer calf and medium-frame yearling steer.

+5% for large-frame bulls.

−10% for medium-frame heifers.

*Extracted from National Research Council: Nutrient Requirements of Beef Cattle, 6th rev ed. Washington, DC, National Academy of Sciences, 1984, pp 38, 39.
†Data from Burroughs W, Nelson DK, Mertens DR: Protein physiology and its application in the lactating cow: the metabolizable feeding standard. J Anim Sci 41:933, 1975.
‡Data from Satter LD, Roffler RE: Nitrogen requirements and utilization in dairy cattle. J Dairy Sci 58:1219, 1975.

to estimate the ME requirement. The ME requirement is converted into equivalent NE_m units. The relationship used to estimate the pregnancy requirement (kcal/day of NE_m equivalent) is based on expected birth weight of the calf and the day of gestation (t). It is assumed that the diet consists of average roughage (ME = 2 Mcal/kg DM). The formula is listed in Table 4. Specific NE_m requirements for small, medium, and large calves in the seventh, eighth, and ninth months of pregnancy are also listed in Table 4.

The energy requirements for milk production have been estimated from the information available for the dairy cow.[28] The requirement can be calculated and expressed in NE_m units, as NE is utilized for lactation and maintenance at similar levels of efficiency. The equation used to calculate the NE_m requirements of lactation for beef cows is listed in Table 4. Accordingly, a beef cow producing 5 kg of 3.5 per cent fat milk/day requires, in addition to her normal maintenance requirement,

$$0.1(3.5) + 0.35(5) = 3.5 \text{ Mcal of } NE_m$$

Special Energy Requirements for Dairy Cattle

The 1988 NRC publication for dairy cattle uses one energy value (NE_L) to express requirements for maintenance, gestation, lactation, and body weight change.[34] Because the methods of derivation of the values of NE_m and NE_l were substantially different, there are some differences in individual values in the nutrient concentration tables.

For dairy cows the NE_L requirement for maintenance only at moderate temperatures is $(0.08 \text{ Mcal } NE_l)(BW/kg)^{0.75}$. The maintenance requirement is modified by activity. The NE_l for maintenance requirement should be increased 5 per cent per mile of travel. To support grazing, maintenance requirements should be increased 10 per cent for good pastures and 20 per cent for sparse pastures.

The influence of cold temperatures on the energy requirements of dairy cows is limited by relatively high heat production caused by high feed intake. When loose housing systems are used, it is probable that some cows will suffer from acute cold stress if winter conditions are severe. It is recommended that under such conditions the NE in the daily ration (maintenance plus production) be increased by 8 per cent.

Few quantitative data are available on the specific energy requirements for gestation in dairy cows. It would seem that the gestation requirements for beef cows listed in Table 5 should be applicable. The 1988 NRC publication for dairy cattle states that the energy required for gestation equals 30 per cent of the energy required for maintenance alone.[34] The equations used to calculate the energy requirements for gestation include 24 kcal NE_l, 40 kcal ME, 46 kcal DE, and 10.6 g of TDN/kg$^{0.75}$ of LW/day.

The NE_l required for milk production is defined as the energy contained in the milk produced. The requirement varies with the milk fat percentage. 4 per cent fat milk contains 0.74 Mcal NE_l/kg. An equation derived to calculate the energy values of milk samples having varying fat contents states that

$$NE_L (\text{Mcal/kg of milk}) = 0.3512 + [0.0962 \text{ (per cent fat)}]$$

Energy requirements for weight changes in growing animals and mature bulls are measured as NE_g. The amount of NE_g required is equal to the energy deposited in the gain. Total energy retained in the tissues is influenced by the animal's rate of gain and stage of growth or LW. The form and exponents of the equations used in the 1984 NRC beef cattle publication[30] are used to calculate NE_g requirements, but the coefficients are adjusted so that the predicted gains approximate those summarized in the 1978 NRC dairy cattle manual.[28] The following equations are used in the 1988 NRC dairy cattle publication[34] to calculate NE_g requirements for growing large-breed dairy heifers, growing large-breed dairy bulls, growing small-breed dairy heifers, and growing small-breed dairy bulls:

Large-breed heifers:
$$NE_g (\text{Mcal/day}) = (0.035 \, W^{0.75})(LWG^{1.119}) + LWG$$

Large-breed bulls:
$$NE_g (\text{Mcal/day}) = (0.025 \, W^{0.75})(LWG^{1.097}) + LWG$$

Small-breed heifers:
$$NE_g (\text{Mcal/day}) = (0.45 \, W^{0.75})(LWG^{1.119}) + LWG$$

Small-breed bulls:
$$NE_g (\text{Mcal/kg}) = (0.035 \, W^{0.75})(LWG^{1.097}) + LWG$$

Energy Measurements for Sheep

ME is the most widely used energy category for measuring energy requirements and feed energy concentrations. DE and TDN are also commonly used. NE is a more accurate measurement for energy in ruminant animals, and the 1985 NRC sheep publication discusses NE in depth.[31]

The NE_m requirement for sheep has been adjusted from an empty body weight (EBW) basis to a live weight (LW) basis by assuming a 6.1-kg fill for a 40-kg sheep and is approximated as 56 kcal $\times (W/kg^{0.75})$ or 0.056 Mcal $\times W/kg^{0.75}$.

Energy requirements for weight change are influenced by the proportions of lipid, protein, and water deposited. Each kilogram of empty body gain (EBG) requires between 1.2 Mcal (mainly protein and water) and 8 Mcal (mainly fat and water). Changes in the LW of sheep also reflect changes in the weight of the contents of the gastrointestinal tract. The weight of these contents can vary between 60 and 540 g/kg of EBW. The caloric densities of EBGs scaled to the EBW raised to the 0.75 power are quite consistent within a specific ovine genotype. Variations in caloric densities of weight gains are significant among different genotypes and range between 300 and 440 kcal/kg gain when expressed as kcal $\times$ EBG $\times$ EBW$^{0.75}$.

The NE_g requirement per unit of gain appears to be closely related to the yearling ram weight of the genotype.[5,8,9] Analysis of the research yields the following equation:

$$NE_g = 644 - 2.61W$$

where NE_g equals Mcal of retained tissue energy per day in EBGs per kg EBG per EBW$^{0.75}$ and W = ram yearling weight of the genotype. For example, if the ram yearling weight is 115 kg, the NE_g density of the EBG equals 644 $-$ (2.61 $\times$ 115) = 344 kcal/kg.

Practical application requires extrapolation from EBG to LWG. LWGs are predicted as 9 per cent higher than EBGs, and EBW is multiplied by 1.195 to predict LW, including gut fill.

Tissue energy retained (NE_g) can be calculated from LWGs and weights. NE_g (kcal $\times$ d-1) = 276 LWG $\times$ W$^{0.75}$ for medium ram weight (115 kg) genotypes. For every 10 kg weight below 115 kg, the energy requirement increases by 7.6 per cent. Conversely, for every 10 kg of weight above 115 kg, the energy requirement decreases by 7.6 per cent.

Rams deposit less energy per unit of gain relative to ewes of the same genotype and equal weights. Some data suggest that caloric density of gains in ram lambs equals caloric density of gains in comparable ewe lambs multiplied by 0.82. Castrated males may also require less energy per unit of gain than comparable females, but no adjustment is recommended at this time. Caloric density in gain is effected by

1. Very slow rates of growth. This is possibly caused by the demand for protein deposition in wool from a limited supply of essential amino acids in the diet.

2. Very high rates of gain in milk-fed lambs have been associated with high fat deposition and thus increased energy density in the gains.

3. High-protein diets in early-weaned, fast-growing lambs have been associated with decreased fat deposition and thus decreased energy density in the gains.

Sheep utilize ME at 12 to 14 per cent efficiency for conceptus development and at 16 to 18 per cent efficiency for uterine and mammary development, as determined by Rattray and associates.[39] The research was done with diets containing 2.4 to 2.6 Mcal ME/kg DM. The NE requirements for pregnancy are listed as NE_y in the 1985 NRC publication for sheep.[31] NE pregnancy requirements above those for maintenance and growth are tabulated for ewes carrying single, twin, and triplet fetuses at different stages of late pregnancy. It has been shown by Rattray and colleagues that the efficiency of utilization of ME for maintenance and gain is not altered by pregnancy.[39] Fetal growth and pregnancy requirements are substantial in the last 6 weeks of gestation. The total maintenance and pregnancy requirements in this period average about 1.5 times maintenance levels for ewes bearing single fetuses and two times maintenance levels for ewes bearing twins.

Few estimates of ME utilization for lactation in sheep are available. The lactation period is short, and the composition and quantity of milk produced by lactating ewes are difficult to determine. It has been estimated that from 65 per cent of ME for ewes suckling single lambs to 83 per cent of ME for ewes suckling twins is converted to milk energy during 12 weeks of lactation. The average value is slightly above that calculated for cattle. The same workers have also estimated that the NE for lactation plus maintenance is 2.3 to 2.4 times maintenance levels for ewes suckling singles and 2.7 to 2.9 times maintenance levels for ewes suckling twins. The NE values (Mcal/kg DM) of feeds commonly used can be closely related to the ME value of the feed (Mcal/kg DM). The relationships are as follows:[18]

$$NE_m = 1.37\ ME - 0.138\ ME^2 + 0.0105\ ME^3 - 1.12$$

$$NE_g = 1.42\ ME - 0.174\ ME^2 + 0.0122\ ME^2 - 1.65$$

Energy requirements for sheep are affected by environmental conditions. Ambient temperatures, thermal radiation, humidity, wind, and precipitation may all have a positive or negative effect on the energy requirement depending on where the animal is in relation to its thermoneutral zone (see NRC[29] for specific information).

Prudent management responds to the condition of the animals used for reproduction. Very thin pregnant ewes can be fed at levels recommended for ewes that are 10 kg heavier, and ewes that are overweight can be fed ration intakes that are recommended for lighter weights during the first 3.5 months of pregnancy without affecting lamb and wool production. The 1985 NRC publication for sheep lists separate energy requirements for replacement ewes and rams.[31] Ewe lamb requirements for maintenance and gain are very similar to those recommended in the tables of that publication. Ram lambs grow more rapidly, have higher feed intakes, and use feed more efficiently than the NRC tables suggest. Gains in intact males are higher in protein and water content and lower in fat content relative to ewe lambs. If ewe lambs or yearlings are to be bred, they should be fed at levels that will result in Finn cross ewe lambs weighing a minimum of 43 kg and larger breeds weighing 50 kg at breeding. Energy for gain, in addition to energy for maintenance, gestation, and lactation, should be provided for growing animals.

Energy for Swine

The energy requirements for swine are expressed as DE and ME values.[35] Relative values are expressed in the following formula:[29]

$$ME = DE \times \left(96 - \frac{[0.202 \times \text{per cent crude protein}]}{100}\right)$$

ME relative to DE decreases if dietary protein is of poor quality or if protein is fed in excess of recommended amounts. Amino acids not used for protein synthesis are deaminated, and the nitrogen (N) is excreted as urea. Energy is required both to synthesize and to excrete urea. Therefore as the nitrogen content of urine increases, the ME concentration in the ration decreases. Sometimes a correction is made for ME values for nitrogen retained by or lost from the body. This is because the energy that is deposited in stored protein cannot be totally recovered by the animal if the amino acids are degraded and used for energy. This type of correction is probably more valid in adult animals than in growing animals, where nitrogen retention is usual. Suggested specific corrections include the following:

6.77 kcal ME/g N[7a]
9.17 kcal ME/g N[26a]
7.83 kcal ME/g N[49a]

The correction is added to determined ME in negative nitrogen balance and subtracted when the ratio is in positive nitrogen balance.

NE is the best measure of the energy available for maintenance and production, but it is difficult to measure and is not commonly used. For pigs fed ordinary diets and maintained at thermoneutral temperatures, the ratio of NE:ME has been shown to range between 0.66:1 and 0.72:1. Research also shows that the efficiency of ME utilization varies from 27 per cent for wheat middling to 69 per cent for corn and 75 per cent for soybean oil. NE values are affected by composition of the feedstuff, level of feed intake, balance of nutrients in the diet, age, breed, sex, environmental conditions, and the percentage of energy retained as protein.

Categories of DE include maintenance (DE_m protein retention [DE_{pr}], fat retention [DE_f], and cold thermogenesis [DEH_c]):

$$DE = DE_m + DE_{pr} + DE_f + DEH_c$$

The DE requirements are affected by environmental temperature, activity level, group size, stress, and body composition.

The DE requirements are usually expressed on the basis of metabolic weight $(W/kg)^{0.75}$. The mean energy costs of the deposition of protein and fat per unit of weight are similar, but lean muscle tissue contains only about 20 to 22 per cent protein. Therefore the energy cost of muscle production is considerably less than the energy cost of adipose tissue production per unit of weight.

Cold thermogenesis influences energy requirements when the ambient temperature is below the lower critical temperature (T_c). The thermoneutral zone for swine is relatively narrow, and the lower T_c for sows is estimated to be about 18 to 20°C. The energy cost of cold thermogenesis is described by the following equation:

$$DEH_c\ (kcal\ DE/day) = 0.326W + 23.65\ (T_c - T)$$

where W is animal weight in kg, T_c is the lower critical temperature, and T is the effective ambient temperature. T_c and T are expressed in degree Celsius.

It is estimated that growing pigs weighing from 25 to 60 kg need an additional 25 g of feed or 80 kcal of ME per day to compensate for each 1°C below T_c. During the finishing period (60 to 100 kg), this requirement increases to 39 g of feed or 125 kcal of ME per day for each 1°C below T_c. Environmental temperatures above the upper T_c will reduce feed intake. It has been suggested that DE intake is reduced by 0.017 per cent for each 1°C that the effective ambient temperature exceeds the upper T_c.[33]

In recent years it has become apparent that the long-term reproductive efficiency of sows is enhanced by minimizing weight and fat loss during lactation. This is achieved by limiting feed intake in the gestation period. Research has suggested that sows should be fed to gain about 25 kg in body tissue in the gestation period.[2] The weight of the products of conception will add another 20 kg to make a total of 45 kg of weight gain during the pregnancy. This rate of gain should be maintained at least for the first three or four parities. Energy intake above 6.0 Mcal DE/day results in increased maternal weight but does not significantly affect litter size. Sows fed ad libitum during pregnancy will be in positive energy balance and become obese. Assuming a DE requirement of 1.10 Mcal/day to support a net weight gain of 25 kg in the 114-day gestation period and an additional 0.19 Mcal DE/day to support the conceptus, the DE required for total gestation weight gain is 1.29 Mcal/day above the maintenance requirement. For each degree below the sow's lower T_c there will be an increase of about 4 per cent in maintenance energy cost.

The daily energy requirements in the lactation period include a requirement for maintenance plus a requirement for lactation. NRC requirement tables assume that the DE_m requirement in the lactation period is the same as in the gestation period (110 kcal/Wkg$^{0.75}$).[35] Some recent reports suggest that the DE_m requirement of lactating sows is 5 to 10 per cent higher relative to gestating sows. The energy requirement for milk is calculated as 2 Mcal DE for each kilogram of milk. The computation is based on an assumption that sow's milk contains 1.3 Mcal DE/kg and a 65 per cent efficiency of feed utilization. The NRC requirement tables assume that weight loss during lactation includes 30 per cent fat, 13 per cent protein, and consequently 4.5 Mcal/kg that is converted into milk energy with an efficiency of 85 per cent.[35]

Practical energy sources for swine are limited. Pigs under 7 to 10 days of age require glucose or lactose. It takes 7 to 10 days for the neonatal pig to begin to produce sufficient disaccharidases and about 2 to 3 weeks to begin to produce sufficient amylases to digest sucrose and starch efficiently.

The addition of fiber to swine diets decreases DE and ME concentrations in the diet. Feed intake will increase as the pig attempts to maintain DE intake, but when the fiber concentration of the diet exceeds 10 to 15 per cent, feed intake will be reduced owing to lack of palatability and excessive bulk. Diets having relatively low energy concentrations are more effective at low ambient temperatures than at thermoneutral or higher temperatures. The large intestine of adult swine includes 35 to 45 per cent of the gastrointestinal tract, and a significant amount of microbial fermentation occurs. The principal end products of microbial fermentation are volatile fatty acids, which account for between 5 and 28 per cent of the DE_m requirements. The influence of crude fiber on protein digestibility is controversial. It seems probable that when the fiber source is high in protein content, increasing fiber will depress protein digestibility. If the fiber source is low in protein content, the effect on protein digestibility may be negligible.

The control of feed intake is influenced by physiologic, environmental, and dietary factors. These factors have been extensively reviewed.[33] Voluntary feed intake formulas for pigs fed balanced corn-soybean diets include the following:

For nursing pigs:
  DE_{intake} in kcal/day = 11.2 days − 151.7 where day is the age of the pig. The intake of dry feed is considered to be negative prior to day 13.5.
For postweaning pigs:
  DE_{intake} (kcal/day) = 108 days − 100 where day means days postweaning.
For pigs in the growing-finishing period (15 to 110 kg):
  DE_{intake} (kcal/day) = $13{,}162(1 - e^{-0.01768W})$.
For sows:
  Because feed intake is restricted during gestation, predictions of DE_{intake} are not applicable.
For lactating sows:
  The voluntary intake responds according to the following relationship: DE_{intake} (Mcal/day) = (13 + 0.596 day) − 0.172 day^2 where day is day postfarrowing.

PROTEIN REQUIREMENT

Dietary protein supplies the animal with amino acids essential to vital synthetic processes in the body. Amino acids are the building units of all animal cells and tissues. In addition, all protein secretions, including enzymes, hormones, mucin, and milk, require specific assortments of amino acids. In ruminant animals all of the required amino acids may be obtained from dietary protein, nonprotein nitrogen (NPN) compounds, and fermentation products of microbial metabolism if all of the required elements are present. Monogastric animals and very young ruminant animals are unable to synthesize endogenously all of the amino acids that compose their specific proteins. The amino acids that cannot be synthesized by monogastric animals include arginine, histidine, isoleucine, leucine, lysine, methionine, phenylalanine, threonine, tryptophan, and valine. For swine, cystine can meet 50 per cent of the methionine requirement and tyrosine can meet 30 per cent of the requirement for phenylalanine.

Crude protein (CP) values for all species are calculated from nitrogen content. Protein averages 16 per cent nitrogen; therefore

$$CP = N \times \frac{100}{16}$$
$$= N \times 6.25$$

Protein for Swine

The NRC publications for the various species differ somewhat in their approach to protein computation.

For swine, optimum performance requires that each essential amino acid be fed at the proper level at the proper time and with the proper level of all other essential amino acids. The nonessential amino acids are obtained from ordinary dietary components or can be synthesized by using amino groups derived from excess amino acids in the diet. The amino acid requirements of growing swine increase as energy concentrations in the diet increase. The NRC amino acid requirements for swine are extrapolated for growing pigs (20 to 35 kg) on the basis of percentages of amino acid in a 16 per cent protein diet.[35]

In corn-soybean diets lysine is the limiting amino acid. If the corn-soybean mixture is adjusted to furnish the recommended percentage of lysine, all other essential amino acids will be furnished in adequate amounts. Table 5 illustrates the percentages of CP and lysine in corn and soybean meal. The recommended percentage of lysine for growing and finishing swine weighing 20 to 50 kg is 0.75 per cent. It is assumed that corn and soybean meal will compose 97 per cent of the DM.

Table 5. LYSINE AND CRUDE PROTEIN VALUES FOR CORN AND SOYBEAN MEAL

Feed	Lysine (%)	Crude Protein (%)
Corn	0.25	8.5
Soybean meal	2.90	44.0

Use a Pearson's square to mix the corn and soybean meal:

```
Corn 0.25                        2.13  = 80.4%
           0.77 Recommended
                                 0.52    19.6%
Soybean meal 2.90                ---- = ------
                                 2.65    100%
```

1. The number in the left corner that is smaller than the recommendation is subtracted from the recommendation, and the difference is recorded in the opposite corner (0.77 − 0.25 = 0.52).
2. The recommendation is subtracted from the number in the left corner that is larger than the recommendation, and the difference is recorded in the opposite corner (2.90 − 0.77 = 2.13).
3. The recorded numbers in the right corners are the proportional parts of the ingredients (corn = 2.13 parts, soybean meal = 0.52 parts).
4. The proportional parts are added together and converted to fractions and percentages.

Therefore the lysine content of the corn-urea portion of the ration is

$$\frac{100}{97} \times 0.75 = 0.77 \text{ per cent}$$

The requirements for pregnant gilts and sows are based on amounts required for satisfactory nitrogen retention in late pregnancy.

The requirements for lactation have been extrapolated from published maintenance requirements for adult female swine plus the amount calculated to support the production of 6 kg of milk daily. Recommended percentages of CP vary from 24 per cent for growing pigs under 5 kg BW to 13 per cent for finishing pigs over 60 kg BW. Lactating gilts and sows require 13 per cent and gestating sows and gilts 12 per cent of CP in the air-dry diet (DM content, 90 per cent).

Best results are obtained when concentrate mixtures are used in which the protein biologic values complement each other (maximum nitrogen retention). Corn and soybean meal presents the classic example. By using these feeds, optimum percentages of both total protein and amino acid balance can be achieved.

Protein for Ruminants (General)

Protein digestion in ruminant animals is complicated by the microbial population in the rumen. Dietary protein is divided into two portions, including (1) degradable protein (converted by microbial enzymes into energy skeletons and ammonia) and (2) bypass or escape protein (escapes to the omasum and abomasum without being degraded in the rumen). Bypass protein will be digested in the abomasum or the small intestine, or both, or will pass, undigested, in the feces. Ammonia and energy skeletons resulting from degradation of dietary protein plus other degraded energy sources (degraded carbohydrate and fat) may be converted to microbial protein (protein constituents of microbes) in the rumen. Microbial protein synthesis includes forming all of the essential amino acids if all of the elementary constituents (including minerals) of these amino acids are available in the diet. Dietary protein sources have been classified according to degree of ruminal degradation.[1, 6, 42] Such classifications include the following:

Low bypass feeds (> 60 per cent degradable)
  Casein
  Soybean meal
  Sunflower meal
  Peanut meal
Medium bypass feeds (40 to 60 per cent degradable)
  Cottonseed meal
  Dehydrated alfalfa meal
  Corn grain
  Brewer's dried grains
High bypass feeds (< 40 per cent degradable)
  Meat meal
  Blood meal
  Feather meal
  Fishmeal
  Formaldehyde-treated proteins

The extent of ruminal protein degradation is affected by feed processing conditions, animal variations, dietary alterations, and changes in the microbial population. At present these effects are not well understood. If a basic ration is limited to high bypass protein sources, NPN supplementation may be needed to provide adequate rumen ammonia to maintain a healthy microbial population. Conversely, if microbial protein is the only source of amino acids, the supply of absorbable amino acids may not be sufficient to meet the maintenance and production objectives. Presentation of a mixture of bypass and microbial protein in the small intestine is apparently desirable. Optimizing this mixture has been the subject of considerable research, and understanding of the total process is not yet complete.

Ruminal microbes can use various sources of nitrogen for amino acid and protein synthesis. Possible sources include ammonia, some amino acids, and some peptides. Energy constituents derived from carbohydrates and fats and some minerals are also necessary for microbial protein formulation.

Ammonia is the primary nitrogen source for microbial growth. When dietary protein is deficient, or degradable protein supplies are low, microbial synthesis will be limited. In these cases the rate and extent of digestion will be impaired and feed intake may be reduced. The minimum concentration of ammonia-nitrogen needed for microbial growth and optimal digestion has been estimated by a variety of procedures.[10, 21, 25, 43, 44] Consensus regarding these procedures is limited.

The following are widely accepted generalities regarding the digestion and absorption of dietary protein in ruminants:

1. Ammonia is the primary supply of nitrogen for microbial protein synthesis in the rumen.
2. Concentrations of ammonia in rumen fluid greater than 5 to 10 mg/100 ml do not contribute to microbial production.
3. Ammonia is derived from the degradation of protein or NPN substances in the rumen.
4. Although most microbial species can survive using ammonia as their sole source of nitrogen, added natural protein may stimulate growth by providing amino acids, essential branched chained fatty acids, and unidentified factors that enhance microbial growth.
5. Typically the least expensive source of ruminal ammonia is some form of NPN. The most common source is urea.
6. Utilization of NPN for incorporation into microbial protein is limited by the energy supply. Best results are obtained by using high-energy–low-CP rations.
7. Ammonia not used in microbial synthesis is absorbed from the rumen and circulated to the liver, where it is combined with carbon dioxide to form urea. Most of this urea is eliminated in urine, but a portion is recycled to the digestive tract in saliva and rumen secretions. It is possible for the outflow of protein from the digestive tract to exceed the dietary intake.

8. NPN should be added to the diet only when the ruminal concentration of ammonia is inadequate for optimal microbial action to digest organic matter or to supply sufficient ammonia for microbial protein synthesis.

Protein for Sheep

The lamb is born with a nonfunctional rumen. Milk or a milk replacer is required in these diets for 6 to 8 weeks. Rumen function develops over this period, and early creep feeding, using dry feed, is desirable to hasten the development of an effective rumen microbial population. When the microbial population in the rumen-reticulum is completely functional, microbial protein accounts for between 40 and 80 per cent of the total protein presented to the absorptive area.

The NRC protein requirements for sheep were determined factorially with the following basic formula:[31]

$$CP \text{ in g/day} = \frac{PD + MFP + EUP + DL + Wool}{NVP}$$

where PD = protein deposited; MFP = metabolic fecal protein; UEP = endogenous urinary protein; DL = dermal loss; and NVP = net protein value. Protein deposited in gain is estimated by the following equation:[30]

PD in g/day = daily gain/kg × (268 − 29.4 × ECOG)

$$\text{when energy content of gain (ECOG)} = \frac{NE_g \text{ in kcal/day}}{\text{gain in g/day}}$$

NE_g values are taken from NRC,[31] Table 3.

Protein deposits for gestation are estimated by the following equations:

For ewes carrying single lambs, early gestation:
PD = 2.95 g/day
For ewes carrying single lambs, last 4 weeks of gestation:
PD = 16.75 g/day

The requirement is increased proportionately for higher lambing rates.

CP requirements for lactation are assumed to equal 47.875 g/kg of milk. Milk production is assumed to equal 1.74 kg/day for ewes nursing single lambs and 2.60 kg/day for ewes nursing twins. Ewe lambs (first parity) are assumed to yield 75 per cent of adult milk production.

MFP* is estimated to equal 3.44 g/kg DM intake
UEP* is assumed to equal 0.14675 × BW in kg + 3.375
DL* is estimated to equal 0.1125 × kgW$^{0.75}$

CP deposited in wool for ewes and rams is estimated to equal 6.8 g/day, assuming an annual grease fleece weight of 4 kg. For lambs, CP deposited in wool is calculated as 3 + (0.1 × protein retained in the fleece-free body). The net protein value is estimated to be 0.561 based on a digestibility coefficient of 0.85 and a biologic value of 0.66.

Use of NPN crude supplements is sometimes practical in sheep nutrition. Urea is the most common NPN source. NPN supplementation is only useful when it is needed to provide a source of ammonia for ruminal microorganisms. Dangers involved in NPN supplementation include decreased feed intake and ammonia toxicity. It is recommended that urea not exceed 1 per cent of dietary DM or one third of the total dietary CP. Urea is utilized most efficiently when thoroughly mixed in high-concentrate, low-protein diets that are fed continuously. When NPN supplementation is used, consequent supplementation of potassium (K), phosphorus (P), and sulfur (S) may be necessary. Sulfur is especially critical because wool protein is high in sulfur-containing amino acids. Attempts to minimize the possibility of ammonia toxicity or improve the utilization of ruminal ammonia, or both, by using NPN sources other than urea (biuret, triuret, and complexes of urea with formaldehyde) have not been uniformly successful.

Protein for Beef Cattle

The CP requirement of cattle can be divided into specific metabolic factors. These include metabolic fecal loss (F), endogenous urinary loss (U), scurf loss (S), tissue growth (G), fetal growth (C), and milk production (M). The complete factorial equation[30] is

$$CP = \frac{F + U + S + G + C + M}{D \times BV \times CE}$$

where D, BV, and CE are decimal figures representing digestibility (D), amount of protein retained in the body (BV), and the efficiency of converting dietary protein to ruminal protein output (CE). The values of the factors in the divisors of the factorial equation are assumed to include D = 0.9, BV = 0.66, and C = 1.0.

Equations to estimate the various specific CP factors (6.25 N) include the following: F = 3.34 per cent of DMI; U = 2.75 W$^{0.5}$; S = 0.2 W$^{0.6}$; G = 268 − (29.4 × energy content of gain in Mcal/kg) (kg daily gain); C = 55 g/day in the last third of pregnancy; and M = 33.5 its milk production in kg.

NE content of gain is estimated from prediction equations listed in Table 4. For example, a medium-frame steer calf whose shrunk weight equals 400 kg and is gaining 1.2 kg/day will deposit

$$0.0557 \times 400^{0.75} \times 1.2^{1.097} = 5.07 \text{ Mcal NE}_g/\text{day}$$

If the above steer calf is consuming 8.3 kg of DM/day, the CP requirement will be

F = 8300 × 0.0334   = 277 g
U = 2.75 × 400$^{0.5}$ = 55 g
S = 0.2 × 400$^{0.6}$ = 7 g
G = 268 − (29.4 × 5.07/1.2) = 173 g

$$\frac{F + U + S + G}{0.9 \times 0.66 \times 1} = 853 \text{ g}$$

Protein for Dairy Cattle

The proteins contained in practical dairy forage and least-cost concentrate sources include fractions of degradable and bypass proteins. These dietary protein sources will supply essential amino acids sufficient to support optimal weight gains in nonlactating cattle and up to 20 kg of milk production per day. As milk production increases beyond 20 kg/day, a substantial amount of additional dietary proteins must escape rumen fermentation. Such proteins must be significantly digested in and absorbed from the small intestine. Many modern dairy herds approach and even exceed 20,000 lb in average yearly milk production. To do this, large numbers of cows must produce in excess of 40 kg (88 lb) of milk per day in the first half of the lactation period. Using the requirements we are about to discuss, a 600-kg cow producing 40 kg of 4 per cent fat milk per day secretes 1400 g of milk protein and 29.6 Mcal of milk energy daily. The modern dairy cow is remarkable in that she can utilize tissue proteins, energy, and some minerals for milk production for a short time at the beginning of lactation without significantly reducing milk production.

The 1988 NRC cattle publication continues to use the

---
*Grams per day.

factorial method to estimate protein requirements,[34] but two changes have been made since the previous edition.[28] First, the unit of protein measurement is absorbed protein (AP) instead of total CP. Second, the fecal metabolic nitrogen requirement is computed separately from the other maintenance components. This is because fecal nitrogen is a function of indigestible dry matter (IDM) excretion. The other maintenance components are functions of LW. The protein requirement consists of three components, including maintenance, fecal metabolic nitrogen, and production. The maintenance requirement includes urinary endogenous protein and surface protein. The production requirement includes the protein needed for growth, the conceptus, and lactation. The specific requirement for each category of net AP is listed in the following equations:

For endogenous urinary protein (UPN):
$UPN = 2.75^{0.5}$
For scurf protein (SPN):
$SPN = 0.2 LW^{0.6}$
For total maintenance protein (MPN):
$MPN = SPN + UPN$ (The efficiency for using MPN = 0.67.)
For the metabolic fecal protein equivalent (FPN):
$FPN = 0.09 \times$ absorbed protein equivalent in indigestible dry matter (FPAIDM)
For conceptus protein (YPN) in g/day after 210 days of gestation:
$YPN = 1.136 \, LW/kg^{0.70}$ (The efficiency of converting absorbed protein units [YPA] to net protein units [YPN] is assumed to be 0.5.)
For protein deposited in growth (retained protein or RPN) as a function of the concentration of NE_g in LWG:
$RPN = [211 - (26.2 NE_g/kgLWG)] \, LWG/1000$
For protein deposited in lactation (LPN/kg milk) in g/day:
$LPN/kg \, milk = [1.9 + (0.4)(milk \, fat, \, per \, cent)]/100$ (This equation should not be applied when milk fat concentrations have been depressed by high-energy, low-fiber diets because protein changes may have a low correlation with fat changes. The efficiency of converting absorbed lactation protein units to net lactation protein units is assumed to be 0.7.)

The use of AP units requires the consideration of the factors that influence the transformation of intake protein (IP) to AP. New equations must be developed to describe the following:

1. The fractionation of IP into degraded intake protein (DIP) and undegraded intake protein (UIP)
2. The net flux as the algebraic sum of the efflux of ammonia from the digestive tract and the influx of urea into the digestive tract
3. The bacterial and protozoal protein (BCP) produced relative to the fermentation energy
4. The bacterial and protozoal true protein (BTP) in the BCP
5. The proportion of digestible bacterial and protozoal protein (DPB) in the BTP and the percent of digestible undegraded intake protein
6. The mobilization of tissue protein

Fractionation of Intake Protein into Degraded Intake Protein and Undegraded Intake Protein

NRC 1985 values,[32] plus more recent values including in situ data, are summarized for some major feeds in NRC[34], Table 7–3.

Ammonia and Urea Fluxes

Current data indicate that under various conditions, the ammonia efflux from the ruminant digestive tract varies between 16 and 80 per cent of nitrogen intake with a mean near 40 per cent. The urea influx has been shown to vary between 10 and 42 per cent with a mean of 23 per cent. Huntington and Reynolds found that 33 per cent of ammonia nitrogen and 65 per cent of urea nitrogen fluxes occurred postruminally in steers.[22]

Bacterial and Protozoal Crude Protein

The efficiency of conversion of rumen available protein (RAP) to BCP is assumed to be 0.9.[32] The proportional rumen influx protein is assumed to equal 15 per cent of the rumen influx protein.[32] These two factors combine in such a way that the protein made available in the small intestine (SCP) can be computed as a linear function of the DIP as a proportion of total IP:

$$SCP \text{ as a proportion of intake protein} = 1 - DIP + 0.9(DIP + 0.15)$$

When DIP = 1, SCP = 1.035. When DIP = 0, SCP = 1.135. The 1984 beef cattle and 1978 dairy cattle NRC publications both assume that the conversion efficiency of dietary protein to postruminal protein is 1.00.[28, 30]

The production of BCP, in grams, is described as a function of NE_l or TDN in the following equations:[32]

For lactating cattle, function of NE_l:
$BCP = 6.25(-30.93 + 11.45 \, NE_l)$

For growing cattle, function of TDN:
$BCP = 6.25(-31.86 + 26.12 \, TDN)$

Bacterial and Protozoal True Protein (Microbial Protein) and Digestible Microbial Protein

The proportion of BTP to BCP is assumed to be 0.8, with a digestibility coefficient also being 0.8. Thus the coefficient of absorption of BCP = $0.8 \times 0.8 = 0.64$.

Mobilization of Tissue Protein

Limited mobilization of labile tissue protein for milk production is possible in early lactation without significantly decreasing daily milk production. Estimates of this labile protein range from 8 to 22 per cent of total body protein. Estimates derived from modern research suggest that the maximum negative nitrogen balance is 30 to 60 g of nitrogen/day. A negative balance of 40 g of nitrogen or 250 g of protein/day for 60 days is equivalent to 15 kg of tissue protein loss.

The 1988 NRC dairy cattle publication assumes that the protein components in weight gains = 320 g/kg gain for CP and 256 g/kg gain for AP.[34]

Special Considerations for Feeding Urea

Use of urea as a CP supplement is similar to feeding DIP. Urea does not provide the branched chained carbon skeletons or the sulfur that is ordinarily supplied by the DIP of the basic ration. Both of these components are necessary for the synthesis of microbial amino acids. It is generally assumed that the efficiency of urea relative to DIP in the rumen is inadequate for the maintenance of the desirable microbial population.

Interaction of Protein and Energy Supply with Milk Production, Live Weight Change, and Reproduction

Maximum milk production, optimum weight changes, and maximum reproductive efficiency require a proper balance of energy DIP and UIP in the diet of the dairy cow. Production energy is required to synthesize microbial protein, absorb excess ammonia from the gut, synthesize urea in the liver, recycle urea, and eliminate urea from the body. Excessive absorption of ammonia from the digestive tract entails an energy cost and the possibility of ammonia toxicity. Insufficient DIP deprives the ruminal microbial population, and insufficient UIP may limit the possibility of replenishing tissue proteins. Predictability of the effects of changing levels of the various categories of dietary protein is still questionable. The 1988 NRC dairy cattle publication lists two methods for calculating the dietary requirements for protein in lactating dairy cow rations.[34] The first is to measure CP using updated recommendations (Table 6–3). The other is to calculate the requirements for DIP and UIP using Table 6–4, Appendix Table 4, and Table 7–3. Caution is advised in using the second method for ration formulation in high-producing cows. Values listed in these tables were calculated from data obtained from sheep, growing cattle, and lactating cows that were eating less feed than normally eaten by high-producing cows. Use of such data to formulate rations for high-producing cows may result in errors in estimating protein degradability and the DIP and UIP requirements.

COMPUTATION OF THE MINERAL REQUIREMENT

Calcium, phosphorus, potassium, sodium, chlorine, magnesium, sulfur, iron, zinc, iodine, copper, cobalt, manganese, selenium, molybdenum, fluorine, chromium, silicon, vanadium, and possibly nickel and tin have been established as essential minerals in the diets of one or more animal species. The mineral requirement tables listed in the NRC manuals are based on data acquired by factorial computation or are experimentally established minimal amounts required to support maintenance plus acceptable production objectives. Daily requirements per animal are listed in NRC tables as grams or milligrams or as recommended percentages of dry or air-dry rations. Concentrations of minerals in feedstuffs are listed as grams or milligrams per kilogram of dry matter or as parts per million in dry matter.

Rations are first balanced for energy and protein and then analyzed for specific mineral content. The mineral content is compared with the requirement tables, and specific mineral supplements are added where deficiencies are indicated. The common mineral supplements are listed in the nutrient concentration tables in the NRC manuals.

The minerals are listed in the NRC tables as specific percentages of the supplement feed DM. For example, the 1984 beef cattle publication lists dicalcium phosphate containing 22 per cent calcium and 19.3 per cent phosphorus.[30] The amount of supplement required equals the grams of nutrient required divided by the percent of nutrient in the supplement listed as a decimal. Thus if the calcium deficiency in the ration = 20 g, it will require 20/0.22 = 90.9 g of dicalcium phosphate to supply the deficiency.

It is generally assumed that sodium and chlorine will be deficient in all basic rations. These deficiencies are often supplied by adding a specific percentage of sodium chloride (NaCl; 0.25 to 0.5 per cent) to the DM ration. If ration iodine is in question, iodized sodium chloride is used. The sodium chloride requirement may also be satisfied by feeding salt or iodized salt free choice. Trace mineral deficiencies are often assumed or may be established by analysis. Analysis is more practical where large numbers of animals are being fed. Generally there is a wide margin of safety between the required amounts of trace minerals and toxic levels. It is often practical to incorporate a portion of the requirements for trace minerals (50 to 100 per cent) in the salt portion of the ration. A number of trace mineral salt preparations are available on the market.

COMPUTATION OF THE VITAMIN REQUIREMENT

Food animals have a need for both fat- and water-soluble vitamins. Consideration in practical ration formulation is usually limited to those vitamins not expected to be adequately supplied by natural feeds, rumen synthesis, or tissue synthesis.

For ruminants, vitamins A, D, and E are usually present in significant amounts in high-quality forage. Members of the B-vitamin group and vitamin K are synthesized in the rumen. Vitamin C is synthesized in the tissues of the common food animal species. There are conditions in which the natural supply may be deficient. Forages may be fed in limited amounts or may be of low quality. Sun-curing of hay may be limiting for vitamin A. Milk replacers for calves and lambs may be deficient in some of the B vitamins. Normally vitamin A is most likely to be limiting. Concentrations of vitamin A precursors (β carotene) are listed in the NRC manuals. For cattle, 1 mg β carotene = 400 IU of vitamin A. Vitamin A palmitate and vitamin A acetate provide inexpensive supplementary sources. These products may be provided in feed or water or they may be injected parenterally.

As with minerals, basic rations are analyzed for vitamin content. Practical assumptions are often made. If deficiencies are established or assumed, specific vitamin supplements are incorporated in the complete supplement, salt mix, or drinking water.

For swine, the 1988 NRC tables list requirements for vitamins A, D, E, K, C, biotin, choline, folacin, niacin, pantothenic acid, riboflavin, thiamine, and vitamins B_6 and B_{12}.[35] Because of micromixing problems, vitamin deficiencies are generally met by feeding complete commercial supplements. When energy and protein needs are met and supplemented by the use of these supplements, the vitamin and mineral needs also will be met.

FORMULATING RATIONS

Ration formulation is similar for all food animal species and classes. The following steps are generally taken:

1. Assess the nutritional needs based on the requirements for maintenance and production (NRC manual current for species).
2. Choose the least expensive available ingredients for the basic energy ration and the complete supplement. The basic ingredients will include the least expensive sources for energy, protein, the limiting bulk minerals (calcium, phosphorus, potassium, and sometimes magnesium and/or sulfur), vitamin A, and a premix of necessary trace minerals. The NRC nutrition manuals contain tables that list nutrient concentrations in specific feeds. It may be expedient to include more than one nutrient source for energy, supplemental protein, and supplemental calcium and phosphorus.

Examples include the situation in which wheat is the least-cost energy source and a urea-concentrate mix is the least-cost supplemental protein source. In these cases some people would recommend that wheat not be used to supply more than 50 per cent of the energy concentrate, and it is widely accepted that urea should not supply more than 25 to 33 per cent of the total nitrogen in the ruminant ration. Consideration must also be given to palatability, nutrient concentration, and transportation costs.
3. Balance the ration for energy.
4. Analyze the basic energy ration for deficiencies of protein, minerals, and vitamins.
5. Formulate the most practical complete supplement to provide for deficiencies of proteins, minerals, and vitamins in the basic energy ration. There are a number of viable approaches.
   a. Formulate a complete supplement and incorporate it into the basic energy ration.
   b. Incorporate the protein supplement into the energy ration and feed the mineral and vitamin supplements in a free-choice mixture either loose or in block form.
   c. Formulate a complete supplement using a liquid carrier and feed in a licker. This is often a good approach if NPN is used as a CP source.
   d. Use a prescribed amount of a preformed commercial supplement. The recommended amount is generally 1 lb/animal day in the as-fed ration. Such supplements supply the recommended amounts of ionophores and chemotherapeutic agents. CP, salt, and calcium will often be supplied in excess. Total requirements for vitamins A and D and trace minerals are generally supplied. Phosphorus and potassium concentrations may be marginal.
6. Formulate the ration to comply with available delivery systems. Blocks, cubes, and loose hay may be fed on the ground. Mangers or bunks with adequate space are necessary if ground, rolled, or pelleted feeds are used.

For an example we will formulate a ration for 250-kg medium-frame steer calves. The expected gain is 1 kg/day, and the average ambient temperature is 0°C.

1. Daily nutritional needs are determined. They include the following:
   a. $NE_m = 250^{0.75} \times \{0.077 + [0.0007 \times (20 - 0)]\} = 5.72$ Mcal.
   b. $NE_g = 0.0557 \times 250^{0.75} \times 1^{1.097} = 3.5$ Mcal.
   c. Dry matter intake (DMI). Assume NE_m concentration of the DM ration to be 1.7 Mcal/kg DM. DMI = $[(0.1493 \times 1.7) - (0.046 \times 1.7^2) - (0.0196)] \times 250^{0.75}$ = 6.37 kg.
   d. CP requirement (from NRC,[30] Table 2). CP requirement for 250-kg medium-frame steer calf gaining 1 kg/day = 720 g/day.
   e. Calcium requirement (from NRC,[30] Table 3). Calcium requirement for 250-kg medium-frame steer calf gaining 1 kg/day = 29 g/day.
   f. Phosphorus requirement (from NRC,[30] Table 3). Phosphorus requirement for 250-kg medium-frame steer calf gaining 1 kg/day = 29 g/day.
   g. Trace mineral salt requirement assumed to equal 0.5 per cent DMI. Trace mineral salt requirement for animal consuming 6.37 kg daily = 6.37 kg × 1000 g/kg × 0.005 = 32 g.
   h. Potassium requirement (from NRC,[30] Table 4) assumed to equal 0.5 to 0.7 per cent of DMI. Potassium requirement for 250-kg medium-frame steer calf consuming 6.37 kg DM/day = 32 to 45 g/day.
   i. Vitamin A requirement (from NRC,[30] p. 25) for feedlot cattle = 2200 IU/kg DMI. Vitamin A requirement for 250-kg medium-frame steer calf consuming 6.37 kg DM/day = 2200 × 6.37 = 14,000 IU/day.
2. The least expensive available ration ingredients are chosen. Generally the basic feeds (roughages and concentrates) that are locally grown will be least cost. This premise may be affected by unfavorable weather in the local area or very high production in another area.

There are limitations to a least-cost feed approach. Examples include the following:
   a. A minimal amount of roughage is required to maintain the health of the digestive tract throughout the feeding period.
   b. The value of protein varies with need. Concentrates with relatively high protein concentrations are more valuable when the protein requirement of the production objective is high (lactating dairy cows and fast-growing young animals).

Estimations of comparative feed values include three basic considerations:
   c. The economic substitution value of the feed.
   d. Analysis of feed cost trends for predicting the most favorable times to buy feeds that can be stored.
   e. Managing ration formulation to allow producers to benefit from feed price changes.

The economic substitution values of feeds assume that the actual value of any feed is the sum of the values of its nutrient constituents. The value of energy expressed as Mcal of "average energy"/unit of as-fed feed and the amount of CP/unit of as-fed feed are the only nutrient constituents that are commonly considered. Nutrient densities are not taken into account, but roughages are compared with roughages, and concentrates are compared with concentrates. The objective of calculating economic substitution values is to determine affordable prices that can be paid for alternative feed sources. The calculation can be made by using the following steps:
   f. Choose one concentrate grain and one natural protein supplement. For our examples we use Number 2 corn and solvent-extracted cottonseed meal (CSM). We will use as-fed concentrations of total protein and energy converted from DM concentrations listed in the 1984 NRC beef cattle publication.[30] We calculate average energy values by adding the listed DM values for NE_g and NE_m and dividing by two. The as-fed value is obtained by multiplying the DM value by the listed DM per cent expressed as a decimal. The as-fed total protein per cent and average energy concentrations are listed in Table 6.
   g. Formulate an equation for each feed that shows the value of the feed to be a function of the energy and protein content. Let X = the market value of 1 ton of total protein, and let Y = the market value of 1000 Mcal of average energy as follows:

Table 6. AVERAGE ENERGY AND TOTAL PROTEIN PER CENT IN AS-FED NUMBER 2 CORN AND SOLVENT-EXTRACTED COTTONSEED MEAL

Feed*	Average NE As-Fed (Mcal/kg)	Total Protein % As-Fed
Number 2 corn	1.67	8.9
Cottonseed meal (CSM)	1.47	41.5

*The assumed market values of these feeds are: corn = $100.00/ton, and CSM = $180.00/ton.

For 1 ton of corn: $0.089X + 1.67Y = \$100.00$
For 1 ton of CSM: $0.415X + 1.47Y = \$180.00$

h. Use the simultaneous equation method to solve for the values of X and Y as follows: Divide the coefficient of X in the CSM by the coefficient of X in the corn equation:

$$\frac{0.415}{0.089} = 4.66$$

Multiply the total corn equation by the quotient that results in part (a) above:

$$4.66\,(0.089X + 1.67Y = \$100.00)$$
$$= 0.415X + 7.78Y = \$466$$

Subtract the CSM equation from the modified corn equation and solve for Y:

$$0.415X + 7.78Y = \$466$$
$$\underline{0.415X + 1.47Y = \$180}$$
$$6.31Y = \$286$$

Y (value of 1000 Mcal average energy) = $286/6.31$ = \$45.32. Substitute calculated value of X for X in the corn equation and solve for X:

X (value of 1 ton of total protein) =
$$\frac{\$100 - (1.67 \times \$45.32)}{0.89} = \$273.21$$

i. Use the calculated values of X and Y to establish the price that we can afford to pay for a unit of an alternative feed.

For example, if a sample of as-fed barley contains 11.9 per cent total protein and 1.54 Mcal average net energy/kg, we can afford to pay $(0.119 \times 273.21) + (1.54 \times \$45.32) = \$102.30/\text{ton}$ for barley if we have use for all of the protein in the basic ration.

j. The values of alternative sources of available concentrates, roughages, and protein supplements can be established by this method. Various alternative sources of specific minerals and vitamins A and D can also be compared in this manner.

3. Feed cost trends are analyzed to determine at what time of year feeds to be stored should be purchased. Generally feed prices will be depressed in the harvest season. Prudent producers develop storage areas to enable them to take advantage of favorable markets. The study of fluctuating markets is called trend analysis and is often reflected in futures listings.

4. The market value of feeds is quite variable. Ration formulation should be flexible to allow for the possibility that alternative feed sources can be used in seasons or years when use of these sources is advantageous. An example is the use of animal fats as energy sources in feedlot rations.

The caloric density of fats is very high, and when feed grain prices are high, fats may provide a less-expensive source of ration energy.

We will now complete our example of ration formulation. So far we have established the following objectives and nutrient daily requirements:

Class of cattle	Medium-frame steer calves
LW	250 kg
Production objective	LWG = 1 kg/day
Average ambient temperature	0°C
NE_m requirement	5.72 Mcal
NE_g requirement	3.50 Mcal
CP requirement	720 g
Calcium requirement	29 g
Phosphorus requirement	16 g
Potassium requirement	32 to 45 g
Trace mineral salt requirement	32 g
Vitamin A requirement	14,000 IU
Estimated DMI	6.37 kg ($\times$ 0.98 for the basic energy ration, DMI in the basic energy ration = 6.47 × 0.98 = 6.24 kg)

We will assume that our least-cost nutrient sources include the following:

Concentrate	Number 2 corn
Roughage	Corn silage
CP supplement	Cottonseed meal, solvent extract
Calcium	Limestone
Phosphorus	Dicalcium phosphate
Trace mineral salt	Mixed so that an amount equal to 0.5 per cent of the DM ration furnishes the complete requirements for sodium, chlorine, and trace minerals.
Vitamin A	Deficiencies, if any, will be supplied by adding vitamin A palmitate to the drinking water

Table 7 summarizes the nutrient content of the least-cost feeds on a DM basis.

Formulation of the Basic Energy Ration

a. Compute a theoretical LWG if the total DM ration (6.24 kg) is fed as corn:

$$6.24 \text{ kg} - \frac{5.72 \text{ Mcal}}{2.20} \times 1.55 \text{ Mcal/kg DM} = 5.64 \text{ Mcal } NE_g$$

b. Compute a theoretical LWG if the total DM ration (6.24 kg) is fed as roughage (corn silage):

Table 7. ANALYSIS OF LEAST-COST NUTRIENT SOURCES (DM BASIS)

Ingredient	DM (%)	NE_m*	NE_g*	CP (%)	Ca (%)	P (%)	K (%)	Carotene†
Corn	89	2.20	1.55	10	0.02	0.35	0.37	0.8
Corn silage	33	1.60	1.03	8	0.23	0.22	0.96	18.0
Cottonseed meal	91	1.90	1.3	45	0.22	1.21	1.39	—
Limestone	100	—	—	—	39.0	0.04	0.06	—
Dicalcium phosphate	97	—	—	—	22.0	19.3	0.07	—
Trace mineral salt‡								

*Mcal/kg DM adjusted for 0°C.
†Vitamin A activity = 1000 IU/k.
‡0.5% in DM ration supplies total sodium, chlorine, trace minerals.

$$6.24 \text{ kg} - \frac{5.72 \text{ Mcal}}{NE_g} \times 1.03 \text{ Mcal/kg DM} = 2.74 \text{ Mcal}$$
$$LWG = 13.91 \times 2.74^{0.9116} \times 250^{-0.6837} = 0.8 \text{ kg/day}$$

c. Use a Pearson's square to mix the concentrate and roughage to achieve a daily LWG of 1 kg.

$$LWG\text{–corn } 1.54 \text{ kg} \quad \frac{0.20}{0.74} = 0.27$$

$$\text{Desired gain} = 1 \text{ kg}$$

$$LWG\text{–corn silage } 0.8 \text{ kg} \quad \frac{0.54}{0.74} = 0.73$$

The basic energy ration will contain $0.27 \times 100 = 27$ per cent corn and $0.73 \times 100 = 73$ per cent corn silage.

d. Check the basic energy ration for CP content:

Feed	DM Ration (%)	DM (kg)	CP (%)	CP (g)
Corn	27	1.68	10	168
Corn silage	73	4.56	8	365
Totals	100	6.24		533

CP requirement = 720 g
CP in ration = 533 g
CP deficiency = 187 g

e. Substitute the least-cost protein supplement (CSM) for corn to satisfy the CP deficiency. Use average energy

$$\frac{(NE_m + NE_g)}{2}$$

to compare energy values at 0°C.

$$\text{Average energy for corn at 0°C} = \frac{2.22 + 1.55}{2} = 1.86 \text{ Mcal/kg}$$

$$\text{Average energy for CSM at 0°C} = \frac{1.90 + 1.30}{2} = 1.6 \text{ Mcal/kg}$$

Thus it will require $1.86/1.6 \times 100 \text{ g} = 116 \text{ g}$ of CSM to replace 100 g of corn to keep the energy levels from changing.

When we exchange 100 g of corn for 116 g of CSM, we gain $(0.45 \times 116) - (0.10 \times 100) = 42 \text{ g}$ of CP.

To supply our CP deficiency we need $187/42 \times 116 = 516$ g of CSM to be added and we need to remove $187/42 \times 100 = 445$ g of corn to maintain the energy level.

The basic DM energy-protein diet now contains the following ingredients:

Feed	DM (kg)
Corn	1.240
CSM	0.516
Corn silage	4.55

f. Check the basic energy-protein DM ration for mineral and vitamin A deficiencies.

Feed	DM (kg)	Ca (g)	P (g)	K (g)	Vitamin A Activity
Corn	1.24	0.25	4.34	4.59	992 IU
CSM	0.516	1.14	4.95	7.17	—
Corn silage	4.55	10.47	10.01	43.68	81,900 IU
Totals	6.31	11.86	19.3	55.4	82,892 IU

Nutrient	Daily Requirement (g)	In Ration (g)	Deficiency
Calcium	29	11.86	17.14
Phosphorus	16	19.30	—
Potassium	32–45	55.44	—
Vitamin A	14,000	82,892	—

g. Formulate a complete supplement including CP, mineral, and vitamin supplements.

Nutrient	Deficiency (g)	Supplement Feed	Grams Required
CP	187	CSM	516*
Calcium	17.14	Limestone (34% Ca)	50.4
Trace mineral salt	0.5% DMI	Trace mineral salt	32.0

Supplement Feed	Grams in Daily Ration	% of Complete Supplement
CSM	516	86.2
Limestone	50.4	8.4
Trace mineral salt	32	5.4

*Includes energy and protein lost in removing 445 g of corn DM plus enough crude protein to satisfy the CP deficiency in the basic energy ration.

h. List final DM and as-fed rations.

Feed	DM (kg)	As-Fed (kg)	% of As-Fed Ration
Corn	1.240	1.41	8.9
Corn silage	13.79	4.55	87.0
Complete supplement	0.598	0.65	4.1

REFERENCES

1. Agricultural Research Council: The Nutrient Requirements of Ruminant Livestock. Commonwealth Agricultural Bureaux. Surrey, The Gresham Press, 1980.
2. Aherne FX, Kirkwood RN: Nutrition and sow prolificacy. J Reprod Fertil Suppl 33:169, 1985.
3. Brody S: Bioenergetics and Growth with Special Reference to the Efficiency Complex in Domestic Animals. New York, Reinhold Publishing, 1945.
4. Burroughs W, Nelson DK, Mertens DR: Protein physiology and its application in the lactating cow: the metabolizable protein feeding standard. J Anim Sci 41:933, 1975.
5. Burton JH, Reid JT: Interrelationship among energy input, body size, age, and body composition in sheep. J Nutr 97:517, 1969.
6. Chalupa W: Rumen bypass and protection of amino acids. J Dairy Sci 58:1198, 1975.
7. Chalupa W, Ferguson JD: The roll of dietary fat in productivity and health of dairy cows. Proceedings, The Application of Nutrition in Dairy Practice. The Dairy Production Medicine Continuing Education Group Annual Meeting. North Carolina State University, Raleigh, American Cyanamid Co, 1988.
7a. Diggs BG, Becker DE, Terrill SW, Jensen AH: The energy value for various feedstuffs for the young pig. J Anim Sci 18:1492, 1959.
8. Drew KR, Reid JT: Compensatory growth in immature sheep. I. Effects of weight loss and realimentation on whole body composition. J Agric Sci 85:193, 1975a.
9. Drew KR, Reid JT: Compensatory growth in immature sheep. II. Some changes in the physical and chemical composition of sheep. J Agric Sci 85:201, 1975b.
10. Edwards JJ, Bartley EE: Soybean meal or starea for microbial protein synthesis or milk production with rations above thirteen percent natural protein. J Dairy Sci 62:732, 1979.
11. Ferguson JD: Feeding for reproduction. Proceedings, The Application of Nutrition in Dairy Practice. The Dairy Production Medicine Continuing Education Group Annual Meeting. North Carolina State University, Raleigh, American Cyanamid Co, 1988.
12. Ferrell CL, Garrett WN, Hinman N, Griching G: Energy utilization by pregnant and non-pregnant heifers. J Anim Sci 42:937, 1976.
13. Fox DG, Black JR: A system for predicting body composition and performance of growing cattle. J Anim Sci 58:725–730, 1984.
14. Galligan DT: Economic aspects of nutritional monitoring. Proceedings, The Application of Nutrition in Dairy Practice. The Dairy Production Medicine Continuing Education Group Annual Meeting. North Carolina State University, Raleigh, American Cyanamid Co, 1988.
15. Garrett WN: Energetic efficiency of beef and dairy steers. J Anim Sci 32:451, 1971.

16. Garrett WN: Influence of roughage quality on the performance of feedlot cattle. Calif Feeder's Day Rep 13:51, 1974.
17. Garrett WN: Energy gain in mature non-pregnant beef cows (abstract). J Anim Sci 34:238, 1974.
17a. Garrett WN: Least cost gain and profit projection. 1. Estimating nutrient requirements. Calif Feeders' Day Rep 15:68, 1976.
18. Garrett WN: Energy utilization of growing cattle as determined in seventy two comparative slaughter experiments. 3. *In* Mount LE (ed): Energy Metabolism. EEAP Publication No. 26. London, Butterworths, 1980.
19. Garrett WN: Factors influencing energetic efficiency of beef production. J Anim Sci 51:1434, 1980.
20. Garrett WN, Hinman N: Revaluation of the relationship between carcass density and body composition of beef steers. J Anim Sci 28:1, 1969.
21. Hespell RB: Efficiency of growth by rumen bacteria. Fed Proc 38:2707, 1979.
22. Huntington GB, Reynolds CK: Blood flow and nutrient flux across stomach and post-stomach tissues of beef steers. Fed Proc 45:606, 1986.
23. Johnson DE, Crownover JC: Energy requirements of feedlot cattle in North Central Colorado: variation in maintenance requirements by the month. Research Highlights of the Animal Science Department, Colorado State University, Experiment Station General Series 948, 1975.
24. Lofgreen GP, Garrett WN: A system for expressing net energy requirements and feeding values for growing and finishing beef cattle. J Anim Sci 27:793–806, 1968.
25. Mehrez AZ, Orskov ER, McDonald I: Rates of rumen fermentation in relation to ammonia concentration. Brit J Nutr 38:447, 1977.
26. Moe PW, Flatt WP, Tyrell HF: Net energy value of feeds for lactation. J Dairy Sci 55:945, 1972.
26a. Morgan DJ, Cole DJA, Lewis D: Energy values in pig nutrition. I. The relationship between digestible energy, metabolizable energy, and total digestible nutrient values of a range of feedstuffs. J Agric Sci (Camb) 84:7, 1975.
27. Moore T: The calorie as the unit of nutritional energy. World Rev Nutr Diet 26:1–25, 1977.
28. National Research Council: Nutrient Requirements of Dairy Cattle, 5th rev ed. Washington, DC, National Academy of Sciences, 1978.
29. National Research Council: Effect of Environment on Nutrient Requirements of Domestic Animals. Washington, DC, National Academy Press, 1981.
30. National Research Council: Nutrient Requirements of Beef Cattle, 6th rev ed. Washington DC, National Academy of Sciences, 1984.
31. National Research Council: Nutrient Requirements of Sheep, 6th rev ed. Washington, DC, National Academy of Sciences, 1985.
32. National Research Council: Ruminant Nitrogen Usage. Washington, DC, National Academy Press, 1985.
33. National Research Council: Predicting Feed Intake of Food Producing Animals. Washington, DC, National Academy Press, 1986.
34. National Research Council: Nutrient Requirements of Dairy Cattle, 6th rev ed. Washington, DC, National Academy of Sciences, 1988.
35. National Research Council: Nutrient Requirements of Swine, 9th rev ed. Washington, DC, National Academy of Sciences, 1988.
36. Owens FN (ed): Symposium, Protein Requirements for Cattle. Oklahoma State University, MP-109, 1982.
37. Owens FN, Bergen WG: Nitrogen metabolism of ruminant animals. Historical perspective, current understanding and future implications. J Anim Sci 57:498, 1983.
38. Rattray PV, Garrett WN, East NE, Hinman N: Net energy requirements for ewe lambs for maintenance gain and pregnancy and net energy values for feedstuffs for lambs. J Anim Sci 37:853–857, 1973.
39. Rattray PV, Garrett WN, East NE, Hinman N: Efficiency of utilization of metabolizable energy during pregnancy and energy requirements for pregnancy in sheep. J Anim Sci 38:383–393, 1974.
40. Rattray PV, Garrett WN, Hinman N, et al: A system for expressing the net energy requirements and net energy content of feeds for young sheep. J Anim Sci 36:115–122, 1973.
41. Rattray PV, Garrett WN, Meyer HH, et al: Net energy requirements for growth of lambs age three to five months. J Anim Sci 37:1386–1389, 1973.
42. Satter LD, Roffler RE: Nitrogen requirements and utilization in dairy cattle. J Dairy Sci 58:1219, 1975.
43. Satter LD, Slyter LL: Effect of ammonia concentration on rumen microbial protein production in vitro. Brit J Nutr 32:199, 1974.
44. Satter LD, Whitlow LW, Beardsly, GL: Resistance of protein to rumen degradation and its significance to the dairy cow. Des Moines, Dist Feed Res Counc Proc 32:63, 1977.
45. Slyter LL, Satter LD, Dinius DA: Effects of ruminal ammonia concentration on nitrogen utilization by steers. J Anim Sci 48:906, 1979.
46. Smuts DB: The relation between the basal metabolism and the endogenous nitrogen metabolism with particular reference to the maintenance requirement of protein. J Nutr 9:403, 1935.
47. Sniffen CJ: Balancing rations for carbohydrates for dairy cattle. Proceedings, The Application of Nutrition in Dairy Practice. The Dairy Production Medicine Continuing Education Group Annual Meeting. North Carolina State University, Raleigh, American Cyanamid Co, 1988.
48. Sniffen CJ, Chase LE: Field application of the degradable protein system. Proceedings, The Application of Nutrition in Dairy Practice. The Dairy Production Medicine Continuing Education Group Annual Meeting. North Carolina State University, Raleigh, American Cyanamid Co, 1988.
49. Webster AJF: Prediction of energy requirements for growth in beef cattle. World Rev Nutr Diet 30:189–226, 1978.
49a. Wu, Ewan RC: Utilization of energy of wheat and barley by young swine. J Anim Sci 49:1470, 1979.

Special Dietary Management in Lactation and Gestation

JOHN C. SIMONS, DVM

MICHAEL S. HAND, DVM, PhD, Diplomate, ACVN

The total nutritional requirement of any reproducing female animal is the sum of the individual requirements for maintenance, physical activity, body weight change, the products of conception, and milk production. The needs for maintenance are related to environmental temperature and wind velocity. The energy and protein requirements per unit of body weight are inversely related to size. The requirements for weight change in any species vary according to rate of gain, age, and sex. Normal weight increase resulting from growth requires a diet that is high in protein and low in energy relative to the diet required for weight increase in excess of normal growth. Weight gain in females requires a diet that is high in fat (and thus energy) relative to that of males of the same species and comparable age, size, breed, and type.

Specific needs for the products of conception are practically negligible for the first two trimesters of gestation. During the third trimester there is a significant increase in the requirement for all nutrients. The deposition of nutrients in the products of conception increases daily. For convenience, we use average deposition over a period of time in nutrient requirement tables, but the actual situation is a dynamic one in which the need for nutrients is steadily increasing. Average gestation requirements for energy, protein, and minerals vary considerably among species.

The nutrient requirements for lactation are substantial and may exceed three times the maintenance requirement for sows nursing large litters or for high-producing dairy cows. The efficiency of feed conversion for milk production is comparable to that of maintenance. Lactating animals may lose weight on what would appear to be maximum amounts of optimum rations.

This article deals with problems encountered in meeting the needs of gestating and lactating food animal species and the consequences of nutritional deficiencies in these animals. In the interest of simplicity, we are using tables and figures derived from the equations and explanations documented in the article Field Calculations for Ration Formulation. Reference to these equations may be necessary for more complete understanding.

BEEF CATTLE

The beef cow is preserved and propagated in the interest of converting plants containing large amounts of cellulose into highly palatable foods that have efficient utility for man. In addition to plants, grains, oil meals, and by-products of food and brewing industries are often fed to beef cattle. The production entities, including growth, gestation, and lactation, can be sustained only after maintenance needs are met. The maintenance ration is the baseline of cow-calf nutrition. The objective is to provide least-cost rations that are adequate to maintain the cow and, in addition, that allow her to produce one calf every 12 months that will, at weaning time, weigh 40 per cent or more of the cow's normal weight. It is expected that the cow will be able to maintain this level of production until she is 8 to 10 years old (total lifetime production equals six to eight calves). It is important that we use feeds that are not otherwise available for consumption by people or monogastric food animals; the latter being more efficient in the conversion of concentrate feeds than are beef cattle.

Of special interest is the utilization of roughages that are not of sufficient quality or concentration, or both, for practical milk production or for high-priced horse forage. Such roughages include the following:

1. Native pastures in mountain, plains, desert, forest, and swamp areas.
2. Crop residues including cornstalks, sugar beet tops, straw, stubbles, and cannery wastes.
3. Medium- to low-quality hay and ensilage, especially if fed between weaning and late gestation.

Concentrates and high-quality roughages are used in beef cow rations in several situations:

1. When transportation costs prohibit exportation to favorable markets.
2. When the market price of high-quality feed is low enough to consider in least-cost formulations.
3. When supplementation of low-quality feeds is necessary to meet practical production objectives.

Nonprotein nitrogen can be used as a protein supplement when the urea fermentation potential of the basic ration is positive.

Normal, well-managed beef cows are either gestating, lactating, or both 100 per cent of the time. Heifers are bred as yearlings or 2 year olds (13 to 27 months), and many heifers produce two calves before they stop growing.

The primary considerations in beef cow nutrition include:

1. A nutritional needs assessment of the maintenance and production requirements.
2. A mathematical analysis of the basic forage ration in terms of consumption and nutrient concentration.
3. The deficiencies of the basic forage ration in meeting the maintenance and production requirements.
4. The most economical sources of the necessary supplements.
5. The most practical delivery system.

Ordinarily beef cows will be offered a free-choice forage ration. This daily intake of forage may include all of the necessary nutrients in excess of maintenance and production objectives (dry cows will gain about 0.45 kg/day on good cornstalks or sugar beet tops).

Most forage rations vary in quality and quantity with season and weather conditions. Cows on high-quality free-choice forage may gain weight during the late lactation and postweaning periods. Overweight cows may lose weight on submaintenance rations in midgestation without harm to the cow or fetus. The quality of late fall and early winter forage is relatively high and decreases in value and availability as the cow's needs increase in late winter. In late gestation and early lactation the basic forage ration is often deficient, and knowledge of what is needed, available, and economical is essential in these periods. Cows should be in good condition at parturition and gaining in the breeding season. Quite naturally, native pastures are at their best in the time of greatest need.

The Need Assessment

The California Net Energy System most accurately describes the energy requirements for maintenance (NE_m) and gain (NE_g). At moderate temperatures, the daily requirement for NE_m in megacalories (Mcal) equals $0.077 \times (BW_{kg})^{0.75}$. This requirement is modified by weather. The Handley formula or the table devised by Johnson and Crownover, or both, can be used to evaluate the effect of the temperature wind index (TWI).*

Net energy for gain must be considered in the case of growing heifers. Table 1 is a reprint of Table 7 in the 1984 National Research Council (NRC) publication for beef cattle[9] and lists net energy requirements for maintenance and gain in 25-kg increments of body weight and varying increments of daily gain.

Net energy requirements for the products of conception can be determined from the following formula:

$$NE_m = \text{calf birth weight (kg)} (0.0149 - 0.0000407t) \times e^{0.05883t - 0.0000804t^2}$$

where NE_m is kcal/day, t is day of gestation, e is the antilog of the natural log of 1 and is approximately equal to 2.72, and a diet of average-quality forage (metabolizable energy [ME] of 2.00 Mcal/kg) is assumed. Thus for a 34-kg anticipated calf birth weight on day 240 of the gestation period, 2300 kcal, or 2.3 Mcal, of NE_m are required for the conceptus. However, total net energy as well as metabolizable energy and total digestible nutrient (TDN) requirements for pregnancy can more readily and practically be obtained from Table 1.

The net energy requirement for lactation is also expressed in Mcal of NE_m. The energy requirements for milk production have been estimated from the information available for dairy cows.[44] Assuming 4 per cent milk fat, the requirement for beef cows is 0.75 Mcal NE_m/kg milk produced (0.34 Mcal/lb milk). Therefore a cow producing 4.54 kg (10 lb) milk/day requires $4.54 \times 0.75 = 3.4$ Mcal NE_m/day for milk production. Total energy requirements for lactation are listed in Table 1.

The gross energy of feed minus fecal energy is termed digestible energy (DE). An approximately equivalent term, TDN measures DE in weight units. TDN can be converted to DE by the relationship 1 kg TDN = 4.4 Mcal DE (or 1 lb TDN = 2 Mcal DE). TDN and DE are easier to measure than NE_m and NE_g. Therefore feed analysis laboratories more commonly represent the energy content of a feed in their reports in terms of TDN and DE rather than NE_m and NE_g. The major weakness of the TDN/DE system is that it overestimates the energy available in roughages and underestimates the energy available in concentrates. The system does adequately model energy metabolism in the beef cow. See Table 1 for TDN requirements at various stages of maturity, gestation, and lactation.

Lack of sufficient energy is probably the most common deficiency in cow-calf nutrition. When feed is limited on farms or overstocked ranges, low energy intake occurs. The results include reduction or cessation of growth, weight loss, failure to conceive, and increased mortality. Range animals on deficient rations are more prone to eat toxic plants and are more susceptible to internal parasites. Usually energy deficiency is accompanied by deficiencies of protein and other nutrients. In spite of these shortcomings, rations deficient in energy are sometimes economically acceptable. Desert and semidesert ranges may be too sparse to supply intake sufficient for optimum production. Supplementation of such rations may be too expensive and inconvenient to justify. Such ranges may support conception and birth rates of 50 to 70 per cent without significant supplementation. Vast acreages of marginal rangeland are controlled by state and federal governments in the western United States. Grazing lease costs for these lands are relatively modest. Generally cattle operations in these areas have been successful when operating costs have been kept at a minimum and below average production objectives have been accepted.

The crude protein requirement of breeding cattle is due to

Table 1. NUTRIENT REQUIREMENTS OF BREEDING CATTLE*

Weight† (kg)	Daily Gain‡ (kg)	Daily DM§ (kg)	Energy Daily				Energy In Diet DM				Total Protein		Calcium		Phosphorus		Vitamin A‖
			ME (Mcal)	TDN (kg)	NE_m (Mcal)	NE_g (Mcal)	ME (Mcal/kg)	TDN (%)	NE_m (Mcal/kg)	NE_g (Mcal/kg)	Daily (g)	In Diet DM (%)	Daily (g)	In Diet DM (%)	Daily (g)	In Diet DM (%)	Daily (1000's IU)
Pregnant yearling heifers—last third of pregnancy																	
325	0.4	7.1	14.2	3.9	8.04	NA**	2.00	55.2	1.15	NA**	591	8.4	19	0.27	14	0.20	20
325	0.6	7.3	15.7	4.3	8.04	0.77	2.15	59.3	1.29	0.72	649	8.9	23	0.32	15	0.21	20
325	0.8	7.3	17.2	4.8	8.04	1.67	2.35	64.9	1.47	0.88	697	9.5	27	0.37	16	0.22	20
350	0.4	7.5	14.8	4.1	8.38	NA	1.99	55.0	1.14	NA	616	8.3	20	0.27	15	0.21	21
350	0.6	7.7	16.5	4.6	8.38	0.81	2.14	59.1	1.28	0.71	674	8.8	24	0.32	16	0.21	22
350	0.8	7.8	18.1	5.0	8.38	1.76	2.34	64.6	1.46	0.88	720	9.3	27	0.35	17	0.22	22
375	0.4	7.8	15.5	4.3	8.71	NA	1.98	54.7	1.13	NA	641	8.2	21	0.27	15	0.19	22
375	0.6	8.1	17.2	4.8	8.71	0.86	2.13	58.8	1.27	0.70	697	8.6	25	0.31	17	0.21	23
375	0.8	8.2	19.0	5.2	8.71	1.86	2.32	64.1	1.45	0.86	743	9.1	27	0.33	18	0.22	23
400	0.4	8.2	16.1	4.5	9.04	NA	1.97	54.4	1.12	NA	664	8.1	22	0.27	16	0.20	23
400	0.6	8.5	18.0	5.0	9.04	0.90	2.12	58.6	1.26	0.69	721	8.5	25	0.30	18	0.21	24
400	0.8	8.6	19.8	5.5	9.04	1.95	2.31	63.8	1.44	0.85	764	8.9	28	0.33	18	0.20	24
425	0.4	8.6	16.8	4.6	9.36	NA	1.96	54.1	1.11	NA	687	8.0	23	0.27	17	0.20	24
425	0.6	8.9	18.7	5.2	9.36	0.94	2.11	58.3	1.25	0.69	743	8.4	26	0.30	18	0.20	25
425	0.8	9.0	20.7	5.7	9.36	2.04	2.30	63.5	1.43	0.84	786	8.8	28	0.31	19	0.21	25
450	0.4	8.9	17.3	4.8	9.67	NA	1.95	53.9	1.10	NA	710	8.0	23	0.26	18	0.20	25
450	0.6	9.2	19.4	5.4	9.67	0.98	2.10	58.0	1.25	0.68	765	8.3	26	0.29	19	0.21	26
450	0.8	9.4	21.5	5.9	9.67	2.13	2.29	63.3	1.42	0.84	807	8.6	28	0.30	20	0.21	26
Dry pregnant mature cows—middle third of pregnancy																	
350	0.0	6.8	11.9	3.3	6.23	NA	1.76	48.6	0.92	NA	478	7.1	12	0.16	12	0.18	19
400	0.0	7.5	13.1	3.6	6.89	NA	1.76	48.6	0.92	NA	525	7.0	13	0.17	13	0.17	21
450	0.0	8.2	14.3	4.0	7.52	NA	1.76	48.6	0.92	NA	570	7.0	15	0.17	15	0.18	23
500	0.0	8.8	15.5	4.3	8.14	NA	1.76	48.6	0.92	NA	614	7.0	17	0.19	17	0.19	25
550	0.0	9.5	16.7	4.6	8.75	NA	1.76	48.6	0.92	NA	657	6.9	18	0.19	18	0.19	27
600	0.0	10.1	17.8	4.9	9.33	NA	1.76	48.6	0.92	NA	698	6.9	20	0.20	20	0.20	28
650	0.0	10.7	18.9	5.2	9.91	NA	1.76	48.6	0.92	NA	739	6.9	22	0.21	22	0.21	30
Dry pregnant mature cows—last third of pregnancy																	
350	0.4	7.4	14.7	4.1	8.38	NA	1.98	54.7	1.13	NA	609	8.2	20	0.27	15	0.20	21
400	0.4	8.2	16.0	4.4	9.04	NA	1.96	54.1	1.11	NA	657	8.0	22	0.27	16	0.20	23
450	0.4	8.9	17.2	4.8	9.67	NA	1.94	53.6	1.10	NA	703	7.9	23	0.26	18	0.21	24
500	0.4	9.5	18.3	5.1	10.29	NA	1.92	53.1	1.08	NA	746	7.8	25	0.26	20	0.21	27
550	0.4	10.2	19.5	5.4	10.90	NA	1.91	52.8	1.07	NA	790	7.8	26	0.25	21	0.21	29
600	0.4	10.8	20.6	5.7	11.48	NA	1.90	52.5	1.06	NA	832	7.7	28	0.26	23	0.21	30
650	0.4	11.5	21.7	6.0	12.06	NA	1.89	52.2	1.05	NA	872	7.6	30	0.26	25	0.22	32
Two-year-old heifers nursing calves—first 3 to 4 months post partum—5.0 kg milk/day																	
300	0.2	6.9	16.6	4.6	9.30††	0.72	2.41	66.6	1.53	0.93	814‡‡	11.8	26	0.38	17	0.25	27
325	0.2	7.3	17.4	4.8	9.64††	0.77	2.37	65.5	1.49	0.90	841‡‡	11.5	27	0.37	18	0.25	28
350	0.2	7.8	18.1	5.0	9.98††	0.81	2.34	64.6	1.46	0.88	866‡‡	11.2	27	0.35	19	0.24	30
375	0.2	8.2	18.9	5.2	10.31††	0.86	2.31	63.8	1.44	0.85	892‡‡	10.9	28	0.34	19	0.23	32
400	0.2	8.6	19.7	5.4	10.64††	0.90	2.29	63.3	1.42	0.84	916‡‡	10.7	28	0.33	20	0.23	34
425	0.2	9.0	20.4	5.6	10.96††	0.94	2.27	62.7	1.40	0.82	939‡‡	10.5	29	0.32	21	0.23	35
450	0.2	9.4	21.1	5.8	11.27††	0.98	2.25	62.2	1.38	0.80	963‡‡	10.3	29	0.31	22	0.23	37
Cows nursing calves—average milking ability—first 3 to 4 months post partum—5.0 kg milk/day																	
350	0.0	7.7	16.6	4.6	9.98††	NA	2.15	59.4	1.29	NA	814‡‡	10.6	23	0.30	18	0.23	30
400	0.0	8.5	17.9	4.9	10.64††	NA	2.11	58.3	1.25	NA	864‡‡	10.2	25	0.29	19	0.22	33
450	0.0	9.2	19.1	5.3	11.27††	NA	2.08	57.5	1.23	NA	911‡‡	9.9	26	0.28	21	0.23	36
500	0.0	9.9	20.3	5.6	11.89††	NA	2.05	56.6	1.20	NA	957‡‡	9.7	28	0.28	22	0.22	39
550	0.0	10.6	21.5	5.9	12.50††	NA	2.03	56.1	1.18	NA	1001‡‡	9.5	29	0.27	24	0.23	41
600	0.0	11.2	22.6	6.2	13.08††	NA	2.01	55.5	1.16	NA	1044‡‡	9.3	31	0.28	26	0.23	44
650	0.0	11.9	23.9	6.6	13.66††	NA	2.00	55.3	1.15	NA	1086‡‡	9.1	33	0.28	27	0.23	46
Cows nursing calves—superior milking ability—first 3 to 4 months post partum—10.0 kg milk/day																	
350	0.0	6.2	18.5	5.1	13.73††	NA	3.00	82.9	2.03	NA	1009‡‡	16.4	36	0.58	24	0.39	24
400	0.0	7.6	21.4	5.9	14.39††	NA	2.80	77.4	1.86	NA	1099‡‡	14.4	37	0.49	25	0.33	30
450	0.0	9.1	23.2	6.4	15.02††	NA	2.56	70.7	1.66	NA	1186‡‡	13.1	39	0.43	26	0.29	35
500	0.0	10.0	24.6	6.8	15.64††	NA	2.45	67.7	1.56	NA	1246‡‡	12.4	40	0.40	28	0.28	39
550	0.0	10.9	25.8	7.1	16.25††	NA	2.38	65.8	1.50	NA	1299‡‡	12.0	42	0.39	30	0.27	42
600	0.0	11.6	27.0	7.5	16.83††	NA	2.32	64.1	1.45	NA	1348‡‡	11.6	43	0.37	31	0.27	45
650	0.0	12.4	28.2	7.8	17.41††	NA	2.28	63.0	1.14	NA	1394‡‡	11.3	45	0.36	33	0.26	48

Source: Reprinted with permission from Nutrient Requirements of Beef Cattle, 6th rev ed. © 1984 by the National Academy of Sciences. Published by National Academy Press, Washington, DC.

*Expressed in metric units.

†Average weight for feeding period.

‡Approximately 0.4 ± 0.1 kg weight gain/day over the last third of pregnancy is accounted for by the products of conception. Daily 2.15 Mcal NE_m and 55 g protein are provided for this requirement for a calf with a birth weight of 36 kg.

§Dry matter consumption should vary depending on the energy concentration of the diet and environmental conditions. These intakes are based on the energy concentration shown in the table and assuming a thermoneutral environment without snow or mud conditions. If the energy concentrations of the diet to be fed exceed the tabular value, limited feeding may be required.

‖Vitamin A requirements per kilogram of diet are 2800 IU for pregnant heifers and cows and 3900 IU for lactating cows.

**Not applicable.

††Includes 0.75 Mcal NE_m/kg milk produced.

‡‡Includes 33.5 g protein/kg milk produced.

several physiologic expenditures. These include metabolic fecal loss (F), endogenous urinary loss (U), scurf loss (S), tissue growth (G), growth of the conceptus (C), and milk production (M). These are represented in a factorial equation for determining crude protein (CP) requirement:

$$CP = (F + U + S + G + C + M) \div (D \times BV \times CE)$$

where D is the percentage of dietary protein that may be absorbed as amino acids, BV is the efficiency of conversion of the absorbed amino acids to body protein (maintenance, gain, or milk), and CE is the efficiency of converting dietary protein to ruminal protein output.

Equations to estimate these various crude protein expenditures (grams) include the following:

1. F = 3 per cent dry matter (DM) intake or 6.8 per cent fecal DM.
2. $U = 2.75 \, W^{0.5}$.
3. $S = 0.2 \, W^{0.6}$.
4. G = daily gain in kg × (268 − 29.4 × energy content of gain in Mcal/kg). The net energy content of the gain = $0.0608 \, W/kg^{0.75}$ (LWG).[1,119] (W is weight in kilograms, and LWG is live weight gain.)
5. C = 55 g/day for the last trimester.
6. M = kg milk/day × 0.0335.

The factors in the divisors of the factorial equation are assumed to be: D = 0.9, BV = 0.66, and CE = 1.0. Thus the daily crude protein requirement for a 364-kg (800-lb) 2-year-old heifer consuming 8 kg (17.6 lb) DM/day, gaining 0.23 kg (0.5 lb)/day, and nursing a 90-day-old calf (4.54 kg, or 10 lb, milk/day) would be

$$CP = (8000 \times 0.03340) + (2.75 \times 364^{0.5}) + (0.2 \times 364^{0.6}) + 0.23 \times [268 - (29.4 \times 5.06)] + (4.54/0.01 \times 0.0335) = 843 \text{ g,}$$
or 1.9 lb (see Table 1)

These calculations have been performed and tabulated for varying stages of maturity, gestation, and production (see Table 1). In nearly all instances these listed values of crude protein requirement will suffice.

Depressed appetite is said to be the primary sign of protein deficiency in beef cattle diets. Diminished appetite for a ration that is complete and balanced at one level of intake will result in a deficiency of all nutrients when intake falls below that level. Irregular or delayed estrus is the primary sign of protein shortage in diets for breeding animals. Abnormal estrus may also result from energy deficiency. Many cows on rations deficient in protein or energy, or both, do not conceive while lactating. After weaning, such a cow will not be subject to the stress of either lactation or late gestation. Her requirement for energy and protein will be reduced and she will probably be gaining in the following breeding season. Thus there is a negative feedback mechanism that enables limited reproduction in marginal nutritive situations. Adequate supplementation of these cows may be frustrating. The cow may prefer to wait until tomorrow rather than work for the forage ration on a marginal pasture. Scattering the supplement over a wide area is very inconvenient, and there is some loss of efficiency. In some cases accepting below-average production objectives, including fewer and smaller calves, may be the most practical answer.

Urea and certain other sources of nonprotein nitrogen may be used as supplemental protein and substituted for as much as 25 per cent of the total nitrogen in the diets of pregnant and lactating cows. Supplemental nonprotein nitrogen expressed as urea equivalents should not exceed 1 per cent of the diet. Nonprotein nitrogen is not as well utilized when fed as a supplement to low-quality roughages. See the article Field Calculations for Ration Formulation for methods of determining urea fermentation potential.

Minerals

In formulating mineral rations for beef cows, practical consideration needs to be given to salt, calcium, phosphorus, and magnesium. The specific requirement for some of these minerals may be affected by the potassium concentration in the diet, and sulfur should be considered if nonprotein nitrogen is used as a crude protein source. Iodine-deficient soils prevail in much of the northern United States. Supplementation of iodine is necessary for cattle grazing in deficient areas. Cobalt supplementation is necessary for cattle grazing in some areas of Florida, Michigan, Wisconsin, Massachusetts, New Hampshire, Pennsylvania, and New York. Both selenium-deficient and toxic areas exist in the United States.

The sodium and chlorine needs are expressed as the salt requirement. No special needs for gestation or lactation are apparent. Requirements for sodium and chlorine appear to be met by including 0.1 per cent salt in the dry matter ration. Salt is commonly self-fed free choice. It is also commonly mixed with other ration ingredients. Intake varies considerably and often exceeds minimum requirements. Grazing cattle will voluntarily consume more salt than those fed dry feeds, and such consumption is increased if the forage is succulent. Salt is often used in beef cattle supplements to control intake of highly palatable supplements. Concentrations may vary from 10 to 50 per cent. Cattle should be gradually introduced to high-salt intakes and should have free access to clean water. Salt deficiency produces an abnormal appetite for salt. Prolonged deficiency results in anorexia, unthrifty appearance, and decreased production.

The calcium requirement for beef cows will generally be exceeded by normal concentrations in the forage ration. The daily requirement varies between 12 g for small dry cows and 42 g for large lactating cows of superior milking ability (see Table 1 for specific requirements). Soils in arid and semiarid climates are ordinarily low in phosphorus. Also, mature forages and crop residues generally contain low levels of phosphorus. Deficiencies may occur in cattle subsisting on dry, mature forage for long periods. The minimum for phosphorus (maintenance, gestation, lactation) is said to be 0.22 per cent of the dry diet (2.2 g/kg DM). This figure might possibly be high. Research workers at Utah State University have failed to produce deficiency symptoms in breeding beef cows over a 5-year period using a straight forage ration (minimum phosphorus content 0.16 per cent). However, it is probably wise to supplement lactating cows grazing on less than excellent forage.

Specifically, the phosphorus requirements vary between 12 g daily for light cows and 31 g daily for heavy lactating cows of superior milking ability (NRC recommendation; see Table 1). If the phosphorus intake is adequate, wide calcium:phosphorus ratios are acceptable. Satisfactory performance has been achieved with calcium:phosphorus ratios as high as 7:1. Both calcium and phosphorus may be deficient in dry, mature range forage consisting mostly of grasses. Phosphorus deficiency causes decreased appetite and milk production. In extreme cases bone changes, lameness, and stiffness may occur. Failure to cycle and conceive is the likely consequence. Calcium deficiency is less common, and specific symptoms are not conspicuous. Bone changes will be apparent in advanced cases.

The magnesium requirement of the beef cow is between 7 and 9 g/day during gestation and 21, 22, and 18 g/day during early, mid, and late lactation, respectively. Most cattle feeds appear to contain adequate amounts of magnesium, but there are some complicating circumstances. Generally magnesium in grains and other concentrates is more available to cattle than is magnesium contained in forages. Also, magnesium in preserved forages is more available relative to pasture forages. Net magnesium absorption is lowest from highly succulent pasture and, in contrast to most nutrients, increases with maturity.

The mean magnesium availability of pasture forage has been calculated to be about 17 per cent. Milk contains a relatively high magnesium level (about 0.08 per cent). Thus the requirement is directly related to milk production. Under practical conditions two types of magnesium deficiency occur. The least prevalent results from feeding a magnesium-deficient diet for an extended period—for example, calves on an all-milk diet. Young calves require 0.07 per cent magnesium in their diet. The second type (hypomagnesemia, or grass tetany) often occurs without any significant depletion of body reserves. Grass tetany can be a major problem when lactating cows are grazing on lush, rapidly growing pastures. Insufficient absorption or mobilization, or both, accounts for the symptoms. Nervousness, incoordination, convulsions, frothing, and sudden death compose the common syndrome. Feeding high-energy range blocks containing 2 to 3 per cent magnesium oxide and 10 to 20 per cent salt (intake control) is an effective preventive measure.

Potassium deficiencies are extremely rare in ordinary beef cattle rations. Lush, rapidly growing pasture may contain up to 3 per cent potassium in the dry matter. Under these conditions, potassium may interfere with magnesium absorption and may complicate the grass tetany problem.

Selenium deficiencies as well as toxicities may occur in beef reproducing beef cattle. Generally soils (and therefore plants) in northwestern, northeastern, and Atlantic coastal states (including Florida) and in areas around the Great Lakes are deficient in selenium. Forages and grains grown on these soils may contain less selenium than the dietary requirement of 0.1 mg/kg. However, in isolated areas throughout the Rocky Mountain–Great Plains regions of the United States, some plants accumulate toxic amounts (>5 mg/kg) of selenium.

The signs of gross deficiency in cows grazing pastures containing inadequate selenium include the production of calves with nutritional muscular dystrophy (white muscle disease). Subclinical deficiencies of selenium are not easily determined and may limit performance. Infertility has been noted in ewes grazing selenium-deficient pastures. Signs of selenium toxicity include partial anorexia, loss of tail hair, and sloughing of hooves. Selenium supplementation is usually accomplished via drenches, injections, feed or salt additives, or selenium in fertilizers applied to pastures. Since selenium can be toxic, supplementation should be done carefully. For selenium-toxic areas, utilize feeds from nonseleniferous areas or rotate cattle through nonseleniferous pastures, or both.

When nonprotein nitrogen is used in beef cow rations, sulfur supplements are probably a practical addition. Three grams of inorganic sulfur to 100 g urea is the recommended amount.

Table 2 lists common sources of supplementary minerals for beef cow rations.

Vitamins

Vitamin requirements will generally be met by the natural feeds plus microbial synthesis in the rumen. The exception is vitamin A when fresh forage or hay containing adequate

Table 2. COMMON SOURCES OF SUPPLEMENTARY MINERALS FOR BEEF COW RATIONS

Mineral Deficiency	Source
Calcium and phosphorus	Dicalcium phosphate (23.13% Ca and 18.65% P)
Sodium, chlorine, and iodine	Iodized salt (40% Na, 60% Cl, and 0.01% I)
Magnesium	Magnesium oxide (50% Mg) or magnesium sulfate (20% Mg)
Sulfur	Magnesium sulfate (27% S) or calcium sulfate (24% S)
Selenium	Sodium selenite (45.6% Se)

concentrations of β-carotene is not available. The need for vitamin A in beef cows varies from 19,000 IU daily for light dry cows to 47,000 IU per day for heavy lactating cows of superior milking ability.

Vitamin A deficiency in breeding bulls may lead to a decline in sexual activity and semen quality. In breeding cows estrus may not be impaired, but conception rates are often decreased. Gestation periods may be shortened, and the incidence of retained placentas is increased. Under practical conditions the following points should be considered: (1) in drought years with prolonged feeding of bleached grasses or hay or when replacement cattle of unknown history have an unthrifty appearance, the body stores of vitamin A may be low; (2) the β-carotene content of dried or sun-cured forages decreases upon storage in direct relation to temperature, exposure to air and sunlight, and length of storage; and (3) vitamin A losses occur during the processing of feeds with steam and pressure or when feeds are mixed with certain oxidizing materials, including some minerals or organic acids. In addition, it should be remembered that synthetic vitamin A supplements (vitamin A acetate or vitamin A palmitate) are generally more stable than vitamin A from natural sources. Vitamin A supplementation is relatively inexpensive. Practical administration procedures include feed supplements, addition to drinking water, and parenteral injection. The specific role of β-carotene in reproduction remains unclear.

Summary for Beef Cattle

Using data from NRC publications, laboratory analysis, and current weather information, requirements for maintenance, gain, late pregnancy, and lactation of beef cattle can be calculated. Use of the 1978 and 1989 NRC publications for dairy cattle[44, 46] to supplement information included in the 1984 NRC publication for beef cattle[9] can be helpful.

1. Energy requirements for maintenance, late gestation, and lactation can all be calculated in terms of net energy for maintenance (NE_m).
   a. Daily maintenance needs are calculated from the equation NE_m (Mcal) = $0.077 \times (BW_{kg})^{0.75}$ in moderate weather conditions. The effects of weather on the net energy requirements for maintenance can be calculated from the equation NE_m (kcal/kg) $(BW^*)^{0.75}$ = (116) − (0.8133 × TWI) (temperature wind index). See the article Field Calculations for Ration Formulation.
   b. Late gestation needs may be assumed to equal maintenance needs plus 1.57 Mcal NE_m/day.
   c. Lactation needs = 0.75 Mcal NE_m/kg milk produced.
   d. Needs for gain in growing heifers and/or adult cows being flushed for breeding can be calculated by the

following equations: for cows: $NE_g = 6.2$ Mcal/kg gain; for growing heifers: $NE_g = (0.0608 \times W^{0.75})(LWG)^{1.119}$.
2. Protein needs are calculated on the basis of crude protein.
   a. Crude protein concentrations in a wide variety of feeds are listed in NRC,[9] Table 8.
   b. Daily requirements of crude protein and digestible protein are listed in Table 1.
3. Daily requirements of calcium and phosphorus are listed in Table 1. Generally salt is fed free choice or at the rate of 0.1 per cent of the dry matter. Seven to 9 g of magnesium are required daily by the gestating cow, and 21, 22, and 18 g/day are needed during early, mid, and late lactation, respectively. The minimum requirement for selenium is 0.1 mg/kg DM, whereas over 5 mg/kg may be toxic.
4. Concentrations of vitamin A expressed as mg/kg of β-carotene per kg DM, and the daily requirements for vitamin A (1 mg β-carotene = 400 IU vitamin A), are also listed in the NRC.[9]
5. The requirements for vitamins D, E, and K and the B vitamins will usually be met by the natural feeds or by microbial synthesis in the rumen.

A number of rules of thumb may be formulated from computation data. (1) Net energy requirements over maintenance increase about 25 per cent in late gestation—from 40 to 80 per cent at peak lactation and from 15 to 20 per cent over maintenance plus lactation in the breeding season for growth and/or gain. (2) Protein requirements over maintenance increase 15 to 30 per cent in late gestation, 100 to 300 per cent in peak lactation, and 10 to 15 per cent over maintenance and lactation for growth and/or gain in the breeding season.

Calcium and phosphorus needs increase about 25 per cent in late gestation and from 100 to 375 per cent in peak lactation. Magnesium needs in gestating cows probably increase by 25 per cent. In lactation these needs probably increase by 50 to 100 per cent. Magnesium absorption is decreased when the cows are eating succulent forage. Excess potassium or nitrogen, or both, may also interfere with absorption. In addition, magnesium deficiencies are more likely to manifest themselves if calcium is deficient. It is practical to feed a salt-controlled, high-energy supplement containing 2 to 3 per cent magnesium oxide or 3 to 5 per cent magnesium sulfate when grass tetany is a problem. Vitamin A requirements increase by 15 to 25 per cent in late gestation and by up to 125 per cent in lactation (average 20 to 25 per cent).

Tall fescue is the major cool season grass grown in the Southeast. Almost all of the tall fescue is infested by an endophyte fungus. This fungus (presumed to be present on fescue grazed during the high ambient temperatures of the summer months) has been incriminated in a number of conditions collectively referred to as the "summer syndrome." These conditions include unthriftiness and sometimes loss of body weight, rough hair coat, panting, and increased body temperature. Cattle being bred in the summer may experience poor reproductive performance (reduced conception rate) if grazing infested fescue. Also, cows grazing tall fescue in the summer produce less milk. Management procedures, which call for rotating cattle out of fescue pastures during the summer or planting clover with fescue, do much to control the problem. New fescue varieties being developed and certified fungus-free seed may offer promise.

Example Ration Outline

I. Data
   Location: Midwestern U.S.
   Class: Conventional 2-year-old heifers, breeding season
   Body weight: 364 kg (800 lb)
   Desired gain: 0.23 kg (0.5 lb) daily
   Estimated milk production: 4.54 kg (10 lb daily)
   Estimated dry matter consumption: 8 kg (17.6 lb) daily
   Temperature wind index: 48 (NE_m requirement = 0.077 × $[BW_{kg}]^{0.75}$)
II. Daily requirements per heifer
   A. NE_m for maintenance plus lactation: 9.8 Mcal (from Table 1)
      NE_g for gain: 0.96 Mcal (from Table 1)
      TDN for maintenance and lactation: 5.1 kg (11.2 lb), or 63.8 per cent of the diet dry matter if consuming at least 2.3 per cent of body weight in dry matter (from Table 1)
   B. Crude protein requirement: 0.86 kg (1.9 lb), or 10.8 per cent of the diet dry matter if consuming at least 2.3 per cent of body weight in dry matter (from Table 1)
   C. Mineral requirement:
      1. Calcium: 17 g (from Table 1)
      2. Phosphorus: 19 g (from Table 1)
      3. Magnesium: 21 g (from text)
      4. Salt (0.5 per cent DM): 40 g (from text)
   D. Vitamin A: 31,000 IU (from Table 1)
III. Forage ration analysis: assume free-choice native short grass in an intermediate stage of maturity
   A. Nutrient concentration per kg DM:
      NE_m: 1.25 Mcal
      NE_g: 0.6 Mcal
      TDN: 650 g
      Crude protein: 110 g
      Calcium: 4.5 g
      Phosphorus: 1.6 g
      Magnesium: 1.4 g
      Salt: none
   B. Total nutrients in forage ration and requirements:
      1. NE_m for maintenance and lactation:
         Requirement: 9.8 Mcal
         Ration supplies 8 × 1.25 = 10 Mcal
         Ration available for gain 10 − (9.8/1.25) = 2.16 kg
      2. NE_g for gain:
         Requirement for 0.23-kg gain = 1.13 Mcal
         Ration supplies 2.16 × 0.6 = 1.30 Mcal
      3. TDN:
         Requirement: 5.1 kg
         Ration supplies 8 × 650 g = 5.2 kg
      4. Crude protein:
         Requirement: 860 g
         Ration supplies 8 × 110 = 880 g
      5. Calcium:
         Requirement: 27 g
         Ration supplies 8 × 4.5 = 36 g
      6. Phosphorus:
         Requirement: 19 g
         Ration supplies 8 × 1.6 = 12.8 g
      7. Magnesium:
         Requirement: 21 g
         Ration supplies 8 × 1.4 = 11.2 g
      8. Salt:
         Requirement: 40 g
         Ration supplies: 0
   C. Deficiencies of the forage ration:
      Phosphorus: 6.2 g
      Magnesium: 9.8 g
   D. Sources of supplements and required amounts:
      1. Phosphorus: 6.2-g deficiency
         Dicalcium phosphate (18.65 per cent phosphorus) 6.2/0.1865 = 33 g (~ 1 oz)

2. Magnesium: 9.8-g deficiency magnesium oxide (60 per cent magnesium)
   9.8/0.6 = 16 g (~0.5 oz)
3. Salt: 40 g
4. Total supplements per day: 89 g

E. Supplement delivery system:
   Supply a free-choice mixture containing:
   dicalcium phosphate 33/89 = 37 per cent
   magnesium oxide 16/89 = 18 per cent
   salt 40/89 = 45 per cent

THE DAIRY COW

The dry matter feed consumption of a lactating cow is equal to between 2 and 4 per cent of her body weight. The great variation is largely due to differences in milk production. An average-sized cow (600 kg, or 1320 lb) producing 25 kg (55 lb) of 4 per cent fat-corrected milk (FCM) will consume about 3 per cent of her body weight (18 kg) in feed dry matter per day.

Energy

The 1989 NRC dairy cattle publication[46] uses one value to express energy needs for maintenance, pregnancy, milk production, and body changes.[38, 39] This value is designated as net energy for lactation (NE_L).

The maintenance requirement of lactating cows was found to be 73 kcal NE_L/kg $(BW)^{0.75}$. An activity allowance of 10 per cent is added, so the maintenance requirement is computed as 80 kcal (0.080 Mcal) NE_L/kg $(BW)^{0.75}$. To support the activity of grazing, allowances for maintenance should be increased by 10 per cent on good-quality pasture and 20 per cent on sparse pasture.

The influence of cold is probably minimized by the normally high heat production of cows consuming large amounts of feed. When loose housing systems are used, it seems advisable to increase feed intake up to 8 per cent in severe winter conditions.

Few quantitative data are available for the energy requirements of gestation. Balance experiments indicated that the total energy requirements for pregnant cows increased markedly in the last 4 to 8 weeks of gestation.[26] It would appear that an additional 3 to 6 Mcal above maintenance are required to meet the need. The requirements for maintenance plus late gestation are currently calculated as 104 kcal (0.104 Mcal) NE_L/kg $(BW)^{0.75}$.

The dry period of a dairy cow is relatively short (usually 6 to 10 weeks). Care should be taken to avoid overfattening, especially with corn ensilage–based diets. Cows in good condition should receive minimal amounts of concentrates throughout most of the dry period. Concentrate levels are increased in the last 2 to 3 weeks of pregnancy to adapt the rumen microorganisms to the high-energy ration that will be required for early lactation. The amount of concentrate, however, should not exceed 40 per cent of the total dry matter intake. Grain feeding does not significantly increase the severity of udder edema.[52]

It is important to bring a cow to full feed as rapidly as possible following parturition to avoid excess weight loss and symptoms of ketosis. High-producing cows are often unable to consume enough feed in early lactation to prevent some loss of body energy, calcium, phosphorus, and perhaps protein. These losses are minimized by feeding maximum amounts, within safety limits, of a properly balanced ration during the first 6 to 8 weeks of lactation. After the first 2 months of lactation, milk yields should be used to calculate the energy requirement. NE_L requirements for milk production are directly related to the fat content of the milk. The requirement for 4 per cent FCM is 0.74 Mcal/kg milk produced. Because the efficiency of milk production compares favorably with the efficiency of maintenance relative to energy consumption, energy deficiency will result in weight loss as well as decreased milk production. Consistent gradual weight loss acts as a negative feedback mechanism that interferes with the normal estrous cycle. It is difficult to maintain a calving interval of less than 380 days for adult cows and 400 days for growing heifers.

Energy utilization in ruminant animals depends to a large extent on microbial fermentation in the reticulorumen. The texture and content of ingested feedstuffs dictate the variety of microflora present in the rumen and, therefore, the nature and amounts of microbial metabolites available to the host animal. These metabolites in turn influence the way energy is used (i.e., milk synthesis versus syntheses of body tissue). In general, rations with high roughage content result in higher acetate-propionate ratios and produce more milk fat than diets high in concentrates. Therefore the roughage content (fiber) and the physical form are important considerations in a lactation ration. The roughage content of the dry cow ration can also have serious herd health ramifications. The feeding of high-fiber rations during the dry period reduces the incidence of displaced abomasum and other postcalving disorders. Minimum crude fiber levels of 15 per cent of ration dry matter for heifers and bulls and 17 per cent for lactating cows and 22 per cent for dry cows are recommended.[46] The paradox most commonly encountered when feeding high-producing dairy cows is feeding enough energy *and* enough fiber.

Protein

The 1989 NRC publication for dairy cattle expresses protein requirements as absorbed protein and crude protein.[46] The absorbed protein requirement is expressed on the basis of ruminally undegradable and ruminally degradable intake protein. The number of values available for protein undegradability of feeds is relatively low and, therefore, for the purposes of this discussion, crude protein requirements are used.

Consideration of ruminally undegradable protein is more important for high-producing milk cows[33] and during early rapid growth. The concept of absorbed protein is more fully discussed in the NRC publication on ruminant nitrogen usage.[45]

Using Table 6–3 from NRC,[46] a 600-kg (1320-lb) cow requires daily: 406 g crude protein for maintenance; 1207 g CP for maintenance plus the products of conception during the last 2 months of pregnancy; and 90 g CP/kg of 4 per cent FCM. Thus a 600-kg cow producing 25 kg (55 lb) of 4 per cent milk requires 406 + (25 × 90) = 2656 g CP/day (2656/18,000 = 0.148, or 14.8 per cent of a dry diet of 18 kg).

The protein concentration in milk can be calculated from the fat concentration (per cent protein = 0.4 × per cent fat + 1.9). Thus milk containing 4 per cent fat should contain 0.4 × 4 + 1.9 = 3.5 per cent protein.

Cows may store protein in blood, liver, and muscle tissue. These reserves will be rapidly depleted in late gestation or lactation if the diet is protein deficient. Chronic protein deficiency results in depressed appetite and, thus, concurrent deficiency of energy and other nutrients. The consequences include depressed milk production, loss of condition, and failure to cycle. The protein content of blood, liver, and muscle is decreased in protein-deficient animals. Protein concentration in blood serum can be used to diagnose the condition. Serum from animals having adequate protein nutrition normally contains 3 to 3.5 g albumin, 4 to 5 g globulins, and 10 to 20 mg urea nitrogen/dl. Serum concentrations of less than 2.5 g albumin and 7 mg urea nitrogen/dl are indicative of protein-deficient diets. Pregnant cows on protein-deficient diets will have smaller than normal calves. Reduced levels of transport proteins, immune proteins, and endocrine secretions may predispose animals to infections and metabolic diseases.

Some consideration should be made to avoid substantial dietary protein excesses. Recent studies indicate that protein excess can also have a negative influence on production. A large excess of dietary protein may decrease the energy supply and reduce milk production.[23, 48] Excess protein must be deaminated to ammonia and, for the most part, transformed back into urea for excretion. The energy cost of synthesizing urea and the energy lost in the excretion of that urea were probably responsible for reduction in milk production in the aforementioned references.

Several reports suggest that feeding excessive protein decreases reproductive performance.[21, 33, 55] In one study in lactating cows, serum luteinizing hormone was directly related to protein feeding and serum progesterone was inversely related to protein feeding.[30] Another report noted that cows with blood urea of greater than 20 mg/dl at breeding were three times less likely to conceive.[25] In a study where workers examined vaginal fluid urea levels, they observed that these levels were related to dietary protein levels. Furthermore, when vaginal fluid urea levels exceeded 40 mg/dl, no cows conceived.[20]

Alert downer syndrome and other metabolic disturbances were observed at an increased rate in a group of cows when the protein concentration was increased from 8 to 15 per cent using soybean meal in the dry period.[32]

The use of urea and other nonprotein nitrogen (NPN) substances in dairy cow rations is quite limited. It is feasible to use NPN to increase crude protein concentrations up to 12.6 per cent for an all-corn grain ration or up to 9.4 per cent for an all-corn silage ration.

If a 600-kg cow consumes 16.8 kg DM/day of an all-corn ration containing 33 per cent corn grain and 67 per cent corn silage and this ration is supplemented with urea to give a urea fermentation potential (UFP) value of 0, the nutrient analysis includes:

NE_L = 29.1 Mcal (will support production of 26 kg 4 per cent FCM)*

CP = 10.5 per cent (will support production of 15.1 kg 4 per cent FCM)†

If milk production and, thus, energy intake are increased, the protein deficiencies of this ration become greater. Thus it would appear that the use of NPN to supplement the rations of cows producing more than 25 kg (55 lb) milk is not practical. If preformed protein supplements or alfalfa is used in significant amounts, the UFP of the total ration will be negative and NPN supplementation will be ineffective. Using Iowa State University criteria, practical use of urea should not exceed 1.18 per cent of total dry matter for an all-corn grain ration. This recommendation is compatible with the 1978 NRC recommendation that urea should not exceed 1 per cent of the ration dry matter.[44]

Minerals

Dairy cows are generally fed mixtures of high-quality roughage and concentrations in amounts necessary to meet substantial production objectives. Mineral deficiencies that are likely to occur include those of calcium when corn ensilage composes the bulk of the forage ration, phosphorus when milk production exceeds about 25 kg milk/cow/day, and magnesium when the cow is producing milk. The unsupplemented ration can probably be depended on to supply the maintenance need.

The calcium requirement for maintenance of mature lactating cows is assumed to be 4 g/100 kg BW. Each kilogram of 4 per cent FCM contains an average of 1.2 g calcium. The calcium content of milk is positively related to the level of protein. Because of the relationship between milk fat and protein, the calcium requirement is expressed in relationship to milk fat percentage. For example, the requirement for production of 4 per cent FCM is 3.2 g calcium/kg milk. Calcium deposited during gestation is low until the last 2 months of pregnancy. About 75 per cent of total fetal calcium is deposited in this period. The requirement for maintenance plus the last 2 months of gestation of mature dry cows is approximately 6.5 g/100 kg BW.

The amount of calcium that is absorbed and, thus, available to the animal is related to an animal's calcium intake, its calcium status and age, the amount of calcium it requires, the chemical form and source of the calcium, and mineral interrelationships. High-fat diets increase fecal calcium losses through the formation of soaps and, thus, increase dietary requirements.

The dietary calcium requirements for maintenance plus milk production in the NRC 1978 edition for dairy cattle were based on 45 per cent availability.[44] The 1989 edition based the dietary calcium requirements for dry pregnant and lactating cows on 38 per cent availability.[46]

The effects of variations in calcium:phosphorus ratios have been overemphasized. Several studies have shown that dietary calcium:phosphorus ratios between 1:1 and 7:1 result in nearly equal performance, provided the animal's phosphorus intake meets its requirement.

Calcium deficiency in dairy cows is manifested by two well-known syndromes:

1. Depletion of calcium reserves in the skeleton results in weakened and fragile bones in mature animals and in rickets in young animals. It is quite common for high-producing cows to lose calcium in early lactation and replace it as production decreases. It is only in extreme cases that significant fragility of bones and decreased milk production occur.

2. Parturient paresis (milk fever) is caused by a disturbance in calcium metabolism. The syndrome is manifested by a marked drop in blood calcium at or near parturition. Calcium intake during the dry period influences the problem. Experimental data indicate that high calcium intake in the dry period aggravates the condition and low calcium intake (8 g/day/450-kg cow) in the last 2 weeks of gestation followed by a calcium-rich diet after parturition tends to prevent the problem. Increasing the quantity of acidogenic minerals in relation to the alkalogenic minerals in prepartum diets also reduces the incidence of milk fever. Some data indicate that the calcium:phosphorus ratio is critical, but other evidence suggests that the absolute calcium level is more important.

The amount of phosphorus absorbed by the animal depends on the source of the phosphorus, the amount of intake, the calcium:phosphorus ratio, intestinal pH, and dietary levels of calcium, iron, aluminum, manganese, potassium, magnesium, and fat. Phosphorus absorption is also dependent on the animal's age. There is an apparent decline in true digestibility of phosphorus relative to increasing age. Experimental data suggest a decline from about 90 per cent digestibility in calves to about 55 per cent in animals weighing over 400 kg.

The 1989 NRC publication for dairy cattle[46] has increased

---
*NRC,[46] recommendation for energy, Table 6–3.
†NRC,[46] recommendation for crude protein, Table 6–3.

the phosphorus requirement by 10 to 22 per cent over the 1978 edition.[44] The requirement for maintenance of mature lactating cows is approximately 2.8 g/100 kg BW. The phosphorus content of milk varies with its fat content. For the production of 4 per cent FCM, 1.98 g/kg milk produced is required in addition to the 2.8 g/100 kg BW for maintenance.

For gestation the requirement is based on slaughter data (a 40-kg calf contains about 300 g phosphorus). About 75 per cent of this deposition takes place in the last 2 months of gestation. The phosphorus requirement for maintenance plus the last 2 months of gestation is 4 g/100 kg BW.

Relative to calcium, plasma phosphorus is not as closely regulated by homeostatic control mechanisms. Thus when inadequate diets are fed, signs of deficiency become evident at an earlier stage than with calcium deficiency. Signs of phosphorus deficiency include increased fragility of bone and anorexia, and blood plasma inorganic phosphorus declines to subnormal levels (below 4 mg/dl). In chronic phosphorus deficiency the animal sometimes develop joint stiffness. Anestrus and low conception rates may be manifested in breeding animals. The phosphorus content of milk does not decline.

The magnesium requirement for lactating cows is about 2 to 2.5 g of available magnesium daily plus 0.12 g/kg milk produced. There are many factors that affect this requirement under practical conditions. It is difficult to select a dietary level that is adequate at all times without having more than is needed part of the time. Since cattle have a good homeostatic control mechanism for eliminating excess magnesium via the urine and relatively poor homeostatic control of mobilizing the skeletal reserves, in the face of deficiency modest errors on the high side are tolerable. The suggested magnesium concentration in the dry diets of lactative cows is 0.2 per cent in cows fed substantially on preserved forages or concentrates, or both. The concentration should be increased to 0.25 to 0.30 per cent in cows fed on lush pasture in cool seasons. Some supplemental magnesium in a readily available form (magnesium oxide) should be supplied in the concentrate or mineral mixture under these conditions. Magnesium toxicity is not known to be a practical problem in dairy cattle.

Magnesium deficiency produces the same syndrome in dairy as in beef cows. It is less likely to occur because substantially more concentrates are fed to dairy cows and conscientious supplementation is more likely to be carried out.

Potassium deficiency is not generally considered to be a practical problem in gestating or lactating cows. As a rule the forage ration contains more than adequate amounts.

It is expected that the sodium, chlorine, and iodine needs will be met by feeding iodized sodium chloride equal to 0.5 per cent of the dry ration. The 1989 NRC recommendation for iodine is 0.6 ppm for the total ration.[46] Iodine toxicosis can manifest when the diet consistently contains 50 to 100 ppm. Herd complaints associated with excessive iodine supplementation include decreased milk production and feed consumption and increased incidence of disease.

Sulfur may be beneficial when significant amounts of NPN are fed. For efficient utilization of urea, a nitrogen:sulfur ratio of 10:1 is suggested.

Vitamins

When high-quality ingredients are fed to meet production objectives, all vitamin requirements are usually met without supplementation. However, there are exceptions.

1. Cows that are kept in the barn all of the time may develop symptoms of vitamin D deficiency.
2. Cows fed less than 3.6 to 4.5 kg (8 to 10 lb) good-quality alfalfa hay may require vitamin A supplementation.
3. There is growing evidence that niacin supplementation (6 to 12 g/day) is of value, particularly in stressed cows, as evidenced by increased feed intake and milk production. The effect my be on microbial protein synthesis and/or reduction of subclinical ketosis in early lactation.[34] It is suggested that supplementation should begin 2 weeks before calving and should be continued for 8 to 12 weeks after calving.

Common Problems

A number of problems related to nutrition continue to plague managers of dairy herds, and better solutions are still being sought.

1. Maintaining a 12- to 13-month calving interval is very difficult for high-producing dairy cows, especially for heifers that are still growing in the first lactation period.
2. The appetites of cows are ordinarily decreased for a short time after parturition. Hypoglycemia and ketosis present special problems. The problems are minimized by adjusting the rumen to concentrate feeds in the last 2 to 3 weeks of gestation.
3. High-concentrate rations tend to propagate lactic acid-producing bacteria. Milk fat content may be lowered by such rations. Finely ground high-quality roughage may cause similar problems. Sodium bicarbonate, magnesium oxide, and/or yeast is commonly fed to lactating cows to prevent the syndrome.
4. Hypocalcemia is a constant problem at or near parturition. Reducing the calcium level in the ration of dry cows in late gestation to deficiency levels (1.1 g/50 kg body weight) while maintaining adequate phosphorus intake is an effective method of preventing milk fever in susceptible cows. This procedure should be undertaken during the last 2 to 4 weeks of gestation. Calcium-rich diets are begun in the immediate postparturient period. The low intake of dietary calcium is believed to stimulate the secretion of parathormone, which catalyzes the formulation of active vitamin D.
5. Grass tetany may occur in cattle grazing rapidly growing succulent pasture or being fed similar green chop. Feeding 28 to 85 g (1 to 3 oz) of magnesium oxide daily in grain or salt will prevent the condition.

Ration Formulation (Adult Lactating Cows)

I. Assumptions:
The energy, protein calcium (Ca), phosphorus (P), salt (NaCl), magnesium (mg), and vitamin A requirements are obtained from NRC,[46] Tables 6–3 and 6–5.
Body weight: 600 kg
Milk production: 25 kg, 4 per cent FCM/cow/day
Dry matter consumption: 18 kg/cow/day
Least-cost nutrients include:
For energy: ground corn 89 per cent DM
For protein: soybean meal (SBM) sol. ext. 89 per cent DM
For roughage (fiber): 60 per cent (DM basis) corn ensilage, 35 per cent DM; 40 per cent (DM basis) alfalfa hay, 89 per cent DM
For Ca and P: dicalcium phosphate
For Na, Cl, and I: iodized No. 4 salt
For Mg: magnesium oxide
Ingredient analysis of dry matter for:
Net energy for lactating cows (NEL): Mcal/kg
Crude protein (CP): g/kg
Crude fiber (CF): per cent
Urea fermentation potential (UFP): g/kg
Ca, P, NaCl, and Mg; per cent of DM

Vitamin A: 1000 IU/kg
II. Needs assessment (daily requirements per cow from NRC,[46] Tables 6–3 and 6–5):
Maintenance: 9.70 Mcal
Lactation: 25 kg × 0.74 Mcal/kg = 18.5 Mcal/28.2 Mcal
Concentration needed in ration dry matter: 28.2 Mcal/18 kg DMI = 1.57 Mcal/kg DM
CP: (406 g for maintenance) + (90 g/kg milk × 25 kg milk) = 2656 g
CF: 17 per cent

Ca: Maintenance: 24.0 g
     Lactation: 3.21 g/kg × 25 kg = 80.25 g
                                    ────────
                                    104.25 g

P: Maintenance: 17   g
     Lactation: 1.98 g/kg × 25 kg = 49.5 g
                                    ────────
                                    66.5 g

NaCl: 0.005 × 18,000 = 90 g
Mg: 0.002 × 18,000 = 36 g
Vitamin A: 49,000 IU

III. Formulation of energy-protein ration (dry matter): Table 3
A. Energy (NE_L):
NE_L concentration in the DM roughage component = (0.6 × 1.59) + (0.4 × 1.25) = 1.45 Mcal/kg DM

NE_L concentration in the concentrate component is estimated to be 1.98 Mcal/kg DM

The Pearson's square is used to determine the relative percentages of the roughage and concentrate components.

1.98   12 parts concentrate percentage = 23 per cent of DM
      ┌──────┐
      │ 1.57 │
      └──────┘
1.45   41 parts roughage percentage = 77 per cent of DM
             ──
             53 parts

18 kg DMI × 77 per cent roughage = 13.86 kg roughage
13.86 kg roughage × 1.45 Mcal/kg DM = 20.1 Mcal from roughage
18 kg DMI × 23 per cent concentrate = 4.14 kg concentrate
4.14 kg concentrate × 1.98 Mcal/kg DM = 8.2 Mcal from concentrate
20.1 Mcal (roughage) + 8.2 Mcal (concentrate) = 28.3 Mcal total
28.3 Mcal ÷ 18 kg DMI = 1.57 Mcal/kg DM

B. Protein (CP):
The total crude protein of the ration will exceed 13 per cent of the dry matter so the total ration UFP will be negative. All of the positive UFP of the corn and corn ensilage will be utilized to synthesize microbial protein.

Total CP available from concentrate (corn):
18 kg DMI × 23 per cent = 4.14 kg corn
4.14 kg × 10 per cent CP = 414 g CP

Total CP available from roughage (ensilage 60 per cent plus alfalfa 40 per cent):
18 kg DMI × 77 per cent = 13.86 kg roughage
13.86 kg × 60 per cent = 8.32 kg ensilage
13.86 kg × 40 per cent = 5.54 kg alfalfa
8.32 kg × 8 per cent CP = 666 g CP ensilage
5.54 kg × 16 per cent CP = + 886 g CP alfalfa
                           1552 g CP roughage
                           + 414 g CP concentrate
                           1966 g CP total ration

CP requirement = 2656 g
Ration CP   = 1996 g
CP deficit   = 660 g

Determine amount of SBM required to meet total ration CP requirement:
660 g/49.6 per cent CP (SBM) = 1.33 kg SBM
Subtract 1.33 kg corn and add 1.33 kg SBM to make up new concentrate mix that contains 32 per cent SBM and 68 per cent corn.

C. Check crude fiber (CF):
8.32 kg ensilage ÷ 18 kg   = 11 per cent
= 46 per cent ration
DM × 24 per cent CF
5.54 kg alfalfa ÷ 18 kg =   = 10 per cent
31 per cent ration DM
× 33 per cent CF
1.33 kg SBM ÷ 18 kg = 7   = 0.5 per cent
per cent ration DM × 7
per cent CF
2.81 kg corn ÷ 18 kg =   = 0.3 per cent
16 per cent ration DM
× 2 per cent CF
Total ration CF   = 21.8 per cent

IV. Formulating mineral–vitamin A ration: Table 4
A. Minerals and vitamins available in energy-protein ration in grams and 1000s of IU
B. Deficiencies:
Calcium, magnesium, and vitamin A are present in adequate amounts.
Deficiency for P: 66.5 − 47.8 = 18.7 g
Deficiency for NaCl: 90 − 10.9 = 79 g
C. Supplements:

Dicalcium phosphate: $\dfrac{18.7}{0.1884}$ = 99 g

NaCl 79 g
Adequate supplementation will best be ensured by adding

$\dfrac{99}{18{,}000}$ = 0.55 per cent dicalcium phosphate and $\dfrac{79}{18{,}000}$

Table 3. FORMULATION OF ENERGY-PROTEIN RATION (DRY MATTER)

Ingredient	NE_Ld (Mcal/kg)	CP (%)	CF (%)	Ca (%)	P (%)	NaCl (%)	Mg (%)	Vitamin A Activity (1000 IU/kg)
Ground corn	2.03	10.0	2	0.03	0.31	—	0.13	1
Soybean meal	1.86	49.6	7	0.36	0.75	0.31 (Na)	0.30	—
Corn ensilage	1.59	8.0	24	0.27	0.20	—	0.28	18
Alfalfa hay	1.25	16.0	33	1.40	0.22	—	0.29	26
Salt	—	—	—	—	—	100	—	—
Dicalcium phosphate	—	—	—	23.7	18.84	2.71	—	—
Magnesium oxide	—	—	—	—	—	—	60	—

CF = crude fiber; CP = crude protein; NE_Ld = net energy for lactation.

Table 4. FORMULATION OF MINERAL–VITAMIN A RATION

Ingredient	Ca (g)	P (g)	NaCl (g)	Mg (g)	Vitamin A Activity (1000 IU)
Corn	0.0003 × 2740 = 0.8	0.0031 × 2740 = 8.5	—	0.0013 × 2740 = 3.6	2.74
Soybean meal	0.0036 × 1400 = 5.0	0.0075 × 1400 = 10.5	0.0031 × 1400 = 10.9	0.0031 × 1400 = 4.3	—
			0.4		
Corn silage	0.0027 × 8320 = 22.5	0.002 × 8320 = 16.6	—	0.0028 × 8320 = 23.3	150
Alfalfa	0.0140 × 5540 = 77.56	0.0022 × 5540 = 22.2	—	0.0029 × 5540 = 16.1	144
Totals	105.9	47.8	10.9	47.3	297

= 0.44 per cent iodized salt to the concentrate component of the ration. Note: the additional 178 mineral (99 g dicalcium phosphate plus 79 g salt) have been ignored in the divisor (18,000 g). The error inserted by this omission is negligible.

V. Final dry matter ration: Table 5.

SOWS AND GILTS

Nutrient requirements for breeding swine are listed in the 1988 NRC publication for swine, Tables 5–3 to 5–7.[60] Nutrient concentrations in various feeds are listed in Table 8 of the NRC publication.

Energy

Energy values are expressed for digestible energy (DE) and metabolizable energy (ME) in kilocalories or megacalories per kilogram of feed and/or per animal per day for various classes and physiologic states. DE values approximate 96 per cent of ME values with some significant variations.

The long-term reproductive efficiency of the sow is best served by minimizing weight and fat loss during lactation. This translates to moderation of weight gains during gestation and adequate feeding during lactation. If pregnant sows are offered feed free choice, they will consume more energy during gestation than they need for maintenance and for the development of the products of conception. The excess will be deposited as body fat and protein. To control weight gain during pregnancy, it is necessary to limit energy intake.

The daily energy requirements for pregnancy include the costs of maintenance, energy required for the deposition of protein and fat in the maternal tissue, and energy requirements of the conceptus. For the first three or four parities, sows should be fed and managed to gain approximately 25 kg throughout gestation.

Increasing feed intake during early gestation does not increase the number of pigs born. In general, an increase in the energy intake of the pregnant sow above 6.0 Mcal DE/day will increase maternal weight gain but will not significantly affect litter size at parturition. Pig birth weights, however, progressively increase when sow energy intake increases during pregnancy. Birth weight increases are seldom significant once the energy intake of sows exceeds 6.0 Mcal DE/day.

The daily energy requirement for intermediate-weight bred gilts and sows is 6.3 Mcal/day.

Energy requirements during lactation include a requirement for maintenance and a requirement for milk production. The daily energy requirement for intermediate-weight lactating gilts and sows is 17.7 Mcal/day.

Protein

The quality of the dietary protein is determined by its ability to supply all of the essential amino acids in adequate amounts and sufficient nitrogen for synthesis of nonessential amino acids. Optimum performance necessitates adequate feed levels of essential amino acids and the appropriate balance of amino acids in feeds. Some variation in crude protein levels is acceptable if these conditions are met.

The NRC requirements for essential amino acids[60] correspond to the requirements for the natural isomer (L) that normally occurs in feeds. Synthetic amino acids composed of other isomers may be used according to their biologic value in relation to that of the natural isomer. DL-Methionine can replace L-methionine completely. D-Tryptophan has a biologic value of about 60 per cent of the L isomer. It is assumed that D-phenylalanine can replace to some extent phenylalanine plus tyrosine, but the efficiency of the inversion is in question. D-Histidine may replace L-histidine to a small extent. Isoleucine, leucine, lysine, threonine, and valine are poorly invertible. Pigs can synthesize arginine to supply about 60 to 70 per cent of their needs. Cystine can supply 50 to 70 per cent of the total need for sulfur-containing amino acids (methionine and cystine), and methionine can supply the entire need in the absence of cystine. Phenylalanine can supply the entire need for phenylalanine and tyrosine.

The nonessential amino acids are either obtained from normal dietary sources or synthesized by using amino groups derived from amino acids supplied in the diet in excess of need.

The protein requirements for pregnant sows and gilts are based on amounts required for satisfactory retention of nitrogen during the late stages of pregnancy. Such amounts must be adequate to support development of a normal litter. Intermediate-weight bred gilts and sows require approximately 230 g CP/day.

Protein requirements for lactation are based on maintenance needs plus amounts required to support the production of 6 kg milk/day. Intermediate-weight gilts and sows require approximately 690 g CP/day for lactation.

Practical swine diets contain between 0.03 and 0.22 per cent of linoleic acid to ensure normal skin condition.

Minerals

Calcium and phosphorus are elements of major importance, and vitamin D is essential for absorption and retention of

Table 5. FINAL DRY MATTER RATION

Ingredient	Percent of DM	DM	As Fed
Ground corn	15.61	2.81 kg	3.16 kg (6.9 lb)
Soybean meal	7.38	1.33 kg	1.49 kg (3.3 lb)
Corn ensilage	46.22	8.32 kg	23.8 kg (52.4 lb)
Alfalfa hay	30.77	5.54 kg	6.22 kg (13.7 lb)
Dicalcium phosphate	0.55	99 g	99 g
Salt	0.44	79 g	79 g

DM = dry matter.

calcium and for normal skeletal development. The phytic acid content of the diet and the level of magnesium intake affect the retention of both calcium and phosphorus. The calcium:phosphorus ratio is less emphasized than formerly, but the most favorable ratio appears to be between 1:1 and 1.5:1. Data on calcium and phosphorus requirements of gestating and lactating sows are limited. In pregnancy the dietary requirement is proportional to the need for fetal growth, reaching maximum levels in the final week of gestation. At recommended levels of dry matter intake, 0.75 per cent calcium and 0.60 per cent phosphorus in the diet are adequate for breeding swine. Current recommendations assume that calcium and phosphorus will be present in forms that are well utilized. In grains, one half to two thirds of phosphorus is in the phytate form. Phytase enzymes in corn and other grains may affect utilization of phytate phosphorus. NRC,[60] Table 6–7, lists phosphorus availability from a variety of plant ingredients. Allowances are made for incomplete utilization of phytate phosphorus in the grain and plant protein portion of the diet. Utilization of phytate phosphorus is influenced by the levels of calcium, vitamin D, zinc, and the pH of the digestive tract.

Sodium, chloride, and iodine requirements are met by feeding iodized salt at a level of 0.4 to 0.5 per cent in the dry diet or by free access to an adequate mineral mixture. Symptoms of salt poisoning occur when intake equals 6 to 8 per cent of the dry diet. As little as 1.0 per cent dietary sodium chloride has produced toxicity signs when water has been restricted.

Cobalt may be a necessary supplement if vitamin B_{12} is limiting. Levels of 0.1 mg/kg of dry diet are often added to swine rations.

Beyond breeding age, natural feedstuffs ordinarily furnish adequate copper for hemopoiesis and other copper-related functions.

Natural feedstuffs usually provide enough iron to supply the needs of swine after the nursing period.

It is suggested that breeding swine diets contain a minimum of 400 mg/kg dry diet of magnesium and a minimum of 10 mg/kg dry diet of manganese.

A deficiency of potassium has not been observed in swine fed natural diets.

Ordinary feeds vary in their content of vitamin E and selenium. Deficiencies may occur in swine fed feed that has been grown on low-selenium soils. Injections of 5 mg sodium selenite or barium selenite every 28 days will prevent symptoms of selenium deficiency. Levels above 5 to 8 mg selenium/kg dry diet are toxic for swine.

Zinc deficiency in swine results in parakeratosis or dermatosis. High levels of calcium increase the zinc requirement. The recommended level is 50 mg/kg dry diet with normal levels of calcium and 100 mg/kg dry diet when excessive calcium is fed.

Vitamins

Any or all of the fat-soluble vitamins may be deficient in natural feedstuffs for swine. Vitamin A requirements can be met by either β-carotene or vitamin A (1 mg β-carotene = 500 IU vitamin A). Bred gilts and sows require 4000 IU vitamin A/kg dry diet. Lactating sows and gilts require 2000 IU/kg dry diet. Except for corn and alfalfa, natural feeds for swine are deficient in vitamin D. The need can be met by feeding vitamin D_2 (irradiated dehydrocholesterol). Unless the pigs are exposed to direct sunlight daily, the diet should be fortified with vitamin D. The listed requirement is 200 IU/kg dry diet daily for gestating and lactating swine. Symptoms of vitamin E deficiency are more likely to develop in sows and gilts fed chiefly on grains grown on soil that is low in selenium. It is suggested that 10 IU of vitamin E/kg dry diet be added to practical swine rations. Symptoms of vitamin K deficiency have been produced by feeding moldy feeds. The symptoms were prevented by feeding 2.0 mg menadione/kg dry diet.

Swine require most of the water-soluble vitamins, but only a few are of practical importance in diets based on natural feedstuffs. Deficiencies of niacin, pantothenic acid, riboflavin, choline, vitamin B_{12}, and possibly biotin may occur in ordinary diets. In practice, identifiable symptoms of a specific deficiency are generally not apparent. The specific natural feeds included in the diet are important in determining whether a deficiency of one or more of these vitamins may occur. Specifics include the following:

1. Niacin occurs in cereal grains in bound form and may be largely unavailable to the pig. Conventional assays may be misleading. The amino acid tryptophan converts to niacin and is important in determining the need and providing a source.
2. Pantothenic acid occurs in practically all feedstuffs but may be present in less than adequate amounts. Calcium pantothenate is the common supplementary source and is frequently marketed as the racemic mixture (DL-calcium pantothenate). Only the D isomer has vitamin activity.
3. 3.5 to 5 mg of riboflavin/kg dry diet are necessary to prevent symptoms of deficiency.
4. The choline requirement is related to the presence of the amino acid methionine. The requirement for bred sows is 2.4 g/day and for lactating sows is 5.3 g/day.
5. Feedstuffs of animal origin contain substantial but highly variable amounts of vitamin B_{12}. Synthesis by intestinal bacteria probably supplements dietary sources. Vitamin B_{12} contains the mineral cobalt, and bacterial synthesis is dependent on the presence of this mineral in the diet. Under some conditions, the reproductive performance of sows has been improved by increasing vitamin B_{12} intake. The response is manifested by an increase in the number and birth weight of pigs. The positive response is not a consistent finding. Biotin is ordinarily synthesized in adequate amounts by intestinal microbes. The vitamin B_{12} requirement for gestation and lactation is 15 μg/kg of dry diet. Vitamin C, thiamine, pyridoxine, and folic acid are generally furnished in adequate amounts by natural feedstuffs or by endogenous synthesis.

Feeding Pregnant Sows and Gilts

Nutrients must be provided for maintenance, normal activity, growth of first-litter gilts and second-litter sows, development of the litter (especially in the last trimester), and nominal gain in the dam (9 to 13.5 kg parity net gain and 23 to 32 kg total gain per gestation).

Feedstuffs commonly used in diets for pregnant sows and gilts include No. 2 yellow corn, ground ear corn, milo grain, oats, barley, solvent-extracted soybean meal, meat and bone meal, alfalfa meal (sun-cured or dehydrated), fish meal, linseed meal, and bulking agents such as ground corn cobs, ground oats, ground oat hulls, and fair- to high-quality alfalfa meal.

Hand feeding and ad libitum feeding are both acceptable practices in the case of gestating swine. The advantages of hand feeding include the possibility of reducing bulk and mixing procedures. Corn, barley, oats, or milo or mixtures of these can compose the major portion of the ration if mixed with appropriate amounts of balanced protein, minerals, and vitamins. The disadvantage of these mixtures is that sows and gilts must be fed individually to control intake. About 1.8 to

2.0 kg air-dry ration is sufficient for bred sows and gilts if properly concentrated and balanced.

If gestating swine are fed in groups, the concentrates must be diluted with bulking agents. Recommended amounts of bulking agents depend on the specific concentrate used: 50 to 60 per cent with ground or cracked corn, milo, or barley; 35 to 45 per cent with ground ear corn; and 25 to 35 per cent with oats.

Commonly used feeds vary widely in essential amino acid, mineral, and vitamin content. No. 2 corn is the basic energy feed. It is low in crude protein but provides a substantial amount of true protein. It provides some vitamin A potency but is practically devoid of calcium. Ground ear corn contains about 20 per cent cob and should be ground through a 6.5-mm (1/4-inch) screen. Milo is similar to corn but has no vitamin A potency. Oats are an excellent dietary component for pregnant swine. Oats can be used as the only grain in a self-fed ration and at levels of up to 15 per cent in hand-fed rations. Barley contains metabolizable energy equal to about 80 per cent of that of corn. It is relatively high in crude protein (12 to 14 per cent) and can supply all or nearly all of the amino acid requirement for pregnant sows and gilts. Barley is very low in calcium and devoid of vitamin A. Solvent-extracted soybean meal (44 or 48.5 per cent protein) is the major source of supplemental protein used to correct the amino acid deficiencies in basic cereal grains.

Meat and bone meal (also meat meal with 55 per cent protein and tankage with 60 per cent protein) is an excellent source of total protein, calcium, and phosphorus. It is variable in vitamin B_{12}, poor in riboflavin and pantothenic acid, excellent in niacin, devoid of fat-soluble vitamins, good to excellent in choline, a desirable, but not essential, component for diets of gestating swine. Meat and bone meal can supply much of the needed calcium and phosphorus to correct deficiencies existing in cereal grains and soybean meal. It may be used as the only source of supplemental protein to barley and as the major source of supplemental protein to corn in hand-fed diets.

Alfalfa meal (sun-cured 17 per cent protein) is a good to excellent source of vitamins except B_{12}. A high-quality product provides significant protein, calcium, and vitamin D. Alfalfa meal may be used in hand-fed diets (10 to 15 per cent) and at levels of up to 45 per cent in self-feeding programs. Fish meal is an excellent source of good to high-quality protein and provides a good to excellent source of calcium and phosphorus. The price, however, is usually prohibitive. Linseed meal may be used in small amounts (3.5 per cent of the dry diet). It improves the laxative nature of the diet but is deficient in lysine.

Feeding levels have some effect on the reproductive performance of sows and gilts. Heavy feeding (flushing just prior to breeding) increases ovulation rates. Heavy feeding just after breeding increases the embryo mortality. Limiting of feed just prior to breeding decreases the ovulation rate, and limiting of feed just following breeding increases embryo survival.

Feeding Sows at Farrowing Time

Farrowing diets should contain at least 12 per cent protein, 0.75 per cent calcium, and 0.60 per cent phosphorus. Vitamin inclusions generally correspond to those used in diets for hand feeding pregnant sows and gilts.

Diets at farrowing time may be of moderate energy content or fairly concentrated. In either case the diet should be somewhat laxative in nature. Wheat bran is a feed of choice for many producers. It contributes bulk to the diet, reduces energy content, and improves the laxative nature of the diet. It generally constitutes from 15 to 25 per cent of the total diet. Wheat bran is relatively high in some B vitamins and phosphorus. It is deficient in vitamin B_{12}, and the niacin content may not be fully available. Linseed meal may be used in lieu of bran to some extent. It provides significant protein and phosphorus. One kilogram linseed meal provides laxative properties equal to 3 kg wheat bran. The farrowing diet should be fed for 4 to 6 days prefarrowing and 5 to 10 days postfarrowing. Intake should be adjusted to the condition of the sow, milk production, and litter size. If sows are confined to farrowing stalls for 3 weeks, it may be advantageous to feed 3 to 5 per cent linseed meal to avoid constipation.

Diets for Lactation

These diets are generally high in energy and contain at least 13 per cent protein, 0.75 per cent calcium, 0.5 per cent phosphorus, and 0.5 per cent salt. Vitamins are included in the same concentrations as in diets for pregnant swine (using the same vitamin premix).

Diets for lactating swine generally do not contain more than 10 per cent ground oats and do not include alfalfa meal, wheat bran, or meat and bone meal. Lactating sows and gilts are usually fed to appetite, but they may be fed to scale to provide adequate nutrients for maintenance and milk production required to support the number of pigs being nursed. Diets fed in the lactation period are often formulated to be acceptable for small pigs. This may be advantageous in training these pigs to consume feed, other than milk, at an early age.

Wheat middlings (shorts) can sometimes be purchased economically in terms of energy and crude protein concentration. They may constitute up to 20 per cent of a total ration.

Common sources of calcium, phosphorus, and sodium chloride are used. It is probably advisable to feed a high-zinc trace mineral salt and the same vitamin premix as that used in the gestation diet.

Lactation diets are generally fed from 3 to 7 days postfarrowing to the end of the lactation period. Feed consumption in terms of energy, protein, minerals, and vitamins is expected to be two and one half to three times the requirement for gestation.

BREEDING EWES

Breeding ewes are kept in a variety of conditions to utilize feeds not readily available to man or other types of livestock. Small flocks (1 to 100 ewes) are often maintained to harvest watercourses, fence corners, woodlots, and crop residues. Larger flocks are maintained on permanent pastures where rainfall is abundant or on irrigated pastures where rainfall is less than adequate, or both. Many purebred breeding sheep are grazed on such pastures, and cured forages (ensilage and hay) are used extensively in winter and early spring. Concentrates are often used on a least cost basis to provide supplementary energy, protein, essential minerals, and vitamins in late gestation and lactation and when stressful environmental conditions dictate. Large flocks of sheep are maintained on western ranges (mountain and desert) on a seasonal basis. Range management in these areas is a unique combination of art and science that has been, and continues to be, studied extensively and that is subjected to stringent regulation on the public lands. There are a number of advantages to sheep husbandry:

1. The stress conditions of late gestation and peak lactation are relatively short.

2. Sheep generally utilize the nutrients in browse more efficiently than do cattle.
3. Sheep are relatively efficient in their utilization of plants growing on rough terrain.
4. Dogs can be used to handle sheep efficiently.

There are also some disadvantages:

1. Sheep are relatively susceptible to predators.
2. Sheep are relatively susceptible to oxalate poisoning, lupine poisoning, and photosensitization.

The best source of information is the 1985 NRC publication for sheep,[109] in which the major nutrient requirements are listed in Table 1 (amounts per animal per day), concentrations of nutrients in diet dry matter in Table 2, and macromineral and micromineral requirements, respectively, in Tables 7 and 8.

Energy

Insufficient energy limits the productive performance of sheep more than any other nutritional entity. Such deficiency results from inadequate intake and overdependence on low-quality feeds. The most important consequences include reproductive failure (particularly during the breeding season), reduced milk production, and short lactation periods. Wool production and quality may be reduced, and the sheep may become more susceptible to internal and external parasites and bacterial infections. Generally energy deficiencies are complicated by deficiencies of protein, minerals, and vitamins. As with cattle, sheep rations that provide adequate energy require only limited supplementation.

1. Metabolizable energy (ME) concentrations recommended in dry diets of farm sheep:
   a. For maintenance and first 15 weeks of gestation: 2 Mcal/kg
   b. For last 4 weeks of gestation and last 4 to 6 weeks of lactation (suckling singles): 2.1 Mcal/kg
   c. For first 6 to 8 weeks suckling singles and last 4 to 6 weeks suckling twins: 2.4 Mcal/kg
   d. For first 6 to 8 weeks suckling twins: 2.4 Mcal/kg
2. Dry matter consumption as percent of body weight:
   a. For maintenance: 1.5 to 2.0
   b. For first 15 weeks of gestation: 1.8 to 2.4
   c. For last 4 weeks of gestation and last 4 to 6 weeks of lactation (suckling singles): 2.2 to 3.2
   d. For first 6 to 8 weeks of lactation (suckling singles) or last 4 to 6 weeks lactation suckling twins: 3.0 to 4.2
   e. For first 6 to 8 weeks lactation (suckling twins): 3.6 to 4.8
3. Metabolizable energy requirements for breeding ewes include:[108]
   a. For maintenance: 98 kcal/(BW)$^{0.75}$ (in kg)
   b. For maintenance plus pregnancy in last 6 weeks of gestation: 1.5 × maintenance for singles
   c. For maintenance plus lactation: 1.3 to 1.4 × maintenance (for singles and for twins: 1.7 to 1.9 × maintenance
4. ME concentrations in ordinary range diets (dry matter) include:[108]
   a. 100 per cent browse: 1.22 Mcal/kg
   b. 100 per cent grass: 2.05 Mcal/kg
   c. 70 per cent browse, 30 per cent grass: 1.47 Mcal/kg
   d. 30 per cent browse, 70 per cent grass: 1.80 Mcal/kg
5. ME concentrations in the dry matter of some ordinary concentrates include:
   a. Corn: 3.31 Mcal/kg
   b. Barley: 3.11 Mcal/kg
   c. Oats: 2.71 Mcal/kg
   d. Soybean meal: 3.00 Mcal/kg
   e. Cottonseed meal: 3.00 Mcal/kg
6. ME concentrations in the dry matter of some ordinary cured forages include:
   a. Alfalfa hay, midbloom, sun-cured: 1.94 Mcal/kg
   b. Praire hay, midbloom, sun-cured: 2.02 Mcal/kg
   c. Corn ensilage, well-eared: 2.49 Mcal/kg

The maintenance requirements of sheep on pasture or range are 10 to 100 per cent higher than those for sheep kept in confinement. The size of the increase depends on the availability of feed and water, the nature of the terrain, and the distance traveled daily.

Protein

Satisfactory production from pregnant ewes (50 to 60 kg) has been realized with a daily intake of 110 to 120 g digestible crude protein (about 9 to 10 per cent of the dry diet). These values are probably minimal in the latter stages of pregnancy for ewes carrying twins. These values are also minimal for optimum wool production unless the diet is relatively high in sulfur-containing amino acids.

Research indicates that protein quality (level and balance of amino acids) is more important than previously thought. The sulfur-containing amino acid methionine is first limiting in microbial protein for both wool production and weight gain. Lysine and threonine may also be limiting. The amount of protein escaping microbial action in the rumen and entering the abomasum intact (bypass protein) can influence the quality of protein that reaches the tissues. Heat treatments and the use of tannic acid or one of several aldehydes to complex proteins and reduce degradation in the rumen have been shown to reduce rumen ammonia levels and increase lamb performance.

Nonprotein nitrogen has limited value in the diets of breeding ewes. Ordinary forage usually carries enough protein to supply maintenance and pregnancy needs. All-grass winter range (crude protein about 5.5 per cent) is an exception. Lactating ewes generally have access to fresh vegetative forage that is adequate in protein for maximum milk production. Nonprotein nitrogen can be utilized in combination with low-quality forage and high-energy supplements that have positive urea fermentation potentials (molasses or corn) for ewes in gestation or lactation. It is recommended that urea constitute not more than 1 per cent of the dry diet.

Symptoms of protein deficiency include reduced appetite and feed intake. The efficiency of total feed utilization is decreased. Reproductive efficiency is impaired, and wool production is decreased in both quantity and quality.

Recommended crude protein levels as a percent of dry diet include:

1. For maintenance: 9.4 per cent
2. For first 15 weeks of gestation: 9.3 per cent
3. For last 4 weeks of gestation or last 4 to 6 weeks of lactation (singles): 10.7 per cent
4. For first 6 to 8 weeks of lactation (singles) or last 4 to 6 weeks of lactation (twins): 13.4 per cent
5. For first 6 to 8 weeks of lactation (twins): 15.0 per cent

Minerals

Fifteen minerals have been determined to be essential for sheep. Major mineral constituents include calcium, phosphorus, sodium, chlorine, magnesium, potassium, and sulfur.

Trace minerals include iodine, iron, copper, molybdenum, cobalt, manganese, zinc, and selenium.

Salt is an almost universal supplement. Range operators commonly provide 220 to 340 g salt/ewe/month. When adding salt to mixed feeds, it is customary to use 0.5 per cent of the dry diet or 1 per cent of the concentrate portion. Salt may be safely used to limit intake of free-choice supplements if adequate water is available. Mixtures containing 10 to 50 per cent salt are commonly used. Trace mineralized salt should not be used for this purpose. Iodized salt is ordinarily used to supply the iodine requirement, especially in iodine-deficient areas.

Most pasture and range forage contains adequate amounts of calcium. Areas where calcium supplement is required on pasture have been reported in Florida, Louisiana, Nebraska, Virginia, and West Virginia.

Mature pasture and range forage in North America are commonly deficient in phosphorus. Sheep are efficient utilizers of phosphorus and recycle considerable amounts through saliva. The phosphorus concentrations of saliva, rumen fluid, and blood serum are related to dietary intake. In some cases sheep recycle more phosphorus per day through parotid saliva than is required in the diet to maintain the body pools. Phosphorus supplementation may be necessary on winter range and is ordinarily supplied by dicalcium phosphate mixed with salt.

Diets that are significantly lacking in calcium or phosphorus, or both, result in abnormal bone development (rickets and osteomalacia). Blood serum levels of calcium below 9 mg/dl and of phosphorus below 4 mg/dl are indicative of deficiencies.

Forage containing 0.06 per cent magnesium is considered to be adequate for sheep. Hypomagnesemia can be a problem in lactating ewes on fresh vegetative forage. Such hypomagnesemia may be accompanied by hypocalcemia and produces symptoms of grass tetany. The need for a continuous supply of magnesium is recognized. The use of intraruminal magnesium alloy pellets (bullets) weighing 30 g has effectively prevented hypomagnesemic tetany in lactating ewes.

Ordinary forage supplies the potassium requirement.

Mature ewes require 0.14 to 0.26 per cent sulfur in the dry diet. Practically all common feedstuffs contain more than 0.1 per cent sulfur, but mature grass and grass hays may not furnish enough for optimum performance. When forages are low in sulfur or when significant amounts of urea are being fed, a sulfur supplement should be fed. Sulfate sulfur, elemental sulfur, or sulfur-containing proteins may be used. Inorganic compounds are generally relatively economical and convenient.

There is no evidence that iron deficiency occurs normally in breeding sheep.

Interactions of copper, molybdenum, and sulfate may produce significant effects on sheep, but the mechanisms involved are obscure. A high molybdenum intake can induce a copper deficiency even when the copper content of forage is quite high. This effect can be prevented by increasing the copper intake. When the pasture provides low intakes of molybdenum, an excess of copper accumulates in the tissues even when the copper intake is moderate. The liver copper concentrations may become very high, and, under certain stress conditions, copper from the liver is mobilized rapidly, increasing the copper content of blood and precipitating a fatal hemolytic jaundice. The disease can be prevented by increasing the molybdenum intake of the animals. These contrasting situations complicate the definition of copper and molybdenum requirements. It is difficult to predict the reactions of animals in any given pastoral situation.

Sheep are very susceptible to copper poisoning relative to cattle, and cattle are much more severely affected than sheep by high molybdenum intake. The dietary concentration of copper should be 7 to 11 ppm of dry matter when molybdenum and sulfate intakes are normal. Merino sheep are less efficient in absorbing copper than are English breeds, and an additional 1 to 2 ppm are recommended. Nutritional copper is adequate in forages over most of the United States. Deficient areas have been reported in Florida and in the coastal plains area of the Southeast. Copper can conveniently be provided by adding 0.5 per cent copper sulfate to the salt ration.

There is some question concerning the role of molybdenum in the diets of livestock. It is believed that molybdenum complexes with copper in the intestine and that copper thus bound is biologically inactive. Research has shown that feeds containing small amounts of molybdenum are more effectively digested and produce more rapid weight gains than do diets not containing molybdenum. An excess of molybdenum in forage in areas of California, Nevada, and England causes diarrhea in sheep. Symptoms become apparent a few days after the sheep are turned on pasture having a high molybdenum content (5 to 20 ppm in the dry diet). If dietary copper levels are below normal, or if sulfate levels are high, molybdenum intakes as low as 1 to 2 ppm may be toxic. Such toxicity is controlled by increasing the dietary copper level by 5 ppm. Complete manufactured feeds in the United States may contain 25 to 35 ppm of copper in the dry matter. These levels of copper can be extremely harmful if the molybdenum levels of the diet are low. An effective treatment for lambs is to drench each lamb daily with 100 mg ammonium molybdate and 1 g sodium sulfate in 20 ml water for a minimum of three weeks. The Food and Drug Administration prohibits the use of molybdenum as a feed additive. Prevention of copper poisoning can often be achieved by eliminating extraneous sources of copper from the diet.

Areas deficient in cobalt have been widely reported in the United States and Canada. Feed or forage containing more than 0.07 ppm in the dry diet has prevented symptoms of deficiency. The recommended intake is 0.1 to 0.2 ppm in the dry diet. A preventive measure suggested for deficient areas is to feed cobalt as cobalt chloride or cobalt sulfate to furnish 12 g cobalt/100 kg salt. Cobalt in excess of 4.5 ppm may be toxic.

Research has shown that 17.4 ppm of zinc in the dry diet are necessary for normal growth of lambs, and 32.4 ppm are necessary for normal reproductive development in ram lambs. Toxic symptoms (reduced feed consumption and gain) are produced when lambs are fed 1 g/kg of diet.

In the northwestern, northeastern, and southeastern parts of the United States, there are extensive areas where the selenium content is below 0.1 ppm in dry forage. This is the level considered adequate for preventing deficiency in sheep. The area between the Mississippi River and the Rocky Mountains produced forage that is in the adequate but nontoxic range. Parts of Wyoming, South Dakota, and Utah produce forage that causes selenium toxicity in farm animals. Selenium deficiency produces serious consequences (reduced growth and white muscle disease) in lamb production. The addition of 26 ppm of selenium as sodium selenite to trace mineralized salt fed free choice to ewes prevents white muscle disease in lambs 2 to 8 weeks of age.

Experimental methods of supplying selenium to sheep include an oral drench, intramuscular or subcutaneous injection, addition to feedstuffs, and application of selenium to the soil. One method is to incorporate selenium in pellets composed of finely divided metallic iron and selenium in a proportion of 10:1. A single pellet in the reticulum has been shown to enhance blood and tissue selenium levels for up to 12 months. The most common method of supplying selenium to deficient lambs is to inject a commercial pharmacologic product containing selenium and vitamin E. Two injections are given: one at birth and one 2 weeks later. The first injection contains 0.25 mg selenium and 68 IU of vitamin E as d-α-tocopherol. The second injection contains 1 mg selenium and 68 IU of vitamin E.

Chronic selenium toxicity occurs when sheep consume seleniferous plants containing more than 3 ppm of selenium over a prolonged period. Toxicity signs include loss of wool, soreness, sloughing of hooves, and marked reduction in reproductive performance. The most practical way to prevent livestock losses from selenium poisoning is to alternate grazing between selenium-bearing and other areas.

Fluorine rarely occurs free in nature, but combines chemically to form fluorides that are toxic in amounts exceeding 60 ppm of fluorine in the dry diet. Forages may be seriously contaminated when grown near manufacturing plants that process minerals containing fluorides. Rock phosphate may contain up to 3 to 4 per cent fluorides and must be defluorinated prior to use for livestock supplementation.

Vitamins

Vitamin deficiencies are not common in breeding sheep fed ordinary diets. Vitamin C is synthesized endogenously. The B vitamins are synthesized in adequate amounts by rumen microflora. Vitamin K_2 is synthesized in large amounts in the rumen. No evidence has been found relating vitamin E deficiency to reproductive failure in sheep. Vitamin D is seldom deficient in sheep on pasture, although the question of adequacy arises if the weather is cloudy for long periods or when sheep are fed indoors. Sheep convert the carotenes to vitamin A with efficiency comparable to that of cattle (1 mg β carotene = 400 to 500 IU vitamin A). Vitamin A values for carotene are lower in the following conditions:

1. When xanthophylls and other carotenes are diluents of β-carotene.
2. When animals are vitamin A deficient.
3. When the diets are of low digestibility.
4. When oxidants are present in the feed, ingesta, or tissues.
5. When goitrogenic agents are present.
6. When the diets are high in phosphorus.
7. When the diets are low in vitamin E.
8. When dietary fat levels are low.

Vitamin A is fat soluble and is stored in the body. It takes about 200 days to entirely deplete liver storage of ewe lambs previously pastured on green plants. It is expected that sheep will perform well on low vitamin A diets for 4 to 6 months if they have grazed on green forage in the normal growing season. Sheep that weigh 32 kg or more and are deficient in vitamin A should receive 100,000 IU by injection, and their diets should be supplemented to provide recommended levels of vitamin A or carotene. Ewes deficient in vitamin A should be given vitamin A orally or by injection prior to breeding. The greatest need is in late pregnancy. NRC vitamin A requirements vary from 2742 IU/kg DM for maintenance to 3306 IU/kg DM for ewes in the last 6 weeks of pregnancy.

Water

Sheep get water from snow, dew, guttation in feed and metabolic water, and by drinking. Voluntary water intake is adjusted to balance body water and is indicative of need. Voluntary water intake is affected by ambient temperature, rainfall, snow, dew coverage, age, breed, stage of gestation, wool covering, respiratory rate, frequency of watering, feed composition, and exercise. Sheep normally drink after consuming feed in a dry lot. In general, water consumption is two to three times dry matter feed consumption. The total water intake to dry matter feed intake ratio (TWI:DMI) increases significantly in late gestation, doubles in the fifth month, and is maintained through the lactation period. Sheep may consume as much as 12 times more water in summer than in winter. On western ranges, snow is often the only source of water in winter. No adverse syndromes result when ambient temperatures are below 21°C.

Frequent watering in summer is sometimes difficult. Watering on alternate days is an acceptable practice when the temperature is below 4°C. Sheep grazing on sagebrush-grass desert range in Utah consumed 2.7 L water/head daily. When they were confined to range growing shadscale, winter fat, or salt brush, their water consumption tripled. The water requirement is increased greatly when sheep graze halogeton (oxalate containing). The increased water consumption enhances the excretion of oxalate and reduces death loss. Breeding ewes can tolerate bicarbonate water in which the total salt concentration is 5000 ppm (0.5 per cent) and chloride water in which the total salt content is 10,000 ppm (1 per cent). Salt concentrations above these levels produce toxicity.

Special Requirements for Range Sheep

The 1975 NRC publication for sheep is the recommended source of information for range sheep (Tables 12, 13, 14, and 16 are especially helpful).[108] Tables 12, 13, and 14 from the 1975 publication are reproduced here as Tables 6, 7, and 8.

A knowledge of the nutritive value of range plants in various stages of growth and the nutrient concentrations according to area is essential to the optimal production of range sheep. Feed intake can be estimated, and balance of nutrients can be evaluated by periodically weighing the animals or assessing the body condition, or both. The cost of activity must also be considered, especially on sparse ranges.

Seasonal functions, including breeding, gestation, and lactation, all present special problems and requirements. Considerable knowledge and careful planning and management are essential to a successful operation.

Research in Utah has demonstrated that range sheep respond to protein, phosphorus, and energy supplements when grazing desert forage in winter. When sheep are required to subsist on forage low in carotene for more than 6 months without intermittent access to green feed, vitamin A supplements are recommended. The intermountain range is deficient in iodine (iodized salt is recommended), but other trace minerals are not known to be deficient. In formulating supplements for range ewes, it is necessary to:

1. Calculate the requirements for metabolizable energy (ME), crude protein (CP), and phosphorus (P).
2. Determine the composition of the forage and estimate the dry matter intake.
3. Compute the deficiencies and formulate the supplement in terms of ME, CP, and P.

A useful working calculation of the diet can be obtained by weighing the percentage of each floral component of the range forage by an index of the animal's preference for each species of forage present. The preferences that have been worked out for sheep are listed in Table 6. This table and Tables 6 and 8 can be used to calculate the nutrient make-up of the diet. The calculations usually include only the estimated forage intake and the energy, protein, and phosphorus concentrations in the forage. When the forage diet has been evaluated, the results may be compared with the sheep's requirements, as illustrated in Table 7. In this table, line 1 states the proposed requirement

Table 6. AVERAGE DEGREE OF UTILIZATION, OR PREFERENCE INDEXES, USED IN CALCULATING A DIET FOR A PARTICULAR SHEEP ALLOTMENT

Plant	(1) Composition of Diet (%)	(2) Preference Index	(3) Plant Composition × Preference Index	(4) Diet* (%)	(5) Mcal ME/kg of Plant†	(6) Mcal ME‡ (7)
Sagebrush, big (*Artemisia tridentata*)	15	40	600	19	1.27	0.241
Sagebrush, bud (*Artemisia spinescens*)	10	20	200	6	2.01	0.121
Saltbrush, shadscale (*Atriplex canescens*)	25	20	500	15	0.88	0.132
Winter fat (*Eurotia* sp.)	24	40	960	30	1.19	0.357
Browse total	74	—	—	70	—	—
Wheatgrass (*Agrophyron cristatum*)	14	40	560	17	2.39	0.406
Galleta (*Hilaria jamesii*)	3	25	75	2	1.31	0.026
Needle and thread grasses (*Stipa comata*)	9	40	360	11	1.65	0.182
Grass total	26	—	—	30	—	—
Grand total	100	—	3225	100	—	1.465§

Sources: Data from National Research Council: Nutrient Requirements of Sheep, 5th ed. Washington, DC, National Academy of Sciences, 1975. Modified from Cook CW, et al: The nutritive value of winter range plants in the Great Basin as determined with digestion trials with sheep. Utah Agr Exp Sta Bull 372, 1954.
*Obtained by dividing each value in column 4 by the total of that column (3255).
†Dry matter basis.
‡Calculated as column 5 times column 6.
§Mcal ME/kg diet.

Table 7. TYPICAL REQUIREMENT, PROBABLE INTAKE, AND DEFICIENCIES FOR 60-kg EWES IN EARLY AND MID-PREGNANCY GRAZING INTERMOUNTAIN WINTER RANGE (100 PER CENT DRY MATTER BASIS)

Line No.		Daily Intake kg	Daily Intake lb	Crude Protein (%)	Metabolizable Energy (Mcal/kg)	Phosphorus (%)
1	Requirement	1.63	3.59	8.5	1.466	0.18
2	If 70% browse and 30% grass as given in Table 6	—	—	9.1	1.47	0.14*
3	If 100% browse	—	—	10.7	1.22†	0.15*
4	If 100% grass	—	—	5.5†	2.05	0.12†
5	If 70% grass and 30% browse	—	—	7.1†	1.80	0.13†

Sources: Data from Table 13, National Research Council: Nutrient Requirements of Sheep, 5th ed. Washington, DC, National Academy of Sciences, 1975 (digestible protein converted to crude protein via Y = 0.929 X = −3.48, where Y = digestible protein and X = crude protein); Cook CW, et al: The nutritive value of winter range plants in the Great Basin as determined with digestion trials with sheep. Utah Agr Exp Sta Bull 372, 1954; and Harris LE, et al: Feeding phosphorus, protein and energy supplements to ewes on winter ranges of Utah. Utah Agr Exp Sta Bull 398, 1956.
*Slightly deficient.
†Deficient.

Table 8. RANGE SUPPLEMENTS FOR SHEEP (DRY MATTER BASIS)*

Feed	Relative Protein Level (%) High	Medium-High	Medium-Low	Low
Barley, grain or corn, dent yellow, grain, grade 2 US, min 54 lb/bu	5	40	75	65
Beet, sugar, molasses, or sugar cane molasses, 48% invert sugar, min 79.5° Brix	5	5	5	5
Cottonseed with some hulls, solvent extracted, ground, min 41% protein, max 14% fiber, min 0.5% fat (cottonseed meal)	66	36	—	16
Soybean, seeds, solvent extracted, ground, max 7% fiber, 44% protein (soybean meal)	10	10	10	10
Urea, technical, 282% protein equivalent	—	—	5	—
Alfalfa, aerial parts, dehydrated, ground, min 17% protein or alfalfa, hay, sun-cured, early bloom	10	5	—	—
Vitamin A (IU/kg)	—	4,000	8,000	8,000
Calcium phosphate, monobasic, commercial	1	1	2	1
Sodium phosphate, monobasic, technical	2	2	2	2
Salt or trace mineralized salt	1	1	1	1
Total	100	100	100	100
Composition†				
Protein (N × 6.25) (%)	33.8	24.3	26.2	17.7
Digestible energy (Mcal/kg)	3.3	3.3	3.3	3.1
Phosphorus (%)	2.0	1.5	0.9	1.2
Carotene (mg/kg)	22.0	10.0	—	—
Vitamin A (IU/kg)	—	4,000.0	8,000.0	8,000.0
Rate of feeding (kg/day)‡	0.1–0.2	0.1–0.2	0.1–0.2§	0.1–0.2§

Source: Reprinted with permission from National Research Council: Nutrient Requirements of Sheep, 6th ed. © 1985 by the National Academy of Sciences. Published by National Academy Press, Washington, DC.
*Feeds mixed and fed in meal or pellet form.
†Molasses and alfalfa hay, sun-cured, early bloom not included.
‡Calculated on as-fed basis for mixing and feeding.
§In emergency situations, up to 0.5 kg may be fed.
gr = grade; mn = minimum; Brix = % solubilized sugar; solv-extd grnd = solvent-extracted, ground; mx = mix; dehy grnd = dehydrated, ground; s-c = sun-cured.

for pregnant ewes under intermountain range conditions. Line 2 indicates that the diet shown in Table 6 is only slightly deficient in phosphorus. Lines 3, 4, and 5 illustrate two basic facts concerning the diets of sheep on intermountain ranges in winter: (1) browse plants are the best sources of protein and phosphorus and are low in metabolizable energy, and (2) the grasses are adequate in energy but are seriously deficient in protein and phosphorus.

Tables 6 and 7 illustrate a basis for intelligent selection of supplements. Examples of physical and chemical composition of supplements are given in Table 8 and are applicable to such corrective measures as are indicated by the forage evaluation, the estimated intake, and the calculated requirements of the sheep. The suggested supplements in Table 8 are only examples and may be modified by availability, costs, and requirements. Feeds listed in Table 8 (and in NRC,[108] Table 16) are listed on a 100 per cent dry basis, and it is necessary to adjust these values to as-fed values in the final computation.

Deficient nutrients may be supplied by increasing ration intake or by using supplements. The normal range of supplementation for breeding ewes is 0.1 to 0.2 kg/day. On a group feeding basis, a rate of 0.1 kg/day is necessary for a practical delivery operation. Rates above 0.2 kg/day will result in reduced intake of range forage.

Supplements to balance diets and provide nutrients during short-term emergencies are added in the form of small quantities of a nutrient or a combination of nutrients. Supplements may be required for energy when forage is covered with snow or to prevent sheep from consuming poisonous plants while being trailed. Except for emergencies, if it is necessary to supplement the sheep with more than 0.2 kg DM/day, the practical value of using the range is questionable. On some public lands, supplementation beyond salt, phosphorus, and trace minerals is prohibited except in emergency situation. There is some danger of seeding range with noxious weeds.

Exceptional skill is required to recognize the physical and nutritional state of the sheep, the range condition, and the need for supplements. Sheep may be divided into flocks on the basis of age, condition, or function to provide an even plane of nutrition according to need. McDonald speaks to the complexities of grazing as follows[105]:

... attention has been drawn to many gaps in our present knowledge of the nutrition of grazing nutrients. It has become clear that a full understanding of the subject cannot be obtained from research on animals handfed in pens; it is necessary to study the many interactions between soil, plant, animal and climate so that the mechanism governing the animal's response within the ecosystem can be elucidated. Knowledge of these mechanisms is essential to permit the effective application of scientific findings to practical husbandry in the pastoral system.

Special Aspects of Nutrition for Breeding Sheep

High-quality forage is more palatable and digestible than low-quality forage and passes through the digestive tract more quickly; hence sheep will consume more high-quality forage than low-quality forage. When sheep are forced to sustain themselves on low-quality forage (low protein, low metabolizable energy, and so on), intake and utilization can be enhanced by adding sources of natural protein or properly formulated nonprotein nitrogen supplements.

There are some advantages to pelleting or cubing forage components of sheep rations, including decreased wastage and convenience in handling and transport. Care must be exercised; parakeratosis (a degeneration of the rumen papilla) may result from feeding pellets, particularly those with a high concentrate content. Breeding animals should not be fed for extended periods on pelleted diets without long or chopped forage.

Flushing is the practice of increasing the nutrient intake of ewes prior to mating. Its purpose is to increase the ovulation rate. Flushing is usually accomplished by providing fresh pastures, supplemental cured forage, or up to 0.25 kg of grain daily. This special feeding begins 2 to 3 weeks prior to, and continues into, the breeding season. Ewes maintained in a high state of nutrition benefit only slightly or not at all from flushing, but thin ewes benefit considerably. Mature ewes respond better than yearlings. Also, flushing is probably more beneficial early and late in the breeding season than during the peak, when ovulation rates are highest.

Early weaning of lambs has some advantages when forage for ewes is limited. Weaning lambs at 5 to 8 weeks of age and feeding them a relatively high concentrate diet in a dry lot is common practice. Weaning ewes from the lambs gradually is a good practice.

Halogeton and greasewood are common poisonous plants that grow in the arid and semiarid regions of the West. They are toxic because of their high content of soluble oxalate (up to 30 per cent). When the oxalate is consumed, it may (1) be degraded by microorganisms, (2) combine with calcium in the rumen, and (3) be absorbed into the blood stream. Intoxication occurs when large amounts are absorbed. Oxalate produces its effect through interference with certain steps of energy metabolism, its affinity for calcium, and its mechanical damage to rumen and kidney tissues as a result of crystal formation. The toxic dose is much lower (about 60 per cent) in a fasted animal, and there is much greater chance that a fasted animal will consume a lethal amount. The lethal dose is increased by about 50 per cent after the animals have been grazing halogeton for 2 to 3 days. This is probably due to increased water intake. Sheep should have access to good feed and water before entering halogeton areas. Supplementing sheep with grain or alfalfa pellets during stress periods of trailing or trucking is a valuable part of management.

Lupine poisoning occurs sporadically in sheep grazing on western ranges, particularly in late summer and fall. The seeds of the plants carry the greatest concentrations of the toxic alkaloids. It is common for sheep to graze on lupine-infested ranges without problems, but occasionally acute and drastic syndromes develop. Mortality rates as high as 50 per cent have been reported. Hungry sheep are particularly susceptible. Prevention is best accomplished by supplementing diets with grain or alfalfa pellets while trailing and avoiding lupine-infested range in late summer and fall, particularly if the range is in poor condition.

Pregnancy disease (ketosis, acetonemia, or pregnancy toxemia) is associated with undernourishment. It occurs in late pregnancy and is more common in ewes carrying twins or triplets. Early symptoms include sluggishness, anorexia, staggering, and nervousness. Advanced symptoms include impaired vision, partial paralysis, and prostration. Ewes that give birth in the early stages generally recover. Pregnancy disease results from a disturbance of carbohydrate metabolism, causing hypoglycemia and acetonemia. Prevention is achieved by assuring adequate feed intake in late pregnancy and avoiding stress. A drench of 200 to 300 ml propylene glycol can be used as an energy source for ewes refusing to eat at the onset of symptoms.

REFERENCES

BEEF CATTLE

1. Chalupa W: Problems in feeding urea to ruminants. J Anim Sci 27:201, 1968.
2. Dunn TG, Ingalls JE, Zimmerman DR, Wiltbank JN: Reproductive

performance of 2 year old Hereford and Angus heifers as influenced by pre- and post-calving energy intake. J Anim Sci 29:719, 1969.
3. Lewis L, Geasler M, Lofgreen G, et al: Bovine nutrition. Preconvention Seminar II, 11th Annual Conference of AABP, Baltimore, MD, 1978.
4. Lofgreen GP, Garrett WN: A system for expressing net energy requirements and feed values for growing and finishing beef cattle. J Anim Sci 27:793, 1968.
5. Moe PW, Flatt WP, Tyrell HF: Net energy values of feeds for lactation. J Dairy Sci 55:945, 1972.
6. National Research Council, Committee on Animal Nutrition: Nutrient Requirements of Dairy Cattle, Washington, DC, National Academy of Sciences, 1971.
7. National Research Council, Committee on Animal Nutrition: Feed Phosphorus Shortage, Levels and Sources of Phosphorus Recommended for Livestock and Poultry. Washington, DC, National Academy of Sciences, 1974.
8. National Research Council, Committee on Animal Nutrition: Nutrient Requirements of Dairy Cattle, 5th rev ed. Washington, DC, National Academy of Sciences, 1978.
9. National Research Council, Committee on Animal Nutrition: Nutrient Requirements of Beef Cattle. Washington, DC, National Academy of Sciences, 1984.
10. National Research Council, Committee on Animal Nutrition: Nutrient Requirements of Dairy Cattle, 6th rev ed, update. Washington, DC, National Academy of Sciences, 1989.
11. O'Kelley RE, Fontenot JP: Effects of feeding different levels of magnesium to dry lot fed, lactating beef cows. J Anim Sci 26:959, 1969.
12. Oltjen RR: Effects of feeding ruminants nonprotein nitrogren as the only nitrogen source. J Anim Sci 28:673, 1969.
13. Pinney DO, Stephens DF, Pope LS: Lifetime effects of winter supplement feed level and age at first parturition on range beef cows. J Anim Sci 34:1067, 1972.
14. Stillings BR, Bratzler JW, Marriot LF, Miller RC: Utilization of magnesium and other minerals by ruminants consuming low and high nitrogen containing forages and vitamin D. J Anim Sci 23:1148, 1964.
15. Swanson EW, Martin GG, Pardue FE, Gorman GM: Milk production of cows fed diets deficient in vitamin A. J Anim Sci 27:541, 1968.
16. Ullrey DE, Covert RL, Wellenreiter RH, et al: Vitamin A injections for wintering beef cows. In Beef Cattle Forage. Research Report 118. East Lansing, Michigan State University, 1970, p. 38.
17. Wiltbank JN: Puberty: the effect of breed and feed. Soc Theriogenol J VII, 2nd ed (reprint), 1976.
18. Wiltbank JN: Influence of nutrition on calf crop. Soc Theriogenol J III, 2nd ed (reprint), 1976.
19. Wiltbank JN, Bond J, Warwick EJ, Davis RE, et al: Influence of total feed and protein intake on reproductive performance in the beef female through second calving. USDA Tech Bull 1314, 1965.

DAIRY CATTLE

20. Carroll DJ, Barton BA, Anderson GW, Grindle BP: Influence od dietary crude protein on urea-nitrogen and ammonia concentration of plasma, ruminal, and vaginal fluids of dairy cows. J Dairy Sci 70(Suppl 1):117, 1987.
21. Chalupa W: Discussion of protein symposium. J Dairy Sci 67:1134, 1984.
22. Clifford AJ, Goodrich RD, Tillman AD: Effect of supplementing ruminant all concentrate and purified diets with vitamins of the B complex. J Anim Sci 26:400, 1967.
23. Danfaer A, Thysen I, Ostergaard V: The effect of level of dietary protein on milk production. I. Milk yield, liveweight gain and health. Research Report No. 492. Copenhagen, Beretning fra Staten, Husdyrbrugs forsog, 1980.
24. Dobson RC, Ward G: Vitamin D physiology and its importance in dairy cattle: a review. J Dairy Sci 57:985, 1974.
25. Ferguson JD, Blanchard TL, Hoshall D, Chalupa W: High rumen degradable protein as a possible cause of infertility in a dairy herd. J Dairy Sci. 69(Suppl 1):120, 1986.
26. Flatt WP, Moe PW, Moore LA: Influence of pregnancy and ration composition on energy utilization by dairy cows. Proceedings, 4th Symposium on Energy Metabolism, Jablonna near Warsaw, Poland. Eur Assn Anim Prod Publ 12:123, 1969.
27. Gullickson TW, Palmer LS, Boyd WL, et al: Vitamin E in the nutrition of cattle. I. Effect of feeding Vitamin E poor rations on reproduction, health, milk production and growth. J Dairy Sci 32:495, 1949.
28. Harris LE, Asplund JM, Crampton EW: An international feed nomenclature and methods for summarizing and using feed data to calculate diets. Utah Agr Exp Sta Bull 479, 1968.
29. Huber JT: Protein and nonprotein nitrogen utilization in practical dairy rations. J Anim Sci 41:954, 1975.
30. Jordan ER, Swanson LV: Serum progesterone and luteinizing hormone in dairy cows fed varying levels of crude protein. J Anim Sci 48:1154, 1979.
31. Jorgenson NA: Combating milk fever. J Dairy Sci 57:933, 1974.
32. Julien WE, Conrad HR, Redman DR: Influence of dietary protein on susceptibility to alert downer syndrome. J Dairy Sci 60:210, 1977.
33. Kaufmann VW: The significance of using special protein in early lactation (also with regard to the fertility of the cow). In Protein and Energy Supply for High Production of Milk and Meat. New York, Pergamon Press, 1982, p 117.
34. Kung L Sr, Gubert K, Huber JT: Supplemental niacin for lactating cows fed diets of natural protein or nonprotein nitrogen. J Dairy Sci 63:2020, 1980.
35. Lofgreen PA, Warner RG: Influence of various fiber sources and fractions on milk fat percentage. J Dairy Sci 53:296, 1970.
36. McGillivray JJ: Biological availability of phosphorus in feed ingredients. Proceedings, Minnesota Nutrition Conference, 1974, pp 15–21.
37. Miller WJ: New concepts and developments in metabolism and homeostasis of inorganic elements in dairy cattle: a review. J Dairy Sci 58:1549, 1975.
38. Moe PW: Energy metabolism of dairy cattle. J Dairy Sci 64:1120, 1981.
39. Moe PW, Flatt, WP Tyrell HF: The net energy value of feeds for lactation. J Dairy Sci 55:945, 1972.
40. Moe PW, Tyrell HF: Estimating metabolizable and net energy of feeds. Proceedings, 1st International Symposium on Feed Composition. Animal Nutrient Requirements and Computerization of Diets. International Feedstuffs Institute, Logan, Utah, 1976.
41. Moe PW, Tyrell HF: Observations on the efficiency of utilization of metabolizable energy for meat and milk production. Univ. Nottingham Nutr Conf Feed Manufact 7:27, 1974.
42. Moe PW, Tyrell HF: The metabolizable energy requirements of pregnant dairy cows. J Dairy Sci 55:480, 1972.
43. National Research Council: Urea and Other Nonprotein Compounds in Animal Nutrition. Washington, DC, National Academy of Sciences, 1976.
44. National Research Council, Committee on Animal Nutrition: Nutrient Requirements of Dairy Cattle, 5th rev ed. Washington, DC, National Academy of Sciences, 1978.
45. National Research Council: Ruminant Nitrogen Usage. National Academy Press, Washington, DC, 1985.
46. National Research Council, Committee on Animal Nutrition: Nutrient Requirements of Dairy Cattle, 6th rev ed. Washington, DC, National Academy of Sciences, 1989.
47. O'Dell GD, King WA, Cook CW: Effect of grinding, pelleting and frequency of feeding of forage on fat percentage of milk production of dairy cows. J Dairy Sci 51:50, 1968.
48. Oldham JD: Protein-energy interrelationships in dairy cows. J Dairy Sci 67:1090, 1984.
49. Owen JB, Miller EL, Bridge PS: A study of the voluntary intake of food and water and the lactation performance of cows given diets of varying roughage content ad libitum. J Agric Sci 70:223, 1968.
50. Ronning M, Berousek ER, Griffith JR, Gallup WD: Carotene requirements of dairy cattle. Okla Agr Exp Sta Tech Bull T-76, 1959.
51. Satter LD, Roffler RE: Nitrogen requirements and utilization in dairy cattle. J Dairy Sci 58:1219, 1975.
52. Schmidt GH, Schultz LH: Effect of three levels of grain feeding during the dry period on the incidence of ketosis, severity of udder edema and subsequent milk production of dairy cows. J Dairy Sci 42:170, 1959.
53. Swanson EW: Factors for computing requirements of protein for maintenance of cattle. J Dairy Sci 60:1583, 1977.
54. Swanson EW, Martin GG, Pardue FE, Gorman GM: Milk production of cows fed diets deficient in vitamin A. J Anim Sci 27:541, 1968.
55. Visek WJ: Ammonia: its effects on biological systems, metabolic hormones and reproduction. J Dairy Sci 67:481, 1984.
56. Ward G, Dobson RC, Dunham JR: Influences of calcium and phosphorus intakes, vitamin D supplement and lactation on calcium and phosphorus balances. J Dairy Sci 55:768, 1972.

SWINE

57. Jurgens MH: Swine feeding guides. In Jurgens MH (ed): Applied Animal Feeding and Nutrition. Dubuque, Kendall/Hunt Publishing, 1974, pp 95–105.
58. Leman AD: Feeding pregnant sows and gilts; feeding sows at farrowing time; diets for feeding during lactation. Soc Theriogenol J VII, 2nd ed, 1976.
59. National Research Council, Committee on Animal Nutrition: The Nutrient Requirements of Swine. 8th rev ed. Washington, DC, National Academy of Sciences, 1979.
60. National Research Council, Committee on Animal Nutrition: The Nutrient Requirements of Swine. 9th rev ed. Washington, DC, National Academy of Sciences, 1988.

SHEEP

61. Armstrong DG, Annison EF: Amino acid requirements and amino acid supply in the sheep. Proc Nutr Soc 32:107, 1973.
62. Asplund JM, Pfander WH: Effects of water restriction on nutrient digestibility in sheep receiving fixed water rations. J Anim Sci 35:1271, 1972.
63. Bailey CB, Hironaka R, Slen SB: Effects of the temperature on the environment and the drinking water on the temperature and water consumption of sheep. Can J Anim Sci 42:1, 1962.
64. Beardsly DW: Symposium on forage utilization: nutritive value of forages

as affected by physical form. 2. Beef cattle and sheep studies. J Anim Sci 23:239, 1964.
65. Bhattacharya AN, Pervez E: Effect of urea supplementation on intake and utilization of diets containing low quality roughages in sheep. J Anim Sci 36:976, 1973.
66. Binns W: Range and pasture plants poisonous to sheep. J Am Vet Med Assoc 164:284, 1974.
67. Bogazoglu PA, Jordan RM, Meade RJ: Sulfur-selenium-vitamin E interrelations in ovine nutrition. J Anim Sci 26: 1390, 1967.
68. Buck WB, Sharma RM: Copper toxicity in sheep. Iowa State Univ Vet 31:4, 1969.
69. Butcher JE: Is snow adequate and economical as a water source for sheep? Nat Wool Grow 60:28, 1970.
70. Calder FW, Nickolson JWG, Cunningham HM: Water restriction for sheep on pasture and rate of consumption with other feeds. Can J Anim Sci 44:266, 1964.
71. Clifford AJ, Goodrich RD, Tillman AD: Effects of supplementing ruminants all concentrate and purified diets with vitamins of the B complex. J Anim Sci 26:400, 1967.
72. Cook CW, Stoddart LA, Harris, LE: Comparative nutritive value and palatability of some introduced and native forage plants for spring and winter grazing. Utah Agr Exp Sta Bull 385, 1956.
73. Cook CW, Stoddart LA, Harris LE: The nutritive value of winter range plants in the Great Basin as determined with digestion trials with sheep. Utah Agr Exp Sta Bull 372, 1954.
74. Coop IE: The energy requirements of sheep for maintenance and gain. 2. Pen fed sheep. J Agr Sci 58:179, 1962.
75. Coop, IE, and Hill, MK: The energy requirements of sheep for maintenance and gain. II. Grazing sheep. J Agr Sci 58:187, 1962.
76. Daniels LB, Muhrer ME, Campbell JR, Martz FA: Feeding heated urea-cellulose preparations to ruminants. J Anim Sci 32:348, 1971.
77. Dewey DW, Lee HJ, Marston HR: Efficacy of cobalt pellets for providing cobalt for penned sheep. Aust J Agr Res 20:1109, 1969.
78. Driedger A, Hatfield EF: Influence of tannins on the nutritive value of soybean meal for ruminants. J Anim Sci 34:456, 1972.
79. Egan DA: Control of an outbreak of hypomagnesaemic tetany in nursing ewes. Ir Vet J 23:8, 1969.
80. Garrett WN, Meyer JH, Lofgreen GP: The comparative energy requirements for sheep and cattle for maintenance and gain. J Anim Sci 18: 528, 1959.
81. Garrigus US: The need for sulfur in the diets of ruminants. In Muth, OH, Olds JF (eds): Symposium: Sulfur in Nutrition. Westport, CT, A.V.I. Publishing, 1970, pp 126–152.
82. Goodrich RD, Tillman AD: Copper sulfate and molybdenum interrelationships in sheep. J Nutr 90:76, 1966.
83. Harris LE, Asplund JM, Crampton EW: An international feed nomenclature and methods for summarizing and using feed data to calculate diets. Utah Agr Sta Bull 479, 1968.
84. Harris LE, Cook CW, Stoddart LA: Feeding phosphorus, protein and energy supplements to ewes on winter ranges of Utah. Utah Agr Exp Sta Bull 398, 1956.
85. Hedrich MF, Elliot JM, Low JE: Response in vitamin B_{12} production and absorption to increasing cobalt intake in sheep. J Nutr 103:1646, 1973.
86. Hinds FC, Mansfield ME, Lewis JM: Early weaning of spring lambs. Ill Res 3:6, 1961.
87. Hogue DE: The nutritional requirements of lactating ewes. In Sheep Nutrition and Feeding (Proceedings of a Symposium). Ames, Iowa State University, 1968, pp 32–39.
88. Holter JA, Reid JT: Relationships between the concentrations of crude protein and apparently digestible protein in forages. J Anim Sci 18:1339, 1959.
89. Hopkins LL Jr, Pope AL, Baumann CA: Contrasting nutritional responses to vitamin E and selenium in lambs. J Anim Sci 23:674, 1964.
90. Huisingh J, Gomez GG, Matrone G: Interactions of copper, molybdenum and sulfate in ruminant nutrition. Fed Proc 32:1921, 1973.
91. Hutchings SS: Managing winter sheep range for greater profit. USDA Leaflet 423, Washington, DC, US Government Printing Office, 1958.
92. Investigation Committee Report: Toxemic jaundice of sheep. Phytogenous chronic copper poisoning. Aust Vet J 32:229, 1956.
93. James LF, Butcher JE, VanKampen, KR: Relationship between Halogeton glomeratus consumption and water intake by sheep. J Range Manage 23:123, 1970.
94. Jensen E, Klein JW, Rauchenstein E, et al: Input-output relationships in milk production. USDA Tech Bull 815, 1942.
95. Jensen R: Diseases of Sheep. Philadelphia, Lea & Febiger, 1974, pp 246–247.
96. Joyce JP, Blaxter KL, Park C: The effect of natural outdoor environments on the energy requirements of sheep. Res Vet Sci 7:342, 1966.
97. Klosterman EW, Bolin DW, Buchanan ML, Dinusson WE: Protein requirements of ewes during breeding and pregnancy. J Anim Sci 12:451, 1953.
98. Kromann RP, Joyner AE, Sharp JE: Influence of certain nutritional and physiological factors on urea toxicity in sheep. J Anim Sci 32:732, 1971.
99. Langlands JP, Corbett JL, McDonald I, Duller JD: Estimates of the energy required for maintenance by adult sheep. 1. Housed sheep. Anim Prod 5:11, 1963.
100. Langlands JP, Corbett JL, McDonald I, Reid GW: Estimates of the energy required for maintenance by adult sheep. 2. Grazing sheep. Anim Prod 5:11, 1963.
101. Lee HJ, Marston HR: The requirement for cobalt of sheep grazed on cobalt deficient pastures. Aust J Res 20:905, 1969.
102. LeRoy RS, Zelter SZ, Francois AC: Protection of protein in feeds against deamination in the rumen. Nutr Abstr Rev 35:444, 1965.
103. Lillie RJ: Air pollutants affecting the performance of domestic animals. In Agriculture Handbook 380. Washington, DC, Agriculture Research Service, USDA, 1970.
104. Marcilese NA, Ammerman CB, Valsecchi RM, et al: Effect of dietary molybdenum and sulfate upon copper metabolism in sheep. J Nutr 99:177, 1969.
105. McDonald IW: The nutrition of grazing ruminants. Nutr Abstr Rev 38:381–400, 1968.
106. Mitchell HH, Edman M: The fluorine problem in livestock feeding. Nutr Abstr Rev 21:787, 1952.
107. Moir RJ, Somers M, Bray AC: Utilization of dietary sulfur and nitrogen by ruminants. Sulfur Inst J 3:15, 1967–1968.
108. National Research Council: Nutrient Requirements of Sheep, 5th ed. Washington, DC, National Academy of Sciences, 1975.
109. National Research Council: Nutrient Requirements of Sheep, 6th ed. Washington, DC, National Academy of Sciences, 1985.
110. Oltjen RR: Effects of feeding ruminants nonprotein nitrogen as the only nitrogen source. J Anim Sci 29:673, 1969.
111. Pierson RE, Aanes WA: Treatment of chronic copper poisoning in sheep. J Am Vet Med Assoc 133:307, 1958.
112. Purser DB: Nitrogen metabolism in the rumen: microorganisms as a source of protein for the ruminant animal. J Anim Sci 30:988, 1970.
113. Ranhotra GS, Jordan RM: Protein and energy requirements of lambs weaned at six to eight weeks of age as determined by growth and digestion studies. J Anim Sci 25:630, 1966.
114. Rattray PV, Garrett WN, East NE, Hinman N: Efficiency of utilization of metabolizable energy during pregnancy and energy requirements for sheep. J Anim Sci 38:383, 1974.
115. Reid RL: The physiopathology of undernourishment in pregnant sheep with particular reference to pregnancy toxemia. In Brandly CA, Cornelius CE (eds): Advances in Veterinary Science. New York, Academic Press, 1968, pp 163–238.
116. Reis PJ: The growth and composition of wool. 4. The differential response of growth and sulfur content of wool to the level of sulfur containing amino acids given per abomasum. Aust J Biol Sci 20:809, 1967.
117. Ross DB: The effect of oral ammonium molybdate and sodium sulfate given to lambs with high levels of copper concentration. Res Vet Sci 11:295, 1970.
118. Sheepman's Production Handbook, Denver, SID, 1970.
119. Subcommittee on Feed Composition, Committee on Animal Nutrition, National Research Council: United States–Canadian Tables of Feed Composition. Washington, DC, National Academy of Sciences, 1969.
120. Subcommittee on Fluorosis, Committee on Animal Nutrition, National Research Council: Effects of Fluorides in Animals. Washington, DC, National Academy of Sciences, 1974.
121. Subcommittee on Selenium, Committee on Animal Nutrition, National Research Council: Selenium in Nutrition. Washington, DC, National Academy of Sciences, 1971.
122. Tomas FM, Jones GB, Potter BJ, Langsford GL: Influence of saline drinking water on mineral balances in sheep. Aust J Res 24:377, 1973.
123. Torrell DT, Hume ID, Weir WC: Flushing of range ewes by supplementation, dry lot feeding or grazing of improved pasture. J Range Manage 25: 357, 1972.
124. Underwood EJ, Somers M: Studies of zinc nutrition in sheep. 1. The relation of zinc to growth, testicular development and spermatogenesis in young rams. Aust J Agr Res 20:889, 1969.
125. VanSoest PJ: Symposium on factors influencing the voluntary intake of herbage by ruminants: voluntary intake in relation to chemical composition and digestibility. J Anim Sci 24:834, 1965.
126. Weir WC, Torrell DT: Supplemental feeding of sheep grazing on dry range. Calif Agr Exp Sta Bull 832, 1967.
127. Wilson AD, Dudzinski ML: Influence of the concentration and volume of saline water on the food intake of sheep and their excretion of sodium and water in urine and faeces. Aust J Agr Res 24:245, 1973.
128. Wright PL, Pope AL, Phillips PH: Pelleted roughages for gestating and lactating ewes. Wis Agr Exp Sta Res Bull 239, 1962.
129. Young BA, Corbett JL: Maintenance energy requirements of grazing sheep in relation to herbage availability. I. Calorimetric estimates. Aust J Agr Res 23:57, 1972.

Protein Nutrition and Nonprotein Nitrogen

H. H. VAN HORN, PhD

Protein is required in animal nutrition in larger quantity than any other nutrient with the exception of the total quantity of carbohydrates and fats, which are required for energy. Carbohydrates and fats contain many chemically different entities, but they all are metabolized in the body to carbon dioxide and water. Any surpluses are stored as adipose tissue. With protein, on the other hand, a different situation exists. The primary units, amino acids, are used for the synthesis of body or secretory proteins. In addition, amino acids can provide energy, as they are catabolized to carbon dioxide, water, and a nitrogenous residue that must be excreted. Thus protein metabolism is more complex than that of either carbohydrate or fat, which are both concerned mostly with energy transfer.

Proteins are large molecules of connected amino acids with molecular weights ranging from 35,000 to several hundred thousand. Since protein is the principal constituent of the organs and soft structures of the animal body, a liberal and continuous supply is needed in food throughout life for growth and repair of tissues. It is also a significant part of important animal products, for example, eggs, milk, and the fetus. Transformation of food protein into body or product protein is a very important part of the nutrition process. In order to be utilized by an animal, protein must be broken down by digestion into its constituent amino acids. Proteins from various sources have different combinations of amino acids. The generalized chemical structure of an amino acid is

$$\begin{array}{c} H\quad H \\ \diagdown\;\diagup \\ N \\ | \\ R-C-C-O-H \\ | \quad\;\; \| \\ H \quad O \end{array}$$

R represents different carbon chains with varying lengths and configurations. Some amino acids can be made within the body from other compounds, but others can be made only by plants and bacteria.

For more than a century it has been known that proteins differ in nutritional value. The variation in nutritional value of proteins for nonruminants has been shown to be due to differences in amino acid content. In ruminants, nutritional value is related to a combination of amino acid content and ability of the protein to escape degradation within the rumen.

Amino acids that cannot be manufactured by the animal's metabolism in adequate amounts are termed "essential amino acids." Simple-stomached animals require dietary sources of these amino acids. Animal nutrition research has identified dietary requirements for most limiting amino acids for poultry and swine. In ruminants, protein researchers now are concerned with whether amino acids delivered from the rumen to the lower intestine for final digestion and absorption satisfy optimum performance requirements. Ruminant research is concentrating on how to get "bypass" protein or specific amino acids through the rumen most efficiently to meet these requirements.

Those amino acids that are essential to the animal and are needed in the diet because the animal body cannot synthesize them fast enough to meet its requirement are

Phenylalanine	Isoleucine	Leucine
Valine	Methionine	Lysine
Threonine	Histidine	Glycine
Tryptophan	Arginine	(for poultry)

Fortunately a ruminant like the cow has billions of microorganisms in its rumen that are capable of synthesizing proteins for themselves from amino acids and nonprotein nitrogen (NPN) derived from the cow's diet. These microbial proteins subsequently are digested and absorbed by the cow, giving her a source of all essential amino acids, even though her initial diet may not have contained adequate amounts. Therefore protein quality is not of as much importance to the ruminant as it is to simple-stomached animals. Cows eating purified diets with all of the nitrogen in the form of urea and ammonium salts not only have survived and maintained themselves but have produced as much as 4500 kg milk in a year and reproduced normally.[11]

These experiments demonstrate that ruminants can live without any preformed protein in their rations so long as nitrogen is available to ruminal microorganisms for protein synthesis. However, the level of milk production is not high by today's standards, indicating that rumen synthesis of amino acids cannot totally meet optimum performance needs of ruminants. Growth has also been enhanced in rapidly growing ruminants by "true protein" supplementation in addition to nonprotein nitrogen.

Of possible detriment to ruminants is the degradation of much (60 per cent is common) dietary true protein in the rumen to peptides, amino acids, and ammonia by microorganisms. Ammonia is used by many species of microorganisms; however, some require preformed peptides or amino acids to survive. If these are not provided in the diet, some microorganisms may disappear from the rumen, changing the balance of species. The total quantity of protein synthesized may thus be altered. There may be a reduction in microbial protein synthesis if ammonia concentration is low, that is less than 8 mg nitrogen/100 ml. When rumen ammonia concentration is low, nonprotein nitrogen may be used as efficiently as protein nitrogen.

The meaning of the term "an essential dietary amino acid" should not be misunderstood. Physiologically all amino acids found in animal tissues are essential. Nonessential amino acids can be synthesized within metabolic pathways of animal cells or by microorganisms in the rumen. However, if optimum animal performance is limited because the animal had to degrade essential amino acids to obtain the amino radicals necessary to synthesize "nonessential" amino acids, then perhaps even the nonessential amino acids become "essential."

Protein (amino acid) deficiencies do not show up as rapidly as deficiencies owing to reduced feed intake (reduced energy intake). However, over time, growth and milk or egg production will be subnormal from protein-deficient diets. Severe protein deficiencies will reduce growth rate in both the fetus (resulting in small animals at birth) and the young animal. Deficiencies of essential amino acids in the diet result in subnormal growth even though there may be an excess of other amino acids available. Restricted growth or limited body stores of protein may also affect production later in life.

ANALYSIS OF FEED FOR PROTEIN

In common with fats and carbohydrates, proteins contain carbon, hydrogen, and oxygen. In addition, they contain a large and fairly constant percentage of nitrogen. Most proteins also contain sulfur, and a few contain phosphorus and iron. Since proteins are unique in containing a large amount of nitrogen (about 16 per cent) while other major nutrients contain no nitrogen, "crude protein" is generally calculated by multiplying the analyzed nitrogen content by 6.25. This figure is derived from the estimated 16 per cent nitrogen content (100/16 = 6.25). This procedure is based on an assumption that is only approximately true. Proteins vary in nitrogen content between 15 and 18 per cent. If precise estimates of protein content are to be made from nitrogen analyses, it is more accurate to multiply by a factor specific for the type of protein if it is known to deviate from 16 per cent. Proteins of nonlegume plant origin show the greatest deviation from 16 per cent, averaging about 17.5 per cent nitrogen. Milk proteins, on the other hand, average only 15.5 per cent. Meat, egg, and fish proteins, and those of legume plant seeds, average 16 per cent nitrogen. Most modern tables of human foods give protein values calculated using the specific nitrogen content for their protein. Tables for animal feeds normally assume 16 per cent nitrogen in the proteins.

Another factor to be considered in protein calculations is that not all nitrogen is a part of protein. Some feeds, particularly green roughages, contain one third or more of their nitrogen as nonprotein nitrogen substances, such as amides, ammonium salts, amino acids, alkaloids, and other nitrogenous compounds. Because of nonprotein nitrogen, multiplication of nitrogen content by 6.25 does not give a true protein content. Crude protein values represent a combination of true protein and nonprotein nitrogen. For ruminant animals that can make use of some nonprotein nitrogen, crude protein is often as good a measure for protein allowances as true protein. Although nonruminants cannot use nonprotein nitrogen, ingredients with appreciable nonprotein nitrogen are not usually part of their diet. Thus estimating protein content of dietary ingredients from analyzed nitrogen content is common for nonruminants too.

DIGESTION AND ABSORPTION OF PROTEINS IN NONRUMINANTS

The biologic availability of dietary proteins is affected by the ability of an animal to digest them to their constituent amino acids, to absorb these amino acids, and to utilize them in the body to synthesize new proteins. Proteins must be hydrolyzed into the constituent amino acids before they can be absorbed. An exception is that some newborn mammals are capable of absorbing certain milk proteins intact during the early hours of life to obtain passive immunity to various diseases.

Protein digestion begins in the stomach in nonruminants with denaturation by hydrochloric acid followed by peptic digestion, which is active at low pH (2.1). Pepsin is an endoenzyme that acts within the peptide chain and cleaves bonds adjacent to an aromatic amino acid. It results in production of large peptides and relatively few free amino acids. In the duodenum several pancreatic enzymes (trypsin, chymotrypsin, carboxypeptidase) act to free individual amino acids by cleaving terminal acids from peptide chains. Smaller peptides are absorbed directly into the intestinal mucosa, where hydrolysis to amino acids is completed by peptidases. No peptides appear in portal blood, indicating that hydrolysis is complete before absorption is complete. Absorption is an active process, similar to that of glucose, in which the cotransport of sodium is involved.[7]

After absorption, which is usually sporadic owing to the interval between meals, amino acids are carried by the blood stream to the liver. The liver synthesizes proteins, supplies amino acids to the circulation when needed, and processes excess nitrogen for excretion. Many chemical reactions take place in protein metabolism within the liver and other tissue cells. Transamination permits the exchange of ammonia from an amino acid to the keto moiety of an alpha keto acid. The ammonia can be transferred through glutamic acid to other chemical structures for synthesis of nonessential amino acids. Deamination reactions are similar to transamination except ammonia is released and is shunted through the urea cycle en route to excretion as urea via the urine. In avian species uric acid is formed instead of urea. After ammonia is removed from excess amino acids (essential or nonessential), the remaining keto acid can be metabolized via the tricarboxylic acid cycle for energy.

Amino acids resulting from absorption or transamination move through the blood to various cells dedicated to the synthesis of specific proteins; for example, to build muscle, milk protein, and egg protein and to replace protein in dead cells. The protein mass of the body is in a continuous state of flux, with tissues constantly being catabolized and resynthesized. As amino acids are released they become available to the general amino acid pool and can either be reused for protein synthesis or be utilized as a source of energy.

Aside from total dietary amino acid content, digestibility of dietary protein is the most important variable affecting the quantity of amino acids absorbed. Research by animal nutritionists on protein digestibility has been extensive. Digestible protein is usually defined as the amount of crude protein consumed minus the crude protein excreted in the feces. In actuality this should be called apparent digestible protein rather than true digestible protein. This is because part of the nitrogen in feces is in the form of metabolic fecal nitrogen. Metabolic fecal nitrogen is not affected by the type of protein consumed; it arises from metabolic functions in the gut, such as residues of bile and other digestive proteins, epithelial cells, and undigested bacterial residues. The amount is primarily dependent on dry matter intake rather than protein intake.

Because metabolic fecal nitrogen is independent of the amount of protein consumed, it contributes a larger proportion of the total fecal nitrogen when low-protein feeds are fed than when high-protein diets are fed. Thus failure to account for metabolic fecal nitrogen artificially reduces digestibility coefficients for low-protein feeds. Since it is very difficult to separate metabolic fecal nitrogen from truly undigested feed nitrogen, and since both represent losses to the animal, digestible protein has come to be synonymous with apparent digestible protein. Some researchers have taken an alternative approach and convert apparent digestibility to estimated true digestibility based on the fact that metabolic fecal nitrogen is proportional to dry matter intake, that is about 2 mg metabolic fecal nitrogen produced per gram of dry matter intake. In avian species it is easier to obtain estimates of metabolizable protein (total nitrogen consumed minus nitrogen in feces and urine) than of digestible protein since kidney excretions containing uric acid and fecal contents are excreted as one intermixed product.

Although the digestibility of proteins from different sources is variable, most proteins are digested to the extent of 75 to 80 per cent unless some inhibitory factor exists that protects the protein from attack by enzymes. Some common inhibitory factors include the presence of protease inhibitors and heat damage to the protein. For example, soybeans contain at least four proteins that inhibit trypsin or chymotrypsin activity (trypsin inhibitors and hemoglutinins). The presence of antitrypsin factor reduces protein digestibility in nonruminants and results in hypertrophy of the pancreas and a reduction in the available energy of the feed.[7] The hemoglutinins agglutinate erythrocytes in vitro, reduce amylase activity, and also cause a severe growth depression. Most other beans contain similar antinutritional factors. Ruminants are not affected, as the rumen fermentation renders the factors ineffective. Heat treatment inactivates these factors.

In the case of commercial production of soybean and other oilseed meals, proper heat treatment is routine. However, if overheating occurs, the protein may be denatured so severely that enzymes cannot attach to cleave the protein. This reduces digestibility drastically, and most of the protein is lost in the feces. Although not usual, nutritional troubleshooting often uncovers ingredients where heat damage has been excessive. Heat damage may need to be checked more often in byproducts other than oilseed meals, such as distiller's dried grains, brewer's dried grains, corn gluten feed, and whey. With ruminants, haylage (high dry matter silage) sometimes gets so hot during the ensiling fermentation that the forage protein becomes heat damaged and digestibility is reduced.

If the correct balance of amino acids is not available to animal tissues for maintenance and productive protein synthesis, the use of absorbed protein is limited by the content of the most limiting amino acid. For example, if absorbed lysine is in short supply, the amount of tissue synthesis of a particular protein will be governed by the available lysine. Other essential amino acids present over and above the amount that can be used with the lysine will then be used as an energy source and the waste nitrogen excreted in the urine. This situation leads to poor performance and low feed efficiency.

In practice an animal normally consumes proteins from several sources in any given meal. Thus the inadequacies of a poor-quality protein in a single ingredient are apt to be balanced out by other proteins of higher quality from other ingredients. In ruminants degradation of dietary protein by rumen microorganisms and synthesis of microbial protein also compensates for poor-quality dietary protein. Supplementing diets with well-digested protein supplements and proper quantities of the limiting amino acid(s) optimizes the efficiency of protein utilization by monogastric animals.

DIGESTION AND ABSORPTION OF PROTEINS BY RUMINANTS

One major difference of ruminants as compared with nonruminants is that they can conserve nitrogen during protein-deficient periods. Nitrogen is recycled through urea secreted into the saliva and is delivered back to the rumen mixed with masticated feedstuffs. In the rumen, urease releases ammonia from urea, and this can be used by microorganisms in protein synthesis. This important mechanism facilitates survival when dietary protein is deficient.

Total tract digestion of true protein does not equate with absorption of amino acids from that protein. Both degradation of dietary true protein and gain of protein synthesized from nonprotein nitrogen by rumen microorganisms occur and have large effects on net quantities of amino acids delivered to the small intestine. Furthermore, a limiting amino acid in the diet does not necessarily mean that amino acid is limiting in the pool of absorbed amino acids, since amino acids from digested microbial cells that passed from the rumen to the small intestine usually supply more than half of absorbed amino acids. Postruminally, protein metabolism is essentially the same as for nonruminants. An abbreviated schematic of crude protein metabolism (true protein plus nonprotein nitrogen) is shown in Figure 1.

Protease activity is quite high in rumen microorganisms, but the proportion of dietary protein that escapes rumen degradation varies tremendously with different dietary ingredients. A major influence is the solubility of protein in the rumen. Heat-denatured proteins that are relatively insoluble resist hydrolysis in the mildly acidic rumen, but most are still readily hydrolyzed by strong acid and pepsin in the abomasum. These proteins have a much higher percentage of their original amino acids absorbed intact from the small intestine than do more-soluble proteins.

Iowa State University researchers were among the first to propose a quantitative model to estimate protein requirements for ruminants in terms of "metabolizable protein," which they defined as the amount of protein (amino acids) absorbed from the gastrointestinal tract.[3] Metabolizable protein is the same as truly digestible protein for nonruminants. Microbial cell growth and protein synthesis are functions of available energy, assuming adequate ammonia is available. Burroughs and colleagues estimated that 0.1044 g microbial protein is formed per gram of total digestible nutrients in the diet (a dietary energy estimate).[3] The feed expense of forming fecal metabolic protein is assumed to be directly related to the quantity of dietary dry matter ingested (15 g protein/kg dry matter).

Table 1 shows estimates of undegraded fractions and of metabolizable protein for a number of common dietary ingredients using Burroughs' equations. Also shown is an estimated urea fermentation potential (UFP), which is an estimate of the potential for protein synthesis from the energy derived from the feedstuff compared with the nonprotein nitrogen released from rumen degradation of the protein. The large negative UFP numbers associated with high-protein feeds show that degradation potential for most ingredients is far greater than potential for protein gain from microbial synthesis. Positive UFP numbers are associated with readily fermented carbohydrate sources.

Table 1 illustrates a number of principles of ruminant protein metabolism. For example, casein (milk protein) is readily soluble and highly degradable within the rumen. Thus although it is a high-quality protein if infused directly into the lower digestive tract, it is similar in value to urea when fed to mature ruminants because of its degradation to amino acids and then to ammonia and volatile fatty acids. Conversely, less-soluble proteins, such as zein (corn protein), may largely escape degradation within the rumen and be digested in the lower digestive system. The value of zein is more dependent on its amino acid composition and the extent of digestion in the lower digestive tract than is the value of a more degradable protein. If proteins escape degradation in the rumen but are of lower quality than microbial protein, little gain is achieved. Ideally, undegraded protein should be fed to supply the limiting amino acids needed to support optimum production by the animal.

The advantage of a metabolizable protein model over crude protein is illustrated in Figure 2, where metabolizable protein intake is shown to have a better relationship to milk yield in dairy cows than does crude protein intake.

Effect of Protein on Dry Matter Intake and Digestibility

Often with high-producing or rapidly gaining cattle, the benefits of supplemental protein have been accounted for through increased voluntary dry matter intake and increased dry matter digestibility.[10] With animals at maintenance level of energy intake, increasing crude protein concentrations beyond 10 to 12 per cent of dry matter has little or no effect on dry matter digestibility. However, with high-producing dairy cows consuming more than 3.0 to 4.0 times maintenance

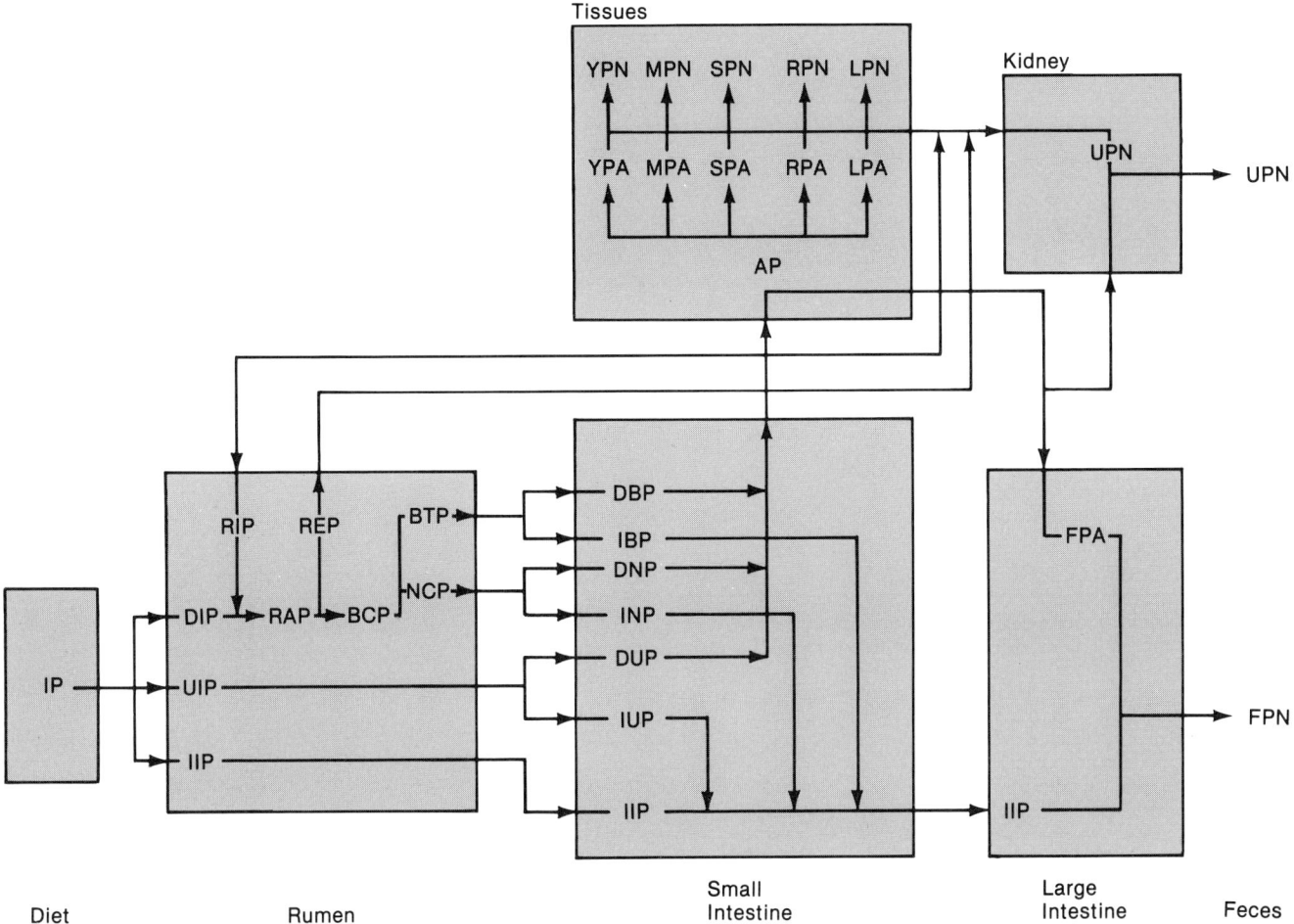

Figure 1. Schematic diagram of nitrogen flow in the ruminant. (From National Research Council: Nutrient Requirements of Domestic Animals No. 3. Nutrient Requirements of Dairy Cattle, 6th ed. Washington, DC, 1988.) BCP = bacterial (and protozoal) crude protein, BTP = true protein; DBP = digestible (true) bacterial (and protozoal) protein; DIP = degraded intake (crude) protein; DNP = digestible nucleic (acid crude) protein (intestine); DUP = digestible undegraded (crude) protein (intestine); FPA = (metabolic) fecal protein (in) absorbed (protein units), FPN = FP net units; IBP = indigestible (true) bacterial (and protozoal) protein; IP = intake (crude) protein; IIP = indigestible intake (crude) protein; INP = indigestible nucleic (acid crude) protein (intestine); IUP = indigestible undegraded (crude) protein (intestine); LPA = lactation protein (in) absorbed (protein units), LPN = LP (in) net units; MPA = maintenance protein (in) absorbed (protein units), MPN = MP (in) net units; NCP = nucleic (acid) crude protein; RAP = ruminally available (nitrogen as) protein; REP = rumen efflux (crude) protein (ammonia if positive, urea influx if negative); RPA = retained protein (in) absorbed (protein units), RPN = RP (in) net units; SPA = surface protein (in) absorbed (protein units), SPN = (in) net units; UIP = undergraded intake (crude) protein; UPN = (endogenous) urinary protein (in) net (protein units); YPA = conceptus protein (in) absorbed (protein units), YPN = conceptus P (in) net units.

energy needs, increasing protein from 11 to 13 per cent of dry matter to approximately 16 per cent of dry matter appears to increase digestibility of dry matter by approximately 4 percentage points. Two important rumen factors that may be influenced by dietary protein, which may affect intake and digestibility, are the retention time of feeds in the rumen and the rate of microbial growth.

Feeding Standards for Ruminants

Minimum recommended allowances for crude protein have been available for all classes of ruminants for many years, with some guidance given on whether supplemental nonprotein nitrogen is useful. More recently standards have been developed using a metabolizable protein model. For example, the 1988 revision of *Nutrient Requirements of Dairy Cattle*, published by the National Research Council (NRC) of the U.S National Academy of Sciences, includes standards for unde-

graded protein and degraded protein.[8] The method estimates total absorbed protein required and then predicts absorbed protein that can be derived from digested bacterial and protozoal crude protein. The difference between total needed and that supplied by bacteria and protozoa is the amount that must be supplied by digested undegraded intake protein. The principles are the same for all ruminants. Examples of steps used by the NRC for dairy cattle follow[8]:

A. Absorbed protein (AP) requirements for milk production or body weight gain are based on estimating net protein in product produced adjusted for assumed efficiency of the use of AP in producing the product. For example, for milk production, NRC assumed the efficiency to be 0.70:

Milk has about 3.3 per cent protein.
AP needed for 40 kg milk   = 40 kg × .033/.70
                           = 1.32 kg/.70
                           = 1.886 kg
                           = 1886 g

Table 1. CALCULATED METABOLIZABLE PROTEIN AND UREA FERMENTATION POTENTIAL

Ingredient	Fractional UP	% of Dry Matter			UFP† (g/kg)
		CP	TDN	Est. MP*	
Ground corn	0.45	10.0	92	10.5	14.6
Wheat	0.30	12.5	92	9.9	3.0
Wheat middlings	0.25	18.7	84	10.0	−18.7
Barley	0.20	13.9	87	8.6	−7.2
Citrus pulp	0.25	6.9	80	7.0	11.2
Cane molasses	0.10	4.3	80	5.9	16.0
Soybean hulls	0.25	12.0	81	8.3	−1.9
Alfalfa hay #1	0.25	20.0	64	8.6	−29.6
Alfalfa hay #2	0.30	15.0	55	7.4	−16.9
Bermuda grass hay	0.25	6.0	48	4.2	1.8
Corn silage	0.30	8.0	72	7.0	6.8
Sorghum silage	0.40	6.2	59	6.0	8.7
Soybean meal (49%)	0.30	54.0	84	20.4	−103.3
Soybean meal (44%)	0.30	49.6	84	19.2	−92.4
Peanut meal	0.25	54.2	80	17.7	−114.9
Cottonseed meal	0.30	44.0	80	17.4	−81.9
Whole cottonseed	0.30	24.9	104	15.3	−23.4
Whole soybean	0.20	41.7	99	14.6	−81.9
Dist. dried grains	0.55	29.8	92	21.2	−13.1
DDGS	0.55	29.5	92	21.1	−13.1
Sunflower meal	0.25	44.1	72	14.7	−91.0
Urea	0	281.0	0	0	0
Casein	0.19	92.7	89	22.1	−234.1

UP = estimated fraction of crude protein that is undegraded in the rumen.
CP = crude protein; TDN = total digestible nutrients; Est. MP = estimated metabolizable protein; UFP = urea fermentation potential in g/kg DM of feed ingredient; DDGS = distillers dried grains plus solubles.
*MP = Burroughs' metabolizable protein,[3] g/kg dry matter (DM) or % = g/kg/10.
$$MP (g/kg\ DM) = [(UP*0.90) + (\{BCP - 15.0\}*0.80)]$$
0.90 = Fraction of undegraded protein truly digested postruminally.
BCP = Bacterial (and protozoal) CP (grams) entering abomasum per kg DM. Estimated to be 0.1044 g MCP/g total digestible nutrients (TDN).
15.0 = Feed expense (g protein/kg DM) of forming fecal metabolic protein
0.80 = Fraction of MCP truly digested postruminally.
†UFP = urea fermentation potential,[3] grams of urea that can be used for microbial protein synthesis per kg of feed ingredient dry matter.
UFP(g/kg DM) = (0.1044*TDNg − DIP)/2.81
0.1044 = Same as described above for MCP.
DIP = Rumen degradable intake protein (g/kg DM) whose ammonia contributes to rumen pool.
2.81 = Urea @ 45% nitrogen has 2.81 times as much nitrogen as an average protein with 16% nitrogen.
Source: Burroughs W, Nelson DK, Mertens DR: J Anim Sci 41:933, 1975.

B. Maintenance crude protein (CP) requirements are based on research measuring endogenous urinary nitrogen excretion in fasting animals and scurf protein lost from the surface of the animal in the form of skin secretions, scurf, and hair. These equations are:

Maintenance urinary CP (g/day) = $2.75 \times$ live weight $(kg)^{0.5}$
For 650-kg cow = $2.75 \times 650^{0.5}$
= 2.75×25.5
= 70.1 g protein equivalent

Scurf CP (g/day) = $0.2 \times$ live weight $(kg)^{0.6}$
For 650-kg cow = $0.2 \times 650^{0.6}$
= 0.2×48.7
= 9.7 g protein equivalent

Maintenance net protein needed = 70.1 + 9.7 = 79.8

Maintenance AP needed if efficiency of use is 0.67 = 79.9/0.67

Maintenance AP (g/day) = 119 g/day

C. Metabolic fecal protein is endogenous debris nitrogen and endogenous water-soluble nitrogen resulting from internal secretions. Expressed in AP units it was assumed to be 0.09 units of AP (for dairy) per unit of indigestible dry matter intake. The NRC committee assumed dry matter digestibility to be 0.67 and, therefore, 0.33 indigested. Thus

Metabolic fecal AP (kg) = $.09 \times$ kg indigestible dry matter

For a 650-kg cow producing 40 kg milk, NRC estimates her dry matter intake to be 22.64 kg

Her metabolic fecal AP (kg) = $0.09 \times 22.64 \times .33$
= 0.09×7.47
= 0.672 kg
= 672 g

D. Total requirements of absorbed protein units for the above functions are 2677 g/day, that is,

Total required AP g = 1886 + 119 + 672 = 2677 g

E. Now we must estimate how the above requirements can be met. The first step is to estimate bacterial and protozoal crude protein (BCP) production and then, by difference, determine how much undegraded intake protein (UIP) must be provided by the diet. BCP production is estimated by NRC as a function of available energy in the rumen assuming adequate nonprotein nitrogen is available. Using Mcal of net energy for lactation (NEL) intake, the equation used to estimate grams of bacterial and protozoal crude protein (BCP) production is

BCP = 6.25 (−30.93 + 11.45 NEL)

For example, the cow described above is estimated to need 37.81 Mcal NEL in the 22.64 kg dry matter consumed. Therefore her total BCP production is estimated to be

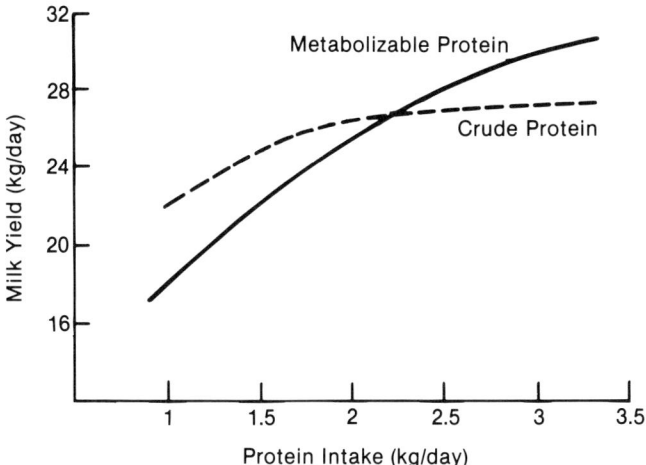

Figure 2. Milk yield response to Burroughs' metabolizable protein intake compared with response to crude protein intake. Both response curves are adjusted to equal feed intake. (Adapted from Briceno JC, Van Horn HH, Harris B Jr, Wilcox CJ: J Dairy Sci 71:1647, 1988.)

$$BCP = 6.25 \, (-30.93 + 11.45 \times 37.81) = 2512 \text{ g}$$

The proportion of BCP to bacterial and protozoal true protein (BTP) is assumed to be 0.80, the remaining being nucleic acid crude protein. The digestibility of BTP is assumed to be 0.80. Thus

$$\text{Absorbed BCP} = 2512 \times 0.80 \times 0.80 = 1608 \text{ g}$$

F. Absorbed UIP needed can now be calculated by difference:

$$\begin{aligned}\text{Absorbed UIP required} &= 2677 \text{ g/day required} - 1608 \text{ g from BCP} \\ &= 1069 \text{ g/day}\end{aligned}$$

If digestion of UIP is 0.80 then

$$\begin{aligned}\text{UIP required} &= 1069/0.80 \text{ g/day} \\ &= 1336 \text{ g/day}\end{aligned}$$

G. The final step of the requirements calculation is to determine the amount of total intake protein (IP) required:

$$\text{IP g required} = \text{UIP g} + \text{degraded protein intake (DIP) g required}$$

Required DIP is the minimum amount of dietary degradable nitrogen necessary for optimum microbial fermentation. NRC designates dietary nonprotein nitrogen and ruminally degraded protein as rumen available protein (RAP). It is estimated that microbial fermentation in the rumen converts 0.90 of the *minimum* RAP to BCP. Therefore

$$BCP \text{ g} = .90 \times RAP \text{ g}$$

For example, in the example shown in E

$$2512 \text{ g BCP} = 0.90 \times RAP \text{ g}$$

or

$$\begin{aligned}RAP \text{ g} &= BCP \text{ g}/0.90 \\ &= 2512 \text{ g}/0.90 \\ &= 2791 \text{ g}\end{aligned}$$

But part of the RAP can be supplied by recycled rumen influx protein coming into the rumen from diffused blood urea and the salivary secretion of urea. NRC estimates rumen influx protein to be 0.15 of total intake protein (IP), which we have not determined yet in our example. Also, the rumen efflux protein has an opportunity to be recycled again. This somewhat dynamic situation was solved algebraically and by assuming that net crude protein delivered to the small intestine equals intake protein so that

$$\begin{aligned}\text{IP g} &= (\text{RAP g} + \text{UIP g})/(1 + \text{influx P/IP}) \\ &= (2791 + 1336)/1 + .15) \\ &= 4127/1.15 \\ &= 3589 \text{ g}\end{aligned}$$

since

$$\begin{aligned}\text{IP g} &= \text{UIP g} + \text{DIP g} \\ 3589 &= 1336 + \text{DIP g}\end{aligned}$$

and

$$\begin{aligned}\text{DIP g} &= 3589 - 1336 \\ &= 2253 \text{ g}\end{aligned}$$

H. In practice it is necessary to evaluate or formulate a ration to determine if it will supply 1336 g UIP and 2253 g DIP in the 22.64 kg of dry matter to be eaten. An alternative often used is to formulate a diet that is estimated to be $1.336/22.64 = .059 = 5.9$ per cent UIP and $2.253/22.64 = 10.0$ per cent DIP and contains the required energy in 22.64 kg dry matter. Estimating dietary UIP involves summing estimated UIP from all diet ingredients.

Ingredient	DM (%)	CP (%)	CP (kg)	UIP Fraction	UIP kg
Corn silage	50.0	8.1	4.05	.31	1.255
Corn meal	22.0	10.0	2.20	.52	1.144
Soybean hulls	6.0	12.1	.73	.25	.182
Whole cottonseed	8.0	23.0	1.84	.35	.644
Soybean meal (49%)	10.9	55.1	6.01	.30	1.802
Mineral supplements	3.1	0	0	0	0
Totals (kg or %)	100.0		14.8%		5.027%

For evaluation let us assume that the following ingredients are being fed with fractional UIP of CP as indicated:

DIP per cent in this diet = CP per cent − UIP per cent = 9.8 per cent. This diet needs more UIP than 5.027 per cent, but it is almost sufficient in DIP. Reformulation should explore the economics of adding additional UIP up to the 5.9 per cent calculated to be needed.

Importance of Amino Acids for Ruminants

Nutritionists have not yet shown benefits from routine supplementation of ruminant diets with specific amino acids. From analysis of the NRC feeding standards shown previously, it is evident that most of the amino acids absorbed postruminally originate from rumen microbial protein (1608 g versus 1069 g from digested undegraded intake protein in the example). Probably the main reason that amino acid content of the diet is not always of critical importance is that the quality of microbial protein for growth and milk production is relatively good. Thus many diets with amino acid imbalance in the component ingredients can be corrected in large part with the microbial protein. Research continues to try to improve the rumen protein model so that limiting amino acids can be identified and supplemented if possible. We are certain to see changes in the rumen model being used by the NRC in the future. One likely change will be to include factors that base estimated microbial protein synthesis on rumen fermentable organic matter rather than total tract dietary energy such as NEL as used in the BCP equation by the NRC shown previously.

With lactating dairy cows consuming a diet consisting primarily of corn, corn silage, and limited amounts of alfalfa-grass hay, lysine and methionine appear to be the first limiting amino acids. Supplying undegraded intake protein with protein sources known to contain higher amounts of amino acids identified to be critical can increase total absorption of those amino acids.[4] However, we still need better definition of specific amino acid requirements and responses to supplementation of specific amino acids.

NONPROTEIN NITROGEN (NPN) UTILIZATION BY RUMINANTS

NPN is of most concern in protein metabolism in ruminant animals since it is only in ruminants that proteins and amino acids derived from microbial fermentation are made available in large quantities to the host animal. Protein may be synthesized from NPN by microorganisms in the large intestine as well (e.g., in the horse), but protein synthesized here is apparently not available for absorption. It is possible that NPN could be of some benefit for nonruminants if essential amino acids were available at adequate levels but nonessential amino acids were not. Then, with available ammonia and proper carbon structures for transamination, nonessential amino acids might be synthesized in the absence of microbial intervention.

If inadequate ammonia is available to maintain rumen nitrogen levels of 8 to 10 mg nitrogen/100 ml, not only will microbial protein synthesis be depressed but digestion of organic matter will also be reduced. Reduction in cellulose digestion is most critical. Associated with reduced digestibility will be a reduction in dry matter intake. The combined effects will greatly inhibit animal production.

Urea is by far the major feed additive used to supply NPN to rumen microorganisms. The major justification for feeding NPN is economics. Generally a reduction in feed costs and increased profits have resulted from inclusion of as much NPN in ruminant rations as possible without depressing growth. In many rations, 3.2 kg shelled corn and 0.45 kg urea are equal in net energy and crude protein to 3.6 kg soybean meal. With this kind of comparison, the projected savings depends directly on the price of soybean meal, urea, and corn.

Complete substitution of NPN for protein in purified diets for ruminants has shown that animals do not perform as well as when some natural protein is provided; growth and feed efficiency are reduced. Ruminants fed diets free of protein have depressed concentrations of branched-chain volatile fatty acids. They also have depressed free blood plasma concentrations of essential amino acids and increased concentrations of glycine and serine. Ruminal synthesis of B vitamins is normal, and cattle raised on purified diets from 84 days of age to 4 years of age have been fertile and reproduced normally. Also, moderate milk production (up to 4500 kg/cow yearly) has been obtained. Benefit from urea supplementation in diets requiring more than 12 per cent crude protein is unlikely because degraded intake protein is then great enough to supply needed crude protein for optimum microbial growth. Ammonia accumulates after microorganisms stop increasing their growth rate.

The metabolizable protein model represented in feed values in Table 1 can be used to estimate when there is a positive urea fermentation potential (UFP). If the estimated synthesis of microbial protein exceeds the estimated amount of degraded protein, then bacteria in the rumen will not have enough ammonia available from protein breakdown to grow optimally. Thus there is a potential to use some urea (positive UFP). The amount depends on the ingredients. For corn (92 per cent total digestible nutrients [TDN], 10 per cent crude protein, and 45 per cent undegraded protein; DM = dry matter):

Microbial protein	= 0.1044 g/kg TDN × 920 g TDN/kg DM = 96.0 g/kg DM
Rumen degraded	= 100 g CP/kg DM × 0.55 = 55.0 g degraded/kg DM
Net g from rumen	= 196.0 g − 55.0 g = 41.0 g/kg DM
Net g nitrogen (N) converted	= 41.0 g protein × 0.16 = 6.56 g N/kg DM
UFP = g urea @ 45% N to supply 5.9 g N	= 6.56/0.45 = 14.6 g/kg DM

Therefore corn, being high in energy and low in rumen-degraded protein, is a good ingredient with which to add urea. A mixture of 1 kg ground corn and 14.6 urea would give a mixture of 14.1 per cent crude protein (100 per cent dry basis). With most mixed diets for ruminants there rarely is a positive benefit from adding urea to diets above 11 or 12 per cent crude protein (100 per cent dry basis). For example, the estimated UFP for 15 per cent crude protein alfalfa hay (55 per cent TDN, 30 per cent undegraded protein) is − 16.9 g urea/kg DM. Combining 1 kg corn with 1 kg hay gives −2.3 g UFP for the mixture: [14.6 g urea + (− 16.9 urea)] = −2.3 g urea for 2 kg DM. Thus there is more than enough rumen ammonia available from the crude protein in alfalfa hay to maximize microbial protein synthesis in the rumen. Urea's main potential dietary benefit is with fattening and some growing diets for ruminants where relatively low dietary protein percentages are required.

Palatability

Concentrates containing over 2 per cent urea result in depressed feed intakes for cattle, even in animals adapted to urea diets. Lower urea levels (1 to 1.5 per cent) can cause feed intake problems when fed as part of high-moisture (>14 per cent) concentrates. This is probably because of partial hydrolysis of urea to ammonia. This can present serious problems when urea-containing feeds are held in storage during warm, humid weather. Adding molasses to diets with high levels of urea improves intake in some cases but not others. Addition of urea to corn silage effectively alleviates palatability problems, probably because ammonia released from urea during ensiling is converted to ammonium salts and also because silage acids mask the taste of urea. Urea should not give palatability problems if it is incorporated at or less than 1 per cent of total ration dry matter or 1.5 per cent of the concentrate portion.

Reproductive Performance

For many years some veterinarians and cattle growers have suggested that feeding rations containing NPN compounds such as urea lower conception rates of cattle. In a Michigan survey of over 600 dairy herds involving 85,281 individual cow lactations and 3157 year-herd observations, no reduction in calving interval was found in herds that were fed urea.[9] Urea was fed in 1709 of the 3157 herd-years, with an average intake per cow of 81 urea/day. This and many other studies show that urea per se is not detrimental to reproduction. Feeding high levels of protein has nearly the same effect on blood urea nitrogen levels as feeding urea. In several recent experiments it has been suggested that feeding protein above 18 per cent of total diet dry matter interferes with reproductive performance. Excess ammonia from either protein or urea at critical tissue sites may interfere with conception. If this is the case, total dietary nitrogen level (crude protein), and particularly total rumen degradable crude protein, will better predict the possibility of tissue ammonia excess. A review of a number of experiments by Ferguson and Chalupa concluded that a high level of dietary protein, particularly highly degradable protein, contributes to poor reproductive performance.[5]

Although detrimental effects of protein on reproduction have been reported with diets where protein was approximately 20 per cent of total diet dry matter, the studies certainly are not conclusive at this point. Two of the studies with the greatest cow numbers did not find that high protein was detrimental to reproduction; milk yield was increased with high protein in both studies (e.g., Howard et al.[6]).

One theory explaining the possible negative impact of high protein is that high intakes may cause excessive ammonia or urea nitrogen concentrations in the reproductive tract leading to a less than optimal environment for conception. Alternatively, high systemic or local urea nitrogen concentrations may reduce luteinizing hormone binding to ovarian receptors on luteal cells, leading to a decrease in progesterone concentration and fertility.[12]

It is good judgement to try to feed a nutritionally balanced ration and to manage feed offerings in such a way as to keep blood levels of urea nitrogen from peaking higher than necessary without compromising the feeding program for optimum milk and meat production. Thus with good management of the sequence and frequency of feeding the desired ingredients, feeding for optimum animal performance still seems compatible with the feeding program necessary for good reproduction.

Relationship to Possible Nitrate Toxicity

Neither logic nor experiment supports the notion that urea and nitrate are additive in their toxic effects. Although both are simple nitrogenous compounds, they are quite different in their physiologic action. Nitrate accumulates in plants grown on soils high in nitrogen, mainly in hot weather, following frosts, or during drought. The nitrogen content of nitrates is relatively small and only a very small proportion is reduced to ammonia. Conversely, oxidation of ammonia to nitrite, which would aggravate a nitrate toxicity, is highly unlikely because the rumen is a reducing environment.

Ammonia Toxicity

It is well known that dietary urea, if consumed in large quantities in a short time, can be toxic. In a Kansas experiment, cattle were dosed with 0.5 g urea/kg body weight, which was added through a rumen fistula.[1] In approximately one half of the cases signs of toxicity were seen. Most of these occurred within 60 minutes of dosing (average time 52.8 minutes). In toxic cases, blood ammonia nitrogen (29 mg/L blood) and rumen pH (7.41) were elevated 60 minutes after dosing.

Signs of toxicity include uneasiness, dullness, muscle and skin tremors, excessive salivation, frequent urination and defecation, rapid respiration, incoordination, stiffness of the front legs, prostration, tetany, and death. Muscle tremors followed by muscle spasms were the most frequently observed symptom (all 125 toxic cases). Bloat was never observed. As tetany became severe, most animals lost muscular coordination and became prostrate. When tetany became severe, any loud noise, such as talking, slamming doors, or dropping metal objects, caused a violent involuntary contraction of the muscles (convulsions), characterized by stiffening of the fore and hind legs.

A common recommendation for treatment has been to inject acetic acid intraruminally. Cattle given approximately 1 mol acetic acid (5 per cent v/v)/mol nitrogen administered to induce toxicity usually showed improvement if it was administered prior to time of tetany. Emptying the rumen contents of animals in severe tetany brought about survival in all animals treated in this way. Following rumenotomy the cattle were left in a quiet place, and signs of tetany would usually cease after about 30 minutes. Respiration and heart rate would also return to normal. After about 60 minutes the animals would stand and appear normal. For severe field cases emergency rumenotomy should be performed and rumen contents evacuated rapidly. In their studies, Bartley and associates added about 4 L warm water to the rumen when the animal stood and appeared normal.[1] Recovery was dramatic, and rumen fermentation was good 48 hours after the experiment.

Ammonia toxicity is not a major concern in relation to utilization of NPN if standard recommendations are followed. Toxicity is only associated with consumption of high levels of urea (over 44 g/100 kg body weight) in a short period by unadapted cattle. Mistakes such as animals breaking into urea supplies or into areas where feed was inadvertently spilled and miscalculation of the intended feeding levels are sometimes found as causes of toxic situations.

Bovine Bonkers Syndrome

Ammoniation of forages to help increase dry matter digestibility and reduce molding is sometimes recommended. However, ammoniation of high-quality forages such as alfalfa, sorghum-Sudan, rye, wheat, oats, brome, or fescue hays may produce 4-methyl imidazole, a toxic compound. Clinical signs from toxicosis from feeding hays containing 4-methyl imidazole (Bovine Bonkers syndrome) include hyperexcitability, wild running, circling, convulsive seizures, and death. The same syndrome has been seen when feeding large amounts of ammoniated molasses.

REFERENCES

1. Bartley EE, Davidovich AD, Barr GW, et al: Ammonia toxicity in cattle. I. Rumen and blood changes associated with toxicity and treatment methods. J Anim Sci 43:835, 1976.
2. Briceno JV, Van Horn HH, Harris B Jr, Wilcox CJ: Comparison of different methods of expressing dietary protein for lactating dairy cows. J Dairy Sci 71:1647, 1988.
3. Burroughs W, Nelson DK, Mertens DR: Protein physiology and its application in the lactating cow. J Anim Sci 41:933, 1975.
4. Clark JH, Murphy MR, Crooker BA: Supplying the protein needs of dairy cattle from by-product feeds. J Dairy Sci 70:1092, 1987.
5. Ferguson JD, Chalupa W: Impact of protein nutrition on reproduction in dairy cows. J Dairy Sci 72:746, 1989.
6. Howard HJ, Aalseth EP, Adams GD, et al: Influence of dietary protein on reproductive performance of dairy cows. J Dairy Sci 70:1563, 1987.
7. Maynard LA, Loosli JK, Hintz HF, Warner RG: Animal Nutrition, 7th ed. New York, McGraw-Hill, 1979.
8. National Research Council: Nutrient Requirements of Domestic Animals No. 3. Nutrient Requirements of Dairy Cattle, 6th ed. Washington, DC, National Academy of Sciences, 1988.
9. Ryder WL, Hillman D, Huber JT: Effect of feeding urea on reproductive efficiency in Michigan Dairy Herd Improvement Association Herds. J Dairy Sci 55:1290, 1972.
10. Van Horn HH, Zometa CA, Wilcox CJ, et al: Complete rations for dairy cattle. VIII. Effect of percent and source of protein on milk yield and ration digestibility. J Diary Sci 62:1086, 1979.
11. Virtanen AI: Milk production of cows on protein-free diet. Science 153:1603, 1966.
12. Visek WJ: Ammonia: its effects on biological systems, metabolic hormones, and reproduction. J Dairy Sci 67:481, 1984.

New Concepts for Measuring Proteins for Cattle

JOHN C. SIMONS, DVM
MICHAEL S. HAND, DVM, PhD, Diplomate, ACVN

Proteins are essential components of both plants and animals. They are necessary to the structure of all cells of all animals. They constitute basic portions of all enzyme systems, antibodies, and part of the hormones. Plasma proteins are necessary to maintain osmotic pressure and water balance. They also assist in the blood clotting process. There are vast numbers of different proteins. Each has a specific structure that permits a specific function.

Proteins are essential in the diets of all animals except those that harbor a microbial population in the digestive tract that is capable of synthesizing proteins from nonprotein nitrogen and energy nutrients.

The levels of dietary protein required by young growing animals are high relative to those of mature animals. The processes of gestation and lactation include protein deposition and thus increase the dietary requirements. If carbohydrates and fats are in short supply, proteins will be metabolized to produce energy. The amino acid components will be deaminated, and the excess nitrogen will be incorporated into urea by the liver. The urea thus produced will be eliminated in urine or recycled to the digestive tract. When energy requirements are met by carbohydrate and fat, excess protein will be deaminated and the energy-containing portions will be incorporated into fat.

Structurally proteins are long polymers of alpha amino carboxylic acids combined by peptide linkages. Each alpha amino acid has a carboxyl group bound to an adjacent (alpha) carbon. The alpha carbon contains an amino group and a specific R group (Fig. 1). There are about 20 different R groups that occur naturally. The R groups differentiate and identify the individual amino acids. In protein molecules the amino group of one amino acid is combined with the carboxyl group of another amino acid to form a peptide bond (Fig. 2).

In synthesis one molecule of water is formed with each peptide linkage formed. Up to 300 amino acids may be linked together in a single molecule of protein. In addition, long polymers of amino acids may link together with hydrogen or disulfide bonds to make sheets and layers of fibrous protein. Also, the protein molecules may be coiled or folded by polar bonds between parts of the molecule. Finally, several protein polymers may be linked to a common chemical entity to make a complex compound such as hemoglobin.

Given access to amino nitrogen and energy nutrients, animals can synthesize most of the amino acids in the cells. Microbial populations maintained in the forestomachs of ruminant animals are capable of synthesizing all of the amino acids if all of the essential elements are available. The amino acids incorporated in the microbial protein are available for digestion and absorption in ruminant animals.

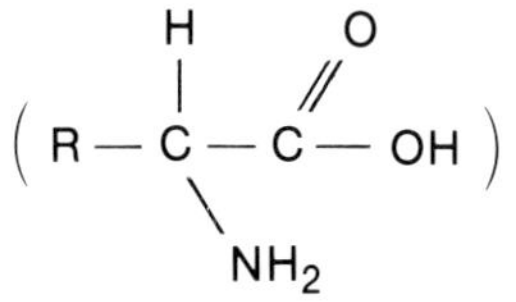

Nine specific alpha amino acids must be present in the diets of monogastric herbivores. These (essential) amino acids cannot be synthesized endogenously by monogastric carnivores or omnivores. Microbial populations in the lower digestive tracts of monogastric herbivores may synthesize all of the amino acids, but microbial protein is not significantly susceptible to digestion and absorption in these animals. These essential amino acids include methionine, threonine, tryptophan, isoleucine, leucine, lycine, valine, phenylalanine, and histidine. Three of the alpha amino acids contain sulfur in the R groups.

Complete protein rations contain all of the amino acids essential to animal nutrition in amounts adequate to meet the maintenance and production requirements of the animal being fed. High-quality food protein is not only complete but contains all of the essential amino acids in amounts proportional to the body's need for them. High quality also implies high digestibility, adsorbability, and utility.

Food protein sources include both animal and plant proteins. Generally the quality of animal protein (eggs, meat, dairy products) is relatively high. All plants contain some protein. Seeds, stems, leaves, and some roots are all potential sources. Combinations of plant proteins using two or more plant sources whose essential amino acid components complement each other may approach animal protein quality.

Commonly used forages (pasture, hay, ensilage) and energy concentrates (grain and tubers) are often deficient in protein required to meet maintenance and production objectives. Feeds classified as protein supplements are used to supply the deficiencies. These are generally high-energy feeds containing more than 20 per cent crude protein. Commonly used plant protein supplements include soybean meal, cottonseed meal, linseed meal, peanut meal, and low-quality beans. Animal-source protein supplements are not widely used in ruminant rations. They are, however, commonly used in poultry and swine rations when the market is favorable. Common animal-source protein supplements include meat meal, fish meal, tankage, and by-products of the dairy industry. Protein supplements formed by combining nonprotein nitrogen compounds with a high-energy carrier (cornmeal-urea) are often used to supplement ruminant rations.

PROTEIN DIGESTION AND ABSORPTION IN MONOGASTRIC ANIMALS

Digestion is the process whereby foodstuffs are taken into the digestive tract and the nutrients are prepared for absorption. The process of digestion begins when food enters the mouth. The food is ground and mixed with saliva. The saliva contains water, mucus, and a starch-splitting enzyme (salivary amylase), which begins to hydrolyze starch. In the stomach the food is mixed with hydrochloric acid, which acts to degrade and separate the nutrients. Also, a proteolytic enzyme precursor is secreted in the stomach. This proenzyme (pepsinogen) is converted by hydrochloric acid into the proteolytic enzyme

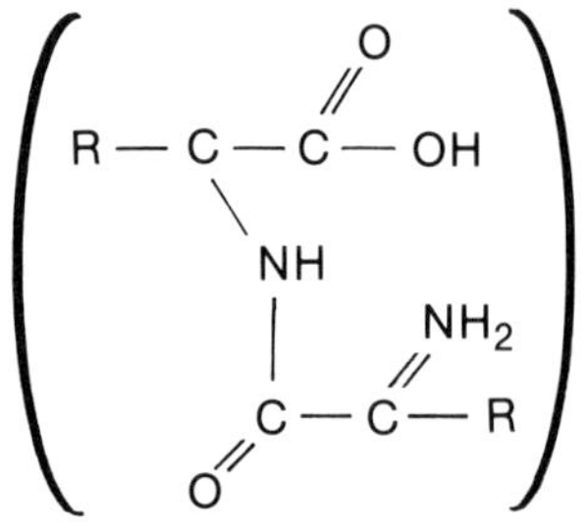

Figure 1. Structure of the alpha carbon.

Figure 2. A peptide bond of a protein molecule.

pepsin, which begins to hydrolyze the food protein into shorter fragments called peptides.

The food passes from the stomach to the small intestine, where it is subject to the pancreatic secretions. These secretions include bicarbonate to neutralize the gastric acid and a number of digestive enzymes, including pancreatic lipase, pancreatic amylase, and three prominent enzyme precursors—trypsinogen, chymotrypsinogen, and propolypeptidase. The trypsinogen is converted by an enteric enzyme, enterokinase, into the active proteolytic enzyme trypsin. Trypsin converts chymotrypsinogen into chymotrypsin and propolypeptidase into polypeptidase. These active proteolytic enzymes hydrolyze proteins and peptides into simple dipeptide molecules. The absorptive cells of the small intestine contain enzymes called dipeptidases that hydrolyze dipeptides into individual alpha amino acids. The amino acids are actively transported or diffused across the absorptive cells and into the capillaries that supply and drain the small intestine. The absorptive surface of the small intestine is multiplied by folds, villi, and the brush borders of the absorptive cells. These structures multiply the absorptive surface of the small intestine about 600 times.

PROTEIN DIGESTION AND ABSORPTION IN RUMINANTS

There are no digestive enzymes in the saliva of ruminant animals. The food is ingested, masticated, and swallowed before significant hydrolysis of complex nutrient molecules begins. The digestive process in the stomach of ruminants differs markedly from that of monogastric animals. The nonglandular portion of the ruminant stomach is very large and is divided into three different compartments, including the rumen, reticulum, and omasum. The rumen and reticulum communicate freely and can be thought of as a single functional entity. This reticulorumen comprises a large fermentation vat that contains a vast and varied microbial population, including bacteria, protozoa, and fungi. A unique symbiotic relationship between the ruminal microbes and the host animal has evolved.

The rumen is not fully developed and functional at birth. Neonate ruminants can be practically regarded as monogastric animals. The rumen becomes functional at 6 to 8 weeks of age, depending on diet. After rumen function is established, the crude protein needs of two systems must be met: nitrogen (crude protein) for microbial protein synthesis in the reticulorumen, and postruminal amino acids for the host animal.[35] The rumen microbes aid in the degradation of cellulytic compounds that are indigestible for monogastric animals. These microbes are also capable of converting nonprotein nitrogen into microbial protein. This microbial protein is utilized by the host animal and furnishes about half of the protein requirements of ruminant animals.[41]

There is general agreement among current investigators regarding the principles involved in the digestion of proteins and proteinaceous materials by ruminants.

1. Degradation in the rumen of a substantial portion of true protein and nonprotein nitrogen substances contained in feedstuffs. The nitrogen content of the degraded material is largely incorporated into ammonia.

2. Bypass or escape of some true protein contained in feedstuffs from the rumen into the lower digestive tract without degradation.

3. Incorporation of ammonia accumulated in the rumen into microbial protein (including synthesis of all of the essential amino acids).

4. Absorption of ammonia not incorporated in microbial protein from the rumen and intestines.

5. Conversion of absorbed ammonia into urea by the liver. Most of this urea is eliminated in urine.

6. Recycling of a portion of the urea synthesized in the liver into the digestive tract via salivary and ruminal secretions.

7. Digestion of bypass and microbial protein in the abomasum and small intestine into alpha amino acids. The abomasum and small intestine of the ruminant are very similar in function to the stomachs and small intestines of monogastric animals.

8. Absorption of alpha amino acids from the small intestine.

ESTIMATING PROTEIN CONTENT IN FEEDS

Protein content in feeds is generally expressed as crude protein (CP). CP is determined by measuring the nitrogen (N) content of the feed and multiplying by 6.25 or dividing by 0.16. Protein is generally considered to contain 16 per cent nitrogen. It is assumed that all of the nitrogen in a feed sample is incorporated in protein, so $CP = N \times 6.25$, or $CP = N/0.16$. The measurement of "apparently digestible protein" is no longer used in National Research Council (NRC) recommendations for beef or dairy cattle. Such computation is dependent on a given value for crude protein and does not improve the accuracy of measuring the protein requirement. Current NRC requirements for protein in beef and dairy animals[35, 38] are derived by factorial methods.[32] The maintenance factors include protein lost in urine (U), fecal material (F), and skin secretions, scurf, and hair (S).[63] The production factors include increase in body weight (G),[35] protein deposited in the products of conception (C),[22] and protein deposited in milk (M or L).[23, 40, 74] The factors for maintenance and production are divided by other factors ($D \times BV \times CE^*$).[35] These factors have been derived from empirical values established by experimentation.

In recent years the accuracy of the factorial method has been called into question. Considerable effort has gone into deriving models and methods to measure metabolizable protein and using them in place of the empirical data that are still in current use.

In November 1980 an international symposium to consider the protein requirements of cattle was held at Oklahoma State University. Current findings concerning protein and nonprotein nitrogen utilization were discussed by a number of experts in the field. The discussions included the presentation of a number of models of nitrogen utilization in ruminants and proposed computations to estimate metabolizable protein requirements in beef and dairy animals.

In his summary of the conference, R. R. Johnson said that "full appreciation of the topics and discussions will come only to those scholars who place the composite information from this conference in perspective with the problems of supplying food and particularly animal protein to a hungry world." He also pointed out that "the role of the ruminant in food production has possibly been debated too often, but even the most casual student of world history and geography will quickly realize that the ruminant was likely one of the first, if not the first, producer of animal protein by domesticated animals and will unquestionably be the one food producing animal which survives the longest in the competition between animals and man for plant foodstuffs."

It was generally expressed at the conference that "traditional systems for calculating ruminant protein requirements are recognized to be of limited value," and that "it is clear that the traditional use of crude protein and digestible protein must

---

*D = digestibility; BV = biologic value; CE = conversion efficiency from rumen to small intestine.

be modified to reflect the intervention of rumen microbes in the digestive process and to recognize the contribution of endogenous nitrogen and microbial residues to the fecal output."

Our primary objective in this article is to illustrate the models and systems that are being designed, studied, and modified to enable a more practical approach to protein utilization. The objectives of these designs, studies, and modifications include the following:

1. Refinement of concepts of biologic happenings.
2. Providing to those associated with food production (producers, allied industries, and extension specialists) a more precise way to perform their tasks.
3. The end result: a system that adequately enables the formulation of ruminant rations before they are fed.

The models and systems outlined at the conference included:

1. Empirical Value of Crude Protein Systems for Feedlot Cattle, R. L. Preston, Washington State University.
2. The Metabolizable Protein Feeding Standard, Allen Trenkle, Iowa State University.*
3. A Metabolizable Protein System Keyed to Ammonia Concentration—The Wisconsin System, Larry D. Satter, University of Wisconsin.†
4. A Net Protein System for Cattle: The Rumen Submodel for Nitrogen, P. J. Van Soest, C. J. Sniffen, D. R. Mertens, D. J. Fox, P. H. Robinson, and U. Krishna Moorthy, Cornell University.‡
5. Foreign Systems for Meeting the Requirements of Ruminants, D. R. Waldo and B. P. Glenn, USDA and University of Maryland.
6. Nebraska Growth System, Terry Klopfenstein, Robert Britton, and Rick Stock, University of Nebraska.
7. Michigan Protein Systems, J. C. Waller, R. Black, and W. G. Bergen, Michigan State University, and D. E. Johnson, Colorado State University.

All of the systems are based on the common assumptions listed earlier. We have selected and outlined three of these systems: the Iowa State System, the Wisconsin System, and the Cornell System. We do not imply superiority for these systems, but they are representative of current thinking and we are limited for space.

The Iowa State System

The use of urea as a source of dietary nitrogen in cattle is extensive. There is a definite need for improving methods of expressing protein requirements of cattle. The Iowa State System outlines a concept that expresses these protein requirements as metabolizable protein (MP).[6] The system also expresses the capacity of a ration to benefit from urea supplementation as the urea fermentation potential (UFP).

Since microbial protein is formed from nonprotein nitrogen (NPN) and energy nutrients, utilization is dependent on (1) the amount of nitrogen in the feed that is reduced to ammonia in the rumen and (2) the amount of digestible energy nutrients that are available in the rumen.

The relationship between the ammonia and the total digestible nutrients (TDN) in the rumen is expressed as the UFP in grams of urea per kilogram of dry matter feed. If the available energy nutrients in the rumen exceed the amount required to convert the entire rumen ammonia pool to microbial protein, the UFP is positive. If there is insufficient energy to convert the entire ammonia pool to microbial protein, the UFP is negative.

---
*The Iowa State System.
†The Wisconsin System.
‡The Cornell System.

Definitions necessary to understand the concept include the following:

1. Degraded protein is that portion of protein or NPN in a feed from which all of the nitrogen (100 per cent) will be reduced to ammonia in the rumen.
2. Undegraded protein is that portion of protein in a feed that is not degraded or digested in the rumen. This portion of protein will not be affected by rumen fermentation but will be digested into amino acids in the abomasum and small intestine. It is sometimes called bypass protein.
3. Microbial protein is the dietary protein incorporated in the cells of the rumen microbes. For a specific feed, microbial protein equals 0.1044 TDN if the UFP is negative, or 100 per cent of the degraded protein if the UFP is positive.
4. The UFP expressed in grams of urea per kilogram of dry matter: $(11.78\ NE_m + 6.85) - (0.0357\ CP \times DEG)$, where NE_m = net energy for maintenance (Mcal/kg); CP = crude protein per cent in the DM; and DEG = degraded protein per cent. The UFP can also be expressed as

$$\frac{(0.1044\ g\ TDN/kg\ DM) - g\ degraded\ protein/kg\ DM}{2.8^*}$$

The Metabolizable Protein Model (Fig. 3)

By way of explanation:

1. Feeds vary in degradability from 52 to 95 per cent.
2. The portion of TDN that will be available for microbial protein synthesis is 10.44 per cent. It is the product of the assumed percentage of TDN digested in the rumen (52 per cent) multiplied by the percentage of TDN used in microbial synthesis (25 per cent) multiplied by the efficiency factor (80 per cent): $0.52 \times 0.25 \times 0.8 = 0.104$.
3. Escaped or bypass protein is assumed to be digested into amino acids and absorbed with an efficiency of 90 per cent.
4. Fifteen grams fecal CP (2.4 g N)/kg DM feed is assumed to be lost from the total microbial protein production. Eighty per cent of the remaining microbial protein is assumed to be digested into amino acids and absorbed.
5. Thus metabolizable protein per kilogram dry matter feed is

$$(P_1 \times 0.9) + ([P_2 - 15][0.8])$$

where P_1 = g bypass protein/kg DM feed, P_2 = g microbial protein produced/kg DM feed, and 15 = microbial protein lost in fecal material/kg DM feed.

6. Estimates of protein degradation and microbial protein passage from the rumen and the digestion coefficients for bypass and microbial protein and fecal protein losses are based on
   a. data published in the literature (various sources),
   b. feeding trials with young growing cattle,[6]
   c. analysis of postruminal digesta by several laboratories,
   d. average true digestion of undegraded feed protein in monogastric species (various sources), and
   e. studies of protein digestibility in sheep.[28]

Feed Analysis

Data concerning feed concentration ingredients pertinent to metabolizable protein computations are listed in Table 1.

---
*2.8 is the crude protein equivalent of urea. Protein contains 16 per cent nitrogen, and urea contains about 45 per cent nitrogen; thus 45/16 = 2.81.

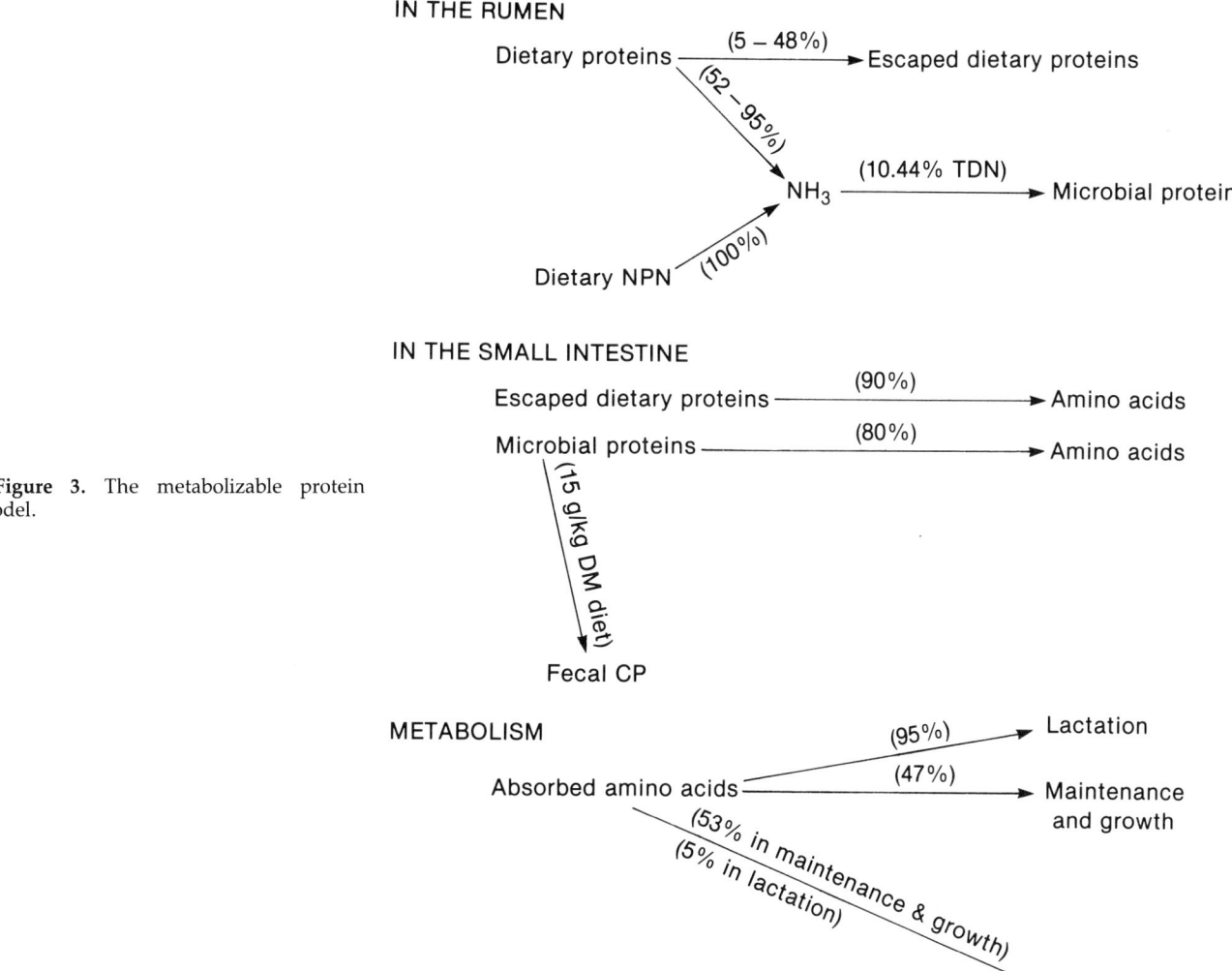

Figure 3. The metabolizable protein model.

Table 1. METABOLIZABLE PROTEIN AVAILABLE FOR BODY PURPOSES PLUS UREA FERMENTATION OF FEEDSTUFFS

			Abomasal Protein		Rumen			
Feed	TDN (% DM)	CP (% DM)	UDG (g/kg DM)	MCB (g/kg DM)	Prot (% DM)	Deg (g/kg DM)	Met Prot (g/kg DM)	UFP (g/kg DM)
Alfalfa (aerial part)	61	19.3	9.6	63.7	95	183	47.6	−42.8
Alfalfa	57	16.3	8.2	59.5	95	155	43	−34
Barley grain	83	13	39	86.6	70	91	92.4	−1.6
Beet aerial + crown	54	12.7	25	56.4	80	102	56	−16.1
Beet pulp	72	10	20	75.2	80	80	66.2	−1.7
Brome grass	68	20.3	10	71	95	193	53	−43.5
Brome grass	65	6.4	16	48	75	48	40.8	+7.1
Buffalo grass	59	9.2	13.8	62	85	78	49.7	−5.9
Corn (ears)	89	9.3	32.6	60	65	60	65.8	+11.6
Corn grain #2	91	10	38	62	62	62	71.8	+11.8
Corn (aerial ensiled)	70	8.1	26	55	68	55	55.4	+6.4
Cotton seed meal (sol. ext.)	75	44.8	112	78	75	336	151.4	−92
Oat grain	76	13.2	39.6	79	70	92	87	−4.7
Prairie grass	50	8.1	12	52	85	69	40.6	−6
Prairie grass	54	4.6	11.5	35	75	35	2.6	+7.8
Sorghum grain	80	12.4	59.5	65	52	65	93	+6.8
Soybean meal (sol. ext.)	81	51.5	129	85	75	386	171.6	−108
Urea	0	280	—	—	—	—	223	—
Wheat grain	88	14.3	42.9	92	70	100	100	−2.9

Source: Data exatrapolated from Burroughs W et al: Metabolizable protein (amino acid) feeding standard for cattle and sheep fed rations containing either alpha amino or nonprotein nitrogen. Iowa State Univ Agr Exp Sta Leaflet R190, 1974, Table 6.

TDN = Total digestible nutrients; CP = crude protein; UDG = undegraded; MCB = microbial protein; Prot = protein; DEG = degraded; Met Prot = metabolizable protein; UFP = urea fermentation potential.

Table 2. ASSUMED PROTEIN DEPOSITION

Body Weight (kg)	Protein Deposition in Gain (g/kg)
150	150
200	140
300	130
400	120
500	110

The Metabolizable Protein Requirement

A factorial system is used to establish the requirements for growth and maintenance.

1. The net protein requirement for maintenance is computed from a formula developed by Smuts.[57] Protein (g/day) required for maintenance = $(0.0125) \times (70.4 \, W/kg^{0.734})$.
2. The net protein requirements for growth are based on the quantity and composition of empty body weight gain. If the gain = 1 kg/day and contains 15 per cent protein, the net protein requirement for gain = 150 g/day.
3. The net protein requirements for lactation equals the protein deposited in milk. If daily milk production = 10 kg milk containing 3.5 per cent protein, the requirement = $10 \times 0.035 = 0.35$ kg (350 g).

These requirements must be subjected to efficiency factors and added together to total the net protein requirement for a specific animal. The maintenance and growth factor is 47 per cent. The lactation factor is 95 per cent. The requirements for MP listed previously should be multiplied by a factor of 1.1 to 1.2 to account for the less than perfect amino acid balance presented for absorption.

The requirements for growth are based on the assumption that cattle of a given weight deposit gain having a constant composition. The percent of protein in gain is inversely proportional to body weight. Table 2 lists the assumed protein deposition in the gain of cattle of various body weights.

This system is under constant surveillance at Iowa State University, and the recommendations are subject to change. Considerations include the following:

1. Recent studies indicate that composition of gain for a given weight of cattle varies with the rate of gain.
2. Some feeding trials seem to indicate that the tabulated UFP values are too low (see the Wisconsin System).
3. There is some argument that the fecal protein computation is too low.

The system is flexible and susceptible to alteration, and we think it is based on practical concepts that will improve as research progresses.

The Practical Application

For an example we will use the Iowa State System to formulate an energy protein ration as follows:

1. Class: Medium-frame steers.
2. Live weight: 300 kg.
3. Metabolic weight ($300^{0.75}$): 72.08 kg.
4. Expected daily gain: 1 kg.
5. NE_m requirement (cold weather) (0.09×72.08): 6.48 Mcal.
6. NE_g requirement (Table 1, NRC[35]): 4.02 Mcal.
7. Metabolic protein requirement (Iowa model):

$$\left(300^{0.734} \times \frac{0.0125 \times 70.4 \times 1.2}{0.47}\right) + \left(\frac{130}{0.47} \times 1.2\right) = 480 \text{ g}$$

8. DM consumption (feed intake equation, NRC[35]): 7.1 kg.
9. Least-cost feed sources (Table 3).
10. Basic energy ration—Table 4 (25 per cent No. 2 corn, 75 per cent corn silage).

    $NE_m = (0.25 \times 2.24) + (0.75 \times 1.63) = 1.78$ Mcal/kg.

    $NE_g = (0.25 \times 1.55) + (0.75 \times 1.03) = 1.16$ Mcal/kg.

    Daily DM consumption = $6.48/1.78 + 4.02/1.16 = 7.1$ kg.
    Total CP in the basic energy ration = 422.5 g (Table 4).
    The MP deficiency = $480 - 422.5 = 57.5$ g.
    122.5 g of MP equivalent from UFP is more than the 57.5 g deficiency, so we will use corn-urea for an MP supplement.

11. Computation of substituting corn-urea for corn in the ration to maintain energy and supply the MP deficiency:
    a. To maintain energy we need to put in 1 kg of corn-urea to replace 0.85 kg of corn.
    b. When we substitute 1 kg corn-urea for 0.85 kg corn we gain $(75 = [143 \times 2.225]) - (0.85 \times 71.8) = 332$ g MP. (Assumes energy will be supplied to convert the negative UFP to microbial protein.)
    c. We need $57.5/332 = 0.173$ kg corn-urea to be added to the ration and $0.173 \times 0.85 = 0.147$ kg corn removed from the ration.

12. The final DM energy protein ration (Table 5). Total MP in energy-protein ration:

$$(1.653 \times 71.8) + (0.173 \times 75) + (0.173 \times 143 \times 2.225) + (5.32 \times 55.4) = 481.4 \text{ g}$$

The Wisconsin System[52]

Most approaches used to estimate metabolizable protein sources and requirements involve the summation of the rumen microbial protein synthesized and the dietary true protein that escapes degradation in the rumen. This is a logical way to proceed, but it is currently susceptible to error owing to lack of information on protein degradability of many feedstuffs and variations in estimates of microbial synthesis.

The approach used by Satter and Roffler is keyed to rumen ammonia concentration.[52] When this concentration gets beyond a critical point, ammonia is absorbed from the digestive tract and does not contribute to microbial synthesis. The

Table 3. LEAST-COST FEED SOURCES

Category	Feed	TDN %	DM %	NE_m	NE_g	MP	UFP	MP Equiv of UFP
Energy	Corn #2	90	88	2.24	1.55	71.8	+11.8	26.26
Fiber	Corn silage	70	30	1.63	1.03	55.4	+6.4	14.24
Protein*	Soybean meal	89	89	2.06	1.40	171.6	−107.7	238.10
Protein†	Corn-urea (85/15)	90	90	1.90	1.32	75	−143	318.20

*Use if MP deficiency > MP equivalent of UFP.
†Use if MP equivalent of UFP > MP deficiency.
TDN = total digestible nutrients; DM = dry matter; NE_m = net energy for maintenance (Mcal/kg DM); NE_g = net energy for gain (Mcal/kg DM); MP = metabolizable protein (g/kg DM); UFP = urea fermentation potential (g/kg DM); MP Equiv of UFP = metabolizable protein equivalent of UFP (g/kg DM).

Table 4. BASIC ENERGY RATION

Feed	DM (kg)	MP (g)	UFP (g)	MP Equiv of UFP (g)
Corn	1.78	(71.8 × 1.78) = 127.8	(11.8 × 1.78) = 21	21 × 2.225 = 46.7
Corn silage	5.32	(55.4 × 5.32) = 294.7	(6.4 × 5.32) = 34	34 × 2.225 = 75.8
Totals	7.10	422.5	55	122.5

critical point is related to TDN and crude protein concentrations in the diet.

The amount of ammonia that can be utilized by the rumen microbes depends on the number of such microbes and how rapidly they are growing. The size of the microbial population and its rate of growth are determined by the amount of fermentable energy nutrients that are available to the microbes. Feeds high in TDN are generally more fermentable than those with lower TDN values. It follows that larger amounts of ammonia and dietary NPN can be utilized by high digestible feeds than by less digestible feeds.

It apparently makes little difference to the animal whether dietary true protein is degraded as long as the rumen microbes can utilize all of the available ammonia. In these cases both dietary and recycled nitrogen end up as protein presented to the intestine for digestion and absorption. When ammonia production exceeds the microbial requirement for protein synthesis, only dietary true protein that escapes degradation in the rumen can contribute to the intestinal amino acid pool. Ammonia produced beyond the capacity of microbial utilization results in ammonia overflow (absorption from the rumen and/or intestines). The ammonia overflow does not contribute to metabolizable protein and is useless to the animal.

The prediction of the point of ammonia overflow in the rumen is important in the determination of practical quantities of NPN that can be used in ruminant rations. Two pieces of information are essential for the prediction: (1) the concentration of ruminal ammonia necessary to support maximal microbial growth and (2) the mean concentration of ruminal ammonia produced by specific rations and feeding conditions. The objective is to relate mean ruminal ammonia concentration to TDN and crude protein content. These are well-understood and readily measured characteristics, and the relationship is used to predict the point of ammonia overflow.

The question of optimal concentrations of ammonia in the rumen to support microbial growth is controversial. Several enzymes are known to be involved. Two of the more important ones are said to be glutamate dehydrogenase (low affinity for ammonia) and glutamine synthetase (high affinity for ammonia). Studies by Baldwin and Denham[2] and Schaefer and associates[55] have provided significant information.

The vast bulk of available evidence suggests that mixed populations of rumen microbes attain maximum yields of cell protein when the rumen fluid has a minimum average concentration of 5 mg ammonia nitrogen/100 ml. This concentration equals 3.6 mmol ammonia/L.[49, 54]

Roffler and Satter studied the influence of ration composition on mean ruminal ammonia concentrations.[48] They col-

lected more than 1000 samples from 211 cattle. The cattle were fed in average groups of six. Thirty-five different rations were used. The rations varied from 8 to 24 per cent CP (N × 6.25) and from 53 to 85 per cent TDN. CP was established by Kjeldahl analysis, and TDN was established by NRC tables. Only natural protein resources were used. A multiple regression equation was formulated as follows:

Ammonia nitrogen (mg/100 ml) = $38.73 - (3.04 \times \% \text{ CP})$
$+ (0.171 \times \% \text{ CP}^2) - (0.49 \times \% \text{ TDN})$
$+ (0.0024 \times \% \text{ TDN}^2), R^2 = 0.92$

A less precise equation has been formulated to predict ruminal ammonia concentration in sheep:

NH_3 (mg/100 ml) = $5.2 + (1.25 \times \% \text{ CP})$
$- (0.18 \times \% \text{ DDM*}), R^2 = 0.76$

Substituting NPN for true protein in the ruminant ration results in a decreasing percentage of true protein escape, and the fraction of dietary nitrogen contributing to the rumen ammonia pool increases. As the NPN content of the ration is increased, the point of zero utilization of NPN is reached at a corresponding lower protein concentration in the ration. Thus the point of excessive ammonia accumulation in the rumen is affected by TDN, percent total protein in the unsupplemented ration, and the NPN added to the ration as a crude protein supplement.

Calculations using these criteria indicate that no benefit will result from NPN supplementation when the TDN per cent of a ration is less than 60 per cent if the CP per cent is greater than 8 per cent. NPN supplementation of rations containing more than 80 per cent TDN may be used to increase the utilizable CP per cent from 8 to 11.6 per cent and from 12 to 13.6 per cent. NPN supplementation will be of no benefit in rations containing more than 13.6 per cent CP. These estimates for limitation of NPN supplementation are comparable to those of Burroughs and colleagues at Iowa State University.[6] The current NRC publication for beef cattle[35] recommends usage of the Satter-Roffler data[52] to establish a relationship that determines the practical limitation for the use of urea as a crude protein supplement.

Urea potential (g/kg dry feed) = $31.64 - (3.558 \text{ CP}) +$
$[(945 \times NE_m - 887 - 179 \times NE_m^2)]^{0.5}$

where CP = crude protein per cent and NE_m = Mcal/kg DM. Thus in a ration containing 9 per cent CP and an NE_m concentration of 1.9 Mcal/kg, the urea potential is

$31.64 - \{(3.558 \times 9) +$
$[(945 \times 1.9) - (887) - (179 \times 1.9^2)]^{0.5}\} = 14.48$ g/kg DM

The following assumptions form the basis for the Wisconsin system of estimating metabolizable protein (Fig. 4). Some of these assumptions are well documented, but others must be considered tentative. All values are averages associated with variance.

1. The amount of nitrogen recycled into the reticulorumen is equal to 12 per cent of dietary nitrogen intake.

Table 5. FINAL DM ENERGY PROTEIN RATION

Feed	kg DM			kg As Fed			% As Fed
Corn	1.78 − 0.147	=	1.653	1.653/0.88	=	1.878	9.5
Corn-urea		=	0.173	0.173/0.9	=	0.192	1.0
Corn silage		=	5.320	5.32/0.3	=	17.733	89.5
Totals			7.146			19.8	100

*DDM = digestible dry matter and is equal to TDN.

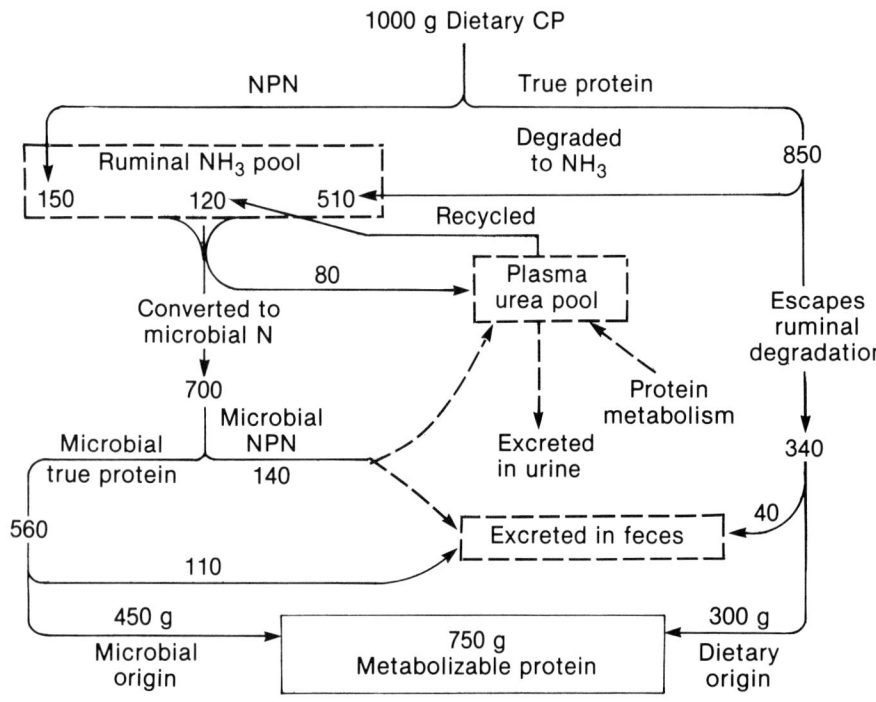

Figure 4. Schematic summary of metabolizable protein calculations.

2. Eighty-five per cent of the dietary nitrogen intake with typical ruminant rations, including protein supplements, is in the form of true protein; 15 per cent is in the form of NPN.

3. An average of 40 per cent of the true dietary protein escapes degradation in the rumen and passes to the abomasum and small intestine intact. About 87 per cent of escaped protein will be absorbed from the small intestine as amino acids. All of the dietary NPN and recycled nitrogen passes through the ruminal ammonia pool.

4. Ninety per cent of all ruminal ammonia produced is incorporated into microbial nitrogen when the ration fed does not exceed the upper limit for crude protein (ruminal ammonia does not exceed 5 mg/100 ml).

5. None of the ruminal ammonia produced in excess of 5 mg/100 ml rumen fluid is incorporated into microbial nitrogen.

6. Eighty per cent of microbial nitrogen is in true protein form and 20 per cent is in the form of NPN and is not available to the animal as amino acid nitrogen.

7. Eighty per cent of the microbial true protein will be absorbed as metabolizable protein.

Under conditions where ruminal ammonia does not exceed microbial use, 1 kg dietary protein produces about 750 g metabolizable protein. Of this amount, 450 g is from microbial origin and 300 g is from bypass protein origin. For the sake of simplicity, all forms of dietary nitrogen are considered to be equal when dietary protein does not exceed the upper limit of microbial utilization.

When the rumen ammonia pool exceeds the upper limit of microbial utilization, the efficiency of amino acid absorption decreases significantly. In these cases only escaped true protein (40 per cent of total CP) is available as a source of amino acids. The metabolizable protein will be limited to $0.75 \times 0.40 = 30$ per cent of dietary CP. It is assumed that the efficiency of tissue deposition will remain the same. Thus the prediction of efficiency for dietary protein utilization above the point where ruminal ammonia concentration exceeds 5 mg/100 ml rumen fluid is $0.75 \times 0.4 \times 0.6 = 0.18$, or 18 per cent.

In summary, the efficiency of dietary protein utilization is $0.75 \times 0.6 = 0.45$, or 45 per cent, when the ruminal ammonia concentration is less than 5 mg/dl, and decreases to 18 per cent when the ruminal ammonia concentration is more than 5 mg/100 ml rumen fluid.

Crude protein concentrations in feeds are established by laboratory analysis (Kjeldahl) or by using tables from current NRC manuals. Perhaps a practical approach is to rely on the tables for concentrate analysis and use laboratory analysis to evaluate roughage.

The daily requirements for metabolizable protein include the following:

1. The maintenance requirement = 2.4 g/kg of body weight ($BW^{0.75}$).

2. The requirement for body weight gain = 0.15 kg per kg gain/0.6.

Such gain includes normal growth, fat deposition, and the products of conception.

3. The requirement for lactation = CP in milk/0.6.

The protein requirement for dairy cows is complicated by the stage of milk production. Generally, high-producing cows will lose 30 to 70 kg body weight in the first 40 days of lactation. This will be followed by a brief period of weight stabilization and then a gradual weight gain for the remainder of the lactation period. Lactation typically peaks about 6 weeks after parturition, and feed consumption peaks about 10 to 12 weeks after parturition. The ordinary diet for lactating dairy cows is high in protein (more than 13 per cent CP); also, supplementary protein will be metabolized at low rates of efficiency. In early lactation, when appetite is less than maximum and milk production is ascending, crude protein requirements in terms of per cent of dry diet are potentially high. Some compensation is achieved because for each kilogram of weight loss, 150 g metabolizable protein are made available for milk production. Undoubtedly some of the tissue protein is used for energy. The amino groups of energy contributing protein are converted to urea in the liver, and some of this urea is released into the digestive tract in saliva and rumen secretions. Such urea is probably useless to the animal owing to high rumen ammonia associated with high protein consumption typical of dairy rations. On the other hand, milk production is an efficient process relative to gestation, growth, and even maintenance. It is quite probable that a significant amount of amino acids liberated by the catabolism of body tissue is incorporated into milk protein.

Practical Application

Examples using the Wisconsin System to compute protein requirements and ration formulation follow.

1. The protein requirements for a 400-kg medium-frame steer calf being fed for maximum gain. The basic energy ration contains 90 per cent flaked corn (NE_m = 2.38 Mcal/kg DM; NE_g = 1.67 Mcal/kg; NE_g = 1.03 Mcal/kg DM; CP = 8 per cent DM). We will assume normal weather. NE_m requirements = 0.077 Mcal/kg $W_{0.75}$.
   a. Metabolic weight of steer: $400^{0.75}$ = 89.44 kg.
   b. NE_m of basic energy ration: $(0.9 \times 2.38) + (0.1 \times 1.6)$ = 2.30 Mcal/kg.
   c. NE_g of basic energy ration: $(0.9 \times 1.67) + (0.1 \times 1.03)$ = 1.61 Mcal/kg.
   d. CP per cent of basic energy ration = $(0.9 \times 11.2) + (0.1 \times 8)$ = 10.88 per cent.
   e. TDN per cent of basic energy ration: $(0.9 \times 95) + (0.1 \times 70)$ = 92.5 per cent.
   f. NH_3 concentration in rumen fluid:
   $38.37 - (3.04 \times 10.88) + (0.171 \times 10.88^2) - (0.49 \times 92.5) + (0.0024 \times 92.5^2)$ = 1.11 mg/100 ml
   g. Urea potential:
   $31.64 - (3.558 \times 10.88) + ([945 \times 2.30] - [179 \times 2.30^2])^{0.5}$ = 11.4 g/kg DM

   We can use NPN to increase the CP per cent of the ration to more than 13 per cent without loss of metabolic efficiency.
   h. The NE_m requirement: $0.077 \times 400^{0.75}$ = 6.89 Mcal.
   i. The dry matter intake (DMI) =
   $[(0.1493 \times 2.3) - (0.046 \times 2.3^2) - (0.0196)] \times 400^{0.75}$ = 7.2 kg[35]
   j. The NE_g available (RE): 7.2 kg $-$ 6.89/2.3 Mcal $\times$ 1.61 Mcal/kg DM = 6.77 Mcal.
   k. Estimated live weight gain (LWG):
   $13.91 \times 6.77^{0.9116} \times 400^{-0.6837}$ = 1.32 kg/day
   l. The CP requirement in grams:
   $$\frac{(2.4 \times 89.44) + (1.32 \times 0.15 \times 1000)}{0.75 \times 0.6} = 917 \text{ g}$$
   m. CP content in the basic energy ration:
   0.1088×7.2 kg = 783 g.
   n. The CP deficiency: 917 $-$ 783 = 134 g.
   Our urea potential (UP) enables us to use NPN beyond the requirement to supply the CP deficiency (UP = 11.4 g/kg DM). Total CP equivalent from UP in the ration = 11.4×7.2 kg $\times 2.25$ = 185 g.
   One method of supplying the CP deficiency is to use a corn-urea mix (85 per cent corn, 15 per cent urea). The corn-urea mix contains about 51 per cent CP. To keep energy levels constant, it will require 100 g corn-urea mix to replace 85 g corn. Such an exchange would produce 51 $-$ (0.112 $\times$ 85) = 41 g net CP gain. We need to use 124/41 $\times$ 100 = 302 g corn-urea mix to replace 302 $\times$ 0.85 = 257 g corn in the basic energy ration. The daily DM consumption is expected to increase from 7.2 to 7.245 kg.

2. The protein requirements of a 600-kg cow in midlactation, producing 30 kg milk/day. The milk is assumed to contain 3.5 per cent fat and 3.3 per cent CP. We will assume a body weight gain of 0.2 kg/day and the NE_l requirement for maintenance to equal $0.08 \times BW^{0.75}$/day. The basic energy ration dry matter contains the following ingredients:

Feed	NE_L Concentration*	NE_g Concentration*	CP (%)	Per cent of Ration DM
Ground corn	2.03	1.42	10	40
Corn silage	1.64	1.03	8.8	30
Alfalfa hay	1.30	0.59	17.2	30

*Mcal/kg.

   a. Metabolic weight of the cow: $600^{0.75}$ = 121.23 kg.
   b. NE_L concentration of basic ration = 1.69 Mcal/kg DM.
   c. NE_g concentration of basic ration = 1.05 Mcal/kg DM.
   d. CP per cent of basic ration = 11.8 per cent of DM.
   e. TDN per cent of basic ration = 74 per cent.
   f. NH_3 concentration in rumen fluid:
   $38.73 - (3.04 \times 11.8) + (0.171 \times 11.8^2) - (0.49 \times 74) + (0.0024 \times 74^2)$ = 3.55 mg/100 ml
   g. The urea potential of the ration:
   $31.64 - (3.558 \times 11.8) + ([945 \times 1.69 - 887 - 179 \times 1.69^2])^{0.5}$ = 3.76 g/kg DM
   Urea can only be used to raise the CP per cent to about 12.6 per cent. The cow's requirement will be considerably higher, so NPN cannot be beneficially used in this ration.
   h. The daily NE_l requirement: $(0.09 \times 121.23) + (30 \times 0.69)$ = 30.4 Mcal.
   i. The daily NE_g requirement: = 1.21 Mcal.[35]
   j. The estimated DM intake:
   $$\frac{30.4}{1.69} + \frac{1.12}{1.05} = 19.14 \text{ kg/day}$$
   k. The estimated DM as per cent of body weight = 19.14/600 = 0.032, or 3.2 per cent, of body weight.
   l. The metabolic protein requirement:
   $$(2.4 \times 121.23) + \frac{(0.033 \times 30 \times 1000)}{0.6} + \frac{(0.15 \times 0.2 \times 1000)}{0.6} = 1991 \text{ g (1.991 kg)}$$
   m. The CP requirement:
   The cow will convert CP to metabolizable protein at about 75 per cent efficiency until the rumen ammonia exceeds 5 mg/100 ml of rumen fluid (CP > 12.6 per cent in the ration DM). This means that the first 2.41 kg CP in the diet will produce 1.81 kg metabolizable protein. It also means that 1.991 $-$ 1.81 kg metabolizable protein must come from escaped true protein. The crude protein necessary to increase metabolizable protein beyond 1.81 kg will be converted to metabolizable protein at 30 per cent efficiency. Thus the total CP requirement will be:
   $$\frac{1.81 \text{ kg}}{0.75} + \frac{1.991 - 1.81}{0.30} = 3.02 \text{ kg}$$
   n. The CP in the final ration should be 3.02/19.14 = 15.8 per cent.
   o. The basic energy ration contains 0.118×19.14 = 2.26 kg CP, which will convert to 2.26×0.75 = 1.69 kg metabolizable protein. We have a deficiency of 3.02 $-$ 2.26 = 0.76 kg CP.

p. One method of supplying the deficiency is to substitute the least-cost, high-energy, true protein supplement for corn. We will assume that soybean meal is that supplement. As most of the energy is used for maintenance and lactation, we can use NE_L concentrations to compare relative energy values: NE_L for corn = 2.03 Mcal/kg DM; NE_L for soybean meal = 1.86 Mcal/kg DM. Thus the NE_L ratio of soybean meal to corn is 1.86/2.03 = 0.92 and it will require 100 g soybean meal to replace 92 g corn.

q. If we make such a substitution, assuming that soybean meal contains 50 per cent CP, we will gain (100 × 0.50) − (92 × 0.1) = 41 g CP. The CP deficiency of our basic energy ration is 0.76 kg, or 760 g. We will need to replace 760/41 × 92 = 1705 g corn with 760/41 × 100 = 1854 g soybean meal (SBM) to supply our CP deficiency and maintain the energy requirement. Our final dry matter ration will include:

Corn (19.41 × 0.4) − 1.705	= 6.06 kg
SBM	= 1.85 kg
Corn silage 19.14 × 0.3	= 5.74 kg
Alfalfa 19.4 × 0.3	= 5.74 kg
	19.39 kg

The total CP = (6.06 × 0.1) + (1.85 × 0.50) + (5.74 × 0.088) + (5.74 × 0.172) = 3.02 kg.

The CP per cent = 3.02/19.29 = 15.6 per cent. Comparing our two examples with NRC recommendations,[33, 35, 37] we get the data that are given in Table 6.

Two tables have been designed for practical application of the Wisconsin System.[52] We have summarized these tables (Tables 7 and 8).

In summary, the results obtained using the Wisconsin System are very similar to those obtained using the factorial systems recommended by the NRC.[33, 35] The advantage of the Wisconsin System is its simplicity. No tables to show degradability of individual or mixed feeds are necessary. The aim of the system is practical application in a variety of situations. From a critical standpoint, the estimation of recycled urea nitrogen (12 per cent) is quite high relative to other systems. Also, the Wisconsin System assumes a constant percentage of protein in gain and a constant percentage of degradability in all feeds and mixtures of feeds. These assumptions differ significantly from those of other systems.

The Cornell System

The Cornell System is possibly the most sophisticated and forward-looking of those reviewed. Other proposed systems are based on static models that assume fixed rates of protein degradation and microbial synthesis in the rumen. They also assume fixed rates of protein digestion and absorption in the small intestine. The Cornell System presents a dynamic model

Table 6. PROTEIN REQUIREMENTS: NATIONAL RESEARCH COUNCIL (NRC) VERSUS WISCONSIN SYSTEM*

Class	BW (kg)	Gain (kg/day)	Milk Prod (kg)	NRC Reqmt CP (kg)	Wisconsin System Reqmt CP (kg)
Beef steer	400	1.5	—	0.978	0.981
Dairy cow	600	0.2	30	3.37	3.02

*NRC requirement = $\frac{(2.75 \times 600^{0.5})}{0.45} + \frac{(0.03 \times 19290)}{0.45} + \frac{(0.2 \times 600^{0.5})}{0.45} + \frac{(0.2 \times 160)}{0.45} + \frac{(30 \times 0.032)}{0.52} = 3374$ g = 3.37 kg.

Table 7. UPPER LIMIT FOR NONPROTEIN NITROGEN (NPN) UTILIZATION

CP % in Basic DM Ration	TDN % 55–60	TDN % 60–65	TDN % 65–70	TDN % 70–75	TDN % 75–80	TDN % 80–85
			(% CP after NPN addition)			
8	NB	10	10.5	10.9	11.2	11.4
9	NB	10.4	10.9	11.3	11.6	11.8
10	NB	10.8	11.3	11.7	12	12.2
11	NB	11.2	11.7	12.1	12.4	12.6
12	NB	NB	12.1	12.5	12.8	13.0

NB = no benefit.

that assumes variations in these criteria caused by differences in feed intake, energy concentrations, diet mixtures, and rates of flow if ingested through the digestive tract.

Rumen Dynamics

Plant cells are degraded (starch and cellulose → short-chain fatty acids) in the forestomachs of ruminant animals. The rate and degree of this degradation are related to feed intake and digestibility.[29] The rate of cell-wall degradation competes with passage from the rumen. Slow rates of degradation and rapid rates of flow from the rumen lead to depressions of digestibility and increases of fecal losses.[67] Depressions of digestibility are characteristic of high feed intake. These depressions appear to be the result of ruminal escape of plant cell wall without degradation.

In ruminants dietary protein is also affected by variable rates of degradation (proteins → volatile fatty acids and ammonia), but the consequences are quite different. Complex carbohydrates that escape degradation in the rumen have reduced chances of digestion and absorption from the small intestine. There are no pancreatic or enteric enzymes that can digest cellulose. In contrast, true protein that escapes ruminal degradation is utilized more efficiently than is microbial protein synthesized in the rumen from the degradation products of carbohydrate, dietary protein, and NPN.

The relative inefficiency of microbial protein utilization results because the rumen microbes may degrade true protein beyond their needs for cell synthesis. The products of excess degradation are ammonia and volatile fatty acids. These are not available to produce amino acids in the abomasum and intestines. In addition, more than 30 per cent of microbial crude protein is in the form of NPN. Such microbial NPN includes RNA, DNA, capsular peptides, and glycoproteins. This microbial NPN is not available for amino acid synthesis and thus is not a source of metabolizable protein for the animal. The chief benefit of rumen microbes is to convert dietary and recycled NPN into microbial protein in the rumen.

The relative efficiency of escaped protein has stimulated research aimed at increasing ruminal escape of dietary protein. It has been assumed that insoluble proteins are less likely to be degraded in the rumen. Heat or formaldehyde is sometimes used to reduce protein solubility in the rumen and thus increase the percentage of relatively efficient escape of bypass protein. This concept can be questioned in several respects.[27, 44]

1. Many feedstuffs contain NPN that is the most soluble crude protein fraction.
2. Most heat- or formaldehyde-treated feedstuffs contain increased amounts of bound unavailable nitrogen.
3. Both forages and concentrations contain buffer insoluble proteins that have very fast rates of degradation in the rumen.
4. Feedstuffs may also contain soluble proteins that have slow rates of degradation.

Treatment to increase bypass protein will not likely have a

Table 8. RELATIONSHIP BETWEEN DIGESTIBLE DRY MATTER AND DIETARY CRUDE PROTEIN AT CONSTANT RUMINAL AMMONIA LEVELS*

Species	DDM % 50–55	DDM % 55–60	DDM % 60–65	DDM % 65–70	DDM % 70–75	DDM % 75–80	DDM % 80–85
			Rumen NH$_3$/100 ml = 5 mg at:				
Cattle	—	—	10.3% CP	11.8% CP	12.6% CP	13.2% CP	13.6% CP
Sheep	7.4% CP	8.1% CP	8.8% CP	9.6% CP	10.3% CP	11.0% CP	11.7% CP

*5 mg NH$_3$/100 ml rumen fluid.
DDM = digestible dry matter; DDM is practically synonymous with TDN.

positive effect if microbial protein synthesis is limited by the treatment.

Animal data suggest that microbial yields vary significantly. In general they are larger with high-quality forage-based diets as compared with high-concentrate diets. Diets producing low microbial yields appear to be fermented or overprotected by heat or formaldehyde. The decreased utilization of fermented feeds may be related to increased percentages of unavailable nitrogen content. Microbial yields may also be limited by the lack of readily available carbohydrate. The capacity of microbes to increase protein quality (synthesize essential amino acids) is also worthy of consideration.

Feed Analysis

The Cornell System classifies feed nitrogen into three biologic groups: soluble nitrogen (fraction A), available true proteins (fraction B), and bound unavailable nitrogen (fraction C).

Fraction C is composed of Maillard products, leather (tannin-protein condensates), and liquefied nitrogen. In fermented feeds fractions A and C may be increased by depletion of fraction B. Use of crude protein values in ration formulation from feeds containing these damaged ingredients may cause underfeeding of usable nitrogen.

The Rumen Model

The rumen model used in the Cornell System is based on the total disappearance of protein from the digestive tract by absorption and passage.[14] Ruminal escape and microbial yield are treated as variables. Figure 5 outlines the rumen submodel. Figure 6 outlines the conceptual model of the net protein system for ration formulation.

Rumen Degradation Rates

The determination of protein degradation rates is complex. The generalities of the procedures include the following:

1. Total nitrogen is determined by the Kjeldahl method.
2. Fraction A is determined as NPN by means of tungstic acid precipitation.
3. Bound unavailable nitrogen (fraction C) is determined as acid detergent fiber nitrogen (ADFN).[18]
4. Fraction B is determined by subtracting fractions A and C from total nitrogen. B = total N − (fraction A + fraction C). Fraction B is referred to as "residual available protein" (RAP).

The individual degradabilities of the various fractions are measured by the use of microbial proteases in a sterile system.

The partition of the available true protein (fraction B) into

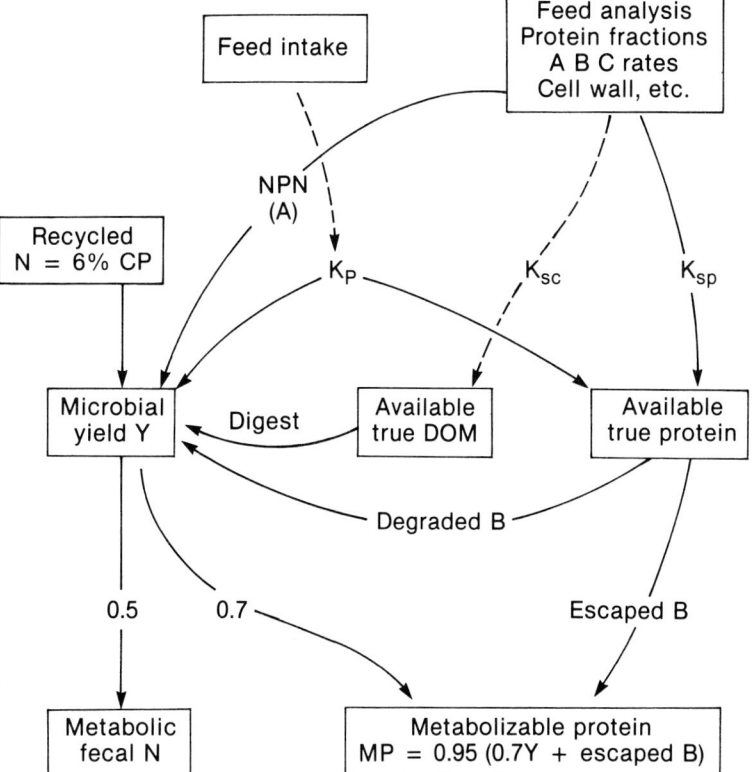

Figure 5. The rumen submodel. K_{sp} is the fractional rate of proteolysis for each protein, and K_{sc} is the fractional rate of digestion of carbohydrate. Dashed lines indicate features for which information is incomplete and more research is needed.

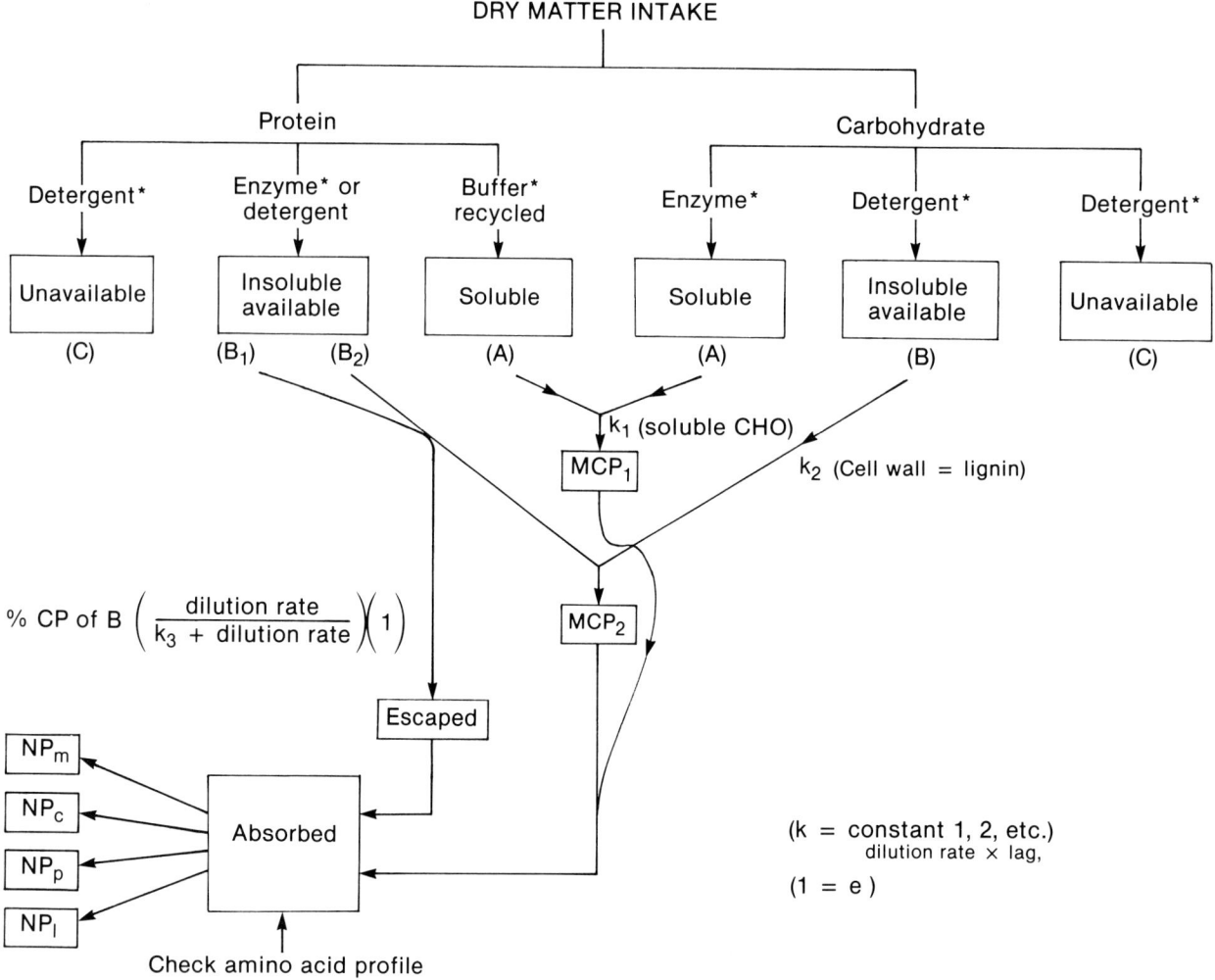

Figure 6. Net protein system for cattle. *Van Soest system of feed analysis. (Data from Fox DG, Sniffen CJ, Van Soest PJ, Robinson PH: Proc Okla Protein Symposium, 1981.)

subfractions and their inherent rates of digestion are obtained from the mathematical analysis of time-sequence digestion measurements. The fractional rate for the NPN fraction (A) is considered to be infinite and is not used in any calculation. The B fractions show considerable variation among the various feedstuffs. For example, corn shows a single slow digesting pool (B_3); soybean meal shows two faster digesting fractions (B_1 and B_2); whereas timothy and brewer's grain show B_1, B_2, and B_3 fractions. The heating of a feedstuff can have substantial effect on proteolytic rates and the distribution of the respective fractions.

Examples of digestion rates calculated from log plots of protease degradation measurements published in the Proceedings of the International Symposium on Protein Requirements for Cattle (Van Soest, 1980) are shown in Table 9.

Potentially Digestible Organic Matter

To simplify the model, all fermentable organic matter constituents are aggregated into a single component called potentially digestible organic matter (PDOM). PDOM is calculated as

$$PDOM = 100 - (2.4 \text{ lignin} + \text{ash})$$

Lignin multiplied by 2.4 represents the indigestible organic matter associated with lignin[29] (P. J. Van Soest and P. H. Robertson, unpublished) and nonstructural carbohydrate.[21]

Rates of passage (K_p) are estimated for each feed ingredient at each intake level.[8, 19, 42] Rates were estimated to be faster for feeds of small particle size and high density (concentrates faster than forages) and for high feed intakes. Liquid turnover rates are estimated from literature values for lactating cows and beef cattle. Rates of passage of liquids vary according to levels of productivity and frame size of the animal.

Rates of passage for liquids are important variables. They are used to estimate microbial protein yield per unit of fermented organic matter. There is significant variability among and within experiments designed to analyze liquid turnover.[8, 19, 42] It does not seem probable that a predictive relationship between liquid turnover and body weight, forage, concentrate, or DM intake can be developed, but some general conclusions can be made.

There appear to be two distinct groups of liquid rates of passage. Animals restricted to DM intakes of less than 2 per cent of body weight had low rates of liquid passage. Animals fed ad libitum with DM intakes of more than 2 per cent of body weight showed more variation in rates of liquid passage. There was a trend toward increase of passage with increased

Table 9. DIGESTION RATES

Feed	% Total Crude Protein	Fraction	% DM	% B
Corn	9.93	A	1.1	—
		B_3	8.3	100
		C	0.5	—
Soybean meal	54.8	A	11.15	—
		B_1	33.6	81
		B_2	7.9	19
		C	2.2	—
Brewers' grains	31.73	A	2.6	—
		B_1	18.3	71
		B_2	7.5	29
		C	3.3	—
Timothy	8.09	A	2.1	—
		B_1	1.5	27
		B_2	1.2	22
		B_3	2.7	51
		C	0.6	—
Wheat middlings	19.07	A	11.54	—
		B_1	4.42	59
		B_2	1.05	14
		B_3	2.03	27
		C	0.63	—

intake, but the r^2 values were low. It is probable that factors other than body weight and intake influence rates of liquid passage.

Mathematical Considerations

1. PDOM = 100 − (2.4 lignin + ash).
2. Fractional escapes:
   a. Digestion and passage rates are proportional to substrate concentration,[29, 71] leading to the general differential equation

   $$\frac{-ds}{dt} = S(K_s + K_p)$$

   where K_s and K_p are rates of digestion and passage, respectively, and S is substrate concentration in the rumen. The proportion of substrate (S) escaping rumen fermentation is a function of the competition between digestion and passage. Theoretically, S is a constant for any given feeding situation.

   b. Each escape function applies only to uniform feed fractions that have similar digestion and passage rates:

   $$E = \frac{K_p}{K_p + K_s}$$

   c. The protein fractions (B_1, B_2, B_3) in the diet will have different digestion rates but possibly similar passage coefficients. Dairy cattle on mixed diets appear to have three main passage pools: liquids, concentrate fiber (may include insoluble proteins and starch), and coarse fiber. The total escape of protein, then, will be the sum of the respective component feed fractions classified according to their particular digestion and passage rates.

   To calculate total true protein escape (TPE), all escape fractions must be multiplied by their respective protein substrate concentrations in the feed (B_i) and the DM intake (A). The total escape is described by the following equation:

   $$TPE = \sum_{i=1} B_i A \left(\frac{K_{pi}}{K_{si} + K_{pi}}\right)$$

3. Lag effects:
   The primary objective of biochemical analysis of feedstuffs is to characterize the limitation of the substrate. Therefore protease measurements must be operated under conditions of limiting substrate (excess enzyme). However, evidence indicates that the rumen may not be substrate limited, especially during fermentation periods, when microbial numbers are low. For this reason a lag function has been introduced into the model[30]:

   $$P_i = eK_{pi} L_i$$

   and

   $$FE_i = L - eK_{pi} L_i$$

   where P_i is the proportion of protein remaining when digestion begins, K_{pi} is rate of passage, L_i is the lag time in hours, and FE_i is the fraction that escapes during the digestion lag. These lag functions are incorporated into the TPE equation as follows:

   $$TPEL = \sum_{i=1} (B_i)(A) \left[\left(\frac{K_{pi}}{K_{si} + K_{pi}}\right)(P_i) + FE_i\right]$$

   where TPEL = total true protein escaped with lag effect.

   Comparison of protease degradation rates with proteolytic activity suggests that adding the lag effect brings the estimate of protein escape into reasonable approximation with in vivo results. The concentration of enzyme used in the protease procedure is the amount required to saturate soybean meal (about 6 mg/ml). About 80 per cent of the soybean protein is hydrolyzed in 1 hour. These rates are much faster than those reported for the rumen using the azocasein technique.[26]

   Assay of rumen fluid measures only the free proteolytic activity in the rumen. If maximum proteolysis occurs when microbes are in close proximity to protein, then it is likely that there is a lag in proteolysis when microbial numbers are low or microbes are not in close association with protein particles.

4. Microbial protein output from the rumen:
   In order to calculate the amount of microbial protein that can be produced during fermentation in the rumen, the amount of potentially digestible organic matter that is fermented in the rumen must be estimated. An equation to measure true fermented organic matter (TFOM) has been derived as follows[30]:

   $$TFOM = (A)\frac{(PDOM)}{100}\left(\frac{K_s}{K_s + K_p}\right)(e^K p^l)$$

   where TFOM = true fermented organic matter, A = DM feed intake, and K_s, K_p, and L = digestion rate, passage rate, and lag time of PDOM, respectively. Microbial protein output (MICP) from rumen fermentation is calculated by multiplying microbial yield (MY) by the amount of TFOM.

   $$MY \text{ in g protein/100 g TFOM} = (6.25)\left(\frac{1}{0.14 + 0.015 K_{Liq}}\right)$$

   where K_{Liq} is the fractional rate of liquid passage from the rumen. Microbial protein output is calculated by the equation MICP = (TFOM)(MY). Fecal metabolic nitrogen loss is calculated as indigestible microbial matter according to Mason and Fredricksen.[28a]

Model Simulation Results

Model simulations predict the following:

1. Milk yields greater than 33 kg/day can be better predicted by dynamic microbial yield and dietary escape estimates than by conventional methods.

2. Microbial yield and rumen escape are confounded in animal responses obtained at higher feed intakes.

3. Animal response to increased metabolizable protein depends on the animal's requirement for amino acid nitrogen being greater than the nitrogen requirement of rumen microbes.

4. The requirements for metabolizable protein of most ruminants are probably lower than the nitrogen required by rumen microbes. Exceptions include very rapidly growing young ruminants and perhaps high-producing dairy cattle.[39]

5. Ruminants with metabolizable protein requirements lower than those required by rumen microbes are energy limited and will respond to monensin or other methanogenic inhibitors that reduce microbial yields.[45] Response to antimethanogens is not expected when animal protein requirements exceed the nitrogen required by rumen microbes.

6. The response to NPN is variable depending on microbial requirements and nitrogen supply. Overprotection of dietary nitrogen will cause rumen fermentation to become nitrogen limiting and theoretically responsive to any level of urea addition. It has been observed that milk production decreases when higher levels of insoluble protein are included in the diet.[9] The exact value for the dietary NPN equivalent for recycled nitrogen is not known. This value is probably reduced when digestible nitrogen sources are lacking, and the basal value is probably about 6 per cent of crude protein equivalent (the level at which digestibility and intake are reduced in low-protein diets).[10, 31]

Alternate Nitrogen Fractionization Systems

Fractionization of protein is an important input to the rumen submodel. There is an alternative to using proteases to measure protein degradation. True protein can be divided into soluble and insoluble parts in acid detergent (AD) and neutral detergent (ND). This scheme avoids the technical expertise and standardization needed for biologic systems. Classifications include the following:

1. Protein soluble in ND is a constituent of cell solubles and would have a fast rate of digestion (B_1).

2. Protein insoluble in ND but soluble in AD is completely available but is digested at a slower rate than the ND soluble fraction and corresponds to the B_2 fraction. This fraction is markedly affected by heating and processing.[44] Protein insoluble in AD is unavailable and represents fraction C. The ND-AD method of measuring protein degradation in the rumen is based on the large range in ND-insoluble nitrogen that is observed in feedstuffs. Also, feedstuffs contain a variable mixture of protein types with differing solubility characteristics. The analysis is simpler than the protease procedure but has less accuracy and theoretical meaning. Also, knowledge is lacking about the proteins that are insoluble in ND. Whatever system is used, the quantitative partition of the nitrogen fraction into A, B_1, B_2, and C rates is applicable only to the B fractions. The rate for A (NPN) is not relevant since it can only be converted into microbial protein, and rumen escape of A has no meaning. The rate for fraction C is assumed to be zero.

Summary

The Cornell model dynamically mimics protein digestion based on rates of passage and digestion. The operation of the system requires a more precise definition of nitrogen fractions than can be obtained from solubility measurements. The model offers the possibility of a more flexible method of predicting responses of ruminants to various diets. However, it generates the need for requisite dietary feed information.

The workers at Cornell have taken a stepwise approach to developing a net protein system that (1) accurately describes the actual net protein needs for maintenance, weight gain, pregnancy, and milk production; (2) allows accurate calculation of the net protein value of individual feedstuffs in a specific diet; and (3) determines supplemental protein needs from chemical analysis of individual feedstuffs in the diet. The developmental steps include:

1. A conceptually correct model that is closely related to physiologic function. Also, the model must lend itself to laboratory analysis to adjust feed values for various field conditions.

2. A computer program for purposes of sensitivity analysis to determine which estimates of physiologic function have the greatest impact and to identify those that need more refinement.

3. Validation of the program with field experimentation.

4. A program for microcomputers that can be used over a wide array of conditions.

ANIMAL REQUIREMENTS

The protein content of tissue or milk determines the dietary protein requirements of each animal. These requirements are met by combining feeds to meet microbial protein needs and provide escaped protein as needed to supplement microbial protein. Amounts and forms of energy consumed and dilution rates of energy substrates in the rumen determine maximum rates of microbial synthesis and growth.

Determining the protein requirement for a specific situation is a stepwise procedure.

1. The first step is to ensure that adequate protein is provided to optimize energy utilization for microbial protein synthesis.
2. Then feed sources high in escape protein are substituted into the diet for highly degraded protein sources if
    a. microbial protein output is maximal, and
    b. tissue or milk requirements are not met.
3. When microbial and tissue needs are met, an amino acid profile can be calculated to check for any deficiencies or imbalances.

The equation of Smuts[57] is used to estimate metabolizable protein required for maintenance (NP_m):

$$NP_m = (70.4 \text{ wt/kg}^{0.735}) (0.0125)$$

The requirements for microbial protein synthesis are assumed to be equal to the maximum microbial protein that can be synthesized each day. The protein available to meet this requirement is dietary NPN, recycled nitrogen (assumed to be equal to NP_m), and degraded fraction B protein. The following input information is required to calculate microbial protein synthesis and feed protein escaping degradation in the rumen:

1. Dry matter intake.
2. Concentrations of the protein subfractions including NPN and protein rapidly available (B_1), intermediate in availability (B_2), slowly available (B_3), and unavailable (C).
3. Concentrations of the energy fractions (available and unavailable fiber, fat, and rapidly available and unavailable carbohydrates).
4. Rates of digestion for each protein and energy fraction.
5. Rates of passage for liquids and solids (see Mathematical Considerations).

Determination of net protein required for weight gain (NP_g) is a two-step procedure as follows:

1. Determine energy allowable gain.

The system described by Fox and Black is used to predict daily gain allowable by the dietary energy intake.[12] This predicted gain becomes the daily gain used to calculate the NP_g requirement. In this system the NRC NE_m requirement equation is adjusted for environmental breed effects. The weight used in the modified equation is called the animal's equivalent weight. The weight of various frame sizes and sexes is multiplied by an adjustment factor to determine the weight of an average-frame steer having the same body composition. This equivalent weight is then used in the NE_g equation to determine the daily NE_g requirement. Use of this procedure eliminates the need for separate equations for each cattle type.

Dry matter intake is assumed to be 100 g/wt $kg^{0.75}$. Actual intake declines linearly after animals achieve about 22 per cent body fat and as net energy concentration in the diet increases above 1.27 Mcal/kg DM feed. Adjustment is made for use of growth stimulants, feed additives, body condition, and environment.[12]

2. Determine protein allowable gain.

The net dietary protein available for weight gain is a summation of absorbed microbial and escaped protein adjusted for metabolic losses. Those who formulated the Cornell System say that "further study is still required to determine if these values are appropriate for all ages and physiological states." Net protein requirements are calculated by the equation (0.235 − 0.00026 W) (DG), where DG = kg expected daily gain and W = equivalent weight in kg.[13] This expression was developed from the body composition equation of Sempfendorfer[56]: $Y = 0.235 X - 0.00013 X^2 - 2.418$, where Y = protein per cent expressed as a decimal and X = body weight in kg.

Validation trials have shown that energy concentrations in the diet influence protein requirements. For example, trials on 144 steer calves showed that protein composition of the gain was 14.2 per cent when ration grain content was less than 50 per cent of DM, 13.1 per cent when ration grain content was 50 to 80 per cent of DM, and 12.8 per cent when ration grain content was more than 80 per cent of DM. The Cornell net protein system was accurate in predicting protein content of the gain when high-silage diets were fed (predicted, 14 to 14.5 per cent; actual, 14.2 per cent). The system overestimated protein gain when cattle were fed high-grain diets continually from weaning (predicted, 14 to 14.5 per cent; actual, 13 per cent). This difference would result in an increase of 0.5 per cent in the crude protein requirements. Thus it would seem that the error in not adjusting body protein gain for feeding high-grain rations is small.

APPLICATION USING A MICROCOMPUTER

The following shows the input/output of computer programs that are being developed at Cornell University to evaluate and test the net protein system described. Field application is also demonstrated. Data from two forms of soybeans were compared (raw versus 135°C heat treatment) when fed to young calves. Alternate runs of the program were used to demonstrate the program operation and how it can be used to evaluate diets. Actual performance is listed next to predicted performance.

1. Enter profile of animal characteristics
   a. Age (1 = calf; 2 = yearling): 1
   b. Sex (1 = steer; 2 = heifer; 3 = bull): 1
   c. Breed (1 = beef; 2 = Holstein cross; 3 = Holstein): 3
   d. Frame size (1 = small; 5 = average; 9 = large): 9
   e. Number of feeding periods (1 to 6): 1
   f. Quality of animals' environment: 7
      (1) = no shelter, extended period of mud/cold
      (5) = no shelter, lot well drained
      (7) = no stress
   g. Body condition (1 = fleshy; 5 = average; 9 = thin): 5
   h. Average weight = 330 lb
   i. Percent of standard intake: 104 first treatment, 110 second treatment
   j. Feed additives and growth stimulants:
      (1) = none
      (2) = antibiotics
      (3) = estrogens (heifers)
      (4) = estrogens or Ralgro* (zeranol) (steers); zeranol (heifers)
      (5) = rumensin
      (6) = rumensin plus antibiotics
      (7) = rumensin plus estrogens (heifers)
      (8) = rumensin plus estrogens or zeranol (steers): 4
2. Enter feedstuff descriptions
   a. This section is for feed data entry. Data for feeds typically used can be stored. Only minor changes are necessary as diets are reformulated. The user can also call in feed from a feed dictionary that includes average values for NE_m, NE_g, ADF, calcium, phosphorus, magnesium, potassium, sodium, chlorine, sulfur, zinc, iron, copper, manganese, selenium, and vitamins A, D, and E. The various energy and protein fraction values outlined previously are included. The user can adjust only the values that can be obtained from feed analysis. The protein profile for two types of soybeans (raw and roasted) is listed in Table 10.
3. Enter ration description (Table 11)
   a. Feeding management for protein supplement: 3
      (1) = once/day
      (2) = twice/day
      (3) = total mixed ration
4. Results of computer analysis
   a. Growth and intake predictions (Table 12)
   b. Comparable gain predictions and actual gains (Table 13)
   c. Protein classification analysis (Table 14)
   d. Daily gains of Holstein calves as influenced by weight, dietary energy, and supplemental protein source (Table 15)

As shown in the protein profile (Table 10), predicted energy allowable gain was about 9 per cent less on the raw soybean–supplemented ration. This results from a 6 per cent lower daily intake. The predicted protein allowable gain was 20 per

---

*Available from Pitman-Moore.

Table 10. PROTEIN PROFILE FOR SOYBEANS

Fraction	% DM	K_s	Lag time (hr)
Raw			
Soluble	18	99	0.3
B_1	5	2.55	0.5
B_2	15.5	0.12	1.5
B_3	0	0	0
Bound	3.5	0	99
Roasted			
Soluble	3.5	99	0.3
B_1	0	0	0
B_2	16.6	0.12	1.5
B_3	2	0	99
Bound	2	0	99

K_s = degradation rate, % hr; Lag time = hours before degradation begins.

Table 11. RATION DESCRIPTION

Ingredient	% of Ration Dry Matter	
	1st Analysis	2nd Analysis
Corn silage	72	72
Supplement 380	3.8	3.8
Raw soybeans	23.2	—
Roasted soybeans	—	23.2
Calcium carbonate	1.0	1.0

cent less with the raw soybean ration. In the raw soybean–supplemented ration actual daily gain was limited by available protein. In the roasted soybean–supplemented ration the protein allowable gain was similar to the energy allowable gain, indicating that neither protein nor energy would be wasted. The object of the program is to analyze the key factors known to affect performance and then supplement at a level that is neither limiting nor wasted.

The protein profile helps identify some of the dietary factors involved in the lower availability of net protein from the raw soybeans. Both diets contained 16 per cent crude protein, but the actual crude protein intake was 5.8 per cent higher with the roasted soybeans because of increased dry matter intake. In addition, net protein intake was 24.8 per cent higher with the roasted soybean–supplemented diet because a higher proportion of the roasted beans escaped degradation in the rumen. One gram of escape protein yields 0.54 g net protein, whereas 1 g microbial protein yields only 0.39 g net protein. However, caution must be taken that the amount of degraded protein available in the rumen is adequate to support the microbial growth that is predicted to be synthesized from the predicted digestible organic matter. The available degraded protein should be equal to or exceed that needed to support microbial growth. Otherwise fiber digestion would be depressed and performance would be reduced.

MODEL EVALUATION

Development and refinement of the protein model continue to be ongoing processes. The biologic systems being described are very complex, and there is a need for more complete data in many areas. Nevertheless a number of general observations can be made based on simulations with the model and evaluations to date.

1. Reducing dietary protein rumen degradability to meet animal protein requirements will have the greatest affect in calves under 270 kg equivalent weight and in dairy cows producing over 33 kg milk/day. This is especially true if the diet contains a high proportion of fermented forage. Table 15 summarizes the results of a series of experiments (D. G. Fox, Cornell University, unpublished data) with young

Table 12. GROWTH AND INTAKE PREDICTIONS

Statistics	1st Analysis Raw Soybeans	2nd Analysis Roasted Soybeans
Animal body weight (lb)	330	330
Energy allowable gain (lb/day)	2.84	3.09
Actual feed DMH (lb/day)		
Corn silage	6.99	7.4
Supplement 380	0.37	0.39
Raw soybeans	2.25	—
Roasted soybeans	—	2.38
Calcium carbonate	0.10	0.10
Totals	9.71	10.27

Table 13. COMPARABLE GAIN PREDICTIONS AND ACTUAL GAINS

Statistics	1st Analysis Raw Soybeans	2nd Analysis Roasted Soybeans
Energy allowable gain (lb/day)	2.84	3.09
Protein allowable gain (lb/day)	2.30	2.96
Actual daily gain (270–440 lb)	(2.28)	(3.04)

light Holstein steers fed with a wide range of diets. Light calves fed all corn silage diets were very responsive to the provision of dietary escape protein. The corn silage–based diet is high in protein fractions that will be degraded in the rumen. Those fed the dry shelled corn diet were more sensitive to reduced ruminal nitrogen when both basal and supplemental protein sources were low in rumen degradability. It is apparent that protein fractions must be balanced to meet both microbial and animal requirements. It is also apparent that a dynamic model that can take into account variation in protein fractions between and within individual feedstuffs and changes in dry matter intake is also essential. The data of Thomas and associates demonstrate the impact of variation in protein fractions in corn silage on performance.[64]

2. The metabolic protein requirements of cattle at later stages of growth or lower levels of milk production will often be met or exceeded if nitrogen requirements of rumen microorganisms are met.
3. Minimum dietary protein concentration needed to maximize rumen fermentation and thus dry matter intake will vary with the diet. For example, model predictions indicate that dietary protein must equal at least 9 per cent in high corn silage diets but only 6 to 7 per cent in hay diets. These predictions agree with protein levels at which dry matter intake is maximized.[25, 31]
4. Cattle should be grouped for feeding according to their stage of growth and level of production. Such grouping is necessary to match both total dietary protein and protein sources required to properly meet both microbial and animal requirements.
5. A complex dynamic biologic model can be applied in the field because of the availability and acceptance of powerful microcomputers by livestock producers.
6. The major area still needing refinement before this model can be directly applied on a wide basis is the rumen submodel. Improved methods are needed to:
   a. identify protein and carbohydrate fractions with routine laboratory analysis,
   b. predict degradation rates and turnover rates for liquids and solids (these are key components necessary to accurate prediction of microbial yield and escaped true dietary protein), and
   c. determine if and how efficiency of use of absorbed nitrogen varies with physiologic state (growth, pregnancy, lactation).

Table 14. PROTEIN CLASSIFICATION ANALYSIS

Category	1st Analysis Raw Soybeans		2nd Analysis Roasted Soybeans	
	Required	Avail	Required	Avail
Net protein (g)	296	246	319	307
Crude protein (g)	?	711	?	752
Rapidly degraded (g)	?	340	?	172
Slowly degraded (g)	?	85	?	96
Total microbial (g)	?	425	?	286
Feed escaped (g)	?	145	?	373

Table 15. DAILY GAINS OF HOLSTEIN CALVES AS INFLUENCED BY WEIGHT, DIETARY ENERGY, AND SUPPLEMENTAL PROTEIN SOURCE

Growth Price* (kg)	Supplemental Protein Source†			
	Urea	Raw SB	50:50	High Roast
Experiment 1 (corn silage–based diet)				
124–242 kg	—	0.99	1.02	1.15
242–548 kg	—	0.97	0.96	0.96
Experiment 2 (corn silage–based diet)				
96–251 kg	0.97	1.07	1.2	1.23
251–423 kg	1.04	1.05	0.97	1.01
Experiment 3 (corn silage–based diet)				
92–275 kg	0.85	1.05	—	1.15
Experiment 4 (high moisture corn–based diet)				
167–243 kg	1.30	1.29	1.35	1.45
243–390 kg	0.91	0.88	0.83	0.90
Experiment 5 (dry shelled corn–based diet)				
102–245 kg	1.15	1.06	—	1.18
245–335 kg	1.35	1.29	—	1.23

Source: DG Fox, Cornell University, unpublished data.
*Each value represents the mean of three pens of four Holstein steer calves each.
†Raw or high roast = form of whole soybeans; high roast = heated to 135°C; 50:50 = one half raw and one half heated soybeans.

Current Applications

In 1985 the NRC published the manual *Ruminant Nitrogen Usage*.[36] This publication suggests recommendations to improve the precision of predicting the protein requirements of growing and lactating ruminants. As weight change or milk production, or both, increases, it becomes important that larger portions of dietary protein escape degradation in the rumen and be digested into absorbable amino acids in the small intestine.

In 1988 the NRC published the sixth revised edition of *Nutrient Requirements of Dairy Cattle*.[37] Some of the concepts recommended in the 1985 edition[36] are incorporated in the Formulation Rations section (chapter 4) of the 1988 edition. See the previous article, Figure 1, for a reproduction of Figure 2–4 from the 1988 edition. Table 16 is a reproduction of Table 2–1 from the 1988 edition.

The unit used to describe the protein requirement for dairy cattle in the 1988 edition is "absorbed protein" and specifically means amino acids absorbed from the small intestine. Crude protein that is degraded in the rumen and absorbed as ammonia is not included in the definition of absorbed protein.

The absorbed protein concept recognizes differences in the portion of dietary protein that escapes rumen fermentation and the portion that is degraded in the rumen and becomes incorporated into microbial protein. The nutritional requirement for protein expressed in absorbed units includes both microbial and escaped protein and will always be equal to or less than the requirement for units expressed as crude protein.

As in the 1978 edition of *Nutrient Requirements of Dairy Cattle*,[34] the factorial method is used to derive the protein requirements of each class of cattle and each physiologic function in the 1988 edition; however, two significant changes have been made: (1) the unit to express the protein requirement is "absorbed protein" (AP) rather than "total crude protein" (TCP) and (2) the fecal metabolic nitrogen requirement is considered separately from the other components of the maintenance requirement because it is a function of indigestible dry matter (IDM) rather than a function of live weight as are the other maintenance components. The total protein requirement is then threefold and includes requirements for maintenance (urinary endogenous protein and surface protein), fecal metabolic nitrogen, and production (conceptus, growth, and lactation). The metabolic fecal protein equivalent is expressed in units of absorbed protein (FPA). It is calculated from IDM excretion. The proportional unit for FPA is $0.09 \times IDM$. The figure 0.09 is slightly less than the 1978 recommendation:

$$\frac{(0.068 \times \text{Total Protein Intake} = 0.088 - 0.113)}{\text{Efficiency factor } (0.6 - 0.77)}$$

To calculate the crude protein requirements, the 1988 edition assumes (1) that the undegraded portion of intake protein is useful only if the tissue need for absorbed protein is greater than the rumen need, and (2) that the degraded portion is useful only if the rumen need is greater than the tissue need. Using these methods, the implied intake protein requirement is about 10 per cent greater than the intake protein requirement listed in the 1978 NRC publication. The increase seems to be unreasonably high relative to the amounts of protein currently used in feeding cows. For this reason the current (1989) NRC[38] recommendation is about 5 per cent below the calculated values and about 5 per cent above the 1978 recommendation.

Using current recommendations for protein, ration formulation is complicated by the inclusion of three protein requirements (crude protein, degraded intake protein, and undegraded intake protein). The requirement for significant amounts of fiber also causes problems. The fiber requirement dictates that the roughage component of the lactating cow ration be quite high to ensure that fat content of milk will be satisfactory and that metabolic upsets are minimized. The protein concentration required in the concentrate component is dictated by the protein concentration in the roughage. When forage quality is low or the forage is composed of low-protein types of roughage, the protein concentration of the concentrate must be relatively high. It is quite possible to formulate a satisfactory ration if access to a variety of high-quality feeds is readily available. Unfortunately roughage quality is subject to weather-caused effects (rain, frost, etc.) and access to some desirable feeds is limited by local production and transportation costs. It is important that the proper amount of undegraded protein be included in the rations of high-producing cows. In many cases it is necessary to exceed expected CP requirements to provide for the undegraded intake protein (UIP) requirement. In these cases degraded intake protein (DIP) is in excess, and the question of ammonia toxicity arises. It is recommended that crude protein concentrations not exceed 18.5 per cent.[59]

Table 16. PARAMETER NAMES FOR DESCRIBING PROTEIN METABOLISM

Fractions or Pools

Term	Meaning	Term	Meaning
ADIN	Acid detergent insoluble nitrogen	LPN	Lactation protein (in) net (protein units)
AP	Absorbed protein	MPA	Maintenance protein (in) absorbed (protein units)
BCP	Bacterial (and protozoal) crude protein	MPN	Maintenance protein (in) net (protein units)
BTDN	Baseline total digestible nutrients (1 × maintenance)	NCP	Nucleic (acid) crude protein
BTP	Bacterial (and protozoal) true protein	RAP	Ruminally available (nitrogen as) protein
DBP	Digestible (true) bacterial (and protozoal) protein	REP	Rumen efflux (crude) protein (ammonia if positive, urea influx if negative)
DIP	Degraded intake (crude) protein (rumen)		
DM	Dry matter	RIP	Rumen influx (crude) protein (urea if positive, ammonia efflux if negative)
DMI	Dry matter intake		
DNP	Digestible nucleic (acid crude) protein (intestine)	RPA	Retained protein (in) absorbed (protein units)
DUP	Digestible undegraded (crude) protein (intestine)	RPN	Retained protein (in) net (protein units)
FP	Fecal (crude) protein	SCP	Small (intestine) crude protein (BCP + UIP)
FPA	(Metabolic) fecal protein (in) absorbed (protein units)	SPA	Surface protein (in) absorbed (protein units)
FPN	(Metabolic) fecal protein (in) net (protein units)	SPN	Surface protein (in) net (protein units)
IBP	Indigestible (true) bacterial (and protozoal) protein	UIP	Undegraded intake (crude) protein
IDM	Indigestible dry matter (total tract)	UP	Urinary (crude) protein
IIP	Indigestible intake (crude) protein (from ADIN or PIN analysis)	UPA	(Endogenous) urinary protein (in) absorbed (protein units)
INP	Indigestible nucleic (acid crude) protein (intestine)	UPN	(Endogenous) urinary protein (in) net (protein units)
IP	Intake (crude) protein	YPA	Conceptus protein (in) absorbed (protein units)
IUP	Indigestible undegraded (crude) protein (intestine)	YPN	Conceptus protein (in) net (protein units)
LPA	Lactation protein (in) absorbed (protein units)		

Transfer Coefficients

Term	Meaning	Term	Meaning
BCPRAP	Bacterial (and protozoal) crude protein/ruminally available (nitrogen as) protein	FPNFPA	Fecal (metabolic) protein (in) net (protein units)/fecal (metabolic) protein (in) absorbed (protein units)
BCPTDN	Bacterial (and protozoal) crude protein/total digestible nutrients	IPDM	Intake (crude) protein/dry matter
BTPBCP	Bacterial (and protozoal) true protein/bacterial (and protozoal) crude protein	LPNKG	Lactation protein (in) net (protein units) calculated from milkfat percentage
DBPBCP	Digestible bacterial (and protozoal true) protein/bacterial (and protozoal) crude protein	LPNLPA	Lactation protein (in) net (protein units)/lactation protein (in) absorbed (protein units)
DBPBTP	Digestible bacterial (and protozoal true) protein/bacterial (and protozoal) true protein	MPNMPA	Maintenance protein (in) net (protein units)/maintenance protein (in) absorbed (protein units)
DIPIP	Degraded intake (crude) protein/intake (crude) protein	NCPBCP	Nucleic (acid) crude protein/bacterial (and protozoal) crude protein
DUPUIP	Digestible undegraded (crude) protein/undegraded intake (crude) protein	RIPIP	Rumen influx (crude) protein/intake (crude) protein
		RPNRPA	Retained protein (in) net (protein units)/retained protein (in) absorbed (protein units)
FPAIDM	Fecal (metabolic) protein (in) absorbed (protein units)/indigestible dry matter	YPNYPA	Conceptus protein (in) net (protein units)/conceptus protein (in) absorbed (protein units)

Source: Reprinted with permission from Nutrient Requirements of Dairy Cattle, 6th rev ed, 1989. © 1988 by the National Academy of Sciences. Published by National Academy Press, Washington, DC.

A major change in the 1989 NRC edition[38] is the use of computer programs to calculate the requirements for most nutrients. A diskette containing these programs is mailed with each volume purchased. Table 11 is a printout of the computed requirements of a 700-kg cow producing 40 kg of 3.5 per cent fat milk 30 days postconception and in her third lactation. Ration formulation consists of the selection, including amounts, of available feeds on a least-cost basis.

The calculation of metabolic or absorbed protein, or both, in ration formulation is not as widely used in beef cattle or sheep as in dairy cattle. Personal experience and conversation with Dr. Mark Peterson at Montana State University indicate that the use of the Wisconsin System[52] is a practical method of computing the limitations of using NPN supplements in beef rations. Recently published research papers indicate the following results:

1. The use of protein supplements formulated for escape protein may influence growth rate in cattle fed mature forage diets.[43]

2. Treatment of soybean meal with 0.3 per cent formaldehyde reduces protein degradability without affecting postruminal digestibility and results in increasing nitrogen utilization.[60]

3. A high escape protein supplement composed of corn gluten meal and blood meal improved performance of yearling steers grazing on actively growing Smooth Brome grass pastures.[1]

4. Growing cattle grazing cornstalks responded positively to protein supplementation. Maximum gain (0.378 kg/day) was achieved when 0.163 kg escape protein was included in the ration.[11]

5. Holstein cows in late lactation did not respond positively to substitution of low degradable, high escape proteins for conventional protein sources.[47]

In conclusion it would seem that further work is necessary to improve our knowledge of protein metabolism and optimum ration formulation. Primary needs might be to improve feed and complete ration analysis for digestible fiber and absorbable bypass protein. Remarkable progress has been made since Wise Burroughs and his associates published their original concepts in 1974.[7] We are indebted to those who have continued to pursue this vital subject.

REFERENCES

1. Anderson JJ, Klopfenstein TJ, Wilkerson VA: Escape protein supplementation of yearling steers grazing Smooth Brome pastures. J Anim Sci 66:237, 1988.
2. Baldwin RL, Denham SC: Quantitative and dynamic aspects of nitrogen metabolism in the rumen: a modeling analysis. J Anim Sci 49:1631, 1979.
3. Blaxter KL: Protein metabolism and requirements in pregnancy and lactation. *In* Munro HN (ed): Mammalian Protein Metabolism, Vol 2. New York, Academic Press, 1964, pp 173–223.
4. Braddy PM, Horton D: Feedlot nutrition. *In* Current Veterinary Therapy: Food Animal Practice. Philadelphia, WB Saunders, 1981, pp 217–227.
5. Brisson GJ, Cunningham HM, Haskell SR: The protein and energy requirements of young dairy calves. J Anim Sci 37:157, 1957.

6. Burroughs W, Nelson DK, Mertens DR: Protein physiology and its application in the lactating cow: the metabolizable protein feeding standard. J Anim Sci 41:933, 1975.
7. Burroughs W, Trenkle WA, Vetter R: Metabolizable protein (amino acid) feeding standard for cattle and sheep fed rations containing either alpha amino or nonprotein nitrogen. Iowa State Univ Agr Exp Sta Leaflet R190, 1974.
8. Colucci RD: Rate of passage of digesta through the gastrointestinal tract of cattle. MS Thesis, Cornell University, 1979.
9. Davis RF: Response of dairy cattle to ration protein of different solubilities. Proc MD Nutr Conf, 1978, pp 116–120.
10. Ellis WC, Lippke H: Nutritional value of forages. In Grasses and Legumes in Texas—Development, Production and Utilization. Texas Agr Exp Sta Res Monog, 1976, pp 26–66.
11. Fernandez-Riveria S, Klopfenstein TJ, Britton RA: Growth response to escape protein and forage intake by growing cattle grazing corn stalks. J Anim Sci 67:574, 1989.
12. Fox DG, Black JR: A system to predict body composition and performance of growing cattle. J Anim Sci 58:725–730, 1984.
13. Fox DG, Crickenberger RG, Bergen WG, Black JR: A net protein system for predicting protein requirements and feed protein values for growing cattle. Mich Agr Exp Sta Rpt 328:141, 1977.
14. Fox DG, Sniffen CJ, Van Soest PJ, Robinson PH: A net protein system for formulating beef rations. Proc Cornell Nutr Conf 1979, pp 57, 62.
15. Fox DG, Sniffen CJ, Van Soest PJ, Robinson PH: Net protein system for cattle. Proc Okla Protein Symp, 1981.
16. Fox DG, Sniffen CJ, Van Soest PJ: Proc Ga Nutr Conf, 1984.
17. Glover J, Duthie DW, French MH: The apparent digestibility of crude protein by the ruminant I. A. Synthesis of the results of digestibility trials with herbage and mixed feeds. J Agr Sci 48:373, 1957.
18. Goering HK, Van Soest PJ: Forage Fiber Analyses (Apparatus, Reagents, Procedures and Some Applications). Agriculture Handbook No. 379. Washington, DC, Agr Res Ser USDA, 1970.
19. Hartnell GF, Satter LD: Determination of rumen fill, retention time and ruminal turnover rates of ingesta at different stages of lactation in dairy cows. J Anim Sci 48:381, 1979.
20. Hogan JP, Weston RH: Quantitative aspects of microbial protein synthesis in the rumen. In Phillipson AT (ed): Physiology of Digestion and Metabolism in the Ruminant. Newcastle-upon-Tyne, England, Oriel Press, 1970, pp 474–485.
21. Hungate RE: The Rumen and Its Microbes. New York, Academic Press, 1966.
22. Jakopsen PE, Sorensen PH, Larsen H: Energy investigations as related to fetus formation in cattle. Acta Agr Scand 7:103–112, 1957.
23. Lamond DR, Holmes JHG, Haydock KP: Estimation of yield and composition of milk produced by grazing beef cows. J Anim Sci 29:606, 1969.
24. Lofgreen GP, Loosli JK, Maynard LA: Comparative study of conventional protein allowances and theoretical requirements of growing Holstein heifers. J Anim Sci 10:171, 1951.
25. Lomas LW, Fox DG: Ammonia treatment of corn silage. I. Feedlot performances of growing and finishing steers. J Anim Sci 55:924, 1982.
26. Mahadevan S, Erfle JD, Sauer FD: A colormetric method for the determination of proteolytic degradation of feed proteins by rumen microorganisms. J Anim Sci 48:947, 1979.
27. Mahadevan S, Erfle JD, Sauer FD: Degradation of soluble and insoluble proteins by Bacteroides amylophylus protease and by rumen microorganisms. J Anim Sci 50:723, 1980.
28. Mason VC: The quantitative importance of bacterial residues in the nondietary faecal nitrogen of sheep. Z Tierphyseol, Tievernahrg. u Futtermittelkde 41:140, 1979.
28a. Mason V, Fredericksen JH: Partition of the nitrogen metabolism in the hindgut and nitrogen excretion. Proc 2nd Int Symp Prot Metab and Nutr 61, 1979.
29. Mertens DR: Application of theoretical mathematical models to cell wall digestion and forage intake in ruminants. PhD Thesis, Cornell University, 1973.
30. Mertens DR: Dietary fiber components, relationship to the rate and extent of ruminal digestion. Fed Proc 36:187, 1977.
31. Milford R, Minson DJ: The relation between crude protein content and the digestible crude protein of tropical pasture plants. J Br Grass L Soc 18:177, 1965.
32. Mitchell HH: The minimum protein requirements of cattle. Nat Res Council Bull 67, 1929.
33. National Research Council: Nutrient Requirements of Beef Cattle. Washington, DC, National Academy of Sciences, 1978.
34. National Research Council: Nutrient Requirements of Dairy Cattle. Washington, DC, National Academy of Sciences, 1978.
35. National Research Council: Nutrient Requirements of Beef Cattle. Washington, DC, National Academy of Sciences, 1984.
36. National Research Council: Ruminant Nitrogen Usage. Washington, DC, National Academy of Press, 1985.
37. National Research Council: Nutrient Requirements of Dairy Cattle, 6th ed. Washington, DC, National Academy Press, 1988.
38. National Research Council: Nutrient Requirements of Dairy Cattle. 6th rev ed. Washington, DC, National Academy Press, 1989.
39. Orskov EV: Factors influencing protein and nonprotein nitrogen utilization in young ruminants. In Cole DJA, Boorman KN, Buttery PJ, et al (eds): Proceedings, 1st International Symposium on Protein Metabolism and Nutrition. EAFA P.P. No. 16. London, Butterworths, 1976, pp 457–476.
40. Overman OR, Garrett OF, Wright KE, Sanmann FP: Composition of milk of brown Swiss cows with summary of data on the composition of milk from cows of other dairy breeds. Ill Agr Exp Sta Bull 457:575, 1939.
41. Owens FN, Bergen WG: Nitrogen metabolism of ruminant animals: historical perspective, current understanding and future implications. J Anim Sci 57(Suppl 2):498, 1983.
42. Owens FN, Kazema M, Galveen ML, Mizwicky KL, Solaiman SG: Ruminal turnover rate. Influence of feed additives, feed intake and roughage level. Olka Anim Sci Res Rpts 1979, p 27.
43. Peterson M, Clanton DC, Britton R: Influence of protein degradability in range supplements in abomasal nitrogen flow, nitrogen balance and nutrient digestibility. J Anim Sci 60:1384, 1985.
44. Pichard G, Van Soest PJ: Protein solubility of ruminant feeds. Proc Cornell Nutr Conf, 1977, p 91.
45. Poos MI, Hanson TL, Klopfenstein TJ: Monensin effects on diet digestibility, ruminal protein bypass and microbial protein synthesis. J Anim Sci 48:1516, 1979.
46. Preston RL: Empirical value of crude protein systems for feedlot cattle, 1980. Proceedings, International Symposium on Protein Requirements for Cattle. Oklahoma State University, 1980.
47. Robinson PH, Kennelly: Influence of rumen (undegradable) protein on milk production of late lactation Holstein cows. J Dairy Sci 71:2135, 1988.
48. Roffler RE, Satter LD: Relationship between ruminal ammonia and nonprotein nitrogen utilization by cattle. I. Development of a model for predicting nonprotein nitrogen utilization by cattle. J Dairy Sci 58:1880, 1975.
49. Roffler RE, Satter LD: Relationship between ruminal ammonia and nonprotein nitrogen utilization by cattle. II. Application of published evidence to the development of a theoretical model for predicting nonprotein nitrogen utilization. J Dairy Sci 58:1889, 1975.
50. Roy JH, Blach CC, Miller EL, et al: Calculation of the N-requirement for ruminants from nitrogen metabolism studies. In Protein Metabolism and Nutrition. Proc 2nd Int Symp, Netherlands. Eur Assoc Anim Prod Pub No 22. Wageningen, Centre for Agr Pub Doc, 1977, p 126.
51. Roy JH, Stobo IJF, Gaston HJ, Greatorex JCP: Nutrition of the veal calf. 2. The effect of different levels of protein and fat in milk substitute diets. Br J Nutr 24:441–457, 1970.
52. Satter LD, Roffler RE: Nitrogen requirements and utilization in dairy cattle. J Dairy Sci 58:1219, 1975.
53. Satter LD, Roffler RE: Relationship between ruminal ammonia and nonprotein nitrogen utilization by ruminants. In Tracer Studies on Nonprotein Nitrogen for Ruminants III. Vienna, International Atomic Energy Agency, 1976.
54. Satter LD, Slyter LL: Effect of ammonia concentration on rumen microbial protein production in vitro. Br J Nutr 32:199, 1974.
55. Schaefer DM, Davis CL, Bryant MP: Ammonia saturation constants for predominant species of rumen bacteria. J Dairy Sci 63:1248, 1980.
56. Sempindorfer S; Relationship of body type and size, sex and energy intake to the body composition of cattle. PhD Thesis, Cornell University, 1974.
57. Smuts BB: The relation between the basal metabolism and the endogenous nitrogen metabolism with particular reference to the maintenance requirement of protein. J Nutr 9:403, 1935.
58. Sniffen CJ: Balancing Rations for Carbohydrates for Dairy Cattle. The Application of Nutrition in Dairy Practice (Proceedings of a Symposium). Dairy Production Medicine Continuing Education Group Annual Meeting, College of Veterinary Medicine, North Carolina State University. American Cyanamid, 1988.
59. Sniffen CJ, Chase LE: Field Application of the Degradable Protein System. The Application of Nutrition in Dairy Practice (Proceedings of a Symposium). Dairy Production Medicine Continuing Education Group Annual Meeting, College of Veterinary Medicine, North Carolina State University. American Cyanamid, 1988.
60. Spears JW, Clark JH, Hatfield EE: Nitrogen utilization and ruminal fermentation in steers fed soybean meal treated with formaldehyde. J Anim Sci 60:1383, 1985.
61. Stobo IJF, Roy JHB: The protein requirement of the ruminant calf. 4. Nitrogen balance studies on rapidly growing calves given diets of different protein content. Br J Nutr 30:113–125, 1973.
62. Swanson EV, Herman HA: The nutritive value of Korean lespedeza proteins and the determination of biological value of proteins for growing dairy heifers. Mo Agr Exp Sta Bull 372, 1943.
63. Swanson EV: Factors for computing requirements for protein for maintenance of cattle. J Dairy Sci 60:1583–1593, 1977.
64. Thomas E, Trenkle A, Burroughs W: Evaluation of protective agents applied to soybean meal and fed to cattle. II. Feedlot trials. J Anim Sci 49:1346, 1979.
65. Trenkle A, Burroughs W: Supplemental protein requirements of finishing yearling heifers. Iowa State University Coop Ext Serv A S Leaflet R291, 1979.
66. Van Es AJH, Bockholt HA: Protein requirements in relation to the lactation cycle. In Protein Metabolism and Nutrition. Eur Assoc Anim Prod Publ 16. London, Butterworths, 1976, pp 441–455.

67. Van Soest PJ: International Ruminant Conference. University of New England Publishing Unit, 1975.
68. Van Soest PJ: Nutritional Ecology of the Ruminant. Corvalis, OR, O and B Books, 1982.
69. Van Soest PJ, Mertens DR: The use of neutral detergent fiber versus acid detergent fiber in balancing dairy rations. Monsanto Tech Symp, Fresno, CA, 1984.
70. Van Soest PJ, Sniffen CJ: Nitrogen fractions in NDF and ADF, vol 39. Distillers and Feed Conference, Cincinnati, OH, 1984.
71. Waldo DR, Smith LW, Cox EL: Model of cellulose disappearance from the rumen. J Dairy Sci 55:125, 1972.
72. Whitlow LW: Rumen microbial degradation of feed protein. PhD Thesis, University of Wisconsin, 1979.
73. Whitlow LW, Satter LD: Evaluation of models which predict amino acid flow to the intestine. Annales de Recherches Veterinaires 10:307, 1979.
74. Williams JH, Anderson DC, Kress DD: Milk production in Hereford cattle. I. Effects of separation interval on weigh-suckle-weigh milk production estimates. J Dairy Sci 49:1498, 1979.
75. Yu Y, Thomas JW: Estimation of the extent of heat damage in alfalfa by laboratory damage. J Anim Sci 42:766, 1976.

Cattle Feeding

DAVID P. HUTCHESON, PhD

The science of feeding cattle has advanced since the early development of the feedlot industry. Feeding standards such as *Nutrient Requirements of Beef Cattle*, published by the National Research Council (NCR),[2] provide a basis for formulating cattle feeding rations.

NUTRIENT REQUIREMENTS

Published nutrient requirements should not be considered the final word on animal nutritional needs, but rather are prepared as an aid in formulating rations and diets. Biologic variation in nutrient requirements for individual animals is a recognized phenomenon. Therefore the limitations of ration and diet formulation should be apparent. However, advantage can be gained from the proper use of the nutrient guidelines.

The specific nutrient needs of beef cattle can be divided into six general categories: protein, carbohydrate, lipids, minerals, vitamins, and water. Energy itself is not a nutrient but is a property of several nutrients. All of these nutrients are needed in the proper amounts for growth and finishing of beef cattle.

Energy

Energy is used by the animal as energy for maintenance or energy for gain, or both. The primary source of energy for feeding beef cattle comes from grains. In growing and finishing cattle, the maximum amount of energy that can be given to the cattle normally results in the least cost per unit of cattle gain.

The Net Energy System

The increased popularity of the net energy system has been due to its improvement in the accuracy of formulating cattle rations. The net energy system allows a more accurate comparison of the energy value of roughages compared with grains. Recent research generally indicates that the total digestible nutrient (TDN) system may slightly overevaluate roughages and underevaluate grains, especially in high-energy diets.

Energy is the largest single component used by animals for growth and production. A system utilizing net energy (NE) was introduced by Lofgreen at the University of California, Davis.[1] The system separated the energy requirements for maintenance from those for body weight gain and expressed a net energy value of the feed for these two functions. The energy content of feedstuffs using the net energy system is stated in terms of calories. A kilocalorie (kcal) is 1000 calories, and a megacalorie (Mcal), or therm, is 1000 kcal. Net energy calculations can be used to determine expected body gains or to formulate rations for certain body gains. Table 1 gives net energy requirements for growing and finishing steers and heifers.

Protein

Protein is nitrogen multiplied by 6.25; however, protein nutrition for ruminants has become more complex. Protein can be divided into two types for ruminants: (1) rumen

Table 1. NET ENERGY REQUIREMENTS OF GROWING AND FINISHING BEEF CATTLE

Weight (lb) NE_m* Required	500 4.51	600 5.17	700 5.80	800 6.41	900 7.00	1000 7.58	1100 8.14
Daily Gain (lb)				NE_g† Required			
				Medium-Frame Steers			
2.50	3.75	4.30	4.83	5.34	5.83	6.31	6.78
2.80	4.25	4.87	5.47	6.04	6.60	7.14	7.67
3.00	4.58	5.25	5.90	6.52	7.12	7.71	8.28
				Large-Frame Steers			
2.50	3.32	3.81	4.27	4.72	5.16	5.58	6.00
2.80	3.76	4.31	4.84	5.35	5.84	6.32	6.79
3.00	4.06	4.65	5.22	5.77	6.30	6.82	7.33
				Medium-Frame Heifers			
2.50	4.63	5.31	5.96	6.59	7.20	7.79	8.37
2.80	5.26	6.03	6.77	7.48	8.17	8.85	9.50
3.00	5.68	6.51	7.31	8.08	8.83	9.56	10.26
				Large-Frame Heifers			
2.50	4.11	4.71	5.28	5.84	6.38	6.91	7.42
2.80	4.66	5.34	6.00	6.63	7.24	7.84	8.42
3.00	5.04	5.77	6.48	7.16	7.83	8.47	9.10

Source: Data adapted and converted from Nutrient Requirements of Beef Cattle, 6th rev ed, 1984. © 1984 by the National Academy of Sciences. Published by National Academy Press, Washington, DC.
*Net energy of maintenance, Mcal.
†Net energy of gain, Mcal.

degradable protein and (2) nondegradable protein. To be of nutritional value a degradable protein must be reformed into microbial protein. The nondegradable protein, or bypass or escape protein, is the protein that escapes digestion in the rumen but that may be digested in the small intestine. When a nondegradable protein is increased in the diet, more ammonia (urea) or degradable protein could be utilized to supply ammonia for maximum rumen function and microbial protein synthesis.

The amounts of digestible protein recommended in the feeding standards for the various classes of livestock are based on the assumption that protein of average quality will be furnished. Protein quality refers to the ratios and levels of essential (indispensable) amino acids in the feed or diet compared with the ratios and levels of essential amino acids required by the animals for efficient protein synthesis (muscle).

The addition of certain nondegradable amino acids to ruminant diets has been beneficial under certain stress conditions. Current knowledge is inadequate to establish requirements for amino acids for cattle feeding.

Minerals

Minerals are inorganic compounds necessary for growth in feedlot cattle. They contribute to bones, teeth, protein, and lipid fractions of the body. Animals have two sources of inorganic elements: the natural feeds they consume or supplementation. Most minerals are absorbed in the small intestines of beef cattle. Minerals are divided into two subgroups: macrominerals and microminerals. The macrominerals are calcium, chloride, magnesium, phosphorus, potassium, sodium, and sulfur. Microminerals are chromium, cobalt, copper, iodine, iron, manganese, molybdenum, selenium, and zinc.

Calcium is required for bone and teeth formation, nerve and muscle tone, and acid-base balance. Calcium deficiency is indicated by abnormal bone development (rickets) in growing cattle.

Phosphorus is necessary for bone formation and utilization of energy. Adequate calcium and phosphorus nutrition requires that (1) an adequate supply of calcium and phosphorus is available, (2) a suitable calcium:phosphorus ratio exists, and (3) an adequate amount of vitamin D is present. The optimum calcium:phosphorus ratio is between 1.2:1 and 2:1.

Magnesium functions in bone formation, muscle tone, and electrolyte balance and is a cofactor in several enzyme systems.

Potassium, sodium, and chloride function in the regulation of osmotic pressure and electrolyte balance. Cattle require 0.6 to 0.8 per cent potassium in the diet; however, our work has indicated that stressed cattle require about 20 per cent more potassium than nonstressed cattle. Salt provides sodium chloride, and the requirement is met with 0.1 to 0.5 per cent salt in the diet.

Sulfur is a component of the sulfur-containing amino acids and is necessary for several metabolic reactions. It is part of the vitamin biotin. Sulfur amounts should be considered when nonprotein nitrogen is added to the diets of beef cattle. A 10:1 (N:S) ratio will allow optimum bacterial synthesis of nitrogen to protein. Sulfur requirements are about 0.12 to 0.15 per cent of the diet.

Copper is essential for the utilization of iron in blood hemoglobin formation and is a coenzyme in several enzyme systems. Deficiency of copper results in anemia and loss of hair pigmentation. Copper requirements are between 8 and 12 ppm.

Iron functions as a component of hemoglobin, and a deficiency results in anemia. It is stored in the liver as ferritin iron. Iron is poorly absorbed—usually from only 3 to 10 per cent of the diet.

Cobalt is required as a component of vitamin B_{12}. When cobalt is supplied in the ruminant diet, B_{12} can be synthesized by rumen microorganisms and the B_{12} requirement is considered met.

Molybdenum is a coenzyme in several enzyme systems of the animal body. The molybdenum requirement has not been established, but it approaches 0.1 ppm on a dry matter basis of feedstuff. Molybdenum is normally considered a toxic element and can produce toxic effects at higher levels. Some interesting interactions occur between copper, molybdenum, and sulphate. High molybdenum in the diet binds copper and can render the animal copper deficient. As molybdenum increases, copper in the diet must be increased.

Iodine functions as a component of thyroxine and is necessary for animal life. It is generally deficient in most pastures and most feeding systems. Iodine is added as iodized salt. The iodine requirement is about 0.1 ppm.

Zinc functions largely, or entirely, in the enzyme systems. Zinc is like iron in that it is poorly absorbed. Zinc deficiency results in decreased growth and reduced feed efficiency. High levels of calcium apparently decrease zinc absorption.

Manganese functions in several enzyme systems and is involved in skeletal growth.

Selenium functions have not been totally determined; however, data indicate that it is an essential element and is required at about 0.1 ppm in the feed. Selenium is involved with muscular dystrophy.

In summary, addition of the following minerals should be considered in feedlot rations: calcium, copper, phosphorus, selenium, and sulfur.

The knowledge of minerals is a dynamic area. Everyday new information is added to our storehouse of data on mineral interrelationships. Many of these interrelationships are more important than the individual dietary mineral levels. The practical role of mineral nutrition is important. Many health problems of cattle may be attributed to deficiencies in mineral nutrition. No longer can a standard trace mineralized salt be added to the diet to meet the mineral demands of beef cattle.

Vitamins

Vitamins are a group of chemically unrelated organic compounds. These compounds are essential for life and normal rate of growth in cattle. Vitamins are generally designated with a letter, such as vitamin A and the B-complex vitamins. Vitamins are divided into two classes: the fat-soluble vitamins, which are A, D, E, and K, and the water-soluble vitamins, which are thiamine, riboflavin, niacin, pyridoxine, pantothenic acid, cobalamin, biotin, and ascorbic acid. Vitamins have many functions; however, all of the biochemical roles, primarily those of the fat-soluble vitamins, have not been established. More biochemical roles of the water-soluble vitamins have been established, particularly because they are water-soluble and occur as components of many enzyme systems. The water-soluble vitamins are absorbed in the small intestine; however, little or no storage occurs. Fat-soluble vitamins are absorbed by the small intestine with lipids and can be stored in quantities in the liver. Therefore the fat-soluble vitamins can be given in doses that would allow for several weeks supply, whereas B vitamins must be supplied more often.

Vitamin A is important to consider in beef cattle nutrition. Vitamin A deficiency can, and does, occur, especially when animals are fed corn silage growing rations for a long period before being fed a finishing ration. It is possible that finishing rations, especially with high amounts of grain and small amounts of roughage, can be predisposing to vitamin A deficiency. It has generally been recognized that heat increases the vitamin A requirement of animals; therefore vitamin A supplementation should be considered during hot weather. Other work has demonstrated that the level of protein of the ration influences vitamin A utilization. As protein becomes low, vitamin A utilization becomes lower. Carotene is a source of vitamin A and is converted to the vitamin by the animal body; in cattle particularly, carotene is one of the major sources of vitamin A. However, various feedstuffs can be involved in the conversion of carotene to vitamin A. Alfalfa seems to enhance this conversion, whereas other feedstuffs depress it. Beta carotene is the form of carotene that is converted to vitamin A with the highest efficiency. Several trace minerals will catalyze the oxidation of both carotene and vitamin A. Thus it is important that stabilized vitamin A is used in mineral mixes. The vitamin A requirement of beef cattle is 1000 IU/100 lb body weight/day for growth with no storage. For growth and adequate storage, the requirement is 2000 IU/100 lb body weight/day. If cattle are showing symptoms of vitamin A deficiency, they should be given three to four times these recommended amounts for approximately 10 days. The deficiency signs for vitamin A are as follows: (1) depressed growth, (2) appetite failure, (3) reduced resistance to parasite infections, and (4) rough hair coats. Classical vitamin A deficiency is xerophthalmia, which is commonly called night blindness.

The other fat-soluble vitamins, D, E, and K, are required by beef cattle. Marginal vitamin E deficiency might be hard to ascertain in beef cattle because the signs are not easily manifest.

It is generally recognized that all eight of the B-complex vitamins are integral parts of various coenzymes that are necessary for growth and reproduction of beef cattle. The B-complex vitamins are components of enzymes that are required for one or more reactions in most of the major metabolic pathways. It is generally agreed that ruminants need only vitamins A, and perhaps E, added to their feeds.

Thiamine (B_1) is an important vitamin for consideration in beef cattle nutrition. Thiamine deficiency in beef cattle results in a central nervous system disorder called polioencephalomalacia. Polioencephalomalacia normally occurs in feedlot cattle fed a high-grain finishing ration. It is theorized that when cattle are fed a high-grain finishing ration, the thiamine-consuming bacteria demand all the thiamine that is produced by the rumen, leaving no thiamine to be used by the animal's body and resulting in a thiamine deficiency. Polioencephalomalacia responds very well to a mass injection of thiamine.

Recent work has indicated that niacin may hasten growth and improve the feed efficiency of ruminants. This work has shown that the growth of bacteria in the rumen is increased by the addition of niacin to the feed. This may lead to several types of hypotheses, from improving microbial protein to improving the homeostasis of the rumen.

In summary, the vitamins that should be considered for supplementation in beef cattle production are vitamin A, perhaps vitamin D in confinement situations with no sunlight, vitamin E, thiamine, and niacin.

The mineral and vitamin requirements for beef cattle are indicated in Table 2.

Table 2. MINERAL AND VITAMIN REQUIREMENTS OF BEEF CATTLE, IN PERCENTAGE OF RATION DRY MATTER OR AMOUNT PER POUND OF DRY RATION

Nutrient	Growing and Finishing Steers and Heifers
Vitamin A activity, IU*	1000
Vitamin D, IU	125
Vitamin E, IU†	7–27
Minerals	
Sodium, %	0.06–0.15
Calcium, %	0.18–1.04
Phosphorus, %	0.20–0.30
Magnesium, %	0.05–0.15
Potassium, %	0.60–0.80
Sulfur, %	0.10–0.20
Iodine, ppm	6
Iron, ppm	100–300
Copper, ppm	8–15
Cobalt, ppm	0.1–0.2
Manganese, ppm	20–40
Zinc, ppm	40–75
Selenium, ppm	0.1–0.3

*May be vitamin A or provitamin A.
†Exact requirement not known.

Table 3. WATER CONSUMPTION OF FEEDLOT CATTLE

	Ambient Temperature		
	40°F (3.3° C)	60°F (15.5° C)	90°F (32.2° C)
Growing cattle (lb)			
400	4.0	5.0	9.5
600	5.3	6.6	12.7
800	6.3	7.9	15.0
Finishing cattle (lb)			
600	6.0	7.4	14.3
800	7.3	9.1	17.4
1000	8.7	10.8	20.6

Data from Winchester CF, Morris MJ: Water intake rates of cattle. J Anim Sci 15:722, 1956.

Water

Water is sometimes the forgotten nutrient; however, water must be in adequate amounts and free of toxins and contamination for cattle to perform well. Most steers on a finishing ration will consume 8 to 10 gal/head/day under normal ambient temperatures. Newly arrived feeder cattle need to consume 4 to 6 gal/day just to maintain their body water balance. Fresh and clean water in adequate amounts should be provided at all times for all cattle. Table 3 illustrates water consumption of feedlot cattle at different ambient temperatures.

REFERENCES

1. Lofgreen GP, Garrett WN: A system for expressing net energy requirements and feed values for growing and finishing beef cattle. J Anim Sci 27:793–806, 1968.
2. National Research Council: Nutrient Requirements of Domestic Animals. No. 4. Nutrient Requirements of Beef Cattle. Washington, DC, National Academy of Sciences, 1984.

Dietary Management of the Beef Breeding Herd

LARRY R. CORAH, PhD

Numerous factors influence the profitability of a commercial beef cattle operation. All of these factors can be grouped into four principal areas:

1. Calf weaning weights.
2. Per cent of cows weaning calves.
3. Cost of maintaining the cow per year.
4. Price of calves.

Many factors influence each of these four areas. Likewise, there is a tremendous interrelationship between the four areas in how they affect the profit potential in the herd.

ECONOMIC CONSIDERATIONS

In analyzing in greater detail the components of each of these four profit areas, feed cost is one of the major items influencing profitability. Obviously, as we focus in the future on low-cost production systems, analyzing feed costs will become a key component. A recent 6-year summary of the Iowa State University Beef Cow Business Record System compared the top one third of the herds in profitability with the bottom one third. The higher-profit producers averaged $296.80 for total cost per cow. The low-profit producers averaged $413.40 per cow. Of this $116.60 difference, differences in feed and pasture alone accounted for 35 per cent. Of particular interest is that even though the more profitable cow producers invested $40 less in feed and pasture costs, their herds produced an average of 121 lb more calf per cow and had a 3.7 per cent higher calf crop.

In attempting to reduce or keep costs of production to a minimum, it is extremely important that a producer evaluate the nutritional needs of the cow herd and how they relate to the forage resources available. The key in any cattle operation anywhere on the North American continent is effectively matching cow requirements to the available forage resources and then understanding how to formulate supplements properly to cover forage deficiencies.

Stage of Production (Tables 1 and 2)

The first consideration in building a nutrition program is understanding the nutritional requirements of the cow. These requirements vary depending on whether the cow is lactating or dry, the size of the cow, the level of milk production, and the stage of production of the cow.

Table 1 illustrates a cow herd nutrition calendar that starts with calving and ends with the production of the next calf 365 days later. Although this nutritional calendar appears to be based on an individual cow, it fits an operation for the whole cow herd. Period 1 begins on the date when the first calf is born. To ensure that a large percentage of the cows are in the same period and, therefore, can be fed similarly, a short breeding season and subsequent calving season must be utilized.

Period 1

To maintain a yearly calving interval, the cow has approximately 80 days from the time of parturition until rebreeding.

Table 1. THE 365-DAY BEEF COW YEAR BY PERIODS

Period 1	Period 2	Period 3	Period 4
80 days (postcalving)	125 days (pregnant and lactating)	110 days (midgestation)	50 days (precalving)

In the case where it is desirable to move late calving cows to an earlier calving date, the cow may have less than 50 days. Because mature cows typically take from 40 to 80 days to recycle and first calf heifers take from 60 to 100 days, proper nutrition during this period is important. Thus Period 1 becomes the most critical, because the cow is maintaining a peak level of lactation and the onset of cyclicity and rebreeding must occur. Nutrition during this period will have a major influence on conception rates.

Period 2

Once the cow is pregnant, the major nutritional needs are to maintain lactation. Also, in most production systems it is advantageous that the cow gain weight during this period, putting on adequate flesh for harsh environmental conditions that may await. This is particularly true for spring calving cows in northern climates.

Period 3

This period has the lowest nutritional requirements. In some environments period 3 is an ideal time to utilize crop residues, lower-quality feeds, or the poorest roughage that is available. However, it is important that the cow not lose excessive weight during this period unless she enters it in fairly good body flesh. If the cow enters in moderate to slightly below average condition, she should maintain weight and possibly even gain some weight.

Period 4

This is the period often overlooked in many cattle operations. It should be kept in mind that during this short period (about 50 days), approximately 65 to 80 per cent of the fetal growth will occur. In cases where typical birth weights are 80 to 85 lb, this means that from 50 to 60 lb of fetal growth may occur during this time. Research has clearly shown that improper nutrition during this period will influence calf birth weight, vigor, and survival. There is no advantage to reducing the cow's plane of nutrition to reduce calf size as a means of alleviating calving difficulty. Poor nutrition during this period will cause a longer postpartum interval, reduce level of milk production, and reduce calf weaning weights.

Table 2. NRC REQUIREMENT FOR A 1100-lb BEEF COW WITH AVERAGE (15 lb/DAY) MILK PRODUCTION

Nutrient	Period 1	Period 2	Period 3	Period 4
TDN (lb/day)	13.3	11.5	9.5	11.2
NE (Mcal/day)	13.5	12.2	9.2	10.3
Protein (lb/day)	2.3	1.9	1.4	1.6
Calcium (g/day)	33	27	17	25
Phosphorus (g/day)	25	22	17	20
Vitamin A (IU/day)	39,000	36,000	25,000	27,000

Source: National Research Council: Nutrient Requirements of Beef Cattle. Washington, DC, National Academy of Sciences, 1984.

Table 3. RELATIONSHIP OF BODY CONDITION AND PER CENT COWS CYCLING 60 DAYS POSTPARTUM

Condition at Calving	Weight Change Precalving	Weight Change Postcalving	Per Cent Cycling 60 Days Postcalving
Good	Lost	Gained	90+
Good	Lost	Lost	90+
Moderate	Gained	Lost	74
Moderate	Lost	Lost	48
Thin	Lost	Gained	46
Thin	Lost	Lost	25

Source: Whitman RD: Ph.D. Thesis, Colorado State University, 1975.

Flesh or Condition of the Cow

In the past 5 years a new term—body condition—has entered the vocabulary of many cattle producers, nutritionists, and veterinarians to describe the nutritional status of cows. The concept is really not new because for years operators of well-managed cow herds have based their feeding program on the idea that "the eye of the master influences the size of the feed bucket." However, research in the last 10 years has clearly quantified the influence of body condition at calving time and breeding time on reproduction function. Table 3 indicates the impact of body condition at calving time on the onset of cyclicity 60 days postpartum.

Besides the impact on cyclicity, research has also shown that cows that are thin at calving time will have weaker and slower-growing calves and will produce less milk.

Body condition scores are numbers used to suggest the relative fatness of the beef cow. The most commonly used system in the United States ranges from 1 to 9, with a score of 1 representing very thin body condition and a score of 9 extreme fatness. A cow with a body condition score of 5 or 6 should look in average flesh and probably represents the target toward which many cattle producers strive. The following list describes the 9-point body condition scoring system:

1. Bone structure of shoulder, ribs, back, hooks, and pins sharp to touch and easily visible. Little evidence of fat deposits or muscling.

2. Little evidence of fat deposition but some muscling in hindquarters. The spinous processes feel sharp to touch and are easily seen with space between them.

3. Beginning of fat cover over the loin, back, and foreribs. Backbone still highly visible. Processes of the spine can be identified individually by touch and may still be visible. Spaces between the processes are less pronounced.

4. Foreribs not noticeable; twelfth and thirteenth ribs still noticeable to the eye, particularly in cattle with a big spring of rib and ribs wide apart. The transverse spinous processes can be identified only by palpation (with slight pressure) to feel rounded rather than sharp. Full but straightness of muscling in the hindquarters.

5. Twelfth and thirteenth ribs not visible to the eye unless animal has been shrunk. The transverse spinous processes feel rounded only with firm pressure (not noticeable to the eye). Spaces between the processes not visible and only distinguishable with firm pressure. Areas on each side of the tail head are fairly well filled but not mounded.

6. Ribs fully covered, not noticeable to the eye. Hindquarters plump and full. Noticeable sponginess to covering of foreribs and on each side of the tail head. Firm pressure now required to feel transverse processes.

7. Ends of the spinous processes can be felt only with very firm pressure. Spaces between processes can barely be distinguished. Abundant fat cover on either side of tail head with some patchiness evident.

8. Animal taking on a smooth, blocky appearance; bone structure disappearing from sight. Fat cover thick and spongy with patchiness likely.

9. Bone structure not seen or easily felt. Tail head buried in fat. Animal's mobility may actually be impaired by excess amount of fat.

Basically body condition allows us to sort cattle or plan a nutrition program. The initial phase of sorting can often be done by age, because many cattle producers keep 2-year-old cows separate from mature cows so that they can feed the younger females at a higher plane of nutrition. Occasionally, mature cows that are thin will be placed with the 2 year olds.

Body condition also can be used to formulate nutritional diets. For a cow to change by one body condition score, she will have to gain or lose 50 to 80 lb and on occasion as much as 100 lb. Thus if you have cows that are body condition score 4 at 60 to 80 days prior to the start of calving and you want to get them to score 5, you have to strive for an additional 60 to 80 lb of weight gain above normal. This means that the cows need to gain 1.5 to 2.0 lb/day to increase their body condition by one score and account for fetal growth.

How much energy (feed) is required to make a one-unit change depends on the starting body condition (Table 4; see also Table 13). Thin cows require considerably less net energy (Mcal/day) than fleshy cows.

Age of Cattle

A good management practice that is used by many cattle producers is to sort cattle by age. The nutritional requirements are different for young heifers being developed than for mature cows. When animals are in a growth stage, it is important to have adequate energy and protein present in the ration to

Table 4. NET ENERGY REQUIREMENT OF MATURE BEEF COWS AS INFLUENCED BY WEIGHT AND LEVEL OF MILK PRODUCTION

Energy Requirements	Cow Weight (lb)								
	1000	1050	1100	1150	1200	1250	1300	1350	1400
NE_m, Mcal/d*	7.57	7.86	8.13	8.41	8.68	8.95	9.22	9.48	9.75
NE_c, Mcal/d for fetal growth†	2.15	2.15	2.15	2.15	2.15	2.15	2.15	2.15	2.15
NE_l, Mcal/d (average milk)‡	3.40	3.40	3.40	3.40	3.40	3.40	3.40	3.40	3.40
NE_l, Mcal/d (superior milk)‡	6.80	6.80	6.80	6.80	6.80	6.80	6.80	6.80	6.80

*NE_m is calculated to be 0.077 Mcal/$kgW^{0.75}$, or 0.072 + allowance for activity.
†Energy required for the conceptus (products of conception) during the last trimester of gestation.
‡Energy required to support lactation. Average milk is 10 lb of milk production/day; superior milk is 20 lb/day. Calculated as lb of milk × 0.34 Mcal/lb. This is added to NE_m during lactation.

Table 5. RELATIONSHIP BETWEEN COW SIZE AND MILK PRODUCTION

Cow Size	Milking Level	lb/Milk/Cow/Day	TDN Needed (lb)*	NE_m (Mcal/Day)*	Crude Protein (lb)*
1000	Average	10	11.5	11.0	2.0
	Above average	15	12.7	12.7	2.2
	Superior	20	13.8	14.4	2.5
1100	Average	10	12.1	11.5	2.0
	Above average	15	13.3	13.2	2.3
	Superior	20	14.5	14.9	2.6
1200	Average	10	14.0	12.1	2.4
	Above average	15	12.8	13.8	2.1
	Superior	20	15.2	15.5	2.7

*1984 NRC requirements.[3]

maintain growth. In contrast, with mature cows, particularly those that enter the fall in "good" condition, some weight loss can occur during the winter with no adverse effect on productivity. One of the keys to having a sound reproductive program with cows is the nutritional management of the replacement heifers. These heifers need to achieve approximately 65 per cent of their mature weight by the time they are bred as yearlings.

Cow Size and Milk Production

To develop a more productive cow, many cow-calf producers have emphasized growth and milk production in their selection process. This has tended to increase cow size and level of milk production. Table 5 shows that a 5-lb increase in milk production per cow per day increased the total digestible nutrient (TDN [net energy]) requirements by 10 per cent and the crude protein requirement by 13 to 15 per cent.

Changes in cow size do not have the same impact on energy requirements that significant changes in milk production do. Each change of 100 lb in cow size changes the maintenance net energy requirements by 6 to 8 per cent.

A common question asked by today's beef producer is, can we maintain reproductive efficiency in higher-producing cows? Actually the question is, will a commercial cattle producer adjust his management program and nutritional philosophies to accommodate the added nutrient demands of a higher-producing cow? Ample research indicates that normal reproductive performance can be maintained in more productive cows if the additional nutrient needs are met. The real dilemma facing the commercial cow-calf producer is that the nutritional needs will be increased, and thus some change in managerial philosophy must occur to accommodate the more productive cow. In making the decision to have a more productive cow, the producer needs to consider the resources available. If there is an ample supply of high-quality feed, a heavier, larger milking cow can often be maintained. If the feed supply is limited or if environmental conditions such as drought, which reduces reproductive rates, frequently occur, then maintaining a slightly smaller, somewhat lower producing cow may be the best choice.

Effect of Environmental Stress

In monitoring the nutritional needs of cattle, keeping an eye on the weather is important. This is true not only during the critical winter months when severe cold is a problem, but also during the spring when wet, damp weather affects the nutritional requirements of cattle.

For cows with a winter hair coat, the critical winter temperature is around 30°F (Table 6). When the temperature drops below the critical level (this is not the actual temperature but the wind chill index), there is an increase in the energy requirement. For each 1°F drop in critical temperature, there is approximately a 1 per cent increase in the TDN, or net energy, required.

To determine the magnitude of cold, critical temperatures are used as a starting point. Estimates of critical temperature for beef cows are shown in Table 7.

Table 8 illustrates the increase in TDN and the amount of hay or grain it would take daily to maintain weight on the cows.

Many cow-calf producers often overlook the effect of spring weather on the nutrient requirements of cows. Cows that have lost weight and are in thin condition are very susceptible to the environmental effects of spring weather. When cattle, even with a winter hair coat, are wet, the critical temperature increases to around 50°F. Thus during wet spring weather when the temperature is around 30 to 35°F, weight loss can occur. In most cases these cows are immediately pre- or postcalving, and weight loss at this time can have a very detrimental effect not only on milk production and calf performance but also on how soon the cow will cycle and rebreed.

Specific Area Deficiencies

Items that any practitioner or nutritionist need to consider in formulating cow diets are specific area deficiencies.

Considerable variation can occur in the quality and composition of forage in a particular region. It is virtually impossible to formulate diets without having some appreciation of the forage protein, energy, and mineral content and how this changes during the season. Unfortunately it is impossible to

Table 6. INCREASED MAINTENANCE ENERGY COSTS FOR CATTLE PER DEGREE (F) COLD

Insulation (C/Kcal/m²/day)	Cow or Heifer Weight (lb)				
	440	660	880	1100	1320
0.010	2.3	2.1	2.0	2.0	1.9
0.015	1.5	1.4	1.4	1.3	1.3
0.020	1.2	1.1	1.1	1.0	1.0
0.025	0.9	0.9	0.8	0.8	0.8
0.030	0.7	0.7	0.7	0.7	0.6

Table 7. ESTIMATED CRITICAL TEMPERATURE—BEEF CATTLE

Coat Description	Critical Temperature	Expected Insulation (C/Kcal/m²/day)
Summer or wet coat	15°C (59°F)	0.010
Fall coat	7°C (45°F)	0.015
Winter coat	0°C (32°F)	0.020
Heavy winter coat	−7°C (18°F)	0.030

Source: Ames DR, Insley LW. Wind-chill effect for cattle and sheep. J Anim Sci 40:161, 1975.

Table 8. EFFECT OF TEMPERATURE ON ENERGY NEEDS

Effective Temperature (°F)	Amount of TDN Increase (%)	Amount of Extra Hay Needed	Extra Grain Needed
50	0	0	0
30	0	0	0
10	20	3.5–4 lb/Cow	2–2.5 lb/Cow
–10	40	7–8 lb/Cow	4–5 lb/Cow

develop tables that can be used nationwide, and thus it is imperative that individuals develop nutritional guidelines for their specific areas. Often an excellent source of information will be either the local extension service or the local feed companies.

Equally important is understanding the regional nutrient deficiencies or even excesses. This particularly applies to trace minerals. As an example, parts of the country are selenium deficient and other parts of the country have excess levels of selenium. As fertilizer practices have changed and the level of productivity of cows has increased, cows have greater demands for specific minerals, which often creates an ideal environment for nutritional interactions that render a specific trace mineral deficient.

NUTRITIONAL DEVELOPMENT OF REPLACEMENT HEIFERS

The replacement heifer is a mixed blessing for most cow-calf operators. On one hand she represents the future profitability and genetic improvement of the cow herd. Thus her selection and development is of paramount importance to the continued success of the operation. On the other hand the replacement heifer is an inconvenience at best. Her smaller size and higher nutritional requirements dictate that she be raised and managed separately from the rest of the herd. Yet because she is essentially nonproductive for the first 2 years of life, she is easy prey for mismanagement. However, the growth and development of the replacement female from birth until she produces her first calf are of critical importance in order for her to become a highly productive part of the cow herd.

The development of replacement heifers can be divided into three phases: (1) preweaning, (2) weaning to breeding, and (3) breeding to calving.

Preweaning

During this phase we largely depend on the dam to nurture and care for the replacement heifer until weaning. However, the influence of a few management practices should be mentioned. Producers are encouraged to individually identify (ear tag, number brand, etc.) both cows and calves so that selection of replacement heifers can be based on objective records of birth dates and weaning weights from consistently early calving, high-producing cows.

The replacement heifer should weigh at least 450 to 600 lb at weaning, depending on breed, frame, and feed supply. It is important that this weight be the result of true skeletal and muscle growth without a substantial amount of fat. Research at several locations has shown that feeding a high-energy creep feed to suckling heifers of British breeding will hinder their subsequent milking ability because of fat deposition in the developing udder. However, a recent summary of large-framed heifers of European breeding showed no effect of creep feeding on subsequent maternal performance. Thus the creep feeding of replacement heifers, when economically feasible, should depend on the breeding and "growthiness" of the calves, with no creep or lower-energy bulky creep feeds being used on smaller-framed heifers.

Weaning to Breeding

Once the replacement heifer is selected at weaning, making sure that she grows and develops properly prior to breeding has a profound impact on her subsequent productivity. Replacement heifers need to weigh about 65 to 70 per cent of their mature weight in order to breed consistently as yearlings. Thus a good nutrition program is essential. Generally heifers should gain 1 to 1.5 lb/day from weaning to breeding, depending on their weaning weight and the length of the feeding period prior to breeding. Usually this means that the average British-bred heifer will need to gain about 250 lb in order to weigh the 650 to 700 lb necessary to begin cycling. With the larger-framed European breeds and crosses, a target breeding weight of 700 to 800 lb is usually necessary.

Puberty in heifers is a function of breed, age, and weight. Recent research has illustrated that the degree of development from weaning to breeding influences not only how soon heifers cycle (reach puberty) as yearlings, but also their productivity and rebreeding rate after they calve as 2 year olds. Research at Kansas State University and Purdue University, as shown in Table 9, indicates the impact of inadequate growth and development during this phase.[2]

It should be emphasized that replacement heifers need to be fed separately from the rest of the herd. Because of their size and age, as well as higher nutritional demands, they simply cannot compete with the rest of the cow herd, nor can they be expected to utilize poorer quality forages efficiently and still breed as yearlings.

Cow-calf operators are encouraged to have their replacement heifers cycling early so that they can be bred 3 to 4 weeks before the rest of the cow herd. The stress of calving is

Table 9. EFFECT OF FIRST-WINTER NUTRITION ON SUBSEQUENT PERFORMANCE OF HEIFERS

Item	Grain (lb) Per Head Fed Daily in Addition to Low-Quality Fescue Hay Fed Ad Libitum		
	0.0	3.0	6.0
Number of heifers	112	113	112
Initial fall weight, lb	496	502	493
Daily gain—winter, lb	0.07	0.50	0.80
Breeding weight, lb	506	577	613
Per cent conceiving as yearlings	69.2	73.9	83.5
Subsequent production			
Per cent rebreeding after first calf	67.3	75.4	87.1
Weaning weight—first calf, lb	405	433	443

Source: Lemenger RP, et al: Effects of winter and summer energy levels on heifer growth and reproductive performance. J Anim Sci 51:837, 1980.

greater on heifers than older cows, and heifers are more likely to have calving difficulty. Thus breeding replacement heifers essentially one heat cycle earlier than the mature cow allows the producer more time to watch the heifers at calving time and gives the heifer the extra time she needs to start recycling and to breed back in sync with the rest of the herd. In addition, the weaning weights of calves from replacement heifers that are bred 3 to 4 weeks early will usually be increased 30 to 45 lb because the calves will be older.

If it is impractical for cow-calf producers to breed replacement heifers prior to the rest of the cow herd, they should then stress a very short breeding season for them. The place to start emphasizing reproductive efficiency in a cow herd is with the replacement heifers. Utilizing a short breeding season (35 to 45 days) ensures that the producer is keeping fertile replacements that conceive promptly. This will also force the heifers into a short calving season so that the producer can give them more attention.

Breeding Until Calving

The final step in the profitable management of the replacement heifer is to ensure her adequate growth and development from breeding until she calves as a 2 year old at about 85 to 90 per cent of her mature weight. During this time the bred heifer should gain about 0.75 to 1 lb/day, or about 250 to 300 lb. Thus British-bred heifers and crossbred heifers of British breeding should go into the calving season weighing 850 to 950 lb, and the larger-framed breeds and crosses should weigh 950 to 1000 lb. It is preferable for the heifer to grow continuously throughout this phase. For spring calving herds, summer pasture is usually adequate for the first half of this period. However, it is important to recognize that most of the fetal growth occurs during the last 50 to 60 days prior to calving. Thus adequate nutrition, especially energy (fed apart from the mature cows), is essential for proper development of the fetus and to prepare the heifer for calving and lactation. To help monitor the status of the heifer's nutritional development, use body condition as a guide, with a body condition score of 6 as the targeted goal.

Research at several agricultural experiment stations has consistently shown that "roughing" the heifer along prior to calving results in lighter, weaker calves at birth without any decrease in calving difficulty; greater calf sickness and mortality; lower milk production; slower return to estrus; and poorer overall reproductive performance. Thus "shorting" the heifer nutritionally prior to calving is an invitation to disaster.

Table 10 shows the major nutritional requirements of replacement heifers from weaning through calving and rebreeding. This information can be used as a guide to feeding these females. However, genetics and environment can substantially influence the heifer's needs. Thus body condition and weight should be used to modify the feeding program.

NUTRITIONAL MANAGEMENT OF BEEF BULLS

Characteristically, when purebred bull calves are weaned and are intended as prospective sires, most producers will nutritionally develop them so that additional genetic information can be collected and used along with expected progeny differences in the selection procedure. The nutritional requirements for bulls of this weight are outlined in Table 11.

In the development of yearling bulls, it is important that skeletal growth be achieved without the cattle being excessively fleshy at the time of use as a yearling. Yearling bulls can and should be used in cattle production systems, but in order to be useful as herd sires they must be properly developed so that they have attained puberty, which is a function of weight, age, and breed. When formulating diets for bulls it is important to recognize that because of the added growth, proper levels of protein and minerals along with energy are needed.

When yearling bulls are used in a production system it is ideal that the breeding periods are not so extended that the bulls are extremely thin when they are removed from pasture. Once a yearling bull is used in a breeding season it is important that he be placed on a plane of nutrition at which he can continue to grow and develop. Mature bulls, when removed from the breeding pasture, also may need to regain some weight and body condition in preparation for the forthcoming breeding season. Bulls should be in moderate flesh when they are turned into a breeding pasture. Typically, mature bulls can be maintained largely on pasture with proper supplementation of additional roughage in areas of harsher environmental climates, but supplemental protein, grain, and minerals are as important as they are with mature cows.

PRACTICAL CONSIDERATIONS

Forage Intake

The fact that virtually all cow nutrition programs are forage based means that at some time during the year cattle will be grazing various types and qualities of forages. The weekly variation that occurs in forage quality and the difficulty in estimating forage intake make precise formulation of cow diets difficult.

The three major factors influencing forage intake are the quantity and quality of available forages and existing environmental conditions. The quantity of available forages is often the first limiting factor. In pastures, crop residue fields, or ranges where abundant available forage exists, animals can selectively graze the most nutritious plant parts that are available. As the quantity, or the quality, declines, the amount of intake per grazing bite tends to decline.

In cattle grazing extremely high quality spring and summer forages, the intake may range as high as 3.5 to 3.8 per cent of the body weight on a dry matter basis when the forage quality is highest. As the plants mature, this declines to intakes of approximately 1.5 per cent of the body weight on a dry matter basis for very mature, low-quality forages. Characteristically, cattle graze at all hours of the day or night. However, evidence exists that the two most common grazing periods are around sunrise and late afternoon, both of which can be affected by environmental temperature and conditions.

Knowing and understanding when cattle graze can have an impact on when supplements are fed. Because supplements should complement the forage, their value is greatest when they are fed at a time that does not disrupt grazing. Research evidence exists that supplemented cattle may not graze for 2 to 4 hours following supplementation. Numerous environmental conditions can have an impact on forage intake. In the northern hemisphere, snow cover often precludes late fall and winter grazing. Up to a point, cold stress will stimulate intake. However, once a certain temperature is reached, actual daily foraging of the cattle will decline. Recent research indicates that as temperatures drop below 0°C, up to a 50 per cent reduction in total daily grazing time occurs.

Table 12 gives a general rule of thumb for expected intakes of cows expressed as a per cent body weight on a dry matter basis.

Table 10. MAJOR NUTRITIONAL REQUIREMENTS OF REPLACEMENT AND FIRST-CALF HEIFERS

Body Weight*	Daily Gain	Crude Protein (lb/Day)	TDN‡ (lb/Day)	ME (Mcal/Day)	Calcium (g)	Phosphorus (g)	Vitamin A (IU/Day)
Replacement Heifers							
400	1.5	1.2	6.9	11.5	20	11	10,000
500	1.5	1.3	8.2	13.7	21	12	12,000
600	1.2	1.3	8.8	15.6	21	13	14,000
700	1.2	1.4	9.9	17.5	20	14	16,000
Bred Yearling Heifers—Last Third of Pregnancy†							
700	1.0	1.3	8.5	13.9	22	14	20,000
800	1.0	1.4	9.2	15.1	22	15	21,000
900	1.0	18.3	9.9	16.2	22	16	23,000

Trace mineralized salt should be provided either free choice in a mineral supplement or mixed into the ration at 0.3% of DM to all cattle.

Source: Some data taken from National Research Council: Nutrient Requirements of Beef Cattle, pp 84–85. © 1984 by the National Academy of Sciences. Published by National Academy Press, Washington, DC.
*Average body weight during feeding period.
†Approximately 0.8 lb gain/day during the last third of pregnancy is made up of fetal growth.
‡The energy (TDN) levels reported are sufficient in relatively mild climates. As a general rule the amount of TDN should be increased by 1 per cent for each 1°F decrease in the wind chill temperature below 30°F for cattle with dry, winter hair or below 55°F for cattle with wet or summer hair coats.

Formulating Diets Using Weight and Body Condition

The calculation of the amount of energy that should be provided a beef cow to meet gain objectives must take into account the cow's weight and body condition status. The "eye of the master" is still an important factor in feeding the cow herd. Weight and body condition are important criteria to monitor in formulating cow diets. The following illustrates how this can be done.[5]

Assumption

A mature cow now weighs 1000 lb but needs to weigh 1150 lb at calving.

Time to calving = 100 days
Body condition score = 4 (thin)
Desired body score = 6 (moderate)
Weight difference between two scores = 150 lb

Procedure

1. Determine the average weight of the cow for the 100-day period. Start with the 1000-lb cow in body condition 2. Add 150 lb to improve a full condition score to 6, or 1150 lb. The average is (1000 + 1150 ÷ 2) 1075 lb.
2. Calculate the average daily gain needed to change a full condition score in 100 days (150 lb ÷ 100 days = 1.5 lb/day).
3. Determine the net energy for maintenance requirement for a 1075-lb cow from Table 5. This is the simple average between the 1050- and the 1100-lb columns (7.86 + 8.13 ÷ 2 = 8.00 Mcal/day).
4. Locate (Table 4) the net energy requirement for fetal growth (2.15 Mcal/day).
5. Add them up. The net energy requirement of 8.00 from step 3 and the fetal growth requirement of 2.15 from step 4 equals 10.15 Mcal/day.
6. Determine the average net energy requirement per pound of gain from Table 13 for a cow going from a condition score of 4 to a condition score of 6 and average these two numbers (1.73 + 2.87 ÷ 2 = 2.30 Mcal/day).
7. Next, calculate the net energy requirement for 1.5 lb/day. The net energy for 1.5 lb of gain is 1.5 lb/day × 2.30 Mcal/lb = 3.45 Mcal/day. This factors in the length of time needed to achieve the desired condition score (100 days).
8. Calculate the net energy for maintenance (NE_m) and net energy for gain (NE_g) values of the ration. These numbers are calculated by multiplying the NE_m and NE_g values (Mcal/lb) of each feed in the ration (using National Research Council [NRC] 1984 feed tables[3]) times the corresponding amount (per cent) of each feed in the ration on a dry matter basis. Sum the products and divide the resulting NE_m and NE_g values by 100.
9. Using the calculated numbers from steps 5 and 7, calculate the amount of ration needed per day to obtain the desired end-point. Divide the net energy for maintenance requirement (10.15 Mcal/day) by the NE_m value (Mcal/lb) of the ration. This will give the amount of ration needed to maintain cow

Table 11. NUTRIENT REQUIREMENTS FOR BULL MAINTENANCE AND FOR REGAINING BODY CONDITION

| Weight* (lb) | Daily Gain (lb) | Daily Energy | | | | Daily Total Protein (lb) | Daily Calcium (lb) | Daily Phosphorus (lb) | Daily Vitamin A (1000s IU) |
		ME (Mcal)	TDN (lb)	NE_m (Mcal)	NE_g (Mcal)				
1430	0.9	24.3	14.8	9.91	2.06	2.0	25	23	48
1430	1.3	26.7	16.3	9.91	3.21	2.1	27	24	49
1430	1.8	28.7	17.4	9.91	4.40	2.2	29	25	50
1540	0.9	25.7	15.6	10.48	2.18	2.1	26	25	51
1540	1.3	28.2	17.2	10.48	3.40	2.2	29	26	52
1540	1.8	30.3	18.5	10.48	4.66	2.3	30	26	53
1760	0	22.6	13.9	11.58	NA	1.9	27	27	50
1760	0.4	25.5	15.6	11.58	1.12	2.1	27	27	53
1980	0	24.7	15.0	12.65	NA	2.1	30	30	55
1980	0.4	27.9	16.9	12.65	1.23	2.3	31	31	58
2200	0	26.8	16.3	13.69	NA	2.3	33	33	60

*Average weight for a feeding period.
NA = not available.

Table 12. INTAKE OF FORAGES OF VARIOUS QUALITIES

Forage Quality	Per Cent Body Weight Intake
Excellent	2.5–3.3
Average	2–2.5
Crop residues and slightly below average quality	1.8–2
Extremely poor quality	1.4–1.8

weight. Next, divide the net energy for gain requirement (3.45 Mcal/day) by the NE_g value (Mcal/lb) of the ration. This is the amount of ration needed to produce 1.5 lb of gain. The sum of the amounts needed for maintenance and gain equals the amount of ration needed by the cow to reach a body condition score of 6 by calving.

Energy Needed	Mcal/day
Maintenance	8.00
Fetal growth	2.15
For weight gain	3.45
Total	13.60

Meeting Protein Needs

The second most expensive nutrient in a cow herd nutrition program is protein. Protein plays a particularly major role during lactation. Likewise it plays a major role by affecting appetite, which alters the level of forage and, therefore, the level of energy that animals will consume. Research has shown that the amount of protein consumed by the cow during the last 60 days precalving was associated with the "weak calf syndrome."[1] Early work linking excess protein levels in the cow diet with increased birth weights has not been supported by subsequent research.

Another important reason to consider protein is that it is often the nutrient most likely to be purchased in a typical cattle operation. Cattle producers need to consider both protein and energy in the initial formulation of cow diets. Some of the common mistakes in feeding protein to beef cows are listed below.

OVERFEEDING DURING MIDGESTATION. A typical 1000-lb cow of average producing ability will need only 1.2 to 1.5 lb of crude protein during the middle part of gestation. However, in many cases producers will feed a roughage of fair quality during this period and also feed a protein supplement, which actually is not needed.

UNDERFEEDING PROTEIN AFTER CALVING. When a cow calves, her requirements for protein double. For a cow producing 15 lb of milk, the requirements are 1.9 to 2.3 lb of crude protein after calving. But when that cow produces 22 lb of milk, the level of protein needed is increased to 2.7 lb.

MISUSE OF NPN OR UREA. Urea is a very cheap source of nitrogen and in many cases can be fed successfully to cattle, particularly feedlot steers. Yet in most cow herd nutrition programs, when forage is often limited or of low quality, urea is poorly utilized because of a lack of available energy. When urea is fed to beef cows under these conditions, a negative response to the high-urea protein supplements can occur, causing a weight loss and subsequent reductions in weaning weights and reproductive performance. In order for urea to be successfully utilized, it must be accompanied by adequate energy and fed to cows being maintained in a positive energy balance.

Vitamin A Considerations

Although many vitamins are known to be important to cattle, the one that is addressed most commonly in cow-calf nutrition is vitamin A. All cattle require a dietary source of vitamin A because it is needed for proper maintenance and function of epithelial tissues of the body.

Research has indicated that cattle are quite capable of protecting or storing large quantities of vitamin A in the liver during periods of high intake. In plants vitamin A occurs in a precursor form as carotene, which is also often stored in body fat. Thus in most systems liver storage is adequate. When depletion does occur and a serious deficiency develops, symptoms include respiratory infection, reproductive disorders, night blindness, rough hair coat, slow growth, muscular incoordination, and even excessively watery eyes.

The requirements for cows at various stages of production are shown in Table 2. The most common ways of supplying vitamin A in cow-calf operations are as follows:

1. The use of forages known to be high in vitamin A, such as alfalfa and other legumes.
2. Inclusion of vitamin A in mineral mixes and even protein supplements that are either self-fed or fed on a daily basis.
3. Injectable vitamin A administered either prior to calving or on occasion twice a year with cows given both fall and spring injections.

Meeting Phosphorus Needs

The key mineral that needs to be considered in formulating a cow-calf nutrition program is phosphorus. In many situations where cows are grazing dry winter grass or crop residue fields, their diet may well be deficient in phosphorus.

Potential for phosphorus deficiency is present anywhere on the North American continent but is particularly prevalent in the Southwest United States, in states such as Texas and Oklahoma. Traditionally the lower the forage quality being utilized in the cow program, the greater the likelihood of a phosphorus deficiency.

There are many ways to meet phosphorus needs. A common method is to buy one of the excellent commercial mixes that are marketed. Some producers choose to mix their own. A

Table 13. ENERGY REQUIRED TO CHANGE BODY CONDITION

Body Condition Score*	Cow Weight (lb)				
	1000	1100	1200	1300	1400
	NE Required for 1 lb of Weight Change, Mcal/lb				
1–3 (very thin)	1.17	1.17	1.17	1.17	1.17
4 (thin)	1.73	1.73	1.73	1.73	1.73
5 (moderate)	2.30	2.30	2.30	2.30	2.30
6–7 (fleshy)	2.87	2.87	2.87	2.87	2.87
8–9 (very fat)	3.44	3.44	3.44	3.44	3.44

Source: Corah LR, Houghton PL, Lemenger RP: Feeding your cows by body condition. Proc KS Focus on Cow Feed Costs. p. 39, 1990.
*Approximately 75 lb difference between condition scores.

Table 14. MINERAL REQUIREMENTS AND MAXIMUM TOLERABLE LEVELS FOR BEEF CATTLE

Mineral	Requirement		Maximum Tolerable Level
	Suggested Value	*Range**	
Cobalt, ppm	0.10	0.07–0.11	5
Copper, ppm	8.0	4–10	115
Iodine, ppm	0.5	0.20–2.0	50
Iron, ppm	50.0	50–100	1000
Magnesium, %	0.10	0.05–0.25	0.40
Manganese, ppm	40.0	20–50	1000
Molybdenum, ppm	—	—	6
Phosphorus, %	—	See Table 1	1
Potassium, %	0.65	0.5–0.7	3
Selenium, ppm	0.20	0.05–0.30	2
Sodium, %	0.08	0.06–0.10	10†
Sulfur, %	0.10	0.08–0.15	0.40
Zinc, ppm	30	20–40	500

Source: Reprinted with permission from Nutrient Requirements of Beef Cattle, 6th rev ed. © 1984 by the National Academy of Sciences. Published by National Academy Press, Washington, DC.

*The listing of a range in which requirements are likely to be met recognizes that requirements for most minerals are affected by a variety of dietary and animal (body weight, sex, rate of gain) factors. Thus it may be better to evaluate rations based on a range of mineral requirements and for content of interfering substances rather than to meet a specific dietary value.

†10 per cent sodium chloride.

popular mix that works very well is a blend of half salt and half phosphorus source like dicalcium phosphate, which contains 18.5 per cent phosphorus. Mixing these equally will provide 50 per cent salt, 11.5 per cent calcium, and 9.3 per cent phosphorus.

It is important to remember that a pregnant cow needs about 18 to 22 g/phosphorus/day, whereas a lactating cow requires from 22 to 26 g/phosphorus/day.

How much phosphorus is supplied by the forage? We will use the example of a cow eating 20 lb of brome hay that on an "as fed" basis contains 0.15 per cent phosphorus (here is where an analysis can be helpful in telling you exactly what the phosphorus content of the feed is). Convert to grams (there are 454 g in a pound, so the 20 lb of feed × 454 = 9080 g total hay fed, which × 0.15 per cent phosphorus = 13.6 g phosphorus). That means that pregnant cows should have at least 6 or 7 additional grams of phosphorus. Eating 0.2 lb of the half salt/half dicalcium phosphate mix would supply 8 to 8.5 g of phosphorus (0.2 lb × 454 g × 9.3 per cent phosphorus = 8.4 g).

A common question that arises in the cattle industry relates to the value of trace minerals. Mineral requirements suggested by the NRC are shown in Table 14. There is considerable discrepancy in the research data around the United States of how important trace minerals are. Much of the research shows very little response; however, there are also indications of isolated areas of trace mineral deficiencies. With the higher-producing cow, it is logical to expect a higher need for specific trace minerals. To be on the safe side, many individuals formulating their own mineral mix will add a well-fortified trace mineral premix to protect against deficiencies. Commercial mineral mixes are generally fortified with various trace minerals.

Water Requirements

The water requirements of cattle are influenced by a number of physiologic environmental factors. These include such things as rate and composition of gain, pregnancy, lactation, physical activity, type of ration, salt, dry matter intake, and environmental temperature. Table 15 estimates daily water requirements of cattle as they relate to month and mean temperature.

Detecting potential problems in water is often difficult. Unfortunately unless you know exactly what to analyze for, water analysis tests may not provide the answer. However, in a number of situations excessive salinity—too high a concentration of dissolved salts—may be one of the more common problems affecting water intake or making water unacceptable to animals. Other factors that may enter into a water evaluation are nitrate contents and alkalinity.

REFERENCES

1. Bull RC: Cow nutrition and calf survival. Proceedings, Range Cow Symposium, 1983.
2. Lemenger RP, et al: Effects of winter and summer energy levels on heifer growth and reproductive performance. J Anim Sci 51:837, 1980.
3. National Research Council: Nutrient Requirements of Beef Cattle. Washington, DC, National Academy of Sciences, 1984.
4. Ames DR, Iusley LW: Wind chill effects on cattle and sheep. J Anim Sci 40:161, 1975.
5. Corah LR, Houghton PL, Lemenger RP: Feeding your cows by body condition. Proc KS Focus on Cow Feed Costs p. 39, 1990.
6. Guyer PQ: Water requirements for beef cattle. Nebraska Neb Guide G77-372, 1977.

Table 15. ESTIMATED DAILY WATER INTAKE OF CATTLE

Month	Mean Temperature (°F)	Cows		Bulls (gal)
		Nursing Calves (gal)*	*Bred Dry Cows and Heifers (gal)*	
January	36	11.0	6.0	7.0
February	40	11.5	6.0	8.0
March	50	12.5	6.5	8.6
April	64	15.5	8.0	10.5
May	73	17.0	9.0	12.0
June	78	17.5	10.0	13.0
July	90	16.5	14.5	19.0
August	88	16.5	14.0	18.0
September	78	17.5	10.0	13.0
October	68	16.5	8.5	11.5
November	52	13.0	6.5	9.0
December	38	11.0	6.0	7.5

Source: Guyer PQ: Water requirements for beef cattle. Nebr Neb Guide G77-372, 1977.

*Cows nursing calves during first 3 to 4 months after parturition—peak milk production period.

Dietary Management of Dairy Cattle

J. T. HUBER, PhD

Milk production in cows is highly dependent on reproduction, which is largely controlled by the endocrine system. Exerting greatest control on reproduction and lactation are secretions from the pituitary, hypothalamus, and ovary, but other secretions have a direct or an indirect influence, with 25 individual hormones that affect growth, reproduction, and lactation of dairy cows.[2]

For optimum milk production a cow must reproduce at least once a year. Endocrine stimulation during gestation prepares the mammary gland for milk synthesis. The normal lactation curve of the cow is largely a reflection of hormonal secretions.

Moreover, hormonal levels are influenced by dietary constituents; hence nutrient deficiencies, excesses, or imbalances can affect endocrine output. Many hormone-diet interrelationships have been shown, but most are not well understood and offer a fertile field for future investigations.

ENERGY MANAGEMENT OF THE LACTATING COW

Mismanagement of energy feeding in dairy rations is probably the most costly error made on dairy farms. The problem manifests itself by undernutrition in early lactation, when propensity for milk production is greatest, and by overfeeding during the late lactation and dry periods, resulting in excessive fattening and consequent metabolic embarrassment. Aside from quantity of energy, form of energy also profoundly affects milk yield and quality. This article will address problems of energy management of the dairy cow during the different phases of lactation and proposed remedies.

Feeding in Early Lactation

For 6 to 8 weeks immediately following parturition (after the cow has had a chance to recover), the milk synthesis machinery of the mammary gland is at optimum function. However, the cow's desire to consume nutrients to make milk is seriously limiting. Mean intakes for cows during the first few weeks of lactation seldom exceed 2.5 per cent of body weight even though highly palatable rations are provided.[13] For high-yielding cows this creates an energy deficit that must be compensated for by mobilization of body tissue. It has been well documented that the early lactation cow has a great capacity for fat mobilization and conversion of that energy to milk.[11] Energy balance studies showed that a cow may incur an energy deficit of as high as 20 Mcal/day (roughly equal to 3 kg body fat) during the first 3 weeks of lactation.[12] For a group of cows consuming all they would eat of a ration containing 40 per cent concentrate and 60 per cent alfalfa hay, the average loss of energy was 7 Mcal/day for the first 66 days of lactation. From 66 to 176 days the cows were essentially at energy equilibrium with a slight positive balance of 0.7 Mcal/day, which increased to 3.4 Mcal/day between 176 and 292 days.

Cows mobilizing fat at too fast a rate in early lactation run a high risk of metabolic disorders, and the practice should be avoided. Solving the appetite problem during early lactation looms as one of the greatest challenges facing dairy nutritionists today.

There are several considerations for maintaining high intakes of cows in early lactation: (1) Rations should be adequately balanced for the necessary nutrients. (2) Sufficient fiber should be available to maintain optimal rumen function. This appears to be 19 to 20 per cent acid detergent fiber (on a dry matter basis). When corn silage is the main forage source, with limited hay, concentrate should not exceed 50 per cent of the total dry matter. When fiber is too low and concentrate too high, erratic consumption and a high incidence of displaced abomasums will result. (3) Texture and sweetness of the concentrate mix are also important. Cows prefer a rough, chewy texture (as with cracked or rolled grains or pellets) to one that is finely ground. They also respond favorably to molasses; generally 4 to 6 per cent in concentrate is sufficient.

On the day of calving, the cow has little desire to eat. Thereafter feed (particularly concentrate) should be increased slowly. Overconsumption will cause digestive upsets. The type of ration received in early lactation should be similar to that received during the last 2 to 3 weeks of the dry period. One system suggested for building up energy intake of the fresh cow is to offer daily about 4 kg concentrate just after calving and increase in increments of 0.7 to 1 kg/day up to a level commensurate with that cow's need for milk production. For most cows it will take 10 to 14 days to build up to the desired concentrate intake.

Body Condition of Dairy Cows

High-producing cows will lose weight during early lactation, when milk yields are greatest and appetite lowest. As mentioned, too rapid a loss in weight causes metabolic disturbances that seriously impair productivity and profitability of the cow for the entire lactation. However, a moderate amount of body fat available for mobilization and milk synthesis is desirable. Large cows can safely lose up to 100 kg body fat during the first 80 days of lactation. This would amount to 12 to 15 per cent of their postcalving weight and should furnish enough energy for production of approximately 650 kg milk. Smaller cows might lose a proportional amount. Body weights, however, do not always reflect tissue loss at this stage of lactation because of changes in gut fill and shifts in body composition (water filling of adipose space).

Restoration of body tissue should occur during mid- and late lactation. If allowed ad libitum consumption, intakes are usually maximized at 50 to 70 days postpartum, and cows reach an energy equilibrium shortly thereafter. As milk production decreases, feeding excessive energy relative to needs allows for regaining lost tissues.

Extra allotment of energy should not usually continue into the dry period because fat accumulated by nonlactating cows is less efficiently converted to milk (about 70 per cent as efficient) than that gained during lactation.[33] Moreover, there is greater danger of excessive fattening if dry cows are allowed to overconsume energy.

Extremely fat cows are more susceptible to ketosis, parturient paresis, mastitis, metritis, displaced abomasum, and poor appetite. The fat cow syndrome, characterized by hyperlipemia and fatty livers and kidneys, results in decreased resistance to pathogenic challenges because of an impaired synthesis of white blood cells.[34] Table 1 lists metabolic diseases encountered in cows calving in a dairy herd over a 4-month period. Approximately 1 year previous to the recorded dates, a reproductive problem occurred in this herd that increased the nonlactating period of many cows. These cows, which were dry for long periods, had a tendency to become excessively fat. Also, energy furnished the herd prior to making ration adjustments on June 1 was about 50 per cent above that recommended by the National Research Council (NRC).[36] The mean white cell count from eight cows with fat cow syndrome, sampled just before ration changes were made, was about 33 per cent of normal (2800 versus 8100 cells/mm^3). For large breeds, feeding sufficient energy to maintain body weight when turned dry, plus that needed for calf and placental growth, appears desirable. Typical rations for dry cows are given in Table 2.

Accurate assessment of body condition of a cow is often difficult. Some cows that might not appear excessively fat may suffer from the fat cow syndrome, and large amounts of internal fat surrounding vital organs might be present. As mentioned, body weight changes do not always indicate gain or loss in body fat because of possible changes in body composition or fill. It is my opinion that weight changes more accurately reflect fat accumulation than loss.

The experienced dairy producer, however, who observes cows day after day is often the best judge of when a cow is

Table 1. DISEASE CONDITIONS AND LOSSES FROM THE FAT COW SYNDROME IN A 600-COW HOLSTEIN-FRIESIAN DAIRY HERD DURING A 4-MONTH PERIOD BEFORE AND AFTER INITIATION OF TREATMENT AND PREVENTIVE PROCEDURES

Time	No.	Disease Condition			Losses		
		Parturient Paresis (%)	Ketosis (%)	Retained Fetal Membranes (%)	Mastitis (%)	Sold (%)	Died (%)
Before prevention* (2/1–5/31)	120	5	38	62	6	3	25
After prevention*	120	2	5	13	2	2	3

Source: Reprinted with permission from Morrow DA, et al: Clinical investigation of a dairy herd with the fat cow syndrome. J Am Vet Med Assoc 174:161, 1979.

*Prevention consisted of decreasing intakes of energy and other nutrients from about 150 per cent to 100 per cent of the recommended allowance.[36] The white blood cell count from eight cows diagnosed to have "fat cow syndrome" averaged just 2800/mm^3.

becoming too fat. Animals that are so heavy that ribs are not visible and hipbones barely protrude above the plane of the back will often suffer postparturient problems. Cows that are dry for long periods, because of a miscalculated breeding date or cessation of lactation, become excessively fat unless energy is restricted.

Many dairy managers, consultants, and veterinarians regularly evaluate body condition of cows during the complete lactation and dry periods. A system widely adopted in the United States is the rating of cows on a scale of 1 to 5 (from very thin to very fat).[43a] This system has since been refined to divide ratings into 0.25 units (i.e., 3.25, etc.). Figure 1 illustrates cows given different scores.

At calving, the body condition score (BCS) of cows should be at least 3.5, and preferably about 4.0, to allow a decrease during the first 70 days of lactation of 1.0 BCS units.[10a] For maximum performance in early lactation, BCS should not drop below 2.5, and a BCS that exceeds 4.0 at parturition might result in depressed dry matter intake during early lactation. A low BCS (<3.0) after 100 days in milk indicates repletion of body tissue at a suboptimal rate. The BCS should increase 0.25 to 0.5 units every 100 days after 70 days postpartum, and a BCS loss exceeding 1.0 for 90 days or longer after calving suggests severe nutritional mismanagement.

Grouping of Cows for Maximum Milk Production

Loose housing units resulting in group feeding of forages and concentrates often cause problems in furnishing the individual cow her nutrient needs. Each cow has specific nutrient requirements related to milk production, body size, age, and stage of gestation. Because of imbalanced rations, social behavior, availability to feed, bunk space, and a variety of other reasons, it is doubtful that a large percentage of the cows in group feeding situations are receiving the most profitable ration.

The practice of grouping cows according to stage of lactation and milk production has worked successfully for many dairy producers. Often unbred animals are placed in one group. This group will usually include all cows up to 90 days after calving. Other cows are divided according to milk production into two or three groups. Dry cows and springing heifers will usually constitute an additional group. Where facilities permit (in larger herds), first- and second-calf heifers would be separated from mature cows to feed for extra growth. Nutrients for the different groups are allotted according to the group needs. Generally energy and protein will be supplied at about 10 per cent in excess of the group's average requirement to accommodate needs of higher-producing cows. Complete rations fed to cow groups will vary from 0 to 60 per cent concentrate to meet nutrient needs at the different stages of lactation. Feeding concentration to late lactation and dry cows is often unprofitable. However, these rations should be properly balanced for protein, vitamins, and minerals.

Where facilities do not permit physical separation of cows, magnet feeders, electronic gates, or transponder feeding units have allowed consumption of extra concentrate by high producers. Magnet feeders are usually the simplest and most economical of the three and are widely used on dairy farms in the United States (Fig. 2). Computerized feeding systems, which electronically control the quantity of feed allowed each cow depending on needs, are in use on some farms. One advantage of these systems over methods mentioned previously is that release of feed is timed so that only the correct cow consumes her own feed. Large expansion of such practices might be expected in the future. Many dairy workers have boosted milk yields and profits by using systems that provide extra feed to high producers. However, if the automated dispensing units are not well managed, they might prove unprofitable.

Milk Production As Related to Forage Quality

Forage quality often makes the difference between profit and loss in a dairy feeding program and is one variable over which the farmer can exert considerable control. Poorly managed, low-quality forages are usually unpalatable and of reduced value in usable nutrients, principally in energy, protein, and minerals.[21]

Maturity at harvest greatly influences the quality of forages.[38] First-cut, cool-season grasses and legumes are highest in energy and protein at the young, vegetative state and decrease in digestible energy by 0.3 to 0.5 per cent/day for each day harvest is delayed. The nutritive value of subsequent cuttings (aftermath) generally decreases at a slower rate than that of first cutting. To achieve maximum crop energy yields and

Table 2. TYPICAL RATIONS FOR DRY COWS BASED ON DIFFERENT FORAGES

Requirement: 14 Mcal NE, 1 kg CP
Type of ration*
  Corn silage (25 kg at 33% DM) + 0.45 kg% 50 CP soybean meal
  Corn silage—urea or ammonia treated (27 kg at 33% DM)
  Sorghum silage (29.5 kg at 33% DM) + 0.68 kg soybean meal
  Sorghum silage—treated with ammonia or urea (32 kg at 33% DM)
  Alfalfa hay† (12 kg)—protein sufficient
  Alfalfa hay (6 kg) + corn silage (13.5 kg)
  Grass hay† (13.5 kg)—may need supplemental protein depending on protein content of hay
  Pasture—protein sufficient

*Mineral supplementation will vary with the ration fed, but all should include TM salt, and calcium:phosphorus ration should be about 1.5:1.
†If forage quality is low, then a limited amount of grain is recommended.

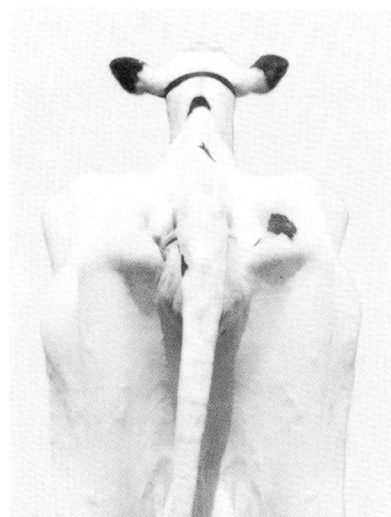

BCS = 1

Deep cavity around tailhead. Bones of pelvis and short ribs sharp and easily felt. No fatty tissue in pelvic or loin area. Deep depression in loin.

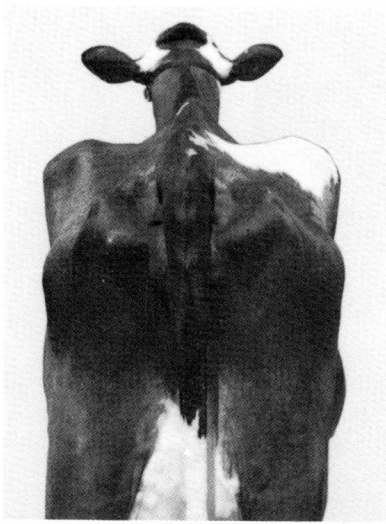

BCS = 2

Shallow cavity around tailhead with some fatty tissue lining it and covering pin bones. Pelvis easily felt. Ends of short ribs feel rounded and upper surfaces can be felt with slight pressure. Depression visible in loin area.

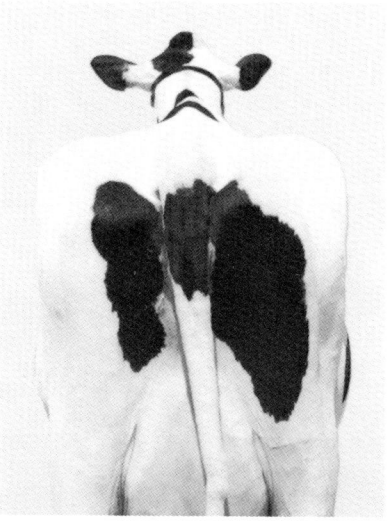

BCS = 3

No cavity around tailhead and fatty tissue easily felt over whole area. Pelvis can be felt with slight pressure. Thick layer of tissue covering top of short ribs which can still be felt with pressure. Slight depression in loin area.

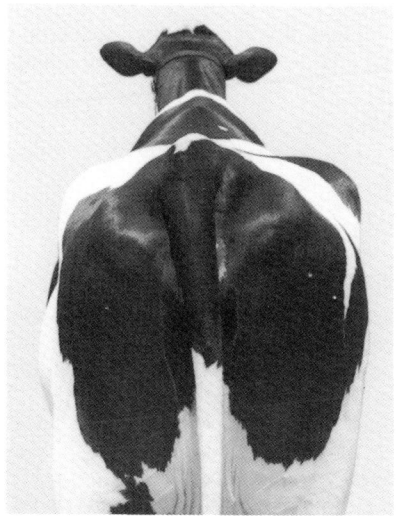

BCS = 4

Folds of fatty tissue are seen around tailhead with patches of fat covering pin bones. Pelvis can be felt with firm pressure. Short ribs can no longer be felt. No depression in loin area.

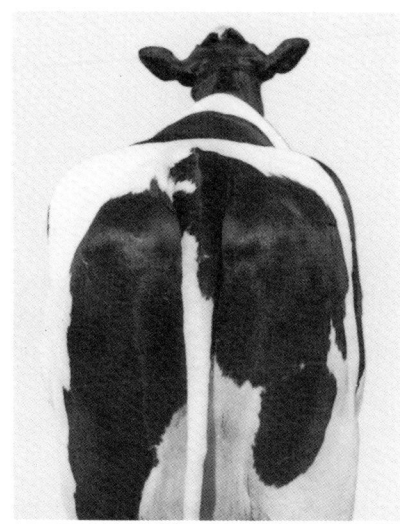

BCS = 5

Tailhead is buried in thick layer of fatty tissue. Pelvic bones cannot be felt even with firm pressure. Short ribs covered with thick layer of fatty tissue.

Figure 1. Rear view photographs of cows possessing body condition scores (BCS) from 1 to 5, with a brief description of each score. (Photos by Craig Johnson provided by courtesy of Elanco Products Co., Indianapolis, IN.)

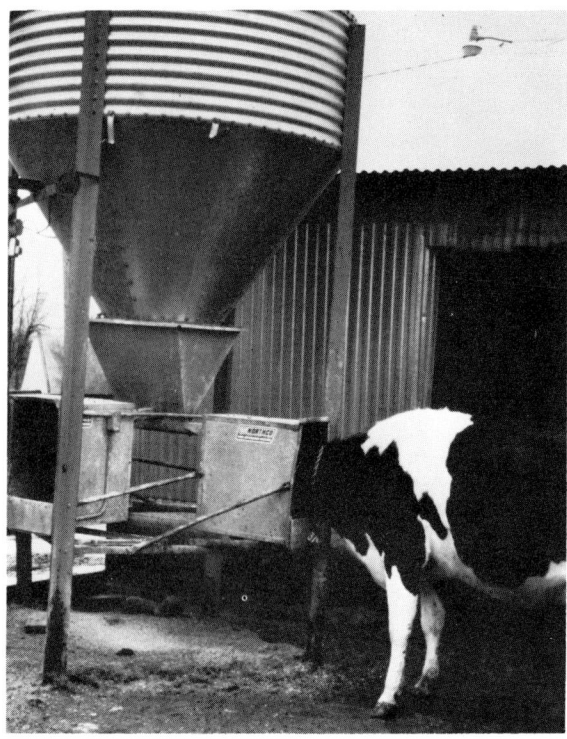

Figure 2. A cow using a magnet feeder on a dairy farm in Michigan.

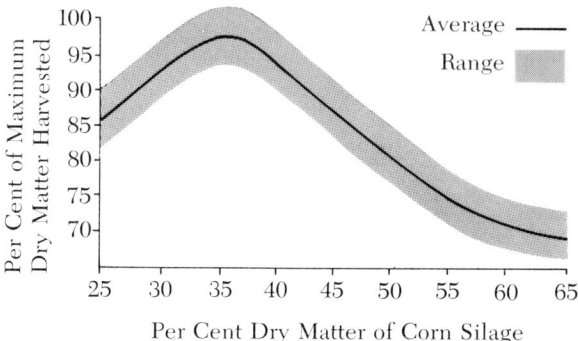

Figure 3. Effect of stage of maturity of corn silage on dry matter harvested per acre. (Summary of research conducted at Michigan, Indiana, and U.S. Department of Agriculture.)

greatest animal productivity, alfalfa and other legumes should be harvested at about 10 per cent bloom, and perennial grasses (orchard grass, timothy grass, rye grass) just prior to budding. Summer annuals (such as Sudan grass and Sudax grass) usually grow at a very rapid rate (if moisture is available) and should be harvested between 90 and 130 cm in height.

Because of starch accumulation in kernels with advanced maturity, the organic matter digestibility of most corn plant varieties changes very little between the tassel and hard dough stages, but nutrient yield is almost doubled during this time.[24] Thus corn should be harvested for silage at approximately the time when starch deposition in the kernels is completed. An easy method for detection of this stage is appearance of a small black layer where the kernel is attached to the cob. Corn harvested at this maturity will possess 33 to 37 per cent dry matter, which is ideal for ensiling in most silo structures (Fig. 3). Fortuitously, corn silage harvested at hard dough (about 35 per cent dry matter) is also more palatable for cattle compared with that harvested earlier (25 per cent dry matter) or later (45 per cent dry matter) and, as shown in Table 3, resulted in higher milk yields in controlled studies.[24] Another disadvantage of delaying harvest is high field loss, particularly in severe weather. Also, with the drier silage, exclusion of oxygen is more difficult and heating and spoiling occur frequently.

The particle size of forages can exert a profound effect on utilization by cows.[20] Forages that are cut too fine (whether grasses, legumes, or grain silages) exit the rumen more rapidly, causing a shift in rumen fermentation toward increased propionate and decreased acetate:propionate ratio. They result in depressed butterfat and a higher incidence of displaced abomasums. An average size of about 7 mm for forage particles should avoid most problems, but minimums might be higher for the denser materials. Silages chopped to achieve a 7- to 12-mm particle size are desirable. On the other hand, silage particles that are too large result in poor packing and a greater chance of spoilage.

Silages inadequately packed or ensiled too dry will undergo excessive heating and a marked decrease in protein and energy availability. Extent of heat damage can be detected by increased fiber-bound nitrogen. Vitamins A and E are heat labile and rendered biologically inactive by excessive heat during storage. This change should be considered when formulating rations for dairy cows fed heated forages to compensate for the lost nutrients.

MEETING THE PROTEIN NEEDS OF LACTATING COWS

Effect of Protein Level on Milk Yields

Protein and energy requirements for lactation vary with the level of milk production and are closely related. National Research Council allowances for a 700-kg cow producing different amounts of milk are shown in Table 4.[36]

Studies during the past 10 years in which protein level has been varied for cows in early lactation (up to 3 months postpartum) have generally shown increased milk production as per cent crude protein increased from 11 to about 18 per cent, but most reports have shown little boost above 18 per cent.[25] Usually when milk yields increased with higher protein, there was also an increase in the amount of feed eaten by cows. Response to higher protein seems mainly to be a

Table 3. INFLUENCE OF MATURITY ON THE FEEDING OF CORN SILAGE

Maturity	Per Cent DM of Silage	Per Cent Total DM as Ears	Milk Yield (lb/day)	Silage DM* Intake (% BW)	TDN in Silage (% DM)
Soft dough	25	37	37.9	1.95	68.2
Medium dough	30	47	40.6	2.13	68.4
Hard dough	33	51	42.1	2.30	68.0

Source: Reprinted with permission from Huber LT, et al: Effect of maturity on the nutritive value of corn silage for lactating cows. J Dairy Sci 48:1121, 1965.
*Cows were fed only corn silage (ad libitum) and soybean meal (1 kg/9.2 kg milk).

Table 4. SUGGESTED PROTEIN AND ENERGY CONCENTRATIONS (INCLUDING UNDEGRADABLE AND DEGRADABLE PROTEIN FRACTIONS) FOR LACTATING COWS (700 KG BODY WEIGHT PRODUCING 3.5 PER CENT FAT MILK)

	Milk Yield (kg/day)					Early Lactation
	12	24	36	49	60	2–3 wk
DM intake (kg/day)	14.9	19.3	23.3	26.7	31.5	AMAF
NE_L intake (Mcal/day)	21.1	29.4	37.2	45.9	54.1	AMAF
TDN intake (kg/day)	9.3	12.9	16.5	20.0	23.7	AMAF
CP (kg/day)	1.83	2.72	3.75	4.35	5.26	—
% (from DMI)	12.2	14.1	16.1	16.3	16.7	—
% (from Summary Table 7)	12	15	16	17	18	19
% of total CP as UIP	37	35	36	35	34	37

Source: Adapted from National Research Council: Nutrient Requirements of Dairy Cattle, 5th rev ed. Washington, DC, National Academy of Sciences, 1989. AMAF = as much as feasible (without causing digestive disturbances).

stimulation in feed intake. In several studies in which intakes were not improved at ration crude proteins higher than 13 per cent, little increase in milk production was noted.[6, 13]

One reason for the higher intakes with increased protein appears to be an increase in the digestibility of the ration the cow is eating, which would increase turnover rate of feed in the digestive tract and allow more space for new feed.[27] Why digestibility is improved with increased protein is not clear, but up to about 14 per cent crude protein it appears related to a more active rumen fermentation. Increased buffering due to greater ammonia release has been proposed as another reason for the higher intakes with increased protein in the diet.

An important observation has been that as level of protein more nearly approached the requirement for maximum milk, response in milk yields per unit protein decreased.[40] Table 5 presents milk yields and intakes of three studies in which protein levels were varied for early lactation cows and shows greater increase in both intakes and milk production when raising protein from 12 to 15 per cent than when raising protein from 15 to 18 per cent.

Special consideration of protein needs should be given to early lactation cows producing high levels of milk that appear to be losing large amounts of body weight. Owing to the normally diminished intakes in these cows, calculations show that as high as 19 to 20 per cent crude protein might be needed to avoid excessive depletion of body protein stores; however, the type of extra protein for these cows should be of low rumen degradability and high biologic value.

Economics of Protein Feeding

The law of diminishing returns in response to protein level is operative in lactating cows.[40] Therefore as ration protein approaches the physiologic requirement, increased milk yields per unit protein decrease. Hence the most profitable amount of protein to feed is often less than that which elicits maximum milk production. Table 6 shows that at low costs for protein supplements, more protein can be profitably added to a dairy ration than at higher costs. Considering present costs of protein supplements, it is doubtful that routine feeding of more than about 18 per cent crude protein would be profitable for most herds, even though early lactation and high-producing cows might respond to as high as 20 per cent.

A factor not considered in Table 6 is the effect of added protein on peak milk production. For each additional kilogram increase in peak production, total lactation yields were increased 200 kg. Hence a protein level that might not show a profit in early lactation but that increases peak yields might be profitable when the complete lactation is considered.

Type of Protein to Feed

Amino acids absorbed from the small intestine are the end-products of protein feeding and directly supply the cow's needs for milk synthesis and tissue replenishment. These amino acids come from microbial protein synthesized in the rumen or from feed protein that escapes rumen degradation. Because of its anaerobic nature, the rumen fermentation is inherently limited in the amount of protein microbes can supply. Estimates are that protein from microbes might be sufficient for the cow's maintenance and 10 to 12 kg of milk production. Hence in high-producing cows a substantial amount of rumen undegraded protein must be available for small intestinal digestion.[25, 39] Early studies of direct infusion of casein into the abomasum showed increased milk yields and milk protein production.[7] Analysis of blood of abomasally infused cows suggested that the amino acids in lowest supply for milk synthesis on typical dairy rations were methionine, lysine, phenylalanine, and threonine.[42] From infusion studies, Wisconsin workers identified lysine and methionine as giving the greatest increase in milk protein production after abomasal infusion.[41]

Increasing undegradable protein has usually yielded positive results in early lactation and high-producing cows. Feeding protected protein during mid- and late lactation has not been as beneficial. Methods for decreasing rumen degradability of protein have included selection of certain protein supplements (such as fish meal, blood meal, corn gluten meal, distillers' grains, or brewers' grains), heat and extrusion processing of protein supplements, and chemical treatment (with formaldehyde).

The approach of formulating rations on the basis of selecting for low protein degradability was commercially developed by a large farmers' cooperative group in the United States. A patent was granted to Braund and associates[4] based on studies showing increased milk production of cows fed a dairy con-

Table 5. MILK YIELDS AND INTAKES IN RESPONSE TO INCREASING PROTEIN IN THREE STUDIES

Location	Protein (% DM)	Milk Yield (lb/day)	Intake (lb DM/day)
Kansas State University[10] (8 cows/treatment, 1–21 wk)	13.0	54.7	40.5
	15.0	62.5	43.2
	17.0	61.4	41.9
Michigan State University[31] (12 cows/treatment, 3–13 wk)	11.3	69.5	36.4
	14.5	74.1	42.0
	17.5	76.3	47.0
New Hampshire University[17] (8 cows/treatment, 2–23 wk)	11.1	60.0	38.5
	13.7	67.4	40.2
	15.7	75.0	41.2
	19.2	73.4	41.7

Table 6. ECONOMICS OF INCREASING PROTEIN FEED

Ration (%)	Change In			Feed Cost—Soybean Meal at		
	Milk Yield (lb/day)	Intake of DM (lb/day)	Milk Value (¢/day)	$200/ton (¢/day)	$250/ton (¢/day)	300/ton (¢/day)
10–12	7.5	4.5	98	39	47	53
12–14	3.9	1.5	51	21	28	36
14–16	2.4	0.7	31	16	24	31
16–18	1.5	0.5	20	15	22	30

Source: Adapted from Satter LD, et al: Supplementing protein to the dairy cow for maximum profit. Proc Distillers Feed Research Council 34:77, 1979.
Note: Prices used were: milk = $13/cwt; grain = 6¢/lb.

centrate of reduced protein solubility (according to methods developed by Wohlt and coworkers[45]) when compared with normal concentrate. Table 7 summarizes this study. The principal change in the supplements to achieve reduced solubility was to increase brewers' and distillers' dried grains and decrease corn gluten feed. More information on rumen bypass protein for lactating cows is needed and should contribute to higher and more efficient milk yields. More exacting studies to assess response to protein quality of the bypass protein are needed.

Combining Undegraded Protein and NPN

The rumen microbes use ammonia for protein synthesis, which is furnished most economically from nonprotein nitrogen (NPN; urea or ammonia). Ideally the most profitable ration for high-producing cows would supply the rumen microbes with ammonia from NPN and would provide the small intestine with "bypass" protein to enhance milk protein synthesis directly. A study by Kung and Huber (Table 8) showed that feeding heated soybean meal resulted in about 1.5 kg more milk per day than the unheated soybean meal, but production was slightly higher and profit was greatest when ammonia-treated corn silage and heat-treated soy were combined in the same diet.[31] The data clearly indicate that in feeding high-producing cows early in lactation, dairy producers can take advantage of savings in feed costs by using NPN while feeding rumen undegraded protein to increase milk production.

Overprotection of the protein from excessive heating or applying too much chemical (such as formaldehyde) results in poor utilization of that protein in the small intestine. Usually, marked increases in fiber-bound protein (acid detergent insoluble nitrogen) indicate overheating. In one study (Table 9) we showed that heating soybean meal for 2 hours at 149°C essentially maximized rumen undegradability with only slight decreases in dry matter digestibility.[31] However, heating for 4 and 6 hours greatly increased the unavailable protein. Insufficient ammonia for optimum rumen function might also occur on rations too high in undegradable protein. The preferred source of nitrogen for 80 per cent of the bacteria in the rumen (particularly the fiber digestors) is ammonia; so a uniform supply of adequate ammonia is necessary for growth of these organisms. Unfavorable results have occurred from incorporation of excessive bypass protein into dairy rations, resulting in insufficient rumen ammonia.

Nonprotein Nitrogen (NPN)

Ruminants possess the unique ability to meet a large percentage of their nitrogen requirements with simple nitrogenous compounds such as urea, ammonia, and others. It was estimated that an annual saving in feed costs of over $500 million is realized by United States livestock producers through feeding NPN to ruminants. In periods of high cost of oilseed meals, savings are greater. Increased profit available to dairy farmers feeding high-energy, low-protein diets who replace about 50 to 60 per cent of the supplemental natural protein fed lactating cows with NPN is about $70 per cow annually.[22]

However, a high level of management is necessary for successful incorporation of NPN into dairy cattle rations, and failure to follow recommended practices might reduce milk yields, making use of NPN unprofitable. Rations ideal for using maximum NPN are low in protein and high in energy, such as those that use liberal quantities of grain and grain silages as is typical in the midwestern and eastern United States. An adaptation period of about 2 weeks is advisable, during which diets are gradually raised in NPN level.

Limits for Feeding NPN

The maximum level at which NPN is profitable in a dairy ration depends largely on the feeding system used.[25] When

Table 8. MILK PRODUCTION, INTAKE, AND ECONOMIC EVALUATION OF DIFFERENT PROTEIN REGIMENS FOR EARLY LACTATION COWS

Corn Silage/Soybean Meal	Protein Type*		
	Normal/Normal	Normal/Heated	Ammoniated/Heated
Milk production (lb/day)	75.2	77.8	78.5
DM intake (lb/day)	45.0	42.6	44.4
Cost of feed ($/day)†	3.33	3.17	3.01
Milk income ($/day)‡	9.85	10.11	10.26
Income over feed cost ($/day)	6.52	6.94	7.25

Source: Adapted from Kung L Jr, Huber JT: Performance of high producing cows in early lactation fed protein of varying amounts, sources and degradability. J Dairy Sci 66:227, 1983.

*Each protein type represents a mean of 24 cows: 12 on 14.5 per cent crude protein and 12 on 17.5 per cent. Treatments were from 3 to 13 weeks of lactation.

†Feed costs ($/ton): hay, 60; corn silage, untreated, 22; high-moisture ear corn (65 per cent DM), 85; normal soybean meal (NS), 300; heated soybean meal (HS), 400.

‡Milk = 13¢/lb.

Table 7. SUMMARY OF DATA OF PROTEIN SOLUBILITY EXPERIMENT

Treatment	Ration Characteristics		Milk Production (lb/day)
	Crude Protein (%)	Soluble Protein (% CP)	
Normal	17.8	38.2	64.2
Low solubility	18.5	21.3	70.2

Source: Reprinted with permission from Braund DG, et al: Method for formulating dairy rations. Pat No 4,188,513. Washington, DC, US Patent Office, 1978.

Note: 20 cows/treatment, from 5 to 15 weeks post partum.

Table 9. SELECTED MEASUREMENTS FOR SOYBEAN MEAL HEATED FOR VARIOUS TIMES

Hours at 149°C	Nitrogen Disappearance from Nylon Bags* (%)	Nitrogen Solubility (%)	In Vitro Dry Matter Disappearance (%)	ADIN/N† (%)
0	76.9	26.5	92.1	1.9
2	36.3	3.9	89.0	4.6
4	38.0	3.8	86.5	8.9
6	37.9	4.1	82.3	19.7

Source: Adapted from Kung L Jr, Huber JT: Performance of high producing cows in early lactation fed protein of varying amounts, sources and degradability. J Dairy Sci 66:227, 1983.
*After 12 hours suspension in the rumen.
†Acid detergent insoluble nitrogen as a per cent of total nitrogen (fiber-bound protein).
Note: Means of 2 to 4 replicates.

urea is added to concentrate fed twice daily, intake should not exceed 200 to 220 g/day (as urea or urea equivalent). Adding NPN to complete rations, to silages, to grain during gelatinization (Starea), or to dehydrated alfalfa during pelletization (Dehy-100) (developed by Conrad and coworkers at Ohio State University) better synchronizes ammonia release from NPN with available energy, which positively affects microbial protein synthesis. These improved methods of NPN delivery allow for greater quantities of NPN to be consumed without depressing milk yields or decreasing feed intakes. The approximate limit of adding urea to dairy concentrate is 1.7 per cent, to complete rations is 1.2 per cent (or equivalent nitrogen), and to silage is 2 per cent of the silage dry matter. When feeding Starea or Dehy-100, the recommended limit is 300 g urea equivalent daily per cow.

Response of High-Producing Cows to NPN

There has been some controversy over feeding NPN-containing rations to high-producing cows, particularly in early lactation. Satter and Roffler suggested that NPN is contraindicated when the crude protein requirement exceeds 11 to 12 per cent.[39] However, experiments (Table 10) show that increased milk yields from adding urea to diets containing 12 to 13 per cent crude protein were about equal to those received from natural protein supplementation. A summary of milk yields of high-producing cows from several Michigan experiments also showed NPN equal to soybean meal for partial protein supplementation of rations up to 14 per cent crude protein.[19]

In contrast, Illinois studies showed that cows fed a 14.5 per cent crude protein diet containing 1.5 per cent urea in concentrate during the entire lactation produced less milk than those fed similar protein from all natural sources.[44] Energy consumption was lower in the cows fed urea, accounting for a large part of the decreased production. These data contrast with those of Holter and colleagues,[18] who showed no difference in milk yields of cows fed urea or soybean meal at levels similar to the ones used in the Illinois study.[44]

In conclusion, data do not warrant excluding NPN from rations for high-producing cows early in lactation. They suggest an efficient utilization of nitrogen from nonprotein as natural protein sources in rations where NPN might be indicated. Adherence to the "Degradable-Undegradable Intake Protein" guidelines in NRC[36] is recommended. Certainly increased profits can be realized by inclusion of more NPN in diets for mid- and late lactation, for dry cows, and for heifers. However, NPN should be used judiciously, and if lowered energy consumption results from feeding NPN to heavily lactating cows, it should be withdrawn.

Adding NPN to Silage

UREA. One of the preferred methods of incorporating NPN into diets for lactating cows is its addition to grain silages.[27] Comparisons of isonitrogenous diets containing urea-treated and control silages have shown milk yields just as high as for the urea silages (Table 11). However, neither urea nor ammonia should be added to silages harvested in excess of 45 per cent dry matter.[26]

AMMONIA. Addition of ammonia to grain silages has been extensively investigated[22] and is a common silage treatment in the United States, Canada, and other countries. A key incentive for development of ammonia treatment was that ammonia nitrogen usually costs about 60 per cent as much as urea nitrogen.

Unlike bound ammonia in ammoniated industrial wastes, which is largely unavailable for rumen microbial use, most of the ammonia from ammoniated silage is in the form of free ammonium salts of organic acids (principally lactic and acetic).[23] These acids keep ammonia from escaping into the atmosphere before feeding.

Ammonia treatment inhibits initial plant respiration and proteolysis, thereby conserving silage energy and natural pro-

Table 10. RESPONSE OF HIGH-PRODUCING COWS IN EARLY LACTATION TO NPN ON NATURAL PROTEIN

Item	Basal Ration (12–13% CP)	Soybean Ration (15–17% CP)	Urea Ration (15–17% CP)
Milk yields (lb/day)	67.6	72.0	71.3
DM intake (% BW)	3.22	3.18	3.23

Source: Pooled from four studies comparing 54 cows per treatment starting 0 to 5 weeks postpartum and continuing to 9 to 20 weeks. Data from Kwan K et al: Use of urea by early postpartum Holstein cows. J Dairy Sci 60:1706, 1977; Murdock FR, Hodgson AS: Effects of protein level and urea on milk production of high performance cows. J Dairy Sci 61(Suppl 1):183, 1978; Clay AB et al: Milk production response to either plant protein or NPN. J Dairy Sci 61(Suppl 1):170, 1978; Foldager J, Huber JT: Influence of protein and source on cows in early lactation. J Dairy Sci 62:954, 1979.

Table 11. RESPONSE OF DAIRY COWS TO UREA-TREATED CORN SILAGE

	Silage Treatment			
	Control	Urea	Urea	Control
CP in concentrate (%)	8.1	8.1	12.3	18.4
CP in total ration (%)	8.2	10.5	13.0	13.5
Milk yield (lb/day)	42.3^a	52.2^b	58.2^c	56.4^c
DM intake (% BW)	2.46^a	2.65^b	3.05^c	2.81^{b,c}
DM digestibility (%)	56.4^a	59.0^{a,b}	65.0^{b,c}	69.2^c

Source: Adapted from Huber JT, Thomas JW: Urea-treated corn silage in low protein rations for lactating cows. J Dairy Sci 54:224, 1971.
$^{a-c}$Treatment comparisons not sharing common letter are different (P < .05).

tein in silages. This protein-sparing action of ammonia was confirmed in nitrogen (^{15}N) studies[23] and was probably responsible for superior results with ammonia-treated silages compared with urea-treated silages when lactating cows were fed large quantities of NPN. Ammonia treatment of silage also inhibits mold and yeast growth (with accompanying heating). This prevention of secondary fermentation is especially beneficial in warm weather and during feeding of silages with large, exposed surfaces. A third benefit of ammonia is preservation of ensiled energy.[25] Studies by Beltsville workers showed that 5 per cent more dry matter and 8 per cent more energy were saved by adding ammonia to corn silage compared with untreated silage.[14a]

SPECIAL PROBLEMS RELATED TO MINERAL AND VITAMIN FEEDING OF LACTATING COWS

There is much confusion regarding feeding minerals to dairy cattle. Farmers are continually bombarded by mineral salespeople whose product is claimed superior to all others. A problem often encountered in the field is that the same mineral is sold regardless of the type of ration the farmer is feeding. Need for supplemental minerals differs greatly depending on the other ration ingredients.

Calcium, Phosphorus, and Vitamin D Relationship to Milk Fever

There may not be one ideal calcium:phosphorus ratio for dairy cows. The optimum ratio probably varies according to the function of the cow (whether milking or dry) and the type of feeds consumed. A ratio of 1.5 to 1.6:1 is calculated from NRC standards.[36] This ratio is probably satisfactory for the dry cow but too narrow for lactating animals. Research has shown that ratios narrower than 1:1 and wider than 2.5:1 tend to increase the incidence of milk fever.[14] High calcium diets just prior to calving stimulate secretion of the hormone thyrocalcitonin, which moves minerals from the blood to the bone, whereas the heavy drain of calcium for milk synthesis requires movement in the opposite direction, from bone through blood to milk. Hence low blood concentrations result in paralysis and death if not corrected.

Just as excess calcium is detrimental to lactating cows, so is excess phosphorus.[5] Primiparous Holstein cows fed phosphorus at 138 per cent of the NRC allowance for the first 12 weeks of lactation yielded an average of 2.7 kg less milk per day for the entire lactation (305 days) than similar cows fed 98 per cent of the suggested phosphorus requirement. The reason for decreased milk production resulting from high phosphorus intake is not known, but these data should discourage the indiscriminate and uncontrolled addition of several phosphorus sources to dairy diets, as has been practiced on some farms.

Heavy supplementation of vitamin D on a routine basis is not desirable, but feeding massive doses (10 to 20 million IU/day) for 7 days before calving has alleviated milk fever, particularly in aged cows.[15] However, feeding for longer than 7 days is dangerous, and it is often difficult to predict calving dates with sufficient accuracy for this treatment to be effective. Research has shown that more biologically active metabolites of vitamin D (hydroxylated cholecalciferols) prevented milk fever when administered in smaller doses.[28] Further study should make their use commercially feasible.

Based on the current state of knowledge, with many questions relating to calcium and phosphorus feeding still unanswered, our current recommendation is to provide phosphorus at 90 to 100 per cent of the allowance recommended by the NRC.[36] Calcium would be calculated from phosphorus to provide a 1.7 to 2.0:1 calcium:phosphorus ratio for milking cows and a 1.5:1 ratio for dry cows. Where corn silage constitutes the main forage for cows, both calcium and phosphorus should be supplemented, whereas only phosphorus is needed in most diets high in legumes.

Sulfur

With supplementation of NPN (urea, ammonia, etc.) in ruminant rations, there is a decrease in natural protein supplements, which contain sulfur amino acids. Also, feeding more of corn silage with less legume hay decreases sulfur intake. Hence dairy diets where heavy corn silage and NPN are employed are likely to be deficient in sulfur.

Sulfur needs of cattle are often expressed in relation to the nitrogen content of the diet. Diets for lactating dairy cows containing about 18 per cent crude protein should have 0.23 per cent sulfur. When corn grain and corn silage are the main components, sulfur usually will not exceed 0.12 per cent, so supplemental sulfur is indicated. Addition to about 2 kg/ton of calcium or sodium sulfate to dairy cattle concentrate should correct a possible sulfur deficiency of high corn silage diets supplemented with NPN. Precautions should be made not to exceed 0.35 per cent sulfur or intakes might decrease.[3] When legume hay is fed in liberal amounts, supplemental sulfur is not needed.

Selenium and Vitamin E

Selenium is an essential nutrient and a constituent part of the enzyme glutathione peroxidase, which, in concert with vitamin E, prevents harmful biologic oxidations.[1] Excessive selenium accumulates in plants in certain areas. Some of these plants have been shown to be toxic (at about 5 ppm). Conversely, soils in large regions of the United States (in the Northwest and eastern Midwest) are deficient in selenium, so rations in those areas require supplementation of up to a required level of 0.2 to 0.3 ppm.

A problem related to low selenium intake on high corn rations is retained placentas in postparturient cows. Julien and coworkers found that injection of 50 mg sodium selenite and 680 mg vitamin E approximately 14 days before calving effectively reduced retained placentas.[29] Vitamin E–selenium injections before calving also decreased retained placentas in herds fed marginal amounts of selenium or vitamin E.

Fluoride

It was generally thought dairy cattle tolerate up to 30 ppm fluoride without adverse effects. However, data reported by Hillman and colleagues showed damaged teeth (mottled and broken) and bone lesions in cattle fed rock phosphates that furnished 15 to 20 ppm fluoride in the total ration.[16] Cornell workers reported fluoride toxicity in cattle exposed to less than 40 ppm fluoride for prolonged periods (3 months of age to adult).[30] Achieving a lower level of fluoride, now required in some states, often requires special processing of phosphate supplements, rendering them more expensive. Until research clearly establishes toxic levels, caution is recommended because bone damage from fluorosis is irreversible.

How to Feed Minerals

Feeding minerals free choice has long been practiced in many dairies. It was thought that if correct minerals were offered free choice, cows would consume according to their needs. However, studies in New York[9] and Minnesota[37] showed no relationship between the amount of minerals needed by ruminants and free-choice consumption.

Minerals should be force-fed by adding them to the concentrate or forage or both. These major feed ingredients are usually consumed in relation to the animals' needs; thus problems of mineral shortages to individual cows would be less likely with force-feeding than free-choice feeding. Force-feeding of minerals prevents overconsumption by cows, whereas free-choice feeding often results in harmful excesses or deficiencies. Silages are ideal carriers of many minerals needed in dairy rations, and in some cases minerals exert a beneficial effect upon fermentation. When cattle are grazing there is usually no good way to force-feed minerals, so offering them free choice on pasture is still recommended.

NUTRIENT REQUIREMENTS FOR DAIRY CATTLE

Table 12 lists feed requirements for heifer calves and growing dairy heifers from birth to 24 months of age, the recommended time of calving. To calculate feed for a specific time, divide totals for 2 months by 60 and allot a little more if age is toward the end of the period. These quantities of feed are for large breeds (Holstein, Brown Swiss, and so on). For the smaller breeds follow recommendations according to body weight, except for milk for the baby calf, which will be about 20 per cent less (mean of 2.75 to 3.0 for small breeds versus 3.50 to 4.0 kg/day for large breeds).

Table 13 gives the recommended nutrient requirements for lactating and pregnant dairy cows as published by the NRC.[36] The NE_l system for feed energy is the most accurate of those listed, but the others are probably satisfactory in any given feeding situation. Successful feeding for high-level milk production is an art as well as a science, and a great deal will depend on the daily observations and contact of the feeder with the cows. These are suggested guides to be used in combination with sound judgment.

Recommended nutrient content of dairy cattle rations is given in Table 14 with suggested concentrations for differing levels of milk production and other functions. Please read the footnotes of this table carefully, because they contain needed information for its successful application.

SUMMARY

The milk synthesizing machinery is at peak function in early lactation, but desire of the animal to consume nutrients lags behind her need for high milk production. Hence large amounts of body fat are mobilized for producing milk until the cow reaches energy equilibrium (8 to 10 weeks postpartum). Caution should be exercised not to build excessive fat reserves in the dry cow so as to avoid a depressed appetite with accompanying ketosis, metritis, mastitis, and displaced abomasum. Restoration of body fat should occur during mid- and late lactation and not while dry because of greater efficiency of conversion to milk from fat accumulated while milking.

Wise energy management of dairy cows includes grouping cows according to milk production and often by age and reproductive status. Harvesting forages at the correct maturity for optimizing nutrient quality and quantity and storing under conditions that prevent deterioration are important for successful dairying. Profits are usually greatest from legumes harvested at 10 per cent bloom, grasses just before the bud stage, corn silage in hard dough or dent, and small grain silage in soft dough.

Protein requirements for lactating cows vary with milk yields. Response in milk production to increased protein diminishes as the diet approaches the theoretical requirement of the cow. Under current prices of protein supplements, diets that exceed 17 to 18 per cent crude protein will probably not increase milk yields enough to pay for the cost of higher

Table 12. APPROXIMATE FEED REQUIREMENTS FOR HOLSTEIN HEIFERS ON ALFALFA HAY OR CORN SILAGE

Age (mo)	Weight (lb)	Liquid Ration (lb)	Grain* (lb)	Hay System† (lb)	Corn Silage Systems† (lb)
1 and 2	90–150	340‡	80	45	—
3 and 4	150–230	0	190	200	—
5 and 6	230–340	0	180	425	995
7 and 8	340–450			600	1400
9 and 10	450–560			880	2060
11 and 12	560–670	—	—	1050	2460
Total to 1 yr		340	450	3200	6915
13 and 14	670–780‖§	0		1180	2760
15 and 16	780–870			1280	3000
17 and 18	870–950			1400	3275
19 and 20	950–1040			1500	3500
21 and 22	1040–1150			1590	3700
23 and 24	1130–1260‖	—	300	1350	3160
Total 1 to 2 yr		0	300	8300	19,395
Total: birth to 2 yr		340	750	11,500	26,310

Source: Data in part from Hillman D, et al: Raising calves. Mich State Univ Ext Bull 412, Nov 1971.
*Grain fed to calves up to 3 to 4 months of age should be a high-energy calf starter containing approximately 16 per cent crude protein and balanced for vitamins and minerals. Feed about 3 lb/day from weaning to 4 months while offering high-quality hay ad libitum.
†Assume corn silage of 35 per cent dry matter supplemented with soybean meal of NPN (urea or ammonia) to contain at least 13.5 per cent crude protein. Feed according to hay system up to 4 months. If hay quality is low during any part of the growth period, grain feeding should be increased to maintain desired energy intake. Corn silage–fed heifers do not need grain during 5 and 6 months. Supplement corn silage with dicalcium phosphate and trace mineralized (TM) salt. Hay systems usually only require TM salt addition.
‡This can be diluted colostrum (2:1 with water), waste whole milk, whole milk, or milk replacer (reconstituted to about 12 per cent solids). Feed approximately 8 lb/day and wean at 5 to 6 weeks when calves are eating about 1.5 lb/day of starter.
§Breed at 14 to 15 months so that heifers will calve by 24 months of age.
‖Weight includes fetus and associative organs (or about 150 lb).
Note: Clean, fresh water should be available at all times.

Table 13. RECOMMENDED NUTRIENT CONTENT OF DIETS FOR DAIRY CATTLE

Cow Weight (kg)	Fat (%)	Weight Gain (kg/day)	Lactating Cow Diets					Early Lactation (wk 0–3)	Dry Pregnant Cows	Calf Milk Replacer	Calf Starter Mix	Growing Heifers and Bulls[a]			Mature Bulls	Maximum Tolerable Levels[b,c]
			Milk Yield (kg/day)									3–6 mo	6–12 mo	>12 mo		
900	5.0	0.50	14	29	43	58	74									
1100	4.5	0.60	18	36	55	73	91									
1300	4.0	0.72	23	47	70	93	117									
1500	3.5	0.82	26	52	78	104	130									
1700	3.5	0.94	29	57	86	114	143									
Energy																
NE$_L$, Mcal/kg			1.42	1.52	1.62	1.72	1.72	1.67	1.25	—	—	—	—	—	—	—
NE$_m$, Mcal/kg			—	—	—	—	—	—	—	2.40	1.90	1.70	1.58	1.40	1.15	—
NE$_g$, Mcal/kg			—	—	—	—	—	—	—	1.55	1.20	1.08	0.98	0.82	—	—
ME, Mcal/kg			2.35	2.53	2.71	2.89	2.89	2.80	2.04	3.78	3.11	2.60	2.47	2.27	2.00	—
DE, Mcal/kg			2.77	2.95	3.13	2.31	3.31	3.22	2.47	4.19	3.53	3.02	2.89	2.69	2.43	—
TDN, % of DM			63	67	71	75	75	73	56	95	80	69	66	61	55	—
Protein equivalent																
Crude protein, %			12	15	16	17	18	19	12	22	18	16	12	12	10	—
UIP, %			4.4	5.2	5.7	5.9	6.2	7.0	—	—	—	8.2	4.4	2.1	—	—
DIP, %			7.8	8.7	9.6	10.3	10.4	9.7	—	—	—	4.6	6.4	7.2	—	—
Fiber content (min.)[d]																
Crude fiber, %			17	17	17	15	15	17	22	—	—	13	15	15	15	—
Acid detergent fiber, %			21	21	21	19	19	21	27	—	—	16	19	19	19	—
Neutral detergent fiber, %			28	28	28	25	25	28	35	—	—	23	25	25	25	—
Ether extract (min.), %			3	3	3	3	3	3	3	10	3	3	3	3	3	—
Minerals																
Calcium, %			0.43	0.51	0.58	0.64	0.66	0.77	0.39[e]	0.70	0.60	0.52	0.41	0.29	0.30	2.00
Phosphorus, %			0.28	0.33	0.37	0.41	0.41	0.48	0.24	0.60	0.40	0.31	0.30	0.23	0.19	1.00
Magnesium, %[f]			0.20	0.20	0.20	0.25	0.25	0.25	0.16	0.07	0.10	0.16	0.16	0.16	0.16	0.50
Potassium, %[g]			0.90	0.90	0.90	1.00	1.00	1.00	0.65	0.65	0.65	0.65	0.65	0.65	0.65	3.00
Sodium, %			0.18	0.18	0.18	0.18	0.18	0.18	0.10	0.10	0.10	0.10	0.10	0.10	0.10	—
Chlorine, %			0.25	0.25	0.25	0.25	0.25	0.25	0.20	0.20	0.20	0.20	0.20	0.20	0.20	—
Sulfur, %			0.20	0.20	0.20	0.20	0.20	0.25	0.16	0.29	0.20	0.16	0.16	0.16	0.16	0.40
Iron, ppm			50	50	50	50	50	50	50	100	50	50	50	50	50	1,000
Cobalt, ppm			0.10	0.10	0.10	0.10	0.10	0.10	0.10	0.10	0.10	0.10	0.10	0.10	0.10	10.00
Copper, ppm[h]			10	10	10	10	10	10	10	10	10	10	10	10	10	100
Manganese, ppm			40	40	40	40	40	40	40	40	40	40	40	40	40	1,000
Zinc, ppm			40	40	40	40	40	40	40	40	40	40	40	40	40	500
Iodine, ppm[i]			0.60	0.60	0.60	0.60	0.60	0.60	0.25	0.25	0.25	0.25	0.25	0.25	0.25	50.00[j]
Selenium, ppm			0.30	0.30	0.30	0.30	0.30	0.30	0.30	0.30	0.30	0.30	0.30	0.30	0.30	2.00
Vitamins[k]																
A, IU/kg			3,200	3,200	3,200	3,200	3,200	4,000	4,000	3,800	2,200	2,200	2,200	2,200	3,200	66,000
D, IU/kg			1,000	1,000	1,000	1,000	1,000	1,000	1,200	600	300	300	300	300	300	10,000
E, IU/kg			15	15	15	15	15	15	15	40	25	25	25	25	15	2,000

Note: The values presented in this table are intended as guidelines for the use of professionals in diet formulation. Because of the many factors affecting such values, they are not intended and should not be used as a legal or regulatory base.

Source: Reprinted with permission from Nutrient Requirements of Dairy Cattle, 6th rev ed, 1989. © 1988 by the National Academy of Sciences. Published by National Academy Press, Washington, DC.

[a]The approximate weight for growing heifers and bulls at 3–6 mo is 150 kg; at 6–12 mo, it is 250 kg; and at more than 12 mo, it is 400 kg. The approximate average daily gain is 700 g/day.

[b]The maximum safe levels for many of the mineral elements are not well defined and may be substantially affected by specific feeding conditions. Additional information is available in *Mineral Tolerance of Domestic Animals* (NRC, 1980).

[c]Vitamin tolerances are discussed in detail in *Vitamin Tolerance of Animals* (NRC, 1987).

[d]It is recommended that 75 per cent of the NDF in lactating cow diets be provided as forage. If this recommendation is not followed, a depression in milk fat may occur.

[e]The value for calcium assumes that the cow is in calcium balance at the beginning of the dry period. If the cow is not in balance, then the dietary calcium requirement should be increased by 25 to 33 per cent.

[f]Under conditions conducive to grass tetany (see text), magnesium should be increased to 0.25 or 0.30 per cent.

[g]Under conditions of heat stress, potassium should be increased to 1.2 per cent (see text).

[h]The cow's copper requirement is influenced by molybdenum and sulfur in the diet (see text).

[i]If the diet contains as much as 25 per cent strongly goitrogenic feed on a dry basis, the iodine provided should be increased two times or more.

[j]Although cattle can tolerate this level of iodine, lower levels may be desirable to reduce the iodine content of milk.

[k]The following minimum quantities of B-complex vitamins are suggested per unit of milk replacer: niacin, 2.6 ppm; pantothenic acid, 13 ppm; riboflavin, 6.5 ppm; pyridoxine, 6.5 ppm; folic acid, 0.5 ppm; biotin, 0.1 ppm; vitamin B$_{12}$, 0.07 ppm; thiamin, 6.5 ppm; and choline, 0.26 per cent. It appears that adequate amounts of these vitamins are furnished when calves have functional rumens (usually at 6 weeks of age) by a combination of rumen synthesis and natural feedstuffs.

Table 14. DAILY NUTRITIONAL REQUIREMENTS OF DAIRY CATTLE

Daily Nutrient Requirements of Growing Dairy Cattle and Mature Bulls

Live Weight (kg)	Gain (g)	Dry Matter Intake[a] (kg)	Energy					Protein			Minerals		Vitamins	
			NE_m (Mcal)	NE_g (Mcal)	ME (Mcal)	DE (Mcal)	TDN (kg)	UIP (g)	DIP (g)	CP (g)	Ca (g)	P (g)	A (1000 IU)	D (1000 IU)
1100	—	14.26	16.43	—	28.52	34.59	7.85	122	1029	1426	45	28	46.64	7.26
1200	—	15.22	17.53	—	30.44	36.92	8.37	115	1113	1522	49	30	50.88	7.92
1300	—	16.16	18.62	—	32.32	39.21	8.89	108	1196	1616	53	32	55.12	8.58
1400	—	17.09	19.68	—	34.17	41.45	9.40	102	1277	1709	57	35	59.36	9.24

Daily Nutrient Requirements of Lactating and Pregnant Cows

Live Weight (kg)	Energy				Total Crude Protein (g)	Minerals		Vitamins	
	NE_L (Mcal)	ME (Mcal)	DE (Mcal)	TDN (kg)		Ca (g)	P (g)	A (1000 IU)	D (1000 IU)
Maintenance of Mature Lactating Cows[b]									
400	7.16	12.01	13.80	3.13	318	16	11	30	12
450	7.82	13.12	15.08	3.42	341	18	13	34	14
500	8.46	14.20	16.32	3.70	364	20	14	38	15
550	9.09	15.25	17.53	3.97	386	22	16	42	17
600	9.70	16.28	18.71	4.24	406	24	17	46	18
650	10.30	17.29	19.86	4.51	428	26	19	49	20
700	10.89	18.28	21.00	4.76	449	28	20	53	21
750	11.47	19.25	22.12	5.02	468	30	21	57	23
800	12.03	20.20	23.21	5.26	486	32	23	61	24
Maintenance Plus Last 2 Months of Gestation of Mature Dry Cows[c]									
400	9.30	15.26	18.23	4.15	890	26	16	30	12
450	10.16	16.66	19.91	4.53	973	30	18	34	14
500	11.00	18.04	21.55	4.90	1053	33	20	38	15
550	11.81	19.37	23.14	5.27	1131	36	22	42	17
600	12.61	20.68	24.71	5.62	1207	39	24	46	18
650	13.39	21.96	26.23	5.97	1281	43	26	49	20
700	14.15	23.21	27.73	6.31	1355	46	28	53	21
750	14.90	24.44	29.21	6.65	1427	49	30	57	23
800	15.64	25.66	30.65	6.98	1497	53	32	61	24
Milk Production—Nutrients/kg of Milk of Different Fat Percentages									
(Fat %)									
3.0	0.64	1.07	1.23	0.280	78	2.73	1.68	—	—
3.5	0.69	1.15	1.33	0.301	84	2.97	1.83	—	—
4.0	0.74	1.24	1.42	0.322	90	3.21	1.98	—	—
4.5	0.78	1.32	1.51	0.343	96	3.45	2.13	—	—
5.0	0.83	1.40	1.61	0.364	101	3.69	2.28	—	—
5.5	0.88	1.48	1.70	0.385	107	3.93	2.43	—	—
Live Weight Change During Lactation—Nutrients/kg of Weight Change[d]									
Weight loss	−4.92	−8.25	−9.55	−2.17	−320	—	—	—	—
Weight gain	5.12	8.55	9.96	2.26	320	—	—	—	—

Source: Reprinted with permission from Nutrient Requirements of Dairy Cattle, 6th rev ed, 1989. © 1988 by the National Academy of Sciences. Published by National Academy Press, Washington, DC.

[a]The data for DMI are not requirements per se, unlike the requirements for net energy maintenance, net energy gain, and absorbed protein. They are not intended to be estimates of voluntary intake but are consistent with the specified dietary energy concentrations. The use of diets with decreased energy concentrations will increase dry matter intake needs; metabolizable energy, digestible energy, and total digestible nutrient needs; and crude protein needs. The use of diets with increased energy concentrations will have opposite effects on these needs.

[b]To allow for growth of young lactating cows, increase the maintenance allowances for all nutrients except vitamins A and D by 20 per cent during the first lactation and 10 per cent during the second lactation.

[c]Values for calcium assume that the cow is in calcium balance at the beginning of the last 2 months of gestation. If the cow is not in balance, then the calcium requirement can be increased from 25 to 33 per cent.

[d]No allowance is made for mobilized calcium and phosphorus associated with live weight loss or with live weight gain. The maximum daily nitrogen available from weight loss is assumed to be 30 g or 234 g of crude protein.

NE_m = net energy for maintenance; NE_g = net energy for gain; ME = metabolizable energy; DE = digestible energy; TDN = total digestible nutrients; UIP = undegraded intake protein; DIP = degraded intake protein; CP = crude protein; NE_L = net energy for lactation.

protein. Feeding NPN can increase profits from dairy cattle. Improved methods of delivering NPN to dairy cattle to better synchronize release of ammonia with the fermentation of energy in the rumen include mixing NPN in complete rations, adding urea or ammonia to corn silage, and feeding modified forms of urea such as Starea or Dehy-100. Investigations showed NPN to be beneficial as natural protein in diets fed to high-producing cows that contained up to 16 per cent crude protein.

For prevention of milk fever, calcium:phosphorus ratios of 2:1 for lactating cows and 1.5:1 for dry cows are recommended. Activated forms of vitamin D (hydroxycholecalciferols) effectively prevented milk fever in susceptible cows when administered 3 to 5 days before calving. This material is safer and more effective than massive doses of vitamin D and will be developed for future commercial use.

Sulfur should be supplemented to dairy cattle diets high in corn and corn silage if they contain NPN. In the areas of low selenium in soils and plants, selenium should be supplemented up to 0.3 mg per cent of the diet dry matter. A reevaluation of fluoride levels that might damage lifetime performance of dairy cattle now appears warranted.

REFERENCES

1. Ammerman CB, Miller SM: Selenium in ruminant nutrition: a review. J airy Sci 58:1561, 1975.
2. Bath DL, Dickerson FN, Tucker HA, Appleman RD: Dairy Cattle: Principles, Practices, Problems, Profits, 2nd ed. Philadelphia, Lea & Febiger, 1978.
3. Bouchard R, Conrad HR: Sulfur requirement of lactating dairy cows. I. Sulfur balances and dietary supplementation. J Dairy Sci 56:1276, 1973.
4. Braund DG, Dolge KL, Goings RL, Steele RL: Method for formulating dairy rations. Pat No 4,188,513. Washington, DC, US Patent Office, 1978.
5. Carstairs JA: Postpartum reproductive and lactational performance of cows relative to energy phosphorus and hormonal status. PhD Thesis, Michigan State University, 1978.
6. Chandler PT, Brown CA, Johnston RP Jr, et al: Protein and methionine hydroxy analog for lactating cows. J Dairy Sci 59:1897, 1976.
7. Clark JH: Lactational responses to postruminal administration of proteins and amino acids. J Dairy Sci 58:178, 1975.
8. Clay AB, Buckley BA, Hasbullah M, Satter LD: Milk production response to either plant protein or NPN. J Dairy Sci 61(Suppl 1):170, 1978.
9. Coppock CE, Everett RW, Merrill WG: Effect of ration on free choice consumption of calcium-phosphorus supplements for dairy cattle. J Dairy Sci 55:245, 1972.
10. Edwards JS, Bartley EE, Dayton AD: Effects of dietary protein concentrations on lactating cows. J Dairy Sci 63:243, 1980.
10a. Ferguson JD, Otto KA: Managing body condition in dairy cows. Proc Cornell Nutr Conf, Syracuse, NY, 1965, p 75.
11. Flatt WP: Influence of pregnancy and ration composition on energy utilization by dairy cows. Proc 4th Symp Energy Metab, Eur Assoc Anim Prod Publ 12:123, 1969.
12. Flatt WP, Coppock CE, Moore LA: Energy balance studies with lactating non-pregnant dairy cows consuming rations with varying hay to grain ratios. Proc 3rd Symp Energy Metab, Eur Assoc Anim Prod Publ 11:121, 1965.
13. Foldager J, Huber JT: Influence of protein and source on cows in early lactation. J Dairy Sci 62:954, 1979.
14. Gardner RW, Park RL: Effects on prepartum energy intake and calcium to phosphorus ratios on lactation response and parturient paresis. J Dairy Sci 56:385, 1973.
14a. Göering HK, Waldo DR: Anhydrous ammonia addition to whole corn plant for ensiling. J Dairy Sci 53:1:183, 1980.
15. Hibbs JW, Conrad HR: Studies on milk fever in dairy cows. VI. Effect of three prepartal dosage levels of vitamin D on milk fever incidence. J Dairy Sci 43:1124, 1960.
16. Hillman D, Bolenbaugh D, Convey EM: Fluorosis from phosphate mineral supplements in Michigan dairy cattle. Mich State Univ Farm Sci Res Rep 365, 1978.
17. Holter JB, Byrne JA, Schwab CG: Crude protein for high milk production. J Dairy Sci 65:1175, 1982.
18. Holter JB, Colovos NR, Urban WE Jr: Urea for lactating dairy cattle. IV. Effect of urea vs. no urea in concentrate on production performance in a high producing herd. J Dairy Sci 51:1403, 1968.
19. Huber JT: Protein and nonprotein nitrogen utilization in practical dairy rations. J Anim Sci 41:1403, 1968.
20. Huber JT: Feeding corn silage to ruminants. Proc 11th Ann Pacific Northwest Nutr Conf, 1976.
21. Huber Jt: The effect of maturity on the digestibility of plant. In Handbook of Nutrition Series. Vol. 111. West Palm Beach, FL, CRC Press, 1979.
22. Huber JT: Nonprotein nitrogen in dairy cattle rations. In Large Dairy Herd Management. Gainesville, FL, University Press of Florida, 1979.
23. Huber JT, Foldager J, Smith NE: Nitrogen distribution in corn silage treated with varying levels of ammonia. J Dairy Sci 61:(Suppl 1):138, 1978.
24. Huber JT, Graf GC, Engel RW: Effect of maturity on the nutritive value of corn silage for lactating cows. J Dairy Sci 48:1121, 1965.
25. Huber JT, Kung L Jr: Protein and nonprotein nitrogen utilization by dairy cattle. J Dairy Sci 64:1176, 1981.
26. Huber JT, Lichtenwalner RE, Thomas JW: Factors affecting response of lactating dairy cows to ammonia-treated corn silages. J Dairy Sci 56:1283, 1973.
27. Huber JT, Thomas JW: Urea treated corn silage in low protein rations for lactating cows. J Dairy Sci 54:224, 1971.
28. Jorgensen NA: Combating milk fever. J Dairy Sci 57:933, 1974.
29. Julien WE, Conrad HR, Moxon AL: Selenium and vitamin E and incidence of retained placenta in parturient dairy cows. II. Prevention in commercial herds and prepartum treatment. J Dairy Sci 59:1960, 1976.
30. Krook L, Maylin GA: Industrial fluoride pollution: chronic poisoning of cattle on Cornwall Island. Cornwall Vet 6(Suppl 8):1, 1979.
31. Kung L Jr, Huber JT: Performance of high producing cows in early lactation fed protein of varying amounts, sources and degradability. J Dairy Sci 66:227, 1983.
32. Kwan K, Coppock CE, Lake GB, et al: Use of urea by early postpartum Holstein cows. J Dairy Sci 60:1706, 1977.
33. Moe PW, Tyrrell HF, Flatt WP: Energetics of body tissue mobilization. J Dairy Sci 54:548, 1971.
34. Morrow DA, Hillman D, Dade AW, Kitchen H: Clinical investigation of a dairy herd with the fat cow syndrome. J Am Vet Med Assoc 174:161, 1979.
35. Murdock FR, Hodgson AS: Effects of protein level and urea on milk production of high performance cows. J Dairy Sci 61(Suppl 1):183, 1978.
36. National Research Council: Nutrient Requirements of Dairy Cattle, 5th rev ed. Washington, DC, National Academy of Sciences, 1989.
37. Pamp DE, Goodrich RD, Meiski JC: Free choice minerals for lambs fed calcium or phosphorus deficient rations. J Anim Sci 45:1458, 1977.
38. Reid JT, Kennedy WK, Turk KL, et al: Effect of growth stage, chemical composition and physical properties upon the nutritive values of forages. J Dairy Sci 42:567, 1959.
39. Satter LD, Roffler RE: Nitrogen requirements and utilization in dairy cattle. J Dairy Sci 58:1219, 1975.
40. Satter LD, Whitlow LW, Santos KA: Supplementing protein to the dairy cow for maximum profit. Proc Distillers Feed Research Council 34:77, 1979.
41. Schwab CG, Satter LD, Clay AB: Response of lactating dairy cows to abomasal infusion of amino acids. J Dairy Sci 59:1254, 1976.
42. Standish JF, Ammerman CF, Simpson FC, et al: Influence of graded levels of dietary iron as ferrous sulfate, on performance and tissue mineral composition of steers. J Anim Sci 29:496, 1969.
43. Vik-Mo L, Huber JT, Bergen WG, et al: Blood metabolites in cows abomasally infused with casein or glucose. J Dairy Sci 57:1024, 1974.
43a. Wildman EE, Jones GM, Wagner PE, Boman RL: A dairy cow body condition scoring system and its relationship to selected production characteristics. J Dairy Sci 65:495, 1982.
44. Wohlt JE, Clark JH: Nutritional value of urea vs. performed protein for ruminants. I. Lactation of dairy cows fed corn based diets containing supplemental nitrogen from urea and/or soybean meal. J Dairy Sci 61:902, 1978.
45. Wohlt JE, Sniffen CJ, Hoover WH: Measurement of protein solubility in common feedstuffs. J Dairy Sci 56:1052, 1973.

Dietary Management in Goats

J. E. HUSTON, PhD

Goats are distributed widely around the world. They are found in environments ranging from deserts to jungles and are a particularly important livestock species to small landholders in developing countries. The goat's small size, high degree of adaptability, high fertility, and appealing nature make it a popular animal in most societies.

The goat's foraging behavior includes an aggressive pursuit of shrubs, trees, seeds, and fruits. This unique dietary preference for the unusual has led many casual observers to the erroneous conclusion that "browse" is essential in goat management. Actually the most significant aspect in the nutritional character of the goat is its adaptability. The goat will eat what it can find as long as it is clean. When given a choice, the goat will sample from the many plant species and parts (leaf, stem, seed, etc.) and seldom will take more than a few bites from any one location.

Goats are observed in all shapes, sizes, and colors. A few breeds have been established that emphasize production of particular commodities (milk, fiber, skins). Many of the goats in the world have no clearly defined physical features, and breeding is largely uncontrolled. The discussion of dietary management will be confined to applications for the Angora, dairy, and meat (and cashmere-producing) goats.

ANGORA GOAT

The Angora is managed primarily for the production of mohair, a luxury fiber that is usually coarser than apparel wool (25 to 40 μm versus 18 to 25 μm in diameter). Mohair possesses a characteristic called luster that gives highlight to fabric, especially to brightly colored apparel. Because mohair is a specialty fiber, the market is volatile and greatly dependent on changing styles.

Perhaps because the Angora has been selected over a long period for a single trait (mohair production), other traits are distinctly inferior. Nutritional requirements are high, whereas growth rate, carcass value, and reproductive rate are relatively low. Recent generations of Angoras have diverged into rather definable breeding lines. Some breeders have selected for larger, hardier ("easy-care") types that produce a good quantity of lower-quality (coarser) mohair. These goats can maintain productivity under marginal nutritional conditions. Others have continued to emphasize mohair production and quality (fineness) at the expense of size and hardiness. Adult size of females ranges from 60 to 120 lb depending on condition (fatness) and stage of production. Reproductive rates range from less than 50 per cent to greater than 100 per cent and are influenced by type of Angora, level of nutrition, and environmental conditions.

Nutrient Requirements

Nutrient requirements for goats were published by the National Research Council (NRC) in a form to be applied to all types and productivity levels of goats.[2] Table 1 was adapted from the NRC nutrient requirement tables. Major nutrients include energy, protein, calcium, phosphorus, and vitamins A and D. Energy is expressed as total digestible nutrients (TDN) in pounds and digestible energy (DE) in megacalories (Mcal). Protein is expressed as crude protein (CP) and digestible protein (DP) in grams. Requirements for calcium (Ca) and phosphorus (P) are reported in grams and vitamins A and D in international units (IU). Body weights are given in both kilograms and pounds. Metabolic functions requiring nutrients include maintenance, body growth, reproduction, hair growth, and milk production. Requirements for the maintenance component were computed to include different amounts of body activity in order that they may apply to the various circumstances in which goats are found throughout the world. The following example (example 1) illustrates the use of Table 1 to calculate the energy (DE) and protein (CP) daily requirements for a 40-kg adult Angora female on rangeland during late pregnancy and producing an annual fleece of 4 kg:

Function	Energy DE (Mcal)	Protein CP (g)
Maintenance	2.97	93
Pregnancy	1.00	57
Mohair	0.15	17
Total	4.12	167

Similarly in a second example (example 2), an Angora kid under pasture management and weighing 20 kg, gaining 100 g/day, and producing an annual fleece of 3 kg (halfway between 2 and 4 kg) would require 2.46 Mcal and 87 g daily DE and CP, respectively.

Feeding Practices

Appropriate approaches to feeding include the very simple to the complex. Perhaps a single feedstuff is available; thus an appropriate question would be, how much alfalfa hay should be fed to an Angora goat? Many books, bulletins, and charts are available that include tables on the nutrient content of feedstuffs, forages, and various by-products. Table 2 includes feed and forage composition data compiled from various sources.[1,2] Alfalfa hay contains 2.49 Mcal/kg DE and 17.9 per cent CP. Therefore 1.66 kg (3.6 lb) alfalfa would provide 4.13 Mcal DE and 0.297 kg (297 g) CP and would be adequate for the pregnant goat (example 1). Similarly, it would require 1 kg (2.2 lb) alfalfa to provide for the energy and protein requirements of the growing kid (example 2). One kilogram of alfalfa would provide 2.49 Mcal DE and 179 g CP, which equals or exceeds the requirements of 2.46 Mcal and 87 g DE and CP, respectively.

Mixed rations are used to balance nutrient composition to meet requirements more accurately without supplying excess (wasting) nutrients. Whereas 1 kg alfalfa would accurately provide the required DE for the kid (2.49 versus 2.46 Mcal), excess CP would be provided (179 versus 87 g). A mixed ration of 25 per cent alfalfa and 75 per cent corn would contain 3.26 Mcal/kg DE and 11.4 per cent CP. In the amount of 0.75 kg (1.67 lb), this mixed ration would provide 2.45 Mcal DE and 86 g CP, which are approximately the energy and protein requirements of the growing kid (example 2). For the pregnant female, a ration comprised of 30 per cent Johnsongrass hay, 30 per cent oats, 35 per cent sorghum grain (milo), and 5 per cent cottonseed meal fed at 1.42 kg/day would provide 4.12 Mcal DE and 166 g CP. Rations can be balanced using a wide array of feed ingredients and optimized for price of ingredients (least-cost formulation).

A major consideration in formulating rations to supply nutrient requirements for goats is intake. How much of a particular feed, forage, or ration will the goat eat? Goats will tend to consume at a level to fulfill their energy requirements. This level will usually range from 2 to 5 per cent of body weight depending on bulkiness of the feed and energy requirements of the current body functions. A goat will consume a medium-bulk feed at a higher level compared with a low-bulk feed, provided that energy requirements are met before body capacity (maximum fill) is reached. Seldom can a goat consume enough of a bulky, low-energy-dense ration to meet energy requirements. However, considerable variation exists between individual animals in voluntary intake. Goats that are growing or lactating will consume approximately twice as much (per cent of body weight) as dry, nongrowing goats. Pregnant goats will eat more of a low- or medium-bulk feed than a similar nonpregnant goat but may reach capacity at a lower intake of a bulky diet, especially late in gestation.

Goats on pasture or rangeland usually will derive most of their required nutrients from consumed foliage. The nutritional

Table 1. DAILY NUTRIENT REQUIREMENTS OF GOATS

Body Weight		Energy		Protein		Minerals		Vitamins	
kg	lb	TDN (lb)	DE (Mcal)	TP (g)	DP (g)	Ca (g)	P (g)	A (1000 IU)	D (IU)
Maintenance Only (Minimal Activity and Early Pregnancy)									
10	22	0.35	0.70	22	15	1	0.7	0.4	84
20	44	0.59	1.18	38	26	1	0.7	0.7	144
30	66	0.80	1.59	51	35	2	1.4	0.9	195
40	88	0.99	1.98	63	43	2	1.4	1.2	243
50	110	1.17	2.34	75	51	3	2.1	1.4	285
60	132	1.34	2.68	86	59	3	2.1	1.6	327
70	154	1.50	3.01	96	66	4	2.8	1.8	369
Maintenance Plus Low Activity (Pasture Management and Early Pregnancy)									
10	22	0.44	0.87	27	19	1	0.7	0.5	108
20	44	0.74	1.47	46	32	2	1.4	0.9	180
30	66	1.00	1.99	62	43	2	1.4	1.2	243
40	88	1.23	2.47	77	54	3	2.1	1.5	303
50	110	1.46	2.92	91	63	4	2.8	1.8	357
60	132	1.67	3.35	105	73	4	2.8	2.0	408
70	154	1.88	3.76	118	82	5	3.5	2.3	462
Maintenance Plus Medium Activity (Rangeland Management and Early Pregnancy)									
10	22	0.52	1.05	33	23	1	0.7	0.6	129
20	44	0.88	1.77	55	38	2	1.4	1.1	216
30	66	1.20	2.38	74	52	3	2.1	1.5	294
40	88	1.48	2.97	93	64	4	2.8	1.8	363
50	110	1.75	3.51	110	76	4	2.8	2.1	429
60	132	2.01	4.02	126	87	5	3.5	2.5	492
*Additional Requirements for Late Pregnancy (for All Sizes of Goats)**									
—	—	0.50	1.74	82	57	2	1.4	1.1	213
Additional Requirements for Growth-Weight Gain at 50 g/day									
—	—	0.22	0.44	14	10	1	0.7	0.3	54
Additional Requirements for Growth-Weight Gain at 100 g/day									
—	—	0.44	0.88	28	20	1	0.7	0.5	108
Additional Requirements for Growth-Weight Gain at 150 g/day									
—	—	0.66	1.32	42	30	2	1.4	0.8	162
Additional Requirements for Mohair Production									
Annual fleece yield (kg)									
2	—	0.04	0.07	9	6	—	—	—	—
4	—	0.07	0.15	17	12	—	—	—	—
6	—	0.11	0.22	26	18	—	—	—	—
8	—	0.15	0.29	34	24	—	—	—	—
Additional Requirements for Milk Production per kg at Different Fat Percentages									
Fat %									
2.5	—	0.73	1.47	59	42	2	1.4	3.8	760
3.0	—	0.74	1.49	64	45	2	1.4	3.8	760
3.5	—	0.75	1.51	68	48	2	1.4	3.8	760
4.0	—	0.76	1.53	72	51	3	2.1	3.8	760
4.5	—	0.77	1.55	77	54	3	2.1	3.8	760
5.0	—	0.78	1.57	82	57	3	2.1	3.8	760

Source: Adapted from National Research Council: Nutrient Requirements of Goats. Washington, DC, National Academy Press, 1981.
*These values have been reduced to correspond with results observed by the author.

value of foliage selected from pasture and range plants is highly variable depending on plant type (annual versus perennial, grass versus legume, winter versus summer-growing, etc.), age of growth (e.g., early, mature, dormant), and environmental conditions. Table 2 lists a few pasture and range plants, illustrating the variability in nutrient content. Whereas legumes (alfalfa), cereal grains, grasses, and even most deciduous trees and shrubs provide good to excellent nutrition while actively growing, they are of somewhat lesser value during slowed growth and of low value during dormancy.

Grazing goats should be fed supplemental feed to provide limiting or deficient nutrients that are not contained in adequate supply in the forage diet. A proper supplement should maximize the value of the forage by providing the deficient nutrients to combine with the forage nutrients to provide a balanced diet. Bulky feeds such as grass hays, hulls, and brans will "substitute" rather than "supplement" the forage diet. Supplemental feeds should be concentrated in energy, protein, phosphorus, and vitamin A. Occasionally other minerals such as potassium, magnesium, selenium, copper, and cobalt will be low.

Supplemental feeding of goats is similar to that of other livestock species. Supplements are commonly fed as loose blends in a trough that is placed strategically in the pasture for convenient access or to enhance proper grazing distribution, or both. Feed limiters such as salt are often included in the blend to allow for free-choice feeding. Salt levels of 10 to 30 per cent are moderately effective at restricting feeding rates to 0.23 to 0.68 kg/head/day (0.5 to 1.5 lb/head/day) depending on forage and water availability and various other conditions. Blended, pelleted feeds and unprocessed feed products (e.g., corn, cottonseed) can be hand-fed either in a feed trough or on the ground. Goats are very efficient at locating and selecting feed particles off the ground. High-molasses liquid or gel feeds and feed blocks are convenient methods for self-feeding animals on rangeland.

Table 2. NUTRIENT COMPOSITION OF SOME FEEDSTUFFS AND FORAGES COMMON IN GOAT DIETS

Feedstuff	Energy		Protein		Minerals*		Carotene* Vitamin A Activity (1000 IU/kg)
	TDN (%)	DE (Mcal/kg)	CP (%)	DP (%)	Ca (%)	P (%)	
Hays and roughages							
Alfalfa hay	57	2.49	17.9	13.7	1.38	0.26	301
Johnsongrass hay	47	2.09	8.5	4.8	0.75	0.25	58
Bermudagrass hay (fertilized coastal)	57	2.53	15.0	10.8	0.43	0.16	193
Pasture-range plants							
Alfalfa, late vegetation	63	2.78	20.0	15.2	2.19	0.33	308
Cereal grain pastures (oats, barley, rye, etc.)	65	2.85	16.6	12.1	0.50	0.36	477
Range grasses							
Lush	66	2.91	11	6.8	0.40	0.17	500
Vegetative	55	2.42	9	5.0	0.55	0.09	167
Winter dormant	32	1.41	4	0.3	0.60	0.05	0
Deciduous shrubs							
Early leaf	65	2.86	15	10.6	+	0.18	+++
Late leaf	52	2.29	8	4.0	++	0.11	+
Evergreen shrubs							
Summer	46	2.02	11.5	2.2	+	0.14	++
Winter	44	1.94	9.2	1.1	++	0.09	+
Energy feeds							
Oats	68	3.02	11.8	8.4	0.07	0.33	0.2
Sorghum grain (milo)	78	3.46	10.2	6.8	0.03	0.28	0.3
Corn	80	3.52	9.2	7.5	0.06	0.24	5.3
Molasses	54	2.37	4.4	1.9	0.75	0.08	—
Protein feeds							
Fish meal	67	2.95	61.1	49.4	5.18	2.89	—
Soybean meal	79	3.48	44.8	41.5	0.30	0.63	0.3
Cottonseed meal	69	3.06	41.2	35.0	0.17	1.10	—
Feather meal	64	2.82	83.2	73.5	0.20	.80	—
Urea	0	0	281.0	281.0	—	—	—

Source: Derived from values published in National Research Council: Nutrient Requirements of Goats. Washington, DC, National Academy Press, 1981; Huston JE et al: Nutritional value of range plants in the Edwards Plateau region of Texas. Texas Agr Exp Sta Bull B-1357, 1981; Landers RQ, unpublished data.
*The calcium and carotene contents of shrubs have not been clearly described. In this table only relative denotations are provided (+ < ++ < +++).

Periods of Critical Nutritional Management

Although Angoras tend to be in continuous nutritional stress, three periods are of particular importance. These are (1) during the developmental period of the young female, (2) at breeding, and (3) from midgestation through the perinatal period.

Early research on the reproductive performance of Angora goats showed that body weight of the yearling Angora female entering the breeding flock (approximately 18 months of age) was highly related to lifetime productivity.[3] Under range conditions, kids weaned at 5 to 7 months of age will weigh 15 to 20 kg (33 to 44 lb). These animals should gain approximately 10 kg (22 lb) during the next 12 months and weigh at least 25 kg (55 lb) at first breeding. Seldom can these young females attain the necessary growth rate under typical range conditions without special attention to health (especially internal parasite control) and supplemental nutrition.

Angoras have a reasonably high capacity for reproduction under ideal conditions yet commonly produce a low kid crop. Low nutrition during the breeding period can result in low ovulation rates and poor conception. Because Angoras have a rigid fall breeding season, diets during late summer and fall are particularly critical. Under typical range conditions in the Southwest United States, diets during late summer (August and early September) are medium to low in quality and Angora females are not able to regain body condition that was lost during the preceding lactation period. Therefore during early fall, which is physiologically the most favorable period for breeding, body condition can restrict breeding success. In underconditioned females, supplemental feeding prior to and during breeding (flushing) can increase pregnancy rate.

Significant additional losses in reproduction in malnourished goats can occur at mid- to late-stage pregnancy from abortion and at the perinatal period. The Angora shows a unique propensity to abort at about 90 to 120 days of gestation if subjected to any type of physiologic (including nutritional) stress. Goats subjected to marginal to poor nutrition as parturition nears often give birth to premature dead or morbid kids. If carried to term, newborn kids may be small and weak and unable to survive, especially during inclement weather.

Examples of Supplements for Angora Goats on Rangeland

Some inclination of the nutritional value of diets selected from the available range vegetation is essential to select appropriate supplemental feeds. Diets of goats grazed on rangelands typically will be of high value in spring, marginal in summer, low to moderately high during early fall (depending on rainfall), and deficient in late fall and winter.[1] The following supplements are examples for the indicated situations.

Adult Angora doe at breeding
  Assume: 40-kg (88-lb) female
         Grazing on rangeland
         Producing 6 kg annual fleece
         Diet quality
           = 2.2 Mcal/kg DE
           = 7 per cent CP
         Intake = 2.5 per cent body weight
           = 1 kg/day
         Nutrient intake from range
           = 2.2 Mcal DE
           = 70 g CP
         Requirements (Table 1)
           = 3.2 Mcal DE
           = 119 g CP

Deficiencies
= 1 Mcal DE
= 49 g CP
Supplement

Ingredient	%
Corn	72
Cottonseed meal	24
Molasses	4

Feeding level
= 0.3 kg (0.66 lb)/head/day
Feeding period
3 weeks before to 3 weeks into breeding season

Adult Angora doe, fourth and fifth months of pregnancy
Assume: 35-kg (77-lb) female
Grazing on rangeland
Producing 6 kg annual fleece
Diet quality
= 2 Mcal/kg DE
= 6 per cent CP
Intake = 3 per cent body weight
= 1.05 kg/day
Nutrient intake from range
= 2.1 Mcal DE
= 63 g CP
Requirements (Table 1)
= 3.90 Mcal DE
= 166 g CP
Deficiencies
= 1.8 Mcal DE
= 103 g CP
Supplement

Ingredient	%
Corn	64
Cottonseed meal	32
Molasses	4

Feeding level
= 0.55 kg (1.2 lb)/head/day
Feeding period
90 days after beginning of breeding season to end of kidding season

Weaned kid growing at 50 g/day
Assume: 20-kg (44-lb) female kid
Grazing on rangeland
Producing 4 kg annual fleece
Diet quality = 2.2 Mcal/kg DE
= 5 per cent CP
Intake = 3.5 per cent body weight
= 0.7 kg/day
Nutrient intake from range
= 1.54 Mcal DE
= 35 g CP
Requirements (Table 1)
= 2.36 Mcal DE
= 86 g CP
Deficiencies
= 0.82 Mcal DE
= 51 g CP
Supplement

Ingredients	%
Corn	66
Cottonseed meal	30
Molasses	4

Feeding level = 0.28 kg (0.6 lb)/head/day
Feeding period: midfall to early spring

No single set of examples can possibly apply to all possible situations. Therefore the reader is encouraged to remain flexible and experiment with various feeds and feeding procedures until the most satisfactory nutritional management program is identified. As a concluding suggestion, when in doubt increase protein level in the diet.

DAIRY GOATS

Compared with Angoras, dairy goats are larger, grow faster, and have higher prolificacy. The five most common dairy breeds are Saanen, Toggenburg, Alpine, La Mancha, and Nubian. Most dairy herds average between 500 and 1000 kg (1100 and 2200 lb of milk) during a 240- to 300-day lactation. The Nubian, perhaps the most popular breed, produces slightly less milk but of higher fat content and combines superior carcass characteristics. Prolificacy in dairy goats is approximately two offspring per doe per year.

Dairy goats have large changes in nutrient requirements, voluntary intake, and body weight during the productive cycle. Mating is accomplished during the last month or two of the previous lactation while the doe is expected to be gaining weight. After termination of lactation and at about 3 months pregnancy, the doe begins a rapid weight gain phase that corresponds with growth of the conceptus. Between breeding and parturition, the doe should gain approximately 12 kg (26 lb), which includes both the conceptus and the stored fat. Shortly after parturition and onset of lactation, fat is mobilized from body stores to support the rapid increase in milk synthesis, which is maximum at about 1 month after onset. Feed intake increases and peaks about 2 months after parturition (1 month after peak lactation). During the 2 months between parturition and maximum intake, the doe is in negative energy balance and drops to its lowest weight during the annual cycle. Thereafter feed intake slightly and increasingly exceeds the demands for maintenance and diminishing milk production and the doe shows a small weight gain until mating. Expected voluntary intake ranges between 2.25 and 4.75 per cent of breeding weight at midpregnancy and 2 months lactation, respectively. Deviations from this typical pattern are common depending on feed resources and genetic potential of the doe.

Feeding the Dairy Goat

Dairy goats can be managed either totally on forages (pasture), in confinement on complete rations, or on a combined system that includes both forages and concentrates. Preferred pastures would include some type of legume (e.g., alfalfa, clover) and a high-quality grass. The nature of the pasture will dictate the need for concentrates of supplemental forage (high-quality hay) to balance nutrient supply and animal requirements. Pasture quality will be high when in early vegetative stage and light to moderately stocked. Mature and overly mature pastures and heavily stocked pastures will not support high lactation. Goats that are not lactating and are less than 15 weeks pregnant can be maintained on average pasture.

Goats managed in confinement can be fed a complete ration or can be fed a harvested forage (greenchop, silage, or hay) and a separate concentrate. A complete ration should contain ample fiber to prevent acidosis and maintain desired fat level in the milk. By-product ingredients such as cereal straw, corn cobs, cottonseed hulls, and peanut hulls are examples of high-fiber ingredients that can be included in mixed rations. It is suggested that no more than 50 per cent of the roughage portion of the ration be made up with these ingredients. At least a matching amount should be a good quality legume or grass hay. Feeding of long or chopped hay with concentrates should be in excess of the desired consumption level, and goats should not be forced to consume all that is offered. Feeding 10 to 25 per cent excess, especially if long hay is fed, allows the goats to refuse the least desired and low-quality portions.

Kids should receive special dietary consideration. Newborn kids should receive colostrum as soon as possible, preferably for 2 or 3 days. Thereafter until at least 2 months of age, a liquid milk replacer that is formulated for goats or lambs (or whole milk) should be fed at a level of 500 g/day up to ad libitum. Beginning at about 1 week a leafy legume hay and a palatable concentrate can be offered. Intake of the dry feed will be low at first but will slowly increase until at weaning (2 to 3 months) the kids will be eating at least 50 g (0.1 lb) hay and 100 g (0.22 lb) concentrate/day. The concentrate should contain 12 to 16 per cent protein. After liquid feeding is discontinued (weaning), intake of hay and concentrate will increase to about 4 per cent of body weight. At about 6 months of age continue feeding a high-quality hay ad libitum and limit feed a 10 to 12 per cent protein concentrate at 250 g (0.55 lb)/day. During the last 6 weeks of gestation, concentrate feeding should be increased gradually to 450 g (1 lb)/day.

Feeding of bucks is less critical than feeding of does. Usually bucks can be maintained on average pastures or on average to good quality grass hay. Special attention is required prior to and during breeding since some breeding bucks drop off in intake. Some concentrate feeding may be required to assure that bucks are in good condition at breeding.

Example Rations and Concentrates for Dairy Goats

The following rations and supplements were formulated using ingredients described in Table 2 to satisfy tabulated requirements (Table 1). Other ingredients can be used if the nutrient compositions are estimated.

Adult dairy goat, complete ration
   Assume: 60-kg (132-lb) female
      3 kg (6.6 lb) milk/day
      4 per cent fat
      Intake = 4.5 per cent body weight
          = 2.7 kg (5.9 lb)/day
      Requirements (Table 1) = 7.27 Mcal DE
          = 302 g CP
          = 12 g calcium
          = 8.4 g phosphorus
   Ration

Ingredients	%
Cottonseed hulls	25
Alfalfa hay	25
Corn	38
Soybean meal	6
Molasses	4
Limestone	0.5
Dicalcium phosphate	0.5
Trace mineral salt	1.0

      Nutrient composition
        of ration = 2.71 Mcal/kg DE
             = 11.8 per cent CP
             = 0.77 per cent calcium
             = 0.31 per cent phosphorus

Adult dairy goat, supplement for pasture
   Assume: 50-kg (110-lb) female
      Grazing/browsing on pasture
      2 kg (4.4 lb) milk/day
      5 per cent fat
      Diet quality (dry matter basis)
        = 2.6 Mcal/kg DE
        = 12 per cent CP
        = 0.5 per cent calcium
        = 0.25 per cent phosphorus
      Intake = 3.5 per cent body weight
        = 1.75 kg/day
      Nutrient intake
        from pasture = 4.55 Mcal DE
             = 210 g CP
             = 8.8 g calcium
             = 4.4 g phosphorus
      Requirements (Table 1) = 7.06 Mcal DE
          = 255 g CP
          = 10 g calcium
          = 7 g phosphorus
      Deficiencies = 2.51 Mcal DE
          = 45 g CP
          = 1.2 g calcium
          = 2.6 g phosphorus
   Supplement

Ingredient	%
Corn	100

      Feeding level = 0.71 kg (1.56 lb)/day
      Mineral shortage = 0.8 g calcium
          = 0.9 g phosphorus
          (Minor: supply with balanced mineral free choice)

Adult dairy goat, supplement for hay
   Assume: 60-kg (132-lb) female
      4 kg (8.8 lb) milk/day
      3.5 per cent fat
      Hay quality = 2.4 Mcal/kg DE
        = 9 per cent CP
        = 0.55 per cent calcium
        = 0.20 per cent phosphorus
      Hay intake = 3 per cent body weight
        = 1.8 kg (4 lb)/day
      Nutrient intake from hay = 4.32 Mcal DE
          = 162 g CP
          = 9.9 g calcium
          = 3.6 g phosphorus
      Requirements (Table 1) = 8.72 Mcal DE
          = 358 g CP
          = 11 g calcium
          = 7.7 g phosphorus
      Deficiencies = 4.4 Mcal DE
          = 196 g CP
          = 1.1 g calcium
          = 4.1 g phosphorus
   Supplement

Ingredients	%
Corn	78
Soybean meal	18
Molasses	4

      Feeding level = 1.27 kg (2.8 lb)/day

Kid goat, weaned at 8 weeks
　Assume: 10 to 20 kg (22 to 44 lb)
　　Daily gain = 150 g/day
　　Requirements (Table 1)
　　　= 2.26 Mcal/day DE
　　　= 72 g/day CP
　　　= 3 g/day calcium
　　　= 2.1 g/day phosphorus
　　Recommendation
　　　Alfalfa hay = 0.2 kg (0.44 lb)/day
　　　Corn = 0.5 kg (1.12 lb)/day
　　　　(plus balanced mineral free choice)

As with the Angora, these examples are not intended to apply to all possible situations. However, the illustrated approaches to calculating proper feed mixtures should be useful once the user becomes familiar with requirements of the goats in the different physiologic stages (Table 1) and nutrient contents of feedstuffs (Table 2). Calcium and phosphorus are more critical considerations in dairy goats than in Angoras. It is suggested that other macrominerals and trace elements be included at low levels in the free-choice mineral mixes. Vitamin A should be included at 2500 to 5000 IU/lb in any feed mixture that does not contain at least 25 per cent legume or bright grass hay.

MEAT (INCLUDING CASHMERE-PRODUCING) GOATS

These goats can be considered similar to milk goats without the extra-high requirements for milk and to Angora goats without the demand for mohair growth. However, meat goats have a higher reproductive rate than Angoras (similar to dairy goats), and this should receive consideration. On the other hand, meat goats that have been selected for cashmere production will have a slightly higher requirement for fiber production compared with dairy goats. The exact requirements of these goats have not been determined. It is suggested that requirements for the lowest level of mohair production (2 kg/year) be used for adult cashmere goats and that fiber growth be ignored for kids.

CONCLUDING COMMENTS

Many management considerations that are not directly nutritional are very important for goat production. Among these are water quality, sanitation, parasitism (especially coccidia), protection from predators and adverse climate, diseases, quality of products, and marketing. It is suggested that readers refer to the other chapters in this volume and other listed references for additional information.

REFERENCES

1. Huston JE, Rector BS, Merrill LB, Engdahl BS: Nutritional value of range plants in the Edwards Plateau region of Texas. Texas Agr Exp Sta Bull B-1357, 1981.
2. National Research Council: Nutrient Requirements of Goats. Washington, DC, National Academy Press, 1981.
3. Shelton M: Factors affecting kid production of Angora does. Texas Agr Exp Sta MP-496, 1961.

BIBLIOGRAPHY

Devendra C, McLeroy GB: Goat and Sheep Production in the Tropics. Intermediate Tropical Agriculture Series. London and New York, Longman Group Ltd, 1982.

Hanlein GFW, Ace DL: Goat Extension Handbook. Newark, DE, Cooperative Extension Service, University of Delaware, 1983.

Morand-Fehr P, Sauvant D: Goats. *In* Jarrige R (ed): Ruminant Nutrition: Recommended Allowances and Feed Tables. Montrouge, France, John Libbey Eurotext, 1989.

Dietary Management in Pigs

ROBERT C. THALER, PhD
ERIC M. WEAVER, MS

Since approximately 65 per cent of the total cost of swine production is feed, a great deal of attention must be paid to the nutritional program of a swine operation. The goal of a successful swine feeding program is to provide all the essential nutrients (amino acids, fatty acids, vitamins, minerals, and water) in the required amounts necessary to maintain proper growth and reproduction. The factor that makes this challenging is the pig's ability to utilize a great many feedstuffs, ranging from corn and soybean meal to alfalfa and sweet potatoes. However, by combining the different ingredients in the proper ratios, the goal can be achieved.

Other factors can also influence the effectiveness of a swine feeding program. Some of them include stage of life cycle, nonnutritive feed additives, and proper feed processing. Sound management practices in these areas, along with the required amounts of amino acids, fatty acids, vitamins, minerals, and water, will ensure a successful swine dietary management program.

ESSENTIAL NUTRIENTS FOR SWINE

Protein

Traditionally protein "requirement" is the requirement most people are familiar with when working with swine rations. However, pigs do not have a protein requirement per se; they have a requirement for 10 essential amino acids and a source of nonspecific nitrogen. The 10 essential amino acids that must be present in the diet are lysine, tryptophan, threonine, methionine, isoleucine, phenylalanine, arginine, histidine, leucine, and valine. In swine diets utilizing natural feedstuffs, the amino acids of concern are lysine, tryptophan, and threonine. Nonspecific nitrogen is used in the synthesis of nonessential amino acids and is usually supplied by transamination of excess amino acids in the diet. As a rule of thumb, as long as the requirements for all the essential amino acids are met, the requirement for nonspecific nitrogen also will be met.

It is also critical that the essential and nonessential amino acids be present in the diet in a specific ratio for optimum performance. If the ratio of the amino acids is grossly out of line, an imbalance or antagonism could occur. Symptoms of an imbalance or antagonism include a reduction in feed intake with a concomitant decrease in growth. However, minor discrepancies will usually not inhibit performance, so various other feedstuff combinations will work as long as the requirements for the essential amino acids are met.

Since an "ideal protein" with all the amino acids present in the correct amounts does not exist, various feedstuffs are mixed to provide an acceptable combination. Typically, when comparing natural feedstuffs, a corn–soybean meal blend provides amino acid ratios closest to that of the ideal protein. In fact, corn–soybean meal diets can be formulated on a protein basis. However, when using other feedstuffs, diets should be formulated on a lysine basis, making sure tryptophan and threonine are present in adequate optimum performance.

With the advent of commercially available amino acids, certain feedstuff combinations can supply an amino acid balance closer to the ideal protein concept, or diet cost can be lowered by decreasing the amount of protein supplement used. It should be remembered, though, that the pig can utilize only the L-isomer of most amino acids. The exceptions are that DL-methionine can completely replace L-methionine, and DL-tryptophan can replace approximately 85 per cent of the L-tryptophan in a diet. All other amino acids must be present in the L-isomer in order to be utilized by the pig. At today's prices, lysine is the only synthetic amino acid that is price competitive. Since the form of commercially available synthetic lysine is L-lysine HCl, it is only 78 per cent L-lysine. For example, 3 lb of L-lysine HCl provides only 2.34 lb of actual lysine. In corn–soybean meal diets, synthetic lysine can decrease percentage protein of a diet by 2 per cent (16 per cent down to 14 per cent) without other amino acids becoming limiting. This can be accomplished by replacing 100 lb of 44 per cent protein soybean meal with 3 lb of L-lysine HCl and 97 lb of corn. The decision to make the switch should be based strictly on the cost of 100 lb of soybean meal compared with that of 97 lb of corn and 3 lb of synthetic lysine.

Perhaps since protein sources are some of the more expensive components in a swine diet, the most common nutrient deficiency is amino acids. Amino acid deficiencies result in increased feed wastage, reduced growth, general unthriftiness, and, in the case of lactating sows, impaired milk production. At the other extreme, excess amounts of protein will cause no ill effects, except perhaps a mild case of diarrhea. However, large excesses of individual amino acids can result in an imbalance, antagonism, or even toxicity.

Amino acid and protein requirements throughout the life cycle of the pig are shown in Table 1. Since these are National Research Council (NRC) recommendations, these values represent the concentration of each nutrient necessary to support normal growth.[4] Because these are minimums, many universities and commercial feed companies recommend nutrient concentrations 10 per cent greater or more than those listed by the NRC in order to establish a safety factor and to achieve maximum instead of normal growth.

Other factors can also influence the amino acid requirements of pigs. Amino acid requirement is dependent on the type of response criteria measured. It takes higher levels of amino acids to achieve maximum carcass leanness than it does to achieve maximum gains. Another factor is gender effect. Since gilts and boars eat less feed and are leaner, they need higher amino acid concentrations than barrows for lean tissue accretion. This difference has led to the development of split-sex feeding in the finisher phase. In this situation, barrows and gilts are sorted into different pens (rooms, barns) that can accommodate feeding two different diets. The barrows are fed a lower protein diet than the gilts, which lessens the diet cost for the barrows without a reduction in performance. Recent work at the University of Kentucky indicates that the lean, rapid-growth genotype pig has a greater amino acid requirement than the "average" genotype pig. Based on this, nutrient levels used in each operation must be determined by how the hog is marketed (live-weight versus carcass merit basis), genotype of pig, and method of feeding (split-sex versus traditional).

Minerals

Swine require minerals for skeletal structure and metabolic functions. Minerals are classified according to relative need into two groups: macrominerals and microminerals. Macrominerals are required in relatively large quantities, whereas microminerals are required in very small quantities. Commonly the minerals added to grain–soybean meal based diets include calcium, phosphorus, sodium, chlorine, iron, zinc, iodine, selenium, copper, and manganese. Traditional feedstuffs usually supply adequate amounts of three additional macrominerals: magnesium, potassium, and sulfur. Levels of specific microminerals are sometimes altered in swine feeds in different geographic locations to eliminate a potential imbalance or deficiency. Generally, excess levels of minerals are not recommended, as they can create an imbalance. Dietary mineral levels that support maximum rate of growth and feed efficiency or that are necessary for maintenance and reproduction are shown in Table 1.

CALCIUM AND PHOSPHORUS. Calcium and phosphorus play major roles in bone mineralization and in vital metabolic reactions. Common feedstuffs of plant origin usually contain limited quantities of calcium and little available phosphorus. For example, corn contains only 0.03 per cent calcium and 0.28 per cent phosphorus. Phosphorus from plants is typically bound in phytates, which limits phosphorus bioavailability to 15 to 30 per cent. Dicalcium phosphate, limestone, and bone meal are common feedstuffs used in fortification of swine diets with calcium and/or phosphorus.

The pig's daily need for calcium and phosphorus is fairly well defined. However, excess calcium competes with phosphorus for absorption, creating a need for a balanced ratio of calcium to phosphorus. A calcium:phosphorus ratio of 1:1 to 1.5:1 is acceptable for swine in all stages of production. A calcium or phosphorus deficiency, or a deviation from the accepted ratio, results in poor growth, lameness, and bone demineralization. High-milk-producing sows frequently exhibit posterior paralysis, or Downer Sow syndrome, as a result of extensive bone demineralization. Improper dietary level of calcium, phosphorus, or vitamin D in either gestation or lactation rations is regularly the cause of an increased incidence of posterior paralysis, but frequently a high level of production and physical stress following weaning are equally important in causing the syndrome.

SODIUM AND CHLORINE. Sodium and chlorine are extracellular electrolytes involved in nerve function. Chlorine is also the anion in hydrochloric acid secreted by the stomach. Both minerals are supplied in swine diets as white salt, so the requirement is usually listed as the per cent of salt in the diet. Salt additions are recommended to be 0.25 per cent for starter, grower, and finisher phases, and 0.5 per cent for gestating and lactating sows. Sodium and chlorine deficiency reduces appetite and growth rates in swine. Swine can tolerate up to 2.0 per cent salt provided that they have free access to water. Salt toxicity can result if access to water is limited or if the water contains salt. Symptoms of salt toxicity are nervousness, weakness, staggering, epileptic seizures, and death.

IRON. Iron is required by the body as a component of hemoglobin, myoglobin, and many other metabolic enzymes. Lack of placental transfer of iron does not allow for substantial iron stores in the liver of the newborn pig. Also, the iron content of sow milk, as lactoferrin, is low, which leaves the young nursing pig susceptible to iron-deficiency anemia. Supplemental dietary iron can be supplied through many sources and methods. Sources of dietary iron include ferrous sulfate, ferrous fumarate, ferric chloride, ferric ammonium citrate, and ferric citrate. Swabbing the udder of the dam, providing clean (pathogen-free) dirt in the crate, oral gavage, and

Table 1. NUTRIENT REQUIREMENTS OF SWINE*

Item	Pig Weight (lb)					
	11–22	22–44	44–110	110–240	Gestation†	Lactation
Feed intake,‡ lb/day	1.01	2.09	4.19	6.85	4.19	11.67
Energy concentration, kcal ME/lb diet	1473	1477	1482	1489	1481	1481
Nutrients§						
Protein, %	20	18	15	13	12	13
Arginine, %	0.50	0.40	0.25	0.10	0.00	0.40
Histidine, %	0.31	0.25	0.22	0.18	0.15	0.25
Isoleucine, %	0.65	0.53	0.46	0.38	0.30	0.39
Leucine, %	0.85	0.70	0.60	0.50	0.30	0.48
Lysine, %	1.15	0.95	0.75	0.60	0.43	0.60
Methionine + cystine, %	0.58	0.48	0.41	0.34	0.23	0.36
Phenylalanine + tyrosine, %	0.94	0.77	0.66	0.55	0.45	0.70
Threonine, %	0.68	0.56	0.48	0.40	0.30	0.43
Tryptophan, %	0.17	0.14	0.12	0.10	0.09	0.12
Valine, %	0.68	0.56	0.48	0.40	0.32	0.60
Linoleic acid, %	0.10	0.10	0.10	0.10	0.10	0.10
Calcium, %	0.80	0.70	0.60	0.50	0.75	0.75
Phosphorus, %	0.65	0.60	0.50	0.40	0.60	0.60
Sodium, %	0.10	0.10	0.10	0.10	0.15	0.20
Chlorine, %	0.08	0.08	0.08	0.08	0.12	0.16
Magnesium, %	0.04	0.04	0.04	0.04	0.04	0.04
Potassium, %	0.28	0.26	0.23	0.17	0.20	0.20
Copper, mg	2.7	2.3	1.8	1.4	2.3	2.3
Iodine, mg	0.06	0.06	0.06	0.06	0.06	0.06
Iron, mg	45	36	27	18	36	36
Manganese, mg	1.82	1.36	0.91	0.91	4.55	4.55
Selenium, mg ‖	0.14	0.11	0.07	0.05	0.07	0.07
Zinc, mg	45	36	27	23	23	23
Vitamin A, IU	1000	795	591	591	1818	909
Vitamin D, IU	100	91	68	68	91	91
Vitamin E, IU	7.3	5.0	5.0	5.0	10.0	10.0
Vitamin K, mg	0.23	0.23	0.23	0.23	0.23	0.23
Biotin, mg	0.023	0.023	0.023	0.023	0.091	0.091
Choline, g	0.23	0.18	0.14	0.14	0.57	0.45
Folacin, mg	0.14	0.14	0.14	0.14	0.14	0.14
Niacin, mg	6.8	5.7	4.6	3.2	4.6	4.6
Pantothenic acid, mg	4.6	4.1	3.6	3.2	5.5	5.5
Riboflavin, mg	1.59	1.36	1.14	0.91	1.70	1.70
Thiamin, mg	0.45	0.45	0.45	0.45	0.45	0.45
Vitamin B_6, mg	0.68	0.68	0.45	0.45	0.45	0.45
Vitamin B_{12}, μg	8.0	6.8	4.5	2.3	6.8	6.8

Source: Reprinted with permission from National Research Council: Nutrient Requirements of Swine, 9th ed. © 1988 by the National Academy of Sciences. Published by National Academy Press, Washington, DC.

*Values represent the concentration of each nutrient necessary to support normal growth. Since these are minimums, many universities and commercial feed companies recommend nutrient concentrations 10 per cent greater or more than those listed by the NRC.

†Gestation values also represent the recommended nutrient concentrations for adult boars.

‡Values listed as % or amount/lb are dependent on the assumption that pigs consume at least the recommended amount of feed/day.

§Nutrient recommendations are given as % or amount/lb of complete feed.

‖ Maximum amount of added selenium allowed by the FDA is 0.14 mg/lb of feed.

supplementing the sow diet while providing the pig access to her fecal material are feasible methods of supplying dietary iron to the young pig.

The most common method of supplying iron is by injection of up to 200 mg of iron dextran, iron dextrin, or gleptoferron. The injection should be made in the neck muscle instead of the ham to prevent paralysis and the staining of a primal cut of pork. Excess iron should not be administered, as unbound serum iron promotes bacterial growth in the blood. Also, a route of excretion of iron is via sloughing of intestinal epithelial tissue, which can also encourage bacterial growth in the gut. Dietary iron levels of 3000 ppm or more are toxic, while a single oral dose of 200 mg of ferric ammonium citrate, ferrous sulfate, or ferric oxide can be toxic in the newborn.

ZINC. Zinc is involved either as a component or as an activator of many enzymes and at least two hormones—insulin and estrogen. Swine diets containing grains and plant proteins are low in available zinc and so require supplementation for prevention of a zinc deficiency. The symptoms of a zinc deficiency include parakeratosis, impaired reproductive function, and depressed growth, including growth following correction of the deficiency. The requirement for zinc is elevated by plant phytates, calcium, copper, cadmium, and histidine. The maximum tolerable level of zinc is 1000 ppm, although lower copper stores have been observed in pigs born of sows fed this level of zinc in gestation.

IODINE. Iodine is required as a component of the thyroid hormones. Similar to other minerals, such as iron and selenium, the concentration of iodine in feedstuffs is dependent on geographic location. Low iodine concentrations exist in the soils of the Great Lakes and Northwest regions of the United States. Hypertrophy of the thyroid, commonly called goiter, results from low dietary iodine concentrations or from substances in the diet lowering the availability of iodine, called goitrogens. Feedstuffs such as rapeseed, soybeans, and peanuts contain moderately high concentrations of goitrogens. Common sources of iodine are calcium iodate, potassium iodate, and iodized salt. Swine have a high tolerance to iodine, but toxicity can occur at 400 ppm.

SELENIUM. Selenium is required by swine as a component of the antioxidant enzyme glutathione peroxidase. Therefore the function of selenium is interrelated with the presence of vitamin E, polyunsaturated fatty acids, and other antioxidants. A deficiency of either vitamin E or selenium in swine diets results in similar deficiency symptoms, including sudden death, liver necrosis, pale skeletal muscle, and a mottled, dystrophic myocardium, frequently with edema and fluid build-up in the pericardial sac. The U.S. Food and Drug Administration approved selenium additions of 0.3 ppm in 1982, but diagnosis of vitamin E–selenium deficiency syndrome has continued to rise (for further discussion see Vitamin E). Regional differences in the selenium content of soils may contribute to incidence of selenium deficiency or, in isolated cases, toxicity.

COPPER. Copper is required as a component of many enzymes involved in collagen, elastin, and myelin synthesis and for hemoglobin formation. Dietary copper levels of 125 to 250 ppm stimulate growth in starter pigs despite a copper requirement of only 6 ppm. The mechanism of the response has yet to be determined but is probably due to an antibacterial action in the gut. The growth response occurs in addition to the growth-promoting effects of other antimicrobials. Copper toxicity can occur when dietary levels exceed 250 ppm. Signs of toxicity include reduced feed intake, anemia, jaundice, increased serum and liver copper concentrations, and death.

MANGANESE. Enzymes involved in mucopolysaccharide formation and energy metabolism contain manganese. Consequently a manganese deficiency can result in varied symptoms, such as slow growth, lameness, impaired reproductive function in adult swine, and ataxia in newborns. A corn–soybean meal based diet will usually meet the pig's requirement of 10 ppm, although supplementation is still quite common. Manganese toxicity occurs with dietary manganese levels of 1000 ppm.

Vitamins

Vitamins are defined as organic compounds other than carbohydrate, protein, or lipids required by organisms in small quantities for normal growth, maintenance, or reproduction. Vitamins are generally classified according to their solubilities, being either fat or water soluble. The fat-soluble vitamins required by swine are vitamins A, D, E, and K. The water-soluble vitamins are the B-complex vitamins and ascorbic acid (vitamin C). The B vitamins include biotin, choline, folic acid, niacin, pantothenic acid, vitamin B_6, vitamin B_{12}, riboflavin, and thiamine. Generally vitamins are required as coenzymes in metabolic reactions. Thus the need for vitamins changes with the physiologic state of the animal. As shown in Table 1, for example, the vitamin D requirement on a grams/day basis of the gestating sow differs from that of the lactating sow owing to the changing physiologic requirement for calcium and phosphorus. In this light, recent work demonstrates that the reproductive performance of the sow can be improved with additional B vitamins (folic acid, riboflavin, and biotin) and β-carotene injections during gestation by improving the nutrition of the fetus. Generally swine diets are supplemented with vitamins A, D, E, and K, riboflavin, niacin, pantothenic acid, choline, and vitamin B_{12}. A grain–soybean meal diet is considered to contain adequate available concentrations of the remaining vitamins.

VITAMIN A. The functions of vitamin A remain unknown, but lesions in the case of a deficiency suggest that vitamin A plays many diverse roles in the pig. Vitamin A deficiency results in defects in bone growth resulting in incoordination and paralysis, poor vision due to impaired rhodopsin formation in the eye, keratinization of epithelial tissue resulting in defects in its growth, and maintenance and reproductive failure.

Plants do not contain vitamin A but do contain its precursor, β-carotene. Beta carotene is oxidized in the presence of heat, moisture, and storage, so vitamin A is supplied in swine diets using an esterified form of retinol (retinyl palmitate or retinyl acetate) for stability in these conditions. The pig readily stores vitamin A in the liver, so vitamin A status is best quantified through determinations of retinol in both plasma and liver tissue. Serum retinol concentrations of less than 10 μg/dl or liver retinol concentrations of 10 μg/g in tissue indicate a deficiency state. High levels of vitamin A supplementation can cause hypervitaminosis A and impair vitamin E status in the pig.

Beta carotene may play a role in reproduction independent of its conversion to vitamin A. Beta carotene injections have been shown to improve embryonic survival, resulting in larger litter sizes in the gilt and sow.

VITAMIN D. Vitamin D functions to maintain calcium and phosphorus homeostasis. Consequently deficiency symptoms include rickets, bone deformities, lameness, and osteomalacia. Exposure of animal to ultraviolet (UV) radiation converts 7-dehydrocholesterol to cholecalciferol (vitamin D_3) in the skin. Ingestion of ergocalciferol (vitamin D_2), the form occurring in plants, is another means of supplying vitamin D. Swine diets are supplemented with either vitamin D_2 or vitamin D_3 due to the limited exposure of the animals to UV radiation in confinement. In addition to the deficiency symptoms, low serum calcium and high alkaline phosphatase concentrations can be used to support a diagnosis of vitamin D deficiency.

Vitamin D toxicity results from a high level of vitamin D supplementation (33,000 IU/kg of feed). Elevated serum calcium concentrations and calcification of soft tissue are signs of vitamin D toxicity.

VITAMIN E. Vitamin E functions as an antioxidant in intracellular membranes in prevention of membrane damage that occurs when membrane lipids become peroxidized. Vitamin E supplementation of grain–soybean meal diets rarely improves pig performance, although an increased incidence of mulberry heart disease and hepatic necrosis might result without supplementation, presumably resulting from peroxidation of lipids in these tissues. The requirement for vitamin E is independent of selenium but is higher in situations that would elevate the level of peroxidation in vivo and oxidation in the diet, such as stress, high levels of polyunsaturated fats, and low dietary selenium and other antioxidant levels.

Vitamin E can be supplemented through injection of d-α-tocopherol or d-α-tocopheryl acetate in an emulsifiable base or by dietary supplementation with an esterified form, d- or dl-α-tocopheryl acetate. Tissue or serum α-tocopherol concentrations are good indicators of vitamin E status. Serum α-tocopherol concentrations less than 0.40 μg/ml or liver α-tocopherol concentrations less than 0.80 μg/g wet tissue can support pathologic evidence of a vitamin E deficiency. Epidemiologic evidence is contradictory concerning the modern condition of mulberry heart disease. This condition may not be a result of vitamin E and/or selenium deficiency.

VITAMIN K. Vitamin K is required for normal blood clotting, but the requirement of the pig can be supplied by the concentrations of vitamin K in common feedstuffs. Field cases of a hemorrhagic syndrome associated with the feeding of grains contaminated with mycotoxins have shown to be responsive to vitamin K supplementation. Bacterial synthesis of vitamin K and subsequent absorption also lower the need for supplemental vitamin K. Menadione is the synthetic form of vitamin K used in supplementation of swine diets.

BIOTIN. Common feedstuffs contain enough biotin to meet the requirement of the growing pig, but the bioavailability is poor in small grains. Generally biotin supplementation of gestating sow diets improves reproductive performance, but no single reproductive parameter has responded consistently to supplementation.

CHOLINE. The choline requirement of the growing pig is supplied in natural feedstuffs. Since choline supplementation of gestating sow diets has been shown to increase the number of pigs born alive, choline is generally added to gestation diets. Signs of choline deficiency in newborn pigs include incoordination, fat infiltration of the liver and kidney, depressed hematocrit, and reduced weight gains.

NIACIN (NICOTINIC ACID). The low niacin availability in common feedstuffs and the importance of niacin as a component of the coenzymes nicotinamide-adenine dinucleotide (NAD) and nicotinamide-adenine dinucleotide phosphate (NADP) mean diets fed to all classes of swine should be supplemented with niacin. Common deficiency signs include diarrhea, anorexia, dry skin, anemia, and inflammation of the cecum and colon. Excess tryptophan can be converted to niacin at the rate of 50 mg of excess tryptophan to 1 mg of niacin.

PANTOTHENIC ACID. Pantothenic acid is one of the few B vitamins not contained in sufficient quantities in grain–soybean meal diets to meet the requirement of the growing pig. A deficiency of pantothenic acid results in an unusual characteristic gait called "goose-stepping," bloody diarrhea, anorexia, poor growth, and reproductive failure. Pantothenic acid is generally supplemented as either d- or dl-calcium pantothenate. The l-form, resulting from synthesis of synthetic pantothenic acid, is not utilized by the pig, so the racemic mixture (dl-) contains only 0.46 mg active pantothenic acid per milligram.

RIBOFLAVIN. Signs of riboflavin deficiency include poor growth, anorexia, cataracts, light sensitivity, and eye-lens opacities. In addition, riboflavin-deficient sows may resorb fetuses, farrow preterm, or discontinue cycling. Consequently riboflavin is supplemented to all classes of swine.

VITAMIN B_{12}. The vitamin B_{12} requirement of the growing pig is estimated to be only 19 μg daily. However, the rapid decline in growth and anorexia observed in the case of a deficiency makes vitamin B_{12} a very important part of a balanced swine diet. There is no clear evidence that microbial synthesis and subsequent absorption of vitamin B_{12} will meet the pig's requirement, so supplementation is essential.

FOLACIN (FOLIC ACID). The pig's folacin requirement for growth and maintenance is met by folacin from the feedstuffs and from bacterial synthesis in the hindgut. However, recent research has shown that folic acid supplementation (1.5 g/ton of complete feed) of gestation and lactation diets increases the number of pigs born alive and pigs weaned.

Fatty Acids

Fatty acids are obtained from the hydrolysis of fats and oils and are essential for the production of several hormones. Since pigs cannot synthesize certain fatty acids such as linoleic and arachidonic acid, they must be provided in the diet. However, since arachidonic acid can be derived in vivo from linoleic acid, only linoleic acid is an essential dietary constituent. The current recommended level of linoleic acid in all swine diets is 0.1 per cent.

Water

Water is probably the most overlooked essential nutrient in swine production. Deprivation of water will result in depressed performance and death more rapidly than a deficiency of any other nutrient. Pigs need approximately 2 to 2.5 lb of water for every pound of feed consumed. Water requirements for the various sizes of pigs are given in Table 2. Also, if using nipple waterers, the water flow rate for pigs less than 40 lb should be 0.25 gal/minute, and 0.5 gal/minute for pigs more than 40 lb.

Not only must water be provided in adequate amounts for optimum performance, it must also be clean, good quality water. Table 3 lists the maximum amounts that various compounds can be present in water without affecting performance. Although little research has shown that water temperature affects the performance of swine, the recommended water temperature is 50 to 55°F.

Table 2. WATER REQUIREMENTS FOR SWINE

Animal Type	Gal/Head/Day
Sow and litter	8
Nursery pig	1
Growing pig	3
Finishing pig	4
Gestating sow	6
Boar	8

NONNUTRITIVE FEED ADDITIVES

Nonnutritive feed additives are compounds added to diets in an attempt to enhance gain, feed efficiency, and reproductive efficiency. Commonly used feed additives include antibiotics, probiotics, flavors, organic acids, anthelmintics, copper sulfate, and enzymes. While some of these compounds do enhance pig performance, not all of them have shown a consistent, positive effect.

Antibiotics, chemotherapeutics, and antibacterials are well-known feed additives that do improve performance. These compounds are thought to affect various metabolic processes, nutrient-sparing in the small intestine, and/or suppression of subclinical or nonspecific diseases. Subtherapeutic use of antibiotics began in approximately 1950, and today over 75 per cent of all hogs raised receive antibiotics in their feed sometime throughout their lives.

The reason for the high usage rate of antibiotics is their effectiveness. However, the magnitude of response observed is dependent on several factors. The younger the pig, the greater the growth response observed. Daily gain and feed efficiency of starter pigs are improved by 15 and 6.5 per cent, respectively, while for grower-finisher pigs they are improved by only 3.6 and 2.4 per cent, respectively. Also, level of production affects the response since the slowest-gaining pigs will show the greatest response when an antibiotic is added to the diet. Environment and health status also affect the magnitude of the response. Pigs housed in a poor environment and/or exposed to a high disease load will show the greatest improvement to dietary additions of subtherapeutic levels of antibiotics. Antibiotics not only enhance growth performance,

Table 3. MAXIMUM AMOUNTS OF IMPURITIES ACCEPTABLE IN WATER

Compound	Maximum Concentration (ppm)
Nitrates	300
Nitrites	100
Sulfates	350
Total dissolved solids	4290
Iron	No limit

they have also been shown to improve reproductive performance. Conception rate, number of pigs born alive, weaning weights, and survival were increased when antibiotics were added at breeding or during lactation. To be fully effective, antibiotics must be matched against the pathogens present on the farm. Also, it is a good idea to review antibiotic usage annually to ensure that they are still efficacious and economical to add. For further information on feed additives, usage levels, and legal requirements, consult the *Feed Additive Compendium* (Miller Publishing Company, 12400 Whitewater Drive, Minnetonka, MN 55343).

Copper sulfate improves growth performance owing to its antibacterial properties. When added at 125 to 250 ppm in the starter diet (1 to 2 lb addition of copper sulfate), gain and feed efficiency are substantially improved. Much like the response to antibiotics, the response to copper sulfate is age dependent. Grower pigs exhibit a smaller response than starter pigs, and finishing pigs show little if any response to copper sulfate additions. Copper sulfate additions have been attributed to dirty pens, but that is because copper turns feces black, so pens only appear dirty.

Anthelmintics are commonly added to swine diets to combat internal parasites. In order to get maximum parasite control, the anthelmintic used must be matched against the spectrum of parasites present in the operation. Also, the parasite control plan must be followed religiously for continuous control.

The response to probiotics and organic acids has been quite variable. These compounds are mainly used in the starter phase, but the results have been inconsistent. These additives should be used if the response to them can be documented in each individual operation. If not, they are not economical to use.

Flavors and enzymes have been promoted as being beneficial in swine diets. However, research indicates that they have little, if any, positive effect on pig performance.

LIFE-CYCLE STAGES

Nutrient requirements for the entire life cycle of the pig are listed in Table 1. Again, since these values represent the minimum value of each nutrient that supports normal growth, many universities and commercial feed companies recommend nutrient concentrations 10 per cent greater or more than those listed by the NRC to ensure optimum performance. Also, the pig requires specific amounts of nutrients, not percentages of nutrients. The requirements are listed in percentages to assist in ration formulation. However, as long as the pig is consuming at least the expected feed intake given, its nutrient requirements will be met. If the pig is consuming less feed than expected, the diet will not provide adequate levels of the essential nutrients.

There are basically five stages in the life cycle of the pig: starter, grower, finisher, gestation, and lactation (boars are included in the gestational feeding program). Besides meeting the nutrient requirements of the animal, other factors must be taken into consideration to guarantee proper performance. These factors will be discussed individually under the appropriate growth phase.

Starter Phase

Starter pig diets are the most expensive and complex diets used in a swine operation. The main problem in this phase is feed consumption. Anything that inhibits feed consumption will adversely affect the young pig. A poor nutritional program in this phase could result in depressed performance for an extended period. Therefore it is critical that the proper nutritional program be used.

With the increased popularity of weaning pigs at 3 weeks of age or less, an increase in "postweaning lag" has been observed. This is not surprising when you compare the pig's diets before and after weaning. Before weaning, the pig receives its feed in 16 equally spaced, highly digestible meals in liquid form. The diet is composed solely of milk products and is 30 per cent protein, 35 per cent fat, and 25 per cent lactose on a dry matter basis. After weaning, the pig receives a low-fat, low-lactose, high-carbohydrate diet composed of grain and soybean meal in dry form. It follows, then, that the young pig does not start eating immediately and that performance is reduced.

In order to alleviate postweaning lag, researchers at Kansas State University have developed a three-phase feeding program. It is designed to initially provide the weaned pig nutrients from sources it currently utilizes such as milk proteins and sugars, and then gradually to switch it over to a grain-soybean meal based diet. The three-phase starter program is as follows:

Phase One: High nutrient-dense diet (fed to pigs up to 15 lb)

Phase Two: 1.25 per cent lysine, whey–corn–soybean meal diet (fed to pigs from 15 to 25 lb)

Phase Three: 1.10 per cent lysine, grain–soybean meal diet (fed to pigs over 25 lb)

A description of the diets is given in the following table.

Pig Size	Phase One (<15 lb)	Phase Two (15–25 lb)	Phase Three (>25 lb)
Protein, %	20–25	18–20	18
Lysine, %	1.5–1.6	1.25	1.10
Soybean oil, %	8–10	3–5	0
Edible dried whey, %	15–25	15–20	0–5
Dried skim milk, %	10–25	0	0
Select fish meal, %	0–3	3–5	0
Copper, ppm	190–260	190–260	190–260
Vitamin E, IU/ton	40,000	40,000	40,000
Selenium, ppm	0.3	0.3	0.3
Antibiotic or antibacterial	+	+	+
Physical form	1/8-inch pellet	1/8-inch pellet	Meal form

The nutrient concentrations are higher than those listed in Table 1 owing in part to the assumption that feed intake is normally lower in newly weaned pigs and to an expectation of a more rapid gain. Also, it is important that only high-quality ingredients be used, especially in the Phase One diet. It does make the diet more expensive, but it represents less than 1 per cent of the feed necessary to get a pig to market weight. This program is also applicable when weaning at later ages. If weaning at 5 or 6 weeks of age, start the heavier pigs on the Phase Two diet and switch to the Phase Three diet when appropriate.

Grower and Finisher Phase

Since pigs in these stages are adjusted to grain–soybean meal diets, little has to be done to alter the diets under normal conditions. However, in times of heat and cold stress, dietary manipulations may improve pig performance.

If temperatures remain above 85°F (29.4°C) during both day and night, the grower and finisher pig will be in a heat-stressed condition. One symptom of heat stress is a reduction in feed intake in an attempt to reduce the heat produced during digestion. Since feed intake is depressed, the pig is not receiving enough total nutrients on a daily basis to support normal performance. In order to alleviate the situation the nutrient density of the diet can be increased. That way, even though the pig is consuming less feed, it is still meeting its nutrient requirements when fed the nutrient-dense diets. The recommended dietary changes in a heat-stress situation are to increase lysine concentration 0.1 per cent with synthetic lysine and add 3 per cent fat to the diet.

In a cold-stress situation, the pig has a higher energy requirement owing to the increased energy requirement for maintaining body heat. In general the pig meets its increased energy requirement by consuming more feed. Even though fat is 2.25 times as energy dense as carbohydrates, it should not be added to the diets of cold-stressed pigs because it gives off less heat during digestion and the cold stress is made even worse. Fiber additions are more practical in cold stress since a great deal of heat is produced during its digestion. However, the increased heat increment is not enough to offset the energy dilution of the diet, so performance stays approximately the same. The decision to increase fiber additions in cold stress should be based on economics, and the fiber then removed when the pig is back in a thermal-neutral environment.

Since the majority of the feed a pig consumes is during the grower and finisher phases, feed efficiency becomes an economically important factor. Feed processing, as will be discussed later, has a tremendous impact on feed efficiency. Fat additions can improve feed efficiency and dust control. Wet feeders also improve performance in the grower and finisher phases, again perhaps through a reduction of dust. However, wet or wet/dry feeders should not be used in the starter phase owing to water's nutrient-diluting action.

Lysine level must be adequate in these phases or carcass merit will suffer. If the producer is selling hogs on a carcass merit basis, a higher lysine level can be fed since the bonus for the leaner carcass should more than offset the additional cost of increasing lysine level. However, if the producer is marketing on a live-weight basis, there is no economic benefit to feeding higher levels of lysine.

Females identified as replacement gilts need to be switched to the gestation diet at least by the time they reach 175 lb. Since the gestation diet is higher in minerals and vitamins than the finisher diet, mineral stores, mainly calcium and phosphorus, will increase for later lactations.

Gestating Females and Boars

Feed intake is probably the most important factor for animals in this phase. Feed needs to be limited to ensure that the animals do not become obese. This could lead to boars with low libido, increased farrowing problems, more crushing of pigs after farrowing, and a delay in estrus after weaning. On the other hand, emaciated animals cannot perform to their full potential either. One recommendation is to feed boars and gestating sows 4 lb of feed/day of a grain–soybean meal mix. This is adequate in a thermal-neutral environment, but if the animals are cold stressed, energy intake needs to be increased. Also, prebreeding condition and genotype affect feed utilization by the sow. Therefore the best recommendation is to feed sows and boars according to their body condition, with an average to moderate condition being most desirable.

There are several methods to limit-feed animals. One common method is floor feeding. In floor feeding, the sows receive, on average, the appropriate amount of feed. However, if there are dominant sows or differences in size of animals within the pen, the dominant and larger sows will overeat while the smaller, more docile gilts will get what little feed is left. This results in both over- and underfed animals in the same pen. The best way to limit-feed is with individual feeding stalls. Feed offered can be controlled on an individual basis, and the producer also has the opportunity to observe each animal every day. This leads to better management. Other alternatives include allowing ad libitum consumption of a high-fiber, low-energy diet or allowing ad libitum consumption of a traditional diet 1 out of every 3 days. These last two methods work well in certain situations but are not recommended as a general rule.

Flushing, increasing energy intake by at least 50 per cent prior to breeding, has been used to increase ovulation rate and, consequently, number of pigs born alive in gilts. However, sows benefit little from flushing. Also, timing of flushing is critical. Increasing feed intake needs to begin 10 to 14 days prebreeding and must stop immediately after mating. If the high plane of nutrition continues after mating, there is an increase in embryonic mortality and the advantage of flushing is lost. Therefore flushing only really works in a hand-mating or artificial insemination situation where the exact breeding date is known and the female then returned to limit-feed. Flushing is not effective in sows or in a pen mating program.

As was previously mentioned, sows that gain too much weight during gestation can have problems in returning to estrus after weaning. This is because the more a sow eats during gestation, the less she will eat during lactation. If the sow is consuming less feed in lactation, body tissue is being catabolized to meet the nutrient requirements for milk production, and she loses a tremendous amount of weight, mostly body fat. This weight loss results in a delay or inability to return to estrus. Therefore it is essential that gestating animals are not overfed so that subsequent performance is not adversely affected. Gestating gilts and sows should gain 125 and 75 lb, respectively, as a rule of thumb.

Lactation

The goal in lactation is to maximize feed consumption for milk production and subsequent rebreeding. The addition of high-fiber feedstuffs to prevent constipation decreases energy intake and is not recommended. If constipation is a problem, chemical laxatives such as potassium chloride or magnesium sulfate should be added to the diet.

Fat additions to increase energy density of the lactation diet have produced mixed results. In herds with a large number of pigs of light birth weight, or a preweaning mortality rate greater than 15 per cent, fat additions are beneficial. In those instances, sows should consume a total of 3 lb of fat spread over 7 days before farrowing, and then at least 7 per cent fat should be added to the lactation diet. However, if high mortality and light-weight pigs are not a problem, fat additions to the lactation diet are not economical.

If feed consumption is reduced due to heat stress, drip coolers will increase feed intake. Also, some producers have found that wet feeders enhance feed intake during lactation.

FEED PROCESSING

Even if a diet is properly formulated and nutritionally sound on paper, it must be processed before it reaches the pig. During processing, acceptable diets can become unacceptable. Feed is ground to increase surface area for improved digestion and improved mixing characteristics. The smaller the particle, the better the digestibility and feed efficiency and the less segregation that will occur. However, if feed is ground too fine, problems such as gastric ulcers, increased dustiness, increased grinding costs, and increased feeder management will occur. Basically, feed ground through a 3/16-inch screen will give the proper particle size.

Pelleting will improve feed efficiency and decrease dust levels. However, due to the cost of pelleting it is not economically feasible except for high nutrient-dense diets or expensive specialty diets.

Portable, on-farm grinder-mixers are responsible for a large number of nutritional wrecks when not used properly. One problem is properly weighing the feedstuffs. Without a scale it is difficult to add the correct amount of grain or soybean meal. This is especially true when the test weights of the feedstuffs vary. By simply adding an extra 10 bushels of corn to a finishing diet, the protein content is reduced from 14.4 to 13.1 per cent. Also, without a set of scales the grinder can be overfilled, resulting in a reduction in mixing efficiency. Therefore scales will greatly reduce the chances of improper mixing.

Probably the most common mistake made in on-farm mixing is inadequate mixing time. It is essential that the mixer run at the proper rpm for at least 15 minutes *after the last* feed ingredient is added. If it is mixed for a shorter time or at a lower rpm, the feed will not be properly mixed and performance could suffer. Also, if the grinder is worn, mixing time needs to be increased. Other common problems include the addition of 5- or 10-lb "add-paks." The smallest addition to a portable mixer should be 75 lb. Amounts less than 75 lb will hang up in augers and not get mixed properly.

BIBLIOGRAPHY

Kansas Swine Field Day Report. Manhattan, KS, Kansas State University, 1986.
McDowell LR: Vitamins in Animal Nutrition. San Diego, Academic Press, 1989.
National Research Council: Mineral Tolerance of Domestic Animals. Washington, DC, National Academy Press, 1980.
National Research Council: Nutrient Requirements of Swine, 9th ed. Washington, DC, National Academy Press, 1988.
Pond WG, Maner JH: Swine Production and Nutrition. Westport, CT, AVI Publishing, 1984.
Pork Industry Handbook. West Lafayette, IN, Purdue University, 1990.

Nutrition for Livestock Grazing Rangelands and Pasturelands

M. M. KOTHMANN, PhD, MS

Classical animal nutrition is based on the concept of determining the nutrient requirements of an animal and the nutritive value of feed. A ration is formulated to meet the requirement of the animal. However, animals grazing rangelands and pasturelands are not fed a ration. The nutritive value of forage consumed is difficult to determine because animals select diets containing various combinations of plant species and plant parts. Also, the nutrient requirements of the animal, especially for energy, may be increased by activity associated with grazing and travel or by environmental stress such as high or low temperatures. Supplements generally provide only a small fraction of the total diet, but they may affect both the intake and the digestibility of grazed forage.

Nutrition for grazing animals must be concerned with management factors such as stocking rates, season of grazing, grazing systems, plant species available, and kinds and classes of animals best suited for the forage resource. Supplements must be formulated to complement grazed forage and alleviate specific nutrient deficiencies. This chapter will consider (1) forage resources, (2) diet selection, (3) nutrient intake from grazed forage, (4) animal units, (5) supplementation of grazing animals, and (6) water requirements.

FORAGE RESOURCES

Principles for nutrition of grazing livestock are the same on rangelands and pasturelands; however, applications may vary for several reasons. Pasturelands generally consist of monocultures or combinations of two plant species selected and planted by the manager. Rangelands consist of complex mixtures of plant species representing grasses, forbs, and woody plants. Fewer cultural inputs are generally applied to rangelands than to pasturelands.

Because of differences in the characteristics and management of the forage resources on rangelands and pasturelands, different management and cultural practices are emphasized to influence nutrition of grazing animals. The most important factors on pasturelands are selection and breeding of improved plant materials, establishment of new stands, fertilization, harvesting and storing forage during periods of excess production, weed control, and grazing management. On rangelands, grazing management and brush control are the primary management practices. Few other cultural practices are applied to rangelands.

Forage Quality and Availability

The nutritive value of forage depends on its nutrient content, the digestibility of the nutrients, and the amount the animal will consume (intake). The influence of forage classes, maturity, availability, and environment on forage quality will be discussed.

Forage Classes

Forage species may be grouped into three classes: grasses, forbs, and browse. Grasses are members of the family Poaceae; forbs are herbaceous annual and perennial dicots and monocots other than grasses; and browse consists of perennial woody shrubs and vines utilized as forage by grazing animals. Characteristic differences exist among classes and within classes. Variation in nutritive value exists among species within a forage class, among individual plants within a species, and between leaf and stem fractions within a plant. The nutrient content and digestibility of stems decline very rapidly with maturity. The quality of live leaves declines more slowly than that of stems, but leaves have a relatively short life-span.

Warm-season perennial grasses have the lowest average digestibility, legumes the highest, and cool-season perennial grasses and annual grasses intermediate. Total dry matter production of these forage groups tends to follow an inverse trend to forage quality. The cost of forage production is generally less for warm-season perennial grasses than for cool-season annual grasses.

Warm-season perennial grasses, for example, lovegrasses, bermudagrasses, and bahiagrasses, are highly digestible at initiation of growth in the spring, but forage quality declines rapidly from spring to summer as plant maturity increases. However, the rate of decline varies among species and varieties. Varieties selected for improved forage quality, such as

Coastcross bermudagrass, maintain higher digestibility but also reach a low point in midsummer. Late-summer rains during most years, combined with reduced temperatures, result in fall growth, which increases forage quality. The suitability of warm-season grasses for different classes of cattle will vary seasonally. Grasses generally cannot provide adequate digestible energy to meet the requirements for high-producing animals, such as lactating dairy cows or young growing animals, whereas a high-quality legume pasture may. Thus it is usually preferable to graze beef cows on warm-season perennial grasses and to utilize higher-quality legume and cool-season annual grass pastures with growing stock or high-producing lactating cows.

Desert ranges in the intermountain region of the western United States support primarily grass-shrub communities with few forbs. They are grazed primarily by dry ewes and cows during the winter, when forage quality is relatively low. Animal diets contain a mix of grasses and browse. Grasses are lower than browse in crude protein (CP) and phosphorus but contain higher levels of metabolizable energy. Diets consisting of all browse would be deficient in energy but would contain adequate levels of CP, phosphorus, and carotene to meet the maintenance requirements of cows and ewes. Diets composed of all grasses would contain adequate energy but would be deficient in CP, phosphorus, and carotene. Where animals can select from both grasses and browse, the need for supplements can be reduced.

Legumes are the only forbs that have received significant attention as forage species for seeded pastures. Evaluation of the nutrient content of some common weed species, for example, redroot pigweed (*Amaranthus retroflexus*), common lambsquarters (*Chenopodium album*), and common ragweed (*Ambrosia artemisiifolia*), revealed that they had nutrient composition and digestibility equivalent to that of high-quality alfalfa (*Medicago sativa*). Thus some of the common weed species found in stands of perennial forages growing in fertile soils do not decrease the nutritive value of hay or pasture if utilized at relatively early stages of maturation. However, generalizations are not possible in comparison of forage quality among "weed" and crop species. Comparisons must be based on specific examples where species and environmental conditions are described.

Maturity

As plants mature, forage quality declines. Several factors contribute to this decline. Growth and senescence occur simultaneously in plants. New growth of forage consists of green leaves. As plants mature and become reproductive, stem growth increases. During the growing season new leaves are produced and older leaves die and accumulate as standing dead forage. Thus during the early part of the growing season pastures have a higher proportion of green leaves, and as the stand matures the proportions of dead leaf and stem increase.

Grazing diverts forage from senescence through consumption of live forage. Apical meristems may also be removed, thus reducing the amount of stem produced. Grazing alters forage quality by changing the relative proportions and average age of plant parts in the standing crop. It may also alter plant growth rates, either increasing or decreasing production depending on the intensity, frequency, and time of grazing.

Average daily gains of sheep and cattle decline as vegetation on spring and summer ranges matures; however, gains of lambs and calves decline less than gains of ewes and cows. This is a common occurrence in the production of lambs and calves from rangelands and represents an important principle. It is not always possible to meet the total energy requirement for lactating cows or ewes from grazed forage, nor will the forage meet the nutrient requirements of young growing animals. However, the cow or ewe meets the nutrient requirements of the young animal through conversion of forage to milk. When the energy intake of the cow or ewe is below its requirement, energy stored as fat can be mobilized to support lactation. It is usually much more economical to store excess energy as fat in the cow or ewe during periods when high-quality forage is available than it is to feed it as a supplement during periods of deficiency.

Availability

Average daily gain of grazing animals is related to both quality and availability of forage. These relationships were examined for six warm-season perennial grasses (Fig. 1). When dry matter digestibility (DMD) of forage was greater than 60 per cent, gains of yearling heifers were not affected until forage availability fell below 500 kg/hectare (ha). As average digestibility of the forage declined, the relation between gains and availability changed. The reason for this was the variability of forage quality within the standing crop. Standing crop is relatively homogeneous when forage is young and digestibility is high. As forage matures and average digestibility of standing crop declines, there is more variation. The obvious conclusion is that stands of uniformly high-quality forage can be grazed closely with less effect on animal performance than can more mature stands that contain dead leaves and stems. Where the quality of forage in the standing crop varies significantly, animal performance will be much more sensitive to grazing intensity.

There is an asymptotic relationship between animal gain and mean pasture availability. A 4- to 6-inch mean height of green leaves is required for cattle to obtain maximum intake.

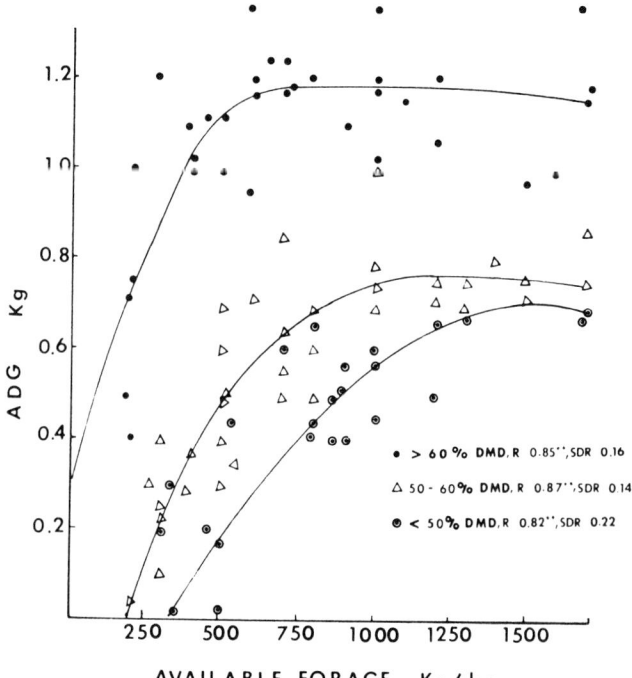

Figure 1. Polynomial regressions, $Y = a + bX + cX^2 + dX^3$, between animal performance (Y) and available forage (X) on warm-season grasses for three ranges of dry matter digestibility (SDR = standard deviation from regression). (From Duble RL, Lancaster JA, Holt EC: Agron J 63:795, 1971.)

Even small increases in green forage, when availability is below 500 lb/acre, will result in significant increases in gain per animal. The critical heights and weights for forage may vary for species having different growth forms, but the management implications would be similar.

Environment

Many environmental factors may affect forage quality, but only temperature, light intensity, moisture, fertility, and leaching will be considered here.

Plant response to temperature and light intensity varies between temperate (C_3) and tropical (C_4) grasses, with species having different optimum levels. C_3 plants are commonly called cool season, and C_4 are warm season. Cool-season grasses and forbs (including legumes) grow during the fall, winter, and spring. Warm-season plants grow only during the frost-free periods.

Low light intensities and temperatures restrict plant growth during the winter. During spring, light intensity and temperature increase, improving conditions for plant growth. During summer, temperature may be above the optimum for plant growth and water is frequently limiting. During fall, light intensity decreases while temperature may remain relatively high. Limited water availability may restrict plant growth during any season.

The effects of temperature, light intensity, and moisture give rise to predictable seasonal changes in forage quality in temperate regions. High light intensities increase water-soluble carbohydrate content, whereas high temperatures and drought will decrease them. In temperate regions spring grass has high CP and low fiber contents; summer grass has low CP and high fiber contents; and fall grass has high CP and average fiber contents. Low light intensities and reduced water availability can result in accumulation of nitrate (NO_3) in plants. In tropical regions forage quality is affected primarily by variations of moisture, stage of maturity, species, and fertility.

Plant response to fertility is primarily reflected in dry matter production, although some changes in chemical composition of forage have been reported. Changes in chemical composition can be confounded with differences in the relative proportion of plant parts (leaf, stem, and inflorescence) and in stage of maturity. High levels of soil nitrogen may alter leaf:stem ratios and retard plant maturity. Crude protein increased, but digestibility of kleingrass (*Panicum coloratum*) and bermudagrasses did not change in response to nitrogen fertilization (Table 1). These data were based on forage harvested at the same stage of maturity. Fertilization may improve animal production by increasing forage growth rates and increasing the ratio of leaf to stem.

Leaching of mature forages is an important factor affecting nutrition of range animals. Young, actively growing plant tissue is relatively immune to loss of mineral nutrients and carbohydrates, whereas more mature tissue approaching senescence and fully mature tissues are very susceptible to leaching. Potassium, calcium, magnesium, and manganese are the inorganic nutrients leached from live plants in largest quantities. Minerals most resistant to leaching are iron, zinc, phosphorus, and chlorine. Of the major organic constituents, carbohydrates are most likely to be leached from live plant material. Quantitative losses of proteins, amino acids, and organic acids from live plant material are slight.

Another major loss of nutrients from foliage as plants mature is translocation. The major elements nitrogen, potassium, and phosphorus, and nonstructural carbohydrates are readily mobilized and translocated from senescing plant tissues. Thus forage quality declines with maturity as a result of the combined effects of reduced nutrient content from translocation and leaching and reduced digestibility of the fiber fraction.

Evaluating Forage Quality by Chemical Analysis

Energy and protein are the major nutrients that need to be evaluated in range forages. The levels of these nutrients are usually positively associated, but the correlation is not extremely high. The gross energy content of forages does not vary greatly among plant species or with plant maturity when expressed on an organic matter (OM) basis. However, digestible energy (DE) varies significantly with plant species and maturity.

Crude fiber, lignin, cellulose, CP, and cell walls (neutral detergent fiber) are chemical constituents that have been used in regression equations to predict DE. Best results are obtained when the regressions are used only with closely related plant species. Lack of fit increases greatly when the equations are extended from warm- to cool-season grasses or from grasses to forbs and browse, or when they are used for different kinds of animals.

In vitro techniques provide a more direct estimate of the DE content of a forage than does use of regression equations. However, considerable variation may occur between different "batches" or analyses with in vitro techniques. Therefore it is advisable to include a standard forage of known digestibility with each batch to correct for this variation. To convert digestible OM to DE, Jeffery[2] developed the equation $DE = 0.218 + 4.92$ DOM ($r = 0.939$), where DOM is the coefficient of digestion for OM and DE is in units of kcal/g. This is very similar to the equation used to convert total digestible nutrients (TDN) to DE.[4]

Table 1. EFFECT OF NITROGEN FERTILIZATION ON CRUDE PROTEIN CONTENT AND ITS LACK OF EFFECT ON DRY MATTER DIGESTIBILITY

| Texas* | | | | | | Homer, Louisiana† | | | Oklahoma‡ | | |
| Kleingrass | | | Coastal Bermuda | | | Coastal Bermuda | | | Coastal Bermuda | | |
N (lb/acre)	CP (%)	DMD (%)	N (lb/acre)	CP (%)	DMD (%)	N (lb/acre)	CP (%)	DMD (%)	N (lb/acre)	CP (%)	DMD (%)
25	5.9	56.1	25	6.7	53.8	0	10.4	51.4	0	11.5	64.9
100	6.6	57.1	100	7.6	54.8	600	15.8	53.1	400	18.4	66.0
200	9.8	55.8	200	10.6	53.4	1200	16.9	52.1	1400	18.9	65.0
300	10.8	57.4	300	10.8	55.1	—	—	—	—	—	—

Source: Ellis CW, Lippke H: Tex Agr Exp Sta Res Monog RM-6c, 1976.
*One application 6 weeks prior to cutting. Data from Buentello JL, Ellis WC: Proc 24th Ann Tex Nutr Conf, 1969.
†Six applications 4 weeks prior to cutting. From Rainwater WA, et al: J Anim Sci 38:214 (abst), 1974.
‡Four applications. In vitro data of Webster JE, et al: Agron J 57:323, 1965.
N = nitrogen; CP = crude protein; DMD = dry matter digestibility.

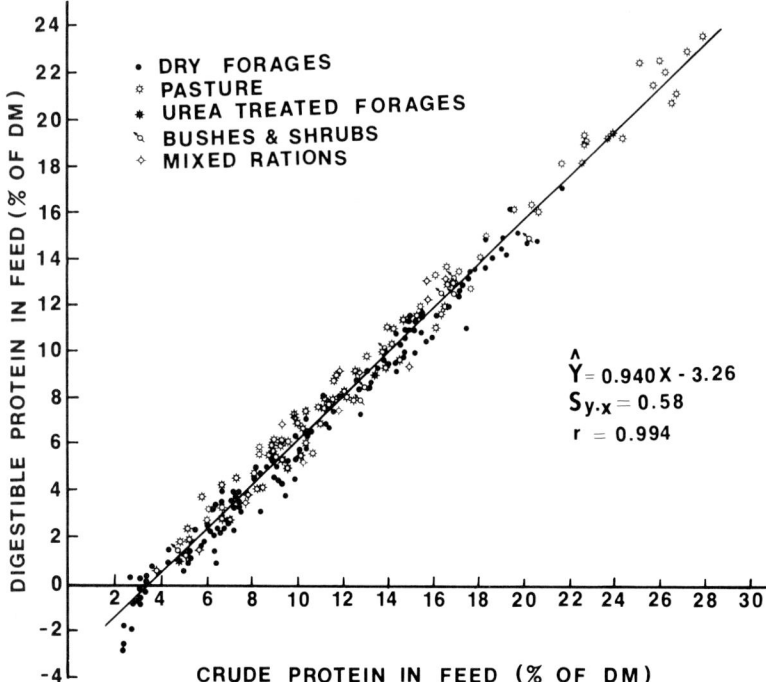

Figure 2. Relationship between the crude protein and apparently digestible crude protein concentration of feeds. (From van Niekerk DGH, Smith DWWQ, Oosthuysen D: Proc S Afr Soc Anim Prod 6:108, 1967.)

Protein may be evaluated as total CP or digestible CP. The relation between the percentage of CP in the diet and digestible CP in the diet was determined to be linear (Fig. 2). The estimated true digestibility of dietary CP is 94 per cent, and metabolic fecal nitrogen is 3.26 g/100 g dry matter consumed. The relationship between CP in the diet (x) and its digestion coefficient (y) was determined to fit the general form y = a + bx^{-1}. Fitting 361 observations from South Africa by least squares techniques produced a realistic equation (Fig. 3) that agreed well with the linear equation. From these data and similar findings by other researchers, it appears that CP is a suitable measure of the protein content of the diet of grazing animals.

Most commercial laboratories that provide nutritional analyses utilize near infrared reflectance (NIR) spectrophotometry. The procedure involves the use of regression equations to relate the composition of samples analyzed by wet chemistry procedures to the reflectance spectrum of the feed. This technique provides a rapid procedure to evaluate samples, but caution must be exercised to see that the samples being analyzed have been represented in the calibration set. Most calibration sets are based on harvested forages and single feeds. Analysis of range diets consisting of mixtures of grasses, forbs, and shrubs with NIR spectrophotometry may result in significant errors.

DIET SELECTION

It is well documented that under almost all circumstances livestock graze selectively on rangelands and pasturelands (Fig. 4). Both animal and forage attributes affect diet selection. Animal attributes include species, class of animal, productive function, prior conditioning, and experience. Forage factors affecting diet selection include chemical composition and physical characteristics such as texture, pubescence, or presence of spines. Preference is a relative value referring to the choice among feeds. Palatability relates to the acceptability of the feed and is measured by the amount the animal will consume.

Absolute values of preference and palatability cannot be assigned to feeds because animals express different forage preferences. For example, characteristics of palatable forage would differ for a goat and a cow.

Certain expressions of forage preference are similar among all kinds of livestock. Leaf is preferred over stem and green tissue is preferred over mature or dead forage. These preferences generally result in the selection of diets having nutritive value higher than the average of the forage available. Heavy grazing pressures will force increased utilization of low-quality forage, reducing nutrient intake of the animal.

The effect of chemical composition of the forage on diet selection is not simply expressed since many chemicals interact with the animal's senses during the grazing process. Plant components such as CP, phosphorus, and carotene and moisture content and digestibility of forage are generally positively associated with palatability. Lignin, cellulose, cutin, silica, cell walls, alkaloids, and various terpenes and essential oils are negatively associated with palatability. Simple classifications of plant palatability based on limited chemical characteristics such as CP, crude fiber, or digestibility are inadequate when applied to the diverse kinds of forages found on rangelands.

Broad generalizations can be made about dietary preferences of cattle, sheep, and goats for forage classes; however, these are subject to the influence of the composition of the available forage. Forage classes are generally selected in proportion to their ability to provide green foliage, with grasses utilized most heavily by cattle, forbs by sheep, and browse by goats. Seasonal shifts in diet are common to all range livestock. These shifts reflect the changing phenology and growth rates of forage species.

Selective grazing is advantageous to the animal but causes a variety of problems for grazing management. Animal performance is enhanced when animals graze selectively. In fact, the average forage quality on many ranges is not adequate to support livestock production, and only by allowing the animals to graze selectively can livestock production be sustained economically. On pastures where the average forage quality is adequate, selective grazing can "stratify" the forage by removing green leaves first and leaving stems and dead leaves,

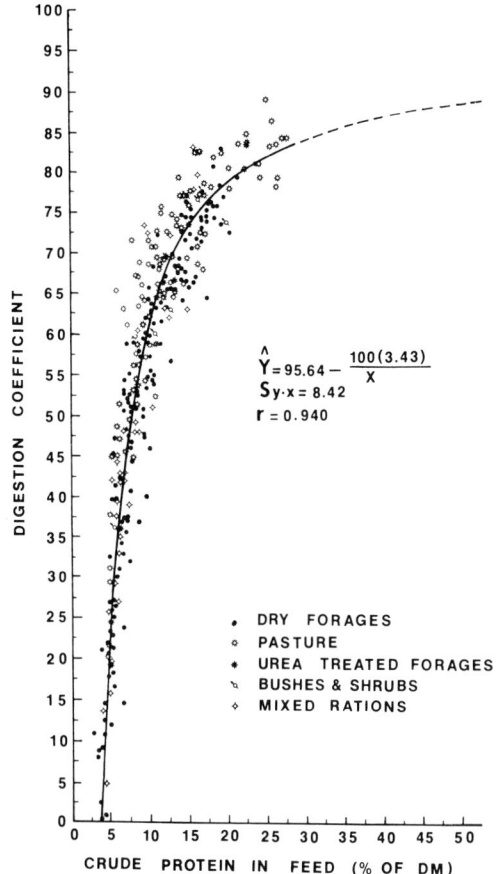

Figure 3. Relationship between the crude protein concentration of feeds and its apparent digestibility. (From van Niekerk DGH, Smith DWWQ, Oosthuysen D: Proc S Afr Soc Anim Prod 6:108, 1967.)

which are not of adequate quality to support livestock production. To avoid this problem on tame pastures, forage can be utilized at an immature stage or can be strip grazed, forcing utilization of all the plant during 1 or 2 days. This maintains the average nutrient intake at an acceptable level and prevents several days of luxury consumption followed by several days of deficient intake, which may occur with longer grazing periods in rotation grazing.

On rangelands the major problems caused by selective grazing are related to species and area selectivity. Most rangelands support diverse floras, with species varying in palatability. Also, topography may be steep and rough, with large paddocks encompassing a variety of soil types. Distance from water to forage may be in excess of 2 miles. All of these factors accentuate selective grazing. Grazing management on rangelands is primarily directed toward alleviating the problems caused by selective grazing. Adjustments of stocking rates and season of grazing and the development of specialized grazing systems are commonly used to alleviate problems of *species selective* grazing. The development of additional water and fencing and the strategic location of mineral supplements and feed grounds are primary methods directed to problems of *area selective* grazing.

NUTRIENT INTAKE FROM GRAZED FORAGE

Nutrient intake is a function of the amount of feed an animal consumes and the content and availability of the nutrients in the feed. The amount of forage a grazing animal will consume is a function of the availability and quality of the forage, the kind of grazing management applied, and the kind, class, and physiologic condition of the animal. We have already considered some of the factors affecting nutrient content of forages and the process of diet selection by the animal. Understanding the interrelationship of plant and animal components in range and pasture systems is vital to providing proper nutrition for grazing animals.

The relation between forage intake and digestibility of forage has been the subject of many investigations (Fig. 5). The relation between intake and diet digestibility is affected by age, size, and physiologic condition of the animal, but certain principles apply generally. Intake control shifts from primarily physical to metabolic control as the concentration of digestible energy increases to a level where the animal's nutritive requirement for energy is met. However, on most ranges and pastures, digestibility or availability of forage limits intake. Thus digestibility of forages has a dual effect on animal performance, as it reflects the availability of energy in the feed and also affects the amount of feed that will be consumed. As digestibility of forage declines, nutrient intake will decline even more rapidly.

The relation between digestibility and intake is affected by the class of forage. For tropical and temperate grasses and legumes, digestibility is a good basis for comparing nutritive value within a forage class but may not be valid when comparing grasses with legumes because of differences in voluntary intake. Voluntary intake of sheep was 13.7 per cent higher for legumes averaging 53.2 per cent DOM than for grasses averaging 63.0 per cent DOM. Voluntary intake was 28 per cent greater for legumes having the same per cent DOM as grasses. This difference was caused by a shorter retention time (17 per cent) and a higher amount of OM (14 per cent) in the rumen digesta from legume diets than from grass diets. There was a close relation (r = 0.96) between daily intake of digestible OM and retention time in the rumen. This relation applied to both temperate and tropical forages.

Voluntary intake of grazing animals is influenced by the composition and growth rate of available forage and forage demand rate. Since animals graze selectively, total standing crop is not an adequate measure of forage availability. Standing crop should be evaluated by species or groups of similar species and separated by leaf/stem and live/dead. This will

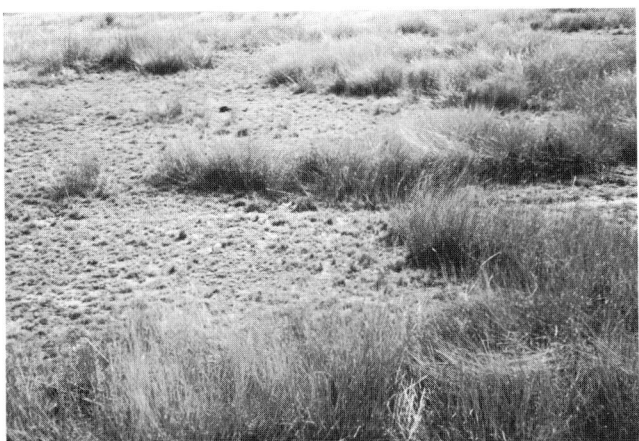

Figure 4. Selective grazing is a major problem in range utilization. Animals graze some plants too closely while leaving other plants undergrazed. This results in inefficient utilization of the forage and leads to deterioration of the range.

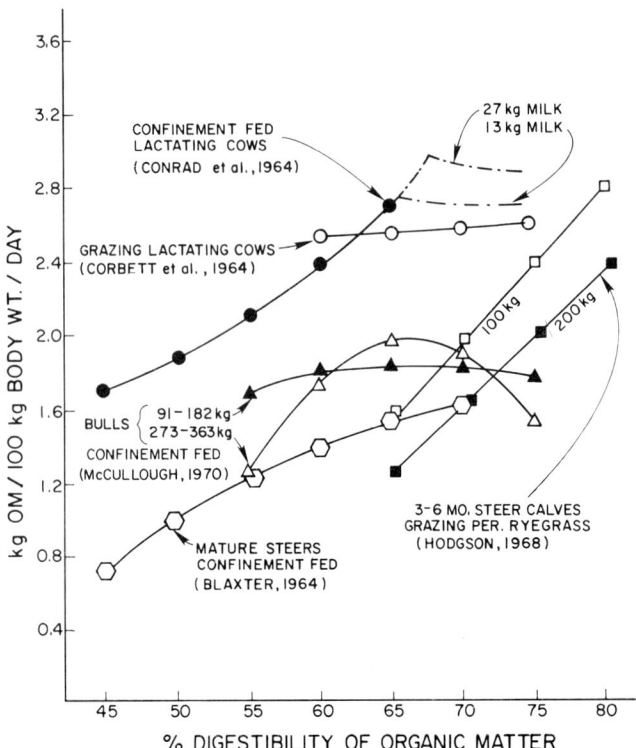

Figure 5. Forage intake is frequently a function of diet digestibility, but the relationship varies with the kind and class of animal and their physiologic status. OM = organic matter. (From Ellis WC: J Dairy Sci 61:1828, 1978.)

allow identification of the sources and extent of nutritional heterogeneity. Growth rate of leaf and stem of the various species should also be estimated. Three general conditions exist for the relationship between forage growth rate (FGR) and forage demand rate (FDR): FGR > FDR, FGR < FDR, FGR = FDR.

If FGR > FDR, standing crop will increase and animals will graze selectively. This produces optimal animal performance as long as the availability of the new growth is not hindered by the accumulation of mature forage. Under this condition, nutrient intake will not be sensitive to the duration of the grazing. However, selective grazing increases nutritional heterogeneity of the stand. If the grazing season on ranges is longer than the growing season, then periods when FGR > FDR will be necessary. The result is great changes in forage quality with resultant change in nutrient intake of animals. Supplementation must be provided to meet the nutrient requirements of animals grazing on mature dormant forage.

When FGR < FDR, standing crop will decline. Selective removal of live leaves results in dead leaves and stems contributing a greater proportion of the standing crop, and sensitivity to grazing pressure increases. The impact on nutrient intake will depend on the nutritional heterogeneity of the standing crop. If nutritional heterogeneity is high, selective grazing will result in a progressive decline in nutrient intake until low forage availability results in a sharp drop in intake. If forage quality of the standing crop is uniform, that is, all green leaves as in winter cereal grains, nutrient intake will be relatively constant until it is restricted by low availability, at which point it will decline sharply.

When FGR = FDR, standing crop should be stable. Nutrient intake will be sensitive to standing crop below some critical level. Above that level there is no relationship between nutrient intake and standing crop. Grazing should be deferred until standing crop is above the critical level; then set demand rate equal to forage growth rate. This grazing strategy offers the most efficient approach to maximizing nutrient intake from a pasture. However, it does not allow for accumulation of forage for use during periods when growth declines, and it assumes a relatively constant growth rate. Where these conditions prevail, as in intensively managed pastures on croplands, it should be considered the preferred management strategy. Unfortunately, on most rangelands the grazing season is significantly longer than the growing season, and growth rates vary throughout the season.

ANIMAL-UNITS

Rangelands are grazed by different kinds and classes of animals, each requiring different amounts of forage. The animal-unit (AU) is a concept designed to allow expression of the forage demand by different kinds of grazing animals, since adding numbers of sheep and steers and cows does not provide a useful figure. The forage requirement of an AU is defined as a constant 8 kg/day. The animal-unit-equivalent (AUE) for any animal may be calculated by dividing that animal's forage demand (kilograms) by 8 kg/AU day. The number of animals multiplied by this AUE will give the number of AUs.

To calculate stocking rates, the time factor must be incorporated. This may be done by multiplying the number of AUs by the number of days they grazed on an area, giving animal-unit-days (AUD). The total number of AUD grazed on an area during a year is the stocking rate. AUD may be converted to animal-unit-months (AUM) or animal-unit-years (AUY) by dividing by 30.5 or 365, respectively.

The AU and AUE should not be confused with substitution ratios or competition indices used for different kinds of animals on ranges. Different kinds of animals have different dietary preferences and grazing behavior. For example, goats and deer will utilize more browse and steeper, rougher topography than cattle. However, cattle will utilize relatively level grasslands more efficiently than goats or deer. Thus the suitability of rangelands for different animal species varies with vegetation, topography, and other factors. The purpose of the AU is simply to express the total forage demand in common units. The suitability of any given range for different kinds of animals must be determined and substitution ratios worked out independently of the AUE.

GRAZING MANAGEMENT

Grazing management should always be one of the first nutritional considerations of the livestock manager. Primary considerations are to select the proper season of grazing, the proper stocking rate, and the most appropriate grazing system.

Season of Grazing

Rangelands are frequently grazed yearlong or throughout the season when grazing is possible. Selective grazing results in the desirable forage species and the most accessible parts of the range receiving the most frequent and intensive grazing. The result is reduced vigor and productivity of these components, and over a period of years less desirable species invade. Thus the effect of continuous grazing, especially at heavy stocking rates, is a long-term decline in productivity of the range.

Two important principles should be considered when making

decisions regarding season of grazing. First, animal production is greatest when forage is grazed soon after it is produced and before it has matured. Second, to obtain range improvement, the desirable forage species must be allowed to reproduce. Thus when range improvement is an important goal, there will generally need to be some reduction in animal production to achieve the improvement. It is obvious that on tame pastures and good condition rangelands where range improvement is not an objective, the grazing plan can be designed to maximize animal production. This is why tame pastures should be fully utilized during the growing season. There is no logical reason to defer use of most tame pastures during the growing season and utilize them during the dormant season. These expensive forages should be grazed to harvest the maximum amount of nutrients for high levels of animal production.

Rangelands generally provide the flexibility in forage systems where they are combined with tame pastures. This means that the tame pastures are grazed when they provide the most nutrients and the rangelands are used to fill the gaps. This not only utilizes the most expensive forage most efficiently, it also can promote range improvement by providing growing season deferment for rangelands. However, it is important that the relative carrying capacity of the range and tame pasture be properly balanced to prevent overutilization of the range.

Range sites may differ significantly in their suitability for grazing during different seasons. Cool-season herbaceous forage and evergreen browse will generally provide better grazing during the winter and early spring, whereas warm-season forages are best suited to use during late spring, summer, or fall. Large pastures with a mix of sites allow animals to rotate their grazing seasonally. Smaller pastures, which contain less variation in vegetation, may require the use of seasonal adjustments in grazing to match the forage.

Stocking Rates

As stocking rate increases, gains per animal decrease but gains per acre increase to a point beyond which further increases in stocking rate reduce both gains per animal and per acre. This general relationship applies to all grazing lands, and the optimum stocking rate will be in the range between the rate producing maximum gain per head and the rate producing maximum gain per acre. This optimum will shift with changing economic conditions. When costs associated with an individual animal are high relative to cost per acre of land, stocking rate should be adjusted to improve gain per animal. Stocking rates should be shifted to increase gain per acre when costs associated with land are high relative to costs per animal.

On tame pastures intensive cultural practices are applied to maintain the productivity of the vegetation, and the land is capable of sustaining intensive agriculture. However, many rangelands are not capable of sustaining intensive agriculture, and heavy stocking rates designed to maximize animal production per unit of land cause deterioration of both vegetation and soil conditions.

If estimates of annual forage production are available, a moderate stocking rate for ranges can be set by allowing four times as much forage per animal as its predicted intake for the year. Allowing two to four times the predicted intake will result in heavy stocking. The author's field experience indicates that on perennial rangelands, approximately one fourth of the total usable forage produced can be consumed by grazing animals under proper stocking. Higher levels of utilization are possible on annual ranges and tame pastures.

The best procedure for arriving at the correct stocking rate is experience combined with records of animal production and vegetation trends. A computer decision aid provides a guide for estimating carrying capacity and adjusting stock numbers to match fluctuations in forage production.[3] This decision aid simplifies this most important and difficult task.

Grazing Systems

Grazing systems have been designed to offset the effects of selective grazing and to enhance range improvement through plant succession. The components of a grazing system are the number of pastures and herds of livestock and the length of grazing and rest periods. Livestock are concentrated on a portion of the land to allow the vegetation on the remaining land in the system to grow for a period of time without grazing. Livestock are rotated among pastures to provide scheduled periods of grazing and rest for each pasture.

To design a grazing system for a given unit of land, the manager must consider three basic aspects of grazing management: (1) *stocking rate*, determined by the number of animals allocated to the system; (2) *stocking density*, determined by the number of pastures and herds for any given stocking rate; and (3) *stocking pressure*, determined by the length of the grazing periods for a given stocking rate and stocking density.

Both stocking density and stocking pressure can be changed in a grazing system without changing stocking rate, but changes in stocking rate will always affect stocking density and pressure. Increasing stocking density will result in more uniform distribution of grazing; thus grazing systems that concentrate animals on smaller portions of the land, that is, more pastures and fewer herds may promote better grazing distribution. Increasing stocking pressure reduces diet quality; thus reducing the length of grazing periods should improve animal performance. Long rest periods that allow significant amounts of forage to mature between grazing periods will reduce animal production unless stocking rates are light. With all of these factors to consider, the design of a successful grazing system that meets both plant and animal requirements is not a simple exercise.

SUPPLEMENTATION OF GRAZING ANIMALS

Livestock grazing on green, actively growing forage generally obtain adequate levels of most nutrients. When they are forced to utilize mature or dormant forage, nutrient deficiencies may be expected.

Supplemental feeding is the practice of providing limited amounts of feed containing concentrated levels of the deficient nutrients. Sometimes supplemental feeding is confused with emergency or maintenance feeding. Emergency feeding should be practiced to meet the total requirement of animals on range or pasture when forage is temporarily unavailable for grazing, for example when covered by snow. Maintenance feeding is required when pastures are overstocked and forage availability drops to levels that restrict intake, resulting in a dry matter deficiency. In emergency and maintenance feeding situations, the objective is generally to feed a balanced diet to carry animals through a stress period. This section will examine the role of supplemental feeding for livestock on range or pasture.

Vitamins and Minerals

Significant body reserves of some nutrients, such as vitamin A and energy, may be accumulated by grazing animals. However, there are small body reserves of most minerals, protein, and water, and the animal's dietary requirements must be met on a regular basis. (Supplementation of vitamins and minerals will not be considered in detail in this chapter.)

Vitamin A is the only vitamin commonly deficient in diets of range livestock. Body reserves may be adequate for 90 to 120 days. Most commercial range supplements contain synthetic vitamin A, and it may also be supplied by injection. Sodium and phosphorus are the minerals that are most widely deficient, and provision should be made to supply them. Sodium should be provided throughout the year. Phosphorus should be provided whenever livestock are grazing mature or dormant vegetation. Phosphorus is required yearlong in some regions that have phosphorus-deficient soils. Recent research indicates that potassium may be deficient in diets of cattle grazing mature dormant forage.

Protein and Energy

Protein and energy are both commonly deficient during certain periods of the year on rangelands. Whenever protein is deficient, animal production will be greatly reduced and utilization of the energy in the forage will be hampered. Growth will be reduced in stocker animals, and reproduction and lactation will be reduced in breeding stock. However, if cows and ewes are provided protein and minerals with an adequate supply of forage, they can, to a limited extent, draw on body reserves of energy (fat) to meet lactation needs without significant losses in production.

The principle of utilizing periods of high-quality forage to store energy reserves for later periods of deficiency has great economic importance. If animals are stocked too heavily or otherwise managed during the growing season to prevent accumulation of energy reserves, the cost of supplemental feeding will increase markedly. It is important to schedule breeding and weaning to try to obtain an optimum combination of the animal's nutrient requirements and the cycles of forage availability and quality.

Not only is it expensive to supplement energy, but intake and digestibility of forage are affected differently by protein and energy supplements. Both intake and digestibility are enhanced by the addition of protein-rich supplements to roughage diets low in nitrogen. Supplemental protein may increase intake of low-quality mature forage by 50 to 100 per cent. The addition of supplements containing large amounts of starch generally depresses cellulose digestion and forage intake. With low-quality forages, the digestibility of nitrogen may also be depressed.

Studies evaluating protein versus energy supplements for sheep on desert winter range in Utah showed that cottonseed meal increased daily intake of range forage but that grain supplements had no effect or tended to decrease daily intake of forage. The quantity of digestible protein consumed daily in the supplement and the range forage was actually decreased by feeding corn or barley in some trials. High-protein supplements substantially increased the levels of metabolizable energy consumed by the sheep. Corn supplements generally increased energy in the daily ration, but barley reduced daily intake of energy because of the reduced daily intake and depressed digestibility of cellulose and other carbohydrates in the range forage. It was concluded that range livestock producers could benefit more from feeding a protein supplement such as cottonseed meal or soybean meal than from feeding energy supplements such as corn and barley because protein supplements enhanced the value of range forage and produced better livestock responses.

WATER REQUIREMENTS

Water consumption by adult livestock of medium weight in a temperate climate may range from 7 to 17.5 gal/day for beef cattle and from 1 to 4 gal/day for sheep and goats.[5] As a general rule, cattle require 8 to 10 gal/day, sheep 0.75 to 1 gal/day, and horses 10 to 12 gal/day. However, these figures should be adjusted to account for the amount that will be lost by evaporation. Cattle and horses should be allowed 12 to 15 gal/day and sheep 1 to 1.5 gal/day.

Sources of water include streams, springs, wells, and stock ponds (earthen tanks). The dependability of a water system should be judged during the dry season. The most common problems related to watering systems include poor distribution of watering places, not having enough water at each place, and poor water quality.

Reducing water intake reduces dry matter intake. The water to dry matter ratio in the rumen remains relatively constant when water intake is restricted. The animal adjusts through a reduction in moisture excreted in urine and feces and by reducing dry matter intake. For this reason cattle should never go longer than 48 hours without water. Reduction of water consumption has also been reported to cause a reduction in CP digestibility.

All mineral elements essential as dietary nutrients are present to some extent in water, and it is generally believed that elements in water solution are available to the animal as much as if they were consumed in dry feed or mineral blocks. Water may contribute part of the animal's requirement of sulfur, iodine, calcium, copper, cobalt, iron, manganese, zinc, and selenium,[1] but the amount contributed is subject to a great deal of variation depending on the kind and class of livestock, the amount of water consumed, and the concentrations of these minerals in the water. In addition, the difference between the minimum requirement and the level at which toxic effects may occur is very small in some cases. For these reasons the NRC suggests that water not normally be relied on as a source of essential minerals.[5]

Of greater importance are the physical, chemical, and biologic properties of the water and their effect on water palatability and animal health. There are a variety of substances suspended or dissolved in livestock water that may influence palatability or be potentially harmful. These include inorganic elements and their salts, biologically produced toxins, parasitic or disease-carrying organisms, and manmade pollutants, particularly fertilizers and pesticides. Concentrations at which these substances render water undesirable are subject to many variables. Turbidity caused by suspended particles of clay and organic matter does not appear to be an important factor in itself with regard to palatability or animal health. Both short- and long-term effects and interactions with other substances must be considered.[1] Substances found in quantities not toxic to the consuming animal may accumulate to levels undesirable for those who consume livestock products. These factors make it difficult to determine safe levels for toxic substances.

Salinity problems are more universal in scope and are more likely to be encountered. Total salt or mineral content (also expressed as total dissolved solids), while not indicating a single contaminating substance, is a common measurement that carries significance in determining livestock water quality. Highly mineralized water can cause physiologic disturbances (and even death) in animals. Even small salt concentrations can result in a decrease in palatability.

From time to time watering places may become infested by "blooms" of blue-green algae that produce toxins, seriously affecting livestock. Toxicity of these blooms is extremely variable depending on which species and strains of algae are present, types and numbers of associated bacteria, growing conditions, animal health, and amount of toxin consumed. Livestock poisonings have also been observed following rapid decomposition of algal blooms. This may be due in part to botulism poisoning resulting from anaerobic conditions accompanying decomposition. Algae can be controlled by use of 1 ppm of copper sulfate added to the water.

The purity of water consumed by livestock has far-reaching implications, and there are many ways in which livestock water can become contaminated. Certain contaminates may hinder livestock directly through losses by death, losses in production, or interference with reproductive processes. They may also contaminate milk and meat to the point that human consumption is undesirable. It is necessary to understand the possible hazards in order to ensure an adequate supply of good quality drinking water for livestock.

REFERENCES

1. Environmental Protection Agency: Proposed Criteria for Water Quality, Vol. I: Water for Livestock Enterprises. Washington, DC, 1973.
2. Jeffery H: Aust J Exp Agr Animal Hus 2:397, 1971.
3. Kothmann MM, Hinnant RT: Grazing Management Stock Adjustments Template, Department of Rangeland Ecology and Management, TAMU, College Station, TX, 1990.
4. National Research Council: United States–Canadian Tables of Feed Composition. Washington, DC, National Academy of Science, Publ 1684, 1969.
5. National Research Council: Nutrients and Toxic Substances in Water for Livestock and Poultry. Washington, DC, National Academy of Sciences, 1974.

Mineral Supplementation for Beef Cattle on Rangeland

J. C. DOYLE, DVM, PhD
J. E. HUSTON, PhD

The American beef cattle operator relies on forage production (pasture and rangeland) to support the cow-calf component of the industry. The limitations imposed on grazing livestock are several, but foremost are the animal's genetic potential and nutrient supply. Recognition of all limitations within any production system is required to maximize efficiency. One of the tenets of nutrition is that none of the nutrients acts in isolation, but that all the nutrients interact within metabolic pathways to maintain homeostasis and promote productivity. Major and trace minerals are required in mammalian cells in numerous biochemical functions, and an inadequate supply of any one can cause a malfunction of the system.

Pasture forage varying in amount and quality must satisfy a majority of the basic physiologic nutrient requirements of grazing livestock. Deficiencies that commonly occur seldom produce simple, well-defined malfunctions. In mineral nutrition, only a few single-element deficiencies are commonly detected by classic clinical signs (e.g., milk fever, grass tetany). However, suboptimal levels of minerals may result from antagonism, chelation, deficiency, or toxicity of both major and trace minerals that alter the biologic process.[1] These marginal deficiencies or imbalances may totally escape notice as a management problem, yet lead to subtle reductions in productivity that have major negative impacts on the economics of an enterprise. Supplementation minimizes the disparity encountered between pastures and animal requirements. The nutrient demands of a cow-calf unit result from maintenance, pregnancy, lactation, and weight gain. Supplementation of minerals should be considered essential since inadequate consumption of various elements may limit productivity of animals on pasture.

AVAILABILITY OF NUTRIENTS FROM PASTURE

Nutrients that animals derive from pasture plants include energy (primarily from carbohydrates), proteins, various vitamin precursors, and variable amounts of the different minerals. Grazing animals are in a dynamic nutrient flux. Nutritional requirements are in a constant state of change with the stage of production,[2] as are forage nutrients with the season.[3] Cows gain or lose tissue (fat and protein) depending on whether intake of nutrients exceeds or is exceeded by the requirements for ongoing metabolic processes. Aligning the animal's major nutrient requirements with the nutrients in forage growth may provide adequate supplies of energy and protein, but some minerals are at minimal levels in the leaves of growing forages[4] and may not satisfy the animal's total requirements.

The translocation of minerals from the soil, through the forage, and finally to the grazing animal does not necessarily proceed without interruption. Seasonal rainfall, climate, day length, and geologic pasture variations have major influences on the levels of plant minerals. Calcareous soils tend to prevent uptake of phosphorus and other individual or groups of minerals owing to high chelation properties.[5] Therefore soil analysis may lead to erroneous conclusions regarding forage content. Different plant species growing on similar soil types and under similar environmental conditions exhibit differences in mineral content.[6] Hartmans reported that copper levels within the soil and plants showed no correlation with copper status of the animal.[7] The presence of minerals in plant matter does not assure their availability to the consuming animal.

Ruminant nutrition includes two unique metabolic systems: the cellular physiology of the animal and the ruminal microbial population. Cellulose is the most abundant carbohydrate in the world, yet may be used only by microbes. Ruminant microbial fermentation includes the conversion of cellulose to volatile fatty acids (VFA) and protein synthesis. The principal function of the major minerals (calcium, sodium, chlorine, phosphorus, potassium, magnesium, and sulfur) in ruminal microbial population is in the regulation of physiochemical properties, including osmotic pressure, buffering capacity, redox potential, and dilution rate. Microbial fermentation and animal tissue cellular function utilize trace elements (i.e., glucose oxidation) as catalysts in enzymatic systems and as metalloenzymes.

Absorption of plant minerals will vary with extent of ruminal fermentation of large molecular compounds followed by changes of pH throughout the digestive tract.[8] Utilization of minerals from the plant may depend on their location within the cell (cell-wall versus non–cell-wall fractions) and the digestibilities of the various cell constituents.[9] Although binding agents such as oxalates may reduce the availability of some elements,[10] minerals from high-quality forages usually will be released extensively for animal metabolism. The rate of forage mineral release in the rumen is greater for potassium, magnesium, and sodium than for calcium and zinc. Rumen solubility of phosphorus and copper vary depending on the forage species.[11,12] Manganese was found to be within the more soluble plant fraction of alfalfa and Sudan hays, whereas copper and zinc were weakly bound to insoluble rumen residue.[13]

Fermentation can either increase or decrease the biologic availability of minerals in the diet. Upon hydrolysis of phytate (inositol hexaphosphoric acid) during ruminal fermentation, phosphorus is released for absorption.[14] The presence of copper, molybdenum, and sulfur in the rumen results in the formation of copper thiomolybdate, a nonabsorbable copper compound.[15] Thus total trace mineral content within plant material will not coincide necessarily with biologically available nutrients for the consumer (ruminal microbe or animal).

FEED INTAKE AND RATE OF PASSAGE

Any nutrient deficiency influences overall animal performance; therefore the complex neurohormonal regulation of dietary intake is critical. The animal's dietary intake and digestion are influenced by thermal, visceral, osmo-, chemo-, and mechanoreceptors. An increased intake generally is accompanied by an increased rate of passage with a decreased digestion coefficient. Thus intake determines the amount of nutrients consumed and influences nutrient digestibilities. Environmental temperatures have a pronounced effect on animal intake and digestibility of various feedstuffs. The heat-stressed animal fed a low digestible diet encounters a slower rate of passage and reduction in consumption.[16] One of the physiologic responses to hyperthermia is sweating, which increases skin loss of sodium, potassium, magnesium, calcium, and chlorine.[17]

Exposure of ruminants to cold environments elicits a variety of physiologic responses that involve minerals. Exposure below the lower critical temperature results in an increased metabolic rate to compensate for heat loss and is accompanied by increased voluntary intake and increased rumen motility. A consistent depression (10.2 versus 4.4 per cent) of apparent digestibility of calcium was observed with exposure to cold temperatures.[18] Exposure to moderately cold temperatures failed to depress plasma magnesium concentrations in fed ewes but did act synergistically with starvation to induce hypomagnesemia.[19]

Absorption of a majority of minerals by the ruminant occurs at the upper gastrointestinal tract (magnesium absorption does occur within the rumen). Thus these minerals undergo ruminal fermentation (microbial metabolism), acidic conditions of the abomasum, and neutralization with entry into the small intestines. The homeostatic control of some minerals (calcium and phosphorus) is well recognized. Trace elements that are cations may share similar absorptive pathways and are known to interact with each other. Thus an excess of one trace mineral may saturate membrane-bound or intracellular carriers that two elements have in common and inhibit the absorption of the other element.[20]

REPRODUCTIVE PERFORMANCE

An important economic loss to a cow-calf operation is the nonpregnant cow; therefore maintaining acceptable reproductive performance is essential. Early embryonic mortality has been estimated to cause 75 to 80 per cent of infertility problems from conception to day 40 in cattle.[21] Recent research has identified several trace elements that affect reproductive efficiency during early embryonic development. Low copper and magnesium during the breeding season increased the number of services for conception and early embryonic death in lactating dairy cows.[22] Elevated levels of manganese (53 ppm versus National Research Council [NRC] requirements of 40 ppm) significantly reduced days to conception (16 versus 34 days) in first-calf heifers and cows.[23]

Body condition at calving to the end of breeding season is clearly associated with return of estrus and conception,[24] but frequently unexplained departures from this generalized cause-and-effect relationship (well-conditioned animals that do not exhibit estrus nor breed) have been noted.[25] Mineral supplementation (phosphorus, copper, manganese, and zinc) on native pasture increased reproductive performance of lactating beef cattle possessing uniform body condition scores without altering serum or liver values.[26] The liver values of these beef cows were within physiologic norms, which may suggest an inadequate tissue response or lack of elemental mobilization to recipient reproductive tissues, or both. Uterine tissue regeneration is mandatory for reproductive response in the postpartum cow. The increase in physiologic response in reproduction to trace mineral supplementation may have been attributed to satisfying the immune system trace element requirements.

The ovum prior to implantation (day 14) is totally dependent on a dynamic oviduct and uterine environment for proper osmolality, nourishment, and defense in order for blastomere division to progress.[27] One of the roles of trace minerals in reproductive performance may be at the endometrium level.[28] The differences of endometrial tissue element levels (elevated at day 1 and depressed at day 12) denote the dynamics of metabolism under hormonal influence. The alteration of copper, manganese, and zinc levels within the endometrium indicates a more sensitive tissue than serum and liver levels to nutritional inputs. The defined roles that copper, manganese, and zinc serve within the endometrium are currently unknown; however, their functions may be both nutritional and protective (detoxification of uterine environment) for the developing ovum.

WEIGHT GAIN

Animals that possess a genetic potential for rapid growth have overall higher maintainance and production requirements. These animals generate more pounds of beef on a per head basis, but many times the cow-calf operator has not realized true genetic potential because of nutritional limitations. Young growing animals will generally encounter energy and protein deficiencies under pasture conditions prior to a limitation of a macro- or trace mineral. The weight gain response observed with mineral supplementation may be a direct fulfillment of a physiologic deficiency or an indirect result of stimulating an increase in forage consumption, thus providing greater quantities of metabolizable energy and protein. Stimulation of intake is well recognized for animals under grazing conditions with supplements of salt, phosphorus, calcium, and cobalt. The use of selenium and cobalt rumen boluses has shown a response in certain geographic regions where these specific trace element deficiencies are encountered.[29, 30] A weight gain response was observed when a balanced mineral supplement was fed to young animals (150 to 200 kg) on pastures marginal to deficient in copper.[31]

The use of steroid implants (anabolic agents) has greatly influenced beef production. Anabolic agents increase the efficiency of utilization of nitrogen from the diet, and ruminants implanted with anabolic agents are faster growing, leaner, and more efficient.[32] Steroid implants have a positive influence on mineral metabolism by improving structural characteristics (cortical width and elasticity) of the bone.[33] When steers were implanted with steroids and fed various levels of zinc in the diet, serum zinc values were not altered whereas hepatic levels were elevated.[34]

Increased condition scores and weights (6.0 versus 4.5, approximately 73 kg difference) were observed when supplemental copper was fed to lactating cows on marginal copper-deficient pastures.[13] An increase in serum copper values was noted for copper-supplemented animals.

BREED INFLUENCE

The NRC mineral recommendations were determined from controlled research studies from several breeds of cattle (primarily British). It should be recognized that many crossbred and exotic cattle breed possessing a greater genetic capacity for production may have an increased requirement of all nutrients. Various breeds have exhibited differences in mineral requirements. The copper requirement of Holstein calves appears to be higher than for beef breeds.[35]

WATER MINERAL CONTENT

The most important physiologic aspect of water as a nutrient is quantity consumed. Depression of water consumption by contaminates (organic or inorganic compounds) is of more importance than an imposed mineral imbalance. Deprivation or reduced water intake depresses dry matter intake, resulting in lowered productivity. Cattle that are moved to different locations should be provided the best quality water for the most rapid rehydration on arrival. Water treatment processes (i.e., filtration, ion exchange, or ozonation) that significantly improve water quality will usually improve consumption and livestock performance. However, water quality is usually considered a function of the concentrations of elemental compounds in solution. This concentration of dissolved elements is referred to as total dissolved solids. Salinity describes the total ionic concentration of salt (NaCl) in water. The term "hardness" is related to the concentration of divalent cations (calcium and magnesium).

The elemental concentration of water is generally inadequate to meet the dietary requirements of ruminants. However, water has the potential to contain elements that can exist at antagonistic or toxic levels. Antagonistic levels of sulfur and molybdenum in solution can interfere with copper metabolism. Substances and elements may vary in toxicity depending on the nature of the suspension (solid or solution) and the chemical forms in which they exist. Copper sulfate is more toxic in solution than when added as a dry form.[36] The total dissolved solid content of water is a valuable tool in detecting elemental excesses that may impose depressed consumption or mineral imbalances.

MACROELEMENTS

Salt (Sodium and Chloride)

Sodium, chlorine, and potassium function in maintaining osmotic pressure and regulating acid-base equilibrium for rumen microbes and animal cells. Both sodium and chlorine are involved with cellular function in basic metabolism, nutrient uptake, and transmission of nerve impulse. Sodium is found in much lower quantities than chlorine in natural feedstuffs. The requirement of sodium is between 0.06 and 0.10 per cent of the diet.[2] The chlorine requirement for beef cattle is currently unknown. The highest physiologic requirement for salt is in lactating cows because of secretions in the milk. Sodium deficiencies are most likely to occur for animals that are growing, exposed to high environmental temperatures, and grazing pastures with high potassium content (rapidly growing forages).

Because grazing beef cattle seek out salt, it is an important component for many free-choice supplements. Along coastal regions or areas with high sodium plant levels, salt-base supplements are not consumed well and alternative attractants may be required (e.g., protein meals, fat, dried yeast products, or molasses) to achieve adequate intake. Excess salt consumption by livestock requires increased water intake for excretion. Caution should be used when using salt to restrict the intake of protein supplements. Salted protein meals can be detrimental to livestock performance. In situations of limited forages (drought conditions) and restricted water intake, energy-deficient animals can consume enough salted protein meal for it to be toxic (approximately 2.2 g salt/kg of body weight).[37]

Potassium

Potassium functions primarily at the cellular level, maintaining osmotic pressure and acid-base equilibrium. In contrast to sodium, it is not stored in the body in appreciable amounts and must be supplied daily. Beef cattle requirements for potassium are between 0.5 and 0.7 per cent.[2] Stressed animals have a higher turnover of potassium and have been shown to respond dramatically to supplementation.[38] The highest physiologic requirement of potassium is in the lactating cow for secretion in the milk. Potassium deficiencies are likely when high-producing animals (lactating dairy cows or feedlot animals) are fed high-grain diets (grains contain less than 0.5 per cent potassium). Forages are high in potassium (1 to 4 per cent) during the growing season, but when dormant may contain inadequate levels (<0.5 per cent) for grazing animals.[39] High potassium levels in plants (small grain pastures) can be antagonistic to magnesium absorption, predisposing to grass tetany.

Calcium and Phosphorus

Calcium and phosphorus are vital to almost all tissues, composing 70 per cent of the total mineral elements in the body. Calcium functions in skeletal formation, blood clotting, cardiac rhythm, neuromuscular transmission, membrane permeability, and enzyme activation. Phosphorus is a constituent of bone, red blood cells, muscle, and nerve tissue and functions in buffering systems in the process of energy exchange. A severe limitation of phosphorus is reflected as a general impairment of health, yet does not directly relate to reproductive performance.[40]

The beef cattle requirements are 0.18 to 1.04 per cent calcium and 0.18 to 0.70 per cent phosphorus for growing heifers and steers, and 0.31 to 0.60 calcium and 0.31 to 0.40 per cent phosphorus for lactating dairy cows. Either calcium or phosphorus, or both, can be deficient for grazing cattle. Forages tend to have higher calcium and lower phosphorus content, and phosphorus deficiencies are the most widespread and of greatest economic importance of all mineral deficiencies for grazing cattle.[41, 42]

Levels of calcium and phosphorus in free-choice mineral mixes that are commercially available are generally in a 1.5:1 to 1:1 ratio. The 2:1 ratio is considered adequate for the total diet, but the high calcium that usually occurs in low-quality forages makes a low calcium:phosphorus ratio in the supplement preferred. The animal's diet calcium:phosphorus ratio can be as high as 7:1, as long as the animal meets its minimal phosphorus requirement.[43] Some phosphorus sources are not palatable, and high levels (i.e., 14 per cent) within a supplement may be economical but poorly consumed. In a free-choice supplement the phosphorus concentration can be 6 to 8 per cent when forages are 0.20 per cent phosphorus or higher. When forages are below 0.2 per cent, a mineral supplement containing 8 to 10 per cent phosphorus would be more efficacious.[44] Higher concentrations of both calcium and phosphorus should be used when forage concentrations are low and when the animal's physiologic requirements are high (i.e., lactation).

The biologic availabilities of calcium and phosphorus in mineral supplements will vary with chemical source. Sources of calcium with high bioavailability include steamed bone meal, monocalcium phosphate, and dicalcium phosphate. Calcium sources with intermediate bioavailability are calcium carbonate (from ground limestone, oyster shells, etc.), defluorinated rock phosphate, and dolomitic limestone. Phosphorus sources with high bioavailability are steamed bone meal, monocalcium phosphate, phosphoric acid, and sodium phosphate. Phosphorus in defluorinated rock phosphate and dicalcium phosphate are intermediate in bioavailability.

Magnesium

Magnesium is found in the skeleton (60 to 70 per cent), and the remainder is found in soft tissues; it functions in numerous enzyme systems. The most critical function under practical conditions is its involvement in neuromuscular activity when low dietary intake or absorption, or both, results in grass tetany (hypomagnesemia). Hypomagnesemia usually occurs on immature pastures with high potassium content, and the incidence may be related to the requirements of different breeds.[45] The digestibility of magnesium was higher for Brangus, Brangus X Holstein, Angus, and Hereford X Holstein than for Hereford, Hereford X Jersey, Brangus X Hereford, Jersey, and Holstein cows. The magnesium requirement is 0.05 to 0.25 per cent,[2] with higher levels required for lactating cows. Older animals are more prone to grass tetany because of the inability to mobilize sufficient magnesium from the bone under higher metabolic requirements (lactation). Animals exposed to pastures where grass tetany may be a problem should be treated prophylactically during that period. The bioavailabilities of magnesium are high for carbonates, oxides, and sulfates.[46] High magnesium supplements used to prevent hypomagnesemia (8 to 14 per cent magnesium) are only successful if adequate intake is achieved. Magnesium is an unpalatable mineral and requires formulation with ingredients (i.e., molasses, protein meals, grains) that induce intake. A complete mineral supplement should contain a minimal level of magnesium (>1 per cent).

Sulfur

Sulfur is an essential component of amino acids (methionine and cysteine), vitamins (thiamine and biotin), hormones (somatostatin and oxytocin), and sulfate polysaccharides (chondroitin). It is involved in numerous metabolic functions, including carbohydrate and fat metabolism, protein synthesis and metabolism, endocrine function, blood clotting, and acid-base balance of intra- and extracellular fluids. Its supplementation has been shown to be beneficial in feedlots when high levels of urea are used in the ration. The proper concentration of sulfur in the diet is in the range of 0.08 to 0.15 per cent. Sulfur is not commonly supplemented under pasture conditions because of its elemental antagonistic properties. High sulfur contents in water have been shown to inhibit absorption and metabolism of copper by the formation of copper sulfide.[2]

TRACE ELEMENTS (Table 1)

Cobalt

The requirement of cobalt is actually for fulfilling the rumen microorganisms' biologic needs and for the ruminal synthesis

Table 1. EXAMPLE OF CONCENTRATIONS OF TRACE MINERALS IN A MINERAL SUPPLEMENT*

Element	Estimated Maximum Requirement (ppm)	Percentage of Minerals in Supplement for Following Per Cent of Requirement:	
		50%	100%
Cobalt	0.10	0.0005	0.001
Copper	8.0	0.04	0.08
Iodine	0.5	0.0025	0.005
Iron	50.0	0.25	0.5
Manganese	40.0	0.2	0.4
Selenium	0.10	0.0005	0.001
Zinc	30.0	0.15	0.3

*This concentration is based on the average of 100 g/day of mineral mixture for beef cattle with a 10 kg consumption of dry matter.

of cobalamin (vitamin B_{12}), necessary for both microorganisms and animal tissues. Vitamin B_{12} is involved in methylmalonyl-CoA isomerase, which is required for hepatic metabolism to glucose. Vitamin B_{12} is also required for the enzyme that catalyzes the recycling of methionine from homocysteine and normal liver folate metabolism. A majority of the cobalt is stored within the muscle (43 per cent) and bone (14 per cent), with small amounts distributed in organ tissues. These stores are not readily passed to the rumen for microbial synthesis of vitamin B_{12}. Of the ingested cobalt, only 3 per cent is converted to vitamin B_{12} within the rumen.[47] Depletion of vitamin B_{12} results in a gradual loss of appetite, followed by anorexia, loss of muscular mass, anemia, and death. Cobalt is required in the diet at 0.07 to 0.11 ppm.[48] Supplemental sources for cobalt that are effective include carbonate, chloride, and sulfate. Generally legumes are higher in cobalt than are grasses. Oilseed meals are good sources of cobalt, whereas cereal grains are poor.

Copper-Molybdenum

Copper imbalances are almost as prevalent as phosphorus deficiencies as limiting factors for grazing livestock in the United States and in tropical regions.[10, 49] Copper acts as a synergistic element for iron absorption and in hemoglobin formation. Ceruloplasmin is a copper protein synthesized in the liver, which serves in the oxidation of iron, permitting it to bind to transferrin (iron transport protein). Achromotrichia, keratinization deficit, and nervous disorders also have been associated with copper imbalances. The reduction in lysyl oxidase (copper protein) activity reduces strength of cardiac and arterial tissues and can lead to aortic aneurysms with rupture. Other enzymes that contain or require copper are cytochrome oxidase, uricase, tyrosinase, glutathione oxidase, catalase, ascorbic acid oxidase, and oxaloacetate decarboxylase.

Copper deficiencies have been categorized into four circumstances: (1) elevated levels of molybdenum (>100 mg/kg); (2) low levels of copper and high levels of molybdenum (<2:1 ratio); (3) low copper concentration (<5 mg/kg); and (4) normal copper and molybdenum concentrations with high intakes of soluble sulfur amino acids.[10]

Liver copper values of pregnant cows decrease during the last 4 months of gestation owing to elemental partitioning to the fetus,[13] and the liver copper content of the bovine neonate is greatly elevated over that of the dam.[50] Stressed, sick, and implanted animals usually have elevated serum copper and depressed zinc values.[51, 52]

General recommendations of copper supplementation cannot be made without reference to other elements that exist within the diet and breed of animal. Copper absorption is inhibited by numerous compounds, including phytates, lignin, calcium carbonate, iron, zinc, cadmium, sulfur, molybdenum, and silver. Elevated levels of molybdenum interfere with copper absorption through the formation of a copper: molybdenum (copper thiomolybdate) complex. The formation of copper sulfide also reduces copper absorption. A proper concentration of copper in the diet is in the range of 4 to 10 ppm when antagonistic elements are minimal. A copper:molybdenum ratio of 2:1 is needed, and lower ratios result in an imbalance.[53] When molybdenum forage levels are greater than 1 ppm, copper supplementation is probably needed. The recommended levels of copper supplementation are in the range of 4 to 10 ppm.[2] Molybdenum is not needed in supplements under most conditions.

The chemical form of copper in the diet and associated dietary ingredients influence the availability of copper to animals.[28, 35, 54, 55] When 1 kg of grain was used as a carrier for supplemental phosphorus, copper levels became elevated within the endometrium, suggesting an increase in the bioavailability of copper. Anionic organic complexes (proteinates) appear to be more readily available than copper sulfate. Bioavailability of copper as a proteinate was greater than copper as a sulfate for calves fed high molybdenum diets. However, both copper sulfate and copper chloride are good inorganic sources.

Iodine

Iodine is required for the synthesis of active thyroid hormones (thyroxine and triiodothyronine), which regulate energy metabolism. Thyroxine functions as the transport form and as the feedback regulator of the thyroid gland. The dietary requirement of iodine is influenced by the efficiency of the thyroid gland and the extent of iodine recycling. Iodine deficiencies may go unobserved for prolonged periods before thyroid gland enlargement (goiter) occurs. Interrelationships that affect iodine metabolism include high arsenic, fluorine, or calcium; deficient or high cobalt; and low manganese.[56]

Goiter can result from animals feeding on Brassicae and Cruciferae plants containing goitergenic substances (e.g., kale, rape, cabbage, soybeans, flaxseed, peas, peanuts, and turnips) as well as from low iodine diets. Thiocyanate-type goitrogens can be overcome by additional iodine, whereas thiouracil types can only be partially suppressed by supplementation. Overall, goitrogens increase the iodine requirement. The recommended level of supplementation of iodine is 0.2 to 2.0 ppm. Supplementation for diets containing 25 per cent goitrogenic feeds require doubling the level of iodine.[57] Sources of supplemental iodine that include calcium iodide, sodium iodide, and potassium iodide (stabilized) are highly available to the ruminant but are unstable because of oxidation. More stable forms of iodine sources include potassium iodate (stable or nonstable) or pentacalcium orthoperiodate. Ethylenediamine dihydroiodide (EDDI) is an organic complex that is used in supplements to treat footrot and lumpy jaw. Current U.S. Food and Drug Administration (FDA) regulations set the maximum limit of iodine supplementation at 10 mg/head/day.

Iron

Iron is an essential component of hemoglobin, myoglobin, cytochromes, and other enzyme systems. Deficiencies in adult cattle are rare compared with those of young calves with higher requirements. Hemopoietic imbalances in cattle are more commonly due to copper imbalances or parasitism. A copper imbalance impairs iron absorption.

The dietary requirement of iron for ruminants is not well established. The suggested requirement for the ruminant is between 30 and 100 ppm.[2] Iron absorption is reduced by high dietary levels of phosphorus because of the formation of an insoluble ferric phosphate and phytate. Excess divalent cations (e.g., copper, manganese, zinc, lead, and cadmium) can interfere with iron absorption because of competition for absorption sites in the intestinal mucosa.[42]

Generally iron is found at high levels in most forages and is a contaminate of many phosphorus sources (1 to 2 per cent). Thus high levels of supplementation with high-iron compounds is not required when contaminated phosphorus sources are incorporated into the supplement. The divalent form of iron (ferrous) is more soluble than the trivalent form (ferric) and is absorbed to a greater extent. Ferrous sulfate has a higher bioavailability than ferrous carbonate. Iron oxide is biologically inert but adds red color to a mineral.

Manganese

Manganese is essential for normal bone development, reproduction, and central nervous system function of the newborn. The functional enzymes that manganese catalyzes include hydrolases, kinases, decarboxylases, and transferases. The manganese body pool is small, and 25 to 50 per cent of the body pool is ingested daily.[58] The manganese requirement for reproduction and normal calf development is higher than for growth.[23, 59, 60] Recent feedlot research showed that higher levels of manganese (80 versus 50 ppm, respectively) depressed average daily gain.[51, 61] Antagonistic agents to manganese absorption include high levels of calcium and phosphorus and alkaloids of lupinus plants.[62, 63] The minimum requirement for manganese is dependent on physiologic function and is in the range of 20 to 50 ppm.[2] Bioavailability of manganese is best achieved with sulfate, followed by oxide and carbonate.[64]

Selenium

Selenium is a constituent of glutathione peroxidase, which aids in protecting cellular and subcellular membranes from oxidative damage.[65] As an antioxidant it destroys peroxides prior to cellular membrane attack and overlaps the functions of vitamin E. The clinical syndrome of selenium deficiency is white muscle disease (WMD) in young animals. Glutathione peroxidase functions in growth, reproduction, and tissue integrity. Other biochemical roles of selenium include adequate immune response, selenoprotein of mitochondria for spermatozoa, RNA synthesis, and prostaglandin synthesis and/or fatty acid metabolism. Selenium exerts a protective function in binding with heavy metals such as arsenic, cadmium, mercury, and silver.[1, 42] Antagonistic agents to selenium absorption are high-sulfur diets (legumes) and the previously mentioned heavy metals. The requirement of selenium is dependent on the animal's previous status, vitamin E status, lipids (rancidity yields peroxides), and antagonistic and agonistic compounds.[66] The NRC recommended level of selenium supplementation is 0.05 to 0.30 ppm.[2] Sources of selenium supplementation are sodium selenate and sodium selenite.

Zinc

Zinc functions as a constituent and catalyst in several hundred enzyme systems (e.g., carbonic anhydrase) and is involved in nucleic acid metabolism, protein synthesis, and carbohydrate metabolism. Maintaining plasma concentrations of vitamin A requires zinc for its mobilization from the liver.[67] Zinc is distributed throughout the body and found in high concentrations in the prostate, pituitary gland, choroid, and iris of the eye. Zinc deficiency results in numerous maladies that usually involve a deficit in epithelial functions (i.e., mucosal epithelial lining, keratinization, and hair growth). Animals are unable to mobilize zinc stores rapidly when the diet is deficient;[28, 68] therefore continuous supplementation may be advised in situations of marginal dietary zinc.

The zinc requirement of an animal is dependent on the animals physiologic function. The requirement for growth is considerably lower than that for testicular development and spermatogenesis.[48] High levels of zinc supplementation protect against hepatic damage caused by fungal toxins of *Pithomyces chartarum*[42] and *Phomopis leptostromiformis*. The suggested level of zinc supplementation is in the range of 20 to 40 ppm.[2] Sources of zinc that are highly available include the carbonate, sulfate, oxide, and proteinate forms.[69]

MINERAL BIOAVAILABILITY

The definition of relative mineral bioavailability refers to the estimated proportion of an ingested source of a trace mineral that is utilized by the animal. The various elemental sources with relative bioavailability are listed in Table 2. The estimates of relative bioavailability in the table do not include chelated forms of trace elements. There is no generally accepted technique for determining percentage chelation of a trace element when it is not synthesized from a reagent grade. The premise of chelated trace elements is to provide an organic metal complex that would be highly available to the animal through digestion and metabolism. The organic compounds that the chelating agent complex include sugars, amino acids, and proteins. The different forms of organic metal complexes vary in structural characteristics, binding properties, charge, and solubility. The value of these products within a diet could be due to protection of vitamin potencies more than to improved absorption rates and/or nutritional value.[71] Both the species and the trace element in question are related to determining the efficacy of chelated agents.[72]

Feeding zinc methionine to feedlot cattle resulted in increased carcass quality grades and higher marbling scores.[52] It was concluded that the response observed was due to either zinc or methionine. Other researchers have found the zinc methionine compound to be of benefit.[73–76] With advanced technology and refined analytic techniques, many such observations will aid in understanding the role of chelated trace elements in animal physiology.

MINERAL IMBALANCES

Mineral deficiency signs can be confusing, as the observed conditions usually involve more than one mineral and can be combined with protein and energy malnutrition, parasitism, toxic plants, and infectious diseases. Clinical signs that are often suggestive of gross mineral imbalances are observed as ill-thrift in the presence of ample forage production. Mineral nutrition disorders range from acute deficiency or toxicity, characterized by well-marked clinical signs and pathologic changes, to mild and transient conditions difficult to diagnose (e.g., unthriftiness, unsatisfactory growth, low reproduction). Rarely does a gross mineral deficiency express itself, but when it does it can be easily diagnosed. Probably the most costly loss in production is the subclinical illness or disease that exists within a production unit.

DETECTION OF MINERAL IMBALANCES

The term "deficient or toxic area" (seen on geographic maps) is designated to a region in which these entities are encountered more frequently. This does not imply that all plants or animals in the region encounter deficiencies or toxicities. The detection of mineral imbalances is derived from the combination of clinical, pathologic, and biochemical status of the animal and chemical analysis of the diet. Mineral deficiencies are best confirmed with response to specific supplementation of a bioavailable element. It is important to recognize limitations of clinical and pathologic data.

Livestock tissue-mineral concentrations portray the contribution of the animal's total environment in meeting its requirement. Unfortunately no mineral concentration of any one tissue will predict true animal status. Animal tissue concentrations are valuable indicators of mineral status but are greatly influenced by many factors. Whole blood, serum, or plasma is used widely in mineral research, yet only values that are significantly and consistently above or below "normal" range provide suggestive, but not conclusive, evidence of dietary excess or deficiency of a particular element. Precautions must be taken in interpreting blood mineral data collected under less than optimal conditions. Extraneous causes for elevated serum or plasma mineral values include collection contaminates (red silicone tube stoppers contribute zinc), stress, hemolysis, temperature, and serum separation time.[77] Hair is a poor indicator of animal mineral status since calcium, phosphorus, and copper do not reflect dietary intake. On the other hand, zinc and selenium concentrations do exhibit some variation with the diet. Chronic consumption of heavy metals such as lead, arsenic, and cadmium has been reflected in hair assays. Enzyme assays for ceruloplasmin (copper) and glutathione peroxidase (selenium) are used regularly as a correlation of mineral status.

MINERAL SUPPLEMENTS

The objectives of a mineral supplementation program must be established when choosing a mineral supplement. Factors for consideration include physiologic stage of animal production, current diet, and mineral imbalances that might potentially occur. These variables will change throughout the year, and it may be economically beneficial to adopt a program that recognizes returns on investments.

A free-choice feeding refers to providing for voluntary consumption of the supplement. The most critical aspect of a free-choice mineral supplement is that it will be consumed in adequate quantitites to meet production demands yet not be wastefully consumed. The characteristics of a "good" free-choice mineral supplement[1] are outlined as follows:

1. Final mixture contains a minimum of 6 to 8 per cent total phosphorus. In areas where phosphorus in forages is consistently lower than 0.20 per cent, mineral supplements in the 8 to 10 per cent range are preferred.
2. Calcium:phosphorus ratio is not substantially over 2:1.
3. Provides a significant proportion (i.e., 50 per cent) of trace mineral requirements of cobalt, copper, iodine, manganese, and zinc. In known trace mineral–deficient regions, 100 per cent of specific trace mineral requirements should be supplied.
4. Composed of high-quality mineral salts that provide the best biologically available forms of each mineral element, and avoids or has minimal inclusions of mineral salts containing toxic elements (e.g., phosphates containing high fluorine concentrations).

Table 2. PER CENT OF MINERAL ELEMENT IN MINERAL SOURCES AND RELATIVE BIOAVAILABILITY

Element	Source of Compound	Per Cent of Element in Compound	Bioavailability
Calcium			
	Steamed bone meal	29.0 (23–37)	High
	Dicalcium phosphate	23.3	High
	Monocalcium phosphate	16.2	High
	Defluorinated rock phosphate	29.2 (19.9–35.7)	Intermediate
	Calcium carbonate	40.0	Intermediate
	Ground limestone	38.5	Intermediate
	Dolomitic limestone	22.3	Intermediate
	Soft phosphate	18.0	Low
	Hay sources		Low
Cobalt			
	Cobalt carbonate	49.6	High
	Cobalt chloride	45.4	High
	Cobalt sulfate	38.0	High
	Cobalt acetate	33.5	Low
	Cobalt oxide	78.6	Low
Copper			
	Cupric chloride	37.2	High
	Cupric sulfate	25.0	High
	Cupric carbonate	53.0	Intermediate
	Cupric oxide	78.6	Low
Iodine			
	Calcium iodinate	63.5	High
	Ethylenediamine dihydroiodide	80.0	High
	Potassium iodide (stabilized)	69.0	High
	Cuprous iodide	66.6	High
Iron			
	Ferrous sulfate	36.8	High
	Ferrous carbonate	48.2	Intermediate
	Ferric oxide	70.0	Unavailable
Magnesium			
	Magnesium carbonate	21.0–28.0	High
	Magnesium chloride	12.0	High
	Magnesium oxide	54.0–60.0	High
	Magnesium sulfate	9.8–17.0	High
Manganese			
	Manganese carbonate	47.8	High
	Manganese sulfate	27.0	High
	Manganese oxide	52.0–62.0	High
Phosphorus			
	Calcium phosphate	18.6–21.0	High
	Phosphoric acid	23.0–25.0	High
	Sodium phosphate	21.0–25.0	High
	Steamed bone meal	12.6 (8.0–18.0)	High
	Dicalcium phosphate	18.5	Intermediate
	Defluorinated rock phosphate	13.3 (8.7–21.0)	Intermediate
	Soft rock phosphate	9.0	Low
	Tricalcium phosphate	18.0	—
	Potassium phosphate	22.8	—
Potassium			
	Potassium chloride	50.0	High
	Potassium sulfate	41.0	High
Selenium			
	Sodium selenate	40.0	High
	Sodium selenite	45.6	High
Sulfur			
	Potassium sulfate	28.0	High
	Potassium and magnesium sulfate	22.0	High
	Calcium sulfate	12.0–20.1	Low
	Sulfur from flowers	96.0	Low
	Anhydrous sodium sulfate	22.0	—
Zinc			
	Zinc carbonate	52.0	High
	Zinc sulfate	22.0–36.0	High
	Zinc oxide	46.0–73.0	High
	Zinc chloride	48.0	Intermediate
	Sodium sulfate	10.0	Intermediate

Source: Ellis GL, et al: *In* Proceedings 17th Annual Conference on Livestock and Poultry in Latin America. Gainesville, University of Florida, 1983, p 841.

5. Formulated to be sufficiently palatable to allow close to adequate consumption in relation to requirements.
6. Backed by a reputable manufacturer with quality control guarantees as to accuracy of mineral supplement label.
7. Has an acceptable particle size that will allow adequate mixing without smaller-size particles settling out.
8. Formulated for the area involved, the level of animal productivity, and the environment (temperature, humidity, etc.) in which it will be fed and is as economical as possible in providing the mineral elements used.

MINERAL REQUIREMENTS AND NEED FOR SUPPLEMENTATION

Mineral ranges are given by the NRC in relation to dry matter (DM) intake (ppm = mg/kg) to fulfill animal requirements. As mentioned previously, these ranges were obtained from controlled research studies from several, primarily British, breeds of cattle. Many of the crossbred and exotic breeds possess a greater genetic capacity for production and will have increased absolute requirements of all nutrients and at times may require higher concentrations in the dry matter. Stage of production and environmental conditions also will influence the animal's basic requirements; thus these ranges should be used only as basic guidelines.

The numerous variables encountered within the animal, diet, and environment suggest the advisability of supplying supplemental minerals to guarantee against imbalances. Major elements (calcium, phosphorus, magnesium) can be predicted for production requirements with some confidence even under pasture conditions and are justified economically. The need for trace minerals is more difficult to predict from forage and animal tissue data. The economics of supplementation often cannot be proven even under carefully controlled research conditions. However, there is credibility to the argument, "to be sure is worth the minor expense required." Supplementing all of the trace minerals at 30 to 100 per cent (100 per cent when known deficiency exists) of the animal's daily requirement is an economic insurance policy against potential imbalances. The potential for toxicity is relatively minor in supplementing all of the trace minerals, and the cost is not excessive in relation to the potential production enhancement. The elements possessing the greatest potential for toxicity are selenium in cattle and copper in sheep. If the history of the circumstances does not suggest these elements to be in dangerously high concentrations, it is probably advisable to supplement all minerals in moderation.

MINERAL SUPPLEMENT TAG

In the United States mineral supplements that claim a concentration are expressed on a per cent basis. Trace elements may or may not be listed as a percentage. The mineral tag should provide the compounds used in the formulation. These compounds can be evaluated for bioavailability and intake enhancers. The following basic units of measurement will be helpful for the proceeding calculations:

$$g = 1000 \text{ mg} \qquad \% = 10,000 \text{ mg/kg}$$
$$kg = 1000 \text{ g} \qquad oz = 28 \text{ g}$$
$$kg = 2.2 \text{ lb} \qquad lb = 454 \text{ g}$$
$$ppm = mg/kg \qquad ton = 2000 \text{ lb}$$

Commercial mineral packages have various levels of elements that should be evaluated for efficacy. An example of contents follows:

$$\frac{\text{Animal requirement (g/day)}}{\text{Elemental contents (g/kg)}} = \text{kg/day mineral consumption required to meet animal daily requirement}$$

Zinc requirement: 30 ppm (30 mg/kg × 10 kg DM consumption = 300 mg or 0.3 g)

Zinc contents: 0.3% or 3.0 g/kg (to convert % to mg/kg, multiply by 10,000) 0.3 × 10,000 mg/kg = 3000 mg/kg

$$\frac{0.3 \text{ g/day}}{3 \text{ g/kg}} = 0.1 \text{ kg/day consumption of mineral is required to meet daily requirement}$$

Generally commercial mineral supplements are formulated for a consumption level of 3 to 4 oz (85 to 113 g) on a per head per day basis. The total dry matter intake for cattle is approximately 2 per cent of the body weight (will vary with forage quality).

For simplicity an average body weight of 500 kg (10 kg of dry matter intake) will be used in the following calculations:

$$\frac{[\% \text{ element in mineral mix}] \times [\text{daily intake of mineral mix (g)}]}{\text{Total daily dry matter intake (g)}}$$

$$= \% \text{ element of the total diet from mineral mix}$$

Example:
Manganese (Mn) in mineral mix (%) = 0.20
Daily intake of mineral mix (g) = 85
Total daily dry matter intake (g) = 10,000

$$\frac{0.2 \times 85 \text{ g/day}}{10,000 \text{ g/day}} = 0.0017\%, \text{ or } 17 \text{ ppm}$$

This mineral mix would provide 42.5% (17 ppm/40 ppm × 100 = 42.5%) of the Mn requirement.

To calculate for the percentage of a mineral compound to provide the desired concentration of a mineral element:

$$\frac{\% \text{ element desired in mixture} \times 100}{\% \text{ element in available compound}} = \% \text{ element containing compound required}$$

Example:
Mn required (%) = 0.40
Mn in Mn sulfate (%) = 27.0

$$\frac{0.4 \times 100}{27.0} = 1.48\% \text{ Mn sulfate required}$$

MEDICATED MINERAL SUPPLEMENTS

Mineral supplements can be used successfully as carriers for medication if a therapeutic dosage is achieved through adequate consumption over the required medication time. The basic goal of a medicated mineral mix is to achieve an effective therapeutic dose within a herd of animals for an extended period. Currently, several classes of feed additives (anthelmintics, antifrothing agents, coccidiostats, and ionophores) are FDA approved for use in mineral supplements. Prior to using any medicated feed additive it is beneficial to consult the *Feed Additive Compendium* for its regulated use and contraindications. Medicated mineral supplements should be mixed and used for their indication to ensure the highest quality of stability of all ingredients and to avoid potential misuse by the client.

Information required for using medicated supplements includes range of animal weights, number of animals, average consumption of the supplement, and required dose and concentration. Usually medicated supplements should be formulated for maximal animal weight within the herd to ensure a therapeutic dose for the heavier animals.

The following is an example of medication required for a herd using minimum, average, and maximal animal weights:

If

D = Medicated dosage/day (active ingredient), g/100 lb
A = Medication activity in feed additive, g/lb
$$\text{cwt} = \frac{\text{Body weight}}{100}$$
C = Herd average consumption of supplement, g/day
% = Per cent of feed additive in supplement

For

D = 0.025 g/100 lb
A = 40 g/lb
$$\text{cwt} = \frac{500 \text{ lb}}{100} = 5$$
C = 200 g/day

Then

$$\% = \frac{[(D \times \text{cwt})/A] \times [454 \text{ g/lb}]}{C} \times 100$$

$$= \frac{[(0.025 \times 5)/40] \times [454]}{200} \times 100$$

$$= 0.71$$

For

6.5 cwt = 0.92%
8.0 cwt = 1.1%

If the average animal weight is used for inclusion of a feed additive (0.92 per cent), the heavier animals (1.1 per cent) will not receive a therapeutic dose. Medicated feed additives are established on a minimal concentration level for biologic response, with a broad dose range for safety from toxicity.

Many feed additives are unpalatable at high concentrations, causing low levels of intake (e.g., 50 g); thus associated ingredients to mask any off-taste should be selected. It is advantageous for medicated supplements to be highly palatable, containing low concentrations of the feed additives to ensure intake and add safety from possible overmedicating. A dose of 1 g/head/day can be administered with a 2 per cent (50-g intake), 1 per cent (100-g intake), and 0.5 per cent (200-g intake) concentration. The inclusion of a protein meal in the 0.5 per cent supplement would add nutritional quality to the supplement. High supplement intake can be achieved with protein meals, dried molasses, bone meal, dried yeast cultures, fat, and flavorings. Animals prefer salt, but it should be limited because changes in forage quality and environment cause inconsistencies in salt consumption.

Classes of Feed Additives

Anthelmintics (fenbendazole and phenothiazine) and coccidiostats (amprolium and decoquinate) should be used strategically during the year for maximal efficacy. Parasite resistance is a problem with many anthelmintics; thus caution is warranted with type and use of an anthelmintic. Ionophores (lasalocid and monensin) must be fed continuously to promote increased rate of gain. These compounds have nutrient-sparing effects but cannot overcome pastures limited in nutrient availability (low digestible energy and protein). Ionophores exhibit greatest response in animals when pasture nutrients are not limited. Lasalocid has been shown to alleviate malabsorption of calcium and magnesium in ruminants, thus decreasing the incidence of hypomagnesemia on small grain pastures.

Antifrothing agents (poloxalene, turcapsol, laureth-23-enproal bloat block) are used in the prevention of legume and wheat pasture bloat. The efficacy of these compounds is based on adequate and continuous intake, which is sometimes difficult to obtain on good quality pastures. Liquid supplements may be more advantageous in achieving continuous intake when mineral supplements are not consumed with regularity.

VITAMINS IN MINERAL SUPPLEMENTS

The inclusion of fat-soluble vitamins (A, D, and E) in mineral supplements can be advantageous when forages are in the dormant stage and vitamins A and E may be limiting nutrients. Vitamins are relatively nontoxic, even when consumed at high levels. Most vitamins are readily oxidized, especially in the presence of several of the trace element compounds within a mineral supplement. Stabilized and protective-coated vitamins are less susceptible to the effects of time, heat, and moisture. However, it is important that mineral supplements that contain vitamins be as freshly mixed as possible and protected from the environment.

MINERAL CONSUMPTION

The hypothesis that "animals eat what they need" or have nutritional wisdom is erroneous. This belief stemmed from observation of cattle with depraved appetites that consumed bones and improved their health. Since bones are good sources of phosphorus, an assumption was made that animals have the ability to select minerals required for their diet. A symptom should not be confused with a diagnosis (rabid animals usually have depraved appetites). Unhealthy animals with depraved appetites will consume many things that are not part of their normal diet (e.g., rocks, noxious plants, or anything else they can find in the pasture). When given a choice of calcium carbonate or calcium carbonate mixed equally with dicalcium phosphate, animals failed to consume adequate amounts of the phosphorus-containing supplement to prevent aphosphorosis.[78] Lactating dairy cows failed to consume adequate amounts of dicalcium phosphate (offered free choice) to meet their calcium and phosphorus requirements.[79, 80] Cafeteria-style mineral supplements (individualized elements in different containers) failed to be an effective means of mineral supplementation.[81] It was concluded that it was nutritionally and economically advantageous to supplement a complete mineral mixture.

Animals will select a palatable diet with little nutritional value in preference to an unpalatable nutritious diet, even to the point of death.[82] Domesticated animals are more responsive to the sensory qualities of feed over nutritive quality.[83] A major problem with free-choice supplements on rangeland is obtaining sufficient intake among individual animals within a herd. Thus the goal is to maintain adequate intake of mineral supplements throughout the year to meet the animal's physiologic requirements.

Factors affecting a free-choice mineral intake have been cited by several authors.[84–86] Soil fertility has been correlated with mineral consumption. Animals consume less minerals on highly fertile soils, whereas on native or poor quality pastures cattle tend to consume more minerals. Supplemental feeding of protein-energy supplements tends to decrease mineral consumption. The salt concentration of plants and water will depress mineral intake if salt is used to enhance acceptance of the supplement. The added physiologic stress of lactation, gestation, and calf crop will increase mineral intake.

An important aspect of any free-choice mineral supplement

program is to monitor intake on a regular basis by the producer. If the minerals are not being consumed in adequate quantities, a palatability factor or appetite stimulator may be mixed into the supplement. Palatability of a mineral supplement is the key to any mineral program. Salt is a very economical and palatable mineral used in many commercial mineral supplements. Alternatives to salt include protein meals, dried molasses, flavoring, fat, or yeast products.

MINERAL FEEDERS

Covered feeders should be used to protect minerals from the environment (water, wind, and other contaminates). Minerals are a feed supplement that can deteriorate in nutritive quality and palatability through changes in pH or oxidation (rancid). The mineral feeder should be at an accessible height for animals of all ages and in an accessible location for all animals. If the mineral supplement is highly palatable its location can be altered within the pasture to distribute animal movement. The act of moving a mineral trough would encourage monitoring mineral consumption for a pasture.

Common questions concerning mineral supplements include the following:

1. Should plain salt be put out with the complete mineral supplement? If animals are given an alternative, they may not consume adequate amounts of the mineral supplement for optimal efficacy.

2. What level of phosphorus should be provided in a mineral supplement? This is dependent on the quality of forage in the pasture and the type of animal production (growth versus lactation). Early forage growth contains higher levels of phosphorus than mature or dormant stage growth. Therefore a lower level of phosphorus can be used in early stages of growth and higher levels in mature and dormant stages.

3. Should one buy the mineral supplement on the basis of the concentration cost of phosphorus in the supplement? Because of the high cost of phosphorus, mineral supplements are at times purchased according to the concentration cost of phosphorus. However, an economical phosphorus source does not assure optimal intake of the mineral supplement.

4. Does a green pasture indicate that a mineral supplement is not needed? No, a green pasture yields more soluble carbohydrates, protein, and phosphorus but does not ensure that all mineral requirements are satisfied.

5. Does a cafeteria-style mineral supplementation really work? This type of supplementation has not been proven to be beneficial over a complete mineral mixture.

6. Do animals consume enough of a block mineral to meet their mineral requirements? Animals usually consume about 10 per cent less from a mineral block (dependent on block hardness) then from a loose form.

REFERENCES

1. McDowell LR: *In* McDowell LR (ed): Nutrition of Grazing Ruminants in Warm Climates. Orlando, Academic Press, 1985.
2. National Research Council: Nutrient Requirements of Beef Cattle, 6th ed. Washington, DC, National Academy Press, 1984.
3. Huston JE, Rector BS, Merrill LB, Engdahl BS: Nutritional value of range plants in the Edwards Plateau region of Texas. Tex Agr Exp Sta Bull 1357, 1981.
4. Loneragon JF: *In* Nicholas DJ, Egan AR (eds): Trace Elements in Soil-Plants-Animal System. New York, Academic Press, 1975, pp 109–134.
5. Buckman HO, Brady NC: The Nature and Properties of Soils, 6th ed. New York, MacMillan, 1962.
6. Kincaid RL, Cronrath JD: J Dairy Sci 66:821, 1983.
7. Hartmans J: *In* Hoekstra WG (ed): Trace Element Metabolism in Animals. New York, University Park Press, 1974, pp 261–271.
8. Bremner I: Br J Nutr 24:769, 1970.
9. McManus WR, Anthony RG, Gout LL, et al: Aust J Agric Res 30:635, 1979.
10. Ward GM: J Anim Sci 46:1078, 1978.
11. Emanuele SM, Staples CR: J Anim Sci 68:2052, 1990.
12. Rooke JA, Akinsoyinu AO, Armstrong DG: Grass Forage Sci 38:311, 1983.
13. Doyle JC: College Station, Texas A&M University, PhD dissertation, 1989.
14. Reid RL, Franklin MC, Hallsworth EG: Aust Vet J 23:136, 1947.
15. Bray AC, Till AR: *In* McDonald IW, Warner ACI (eds): Digestion and Metabolism in the Ruminant. Henniker, NH, University of New England Press, 1975, pp 243–260.
16. Collier RJ, Beede DK: Thermal stress as a factor associated with nutrient requirements and interrelationships. *In* McDowell LR (ed): Nutrition of Grazing Ruminants in Warm Climates. New York, Academic Press, 1985, pp 59–70.
17. Jenkinson DM, Mabon RM: Br Vet J 129:282, 1973.
18. Kennedy PM, Christopherson RJ, Milligan LP: *In* Milligan LP, Grovum WL, Dobson A (eds): Control of Digestion and Metabolism in Ruminants. Englewood Cliffs, NJ, Prentice-Hall, 1985, Chapter 15.
19. Terashima Y, Tucker RE, Deetz LE, et al: J Nutr 112:1914, 1982.
20. Hill CH, Matrone G: Fed Proc Fed Amer Soc Exp Biol 29:1474, 1970.
21. Betteridge K, Miller RB: Proceedings 28th American Association of Bovine Practitioners Annual Conference. Buffalo, NY, 1985.
22. Kappel LC, Ingraham HH, Morgan EB, Shrikandakumar A: J Dairy Sci 70:167, 1987.
23. DiCostanzo A, Meiske JC, Plegge SD: Minnesota Beef Cow-Calf Report. Minn Agr Exp Ser AG-Bu-2310, 1985, pp 27–30.
24. Dunn TG, Ingalls JE, Zimmerman DR, Wiltbank JN: J Anim Sci 29:719, 1969.
25. Huston JE: Unpublished data, 1988.
26. Doyle JC, Huston JE, Spiller DW: J Anim Sci 66:579 (Abstr), 1988.
27. Rowson LEA, Lawson RAS, Moor RM, Baker AA: J Reprod Fertil 28:427, 1972.
28. Doyle JC, Huston JE, Thompson PV: Theriogenology 34:21, 1990.
29. Phillips JM, Brown AH, Parham RW: Lenexa, KS, Vet Med Publications, 1988, pp 20–24.
30. Lee LH, Marston HR: Aust J Agric Res 20:905, 1969.
31. Hutcheson D: Unpublished data, 1986.
32. Heitzman RJ: Mode of action of anabolic agents. *In* Forbes FJM, Lomax MA (eds): Hormones and Metabolism in Ruminants. London, Agricultural Research Council, 1981, p 129.
33. Turner ND, Greene LW, Hurley LA, Byers FM: J Anim Sci 68(Suppl 1):206 (Abstr), 1990.
34. Greene LW: Unpublished data, 1987.
35. Mills CF: Biochem J 63:187, 1976.
36. Chapman HL Jr, Nelson SL, Kidder RW, et al: J Anim Sci 21:960, 1962.
37. *In* Osweiler GD, Carson TL, Buck WB, Van Gelder GA (eds): Water Deprivation—Sodium Salt. Clinical and Diagnostic Veterinary Toxicology, 3rd ed. Dubuque, Kendall/Hunt, 1985, pp 167–170.
38. Hutcheson D: Anim Nutr Health 34:11, 1979.
39. Lander RQ Jr: Unpublished data, 1990.
40. Call JW, Butcher JE, Shupe JL: Am J Vet Res 47:475, 1986.
41. McDowell LR: *In* Smith AJ (ed): Beef Cattle Production in Developing Countries. Edinburgh, University of Edinburgh Press, 1976, pp 216–244.
42. Underwood EJ: The Mineral Nutrition of Livestock. London, Commonwealth Agricultural Bureaux, 1981.
43. Rickets RE, Campbell JR, Weinman DE, Tumbleson ME: J Dairy Sci 53:898, 1970.
44. McDowell LR, Conrad JH, Ellis GL, Loosli JK: Mineral for Grazing Ruminants in Tropical Regions. University of Florida and U.S. Agency for International Development (84-70238), 1983, p 60.
45. Greene LW, Solis JC, Byers FM, Schelling GT: Tex Agr Exp Sta Tech Rept No 86-1, 1986.
46. Ammerman CB, Chicco CF, Loggins PE, Arrington LR: J Anim Sci 34:122, 1972.
47. Smith RM, Marston HR: Br J Nutr 24:857, 1970.
48. Underwood EJ, Somers M: Aust J Agric Res 20:889, 1969.
49. McDowell LR, Conrad JH, Ellis GL: *In* Gilchrist FMC, Mackie RI (eds): Symposium on Herbivore Nutrition in Sub-Tropics—Problems and Prospects. Craighall, South Africa, 1984, pp 67–88.
50. Hidiroglou M, Knipfel JE: Can J Anim Sci 69:141, 1981.
51. Hutcheson D: Unpublished data, 1988.
52. Greene LW, Lunt D, Byers F, et al: J Anim Sci 66:1818, 1988.
53. Miltimore JE, Mason JL: Can J Anim Sci 51:193, 1971.
54. Mills CF: Soil Sci 85:100, 1958.
55. Kincaid RL, Blauwiekel RM, Cronrath JD: J Dairy Sci 69:160, 1986.
56. Underwood EJ: Trace Elements in Human and Animal Nutrition. London, Commonwealth Agricultural Bureaux, 1977.
57. Miller WJ: Dairy Cattle Feeding and Nutrition. New York, Academic Press, 1979, pp 74–180.
58. Lassiter JW, Miller WJ, Pate FM, Gentry RP: Proc Soc Exp Biol Med 139:345, 1972.

59. Rojas MA, Dyer IA, Cassatt WA: J Anim Sci 24:664, 1965.
60. Anke M, Groppel B, Reissig W, et al: Arch Anim Nutr 23:197, 1973.
61. Lomax DA: Lubbock, Texas Tech, MS thesis, 1990.
62. Hawkins GE, Wise GH, Matrone G, et al: J Dairy Sci 38:536, 1955.
63. Howes AD, Dyer IA, Haller WH: J Anim Sci 37:455, 1973.
64. Black J: Gainesville, University of Florida, PhD dissertation, 1983.
65. Rotruck JT, Pope AL, Ganther HE, et al: Science 179:588, 1973.
66. Ammerman CB, Miller SM: J Dairy Sci 58:1561, 1975.
67. Smith CJ, McDaniel EG, Fan FF, Halsted JA: Science 18:954, 1973.
68. Miller WJ: J Dairy Sci 53:1123, 1970.
69. Hutcheson D: Unpublished data, 1989.
70. Ellis GL, McDowell LR, Conrad JH: In Proceedings 17th Annual Conference on Livestock and Poultry in Latin America. Gainesville, University of Florida, 1983, p 841.
71. Albin B: Amarillo, Plains Nutrition Council, 1988.
72. Stakes PE: Feedstuffs 49:21, 1977.
73. Martin J, Strasia C, Gill D, et al: J Anim Sci 65(Suppl 1):500 (Abstr), 1987.
74. Rust S: J Anim Sci 61(Suppl 1):482 (Abstr), 1985.
75. Spears J, Samsell L: J Anim Sci 63(Suppl 1):402 (Abstr), 1986.
76. Stobart R, Medeivors D, Riley M, Russell W: J Anim Sci 65(Suppl 1):500 (Abstr), 1987.
77. Fick KR, McDowell LR, Miles PH, et al: Methods of Mineral Analysis for Plant and Animal Tissue, 2nd ed. Gainesville, University of Florida, 1979.
78. Gordon JG, Tribe DE, Grahman TC: Br J Anim Behav 2:72, 1954.
79. Coppock CE, Everett RW, Merrill WG: J Dairy Sci 55:245, 1972.
80. Coppock CE, Everett RW, Belyea RL: J Dairy Sci 59:571, 1976.
81. Pamp DE, Goodrich RD, Mieske JC: J Anim Sci 45:1458, 1977.
82. Arnold GW: Proc Aust Soc Anim Prod 5:258, 1964.
83. Maller O: In Kare MR, Maller O (eds): The Chemical Senses and Nutrition. Baltimore, John Hopkins Press, 1967.
84. Cunha TJ, Shirley RL, Chapman HL Jr, et al: Fla Agr Exp Sta Bull 683, 1964.
85. Cunha TJ: Anim Nutr Health 35:11, 1980.
86. Coppock CE: Proc Cornell Nutr Conf Feed Manuf, 1970, pp 29–35.

SECTION 5 ☐ ☐ ☐ ☐ ☐ ☐
Metabolic Disorders

IVAN W. CAPLE, BVSc, PhD, Consulting Editor

Parturient Paresis (Milk Fever) and Hypocalcemia (Cows, Ewes, and Goats)

WILLIAM MAURICE ALLEN, DVSc, PhD, MSc, MRCVS

BERNARD FREDERICK SANSOM, DPhil, MA

Milk fever, or parturient paresis, is one of the most common metabolic disorders of food animals, and it has been given many alternative names, including paresis puerperalis, eclampsia, and parturient apoplexy. It occurs principally in cattle and to a smaller extent in sheep and goats. The disease is associated with hypocalcemia and in cattle occurs at or close to parturition, as a result of an acute imbalance between the output and input of calcium. In sheep the disease associated with hypocalcemia is less related to parturition and is more common during late pregnancy and early lactation.

OCCURRENCE

In cattle milk fever is one of the most economically important diseases because it occurs widely and often leads to complications such as the downer cow syndrome. The incidence of milk fever appears to increase as the average milk production increases. For example, in the United Kingdom in 1975, the annual milk fever incidence in dairy cattle was 9.0 per cent, whereas in 1960 it had been only 3.4 per cent. During the same period, average lactation yields had risen by approximately 30 per cent. In Finland, Sweden, and Norway, the annual rates have recently been approximately 10 per cent, 8 per cent, and 7.5 per cent, respectively, whereas in Denmark during 1973, the incidence was only 4 per cent. On 64 farms in Australia (southwestern Victoria), the frequency of the disease in cows after their first lactation was reported to be more than 3 per cent. In these assessments of the national averages, there has been no estimate of the 'between-year' and 'between-farm' variations. In the United Kingdom, the occurrence of the disease on different farms can vary in a single year from 0 to more than 60 per cent, and similarly the average incidence on 8 farms has been observed to change from 16 per cent in one year to 34 per cent in the next year.

Estimates of the cost of the disease must allow not only for the costs of treatment and prevention but also for the losses due to animals that fail to respond to treatment and become downer cows. The prognosis for these cows is poor, and they often die or have to be slaughtered. Estimates of the proportion of cows with milk fever that become downer cows have varied from 4 to 28 per cent, and estimates of the proportion of downer cows that subsequently die or have to be slaughtered vary from 20 to 70 per cent.

Several important predisposing factors influence the occurrence of parturient paresis.

AGE OF COW. As the age and parity of cows increases, the incidence of the disease rises. It is rare, but certainly not unknown, for parturient paresis to occur in heifers, but the frequency gradually increases with parity, so that by the sixth lactation and onward it is common for more than 20 per cent of cows to succumb. This change is mainly due to the gradual decrease in the cow's ability to mobilize its own body stores of calcium when there are either sudden increases in the demand for calcium, such as occur at the onset of lactation, or decreases in the input of calcium, such as occur during transient starvation. In addition to this decreased ability to mobilize calcium, the milk yield of the cow also increases with parity, particularly up to the fourth lactation. Thus the cow's requirements for the output of calcium increase with age and tend to exacerbate the imbalance.

BREED OF COW. The particular susceptibility of the Jersey breed to parturient paresis is well known, but its physiologic basis is still unexplained. It may be related to the relatively high productivity of this small breed of cow.

NUTRITIONAL FACTORS. These include both long-term and short-term factors and are discussed in the section on prevention.

SEASONAL FACTORS. It is important not to confuse apparent seasonal variations in the incidence of the disease with the effect of a seasonal calving pattern. There nevertheless is some evidence that the incidence of the disease is higher at the end of the grazing season. This effect may be due to the limitations on nutritional input, and particularly to the limitations on magnesium intake from autumn grazing.

ETIOLOGY AND PATHOGENESIS

In all ruminants, milk fever is characterized by severe hypocalcemia. Some degree of hypocalcemia occurs normally in cows at and close to calving, but only when hypocalcemia becomes severe does disease occur. Frequently, hypocalcemia is accompanied by hypophosphatemia and hypermagnesemia. Hyperglycemia, associated with reduced concentrations of insulin, is also often observed.

The normal concentration of calcium (Ca) in plasma (and the extracellular fluid) lies within the range of 2.2–2.6 mmol/

L(8.8–10.4 mg/100 ml). This normal range of calcium concentration is maintained by balancing the rates at which calcium enters and leaves the plasma.

Entry, or input, into the plasma depends upon two processes: (1) the absorption of calcium from the diet across the intestinal wall and (2) the resorption or mobilization of the stores of calcium within the skeleton. The absorption of calcium from the diet varies with the animal's requirements and with the amount of calcium available in the diet. The provision of additional calcium to maintain a balance depends on the mobilization of calcium from the skeletal stores. The processes of absorption and mobilization are subject to control mechanisms that are mediated through parathyroid hormone, calcitonin (produced in the thyroid C cells), and vitamin D and its metabolites.

The total rate of output of calcium from the plasma is the sum of the rates of output due to the following processes:

1. Endogenous (or obligatory) loss of calcium in feces
2. Smaller endogenous losses in urine
3. Calcium requirements for the growth of the fetal skeleton and the placenta during pregnancy
4. Calcium secreted in milk (approximately 1.2 gm/L) during lactation
5. Calcium accreted into the skeleton of the cow

Disease usually occurs when there are sudden changes in these requirements for output and when the input processes fail to adapt rapidly enough. During the last stage of pregnancy, the calcium requirements of the cow consist of approximately 10 g Ca/day for the endogenous losses in feces and urine and up to 10 g Ca/day for the growing fetus. Immediately after calving the endogenous loss of 10 g Ca/day is maintained, but the demand for calcium for the production of colostrum increases to 30 g/day. Thus, the total output of calcium rises at least 2-fold within a few hours. To maintain the homeostatic balance, the rate of absorption of calcium from the gut must be substantially increased, calcium stores must be mobilized from the skeleton, or both. These adaptations must occur quickly because the amount of calcium that can be mobilized very rapidly from body stores has been estimated to be between only 10 and 20 g and thus may provide less than 50 per cent of 1 day's requirements. When the processes of adaptation fail, hypocalcemia becomes inevitable, and as it deepens, the concentration of calcium in tissues declines, and normal neuromuscular function is impaired.

In a healthy cow, the processes of adaptation protect her against severe hypocalcemia. At the onset of hypocalcemia, the secretion of parathyroid hormone (PTH) is stimulated. In turn PTH stimulates the production of a hydroxylase enzyme in the kidney that synthesizes the active form of vitamin D_3, 1,25-dihydroxycholecalciferol ($1,25[OH]_2D_3$) from 25-hydroxycholecalciferol ($25[OH]D_3$). The production of $25(OH)D_3$ in the liver from vitamin D_3 is not subject to a similar hormonal control mechanism. The $1,25(OH)_2D_3$ stimulates the absorption of calcium from the intestine through the synthesis of a calcium-binding protein. It can also mobilize calcium from the skeleton, in which it promotes osteoclast activity. At calving the concentrations of both PTH and $1,25(OH)_2D_3$ increase in all cattle, and the increases are larger in cows with severe hypocalcemia. Thus although the hormonal mechanisms for preventing hypocalcemia appear to be operating, in some cows disease still occurs. It has been suggested that one reason for this failure to prevent severe hypocalcemia is a rise in the rate of secretion of thyrocalcitonin. This hormone is secreted from the thyroid C cells in response to hypercalcemia and acts to decrease the rate of resorption of calcium from bone, thus reducing the rate of input of calcium into the plasma. However, there has been no recent evidence to support the role of thyrocalcitonin as a cause of milk fever. It seems more probable that the adaptation of the hormonal mechanisms and synthesis of $1,25(OH)_2D_3$ fails to stimulate the target organs of gut and bone rapidly enough to increase the rate of input of calcium. Furthermore, it has been reported that in those cases of milk fever failing to respond to initial treatment with calcium, the increase in the concentration of $1,25(OH)_2D_3$ is delayed for some 24 to 48 hours.

Other factors may also influence the speed and extent of the response. Age has already been mentioned, older animals being less able to mobilize skeletal stores of calcium. Estrogens also inhibit calcium mobilization, and the concentration of estrogens increases at parturition and again, cyclically, later in lactation. The elevation of plasma estrogen concentrations associated with estrus may in part explain those few cases of milk fever that occur later in lactation. Another important factor that can reduce the mobilization of calcium is subclinical hypomagnesemia. Although at calving slight hypermagnesemia often occurs, the cow's diet during the last few weeks of pregnancy may have induced a sufficent degree of hypomagnesemia to prejudice the mobilization of calcium at parturition.

CLINICAL SIGNS

The clinical signs can be divided into three stages that are approximately related to the severity of the hypocalcemia. In the first stage, the cow loses her appetite and becomes dull and lethargic. She is afebrile, and her ears may be cold. In some cases, the pupil of the eye is dilated even during this early stage. In the second stage, as the hypocalcemia becomes more severe, she stands with her hocks straight and paddles from one hind foot to the other. There may be tremors of the muscles, particularly of the head and limbs. She sometimes grinds her teeth, and she eventually becomes incoordinated. Sometimes she becomes very excitable and hypersensitive when approached and as a result becomes difficult to restrain and sweats profusely. Finally, in the third stage, she becomes recumbent with a drowsy appearance and flaccid paralysis. At first she lies on her sternum, often with a characteristic curvature of the neck, and may struggle to rise. Eventually, she lies on her side and becomes comatose, with dilated pupils and a dry muzzle. She does not pass urine or feces, and the anal reflex is lost. The rumen becomes tympanitic, and its contents may be regurgitated. Unless she is treated, the cow will die of respiratory failure either as a result of the ruminal tympany or as a result of the inhalation of rumen contents. As the third stage of the disease progresses, the body temperature tends to decrease, and the intensity of the heart sounds also decreases. The heart rate remains at about 60 to 80 beats/min, and the respirations are shallow and slow, the pupillary reflex to light is absent, and the pupil is frequently dilated to the maximum. The stasis of the rumen and alimentary tract severely reduces the absorption of calcium from the intestine and so increases the severity of the hypocalcemia. As the hypocalcemia progresses to the terminal stage, the heart rate and breathing become more irregular, and respirations sometimes end with a forced expiratory grunt. The progress to the final stages may take 24 hours. Cows at pasture that have died of milk fever are often found trapped in a ditch or drowned in a stream.

An important consequence of the disease when it occurs before calving is the associated uterine inertia. The process of calving may stop, there is no straining of voluntary muscles, and dystocia may remain undetected. If calving does occur, a prolapse of the uterus is common in severely hypocalcemic cows.

CLINICAL PATHOLOGY

Measurement of the calcium concentration in plasma is the best method of confirming the disease. The normal range of calcium concentrations is between 2.2 and 2.6 mmol/L (8.8–10.4/100 ml), but close to parturition the concentration almost always declines to some extent. However, clinical disease is rarely seen unless the concentration of calcium falls below 1.5 mmol/L (6 mg/100 ml). In some cows, the calcium concentration may fall below this level without the cows showing clinical signs. In cows with the disease, the calcium concentration may be as low as 0.25 mmol/L.

Phosphorus concentrations also decrease. The normal range of concentrations is between 1.40 and 2.48 mmol/L (4.3–7.7 mg/100 ml), and in cows with milk fever, the concentration may fall to 1 mmol/L or less. Magnesium concentrations usually increase to slightly above the upper limit of the normal range (0.85–1.25 mmol/L or 2–3 mg/100 ml), although occasionally they decrease. Hyperglycemia is usual during milk fever, unless the cow is also ketotic, when the concentration of glucose in plasma is low, but this is rare.

At parturition changes in the white blood cell counts of all cows include neutrophilia, lymphopenia, and eosinopenia. These changes resemble the response to stress, adrenocortical hyperactivity, or both.

In fatal cases of uncomplicated milk fever, there are no characteristic gross or histologic post-mortem lesions that can be ascribed specifically to the disease. There is often bruising of subcutaneous tissue and muscles due to the localized trauma associated with collapse, recumbency, and incoordinated struggling. There may also be gross lesions of the genital tract associated with calving. In some animals, the liver may be infiltrated with fat; this infiltration may be gross, with yellow discoloration, and may affect other organs, including the kidney and heart.

DIAGNOSIS

Diagnosis of milk fever in the field is based on observation of the clinical signs, particularly paresis in cows close to calving. Quick, practical confirmation is often provided by a rapid response, sometimes within minutes, to treatment with calcium borogluconate solutions. Blood analysis can only confirm the diagnosis retrospectively.

The differential diagnosis of milk fever and other conditions that cause similar clinical signs must however be considered on every occasion. These conditions, which may arise as a sequel to milk fever, are discussed in detail next and include

1. Downer cow syndrome
2. Severe toxemia
3. Physical injury (e.g., obturator paralysis, fracture of leg bones, pelvic rupture, and ruptured gastrocnemius tendon)
4. Hypomagnesemia
5. Fat cow syndrome

DOWNER COW SYNDROME. A downer cow has been defined as a cow that has been in sternal recumbency for more than 24 hours. In the early stages, she appears bright and usually eats, drinks, defecates, and urinates normally. However, the condition may persist for 1 to 2 weeks, possibly resulting in damage due to pressure on the muscles, especially of the hind limbs. After only a few hours of recumbency, this damage can be so severe that muscles degenerate and the ligaments rupture. At this stage, the damage becomes irreversible and results in mortality of up to 60 per cent.

The downer cow syndrome may arise because a cow fails to respond satisfactorily to the correct treatment for milk fever. However, it more often arises as a sequel to uncomplicated cases of milk fever that have either been treated too late or have been inadequately cared for during the period of incoordination and recumbency.

The condition can be diagnosed initially from the appearance of the clinical signs. The diagnosis can be confirmed by measuring the plasma concentration of those enzymes that are released from damaged muscle tissue. Two enzymes are suitable for measurement—creatine kinase (CK) and aspartate aminotransferase (AST). In downer cows, the activity of these enzymes in plasma may be increased by several thousandfold, and daily measurements can be used to assess the progress of the disease and its likely prognosis. If the activities of the enzymes continue to increase, the prognosis is extremely poor.

SEVERE TOXEMIA. Severe toxemia can easily be confused with the third stage of milk fever. The affected cow is drowsy, recumbent, and will not eat. She may lie with her head on her flank and make expiratory grunts. However, on clinical examination she may have acute mastitis or metritis. In spite of this infection, the cow frequently does not show a febrile response and body temperature is normal, as in a cow with milk fever. Usually the cow's heart rate is increased—up to 120 beats/min—her pulse is weak, and she also has severe leukopenia.

PHYSICAL INJURY. At calving a cow may suffer injuries, such as fracture of the pelvis, or damage to the obturator nerve or sciatic plexus, or both, which may make her recumbent. She may not have been provided with adequate bedding on slippery surfaces, and her legs may have been severely abducted or fractured by a serious slip. The animal will probably eat and drink normally, and her heart rate and gastrointestinal function will be normal. A careful physical examination of the recumbent animal is necessary in an attempt to define the site of the lesion. An assay of plasma CK or AST activities can be used to assess the approximate extent of the muscle damage.

HYPOMAGNESEMIA. Hypomagnesemia can affect cattle of all ages, and dairy cattle can be affected at any time during pregnancy and lactation. It can occur as a complication of milk fever. The clinical signs are a state of excitement and hypersensitivity followed by sudden collapse, frequently in tetanic spasms. The heart rate is generally increased, and the heart sounds are extremely loud.

A clinical diagnosis can be confirmed by measuring the concentration of magnesium in blood plasma. Concentrations below 0.65 mmol/L are abnormal, but in clinical cases, the level may be much less.

FAT COW SYNDROME. In dairy cattle that are excessively fat during pregnancy, the incidence of milk fever and other periparturient disease is higher. Some of these cows with milk fever fail to respond to treatment—the cow remains recumbent while subcutaneous fat is mobilized and then deposited in many tissues of the body, including the liver and skeletal muscle. The deposition of fat may be so great that the cow becomes severely ketotic and eventually dies.

These five conditions are some of the differential diagnoses that need to be considered during a clinical examination of a cow suspected of having milk fever.

TREATMENT

Treatment should be given as soon as possible after the clinical signs have been observed. The best treatment is to administer a solution of calcium borogluconate intravenously. Most cows with milk fever recover after a single intravenous dose of between 8 and 12 g of calcium. A total of 12 g of calcium can be administered in 400 ml of a 40 per cent solution of calcium borogluconate that should be infused over a 5 to 10 minute period. The muscles of recumbent animals may twitch during treatment, and the animals may pass feces and urine and eructate rumen gases.

Treatment with solutions that contain magnesium and phosphorus as well as calcium has also been advocated. However, in uncomplicated cases there is no evidence of a higher rate of recovery among cows treated with solutions containing magnesium (1.03 g) and phosphorus (2.6 g) in addition to calcium (8 g). When subclinical hypomagnesemia (plasma magnesium <0.85 mmol/L) is observed during the last month of pregnancy the addition of magnesium to the solution of calcium borogluconate is advisable. Similarly, when there is evidence of either hypophosphatemia (blood phosphorus <1.35 mmol/L) among cows in late pregnancy or of persistently low phosphorus among cows in relapse, the inclusion of phosphorus is advisable (Table 1).

The administration of intravenous calcium rapidly increases the concentration of calcium in plasma and causes transient hypercalcemia. However, 8 to 12 g of calcium is only a small amount, comparable with the pool of readily exchangeable calcium in the animal's body and is considerably less than the amount excreted in the milk during 24 hours. The treatment cannot therefore be considered as substitution therapy. The short period during which plasma calcium concentrations are restored to normal or above appears to be sufficient to allow the re-establishment of the normal homeostatic mechanisms, and possibly the most important effects are to re-establish normal gut function and to stimulate the cow's appetite. Nevertheless, subclinical hypocalcemia persists in many cows for 24 hours or longer after they have been successfully treated for milk fever. If a cow does not recover within 5 to 8 hours of a single intravenous dose of calcium, the cow should be re-examined and treated with calcium again, provided that the diagnosis suggests that the problem remains an uncomplicated case of milk fever.

It is a common practice to administer calcium borogluconate subcutaneously at the same time as the single intravenous injection of calcium, and this subcutaneous injection can also contain magnesium and phosphorus. Although the total amount of calcium administered may then be as much as 18 g, it has been demonstrated that these auxiliary subcutaneous injections do not reduce the likelihood of a cow relapsing after an initial recovery.

In addition to specific treatment with calcium, it is essential to provide the cow with adequate nursing and care. The calf should be removed, and the cow should not be milked out. If the cow is in lateral recumbency, she should be propped into the sternal position to prevent her from regurgitating rumen contents and running the risk of aspiration pneumonia. She should be turned from side to side at regular intervals and certainly not less than four to five times daily to prevent pressure damage to muscles. If she is lying on concrete or a similarly hard and slippery surface, it should be generously covered with sand, straw, or farmyard manure.

If a cow is recumbent for longer than 48 hours, the prognosis is guarded. It is advisable either to hoist her with a hip sling or to raise her on inflatable cushions so that she can stand for a short period and her ability to move her limbs can be assessed. Such equipment is available from veterinary suppliers. The extent of muscle damage can be assessed by the measurement of CK activity in plasma. If, after 2 days of recumbency, the cow is dull and is neither eating nor attempting to rise, the prognosis for recovery is extremely poor.

PREVENTION

The ability to prevent milk fever depends upon a knowledge of the etiology of the disease. However, the etiology of individual cases of milk fever may vary because one or more of a variety of predisposing factors may be involved. As a result, preventive measures must be designed to reduce the adverse effects of as many of these predisposing factors as possible. They include age, breed, nutritional and husbandry systems, and body condition score at parturition.

Older cows, especially in certain breeds, are more susceptible to disease and need particular attention in order to avoid hypocalcemia.

Several nutritional factors affect the likelihood of the occurrence of disease. They can be divided into those that are important in the long term—that is, during the dry period—and those that are particularly important in the short term—between 48 hours before and 48 hours after calving. The long-term factors affect the cow's body condition at calving and also influence the way in which her calcium and vitamin D metabolism is primed to respond to the sudden increase in demand for calcium at calving. The short-term factors affect the ability of the cow to maintain a sufficient intake of calcium at the onset of lactation.

LONG-TERM FACTORS. During the dry period, and particularly during the last month of pregnancy, it is important to maintain the concentration of magnesium in plasma above 0.65 mmol/L, and if the concentration falls below this level, the cow can be considered to be subclinically hypomagnesemic. In the Northern Hemisphere, there are two periods during the

Table 1. DRUG THERAPY FOR PARTURIENT PARESIS AND HYPOCALCEMIA

Drug[1]	Company and Address[2]	Animal	Dose
Vitamin D	Duphar Veterinary Ltd, Southampton SO3 4QH, UK	Cattle	10^7 IU between 8th and 2nd days before calving
Vitamin D_3			
Calcium borogluconate			
20% wt/vol	Crown Chemical Co Ltd, Lamberhurst, Kent, UK	Cattle	Up to 800 ml IV or SC (12 g Ca)
		Sheep and Goats	50–150 ml IV or SC
40% wt/vol	Willows Francis Veterinary, Horsham, West Sussex, RH13 5QP, UK	Cattle	Up to 400 ml IV or SC
		Sheep and Goats	Up to 100 ml IV or SC
20% or 40% wt/vol	Dales Pharmaceuticals, Skipton, N Yorks, BD 23 2RW, UK	Cattle	Up to 450 ml IV or SC
+ Mg 0.3–0.7% wt/vol		Sheep	Up to 100 ml IV or SC
+ P 0.9–1.1% wt/vol			

[1]20% glucose and 5 to 20% dextrose may be added.
[2]Consult publications such as Veterinary Pharmaceuticals and Biologicals, 6th Edition, Veterinary Medicine Publishing Co., Lenexa, KS, 1989/1990 for current suppliers of these drugs in the United States.
IV = intravenous; SC = subcutaneous.

year when dry cows at pasture are most likely to become hypomagnesemic: in the spring, when dry matter intake is likely to be low and the availability of magnesium in pastures (particularly if they have been heavily fertilized with potassium and nitrogen) is also low, and in the autumn, when similar constraints can affect the supply of magnesium. Spreading large volumes of slurry onto pastures also increases their potassium content. In the spring, the shortage of magnesium may be exacerbated because grasses contain less magnesium than clovers and other legumes, whose growth is slower than grasses in spring. In the Southern Hemisphere, cows are likely to become hypomagnesemic in autumn or winter (see Ruminant Hypomagnesemic Tetanies).

Unfortunately, it is not easy to correct hypomagnesemia in dry cows. Cake or concentrate can be supplemented with calcined magnesite (MgO) but even 50 g/day of MgO does not always appear to provide the necessary intake of magnesium. The addition of magnesium acetate to the drinking water is effective, provided that the cows have access only to a controlled water supply and that the weather is not so wet that the cows drink little water. Wet weather also reduces the effectiveness of dusting the pastures with magnesian limestone, because rain washes the powdered material off the leaves and into the soil.

The intake of calcium during the dry period is also important, and ideally the ration should contain as little calcium as possible until a few days before parturition. The optimum benefit of a low calcium diet occurs with diets supplying <20 g Ca/day. Unfortunately, practical diets, especially those based on forage, rarely contain less than 50 g Ca/day, and their protective effect is probably small. Nevertheless, the calcium content of the diet should be kept as low as is practicable and certainly below 100 g/day. The beneficial effect of a low calcium intake is considered to be derived from the stimulation of $1,25(OH)_2D_3$ synthesis, which in turn increases the rates of mobilization and absorption of calcium at parturition. This process also probably explains the desirability of maintaining a low Ca:P ratio in the diet of dry cows when the percentage of the calcium absorbed from the diet increases. As well as containing a small amount of calcium, the phosphorus content of the diet for the dry cow should not be excessive. Diets containing more than 80 g phosphorus as phosphate per day may increase the incidence of disease. This high intake tends to increase blood phosphate, which in turn probably inhibits renal hydroxylase activity and the formation of $1,25(OH)_2D_3$. Such a high phosphorus content would be likely only because of excessive supplementation.

Another procedure that has been advocated is the alteration of the ionic balance of the diet (the acidity:alkalinity of the diet). The important determinants of acidity and alkalinity are considered to be ($SO_4^{-2} + Cl^-$) and ($Na^+ + K^+$), respectively. The "acidity" of hay diets was increased by the addition of Cl^- and SO_4^{-2} as calcium chloride and aluminum and magnesium sulfate, and these diets were fed for the last 4 weeks before calving. Such "acid" diets, based on silage preserved with mineral acids, may reduce the incidence of milk fever. Feeding diets for 45 days prepartum that contained more of the anionic components ($Cl^- + S^-$) than the cationic components ($Na^+ + K^+$) reduced the incidence of milk fever from more than 40 per cent to none. In practical terms, a potassium-rich grass or legume diet would thus be expected to favor the onset of milk fever, whereas the addition of calcium chloride or other chlorides and a variety of sulfates would shift the diet toward acidity. It does not appear that this effect is related to the concentration of calcium in the diet. The effect of the acidic diet is thought to operate by inducing a slight metabolic acidosis, which increases the size and throughput of the available calcium pool, and increases bone resorption and intestinal absorption of calcium. A higher concentration of $1,25(OH)_2D_3$ is observed in cows on these acidic diets.

SHORT-TERM FACTORS. It is essential that the cow's appetite remain high at and around the time of parturition. If a cow has received a ration rich in concentrates during the dry period and if her body condition score is too high, her intake of dry matter will decline as parturition approaches, and the incidence of milk fever will be likely to increase. The effect of inappetence at this critical time, when increased supplies of calcium are needed, resembles temporary starvation. A similar mechanism may explain some of the increasing number of cases of a milk fever–like syndrome reported in higher yielding cows later on in lactation. These cows may become temporarily starved either while they are being transported or before embryo transfer techniques are applied or through inappetence at estrus. Because the normal requirement for calcium from the diet for secretion into milk is so large and begins so rapidly, even brief starvation may result in an imbalance.

When parturition is imminent, calcium intake should be increased as rapidly as possible to provide for the cow's greater requirement of calcium. However, the use of readily absorbed calcium salts for this purpose is not easy. In one trial, this routine reduced the incidence of milk fever from 46 per cent to 23 per cent, but it is not easy to administer calcium chloride (150 g/animal) by drenching on the day before calving and for 4 days therafter, and the method has not always proved effective. The beneficial increase in calcium absorption that occurs when the calcium content of the diet is increased has been demonstrated to persist for only a few days. This short-term response and the need to provide the dry cow with <20 g Ca/day may explain the conflicting results obtained from different trials.

There is more recent evidence that feeding roughage as either silage or hay alone during the last days of pregnancy can reduce the incidence of milk fever. In these cases, excretion of large amounts of salivary bicarbonate may induce a subclinical acidosis that effectively increases the calcium pool and its turnover, as described previously.

The administration of vitamin D in pharmacologic doses 5 to 10 days before calving can be beneficial. Recently acquired knowledge of the biochemical pathways of the vitamin, together with the chemical synthesis of its metabolites and their analogues, have provided opportunities for new prophylactic approaches to milk fever.

Feeding 20 to 30 $\times$ 10^6 IU of vitamin D_3 (cholecalciferol) daily for a maximum of 7 days, starting 3 to 4 days prepartum has been claimed to reduce the incidence of milk fever. A single intramuscular injection of 10 $\times$ 10^6 IU (250 mg) vitamin D_3 approximately 10 days before calving has also been said to lower the incidence of the disease, although its protective effect has been questioned. Some of the limitations of its therapeutic effect are probably due to the necessity for further metabolism via kidney hydroxylation to form the active metabolite. In order to overcome this limitation, analogues of vitamin D_3 metabolites, including doses of 350 to 500 μg 1α-hydroxycholecalciferol (1α-HCC) and $1,25(OH)_2D_3$ (the active vitamin), have been used in trials to protect cows against milk fever. The results confirm that they can significantly lower the incidence of disease provided that they are administered at least 24 hours and not more than 5 to 7 days before calving. The difficulty of predicting parturition in the cow has been overcome in some trials by combining the vitamin treatment with induction of parturition. However, this procedure can seriously increase the incidence of retained placenta. Thus, the use of 1α-HCC has not become widespread. It has been available for prophylactic treatment in Israel and the Netherlands for a few years and has only recently been available for use in Great Britain.

HYPOCALCEMIA IN EWES

In sheep, hypocalcemia (and hypophosphatemia) are more likely to occur during the last month of pregnancy than at lambing, partly because the calcium requirement of the fetuses is proportionally higher in the sheep than in the cow, and partly because there is not such a rapid increase in the ewe's requirement for calcium at the beginning of lactation. Hypocalcemia is rare at lambing, but it can occur during lactation, most commonly during the first 6 weeks. The likelihood of clinical disease is increased by factors such as sudden inclement weather, strenuous exercise, and temporary starvation.

The clinical signs of disease are similar to those of cattle. Muscle tremors, however, are more common, and the clinical signs may easily be confused with those of hypomagnesemia.

The best method of treatment is by intravenous injection of 50 ml of a 40 per cent solution of calcium borogluconate, and more calcium can be provided subcutaneously. When hypomagnesemia is suspected, a mixture of calcium, magnesium, and phosphorus may be administered instead of calcium alone (Table 1). The frequency of relapses after a single treatment is greater in sheep than in cattle, and repeated treatments may be necessary.

When nursing affected animals, it is as important with sheep as it is with cattle to maintain them in sternal recumbency in order to avoid regurgitation of ruminal contents; however, there is less danger of necrosis of muscles, presumably because of the sheep's lower body weight.

In order to prevent disease during the last 6 weeks of pregnancy, it is important to ensure that the ewe is receiving a continuously rising plane of nutrition. This will ensure that her greater requirement for calcium is provided by the increased intake of calcium from the diet. During pregnancy and lactation, it is also important to maintain the ewe's feed intake, to provide her with shelter from inclement weather, and to avoid stressing her with severe or unaccustomed exercise.

HYPOCALCEMIA IN GOATS

The epidemiology of milk fever in goats is similar to that in cows. The disease is most common close to parturition, and the principles for its prevention, treatment, and care are similar.

Acute cases should be treated by the administration of 25 ml of 40 per cent calcium borogluconate intravenously, together with 75 ml of a 20 per cent solution subcutaneously. However, as a 40 per cent solution of calcium borogluconate can cause severe local reactions at the site of administration, it would be wise to administer solutions of no greater concentration than 20 per cent wt/vol (Table 1).

BIBLIOGRAPHY

Oetzel GR: Parturient paresis and hypocalcaemia in ruminant livestock. Vet Clin North Am 4:351–365, 1988.
Block E: Manipulating dietary anions and cations for prepartum dairy cows to reduce incidence of milk fever. J Dairy Sci 67:2929–2948, 1984.

Acetonemia
IVAN W. CAPLE, BVSc, PhD
J. G. McLEAN, BVSc, PhD

Acetonemia, or bovine ketosis, is a disease of lactating cows characterized by nervous signs, loss of body weight, reduced milk yield, and ketones in the urine and milk. Many of the biochemical changes are similar to those in other ketotic conditions of ruminants, including pregnancy toxemia of sheep, goats, and beef cows, and fatty liver syndrome in dairy cows. There is no single specific metabolic lesion causing ketosis, and the biochemical changes include hypoglycemia, an accumulation of ketone bodies in body fluids, and increased plasma free fatty acids and liver fat, together with decreased liver glycogen. These changes are associated with an inadequate supply of nutrients necessary for the normal carbohydrate and fat metabolism associated with the high milk production usually seen in early lactation.

OCCURRENCE

Acetonemia may occur in dairy cows housed during the winter and also in dairy cows at pasture. Cows of any age, including heifers, may be affected, and ketosis is not confined to those in poor body condition. When there is a high incidence of the disease, it becomes a major economic problem because of the loss of milk production and the failure to return to full production after recovery.

Acetonemia is most prevalent within 6 weeks after parturition when high-producing cows have difficulty adjusting their dietary intake to the production demand. Maximum milk yield usually occurs during the third week after parturition, but maximum intake of metabolizable energy may not be achieved until the seventh week. A cow can maintain a high yield for a limited period, even when dietary intake is inadequate, but loses weight because body reserves of protein and fat are utilized to overcome the energy deficit caused by the continuing synthesis of milk components. Subclinical ketosis can occur when apparently normal cows continue in this state of negative energy balance, and these cows may excrete ketones in urine and milk but do not develop clinical signs. This delicate metabolic balance can rapidly deteriorate into a severe clinical ketosis, however, if any condition causes further reduction of the cow's dietary intake.

Primary spontaneous ketosis may still develop in cows being fed a high-energy diet in early lactation. Factors considered to influence the occurrence of the disease are excessive feeding of silage containing a high content of butyric acid, inadequate exercise, excessive fatness at parturition, and digestive upsets, often caused by inadequate fiber intake when concentrates are fed.

Acetonemia can be found in cows grazing lush, rapidly growing grass pastures if they are unable to obtain sufficient nutrients because of the high water content of the diet. Specific dietary deficiencies of minerals, such as phosphorus, sodium, magnesium, and cobalt, in addition to a reduced food intake, may be associated with a high incidence of ketosis. Cobalt is required for rumen microbial synthesis of vitamin B_{12} and is also essential for adequate utilization of propionic acid.

Secondary ketosis can result from any disease causing a reduction in appetite during early lactation. Diseases frequently encountered are abomasal displacement, metritis, mastitis, and traumatic reticulitis.

ETIOLOGY AND PATHOGENESIS

The ruminant is always in a somewhat precarious position with respect to its carbohydrate metabolism. Very little glucose is obtained directly from the diet, as about 80 per cent of the ingested carbohydrates are fermented by the rumen microflora into volatile fatty acids—acetic, propionic, and butyric acids—which are then absorbed. Acetate may be oxidized by a variety of tissues or incorporated into milk fat by the mammary gland.

Glucose, which is essential for function of the central nervous system, for maintenance of cellular osmotic environment, and for production of lactose in the mammary gland and fructose in the fetus, is synthesized by the liver and renal cortex by way of the gluconeogenic pathway (Fig. 1). Approximately half of the cow's glucose is normally derived from dietary propionic acid, which is incorporated into the tricarboxylic acid (TCA) cycle and then converted into glucose by gluconeogenesis. Glucogenic amino acids, lactic acid, and glycerol can also be converted into glucose by this process. Any condition reducing the amount of propionic acid in the rumen can result in inadequate glucose production and a consequent lowering in blood glucose level. Hypoglycemia leads to a mobilization of free fatty acids and glycerol from fat stores. This mobilization is mediated by a number of factors, including the sympathetic nervous system and hormones such as epinephrine, glucagon, adrenocorticotropic hormone, glucocorticoids, and thyroid hormones. Tissues such as skeletal muscle and heart can utilize fatty acids for energy production when glucose is deficient. However, the liver has a limited ability to oxidize fatty acids because acetyl-CoA, which is the endproduct of fatty acid oxidation, cannot be adequately incorporated into the TCA cycle because of low levels of oxaloacetate, resulting from the active gluconeogenesis. The excess acetyl-CoA is converted into the ketone bodies, acetoacetate, and β-hydroxybutyrate plus a smaller amount of acetone. Ketone bodies are readily oxidized by tissues other than liver, particularly muscle. If the production of ketone bodies by the liver exceeds the utilization by the peripheral tissues, they accumulate in the body, and pathologic ketosis results. Ketone bodies are excreted principally by the way of the urine and milk. The total amount excreted usually does not exceed 10 per cent of the amount produced.

Because acetoacetate and β-hydroxybutyrate are strong acids, excessive accumulation in the body can produce acidosis, but this is not common in cows with acetonemia. Hypoglycemia is the major factor involved in the onset and development of the clinical signs.

CLINICAL SIGNS

Acetonemia in dairy cows is manifest by a range of syndromes in which loss of body condition is most common. Variable nervous signs are present. There is a gradual but moderate decline in milk yield over 2 to 4 days. Cows may first refuse to eat grain, then silage, but continue to eat hay. The dairyworkers may have noted that the cow has not eaten the concentrates provided during milking. Body weight is lost rapidly once appetite has decreased, leading to utilization of body stores and dehydration. Cows often appear depressed and disinclined to move, their hair coat appears roughened, and their eyes appear "glazed" or "lackluster." Temperature and heart and respiratory rates are usually normal. The ruminal movements are commonly normal unless the condition is of long duration; then, they may be decreased or even absent. The odor of acetone may be detected on the breath. Some cows may stagger and may appear partially blind. Other nervous signs that are seen in a small number of cows include excessive salivation, abnormal chewing movements, and exaggerated licking. Muscles, particularly in the shoulder and midflank regions show trembling, and cows have a staggering or swaying gait, appearing incoordinated and apparently blind. Hyperesthesia may be detected. Some cows may charge blindly if disturbed and can injure themselves during these recurrent nervous episodes.

CLINICAL PATHOLOGY

Field tests for ketosis are based on the qualitative detection of ketones in urine and milk by their reaction with sodium nitroprusside (Rothera's reaction) to form a pink to purple color (Acetest tablet, Ketostix and Labstix test strips[1]). The primary value of the urine test is the ability to rule out ketosis if the test is negative. Urine normally contains higher ketones levels than milk, and a positive urine test can be regarded as evidence of ketosis only when the milk is also positive.

Hypoglycemia, hyperketonemia, and excretion of ketones in urine and milk are characteristic of the disease, and plasma free fatty acids and blood glycerol levels are elevated. The blood levels of glucose and ketones are the best measure of the severity of ketosis. Although quantitative chemical estimations of blood ketone levels are often impractical, plasma may react with Rothera's reagent. Blood glucose concentrations are reduced from normal levels of 40 to 50 mg/100 ml (2.2 to 2.8 mmol/L) to less than 25 mg/100 ml (1.4 mmol/L) and are usually lower in cases of primary ketosis than in cases of secondary ketosis. Total blood ketone levels are elevated from a normal value of <10 mg/100 ml (1.75 mmol/L) to >30 mg/100 ml (5.0 mmol/L).

In herds with energy deficiency and subclinical ketosis, cows in the first 6 weeks of lactation often have serum β-hydroxybutyrate concentrations >10 mg/100 ml (1.75 mmol/L). Blood urea nitrogen values may vary, but urinary ammonia concentration may be elevated.

Some cows have hypocalcemia with acetonemia, and severely affected cows may show an increase in serum aspartate

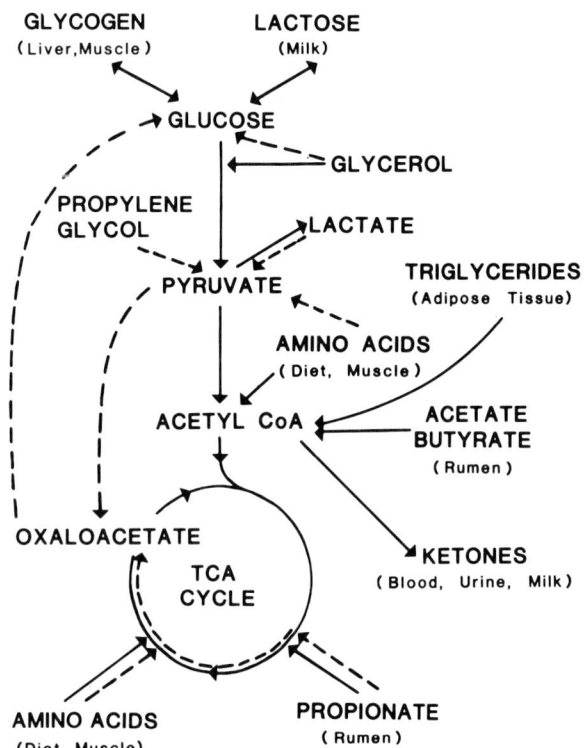

Figure 1. Pathways of glucose synthesis and ketone body production in ruminants. The gluconeogenic pathways are shown by the broken lines.

---
[1]Available from Ames Company, Division of Miles Laboratories, Inc., Elkhart, Indiana, and Mulgrave, Australia.

aminotransferase (AST) activity that is related to the extent of anorexia and liver damage. Although cows with acetonemia do not usually die, necrotic lesions consisting of fatty infiltration and degeneration of the liver and secondary changes in the anterior pituitary gland and adrenal cortex may be present.

DIAGNOSIS

Diagnosis of acetonemia is based on the presence of ketones in the urine and milk, the history related to the time of parturition, feeding program, signs associated with wasting and nervous dysfunction, together with elimination of other conditions that could lead to temporary reduction of appetite. Clinical indications of other diseases include increased temperature, increased heart and respiratory rates, and a rapid drop in or cessation of milk yield, as well as signs specific for conditions such as traumatic reticulitis, metritis, mastitis, abomasal displacement, indigestion, and constipation.

Acetonemia without complications is never fatal, and the nervous dysfunction is transient, which distinguishes it from listeriosis, in which there is a fever. In comparison with acetonemia, rabies is characterized by mania and ascending paralysis and is always fatal. With acetonemia there are no tetanic convulsions, and the condition responds rapidly to treatment. Cows that have ketosis and hypocalcemia concurrently may have a reeling staggering gait, hyperesthesia, and feeble paddling of the limbs when in lateral recumbency. These cows may show a clinical response to calcium therapy but usually have a poor appetite following treatment.

TREATMENT

The basis of treatment is as follows: (1) to immediately increase the glucose supply to organs where metabolic pathways are dependent on glucose availability, (2) to replenish the depleted intermediates of the TCA cycle in the liver so that fatty acids mobilized from fat stores are oxidized completely and the rate of ketone body formation is decreased, and (3) to increase the availability of dietary propionic acid and other glucogenic precursors (Table 1).

An intravenous injection of glucose (500 ml of 40 or 50 per cent solution) causes a transient hyperglycemia for about 2 hours and alleviates the clinical signs. Milk production is stimulated, but as lactose is lost in the milk, relapses commonly occur unless repeated or continuous infusions are given. The necessity for repeated injections of glucose can be overcome by the oral administration of glucose precursors, such as propylene glycol. The recomended dosage is 125 to 250 g twice daily mixed with an equal volume of water. Propylene glycol is more effective than sodium propionate or glycerol, as it is not fermented in the rumen and provides a substrate for gluconeogenesis in the liver. High doses of propionate may cause digestive disturbances, and glycerol has the disadvantage of being converted to ketogenic acids as well as propionic acid in the rumen. Cobalt salts are added to propylene glycol to provide at least 100 mg cobalt/day in cases in which cobalt is deficient.

Glucocorticoids are effective when used alone, when used with glucose therapy, or when followed by oral administration of glucose precursors. However, glucocorticoids may be contraindicated when infectious conditions predispose to secondary ketosis. Glucocorticoid treatment is accompanied by a reduction in ketone body formation owing to greater utilization of the acetyl-CoA derived from fatty acid oxidation and an increase in blood glucose concentration due to a greater availability of glucose precursors in the liver. Most commercial preparations of synthetic glucocorticoids such as dexamethasone and betamethasone are effective, and a single dose is given (see Table 1). Excessive administration of glucocorticoids should be avoided, because it may reduce appetite and milk yield.

Table 1. DIAGNOSTIC TESTS AND DRUG THERAPY FOR ACETONEMIA

Test[1] or Drug[2]	Species	Dose
Acetest tablets	Bovine	
Ketostix		
Glucose solution (40%)		500 ml (IV)
Propylene glycol (with mixtures containing cobalt available)		125–250 g (orally twice daily)
Glucocorticoids		
Dexamethasone preparations		5–20 mg
Betamethasone		10–30 mg
Flumethasone		2.5–5 mg
Triamcinolone acetonide		2.5–10 mg
Anabolic steroids		
Trienbolone acetate		125–250 mg
Dihydrotestosterone undecyclenate		125–250 mg

[1]Division of Miles Laboratories, Inc., Elkhart, Indiana and Mulgrave, Australia.
[2]These preparations are available under a variety of trade names. Consult publications such as Veterinary Pharmaceuticals and Biologicals, 6th Edition, Veterinary Medicine Publishing Co., Lenexa, KS, 1989–1990.

Anabolic steroids also produce a decrease in the levels of blood ketones and free fatty acids and an increase in the concentrations of intermediates of the TCA cycle in the liver. Unlike glucocorticoids, anabolic steroids do not produce hyperglycemia in ketotic cows. Anabolic steroids stimulate appetite, which is beneficial in ensuring an increased supply of glucogenic precursors.

Chloral hydrate has long been used to treat the nervous form of acetonemia. The dosage is 28.5 g in water or by capsule twice daily for 3 to 5 days.

It is important to ensure that the cow's food intake returns to normal as quickly as possible, and this is best achieved by the dairyworker who can entice the cow to eat by offering differing diets, such as hay and whole oats, until she consumes the full amount of her normal diet.

PREVENTION

Acetonemia in dairy cows occurs in housed cows in the Northern Hemisphere and in pastured cows in the Southern Hemisphere. The most successful control of the problem is through attention to feeding and management to ensure that cows have an adequate energy intake (see Special Dietary Management in Lactation and Gestation, Section 4). Cows should not be in poor condition or excessively fat at calving. The ration to be used in lactation should be reduced at least 2 weeks before parturition to permit the rumen microflora to adapt to the change in diet. During the first 3 months of lactation, high-yielding cows should not be subjected to sudden changes in ration. The ration fed during early lactation should provide maximum glucose precursors with the minimum of ketogenic materials, such as hay crop or silage high in butyric acid, and at the same time give maximum energy without reducing food intake. Particular attention must be paid to providing good-quality roughage that composes a minimum of one third of the ration. A good practice is to include good quality alfalfa (lucerne) hay in the diet. If concentrates are used, the carbohydrate should be readily digestible (e.g., ground maize), and the ration should contain adequate amounts of vitamins and minerals. If high-concentrate diets are fed, the daily ration should be divided into four feeds. Cows that are housed should get some exercise each day. In problem herds, the prevalence of ketosis can be assessed from milk production records together with the monitoring of ketone levels in blood or milk. Blood glucose (<1.5 mmol/L) and β-hydroxybutyrate (<1.0 mmol/L) levels from metabolic profiles, and milk acetone concentrations >1.0 mmol/L are useful in detecting subclinical cases, while other data may define the mineral and trace element status. The diet of susceptible cows should be supplemented with propylene glycol.

BIBLIOGRAPHY

Herdt TH: Fuel homeostasis in the ruminant. Vet Clin North Am: Food Animal Practice 4:213–231, 1988.
Hibbitt KG: Bovine ketosis and its prevention. Vet Rec 105:13–15, 1979.
Littledike ET, Young JW, Beitz DD, et al: Common metabolic diseases of cattle: ketosis, milk fever, grass tetany and downer cow complex. J Dairy Sci 64:1465–1482, 1982.

Pregnancy Toxemia

IVAN W. CAPLE, BVSc, PhD
J. G. McLEAH, BVSc, PhD

Pregnancy toxemia is primarily a metabolic disorder of ewes. A comparable condition is also seen in goats and cows. It is characterized principally by hypoglycemia and hyperketonemia and is manifested clinically by nervous signs and recumbency. The disorder arises when synthesis of glucose by the liver is insufficient for metabolic requirements. This occurs when dietary intake is inadequate and utilization of glucogenic precursors from maternal reserves cannot compensate for the energy demands of the developing fetus. There is also a substantial mobilization of body fat reserves.

PREGNANCY TOXEMIA IN EWES

Occurrence

Pregnancy toxemia in ewes occurs during the last 6 weeks of pregnancy when there is a large demand for glucose by the developing fetus. The condition is seen in ewes with a single fetus, but ewes carrying multiple fetuses are most susceptible. It is very often a fatal disease and is usually seen as an outbreak when there is inadequate nutrition available or when there is a reduction in the voluntary food intake.

Inadequate nutrition arises when ewes are placed on low-quality fibrous diets such as crop stubbles or on pastures that decline in nutritive value owing to seasonal or climatic conditions. The most variable factor in the nutrition of the pregnant ewe, however, is voluntary food intake. This declines in overfat ewes because intra-abdominal fat and the enlarging uterus decrease the capacity of the digestive tract. Transport of ewes to a new environment, change of diet such as introduction to grain feeding, and intercurrent diseases such as foot abscess, foot rot, and intestinal parasitism also diminish voluntary food intake. Starvation and hypocalcemia associated with management procedures, such as transport, yarding, shearing, and dipping, also contribute to many outbreaks.

Pathogenesis

A gradual or sudden reduction in food intake is all that is required to produce pregnancy toxemia. The nutrient requirements of a ewe with twin fetuses rise to nearly twice the maintenance level during the last 2 months of pregnancy when the fetuses are growing rapidly. Although inadequate energy and protein intake is the main predisposing factor, deficiencies of other nutritional factors, including choline and biotin, may contribute to the development of pregnancy toxemia.

The ewe cannot regulate the glucose demand of the fetus and must draw on body reserves to supply the demands that cannot be met by food intake alone. The ewe does not obtain the glucose essential for the fetus, central nervous system, eyes, erythrocytes, and mammary glands from its alimentary tract but must synthesize this glucose. More than half the glucose required is normally synthesized in the liver and kidney cortex from the propionic acid produced in the rumen by microbial fermentation of ingested carbohydrates. The remainder is obtained by gluconeogenesis from amino aids, lactic acid, and glycerol released from body fat stores.

In pregnancy toxemia, the propionic acid and glucogenic precursors derived from the diet and body reserves are unable to maintain glucose requirements. Hypoglycemia occurs, and this leads to depression of the central nervous system. Fatty acids, which are rapidly mobilized from fat stores under hormonal influence, enter the liver and are oxidized with the production of acetylcoenzyme A (acetyl-CoA). When there is a deficiency of glucose precursors, there is a reduction in intermediates of the tricarboxylic acid (TCA) cycle, particularly oxaloacetate, which is required if acetyl-CoA is to be utilized by the TCA cycle. Acetyl-CoA accumulates and is diverted into the production of ketone bodies.

Excessive production of ketone bodies produces acidosis, because acetoacetate and β-hydroxybutyrate are strong acids, and prolonged urinary excretion results in loss of sodium and potassium ions and lowering of the plasma alkali reserve. Ketoacidosis leads to dyspnea and exacerbates the central nervous system depression, progressing to the irreversible stage in which there is dehydration, uremia, and loss of consciousness. The entry of fatty acids into the liver results in synthesis and accumulation of triglycerides, and this is responsible for the characteristic fatty liver.

Clinical Signs

In an affected flock, the disease usually appears as a prolonged outbreak that may extend over several weeks, with a few ewes developing clinical signs each day. Although the course of the disease is as long as 7 days, affected ewes are frequently observed only in the latter stages. There is progressive development of clinical signs from an initial depression of consciousness; through muscular disturbances with abnormal posture, loss of muscle tone, balance, and locomotion; and then finally recumbency, coma, and death.

Affected ewes lag behind the flock when it moves. The ewes appear blind; they can still hear and will face humans and dogs when approached but seldom move away. If forced to move, they do so in an aimless manner with a staggering gait and will often lean awkwardly against obstacles. The pupillary light reflex is diminished, and the eye preservation reflex is absent. Temperature, heart rate, respiratory rate, and ruminal movements are mostly normal. As the condition progresses, ewes become more listless.

Neuromuscular disturbances appear as fine tremors of the muscles of the head with twitching of the ears and lips, and some ewes show convulsions. In the latter stages, ewes adopt abnormal postures and jaws are elevated—"stargazing." There may be grinding of the teeth and champing of the jaws. Ewes remain in sternal recumbency, with the head round near the flank, or in lateral recumbency. They become comatose, show labored breathing, and die after 3 to 4 days.

Occasionally, the fetus dies and the ewe experiences a transient recovery, but the ewe relapses as a result of toxemia if the fetus decomposes and is not aborted. Affected ewes commonly have difficulty during lambing. Some may pass a dead fetus and recover. Overfat ewes subjected to a period of acute starvation develop clinical signs more rapidly and die before the condition progresses to the comatose stage. These ewes usually have hypocalcemia as well as ketosis.

Clinical Pathology

In the early stages of pregnancy toxemia, there is hypoglycemia, elevated plasma fatty acid and blood glycerol levels, and hyperketonemia, often with ketonuria. The presence of ketone bodies (acetoacetate and acetone) in the plasma and urine may be detected using sodium nitroprusside reagents (Rothera's test, Acetest tablets, and Ketostix test strips[1]). Plasma cortisol levels are increased. In animals with advanced cases of acidosis and renal failure, plasma bicarbonate concentration may be reduced by 50 per cent, and blood urea nitrogen level may be elevated. In the terminal stages, comatose ewes may even have hyperglycemia.

Necrotic lesions are often minimal. Usually twin fetuses or a large single fetus is present. The lambs may be dead, and a few may show varying stages of decomposition. The liver is enlarged, light yellow in color, and friable, and the cut surface is greasy. Fatty infiltration and degenerative changes may be seen in the adrenal glands, kidneys, and heart.

Diagnosis

Pregnancy toxemia is characterized by nervous signs and is often associated with a history of undernutrition or error of management. Ewes are affected in the last weeks of pregnancy and die in 3 to 5 days.

The disease has to be differentiated from hypocalcemia, which is characterized by paralysis and the "frog-leg" posture of recumbent ewes in which the hind limbs are extended. Hypocalcemia has a much shorter course (12 to 24 hrs) than pregnancy toxemia and affects more ewes in the flock. Hypocalcemia is seen after sudden deprivation of food or after exertion and responds rapidly within minutes to treatment with calcium salts.

Treatment

Treatment is successful only in ewes that show initial signs of pregnancy toxemia and are able to stand. Recumbency or comatose ewes usually die despite treatment. Glucose administered parenterally as a hypertonic solution (40 per cent) is not usually effective, and it is impractical to administer to large numbers of ewes at frequent intervals.

Oral rehydration solutions containing glucose, electrolytes, and glycine, administered to ewes every 4 to 8 hours, have

Table 1. DIAGNOSTIC TESTS AND DRUG THERAPY FOR PREGNANCY TOXEMIA

Test[1] or Drug[2]	Species	Dose
Acetest tablets	Bovine	
Ketostix	Ovine	
Labstix		
Glycerol (50% solution)	Ovine	200 ml (orally twice daily)
Propylene glycol (50% solution)	Ovine	200 ml (orally twice daily)
Anabolic steroids	Ovine	
Trenbolone acetate		30 mg
Glucocorticoids	Ovine	
Dexamethasone 21-isonicotinate		10 mg
Glucose (40% solution)	Bovine	500 ml (IV)
Propylene glycol	Bovine	500 ml (daily)
Anabolic steroids	Bovine	
Trenbolone acetate		125–250 mg
Dihydrotestosterone undecyclenate		125–250 mg

[1]Ames Company, Division of Miles Laboratories. Inc., Mulgrave, Australia and Elkhart, IN.
[2]Many of these preparations are sold under a variety of trade names. Consult publications such as Veterinary Pharmaceuticals and Biologicals, 6th ed., Lenexa, KS, Veterinary Medicine Publishing Co, 1989–1990.

been reported to increase rates of recovery from pregnancy toxemia. When intensive therapy can be given to a valuable animal, glucose should be incorporated into the electrolyte solutions given by intravenous infusion (see Fluid Therapy, Section 1). The object of treatment is to

1. Increase the availability of glucose precursors by increasing dietary intake, supplying glucogenic precursors, or causing their mobilization from body stores (Table 1).
   a. Supplementary feed should be provided. A 50-kg ewe with twin fetuses will require 2 kg of oats/day if no other pasture is available. Ewes fed mainly on grain should receive at least 100 g of hay per day. When pregnancy toxemia occurs in flocks being fed grain as a supplement to pasture, it is often advisable to reduce the stocking rate as well as to increase the supplementary feed.
   b. Affected ewes should be given 200 ml of a warm 50 per cent glycerol solution or propylene glycol orally twice daily until normal appetite returns completely.
   c. The anabolic steroid trenbolone acetate (Finajet)[2] (30 mg intravenously or intramuscularly) stimulates appetite of affected ewes and reduces blood ketone and fatty acid concentrations.
2. Decrease the metabolic drain on the ewe by removing the fetus by cesarean section or by inducing parturition. Cesarean section is a successful procedure for affected ewes that do not show severe acidosis and renal failure. Induction of parturition with 10 mg dexamethasone-21-isonicotinate (Voren),[3] has resulted in higher survival rates of ewes and lambs in flocks predisposed to pregnancy toxemia by outbreaks of foot abscess or foot rot, which suddenly limit their ability to graze. Ewes subjected to prolonged undernutrition have had unreliable responses to glucocorticoids, and higher doses may be required.

Prevention

Ewes need to be watched closely during the last weeks of pregnancy. In flocks in which some ewes show pregnancy toxemia, other ewes may not be affected, at the expense of

---

[1]Available from Ames Company, Division of Miles Laboratories, Inc., Elkhardt, IN, and Mulgrave, Australia.

[2]Available from Hoechst Animal Health, UK.
[3]Available from Bio-Ceutic Laboraboaries, St. Joseph, MO.

growth and development of the fetus and mammary glands. This circumstance may lead to greater mortality in lambs with low birth weights and to poor growth of survivors because of reduced milk production by ewes.

Pregnancy testing may be used to determine those ewes potentially at risk in a flock. A blood glucose concentration profile obtained in midpregnancy can assist in selecting ewes that are at risk. An overnight fasting blood glucose concentration is determined in samples collected from ewes 90 days after mating, and those with levels below the median are considered to be at greater risk and should be managed accordingly. Plasma β-hydroxybutyrate concentration can be used as a guide to adjust supplementary feeding of flocks in the last few weeks of pregnancy. Ten per cent of the flock is sampled, and feeding is increased when the mean concentration of plasma β-hydroxybutyrate rises above 4.8 mg/100 ml (0.8 mmol/L).

If ewes are being fed a diet fulfilling all requirements during the last 3 months of pregnancy, they should gain at least 4 kg of body weight if carrying a single lamb and 7.5 kg of body weight if carrying twins.

When ewes are overfat (condition score 4 or greater on a 0-to-5 scale) at mating, their body weight should be decreased gradually by 20 per cent with restricted feeding in the first 2 months of pregnancy, and then the food supply should be increased for the next 3 months. Supplementary feed is given when necessary.

Ewes that are overfat in late pregnancy should be exercised by driving them slowly for about 1 mile each day. Concentrates can be given to increase energy intake. Shelter and additional feed should be provided during inclement weather. Intercurrent diseases such as parasitism and infections must be treated.

Under grazing or range conditions, lambing should be timed to coincide with maximum pasture growth. Ewes in the last month of pregnancy need to be grazing pastures with greater than 1000 kg (dry matter per hectare [ha]) available green feed to enable them to meet their requirements. Aged ewes with incomplete dentition should be removed from the breeding flock.

PREGNANCY TOXEMIA IN BEEF COWS

Occurrence

Pregnancy toxemia, or ketosis, occurs in pastured and housed beef cows when nutrition is inadequate during the last 2 months of pregnancy. Cows of all ages are affected, and overfat animals and those bearing twin calves are particularly susceptible. Cows given unlimited access to spring pastures during the dry period become overfat, and they are predisposed to the toxemic condition when pastures decline in nutritive value during the summer or when they are placed on stubble pastures after cropping. The disease in beef cows has many similarities to pregnancy toxemia in ewes and to the fat cow syndrome in dairy cows. Pregnancy toxemia can be reproduced experimentally by not providing adequate nutrients for overfat cows during the last 6 weeks of pregnancy.

Clinical Signs

The clinical signs and the rates of progress of the condition are associated with the stage of pregnancy and the degree of nutritional stress.

Those cows that become affected between 7 and 9 months of pregnancy initially show lethargy and depression, stop foraging for food, and separate from the rest of the herd. Acetone can often be detected on the breath of most cows in an affected herd, but only a few cows have other clinical signs such as reduced appetite, rapid deterioration of body condition, and eventual recumbency. Recumbent cows often have a forced expiratory grunt and increased respiratory rate, and there is usually a clear nasal discharge and muzzle epithelium flaking. Feces are sparse, hard, and dry in the early stages and are often covered with mucus that sometimes contains blood. Rectal temperatures range from 38 to 41°C. Affected cows become recumbent 3 to 14 days before they die, and although some remain in sternal recumbency, most fall into lateral recumbency after 2 days.

Cows affected within a few days before parturition show excitability, an uncoordinated and high-stepping gait, and constipation. Experimentally, these signs can be produced in overfat cows with 2 days of starvation. Initially, they appear bright and alert, but they gradually become depressed, recumbent, unable to rise, and anorectic. Some cows may die during parturition, and others die within 30 days after calving. The condition in lactating beef cows is similar to the fatty liver syndrome in lactating dairy cows.

Clinical Pathology

In herds with clinical cases, cows with no obvious signs have hypoglycemia (blood glucose level <30 mg/100 ml or 1.7 mmol/L), hyperketonemia, and ketonuria. In cows with clinical signs, blood ketone concentrations are more elevated (acetoacetate up to 16 mg/100 ml or 1.5 mmol/L and β-hydroxybutyrate up to 125 mg/100 ml or 10 mmol/L). Cows affected near parturition have hypocalcemia, and serum magnesium levels are either normal or low (<0.65 mmol/L). Recumbent cows in the terminal stages have hyperphosphatemia (phosphate level up to 20 mg/100 ml or 5.00 mmol/L) and hyperglycemia (blood glucose level up to 160 mg/100 ml or 9.0 mmol/L). Serum aspartate aminotransferase (AST) activity is elevated. Urinalysis shows ketonuria, and in the terminal stages, proteinuria and hematuria are evident. At necropsy, lesions consist of an enlarged, yellow, fatty liver and fatty changes in the kidney and adrenal cortex. Histologic examination of the liver of cows with extreme cases shows gross fatty infiltration with an appearance resembling adipose tissue. Thrombi associated with infarcts are commonly present in the pulmonary, splenic, and portal veins.

Diagnosis

Usually only 1 or 2 cows show clinical signs before a veterinarian is consulted. General consideration of the history, stage of pregnancy, and nutritional status often enables a tentative diagnosis to be made on the basis of the clinical signs. Clinical pathologic tests will confirm elevated ketone and decreased calcium levels in urine and blood.

Differential diagnosis in individual animals includes traumatic reticulitis, pyelonephritis, ephemeral fever, and lead poisoning.

Treatment

Response to treatment depends on the duration and severity of the condition, and there is a high mortality rate.

Replacement therapy with intravenous solutions of glucose (500 ml of 40 per cent solution) or with combined solutions (500 ml of 20 per cent calcium borogluconate with phosphorus, magnesium, and 20 per cent glucose) is of value only in mild cases. Treatment with oral propylene glycol (500 ml daily) and fluids (see Fluid Therapy, Section 1) is aimed at supplying glucogenic precursors and correcting dehydration. Anabolic steroids (200 to 300 mg of 1-dihydrotestosterone undecyclenate [Vebonol][4] and 125 to 250 mg of trenbolone acetate [Finajet][5] are given to stimulate appetite in affected cows. They also cause mobilization of glucogenic precursors that decrease ketone body production in the liver. Immediate removal of the calf by cesarean section decreases the metabolic drain on the cow and may save a valuable animal. Induction of parturition using glucocorticoids is not satisfactory in recumbent cows because of the delay in response.

Treatment of a herd is by provision of supplementary feed, such as good quality hay.

Prevention

Since fat cows are particularly susceptible, cows should not be in this condition in the later half of pregnancy, but neither should they be subjected to periods of starvation. Supplementary feed should be provided for cows when there is inadequate pasture available in the last 2 months of pregnancy. Changes in body weight of pregnant and lactating cows can be used as a guide to the need for supplementary feeding of the herd. When any pregnant cow shows a weight loss of 30 kg or more, or when a lactating cow shows a weight loss of 50 kg or more in 14 days, supplementary feed should be given.

BIBLIOGRAPHY

PREGNANCY TOXEMIA IN EWES

Buswell JF, Haddy JP, Bywater RJ: Treatment of pregnancy toxemia in sheep using a concentrated oral rehydration solution. Vet Rec 118:208–209, 1986.
Heitzman RJ, Herriman ID, Austin AT, et al: The response of sheep with pregnancy toxemia to trenbolone acetate. Vet Rec 100:317–318, 1977.
Reid EL: The physiopathology of undernourishment in pregnant sheep, with particular reference to pregnancy toxemia. Adv Vet Sci 12:163–238, 1968.

PREGNANCY TOXEMIA IN COWS

Caple IW, Pemberton DH, Harrison MA, et al: Starvation ketosis in pregnant beef cows. Aust Vet J 53:289–291, 1977.
Kingrey BW, Ludwig VD, Monlux WS, et al: Pregnancy disease of cows. N Am Vet 38:321–322, 1957.
Spence AB: Pregnancy toxemia of beef cows in Orkney. Vet Rec 102:459–461, 1978.

---

[4]Available from Ciba-Geigy Agrochemicals, UK Ltd., Basel, Switzerland.
[5]Available from Hoechst Animal Health, UK.

Fat Cow Syndrome and Subclinical Fatty Liver

C. JEREMY ROBERTS, BVSc, PhD, MRCVS
IAN M. REID, BSc, MNS, PhD, MRC PATH

The fat cow syndrome (FCS), or fatty liver syndrome, occurs particularly in high-yielding dairy cows when overfeeding during late lactation and the dry period results in overfat cows at calving. Depressed appetite and consequent energy deficit after calving result in mobilization of adipose tissue, a rapid loss of body weight, and an accumulation of intracellular fat in various organs, including the liver. The clinical syndrome is associated with a higher incidence of metabolic, infectious, and reproductive disorders, such as ketosis, milk fever, mastitis, and retained placenta.

OCCURRENCE

FCS is a clinically recognizable entity in various countries, including the United States, Hungary, France, the republics of the former Soviet Union, Australia, and the United Kingdom. Dairy cows may be affected by subclinical forms of the syndrome.

FCS in its clinical and subclinical forms arises sporadically, as a result of faulty feeding in late lactation and the dry period. It is most frequently observed in loose housing where cattle in all stages of the reproductive cycle are fed and managed as one group. Cows with long dry periods owing to infertility problems are particularly at risk of becoming overfat. Feeding high quality forage such as maize silage or lush grass freely in the dry period will also result in overfat cows.

The syndrome affects all breeds and all ages, although heifers are less at risk under most farming practices. FCS in dairy cows is most commonly seen in the first 2 weeks of lactation, but cases may occur before and as late as 1 month after calving.

INCIDENCE

FCS results from a herd feeding problem, and the incidence within the herd will depend to a large extent on the overall fatness of the herd and the severity of the postcalving energy deficit. Morbidity may be as high as 50 to 90 per cent of newly calved cows, and mortality may reach 25 per cent.

The use of liver biopsy techniques in large numbers of cows in the United Kingdom has shown that the subclinical form of the syndrome is much more common than was previously realized. About one third of dairy cows with milk yields greater than 5500 kg are affected, and the incidence in different herds ranges from 10 to 50 per cent.

PATHOGENESIS

Dairy cows in early lactation commonly are in negative energy balance, because feed intake is insufficient to meet the nutritional demands for maintenance and lactation. As a result of this energy deficiency, cows mobilize body reserves of fat and muscle and so lose body weight and condition.

The mobilization of body reserves involves the release into the blood of fatty acids from subcutaneous and internal fat depots and glucogenic amino acids from protein stores. The fatty acids are transported in the blood to various organs, such as liver, kidney, and muscle, where they are deposited as intracellular droplets of triglyceride. Even before calving, fat is mobilized from body reserves as shown by the rise in liver fat per cent, which increases from around 0.5 per cent 8 weeks before calving to between 4 and 8 per cent 2 to 3 weeks before calving. The greater mobilization of body reserves after calving is reflected in the accumulation of higher levels of fat, up to 24 per cent and 15 per cent in the liver at 1 and 4 weeks after calving, respectively. This fat mobilization is probably brought about by the changing hormonal environment as the cow approaches calving.

The extent of fat deposition in liver and other organs after calving is determined by a number of predisposing factors, including high milk yield potential, condition at calving, and loss of condition after calving.

At the biochemical level, two mechanisms appear to be responsible for the development of fatty liver. The first is greater hepatic uptake of fatty acids as a direct result of raised serum levels resulting from fat mobilization. The second is inadequate hepatic secretion of triglycerides. This may be the result of suboptimal apolipoprotein production in the hepatocyte because of the inadequate supply of necessary amino acids. The extensive deposition of fat in tissues other than the liver suggests that failure of apolipoprotein production in the liver is important in the syndrome because other tissues depend on apolipoprotein synthesized in liver for construction of secretory lipoproteins.

CLINICAL SIGNS

The most useful signs in an affected herd are the presence of very fat cows (condition score greater than 4) in the dry cow group together with the presence of thin cows (condition score less than 2.5) in the freshly calved group, indicating excessive loss of condition in the period immediately after calving. The herd may have either a history or clinical signs of decreased resistance to infection—for example, an increase in mastitis, metritis, or salmonellosis—and an increased incidence of metabolic diseases—for example, ketosis and milk fever.

Specific signs to be observed in individual cows include depression, anorexia, ketonuria, decrease in milk output, and extensive loss of condition. The enlarged liver may sometimes be palpated posterior to the last rib in the right sublumbar fossa.

Any combination of these conditions in the herd with an absence of overtly sick animals may indicate the presence of subclinical fatty liver. In particular, the poor response to treatment of cases that would normally be expected to respond well is a useful aid in recognizing the presence of the syndrome.

CLINICAL PATHOLOGY

A number of blood constituents are significantly altered 1 week after calving in cows with fatty liver (Table 1). The changes in blood concentrations of albumin, bilirubin, and aspartate aminotransferase (AST) may all reflect alterations in liver function associated with hepatic fat accumulation. AST, however, is an enzyme that occurs not only in liver but also in muscle, kidneys, small intestines, and brain. The elevation of AST in the blood of cows with fatty liver may indicate damage to other tissues, such as kidneys and muscle as well as liver. Liver specific enzymes, such as ornithine-carbamoyltransferase (OCT) and glutamate dehydrogenase (GDH), do not appear to be reliable indicators of the presence of fatty liver.

The low blood magnesium concentrations in cows with fatty liver are probably related to the high nonesterified fatty acid concentrations and may be important in increasing the susceptibility of cows with fatty liver to milk fever, since hypomagnesemia reduces the ability to mobilize calcium in early lactation.

The white blood cell count is lowered in cows with fatty liver and may fall to as low as 3×10^9/L in cows with severe clinical FCS. The reduced count is largely due to reductions in neutrophils and lymphocytes.

PATHOLOGY

Post-mortem findings depend on the degree of fat deposition, the presence or absence of other diseases, and any therapy received prior to death or slaughter. Most cows dying of FCS have large deposits of fat around the heart, kidneys, and in the omentum. These large deposits are usually present even if most subcutaneous fat depots have been depleted very quickly, and evidence of fat necrosis may be present, particularly in the perirenal adipose tissue.

The liver will show gross evidence of fat deposition by its large size, round edges, and pale color. Fat deposition is not easily detected macroscopically in other organs, although the kidney cortex and cardiac muscle may appear very pale and greasy. When making an assessment of the carcass, treatment of the animal prior to death should be borne in mind because certain agents such as choline and steroid hormones may have reduced the amount of fat in tissues without improving the underlying cause of the deposition.

Microscopically, the fat deposited in tissues may be detected most easily by the use of specific neutral fat stains (see Diagnosis). In the liver the fat is deposited as globules of triglycerides within the hepatocyte cytoplasm. The extent of deposition may be as great as 70 per cent of the total hepatocyte volume. In addition, fatty cysts may occur, and evidence of damage to mitochondria and of diminished protein synthetic capacity exists. These changes however are all reversible in subclinical and nonfatal clinical cases with no evidence of long-term damage to the liver.

Fat also accumulates in the form of intracellular droplets of triglycerides in a number of other tissues, including proximal tubular cells of the kidney, cortical cells of the adrenal gland, type 1 (slow, red, oxidative) skeletal muscle fibers, and cardiac muscle fibers. This highly specific distribution of the deposited fat suggests that in FCS fat is deposited throughout the body in those cells that normally utilize fatty acids for energy metabolism.

It is important to recognize that some of the changes described here will be seen in animals that have been subjected to feed deprivation of more than 24 hours. Post-mortem findings can only assist in a diagnosis of FCS or subclinical fatty liver when used in conjunction with the herd's history and clinical pathology.

DIAGNOSIS (Table 2)

There are three elements to be considered in the diagnosis of FCS or subclinical fatty liver: history, clinical pathology, and liver biopsy results. If the evidence from the history, including herd appraisal, is sufficiently strong, confirmatory evidence from blood sample test results or biopsy specimen findings may not be necessary. However, in cases of suspected

Table 1. ALTERATIONS IN BLOOD CONSTITUENTS IN COWS WITH FATTY LIVER ONE WEEK AFTER CALVING

Blood Constituent	Alteration
Nonesterified fatty acids Bilirubin Asparate aminotransferase (AST) β-Hydroxybutyrate	Increased
Glucose* Cholesterol Albumin Magnesium Insulin White blood cell count	Decreased

*May be elevated in severe or terminal cases.

Table 2. LIVER FAT VALUES FOR DIAGNOSIS OF FATTY LIVER

Method	Normal	Fatty
Chemical		
Total lipid (mg/g)	≤100	>100
Triglyceride (mg/g)	≤50	>50
Histologic		
Toluidine blue (% fat)	≤20	>20
Oil red O (% fat)	≤24	>24

subclinical fatty liver, diagnosis may only be possible by carrying out liver biopsy sample examinations on freshly calved cows.

HISTORY. Important diagnostic features are fat cows in the dry cow group, thin cows in early lactation, evidence of increased infectious and metabolic diseases with poor response to treatment, and reduced fertility.

CLINICAL PATHOLOGY. The major changes in blood chemistry profiles are shown in Table 1. Using an equation based on blood concentrations of nonesterified fatty acids, glucose, and AST at 7 to 13 days after calving, it has been possible to correctly diagnose fatty liver in 3 out of 4 cows. The equation is as follows:

$$y = -0.51 - 0.0032 \text{ NEFA } (\mu mol/L) + 2.84 \text{ glucose } (mmol/L) - 0.0528 \text{ AST } (IU/L)$$

if y <0, the cow has fatty liver.

The validity of this equation has been tested in a small number of herds in the United Kingdom and needs further testing before its routine use can be advised. It does however form a useful guide for application in situations other than those in which the equation was formulated.

LIVER BIOPSY. Samples of liver can be obtained from cows by percutaneous needle biopsy under local anesthesia. The procedure is quick (with practice about 16/hr) and has no measurable effect on milk yield. Fat content of biopsy samples can then be estimated by one of a number of chemical and histologic methods. Clinically ill cows with liver fat concentrations greater than 35 per cent have a poor prognosis.

Chemical Methods. These generally involve estimation of either hepatic total lipid or triglyceride content. In our view, triglyceride estimation is the chemical method of choice.

Histologic Methods. Histologic methods of estimating liver fat content may be more suitable for laboratories with routine histologic facilities. The percentage of fat in the liver may be estimated by point-counting methods, using plastic sections stained with toluidine blue or frozen sections stained with oil red O (ORO). In our view, fat estimation using frozen sections stained with ORO is the histologic method of choice for most routine purposes.

Buoyancy and Needle Biopsy. Another method suitable for estimating liver fat content in the field has been suggested. In the United States, liver fat content is based on buoyancy of needle biopsy samples in water or copper sulfate solutions. Samples that float in water have greater than 35 per cent fat on a wet weight basis.

Threshold values for the diagnosis of fatty liver, using the chemical and histologic methods described, are given in Table 2.

TREATMENT

Various empirical treatments for fatty liver and FCS have been suggested, but there has been very little controlled research. Choline, at 50 g/day for several days, has been used with limited success, indicating that methyl group donors may be of some value in this condition. Glucose by intravenous infusion at about 60 g/hr has also been used but with little recorded evidence of success. We have examined the usefulness of niacin supplementation in feed, and although our experiment showed evidence of a reduction in lipolysis in treated animals, there was no reduction in the severity of fatty liver.

More promising results have been obtained with the use of hormones, particularly glucocorticoids and anabolic steroids. The use of these compounds is rational because the pathogenesis of fatty liver indicates that a shortage of gluconeogenic and protein synthetic capacities are major contributors to the syndrome. Increasing the glucose supply by administration of glucose, glycerol or propionate, and a short-acting glucocorticoid, followed by stimulation of protein synthesis by administration of an anabolic steroid appears to be the most logical way of restoring metabolic control.

At present, there is no evidence that "tonics," vitamins, or minerals will have a significant effect on the prognosis of the syndrome, except in those cases in which blood levels of calcium or magnesium or both are severely depleted.

PREVENTION

Fatty liver is a problem of high-producing cows that undergo substantial body weight losses in early lactation. We believe that the fatty liver is a *symptom* rather than a cause, i.e., it is a convenient measure of the success with which the cow's metabolism has adapted to the demands of lactation. The degree of success in that adaptation is genetically determined in part but, in considerable measure, can be influenced by the feeding strategy adopted for late pregnancy and early lactation.

To reduce the incidence of fatty liver, it is most important to prevent cows from being overfat (condition score greater than 4 on a 0-to-5 scale) at calving and to maximize their feed intake after calving. There are several ways of helping to achieve reduction of fatty liver incidence.

1. Cows calving in a lean condition (condition score 2.5 to 3.0) have a higher potential for feed intake. If the feeding system and the feed quality help exploit this fact, then a minimum loss of body condition and less fatty liver need occur.

2. To reach high dry matter intake rapidly after calving, forage of good quality should be more freely available. Concentrates should be fed in small amounts and often so that a rapid increase in intake can be achieved without disturbing the rumen.

3. It is important to supply adequate quantities of correctly balanced protein in the diet. Many diets for high-producing cows in early lactation are deficient in nondegradable protein. A protein supplement of low degradability often improves production and may help to reduce the incidence of fatty liver.

BIBLIOGRAPHY

Herdt TH: Fatty liver in dairy cows. Vet Clin North Am: Food Animal Practice 4:269–287, 1988.
Morrow DA: Fat cow syndrome. J Dairy Sci 59:1625–1629, 1976.
Reid IM, Roberts CJ: Fatty liver in dairy cows. In Practice. 4 (Suppl) to Vet Rec 164–168, 1982.

Ruminant Hypomagnesemic Tetanies

IVAN W. CAPLE, BVSc, PhD
DAVID M. WEST, BVSc, PhD, FACVSc

In ruminants, a reduction in the concentration in the ventricular cerebrospinal fluid of magnesium below 0.5 mmol/L leads to hyperexcitability, muscular spasms, convulsions, and death from hypomagnesemic tetany. The disorder occurs following a decrease in plasma magnesium concentration when absorption of dietary magnesium is unable to meet the requirements for maintenance and lactation in cows, ewes, and does fed on either lush grass pastures or young green cereal crops of oats, barley, or wheat. Lactating ruminants are most susceptible owing to loss of magnesium in milk (120 to 170 mg/L), but occasional losses are recorded in nonlactating cows and also bulls and stocker calves.

HYPOMAGNESEMIC TETANY IN CATTLE

Hypomagnesemic grass tetany in lactating cattle often appears as a complex disorder owing to the variety of circumstances that can lead to a reduction in magnesium absorption. Throughout the world, there are several types of hypomagnesemic tetany syndromes, which can be diagnosed according to the ages of cows affected and the etiologic factors inducing the fatal nervous disorder. In beef herds, cows older than 6 years, if they are overfat at calving (body condition scores 4 to 5 on a 1-to-5 scale), and lose liveweight (up to 1 kg/day) during lactation, are more commonly affected with grass tetany than younger cows. Younger cows, two- and three year-olds, may also be affected in herds with more complex types of grass tetany syndromes associated with low magnesium and high potassium intakes, and low sodium and phosphorus nutrition. Determining which factors are likely to be important in reducing magnesium absorption in ruminants at a specific location enables recommendation of cost-effective management strategies to prevent hypomagnesemic tetany.

Hypomagnesemic tetany also occurs in young calves fed for several months on whole milk or milk-replacer diets, which provide inadequate magnesium for their requirements for maintenance and growth.

OCCURRENCE

Hypomagnesemic tetany occurs when lactating cows graze lush green pastures or cereal crops with magnesium concentrations less than 0.2 per cent magnesium, calcium less than 0.3 per cent, sodium (Na) less than 0.15 per cent magnesium, and potassium greater than 3.0 per cent on a dry matter (DM) basis. The disorder occurs more frequently when pastures have been fertilized with potassium and nitrogen and when soils are naturally high in potassium (K) and low in sodium. Young green cereal crops, and short rotation ryegrass pastures used for winter grazing by cattle and sheep often contain low magnesium (<0.2 per cent DM), low calcium (<0.2 per cent DM), and high potassium and nitrogen (N) concentrations (up to 5.0 per cent DM).

In countries where cattle are housed during winter, grass tetany occurs most commonly when lactating cows are turned out to graze lush, grass-dominant pastures in spring. The disorder has occurred in lactating dairy and beef cows fed indoors mainly on silage containing less than 0.1 per cent magnesium DM basis and minimal amounts of concentrates were fed.

The occurrence of hypomagnesemic tetany is seasonal, and its prevalence varies from year to year, depending largely on climatic conditions, pasture availability, the proportion of dry residues in winter pastures, and the clover and grass composition of green herbage. Inclement weather and management procedures such as yarding and transport, which result in reduced magnesium intakes, predispose lactating cows to the disorder. Commonly, hypomagnesemic tetany occurs when cattle recommence grazing lush pastures or cereal crops after being fed on hay during inclement weather.

Hypomagnesemic tetany also occurs when low herbage availability (less than 1000 kg DM per hectare [ha] for lactating cows and less than 600 kg DM/ha for lactating ewes) results in liveweight losses during lactation. Essentially no magnesium is obtained from body tissues mobilized during loss of liveweight to support lactation.

Deaths from hypomagnesemic tetany may be as high as 50 per cent in groups of lactating cows on farms. In southeastern Australia losses of 0.5 per cent of cows in dairy herds, and 3 per cent of cows in beef herds have been recorded on a district basis in grass tetany seasons.

Etiology and Pathogenesis

The normal plasma magnesium concentration in ruminants ranges between 0.75 and 1.3 mmol Mg/L. There are no hormonal systems directly controlling plasma magnesium concentrations, and magnesium homeostasis depends on a continual absorption of magnesium from the gut to provide the amounts lost in milk, feces, and urine. Magnesium absorbed in excess of requirements is excreted in the urine.

Cerebrospinal fluid (CSF) magnesium concentrations are maintained in relative constancy despite wide variations in plasma magnesium concentrations. Plasma magnesium concentrations below 0.4 mmol/L may result in a decrease in the concentration of magnesium in CSF below 0.5 mmol/L and lead to hyperexcitability, muscular spasms, convulsions, and death from hypomagnesemic tetany. More commonly, sudden decreases in plasma magnesium and calcium (Ca), and an increase in plasma potassium concentrations precipitate the disorder by causing a rapid decrease in CSF magnesium concentrations.

In ewes, clinical signs of hypomagnesemic tetany do not occur unless there is concomitant hypocalcemia (plasma Ca <2.0 mmol/L). In sheep, lowering both the concentration of magnesium and calcium in the CSF produces more severe convulsions than reducing magnesium concentration alone.

Lush pastures and green cereal crops that have an excess of fixed cations over anions ($Na^{+1} + K^{+1} - Cl^{-1}$) >500 mEq/kg diet dry DM predispose older cows and ewes to metabolic alkalosis and decreased bone mobilization, thereby increasing the risk of hypocalcemia and hypomagnesemia in late pregnancy and early lactation.

There are differences between animals in their ability to absorb magnesium, and the absorption of magnesium from different diets is extremely variable. Most of the variation is due to changes in absorption from the rumen, the main site of absorption in adult ruminants. There is net secretion of magnesium into the small intestine, and this increases as plasma magnesium increases in the normal range. Magnesium is absorbed from the large intestine, but the amounts absorbed are only significant on high magnesium intakes.

The main factors controlling magnesium absorption from

the reticulorumen are its concentration in the liquid phase of the digesta and changes in the rate of active magnesium transport through the rumen wall caused by factors such as potassium. Increasing potassium concentrations in the reticulorumen from 10 to 30 mmol/L in cattle and from 30 to 60 mmol/L in sheep reduces magnesium absorption by increasing the transcellular potential difference across the rumen wall. Intraruminal potassium concentrations increase following ingestion of herbage with high potassium (greater than 0.3 per cent DM), and low sodium (less than 0.15 per cent sodium DM) concentrations when cattle are deficient in sodium and when the diet is changed from hay or dry feed to lush pasture and salivation and sodium entry into the rumen decreases.

High intraruminal ammonium ion concentrations (30 to 70 mmol/L) also reduce magnesium absorption, and this effect is additive and independent of that of potassium. High intraruminal ammonium ion concentrations occur following ingestion of herbage with high nitrogen (4 per cent nitrogen DM) and low soluble carbohydrate concentrations.

Low magnesium concentrations (0.5 to 1.5 mmol/L) in ruminal fluid associated with low magnesium intake, high potassium concentrations (greater than 30 mmol/L), and high rumen ammonium ion concentrations (greater than 30 mmol/L) are more important in restricting magnesium absorption from most herbage diets than binding of magnesium to organic moieties in the rumen contents.

The important etiologic factors in grass tetany include

1. Low magnesium intake, which can arise simply through a reduction in food intake when cows are grazing short grass dominant pastures containing less than 0.2 per cent magnesium (DM basis).
2. High potassium and low sodium intakes, which have important implications for magnesium absorption from the rumen. Soils naturally high in potassium or fertilized with potash and low in sodium are high-risk areas.
3. The cow's ability to maintain calcium homeostasis. Most cows with hypomagnesemia (less than 0.65 mmol magnesium/L) do not develop grass tetany until blood calcium levels decrease below 2.0 mmol/L. Hay feeding is an important control measure in herds in which hypocalcemia precipitates hypomagnesemic grass tetany in older hypomagnesemic cows. Phosphorus deficiency and low intraruminal phosphorus concentrations exacerbate the effects of high potassium intakes on magnesium absorption from the rumen.

Other epidemiologic factors in hypomagnesemic tetany include grazing management, provision of shelter, and husbandry procedures that involve a reduction of food intake in high-risk cows. The incidence is usually higher in thin and fat cows than in cows in moderate body condition. Fat cows maintain higher milk yields through loss of liveweight in early lactation. Thin cows with chronic hypomagnesemia due to underfeeding are more susceptible to tetany during inclement weather.

Clinical Signs

In the initial stages, cows and ewes appear to become restless, separate themselves from the herd or flock, and stop grazing. They seem unusually alert and may suddenly walk or run for no apparent reason. When affected animals are disturbed, they may walk with a high-stepping action of the forelimbs and bellow continuously. They may either attempt to run away or attack when approached. The animal runs with a stiff gait, becomes uncoordinated, staggers, and falls with the limbs showing tetanic spasms interspersed with bouts of clonic convulsions. During the convulsions, the eyeballs appear distended with retraction of the eyelids, and eye movements are erratic and indicative of nystagmus. Fine muscle trembling is present with champing of the jaws and fine frothy saliva around the mouth. The violence of the muscular activity is associated with a very rapid heart rate up to 150 beats/min, and the force of the beats may make the heart sounds audible up to 2 meters away from the cow. The respiratory rate is increased, up to 60/min, and the rectal temperature may be elevated up to 40.5°C with the increased muscular activity. Between convulsive episodes, the animal often relaxes in lateral recumbency, but stimulation such as the insertion of a hypodermic needle for therapy may trigger another bout of tetanic and clonic convulsions. It is not uncommon for cows to die suddenly during a convulsion.

When cows are found dead from hypomagnesemic tetany at pasture, there are usually signs of scuff marks on the ground around the cow caused by her legs and feet during the tetanic convulsions.

SUBACUTE HYPOMAGNESEMIC TETANY. The subacute form resembles the initial stages of an acute attack and is commonly seen in dairy herds yarded for milking after grazing pastures fertilized with potassium and nitrogen. It may also be observed in beef cows during mustering. Signs include frequent urination and defecation and flinching around the head, with the animal acting as though it is going to be struck. Animals may be aggressive during this stage. The pulse and respiratory rates are rapid, and ruminal movements are reduced. Unless affected animals are treated and herds are supplemented with magnesium, losses from clinical hypomagnesemic tetany can be expected.

CHRONIC HYPOMAGNESEMIA. The chronic form is associated with a vague change in temperament and a loss of appetite and body condition. The mean serum or plasma magnesium concentration in 10 randomly selected cows from affected herds is usually less than 0.65 mmol/L. Affected dairy herds show increases in milk fat production following oral supplementation of magnesium oxide. It has been observed that hypomagnesemic cows in herds tend to be less aggressive, and their reduced production has been attributed to reduced grazing activity.

HYPOMAGNESEMIC TETANY IN EWES AND GOATS

The clinical signs of hypomagnesemic tetany in sheep is almost identical to the disease in cattle. Lactating ewes grazing young green cereal crops are most susceptible. When cases occur on grass pastures, hypomagnesemia is usually associated with undernutrition (herbage availability less than 600 kg DM per ha) when grain supplementation ceases following the first rains of autumn.

Older, twin-rearing ewes in better body condition and producing the most milk are most at risk.

In goats, clinical signs are similar to those reported in cattle, and acute, subacute, and chronic forms of the disease have been recorded.

Clinical Pathology and Lesions

Plasma or serum magnesium concentrations less than 0.65 mmol/L indicate hypomagnesemia, and animals with concentrations of less than 0.4 mmol/L are at risk to tetany. There may be concomitant hypocalcemia (<2.0 mmol Ca/L), and hyperkalemia (>7 mmol K/L). Following tetany there is a transient increase in serum aspartate aminotransferase (AST) and creatine phosphokinase (CPK) activities.

Ventricular cerebrospinal fluid magnesium concentrations

less than 0.5 mmol/L are associated with hypomagnesemic tetany and are reliable indicators for up to 12 hours after death. Vitreous humor magnesium concentrations of less than 0.4 mmol/L are associated with hypomagnesemia, and the concentrations provide a reliable indication for up to 48 hours after death, provided that environmental temperatures do not exceed 23°C after 24 hours.

Urine concentrations provide better information on magnesium status and magnesium supply of cattle than blood plasma or serum concentrations. Correction for the variation in urine water excretion is made by dividing the urine magnesium concentration by urine solute concentration (osmolality) or creatinine concentration. When an osmometer or creatinine assays are unavailable, urine solute concentration can be assessed from urine specific gravity measured with a refractometer. The equation

$$\frac{\text{urine mineral concentration (mmol/L)} \times 0.03}{\text{specific gravity} - 1.000}$$

gives similar values to using osmolality measurements on urine samples with specific gravities greater than 1.010.

Urine values >2 μmol Mg/mOsm or 1.5 mmol Mg/mmol creatinine indicate adequate magnesium status, since cattle with these levels are usually in positive magnesium balance. In cattle with hypomagnesemia (plasma Mg <0.65 mmol/L), urine magnesium concentrations are often undetectable. A commercial kit[1] is available to measure urine magnesium.

Urine samples are also used to assess the sodium status of cattle, because sodium deficiency can predispose cattle to hypomagnesemia. A mean urine sodium concentration less than 10 μmol sodium/mOsm from 10 to 20 cows indicates the herd is in negative sodium balance. Sodium deficiency can be confirmed from samples of parotid saliva having a Na:K ratio of less than 5.

Dairy cows in herds with mean blood magnesium concentrations of less than 0.6 mmol/L have shown increases in milk production when supplemented with magnesium. Low plasma concentrations in cows lead to a reduction in the amounts of calcium that can be mobilized in response to hypocalcemia and may predispose milk fever in cows around parturition.

Diagnosis

A history in which lactating cows or ewes grazing lush grass–dominant pasture or green cereal crops have died suddenly after showing signs of tetany and convulsions is suggestive of hypomagnesemic tetany. Recovery of clinically affected animals following treatment with combined solutions of calcium and magnesium and no deaths after Mg supplements are fed may provide confirmatory evidence.

When losses continue despite magnesium supplementation, low sodium nutrition should be suspected, particularly when potassium fertilizers have been applied to sandy soils. Potassium fertilization results in decreased sodium uptake by plants, and dairy cows can develop sodium deficiency after about a month of grazing on pastures containing less than 0.1 per cent sodium DM. The possibility of sodium deficiency should be considered when water is provided from surface storages and streams rather than from bores and when no salt supplements are provided. With sodium deficiency, sodium in saliva decreases and potassium concentrations in rumen fluid become elevated and reduce magnesium absorption.

In cattle, acute lead poisoning produces clinical signs similar to those of hypomagnesemic tetany, but there is usually a history of access to lead, and there may be blindness and mania. Rabies usually includes ascending paralysis, anesthesia, and absence of tetany. Nervous ketosis is characterized by ketonuria and absence of convulsions and tetany. Lightning strike, plant poisoning, and meningitis need to be considered, but the acute clinical case of hypomagnesemic tetany is fairly easy to recognize. Paspalum staggers *(Claviceps paspali)* poisoning is a fairly important differential diagnosis but occurs only when cattle have access to ergots.

When a dairy herd grazing winter and spring pasture shows suboptimal production, hypomagnesemia must be considered. Other diseases causing similar signs include inadequate available herbage, mastitis, parasitism, and deficiencies of copper and cobalt.

Treatment

In clinically affected animals, combined solutions of magnesium and calcium salts are administered by slow intravenous injection. Intravenous injection of magnesium plus calcium reduces the likelihood of inducing cardiac irregularities, medullary depression, and respiratory failure, all of which may occur when magnesium salts alone are administered intravenously. Since relapses often occur after about 6 hours when intravenous calcium and magnesium therapy is given, it is advisable to administer solutions of magnesium sulfate subcutaneously as well. As a guide, 350 ml of a combined solution of calcium borogluconate (25 per cent wt/vol) and hypophosphite (5 per cent wt/vol) is given intravenously, and 100 to 200 ml of a 50 per cent solution of magnesium sulfate is injected subcutaneously.

To prevent relapses in cows treated under range conditions, we also administer orally a slurry of 100 g magnesium oxide, 100 g dicalcium phosphate, 50 g calcium carbonate, and 50 g sodium chloride. Alternatively, 60 g magnesium chloride ($MgCl_2$) or magnesium sulfate ($MgSO_4$) in 200 ml water can be given as an enema. The herd is supplemented with hay at the rate of 4 kg/cow/day, and magnesium oxide (MgO) (60 g daily or 120 g every second day) is added to the hay.

For parenteral therapy, sterile solutions of 10, 20, and 50 per cent wt/vol magnesium sulfate are available from a number of sources. Also available are combined solutions of either calcium borogluconate (25 per cent wt/vol), dextrose (25 per cent wt/vol) with magnesium chloride (4 per cent wt/vol), or hypophosphite (5 per cent wt/vol), or simply calcium borogluconate (25 per cent wt/vol) and ($MgCl_2$) (4 per cent wt/vol). Other combinations include magnesium as the citrate and varying combinations of ingredients. Packaging is 100 ml for sheep and goats and includes 200-, 300-, 350-, 500-, and 1000-ml sizes for cattle.

Response to therapy is variable and is related to the interval between the onset of tetany and the commencement of therapy. Most cattle respond within an hour, the delay in response being related to the time taken to restore CSF magnesium concentrations.

Care should be taken to avoid unnecessary disturbance of clinically affected cows while they are being treated. In cows at risk of severe injury from continuous convulsions, the use of sedatives and tranquilizers has been recommended.

Prevention

Since there is no readily available store of magnesium in the body, supplementation has to be given daily to animals at risk of hypomagnesemic tetany. Most magnesium salts are quite unpalatable, and an important practical aspect in supple-

---

[1] Equipment: Magnesium in Bovine Urine, no 11005. E. Merck, Rahway, NJ, and Darmstadt, Germany.

mental feeding is combining magnesium with other palatable ingredients such as molasses, concentrates, and hay.

Feeding hay alone may be all that is required to prevent hypomagnesemic tetany in some herds in which only old cows are affected. Other herds may require the addition of magnesium, sodium, and phosphorus. Correction of sodium deficiency aids prevention of hypomagnesemic tetany, but provision of salt to cows receiving adequate sodium intakes may be detrimental.

There are several ways of providing magnesium supplements for ruminants, including individual drenching, treatment of hay, pasture topdressing, water trough treatments, and magnesium licks. It is desirable that the magnesium supplement be readily soluble in the rumen liquor and be sufficient to prevent the development of hypomagnesemia in any individual animal in a herd.

Individual dairy cows may be drenched daily with 20 MgO or 100 g $MgSO_4 \cdot 7H_2O$ or 100 g $MgCl_2 \cdot 6H_2O$ to provide 10 g magnesium. Micronized (<300 mesh) magnesium oxide can be suspended in water and 20 g can be administered by drenching guns provided it is constantly mixed to maintain the suspension.

Magnesium oxide may also be added to hay at the rate of 50 g MgO/cow/day.

Pastures may be dusted with magnesium oxide (calcined magnesite, 60 mesh) at the rate of 500 g/cow just prior to grazing. One treatment at weekly intervals usually suffices, but if rainfall exceeds 40 to 50 mm within 2 to 3 days of dusting, the pastures will require re-dusting.

Addition of magnesium chloride or magnesium sulfate to water is usually an unreliable method of supplementing cows, because water intake by cows is generally low when they are tetany-prone through grazing lush pastures.

Magnesium licks are considered unreliable for 100 per cent protection, because some cows are not good lickers, and licking behavior may be intermittent. More cows accept licks if they have been exposed to licks as calves. Homemade recipes for extensive grazing situations include 1:1 magnesium oxide:molasses, 5:3:2 salt:molasses:magnesium oxide, and 2:2:2:2:2 salt:calcium carbonate:dicalcium phosphate (DCP):molasses:magnesium oxide. Most commercial magnesium licks and blocks contain up to 80 per cent molasses. Licks and blocks should be placed near watering points or stock camping areas. Crusts that develop on licks should be removed, and licks should be moistened before cows are allowed access.

Intraruminal magnesium devices (Sire Sign Magnesium Capsules),[1] which release about 1.5 g Mg/day for 90 days after a stabilizing period of 1 week are marketed as an aid to grass tetany prevention in cattle. Magnesium alloy boluses (Rumbul bullets),[2] weighing 100 g and containing 86 per cent magnesium have also been used. Usually these intraruminal devices do not increase serum magnesium concentrations above those of untreated cows. It is recommended that cattle receiving these devices be also fed hay and the devices be used as an alternative to adding magnesium oxide to the hay.

Magnesium fertilizers are useful in increasing herbage magnesium concentrations on acid, sandy soils with low cation exchange capacity but are not recommended for fine-textured soils of high-cation exchange capacity or calcareous soils. When magnesium fertilizers are contemplated for prevention of hypomagnesemic tetany, trials should be done to assess their effectiveness in increasing herbage magnesium.

Older lactating cows should not be grazed on short green pastures on paddocks that have been fertilized with potassium fertilizers.

HYPOMAGNESEMIC TETANY IN MILK-FED CALVES

In young ruminants, magnesium is absorbed from the small intestine, whereas in adult ruminants the small intestine is a site of net magnesium secretion. The rumen becomes the major site of absorption once it develops; the large intestine is also a site of net magnesium absorption, although of lesser importance than the rumen. Magnesium is absorbed efficiently (0.9) from milk by young calves. The coefficient of absorption decreases rapidly with age, and in calves fed milk on fibrous bedding, the values decrease to 0.12 at 14 weeks of age. Calves fed milk diets deficient in magnesium for extended periods show poor growth, calcification of soft tissue, increased irritability, tetany, and convulsions.

Hypomagnesemic tetany in calves must be differentiated from acute lead poisoning, tetanus, strychnine poisoning, polioencephalomalacia, and enterotoxemia caused by the toxin of *Clostridium perfringens*. Analysis of bone calcium and magnesium provides a useful aid to diagnosis. Normal bone has a ratio of calcium:magnesium of 70:1, and in hypomagnesemic calves this ratio may exceed 90:1.

Affected calves should be treated with 100 ml of 10 per cent wt/vol magnesium sulfate solution subcutaneously and should be given oral treatments of magnesium oxide. Suggested dosages are 1, 2, and 3 g magnesium oxide daily for calves up to 5 weeks, from 5 to 10 weeks, and from 10 to 15 weeks of age, respectively. Provision of good quality legume hay and a starter ration from 2 weeks of age prevents the disorder.

BIBLIOGRAPHY

Reinhardt TA, Horst RL, Goff JP: Calcium, phosphorus and magnesium homeostasis in ruminants. Vet Clin North Am: Food Animal Practice 4:331–350. 1988.

Robinson DL, Kappel LC, Boling JA: Management practices to overcome the incidence of grass tetany. J Anim Sci 67:3470–3484, 1989.

Downer Cow Syndrome
JAKOB MALMO, BVSc, FACVSc

The term *downer cow syndrome* is widely used in cattle medicine but is not clearly defined. Definitions have varied from "any cow that does not rise within 10 minutes after administration of one calcium treatment" to "a cow that remains in sternal recumbency for 24 hours after initial recumbency."

A typical downer cow appears bright and alert but is unable to rise. In practice, many downer cows have remained recumbent after treatment for hypocalcemia. Many conditions can lead to recumbency in cattle. Careful examination of the history and findings of a complete clinical examination are necessary to diagnose the etiology of recumbency in the animal being assessed.

OCCURRENCE

The incidence of the downer cow syndrome in dairy and beef herds depends on a number of factors, including

---

[1]Manufactured by Cheetham Rural, Wacol, Qld, Australia under license from CSIRO.
[2]Pitman-Moore Animal Health Ltd., 1025 Tremaine Ave, Palmerston North, New Zealand.

- Criteria used to define the condition
- Incidence of milk fever and the interval between onset of recumbency and treatment
- Body condition score of cows at parturition
- Size and breed of animals—following hypocalcemia, the syndrome is more likely to occur in larger cows than in smaller cows

An incidence of 21.4 cases per 1000 cow years was determined for Minnesota dairy herds, using the criterion of 24 hours of paradoxical sternal recumbency to define a downer cow. Of these recumbent cows, 33 per cent recovered, 23 per cent were slaughtered, and 44 per cent died or required euthanasia.

Downer cows are most commonly seen in the interval from 2 days before to 10 days after parturition. Downer cows are usually between 5 and 8 years of age and are high producers. Many have a history of parturient paresis.

ETIOLOGY AND PATHOGENESIS

The downer cow syndrome is most commonly seen as a sequel to parturient paresis. It has been observed that the incidence of the downer cow condition increases with time between the onset of milk fever and the initiation of calcium therapy.

Evidence of the role of pressure damage in the pathogenesis of the downer cow condition has been derived from experiments in which cows were positioned in sternal recumbency with the right hind leg under the body. Halothane anesthesia was used to maintain this position for 6 to 12 hours. After recovery from anesthesia, 8 out of 16 animals were unable to stand and became permanent downers. When the animals attempted to stand the right hind leg was weaker than the noncompressed left hind leg.

MUSCLE DAMAGE WITH OR WITHOUT COMPARTMENT SYNDROME. Prolonged recumbency leads to muscle damage with or without compartment syndrome. The local damage caused by compression of muscles during recumbency may lead to increased pressure within an osteofascial compartment. Internal filling of the compartment with blood or edematous fluid may also cause increased pressure within an osteofascial compartment. A combined effect arises when external compression causes ischemia, leading to "leaky" blood vessels and postcompression swelling. Muscles such as the semitendinosus, which has thick fascial boundaries, are susceptible to pressure-induced compartment syndrome. However, the large thigh muscles of the cow are each surrounded by thin elastic fascia and may not be as susceptible to compartment syndrome. In these large thigh muscles, irregular areas of ischemic necrosis are found in cows that have been in prolonged recumbency.

The term *crush syndrome* is used to describe the systemic effects of muscle damage. These systemic effects are largely attributable to absorption of muscle breakdown products into the circulation. Brown discolored urine (due to myoglobin) and extremely high serum or plasma creatine kinase (CK) values are common in downer cows.

Most pressure-induced lesions in downer cows are in the hamstring (biceps femoris, semitendinosus, and semimembranosus muscles) and adductor regions of the thigh, where large muscle masses may be affected.

NERVE DAMAGE. Distal to the greater trochanter, the sciatic nerve of recumbent cattle is compressed against the caudal aspect of the femur just distal to the point where the sciatic nerve traverses the hip joint. In 1982 Cox and colleagues concluded that since there were no significant differences in serum CK activity between downer and ambulatory cows 12 hours after induced recumbency, the clinical differences were due to sciatic nerve damage.

The peroneal nerve is vulnerable to compression damage on the lateral side of the stifle joint, where it passes over the proximal end of the fibula. When there is peroneal paralysis, the cow knuckles over on the fetlock when attempting to walk.

SKELETAL DAMAGE. Pelvic fractures occur most commonly following falls on hard surfaces or following "riding" by other cows. Fractures of the femoral neck and coxofemoral dislocations may occur in recumbent cows struggling to stand, particularly in cows with moderate degrees of calving paralysis.

METABOLIC DISORDERS. Complex metabolic disorders may arise during prolonged recumbency secondary to parturient paresis and include hypophosphatemia, hypomagnesemia, hypokalemia, hypoproteinemia, cerebral edema, and ketosis with liver failure.

Cows initially recumbent as a result of hypomagnesemia, generalized systemic illness (e.g., mastitis, metritis, peritonitis), calving paralysis, spinal injury, or paralysis caused by lymphosarcomatous lesions in the vertebral column may subsequently suffer muscle, nerve, or skeletal damage.

CLINICAL SIGNS

Typically, downer cows are bright and alert and will eat and ruminate, although their appetite may be reduced. Temperature and heart and respiratory rates are usually within the normal range. Defecation is normal, but proteinuria is common. Affected cows sit in sternal recumbency and when stimulated to rise they either will not try or, if they do, they are unable to extend their hind limbs to reach a standing position. Some cows make frequent attempts to rise, resulting in the cow "creeping" or "crawling" along the ground with both hind limbs flexed and displaced posteriorly.

Downer cows affected more severely may sit in sternal recumbency and appear almost normal when supported, but when left unattended they move into lateral recumbency. Some exhibit expiratory moaning and most develop mucoid feces that may contain spots of blood. These animals are referred to as nonalert downer cows.

CLINICAL PATHOLOGY

Serum calcium and phosphate levels normally rise when cows recover from parturient paresis following treatment with calcium, but in cows that remain downers, phosphorus concentrations often remain low. Serum potassium levels have been reported to be low (<3.0 mmol/L) in "creeper" cows that are able to control their forelimbs following calcium therapy but are unable to use their hind limbs.

Serum asparate aminotransferase (AST) and CK levels are usually elevated and indicate muscle damage. The half-life of CK enzyme in blood is short. In cows with induced downer cow syndrome, the maximum serum CK activity occurs after 48 hours and then falls rapidly, even though cows remained recumbent. Plasma AST increases more slowly than plasma CK following recumbency and remains elevated for longer.

A marked proteinuria is usually present 24 hours after the onset of recumbency. In severe cases, the urine may be brown because of severe myoglobinuria. Ketonuria and bilirubinuria may also be present in complicated cases.

There are no specific lesions at necropsy, but hemorrhage and degeneration can be found in the upper hind leg musculature (particularly the medial thigh muscles) and nerves of most downer cows. Some have myocarditis.

DIAGNOSIS

The clinical sign of recumbency 24 hours after its onset is the basis of diagnosis of the downer cow syndrome. It is essential to conduct a systematic and thorough clinical examination to obtain an informed differential diagnosis. Special attention should be paid to the caudal part of the spine, including the tail, the pelvic ring, and the hind legs. Rectal examination is essential. Painful reactions to manipulation, abnormal mobility, lack of motor and sensory responses, or audible crepitation may reveal the site and nature of the physical injuries responsible for prolonged recumbency.

Diagnosis of the downer cow syndrome is made largely by eliminating the other possible causes of continued recumbency. Conditions that must be excluded include

- Maternal obstetrical paralysis
- Systemic disease such as coliform mastitis, acute metritis, acute diffuse peritonitis, ephemeral fever, or lymphosarcomatous lesions in the vertebral canal causing spinal compression
- Physical injuries such as pelvic or limb fractures, coxofemoral dislocations, spinal injuries, rupture of the gastrocnemius muscle, and radial paralysis

TREATMENT

The first approach must be to ensure that the affected animal has been adequately treated for hypocalcemia. A slow intravenous injection of a solution containing calcium, magnesium, phosphorous, and dextrose is given while the rate, rhythm, and intensity of heart sounds are carefully monitored. This may be followed by intravenous injection of a phosphorus-containing solution (e.g., 30 g of sodium acid phosphate [Sodaphos[1]] in 300 ml of water or 20 to 40 ml of butaphosphan [Coforta 5%[2]] injectable phosphorus solution). The rationale for this treatment is that downer cows often have persistent hypophosphatemia. Tripelennamine hydrochloride (Vetibenzamine), given at a dose rate of 10 to 15 ml intravenously, appears to act as a potent, temporary central nervous stimulant in cattle and is usually given before attempting to get the affected animal to rise. Before any of these attempts, it is essential that the cow be moved and positioned so that she has a reasonable footing should she attempt to rise. It is essential to move downer cows from concrete floors or slippery, muddy yards before attempting to get them to stand.

Downer cows may be stimulated to rise by using a cattle goad. When the cow attempts to rise, assistance can be given by lifting strongly on her tail. If this is unsuccessful, another approach is to restrain the cow in lateral recumbency and electrically stimulate (using a cattle goad) the tibial and peroneal nerve of the uppermost limb several times. This will cause the cow to kick the stimulated leg vigorously. The cow is then rolled on to the other side and the stimulation is repeated. The cow is allowed to rest for several minutes; then another attempt is made to urge the cow to rise, again assisting by lifting strongly on her tail. Under no circumstances should downer cows be lifted by the tail when they do not attempt to stand.

In animals that cannot rise following this therapy, lifting devices can be of considerable use. This applies particularly to larger cows that try to get up when encouraged but cannot stand with manual assistance. Bagshawe's hip clamps, which fit over the tuber coxae, are most useful in lifting recumbent cows that can nearly stand. Some cows resent their use and either simply hang in them or throw their head and shoulders onto the ground. In this situation, use of hip clamps should be discontinued. Effective slings and pneumatic bags have been developed. The slings have adjustable webbing straps and are designed to reduce pressure on the abdomen. These slings and pneumatic bags can support downer cows safely for longer than hip clamps. However, any lifting device, inappropriately used, can be counterproductive.

If the downer cow still cannot be made to stand, it should be moved to a clean dry area and sheltered from inclement weather. Affected cows should be kept in sternal recumbency, changed from side to side at least every 3 hours, and regularly fed and watered. Adequate bedding is necessary to protect the bony prominences. Lifting devices, if used at all, should be used sparingly. It must be stressed to the animal attendant that downer cows need careful nursing, which can be time-consuming.

My experience has been that, provided they remain bright and alert and continue to eat and drink well, many of these cows will get to their feet within 2 weeks. Complications such as acute mastitis or coxofemoral dislocation lead to a much more guarded prognosis.

PREVENTION

As most downer cows have previously been recumbent from parturient paresis, the prevention of milk fever will markedly reduce the incidence of downer cows. The article on parturient paresis details its treatment and prevention.

Animal supervision is important in the prevention of downer cows. The time interval between the onset of recumbency and treatment for parturient paresis should be as short as possible. The aim is to prevent prolonged recumbency and muscle damage. Treatment for parturient paresis must ensure that animals receive sufficient calcium. The amount of calcium required to effect a recovery seems to vary, but at least 12 g of calcium (Ca) given intravenously may be required to effect a cure. A solution of 25 per cent calcium borogluconate contains 10.4 g Ca/500 ml. Underdosing increases the risk of incomplete recovery and continued recumbency. Cows should be observed closely after treatment for possible relapse.

Provision of adequate bedding for cows housed during parturition and supervision of cows to minimize prolonged dystocia are important measures to prevent traumatic nerve and muscular damage.

BIBLIOGRAPHY

Cox VS: Nonsystemic causes of the downer cow syndrome. Vet Clin North Am: Food Animal Practice 4:413–433, 1988.
Cox VS, McGrath CJ, Jorgensen SE: The role of pressure damage in pathogenesis of the downer cow syndrome. J Am Vet Res 43:26, 1982.
Kikta MJ, Meyer JP, Bishara RA, et al: Crush syndrome due to limb compression. Arch Surg 122:1078, 1987.
Stober M, Dirksen G: The recumbent cow: differential diagnosis and differential therapy. Vet Ann 22:81–94, 1982.

Postparturient Hemoglobinuria

CHRISTOPHER J. McCAUGHAN, BVSc, MACVSc

Postparturient hemoglobinuria of dairy cows is characterized by intravascular hemolysis, hemoglobinuria, and anemia. The disorder is associated with a variety of factors and has been observed in many countries. It is not common and causes

---
[1]Available from Parnell Laboratories.
[2]Available from Bayer Co.

minor economic losses. Usually only 1 or 2 cows in a herd are affected, although prevalences up to 40 per cent have been recorded, and up to 50 per cent of affected cows may die.

OCCURRENCE

The disease in mature cows usually occurs within 6 weeks of parturition, when cows housed during the winter are turned out to graze on grass in spring and summer. When cows are kept at pasture, the disease occurs in the winter, especially if it is preceded by a dry summer and fall. Generally, affected cows have been fed hay and have limited access to grass pasture in the dry period, then allowed unlimited access to lush grass pasture during early lactation. In Australia it has been proposed that the disease follows recovery from preparturient ketoacidosis caused by undernutrition in late pregnancy, but this association is not always so clear.

Phosphorus deficiency has long been associated with the occurrence of the condition in cows, as has the ingestion of green oats; lush perennial rye grass; newly established subterranean clover; and turnips, rape, kale, and other cruciferous plants. Anemia and hemoglobinemia may occur in sheep and cattle grazing cruciferous and other plants and may not be related to the postparturient period. In New Zealand, predisposition of younger cows to the condition has been attributed to a copper deficiency associated with excessive application of molybdenum fertilizer and lime to pastures.

ETIOLOGY AND PATHOGENESIS

The mechanisms operating to cause intravascular hemolysis are unknown and may vary, depending on the nature of the predisposing factors. Not all outbreaks can be associated with phosphorus deficiency, molybdenum-induced copper deficiency, or cruciferous plant feeding. Hemolytic factors present in some diets may produce oxidative damage to hemoglobin, whereas other diets may render the erythrocytes more susceptible to oxidant challenge. Protection against peroxidation in erythrocytes depends on adequate levels of nicotinamide-adenine dinucleotide phosphate (NADPH reduced form) and reduced glutathione, on the function of the pentose phosphate pathway, and on an adequate supply of glucose.

Inorganic phosphate is a cofactor necessary for activity of glyceraldehyde-3-phosphate dehydrogenase, which plays a key role in erythrocyte glycolysis and the formation of adenosine 5′-triphosphate (ATP). ATP controls erythrocyte shape and plasticity by enabling active extrusion of sodium. Hemolysis associated with ATP depletion can occur with metabolic acidosis and severe hypophosphatemia.

In metabolic acidosis, phosphorus moves from within cells to plasma, and phosphorus excretion in urine is increased. Following restoration of acid-base balance, phosphorylated carbohydrates are re-formed within the cell. This requires a large phosphorus input from the serum pool and may precipitate a profound and rapid hypophosphatemia. Even with an adequate dietary intake of phosphorus, cows grazing on lush green pastures may suffer a net phosphorus depletion as a result of lack of phosphorus flow into the rumen with reduced salivary input and excessive excretion of phosphorus in urine.

Hypophosphatemia depresses glycolysis and lowers the concentration of ATP in bovine erythrocytes. Below a critical point for phosphorus, erythrocytes become spherocytic and rigid. As they pass through capillary beds, erythrocytes may rupture and the onset of hemoglobinuria follows. Highly productive milk cows may be the most at risk, because they excrete more phosphorus in milk, but in practice it appears that the metabolic processes are more important than excretory loss because many cases have been reported in which low- as well as high-yielding milk cows have been affected.

The erythrocyte is also protected from oxidant injury by the actions of the copper-containing enzyme superoxide dismutase; largely by the glutathione system, of which the selenium-containing enzyme glutathione peroxidase is a component; and by vitamin E. Activity of these antioxidants in the erythrocytes is determined, respectively, by the copper, selenium, and vitamin E intake of the cow. Cattle low in these dietary factors are more prone to Heinz-body hemolytic anemia. Hemolytic anemia in cattle of low selenium status has been corrected by selenium supplementation. The importance of various nutritional factors in the pathogenesis of hemolysis and in the predisposition of cows to postparturient hemoglobinuria awaits full definition.

The hemolytic anemia of kale poisoning is due to S-methylcysteine sulfoxide that is converted in the rumen to a secondary hemolysin, dimethyl disulfide. The onset of the hemolytic crisis is indicated by increased Heinz-body counts and erythrocyte osmotic fragility and decreased hemoglobin and blood glutathione. An increase in Heinz bodies indicates exposure to sulfhydryl reactive agents. They occur as breakdown products formed as a result of oxidative damage to hemoglobin that precipitate as coccoid granules, binding to the erythrocyte membranes.

Other dietary oxidants suggested to be involved are nitrates yielding hydroxylamine, unsaturated fatty acids, aromatic amines, and hydropteridines.

Heinz-body anemia is the main feature of postparturient hemoglobinuria associated with molybdenum-induced copper deficiency in dairy cows in New Zealand. This disorder is not related to phosphorus deficiency, and there is no increase in erythrocyte osmotic fragility. Heinz bodies have not been a consistent finding in outbreaks associated with phosphorus deficiency elsewhere or when cows have developed the disorder on ryegrass or clover pastures.

CLINICAL SIGNS

The onset of clinical signs is usually rapid, and the disease runs an acute course of 3 to 5 days. Sickness is first indicated by weakness and staggering gait, lowered milk production, and hemoglobinuria characterized by dark red-brown to black urine, which is often moderately turbid. In less acute cases, appetite and milk yield may be unaffected for 24 hours after hemoglobinuria is observed. In severe cases, milk production ceases, and the cow may lose weight and become dehydrated. The heart rate is increased (50 to 130 beats/min), and the jugular pulse is more pronounced. Respiratory rate is increased, and rectal temperature is often slightly elevated (39° to 40°C) in the first stage of the disease, but usually it is normal or subnormal.

As the condition progresses, the visible mucous membranes are pale, indicating anemia, and the cow becomes dehydrated, weaker, and recumbent. Jaundice is observed if the cow lives long enough. Photosensitization, gangrene, and sloughing of the teats, the tip of the tail, and the digits have occasionally been observed, as has diarrhea. Intercurrent disease such as mastitis and a history of forced exercise is often associated with fatal cases. In nonfatal cases, ketosis commonly occurs concurrently, and convalescence takes from 3 weeks to 2 months. A number of other clinical signs are observed with the predisposing factors. Pica, osteomalacia, lameness, predisposition to botulism, and foreign body obstructions in the alimentary tract are evident only if phosphorus deficiency has been induced by a dietary lack of phosphorus. Anemia is common in cows fed cruciferous plants and in cows in copper-deficient areas.

CLINICAL PATHOLOGY

Hemoglobinuria needs to be differentiated from myoglobinuria. The presence of hemoglobin in the urine can be determined by its reaction with reagent strips (Labstix; see note, Table 1, for source), and absence of erythrocytes on microscopic examination of urine confirms hemoglobinuria. Hematologic examination shows a low hemoglobin value (<8 g/100 ml), and a low erythrocyte count (<5 × $10^6/\mu L$), together with evidence of bone marrow response to anemia-anisocytosis, macrocytosis with polychromasia, basophilic stippling of erythrocytes, and higher numbers of nucleated erythrocytes. Heinz bodies may be demonstrated by mixing whole blood (or sedimented cells retrieved from a clotted sample) with 4 volumes of 0.5 per cent methyl violet in 0.85 per cent saline. The mixture is left to stand for 10 minutes, is centrifuged at low speed, and a film is made from the deposited cells. Heinz bodies are intensely purple-stained intracorpuscular structures near the edges of the erythrocytes in 3 to 50 per cent of cells.

In phosphorus-deficient areas, normally lactating cows have low serum concentrations of inorganic phosphate (2 to 3 mg/100 ml or 0.6 to 0.9 mmol/L), and affected cows have levels of 0.3 to 1 mg/100 ml (0.09 to 0.3 mmol/L). When a copper deficiency exists, blood copper concentration is usually less than 30 µg/100 ml, and liver copper concentration is less than 5 mg/kg on a dry matter basis. Elevated serum bilirubin and blood urea nitrogen levels are found in cows during the advanced stages of the disorder.

At necropsy, lesions observed are a general jaundiced condition of the carcass, a pale swollen liver with centrilobular necrosis attributed to anemic anoxia, and hemoglobinuric nephrosis of the kidneys.

DIAGNOSIS

Laboratory examination is needed to confirm the diagnosis of postparturient hemoglobinuria. An acute hemolytic anemia and hemoglobinuria in cows in the first 6 weeks of lactation is only suggestive of the disease. Postparturient hemoglobinuria is usually afebrile. Other causes of afebrile hemoglobinuria include feeding on cruciferous plants, chronic copper poisoning, blood transfusion reactions, porphyria, facial eczema caused by the ingestion of sporidesmin-coated spores of *Pithomyces chartarum,* and poisoning due to blue-green algae, *Allium* or *Xanthorrhoea* species. Febrile hemoglobinuria may occur with leptospirosis, babesiosis, theileriosis, bacillary hemoglobinuria, septicemic pasteurellosis, and pyelonephritis. Some plants contain phenolic compounds that when eaten by cows lead to the formation of red, brown, or black urine. Drugs that have caused Heinz-body hemolytic anemia in animals include phenothiazine, methylene blue, paracetamol, and propylene glycol. In humans, oxidant drugs such as sulfonamides, nitrofurans, aspirin, and phenacetin have also induced Heinz-body formation and hemolysis with erythrocyte glucose-6-phosphate dehydrogenase deficiency.

TREATMENT

Because the cause of the condition is unknown, supportive therapy is given to combat acute hemolytic anemia and dehydration, and the predisposing causes are eliminated. At least 5 to 10 L of whole blood should be given to severely affected cows, and additional fluids can be administered orally. When phosphorus deficiency is considered to be a predisposing cause, intravenous injection of 60 g of sodium acid phosphate in 300 ml of sterile distilled water and a similar subcutaneous dose are given, followed by further injections at 12-hour intervals for 3 treatments (Table 1). All cows are drenched with 30 g sodium acid phosphate or 150 g bone meal or fed 100 g/day of dicalcium phosphate (DCP). In view of the importance of an adequate supply of glucose in preventing hemolysis of erythrocytes, glucose should be included in solutions given intravenously. Caution should be exercised with IV infusion if hypertonic solutions are to be used. Calcium hypophosphite (30 g in 100 ml of 10 per cent glucose) has been used to treat affected cows. Methylene blue administered intravenously as an antioxidant should prove beneficial for treatment, because it drives erythrocyte glucose metabolism through the pentose phosphate shunt. It should be used warily if renal disease is present. Glucocorticoids (20 mg dexamethasone intramuscularly) and oral treatments for ketosis are also beneficial.

In copper-deficient areas, cows are given copper glycinate subcutaneously to provide 120 mg of available copper, or 20 g oxidized wire needles orally. Other cows should be treated

Table 1. TESTS AND DRUG THERAPY FOR POSTPARTURIENT HEMOGLOBINURIA

Test or Drug	Supplier[5]	Species	Dose
Labstix	Ames Division[1]	Bovine	—
Sodium acid phosphate	Parnell[2]	Bovine	60 g in 300 ml H$_2$O (IV) (e.g., Sodaphos)
Calcium hypophosphite	—	Bovine	30 g in 100 ml 10% glucose (IV)
Glucocorticoids	Many	Bovine	5 mg/100 kg (IM)
Copper			
oxidized wire (Cuprax)	Pitman-Moore[3]	Bovine	20 g orally
Copper glycinate (Cuprate)	Burns-Biotec[4]	Bovine	2 ml (SC) containing 120 mg Cu
Methylene blue	Parnell[2]	Bovine	2–4 mg/kg (IV)

[1]Miles Australia Pty, Ltd., Wellington Rd, Mulgrave, Victoria 3170, Austrl.
[2]Parnell Laboratories (Austrl) Pty, Ltd., 21/28 Vore St, Silverwater, NSW 2141, Austrl.
[3]Coopers Pitman-Moore, 71 Epping Road, North Ryde, NSW 2113, Austrl.
[4]Division of Chromalloy Pharmaceuticals, Inc., Oakland, CA.
[5]Many of these preparations are sold under a variety of trade names. Consult publications such as Veterinary Pharmaceuticals and Biologicals, 6th ed, Veterinary Medicine Publishing Co, Lenexa, KS, 1989–1990.
Cu = Copper; IM = intramuscular; IV = intravenous; SC = subcutaneous.

within 48 hours of calving to prevent the condition. Cruciferous plants should be removed from the diet, and the cows should be fed good quality hay. Hematinics, including iron supplementation, folic acid, and vitamin B_{12} have been given to affected cows, but their therapeutic value has not been evaluated. Any intercurrent disease may also require treatment.

PREVENTION

An adequate dietary intake of phosphorus in early lactation is essential in phosphorus-deficient areas. This can be ensured by supplementation with sodium acid phosphate (30 g/cow/day), DCP (100 mg/cow/day), bone meal (100 g/cow/day), or bone meal licks. In copper-deficient areas, pastures can be topdressed with copper or cows can be given copper glycinate subcutaneously in the month before parturition to provide 120 mg of available copper. Alternatively, cows may be dosed with 20 g oxidized wire needles. Selenium supplements can be provided through fertilizer application or oral or parenteral treatments to cattle. Restricting the intake of cruciferous plants to less than 1.5 kg/day, and restricting the intake of turnips and beet pulp during the first 2 months of lactation is advisable. Exposure to the predisposing factors should be avoided.

BIBLIOGRAPHY

Ellison RS, Young BJ, Read DH: Bovine post-parturient haemoglobinuria: two distinct entities in New Zealand. NZ Vet J 34:7–10, 1986.

Jubb TF, Jerrett IV, Browning JW, Thomas KW: Haemoglobinuria and hypophosphataemia in post-parturient dairy cows without dietary deficiency of phosphorus. Austr Vet J 67:86–89, 1990.

Madsden DE, Nielson HM: Parturient hemoglobinemia of dairy cows. J Am Vet Med Assoc 47:577–586, 1939.

SECTION 6
Physical and Chemical Disorders

JOHN C. HALLIBURTON, DVM, PhD, Diplomate, ABVT, Consulting Editor

Feed-Related Toxicoses

Ammoniated Feed Toxicosis

SANDRA E. MORGAN, DVM, MS

Ammoniated feed syndrome, bovine bonkers, and bovine hysteria are all names that have been associated with hyperexcitability sometimes seen in cows and calves that have ingested ammoniated hay, molasses, or silage and molasses-urea-protein blocks. The common factors in these feedstuffs are ammonia (either directly from the ammoniation process or indirectly from the urea), moisture, heat, alkaline pH, and carbohydrates that provide a source of soluble reducing sugars.

Ammoniation of feed has become a popular inexpensive way to replace 30 to 40 per cent of the protein-derived nitrogen in the diet with nonprotein nitrogen, improve the palatability of the ration, increase the digestibility (particularly of crude protein and crude fiber), and increase the rate of gain and efficiency of feed utilization.

The forages most often reported with this toxicity syndrome have been high-quality hays such as sudan, wheat, alfalfa, Bermuda grass, fescue, orchard grass, and forage sorghums. Although rice straw and wheat straw have been associated with this toxicity problem, the incidence is much lower. Corn stalks, corn silage, and most small grain straws have low levels of soluble sugars and should not cause problems.

When there is excessive environmental heat during the ammoniation process, moisture greater than 20 per cent, ample soluble sugars, and excessive rates of anhydrous ammonia application (greater than 3 per cent of the forage dry matter), toxic substances called imidazoles are formed.

CLINICAL SIGNS

The most notable characteristic of this syndrome is the sudden onset of symptoms in an apparently healthy animal and the equally sudden termination of them. A resting animal may jump up, stampede wildly, bellow, and run into fences or any object in its way as if it did not see them. Often the only things a rancher finds are a torn up fence and animals with broken legs or other injury. Other observations have been restlessness, frequent urination and defecation, involuntary ear twitching, rapid blinking, dilation of the pupils, impairment of vision, trembling, rapid respiration, loss of balance, salivation, frothing at the mouth, sweating, bellowing, and convulsions. All ages of cattle exhibit similar symptoms, but some die whereas others recover spontaneously if they have not injured themselves seriously.

PATHOLOGY

There have been no gross or microscopic lesions associated with this syndrome. Excessive bruising, abrasions, and broken bones are often the only findings after an episode of stampeding.

DIAGNOSIS

A diagnosis can be made by a combination of clinical signs associated with ingestion of ammoniated forages, ammoniated molasses, or molasses-urea-protein blocks. Imidazoles, in particular 4-methylimidazole, have been found in toxic forages when samples were sent to diagnostic laboratories.

TREATMENT

There is no known treatment or antidote for this toxicity problem. The feed should be removed immediately from cattle exhibiting symptoms. Some calves that reportedly survived were sedated with acepromazine (0.045 mg/kg intravenously and 0.045 mg/kg intramuscularly) for prevention of self-mutilation and given thiamine hydrochloride (1.14 mg/kg intravenously and 1.14 mg/kg intramuscularly), but others never responded to any treatment.

PREVENTION

The best prevention is to try to get clients to follow these guidelines when they ammoniate forages: ammoniate poor-quality roughage; calculate the amount of ammonia carefully so it will not be more than 3 per cent of the dry weight of the straw; and ammoniate during the cooler seasons because hay closest to the black plastic was found to be toxic whereas hay underneath was not.

If a feedstuff has caused symptoms, the choices are to remove it immediately or dilute it and mix it with other forages. Avoid feeding it to cows nursing calves and within 1 week before calving. There is evidence that the toxin may be passed in the milk.

BIBLIOGRAPHY

Haliburton JC, Morgan SE: Nonprotein nitrogen induced ammonia toxicosis and ammoniated feed syndrome. Vet Clin North Am [Large Anim Pract] 5:237–249, 1989.

Kerr LA, Groce AW, Kersting KW: Ammoniated forage toxicosis in calves. J Am Vet Med Assoc 191:551–552, 1987.

Morgan SE, Edwards WC: Bovine bonkers: new terminology for an old problem. Vet Hum Toxicol 28:16–18, 1986.

Sodium Ion Toxicosis

ROBERT H. POPPENGA, DVM, PhD,
DIPLOMATE, ABVT

CIRCUMSTANCES OF TOXICOSIS

Sodium ion toxicosis occurs most frequently in swine and poultry, although it is reported to occur in other livestock species such as cattle and sheep. Ingestion of excessive sodium alone is not necessarily hazardous if sufficient fresh water of low salinity is available. However, if fresh water is not available or water intake is restricted in some fashion, otherwise safe dietary concentrations of sodium can cause toxicosis. As an example, feeds containing recommended concentrations of sodium chloride of 0.5 to 1.0 per cent (0.2 to 0.4 per cent sodium) can be hazardous to swine if water intake is restricted, whereas feeds containing up to 13 per cent sodium chloride (5.1 per cent sodium) can be tolerated if adequate fresh water is available. The situation in which sodium causes toxicosis secondary to water restriction has been referred to as *indirect* sodium toxicosis. Scenarios in which toxicosis may occur include human error or neglect, mechanical malfunctions of automatic watering equipment, freezing of water sources, inclusion of medications in water that affect palatability, overcrowding, or introduction of animals into unfamiliar environments. Sodium salt added at high concentrations to rations of range animals for restriction of feed consumption may be particularly hazardous if water is not readily available. Other sodium salts, such as the sulfate, carbonate, propionate, and sulfonamide salts, are also potentially toxic.

Direct sodium ion toxicosis is less common. This occurs primarily from the consumption of water or liquid diets containing high concentrations of sodium. Direct sodium ion toxicosis may occur after the ingestion by livestock of brine associated with oil production or milk replacers containing whey.

PATHOGENESIS

The precise mechanism of sodium ion toxicosis is not clear. A currently accepted hypothesis is based on alterations of sodium ion concentrations in the plasma, brain, and cerebral spinal fluid (CSF) with resultant shifts of body water. Water deprivation or excessive sodium ingestion results in elevated plasma sodium concentrations. Plasma sodium passively diffuses into other extracellular fluid compartments including the CSF, although diffusion into the CSF is relatively slow compared with other extracellular fluid compartments owing to a relative impermeability of the blood-brain barrier to sodium. Sodium is believed to be transported from the CSF back into plasma by an energy-dependent active transport process. However, high sodium concentrations in the brain and CSF interfere with the production of energy necessary for active transport to occur. If the plasma sodium concentration is lowered through subsequent water intake or renal elimination of sodium, an osmotic gradient results that favors the movement of water into the brain and CSF. This results in brain edema and increased CSF pressure, which may be responsible for many of the clinical signs noted.

It has been postulated that edema compromises blood flow to the brain and results in anoxia. This may explain the distribution of brain lesions in affected animals, with blood flow to affected regions being more severely compromised. Impaired energy production resulting from high brain sodium concentration also may contribute to the lesions noted.

Young animals are more susceptible to sodium ion toxicosis than are adults. This sensitivity may be due to smaller reserves of body water available for sodium elimination.

CLINICAL FINDINGS

In swine, early clinical signs of indirect sodium ion toxicosis such as constipation, thirst, and pruritus are subtle and may be overlooked. These signs are followed by a rather distinct nervous syndrome. Initially there is apparent blindness, deafness, insensitivity to environmental stimuli, aimless wandering or running, head pressing, circling, and pivoting around one leg. This is followed by tremors of the snout, which progress to clonic spasms of the neck muscles. Animals may exhibit retropulsion, sit on their haunches, and develop opisthotonos. A generalized clonic seizure follows, with the animal falling over and becoming laterally recumbent. Jaw chomping, hypersalivation, and respiratory distress may occur during the seizure. Seizures that initially occur at regular intervals increase in frequency until they become continuous. Death may ensue as a result of respiratory failure, or the animal may appear comatose for a short time, revive, and wander aimlessly before another seizure. The clinical course may vary from a few hours to several days. Clinical pathologic findings may include eosinopenia and elevations of serum osmolality, sodium, total protein, albumin, and urea nitrogen although the absence of these changes does not rule out toxicosis.

Sodium ion toxicosis in poultry is manifested by increased thirst, dyspnea, discharge of fluid from the beak, wet droppings, and limb paralysis.

In cattle, emesis, diarrhea, mucoid feces, abdominal pain, anorexia, thirst, salivation, and polyuria may be seen. Nervous system signs include knuckling, blindness, muscular spasms, paresis, and seizures. Veal calves with serum sodium concentrations above 200 mEq/L reportedly exhibited hyperesthesia, opisthotonos, nystagmus, muscle twitching, and intermittent seizures. A sequela to toxicosis in cattle is dragging of the rear feet while walking or knuckling of the fetlock joints.

PATHOLOGY

In pigs, indirect sodium ion toxicosis results in gross and microscopic lesions that are generally restricted to the brain. Lesions consist of laminar loss of cortical neurons and malacia. Infiltration of eosinophils into the meninges and perivascular spaces is characteristic. Whereas eosinophil infiltration into the brain can occur in pigs with other diseases, the combination of laminar lesions and eosinophil infiltration is considered to be pathognomonic for sodium ion toxicosis. However, eosinophils may not be found in animals dying from sodium ion toxicosis, so the absence of an eosinophil infiltration does not necessarily rule out toxicosis. Vascular endothelial proliferation, perivascular lymphocytic infiltration, and microgliosis have been noted in experimentally intoxicated pigs. Blood-filled, pinpoint ulcers and congestion and inflammation of the gastric mucosa may be noted.

Brain lesions in cattle and sheep suspected of dying from sodium ion toxicosis are similar to those reported to occur in ruminants due to thiamine deficiency. In poultry, lesions include ascites, enlarged hearts, subcutaneous edema, and glomerulosclerosis.

In direct sodium ion toxicosis, gross post-mortem lesions are generally restricted to the gastrointestinal tract. There is severe congestion of the mucosa of the abomasum, and the intestines may be filled with dark, fluid contents. Cattle surviving for several days may develop moderate anasarca.

DIAGNOSIS

Diagnosis of sodium ion toxicosis is based on history; clinical signs; sodium determinations on feed, water, serum, and CSF samples; and post-mortem lesions. A history of water deprivation is valuable but not always obtainable. Examination of the premises is important to determine if watering procedures and equipment are adequate. The time of year may be important because freezing temperatures may prevent access to otherwise adequate water supplies. The number of animals in relation to the available water supply may be an important consideration.

Clinical signs in affected pigs are characteristic, although pseudorabies, viral or bacterial encephalitides, gut edema, hog cholera, and chlorinated hydrocarbon toxicity should be included in a differential diagnosis. In cattle, a differential diagnosis includes thiamine-responsive polioencephalomalacia, hypomagnesemia, lead, chlorinated hydrocarbon toxicity, and enterotoxemia.

Measurement of elevated serum and CSF sodium concentrations is indicated in suspected cases. Serum or CSF sodium concentrations above 160 mEq/L are considered to be strongly suggestive of sodium ion toxicosis. In pigs, measurement of both serum and CSF concentrations may be indicated because in sodium ion toxicosis, the CSF sodium concentrations are consistently higher than the serum concentrations are. This is the reverse of that found in pigs dying from other causes. Although measurement of brain, stomach, or rumen sodium concentrations or tissue chloride concentrations has been suggested as an aid in diagnosis, they are less reliable than are serum and CSF sodium determinations.

In pigs, microscopic demonstration of laminar cortical malacia and eosinophil infiltration is considered to be pathognomonic for sodium ion toxicosis. However, in ruminants, microscopic lesions are not pathognomonic.

TREATMENT

Treatment of symptomatic animals is generally unrewarding. Initially, affected animals should not be allowed unrestricted access to water. This may worsen the clinical signs in symptomatic animals or precipitate clinical signs in nonsymptomatic animals because of sudden shifts of water into the brain causing edema. Fluid volumes of 0.5 per cent of body weight can be offered at 30- to 60-minute intervals if the animal is stable. Symptomatic therapy for control of seizures may be tried. Recovery of affected animals may take several days with mortality rates of 50 per cent or greater likely.

PREVENTION

The best prevention for indirect sodium ion toxicosis is the provision of adequate fresh water. Automatic watering equipment should be checked frequently and a source of unfrozen water provided to animals during winter months.

Direct sodium ion toxicosis is best avoided by providing water or liquid diets sufficiently low in sodium or total salt content. In terms of water quality, total salt content is more important than is sodium content alone. Calcium and magnesium salts also contribute to the salinity of water. The following maximum recommended concentrations of total salts for different livestock species can be used as guidelines: dairy cattle, 0.7 per cent; beef cattle, 1.0 per cent; sheep, 1.3 per cent; swine, 0.43 per cent; and poultry, 0.286 per cent. It has been suggested that drinking water for all classes of livestock should not contain more than 0.5 per cent sodium chloride. Milk production of lactating dairy cows may be decreased by 0.25 per cent sodium chloride in the drinking water. Variables such as age, sex, pregnancy, stage of lactation, exercise, environment, diet, availability of other water sources, and adaptation to available water may influence susceptibility to toxicosis.

BIBLIOGRAPHY

Blood DC, Radostits OM: Veterinary Medicine, 7th ed. London, Bailliere-Tindall, 1989.
Jubb KVF, Kennedy PC, Palmer N: Pathology of Domestic Animals, 3rd ed. Orlando, FL, Academic Press, 1985.
Osweiler GD, Carson TL, Buck WB, Van Gelder GA: Clinical and Diagnostic Veterinary Toxicology, 3rd ed. Dubuque, IA, Kendall/Hunt Publishing Co, 1985.

Ionophores: Monensin, Lasalocid, Salinomycin, and Narasin

C. PAT McCOY, DVM, MS

Monensin, lasalocid, salinomycin, and narasin are ionophores that are approved for use as coccidiostats and to improve feed efficiency. Some ionophores are sometimes used to reduce incidences of atypical interstitial pneumonia, bloat, ketosis, and lactic acidosis in cattle. Ionophores are chemicals that can transport ions through biologic membranes. Preferential transport of specific ions results in altered ionic gradients and disturbed cellular physiology.

Monensin is approved for use as a coccidiostat in chickens and turkeys (Coban*) and for use to improve feed efficiency in cattle (Rumensin*). Lasalocid is approved for use to improve feed efficiency and for control of coccidiosis in cattle and sheep (Bovatec†) and in chickens (Avatec†). Salinomycin (Bio-Cox‡) and narasin (Monteban†) are approved for control of coccidiosis in chickens.

TOXICITY

The toxicity of ionophores varies considerably among species, with horses being the most sensitive. The acute oral LD_{50}

---
*Elanco Products Co., Division of Eli Lilly & Co., Indianapolis, IN 46285.
†Hoffman-La Roche Inc., Nutley, NJ 07110.
‡Agri-Bio Corp., P.O. Box 897, Gainesville, GA 30503.

for monensin in the following species is horse, 2 to 3 mg/kg; cattle, 20 to 80 mg/kg; chicken, 200 mg/kg; dog, >20 mg/kg; pig, 20 mg/kg. The acute oral LD_{50} for salinomycin and lasalocid in the horse is 0.6 mg/kg and 21.5 mg/kg, respectively. Toxicoses sometimes result when sensitive species ingest ionophore-containing feed formulated for other species. Poisonings also occur when errors in feed mixing result in higher ionophore feed concentrations or when animals gain access to concentrated premixes. The toxicity of some ionophores is potentiated by various antibiotics such as tiamulin, oleandomycin, chloramphenicol, erythromycin, and sulfonomides when they are administered concurrently.

Poisoning by monensin has been investigated more thoroughly than has poisoning by the other ionophores. Limited toxicity studies and field reports of poisonings by ionophores other than monensin suggest that clinical signs and lesions resemble those of monensin poisoning.

CLINICAL SIGNS

Horses suffering from acute monensin poisoning show signs of anorexia, depression, weakness (predominantly in the hindquarters), intermittent sweating, ataxia, congested mucous membranes, progressive respiratory distress, polyuria progressing to anuria, hematuria, abdominal discomfort, and recumbency with thrashing and attempts to rise. Signs begin within 12 hours and may result in death in 24 to 36 hours.[2] Sublethal doses may result in myocardial fibrosis with poor performance, unthriftiness, and subsequent cardiac failure when the animal is stressed.

Changes in clinical chemistry determinations seen in horses with acute monensin poisoning reflect injury to skeletal and cardiac muscle, injury to kidneys, and increased erythrocyte fragility and include the following: alkaline phosphatase increases 3 to 4 times (isoenzyme primarily of bone origin); indirect bilirubin increases 3 to 5 times; blood urea nitrogen increases to 2 times; calcium decreases 1 to 2 mg/dl; creatine phosphokinase increases 2 to 1000 times (isoenzyme mostly of skeletal muscle origin); creatinine increases 2 to 3 times; hematocrit increases 10 to 200 per cent; lactate dehydrogenase increases 2 to 6 times (isoenzymes mostly of cardiac muscle and erythrocyte fraction); potassium decreases 1 to 2 mEq/L; serum osmolality increases; aspartate aminotransferase (formerly SGOT) increases 2 to 10 times, and urine pH declines to neutral or slightly acidic. Erythrocyte fragility increases with substantial lysis at 0.5 per cent salinity. Horses that die after 48 hours or more of illness may have elevated concentrations of creatine kinase and lactate dehydrogenase in the pericardial fluid.[1]

Post-mortem examination of horses acutely poisoned with monensin may suggest myocardial injury with focal to locally extensive areas of cardiac muscle palor and epicardial and endocardial hemorrhages. Pulmonary congestion and serous effusions due to generalized heart failure are sometimes present.

On histologic examination, the heart shows scattered areas of degeneration and necrosis with swollen and shrunken myocardial fibers with dense acidophilic cytoplasm, loss of striations, granulation of sarcoplasm of affected cells, and pyknotic and karyorrhectic nuclear material. These changes may not be seen in horses that die within 18 to 24 hours of poisoning. Inflammatory infiltrates and fibroplasia can be seen in horses that survive several days or more. Myopathy of active skeletal muscles such as the diaphragm is usually present and resembles the changes described in the myocardium; however, regeneration is more complete and fibrosis is minimal in skeletal muscles. Myocardial fibrosis may result in reduced performance or congestive heart failure in surviving animals. Other microscopic lesions seen in the tissues of horses acutely poisoned with monensin include vacuolar change of centrilobular hepatocytes and mild nephrosis.

Cattle poisoned with monensin develop anorexia, lethargy, and diarrhea within 1 day and may develop dyspnea, mild hindlimb ataxia, and myoglobinuria with death due to congestive heart failure in the following days to several weeks.

On necropsy, cattle dying in the acute phase of illness have hydrothorax, ascites, pulmonary edema and congestion, and petechia and pale yellow-brown to gray areas of necrosis in cardiac and skeletal muscles. On microscopic examination, these animals have lesions in the heart and active skeletal muscles similar to those described in the horse. Centrilobular hepatocellular vacuolar change and necrosis due to passive congestion may be seen. Also, acute rumenitis and degranulation of pancreatic acinar cells have been reported.

Sheep poisoned acutely with monensin display lethargy, stiffness, muscular weakness, stilted gait, mild to moderate dyspnea, mild mucoid diarrhea, and recumbency. Gross necropsy lesions may not be evident or may consist of indistinct pale foci and streaks in the myocardium and quadriceps muscle group. Light microscopic changes in the heart and skeletal muscles may be absent in acute poisoning or may consist only of vacuolation of myofibers and proliferation of muscle capillary endothelial cells. Evidence of muscle injury and repair is more prominent in sheep that survive 5 days or more and is more severe in skeletal muscle than in cardiac muscle.[3] Surviving sheep have muscle atrophy of the hindquarters.

Pigs poisoned with monensin show anorexia, lethargy, hypermetria, hindlimb ataxia and paresis, knuckling, myoglobinuria, and reluctance to stand and move. On necropsy, bilaterally symmetric white dry areas are seen in muscles of the thigh, shoulder, and loin. Microscopic changes in muscles are similar to those seen in other species except that heart lesions in pigs are often confined to the atria.[5]

Turkeys and chickens poisoned with ionophores show reduced feed intake, weight loss, fever, weakness, dyspnea, ataxia, paralysis, and death. Adult birds seem to be more sensitive to the toxic effects of ionophores than are poults and growing birds.[4]

DIAGNOSIS

A suspected diagnosis of ionophore poisoning based on the signs, laboratory tests, and lesions described in the preceding is best confirmed by analysis of the suspect feed. Several pounds of feed should be collected for analysis. Contents of the gastrointestinal tract and various tissues should be submitted but may contain below-detectable limits in animals with ionophore poisoning.

TREATMENT

There is no specific antidote or tested treatment regimen for animals that have recently ingested a significant amount of an ionophore; however, general management procedures of a poisoned patient including administration of an emetic (small animals only) and activated charcoal along with a saline cathartic are recommended. Electrolytes should be monitored, and limited fluids should be given to minimize renal injury and to prevent shock. Horses recovering from monensin poisoning should have 6 to 8 weeks of stall rest to allow completion of the repair processes. Permanent scarring of the myocardium may prevent return to full performance in athletic animals.

REFERENCES

1. Amend JF, Nichelson RL, King RS, et al: Equine monensin toxicosis: useful ante-mortem and postmortem clinicopathologic tests. Toronto, Proceedings of the Thirty-first Annual Convention of the American Association of Equine Practitioners, 1986, pp 361–371.
2. Amend JF, Mallon FM, Wren WB, Ramos AS: Equine monensin toxicosis: some experimental clinicopathologic observations. Compend Contin Educ 11:S173–S183, 1981.
3. Confer AW, Revis DI, Panciera RJ: Light and electron microscopic changes in cardiac and skeletal muscle of sheep with experimental monensin toxicosis. Vet Pathol 20:590–602, 1983.
4. Halvorson DA, Van Dijk C, Brown P: Ionophore toxicity in turkey breeders. Avian Dis 26:634–639, 1982.
5. Van Vleet JF, Ferrans VJ: Ultrastructural alterations in atrial myocardium of pigs with acute monensin toxicosis. Am J Pathol 114:367–379, 1984.

Gossypol Toxicosis

SANDRA E. MORGAN, DVM, MS

Cottonseed is widely used in the animal feed industry because of its high protein, high fiber, high digestibility, and affordability. It is also known to be deficient in vitamin D, carotene (vitamin A value), and calcium; to be low in lysine and tryptophan; and to contain high levels of phosphorus and varying amounts of gossypol. In the past, cottonseed toxicity was often attributed to vitamin A deficiency in cattle. Monogastrics such as pigs were known to suffer from gossypol toxicosis, and swine feed was regulated to contain no more than 100 ppm free gossypol. Ruminants were considered to be resistant. With the increase in the amount of concentrate fed, an increase in creep feeding, and a change in the extraction techniques of oil from cottonseed, a significant number of cases of gossypol toxicosis have been reported in ruminants in the past few years.

Gossypol is a toxic yellow pigment found in glands in various parts of the cotton plant (such as hulls, stem, and root), but it is most concentrated in the seed. Gossypol is responsible for the insect resistance of the plant. A variety of factors influence the amount of gossypol in the plants, such as species of cotton plant, climate, soil conditions, length of growing season, fertilizer, and others.

Cottonseed meal is a by-product of cottonseed oil extraction. The old hydraulic and screw press methods produced cottonseed meal with less gossypol because the gossypol glands resist pressure. The glands are ruptured by water or compounds in aqueous solution, which releases gossypol from them. Now, because of improved oil extraction techniques, the solvent method is used, which ruptures more glands. Therefore, almost 10 times as much free gossypol is in the meal as there would have been from the old method. That is why farmers, who insist they are feeding livestock the same way they always have, never had a problem until now.

Gossypol is primarily a cardiotoxin causing gradual destruction of the cardiac musculature, possibly by interfering with the conduction system. This may help explain why some animals have no lesions. Gossypol is also known to cause reproductive problems. Its mechanism of action is uncertain, but adult ruminants are able to detoxify large quantities by binding them to proteins in the rumen, whereas young ruminants are more like monogastrics and are unable to bind as much free gossypol. Low levels of free gossypol can cause illness and death in young ruminants.

CLINICAL SIGNS

Gossypol toxicosis manifests clinically as sudden death in apparently healthy animals or a chronic labored respiratory syndrome accompanied by depression, anorexia, occasionally hemoglobinuria, and death. The highest death losses have been reported in bottle calves whose starter rations and creep feeds used cottonseed meal as their protein source. These animals do not respond to any treatment. The same syndrome has been reported in lambs, particularly those in feedlots or show lambs. These deaths were often misdiagnosed as "overeating" or pneumonia. The producers are often buying what they believe is the highest quality feed available. Research has shown that these young ruminants do not function like adult ruminants and in fact can only tolerate levels similar to monogastrics. It is recommended that ruminants less than 4 months of age have 100 ppm or less free gossypol in their concentrate ration, which is the level approved for swine.

Whereas it takes much higher levels to cause clinical symptoms in an adult ruminant, the signs are similar. Mortality is uncommon in adult ruminants, but reproductive problems are seen. Sterility has been well documented in bulls; decreased conception rates have been reported in cows. In most instances, sterility was reversible after the gossypol was removed from the diet. Chronically affected cattle have also been reported to have decreased heat tolerance, hemoglobinuria, abomasitis, and anorexia.

PATHOLOGY

Necropsy findings of animals that have died from gossypol toxicosis can be quite varied. Some animals have none to minimal lesions, whereas others exhibit severe gross and histopathologic lesions. Chronically affected animals that have exhibited dyspnea usually have uniformly heavy wet congested lungs that may appear pneumonic but on palpation are soft. This is usually accompanied by excessive fluid in the thoracic and abdominal cavities and the pericardial sac. The color and consistency have ranged from clear yellow to dark red with fibrin clots in it. Lymph nodes, mesentery, intestines, and other organs may have mild to excessive edema. The heart may be pale, mottled, streaked, flabby, and enlarged with dilated ventricles. The valves may be edematous. Swollen, nutmeg, friable livers are often seen, which may range from pale mottled to golden in color. Some animals may be icteric. Abomasitis, pale skeletal muscles, red urine, and congestion of kidneys and spleen may be other findings.

Histopathologic lesions consist primarily of myocardial degeneration, pulmonary edema, and congestion with centrilobular hepatic congestion and necrosis. Mild focal tubular necrosis of the kidney, abomasitis, and enteritis can be other findings.

DIAGNOSIS

A diagnosis of gossypol toxicosis can be made by a combination of factors. A history of cottonseed in the diet usually over a period of several weeks to several months is needed. Clinical signs, necropsy findings and histopathologic lesions must be compatible with those previously described. Because anything that causes heart lesions—such as monensin, lasalocid, vitamin–E–selenium deficiency, and toxic plants like *Cassia*—can cause similar signs and lesions, these must be ruled out by feed and tissue analysis and accessibility. Usually more than 1 animal is affected, and there is no response to any treatment. The most important factor is to have the feed tested at an official cottonseed testing laboratory and have the results interpreted by a veterinarian who has dealt with these types of cases. The problem with interpretation is that there are no set levels because of the different ages of livestock, duration of feeding, rumen development, and binding of gossypol to proteins. In general, a level of 400 ppm or less has been known to cause death in very young calves and lambs, whereas older ones can tolerate higher levels; 800 to 1200 ppm free gossypol can be quite toxic to older calves and lambs but may not have any noticeable effect on adults. Some adults have been fed levels greater than 10,000 ppm with no proven side effects.

TREATMENT

There is no treatment at this time for gossypol toxicosis. When gossypol toxicosis has been confirmed or suspected, the gossypol must be removed from the diet. Animals in the same group should not be hauled or stressed in any way. Deaths from gossypol toxicosis have been reported 2 weeks after the feed was removed. The ability to recover is dependent on the severity of damage to the heart. Severely affected animals may always be poor-doers, whereas others may be able to recover completely. Because cottonseed is deficient in vitamin A, vitamin D, and calcium, a balanced ration with plenty of roughage is recommended.

PREVENTION

The best prevention is either to test the feed or to avoid feeding cottonseed meal to animals under 4 months of age. Testing feed is impractical unless it is bought in bulk and random samples are taken from different areas. When the amount of free gossypol is known, a ration can then be formulated that should be safe for the age group needed to be fed. Diluting out the cottonseed and mixing it with other protein sources can help prevent gossypol toxicosis.

BIBLIOGRAPHY

Kerr LA: Gossypol toxicosis in cattle. Compend Contin Educ Pract Vet 11:1139–1146, 1989.

Morgan SE: Gossypol as a toxicant in livestock. Vet Clin North Am [Large Anim Pract] 5:251–262, 1989.

Mycotoxicoses

Trichothecenes

VAL R. BEASLEY, DVM, PhD

The trichothecene mycotoxins, also termed 12,13-epoxytrichothecenes, are a group of over 50 compounds of widely varying toxicity. Toxic concentrations often occur in grains exposed to wet weather and fluctuating temperatures, such as may occur in temperate climates when wet weather delays harvests. Once produced, the toxins are relatively stable.

Trichothecenes that adversely affect farm animals include deoxynivalenol (vomitoxin), nivalenol, T-2 toxin, diacetoxyscirpenol (DAS), the macrocyclic trichothecenes such as roridin A and verrucarin A, and others. The most commonly encountered trichothecene in the United States and Canada is deoxynivalenol. It also occurs in South America, Europe, Asia, Australia, and Africa. T-2 toxin and diacetoxyscirpenol cause problems in North America much less often, but T-2 toxin caused epidemics in farm animals and humans in the Soviet Union and was associated with problems in horses in northern Japan. It, too, is known to occur almost worldwide. The macrocyclic trichothecenes are extremely potent and have caused serious outbreaks of toxicosis in horses of Eastern Europe. Highly toxic macrocyclic trichothecenes have also been isolated from *Baccharis coridifolia*, a plant highly toxic to newly introduced cattle and sheep in areas of Brazil, Argentina, Paraguay, and Uruguay.

Trichothecenes are produced in feedstuffs by several genera of fungi including *Myrothecium, Trichoderma, Trichothecium, Cephalosporium, Cylindrocarpon, Gliocladium, Stachybotrys, Verticimonosporium,* and especially *Fusarium. Fusarium graminearum (Giberella zeae)* is an important producer of deoxynivalenol, zearalenol, and zearalenone in corn and wheat. Thus, these (estrogen-like) compounds are sometimes detected in grain containing deoxynivalenol. T-2 toxin is produced especially by *F. sporotrichoides*, frequently identified in the past as *F. tricinctum*. The detection of a given trichothecene should alert the clinician that other related (or unrelated) mycotoxins, especially those from *Fusarium*, may also be present. Often, mycotoxin assays are directed only toward specific compounds, and toxins not included in the analytical screen will be missed. Consequently, trichothecene screening tests capable of detecting a wide range of the compounds are strongly favored over those that identify a few specific toxins. The recent discovery of fumonisins warrants consideration because fumonisin B1 seems to be particularly toxic to horses and, to a somewhat lesser degree, swine. Unlike the trichothecenes, however, the primary effects on swine include liver damage and pulmonary edema. Nevertheless, it is possible that some previous reports involving foodstuffs naturally contaminated with trichothecenes may have been complicated by the presence of fumonisins. Diagnostic challenges in trichothecene mycotoxicoses are aggravated further by wide variation in toxin contamination of various subsamples of a batch of feed, varying inherent sensitivity of the animals, and different types of other stressors. Such considerations make it quite challenging to recommend concentrations that may be fed without presenting a risk to the animals.

Deoxynivalenol is not among the more highly toxic trichothecenes, but neither is it innocuous. Its synonym, vomitoxin, is something of a misnomer because affected animals rarely vomit. In swine, ingestion of sufficient deoxynivalenol more often results in feed refusal and especially reduced intake.

Less often, soft stools and sometimes diarrhea occur. Pigs experimentally fed for 3 weeks on a ration containing deoxynivalenol at 10.5 ppm from corn inoculated with toxigenic *F. graminearum* developed modest reductions in hematocrit, hemoglobin, serum glucose, and serum phosphorus. Similar effects were observed in pigs pair fed to approximate the intake of the deoxynivalenol-exposed pigs, which suggested that these changes were due largely to reduced feed consumption. Individually or together, these may cause younger animals to fail to thrive and may increase the adverse effects of other insults such as infection, parasitism, and nutritional imbalance. Marked increases in death losses are unlikely in uncomplicated outbreaks of deoxynivalenol-associated disease. Furthermore, specific lesions are not likely to be found, although mild thickening of the squamous (esophageal) mucosa of the stomach was noted in feeding studies with pigs. In some instances, pigs eventually overcome most aspects of deoxynivalenol toxicosis and begin to catch up with nonexposed pigs, despite continued intake of deoxynivalenol.

As in the case of zearalenone, swine are among the species most sensitive to deoxynivalenol. Experimentally, deoxynivalenol in feed, at approximately 4 ppm, caused a 20 per cent reduction in feed intake, and at 40 ppm, 90 per cent refusal occurred. Limited studies suggest that ruminants may be somewhat less sensitive to both of these *F. graminearum* mycotoxins. For example, lambs tolerated a ration containing deoxynivalenol at 15.6 ppm with no evidence of illness. Nonlactating dairy cows tolerated a grain supplement containing deoxynivalenol at 6.4 ppm. However, this resulted in a daily exposure of only about 0.07 mg of deoxynivalenol per kilogram of body weight. Thus, the generally lower intake by cattle of grain may contribute to a perception of lesser relative sensitivity to trichothecenes than actually exists. Broilers are apparently somewhat more resistant.

In one survey based on problem feeds and feed components submitted to a regional diagnostic laboratory, far more instances of rectal and vaginal prolapses, abortions, and infertility in swine were associated with the finding of deoxynivalenol than with the detection of zearalenone. This reflects the ubiquitousness of deoxynivalenol in some years and suggests that it may serve as a marker for growth of *F. graminearum* and associated production of estrogenic toxins possibly including zearalenone and zearalenol in other portions of the feed. Deoxynivalenol alone does not have estrogenic properties.

T-2 toxin, diacetoxyscirpenol, and the macrocyclic trichothecenes are far more toxic than is deoxynivalenol. Feed refusal, decreased feed consumption, and "failure to thrive" are again significant aspects of subacute or chronic forms of these toxicoses. Hemorrhages have been reported in field outbreaks in swine and cattle. Although reductions in clotting factors, thrombocytopenia, and platelet dysfunction have been demonstrated in various studies, bleeding has been difficult to reproduce experimentally except after singular or repeated injections of comparatively large doses.

These more highly toxic trichothecenes also induce local "cytotoxic" effects (potentially mediated through effects on the underlying vasculature) that may be associated with lesions on the snout, muzzle, lips (especially the buccal commissures), tongue, palate, pharynx, and prepuce.

T-2 toxicosis in swine, calves, and other species causes defects in immune function, potentially resulting in increased incidence of opportunistic infections. Reductions in lymphocyte numbers and function may occur. In calves fed T-2 toxin for up to 6 weeks, the most striking and consistent lesion was atrophy of the thymus. Some animals become anemic. Similar cytotoxic, immunologic, and hematopoietic effects should be anticipated with exposure to other highly toxic trichothecenes (i.e., diacetoxyscirpenol, HT-2 toxin, macrocyclics, and others).

Reproductive effects of T-2 toxin at 12 ppm in sow rations included repeat breeding and small litter size. Embryotoxic and embryolethal effects of trichothecenes have been documented primarily at doses with toxic effects on the dam.

Even with these highly toxic trichothecenes, acute manifestations are not nearly as likely to be encountered as are subacute or chronic toxicoses. Experimentally, swine and cattle have tended to refuse to eat lethal doses of T-2 toxin in feeds. Rarely, after massive oral exposure, swine may die after developing vomiting, abdominal rigidity, weakness especially in the rear legs, and cardiovascular shock. Lesions in such animals may include extreme gastric hyperemia and severe congestion of the intestinal tract, which increases in severity as one proceeds from the duodenum to the terminal ileum. The most striking histologic lesion of overwhelming, acute toxicosis is lymphoid necrosis. Necrosis of the gastrointestinal mucosae, bone marrow, and pancreas as well as degeneration in the myocardium may also be noted. Massive oral doses in cattle cause cardiovascular shock, diarrhea, weakness, extreme somnolence, and similar mucosal and lymphoid damage. In survivors, most effects of a single massive dose tend to resolve by 48 hours.

When swine were concurrently exposed via the feed to aflatoxin in combination with T-2 toxin or deoxynivalenol, effects were either additive or less than additive.

DIAGNOSIS

A definitive diagnosis of trichothecene mycotoxicoses is based on appropriate signs and sometimes lesions, in association with analytical detection of a sufficient concentration of a trichothecene in the feed. The clinician or pathologist who encounters reduced feed intake and failure to thrive should include trichothecene mycotoxicosis in a list of differential diagnoses. Oral inflammatory or necrotic lesions suggest a need to test for the more toxic trichothecenes. Reproductive failure, digestive upset, and immunosuppression as well as decreased hemostasis may also warrant consideration of the more highly toxic trichothecenes. T-2 toxin and diacetoxyscirpenol may be detectable in stomach contents, but they are unlikely to be found in tissues. Metabolites of these toxins may be present in tissues, serum, and urine, but few laboratories offer such analyses. By contrast, deoxynivalenol may be found not only in stomach contents but also in urine shortly after exposure. Unfortunately, concentrations consistent with a diagnosis of toxicosis have not yet been established for urine specimens. Generally, 5 kg of feed that has been collected as a composite from multiple areas of the feed bin and shipped for arrival without further mold growth is requested.

Cultural identification of offending fungi, although sometimes meaningful to the mycologist or toxicologist, cannot be relied upon for diagnosis. A given species known to produce trichothecenes may or may not produce significant concentrations of toxin even when subjected to conditions believed to favor maximal toxin production.

TREATMENT

There are no specific antidotes for trichothecene mycotoxicoses. Supportive and symptomatic treatment in conjunction with a change of diet is indicated. The feed should be essentially free of mycotoxin contamination and of slightly elevated protein content. If animals have oral lesions, a nonirritating diet should be chosen. Stress should be minimized and contact with other groups of animals avoided. If animals have been exposed recently to quite high concentrations of the toxin, activated charcoal may be given as an adsorbent.

PREVENTION

Fungal growth and trichothecene contamination can be limited by proper grain drying and handling. However, significant toxin production may occur preharvest. Whenever possible, it is critical to avoid leaving grain over winter in the field. In any case, extremely moldy feedstuffs should be avoided. When analyses for trichothecenes reveal concentrations deemed marginally toxic or subtoxic, a small test group of animals may be fed the grain. If no adverse effects occur, the feed may be used, but it is probably best to avoid feeding it to breeding stock or to young animals. Feeds containing comparatively low concentrations of trichothecene toxins, particularly deoxynivalenol, can generally be fed to broilers with fewer or no toxic effects anticipated. Despite analysis, some trichothecene or non-trichothecene mycotoxins may go undetected. Also, fungal growth may deplete nutrients in the feed. Thus, negative results on mycotoxin analysis do not guarantee a safe ration.

Roasting of grain can be used to diminish concentrations in grain of deoxynivalenol to a modest degree and of zearalenone to a somewhat greater degree. Roasting has the additional benefit of killing fungal elements and producing conditions unfavorable to further fungal growth. A loss of palatability due to roasting, however, may offset the benefit from the reduction in deoxynivalenol content. Some of the more potent trichothecenes (i.e., T-2 toxin) seem to be even less affected by roasting. Another option for reducing deoxynivalenol and possibly zearalenone content is to float corn or barley in water or various types of aqueous solutions followed by removal of the floating damaged kernels and excess water containing water-soluble toxins. To the author's knowledge, however, practical systems for large-scale utilization of this approach are not yet commercially available.

BIBLIOGRAPHY

Beasley VR (ed): Trichothecene Mycotoxicosis: Pathophysiologic Effects, vols I and II. Boca Raton, FL, CRC Press, 1989.
Beasley VR, Swanson SP, Reynolds RD, et al: Current status of toxicokinetics and residue detection of trichothecene mycotoxins in swine, cattle and feedstuffs. Proceedings, U.S. Animal Health Association, 1982.
Hamilton PB: Fallacies in our understanding of mycotoxins. J Food Protection 41:404–408, 1978.
Lun AK, Young LG, Lumsden JH: The effects of vomitoxin and feed intake on the performance and blood characteristics of young pigs. J Anim Sci 61:1178–1185, 1985.
Prelusky DB, Hartin KE, Trenholm HL, Miller JD: Pharmacokinetic fate of ^{14}C-labeled deoxynivalenol in swine. Fundam Appl Toxicol 10:276–286, 1988.
Trenholm HL, Thompson BK, Hartin KE, et al: Ingestion of vomitoxin (deoxynivalenol)–contaminated wheat by nonlactating dairy cows. J Dairy Sci 68:1000–1003, 1985.
Vesonder RF, Hesseltine CW: Metabolites of Fusarium. In Nelson TE, Toussoun TA, Cook RJ (eds): Fusarium: Diseases, Biology and Taxonomy. University Park, Pennsylvania State University, 1981, pp 350–364.
Weaver GA, Kurtz HJ, Mirocha CJ, et al: Acute toxicity of the mycotoxin diacetoxyscirpenol in swine. Can Vet J 19:267–271, 1978.
Weaver GA, Kurtz HJ, Mirocha CJ, et al: Effect of T-2 toxin on porcine reproduction. Can Vet J 19:310–314, 1978.

Ergotism
GARY D. OSWEILER, DVM, PhD, MS

Ergotism is an acute or chronic disease of livestock affecting primarily cattle and occasionally swine. The causative agents, *Claviceps* spp., are parasitic fungi that attack the developing ovary of various grasses, especially certain cereal grains. Rye is most commonly infected, but other cereal grains and pasture grasses are also infected, especially barley and oats. Common pasture grasses may be infected if they are overgrown and mature seed heads develop.

NATURAL OCCURRENCE

Growth of the ergot fungus is promoted by warm, moist conditions. Spores are spread by wind and serve as the primary infective source. A sticky exudate known as "honeydew" is also a vehicle for spores that are spread when insects are attracted to the nectarlike secretion. In late summer, the mass of fungal tissue enlarges to form a dry compact mass called the sclerotium. Sclerotia completely replace the ovary in the grass plant, and their physical appearance is characteristic for each species of ergot. The principal species of veterinary importance are *C. purpurea* and *C. paspali*. Common cool-season grasses and small grains are invaded primarily by *C. purpurea;* Dallis grass *(Paspalum dilatatum)* is the usual host for *C. paspali*. *C. purpurea* is commonly associated with gangrenous ergotism and agalactia, whereas *C. paspali* causes a nervous syndrome known as paspalum staggers.

The toxicity of ergot sclerotia is due to their content of ergot alkaloids. The type and quantity of alkaloid may vary with season, region, year, and type of grain. Generally, alkaloid content increases as grain reaches maturity. Ergot alkaloid concentrations are mainly from ergotamine and the ergotoxine group, and total ergot alkaloid concentration commonly ranges from 0.2 to 0.6 per cent of sclerotia weight. United States Department of Agriculture tolerance for ergot sclerotia in grain is 0.3 per cent.

Ergot sclerotia are commonly removed from cereal grains during cleaning. The "screenings" from such grain, heavily contaminated with sclerotia, may be mixed or milled into feeds given to livestock. Once grinding or milling has occurred, ergot can be recognized only by microscopic examination or chemical analysis for ergot alkaloids. Ergotism is reported sporadically from many locations in North America. Morbidity within a herd is generally low, and unless exposure continues, recovery or salvage of affected animals is possible.

PATHOGENESIS

Gangrenous ergotism is reportedly due to alkaloid-induced smooth muscle stimulation of arterioles. Natural ergot alkaloids produce α-adrenergic blockade and also antagonize 5-hydroxytryptamine. A rise in blood pressure results from peripheral vasoconstriction. Ergotamine is especially potent as a vasoconstrictor. Vasoconstriction results in congestion proximal to the lesion and ischemia distal to the arteriolar spasm. Endothelial swelling and degeneration develop in affected vascular beds. The combined effect of vasoconstriction and endothelial damage results in localized ischemia, vascular stasis, thrombosis, pain, lameness, and eventual necrosis or gangrene. Because venous and lymphatic drainage remain intact, the gangrene is "dry" in nature.

Nervous ergotism from *C. purpurea* is relatively rare. Intense vasoconstriction and cerebral ischemia are sometimes considered responsible for the neurologic signs seen in nervous ergotism occasionally associated with *C. purpurea*. Nervous ergotism in cattle consuming *C. paspali*–infected Dallis grass appears associated with a group of tremorgenic substances with neurotoxic properties expressed as paspalum staggers. One tremorgen has been identified chemically and named paspalinine. Paspalinine is similar to some of the tremorgens isolated from various species of *Penicillium* and *Aspergillus* (see Tremorgenic Toxins).

Agalactia from consumption of ergotized grain can occur in most classes of livestock. Swine appear to be highly susceptible. Ergot alkaloids decrease or prevent the prolactin surge that normally occurs in late gestation. Apparently they act at the hypophyseal level as a prolactin release inhibitor.

CLINICAL SIGNS

The toxicity of ergot alkaloids in feeds has often been expressed as the percentage of ergot sclerotia by weight in a given grain. This value is subject to wide variance, depending on the amount of grain consumed by different animals as well as the specific alkaloid content of ergot sclerotia. Based on limited studies, ergot alkaloid content in sclerotia may range from 0.2 to 0.6 per cent of total sclerotic weight. Approximately 0.5 per cent of ergot in cattle rations is associated with reduced weight gain, poor feed consumption, rough hair coat, and some nonspecific signs. Ergot dietary contamination for several weeks ranging between 0.3 per cent and 1 per cent has been associated with gangrenous ergotism.

Early typical signs of gangrenous ergotism in cattle are lameness or apparent pain or both. Hindlimbs are often affected first. Swelling may occur just above the coronary band and extend upward past the fetlock. Affected cattle appear nervous and may walk with an ataxic or abnormal gait. Temperature, pulse, and respiration are sometimes increased, and milk production or body weight may drop drastically. Feed grains containing ergot alkaloids may be unpalatable and hence are eaten poorly or refused by animals. A toxic dose of ergot is difficult to establish owing to variability of alkaloid content. Any diet containing in excess of 0.25 per cent ergot sclerotia should be considered suspect. On a body weight basis, 40 to 60 mg/kg of ergot alkaloid has been considered toxic. In sheep, there are reports of salivation, nausea, and diarrhea. Abortion is infrequently reported as a consequence of ergot ingestion by ruminants. Field and experimental results are conflicting, but generally a strong case cannot be found for ergot-induced abortions.

In swine, feeding of ergot-containing grains often results in partial or complete feed refusal with decreased weight. Gangrene is infrequently reported, although the author has seen several cases involving loss of margins of ears or tips of noses associated with ergot-containing grain and cold weather. A serious ergot-related problem in swine occurs in late gestation and early lactation. Gestation may be shortened by 3 to 5 days, and newborn piglets are smaller than normal. Abortion rarely occurs. When ergot is fed in the last 2 to 4 weeks of gestation, udder development does not occur, and lactation is inhibited or absent. The resulting agalactia can generally be differentiated from the MMA (metritis-mastitis-agalactia) complex by general good health of sows, lack of fever, and absence of congestive or inflammatory lesions of the udder. If affected sows are removed from the ergot-containing diet within a few days, many will lactate within 5 to 7 days. Usually this is not soon enough to prevent losses from starvation in piglets. The agalactia syndrome has been induced by diets containing from 0.1 to 1 per cent ergot. Results vary greatly depending on alkaloid content.

The first signs of nervous ergotism are hyperexcitability and tremors that are intensified by excitement upon forced movement. At rest, the animals may stand with the rear legs extended and exhibit swaying motions. When made to run, they exhibit exaggerated flexure of the forelegs and incoordination that often becomes severe enough to cause the animals to fall. Once down, cattle usually lie for a short time, the severity of the signs decreases, and they regain their upright position and walk off slowly. In severely affected animals, extensor rigidity, opisthotonos, and clonic convulsions occur when they are down. When animals are left alone, the trembling and incoordination usually are minimal, and animals are able to move about slowly and graze.

CLINICAL PATHOLOGY AND LESIONS

There are no distinctive clinical pathologic lesions to confirm ergotism. Gross lesions of gangrenous ergotism may range from mild swelling, ischemia, and edema to severe ischemia, necrosis, and characteristic gangrene of the extremities that is sharply demarcated from unaffected tissue. The lesion is deep as well as superficial, and the entire appendage may slough. Microscopic lesions of necrosis, edema, endothelial damage, and thrombosis are seen.

There are no reports of clinical pathologic alterations in paspalum staggers. Apparently no characteristic gross or microscopic changes are associated with the disease.

DIAGNOSIS

Gangrenous ergotism should be differentiated from infectious pododermatitis (footrot), fescue toxicosis, frostbite, trauma, and perhaps the vesicular diseases. The lesion is distinctive and should alert one to inspect the feed and forage for ergot sclerotia. These are dark purple to black bodies, which are slightly larger than the grain or grass seed that they replace. They are elongated and roughly resemble a banana in shape. If grain has been milled, gross identification is nearly impossible. Representative feed samples should be submitted to a laboratory for microscopic or chemical analysis. Identification of ergot alkaloids or ricenoleic acid (in the absence of castor bean meal) is confirmatory of exposure to ergot. In swine, differentiation from mastitis or MMA syndrome is of most concern. Ergot-poisoned sows probably will respond poorly or not at all to parenteral oxytocin.

The diagnosis of nervous ergotism is based primarily on observing typical signs in cattle grazing pastures where mature sclerotia are present in the flowers of the grass. The problem usually occurs in late summer or early fall. Rye grass staggers and Bermuda grass tremors have similar clinical manifestations. Differentiation rests primarily on the type of pasture to which the animals have access. *C. paspali* sclerotia on Dallis grass are rough-surfaced, nearly spherical, buff to brown, and 2 to 4 mm in diameter. The toxic fungal metabolites are found predominantly in the mature sclerotia.

TREATMENT AND PREVENTION

The only effective treatment for gangrenous ergot poisoning is removal of the source. If agalactia is not advanced or if gangrene is not present, the prognosis is guarded to good.

Animals with gangrenous ergotism should be protected from cold, damp conditions, and if circumstances allow, hot packs should be applied to enhance circulation. Because little is known of the absorption and excretion of ergot alkaloids, specific therapy to enhance excretion cannot be recommended. A broad-spectrum antibiotic such as oxytetracycline hydrochloride (Liquamycin LA-200) at 6 to 11 mg/kg (3 to 5 mg/lb) or a long-acting penicillin combination such as benzathine penicillin G at 2000 units/lb (4400 units/kg) and procaine penicillin G at 2000 units/lb (4400 units/kg) should be used to control secondary infections.

Treatment of nervous ergotism consists of removing animals from affected pastures. Because death is generally accidental, care should be taken to avoid undue excitement in handling and moving cattle.

The time of greatest risk is in late summer or early fall when the pasture grasses have developed seed heads. Cattle may selectively graze grass heads containing sclerotia, thus obtaining a concentrated amount of toxic material. Control can be effected by grazing forage before it reaches the seed head stage or by clipping the heads as they form. Hay made from such pastures is potentially toxic, but sclerotia usually drop out as the hay is handled.

BIBLIOGRAPHY

Blood DC, Radostits OM, Henderson JA: Diseases Caused by Chemical Agents. II. Veterinary Medicine. London, Bailliere-Tindall, 1983, pp 1153–1156.
Burfening PJ: Ergotism. J Am Vet Med Assoc 163:1288, 1973.
Cole RJ, Dorner JW, Lansder JA, et al: Paspalum staggers: isolation and identification of tremorgenic metabolites from sclerotia of *Claviceps paspali*. J Agri Food Chem 25:1197–1202, 1977.
Coppock RW, Mostrom MS, Simon J, et al: Cutaneous ergotism in a herd of dairy calves. J Am Vet Med Assoc 194:549–551, 1989.
Holliman A: Gangrenous ergotism in a suckler herd. Vet Rec 124:398–399, 1989.
Mantle PG: Ergotism in cattle. Ergotism in swine. *In* Wyllie TD, Morehouse LG (eds): Mycotoxic Fungi, Mycotoxins, Mycotoxicoses. An Encyclopedic Handbook. New York, Dekker, 1977, pp 145, 273.
Mantle PG, Mortimer PH, White EP: Mycotoxic tremorgens of *Claviceps paspali* and *Penicillium cyclopium*: a comparative study of effects on sheep and cattle in relation to natural staggers syndromes. Res Vet Sci 24:49–56, 1977.
Osweiler GD, Carson TL, Buck WB, Van Gelder GA: Mycotoxicoses. *In* Clinical and Diagnostic Veterinary Toxicology. Dubuque, IA, Kendall Hunt, 1985, pp 428–433.

Ochratoxin

JOHN M. SULLIVAN, DVM, MS
WILLIAM W. CARLTON, DVM, PhD
PALLE KROGH, DVM, PhD*

Ochratoxins are potent nephrotoxic isocoumarin derivatives of phenylalanine produced by various fungi including *Aspergillus ochraceus* and *Penicillium viridicatum*. Nine ochratoxins have been identified, but only ochratoxin A (OA) is commonly detected in naturally contaminated products. Ochratoxin A is a contaminant of grains, principally barley, in the temperate climates of northern Europe and North America; it has also been detected in wheat, oats, corn, rye, rice, white beans, peanuts, hay, coffee beans, and mixed processed meats. Ochratoxicosis is primarily a disease of monogastric animals including swine, horses, poultry, and nonfunctional ruminants.

*Deceased.

Tissue residues are commonly encountered in pigs in Europe with porcine nephropathy. Stringent controls on human exposure to OA in Denmark require abattoirs to quantitate OA in all swine carcasses with nephropathic lesions. Any detectable quantity (1 ppb) results in condemnation.

NATURAL OCCURRENCE

The frequency of OA-contaminated grain is highly variable between locations and years. Prolonged storage of grain significantly increases the risk of contamination. Ochratoxin production is favored in grain when moisture content is greater than 16 per cent, preferentially 19 to 22 per cent, and ambient relative humidity is greater than 85 per cent. Highest mycotoxin production occurs at 12 to 25° C, but significant contamination can occur as low as 4° C. Concentrations up to 27.5 ppm have been reported in grain, but most significant naturally occurring contaminations range from 0.2 to 5 ppm.

Acute toxicosis is reported in swine ingesting 1 ppm in the ration. As little as 0.2 ppm can cause nephrotoxicity after being fed for several weeks. Cattle can generally tolerate from 2 ppm to 13 ppm in the ration, depending on age and rumen function. Young calves with nonfunctional rumens may be as sensitive as monogastrics are.

Serum, urine, kidneys, and possibly liver and fat are adequate diagnostic samples for detecting OA. After ingestion, OA is rapidly distributed within the central compartment (blood and extracellular fluid) because of its high binding affinity for serum proteins. The results of radiolabeling studies with radioactive OA in rodents, using a dose equivalent to 4 ppm in the ration, were that intestinal concentrations remained high for at least 48 hours; OA was rapidly distributed into adipose tissue, and adipose tissue had the highest concentration of tissues sampled at 48 hours. Ochratoxin is excreted in the milk but, at naturally occurring concentrations, probably presents no significant hazard to suckling piglets.

CLINICAL SIGNS AND PATHOLOGIC FEATURES

The kidneys are the principal target organs in naturally occurring exposures, although periacinar hepatic necrosis, enteritis, lymphoid necrosis, and teratogenicity are reported at experimental doses. Ochratoxins have an affinity for numerous enzyme systems, inhibiting protein synthesis and disrupting normal carbohydrate metabolism. Additionally, they may be activated by NADPH-dependent cytochrome P-450 reductase in the presence of iron to produce free radicals important in lipid peroxidation.

Often the first presenting sign in swine is poor growth and, at higher concentrations, feed refusal. Clinical signs in toxicosis are consistent with inadequate renal function including polyuria, glucosuria, and elevated serum urea nitrogen and serum creatinine. Leucine aminopeptidase, an enzyme of the brush border of renal tubular epithelium, can be detected very early after acute exposures.

At post-mortem examination, the lesions include pale and enlarged kidneys with a rough capsular surface and a few small subcapsular cysts. Marked perirenal edema is reported in pigs with greater exposures. Microscopic lesions include degeneration of the proximal tubules, loss of epithelial brush borders, and swelling and disorganization of mitochondria and endoplasmic reticulum. Chronic exposure causes cortical interstitial fibrosis and, at later stages, atrophic and sclerotic glomerular tufts.

Ruminants are generally resistant to ochratoxicosis because of degradation of OA by rumen protozoal flora. Toxicosis can occur in young ruminants with a nonfunctional rumen at dietary concentrations reportedly as low as 2 ppm. Poultry are sensitive to OA at 2 ppm in the ration. They develop typical nephrotoxicosis and, additionally, can have visceral gout and marked osteopenia characterized by thinning of the diaphysis of endochondral bone.

DIAGNOSIS, TREATMENT, AND CONTROL

Ochratoxicosis should be considered a possible disease diagnosis in monogastric animals, particularly swine, with poor weight gain, feed refusal, and signs of renal insufficiency. Postmortem examination of the kidneys for typical lesions including subcapsular cysts and interstitial fibrosis will provide a presumptive diagnosis that can be confirmed by detection of OA in feed samples and tissue samples. Tissues useful for analysis include serum, urine, kidney, liver, and adipose tissue. Samples can be analyzed for OA by use of thin-layer chromatography and high-performance liquid chromatography. Enzyme-linked immunosorbent assay (ELISA) techniques are available for detecting part per billion quantities in tissues. Slaughter checks provide an effective means of monitoring kidneys for characteristic lesions.

Renal lesions of ochratoxicosis are similar to those produced by *Amaranthus retroflexus* (redroot pigweed) and mycotoxicosis caused by citrinin (often found as a current contaminant with OA). Feed refusal is a nonspecific sign commonly reported with trichothecene mycotoxin contamination (particularly deoxynivalenol).

No antidotes are available. Experimental evidence of prolonged retention of OA in the intestinal tract indicates the use of activated charcoal and a saline cathartic such as magnesium sulfate or sodium sulfate may be advised in extreme acute exposures for limiting absorption.

Prevention is best achieved by ensuring adequate drying of grain to limit fungal growth in storage. Particular care should be taken in wet harvesting conditions when significant fungal contamination may be a problem.

BIBLIOGRAPHY

Cheeke PR, Shull LR: Natural Toxicants in Feeds and Poisonous Plants. Westport, CT, A. V. I. Publishing Co, 1985, pp 425–461.
Duff SRI, Burns RB, Dwivedi P: Skeletal changes in broiler chicks and turkey poults fed diets containing ochratoxin A. Res Vet Sci 43:301–307, 1987.
Harvey RB, Kubena LF, Lawhorn DB, et al: Feed refusal in swine fed ochratoxin-contaminated grain sorghum: Evaluation of toxicity in chicks. J Am Vet Med Assoc 190:673–674, 1987.
Madsen A, Mortensen HP, Hald B: Feeding experiments with ochratoxin A contaminated barley for bacon pigs. Acta Agr Scand 32:225–238, 1982.
Rahimtula AD, Bereziat JC, Bussacchini-Griot V, et al: Lipid peroxidation as a possible cause of ochratoxin A toxicity. Biochem Pharmacol 37:4469–4477, 1988.

Citrinin

JOHN M. SULLIVAN, DVM, MS
WILLIAM W. CARLTON, DVM, PhD

Citrinin, a nephrotoxic mycotoxin, was first isolated from a culture of *Penicillium citrinum* and since has been obtained from many other *Penicillium* spp. and from a few *Aspergillus* spp. Of the several fungal producers of citrinin, *P. viridicatum* may be of greatest significance in regard to contamination of grains with the mycotoxin. Other mycotoxins including ochratoxin A (OA), patulin, penicillic acid, aflatoxin, and oxalic acid are usual co-contaminants with citrinin in infected grain, which makes assessment of the significance of citrinin in field cases difficult. Citrinin probably functions additively with other mycotoxins in the ration, particularly with OA in producing porcine nephropathy and nephropathy in poultry.

Chemically, citrinin is a *p*-quinone methide, structurally similar to the unsubstituted isocoumarin ring structure of ochratoxin. It is very sparingly soluble in water but is soluble in dilute sodium hydroxide, sodium bicarbonate, and sodium acetate solutions and in many organic solvents.

NATURAL OCCURRENCE

Penicillium spp. are generally responsible for citrinin production and they prefer cooler conditions than do *Aspergillus* spp. This coincides with increased prevalence of citrinin in the upper midwestern United States, Canada, and Europe. It has been isolated from barley, wheat, rye, and corn. As with OA, the optimal condition for citrinin production is 25° C with high relative humidity; however, significant production occurs at temperatures as low as 5° C. Citrinin has been found in Canadian wheat at concentrations of 80 ppm, but usual concentrations in contaminated grain are much lower, probably largely owing to the environmental instability of the mycotoxin.

CLINICAL SIGNS AND PATHOLOGIC FEATURES

Experimentally, citrinin produces lesions similar to those of OA, but the toxic dose is roughly 50 to 100 times greater than for OA. Swine fed 20 mg/kg body weight develop nephropathy within several weeks. Typically, pigs have reduced weight gain and develop proteinuria and glucosuria with elevated serum urea nitrogen and serum creatinine. Grossly, the kidneys are enlarged with a rough capsular surface and subcapsular cysts. On microscopic examination, proximal tubular nephrosis with occasional tubular mineralization is reported. Degenerative and necrotic changes are present in the proximal renal tubules accompanied by dilation of tubules, thickening of tubular basement membranes, and interstitial fibrosis.

DIAGNOSIS, TREATMENT, AND CONTROL

Citrinin mycotoxicosis may be included in the differential diagnosis of tubular nephrosis in swine and poultry, especially if lesions are absent from other tissues. There are no reports of naturally occurring citrinin toxicosis in ruminants. Diagnosis would depend on detection of significant concentrations of citrinin in grain (generally >50 to 100 ppm) by use of high-performance liquid chromatography. Dietary concentrations greater than 130 ppm are required to produce renal lesions in poultry. Suspect rations should be tested for additional mycotoxins, particularly OA and aflatoxin, because their effects could be additive.

Proper grain storage and harvesting practices with mycotoxin testing of suspect grain can limit exposure to sensitive species.

BIBLIOGRAPHY

Carlton WW, Tuite J: Metabolites of *Penicillium viridicatum:* toxicology. *In* Rodricks JV, Hesseltine CW, and Mahlman MA (eds): Mycotoxins in Human and Animal Health. Park Forest South, IL, Pathotox Publishers, Inc, 1977, pp 527–541.

Cheeke PR, Shull LR: Natural Toxicants in Feeds and Poisonous Plants. Westport, CT, A. V. I. Publishing Co, 1985, pp 442–445.

Hanika C, Carlton WW, Tuite J: Citrinin mycotoxicosis in the rabbit. Food Chem Toxicol 21:487–494, 1983.

Slaframine (Slobber Factor)

EUGENE B. SMALLEY, PhD
JULIE M. SANDERSON, MS

The salivary syndrome, characterized by excessive salivation, results from the consumption of legume forages, particularly red clover *(Trifolium pratense)*, parasitized by the fungus *Rhizoctonia leguminicola*. Ingestion of a single nonlethal dose of infested forage causes salivary episodes lasting from 6 to 8 hours in small animals and to over 3 days in cattle. The parasympathomimetic idolizidine alkaloid slaframine (1-acetoxy-6-aminooctahydroindolizine) has been isolated and chemically characterized from pure cultures of *R. leguminicola* (Fig. 1). The alkaloid has also been isolated directly from dried toxic red clover hay or haylage from the field at concentrations ranging from less than 1 ppm to as high as 400 ppm. When activated by liver microsomes to a ketoimine, it induces much of the natural disease syndrome in experimental animals and is considered the salivary factor. Greater detail concerning various aspects of the salivary syndrome and slaframine can be found in several review articles.[1-5]

Swainsonine (1,2,8-trihydroxyoctahydroindolizine) is another indolizidine alkaloid produced by *R. leguminicola* (Fig. 2). This alkaloid was originally found in Darling pea *(Swainsona canescens)* and has recently been found in spotted locoweed *(Astragalus lentiginosus)* and *Oxytropis*. Ingestion of *S. canescens* or *A. lentiginosus* induces *Swainsona* toxicosis or locoism, respectively. Symptoms that are common to both of these diseases are neurologic disturbances, loss of body weight, addiction to the plants, and vacuolation of tissue cells as a result of lysosomal storage of mannose-rich oligosaccharides. Mannosidosis, a genetic deficiency of α-mannosidase, is also characterized by neurologic disturbance and cell vacuolation. Swainsonine is thought to act as a mannosidase inhibitor in both swainsonine toxicosis and locoism. The specific mechanisms of swainsonine biosynthesis in higher plants apparently have not been elucidated. Swainsonine, along with slaframine, has been identified in *R. leguminicola*–infested red clover hay in North Carolina, Iowa, Wisconsin, and elsewhere. Sanderson[5] identified swainsonine concentrations as high as 16 ppm in dried infested hay made from *R. leguminicola*–inoculated field-grown red clover.

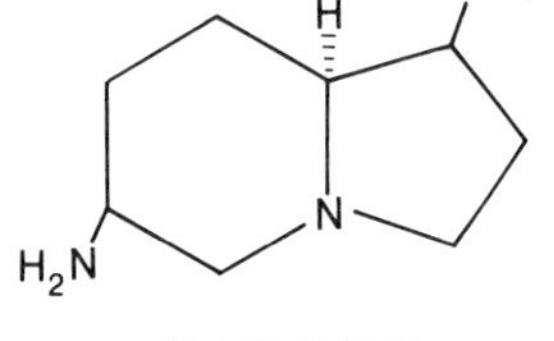

Figure 1. Slaframine, the salivary factor.

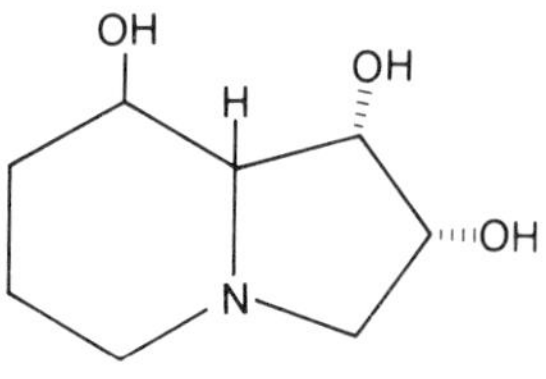

Figure 2. Swainsonine, mannosidase inhibitor.

OCCURRENCE

The salivary syndrome has been observed in cattle, sheep, goats, and horses in many parts of the eastern and central United States and in Japan. The disease of red clover induced by *R. leguminicola*, black patch, is similarly distributed and has also been found in Alberta, Canada. Although the syndrome cannot be considered a major mycotoxic problem, the potential for serious outbreaks is present whenever red clover is grown for forage. Red clover is the major host of *R. leguminicola*, but black patch disease has also been reported on other legumes (white clover, soybeans, kudzu, cowpea, blue lupine, alsike clover, alfalfa, Korean lespedeza, black medick, sainfoin, and cicer milk vetch), and these hosts are potential inducers of the salivation syndrome. *R. leguminicola* overwinters on infested straw and survives at least 2 years on infested seed. It develops most severely during periods of wet weather and high humidity, and farmers often confuse the development of dark-brown infected plant parts with normal plant maturation. Because of this, red clover may be cut, dried, and baled as normally cured hay but still induce severe salivary episodes when it is fed to farm animals. The fungus appears to continue development during drying in baled hay, and the highest naturally occurring concentrations (e.g., >400 ppm) are often found in the centers of heavily infested bales.

CLINICAL SIGNS

Cattle, the principal farm animals affected, begin salivating 30 minutes to 1 hour after eating infested hay. The response from a single exposure intensifies up to 24 hours, at which time the animal ceases to eat, urinates frequently, and develops watery diarrhea. Lacrimation occurs periodically but is rarely intense. Signs diminish after 48 hours, and recovery is usually complete in 96 hours. Other signs after longer field exposures are diminished milk production, bloat, stiffened joints, abortion, and occasionally death. Slaframine, administered as a semipurified culture concentrate on day 19 of gestation, caused uterine hemorrhaging, abortion, and occasional death in pregnant rats and guinea pigs. It seems probable that slaframine alone in contaminated forage or crude culture extracts is not the total cause of clinical signs of the salivary syndrome, because other alkaloids such as swainsonine may also be present. Purified slaframine administration to experimental animals does not induce all of the clinical signs seen in reacting animals in the field. In guinea pigs, in swine, and in probably all animals that react to slaframine, mild to severe respiratory difficulties are associated with the salivary response (Fig. 3). Suffocation, accompanied by severe emphysema, appears to be the most probable cause of death from lethal doses of slaframine. The syndrome appears to be quite similar to that induced by acetylcholine, and studies indicate that activated slaframine binds to acetylcholine receptors.

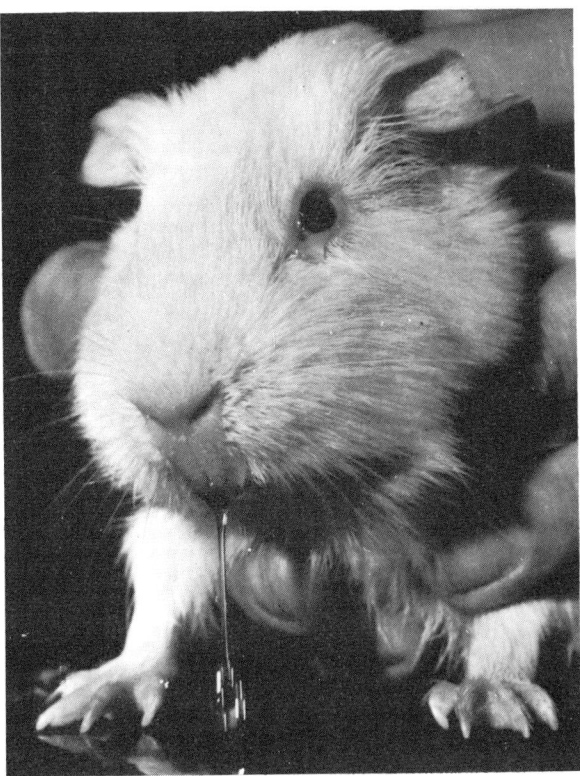

Figure 3. Salivation, lacrimation, and piloerection in guinea pig force-fed blended mycelium of *Rhizoctonia leguminicola*.

PHYSIOLOGY

A delay between the time of oral dosing and the onset of salivation (10 to 60 minutes) results because of the time necessary for the bioactivation of slaframine by liver microsomes. Photochemical activation of slaframine is also recognized. Although slaframine causes specific stimulation of exocrine glands, particularly the salivary glands and the pancreas, other effects include decreased heart and respiration rate, decreased body temperature, and increased peristalsis and uterine motility. Slaframine administration results in sustained increases in pancreatic fluid secretion, accompanied by pancreatic weight increase and decreased lipase activity in the digesta (in poultry). Increased growth hormone production in steers and chickens may also result.

CLINICAL PATHOLOGY

Farm animals reacting to slaframine usually recover completely when the contaminated hay or toxin is withheld. A chronic 3-week exposure of guinea pigs to sublethal doses of slaframine failed to induce observable gross or histologic change. Occasional deaths in cattle and abortions in horses have been reported, however, which suggest more complex pathologic changes. Post-mortem examination of guinea pigs given lethal doses of slaframine revealed that the blood vessels in the thoracic and abdominal cavities had become engorged with blood. The lung surface was pale and dry, with many small hemorrhagic areas, and lung sections revealed large areas of emphysema. Both the liver and kidney were congested, and the submucosal glands of the trachea appeared extremely active, with many eosinophils in the submucosa.

DIAGNOSIS

Diagnosis of slaframine-induced excessive salivation can be based tentatively on the distinctive symptoms (e.g., extreme salivation, lacrimation, diarrhea, frequent urination, and anorexia) after ingestion of legume forage, usually second-cutting red clover hay. Confirmation can be made by identification of the fungus *R. leguminicola* in the suspect forage. The fungus survives for many months in infested dried hay and can readily be isolated in pure culture. Chemical assays for slaframine and swainsonine are not usually necessary for diagnostic purposes because of the unique nature of the clinical signs and the obvious presence of the dark brown (coarse or hairlike) mycelium of the fungus in great abundance throughout the cured hay. However, a gas chromatographic method has been developed for direct identification of slaframine in toxic hay. Detailed methods for quantitative analysis of slaframine and swainsonine (thin-layer chromatography, gas chromatography, and gas chromatography mass spectrometry [GCMS]) have been described.[4,5]

TREATMENT

Although ruminants usually recover without treatment when the toxic legume forage is withheld, reactions can be expected to continue for 1 or 2 days after the toxic feed is withdrawn. In cases of severe intoxication, atropine therapy may be useful but will not be entirely effective. In a trial using guinea pigs, simultaneous administration of atropine with a lethal dose of slaframine prevented signs of toxicosis for 5 hours, after which mild salivation appeared. When atropine was administered 2 or 4 hours after a lethal dose of slaframine, the salivation response was intense, but no fatalities occurred.

PREVENTION

Control of the black patch disease of red clover could provide a major means for prevention of the salivary syndrome. However, fungicides applied before flowering do not reduce seed infection, and ground sprays at the time of renewed growth in the spring and immediately after the first cutting do not reduce foliar symptoms. Chemical seed treatments for eradication of the seed-borne phase of the disease provide an excellent means of control in locations free of the disease. Red clover varieties also vary greatly in their susceptibility to infection by *R. leguminicola*, and the use of highly susceptible varieties such as Norlac should be avoided. In comparative trials in Wisconsin, Redland II proved to be the variety most resistant to infection, and hay cut from inoculated plants contained the least slaframine and swainsonine.[5] Careful use of red clover forage in ruminant feed programs seems mandatory in areas of endemic black patch infection. Precautionary feeding of red clover forage to a few animals before general feeding is useful in preventing extensive outbreaks of salivary syndrome.

REFERENCES

1. Smalley EB: Salivary syndrome in cattle. *In* Wyllie TD, Morehouse LG (eds): Mycotoxic Fungi, Mycotoxins, and Mycotoxicoses. New York, Dekker, 1978, pp 121–141.
2. Smalley EB: Chemistry and physiology of slaframine. *In* Wyllie TD, Morehouse LG (eds): Mycotoxic Fungi, Mycotoxins, and Mycotoxicoses. New York, Dekker, 1977, pp 449–458.
3. Broquist HP: Livestock toxicosis, slobbers, locoism, and the indolizidine alkaloids, Nutr Rev 44:317, 1986.

4. Hagler WM, Croom WJ Jr: Slaframine: occurrence, chemistry, and physiological activity. In Cheeke PR (ed): Toxicants of Plant Origin, vol I. Alkaloids. Boca Raton, FL, CRC Press, 1989, pp 257–279.
5. Sanderson JM: *Rhizoctonia leguminicola*: studies on the production of slaframine and swainsonine in the field, host plant susceptibility, and isolate variability. M.S. Thesis, University of Wisconsin-Madison, 1985.

Stachybotryotoxicosis

JOHN M. SULLIVAN, DVM, MS
WILLIAM W. CARLTON, DVM, PhD

Stachybotryotoxicosis is a naturally occurring disease of sheep, horses, cattle, zoo-confined ruminants, swine, and humans exposed to forage infected by *Stachybotrys atra* and subsequently contaminated with various group C[1] macrocyclic trichothecene mycotoxins (stachybotryotoxins). Toxicosis is most commonly diagnosed in Russia and Middle Europe with a history of exposure of susceptible animals to straw or poor-quality hay infected by *S. atra* (synonyms: *S. alternans, S. chartarum*) and possibly *Myrothecium* spp. Stachybotryotoxins commonly recovered from cultures of field isolates of *S. atra* include satratoxin H, G, and F; roridin E; and verrucarin J. The disease is more commonly observed among confined animals in poorly ventilated stalls where moisture and low ambient temperature contribute to mold growth on straw or hay. Although the syndrome has been described most completely in horses, it probably occurs more frequently in sheep, because sheep are typically fed poorer quality roughages, which are the preferred substrate of the fungus. Outbreaks of stachybotryotoxicosis have not been reported among farm animals of North America. *Stachybotrys atra* grows best on a matrix high in cellulose where there is less competition from other ubiquitous fungi (*Aspergillus* spp. and *Penicillium* spp.); it is rarely found in cereal grains. High concentrations of conidia are detected in cottonseed oil plants, other grain processing facilities, and textile mills.

Stachybotryotoxins cause dermatitis in humans from direct epidermal contact and pulmonary dysfunction after exposure to aerosolized hyphal elements and conidia that contain measurable quantities of satratoxin H. Heavily infected ceiling material, insulation, and jute-backed carpets have been incriminated in maladies in people in Europe and a family in Chicago, Illinois.

Stachybotryotoxins are potent inhibitors of protein synthesis at the ribosome, interfering with initiation, elongation, and termination steps in protein synthesis. Mechanisms involved include polysome disruption by an unknown mechanism and inhibition of peptidyl transferase. Rapidly dividing tissues including intestinal mucosa, bone marrow, and thymus are most affected.

CLINICAL SIGNS

The clinical signs and course of the disease depend on the degree of infection of consumed forages and the duration of exposure. All species typically develop similar signs including anorexia, diarrhea, and decreased production after the consumption of moldy feedstuffs for several weeks. In common with syndromes produced by other trichothecene mycotoxins, stachybotryotoxicosis is characterized by epithelionecrosis resulting in edema, petechiation, and ulceration of the lips, tongue, and buccal mucosa. Fever, conjunctivitis, and serohemorrhagic nasal discharge follow. As the syndrome progresses in severity, necrosis of the mucosa of the gastrointestinal tract results in a secondary enteritis with such signs as bloody diarrhea and emaciation. Systemic suppression of both humoral and cellular immunity allows the secondary infections; in sheep, pneumonia associated with *Pasturella* spp. is common after the feeding of contaminated forages.

Animals usually become anemic, thrombocytopenic, and leukopenic. Hemorrhagic diathesis is reported in calves and swine. Stachybotryotoxicosis may be manifested as focal necrotizing dermatitis, particularly around the teats of lactating sows and the lips of suckling piglets. Abortions are reported in sows. Cardiac arrhythmias and myopathy are additional signs reported in horses.

Ingestion of highly toxic forage causes acute toxicosis characterized by neurologic signs similar to those produced by T-2 toxin, including ataxia, vomiting, salivation, marked depression, muscular tremors, paresis, visual impairment, circulatory dysfunction, and death.

PATHOLOGIC FEATURES

The principal post-mortem findings in sheep, horses, cattle, and swine are similar and characteristically consist of hemorrhagic and necrotic lesions in many tissues. Hemorrhages varying from petechiae to extravasations occur in serous membranes, skeletal musculature, the gastrointestinal tract, lymph nodes, lungs, and the central nervous system. Foci of necrosis are found in the mucosa of most regions of the alimentary tract but are seen principally affecting the buccal structures, the stomach (abomasum), and the large intestine. Lymph nodes, especially the mesenteric and pharyngeal, are enlarged and hemorrhagic. In acute cases with neurologic signs, the periventricular neuropil adjacent to the third ventricle should be examined for neuronal degeneration and necrosis.

DIAGNOSIS, TREATMENT, AND CONTROL

The clinical signs and post-mortem lesions, although suggestive of stachybotryotoxicosis, are not diagnostic, and various signs can be confused with those of other diseases. This is especially true of certain mucosal diseases of cattle and other trichothecene mycotoxicoses. Presumptive diagnosis is aided by demonstrating that animals were exposed to straws and hays infected by a black sooty mold. Such materials examined microscopically will contain the black mycelia and typical conidiospores. Group C macrocyclic trichothecenes including the satratoxins, roridin E, verrucarin J, and verrucarol can be quantitated by use of thin-layer chromatography, high-pressure liquid chromatography, and gas-liquid chromatography. Because the toxic principles have not been firmly established in the disease syndrome, a tentative diagnosis requires identification of *S. atra* in the suspect forage and quantification of stachybotryotoxins. From cultures of isolates of *S. atra*, satratoxin H has been the predominant mycotoxin isolated. This toxin is reportedly lethal in farm animals at 0.2 to 0.4 mg/kg. All the group C trichothecenes in a sample can be hydrolyzed to verrucarol with use of sodium methoxide for obtaining an estimate of the total stachybotryotoxin concentration.

Specific antidotes are not available. Removal of suspect forages from the affected animals would be the first logical

---

[1] Trichothecene mycotoxins are placed into four groups (A, B, C, and D) by the nature of the substituents on the tetracyclic sesquiterpenoid ring structure. Group C includes the macrocyclic substituted forms produced by *Stachybotrys* spp. and *Myrothecium* spp. but not by *Fusarium* spp.

procedure. Broad-spectrum antibiotics combined with supportive care and blood transfusions might be recommended for especially valuable animals. Control is achieved by preventing exposure of animals to hays and straws with extensive growth of *S. atra*. Proper ventilation of stalls reduces additional mold growth in bedding and elaboration of mycotoxins.

BIBLIOGRAPHY

Bata A, Harrach B, Ujszaszi K, et al: Macrocyclic trichothecene toxins produced by *Stachybotrys atra*: strains isolated in Europe. Appl Environ Microbiol 49:678–681, 1985.
Cheeke PR, Shull LR: Natural Toxicants in Feeds and Poisonous Plants. Westport, CT, A. V. I. Publishing Co, 1985, pp 425–461.
Croft WA, Jarvis BB, Yatawara CS: Airborne outbreak of trichothecene toxicosis. Atmos Environ 20:549–553, 1986.
Jarvis BB, Lee Y, Comezoglu SN, et al: Trichothecenes produced by *Stachybotrys atra* from Eastern Europe. Appl Environ Microbiol 51:915–918, 1986.
Sorenson WG, Frazer DG, Jarvis BB, et al: Trichothecene mycotoxins in aerosolized conidia of *Stachybotrys atra*. Appl Environ Microbiol 53:1370–1375, 1987.

Evaluation of Heat- or Mold-Damaged Ensiled Feeds and Their Effects on Livestock

WILLIAM G. OLSON, DVM, PhD

Feeding animals damaged feeds is risky and should be done only after assessment of the feed, testing or feeding at a diluted rate, and weighing all of the animal health and economic risks. The potential losses from reduced productivity, illness, or death can far outweigh the value of the feed if it were simply thrown out and new feed purchased. Some owners in economic distress may not have a choice. Properly stored, dry or ensiled feeds or forages will be stable for many years provided the conditions for mold growth or aerobic degradation are totally excluded (frozen, dry, or wet ensiled feeds kept sealed so that no oxygen can access and penetrate the stored mass of material).

The principles of dry storage or frozen storage are simply that molds and bacteria do not grow in those states. If microbial degradation is taking place, the principles have not been maintained for whatever reason. In the ensiling process, anaerobic bacteria convert 6 carbon sugars into organic acids (primarily lactic, and some acetic and propionic). When the acidity becomes strong enough (pH of about 4), microbial activity is inhibited, and as long as anaerobic conditions are maintained, the ensiled feedstuffs will remain stable for many years (like wine or sauerkraut).

Types of Oxidative Damage to Stored Feeds

1. Visible mold growth with little or no heating
2. Visible mold growth with extensive heating
3. Heating, slight to spontaneous combustion
4. Invisible losses: destruction of nutrients, loss of dry matter, and production of various toxins
5. Any combination of all of the above

Conditions Necessary for Heating or Molding to Occur on any Feedstuff

1. Optimal temperature for "wild" microbes or fungi: 0° C to 70° C depending on species and time

2. Moisture greater than 15.5 per cent; relative humidity above 65 per cent
3. Microorganisms, ever present in the environment
4. Oxygen greater than 0.1 per cent in infused air, which results in discoloration of 28 per cent moisture grain and a change in fat content

DETERIORATION OF MOIST FEEDS ACCESSED BY OXYGEN

The deterioration of silage and high-moisture grains ranges from slight discoloration to visible mold to a dark tobacco color to black to spontaneous combustion. Nutritional changes include loss of dry matter, combustion of simple carbohydrates (decline in net energy), oxidation of fat-soluble vitamins, binding of protein to carbohydrates (resulting in an undigestible complex), and production of mycotoxins and many other unknown by-products of microbial degradation of feedstuffs.

MEASURING THE EXTENT OF DAMAGE TO FEEDS CAUSED BY OXYGEN ACCESS

Visual Observations

Visible mold is of many different colors, and there is change in color of the feed from the normally expected color. For example, corn changes from yellow to dark yellow to brown to black; green forages will become greenish to light brown when they are properly ensiled, but damage from oxygen results in color changes from brown to dark brown to black depending on the temperature attained in the feed mass and the length of time that the feed is held at the elevated temperature.

Olfactory Characteristics

Although the smell of normal silage is difficult to describe, it is often characterized as a sweetly acidic smell. High-moisture grains smell similar, but sometimes they smell like acetone. Any deviation from this should be considered abnormal. Moldy or musty smells, sour or butyric acid smells, or a sweet or sweet caramelized to tobacco to a burnt smell should be considered grossly abnormal.

Temperature

Normal fermentation results in achieving a 20° F rise in temperature. If feedstuffs go into a silo at 75° F, the expected temperature rise would be to 95° F in 1 or 2 days. When the oxygen is used up, the temperature plateaus and starts to fall to near-ambient temperature, depending on the depth and thickness of the mass of the silage. The insulating quality of alfalfa is high; thus, the larger diameter silos loose heat at a slower rate. In any event, temperatures above 95° F must be avoided to reduce dry matter losses and to prevent binding of protein and the concomitant loss of energy density.

INHERENT PROBLEMS IN VARIOUS STORAGE STRUCTURES

Because of the principles of oxygen exclusion and avoidance of temperature increases, rapid consolidation of the mass of feed to be fermented and adequate moisture to allow fermentation and absorb the heat of fermentation are necessary.

Higher moisture feeds aid in packing and will result in a higher specific heat, that is, require more heat input per degree temperature rise. Too much water (moisture percentage) can result in abnormal fermentation (butyric acid production, clostridial growth), which may increase the incidence of ketosis. Silage that is harvested too wet may reduce dry matter intake in high-producing dairy cows. In top-unloading or bunker silos, the guidelines call for feed material being chopped to 1/4 to 3/8 inch cut and between 55 and 70 per cent moisture, but not so that moisture seeps from the silo and it is filled rapidly. Fifty-five to 65 per cent moisture is generally the optimal range, with 60 per cent near ideal. A silo should be completely filled in a couple of days, and in the case of bunker or trench silos, heavy tractors and equipment should be used to achieve maximal packing. Higher moisture silages tend to freeze more severely, which may cause problems with certain unloaders. Any time moisture is less than 50 per cent, heating and molding can be expected to become significant in unsealed structures because of oxygen penetration. In concrete top-unloading structures, cracks and very rough surfaces can allow oxygen penetration, especially if moisture and packing are borderline. For preventing aerobic deterioration of ensiled feed, the surface should be removed daily to a depth of at least 2 inches in cold weather and from 4 to 6 inches daily in warm weather. Mold has been observed growing ahead of unloaders in top-unloading structures and the fresh surface of bunker silos on many occasions.

Bottom-unloading silos present additional risks to stored feeds. Some risks are obvious. First, moisture content must be under 50 per cent in most bottom-unloading silos because the wetter the feed, the heavier it is and the more densely it packs, which makes unloading more difficult. Second, as feed is taken out of the bottom, there is an "unpacking tendency," and as the silo empties, the mass becomes naturally less dense. Third, oxygen-limiting silos (oxygen-limiting is a term introduced by A.O. Smith Harvestore Products, Inc., in 1965) are sealed and have breather bags to compensate for increasing air pressure or partial vacuum. If the vacuum/pressure limits are exceeded, implosions/explosions may occur. A safety valve or breather valve will let air in or out to protect the oxygen-limiting silo from excessive pressure or vacuum.

Additional risks inherent in oxygen-limiting silos include the following.

1. The breather bags do not afford protection to the entire void volume of the oxygen-limited silo; therefore, a breather (safety) valve to let air in or out is provided. In larger silos, the breather bags protect only the top 1/3 to 1/2 of the silo volume.

2. As stated in a United States patent held by A.O. Smith Harvestore Products, Inc., July 25, 1967:

It has been found that in the early morning, the silo is normally at a negative pressure with respect to the atmosphere so the breather bag is in an expanded condition. When the door of the unloader is opened to discharge silage, air flows in through the door to equalize the pressure between the interior of the silo and the exterior, and as the pressures are equalized, the bag tends to collapse. As the breather bag has a substantial volume, generally in the neighborhood of 300 to 600 cubic feet, the volume occupied by the expanded bag is replaced by air coming in through the unloader discharge door. Thus, as the bag collapses, a substantial quantity of air is drawn into the silo through the unloader discharge door and the entry of air will tend to destroy the desired oxygen-free gas composition in the silo.

Then when the door is sealed shut again and solar heating expands the air within, air may be expelled out the breather valve when the critical pressure is achieved. Therefore, air comes in the bottom when it is unloading and may be forced out the top when it is sealed. This ability of air to move through the feed mass is indicative of inadequate packing of the mass of feed.

3. The chain type unloader acts as an air pump: feed is pulled out one side, and the paddles move back in, in a continuous fashion. Also, the physical principle of rapid diffusion of gases will result in increasing oxygen concentration to atmospheric conditions within a short time (5 to 20 minutes or longer) depending on the size of the dome (air space) above the unloader and whether partial vacuum or pressure exists when the door is opened. The dome has been observed to be 40 feet high in 25-foot diameter bottom-unloading oxygen-limiting silos.

ASSESSMENT WITH LABORATORY ANALYSIS

Traditional nutrient analysis of feed is generally unrewarding in assessing damage to feeds. Mycotoxin analysis is a highly sensitive testing procedure detecting parts per billion with predictable accuracy. The unfortunate part of such assays is that there usually are pockets of mold in ensiled feeds, and there are usually mixed growths of mold in a silo. Therefore, the test is only of the sample taken and not of the unsampled feed. Thoroughly mixing the feed mass is impossible and may not be desired because dilution would then take place. Common sense must prevail in setting up a protocol for assessing silos of feed for mycotoxin analysis. Specific mycotoxin information and analysis is given elsewhere in this text. Mold and yeast counts may be helpful in determining the fitness of the feed, but if the samples are not preserved properly, artificially high or low counts can be produced. High mold and yeast counts do indicate abnormal fermentation. In good-quality silage, the counts probably should be below 100,000 per gram. In abnormal silage reports, counts have been in the millions.

Nutrient analysis of damaged feeds can be rather unrewarding, especially if the investigator has little or no knowledge of the quality or type of feed that was ensiled for storage or how long the feed was in storage. Generally, the nutrient parameters that are adversely affected by spoilage are decreased energy, increased unavailable (ADF-N) protein, increased acid detergent fiber (ADF) and neutral detergent fiber (NDF), increased lignin, and increased ash. The magnitude of these changes may be from a few percentage points to 50 per cent or more. One cannot predict from looking at the feed and assessing the feed tests what the effects are going to be on the animals consuming such feeds. The main test that is utilized in assessing heat-damaged forages is the ADF-N (acid detergent fiber nitrogen). Early cut alfalfa will usually have about 5 to 6 per cent of the protein in the ADF-N. Mature alfalfa and grasses may go as high as 10 to 15 per cent ADF-N. Alfalfa haylage stored at 95° F for 21 days will increase 1 to 2 per cent; haylage at 140° F will increase to 10 per cent ADF-N or more. Temperatures from 75° to 160° F have been recorded in bottom-unloading silos under field experimental conditions. Silos of all types have had higher temperatures resulting in spontaneous combustion. Actual field surveys have found ADF-N to increase to 25 to 50 per cent bound protein and greater. Whereas some of the bound protein can be made up by supplementing additional protein, the energy loss and the reduced palatability render the affected feed unfit for cattle attempting to produce milk or gain weight efficiently to their genetic potential, unless it makes up a minor portion of the ration.

The magnitude of losses in terms of milk production or reduced rates of gain is not predictable on the basis of feed tests or observations of the feed. When extensively damaged feeds have been fed for months or years at a time, the losses have been variable, ranging from none to over a 50 per cent drop in milk production or a drop in rate of gain from 2.5 lb/day to 0.5 lb/day. Such drops in production have dire economic consequences. Equally or more important, lactating animals will lose weight and may exhibit none, any, or all of the following complications: (1) unthriftiness; (2) lameness due to laminitis; (3) digestive disturbances including increased incidence of displaced abomasum, diarrhea, and off feed; (4) higher incidence of abortions; (5) reduced breeding efficiency (silent heats, anestrus, more repeat breeders); and (6) increased incidence of infections by opportunistic organisms (pneumonia, metritis, mastitis) because of lowered resistance by the animal.

The difficult problem facing anyone investigating a damaged feed episode is working up the case as completely as possible, so that the investigator can assess all of the management factors that could confound the ultimate diagnosis. The investigator must rule out the other causes of production loss and all of the signs and symptoms listed. This is often a formidable problem for investigators not trained in or familiar with all of the management practices that go into a livestock operation.

FEEDING RECOMMENDATIONS

Do not feed moldy or heat-damaged feeds to animals. Obviously there are circumstances when the livestock owner has no choice but to feed some damaged feeds. The main point to determine is whether the suspect feed is causing a problem. One has simply to work through a process of feeding or withdrawal of the feed and observe the response in terms of performance of the animals. Large feedlots will buy damaged feeds at a lower price and feed the damaged feed at a certain percentage (depending on degree of damage, 5 to 10 per cent or more). The risk of lower production versus lower feed cost must be weighed carefully. If a dairy has all of its feed damaged, then there are very obvious choices to weigh.

Ammoniation of the damaged feed and the use of buffers may have limited value in treating damaged feeds. Ammoniation may neutralize some toxins, and buffers may reduce rumen insults, but they will *not* have any effect on the occurrence of other damage. The use of preservatives may be helpful in the ensiling process, but they will *not* substitute for the principles of proper silage making and storing: *rapid filling, maximal consolidation, proper moisture, sealing to ferment and stabilize until feedout begins, and rapid removal to minimize or avoid aerobic deterioration.*

TREATMENT OF AFFECTED ANIMALS

Affected animals must be taken off the damaged feed. All of the health and body condition effects must be considered, and rational symptomatic treatments may be given. Often the recommendation will be to sell the animals for salvage. The ultimate test is to determine if the animals will respond (in terms of health and production) to a high-quality, well-balanced diet.

BIBLIOGRAPHY

Gracia AD, Olson WG, Otterby DE, et al: Effects of temperature, moisture, and aeration on fermentation of alfalfa silage. J Dairy Sci 72:93–103, 1989.
Goering HK, Adams RS: Frequency of heat damaged protein in hay, haycrop silage, and corn silage. J Anim Sci 37:295, 1973.
Marasus WFO, Smalley EB: Microflora toxicity and nutritive value of moldy maize. Onderstepoort J Vet Res 39:1–10, 1972.
McCullough ME (ed): Fermentation of Silage, A Review. West Des Moines, IA, National Feed Ingredients Association, 1978.
McGilliard ML, Crowgey JH III, Pessok SR, et al: Comparisons of costs after tax of storing silages in four types of structures. J Dairy Sci 70:724–731, 1987.
Janicki FJ, Stallings CC: Nitrogen fractions of alfalfa silage from oxygen-limiting and conventional silos. J Dairy Sci 70:116–122, 1987.
Thomas C (ed): Forage Conservation in the 1980's. European Grassland Federation Symposium No. 11, 1980.
Woolford MK: The determined effects of air on silage, a review. J Appl Bacteriol 68:101–116, 1990.

Plant Toxicoses

Poisonous Plants in Harvested or Prepared Foods

MURRAY E. FOWLER, DVM

Hundreds of plants are potentially toxic to cattle, sheep, goats, and swine. Many of these plants are native plants or weeds of wastelands or ranges used to graze livestock. Such plants are rarely found in harvested or processed feedstuffs. Plants that grow along fencerows or irrigation ditches may be inadvertently included in the border swath of harvested forage. Swathing is frequently carried out by nonowners. Operators may be ignorant of the hazard of including the extra plant material on the border.

Any plant containing a toxin that is stable through the drying process is potentially capable of being included in harvested feed. The "back-to-nature" movement has put non-agriculturally informed individuals in the business of caring for a few head of livestock. They may harvest meadows or marginal lands and be oblivious to the hazards posed by some of the plants growing in the area.

Many livestock producers now buy feed from commercial growers, thus having minimal control over feed quality. With modern methods of feed preparation (grinding, pelleting, and cubing), it may be impossible to detect or prevent the inclusion of poisonous plants unless quality control is rigidly practiced from the field of forage to the feeding of the animal.

Agricultural regulations are designed to maintain quality standards for grains, hays, and mixed feeds entering into commercial trade. For instance, it is illegal to sell hay in California that is known to contain poisonous or deleterious substances. This is probably the case in most states. Yet hay has been sold in California containing as much as 80 per cent common groundsel, *Senecio vulgaris*, with a pyrrolizidine alkaloid content of approximately 0.08 per cent.

In spite of legal action, it has been extremely difficult for the livestock owners to realize compensation for losses. To date, the only protection an animal feeder has is to buy hay and other prepared feeds from a reliable source.

POISONOUS PLANTS FOUND IN PREPARED FEEDS

Table 1 lists some of the more important poisonous plants or biotoxins likely to be found in feeds in the United States. Because many more plant species may be found in feed grown in a particular local area, the list is far from exhaustive. A discussion of a few of these plants may serve to illustrate some of the types of problems that arise.

MYCOTOXINS

Diagnosis of mycotoxicosis is becoming more and more common as sophisticated diagnostic tests are developed. Mycotoxins are produced by molds that are most likely to develop maximally on improperly stored feeds. Feed producers and animal feeders must be continually alert to guard against mold contamination of feeds. Some states are now screening livestock feeds for the presence of mycotoxins. This trend is likely to continue.

NITRATE ACCUMULATOR PLANTS

Nitrite poisoning caused by the ingestion of excessive nitrates is a serious problem in ruminants, particularly cattle. Harvested and prepared feeds are a common source of excessive nitrates. From an economic viewpoint, nitrite poisoning may be the most important plant poisoning problem involving harvested forages. Unfortunately, some important forage crops tend to accumulate nitrates when they are pushed with heavy fertilization for maximal production.

Sudan grass (*Sorghum vulgare* var. *sudanensis*) may be involved with both cyanide and nitrite poisoning. Nitrite poisoning is the more likely to occur because of the amount of nitrogen applied to the soil in order to obtain maximum yields. In sudan grass, fed either as green chop or as hay, accumulated nitrates may cause poisoning under certain conditions.

Stocker cattle and growing stock are frequently at risk. Generally, poor-quality hays are fed to these animals, and supplements are rarely added. In 1 instance, 18 of 20 heifers died from nitrite poisoning after being fed a weedy "hay" consisting of 90 per cent lambsquarter, *Chemopodium album*. The "hay" contained 6 per cent potassium nitrate.

In this regard, it is important to recognize that well-nourished cattle can tolerate higher levels of nitrate in the diet than can poorly nourished cattle. Healthy animals may consume up to 5 per cent nitrate for a short period without apparent ill effects, if the ration is also high in carbohydrates and complete protein.

Truck-garden trimmings (lettuce, celery, broccoli) may contain high amounts of nitrates. Many forage crops and weeds are capable of accumulating nitrates under special circumstances.

CYANIDE POISONING

Cyanide toxicosis is generally seen in pastured ruminants. Cyanogenic glycosides are volatile, so drying usually renders the forage nontoxic. There are, however, 2 situations in which cattle, sheep, or goats may be poisoned with cyanide in harvested feeds. The first is the feeding of green chop. If sudan grass or sorghum is fed as green chop in the fall after frost or early in the season before frost ends, the harvested feed may contain toxic levels of cyanide.

Arrowgrass (*Triglochin maritima*) grows in wet meadows that may be harvested for hay. The glycoside in this plant is not detoxified during the drying process.

Differentiation between nitrate and cyanide toxicosis is crucial, because antidotes for cyanide poisoning exacerbate nitrate toxic effects. A venous blood sample provides a quick, accurate test. The venous blood from an animal with cyanide toxicosis is bright red, whereas that of an animal with nitrate toxicosis is dark or even brownish in color.

PYRROLIZIDINE ALKALOIDS

Pyrrolizidine alkaloid toxicosis is described in the article on hepatotoxic plants. Pyrrolizidine alkaloids are produced by 5 or 6 plant species, but only 2 species occur frequently in harvested feeds: fiddleneck or fireweed (*Amsinckia intermedia*) and common groundsel (*Senecio vulgaris*). Both of these plants are weeds of hay fields growing in California and possibly other states. New plantings of alfalfa may be overgrown with weeds. The first cutting may contain 10 to 50 per cent weeds. Alfalfa stands weakened by heavy infestations of weevils may also allow weeds to take over. Oat hay may also be contaminated with these weeds.

Both plants are readily identifiable in baled hay, but it is virtually impossible to ascertain the presence of poisonous plants in weedy hay that is cubed or pelleted (not an uncommon practice). The fact that the clinical signs of pyrrolizidine alkaloid poisoning do not appear until 2 to 8 months after ingestion complicates correlation of plant consumption and disease. This delay in effect again stresses the importance for the feeder to know the source of harvested feeds.

The seeds of fiddleneck and crotalaria (*Crotalaria* spp.) are a concentrated source of the alkaloid. Swine and poultry fed screenings containing weed seeds have been poisoned.

OLEANDER POISONING

Oleander is a popular ornamental plant that may border hay fields. The plant is extremely toxic, and high mortality may occur when hay containing dropped leaves or plant trimming is fed to livestock.

MILKWEED POISONING

Plants of the genus *Asclepias* contain toxic resins and glycosides. These plants may be found in harvested hays and are

Table 1. PLANTS AND TOXICANTS IN HARVESTED OR PREPARED FEEDS

Nitrates (numerous species including sorghum)
Cyanides (*Sorghum* spp., *Triglochin maritima*)
Pyrrolizidine alkaloids (*Senecio* spp., *Amsinckia* spp., *Crotalaria* spp.)
Mycotoxins
Oleander (*Nerium oleander*)
Milkweed (*Asclepias* spp.)
Nightshade (*Solanum* spp.)
Tree tobacco (*Nicotiana glauca*)
Sweet pea (*Lathyrus* sp.)
Jimsonweed seed (*Datura* spp.)
Yew (*Taxus* spp.)

toxic in the fresh or dry state. Milkweeds are cosmopolitan in distribution throughout the United States. Different species have different habitats, but all must be considered to be potentially poisonous. The clinical syndrome associated with milkweed poisoning may involve the gastrointestinal system or the nervous system.

LATHYRISM

Lathyrism is a rare disease that is periodically reported in various areas of the United States. Lathyrism is caused by dipeptides in plants of the genus *Lathyrus*; posterior spinal cord neuronal degeneration results. Lathyrism in humans was recognized before the birth of Christ and still occurs in areas of the world where pulses are the staple diet. Ornamental sweet peas, caley peas, or rough peas are species of *Lathyrus*, which are leguminous plants closely related to and sometimes confused with vetch, *Vicia* sp. Even vetch has been incriminated in rare cases of poisoning similar to lathyrism.

In 1 instance, a field was planted with what was assumed to be vetch but was instead a species of *Lathyrus*. The plants grew and were cut and baled as vetch hay. Cattle and horses fed the "vetch" hay for 2 to 3 weeks developed neurolathyrism.

The clinical syndrome approximates the "tying up" syndrome of horses. Animals have a stilted gait. The center of gravity is pushed forward over the front legs, giving the appearance that the animal is balancing on the front legs and using the hindlegs to move forward in short mincing steps. The muscles over the back, rump, and hindlegs are *not* hot, swollen, or painful, which differentiates this condition from "tying up" syndrome.

Animals removed from the hay soon after being affected may return to normal. Continued ingestion of *Lathyrus* results in permanent neuronal damage and posterior paresis. No specific treatment is known.

Principal Poisonous Plants in the Western United States*

LYNN F. JAMES, PhD

KIP E. PANTER, PhD

Approximately 835 million acres of rangeland are in the 48 contiguous states. Nearly 82 per cent of the rangeland of the United States is located in 17 western states. Rangelands are, and have been, of great economic importance since the West was first settled. They supply forage for millions of breeding cows yearlong; and, with proper management, this number could be increased. Poisonous plants are one of the serious impediments to the proper use and productivity of these ranges and pastures.

From the beginning of the grazing of livestock on western ranges, poisoning of livestock by plants has been an important cause of economic loss to the livestock industry. This is also true today. Losses are caused by things such as death, chronic illness and debilitation, photosensitization, reproductive failure, abortions, and birth defects. In addition, poisonous plants increase costs to land managers and livestock owners, in that these costs are associated with management of rangelands and pastures. These costs include fencing, lowered forage production and utilization, altered grazing programs, nonuse of some infested range areas, and, in some cases, supplemental feeding programs and added veterinary expenses.

Losses of livestock due to poisoning by plants vary greatly from year to year and from region to region. Some poisonous plants grow only in localized and well-defined areas, whereas others seem to be omnipresent, but they all may be affected by environmental factors such as temperature and moisture and, as a result, may be more abundant and hazardous in one year than in another. Other factors, such as the previous year's grazing pressure, may also affect their abundance. Also, some plants are only seasonally toxic. Therefore, in considering poisonous plants or in attempting to diagnose or predict a poisonous plant problem, one should be familiar with the poisonous plants likely to be encountered and the condition under which livestock may be poisoned by them. Often, livestock owners, knowing of the presence of poisonous plants on their range, become lax regarding preventive strategies because their animals have not been poisoned recently. Then, when conditions and circumstances become ideal for poisonous plants, the owners may suffer huge losses. Losses of livestock due to a great variety of poisonous plants have had devastating effects in many sections of the western United States.

Management errors have contributed heavily to this problem. Indeed, management practices used by the range livestock industry in many cases are conducive to the poisoning of livestock by plants. For example, lupine is more toxic to cattle than to sheep on a weight basis, yet literally thousands of sheep, but few cattle, have died from eating this plant. Halogeton is equally poisonous to cattle and to sheep; however, many sheep have died from halogeton poisoning, yet it has clinically affected relatively few cattle. The differences observed may be due to the way cattle and sheep are managed. Range sheep are usually kept in large flocks and moved from place to place as deemed necessary by the sheep herder. Cattle, however, are left to move freely about a range, limited only by fences and natural barriers. Sheep are normally given water and provided with new forage only when it is allowed by the herder, but cattle are usually free to search out water and forage as needed. Often sheep that are hungry may be driven through, bedded in, or unloaded from trucks into heavy stands of poisonous plants and thus are exposed to plants that they would not normally graze.

Many poisonous plants are not palatable to livestock and are eaten only in stressful situations. Plants eaten under these conditions are death camas, copperweeds, milkweeds, and rubberweeds. Other plants such as lupine, halogeton, and greasewood are palatable and may form an important and beneficial part of a range animal's diet. We need to recognize that plants with toxic properties do not always kill or otherwise harm animals when they are eaten. Death or serious damage often occurs when excessive amounts of toxic plants are consumed over short periods of time.

The cost of eliminating poisonous range plants where infestation is widespread is usually economically prohibitive and nearly physically impossible. Furthermore, chemical or mechanical treatment may be undesirable because of the adverse effects on desirable plants, and often both methods are inadequate.

Medical treatment of livestock poisoned by plants is generally of little value because of the time interval between intoxication and treatment. In addition, the number of animals involved is usually large. Therefore, the most logical approach to prevention of livestock poisoning by plants is proper management—management concerned not only with health of the livestock but also with pasture and range resources. Resource people, such as veterinarians, county agents, and range managers, can render valuable assistance in the development of

---

*All material in this article is in the public domain, with the exception of any borrowed figures or tables.

managerial procedures for the prevention of poisoning of livestock by plants.

POISONOUS PLANTS

Space does not allow a detailed discussion of all plants toxic to livestock. The plants discussed are those considered to be of greatest importance in the western United States.

Lupine (*Lupinus* spp.)

Lupine (*Lupinus* spp.) has been one of the most devastating of the range plants poisonous to sheep. Poisoning results most often when hungry sheep are given access to lupine that is in the seed stage of growth. The signs of poisoning in sheep include nervousness, depression, stiffness and reluctance to move, difficulty in breathing, twitching of muscles, loss of muscular control, convulsions, coma, and death. No effective treatment for lupine poisoning is known. Affected animals should not be disturbed until signs of poisoning have subsided. There are no characteristic lesions.

Losses can be minimized by preventing hungry sheep from grazing in heavy stands of lupine, especially when the plant is in the seed stage. Lupine poisoning is most frequently associated with the handling of animals during trucking or trailing. A plan should be developed for grazing and handling animals so that they can avoid grazing lupine during these periods of stress. There are some species of lupine, such as *Lupinus leucophyllus*, that should be avoided and not grazed at all.

The several species of lupines vary considerably in toxicity. Those concerned should be aware of this fact and be familiar with the toxicity of the species the animals are likely to encounter.

A congenital skeletal malformation ("crooked calf") has been associated with cows grazing lupine during the early part of pregnancy. This condition can be avoided by changing the grazing or breeding season or both, so that grazing of lupine is not allowed during the 40th to 70th days of pregnancy.

Larkspur (*Delphinium* spp.)

Larkspur (*Delphinium* spp.) is one of the principal poisonous plants affecting cattle in the western range states. Cattle graze larkspur even when there is an abundance of good forage available.

All species of larkspur are poisonous. The 2 general types of larkspur are (1) tall, which grows in moist areas at the higher elevations, 1829 to 3353 m (6000 to 11,000 ft), and (2) low, which grows in dry foothills and plains areas. Toxicity of the larkspurs is high during the early vegetative stages and is lowered as the plant matures, except in the seed stage.

The animal may be poisoned when it eats a relatively small amount of larkspur in a short period of time. Signs of poisoning appear in a few hours and include nervousness, staggering, incoordination, collapse, excessive salivation, frequent swallowing, muscle twitching, bloating, vomition, rapid irregular heart beat, respiratory paralysis, and death. There are no significant characteristic gross or microscopic lesions. No specific treatment is known, except to relieve bloating. Affected animals should not be disturbed. Larkspur is less toxic to horses and sheep.

Management to prevent poisoning consists of keeping animals away from the larkspur during growth stages up to flowering.

Death Camas (*Zygadenus* spp.)

Death camas (*Zygadenus* spp.) is an herb with grasslike leaves and an underground bulb. Several species of death camas have various degrees of toxicity. This group of plants is found principally in the western range states.

Death camas is one of the first plants to begin growth in the spring. Animals are usually poisoned at this time, when there is a shortage of good, desirable forage. Poisoning often occurs when a spring snow covers other forage and the death camas protrudes above the snow.

Signs of poisoning are increased respiration rates, excessive salivation, apparent nausea, weakness and staggering, convulsions, coma, and death. No treatment is known for death camas poisoning. Severely poisoned animals usually die, whereas those less affected may recover. Animals poisoned on death camas should not be disturbed.

Prevention lies in avoiding grazing areas infested with death camas in the early spring. As other forage becomes available, livestock are less likely to graze the death camas.

Hemlocks (*Cicuta* spp. and *Conium maculatum*)

Water hemlock and poison hemlock are common poisonous plants often confused because of their similar names and appearance.

Water hemlock (*Cicuta* spp.) grows only in areas that are wet at least part of the time, such as stream banks and swamps. Its main distinguishing features are fascicled tuberous roots and chambered and swollen rootstocks. It is toxic to all classes of livestock, and poisoning in humans is not uncommon.

Cicutoxin, the poisonous principle of water hemlock, is one of the most toxic of all pant toxins. The toxin is concentrated, especially in the tubers. The leaves and stems contain the toxin, but they decrease in toxicity as the plant matures. The toxin acts directly on the central nervous system, causing grand mal seizures and death from respiratory paralysis.

The signs of poisoning are muscle twitching, increased pulse rate and respiration, tremors, convulsions, dilation of pupils, salivation, coma, and death. Affected animals usually die rapidly. No satisfactory field treatment is available for water hemlock poisoning. See Effects of Plant Toxins on the Central Nervous System for details of pathology.

Prevention of poisoning involves either controlling the plant with the appropriate herbicides or keeping animals from grazing it. Animals are most often poisoned in the spring when the plant is young, and they have been poisoned when the roots are exposed during the cleaning of ditches. Water hemlock is a much more important poisonous plant than is generally thought.

Poison hemlock (*Conium maculatum*) is less toxic than is water hemlock but, nevertheless, is responsible for numerous livestock losses. One of the distinguishing features of poison hemlock is the purple spots on the lower part of the stem, and the root is an unbranched taproot. Poison hemlock has a mousey odor.

The toxic principles, coniine and γ-coniceine, volatile alkaloids, are toxic to all livestock and to humans. Signs of poisoning are nervousness, trembling, ataxia, dilation of pupils, weak and slow heart beat, coldness of extremities, coma, and death. Poison hemlock can induce skeletal birth defects in calves, pigs, lambs, and goats.

Poison hemlock intoxication is usually associated with heavily grazed pastures and occurs during early spring. Prevention involves controlling the plant and proper grazing practices.

Halogeton (*Halogeton glomeratus*)

Halogeton (*Halogeton glomeratus*) is an annual plant that grows on the colder, arid, saline ranges of the West. The toxic principle is an oxalate that has been responsible for the death of many sheep and some cattle. This plant competes poorly with other vegetation, so ranges infested with halogeton should be expected to respond well to good range management practices. See Oxalate Accumulators for a more complete discussion.

Greasewood (*Sarcobatus vermiculatus*)

Greasewood (*Sarcobatus vermiculatus*) is an oxalate-producing shrub that grows in the colder, saline, arid and semiarid regions of the western United States. It has been responsible for the deaths of numerous cattle and sheep.

Prevention of losses consists primarily of proper management. The plant sprouts from the crown and does not respond well to herbicide control. Most of the area where it grows is not adapted to the use of herbicides or mechanical treatment.

Greasewood can form a useful part of the diet of sheep and cattle if it is properly managed.

See Oxalate Accumulators for more detail.

Chokecherry (*Prunus virginiana*)

Chokecherry (*Prunus virginiana*) is a low-growing shrub or tree on the western ranges. It contains toxic amounts of hydrocyanic acid. When sheep or cattle graze considerable amounts of chokecherry, they may become poisoned.

Prevention of chokecherry poisoning in animals on western ranges involves proper management procedures. Ruminants can graze large amounts of chokecherry without harm. Poisoning occurs when they graze large amounts of plant rapidly. Therefore, hungry animals should not be allowed to graze chokecherry. Chokecherry is difficult to eliminate from the ranges.

Arrowgrass (*Triglochin* spp.)

Arrowgrass (*Triglochin* spp.) produces hydrocyanic acid under stressful conditions. Arrowgrass grows on wet, heavy, alkaline soil. Prevention involves keeping livestock from grazing this plant after drought or frost.

Senecio, *Amsinckia*, and *Crotalaria* spp.

Certain species of *Senecio*, *Amsinckia*, and *Crotalaria* contain pyrrolizidine alkaloids. These alkaloids are primarily hepatotoxic. They may cause an acute toxicosis that results in rapid death, but they usually cause a chronic cirrhosis-like condition of the liver that may not be manifest until months after the plants have been ingested. Horses and cattle are most susceptible to these alkaloids. Pyrrolizidine alkaloid toxicosis is discussed more fully in the article Hepatotoxic Plants.

Selenium-Accumulating Plants

Several species of plants that grow on seleniferous soils accumulate selenium in such amounts that they become toxic to livestock grazing them. These plants are discussed in the article Selenium Accumulators.

Ponderosa Pine (*Pinus ponderosa*)

Ponderosa pine (*Pinus ponderosa*), when grazed by cows during the last trimester of gestation, can cause abortions. Ponderosa pine grows in all states west of the plains area and in western Canada. There are some abortions in those cattle that ingest pine needles in all of these states, and there are larger numbers of abortions in cattle of Arizona, Colorado, Idaho, Montana, New Mexico, Oregon, South Dakota, Washington, Wyoming, Minnesota, and western Canada.

Abortions can result when pregnant cows eat dried, wilted, or green ponderosa pine needles. Cattle in areas where the ponderosa pine grows generally have yearround access to the needles; however, the animals usually abort during the late fall, winter, and early spring. Several factors apparently cause the cattle to eat pine needles: sudden weather changes such as cold winds and snowstorms, hunger, changes in feed, and other stressful conditions. They will eat ponderosa pine needles even when good forage is available.

Some animals may abort within 48 hours after they ingest pine needles, and other animals may abort as long as 2 weeks after they are removed from access to the needles.

There are generally few signs of impending abortion. The abortion is characterized by weak parturition contractions, excessive uterine hemorrhage, and incomplete dilation of the cervix. A calf that is delivered near term when the needles are eaten generally survives. If the calf survives, as it often does in cows near term, the condition cannot be termed a true abortion but is a premature birth. A cow may show swelling of the external genital organs and filling of the udder if she grazes the needles over a period of time before the abortion.

Persistent retained placentas are a constant finding, regardless of stage of gestation of the abortion. Septic metritis often follows the abortion, and unless the animal is properly treated, generalized septicemia may follow. In acute cases, the cow appears to have toxemia and may die before or soon after she aborts. In such cases, there may be ecchymotic hemorrhages on the peritoneum, pleura, and viscera. There are no specific characteristic lesions in the aborted calves as a result of pine needle ingestion.

Prevention involves keeping the cows from grazing pine needles during the last trimester of gestation. Although cattle may graze in areas with ponderosa pine during the critical stage of gestation and not eat the needles, there is always the risk that they may.

Broomsnakeweed

Broomsnakeweed, *Gutierrezia* spp., is an herbaceous plant that branches near the top of the ground. The branches are topped by yellow composite flowers. The leaves are small, alternate, and filiform.

Signs of poisoning include anorexia, rough hair coat, listlessness, and loss of weight. They may develop diarrhea or may become constipated. There may be a vaginal discharge and also bloody urine.

Pregnant cows, principally in the last trimester of pregnancy, may develop signs of an impending parturition (e.g., swelling of the external genital organs and filling of the udder). Abortion will generally follow. Most cows have a retained placenta. The cow may die of a toxemia associated with the abortion. In excess of 60 per cent of cows grazing broomsnakeweed may abort. The calves of those near term may survive but are small and weak and need supportive care.

Cows grazing in excess of 20 pounds of plant are at risk for an abortion. Cows grazing broomsnakeweed growing on sandy soils are more apt to abort than are cows grazing plants on limestone or hard soils.

Cows are most apt to graze broomsnakeweed after a snowstorm or other adverse weather conditions and during time of forage shortages.

Sheep and goats are also said to suffer abortion after the grazing of broomsnakeweed.

Broomsnakeweed appears to be increasing in amount in

areas farther north, such as Utah and Idaho, than where it has been traditionally a problem in range livestock production.

Milkweeds (*Asclepias* spp.)

Milkweeds (*Asclepias* spp.) are widespread on many ranges of the western United States. They are perennial herbs that contain milky juice, stand erect, and have opposite or whorled leaf arrangements. The milkweeds are divided into 2 groups, the narrow-leaf milkweeds and the broadleaf milkweeds. Not all species of milkweeds are toxic. The principal poisonous species in the West are *A. labriformis*, *A. subverticillata*, *A. eriocarpa*, and *A. fascicularis*. *A. labriformis* is among the most toxic of range plants. Cardiac glycosides (cardenolides) are the toxic principles of these plants. Milkweeds are unpalatable and usually eaten only by hungry animals. They may also be harvested with hay or green chop and thus cause poisoning as a forage contaminant.

The signs of poisoning include muscular incoordination, spasms, bloat, rapid weak pulse, respiratory difficulty, and death.

No treatment is known for animals poisoned on milkweed. Losses from milkweed can be reduced by maintaining ranges and pastures in good condition. Livestock that are hungry should not be allowed to graze in milkweed-infested areas. Milkweed should not be harvested with hay and other forages.

Horsebrush (*Tetradymia* spp.)

Horsebrush (*Tetradymia* spp.) is a shrub growing in the drier range areas of the West. These plants are principally a problem to sheep in the early spring. This plant is discussed in more detail in the article Plants Producing Dermal Injury.

Oak (*Quercus* spp.)

Oak (*Quercus* spp.) is poisonous primarily to cattle. Oaks of the West are low-growing shrubs or small trees. Oak grows in dense stands, and growth starts early in the spring before most other range plants. It is most toxic during the bud and early leaf stage. As the leaves mature, they decrease in toxicity. Large amounts of oak must be eaten for cattle to be poisoned.

The signs of poisoning are rough hair coat, gaunt appearance, emaciation, edema, constipation or diarrhea, mucus or blood (or both) in the feces, dark brown urine, and death.

Lesions include gastroenteritis and edema of the intestinal walls. The kidney may have petechia, subcutaneous edema, and ascites.

Prevention consists of keeping cattle away from the oak brush during the period when oak is in the early bud stage, especially during times of feed shortage. This treatment may involve the development of a range or pasture free of oak brush.

Locoweed (*Astragalus* and *Oxytropis* spp.)

Locoweed (*Astragalus* and *Oxytropis* spp.) can affect all classes of livestock. Species of these plants grow throughout most of the range states and have the potential of poisoning animals where conditions favor their growth. More than 350 species of *Astragalus* grow in North America. About 12 of these cause classic locoism in livestock.

Locoweed poisoning is a chronic type of intoxication. An animal must graze the plant for about 30 days before signs of poisoning appear. The length of time between ingestion and appearance of signs is dependent on the rate of consumption and, to a lesser extent, on the species of plant.

The signs of locoweed poisoning are rough hair coat, dull eyes, emaciation, depression, and irregular gait. High incidence of abortions and birth defects has been associated with locoweed poisoning.

Locoweed, when it is grazed at higher elevations, causes a marked enhancement of congestive right-sided heart failure in cattle.

There are no specific or characteristic gross post-mortem lesions. Microscopic lesions are general neurovisceral cytoplasmic vacuolations.

Animals that have become poisoned on locoweed may recover to varying degrees with proper care. However, locoweed can induce permanent damage, so an animal may show signs of poisoning throughout its lifetime. Locoweed is also habit-forming. Once an animal starts to graze locoweed, it will continue to do so at the exclusion of other forage. If removed from and then exposed to locoweed at a later date, it may start grazing the plant again.

Prevention consists of keeping animals away from areas heavily infested with locoweed. If livestock must graze in such areas, they should be observed closely, and those starting to graze locoweed should be removed immediately. Dried locoweed plant is also toxic, and in several instances, livestock ranchers have sustained heavy losses when their livestock grazed dried locoweed plant.

Timber Milkvetch (*Astragalus miser*)

Timber milkvetch (*Astragalus miser*) and other *Astragalus* plants, such as *A. emoryanus*, *A. pterocarpus*, and *A. canadensis* that contain 3-nitro-1-propanol or 3-nitro-1-propionic acid as a toxic constituent, grow in most of the 11 western states and Canada.

Depending on the rate at which it is eaten by livestock, this group of plants may induce acute or chronic poisoning. Acute intoxication is characterized by nervousness, irregular gait, general body weakness, rapid weak pulse, coma, and death. Some animals may show indications of blindness. Lesions include lobular alveolar pulmonary emphysema, collapsed or constricted bronchioles, and interlobular edema. Some cases have widespread focal hemorrhage in the central nervous system.

Chronic intoxication is characterized by dullness, incoordination of the hindlegs when walking, and goose stepping. The animals may have cocked ankles and may fall when they run. There may be respiratory distress and posterior paralysis if the condition progresses to advanced stages. With proper care, poisoned animals may recover. However, animals grazing the plant usually die if they are not removed from the plant.

The post-mortem lesions are not pathognomonic. The liver may be swollen, and the pericardial fluid may be increased; varying degrees of wallerian degeneration of the spinal cord and varying degrees of pulmonary emphysema are regularly observed.

Poisoning can best be prevented by not allowing animals to graze this plant over extended periods of time. Intoxication in areas where this plant is a problem seems to be more severe in periods of drought. Nursing cows are more often affected than are dry cows. Cows poisoned on this plant should be handled carefully and should not be exposed to stressful conditions.

Rayless Goldenrod (*Haplopappus heterophyllus*)

Rayless goldenrod (*Haplopappus heterophyllus*) is common in the dry rangelands of the Southwest. It is an erect, unbranched perennial shrub with yellow flowers that grows from

61 to 122 cm (2 to 4 ft) tall. The poisonous principle is tremetol, a higher alcohol. It is toxic to all classes of range livestock. If animals that are grazing this plant are not removed from it, they will die. The toxin is excreted in the milk, so the nursing offspring will be intoxicated before the dam.

The signs of poisoning are lassitude and depression, a humped-up posture, and stiff gait. The body may tremble, especially about the head and shoulders. Signs of poisoning may be accentuated by forced exercise. Post-mortem findings are not characteristic. The liver may be pale, and the abomasum and intestines may be congested.

Eupatorium rugosum contains the same toxin as does rayless goldenrod. It has been shown that horses grazing white snakeroot may develop heart and skeletal muscle necrosis.

Prevention consists of eradication of the plants or not allowing livestock to graze them.

Sneezeweed (*Helenium hoopesii*)

Sneezeweed (*Helenium hoopesii*) grows on moist slopes and well-drained meadows at elevations from 1524 to 3048 m (5000 to 10,000 ft) throughout most of the 11 western states. Sneezeweed is an herbaceous perennial with yellow flowers, and it grows from 30 to 90 cm (1 to 3 ft) tall. It is primarily a problem in range sheep. Animals are poisoned after grazing the plant for about 10 days, most often in the late summer and early fall when better forage is gone or dried up. Signs of poisoning are depression, stiffness, weakness, coughing, chronic vomiting (which leaves the area around the mouth stained green), and bloating. If the animals continue to graze the plant until vomiting starts, they usually waste and die.

The principal lesions of sneezeweed poisoning are gastroenteritis, edema of the stomach walls, excessive fluid in the pericardial cavity, and ascites.

Prevention consists of control of the plants or removing the sheep from sneezeweed-infested ranges at frequent intervals.

Rubberweed (*Hymenoxys richardsonii*)

Rubberweed or pingue (*Hymenoxys richardsonii*) is a perennial herb with yellow flowers that grows from 15 to 46 cm (6 to 18 in) tall. It grows principally on dry foothill areas from 1220 to 3048 m (4000 to 10,000 ft) of elevation. Rubberweed is principally a problem in range sheep. Heavy infestation of rubberweed indicates overgrazing. Signs of poisoning are salivation, anorexia, rumen stasis, apparent abdominal pain, uneasiness, weakness, and prostration. Lesions are associated with gastrointestinal irritation and hepatic degeneration.

Rubberweed is distasteful; therefore, the animal is poisoned primarily during trailing and during grazing of ranges heavily infested with the plant.

PREVENTION AND MANAGEMENT

Poisoning of livestock by plants that are part of their normal diet is uncommon. Livestock poisoning on the range usually becomes a problem because of a shortage of nonpoisonous plants or because of an increase in poisonous plants, which results when the more desirable plants have been completely grazed. In general, the prevention of loss from poisonous plants is largely a problem of proper animal and range management. Most poisonous plants are distasteful to livestock. Exceptions are plants such as larkspur and, under some conditions, locoweeds.

Some general rules for preventing livestock poisoning by plants are as follows.

1. Know the poisonous plants, especially those of local significance.
2. Know how poisonous plants affect livestock and the conditions under which they are toxic.
3. Avoid areas infested with poisonous plants during holding, trailing, or unloading of animals. If these situations cannot be avoided, special preventive procedures should be considered.
4. Avoid grazing hungry animals in areas infested with poisonous plants. Animals may become hungry by withholding feed or water and by overgrazing. Provide animals with water and adequate forage of good quality.
5. Provide adequate salt and mineral supplements.
6. Where possible, control or eradicate poisonous plants, especially from problem areas.
7. Develop and practice proper grazing procedures.
8. Keep the range in good condition. Avoid overgrazing.
9. Good management practices will prevent most cases of plant poisoning in livestock.

BIBLIOGRAPHY

James LF, et al: Plants poisonous to livestock in the western United States. USDA Agricultural Information Bulletin 415, 1988, p 90.
James LF: Symposium on poisonous plants. J Range Manage 31:324–360, 1978.
James LF, Johnson AE: Some major plant toxicities of the western United States. J Range Manage 29:356–363, 1976.
Keeler RF: Toxins and teratogens of higher plants. Lloydia 38:56–86, 1975.
Keeler RF, Van Kampen KR, James LF (eds): Effects of Poisonous Plants on Livestock. New York, Academic Press, 1978.
Kingsbury JM: Poisonous Plants of the United States and Canada. Englewood Cliffs, NJ, Prentice-Hall, 1964.

Principal Poisonous Plants in the Midwestern and Eastern United States

GEORGE E. BURROWS, DVM, PHD
ARTHUR A. CASE, DVM, MS*

The nonspecificity of many syndromes caused by toxic plants often makes it difficult to implicate plants as a cause. It also renders difficult the recognition of the overall role of toxic plants in animal health. Gastrointestinal disorders are among the most common manifestations of many diseases, including those caused by toxic plants, yet because the signs are so common, there may be no justification to incriminate specific plants or other causes. Thus, we are unable to assess the potential importance of such plants as threats to livestock health.

Because of the wide geographic area represented in this discussion, there are of necessity a large number of plants included as toxic (Tables 1 to 3). However, there are only a limited number that are significant threats to livestock health despite the recognition that serious problems are caused by the same genera and species in other regions of the United States (Tables 1 to 3). Factors prevailing in the Midwest and East that reduce the threat of intoxication due to plants, compared with other regions of the United States, include (1) relatively greater abundance of vegetation such as grasses,

---
*Deceased.

Table 1. IMPORTANT TOXIC SHRUBS AND FORBS

Plant	Habitat/Distribution	Toxin
Amaranthus spp. (pigweeds, carelessweed)	Widespread, especially in waste areas	Nephrotoxin and nitrate accumulation
Asclepias spp. (milkweeds)	Wide variety of habitats throughout the region	Cardenolides or neurotoxins
Calycanthus (sweet shrub, allspice)	Woodlands and watersides throughout the Southeast	Neurotoxic alkaloid
Cassia spp. (senna)	Open woodlands and fields especially in sandy areas of the South	Quinone cathartics and unknown myotoxins
Cicuta maculata (water hemlock)	Moist, shaded areas throughout the region	Oily, resinous, neurotoxic alcohol
Crotalaria spp. (rattlepod)	Moist, sandy sites throughout the region	Hepatotoxic pyrrolizidine alkaloids
Eupatorium rugosum (white snakeroot)	Woodlands and bottomlands throughout the region	Alcoholic complex, tremetol, acting as metabolic and hepatic toxicants
Gelsemium sempervirens (yellow jessamine)	Open woodlands and fencerows throughout the South	Neurotoxic alkaloids
Helenium spp. (sneezeweeds)	Open pastures throughout the South or moist areas throughout the regions	Sesquiterpene lactone metabolic toxins
Perilla frutescens (purple mint)	Variety of sites, especially open woodlands throughout the regions	Pulmonotoxic aromatic ketones
Pteridium aquilinum (bracken fern)	Well-drained open woodlands throughout the region	Lactone marrow toxin, ptaquiloside
Rhododendron spp. (rhododendrons) also *Kalmia* (laurels), *Leucothoe* (fetterbush), and *Lyonia* (maleberry)	Woodlands, South and East	Diterpenoid neuromuscular grayanotoxins
Senecio spp. (ragwort, groundsel)	Open prairies and woodlands throughout the regions	Hepatotoxic pyrrolizidine alkaloids
Sesbania spp. (rattlebox, bladderpod)	Moist open areas throughout the south	Gastroenteric toxic saponins
Taxus spp. (yew)	Ornamental, throughout the regions	Cardiac conduction inhibitor, taxine
Xanthium strumarium (cocklebur)	Sandy areas subject to flooding throughout the regions	Metabolic toxin, carboxyatractyloside

Table 2. TOXIC PLANTS OF MINOR IMPORTANCE

Plant	Habitat/Distribution	Toxic Effect	Plant	Habitat/Distribution	Toxic Effect
Actaea spp. (baneberry)	Eastern US	GI irritation	*Digitalis* (foxglove)	Ornamental	Cardiac arrhythmias
Allium spp. (onions)	Widespread	Hemolysis	*Euphorbia* spp. (spurge)	Widespread waste areas	GI irritation
Amianthum muscaetoxicum (stagger grass)	Southeastern US	Neurologic	*Hedera helix* (English ivy)	Ornamental	GI irritation
Apocynum spp. (dogbane)	Widespread	Cardiac arrhythmias	*Hordeum vulgare* (barley)	Cultivated	Photosensitization
Baccharis spp. (baccharis)	Widespread, open moist sandy areas, especially coastal plains	Neurologic/cardiac arrhythmias	*Hyacinthus orientalis* (hyacinth)	Ornamental	GI irritation
			Hydrangea spp. (hydrangea)	Ornamental	GI irritation
Beta spp. (beets)	Cultivated	Nephrosis, oxalates	*Hypericum* spp. (St. Johnswort)	Widespread, open woodlands	Photosensitization
Brassica spp. (Kale, rape)	Widespread	GI irritation	*Ilex* spp. (holly)	Ornamental	GI irritation
Buxus spp. (box)	Ornamental	GI irritation	*Iris* spp. (iris)	Ornamental	GI irritation
Celastrus scandens (bittersweet)	Eastern US	GI irritation and cardiotoxic	*Kochia scoparia* (burning bush)	Waste areas, field edges	Neurologic and photosensitization
Cestrum spp. (jessamine)	Ornamental, far South	GI irritation and neurologic	*Lantana camara* (lantana)	Ornamental	Hepatopathy and GI irritation
Conium maculatum (poison hemlock)	Widespread	Neurologic and teratogenic	*Lathyrus* spp. (wild pea)	Widespread	Neurologic and teratogenic
Convallaria majalis (lily of the valley)	Ornamental	Cardiac arrhythmias	*Ligustrum* spp. (privet)	Ornamental	GI irritation
Corydalis spp. (scrambled eggs)	Waste areas to open woods	Neurologic	*Lobelia* spp. (lobelia)	Widespread but not abundant, in moist areas	Neurologic
Daphne spp. (laurels)	Ornamental	GI irritation	*Lotus corniculatus* (bird's-foot trefoil)	Cultivated	Hepatic failure
Datura spp. (thornapples)	Widespread	Neurologic	*Lycopersicon esculentum* (tomato)	Cultivated	GI irritation, neurologic
Delphinium spp. (larkspur)	Moist woodlands and ornamental	Neurologic	*Melanthum virginicum* (bunchflower)	Widespread	Neurologic
Dicentra spp. (Dutchman's breeches)	Moist open woodlands	Neurologic	*Menispermum canadense* (moonseed)	Widespread	Neurologic

Table continued on opposite page

Table 2. TOXIC PLANTS OF MINOR IMPORTANCE Continued

Plant	Habitat/Distribution	Toxic Effect	Plant	Habitat/Distribution	Toxic Effect
Modiola caroliniana (ground ivy)	Waste areas of the South	Neurologic	*Ricinus communis* (castor bean)	Ornamental	GI irritation
Nandina domestica (heavenly bamboo)	Ornamental	Cyanogenic	*Rumex* spp. (dock)	Widespread	Nephrosis, oxalates
Nicotiana spp. (tobacco)	Cultivated	Neurologic, teratogenic	*Sambucus canadensis* (elderberry)	Widespread	GI irritation
Nerium oleander (oleander)	Ornamental	Cardiac arrhythmias	*Secale cereale* (rye)	Cultivated	Photosensitization
Phoradendron spp. (mistletoe)	Widespread	GI irritation	*Solanum* spp. (nightshade)	Widespread	GI irritation, neurologic
Phytolacca americana (pokeweed)	Widespread, waste areas	GI irritation	*Trifolium* spp. (clover)	Cultivated	Photosensitization, estrogenic, cyanogenic
Podophyllum peltatum (mayapple)	Moist meadows, woodlands	GI irritation	*Triticum aestivum* (wheat)	Cultivated	Photosensitization
Ranunculus spp. (buttercup)	Moist open pastures, woodlands	GI irritation	*Wisteria* spp. (wisteria)	Ornamental	GI irritation
Rheum raponticum (rhubarb)	Cultivated	Nephrosis, oxalates	*Zygadenus* spp. (death camas)	Widespread	GI irritation, neurologic

GI = gastrointestinal.

Table 3. TOXIC TREES, MAJOR AND MINOR

Tree	Habitat/Distribution	Toxin
Major		
Aesculus spp (buckeye); also *Hippocastaneum* (horse chestnut)	Woodlands and bottomlands throughout the regions	Neurotoxin
Prunus spp. (cherry)	Woodlands and flood plains throughout the regions	Cyanogenic glycosides
Quercus spp. (oak)	Variety of sites throughout the regions	Nephrotoxic gallotanins
Robinia pseudoacacia (black locust)	Variety of sites in Southeast and cultivated elsewhere	GI irritation, neurotoxin
Minor		
Gymnocladus dioica (Kentucky coffee tree)	Woodlands, flood plains throughout the regions	GI toxin-alkaloid
Laburnum anagyroides (golden chain tree)	Northern portion of region, ornamental	Nicotine-like alkaloid
Melia azedarach (chinaberry)	Woodlands and flood plains throughout the South	GI irritation
Persea americana (avocado)	Florida	Irritant-mastitis

GI = gastrointestinal.

Table 4. POISONOUS SEEDS IN HAY AND GRAINS

Toxic Species	Adulterated Feedstuff	Susceptible Animals
Crotalaria spp.	Cereal grains and sorghums (milo)	All species, especially swine
Corn cockle, cow cockle (*Agrostemma* spp., *Saponaria* spp.)	Cereal grains, especially spring-planted, late-harvested; occasionally hay	All species, especially swine; LD is about 0.01 g/kg of the powerful sapotoxins
Cocklebur (*Xanthium* spp.)	Corn, soybeans, late-cut hay, silage, or fresh chop	All species; if cocklebur is milled, it is very toxic in small amounts
Ergots (*Claviceps* spp.)	Ergot sclerotia are often found in rye, wheat, oats, triticale, and grass hays harvested in the seed stage or later	All species are susceptible to ergotism; acute from large amounts over a short time; chronic from small amounts over a long time
Morning glories (*Ipomoea* spp.)	Corn, soybeans, and occasionally milo or other fall-harvested grains; silage and green chop	Swine are at greatest risk, but cattle, sheep, and goats are also sensitive to lysergic acid
Solanaceae Jimsonweed (*Datura*) Nightshades (*Solanum*)	Seed and fruit are often included in corn, soybeans, fresh chop, silage, or hay; approx. 1000 jimsonweed seeds/kg diet reported as toxic to cattle	The powerful solanaceus toxins will poison any animal eating enough of them; swine are most often affected; calves and lambs as well as kids are susceptible
Mustard family (*Thlaspi arvense*)	Mustard seeds contain isoallyl thiocyanates and other toxic principles; in threshed grain or first-cut hay	All species are susceptible, but swine, lambs, and calves are most likely to be poisoned by mustard seeds
Sneezeweeds (*Helenium* spp.) (*Senecio* spp.)	Seed heads of sneezeweeds or bitterweeds contaminate grain, hay, and fresh chop	All species, with swine, calves, lambs, and kids being most susceptible, especially over time

which makes the animals less likely to consume toxic plants; (2) greater number of plant species available at any one time, which increases the opportunity for animals to eat small amounts of a greater variety of plants; and (3) greater competition between plants, especially grasses, which reduces the likelihood of abundant growth for many of the poorly competitive toxic plants. Because of these factors, very unusual circumstances may need to prevail locally for the appropriate conditions to be provided for intoxication to occur.

Weather often determines whether plant-related problems will occur in a given season or year. Generally, the Midwest and East receive plentiful moisture, compared with the southwestern desert areas; however, there may be extended dry periods or unseasonably hot or cool periods, which will have a significant impact on plant-related toxicoses. Cultivated crops such as corn (*Zea mays*), sorghum, and clover may become toxic because of various influences during growth. Intensive farming areas typically no longer have many native toxic plants, but aggressive weeds, such as cocklebur (*Xanthium* spp.), pigweeds (*Amaranthus*), milkweeds (*Asclepias*), and dogbane (*Apocynum*), several species of the solanaceous plants, morning glory, and bindweeds are likely to invade crop fields. Many such weeds are toxic, have toxic seeds, or concentrate oxalate, nitrate, or toxic minerals (Table 4). There are marked seasonal variations in incidence of many plant-related intoxications; however, because of the geographic scope of the discussion, this will not be addressed in most cases. Intoxications due to oak are an example of the geographic differences; in the South, early spring (April and May) is the high-risk season, whereas farther north this may occur later because of later foliage development or be due to acorn ingestion rather than foliage.

Two of the most serious problems associated with plants are nitrate-nitrite and cyanide intoxication. There are numerous plants capable of causing these problems, many of which are listed in the tables. Nitrates are among the most common chemicals in plants because nitrate salts are the principal form of nitrogen taken up from the soil. There is probably little to be realized from listing all of the plants capable of accumulating nitrate because few are ever associated with intoxication. Nitrate as a serious intoxication problem occurs primarily in the range of sorghums as forage crops, secondarily in areas of other cereal grains including oats and corn, and occasionally in association with weedy plants such as pigweed (*Amaranthus* spp.). The primary factor is rate of intake of the nitrate salt and subsequent rate of conversion to the ultimate toxicant, nitrite. Typically, nitrate intoxication involves feeding of hay made from a nitrate-accumulating forage. Cyanide in many ways is similar to nitrate as a toxicant, often involving the same plants, under different circumstances, especially the sorghums including Johnson grass (*S. halapense*). However, there are many other plants including the wild cherries that may present a serious hazard owing to the presence of cyanogenic glycosides. In most cases, the forage will be fresh, and rate of intake is again a major factor.

Of the important toxic plants listed in Table 1, those of greatest risk in this region include purple mint (*Perilla*) in the fall, yew (*Taxus*) in winter or spring, and cocklebur (*Xanthium*) in late spring or early summer. The other plants are important, but conditions are rarely present that will result in ingestion of amounts sufficient to cause intoxication. In many cases, toxic plants are not palatable (many *Asclepias*, *Helenium*, *Senecio*) and are eaten only in the necessary quantities in the absence of alternative forages. In addition, large amounts of forage may be required, and the species may flourish for only a limited period (*Senecio* spp.).

BIBLIOGRAPHY

Case AA: Toxicologic problems in large animals. J Am Vet Med Assoc 149:1714–1719, 1966.
Cole RJ, Stuart BP, Lansden JA, Cox RH: Isolation and redefinition of the toxic agent from cocklebur (*Xanthium strumarium*). J Agri Food Chem 28:1330–1332, 1980.
Evers RA, Link RP: Poisonous Plants of the Midwest. Special Publication No. 24. Urbana-Champaign, College of Agriculture, University of Illinois, 1972.
Freeman JD, Moore HD: Livestock Poisoning by Vascular Plants of Alabama. Bulletin 460. Auburn, AL, Agriculture Experimental Stations, 1974.
Gress EM: Poisonous Plants of Pennsylvania. Department of Agriculture. Bulletin 531. Pennsylvania Department of Agriculture, 1935.
Hulbert LC, Dehme FW: Plants Poisonous to Livestock, 3rd ed. Manhattan, KS, Kansas State University Printing Service, 1968.
Keeler RF, Van Kampen KR, James L: Effects of Poisonous Plants on Livestock. New York, Academic Press, 1978.
Kingsbury JM: Poisonous Plants of the United States and Canada. Englewood Cliffs, NJ, Prentice-Hall, 1964.
Miller JF, Kates AH, Davis DE, McCormach J: Poisonous Plants of the Southern United States. Athens, GA, Cooperative Extension Service, University of Georgia College of Agriculture, 1980.
Radeleff RD: Veterinary Toxicology, Poisonous Plants, 2nd ed. Philadelphia, Lea & Febiger, 1970, pp 42–157.

Cardiotoxic Plants
MURRAY E. FOWLER, DVM

Few species of plants contain toxic substances that primarily affect the cardiovascular system, but consumption of any of these few species of plants produces dramatic effects.

POISONOUS PRINCIPLES

Cardioactive glycosides are the principal agents producing cardiotoxic effects. Many different cardioactive glycosides are found in plants. The concentration of glycosides within the plant varies with season, stage of maturity, part of the plant, and environmental conditions. The toxic effects of the various glycosides are generally similar, differing mostly in degree of severity and persistence of debility. Most species of mammals and birds are susceptible to the toxic effects of cardioactive glycosides, but a few wild animals can consume cardioactive glycosides with impunity.

Many South African plants contain cardioactive glycosides. A few of the more potent species were used by native Africans to poison arrows for hunting. Rarely will these plants be of concern to North American livestock owners, unless they are planted as ornamentals in North American gardens. The ornamental succulent *Cotyledon orbiculata* killed sheep when prunings were thrown into a sheep pasture.

A number of drugs that have action on the autonomic nervous system also produce effects on cardiac function. Many of these, although synthesized now, originated in a plant species (Table 1). Wild or commercial tobacco and the poi-

Table 1. PLANT-DERIVED DRUGS AFFECTING AUTONOMIC NERVOUS SYSTEM

Atropine	*Atropa belladonna*, *Datura* sp.
Muscarine	*Amanita muscaria*
Ephedrine	*Ephedra* sp.
Ergotamine	*Claviceps purpurea*
Nicotine	*Nicotiana* sp.

Table 2. PLANTS CONTAINING CARDIOACTIVE GLYCOSIDE CAPABLE OF POISONING LIVESTOCK IN NORTH AMERICA

Oleander	*Nerium oleander*
Foxglove	*Digitalis purpurea*
Indian hemp	*Apocynum cannabinum*
Lily of the valley	*Convallaria majalis*
Milkweed	*Asclepias* sp.
Ornamental succulent	*Cotyledon orbiculata*

sonous mushroom *Amanita muscaria* may poison livestock species. Alkaloids found in yews have both direct and indirect cardiac effects.

PLANTS

Detailed taxonomic descriptions of cardiotoxic plants are not possible here. The reader is referred to a standard text for aid in plant identification.[1,2] Table 2 lists the important cardiotoxic plants of North America. A short discussion of poisoning by a few species follows.

Oleander

The plant most often responsible for cardiotoxicosis is oleander (*Nerium oleander*). Oleander, a shrub or a small tree, is grown as an ornamental in the southern United States and throughout much of California. It may be kept as a potted plant in more northern climates. Thus, oleander toxicity is a potential hazard almost anywhere in North America.

Oleander contains a potent cardioactive glycoside. All parts of the plant, including leaves, roots, flowers, and bark, either dry or green, are dangerous. The glycoside is stable in boiling water. The lethal dose of oleander is approximately 110 mg of green or dry leaf per kilogram of body weight. Thus, 55 g are fatal to a 500-kg animal.

Oleander leaves have a bitter taste and are unpalatable. If leaves fall from the shrub and wilt or dry, they are apparently more readily accepted by livestock, especially if they become mixed with grass clippings. Cattle housed in corrals surrounded by oleander plants seldom eat the shrub, but toxicosis may result if cuttings of the shrub are left to wilt in a pasture or are placed in an area where cattle normally feed. Extremely hungry cattle, sheep, and goats have been poisoned when they grazed a strange pasture containing little forage but oleander.

Hay may be a source of the plant. Cattle and sheep have died after ingestion of baled hay harvested from a field bordered by oleander shrubs.

Purple Foxglove

Digitalis purpurea is an ornamental grown in cool, moist climates in the United States. It has become a naturalized weed in north coastal California and Oregon.

Indian Hemp or Dogbane

Apocynum cannabinum is a short shrub of waste places (e.g., vacant lots, roadsides, unused fields).

Table 3. ADDITIONAL PLANTS CONTAINING TOXINS AFFECTING CARDIAC FUNCTION IN LIVESTOCK

Yew	*Taxus* sp. (alkaloid)
False hellebore	*Veratrum* sp. (alkaloid)

Lily of the Valley

Convallaria majalis is an ornamental ground cover. Cuttings and prunings may be unknowingly placed where livestock can consume the material.

Milkweed

A cardioactive glycoside is one component of the toxic agent of milkweed plants of the genus *Asclepias*. Although cardiac effects may accompany the clinical syndrome produced by consumption of milkweeds, other chemicals produce the major effects.

Yew (Table 3)

Taxus sp. is an ornamental evergreen shrub or small tree. In general appearance it resembles a conifer, but its fruit is a small fleshy berry instead of a cone. The poisonous principle is an alkaloid affecting both the nervous system and the heart. The cardiac effects are bradycardia and cardiac arrest. Neural signs are depression, trembling, dyspnea, collapse, and sudden death. Subacute toxicosis, as seen in cattle, is characterized additionally by gastroenteritis and diarrhea.

False Hellebore (Table 3)

Plants of *Veratrum* sp. contain alkaloids that cause cardiac irregularities and potential death. Common syndromes associated with these plants are teratogenic effects of central nervous system derangement.

CLINICAL SIGNS

Cardioactive Glycoside Poisoning

Clinical signs of cardioactive glycoside poisoning develop 4 to 12 hours after ingestion of the plant. Ingestion of lethal quantities results in death within 12 to 24 hours. Clinical signs may persist for 2 or 3 days with ingestion of a sublethal dose. In cattle, continued release of glycosides in the rumen may prolong the syndrome or cause exacerbation after an apparent improvement. As the disease progresses, the animal becomes depressed and weak. Localized muscle fasciculation may occur, or generalized trembling can progress to terminal anoxic convulsions. Cattle commonly become weak and comatose.

Toxic doses of cardioactive glycosides exaggerate the therapeutic effects of these agents. During the course of a poisoning episode, a variety of cardiac conduction abnormalities are seen, such as bradycardia, tachycardia, dropped beats, heart block, atrial fibrillation, ventricular tachycardia, and ventricular fibrillation. There seems to be no set pattern to the sequence of development of irregularities except that fibrillation is usually a terminal sign. At any one moment, the heart rate and rhythm may sound normal. Auscultation over a period of minutes is necessary to detect cardiac irregularities.

Many clinical signs are a direct result of hypoxia caused by inability of the heart to circulate blood. Extremities are cold. Rectal temperature may be normal or slightly subnormal. The pulse is usually rapid and weak. Respiratory rate and depth are increased. Hemorrhagic nasal discharge and open-mouth breathing are seen in severely affected animals. Mucous membranes may be cyanotic.

Cardioactive glycosides (but not yew alkaloids) also produce gastrointestinal signs, such as colic and catarrhal or hemorrhagic diarrhea. In fact, signs of gastroenteritis may be the first symptoms noted. Swine may exhibit nausea and vomiting.

NECROPSY

The most consistent lesions are those of catarrhal or hemorrhagic gastroenteritis. Many organs are congested because of poor tissue perfusion. Petechial hemorrhages may be seen on serosal surfaces in the abdomen and the thoracic cavities. Blood-stained fluids are frequently found in body cavities. Usually no lesions are associated with yew poisoning.

DIAGNOSIS

Clinical signs are suggestive. Prolonged auscultation of the heart is a reliable diagnostic tool. Electrocardiographic examination is helpful but not required. A history of possible consumption of plants known to contain cardioactive glycosides is an aid and, in some cases, is necessary to make a definitive diagnosis. Necropsy lesions are not pathognomonic. Gastroenteric lesions are not easily differentiated from those caused by infectious agents.

Radioimmune assay procedures are available for detecting specific cardioactive glycosides such as digoxin or ouabain in human blood. Such tests are host- and glycoside-specific and are not practicable for evaluating suspected animal poisoning.

Examination of rumen contents for plant segments may be very helpful. Oleander has characteristic leaves. Secondary veins branch from the main longitudinal vein in a parallel fashion. A diagnosis of oleander poisoning would be justified by the presence of any oleander plant segment in the rumen contents. Yew leaves are also distinctive but require close observation for distinguishing them from other forage materials in the rumen.

A differential diagnosis should include infectious enteritis and other toxicoses, such as castor bean (*Ricinus communis*) or arsenic poisoning.

TREATMENT

The most effective treatment is to rid the gastrointestinal tract of residual plant material. In swine, an emetic should be administered followed by intubation and administration of activated charcoal (1 to 3 g/kg) and sodium or magnesium sulfate (1 g/kg). Ruminants are more difficult to treat. If an ante-mortem diagnosis has been made, a rumenotomy is indicated. All of the rumen contents must be extracted, and preferably the rumen should be washed. Any residual plant material is potentially lethal. A rumen content transplant from an animal with no possible exposure to the toxic substance may be required in order for proper rumen function to resume.

General nursing care is indicated. No specific antidotal agents are effective in food animals, but stomach intubation and the administration of laxatives plus activated charcoal should be attempted (2 g/kg).

All access to continued ingestion of plants containing cardioactive glycosides must cease. In one case, lawn and garden clippings containing oleander had been dumped where cattle could reach through a fence and consume them. The farmer was advised to remove the pile of leaves and grass. Losses continued. Finally it was ascertained that he had cleaned up the pile with a 4-tine pitchfork, leaving a few leaves at the site. With oleander, a few leaves can be lethal.

REFERENCES

1. Joubert JPJ: Cardiac glycosides. *In* Checke PR (ed): Toxicants of Plant Origin, vol II. Glycosides. Boca Raton, FL, CRC Press, 1989, pp 61–96.
2. Kingsbury JM: Poisonous Plants of the United States and Canada. Englewood Cliffs, NJ, Prentice-Hall, 1964.

Hepatotoxic Plants
MURRAY E. FOWLER, DVM

Some plant toxins produce deleterious effects on the liver. The liver is a multiple-function organ, and derangement may produce one or more malfunctions. The clinical syndrome produced by a particular toxin varies according to the function affected. Table 1 lists those plants of the United States and Canada that produce hepatotoxicity as a major effect when they are ingested by livestock.

PLANT TOXINS

Pyrrolizidine Alkaloid Poisoning

Although over 100 pyrrolizidine alkaloids are known,[1] only a few are toxic. Plants containing toxic alkaloids were recognized as hazardous to livestock as early as 1787. Pyrrolizidine alkaloid poisoning (PAP) occurs worldwide, causing extensive livestock losses.

Lesion Pathogenesis

Pyrrolizidine alkaloids (PAs) may undergo some degradation in the rumen of certain species, but in most species, PAs are absorbed and transported to the liver. Before toxic lesions are produced, PAs must be converted to pyrroles. The metabolic process that converts PAs to pyrroles may vary in efficiency and rate between species. It is presumed that liver microzyme action is responsible.

The liver parenchyma is bathed with the pyrrole, and hepatocytes are diffusely affected. With large doses, necrosis of the hepatocyte occurs. More characteristically, the cell is affected by a metabolic lesion that prevents the hepatocyte from undergoing normal binary fission to regenerate hepatocytes. Unable to divide, the cell continues to grow. Both the nucleus and cytoplasm expand, sometimes as much as 10-fold (hepatocytomeglia, karyomeglia). Ultimately, the cell reaches a critical mass and dies. If a few cells die simultaneously, the histopathologic process will appear as parenchymal atrophy

Table 1. HEPATOTOXIC PLANTS IN THE UNITED STATES

Plants Containing Pyrrolizidine Alkaloids
Senecio spp. (ragwort, groundsel, many other species)
Amsinckia intermedia (fiddleneck, fireweed)
Crotalaria sp. (rattlebox, rattleweed, wild pea)
Heliotropium europaeum (heliotrope)
Symphytum officinale (comfrey)
Echium sp.
Cynoglossum officinale (hound's tongue)
Plants Causing Photosensitization
Agave lechuguilla (century plant)
Brassica napus (rape)
Nolina texana (sacahiuste, bear grass)
Tetradymia sp. (horsebrush)
Lantana sp. (lantana)
Blue-green algae (water bloom)
Others
Aspergillus flavus (fungus)
Amanita phalloides (death cap mushroom)

with hepatocytomeglia. If large numbers of cells die simultaneously (as might occur with a moderate dose), the necrotic cells will elicit a corrective tissue response, accompanied by bile duct proliferation. The 3 primary lesions of PAP are hepatocytomeglia, fibrosis, and bile duct proliferation. Hepatocytomeglia is always present. The presence of the other 2 lesions is dependent on the dose ingested and the rapidity of lesion maturation. A single dose of the alkaloid may elicit the response, or the liver may be continually exposed to the alkaloid over days, weeks, or months before the response is elicited.

Hepatocyte degeneration and loss cause decreased hepatic function. The liver has tremendous reserve capacity that enables an animal to continue to function normally for many weeks or months, even though the liver may be slowly degenerating. Ultimately, liver function collapses, and the animal suffers from a generalized hepatic insufficiency syndrome.

Discussion

Species susceptibility to PA poisoning is highly variable. Birds and most rodents are highly resistant. Cattle, horses, and rats are highly susceptible. Goats are 40 times less susceptible than are cattle, and sheep are 100 times less susceptible.[2]

Some unique characteristics of PAP must be understood by those dealing with the problem. First, development of the clinical syndrome occurs 2 to 8 months after ingestion of the alkaloid. The delay makes it extremely difficult to obtain feed samples to examine for presence of a suspect plant. Thus, obtaining a satisfactory history of ingestion becomes almost impossible. This fact seriously complicates attempts to adjudicate suspected losses in the courts. Second, pyrrolizidine alkaloids and metabolites are rapidly excreted in body fluids such as urine and milk. Because certain pyrrolizidine alkaloids are considered to be carcinogens, this fact poses a potential public health problem.[2]

Young, growing animals are more susceptible to the hepatotoxic effects of the alkaloid than are adults. Furthermore, alkaloids can pass through the placenta and affect the fetus. In one herd, calves were affected with PAP. The hay source was identified, but because no adult stock had been affected, the decision was made to continue feeding the hay to adult stock and to provide young stock with clean hay. Calf losses continued through the next year until it was recognized that fetuses had been affected in utero.

Comfrey has been recognized in recent years to contain PAs. This plant is commonly used by herbalists, and cases are on record of human poisoning from comfrey. Persons inclined to use comfrey themselves may feel that their animals would benefit as well.

The public health implications of PAs in milk should be considered carefully. Although studies on cattle and goats have shown that calves and kids failed to develop lesions of PAP while nursing dams to which PAs were being administered,[2] this does not negate the possibility that children (particularly infants) drinking that milk may be affected.

It is known that goats are resistant to PAP, and they are sometimes used to control tansy ragwort in marginal pastures. If goats graze tansy ragwort, there will be PAs in the milk. Goat milk is frequently used by families who are involved in a back-to-nature situation. Such families should understand the possible hazard.

Recent work has demonstrated a protective effect against the effects of PA by administration of cobalt boluses, which are retained in the rumen.

PHOTOSENSITIZATION

Photosensitization is a disease caused by the presence of a photodynamic agent in the skin that sensitizes the epithelium to ultraviolet radiation. A lesion similar to that produced by sunburn results.

Three mechanisms may be involved. First, the photodynamic agent may be preformed in the plant ingested by an animal (primary photosensitization). A second mechanism is aberrant pigment synthesis by the animal. This tends to be a genetically controlled trait; congenital porphyria in cattle is an example. The third mechanism operates through hepatogenous photosensitization as a result of ingestion of plants containing toxins that damage the hepatic parenchyma (see Table 1).

One of the metabolites of chlorophyll metabolism is the photodynamic chemical phylloerythrin. Normally, the liver degrades phylloerythrin, which keeps serum levels negligible. When the hepatic parenchyma is damaged, higher concentrations of phylloerythrin in the serum may cause photosensitization in light-skinned animals exposed to sunlight.

Horsebrush (*Tetradymia* sp.) causes heavy losses in sheep in Utah and surrounding states. There is now evidence that the liver damage does not occur unless the animal has ingested black sage (*Artemesia nova*) for a few days before ingesting the horsebrush.[3]

AFLATOXICOSIS

Toxins produced by the fungus *Aspergillus flavus* are highly hepatotoxic.

MUSHROOM TOXICITY

There are numerous species of poisonous mushrooms, but they are rarely consumed in sufficient quantity to produce clinical toxicosis in livestock. One species, however, *Amanita phalloides* (death cap), contains alkaloids or polypeptides or both that are highly hepatotoxic. Consumption of 50 to 100 g of these mushrooms may be sufficient to kill a calf, sheep, or pig.

The toxins in death cap mushrooms produce a massive diffuse necrosis of the hepatic parenchyma, with inevitable death.

HEPATIC INSUFFICIENCY SYNDROME[4]

This syndrome is not pathognomonic for any particular etiologic agent. Signs vary slightly from one species of animal to another.

Clinical Signs

An affected animal may experience some weight loss but need not be emaciated. Icterus is usually present. Light-skinned animals exposed to sunlight may develop photosensitization. Cattle characteristically show gastrointestinal signs consisting of colic, tenesmus, diarrhea, and rectal prolapse. Ascites may be due to hypoproteinemia or portal hypertension. A hemogram may be normal or may indicate low-grade anemia, leukocytosis, left-shift differential leukocyte count, and elevated icteric index.

Caution is important in evaluating serum chemistry parameters. Serum enzyme studies may be within normal limits in animals suffering from hepatic insufficiency caused by PAP, because cellular necrosis does not necessarily take place at the same time as the signs of clinical disease appear. Plants such as *Lantana camara* and *Amanita phalloides*, which cause hepatic necrosis, produce markedly elevated serum enzyme levels.

Signs of acute hepatic insufficiency develop after a latent period of 6 to 24 hours after ingestion of the plant. Acute hepatic insufficiency caused by *A. phalloides* ingestion is characterized by vomiting, diarrhea, dehydration, muscle cramps, hypovolemic shock, hypoglycemia, hyponatremia, and leukocytosis with a left shift. Liver failure allows invasion of the host by enteric bacteria, with septicemia and fever resulting.

Hepatoencephalopathy

Signs of central nervous system depression are usually seen in hepatic insufficiency cases. The inability of the liver to detoxify nitrogenous waste products of the blood results in a plasma build-up, which causes direct effects on the brain. Cattle become depressed. They may stand in awkward positions with legs crossed or fetlocks knuckled. If forced to move, they are uncoordinated and may wander aimlessly or walk in circles. Occasionally, cattle will push against obstacles in their path, but this sign is much more common in horses than in cattle. The animal may be found in a comatose state and remain so for hours only to revive and appear normal for a time.

Livestock generally do not exhibit the aggressive signs seen in horses, such as biting themselves, other animals, or the ground. Convulsions are also rare in cattle.

Diagnosis

Differential diagnosis must include infectious hepatitis, parasites, biliary obstruction, chemical hepatic necrosis (carbon tetrachloride, clay pigeon poisoning), rabies, other encephalomyelitis, brain abscesses, tumors, and hemorrhages. Antemortem diagnosis of the hepatopathies is based on clinical signs, clinical pathologic examination, and liver biopsy.

Necropsy

On gross examination, the liver may be swollen, atrophic, fibrotic, yellowish, or mottled. Hepatic insufficiency cannot be evaluated on the basis of gross lesions. Even with histologic examination, a diagnosis cannot always be made except in the case of pyrrolizidine alkaloid toxicosis or aflatoxicosis.

Treatment

When an animal shows clinical signs of PAP, the prognosis is grave and therapy is useless. For other hepatopathies, affected cattle should be kept out of direct sunlight so that photosensitization is avoided. Supportive treatment with broad-spectrum antibiotics and administration of fluids (particularly 10 per cent glucose) and essential fatty acids are helpful. The prognosis is guarded in all cases of hepatopathy.

REFERENCES

1. Bull LB, Culvenor CCJ, Dick AT: The Pyrrolizidine Alkaloids. Amsterdam, North-Holland Publishing Co, 1968.
2. Cheeke PR: Pyrrolizidine/alkaloid/toxicity and metabolism in laboratory animals and livestock. *In* Cheeke PR (ed): Toxicants of Plant Origin, vol I. Boca Raton, FL, CRC Press, 1989, pp 1–40.
3. Johnson AE: Tetradymia toxicity, a new look at an old problem. *In* Keeler RF, Van Kampen KR, James LF (eds): Effects of Poisonous Plants on Livestock. New York, Academic Press, 1978, pp 209–216.
4. Zimmerman HJ: Hepatotoxicity. New York, Appleton-Century-Crofts, 1978, p 326.

Effects of Plant Toxins on the Central Nervous System*

LYNN F. JAMES, PhD
KIP E. PANTER, PhD

There are many plants ingested by animals that induce profound effects on the central nervous system (CNS). These effects may be manifested acutely (sudden death), be accumulated during prolonged daily ingestion (wasting and debilitation), or be fetotoxic. The toxic effect will vary with the level of toxin contained within the plant, the amount ingested, the duration of ingestion, and the species of animal eating the plant.

Plants inducing CNS signs in animals may have a variety of physiologic effects or cause morphologic lesions. Many of the genera and common names of poisonous plants affecting the

---

*All material in this article is in the public domain, with the exception of any borrowed figures or tables.

Table 1. TOXIC PLANTS AFFECTING THE CENTRAL NERVOUS SYSTEM

Genus	Common Name
Atropa	Belladonna, deadly nightshade
Datura	Jimsonweed, thornapple
Hyoscyamus	Black henbane
Cestrum	Jessamine
Solanum	Nightshades, potato
Lycopersicon	Tomato
Veratrum	False hellebore, skunk cabbage
Kalmia	Lambkill, mountain laurel
Ledum	Western Labrador tea
Leucothoe	Sierra laurel, black laurel
Ericaceae	Heath family
Zygadenus	Death camas
Amianthium	Staggergrass
Lupinus	Lupine, blue bonnet
Lobelia	Indian tobacco, cardinal flower
Nicotiana	Tobacco, tree tobacco
Conium	Poison hemlock, hemlock
Delphinium	Larkspurs
Aconitum	Monkshood, aconite
Asclepias	Milkweeds
Cicuta	Water hemlock, cowbane
Corydalis	Fitweed
Dicentra	Dutchman's breeches, bleeding heart
Aesculus	Horse chestnut, buckeye
Notholaena	Jimmy fern
Gelsemium	Carolina jessamine
Astragalus	Locoweeds, vetches
Oxytropis	White locoweed
Swainsona	Darling pea
Paspalum	Dallis grass
Cynodon	Bermuda grass
Eupatorium	Snakeroots, white snakeroot
Haplopappus or Isocoma	Rayless goldenrod, jimmy weed
Cycas	Cycad palms
Acacia	Guajillo
Cassia	Sennas
Karwinskia	Coyotillo
Centaurea	Knapweeds, yellow star thistle
Sophora	Mescalbean
Strychnos	Poisonnut
Thermopsis	Mountain thermopsis, thermopsis

Source: Adapted from Bailey EM: Physiological response of livestock to toxic plants. J Range Manage 31:343–347, 1978.

CNS are listed in Table 1.[1] This list is not meant to be a complete listing. Some of the more important plants causing greatest loss to the food animal–producing industry are discussed in more detail.

ANNUAL RYEGRASS (Lolium rigidum)[2]

Annual ryegrass (*Lolium rigidum*) or Wimmeria ryegrass often becomes infested with a nematode. *Anguina colii* bores into the developing flower carrying a bacterium (*Corynebacterium rathayi*), which results in the development of a seed gall that is extremely toxic to sheep. Sheep grazing the toxic grass, if disturbed, develop a staggering, stiff-legged gait and collapse with convulsions.

A similar disease has been reported in sheep in Oregon grazing *Festuca rubra commutata* infested by *Anguina agrostis* and a bacterium thought to be a corynebacterium.

Lesions described in sheep poisoned with annual ryegrass include pale, friable liver, congestion of the lungs, and hemorrhage into various organs. Culvenor and associates[2] have reported isolation of a toxin from the seedheads of ryegrass. The toxin has been identified as a glycolipid corynetoxin.[3]

PERENNIAL RYEGRASS (Lolium perenne)[4]

Ryegrass staggers, a neuromuscular disorder primarily affecting sheep but also reported in cattle and horses, has been observed in New Zealand, Australia, England, and the United States. The clinical signs of this disease include head shaking, incoordination, abnormal staggering gait, and eventually collapse. The sheep may have severe muscular spasms followed, after a period of time, by the animal's righting itself and walking away. The onset of these clinical signs is preceded by disturbance or excitement of the animal. Morbidity can be as high as 80 per cent, but mortality is low.

Lesions associated with this disease are not pathognomonic, but degeneration of Purkinje cells and status spongiosus of the cerebellum have been reported. Prolonged recumbency of the animal may result in focal areas of muscular degeneration thought to be a secondary change.

Investigators believe the clinical syndrome is related to tremorgenic *Penicillium* inhabiting the soil beneath the ryegrass. It is evident that a number of tremorgenic compounds may be involved in the syndrome; however, 2 major fungal neurotoxins have been isolated, lolitrem A and B.

LOCOWEEDS (Astragalus and Oxytropis)

The locoweeds (species of *Astragalus* and *Oxytropis*) have worldwide distribution in the temperate zones, especially in the mountainous arid and semiarid areas. Poisonous astragali have been divided into 3 categories according to the clinical manifestation of their toxic properties. These classes are (1) nitro-bearing plants, (2) locoweeds, and (3) selenium accumulators.[5] *Swainsona* spp., which produce an intoxication similar to the locoweeds, are confined to Australia. Swainsonine is the neurotoxin in these plants. The toxin produces neurovisceral cytoplasmic foamy vacuolation.

Locoweed poisoning affects primarily cattle, sheep, and horses, although there are some reports of wild ruminants and insects becoming poisoned. The clinical signs include rough dry hair coat, emaciation, visual impairment, neurologic abnormalities, birth defects, and abortion. The most significant neurologic problem is that animals may have exaggerated movements or become hyperexcitable when they are stressed. Exaggerated movements of mastication may result in slobbering or loss of ruminated ingesta. Intoxicated horses become totally unusable because of the neurologic damage.[5, 6]

The morphologic lesions are not confined to the CNS but are described as neurovisceral vacuolations of the cellular cytoplasm. Neurons in the CNS and autonomic ganglia, glia cells, and endothelial cells in the CNS may be affected by the vacuolar process. The vacuoles are single and membrane-bound, resembling enlarged lysosomes. These lysosomes become distended, coalesce, and may cause rupture of the cytoplasmic membranes, with resultant destruction of the cells. When neurons are affected, there may be permanent damage to the CNS, especially in horses.

Livestock poisoned on locoweed may recover insofar as most functions are concerned but will show signs of poisoning if they are stressed.[7]

NITRO–BEARING PLANTS (Astragalus miser) AND RELATED SPECIES[8, 9]

Certain *Astragalus* (263 species or varieties) contain aliphatic nitro compounds that are catabolized to 3-nitro-1 propanol (3-NPOH) and 3-nitropropionic acid (3-NPA) in the digestive tract of ruminants. 3-NPOH is more toxic than is 3-NPA per milligram of nitrate ingested because it is absorbed more readily from the digestive tract. Acutely poisoned animals may die from cardiac and respiratory failure 4 to 20 hours after the poisoning. Signs of intoxication include emphysema and locomotor disturbances. Acutely poisoned animals develop methemoglobinemia, but the cause of death is not associated with this change.

Chronic poisoning by nitro-bearing *Astragalus* results in permanent impairment of the hindquarters with knuckling of the fetlocks and interference of the hocks when the animals are made to move. Microscopic lesions include interlobular fibrosis, edema, and alveolar emphysema in the lungs; widespread focal hemorrhage of the CNS; and wallerian degeneration of the posterior spinal cord and sciatic nerves.[9]

CYCAD POISONING (Cycas spp., Bowenia spp., and Macrozamia spp.)[10]

The cycads are palmlike plants found in the tropical areas of the world within well-defined geographic locations. The toxins from these plants cause hepatic and gastrointestinal disturbances, ataxia, and radiomimetic or carcinogenic effects upon the liver or intestines.

Cattle, sheep, horses, and pigs have been affected by the cycad-induced ataxia. The primary clinical sign is a loss of proper control over the movement of the hindlimbs. Early in the disease, there is hyperextension of the rear limbs with a "goose-stepping" gait. Later, incomplete extension occurs, and the limbs "knuckle over" at the phalanges.

The morphologic lesions of the CNS described with this disease include bilateral symmetric degeneration of nerve fibers in the fasciculus gracilis up to the nucleus gracilis and the dorsal spinocerebellar tract and possibly the ventral spinocerebellar tract up the cerebellum through the posterior cerebellar peduncle. Morphologic lesions have been compared with amyotrophic lateral sclerosis, a disease that occurs in people living in the tropics who consume the cycad plants.

WATER HEMLOCK (*Cicuta* spp.)[11]

The toxin of water hemlock (cicutoxin) acts on the CNS, causing severe violent grand mal seizures. It is considered the most violently toxic plant in the United States and Europe. Water hemlock poisoning usually occurs in early spring when livestock graze the new growth along streams, ditches, and marshes. Although the first new growth is considered poisonous, the most danger lies in the tuber, which is easily pulled from soft wet soil. The dose between minimal signs of poisoning and grand mal seizures resulting in respiratory paralysis and death is very small (1.1 g/kg fresh tuber and 1.2 g/kg, respectively, for *C. maculata* in sheep). Pathologic and microscopic lesions are those of severe tetanic contracture of the skeletal and cardiac musculature. Microscopic lesions in the heart of animals ingesting water hemlock include multifocal, acute, moderate myocardial degeneration characterized by granular degeneration of myofiber cytoplasm. Grossly pale areas of the heart may be observed. Animals recovering from the intoxication after having experienced grand mal seizures will show a 10-fold to 1000-fold increase in lactic dehydrogenase, aspartate aminotransferase, and creatine kinase because of muscle damage secondary to the seizures. Necropsy 3 to 7 days after recovery from intoxication showed gross lesions of multifocal, pale areas (1 to 5 mm) of the left, right, and interventricular myocardium.[11] Microscopic lesions are confined to the heart and long digital extensor muscles. The heart had multifocal, subacute to chronic, moderate random myocardial necrosis and replacement fibrosis and locally extensive areas of stroma lacking myofibers. There was bilaterally symmetric, subacute to chronic, moderate myofiber degeneration and necrosis of the long digital extensor muscle group. The grand mal seizures may be controlled by intravenous administration of barbiturate anesthetics (pentobarbital) with complete and uneventful recovery and no lesions, gross or microscopic, in the heart or long digital extensor muscle groups. Death and signs of clinical toxicity of 5 to 10 times the lethal dose have been prevented by this method with full recovery; however, because of the rapid onset of clinical signs followed by death, this treatment is not field practical. Good management and avoiding exposure of animals to water hemlock is still the best method of preventing losses.

LUPINE, *CONIUM*, AND TOBACCO[12]

These plants contain piperidine or quinolizidine alkaloids, which cause initial stimulation followed by depression of the CNS. Clinical signs of toxicosis include ataxia, muscle fasciculation, incoordination, depression, muscular weakness, collapse, and death. All species of livestock are similarly affected by *Conium*, tobacco, and the piperidine-containing lupines; however, sheep and goats are resistant to the quinolizidine-containing lupines. This is believed to result from metabolic differences in the rumen of cows versus sheep and goats. Cows are thought to metabolize the quinolizidine alkaloids to complex piperidines. This apparently does not occur or occurs more slowly in sheep and goats. This same phenomenon apparently accounts for differences in teratogenic effects, which are discussed by Keeler et al. in a separate article.

Animals poisoned on these plants will generally recover unless large quantities are ingested over a short period of time. Undisturbed animals have a better chance for recovery than do animals forced to move. Because of the rapid onset and course of this type of poisoning, treatment is usually futile; however, methods slowing absorption, such as activated charcoal, and artificial respiration or respiratory stimulants may provide some benefit.

FALSE HELLEBORE (*Veratrum californicum*)[12]

Ingestion of this plant on the 14th day of gestation by a pregnant ewe may result in neurologic damage to the developing embryo. The clinical manifestation of poisoning may be a return to estrus by the ewe owing to death of the embryo; the ewe may be prolonged in gestation, carrying "monkey-faced" lambs; or the ewe may deliver an abnormal fetus born twin to a normal fetus.

The damage to the CNS of the embryo is caused by the circulation of steroidal alkaloids from the plant within the gravid uterus. Keeler[12] has isolated and identified 3 compounds, all of which induce teratogenesis. These are jervine, cyclopamine, and cycloposine. These compounds cause severe craniofacial malformations, including anencephaly, hydranencephaly, hydrocephalus, and fusion of the cerebral hemispheres.

REFERENCES

1. Bailey EM: Physiological response of livestock to toxic plants. J Range Manage 31:343–347, 1978.
2. Culvenor CCJ, Frahn JL, Jago MV, Lanigan GW: The toxin of *Lolium rigidum* (annual ryegrass) seedheads associated with nematode-bacterium infection. In Keeler RF, et al: Effects of Poisonous Plants on Livestock. New York, Academic Press, 1978, pp 349–352.
3. Vogel P, Petterson DS, et al: Isolation of a group of glycolipid toxins from seed heads of annual ryegrass (*Lolium rigidum* Gaud.) infected by *Corynebacterium rathayi*. Aust J Exp Biol Med Sci 59:455–467, 1981.
4. Gallagher RT, White EP, Mortimer PH: Ryegrass staggers: isolation of potent neurotoxins lolitrem A and lolitrem B from staggers-producing pastures. NZ Vet J 29:189–190, 1981.
5. James LF, Hartley WJ, Van Kampen KR: Syndromes of Astragalus poisoning in livestock. J Am Vet Med Assoc 178:146–150, 1981.
6. Van Kampen KR, Rhees RW, James LF: Locoweed poisoning in the United States. In Keeler RF, et al: Effects of Poisonous Plants on Livestock. New York, Academic Press, 1978, pp 465–474.
7. Van Kampen KR, James LF: Pathology of locoweed poisoning in sheep. Pathol Vet 6:413–423, 1969.
8. James LF, Hartley WJ, Williams MC, Van Kampen KR: Field and experimental studies in cattle and sheep poisoned by nitro-bearing astragalus on their toxins. Am J Vet Res 41:377–382, 1980.
9. Williams MC, James LF: Livestock poisoning from nitro-bearing Astragalus. In Keeler RF, et al: Effects of Poisonous Plants on Livestock. New York, Academic Press, 1978, p 379.
10. Hooper PT: Cycad poisoning in Australia: etiology and pathology. In Keeler RF, et al: Effects of Poisonous Plants on Livestock. New York, Academic Press, 1978, pp 337–348.
11. Panter KE, Keeler RF, Baker DC: Toxicoses in livestock from the hemlocks (*Conium* and *Cicuta* spp.). J Anim Sci 66:2407–2413, 1988.
12. Keeler RF: Alkaloid teratogens from *Lupinus*, *Conium*, *Veratrum*, and related genera. In Keeler RF, et al: Effects of Poisonous Plants on Livestock. New York, Academic Press, 1978, pp 397–408.

Sweet Clover Poisoning

HOWARD H. CASPER, PhD
ARNOLD D. ALSTAD, DVM, PhD

White sweet clover (*Melilotus alba*) and yellow sweet clover (*M. officinalis*) grow readily throughout the central and northern United States and southern Canada. Sweet clover compares favorably with alfalfa (*Medicago sativa*) in terms of quality, utility, and economics.[1] The pleasant odor of unspoiled sweet clover plants is attributable to coumarin. Coumarin is nontoxic but can be converted to the anticoagulant dicumarol when molds grow on clover hay or silage. Pastures are not affected, but moldy hays or silages retain their toxicity for several years. The spoiled, moldy, upper layers (1 to 2 ft) of silage piles can be very toxic.

Sweet clover poisoning is a coagulopathy; cattle and sheep are the animals most often affected. The anticoagulant action of dicumarol is as an antagonist to vitamin K, which results in interference with synthesis in the liver of vitamin K–dependent clotting proteins prothrombin (factor II), factor VII, factor IX, and factor X. The probability that sweet clover poisoning will occur depends on the dicumarol level in the forage and the length of time animals are eating moldy sweet clover.[2] Sweet clover hay with different levels of dicumarol was experimentally fed to 500- to 600-pound steers, and dicumarol concentrations of 60 to 70 ppm resulted in clinical signs after 17 to 23 days. Feeding sweet clover hay with 20 ppm of dicumarol failed to produce the disease. Research and field observations indicate that dicumarol levels below 20 ppm are generally safe, and levels of 40 ppm or greater can be dangerous to livestock.

CLINICAL SIGNS

In typical field cases, problems usually occur 3 to 6 weeks after the start of sweet clover feeding. Sudden death may occur owing to massive hemorrhage, but normally the clinical signs are more prolonged. Hemorrhage may occur in any tissue, and hematomas of varying size are common in the neck, flanks, hips, or legs. Hemorrhage in muscles, joints, and nervous tissue can result in lameness or paralysis. Excessive bleeding, leading to death, may also occur after routine surgical procedures. Some animals may have nosebleeds or bloody stools. Anecdotal observations suggest an association between moldy sweet clover and abortion. Dams fed moldy sweet clover may give birth to calves with impaired clotting mechanisms, with resultant neonatal death.

The diagnosis of moldy sweet clover poisoning is based primarily on clinical signs and necropsy findings associated with coagulopathy, when the animals have eaten moldy sweet clover hay or silage. Clinical pathologic examination reveals low hematocrit, decreased hemoglobin, elevated prothrombin time, elevated partial thromboplastin time, and elevated activated clotting time.[4] Forage dicumarol levels in excess of 30 ppm and liver dicumarol levels of 0.5 ppm or more are supportive evidence for sweet clover poisoning.

TREATMENT

Treatment of sweet clover poisoning should start with the immediate and complete removal of sweet clover from the animal's diet. Quality alfalfa is the substitute of choice. Animals should be handled with care for preventing exacerbation of anemic hypoxic shock and further hemorrhage. Moderately affected animals often recover and have a normal prothrombin time 5 to 6 days after removal of the sweet clover. Severely affected animals will show immediate response to a blood transfusion (1 L blood per 100 k body weight). An alternative treatment is vitamin K_1 injection. Animals will respond within 24 hours after 1 treatment with vitamin K_1* (phytonadione) at a dose of 1 to 3 mg/kg body weight.[3] The vitamin K_1 should be administered intramuscularly, in divided doses, with a small-bore needle. Vitamin K_3 (menadione) is of no benefit in treating sweet clover poisoning.[3]

PREVENTION

Prevention of sweet clover poisoning includes the proper harvesting of sweet clover for limiting the growth of molds. Experimental data indicate that feeding toxic sweet clover for a week and then feeding an alternative forage for 2 weeks will reduce the risk of poisoning. As a general practice, sweet clover of any kind should not be fed for at least 7 to 10 days before castration, dehorning, implanting, surgery, or other medical/management practices. Similarly, sweet clover should not be fed during the last month of gestation in cattle. Dietary supplementation with vitamin K_3 is useless for the prevention of sweet clover poisoning.[5]

REFERENCES

1. Benson ME, Casper HH, Johnson LJ: Occurrence and range of dicumarol concentrations in sweet clover. Am J Vet Res 42:2014–2015, 1981.
2. Casper HH, Alstad AD, Monson SB, Johnson LJ: Dicumarol levels in sweet clover toxic to cattle. Proceedings, 25th Annual Meeting, American Association of Veterinary Laboratory Diagnosticians. Nashville, TN, 1982, pp 41–48.
3. Alstad AD, Casper HH, Johnson LJ: Vitamin K treatment of sweet clover poisoning in calves. J Am Vet Med Assoc 87:729–731, 1985.
4. Schalm OW, Jain NC, Carrol EJ (eds): Veterinary Hematology, 3rd ed. Philadelphia, Lea & Febiger, 1975.
5. Casper HH, Alstad AD, Tacke DB, et al: Evaluation of vitamin K_3 feed additive for prevention of sweet clover disease. J Vet Diagn Invest 1:116–119, 1989.

Plants Teratogenic in Livestock

RICHARD F. KEELER, PhD
KIP E. PANTER, PhD
J. L. SHUPE, DVM

The range forage of grazing domestic livestock is variable in nutritional value, varied in distribution, and in some cases potentially toxic. Many of the commonly ingested range plants have a toxic or teratogenic effect in livestock. Plant-induced congenital malformations are believed to represent, possibly, ⅓ of all spontaneous malformations in range livestock; the other ⅔ are induced primarily by infectious disease or genetic causes based on information accumulated at the authors' laboratory during the past 30 years.

The concepti of domestic livestock are subject to teratogenic insult for many reasons. Teratogens ingested by pregnant animals are not necessarily detoxified immediately or excreted. Some teratogens pass the placenta more readily than was once thought and thus enter the circulatory system of the conceptus.

Certain factors determine whether a teratogen, from a plant or other source, will induce a congenital defect. Wilson (1977) detailed 6 Principles of Teratology that govern the induction of congenital defects by teratogens. Consideration of these principles suggests reasons for the variability in teratogenic effects induced in livestock by poisonous plants. The principles are the following:

---

*Wendt Professional Laboratories, P.O. Box 128, Belle Plaine, MN 56001 (1–800–328–5890).

1. Conceptus genotype determines susceptibility.
2. The teratogen, or its influence, must reach the conceptus.
3. Deformities are dose-dependent.
4. Teratogens can produce death rather than deformity.
5. The conceptus must be exposed at a susceptible embryologic period.
6. Teratogens exert their effects by specific mechanisms.

Thus, we can expect variation in susceptibility among species, breeds, and strains of livestock; variation in incidence or severity due to dose effects or differential metabolism in rumen or liver; possible associated increases in abortions or resorptions seen as a decreased lamb or calf crop; variation in effect and incidence due to gestation age at the time of insult; and, finally, conditions with similar clinical signs induced by unrelated plants containing different teratogens.

Cited here a few of the congenital defects known to be induced in livestock by plants; the signs, diagnosis, epidemiology, compounds responsible, factors that influence incidence, and strategies for prevention are discussed.

KNOWN TERATOGENIC PLANTS

Loco

Some loco plants (*Astragalus lentiginosus* and *Astragalus pubentissimus*) induce congenital deformities and abortions in addition to classic locoism. Deformed lambs have increased incidence of malpositioning, malalignment, or rigidity of joints; excessive carpal flexure; tendon contracture; anterior flexure and hypermobility of the hock; or a combination of these signs. Gestational susceptibility is broad. The conceptus can be deformed under natural and experimental conditions at almost any period of gestation. Results of experimental trials proved the plant to be the cause. Incidence on the range is sporadic because of variable plant abundance. In years of great abundance, the incidence of abortion may approach 60 per cent, and up to 30 per cent or more of the lambs alive at birth may be deformed. Teratogen identity is unknown but may be swainsonine, the compound that induces neurologic locoism. Seeds of some loco plants are viable in soil for many years. Plant abundance evidently is governed by the amount of moisture available to initiate germination and early growth and by subsequent seedling competition. Removal of juniper and sagebrush by dragging anchor chains on ranges has often increased the abundance of loco for a period of time.

Cultivated Tobacco

A teratogenic effect occurs in offspring from sows that graze tobacco stalks (*Nicotiana tabacum*) during gestation. In some midwestern tobacco-raising areas, farmers allow pigs to graze the tobacco stalks discarded in the field after the leaves have been removed for curing. Twisting of the forelimbs or hindlimbs and dorsal flexure of the hindlimb digits are common in the offspring. Breeding records were used to rule out genetics as the cause, and feeding trials have established that the plant is responsible. The susceptible period was once believed to be between days 10 and 30 of gestation on the basis of epidemiologic observations. However, feeding trials have established that susceptibility extends well beyond day 30 and may even be exclusively beyond day 30. The teratogen is likely anabasine or a closely related pyridino-piperidine (see wild tobacco).

Wild Tobacco

Nicotiana glauca (wild tree tobacco) induces limb and palate defects in livestock. Cattle, sheep, and pigs are known to be susceptible from feeding trials. Susceptibility extends from about days 40 to 75 in cattle, days 30 to 60 in sheep and goats, and days 30 to 60 in pigs. Experimental work with *N. glauca* was undertaken to help elucidate details of the deformity induced by common tobacco (*N. tabacum*) described in the preceding. Spontaneous congenital deformities in livestock from *N. glauca* are not known, probably because of the limited distribution of the plant and its unpalatable nature. The teratogen is the piperidine alkaloid anabasine.

Lupine

Ingestion by cows of certain lupine plants during pregnancy induces crooked calf disease. The disease is common. Up to 30 per cent or more of the calves in some areas are born with twisted or bowed limbs with malalignment, malpositioning, or rigidity of joints; spinal curvature; twisted neck; cleft palate; or a combination of these deformities resulting from maternal lupine ingestion. Similar effects are induced by other causes as well, but the major outbreaks are usually due to lupine. The principal susceptible period is between the 40th and 70th days of gestation. The condition has been induced experimentally by feeding a purified alkaloid fraction from the plant containing very high levels of the quinolizidine alkaloid anagyrine. Available evidence suggests anagyrine is the cause. Among the many hundreds of lupines, a few contain the compound: *Lupinus sericeus*, *Lupinus caudatus*, and *Lupinus laxiflorus* are among them.

Concentration of all alkaloids including anagyrine is high in early plant growth and decreases markedly with maturity. Concentration is also high for a brief period while mature seeds remain in the pods. Therefore, teratogenic hazard is minimal when lupine in early flower or post-seed stage is grazed by cows whose average stage of gestation is either earlier than the 40th or later than the 70th day. The degree and incidence of malformations are not necessarily related to the severity of clinical signs (such as tremors, irregular gait, recumbency) in the dam because of the variable concentration of the various toxic alkaloids in lupine.

Whereas most lupines contain only quinolizidine type alkaloids, a few contain piperidine alkaloids related to the teratogens from *Nicotiana* and *Conium*. One of those is *Lupinus formosus*. In feeding trials, it induced severe deformities in calves and goats. The piperidine alkaloid ammondendrine is believed to be responsible.

Poison Hemlock

Ingestion of poison hemlock (*Conium maculatum*) by pregnant cows or sows may induce congenital deformities in calves or piglets. Sheep and goats appear to be resistant to the teratogenic effects of the plant. However, *Conium* seed induced cleft palate and severe skeletal deformities in newborn goats when it was fed to their mothers during the 30th to the 60th days of gestation. The deformities in calves are similar to those induced by lupine. Incidence is much lower than the lupine-induced condition because poison hemlock is less abundant and less palatable than is lupine. Twisted limbs and spinal curvature are the typical signs. In piglets, both limb deformities and cleft palate are induced by the plant. The hazard period for cows is in the 40th to the 70th days of gestation, and for pigs in the 30th to 60th days. The teratogenic compounds in the plant are simple piperidine alkaloids. Feeding trials have shown that coniine and probably γ-coniceine induce the conditions. Concentration of these alkaloids in the plant is highly variable. The plants usually grow in restricted areas, mainly along fences, in waste places, and in overgrazed pastures.

The clinical signs of toxicity and malformations are similar for the tobaccos, lupines, and conium in the susceptible species thus far tested. Ultrasound observations of pregnant goats fed *Nicotiana glauca, Lupinus formosus,* and *Conium maculatum* suggests that the malformations (both cleft palate and skeletal) result from a similar mechanism induced by the piperidine alkaloids of the plants. The putative alkaloids apparently pass the placental barrier to the fetus, causing a reduction in fetal movement that if sustained over the critical developmental period will result in the malformation.

Veratrum

Epidemics of cyclopia and related facial deformities sometimes occur in newborn lambs. Incidence has exceeded 25 per cent of lambs from some ranches. The deformed offspring are often single- or double-globe cyclopics. Ewes may undergo prolonged gestation, and lambs become too large for normal delivery. Lambs that are born are usually dead at birth or die shortly thereafter. Feeding trials showed that *Veratrum californicum* was responsible for the condition when it was ingested by pregnant ewes on the 14th day of gestation. The main compound in the plant responsible for cyclopia is cyclopamine, a steroidal alkaloid. The concentration of cyclopamine in the above-ground or foraged parts of the plant decreases as the plant matures during the summer.

The plant also induces severe limb and tracheal defects and induces early embryonic death. The insult periods for all these effects are before the 32nd day of gestation.

PREVENTION

Therapy is not available for these conditions, and total prevention is not practical because of the logistics of grazing pregnant animals on the range. However, incidence can be significantly reduced in most instances by certain management strategies. They relate to the Principles of Teratology: use of genotypes low in susceptibility, reduction of dose by selective herding, grazing at periods when plant teratogen concentration is low, reduction of plant abundance, and reduction of conceptus exposure during susceptible gestational periods.

Cows mainly seem to be affected by the *Lupinus* teratogen, whereas sheep, but not cows, mainly are affected by the *Veratrum* teratogen.

Cyclopia in sheep from *Veratrum* develops only by insult on the 14th day of gestation. Selective herding of sheep bands to keep them away from *Veratrum* patches until all ewes have passed the 14th day of gestation can eliminate the cyclopia and other facial deformities induced by the plant; but for prevention of other *Veratrum*-induced effects, such as limb and tracheal defects and early embryonic death, plant ingestion must be avoided until all ewes have passed the 32nd or 33rd days of gestation.

In *Lupine*-induced crooked calf disease, susceptibility is mainly between the 40th and 70th days of gestation. The plants are most hazardous while young or while mature seeds are present. During flowering and after seed drop, plants are less hazardous. Consequently, restricting access of cows during the 40th to 70th days if plants are very young or with mature seeds reduces incidence. Sometimes exposure to hazardous plants can be reduced simply by shifting herd breeding periods.

Incidence in *Conium*-induced calf deformities has been reduced by lowering plant abundance by tillage. Similar results might be expected from herbicide treatment. Both are feasible because *Conium* is most abundant on cultivated rather than in native grazing lands.

Management can eliminate the deformity problem in pigs from maternal tobacco stalk ingestion. Sows can be provided feed that does not include tobacco stalks.

Loco-induced deformity problems seem to be almost intractable in "bad" loco years. The conceptus is susceptible at almost any gestational period, so no grazing period is "safe." The dose cannot be reduced by ensuring adequate supplemental feed because ewes appear to become habituated to the loco and seek it out, and careful herding in loco-infested areas is not fruitful. In "bad" loco years, plants are abundant on thousands of square miles of native range. Tillage or herbicide treatment is impractical and inadequate because of seed viability.

BIBLIOGRAPHY

Crowe MW: Tobacco: a cause of congenital arthrogryposis. *In* Keeler RF, Van Kampen KR, James LF (eds): Effects of Poisonous Plants on Livestock. New York, Academic Press, 1978, pp 419–427.
Keeler RF: Teratogens in plants. J Anim Sci 58:1029–1039, 1984.
Keeler RF: Naturally occurring teratogens from plants. *In* Keeler RF, Tu AT (eds): Handbook of Natural Toxins, vol 1. New York, Marcel Dekker, 1983, pp 161–199.
Keeler RF, Panter KE: Piperidine alkaloid composition and relation to crooked calf disease: inducing potential of *Lupinus formosus*. Teratology 40: 423–432, 1989.
Keeler RF, Stuart LD, Young S: When ewes ingest poisonous plants: the teratogenic effects. Vet Med 81:449–454, 1986.
Panter KE, Bunch TD, Wierenga TL: Ultrasonographic studies on the fetotoxic effects of poisonous plants in livestock. *In* Keeler RF, Tu AT (eds): Handbook of Natural Toxins. Vol 6. New York, Marcel Dekker, 1990, pp 589–610.
Shupe JL, Keeler RF: Crooked calf syndrome. *In* Amstutz HE (ed): Bovine Medicine and Surgery, 2nd ed, vol 1. Santa Barbara, CA, American Veterinary Publications, 1980, pp 489–492.
Wilson JG: Current status of teratology: general principles and mechanisms derived from animal studies. *In* Wilson JG, Fraser FC (eds): Handbook of Teratology, vol 1. New York; Plenum Press, 1977, p 47.

Plants Producing Dermal Injury

LOYD D. ROWE, DVM
A. EARL JOHNSON, MS

In the following discussion, plants that may cause damage to the skin of livestock are divided into 3 categories: (1) plants causing mechanical injury, (2) plants causing localized reactions after external contact, and (3) plants causing injury to the skin after oral ingestion. Many of the toxic constituents of plants of category 3 cause photosensitization and may act directly after reaching the skin by means of normal physiologic processes or act indirectly by causing hepatobiliary dysfunction.

PLANTS CAUSING MECHANICAL INJURY

Plants only occasionally produce significant mechanical injury to the skin of animals. Awns, spines, thorns, or any other plant part that can penetrate the skin may cause physical damage. Awn-producing grasses can be particularly troublesome. Awn damage most often affects the mouth, internal ear, or eyes rather than the skin. Representative irritating grasses are needlegrasses (*Stipa* spp.) and field sandbur (*Cenchrus pauciflorus*). Needlegrasses may cause severe irritation resulting in permanent damage to the hide. Burs of sandbur and puncture vine (*Tribulus terrestris*) usually do not penetrate the deep layers of the skin, but they often cause troublesome irritation around the hooves. Diagnosis is relatively easy, and treatment usually involves removal from the source of irritation and topical use of a soothing antiseptic or antibiotic preparation.

PLANTS CAUSING CONTACT DERMATOSES

There are few plants that cause dermatitis in animals after direct contact with the skin. Stinging nettles (*Urtica urens, U. dioica*) may cause rashes and discomfort in pigs similar to that seen in humans. Hairs of bull nettle (*Cnidoscolus stimulosus*) are covered with irritants that cause pain in humans, but the effect of these irritants on the skin of livestock is not known. Poison ivy (*Toxicodendron radicans*) and poison oak (*Rhus toxicodendron*) are classic examples of plants causing allergic contact dermatitis in humans, but these plants do not cause significant problems in livestock.

Although uncommon, localized cutaneous photosensitization may result from absorption of phototoxic plant constituents through the outer layers of the skin after dermal contact. Linear furanocoumarins (psoralens) are compounds produced by a number of plants, particularly those belonging to the parsley (*Umbelliferae*) and citrus (*Rutaceae*) families. Some of these compounds possess potent phototoxic activity in humans and animals after topical, oral, or parenteral exposure. Phototoxic furanocoumarins from celery (*Apium graveolens*) have produced contact photodermatitis on the hands of field and grocery workers handling this vegetable. Outbreaks of vesiculobullous disease in swine, with lesions that resembled those of foot and mouth disease, have been attributed to photosensitization resulting from contact of the snouts and feet of pigs with phototoxic furanocoumarins from parsnips (*Pastinaca sativa*) and celery in vegetable wastes given as feed. This diagnosis was supported by failure to demonstrate the presence of infectious disease and reproduction of the lesions by rubbing parsnip leaves or fungus-damaged celery on the snouts and feet of white pigs followed by exposure to long-wave ultraviolet light.[1]

PLANTS CAUSING SKIN INJURY AFTER INGESTION

By far the most important skin disorder of livestock resulting from ingestion of plants is cutaneous photosensitization. Plants that contain phototoxic agents or cause phylloerythrin to appear at elevated levels in the dermal circulation induce photosensitization when the skin is irradiated by sunlight. Areas affected are usually light-colored and unprotected areas of skin, because skin pigmentation or dense hair may screen out sunlight.

Some phototoxic compounds require the presence of oxygen to produce their phototoxic action. Such compounds are said to be *photodynamic*. When photodynamic compounds are excited by light energy, they either (1) react directly with a substrate molecule (e.g., an amino acid) to give free radical forms of the 2 reactants, which then react with oxygen, or (2) react directly with oxygen to form singlet oxygen, which then reacts with the substrate to form an oxidized product. Phototoxic furanocoumarins are not photodynamic because they do not require oxygen for activity. Their action appears to result from the light-dependent formation of adducts with the pyrimidine bases of DNA.[1] All of these reactions produce cellular damage and inflammation that give rise to the typical signs of photosensitization. Erythema, swelling, pruritus, and photophobia appear first. Edema may become severe, and there may be serous exudation with or without vesiculation. Necrosis may extend into the deep layers of skin. Lips, eyelids, and ears may slough or be permanently deformed. In sheep, wool may be lost permanently, and large areas of light-colored skin may slough in hard, leather-like sheets. Few animals die from photosensitization per se; however, death may occur owing to secondary infection or starvation.

In 1952, Clare[2] identified 3 classifications of photosensitivity disease in livestock: (1) primary—independent of any pre-existing disease process, the phototoxic agent from the plant is absorbed from the digestive tract and reaches the skin via the peripheral blood circulation; (2) endogenous synthesis of aberrant pigment; and (3) secondary (hepatogenous)—the phototoxic agent is phylloerythrin, a degradation product of chlorophyll, which accumulates in the body as a result of compromised hypatobiliary function. All plant-induced photosensitization is of either the primary or secondary type.

Primary Photosensitization

St. Johnswort (*Hypericum perforatum*) is widely known to cause primary photosensitization in livestock. This plant contains a photodynamic, fluorescent, red pigment named hypericin. St. Johnswort grows in many parts of the world and was introduced into the eastern United States. It may now be found throughout the United States except in some arid areas of the West and Southwest. St. Johnswort has caused economic problems to owners of cattle, sheep, and horses. Particularly severe losses have occurred in the western coastal states, but these losses have been greatly reduced by development of methods of controlling the weed. Cattle are more susceptible to hypericin than are other livestock and may react to such an extent that large sheets of leather-like skin in white or light-colored areas slough. Animals that are removed from access to the plant, protected from direct exposure to sunlight, and treated according to symptoms usually recover, although permanent damage to the hide or wool may occur. Other *Hypericum* species also produce photosensitization, but they are not important problems in this country.

Primary photosensitization in sheep, cattle, goats, pigs, and horses resulting from ingestion of buckwheat (*Fagopyrum esculentum*) is also well known. Fagopyrism, or buckwheat rash, has been known since the late 1800s. The condition is less common in cattle than in sheep or pigs. Fresh, green plant, especially that in the growth stage containing blossoms, is considered most toxic to animals. The straw, grain, bran, and chaff of buckwheat may also cause photosensitization if it is eaten in sufficient quantity. Two compounds closely related to hypericin, fagopyrin and photofagopyrin, have been identified as the photosensitizing substances.[3] Lesions of fagopyrism most often appear on the face, ears, eyelids, and neck. Degree of skin damage is dependent on the amount of plant ingested and the amount of sunlight to which the animal is exposed. In mild cases, only erythema, slight swelling, and pruritus may be evident. In more severe cases, vesicles develop and rupture, giving rise to crusty areas on affected skin. Treatment of fagopyrism is the same as for primary photosensitization due to other causes: removal of animals from access to the plant, protection of animals from direct sunlight, and provision of food and rest. Antiseptic or antibiotic ointments may be applied if needed.

Spring parsley (*Cymopterus watsonii*), a small perennial umbelliferous plant that grows in desert areas of Nevada and southern Utah, causes primary photosensitization in livestock, particularly in sheep.[4] Van Kampen and coworkers[5] demonstrated that spring parsley causes photosensitization in chickens that can result in deformities. With the exception of *Cymopterus longipes*, other species of *Cymopterus* are not known to be phototoxic in fowl. However, other *Cymopterus* species are suspected of causing serious photosensitization in cattle. Two highly phototoxic furanocoumarin compounds, xanthotoxin and bergapten, have been isolated from spring parsley.[6]

Ewes that graze *C. watsonii* in early spring, when there may be a scarcity of other forage, become photosensitized in areas of the body not covered by wool (i.e., lips, udder, and vulva). These areas become erythematous, swollen, and extremely sore. Further development of the condition results in vesicle and crust formation. Affected ewes will not allow their lambs to nurse because of the tenderness of their udders. In such cases, death of lambs due to starvation and dehydration may approach 25 per cent.

The furanocoumarin-containing plant Bishop's weed (*Ammi majus*) has produced photosensitization of the primary type in cattle, sheep, ducks, geese, and turkeys when it was accidentally or experimentally included in their diet. Although it is present in the United States, there is no evidence that Bishop's weed is a significant hazard to livestock in this country.[1]

Consumption of the dead, moldy-appearing leaves of giant rain lily (*Cooperia pedunculata*) causes photosensitization of the primary type in cattle and deer in southeastern Texas during the winter and spring almost every year. Major outbreaks have involved 15,000 head of cattle in one county alone. The teats, udder, eyes, and muzzle are most seriously affected. Except for mild scarring of the cornea, recovery is virtually complete. Economic losses are due primarily to failure of cows to nurse their calves and costs associated with provision of shade, alternative feed, and veterinary care. The phototoxic agent associated with this condition is unknown.

Secondary (Hepatogenous) Photosensitization

Secondary (hepatogenous) photosensitization is caused by the presence of elevated levels of phylloerythrin in the dermal circulation. Phylloerythrin is formed during microbial degradation of chlorophyll in the rumen, absorbed into the blood, rapidly removed from the circulation by the liver, and excreted in the bile. A liver incapable of efficiently excreting phylloerythrin permits increased levels of this compound to reach the peripheral circulation, where it may be activated by sunlight. Any disorder that results in increased levels of phylloerythrin in the circulation produces photosensitivity of the secondary type. Ligation of the common bile duct and exposure to sunlight results in photosensitization of ruminants consuming chlorophyll. Similarly, biochemical or membrane dysfunction at the cellular level may also result in retention of phylloerythrin.[1] The basic mechanisms involved in phylloerythrin excretion and factors that influence this process are not fully understood. A conspicuous birefringent crystalloid material in bile ducts, Kupffer cells, and hepatocytes (crystalloid cholangiohepatopathy) is seen microscopically in 4 hepatotoxicities that induce photosensitization in sheep and goats. These conditions are geeldikkop (*Tribulus terrestris* photosensitivity) and dikoor (*Panicum* spp. photosensitivity) in South Africa, and lechuguilla (*Agave lechuguilla*) and sacahuista (*Nolina texana*) poisonings in the southwestern United States. Similarly, ovine and caprine hepatogenous photosensitization with biliary microliths has been associated with the presence of a highly toxic fungus (*Drechslera campanulata*) on green oats (*Avena sativa*).[8] In the case of lechuguilla poisoning, this crystalloid material is thought to be a steroidal sapogenin. The biliary microliths formed by this crystalloid material are considered to be the principal occluding mechanism responsible for retention of phylloerythrin in the diseases in which their presence has been demonstrated.[1]

Johnson[9] and Keeler and associates[10] have shown that photosensitization in sheep caused by *Tetradymia* species can be potentiated by certain sagebrush species. Studies by Horsley[11] also suggest that secondary factors can enhance the effects of other photosensitizers, such as hypericin. Other investigators have found the experimental production of secondary photosensitization in livestock difficult and unpredictable, which indicates that unknown predisposing factors may be important. Livestock owners find that exposure of their stock to plants capable of inducing secondary photosensitization does not always result in the appearance of the disease. This may give some producers a false sense of security, causing them to become careless in the management of their livestock in areas where photosensitizing plants are present. The result is often a sudden outbreak of photosensitization involving many animals.

Plants known to cause secondary photosensitization are numerous. Table 1 presents a list of some important plants causing the condition and the species of animals most frequently affected. An extensive listing of North American plants causing photosensitization in livestock has recently been published.[1]

Treatment of the dermal component of hepatogenous photosensitization is identical to that of primary photosensitization (e.g., shade, antibiotics); however, treatment of the visceral component may be required if severe hepatotoxic disease is present. Correction of dehydration and oral activated charcoal (5 g/kg body weight in 10 to 20 L water) has been reported to be effective treatment for the hepatic component of lantana poisoning and shortens the period of clinical recovery.[12]

Numerous other plants, including some common livestock feeds, have been associated with sporadic outbreaks of photosensitization. These plants include spotted spurge (*Euphorbia maculata*), smartweeds (*Polygonum* spp.), sudan grass (*Sorghum sudanense*), vetches (*Vicia* spp.), field pennycress (*Thlaspi arvense*), oats, rye, alfalfa, and clovers. Because the etiologic agents and pathogenesis of these outbreaks are unknown or poorly understood, the conditions remain unclassified and are said to be of uncertain etiology.[1]

Nonphotosensitizing Plants Affecting the Skin

A syndrome characterized by dermatitis, conjunctivitis, anorexia, weight loss, elevated temperature, and diarrhea is

Table 1. PLANTS COMMONLY INVOLVED IN THE PRODUCTION OF SECONDARY PHOTOSENSITIZATION OF LIVESTOCK

Scientific Name	Common Name	Livestock Frequently Affected
Astragalus cicer	Cicer milkvetch	Cattle and sheep
Agave lecheguilla[1]	Lechuguilla	Sheep and goats
Brassica napus	Cultivated rape	Cattle
Kochia scoparia	Summer cypress	Cattle and sheep
Lantana spp.	Lantana	Cattle and sheep
Nolina texana[1]	Texas sacahuista	Cattle, sheep, and goats
Panicum coloratum[1]	Kleingrass	Lambs
Phyllanthus abnormis	Abnormal-leaf flower	Cattle
Tetradymia glabrata	Littleleaf horsebrush, coal oil brush	Sheep
Tetradymia canescens	Spineless or gray horsebrush	Sheep
Tribulus terrestris[1]	Puncture vine	Sheep

[1]Associated with the production of crystalloid cholangiohepatopathy.

known in cattle pastured for 2 to 3 weeks on hairy vetch (*Vicia villosa*). Unlike photosensitization, skin lesions are not restricted to unpigmented areas. Indeed, most reported cases have involved cattle with black coats. In this condition, plaques develop on the skin of the udder, tail, head, neck, face, trunk, and limbs. These may enlarge to form diffuse lesions covered by a yellow-brown crust. Pruritus and considerable alopecia are common features. In hairy vetch poisoning, morbidity is generally less than 10 per cent, and mortality is approximately 50 per cent. The predominant microscopic lesion is an infiltration of multiple visceral organs with macrophages, lymphocytes, plasma cells, multinucleated giant cells, and eosinophils.[13]

Alopecia may be seen in leucaena (*Leucaena leucocephala*) toxicosis in ruminants. Additional clinical findings may include anorexia, reduced weight gain (or weight loss), excessive salivation, esophageal lesions, thyroid enlargement, and low levels of circulating thyroid hormones.[14]

Occasionally, consumption of feedstuffs such as potatoes, potato waste products, malt, coconut cake, beet pulp, palm oil cake, rice bran, adulterated linseed meal, cottonseed cake, and corn cake have been associated with the occurrence of skin rashes in different species of livestock. These rashes may occur on almost any part of the animal's body.[15]

REFERENCES

1. Rowe LD: Photosensitization problems in livestock. Vet Clin North Am [Food Anim Pract] 5: 301–323, 1989.
2. Clare NT: Photosensitization in Diseases of Domestic Animals. Review Series No. 3 of the Commonwealth Bureaux of Animal Health, Farnham Royal, England, Commonwealth Agricultural Bureaux, 1952.
3. Brockmann H: Photodynamically active plant pigments. Proc Chem Soc 304–312, 1957.
4. Binns W, James LF: *Cymopterus watsonii*: a photosensitizing plant for sheep. Vet Med Small Anim Clin 59:4, 1964.
5. Van Kampen KR, Williams MC, Binns W: Deformities in chickens photosensitized by feeding spring parsley (*Cymopterus watsonii*). Am J Vet Res 30:9, 1969.
6. Williams MC: Xanthotoxin and bergapten in spring parsley. Weed Sci 18:4, 1970.
7. Rowe LD, Norman JO, Corrier DE, et al: Photosensitization of cattle in southeast Texas: identification of phototoxic activity associated with *Cooperia pedunculata*. Am J Vet Res 48:1658–1661, 1987.
8. Collett MG, Spickett AM: Unusual hepatic parenchymal crystalloid material and biliary microliths in goats. J S Afr Vet Assoc 60:134–138, 1989.
9. Johnson AE: Predisposing influence of range plants on tetradymia-related photosensitization in sheep: work of Drs. A. B. Clawson and W. T. Huffman. Am J Vet Res 35:12, 1974.
10. Keeler RF, Van Kampen KR, James LF: Effects of Poisonous Plants on Livestock. New York, Academic Press, 1978, p 209.
11. Horsley CH: Investigation into the action of St. Johnswort. J Pharmacol Exp Ther 50:310, 1934.
12. McLennan MW, Amos ML: Treatment of lantana poisoning in cattle. Aust Vet J 66: 93–94, 1989.
13. Panciera RJ, Johnson L, Osburn BI: A disease of cattle grazing hairy vetch pasture. J Am Vet Med Assoc 138:804–808, 1966.
14. Hammond AC, Allison MJ, Williams MJ, et al: Prevention of leucaena toxicosis of cattle in Florida by ruminal inoculation with 3-hydroxy-4-(1H)-pyridone–degrading bacteria. Am J Vet Res 50:2176–2180, 1989.
15. Kral E, Schwartzman RM: Veterinary and Comparative Dermatology. Philadelphia, JB Lippincott, 1964, p 94.

Oxalate Accumulators*

LYNN F. JAMES, PHD
KIP E. PANTER, PHD

Oxalic acid and oxalate poisonings are of considerable importance throughout the world. Not only are domestic animals affected, but so are household pets and humans. Oxalic acid, an organic dicarboxylic acid, has a great affinity for calcium and magnesium, and the resulting salts are virtually insoluble in water. This acid forms soluble salts with sodium, potassium, and ammonium. Oxalic acid is both a corrosive and a systemic poison. Under natural conditions, soluble oxalates are toxic primarily because of their systemic effects.

Oxalic acid occurs naturally in plants in the form of soluble and insoluble oxalates. Oxalate intoxication in livestock results primarily from the ingestion of plants containing the oxalates. Plants producing high levels of oxalates (generally considered to be 10 per cent or more anhydrous oxalic acid on a dry weight basis) are worldwide in distribution. Some plants may have in excess of 30 per cent oxalate on a dry weight basis. Examples of such plants are halogeton (*Halogeton glomeratus*) and greasewood (*Sarcobatus vermiculatus*) of the Chenopodiaceae family, soursob (*Oxalis pes-caprae*) and the sorrels of the Oxalidaceae family, and certain of the *Rumex* species of the Polygonaceae family.

Some plants with oxalate levels of less than 10 per cent, including some grasses consumed by cattle, can cause problems. Under certain conditions, the fungi *Aspergillus niger* and *A. flavus* can produce large amounts of oxalates on feeds and on moist straw. Livestock poisoning has been reported involving such feeds.

The plants producing high oxalate levels can be divided into 2 groups:

1. Plants such as soursobs and some species of *Rumex* that have a sap pH of about 2. The oxalate anion is chiefly found as the acid oxalate ($HC_2O_4^-$).
2. Plants such as halogeton that have a sap pH of about 6. The oxalate anion is chiefly found as the oxalate ion ($C_2O_4^{2-}$).

The oxalate in group 1 is present chiefly as acid potassium oxalate, and the oxalate in group 2 is present chiefly as soluble sodium oxalate and insoluble calcium oxalate. Certain species of grass, such as *Setaria sphacelata* in Australia and *Pennisetum clandestinum* in Hawaii, produce oxalate at low levels and have caused intoxication in horses and cattle. The oxalate in these grasses causes nutritional secondary hyperparathyroidism and oxalate poisoning. Some of these grasses have caused a negative calcium balance and intoxication in cattle.

Two of the principal oxalate-producing plants of the world are soursob of Australia and halogeton of the western United States. Both of them are introduced plants.

Most oxalate-containing plants are palatable to livestock; therefore, livestock with access to this group of plants must be managed carefully.

EFFECTS OF OXALATES IN THE DIETS OF RUMINANT LIVESTOCK

When a ruminant eats an oxalate-containing plant, 3 things can occur: (1) the soluble oxalates may be detoxified by the metabolic activity of the rumen bacteria; (2) the soluble oxalates may react with calcium in the digestive system to form insoluble calcium oxalate that is excreted in the feces; or (3) the soluble oxalates may be absorbed, which results in intoxication.

Certain microorganisms in the rumen can detoxify the oxalate ion. Ingestion of sublethal levels of soluble oxalate may gradually increase the rate at which rumen microorganisms detoxify the oxalate. This change in rumen microflora can increase the amount of soluble oxalate a ruminant can safely ingest by about 75 per cent. Allowing ruminants to graze small amounts of oxalate-producing plants permits the oxalate-metabolizing bacteria to increase, thus providing increased protection against oxalate poisoning.

---

*All material in this article is in the public domain, with the exception of any borrowed figures or tables.

If the soluble oxalates are ingested rapidly, as when an animal is hungry, the microflora may not be able to detoxify them, and the soluble oxalates are absorbed into the blood stream. If absorption is in large enough amounts, the animal becomes intoxicated. The oxalate combines with tissue calcium and forms crystals that are deposited in the wall of the rumen and in the renal tubules. Hypocalcemia may result. Oxalate also interferes with the enzymes lactic dehydrogenase and succinic dehydrogenase, both of which are essential for energy metabolism. Thus there is interference with energy metabolism, which probably is the cause of death after consumption of large amounts of high-oxalate plants.

Oxalate intoxication in an animal is a complex phenomenon influenced not only by the previously mentioned reactions but by the following factors as well:

1. Amount of oxalate-containing plant ingested
2. Rate of consumption
3. Concentration of soluble oxalate in the plant
4. Amount of other feed in the rumen (dilution factor)
5. Recent exposure to oxalate-containing plants

A ruminant may consume a large quantity of oxalate-containing plants without harmful effects if it is ingested slowly over the grazing period, whereas the same amount may prove lethal if it is ingested rapidly. Oxalate poisoning occurs primarily when hungry animals are allowed to graze on heavy stands of plants with a high oxalate content. A full rumen not only dilutes the oxalate and decreases the rate of absorption, but it also discourages the animal from eating too much. Therefore it is advisable to manage sheep grazing areas containing high-oxalate plants so that the animals are prevented from becoming hungry.

Oxalate-producing plants are high in soluble salts; thus diets containing an abundance of these plants increase water consumption because water is needed to excrete the salts.

Water intake is influenced by dry matter consumption, salt intake, and ambient temperature. As any of these factors increase, water intake increases. If water is withheld, feed consumption decreases so that an animal can become hungry by withholding feed or water. When water is withheld and an animal becomes hungry, it will eat immediately after it has been given water. At such times, animals are much less discriminating about what they eat. If animals are hungry and are feeding on sites infested with oxalate-producing plants such as halogeton, the animals may become intoxicated. Oxalate poisoning often occurs in sheep after trucking or extensive handling because they are hungry.

DIAGNOSIS

Ruminants are more commonly poisoned on oxalates than are other grazing animals, and more sheep than cattle have been poisoned, perhaps because of differences in management practices. Two clinically distinct conditions exist from oxalate ingestion—acute and subacute poisoning and chronic poisoning as reported in Australia, whereas only acute poisoning has been reported in the United States.

Signs of poisoning are rapid and include labored respiration, depression, weakness, coma, and death. There is stasis of the gastrointestinal tract. Mild tetany may be observed in a few individuals. Gross pathologic conditions are hemorrhage and edema of the rumen wall, hyperemia of the abomasal wall and intestinal mucosa, and ascites. Histopathologic changes include hemorrhage and calcium oxalate crystal formation in the rumen wall and oxalate crystals and accompanying cellular damage in the renal tubules of the kidney. The animals can die within 1 to 2 hours or as long as several days after eating a lethal dose of halogeton. When death is rapid, few lesions are observed. Serum calcium levels decrease, and plasma urea nitrogen, aspartate aminotransferase, and lactic dehydrogenase levels all increase. The extent of the changes is dependent on the acuteness of the intoxication.

Subacute and chronic poisonings in sheep grazing soursobs in Australia have been reported. These animals develop a stiffness of gait and eventually collapse. They usually remain bright, continue to eat, and may remain in this condition for weeks until they either die or recover gradually. The kidneys of these animals become fibrotic. The difference observed between soursob poisoning in Australia and halogeton poisoning in the United States is believed to be due to the difference in the chemical form of the oxalate in the plants.

Cattle fed straw that contains low levels of oxalate have been reported to develop a negative calcium balance. Horses grazing the grass *Setaria sphacelata*, which contains low levels of oxalate, develop secondary nutritional hyperparathyroidism. Cattle grazing halogeton may develop a stiffness of the limbs when they are driven. If forced to walk, these animals may become recumbent, but usually they recover with proper treatment.

TREATMENT

There is no treatment for oxalate poisoning.

PREVENTION

Prevention of oxalate poisoning lies principally with proper management. The following practices will help minimize losses in livestock due to oxalate poisoning:

1. Avoid overgrazing pastures and ranges to the extent that perennial vegetation is removed or depleted.
2. Develop a grazing program that will allow ranges and pastures to improve.
3. Supply adequate water and a good variety of forage.
4. Develop a grazing plan. Know what your animals are eating.
5. Allow livestock (ruminants) time to adapt to oxalate in the diet by grazing safe amounts of oxalate-producing plants. Introduce animals slowly into areas with heavy growth of oxalate plants.
6. Do not unload, drive, or bed livestock in areas with dense populations of oxalate-producing plants unless the animals have been well fed and watered.
7. Do not allow hungry animals to graze in dense stands of oxalate-producing plants.

BIBLIOGRAPHY

Cook CW, Stoddard LA: The halogeton problem in Utah. Utah Agri Exp Stn Bull 364, 1953.
Everist SL: Poisonous Plants of Australia. Sydney, Australia, Angus and Robertson, 1974.
James LF: Oxalate toxicosis. Clin Toxicol 25:231–243, 1972.
James LF, Cronin EH: Management practices to minimize death losses of sheep grazing halogeton-infested ranges. J Range Manage 27:424–426, 1974.
James LF, Johnson AE: Prevention of fatal *Halogeton glomeratus* poisoning in sheep. J Am Vet Med Assoc 157:437–442, 1970.
Kingsbury JM: Poisonous Plants of the United States and Canada. Englewood Cliffs, NJ, Prentice-Hall, 1964.
McKenzie BA: Poisoning of horses by oxalate in grass. In Seawright AA, Hegarty MP, James LF, Keeler RF (eds): Plant Toxicology. Published by Queensland Poisonous Plant Committee, Brisbane, Australia, 1988.

Van Kampen KR, James LF: Acute halogeton poisoning in sheep: pathogenesis of lesions. Am J Vet Res 30:1779–1783, 1969.

Selenium Accumulators*

LYNN F. JAMES, PhD
KIP E. PANTER, PhD

Selenium is present in certain soils at levels that may produce plants toxic to livestock. These plants growing on seleniferous soils may accumulate selenium in quantities from less than 1 ppm to several thousand ppm. Plants capable of accumulating high levels of selenium (>1000 ppm) are included in some species of *Astragalus* (Fig. 1), *Stanleya, Haplopappus,* and *Machaeranthera*. These plants are often referred to as selenium accumulator or indicator plants because of their preference for seleniferous soils and their ability to accumulate high levels of selenium. Such plants normally have an unpleasant odor and are unpalatable to livestock. Animals are poisoned by these plants only when they are forced to graze them because of a shortage of good forage.

Many species of *Aster, Atriplex, Castilleja,* and *Gutierrezia* accumulate less selenium than do the major accumulator plants—rarely more than a few hundred ppm. Many weeds, most crop plants, and grasses can accumulate up to 50 ppm of selenium when they are grown on seleniferous soils. Pigs and chickens fed seleniferous small grains and grazing animals ingesting these selenium-accumulating forages can be poisoned. Most problems associated with selenium poisoning are related to the consumption of plants having about 10 ppm selenium.

The distribution of selenium, primarily as selenate, throughout the soil profile is important because it relates to the selenium content of the plants. Selenium that has been leached into the deeper soil profiles is available to the deep-rooted plants. Essentially all of the selenium indicator plants are deep-rooted and therefore accumulate selenium at high levels in their tissue from the deeper soil profiles.

Selenium in small grains (harvested forage and grass) is present in association with protein, whereas the selenium in the indicator plants is largely in water-soluble form that suggests its occurrence in some form other than protein.

---

*All material in this article is in the public domain, with the exception of any borrowed figures or tables.

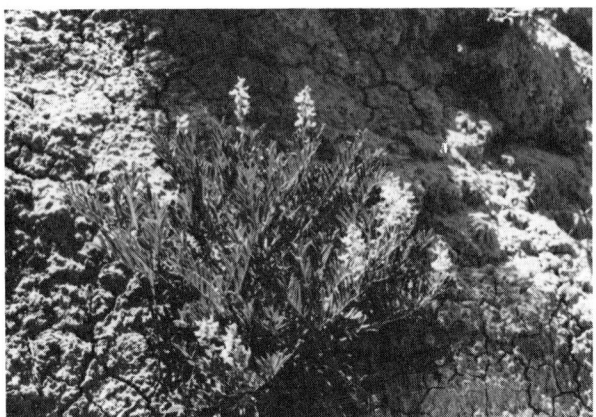

Figure 1. *Astragalus bisulcatus.* One of the principal selenium accumulating plants.

Selenium in plants occurs in a variety of chemical forms. The comparative toxicity of these various compounds has not been elucidated; therefore evaluation of the toxicity of these plants based on total selenium content can be misleading. Total selenium content should serve only as a guide to the toxicity of the plant.

CLINICAL SIGNS

Selenium poisoning in livestock can occur in acute or chronic forms. Animals suffer acute poisoning when they ingest sufficient quantities of selenium accumulator plants or some other source of selenium at high levels. Because of the unpalatability of selenium accumulator plants, acute toxicosis from this source is uncommon.

The signs of acute selenium-induced poisoning are either sudden death or severe distress, labored breathing, abnormal movement and posture, frequent urination, diarrhea, prostration, and then death. Sheep exhibit increased rate of respiration and sudden death. Animals may die within a few hours or not for several days with very few signs.

Two types of chronic intoxication have been described. These are "blind staggers" and "alkali disease." Chronic selenium intoxication of the blind staggers type is said to result from the consumption of accumulator plants in limited amounts over an extended period. The blind staggers type is characterized by inappetence, impairment of vision, wandering (often in circles), weakness, partial or entire paralysis of tongue and swallowing mechanism, abdominal pain, excessive salivation, and death. Although for many years blind staggers has been associated with selenium poisoning, some investigators now question this. The blind staggers type of selenium poisoning has not been verified through research. It is now generally thought that blind staggers is not caused by selenium poisoning but by some other etiologic agent. The term "blind staggers," used to describe animals that appear blind and show evidence of previously listed signs of poisoning, is probably a complex of disease syndromes included in the etiology of polioencephalomalacia. In the past, many of these problems have probably been incorrectly diagnosed as selenium poisoning.

Chronic selenium poisoning of the alkali disease type results from ingesting forage containing from 5 to about 40 ppm selenium for a prolonged period. The time and amount of selenium necessary for poisoning varies considerably with individual animals. Signs of poisoning in cattle and horses include lameness, hoof alterations, emaciation, and loss of long hair from the mane and tail. Sheep do not respond to chronic selenium poisoning as do cattle and horses in that they do not show hoof or wool effects.

Signs of poisoning vary with animal species. Pigs fed diets containing 25 ppm selenium or more have developed severe spinal cord lesions (poliomyelomalacia), which ultimately led to varying degrees of paralysis. These lesions may be preceded by loss of hair and hoof lesions (Fig. 2). Decreased hatchability of chicken eggs has been observed. A reduction in reproductive performance is probably the most significant economic effect of chronic selenium poisoning in livestock. Reproduction may be depressed rather severely without the animals showing typical signs of poisoning.

Although selenium poisoning is classified according to severity, the toxic effects of selenium increase in severity as selenium intake increases, which makes differentiation between the forms difficult. Young animals are more susceptible to selenium poisoning than are older ones. Many species of selenium-accumulating *Astragalus* also contain the locoweed toxin swainsonine.

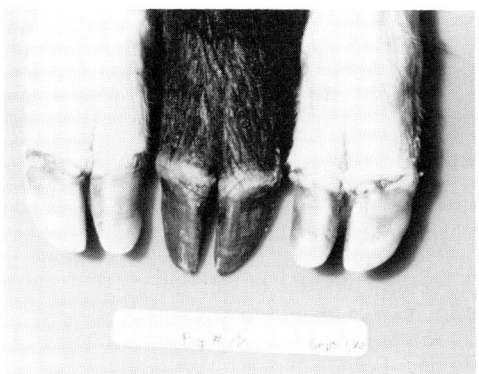

Figure 2. Feet of a pig poisoned by selenium. Note the separation of the hoof at the coronary border.

DIAGNOSIS

Diagnosis of selenium poisoning is discussed for the acute and chronic (alkali disease syndrome) forms. In view of the questionable status of the so-called blind staggers disease, additional discussion of this problem should await further clarification.

Acute selenium poisoning is rare and associated with the accidental ingestion of selenium-containing feedstuffs with the grazing of plants, such as the selenium-accumulating *Astragalus* plants in which selenium levels can vary from a few hundred to several thousand ppm. If animals die from acute selenium poisoning, forage that is high in selenium is probably located in the general area where the animals have been grazing. Signs observed relate to the level of selenium in the plant and rate of consumption. Animals may die rather quickly with few signs, or when intake has been lower, they may linger for a few days. If animals linger, there may be abnormal posture, diarrhea, frequent urination, respiratory distress, prostration, and death. Post-mortem examination reveals primarily a marked congestion of the lungs and hyperemia of the gastrointestinal tract. Microscopic examination of the tissues substantiates the gross lesions listed.

Chronic poisoning accompanies the grazing of seleniferous forage of 5 to 40 ppm (mostly at the lower end of this range) over a prolonged period. Chemical analysis of vegetation in the area where the animals have been grazing or of forage fed to the animals should reflect such selenium intake levels. Not all vegetation in all the areas where animals have grazed will contain the same amounts of selenium.

Horses, cattle, and pigs show the adverse changes in hair coat and hooves and emaciation as described. Reproductive performance declines in all species of farm animals exposed to excessive levels of selenium.

Anemia, cirrhosis and atrophy of the liver, and atrophy of the heart have been observed in cattle and horses with chronic selenium toxicosis. The only known chronic effect of selenium poisoning in sheep is a severely reduced rate of reproduction.

The guidelines in Table 1 have been set by the South Dakota Agricultural Experiment Station for the selenium content of blood and hair.

Some selenium accumulator plants such as *Astragalus bisulcatus* may contain toxins other than selenium (swainsonine, the loco toxin), and in case of chronic toxicosis involving these plants, toxins other than selenium may be involved.

TREATMENT

There is no known treatment for acute selenium poisoning. Chronically poisoned animals should be removed from seleniferous forage. The rate, extent, and incidence of recovery depend on the severity of toxicosis.

PREVENTION

The prevention of chronic selenium poisoning requires the limiting of selenium intake. Control measures should be based on management. Management procedures require, in the case of range animals, a mapping of the range area based on geology and plant analysis. On the basis of the selenium content of the vegetation from the various sites of a range, grazing procedures are established to regulate selenium intake within safe limits when both time and selenium content of the forage are considered.

BIBLIOGRAPHY

Anderson MS, Lakin HW, Beeson KC, et al: Selenium in agriculture. United States Department of Agriculture Handbook 200, 1961.
Moxon AL: Alkali disease or selenium poisoning. SD St Agri Exp Sta Bull 311, 1937.
National Research Council: Medical and biologic effects of environmental pollutants: selenium. Washington, DC, National Academy of Sciences, 1976.
Olsen O, Keeler RF, Van Kampen KR, James LF (eds): Selenium: a cause of poisoning. *In* Effects of Poisonous Plants on Livestock. New York, Academic Press, 1978.
Rosenfeld I, Beath OA: Selenium: Geobotany, Biochemistry, Toxicity, and Nutrition. New York, Academic Press, 1964.

Cyanogenic Plants
STEVEN S. NICHOLSON, DVM

SOURCES

Compounds that release cyanide gas are used in predator control as toxic baits delivered by piston-released cartridges, as fumigants in grain storage, in certain industrial processes involving metallurgy, and in some countries for the recovery of gold from low-grade ore. Plants containing cyanogenic glycosides account for most cyanide toxicoses in farm and ranch animals. Hydrocyanic acid poisoning from plants occurs primarily in ruminants, with cattle being slightly more sensitive than sheep. Monogastrics are seldom involved.

MECHANISM OF ACTION

Hydrogen cyanide is highly soluble and is rapidly absorbed across the digestive tract mucosa. Cyanide combines with the cytochrome oxidase enzyme system, blocking oxygen transport

Table 1. TOXIC LEVELS OF SELENIUM IN BLOOD AND HAIR

Blood (ppm)	Hair (ppm)	Comments
<1.0	<5.0	Chronic selenium poisoning not expected
1.0–2.0	5.0–10.0	Borderline problem
>2.0	>10.0	Selenium intake excessive, and selenosis should be expected; animals at this level may not show signs of toxicosis

to tissues, which results in histotoxic anoxia. Release of the gas from plant material occurs when the leaves are chewed, which allows glycosidase enzymes in the plant to hydrolize the glycoside to hydroxynitrile and a sugar. The hydroxynitrile then breaks down, liberating hydrocyanic acid and an aldehyde or ketone characteristic of the original glycoside. With some plants, a bitter almond or "cherry-coke" odor may be detected during liberation of hydrocyanic acid.

Animals can safely convert some cyanide to thiocyanate and excrete it in the urine. An intake of 2 mg/kg in a single dose or consumed in forage within a few minutes constitutes the minimum lethal dose in ruminants. Johnson grass (*Sorghum halepense*), sudan grass (*S. sudanenese*), sorghum (*S. vulgare*), and various hybrids are examples of forages that ordinarily may have hydrocyanic acid levels of 50 ppm or less and do not pose a significant hazard. Conditions known to increase cyanogenic glycoside in these plants to dangerous levels include rapid growth of immature plants well fertilized with nitrogen. Insufficient soil phosphorus is said to enhance glycoside production.

Immature plants wilted by trampling, frost, dry soil, or herbicide damage may have increased levels of glycoside upon resuming growth. Plants containing 200 ppm or more are considered hazardous. A dose of hydrocyanic acid of 2 mg/kg, eaten within a few minutes, could be delivered to a 450-kg cow in 4.5 kg of Johnson grass containing 200 ppm.

Forages cut for hay and ensilage generally lose their hydrocyanic acid potential before feeding. If forages high in hydrocyanic acid were cut, chopped, and delivered fresh to ruminants as "green chop," the conditions would be right for a rapid kill.

Certain ornamental plants including the cherry laurel (*Prunus laurocerasus*), flowering quince (*Chaenomeles* spp.), Christmas berry (*Nandina domestica*), and *Photina* spp. are potential sources of hydrocyanic acid. The cherry laurel is a shrub or tree found in wooded areas in the Southeast. It is an evergreen, and the dark green leaves, when thoroughly crushed, release a very pronounced bitter almond odor. As little as 50 g of leaves has induced cyanide toxicosis in a 27-kg goat. Cattle have died within 15 minutes of gaining access to cuttings.

In the western United States, chokecherry (*Prunus virginiana*) and mountain mahogany (*Cercocarpus mountanus*) provide valuable browse for livestock and wildlife. Mountain mahogany is considered a premier browse for sheep, cattle, and mule deer in southern Utah, although earlier references incriminated it in livestock losses. Chokecherry has caused losses due to cyanide toxicosis when cattle or sheep ate large amounts of leaves and twigs.

CLINICAL SIGNS

Within a few minutes after ingestion, there is sudden onset of polypnea accompanied by an apprehensive expression, tremors, staggering, then collapse into lateral recumbency and paddling. Mucosae are bright pink and the blood is bright red initially, but these darken as respiratory failure occurs well before the heart stops. Death may occur within 2 to 3 minutes after onset. Animals alive an hour after signs develop often recover.

Horses and cattle grazing sorghum hybrids have developed axonal neuropathy of the spinal cord, which presents as posterior ataxia and paralysis of the urinary bladder. The cause is thought to be due to a nitrile compound.

DIAGNOSIS AND TREATMENT

The presence of an acute anoxic condition in ruminants known to have ingested plants with a high cyanide potential would strongly suggest the need to treat affected animals promptly. Animals with a similar history that are found dead may have bright red blood if death was almost instantaneous. More often the blood is dark red owing to anoxemia, and there are hemorrhages on the epicardium. The "bitter almond" odor is not present in all cases. Nitrite toxicosis resembles cyanide toxicosis, but the blood often has a brown color. *Sorghum* sp. may be high in nitrates.

Cyanide will be quickly lost from rumen contents and liver, but the brain, skeletal muscle, and cardiac muscle retain it longer. Samples should be sealed airtight and refrigerated or covered with 1 to 3 per cent mercuric chloride for delivery to the diagnostic laboratory. Negative tests may occur in actual poisonings because cyanide is so volatile. Leaves of the suspected plant can be tested for confirmation of their toxic potential in the field with use of the picrate test.

Treatment traditionally involved the rapid intravenous injection of a commercial antidote containing sodium nitrite and sodium thiosulfate. A safe and effective treatment is the intravenous injection of 660 mg/kg of sodium thiosulfate in a 30 per cent solution, which can be given rapidly through a 12- or 14-gauge needle.

PREVENTION

Hungry ruminants should not be allowed access to *Sorghum* sp. that are less than 2 feet tall or immature forage that is wilted from drought, frost, or physical damage. Branches and clippings from *Prunus* sp. such as chokecherry and cherry laurel must not be made available to them.

BIBLIOGRAPHY

Burrows GE: Plants causing sudden death in livestock. Vet Clin North Am Food Anim Pract 5:272–273, 1989.

Perilla Frutescens (Purple Mint) Toxicosis in Cattle
LARRY A. KERR, DVM, MS

Interstitial pneumonia is a commonly observed, complex respiratory condition in cattle. This syndrome has multiple etiologic factors including toxic, bacterial, viral, and parasitic. Approximately 35 agents are known to produce this condition, the majority of which are toxic. In the southeastern part of the United States, *Perilla frutescens* or purple mint is perhaps the primary cause of interstitial pneumonia in the bovine.

Perilla frutescens, also known as perilla, purple mint, wild coleus, and beefsteak plant, is a weed found in much of the southeastern United States. Originally introduced from Asia as an ornamental plant, perilla has escaped cultivation and is now found along wood lines, along roadsides, and in waste areas where it does not have to compete with perennial grasses. Perilla is an erect, branching, herbaceous annual that grows from 0.3 to 2 m in height. This plant appears to thrive in the summer when many plants are heat dormant. The leaves of perilla, approximately 5 to 10 cm long and 4 to 8 cm wide, often attain a purple tint late in the season. The plant is a member of the Labitae (mint) family that is characterized by square stems and opposite aromatic leaves.

Perilla frutescens contains 3-substituted furans—perilla ketone, egomaketone, and isoegomaketone—all similar chemically to ipomeanol, the pneumotoxic agent in moldy sweet potatoes. Perilla ketone and, to a lesser extent, egomaketone and isoegomaketone are the agents in perilla that produce interstitial pneumonia in cattle.

CLINICAL SIGNS

Perilla-related interstitial pneumonia of cattle is usually seen in the fall of the year when the plant reaches the flowering stage. The 3-substituted furan concentration of the plant is highest in the seed parts. Because it flowers from August to October, perilla is most toxic during this interval. This time period often corresponds to a period of reduced pasture grass for cattle, which forces them to eat plants they would otherwise avoid. Once ingestion is initiated, cattle often develop a liking for the plant and will return to eat it even after better forage is made available. As little as 5 pounds of the wet plant may produce a fatal pneumonia in cattle under certain circumstances. Although not as toxic as the green material, dried perilla mint has occasionally produced toxicosis in cattle when the very volatile 3-substituted furans have been trapped, such as in large bales of hay.

Clinical signs may develop as early as 12 hours after initial ingestion, and death can occur within 24 hours. Other animals may linger for several days. Characteristic clinical signs of perilla toxicosis include a sudden onset of severe dyspnea with an expiratory grunt. Both beef and dairy cattle are affected, but owing to increased exposure, most cases are observed in beef animals. Affected cattle are usually apart from the remainder of the herd with their heads extended and having breathing difficulties. Body temperatures are usually normal or slightly elevated, pulse and respiratory rates are increased, intestinal peristalsis is reduced or absent, and constipation is common. Froth is often apparent around the mouth and nose of affected animals. The condition usually has a rapid course of 1 to 3 days, and animals may be found dead that were apparently normal 24 hours earlier. Death occurs much more rapidly if affected animals are forced to exert themselves.

NECROPSY

Lesions from perilla toxicosis include lungs swollen to the extent that on opening of the thoracic cavity, an imprint of the ribs is sometimes observed on the lungs. The affected lungs are heavy and do not collapse. Emphysema is often prominent not only in the lungs but also in the mediastinum and the cervical, thoracic, and lumbar subcutaneous areas. The lungs, firmer and darker than normal, often have a marbled appearance. Edema and froth in the trachea and bronchial passages are frequently observed. The interstitial septa are very distinct, being filled with fluid and gas, and thus the lobules separate quite easily.

On histologic examination, cuboidal cells line many of the alveoli, giving the lung a very cellular appearance. These cuboidal cells are referred to as type II pneumocytes in contrast to the flat, squamous epithelial cells (type I) that normally line the alveoli. Infiltrations of neutrophils and eosinophils into the interstitial tissue are commonly observed. These lung changes are distributed throughout the lung, in contrast to bronchopneumonia, which has a more cranioventral distribution.

DIAGNOSIS

Diagnosis of perilla toxicosis is made on the basis of clinical signs and finding evidence of mint ingestion. A sudden onset of severe dyspnea, an expiratory grunt, froth from the mouth, and crackles and consolidated areas upon auscultation are characteristic findings. Evidence of mint ingestion, especially of the flowering plant tops, aids a diagnosis. Post-mortem lesions previously described and finding square stem material in the rumen contents confirm the diagnosis. Differential diagnosis should include other common causes of interstitial pneumonia such as L-tryptophan–3-methylindole of lush pastures, moldy sweet potatoes, turnip tops, *Fusarium semitectum* of beans, and bovine respiratory syncytial virus (BRSV), and a sequela of *Pasteurella* infection.

TREATMENT

Many therapeutic agents have been employed for perilla toxicosis, including antihistamines, corticosteroids, antibiotics, diuretics, antiprostaglandins, and atropine, but with unremarkable results. In fact, stressing affected cattle by herding them through chutes for administering medication may do more harm than benefit because these cattle are already in a compromised condition. If cattle can be given antihistamines, steroids, or furosemide without extreme stress, some beneficial results may be noted. However, if extreme stress is unavoidable, removing the perilla without treating the cattle should be considered. Regardless of the treatment employed, approximately 1 to 2 weeks are needed for clinical signs to abate because the type II pneumocytes must resolve into squamous epithelial (type I) cells. In severe cases, permanent fibrosis of the lungs may result.

PREVENTION

As with many plant toxicoses, prevention of perilla toxicosis is much more beneficial than is treating those already affected. Pasture management is extremely important by avoiding overgrazing. If large areas of purple mint are observed in pasture fields, cutting it before it reaches the flowering stage will reduce the likelihood of animals ingesting mint during its most toxic period.

BIBLIOGRAPHY

Kerr LA, Johnson BJ, Burrows GE: Intoxication of cattle by *Perilla frutescens* (purple mint). Vet Hum Toxicol 28:412–416, 1986.

Linnabary RD, Wilson BJ, Garst JE, et al: Acute bovine pulmonary emphysema (ABPE). Perilla ketone, another cause. 20th Annual Proceedings, American Association of Veterinary Laboratory Diagnosticians. Minneapolis, MN, 1977, pp 323–326.

Peterson DR: Bovine pulmonary emphysema caused by the plant *Perilla frutescens*. In Proceedings, Symposium on Acute Bovine Pulmonary Emphysema (ABPE), Laramie, Wyoming, 1965.

Wilson BJ, Garst JE., Linnabary RD, et al: Perilla ketone: a potent lung toxin from the mint plant, *Perilla frutescens* Britton. Science 197:573–574, 1977.

Fescue Toxicosis

LARRY A. KERR, DVM, MS

Tall fescue (*Festuca arundinacea Schreb*), a major forage grass, is grown on approximately 35 million acres of land in the United States, primarily in the Southeast. Fescue is popular because it is adaptable to a wide range of soil and climatic conditions, is easily established, is persistent year after year, is tolerant of poor grazing management, and can be grazed throughout much of the winter. Nearly all of the tall fescue in the Southeast is the Kentucky 31 variety. Tall fescue is believed to have been introduced to the United States from Europe in the 1800s. However, its first official recognition in this country occurred on a hillside in Kentucky in 1931, hence the variety name Kentucky 31.

Indicators of forage quality such as digestible dry matter, crude protein, cell wall content, and minerals show that tall fescue is of high quality and should produce good performance in grazing animals. The chemical composition of fescue compares favorably with orchard grass, timothy, and brome grass. Whereas tall fescue has excellent agronomic properties and theoretically should produce good animal performance, the actual results have been disappointing because of the forage's toxic properties. These toxic properties manifest themselves in cattle in three syndromes: fescue foot, poor performance (summer slump), and fat necrosis. A single syndrome or combinations of all three may be observed in cattle ingesting toxic fescue over long periods of time. In mares, reproductive problems including prolonged gestation, abortions, thickened placentas, agalactia, and high foal mortality have occurred with grazing of this forage.

Fescue foot has been recognized in cattle since the late 1940s. This syndrome usually develops during the late fall or winter months and is characterized by necrosis of the extremities, usually the hindfeet, tips of the ears, or tail switch. In contrast, poor performance, probably the most costly fescue problem, is characterized by reduced rate of weight gain, decreased milk production, diarrhea, reduced feed intake, poor shedding of winter hair coat, poor reproductive performance, and high body temperatures. These signs are most pronounced in late summer when environmental temperatures are high but can occur at any time of year. Fat necrosis or lipomatosis is the presence of hard masses of necrotic fat in adipose tissue of the abdominal cavity.

During the past decade, extensive research has been conducted to determine the cause and practical solutions to the fescue problem. To date, however, the toxic agent and the mechanism of action of this agent remain unknown. An association has been observed between fescue infested with an endophyte fungus, *Acremonium coenophialum* (formerly *Epichloe typhina*), and the toxic syndrome. Unlike most fungi, *Acremonium coenophialum* grows inside the plant in the intercellular spaces and cannot be detected without special laboratory procedures. Some investigators speculate that this fungus may trigger the formation of various alkaloids (ergot) in the plant that adversely affect the ingesting animal's ability to form some essential hormones. Decreased serum prolactin concentrations and increased rectal temperatures have been demonstrated in animals ingesting endophyte fungus–infested fescue grass and hay.

Prolactin has a primary role in mammary gland differentiation necessary for the biochemical mechanisms involved in milk synthesis. This hormone also influences body growth and reproductive functions. Ergot alkaloids, a group produced by the fungus *Claviceps* spp., are believed to exert their biologic effects by stimulating dopamine receptors in the adenohypophysis and by antagonizing serotonin receptors. Both of these actions decrease prolactin concentrations. The way in which fescue fits into this scheme remains unknown. Because the endophyte fungus of fescue, *Acremonium coenophialum*, is closely related to *Claviceps* spp. (they belong to the same family, *Clavicipitaceae*), it may also produce ergot type alkaloids. Ergot alkaloids could be responsible for all 3 syndromes of fescue toxicosis.

CLINICAL SIGNS

Clinical signs of fescue toxicosis depend on which of the 3 syndromes is involved. Fescue foot usually occurs in late fall or winter, although the condition can occur at any time. This syndrome is characterized by weight loss, lameness of the hindlimbs, and gangrene of the feet and tail. Early signs of fescue foot include a tendency by the animal to shift weight from one rear foot to the other, a slight arching of the back, and soreness in the rear limbs. Often the left rear leg is the first affected. Knuckling of the pastern joint is sometimes observed early in the syndrome. As the condition progresses, reddening and swelling of the coronary band become apparent. Lameness worsens, and the animal becomes unthrifty and reluctant to move. In advanced cases, the swelling above the hoof becomes much more severe, and necrotic tissue is visible just below the swelling. Sloughing of the rear hooves often follows the appearance of this ischemic necrosis. In other cases, the tail switch or tips of the ears may be lost. Emaciation is common in animals suffering moderate to severe signs because these animals are reluctant to move in search of feed.

Poor performance or summer slump appears to be the most common of the 3 fescue syndromes and also the most important in terms of economic loss. The occurrence of this fescue syndrome corresponds to high environmental temperature and high humidity, although the condition may occur anytime animals are on fungus-infested fescue grass or hay. This syndrome is characterized by reduced feed intake, decreased weight gain or an actual weight loss, decreased milk production, reproductive problems, a failure to shed rough winter hair coat, diarrhea, elevated body temperature, increased respiratory rate, and hypersalivation. Animals with the poor performance syndrome spend less time grazing and more time in the shade or in farm ponds attempting to stay cool. Sheep and goats are also affected by the poor performance syndrome by having a marked reduction in milk production while grazing fungus-infested fescue. Conception rates in cattle and sheep may be significantly lower with grazing of toxic fescue as opposed to endophyte-free fescue, orchard grass, or legume pastures.

Fat necrosis or lipomatosis is the presence of hard necrotic fat in the adipose tissue of the abdominal or pelvic cavity. Necrotic fat is very hard, yellowish or chalky white, and often found in the mesentery surrounding the intestine in animals pastured on toxic fescue. This syndrome is probably much more common than is presently recognized because few clinical signs are observed unless the fat masses exert physical pressure on a segment of intestine or gravid uterus. This condition has usually been associated with long-term ingestion of fungus-infested fescue that has been heavily fertilized with nitrogen or chicken litter. Digestive disturbances such as chronic bloating, decreased ruminations, reduced feed intake, weight loss, and scanty feces are often observed in animals affected with this fescue syndrome. In severe cases, these animals may become emaciated and die, whereas others may become chronic poor doers. In pregnant cattle, large masses of necrotic fat may block the pelvic inlet, with resultant dystocia. Cesarean sections are sometimes necessary to deliver this fetus.

DIAGNOSIS

Diagnosis of fescue toxicosis is dependent on observing a clinical syndrome in affected animals similar to fescue foot, poor performance, or fat necrosis and a history of these animals having ingested fungus-infested fescue grass or hay for several weeks or months. Serum prolactin concentrations may be helpful; a relationship apparently exists between serum prolactin and the appearance of signs of fescue toxicosis. In a recent study, a group of steers on fungus-free fescue hay had a mean prolactin concentration of 67.51 ng/ml; a corresponding group of steers on endophyte fungus–infested fescue hay had a mean prolactin concentration of 11.55 ng/ml. The latter group of steers was showing signs consistent with the poor performance syndrome.

Differential diagnoses for fescue foot include ergot and selenium toxicoses, foot rot, frostbite, and trauma. Differential diagnoses for the poor performance syndrome include molybdenum and chronic organophosphate toxicoses, internal parasites, and nutritional deficiencies. Differential diagnoses for fat necrosis include lymphoma, peritonitis, intussusception, and gastrointestinal blockage or torsion. Diagnosis of the last condition can sometimes be aided by the rectal palpation of large, hard masses in the abdominal or pelvic cavity and the history of having applied fertilizer or chicken litter to fungus-infested fescue grass.

TREATMENT AND PREVENTION

Treatment of fescue toxicosis regardless of the syndrome involves removing animals from fungus-infested fescue grass or hay and placing them on a good alternative feed source. Those cattle with advanced fescue foot or cattle with large masses of necrotic fat blocking the intestinal tract or uterus should be considered for slaughter. Many animals exhibiting the poor performance signs will gradually return to normal when better forage is supplied.

Fescue toxicosis could be prevented by grazing animals on forages other than fescue. However, because fescue is the primary established forage in the Southeast, limiting its consumption is usually not possible or practical. If tall fescue is the predominant grass, it should be tested for determining whether the endophyte fungus is present and in what amount. Because endophyte-infested fescue exhibits no external signs of the fungus, detection is dependent on either microscopic examination or serologic testing of plant tissue samples. The microscopic test involves staining thin slices of recently harvested seed or plant tissue and observing the fungus with a microscope. The serologic test employs the use of an enzyme-linked immunosorbent assay (ELISA). An antibody reaction to the presence of the fungus in freshly harvested seed or fresh plant samples is the basis of the ELISA test. Neither of these procedures distinguishes between live and dead fungus in seeds. Because the endophyte fungus is primarily seed transmitted, a seed analysis before planting can help prevent further spread of the toxic fescue. Although the fungus in stored seed probably remains viable for approximately a year, a grow-out process is often used to determine the viability of the fungus in seed. This test involves planting stored seed and establishing plants in a greenhouse. When the seedlings are large enough, the microscopic test may be used to detect the presence of the fungus.

A few alternatives are available for fescue pastures heavily infested with fungus. The concentration of the fescue can be diluted with a legume. However, this process has not been overwhelmingly successful because the highly competitive nature of the tall fescue makes it difficult to maintain legumes in association with fescue. The use of fungicides on fescue pastures and in animals grazing these pastures has not been successful to date. A fairly radical alternative is plowing under or applying herbicides to existing fungus-infested fescue and replanting with a different grass or with a fungus-free variety of fescue. New fescue varieties from certified fungus-free seed are now becoming popular.

BIBLIOGRAPHY

Hemken RW, Bull LS, Boling JA, et al: Summer fescue toxicosis in lactating dairy cows and sheep fed experimental strains of ryegrass: tall fescue hybrids. J Anim Sci 49:641–646, 1979.
Kerr LA, McCoy CP, Boyle CR, et al: Effects of ammoniation of endophyte fungus–infested fescue hay on serum prolactin concentration and rectal temperature in beef cattle. Am J Vet Res 51:76–78, 1990.
Porter JK: Chemical constituents of tall fescue associated with toxicity. In Proceedings, Tall Fescue Toxicosis Workshop, Athens, GA, 1983, pp 27–33.
Stuedmann JA, Rumsey TS, Bond J, et al: Association of blood cholesterol with occurrence of fat necrosis in cows and tall fescue summer toxicosis in steers. Am J Vet Res 46:1990–1995, 1985.
Wallner BM, Booth NH, Robbins JD, et al: Effect of an endophytic fungus isolated from toxic pasture grass on serum prolactin concentrations in the lactating cow. Am J Vet Res 44:1317–1322, 1983.

Taxus (Yew) Poisoning

MERL F. RAISBECK, DVM, PhD, MS
JOE D. KENDALL, DVM, MS

The ornamental yews are hardy, evergreen (gymnospermous) shrubs with reddish-brown scaly bark, flat linear leaves 0.5 to 1 inch long with a prominent ventral midrib, and bright red, ovoid, fleshy fruit. The most commonly cultivated species include English yew (*T. baccata*), Japanese yew (*T. cuspidata*), and various hybrids. As a class, the yews will thrive in virtually any type of soil and are widely used as ornamental shrubs and hedges in cold-temperate regions of Europe and North America. *Taxus* sp. native to North American (western yew and ground hemlock) are reportedly much less toxic than are cultivated species.

The toxicity of *Taxus* shrubs has been recognized since pre-Christian times, yet, paradoxically, yew remains one of the most common sources of livestock intoxication in areas where it is cultivated. With the possible exception of the flesh of the fruit, all parts of the plant are toxic. Limited research indicates that the most toxic part of the plant is mature leaves collected in the spring and that toxicity is not markedly affected by drying. Nonetheless, yews are potentially poisonous throughout the year, and the authors have seen intoxications in all seasons. In one experiment, 200 g of dried leaves collected in the late autumn was sufficient to fatally poison a 550-kg steer.

MECHANISM OF ACTION

The toxicity of *Taxus* sp. is commonly attributed to taxine, a mixture of alkaloids first isolated more than 100 years ago. The identity of individual components of this mixture and the contribution of each to toxicity is still the source of some controversy. Crude extracts (i.e., taxine) produce arrhythmias ranging from decreased chronotropic and inotropic effects to ventricular tachycarida or fibrillation. Electrocardiographic abnormalities such as QRS widening in experimental animals and various in vitro experiments indicate that the cardiotoxicity of taxine is the result of inhibition of both sodium and calcium currents in cardiac myocytes.

CLINICAL SIGNS

Under field conditions, *Taxus* intoxication usually presents as sudden death with no prodromal signs during the late winter or early spring as the result of gates left open or hedge trimmings left in a pasture. Although the plant is reportedly unpalatable, the authors have seen well-fed cattle actively seek it out on several occasions. In experimental intoxications, there may be a very brief period of ataxia for a few minutes before collapse and death. The stress of moving or handling cattle often precipitates acute collapse and death. Post-mortem examination will reveal an enlarged, globular heart (diastole) and possibly pulmonary edema. Gastroenteritis occurs in rodents and human beings and has become ingrained in the veterinary literature. In the authors' experience, however, it seldom if ever occurs in ruminants.

DIAGNOSIS

Diagnosis of *Taxus* intoxication in food animals and horses hinges upon obtaining a history of exposure, observing cardiac arrhythmias such as ventricular tachycardia, finding the heart in diastole at post mortem, and demonstrating the presence of yew leaves in the gastrointestinal tract. Chemical analysis of ingesta for taxine is possible but requires direct insertion probe mass spectrometry and is thus presently beyond the capability of most veterinary laboratories. Other possible causes of sudden death such as cyanide or nitrate intoxication should be eliminated on the basis of appropriate chemical and pathologic tests.

TREATMENT

Parenteral atropine was reported to be beneficial in one clinical report of *Taxus* intoxication. Oral potassium permanganate, saline cathartics, and activated charcoal theoretically limit uptake of alkaloid from the gut of affected animals. In animals that are accustomed to being handled (e.g., dairy cattle), a combination of these treatments may be beneficial. Given the practical difficulty of administering these remedies to beef cattle or sheep under field conditions without causing excitement that may precipitate collapse and death, the most practical approach to therapy is simply clean feedstuffs, water, and rest. It might be possible to make meat animals dose themselves by incorporating activated charcoal into a mineral or "sweet feed" supplement. In this case, the typical ruminant should receive 0.5 to 1 g/kg body weight.

RESIDUES

The residue potential of taxine in milk of dairy cattle after *Taxus* ingestion is uncertain. On 2 occasions, the authors have investigated herdwide episodes of *Taxus* intoxication in which calves nursing both fatally poisoned and clinically normal cows were not affected. The apparent implication of this observation (i.e., that *Taxus* alkaloids are not excreted in hazardous concentrations in milk) needs to be confirmed experimentally before firm recommendations can be made regarding dairy cattle that have been recently exposed to *Taxus* leaves.

BIBLIOGRAPHY

Alden CL, Fosnaugh CJ, Smith JB, Mohan R: Japanese yew poisoning of large domestic animals in the midwest. J Am Vet Med Assoc 170:314–317, 1977.
Tekol Y: Negative chronotropic and atrioventricular blocking effects of taxine on isolated frog heart and its acute toxicity in mice. Planta Med 5:337–1360, 1985.
Yersin B, Frey JG, Schaller MD, et al: Fatal cardiac arrhythmias and shock following yew leaves ingestion. Ann Emerg Med 16:1396–1397, 1987.

Oak Poisoning

BILLY R. CLAY, DVM, MS, Diplomate, ABVT
DEENA G. GREGORY, DVM

Oak (*Quercus spp.*) poisoning has been recognized as a condition of livestock wherever oaks are found and consumed in the world. In North America, where more than 60 species of oaks are found, the toxic effects are more commonly seen in situations in which mismanagement factors come into play along with changes in climatic conditions. Cattle, sheep, and perhaps deer are affected, but goats and swine tend to exhibit tolerance.

The apparent seasonal occurrence coincides with the times of the year when oak buds or leaves may be the predominant forage or when an abundant acorn and leaf crop drops to the ground in the fall. Occasionally, premature shedding of green acorns or leaves after wind or hail may create the setting for poisoning, especially if forage is limited.

The gallotannins found in all parts of the oak are metabolized to nephrotoxic polyhydroxyphenolics such as tannic acid, gallic acid, and pyrogallol. The black oaks contain higher concentrations of these than do the white oaks, and the concentration tends to decrease with maturity of the plant parts in both groups. Most oak species contain toxic amounts, except perhaps the live oak (*Q. virginiana*) and Mohr oak (*Q. mohriana*), which are readily consumed without ill effects by livestock. Freezing or drying does not alter the toxins.

The younger and malnourished animals appear to be more susceptible to the effects of the phenolic compounds. This may reflect pica and inadequate dilution with less offensive forages. Some observers have noted that oak poisoning is uncommon in cattle more than 2 years of age. However, as pasture and climatic conditions become more severe, the older, more experienced animals may become affected as well.

The nursing animal should not directly affected by oak tannins in that little is passed through the milk. However, the nursing dam consuming the toxins will sacrifice milk production as the poisoning progresses, and this may in turn encourage the more susceptible young to select oak forage and become poisoned.

Morbidity in herd cases of oak poisoning has been variable, but mortality may be as high as 80 per cent of those exhibiting signs. The toxicosis may be manifest as an acute disease with a variable course of 2 to 14 days or a lingering debilitating condition that lasts for several weeks.

The low-growing oaks of the West and Southwest cause

significant economic losses annually, whereas the upright oaks cause more sporadic losses. Regardless of the oaks involved, the disease is costly to the livestock owner and deserves to have attention given to its management and prevention.

PATHOGENESIS

The hydrolyzed products of gallotannins are believed to cause damage through hydrogen bonding to the peptide linkages of proteins. This effect is relied upon by the tanning industry in the production of leather. The hydrolysis readily occurs in the rumen where the phenolic moieties may bind directly to mucous membrane epithelium or to salivary mucin and ingesta. In the abomasum, the bound phenolics are once again disassociated owing to the lowered pH. Additional mucosal damage may occur there before gastrointestinal absorption. Plasma proteins bind to the tannins in the circulating blood, allowing transport to all tissues, where resultant endothelial damage occurs and permits leakage of fluids. Glomerular capillary damage results in interstitial edema and tubular necrosis with formation of casts. Renal function becomes decreased with resulting electrolyte imbalances and circulatory accumulation of metabolic products. Anuria or oliguria follows with associated elevations in blood urea nitrogen, serum creatinine, and potassium. The urine produced will be diluted and sometimes contains blood cells, protein, or glucose.

Anorexia occurs as the poisoning progresses with resultant azotemia, hypocalcemia, and hyperphosphatemia. Owing to capillary damage and reduced cardiac and renal function, there may be hemorrhage and fluid loss into the body cavities and interstitial spaces. All contribute to depression, ataxia, and death in the severely poisoned.

CLINICAL SIGNS AND PATHOLOGY

Cattle are frequently affected from consumption of oak plant parts; the incidence is higher in younger than in older animals. Sheep may also become poisoned. When poisoning occurs, the clinical signs are progressive, depending on the dose and duration of intake of gallotannins. Signs may appear as early as 4 days with constipation, depression, and anorexia followed by hemorrhagic diarrhea. Some will not become constipated, and a dark tarry stool will remain prominent. Tenesmus may occur in some. Emaciation and dehydration become apparent, and most will remain in the vicinity of water where they attempt to drink often. Any urine voided will be diluted and perhaps blood-tinged. Edema may be apparent subcutaneously, and ruminal atony with a doughy consistency upon palpation is common. Weakness progresses to recumbency and death within 3 to 7 days.

The cadaver may show evidence of epistaxis having occurred before death and the prominent tarry stool. Ascites, hydrothorax, hemorrhage, and perirenal edema are the most consistent features. Gastritis and enteritis range from catarrhal to hemorrhagic. Muscosal ulceration (including pharyngeal and esophageal) is common in those that die as a result of the toxic nephritis.

Petechial hemorrhages are frequently found in the kidneys, epicardium, endocardium, peritoneal tissues, mesenteries, and sometimes subcutaneous tissues. Edema may accompany the hemorrhages with prominent accumulations of fluid perirenally and subcutaneously along the ventral body wall and extremities.

On histologic examination, there is the presence of eosinophilic (by hematoxylin and eosin staining) debris in the lumen of numerous proximal convoluted and ascending kidney tubules. The luminal material is believed to be destroyed epithelial cells and neutrophils associated with proteinaceous urinary precipitates. Some tubules may remain intact with a normal appearance, whereas others may have the appearance of hydropic degeneration. In a few cases, there may be mononuclear cells scattered in interstitial tissues without evidence of a distinct inflammatory response.

Animals chronically affected or recovering may show scattered areas of tubular regeneration and compensatory function. Evidence of secondary disease may also be apparent. Blood and urine analyses will reveal constituent concentrations similar to those shown in Table 1. These findings generally follow anorexia, renal failure, and tissue necrosis.

DIAGNOSIS

Clinical signs of anorexia, rapid weight loss, polydipsia, polyuria, hemorrhage, or edema along with evidence of consumption of oak are sufficient to support a tentative diagnosis of oak poisoning. Clinical and pathologic changes of blood and urine similar to those shown in Table 1 are also helpful. Blood urea nitrogen, creatinine, and urine specific gravity have proved to be the most beneficial measurements.

If dead animals are available for necropsy, gross pathologic lesions of digestive system mucosal ulceration and hemorrhage, perirenal edema, fluid in body cavities, and subcutaneous edema are typical diagnostic findings. Rumen contents may reveal a preponderance of oak plant parts. If a small amount of the solid rumen content is mixed with a drop of water on a microscope slide, a characteristic stellate (star-shaped) structure present in leaf tissues can often be visualized with use of a low-power magnification. Finding these structures can help confirm a diagnosis of oak toxicosis (Fig. 1).

The gastritis and enteritis with associated ulceration of mucosa and hemorrhage require a differentiation of this disease from those caused by common viruses, heavy metals, other nephrotoxic plants, and some mycotoxins (e.g., stachybotryotoxin). These may be eliminated by appropriate history and diagnostic tests of blood, other tissues, and digestive contents.

Microscopic renal lesions consistent with gallotannin tubular damage aid in confirming the diagnosis when other evidence is supportive. At least one study (Spier et al, 1987) has

Table 1. BLOOD CHEMISTRY AND URINALYSIS RESULTS TYPICAL OF SUBACUTE OAK POISONING

Hematology	
Albumin (g/dl)	<3.5
Fibrinogen (mg/dl)	>700
Blood urea nitrogen (mg/dl)	100–200
Creatinine (mg/dl)	5–10
Sodium (mEq/L)	<132
Potassium (mEq/L)	1.5–7.5
Calcium (mg/dl)	<9.0
Phosphorus (mg/dl)	>6.0
Urinalysis	
Specific gravity	<1.020
Blood	Trace to 2+
Bilirubin	Negative
Ketones	Negative to 1+
Glucose	Negative to 2+
Protein	Trace
Leukocytes (HPF)	0–8
Epithelial cells (HPF)	1–2
Casts (HPF)	Negative

HPF = high-power field.

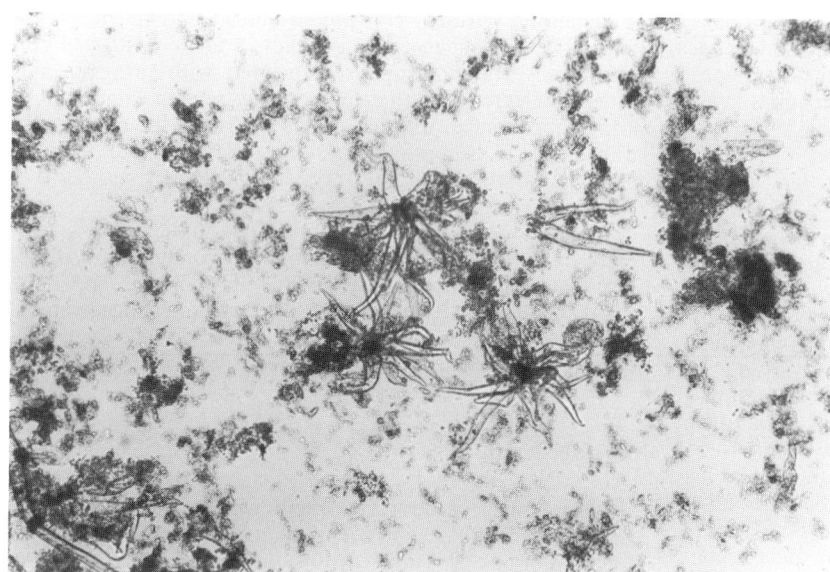

Figure 1. Stellate structures found in oak leaf tissues shown at 110× magnification.

suggested that these lesions are pathognomonic for oak poisoning.

The prognosis is guarded in those with obvious clinical signs. Tubular regeneration and recovery is possible if immediate adjustments in management are made and appropriate therapy is offered to those affected.

TREATMENT AND RECOVERY

Treatment should focus on restoring the nutritional status of the animal, removing the offending toxin, and alleviating the effects of kidney failure. Affected animals should be removed from the offending pasture immediately and provided fresh, familiar forage initially, with 1 to 2 pounds of concentrate offered on the second and succeeding days until the appetites are restored. Severely affected animals may require a rumenotomy for removal of toxic ingesta or cathartics such as mineral oil (1 L/400 kg) or sodium sulfate (1 kg/400 kg). Harsh or irritant cathartics should be avoided. These animals may require rehydration therapy as well. The initial anuric phase may bring about lowered blood pH and hyperkalemia. Hypokalemia may also develop as a result of anorexia. All should be monitored and corrected as a part of the rehydration. Some animals will develop a polyuric phase of the disease. This may last for 2 to 3 weeks and end in either death or recovery after tubular regeneration.

These chronically affected animals may perform poorly after recovery, but those that respond promptly can be expected to perform similarly to nonpoisoned counterparts. In fact, the weight lost during convalescence may even be recouped in the feedlot so that the final weight is equal to or better than that of comparable herdmates.

PREVENTION

Because of a seasonal incidence, livestock should be managed so that adequate nutrition is guaranteed during the critical periods (fall in the North and spring and summer in the South). Many producers reduce or eliminate supplemental feed in the spring with the first sight of annual grasses. Although there may be adequate forage during that time, the water content of that forage may be excessive and result in a depraved appetite. Likewise, during drought, the low-growing oaks become an easily accessible vegetation.

Where acorns are a problem, removal from the pasture may be necessary in years of abundant production. Even with plentiful forage, some animals will select acorns, but that is not to be expected as a rule.

In situations in which removal is impractical, supplemental feed containing 10 per cent calcium hydroxide may help prevent poisoning (2 kg/day for cows and 1 kg/day for calves).

Eradication of the oaks is the only solution in some situations. This may be accomplished through the appropriate use of herbicides. Dichlorprop (1 to 2 lb/acre [A]), Grazon ET (1 to 2 pt/A), or Spike 20P (10 to 20 lb/A) may be used for tall upright oaks; Grazon ET at ½ to 1 pt or Spike 20P at 5 to 15 pounds is more appropriate for the low-growing oaks.

BIBLIOGRAPHY

Ostrowski SR, Smith BP, Spier SJ, et al: Compensatory weight gain in steers recovered from oak bud toxicosis. J Am Vet Med Assoc 195:481, 1989.

Osweiler GD: Nephrotoxic plants. In Howard JL: Current Veterinary Therapy: Food Animal Practice. Philadelphia, WB Saunders, 1986, p 401.

Osweiler GD, Carson TL, Buck WB, Van Gelder GA: Chemical and Diagnostic Veterinary Toxicology, 3rd ed. Dubuque, IA, Kendall/Hunt Publishing Co, 1985.

Spier SJ, Smith BP, Seawright AA, et al: Oak toxicosis in cattle in northern California: clinical and pathologic findings. J Am Vet Med Assoc 191:958, 1987.

Water Quality

Water Quality for Livestock

T. L. CARSON, DVM, PHD, MS

Some have called water the most important nutrient for livestock. The availability of quality water in adequate quantity can be a limiting factor to a livestock enterprize. Increased physical concentrations of livestock, combined with heightened emphasis on nutrition and health, have raised the number of inquiries about water quality. The following discussion summarizes some of the major parameters of water quality for livestock.

PALATABILITY

Palatability directly affects water consumption. A restricted water intake is soon followed by reduced feed consumption and thus reduced productive efficiency.

The palatability of water and its acceptance by livestock is affected by salinity, bacteria, iron, copper and other minerals, odors, pesticides, the amount of dissolved carbon dioxide, and other factors that may not be fully understood.

The milk production of lactating animals is especially affected by reduced water consumption. For example, dairy cattle consuming water containing 4300 mg total dissolved solids per liter consumed less water and less feed and produced less milk than did control cows on water with 430 mg/L total dissolved solids.[1]

MICROBIOLOGIC STANDARDS

Microbiologic examination of water samples will reveal the general sanitary quality and the degree of contamination from human and animal sources.

In general, these examinations are done not to isolate pathogenic bacteria but to detect the presence of indicator organisms. The coliform group of bacteria has traditionally been the indicator used to assess the degree of water pollution and thus the sanitary quality of the particular sample. A recent advance in the microbiologic examination of water, the differentiation of fecal coliforms as a subgroup within the general category of coliforms, is encouraging. The United States Environmental Protection Agency (EPA) proposed in 1973 that acceptable limitations for water to be used directly by livestock should not exceed 5000 coliforms/100 ml, and the monthly arithmetic density of fecal coliforms should not exceed 1000 coliforms/100 ml.[2] Many believe, however, that as long as animals are allowed to range freely and drink surface waters, these proposed limits would be unenforceable and of doubtful value.

The standard plate count, which enumerates the number of bacteria multiplying at 35° C, is of questionable significance in evaluating livestock water sources other than in helping to judge the efficiency of various water treatment processes.

HARDNESS

Water hardness has been understood to indicate the tendency of water to precipitate soap or to form scale on heated surfaces. Hardness is generally expressed as the sum of calcium and magnesium concentrations reported in equivalent amounts of calcium carbonate. Hardness is sometimes confused with salinity, but the two are not necessarily correlated. Waters containing high levels of sodium salts and therefore having high salinity can be very soft if they contain low levels of calcium and magnesium. Most ground waters generally have hardness values of less than 2000 mg/L, but in some arid regions these values may be higher. Hardness, sometimes reported as grains per gallon (1 grain per gallon equals 17.1 mg/L), is in itself not a problem in livestock drinking water from a health issue but may affect mineralization of pipes, valves, water heaters, and other mechanical devices.

SALINITY

Salinity is defined as the total concentration of solids in water after all carbonates have been converted to oxides, all bromides and iodides have been replaced by chloride, and all organic matter has been oxidized. In more general terms, salinity is an expression of the amount of dissolved salts in a particular water sample. The ions most commonly involved in highly saline waters are calcium, magnesium, and sodium in the bicarbonate, chloride, or sulfate form.

Cattle appear to tolerate up to 2500 mg/L dissolved salts (as either sulfate or sodium chloride) without adverse effects.[3,4] Experimental evidence shows no significant effects in swine consuming water containing up to 3000 mg/L dissolved salts.[5,6]

The general recommendations for the use of saline water for livestock are presented in Table 1.

Table 1. A GUIDE TO THE USE OF SALINE WATERS FOR LIVESTOCK

Total Soluble Salt Content of Water (mg/L)	Comments
Less than 1000	A relatively low level of salinity with no serious burden for any class of livestock
1000–2999	Satisfactory for all classes of livestock; they may cause temporary and mild diarrhea in livestock not accustomed to them, but should not affect health or performance
3000–4999	Satisfactory for livestock, although they might cause temporary diarrhea or refusal at first by animals not accustomed to them
5000–6999	Reasonably safe for dairy and beef cattle, sheep, swine, and horses; it may be well to avoid the use of those with higher levels for pregnant or lactating animals
7000–10,000	Probably unfit for swine; considerable risk may exist in using them for pregnant or lactating cows, horses, sheep, the young of these species, or any animals subjected to heavy heat stress or water loss; in general, their use should be avoided, although older ruminants, horses, and even swine may subsist on them for long periods under conditions of low stress
More than 10,000	The risks with these highly saline waters are so great that they cannot be recommended for use under any conditions

Source: Adapted from National Academy of Sciences Subcommittee on Nutrient and Toxic Elements in Water: Nutrients and toxic substances in water for livestock and poultry. Washington, DC, National Academy of Sciences, 1974.

TOXIC ELEMENTS

A number of elements found in water seldom offer any problem to livestock because they do not occur at high levels in soluble form or because they are toxic only in excessive concentrations. Examples of these are iron, aluminum, beryllium, boron, chromium, cobalt, copper, iodide, manganese, molybdenum, and zinc. Also, these elements do not seem to accumulate in meat, milk, or eggs to the extent that they would constitute a problem in livestock drinking waters under any but the most unusual conditions. Proposed acceptable limits for these elements in livestock water are presented in Table 2.

Because arsenic, cadmium, fluorine, lead, mercury, and selenium may under some circumstances present a hazard to livestock, these elements should be evaluated on an individual case basis (Table 2).

NITRATE AND NITRITE

The nitrate ion (NO_3^-) is both a product and a reactant in the chain of animal and plant nitrogen metabolism. The nitrate ion can be reduced to form the nitrite ion (NO_2^-). Decaying animal or plant protein, animal metabolic waste (urea and ammonia), nitrogen fertilizers, silage juices, and soil high in nitrogen-fixing bacteria may be sources of nitrates and nitrites. Nitrates and nitrites are water-soluble and thus, if added to soil, may be leached away, moving with the ground water into the water table. The likelihood of high levels of nitrate contamination to a well or reservoir is much greater when the source of the nitrate is nearby. The most common source of contamination to wells is surface water run-off into shallow, poorly cased wells. Ponded water that collects feedlot or fertilizer run-off may contain toxic levels of nitrates.

Levels of nitrates in water may be expressed in a number of ways. Each of these expressions can be converted to the other (Table 3). One must be cognizant of these distinctions when evaluating laboratory data.

Table 2. RECOMMENDED LIMITS OF CONCENTRATION OF SOME POTENTIALLY TOXIC SUBSTANCES IN DRINKING WATER FOR LIVESTOCK

Element	Safe Upper Limit of Concentration (mg/L)		
	US EPA[7] (for humans)	US EPA (for livestock)	NAS[8] (for livestock)
Aluminum		5.0	
Arsenic	0.05	0.2	0.2
Barium	1.0		NE*
Beryllium		No limit*	
Boron		5.0	
Cadmium	0.01	0.05	0.05
Chromium	0.05	1.0	1.0
Cobalt		1.0	1.0
Copper		0.5	0.5
Fluoride	4	2.0	2.0
Iron		No limit	NE
Lead	0.05	0.1	0.1
Manganese		No limit	NE
Mercury	0.002	0.001	0.01
Molybdenum		No limit	NE
Nickel			1.0
Nitrate	45	100	440
Nitrite		33	33
Selenium	0.01	0.05	
Vanadium		0.1	0.1
Zinc		25.0	25.0

*Not established or no limit. Experimental data available are not sufficient to make definite recommendations.

Table 3. NITRATE AND NITRITE EXPRESSIONS AND CONVERSION FACTORS FOR CONVERTING FROM ONE EXPRESSION TO ANOTHER*

Form A	Form B				
	N	NO_2^-	NO_3^-	KNO_3	$NaNO_3$
Nitrate-nitrogen (N)	1.0	3.3	4.4	7.2	6.1
Nitrite-nitrogen (N)	1.0	3.3	4.4	7.2	6.1
Nitrate (NO_3^-)	0.23	0.74	1.0	1.63	1.37
Nitrite (NO_2^-)	0.3	1.0	1.34	2.2	1.85
Potassium nitrate (KNO_3)	0.14	0.64	0.61	1.0	0.84
Sodium nitrate ($NaNO_3$)	0.16	0.54	0.72	1.2	1.0

*To convert Form A to the equivalent amount of Form B, multiply A by the appropriate conversion factor: (Form A × conversion factor = Form B).[9]

The nitrate ion itself is not particularly toxic. However, nitrite, the reduced form of nitrate, is readily absorbed into the blood, where it reacts with hemoglobin to form methemoglobin. Compared with monogastric animals, ruminants are generally more susceptible to nitrate toxicosis because the bacteria in the rumen readily reduce the nitrate to nitrite.

Acute nitrate poisoning in animals may be expected when nitrates exceed 500 mg/L in the water or 1 per cent nitrate (dry weight basis) in the forage.[9] One report[10] indicates that water containing 2000 mg/L nitrate can be fed at 10 per cent of body weight to cattle for as long as 17 days with no indication of acute toxic effects. However, 3000 mg/L given to cattle for 3 days resulted in death from acute nitrate poisoning. A study of 86 dairy cows over a 35-month period concluded that drinking water containing up to 400 ppm nitrate had no significant effect on reproduction, milk production, or general health of the cows.[11]

The effects of feed and water nitrate levels are additive, and both must therefore be considered in evaluating a potential nitrate problem.

The EPA maximal limit for nitrate in water that is to be used for preparation of human baby formula is 45 mg/L and is set to prevent the methemoglobinemia or "blue baby" syndrome. It has been suggested that neonatal swine are also quite susceptible to elevated levels of nitrates, but Emerick and associates[12] have concluded that pigs 1 week old are no more susceptible to nitrate-induced methemoglobinemia than are older pigs.

PESTICIDES

Pesticides enter water from soil run-off, drift, infall, direct application, accidental spills, or faulty waste disposal techniques. Concern is frequently raised regarding the effects of these water-borne pesticides on livestock. In general, however,

Table 4. MAXIMAL ALLOWABLE CONCENTRATIONS OF PESTICIDES IN HUMAN DRINKING WATER

Pesticide	Maximal Concentration (mg/L)
Aldrin	0.001
DDT	0.05
Dieldrin	0.001
Chlordane	0.003
Endrin	0.0002
Heptachlor	0.0001
Heptachlor epoxide	0.0001
Lindane	0.004
Methoxychlor	0.1
Toxaphene	0.005
2,4-D	0.1
2,4,5-T	0.01

there are not sufficient data available, considering the great number of pesticides, the variability of species response, and the dilution of factors usually present, to make hard and fast recommendations on allowable limits for livestock water.

The EPA[7] has, however, set maximal allowable concentrations of several pesticides in human drinking water (Table 4) and has recently proposed Lifetime Health Advisory levels of numerous pesticides and chemicals in human drinking water.[13]

SUMMARY

In animal husbandry, it is sometimes easy to incriminate the water as the cause of poor performance and nonspecific disease conditions in livestock. It is imperative that attempts to evaluate water quality in the face of animal health problems include obtaining a thorough history, making astute observations, and asking intelligent questions. A thorough laboratory examination of animal specimens and water samples should be evaluated in view of existing standards for livestock water quality.

Basic laboratory evaluation of water quality should include measurement of total dissolved solids, nitrate-nitrite, and coliform count. Supplementary water tests would include sulfate, sodium, magnesium, chloride, calcium, potassium, manganese, and pH.

REFERENCES

1. Challis DJ, Zeinstra JS, Anderson MJ: Some effects of water quality on performance of high yielding dairy cows. Vet Rec 120:12–15, 1987.
2. United States Environmental Protection Agency: Proposed criteria for water quality. I. Quality of water for livestock. Environ Rep 4:663, 1973.
3. Digesti RD, Weeth HJ: A defensible maximum for inorganic sulfate in drinking water of cattle. J Anim Sci 42:1498–1502, 1976.
4. Jaster EH, Schuh JD, Wegner TN: Physiologic effects of saline drinking water on high producing dairy cows. J Dairy Sci 61:66–71, 1978.
5. Anderson DM, Strothers SC: Effects of saline water high in sulfates, chlorides, and nitrates on the performance of young weanling pigs. J Anim Sci 47:900–907, 1978.
6. Paterson DW, Wahlstrom RC, Libal GW, Olson OE: Effects of sulfate in water on swine reproduction and young pig performance. J Anim Sci 49:664–667, 1979.
7. United States Environmental Protection Agency, National Primary Drinking Water Standards, 1989.
8. National Academy of Sciences Subcommittee on Nutrient and Toxic Elements in Water: Nutrients and toxic substances in water for livestock and poultry. Washington, DC, National Academy of Sciences, 1974.
9. Osweiler GD, Carson TL, Buck WB, VanGelder GA: Clinical and Diagnostic Veterinary Toxicology, 3rd ed. Dubuque, IA, Kendall/Hunt Publishing Co, 1985.
10. Dollahite JW, Rowe LD: Nitrate and nitrite intoxication in rabbits and cattle. Southwest Vet 27:246, 1974.
11. Crowley JW, Jorgensen NA, Kahler LW, et al: Effect of nitrate in drinking water on reproductive and productive efficiency of dairy cattle. Tech Rep WS WRC 74-06, 1974.
12. Emerick R, Embry LB, Seerly RW: Rate of formation and reduction of nitrate induced methemoglobin *in virtro* and *in vivo* as influenced by diet of sheep and age of swine. J Anim Sci 24:221–230, 1965.
13. United States Environmental Protection Agency, Office of Drinking Water, Drinking Water Regulations and Health Advisories, 1989.

Toxicants in Geothermal Waters, Cooling Waters, and Mine Tailings

J. L. SHUPE, DVM
C. V. BAGLEY, DVM
H. B. PETERSON, PhD
A. E. OLSON, MS

Animals may be exposed to natural or synthetic toxic substances. The major sources of these toxic or potentially toxic agents for animals, both domestic and wild, are vegetation, water, soil, and volcanic dusts. Toxins also exist in industrial wastes, rodenticides, insecticides, fungicides, herbicides, feed additives, fertilizers, biotoxins, emissions from internal combustion engines, and by-products from the commercial conversion and public use of energy. Some so-called toxicants or pollutants are essential (in proper amounts) for animal health and growth.

As human populations increase, so do the numbers and complexities of toxicologic problems. These problems are frequently induced by a combination of factors, sometimes from multiple sources, as illustrated in Figure 1. The potential additive or synergistic influence of a combination of toxicants from multiple sources is a major concern.

One way of estimating and evaluating the interactions that affect animal health is to identify the toxicants or pollutants and to determine their environmental pathways, ecologic aspects, and health effects. This is particularly important with the ever-increasing demand for new sources of energy (e.g., geothermal waters or coal conversion plants), mining and smelting operations, and related industries.

COMPOSITION

Geothermal Waters

Geothermal waters are usually contaminated with some elements of underground origin. The concentrations of these elements may vary from a few hundred to many thousands of milligrams per liter. The most common elements or combinations of elements are sodium, potassium, lithium, calcium, magnesium, ammonium, silica, chloride, fluoride, borate, sulfate, carbonate, bicarbonate, hydrogen sulfide, and carbon dioxide. Other common elements of particular toxicologic concern include arsenic, molybdenum, selenium, and heavy metals. Of the potential toxicants, fluorides are the most often present in toxic concentrations.

These toxic or potentially toxic substances may occur as suspended solids, in solution, or in combination. They may be accessible to livestock in drinking water or after application to forage crops via irrigation water.

Cooling Waters

When electricity is generated by use of fossil fuels, water is utilized to cool and clean the effluent. It is customary to cycle the water repeatedly through cooling and scrubbing towers. This concentrates the soluble constituents, so any potential pollutant or toxic substance may be concentrated 5 to 20 times.

Published with the approval of the Utah State University Agricultural Experiment Station, Logan, UT, as Journal Paper No. 4007.

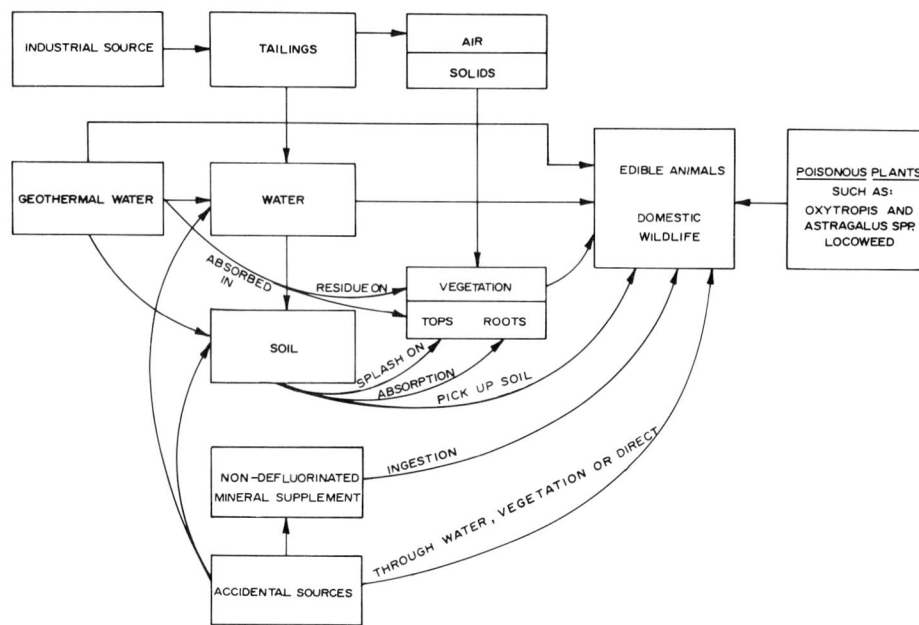

Figure 1. Possible routes of toxicants in geothermal waters and in mine tailings.

For example, water safe for consumption that contains 0.2 mg/L fluoride may contain 2 to 4 mg/L fluoride as effluent water. Animals may drink the effluent water or eat forage contaminated by sprinkle-irrigation with effluent water.

Tailings

Tailings are finely ground rock and minerals that have been processed to remove the desirable ores. Tailings differ greatly in their physical and chemical characteristics. The variability may be influenced by the type of mining operation, composition of the ore body, amounts of pyrites present, type of milling process, and composition of the water used to transport the tailings to the tailing pile. Excessive concentrations of soluble salts are often present. The toxicants may be leached out of tailing piles into animal drinking water supplies.

Tailing piles, which are poor sustainers of vegetation, do not act like normal agricultural soils. They are normally low in water-holding capacity, devoid of plant nutrients, and subject to wind erosion. The wind erosion of a tailing pile may contaminate nearby forage crops with particulate toxic materials.

Most mine tailings contain many kinds of sulfides that, when oxidized, form acids, lower the pH, and increase the availability of soluble heavy metals. The relation between pH and soluble heavy metals is illustrated by the data in Table 1. Drainage waters from waste piles having low pH values could pollute a water supply for animals. The hazard of pollution with heavy metals, therefore, increases as the tailing waters age by oxidation. However, molybdenum compounds, if present, are more soluble at near-neutral pH, so potential pollution by these compounds is greater from waste piles of pH 6 to 8 than from acid piles. As illustrated in Figure 1, animals may obtain pollutants from routes other than directly from contaminated water.

COMPLEXITY OF PROBLEM

There are many complex hazards for livestock associated with the utilization of geothermal waters, industrial cooling or effluent waters, or water exposed to mine tailings.

Little information has been obtained under rigid experimental conditions about the effects of the amounts of different combinations of chemical elements in drinking water and feed. Some elements may be either antagonistic or synergistic to the other elements present in feeds, water supplies, or even mineral supplements. All of these interrelationships must be considered and determined insofar as possible when an actual or potential toxicosis is investigated.

Digestion processes may markedly alter the availability of certain chemicals to an animal. Other factors that should also be evaluated are duration of intake (short-term compared with long-term intake), age and health of animals, rate of water consumption, composition of diet, physiologic demands, and differences among species.

Based on past experience and present knowledge, the many variables and possible interactions make it difficult—if not impossible—to determine exact critical toxic levels of many of these chemical combinations.

DIAGNOSIS

Every available means of obtaining an accurate differential diagnosis should be utilized. In many cases, much effort and laboratory assistance will be required to support or substantiate a tentative clinical diagnosis.

Table 1. ANALYSIS OF WATER EXTRACTS OF TAILINGS MATERIALS*

Sample Source	pH Extract	Concentration of Saturation Extract (mg/L)				
		Cu	Fe	Mn	Zn	Pb
Copper tailings						
New Mexico	2.2	>600	3000	21	21	<5
Montana	7.6	<1	<0.5	0.6	0.2	<5
Uranium tailings						
Utah	1.9	>600	>5000	1005	77	30
Colorado	8	<1	<0.5	<0.2	0.2	<5

*Each material was wet to saturation and the water extracted by suction. Determination of the content was made with a Jarrell-Ash Direct Reading Spectrophotometer.

History

A complete history, including changes in management, recent storms, recent access to new range areas or water sources, and other possible factors, is necessary; all factors should be considered and studied.

Limited amounts of drainage water from tailing piles may pollute the water supply of animals and induce chronic toxicosis. Acute toxicosis may result when large amounts of soluble pollutants are released owing to pond failure and discharge of polluted waters or from tailing piles during a heavy rain or flood.

Clinical Signs

Close observation of live animals may lead to a positive diagnosis. Bovine dental fluorosis induced by prolonged consumption of geothermal water and forage that was sprinkle-irrigated with the same water source is shown in Figure 2.

Necropsy Findings

If animals have died or have been sacrificed, a complete necropsy should be performed. If toxicoses of any specific type are suspected, observe for lesions characteristic of those toxicoses. The presence of any lesion should be noted, however, because lesions may mimic toxicant interactions or other causes of death. Tissues and specimens should be properly collected for chemical, microbiologic, and histologic evaluations. It is important that the clinical signs and lesions be properly correlated before a diagnosis is made. A diagnosis should never be based merely on casual observations. The animals themselves are the best indicators of their own state of health, and the clinician should accurately observe and evaluate each animal's clinical signs and lesions.

Laboratory Findings

Clinical and necropsy findings should be substantiated or dismissed by reliable laboratory tests.

Particularly examine and sample those tissues primarily involved in detoxification, such as liver and kidney. Gastrointestinal contents and lesions may help determine the presence or absence of many toxic elements and aid in diagnosing the cause. Lymph nodes are important as filters and should be examined. Body fluids, both blood and urine, should be examined as to color, physical characteristics, and chemical content.

Because of the expense involved in complete chemical analyses for some elements and chemicals, evaluate history, clinical signs, and lesions for limiting laboratory tests to those toxicants most likely involved. Some special cases, however, may warrant extensive chemical analyses and laboratory support.

In addition to tests of animal tissues, all possible sources of toxic substances should also be considered and checked when indicated. Analyze all possible sources of drinking water, forage, or other feed sources and mineral supplements for suspected toxicants. Also analyze soil samples, and especially any mine tailings, to determine levels of suspected toxicants.

TREATMENT

Until a definite diagnosis is made, treatment of affected animals can only be symptomatic and supportive. After a definitive diagnosis is made, follow prevailing recommended medical therapy and treatment.

PREVENTION

The most practical approach to preventing or alleviating future toxicologic problems may vary. The major objective is to prevent or limit the access of animals to the toxicant's source. Monitor their health closely to enable early detection of deleterious effects. Animals may be removed from the source or replaced with species less susceptible to the particular toxicant involved.

If animals must be exposed to environmental toxicants, then efforts should be made to eliminate other stresses on those animals. In cool areas, animals prefer warm geothermal water rather than cold water. However, they should not be allowed to drink geothermal water if other sources are available. Animals that must drink geothermal waters with high fluoride content should be fed roughage with low fluoride content. Roughage with a high calcium level, such as alfalfa and clover, is of added benefit because the calcium will bind with the fluoride and further reduce its effect. There should be adequate feed of good quality to prevent overgrazing. This will be particularly helpful when the offending elements are present at high levels in the soil or tailing piles. Overgrazing promotes ingestion of larger quantities of soil with the feed. Also, the roots and crowns of the vegetation may contain particularly high concentrations of heavy metals.

Provide adequate and balanced mineral supplementation when either tailings or geothermal waters are involved. Either source may contain some of the essential mineral elements, but the animals may also ingest excessive detrimental amounts of other unwanted toxic elements. Depraved mineral appetites or salt hunger may induce animals to ingest toxic quantities of undesirable compounds.

Efforts should be made to cultivate tailing areas with vegetation to prevent wind or water erosion of these tailings into water supplies or onto forage crops. Vegetation planted on these areas, however, should be unpalatable to livestock. Such plant species will be left to flourish and thereby hold the tailings together, because animals will not be likely to graze in the hazardous areas.

Consider alternative land uses for areas where toxic elements in the soil create hazards for livestock. Other productive agricultural uses may be made of such land. The area, if properly managed, may have recreation potential with complete removal of livestock. However, consider any potential hazards that the area may pose for people.

If the area is suited only for livestock grazing, fence animals

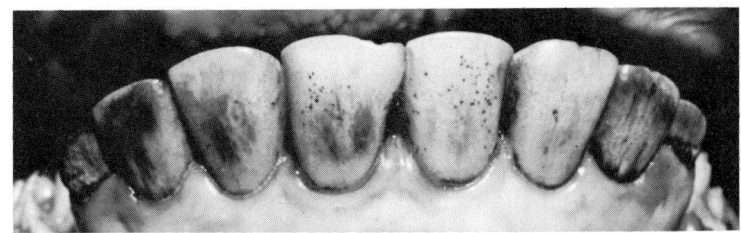

Figure 2. Permanent bovine incisor teeth with dental fluorosis induced by drinking geothermal water and eating forage that was sprinkle-irrigated with the same water source. Note chalkiness and discoloration of enamel and bilateral nature of lesions.

out from known toxic sites and toxic water supplies. Avoid overgrazing and be aware of the consequences of sudden heavy rainfalls, especially in more arid areas.

More needs to be learned about the effects of exposure of livestock to chemicals in their environment. Chronic toxicosis is often more difficult to diagnose and may have greater economic importance than do the more alarming and publicized acute toxicoses. The concerns and warnings about the potential toxicants in geothermal waters and mine tailings also apply to many other toxicants that are not properly handled and managed. Today, there is an urgent need for proper interpretation of existing information, as well as the development of essential data regarding the effects of the combination or interaction of toxicants under conditions that would simulate (as closely as possible) field conditions. Preventive measures are more important than are curative procedures in most cases of toxicoses induced by geothermal or industrial cooling waters and mine tailings.

BIBLIOGRAPHY

Buck WB, Osweiler GD, Van Gelder GA: Clinical and Diagnostic Veterinary Toxicology, 3rd ed. Dubuque, IA, Kendall/Hunt Publishing Co, 1985.

Peterson HB, Nielson RF: Toxicities and Deficiencies in Mine Tailings. Ecology and Reclamation of Devastated Land, vol I. New York, Gordon and Beach Co, 1973, pp 15–25.

Shupe JL: Diagnosis of fluorosis in cattle. *In* Fourth International Meeting of the World Association for Buiatrics. Publ. No. 4. Zurich, Switzerland, 1967, pp 15–30.

Pesticides, Rodenticides, and Herbicides

Chlorinated Hydrocarbon Insecticides

JOE D. KENDALL, DVM, MS
MERL F. RAISBECK, DVM, PhD

The chlorinated hydrocarbon insecticides (CHIs) comprise a group of compounds characterized by two properties: they are lipophilic and highly persistent in the environment. Although persistence following a single application is a desirable characteristic for an insecticide, this same property results in bioaccumulation in the environment, humans, domestic animals, and wildlife. As a result of persistence and bioaccumulation, use of CHIs is highly restricted in most countries. Nevertheless, domestic animals may still be exposed to CHIs as a result of improperly used organochlorine-treated products, chemical wastes, and stockpiled insecticides. For the purposes of diagnosis and treatment, organochlorine insecticide exposure can be divided into two categories: acute toxicity and residues.

CLINICAL SIGNS AND DIAGNOSIS OF ACUTE TOXICITY

As a group, the cellular mechanism of action of CHIs is not completely understood; however, they are all central nervous system stimulants. Domestic mammals exposed to an acutely toxic dose of a CHI initially exhibit apprehensive behavior and hypersensitivity. These signs are followed by muscle fasiculations of the face, head, and neck, which progress caudally. Other common signs of acute toxicity include continuous chewing movements, abnormal posturing, spastic gait, and vomiting. Terminally there may be tonic-clonic seizures, possibly interspersed with intermittent depression, leading to coma and death. There is no specific antidote for CHI intoxication. Barbiturates and muscle relaxants are indicated to control seizures. Intestinal absorbants such as activated charcoal should be administered in cases of oral exposure. Dermal exposure requires thorough washing with soap and water.

Postmortem lesions of acute CHI toxicity are nonspecific. There may be evidence of trauma, hyperthermia, or both due to convulsions. There may also be histologic evidence of renal and hepatic degeneration. Confirmation of CHI toxicity requires that samples of brain, liver, blood, and suspected source of exposure be submitted to an appropriate laboratory in *clean glass or metal containers*. Differential diagnoses that should be considered in animals exhibiting convulsions without parasympathomimetic signs include nervous coccidiosis, lead toxicosis, sodium ion toxicosis, rabies, polioencephalomalacia, infectious encephalomyelitis, and tremorgenic mycotoxins.

CHLORINATED HYDROCARBON RESIDUES

The primary problem associated with CHIs today results from their bioaccumulation effect and the regulatory guidelines concerning chemical residues in food products. The condemnation of meat and dairy products due to CHI contamination is of far greater economic significance than acute toxicity. An in-depth discussion of the various decontamination strategies is beyond the scope of this article, but the following brief overview should be useful to the practitioner faced with a contaminated herd. The reader is referred to the bibliography at the end of this article for a detailed discussion of decontamination strategies.

The high lipid solubility of the CHI results in rapid absorption and transfer to adipose tissue. Once in adipose tissue, the CHIs are not exposed to further metabolism and elimination processes. The only exception to this rule is elimination via milk fat. The rate of elimination of CHI is determined by a variety of factors, including compound involved, dose, duration and route of exposure, species of animal, and stage of lactation. Residues from larger doses and shorter exposure tend to be smaller in proportion to total dose and are eliminated more quickly than those resulting from longer exposure and smaller doses.

The elimination of CHI is multiphasic. After exposure ceases there is a rapid initial decline in body burden followed by an extended period of slower elimination. As a *very rough* rule of thumb, the half-life of persistent CHIs such as heptachlor and chlordane in animals is approximately 180 days for non-lactating cattle and 60 days for lactating animals.

Decontamination strategies previously used have involved attempts to promote excretion by modifying metabolism of the CHI, modifying enterohepatic recirculation of the contaminant, and modifying the nutritional and hormonal status of the animal.

Attempts to increase the metabolism of CHIs have utilized compounds known to increase hepatic enzymatic activity such as phenobarbital, pentobarbital, diphenylhydantoin, butylated hydroxyanisole, and trans-stilbene oxide. While phenobarbital appears to increase elimination of dieldrin and dichlorodiphenyl trichloroethane (DDT) in cattle, it has not been successful with other chlorinated hydrocarbons. In fact, no metabolic inducer has proven successful with all chlorinated hydrocarbons or in all species of animals. This is probably because CHI residue problems are usually not recognized until after the majority of the residues are stored in fat and therefore no longer exposed to hepatic metabolism.

Attempts to decrease enterohepatic recirculation of chlorinated hydrocarbons utilizing intestinal absorbants such as activated charcoal, cholestyramine, or mineral oil have likewise met with mixed success. Mineral oil increased the fecal excretion of dichlorodiphenyl ethylene (DDE) in dairy cattle, mirex in dairy goats, and hexochlorobenzene in sheep by two- to threefold. However, mineral oil failed to decrease heptachlor body burdens in dairy cattle and swine significantly or to increase fecal excretion of heptachlor in sheep. While activated charcoal is useful in cases of acute exposure, it does not significantly decrease body burdens of the CHI once it is in the adipose tissue.

Nutritional strategies of decontamination have met with somewhat greater success. Forced weight loss followed by refattening has been used successfully with dieldrin-contaminated turkeys and steers, DDT-contaminated sheep, and heptachlor-contaminated dairy cattle. This strategy requires careful monitoring of the herd to avoid infectious or nutritional diseases as a result of stress. The value of the animals involved must be considered before this expensive and time-consumingstrategy is employed. Administration of thyroprotein in DDT-, polybrominated biphenyls (PBBs), and heptachlor-contaminated dairy cattle initially increased elimination of these compounds; however, the rate of elimination decreased rapidly. At the end of lactation there was no difference between treated and control animals.

Administration of ovine growth hormone to heptachlor-contaminated lactating sheep had no significant effect on its elimination in the milk or excreta when compared with the control animals. Sheep, however, seem to differ from other species in that significantly more heptachlor is excreted in urine as metabolites. There is no published study detailing use of either bovine or porcine growth hormone in these species after contamination with CHIs. One possible use of CHI-contaminated milk is defatting the milk and feeding it to calves. Natural elimination and dilution caused by growth will further decrease the concentration of CHIs by maturity.

In short there is no simple protocol for the decontamination of livestock. Each case must be evaluated on a situational basis as to the compound(s) involved, the residue level present, and the type and value of livestock affected.

BIBLIOGRAPHY

Cook R, Wilson K: Removal of pesticide residues from dairy cattle. J Dairy Sci 54:712–718, 1971.
Holcombe D, Smith G, Khan M, et al: Elimination of [14C] heptachlor from body stores of lactating ewes treated with ovine growth hormone. J Anim Sci 66:2200–2208, 1988.
Osweiler G, Carson T, Buck W, Van Gelder G: Clinical and Diagnostic Veterinary Toxicology, 3rd ed. Dubuque, Kendall/Hunt, 1985.
Raisbeck M, Kendall J, Rottinghaus G: Organochlorine insecticide problems in livestock. Vet Clin North Am 5(2):391–410, 1989.
Raisbeck M, Rottinghaus G, Satalowich F, et al: Heptachlor contamination of dairy, beef, and swine: the experience in Missouri. Proc Am Assoc Vet Lab Diag 29:161–182, 1986.
Rozman K, Rozman T, Greim H, et al: Use of aliphatic hydrocarbons in feed to decrease body burdens of lipophilic toxicants in livestock. J Agric Food Chem 30:98–100, 1982.

Organophosphorus and Carbamate Insecticides

T. L. CARSON, DVM, PhD, MS

The production of both livestock and crops on the same premises provides a unique opportunity for exposure of livestock to agricultural chemicals. Among the chemicals presenting the greatest potential hazard of livestock poisoning are the organophosphorus (OP) and carbamate insecticides.

Poisoning often occurs when these insecticides are accidentally incorporated into livestock feed. Discarded or unlabeled portions of granular insecticides can be mistaken for dry feed ingredients and mixed into animal feeds. When farm equipment used for feed handling is also used for insecticide transportation, contamination of this equipment may result in insecticides being inadvertently mixed into animal feeds. In addition, animals may have accidental access to insecticides where they are stored, discarded, or spilled on the farm premises. Improperly operating back rubbers and oilers may provide additional sources of these insecticides for livestock.

Miscalculation of insecticide concentration in spraying, dipping, and pour-on procedures may also result in toxicosis. Retreating animals with OP or carbamate preparations within a few days may cause poisoning.

Differences in susceptibility to insecticides (because of breed, sex, or both) used for external parasite control have resulted in restricted use of famphur (Warbex*) on Brahman or Brahman-cross cattle and of chlorpyrifos (Dursban†) on exotic breed beef cattle and mature bulls. Very young or stressed livestock generally should not be treated with insecticides.

The OP and carbamate insecticides are discussed together because of their similar mechanism of action and clinical effects. Several of these insecticides are highly toxic to livestock, with the capability of producing lethal effects at oral doses of less than 10 mg/kg (see Table 1). Therefore in many instances ingestion of only a few grams of commercial material may result in toxicosis. For example, only 4 g of commercial Thimet (phorate; 15 per cent active ingredient) would provide a toxic dose to a 400-kg bovine.

MECHANISM OF ACTION

Cholinergic nerves utilize acetylcholine as a neurotransmitter. Under normal conditions, acetylcholine released at the synapses of parasympathetic nerves and myoneural junctions

---

*Available from American Cyanamid Co., Princeton, NJ 08540.
†Available from Ft. Dodge Laboratories, Fort Dodge, IA 50501.

Table 1. TOXICITY OF GRANULAR INSECTICIDES COMMONLY USED FOR CORN ROOTWORM CONTROL

Trade Name	Common Name	Rat Oral LD$_{50}$ (mg/kg)	Toxic Dose In Cattle (mg/kg)
Counter	Terbufos	4	3.0
Diazinon	Diazinon	250	25.0
Dyfonate	Fonofos	8	1.3
Furadan	Carbofuran	8	4.5
Lorsban	Chlorpyrifos	97	—
Mocap	Ethoprop	61	5.0
Thimet	Phorate	1	1.5

is quickly hydrolyzed by cholinesterase. The OP and carbamate insecticides bind with cholinesterase and inhibit its action. With the hydrolyzing enzyme inhibited, the continued presence of acetylcholine maintains a state of nerve stimulation and accounts for the clinical signs observed with poisoning from these insecticides. In general, inhibition of these enzymes by the OP insecticides tends to be irreversible, while inhibition of the enzymes by the carbamates tends to be reversible.

CLINICAL SIGNS

The key clinical signs that aid in the recognition of acute OP and carbamate toxicosis are characterized by overstimulation of the parasympathetic nervous system and skeletal muscles. The onset of clinical signs in cases of acute poisoning may be as short as a few minutes to several hours after exposure. Earliest clinical signs of acute poisoning frequently include muscle tremors and stiffness, mild progressing to profuse salivation, frequent defecation and urination, emesis (common in swine), and general uneasiness. As the syndrome progresses, profuse salivation, gastrointestinal hypermotility resulting in severe colic and abdominal cramps, diarrhea, excessive lacrimation, sweating, miosis, dyspnea, cyanosis, urinary incontinence, and muscle tremors of the face, eyelids, and general body musculature can be observed. Hyperactivity of the skeletal muscles is generally followed by muscular paralysis, as the muscles are unable to respond to continued stimulation.

Cattle, sheep, and swine may exhibit increased central nervous system stimulation but rarely, if ever, exhibit convulsive seizures. More commonly, central nervous system depression occurs.

Death usually results from hypoxia due to excessive respiratory tract secretions, bronchoconstriction, and erratic slow heartbeat. In severe poisoning, death can occur from a few minutes to several hours after the first clinical signs are observed.

POST-MORTEM LESIONS

Post-mortem lesions associated with acute OP or carbamate toxicosis are usually nonspecific. Excessive fluids in the mouth and respiratory tract as well as pulmonary edema may be observed.

DIAGNOSIS

A history of exposure to OP or carbamate insecticides associated with clinical signs of parasympathetic stimulation warrants a tentative diagnosis of poisoning.

Submission of appropriate specimens to a diagnostic laboratory is important in confirming a diagnosis. After collection and during shipping, whole-blood and brain samples should be well chilled for obtaining best laboratory results.

Chemical analysis of the stomach or rumen content, as well as the feed or other suspect material, for the presence of OP or carbamate insecticides can be valuable. However, tissue residues of these compounds are usually negligible and are of little diagnostic value.

In addition, measuring cholinesterase enzyme activity in whole-blood or brain tissue can help support a diagnosis of poisoning. A reduction of cholinesterase activity to less than 25 per cent of normal is indicative of excessive exposure to these insecticides.

The syndrome of acute OP and carbamate insecticide poisoning must be differentiated from acute urea or other nonprotein nitrogen toxicosis and acute grain overload. In addition, hypomagnesemia (grass tetany), nitrate toxicosis, cyanide poisoning, and acute bloat may be clinically similar to insecticide poisoning.

TREATMENT

The treatment of animals poisoned by OP and carbamate insecticides should be considered on an emergency basis because of the rapid progression of the clinical syndrome.

Initial treatment is with atropine sulfate at approximately 0.5 mg/kg body weight. This initial dose should be divided, with about one fourth of the dose administered intravenously and the balance administered subcutaneously or intramuscularly. Atropine sulfate does not counteract the insecticide-enzyme bond, but rather blocks the effects of accumulated acetylcholine at the nerve endings. Although a dramatic cessation of parasympathetic signs is generally observed within a few minutes after administration of atropine, it will not affect the skeletal muscle tremors. Repeated doses of atropine at approximately one half the initial dose may be required, but should be used only to counteract parasympathetic signs. Caution should be observed with continued atropine therapy, as rumen atony may be a complicating side effect in cattle and sheep.

Oral activated charcoal is very beneficial for treatment of any ingested insecticide. The early use of activated charcoal to adsorb OP or carbamate insecticides in the gastrointestinal tract is especially important in ruminants that continue to absorb insecticide from the rumen contents. The effective dose of activated charcoal ranges from 0.5 kg for sheep to 0.9 kg for adult cattle. A water-charcoal slurry mixed with sodium or magnesium sulfate (1 g/kg) or commercially prepared charcoal-kaolin (Toxiban*), may be pumped intraruminally with a stomach tube after initial respiratory distress has been alleviated with atropine.

Dermally exposed animals should be washed with soap and water to prevent continued absorption.

The oximes, such as TMB-4, 2-PAM, and pralidoxime chloride, are drugs that act specifically on the organophosphorus-enzyme complex, freeing the enzyme. The use of the oximes in large animals, though efficacious, may be economically unfeasible. Pralidoxime chloride is recommended at a dose of 20 mg/kg in small animals and at a dose of 10 mg/kg in large animals. The oximes are of no benefit or harm in treating carbamate toxicoses.

Morphine, succinylcholine, and phenothiazine tranquilizers should be avoided in treating OP poisoning.

BIBLIOGRAPHY

Haas PJ, Buck WB, Hixon JE, et al: Effect of chlorpyrifos on Holstein steers and testosterone-treated Holstein bulls. Am J Vet Res 44:879–881, 1983.

---

*Available from Vet-A-Mix, Shenandoah, IA 51601.

Osweiler GD, Carson TL, Buck WB, and Van Gelder GA: Clinical and Diagnostic Veterinary Toxicology, 3rd ed. Dubuque, Kendall/Hunt, 1985.

Palmer JS: Toxicity of famphur to young Brahman heifers and bulls. J Amer Vet Med Assoc 159:1263–1265, 1971.

Radeleff RD: Veterinary Toxicology, 2nd ed. Philadelphia, Lea & Febiger, 1970.

Rodenticides

MICHAEL J. MURPHY, DVM, PhD, Diplomate, ABVT

Rodenticides are products that are marketed to kill rodents. These products may be labeled to control rats, mice, rabbits, gophers, voles, or, less commonly, other similar pests encountered on farmsteads or around grain storage areas. Several rodenticides are currently marketed in the United States. Although sales of others have been discontinued, they may still be encountered on farmsteads. Anticoagulant, strychnine, and cholecalciferol-containing rodenticides make up more than 90 per cent of the products currently sold in the United States, so they are most likely to be encountered in toxicosis situations. Products such as zinc phosphide, thallium sulfate, and red squill may still be sold in some areas. On the other hand, ANTU (α-Naphthyl thiourea), calcium cyanide, 1080 (fluoroacetate), phosphorus, and vacor either are no longer sold or are severely restricted in sales in most parts of the United States. Occasionally insecticides or other pesticides are used on an individual farm for rodent control purposes.

In poultry, swine, and dairy confinement operations, animals are most likely to be exposed to rodenticides either through a feed mixing error or due to their use within the housing unit. In some instances when penned or stanchioned animals are moved, they gain access to previously inaccessible rodenticides. In nonconfinement operations, animals commonly enter an enclosure where the products are being used or stored. Much less commonly, feed mixing errors are a possible cause for exposure.

When available, the toxicity of the products to food animals is listed under the appropriate following section. Unfortunately in many instances the toxicity of these products to food animals is not reported. In these cases the toxicity rating (Table 1) may be used as a general guideline. In general, ingestion of significant amounts of products having a toxicity rating of I would be of concern, while those with ratings of III or IV may be less likely to induce toxicosis in most food animals unless very large quantities are ingested.

Where specific therapeutic agents are indicated, they are discussed under the appropriate section. However, most of the toxins listed herein have no specific therapeutic agents, so general and symptomatic therapy is indicated. General therapy includes reducing absorption of the toxin and hastening its passage through the gastrointestinal tract. Reduced absorption is commonly accomplished with activated charcoal. For ruminants, 2 to 9 g/kg may be administered orally in water at a concentration of 1 g charcoal/3 to 5 ml water. Elimination from the gastrointestinal tract is commonly accomplished with mineral oil. For this purpose 1 to 4 L is commonly used in cattle, 100 to 500 ml in sheep and goats, and 50 to 100 ml in swine.

ANTICOAGULANT RODENTICIDES

The anticoagulant rodenticides constitute the largest volume of annual rodenticide sales in the United States. Common chemical names of these compounds include brodifacoum, bromadiolone, chlorophacinone, coumafuryl, coumatetralyl, difenacoum, diphacinone, flocoumafen (outside the United States), pival, valone, and warfarin. Trade names are listed in Table 1.

The toxicity of this group ranges from approximately 50 to 0.3 mg/kg acute oral LD_{50} in the rat. Unfortunately LD_{50} and/or minimum lethal dose data are largely unavailable for food animal species. Available data are summarized in Table 2. Ruminants ingesting sweetclover may be more susceptible to anticoagulant rodenticide poisoning than these numbers indicate.

All anticoagulant rodenticides act by inhibiting the "recycling" of vitamin K_1 by the vitamin K_1 epoxide reductase activity in the liver. Depletion of active vitamin K_1 diminishes synthesis of Factors II, VII, IX, and X. Coagulopathies are observed clinically following the normal consumption of these factors in circulation. Depletion of active vitamin K_1 and the existing clotting factors generally occurs 3 to 5 days after exposure to a toxic dose of these products. Thus clinical signs are often not observed for 2 to 3 days following exposure to the anticoagulant rodenticides.

Classical signs of coagulopathy such as melena, epistaxis, hematemesis, and hematoma formation are occasionally observed in cases of toxicoses from these compounds. Less classical signs of dyspnea, lameness, lethargy, excessive periparturient hemorrhage, and death are more commonly observed due to hemorrhage into the thoracic cavity, lungs, joints, or abdomen. Table 3 lists some clinical signs of rodenticide toxicosis and the toxins likely to produce them.

Observance of these clinical signs with a history of availability is commonly used to reach a field diagnosis of anticoagulant rodenticide toxicosis when on-farm mistakes occur. In those cases in which a more conclusive diagnosis is required, laboratory testing is necessary. Serum or liver samples can be analyzed by some diagnostic laboratories to demonstrate the presence of the anticoagulant rodenticides. Additionally, some laboratories can test hay or liver for the presence of dicoumerol to rule out moldy sweetclover poisoning if required.

Vitamin K_1 is the specific therapy of choice for animals suffering from anticoagulant rodenticide toxicosis. Although Aquamephyton* may be administered at a dose of 1 to 2 mg/kg subcutaneously, such therapy is commonly cost-prohibitive for the average food animal. Since vitamin K_3 has been shown to be ineffective in treating cases of moldy sweetclover poisoning in cattle, its efficacy in these cases is questionable. Diets high in vitamin K_1, such as those containing alfalfa, may be a practical alternative to Aquamephyton therapy when cost is a factor.

CHOLECALCIFEROL

Rodenticides containing cholecalciferol include Rampage, Quintox, and Ortho Mouse-B-Gon. All contain 0.075 per cent cholecalciferol. Although toxic doses of these rodenticides have not been reported for food animals, toxic doses of cholecalciferol in feed have been. Adverse production effects and death have been reported in swine consuming 22,000 to 44,000 and 473,000 IU cholecalciferol/kg body weight, respectively. Reduced milk production has been reported in dairy cattle consuming 80,000 IU cholecalciferol/kg/day. One IU equals 0.025 µg cholecalciferol. Thus, 0.26 and 5.5 oz of

---
*Available from Merck & Co., Inc., Rahway, NJ 07065.

Table 1. TRADE NAMES AND TOXICITY CLASSES OF SOME RODENTICIDES

Trade Name*	Common Name	Toxicity Class	Trade Name*	Common Name	Toxicity Class
1080	Fluoroacetamide	I	Pindone	Pival	III
Actosin C	Chlorophacinone	III or II	Pivacin	Pival	III
A-Dust	Calcium cyanide	I	Pival Parakakes	Pival	III
Al-Phos	Aluminum phosphide	I	Pivalyn	Pival	III
Assault	Bromethalin	III	PMP Tracking Powder	Valone	II
A-dust	Calcium cyanide	I	PP 581	Brodifacoum	III
Baran	Fluoroacetamide	I	Promar	Diphacinone	III
Bay 25634	Coumatetralyl	III	P.C.Q. Rodent Cake	Diphacinone	III
Bay ENE 11183B	Coumatetralyl	III	P.C.Q.	Diphacinone	III
Blue-ox†	Zinc phosphide	I, II, or III	Pyriminil†	Vacor	III
Boot Hill	Bromadiolone	III	Quickphos	Aluminum phosphide	I
Bromone	Bromadiolone	III	Quintox	Cholecalciferol	III
Caid	Chlorophacinone	III or II	Ramik	Diphacinone	III
Calcium Cyanide A-Dust	Calcium cyanide	I	Rampage	Cholecalciferol	III
			Ramucide	Chlorophacinone	III or II
Canadien 2000	Bromadiolone	III	Ratak	Difenacoum	III
Celphine	Aluminum phosphide	I	Ratak Plus	Brodifacoum	III
Celphos	Aluminum phosphide	I	Ratimus	Bromadiolone	III
Contrac	Bromadiolone	III	Ratol	Zinc phosphide	I, II, or III
Cov-R-Tox	Warfarin	III	Ratomet	Chlorophacinone	III or II
Co-Dax	Warfarin	III	Raviac	Chlorophacinone	III or II
Co-Rax	Warfarin	III	RAX	Warfarin	III
Cyanogas	Calcium cyanide	I	Redentin	Chlorophacinone	III or II
Dethdiet	Red squill (scilliroside)	III	RH-787†	Vacor	III
Diphacin	Diphacinone	III	Ridall-Zinc	Zinc phosphide	I, II, or III
Ditrac	Diphacinone	III	Rodent Cake	Diphacinone	III
d-Con	Warfarin	III	Rodent pellets	Zinc phosphide	I, II, or III
d-Con Mouse Pruf II	Brodifacoum	III	Rodex	Warfarin	III
DLP-87†	Vacor	III	Rodex	Fluoroacetamide	I
Drat	Chlorophacinone	III or II	Rodex-Blox	Warfarin	III
Enforcer Mouse Kill	Brodifacoum	III	Rodine	Red squill (scilliroside)	III
Fluorakil 100	Fluoroacetamide	I	Rozol	Chlorophacinone	III or II
Fumitoxin	Aluminum phosphide	I	Silmurin	Red squill (scilliroside)	III
Gastoxin	Aluminum phosphide	I	SuperCaid	Bromadiolone	III
Gopha-rid	Zinc phosphide	I, II, or III	Sup'operats	Bromadiolone	III
Ground Force	Chlorophacinone	III or II	Talon	Brodifacoum	III
Havoc	Brodifacoum	III	Temus	Bromadiolone	III
Just-One-Bite	Bromadiolone	III	Topitox	Chlorophacinone	III or II
Kill-Ko Rat	Fumarin	III	Tox-Hid	Warfarin	III
Kill-Ko-Rat-Killer	Diphacinone	III	Tri-ban	Pival	III
Klerat	Brodifacoum	III	Trounce	Bromethalin	III
Kypfarin	Warfarin	III	Vengeance	Bromethalin	III
Liphadione	Chlorophacinone	III or II	Volid	Brodifacoum	III
Liqua-Tox	Warfarin	III	Warfarin	Warfarin	III
LM 91	Chlorophacinone	III or II	Warfarin Dust	Warfarin	III
Maki	Bromadiolone	III	Warfarin Plus	Warfarin	III
Microzul	Chlorophacinone	III or II	Warfarin Q	Warfarin	III
Mouse Blues	Fumarin	III	WBA 8107	Difenacoum	III
Navron	Fluoroacetamide	I	WBA 8119	Brodifacoum	III
Neosorexa PP 580	Difenacoum	III	Weather-Blok	Brodifacoum	III
Ortho Mouse-B-Gon	Cholecalciferol	III	Yanock	Fluoroacetamide	I
Phostoxin	Aluminum phosphide	I	Zinc-tox	Zinc phosphide	I, II, or III
Phosvin	Zinc phosphide	I, II, or III	ZP-Rodent Bait	Zinc phosphide	I, II, or III

*As listed in Farm Chemicals Handbook, Willoughby, OH, Meister Publishing Co, 1988.
†Discontinued.
Note: Specific trade names are listed in the interest of assisting the practitioner in providing appropriate therapy to animals inadvertently exposed to rodenticides. The presence or absence of a product listing in no way implies endorsement or lack of support for that product.

Table 2. TOXICITY OF SOME COMMON RODENTICIDES TO FOOD ANIMALS

Product	Bait Concentration (ppm)	Oral Toxicity					
		Compound (mg/kg)			Finished Bait (oz/kg)		
		Porcine	Bovine	Poultry	Porcine	Bovine	Poultry
Warfarin	250	3*	200†	~0.5	0.42	28.2	0.0071
Brodifacoum	50	0.5–2.0*		10–100	0.7		7.0
Bromadiolone	50	1‡			0.7		
Strychnine	5000	0.5–1.0	0.5	5.0	0.0035	0.0035	0.35

*Single exposure.
†Daily exposure for 12 days.
‡No effect level.

Table 3. SOME CLINICAL SIGNS OR LESIONS ASSOCIATED WITH RODENTICIDE TOXICOSIS

Sign	Toxin	Sign	Toxin
Abdominal pain	Phosphorus	Hemorrhages	Anticoagulant rodenticides
Alopecia	Thallium	Hemorrhagic diarrhea	Anticoagulant rodenticides
Anemia	Anticoagulant rodenticides		Phosphorus
Anorexia	Red squill		Thallium
Apprehension	Strychnine	Hemorrhagic enteritis	Thallium
Cardiac arrhythmias	Fluoroacetate	Hepatic failure	Phosphorus
	Red squill	Hydrothorax	ANTU
Colic	Phosphorus	Hyperesthesia	Strychnine
	Vacor	Hyperreflexia	Strychnine
	Zinc phosphide	Icterus	Phosphorus
Collapse	Fluoroacetate	Lameness	Anticoagulant rodenticides
Coma	Phosphorus	Lethargy	Anticoagulant rodenticides
Conjunctivitis	Thallium		Cholecalciferol
Cyanosis	ANTU	Melena	Anticoagulant rodenticides
Death	Anticoagulant rodenticides	Moist rales	ANTU
	ANTU	Muscle necrosis	Thallium
	Calcium cyanide	Muscle tremors	Strychnine
	Cholecalciferol		Calcium cyanide
	Fluoroacetate	Nausea	Vacor
	Phosphorus	Nervousness	Strychnine
	Red squill	Periparturient hemorrhage	Anticoagulant rodenticides
	Strychnine	Pulmonary edema	ANTU
Defecation	Calcium cyanide	Rapid onset of rigor	Strychnine
Depression	Phosphorus	Rapid weak pulse	Fluoroacetate
	Zinc phosphide	Renal failure	Phosphorus
Dermatitis	Thallium	Salivation	Calcium cyanide
Diarrhea	Cholecalciferol	Seizures	Calcium cyanide
	Red squill		Fluoroacetate
Disorientation	Vacor		Strychnine
Dyspnea	Anticoagulant rodenticides		Zinc phosphide
	ANTU	Subcutaneous hematomas	Anticoagulant rodenticides
	Calcium cyanide	Tetanic seizures	Strychnine
	Cholecalciferol	Tremors; seizures	Thallium
	Thallium	Urination	Calcium cyanide
	Zinc phosphide	Ventricular fibrillation	Fluoroacetate
Epistaxis	Anticoagulant rodenticides	Vomiting	ANTU
Excitement	Calcium cyanide		Cholecalciferol
Fever	Thallium		Fluoroacetate
Full stomach	Strychnine		Phosphorus
Gastroenteritis	Thallium		Red squill
Gastrointestinal necrosis	Thallium		Thallium
Gingivitis	Thallium		Vacor
Hematemesis	Anticoagulant rodenticides		Zinc phosphide
Hematoma formation	Anticoagulant rodenticides	Weakness	ANTU

ANTU = α-naphthyl thiourea.

finished bait per kilogram body weight in swine would be expected to cause production loss and death, respectively. Approximately 0.5 oz of finished bait per kilogram body weight would be required for milk production losses in dairy cattle.

Cholecalciferol toxicosis is characterized by hypercalcemia. Synthesis of 25-hydroxycholecalciferol occurs in the liver and 1, 25-dihydroxycholecalciferol in the kidney. Significant elevations of either metabolite in circulation may induce hypercalcemia. Signs of lethargy, diarrhea, vomiting, respiratory distress, and death have been reported in cases of porcine cholecalciferol toxicoses following feed mixing errors.

Ingestion of toxic amounts of cholecalciferol containing rodenticides is likely only in small food animals. In these instances the availability of the rodenticide, the clinical signs discussed, and the appropriate histologic findings support a diagnosis. Acute myocardial necrosis with dystrophic calcification, acute gastrointestinal necrosis and hemorrhage, severe nephrosis, and mineralization of the vasculature and pulmonary parenchyma have been observed histologically in fatal porcine toxicosis cases. Analysis of feed and liver for cholecalciferol and its metabolites would likely provide a conclusive diagnosis if one is required.

No specific therapeutic agent exists for cholecalciferol toxicosis, so the general and symptomatic treatment mentioned earlier is indicated. In companion animals, glucocorticoids and furosemide are used to enhance renal calcium elimination. Doses of 2 to 6 mg prednisone/kg s.i.d. and 2.5 to 4.5 mg furosemide/kg PO t.i.d. to q.i.d. are recommended to be continued for approximately 2 weeks in cholecalciferol-poisoned dogs.

STRYCHNINE

Strychnine is an indole alkaloid that acts by inhibiting the normal inhibitory effect of glycine on postsynaptic sites in the spinal cord and medulla. It is generally available in baits containing 0.5 per cent strychnine. The toxicity of these baits to some food animals is summarized in Table 2. Animals experiencing strychnine toxicosis demonstrate nervousness, apprehension, and muscle stiffness, which progresses to tetanic seizures. Death occurs due to anoxia or exhaustion during a seizure. Stomach contents or urine may be readily analyzed to reach a diagnosis of strychnine toxicosis. Lesions are not commonly observed. No specific therapeutic agent exists for strychnine toxicosis. Therapy is generally aimed at controlling the seizures until the animal is able to metabolize the toxin. Such metabolism commonly requires 12 to 48 hours. Barbiturates are commonly used to control seizures. General therapy with activated charcoal is recommended after the animal is controlled to attempt to absorb any remaining strychnine in the gastrointestinal tract.

ZINC PHOSPHIDE

Zinc phosphide is a rodenticide, whereas aluminum phosphide is registered as an insect fumigant. Zinc phosphide is marketed under the names Gopharid, Phosvin, Ratol, Ridall-Zinc, Rodent Pellets, Zinc-tox, and ZP-Rodent Bait. It is available as a bait, pellets, or a tracking powder. The tracking powder is available in an 80 per cent formulation, whereas the finished bait contains 1.88 per cent active ingredient. This variety of formulation explains the toxicity rating of I, II, or III. The lethal dose for ruminants and swine is 20 to 40 mg zinc phosphide/kg body weight. Upon exposure to an acid environment, zinc phosphide releases phosphine, which causes direct irritation of the intestinal tract. Animals become depressed, dyspneic, colicky, and may vomit. Occasionally convulsive seizures are observed. Treatment is symptomatic. Alkalinizing agents may be given in an attempt to neutralize the acidity of the stomach. Sodium bicarbonate (2 mEq/kg) may be given intravenously to control systemic acidosis. Treatment is not often rewarding. Conclusive diagnosis is difficult owing to the liberation of phosphine, but frozen stomach contents are the specimen of choice for analysis. The liver may be analyzed for zinc content.

THALLIUM SULFATE

Toxic doses of thallium sulfate in cattle and sheep are 12 to 16 and 9 to 20 mg/kg, respectively. Thallium interacts with sulfhydryl groups, causing gastrointestinal and muscular necrosis. Dyspnea, fever, vomiting, and/or hemorrhagic enteritis may be seen 2 to 3 days postexposure. Alopecia may be seen 7 to 10 days postexposure. The presence of significant concentrations of thallium in liver, kidney, or urine is diagnostic.

PHOSPHORUS

White or yellow phosphorus may cause vomiting, colic, and hemorrhagic diarrhea, progressing to icterus, coma, and death in 2 to 3 days. Toxic doses of 0.5 to 2 g and 0.005 to 0.3 g have been reported for cattle and swine, respectively. Phosphorus may occasionally be detected in the gastrointestinal tract for diagnostic purposes.

ANTU (α-NAPHTHYL THIOUREA)

ANTU is rarely encountered. It acts by significantly increasing the permeability of pulmonary capillaries, resulting in a fatal pulmonary edema. Lethal doses of 25 to 50 mg/kg are reported for pigs. Rarely the compound is found in the stomach. More commonly confirmation is made by histopathology and determining the presence of ANTU in the bait.

1080 (FLUOROACETATE)

1080 is a restricted-use pesticide. It acts via conversion to fluorocitrate, inhibiting aconitase in the Krebs cycle. Acute oral LD_{50} values of 0.39, 0.22, 0.25 to 0.5, and 0.4 to 1.0 mg/kg have been reported for cattle, calves, sheep, and swine, respectively. Cardiac arrhythmias and ventricular fibrillation with collapse and death are observed in herbivores. In addition to these signs, swine may show vomiting and seizures. Analysis of the bait, liver, and/or stomach contents is useful for a diagnosis.

CALCIUM CYANIDE

Calcium cyanide also is a restricted-use pesticide. Cyanide reacts with cytochrome oxidase, halting cellular respiration and producing a cytotoxic anoxia. Animals poisoned with cyanide are generally found dead. If clinical signs are observed, they may include excitement, muscle tremors, dyspnea, salivation, defecation, urination, convulsions, and death. Treatment of cyanide-poisoned animals is rarely possible. Treatment with 10 to 20 mg sodium nitrite/kg body weight followed by 500 mg sodium thiosulfate/kg body weight as needed is recommended for treatment of ruminants with cyanide poisoning. The detection of cyanide from frozen rumen or stomach contents is strongly supportive of cyanide poisoning.

VACOR

Vacor antagonizes nicotine adenine dinucleotide, causing disruption of normal oxidation reduction reactions in cells. LD_{50} doses of 300 mg/kg are reported for calves and pigs. Vomiting, colic, and disorientation may be observed.

RED SQUILL (SCILLIROSIDE)

Red squill is the powdered bulb of *Urginea maritima (U. scilla)*, a plant from Mediterranean countries. The most toxic of several glycosides in red squill is scilliroside. Poisoning from red squill is now quite rare. Animals receiving a toxic dose of cardiac glycosides are commonly found dead, so clinical signs may not be observed. If observed, signs may include anorexia, vomiting, diarrhea, terminal arrhythmias, and death. Cardioglycosides are believed to interfere with the NA^+/K^+-ATPase system, resulting in a decrease in intracellular potassium. Effectively, a marked high-grade block occurs progressively, interfering with electrical conductivity until asystole ensues. Treatment is rarely possible. Specific therapeutic agents are not available, so general and symptomatic treatment is indicated. Calcium-containing solutions are contraindicated.

BIBLIOGRAPHY

Osweiler GD, Carson TL, Buck WB, and Van Gelder GA: Clinical and Diagnostic Veterinary Toxicology 3rd ed. Dubuque, Kendall Hunt, 1987.
Osweiler GD Hook BS: Rodenticides. *In* Howard JL (ed): Current Veterinary Therapy 2, Food Animal Practice. Philadelphia, WB Saunders, 1986.

Organic Herbicides*
LOYD D. ROWE, DVM

Farm animals may be poisoned by herbicides when they consume concentrate or sprays to which they are accidentally or imprudently allowed access; when there is contamination of feed or water; or when allowed to graze plants recently

---
*All material in this article is in the public domain, with the exception of any borrowed figures or tables.

sprayed with toxic amounts of chemical. Animals may be secondarily affected if treatment of poisonous plants with herbicide leads to increased accumulation of harmful amounts of nitrate, cyanogenic glycosides, or other toxic plant constituents, or if normally unpalatable toxic plants are rendered palatable.

Most organic herbicides are of low toxicity to livestock. There are notable exceptions, for example, the organoarsenics. When poisoning due to organic herbicides does occur, it is usually associated with human error or accident. Poisoning of livestock is unlikely if herbicides are properly applied and recommended withholding times observed. The likelihood that animals may be poisoned by a herbicide consumed while grazing treated forage depends primarily on the rate of application and the toxicity of the chemical in question. The minimum toxicity of some organic herbicides to cattle and sheep is presented in Table 1. This data and the corresponding signs and lesions of toxicosis to be described are primarily the results of toxicity trials in which cattle and sheep were given daily oral doses of the herbicides listed.[8-10] In these studies the minimum response considered to be an expression of toxicity was a 5 per cent or greater loss of body weight or other obvious signs of poisoning following daily treatment for a period that was generally 10 or fewer days in length.

ACETAMIDES

These materials are relatively toxic. All acetamide herbicides listed in Table 1 produced anorexia. Salivation and depression were observed with poisoning by N,N-diallyl-2-chloroacetamide (CDAA). Signs of diphenamid toxicosis included diarrhea, muscular spasms, lameness, and ataxia. Severe poisoning with CDAA or diphenamid resulted in prostration. The only signs of toxicity in animals given CDAA plus trichlorobenzyl chloride (TCBC) were anorexia and weight loss. Propachlor poisoning produced diarrhea, depression, and ataxia. Signs of poisoning in cattle and sheep given a single dose of propanil at 250 mg/kg body weight included depression, ataxia, and prostration; these signs were observed over a period of 2 hours. Anorexia was the only sign observed in a sheep given propanil at a daily dosage of 100 mg/kg body weight for 10 days. Cattle given propanil at 100 mg/kg body weight/day for 10 days showed no ill effects.

Postmortem findings in cattle and sheep poisoned with diphenamid included enlargement of the liver and adrenal glands, pallor of the liver, congestion of the kidneys, and undigested rumen contents. Brown-tinged urine and a subcutaneous yellow gelatinous material were seen at necropsy in a sheep poisoned with diphenamid. Gross lesions observed in animals poisoned with CDAA included gastrointestinal hemorrhage; petechial hemorrhages in the bladder mucosa; enlarged kidneys; and congestion of the kidneys, lungs, and respiratory mucosa. Similar lesions were present in animals fatally poisoned by CDAA plus TCBC. In animals poisoned with propachlor, the liver was congested and friable and there was reddening of the intestinal mucosa.

ALIPHATICS

Sodium trichloroacetate (TCA) and dalapon are of relatively low toxicity. Signs of poisoning in cattle and sheep included weight loss, anorexia, lethargy, depression, dull hair coat, diarrhea, and ataxia. Recovery was rapid and uneventful once exposure was terminated. Acute sodium monochloroacetate (SMCA) poisoning in cattle produced stiffness, ataxia, lateral recumbency, extensor paralysis of the limbs, tremors, convulsions, and death. One affected heifer showed hyperexcitability and aggressiveness before collapse and death. At necropsy of cattle poisoned with SMCA, there was severe venous congestion of the ventral neck and thorax. Multiple small subcutaneous hemorrhages that extended into the muscle layers were present in the same regions. The heart was congested, and there were multiple epicardial and endocardial hemorrhages.

BENZOICS

This group of herbicides is relatively nontoxic to cattle and sheep. Chloramben produced no other ill effect than a 5 to 6 per cent weight loss at the minimum toxic dosage (Table 1). Both cattle and sheep tolerated higher treatment levels (cattle, up to 250 mg/kg/day for 10 days; sheep, up to 500 mg/kg/day for 10 days) without ill effects. Signs of poisoning in cattle and sheep given dicamba included bloating, convulsions, and prostration. Weight loss and sudden death were the only signs of poisoning in sheep given 2,3,6-trichlorobenzoic acid (TBA) at 250 mg/kg/day for 10 days. Diarrhea and lameness were observed in a steer after two doses of 2,3,6-TBA at 500 mg/kg/day; however, improvement occurred despite continued dosing for 6 more days. Lymph nodes throughout the body were enlarged and hemorrhagic in dicamba-poisoned sheep. Subepicardial hemorrhages, congestion of the liver and kidneys, enlargement of the spleen, and redness of the intestinal mucosa were also observed. Gross lesions observed in sheep fatally poisoned with 2,3,6-TBA included congestion of the lungs, kidneys, intestinal mucosa, and respiratory mucosa; edema in the pericardium, peritoneal cavity, and tissues surrounding the upper respiratory tract; and petechial hemorrhages on the surface of the kidneys.

BIPYRIDYLIUMS

Diquat and paraquat are highly toxic to cattle and sheep; however, it is considered unlikely that these herbicides will produce serious harm with proper use. The relatively low hazard of these chemicals to grazing stock despite high toxicity under laboratory conditions may be due to factors such as photodecomposition by ultraviolet light, rapid inactivation by soil, and reduced absorption when ingested on herbage versus direct administration as a single daily dose. Once bound to clay particles in the soil, these herbicides are completely unavailable for biologic interaction with plants or animals. Soil capacity for these chemicals is vastly greater than the application rate. Signs of acute poisoning included anorexia, depression, ataxia, diarrhea, accelerated and labored breathing, weakness, recumbency, convulsions, and coma. Necropsy findings included abomasitis (which may be intense); hemorrhage in the intestinal mucosa, heart, adrenal glands, and thyroid; and congestion of the lungs, liver, and kidneys. A highly colored green fluid has been reported in the abomasum of diquat-poisoned ruminants, which is the colored stable free radical of diquat formed by bacterial action in the gut. Similarly, paraquat forms a bluish-green stable free radical. Fibrosing pneumonitis as occurs in humans following paraquat ingestion apparently has not been reported in sheep or cattle.

CARBAMATES

Anorexia was the most prominent sign of poisoning with barban and chlorpropham. Salivation also was observed in

Table 1. MINIMUM TOXICITY OF SOME ORGANIC HERBICIDES IN CATTLE (9 TO 15 MONTHS) AND SHEEP (MATURE)

Common Name	Chemical Name (IUPAC)	Minimum Toxicity C(attle) and S(heep)		Estimate of Corresponding Application Rate (lb AI/acre)†
		(mg/kg/day)	(days)*	
Acetamides				
CDAA	N,N-Diallyl-2-chloroacetamide	C 25	1	3.6
		S 25	4	3.6
CDAA and TCBC	N,N-Diallyl-2-chloroacetamide (30%) and	C 50	2	7.1
	trichlorobenzyl chloride (70%)	S 25	5	3.6
Diphenamid	N,N-Dimethyl-2,2-diphenylacetamide	C 250	3	35.7
		S 250	7	35.7
Propachlor	2-Chloro-N-isopropylacetanilide	C 25	3	3.6
		S 10	9	1.4
Propanil	3′,4′-Dichloropropionanilide	C 250	1	35.7
		S 100	10	14.3
Aliphatics				
Dalapon	Sodium 2,2-dichloropropionate	C 1000	5	142.9
		S 500	7	71.4
TCA	Sodium trichloracetate	C 375	3	53.6
		S 175	2	25.0
Benzoics				
Chloramben	3-Amino-2,4-dichlorobenzoic acid	C 175	10	25.0
		S 25	1	3.6
Dicamba	3,6-Dichloro-o-anisic acid, dimethylamine salt	C 250	2	35.7
		S 500	1	71.4
2,3,6-TBA	2,3,6-Trichlorobenzoic and related acids, dimethylamine salts	C 500	2	71.4
		S 250	10	35.7
Bipyridyliums				
Diquat dibromide	1-1′-Ethylene-2-2′-dipyridylium dibromide	C 5	8	0.7
		S 25	3	3.6
Paraquat	1,1′-Dimethyl-4,4′-bipyridium methyl sulfate	C 10	10	1.4
		S 10	10	1.4
Carbamates				
Barban	4-Chlorobut-2-ynyl-3-chlorocarbanilate	C 25	1	3.6
		S 10	2	1.4
Chlorpropham	Isopropyl-3-chlorocarbanilate	C 100	2	14.3
		S 100	10	14.3
Dinitroanilines				
Benfluralin (benefin)	N-Butyl-N-ethyl-α,α,α-trifluoro-2-6,dinito-p-toluidine	C 25	6	3.6
		S 50	2	7.1
Nitralin	4-Methylsulfonyl-2-6-dinitro-N-N-dipropylaniline	C 250	2	35.7
		S 375	2	53.6
Trifluralin	α,α,α-Trifluoro-2,6-dinitro-N,N-dipropyl-p-toluidine	C 175	2	25.0
		S 175	2	25.0
Nitriles				
Chlorthiamid	2,6-Dichlorothiobenzamide	C 10	2	1.4
		S 25	10	3.6
Dichlobenil	2,6-Dichlorobenzonitrile	C 50	1	7.1
		S 25	4	3.6
Organoarsenics				
Dimethylarsinic acid (cacodylic acid)	Dimethylarsinic acid	C 25	8	3.6
		S 25	10	3.6
DSMA	Disodium methylarsonate	C 25	2	3.6
		S 25	5	3.6
MSMA	Sodium hydrogen methylarsinate	C 10	2	1.4
		S 50	3	7.1
Phenols				
Nitrofen	2,4-Dichlorophenyl-4-nitrophenyl ether	C 100	3	14.3
		S 100	3	14.3

Table 1. MINIMUM TOXICITY OF SOME ORGANIC HERBICIDES IN CATTLE (9 TO 15 MONTHS) AND SHEEP (MATURE) *(Continued)*

Common Name	Chemical Name (IUPAC)	Minimum Toxicity C(attle) and S(heep)		Estimate of Corresponding Application Rate (lb AI/acre)†
		(mg/kg/day)	(days)*	
Phenoxys				
2,4-D	(2,4-Dichlorophenoxyl)acetic acid, dimethyl amine salt	C 100 (6–8 wk old)	1	14.3
		C 100	10	14.3
		S 175	2	25.0
	(2,4-Dichlorophenoxy)acetic acid, ethanol amine and isopropanolamine salts	C 250	15	35.7
		S 100	8	14.3
	(2,4-Dichlorophenoxy)acetic acid, propylene glycol butyl ether ester	C 250	3	35.7
		S 250	2	35.7
	(2,4-Dichlorophenoxy)acetic acid, 2-ethyl hexyl ester	C 250	6	35.7
		S 50	10	7.1
2,4-DB	4-(2,4-Dichlorophenoxy)butyric acid, dimethylamine salt	C 100	2	14.3
		S 50	5	7.1
MCPA	Sodium (4-chloro-p-2-methylphenoxy)acetate	C 175	3	25.0
		S 250	5	14.3
	(4-Chloro-2-methylphenoxy)acetic acid, dimethylamine salt	C 175	10	25.0
		S 100	10	14.3
	(4-Chloro-2-methylphenoxy)acetic acid, ethanolamine and isopropanolamine salts	C 500	8	71.4
		S 250	10	35.7
MCPB	Sodium 4-(4-chloro-2-tolyloxy)butyrate	C 100	1	14.3
		S 50	5	7.1
Mecoprop	(*RS*)-2-(4-Chloro-*o*-tolyloxy)propionic acid, diethanolamine salt	C 175	5	25.0
		S 250	2	35.7
Fenoprop (silvex)	(±)-2-(2,4,5-Trichlorophenoxy)propionic acid, propylene glycol butyl ether ester	C 100	19	14.3
		S 100	9	14.3
2,4,5-T	(2,4,5-Trichlorophenoxy)acetic acid, triethylamine salt	C 100	10	14.3
		S 50	5	7.1
	(2,4,5-Trichlorophenoxy)acetic acid, propylene glycol butyl ether ester	C 250	4	35.7
		S 100	3	14.3
	(2,4,5-Trichlorophenoxy)acetic acid, 2-ethyl hexyl ester	C 100	10	14.3
		S 50	10	7.1
Phthalamic Acids				
Naptalam	Sodium *N*-1-naphthylphthalamiate	C 175	6	25.0
		S 100	3	14.3
Naptalam and dinoseb	*N*-1-Naphthylphthalamic acid (66%) and 2-*sec*-butyl-4,6-dinitrophenol (34%)	C 25	8	3.6
		S 25	10	3.6
Thiocarbamates				
Diallate	S-2-3-Dichloroallyl di-isopropyl(thiocarbamate)	C 25	1	3.6
		S 25	1	3.6
EPTC	S-Ethyl dipropylthiocarbamate	C 50	1	7.1
		S 100	2	14.3
EPTC and 2,4-D	S-Ethyl dipropylthiocarbamate (57%) and 2,4-D iso-octyl ester (43%)	C 25	10	3.6
		S 100	4	14.3
Molinate	S-Ethyl *N*,*N*-hexamethylenethiocarbamate	C 50	1	7.1
		S 75	1	10.7
Pebulate	S-Propyl butyl(ethyl)thiocarbamate	C 50	1	7.1
		S 175	3	25.0
Triallate	S-2,3,3-Trichloroallyl di-isopropylthiocarbamate	C 25	5	3.6
		S 50	2	7.1
Vernolate	S-Propyl dipropylthiocarbamate	C 100	3	14.3
		S 250	8	35.7
Triazines				
Atrazine	2-Chloro-4-ethylamino-6-isopropylamino 1,3,5-triazine	C 25	2	3.6
		S 5	10	0.7
Prometone	2,4-*bis*(Isopropylamino)-6-methoxy-1,3,5-triazine	C 10	8	1.4
		S 25	4	3.6
Prometryn	2-4-*bis*(Isopropylamino)-6-(methylthio)-1,3,5-triazine	C 50	2	7.1
		S 100	6	14.3

Table continued on following page

Table 1. MINIMUM TOXICITY OF SOME ORGANIC HERBICIDES IN CATTLE (9 TO 15 MONTHS) AND SHEEP (MATURE) *(Continued)*

Common Name	Chemical Name (IUPAC)	Minimum Toxicity C(attle) and S(heep)		Estimate of Corresponding Application Rate (lb AI/acre)†
		(mg/kg/day)	*(days)**	
Propazine	2-Chloro-4,6-*bis*(isopropylamino)-1,3,5-triazine	C 25	3	3.6
		S 25	5	3.6
Simazine	2-Chloro-4,6-*bis*(ethylamino)-1,3,5-triazine	C 25	3	3.6
		S 50	10	7.1
Triazoles				
Amitrole	1*H*-1,2,4-Triazole-3-amine	C 25	3	3.6
		S 10	10	1.4
Uracils				
Bromocil	5-Bromo-3-*sec*-butyl-6-methyluracil	C 250	1	35.7
		S 50	10	7.1
Isocil	5-Bromo-3-isopropyl-6-methyluracil	C 50	7	7.1
		S 100	1	14.3
Ureas				
Chloroxuron	3-[*p*-(*p*-Chlorophenoxy)phenyl]-1,1-dimethylurea	C 25	5	3.6
		S 25	8	3.6
Diuron	3-(3,4-Dichlorophenyl)-1,1-dimethylurea	C 100	10	14.3
		S 100	2	14.3
Fenuron	1.1-Dimethyl-3-phenylurea	C 500	2	71.4
		S 100	8	14.3
Fluometuron	1,1-Dimethyl-3-(α,α,α-trifluoro-*m*-tolyl) urea	C 100	2	14.3
		S 50	6	7.1
Linuron	3-(3,4-Dichlorophenyl)-1-methoxy-1-methylurea	C 50	10	7.1
		S 50	1	7.1
Metobromuron	3-(4-Bromophenyl)-1-methoxy-1-methylurea	C 500	2	71.4
		S 100	8	14.3
Monuron	3-(4-Chlorophenyl)-1,1-dimethylurea	C 500	1	71.4
		S 100	4	14.3
Norea	3-(Hexahydro-4,7-methanoindan-5-yl)-1,1-dimethylurea	C 175	2	25.0
		S 250	5	35.7
Miscellaneous				
Bensulide	Di-isopropyl S-2-phenylsulphonylaminoethyl phosphorodithiaoate	C 50	2	7.1
		S 100	3	14.3
Chlorfenac (fenac)	Sodium(2,3,6-trichlorophenyl)acetate	C 50	1	7.1
		S 175	2	25.0
Chloridazon (pyrazon)	5-Amino-4-chloro-2-phenylpyridazin-3(2II)-one	C 100	3	14.3
		S 25	10	3.6
Chlorthal-dimethyl (DCPA)	Dimethyl tetrachloroterephthalate	C 250	5	35.7
		S >500	10	>71.4
Endothal (endothall)	7-Oxabicyclo[2.2.1]heptane-2,3-dicarboxylic acid, potassium salt	C 25	2	3.6
		S 10	10	1.4
Glyphosate	*N*-(Phosphonomethyl)glycine, isopropylamine salt	C 206	5	29.4
Picloram	Potassium 4-amino-3,5,6-trichloropyridine-2-carboxylate	C 500	8	71.4
		S 250	9	35.7
Triclopyr	(3,5,6-Trichloro-2-pyridyloxyacetic acid), triethylamine salt or ethylene glycol butyl ether ester	C 75 (2-yr-old steers)	3	10.7

Source: Data compiled primarily from Palmer JS, Radeleff RD: The toxicity of some organic herbicides to cattle, sheep, and chickens. USDA Production Research Report No. 106, 1969; Palmer JS: The toxicity of 45 organic herbicides to cattle, sheep, and chickens. USDA Production Research Report No. 137, 1972.

*Least number of daily oral doses causing 5 per cent or greater body weight loss or other obvious signs of poisoning for experimental exposure periods of less than 20 days.

†Application rate directly on forage theoretically capable of providing a daily dosage equivalent to the minimum reported toxicity (see text for method of estimation).

IUPAC = International Union of Pure and Applied Chemistry; AI = active ingredient.

sheep poisoned with barban. Death without forewarning signs was seen in a sheep given chlorpropham for 5 days at 250 mg/kg/day. Necropsy findings in this animal included congestion of the lungs, liver, kidneys, spleen, and gastrointestinal mucosa. In sheep fatally poisoned with barban, the liver was abnormally firm and pale, there was hemorrhage on the surface of the liver and kidneys, and the spleen was engorged with dark-colored blood.

DINITROANILINES

Poisoning of cattle and sheep with benfluralin (benefin) or trifluralin produced anorexia and weight loss. Trifluralin also produced diarrhea. Resolution of clinical signs and attainment of original body weight required about 1 month for animals poisoned with trifluralin. Sheep severely poisoned with benfluralin exhibited bloating, depression, and prostration before death. A yearling calf given nitralin showed anorexia, depression, weakness, and death. Signs of nitralin poisoning in sheep were weakness, bloating, tachypnea, and ataxia.

Postmortem findings in sheep poisoned with benfluralin were congestion of the abomasum and intestine. Lymph nodes associated with the gastrointestinal tract were swollen, and the liver was enlarged and friable. Similar gross lesions were observed in nitralin-poisoned animals.

NITRILES

Cattle and sheep poisoned with chlorthiamid showed anorexia accompanied by weight loss; cattle also became depressed and weak. Signs of dichlobenil toxicosis in cattle and sheep were increased salivation, anorexia, and depression. Convulsions occurred in some animals.

In fatal chlorthiamid poisoning there was congestion of the liver and kidneys, distended cranial vessels, and swollen lymph nodes related to reddening of the intestinal mucosa. At necropsy of animals poisoned with dichlobenil, lesions were extensive as in generalized toxemia. There were swollen, hemorrhagic lymph nodes throughout the body. Hemorrhages in muscles were seen chiefly in the thoracic and cervical areas. Epicardial hemorrhages (petechiae) were present, and congestion of the lungs and upper respiratory tract was common. The liver and kidneys were swollen and congested, and the mucosa of the abomasum and intestinal tract was congested to markedly inflamed depending on the acuteness of poisoning. In cases where survival was more prolonged, the liver was pale and friable and the kidneys were firm and reduced in size.

ORGANOARSENICS

Consumption of forage treated with arsenic herbicides should always be considered extremely hazardous. The persistence of arsenic compounds in the soil and their accumulation in plants may present problems where heavy or repeated application is practiced. The clinical effects and postmortem findings in cases of poisoning by organoarsenic herbicides are similar to those described for inorganic arsenic poisoning. The organoarsenic herbicides commonly produce necrotic lesions in the rumen, reticulum, and omasum in addition to the lower gastrointestinal tract.[1]

PHENOLS

Signs of poisoning by nitrofen in cattle and sheep included anorexia, diarrhea, hematuria, depression, and ataxia. At necropsy the kidneys were congested and the spleen was enlarged. Epicardial hemorrhages were present, and clotted blood and edema fluid were found in the pericardial sac. The upper respiratory tract contained edema fluid and froth.

PHENOXYS

The phenoxy herbicides are comparatively harmless and present little hazard to livestock except by way of accidental ingestion of concentrates or sprays. The danger of chronic toxicosis is very low. Continuous high dosage over a period of months was required to produce severe poisoning. Signs of intoxication included anorexia, depression, rumen atony, unthrifty appearance, and weakness (especially in the hind limbs). Animals may gradually become emaciated and moribund. Less frequently observed signs were diarrhea and bloating. Postmortem findings were congestion and enlargement of the liver; reddening of the intestinal and abomasal mucosa; undigested feed in the rumen; and enlarged, hyperemic lymph nodes. Although of low toxicity, the phenoxy herbicides may constitute an indirect hazard to livestock by increasing the toxicity and/or palatability of poisonous plants.

PHTHALAMIC ACIDS

Signs of naptalam poisoning in cattle and sheep included anorexia, diarrhea, and weight loss. Loss of body weight was the only evidence of toxicosis in two sheep during and for a period of time after treatment. One of these sheep became moribund and was sacrificed 12 days after the last dose. Signs of poisoning in cattle and sheep poisoned with naptalam and dinoseb were usually anorexia and lethargy, accompanied occasionally by tympany. One sheep lost weight but otherwise appeared normal throughout the trial.

Necropsy of the sacrificed sheep given naptalam revealed reddening of the intestinal mucosa and congestion of the liver and kidneys. Postmortem findings in cattle and sheep given naptalam and dinoseb included congestion of the lungs and kidneys and enlargement of the adrenals; the liver was pale and friable.

THIOCARBAMATES

These herbicides are moderately toxic to cattle and sheep. Signs of poisoning included anorexia, weight loss, diarrhea, depression, ataxia, muscle spasms, and prostration. Molinate and pebulate produced salivation and occasionally bloating. Anorexia was the only sign observed in most animals poisoned with S-ethyl dipropylthiocarbamate (EPTC) or vernolate. Signs of triallate poisoning were often limited to weight loss followed by a long recuperative period. A delayed, partial to complete alopecia occurred up to 60 days following nonfatal poisoning of cattle or sheep by diallate. Lesions at necropsy were congestion of the lungs, kidneys, and thyroid. The liver was often enlarged, friable, and pale, and the gastrointestinal mucosa was reddened or hemorrhagic.

TRIAZINES

Triazine herbicides are considered to be relatively toxic to cattle and sheep; however, little evidence of spontaneous poisoning has resulted from their use. Experiments in which atrazine or prometone was fed on treated forage to calves and sheep for 27 days produced neither signs of poisoning nor gross nor histopathologic lesions.[5] In these studies daily atrazine intake peaked during the second week of feeding at 69 mg/kg body weight for both cattle and sheep. Peak prometone intake also occurred during the second week of feeding (108 mg/kg/day for cattle; 75 mg/kg/day for sheep). The absence of toxicity of atrazine and prometone in these experiments compared with data in Table 1 may be due to the different modes of administration used (eaten on forage versus direct oral doses). In contrast, clinical signs consistent with triazine herbicide poisoning and 20 per cent mortality have been reported in sheep grazing nonpoisonous weeds during and soon after spraying with a mixture of simazine (2.6 lb/acre) and amitrole (0.9 lb/acre).[3]

Signs of poisoning from direct oral dosing with triazine herbicides included anorexia, depression, muscle spasms, ataxia, and weakness. Muscle spasms produced by atrazine varied in intensity and were restricted to the hindquarters. The clinical condition of two sheep poisoned with atrazine (100 mg/kg/day) appeared to improve despite continued administration of the herbicide; these animals then died unexpectedly after 8 to 10 doses. Increasing dyspnea was an additional observation with simazine poisoning. Heifers given a single oral dose (500 mg/kg body weight) of an atrazine formulation (AAtrex 80W) containing 80 per cent atrazine developed a slight increase in body temperature and marked elevation of pulse and respiratory rates. Diarrhea was present 12 hours after dosing followed by ataxia, stiffness, salivation, and terminal signs.[6] Signs of prometone poisoning were somewhat different from those of the other triazines; these consisted of anorexia, increased salivation, and diarrhea.

Lesions seen at necropsy in animals poisoned by triazine herbicides consisted of congested lungs, liver, and kidneys; pale, friable, and sometimes enlarged livers; enlarged adrenals; and subepicardial petechial hemorrhages. At necropsy of the heifers poisoned by AAtrex 80W, there was diffuse subcutaneous hemorrhage and hemorrhages in the thymus, thyroid, and heart muscle. The liver was enlarged, and the mucosa of the forestomachs appeared black. Pulmonary edema and excessive amounts of fluid in the thoracic and abdominal cavities were seen in sheep chronically poisoned with propazine.

TRIAZOLES

Amitrole is relatively toxic to cattle and sheep, producing anorexia, ataxia, weakness, and loss of weight. Loss of body weight was the only sign of poisoning observed in some sheep given the herbicide at low dosage (10 to 25 mg/kg/day) for 10 days. At necropsy there was congestion of the lungs and kidneys, an enlarged friable liver, and hemorrhages of the abomasal and intestinal mucosa.

URACILS

Cattle and sheep poisoned with bromocil or isocil exhibited anorexia, depression, loss of body weight, and occasionally ataxia and bloat. Enlarged hemorrhagic lymph nodes, congested lungs, and subepicardial hemorrhage were seen at necropsy.

UREAS

Signs of poisoning, some of which appear suddenly, included anorexia, depression, ataxia, dyspnea, and weight loss. Additional signs seen in linuron poisoning were increased salivation, marked weakness (cattle), and hematuria (sheep). Vomiting and diarrhea were observed in cattle poisoned with norea. Additional signs observed in sheep poisoned with monuron were excitability and torticollis. Mild poisoning of cattle and sheep with fluometuron produced only anorexia and diarrhea. Metobromuron produced only anorexia and weight loss in cattle and severe depression and hematuria in sheep.

Necropsy findings included congestion of various internal organs. Commonly involved were the kidneys, intestinal mucosa, meninges, lungs, and liver. Animals poisoned with fluometuron and linuron had friable and sometimes pale livers. Excessive amounts of pericardial fluid and hemorrhages associated with the epicardium, bladder mucosa, and muscle fascia were found in sheep poisoned with linuron. Subepicardial hemorrhages were also present in sheep poisoned with fenuron. Enlargement of the liver (fenuron, monuron) and kidneys (monuron) was present in poisoned sheep.

MISCELLANEOUS HERBICIDES

The only signs of illness reported for sheep poisoned with bensulide were anorexia and death. Bensulide poisoning in cattle produced salivation, diarrhea, ataxia, and prostration. Congestion of the lungs, kidneys, pancreas, and intestinal mucosa was observed in bensulide-poisoned sheep at necropsy. Chlorthal-dimethyl (DCPA) produced anorexia and weight loss in cattle at a daily dosage of 250 mg/kg body weight for 10 days. Sheep given DCPA at a daily dosage of 500 mg/kg body weight for the same period of time remained clinically unaffected. Endothal, chlorfenac (fenac), and glyphosate produced diarrhea, ataxia, and weight loss. Dyspnea was seen in sheep and cattle poisoned with chlorfenac and cattle poisoned with glyphosate. Alopecia occurred in one sheep 30 days after the last treatment with chlorfenac. Necropsy of animals poisoned with endothal revealed congestion of the kidneys and adrenal glands, enlargement of the liver and adrenal glands, excessive peritoneal fluid, and gastrointestinal hemorrhage. Sheep poisoned with chlorfenac had congestion of the liver, kidneys, and meninges; enlargement of the spleen; and petechial hemorrhages subcutaneously. No lesions were observed at necropsy of cattle poisoned with a formulation of glyphosate; however, mild to marked renal tubular vacuolization was seen microscopically. Prominent signs of toxicosis observed in cattle and sheep poisoned with picloram were anorexia, depression, and weakness. Fatally affected animals died 6 to 7 days after the appearance of signs of poisoning. Postmortem lesions in these animals included congestion of the lungs, liver, kidneys, adrenal glands, and intestinal mucosa. Lymph nodes of the anterior half of the body were swollen and hemorrhagic. The liver and adrenal glands were enlarged, and the rumen was filled with undigested feed.

Chloridazon (pyrazon) intoxication produced weight loss, lethargy, and convulsions in both cattle and sheep. Convulsions and death were observed in two sheep 90 days after the last dose of pyrazon had been given. Prominent lesions in acutely poisoned animals were congestion of the kidneys and meninges; hemorrhage of the intestinal mucosa; and a pale, friable liver.

Cattle poisoned with triclopyr exhibited anorexia, depression, weakness, ataxia, tremors, and dyspnea. Constipation, sometimes followed by diarrhea, was a prominent feature of poisoning. Findings at necropsy were enlargement of the kidneys, adrenal glands, and spleen. The liver was enlarged, pale, and friable; the colon was congested or hemorrhagic.

Mild toxic tubular nephrosis and hepatosis were seen microscopically.

DIAGNOSIS

Clinical signs and lesions produced by many organic herbicides are nonspecific, requiring that other evidence be considered. Diagnosis usually depends on quantitative evidence of exposure with the presence of compatible clinical effects. If possible, an estimate of the degree of exposure should be made and compared with known toxicity data such as are presented in Table 1 to establish the likelihood of poisoning.

The method of assessing the potential hazard for the herbicides presented in Table 1 involved (1) the experimental determination of the minimum toxic dosage by daily oral administration of herbicide to cattle and sheep and (2) comparison of that rate of administration to the theoretical daily dosage obtained by an animal grazing treated forage. A realistic yield of 0.1 lb/ft^2 of air-dried forage is assumed. This value represents a high-quality, improved pasture yielding approximately 2 tons/acre of forage. In these calculations, neither the influence of environmental factors nor the rate of decomposition of herbicides is considered. Further assumptions are: (1) a grazing animal would consume, as dry forage, 3 per cent of its body weight each day and (2) all of the applied chemical adheres to and is evenly distributed on vegetation available for grazing. Although the latter is never actually the case, this assumption gives the maximum exposure to be expected. An application of 1 lb/acre (1.12 kg/ha) of active ingredient (AI) provides 10.4 mg/ft^2 and a daily dosage of 7 mg AI/kg body weight to grazing animals under the assumed conditions.

In addition to an estimate of the minimum toxicity of a number of herbicides to cattle and sheep, Table 1 also includes the application rate (calculated using the approach described above) necessary to provide an equivalent daily dosage from grazing treated forage. It should be remembered that the data in Table 1 resulted from the direct oral administration of herbicides (rather than ingestion on forage) to a limited number of animals and calculations based on several conservative assumptions. Therefore this data may not be fully representative of conditions present in a particular case of alleged poisoning. If analytic confirmation or quantitation of a herbicide is desired, samples to be submitted for analysis should include suspected forage, feed, or water. Samples from fatally affected animals should include liver, kidney, muscle, fat, rumen contents, urine, and feces. The presence of herbicide residues in animal tissues or ingesta will confirm that exposure has occurred but will not necessarily be indicative of poisoning. Since many herbicides are rapidly eliminated from the body, the absence of residues may not exclude the possibility that poisoning has occurred, especially if death is delayed. Interpretation of the results of quantitative chemical analysis of animal tissues may be difficult in the absence of data concerning the kinetics of these residues and the levels of residues indicative of poisoning.

POISONOUS PLANTS

Treatment with herbicides may elevate or reduce the hazard of poisonous plants to livestock by increasing or decreasing (1) the concentration of toxic constituents within the plant and/or (2) the plant's palatability. The hydrocyanic acid (HCN) content of *Sorghum halapense* (Sudangrass) has been observed to increase 4 days after treatment with 2,4-dichlorophenoxyacetic acid (2,4-D). Nitrate concentration increased in *Amaranthus retroflexus* (redroot pigweed), *Impatiens biflora* (impatiens), and *Polygonum convulvulus* (wild buckwheat) following herbicide treatment. Reduced levels of nitrate occurred in *Polygonum persicaria* (ladythumb) and *Ambrosia artemisiifolia* (common ragweed). The toxic alkaloid content of *Delphinium barberi* (Barbey larkspur) markedly increased for 3 weeks following treatment with silvex or 2,4,5-trichlorophenoxyacetic acid (2,4,5-T), indicating that areas containing herbicide-treated larkspur should not be grazed for at least 4 weeks, or until the plants have died and become unpalatable. Disruptions in plant carbohydrate metabolism by herbicides, particularly the phenoxy compounds, may increase the content of sugars and render plants more palatable. Increased palatability of normally unpalatable poisonous plants could increase their hazard to livestock despite the absence of change in concentration of toxic constituents.[14]

TREATMENT

Poisoning by the organoarsenic herbicides should be treated in the same manner as inorganic arsenic poisoning. No specific antidotes are available for poisoning by other organic herbicides. Animals with excessive oral exposure to most organic herbicides should be treated with activated charcoal (1 to 3 g/kg body weight) mixed in an aqueous slurry with a saline cathartic (1 g/kg body weight). Treatment with activated charcoal should be done as soon as possible after herbicide exposure and, at least in the case of atrazine, should be repeated daily for 4 days. Forced diuresis and supportive therapy for hepatic and renal functions may also be useful.

PREVENTION

Prevention of herbicide poisoning in livestock involves controlling or eliminating sources of exposure. Following label instructions with regard to application rates and grazing of treated forage will avoid poisoning as well as illegal residues in animal products. If increased toxicity or palatability of poisonous plants is a concern, grazing of treated areas should be discontinued until these plants are dead and no longer palatable. Care should be taken to prevent the access of animals to concentrated herbicide held in storage, spraying equipment, accidental spillage, or contaminated feed or water.

REFERENCES

1. Casteel SW, Bailey EM, Murphy MJ, et al: Arsenic poisoning in Texas cattle: the implications for your practice. Vet Med 81:1045–1049, 1986.
2. Cox JH, Oehme FW: Synthetically manufactured chemicals causing toxicity. *In* Smith BP (ed): Large Animal Internal Medicine. St. Louis, CV Mosby, 1990, pp 1632–1634.
3. Egyed MN, Shlosberg A: Some considerations in the evaluation of a herbicide (simazine-aminotriazole) poisoning in sheep and horses. Vet Human Toxicol 19:83–84, 1977.
4. Humphreys DJ: Veterinary Toxicology, 3rd ed. Philadelphia, Bailliere Tindall, 1988, pp 134–140.
5. Johnson AE, Van Kampen KR, Binns W: Effects on cattle and sheep of eating hay treated with triazine herbicides, atrazine and prometone. Am J Vet Res 33:1433–1438, 1972.
6. Kobel W, Sumner DD, Campbell JB, et al: Protective effect of activated charcoal in cattle poisoned with Atrazine. Vet Hum Toxicol 27: 185–188, 1985.
7. Osweiler GD, Carson TL, Buck WB, et al: Clinical and Diagnostic Veterinary Toxicology, 3rd ed. Dubuque, Kendall/Hunt, 1985.
8. Palmer JS: Toxicity of a 4-chloro-2-butynyl-m-chlorocarbanilate (barban) formulation to cattle, sheep, and chickens. J Am Vet Med Assoc 160:338–340, 1972.

9. Palmer JS: The toxicity of 45 organic herbicides to cattle, sheep, and chickens. USDA Production Research Report No. 137, 1972.
10. Palmer JS, Radeleff RD: The toxicity of some organic herbicides to cattle, sheep, and chickens. USDA Production Research Report No. 106, 1969.
11. Quick MP: Sodium monochloroacetate poisoning of cattle and sheep. Vet Rec 113:155–156, 1983.
12. Radeleff RD: Veterinary Toxicology, 2nd ed. Philadelphia, Lea & Febiger, 1970, pp 264–292.
13. Seawright AA: Animal Health in Australia, Volume 2, Chemical and Plant Poisons. Canberra, Australian Govt Pub Ser, 1982.
14. Williams MC, James LF: Effects of herbicides on the concentration of poisonous compounds in plants: a review. Am J Vet Res 44:2420–2422, 1983.

Heavy Metals and Trace Elements

Arsenic Toxicosis

FRANCIS D. GALEY, DVM, PhD, DIPLOMATE, ABVT

Arsenic is ubiquitous in nature and may be found in many industrial products. The element can exist in multiple forms that exert different, occasionally species-specific effects on animals. The toxicity of arsenic depends not only on its form but also on valence, particle size, dose, rate and route of exposure, toxicokinetics, species, and the preexisting health condition of exposed animals.

Arsenic can be classified in three general groups based on molecular form (inorganic and organic, phenylarsonics, and arsine gas). Additionally, the metal may be present in a pentavalent or a trivalent valence form. The form of arsenic determines the type of toxicosis that is produced. Therefore inorganic and organic arsenic toxicosis along with arsine gas will be considered separately from the phenylarsonics.

INORGANIC AND ORGANIC ARSENIC COMPOUNDS

Sources

Inorganic and organic arsenic are found everywhere in nature. The largest hazard to food animals from arsenic, however, results from exposure to arsenic used industrially, medicinally, or as a pesticide.

Arsenic trioxide and other forms of arsenic, such as lead arsenate, have been used as insecticides. The residues from those insecticides may persist for long periods. For example, cattle developed arsenic toxicosis after exposure to soil from old orchards that had been treated with arsenicals. Other forms of arsenic, such as monosodium methane arsenate (MSMA) and the disodium version (DSMA) (both pentavalent arsenicals), are herbicides and defoliants. Arsenic salts with copper and chromium are effective wood preservatives (e.g., copper chromium arsenate [CCA]-treated wood). Properly dried, CCA-treated wood is not hazardous to animals *unless* it has been burned, because it is both in the pentavalent form (less toxic than trivalent) and tightly bound to the wood. Burning converts the pentavalent to a trivalent form and concentrates the arsenic, thereby increasing the hazard to animals.

Arsenicals historically have been used in medicines. Fowler's solution consists of sodium arsenite, a potentially toxic, trivalent arsenical. Arsenic compounds have been used as rumenatorics, parasiticides for dogs (caparsolate), and treatments for various human maladies. Arsenic has been implicated as a contaminant in a veterinary preparation.

Industrially, arsenic can be found in paints, coal- and waste-burning sites, semiconductors, photocells, and as a by-product of ore refining. Arsine gas was developed as a war gas during World War I, leading to the development of British anti-lewisite (BAL), commonly used in the treatment of arsenic toxicosis. Arsine is now used by the semiconductor industry.

Arsenic toxicosis in food animals can result from exposure to grass clippings (exposed to arsenicals), burned CCA-treated wood, dipping vats, old orchards, and industrial sites. Most common arsenicals present little risk to the food supply, as arsenic does not tend to accumulate in nontuber plant material or animal tissue. It is possible, however, for arsenic to be passed in the milk of cows with arsenic toxicosis.

Toxicity and Mechanism

Trivalent arsenic is generally the more toxic when compared with pentavalent arsenic (2 to 10 times, depending on the solubility and other chemical characteristics). All species of animals are sensitive to arsenic. Weak and dehydrated animals are especially sensitive to the effects of arsenicals, probably owing to reduced renal excretion.

After absorption, trivalent arsenic compounds are distributed to highly perfused areas of the body. Trivalent arsenic acts by formation of a stable complex with sulfhydryl groups in enzymes and cofactors. The binding in lipoic acid (essential for the functioning of the Krebs cycle) significantly inhibits cellular respiration in major capillary beds of oxidative organs, leading to tissue necrosis. The splanchnic and renal capillary beds are the most sensitive to arsenic, although the lungs and other well-perfused organs may also be affected. Trivalent arsenicals are largely detoxified by methylation and rapid elimination in bile and urine.

Pentavalent arsenicals can cause toxicosis after being converted to the trivalent form. Pentavalent arsenic may also uncouple oxidative phosphorylation. Pentavalent arsenic is eliminated rapidly in the feces and urine or converted to trivalent forms and handled accordingly in the body.

Arsine gas denatures protein, ultimately leading to red blood cell hemolysis. Arsine is slowly converted to arsenic trioxide prior to elimination. Organic arsenicals, such as methylated compounds, are very rapidly eliminated in the urine. Therefore such compounds are relatively less hazardous to animals unless renal function is compromised.

Clinical Effects

Acute arsenic toxicosis is associated with high morbidity and high mortality. Affected animals develop abdominal pain within hours of exposure. Shortly after the onset of abdominal pain, ataxia, weakness, and tremors appear. Pigs, and sometimes cattle, will develop vomiting, increased salivation, gut atony (especially rumen), and diarrhea. Signs progress to a fast weak pulse, prostration, dehydration with hemoconcentration, oliguria, and death (within 2 to 3 days of exposure).

Clinical signs of subacute arsenic toxicosis consist of depression, anorexia, and a watery diarrhea. The watery feces may contain shreds of mucosa. Polyuria, present early in the syndrome, may change to anuria as the kidneys fail. As the syndrome progresses, animals will develop dehydration, polydipsia, weakness, tremors, and death. Rarely convulsions may be present prior to death.

Chronic arsenic toxicosis, although rare, consists of a general loss of condition and a rough haircoat. Percutaneous arsenic exposure may lead to blistering and edema of the affected skin.

Lesions

Postmortem, animals with acute arsenic toxicosis will have reddening of the gastrointestinal mucosa (especially rumen, gastric, and duodenal mucosae) with large amounts of fluid, foul-smelling, bloody gut contents. Perforation of the gut, secondary to necrosis, may be present. Occasionally the liver may be pale yellow and the lungs may be red and edematous. Peracutely affected animals may die before the development of any lesions.

Histologic sections of gut will have wide areas of mucosal and submucosal edema and necrosis with extensive mucosal sloughing. Less commonly, glomerular sclerosis and renal tubular necrosis will be evident. Fatty hepatocyte degeneration may be noted in some animals. The predilection of arsenic-associated lesions in the gut, liver, and kidney belies the extensive nature of the splanchnic capillary beds in those organs. Cutaneously exposed animals will have dry, leathery, peeling skin and histologic evidence of epidermal and dermal necrosis.

Diagnosis

A diagnosis of inorganic/organic arsenic toxicosis is suggested when animals develop a rapid outbreak of gastroenteritis with copious amounts of fluid in the gut, weakness, prostration, and a rapid death. Liver and kidney arsenic analysis may reveal concentrations of arsenic greater than 8.0 ppm on a wet-weight basis. Gut contents and urine may contain 2 to 100 ppm of arsenic. Owing to the rapid elimination of arsenic from the body, tissue arsenic concentrations will rapidly decline over several days to levels of 2 to 4 ppm or less. Animals that have been affected for a period of several days or more may have normal tissue arsenic concentrations. Therefore quantification of arsenic in tissues should be done as soon as possible after exposure. In those cases it is especially important to test the possible sources of arsenic exposure.

The differential diagnosis for arsenic toxicosis includes other causes of diarrhea (e.g., infectious or organophosphorus insecticide poisoning) and sudden death in food animals. Lead toxicosis may also be confused with arsenic toxicosis. Lead toxicosis, however, has a more prominent neurologic component and will not be presented with the severe gastrointestinal lesions associated with arsenic toxicosis.

Treatment

Acute arsenic toxicosis carries a poor prognosis unless treatment is quickly initiated. Initially gastric lavage can be used to remove the arsenic. Vigorous lavage is contraindicated, however, once signs have developed because of the risk of gut perforation. Oral (30 to 60 g every 6 hours for 3 to 4 days) and intravenous (30 to 60 g as a 10 to 20 per cent solution) sodium thiosulfate administration has been suggested (to bind the arsenic). Although the efficacy of that treatment remains to be proved, sodium thiosulfate is relatively nontoxic and thus may be useful. Once signs have developed, aggressive therapy to replace losses in fluids and electrolytes must be done to treat shock. The fluid of choice is lactated Ringer's solution, although dextrose may be needed to increase urine flow in anuric patients. B vitamins may be helpful additives to the fluids. Kaolin-pectin solutions may be used orally to soothe the gut. Convalescent animals should be placed on a high-protein, low-residue diet to minimize gastrointestinal stress.

Chelation therapy can be valuable for treatment of arsenic toxicosis. The chelating agent of choice in the United States is BAL. This compound has multiple sulfhydryl groups to bind with the arsenic. Unfortunately the prohibitively high cost and toxicity of BAL limits its use in food animals. If used, BAL should be given via intramuscular injection at a loading dose of 4 to 5 mg/kg body weight, followed by q.i.d administration of 2 to 3 mg/kg body weight for 1 day and by q.i.d dosing with 1 mg/kg body weight for 2 more days. Thioctic acid (exogenous lipoic acid; 50 mg/kg body weight t.i.d.) may be useful for treatment of arsenic toxicosis in food animals. The chelating agents, dimercaptosuccinic acid (DMSA) and 2, 3-dimercapto-1-propanesulfonic acid (DMPS) (suggested dose for each is 20 mg/kg body weight), are more efficacious and have a wider therapeutic index than BAL. Unfortunately DMSA and DMPS are not approved for use in the United States. Milk from exposed cows should be discarded (calves have been poisoned by milk from cows with arsenic toxicosis).

PHENYLARSONIC COMPOUNDS

Sources

The phenylarsonics are used in swine and poultry rations to improve feed efficiency and to control swine dysentery. Examples include arsanilic acid, 3-nitro 4-hydroxy phenylarsonic acid (3-nitro or Roxarsone), and 4-nitrophenylarsonic acid (Nitarsone). Arsanilic acid is used at levels of from 50 to 100 ppm to increase weight gain and improve feed efficiency in chickens, turkeys, and swine and is used at concentrations up to 400 ppm for 5 days to combat swine dysentery. Gestating sows should not be fed over 45 ppm in the diet of arsanilic acid owing to increased risk from increased feed consumption. 3-Nitro is used to improve feed efficiency and weight gain in concentrations of up to 37.5 ppm in swine rations and 50 ppm in poultry rations. Treatment of swine dysentery with 3-nitro requires 200 ppm in the diet for 5 to 6 days. 4-Nitrophenylarsonic acid is fed to poultry at 188 ppm to control blackhead.

Toxicity and Mechanism

The hazard from phenylarsonics results from misformulation, feeding accidents, prolonged feeding at levels used for therapy of dysentery, and feeding the compounds to sick, debilitated, and dehydrated animals. Clinical signs of toxicosis may result from feeding arsanilic acid to swine at concentrations greater than 250 ppm for 3 to 6 weeks. Concentrations of 1,000 ppm may cause toxicosis in swine in 3 to 10 days. The maximum safe level to feed to turkeys is 400 ppm of arsanilic acid.

3-Nitro is more toxic than arsanilic acid. Concentrations of 250 ppm may cause signs in swine in as little as 3 days. After

3 weeks of feeding, 100 ppm may be toxic to pigs. Poultry rations should not exceed 75 ppm to avoid toxicosis.

The phenylarsonic compounds are not well absorbed by the gut. That which is absorbed is rapidly excreted by the kidneys. Thus dehydration or renal impairment increases the risk for developing phenylarsonic toxicosis.

The mechanism of action of the phenylarsonics in swine and poultry is not completely understood. Ultimately the compounds can cause demyelination and gliosis of peripheral nerves. Suggested mechanisms include interference with B vitamins or uncoupling of oxidative phosphorylation. Ruminants metabolize phenylarsonics to inorganic arsenic, and thus overdose of phenylarsonics in those species can result in signs of gastroenteritis typical of inorganic arsenic poisoning. Cattle are resistant to phenylarsonic poisoning when compared with swine.

Clinical Effects

Acute phenylarsonic toxicosis may result after 3 to 5 days of feeding extremely high concentrations to swine. Initial signs include roughened haircoats and diarrhea. Ataxia and hyperesthesia develop, quickly followed by paralysis. Arsanilic acid, unlike 3-nitro, will cause blindness in swine. Chronic feeding of slightly lower toxic levels of phenylarsonics to swine will result in a more gradual onset of paralysis. Initial signs may be insidious, with gradual development of knuckling and goose-stepping. Ultimately blindness (arsanilic acid) and paralysis will develop. Lightly pigmented animals may have a reddened skin and can be hypersensitive to sunlight. Regardless of speed of onset, animals will continue to eat and drink as long as possible.

Poultry with 3-nitro toxicosis develop incoordination and ataxia. Arsanilic acid will cause anorexia, depression, coma, and death in chickens and turkeys.

Lesions

Few gross lesions are present in animals with phenylarsonic toxicosis. Occasionally skin erythema and a full bladder will provide clues. Histologic lesions consist of demyelination of peripheral and optic nerves. Necrosis of myelinating cells, secondary axonal degeneration, and gliosis near neural tubes may also be present. The lesions are progressive and may take from 6 to 10 days to develop (arsanilic acid). Therefore acute cases may be presented with few histologic lesions. Lesions from animals with 3-nitro toxicosis are also progressive, may take 11 to 15 days to develop, and involve the spinal cord as well as peripheral nerves. No meaningful lesions have been reported in brain tissue. The severity of signs is proportional to the severity of clinical effects.

Diagnosis

Phenylarsonic toxicosis is suspected when swine and poultry with a history of being fed phenylarsonics develop progressive paresis, with or without blindness, while retaining the ability to eat and drink. Morbidity is high and mortality rates are low. The diagnosis is supported by histologic findings of demyelination and gliosis. Tissue arsenic quantification may not detect elevated arsenic concentrations because the kidneys so readily excrete the offending compounds. If animals are still exposed to high concentrations of phenylarsonics, 3 to 10 ppm (on a wet-weight basis) of arsenic may be found in kidney and liver tissue and 1 to 2 ppm of arsenic may be found in blood. It is usually necessary to identify excessive concentrations of the phenylarsonic compounds in samples of the suspected feed (see earlier for toxic levels). The differential diagnosis for arsenic toxicosis includes nitrofuran and mercury poisoning, water deprivation/salt toxicosis, pseudorabies, and B-vitamin deficiency.

Treatment

Treatment for phenylarsonic acid toxicosis is nonspecific. Clean feed and water should be provided in such a manner as to be accessible to paralyzed animals. Administration of B vitamins has been suggested, although that therapy has not been demonstrated to be effective. Affected animals should be protected from sunlight. Acutely affected animals can spontaneously recover if quickly removed from the source of phenylarsonic. The prognosis is poor if signs are prolonged, blindness has appeared, or paralysis has developed (suggesting axonal damage).

Although useful, phenylarsonic compounds should always be considered to be potentially toxic. Therefore mixing concentrations and feeding times should be closely monitored and label directions should be closely followed whenever such compounds are to be used.

BIBLIOGRAPHY

Animal Health Institute: Feed Additive Compendium. Minnetonka, MN, Miller Publishing, 1989.
Arnold W: Arsenic. In Seiler HG, Sigel H, Sigel A (eds): Handbook on Toxicity of Inorganic Compounds. New York, Marcel Dekker, 1988, pp 79–93.
Furr A, Buck WB: Arsenic. In Howard JL (ed): Current Veterinary Therapy: Food Animal Practice, 2nd ed. Philadelphia, W B Saunders, 1986, pp 435–437.
Hatch RC: Poisons causing abdominal distress or liver or kidney damage. In Booth NH, McDonald LE (eds): Veterinary Pharmacology and Therapeutics, 6th ed. Ames, IA, Iowa State University Press 1988, pp 1102–1125.
Hatch RC, Clark JD, Jain AV: Use of thiols and thiosulfate for treatment of experimentally induced acute arsenite toxicosis in cattle. Am J Vet Res 39:1411–1414, 1978.
Hindmarsh JT, McCurdy RF: Clinical and environmental aspects of arsenic toxicity. CRC Critical Reviews in Clinical Laboratory Sciences 23:315–347, 1986.
Osweiler GD, Carson TL, Buck WB, Van Gelder GA (eds): Clinical and Diagnostic Veterinary Toxicology, 3rd ed. Dubuque, Kendall/Hunt, 1985.
Thatcher CD, Meldrum JB, Wikse SE, Whittier WD: Arsenic toxicosis and suspected chromium toxicosis in a herd of cattle, J Am Vet Med Assoc 187:179–182, 1985.

Copper-Molybdenum Toxicosis

LARRY J. THOMPSON, DVM, Diplomate, ABVT
WILLIAM B. BUCK, DVM, PhD, Diplomate, ABVT

Copper is an essential trace element for plants and animals, and molybdenum is essential for plant life. Although molybdenum has been shown to be essential in laboratory animal experiments, a deficiency has not been shown to occur under natural conditions. Copper has a complex relationship with molybdenum and sulfur, as well as other dietary components, and when a high dietary concentration of molybdenum is present relative to that of copper, a progressive copper depletion occurs. In the rumen, molybdenum and sulfur combine to form thiomolybdates, which can be absorbed and can combine with copper to hold it in a biologically unavailable form. Thus ruminants are more sensitive to dietary molybdenum excesses than are nonruminants. Different species of animals show varying responses to dietary copper, with cattle being sensitive to deficiencies of copper while sheep are more sensitive to copper excesses on both an acute and a chronic basis. The optimum dietary copper:molybdenum ratio is between 6:1 and 10:1. A copper:molybdenum ratio less than 2:1 will result in a copper deficiency, while increasing the ratio above 10:1 will increase the risk of developing copper toxicosis.

Zinc and iron also interact with copper and are more important in nonruminant species such as swine, poultry, and laboratory animals. Both zinc and iron have been shown to protect swine from the adverse effects of high levels of dietary copper. Similarly, zinc and iron deficiencies tend to exacerbate copper toxicity in swine.

Copper in livestock feed is generally recognized as safe (GRAS) by the U. S. Food and Drug Administration and most animals require approximately 10 ppm in the diet. In 1987 the FDA approved molybdenum as a substance that, when added to animal feed as a nutritional dietary supplement, is GRAS when added at levels consistent with good feeding practice, which is considered to be 5 ppm. This approval allows the addition of molybdenum to obtain a proper dietary copper:molybdenum ratio and has made molybdenum supplements available through most feed manufacturers.

COPPER DEFICIENCY

A variety of disorders in animals have been associated with deficient copper, and deficiencies may be primary or secondary. A primary copper deficiency can occur from an inadequate dietary intake of copper. A secondary copper deficiency can occur when there is adequate copper in the diet but the absorption and utilization of the copper are inhibited. Most commonly this is due to excess molybdenum or sulfur in the diet, or both. Other sources of sulfur, such as the sulfate ion in water, can also interact with copper.

Disorders that have been associated with a relative copper deficiency in various animal species include anemia, depressed growth, bone disorders, depigmentation of hair or wool, abnormal wool growth, neonatal ataxia, impaired reproductive performance, heart failure, cardiovascular defects, and gastrointestinal disturbances. Many factors influence the severity of these problems, including species, age, sex, environment, and breed or strain characteristics. Anemia associated with copper deficiency occurs in most species and is characteristic of the anemia associated with iron deficiency. A decrease in the synthesis and activity of the copper-containing enzyme ceruloplasmin will interfere with the proper utilization of iron. Bone abnormalities associated with copper deficiency have been reported in rabbits, mice, chicks, dogs, pigs, foals, sheep, and cattle. In ruminants, osteoporosis and spontaneous bone fractures are usually associated with excess dietary molybdenum and thus a secondary copper deficiency. Sheep suffering from primary copper deficiency or excess molybdenum or both also develop depigmentation of dark wool together with loss of crimp and quality of their fine wool. In Australia a syndrome called "enzootic ataxia" and in the United Kingdom a similar condition called "swayback" are associated with severe copper deficiency. Pregnant ewes become anemic with stringy wool, and neurologic signs subsequently develop in their lambs, usually before 1 month of age. Affected lambs are severely uncoordinated, have a prominent hind-limb ataxia, and are sometimes blind. Death is the result of exposure, starvation, or pneumonia. Swayback has been reported in the United States and can affect goats. Lesions associated with enzootic ataxia and swayback in lambs are characterized by lysis of the white matter of the cerebrum and degeneration of motor tracts of the spinal cord.

The excess molybdenum syndrome is characterized by emaciation, liquid diarrhea full of gas bubbles, swollen genitalia, anemia, and achromotrichia. Poor weight gains and death from prolonged purgation usually occur. Osteoporosis and bone fractures have been reported in prolonged cases. Copper deficiency–like syndromes have resulted from feeding of forages and grains grown on soils naturally high in molybdenum or low in copper or both. In the United States such soils have been found in California, Oregon, Nevada, and Florida. Cattle grazing pastures on muck or shale soils in England, Ireland, New Zealand, and Holland have suffered severe molybdenosis.

When the copper levels of feed or forages are in the normal range of 8 to 11 ppm, cattle can be poisoned on molybdenum levels above 5 to 6 ppm and sheep can be poisoned on levels above 10 to 12 ppm. When the dietary copper level falls below 8 to 11 ppm, or when the sulfate ion level is high, even 1 to 2 ppm molybdenum may be toxic to cattle.

Treatment

The diet should be analyzed for both copper and molybdenum content. Copper sulfate ($CuSO_4$) may be added to the diet to obtain a proper copper:molybdenum ratio. Other formulations of salt mineral mixture to provide approximately 1 g copper sulfate daily for an adult cow can also be used. Copper glycinate can be given subcutaneously at a rate of 60 mg for calves and 120 mg for mature cattle. This treatment may need to be repeated during a season and should be administered in the brisket due to the swelling and edema that commonly occur at the injection site. Copper disodium ethylenediaminetetraacetic acid (EDTA) generally causes less localized reaction but is potentially more toxic than copper glycinate. Copper-containing glass pellets and copper oxide needles are given orally and remain in the gastrointestinal tract to slowly release copper. For all sources, response to copper therapy is usually good.

COPPER TOXICOSIS

Acute copper poisoning may occur in any species, associated with the use of copper compounds for therapeutic and pesticidal purposes. Cattle may be poisoned by 200 to 800 mg copper sulfate/kg body weight, and sheep may be poisoned by 20 to 100 mg single dose. Copper chloride ($CuCl_2$) is two to four times more toxic than copper sulfate, and when dissolved in water copper sulfate is more toxic than an equal amount in the dry crystalline form. Clinical signs associated with large oral doses of copper formulations include vomiting, excess salivation, abdominal pain, diarrhea (greenish tinged), collapse, and death within 24 to 48 hours. Postmortem findings may include congestion and hemorrhages in the gastrointestinal tract and a blue-green coloration of the gut contents.

The most common form of copper toxicosis results from chronic exposure to diets containing either excess copper or improper copper:molybdenum ratios. Chronic copper toxicosis in sheep may develop over a period of weeks to months, but the onset of clinical signs is usually very rapid. With dietary excess, copper will slowly accumulate in the liver until damage occurs; with stress a sudden release of copper into the bloodstream will occur, causing hemolysis, methemoglobinemia, hemoglobinuria, and kidney damage. Clinical signs will include depression, anorexia, icterus, and rapid respiration. Occasionally an animal may have only pale mucous membranes without icterus and hemoglobinemia. Other liver insults or preexisting liver dysfunction will cause increased sensitivity to elevated dietary copper. Although the morbidity is usually less than 5 per cent, the mortality is usually over 75 per cent.

A diagnosis of chronic copper poisoning is based on a history of compatible clinical signs, chemical analysis of tissues and blood of affected animals, and necropsy findings, which include icterus, swollen gunmetal-blue or black colored kidneys, and pale or yellow liver. For ruminants the dietary levels of copper and molybdenum should be determined, and for swine, in addition to copper, the levels of iron and zinc in the diet and tissues may also be important. Normal serum concentrations of copper in most species are in the range of 0.7 to 2.0 ppm. Concentrations above this are often associated with copper poisoning. Liver concentrations associated with copper poisoning are usually greater than 150 ppm on a wet-weight basis, whereas kidney concentrations are usually greater than 15 ppm.

Copper has been used as a feed additive for swine because of its growth promotant effects. If adequate zinc and iron levels are present in the diet, 125 to 250 ppm copper sulfate may be beneficial. On the other hand, if iron and zinc concentrations are low in the diet, 250 ppm copper sulfate may result in chronic toxicosis in swine. Waste from poultry or swine may be sources of excess copper, as both these species are often supplemented with high dietary levels of copper.

Diseases that should be differentiated from chronic copper poisoning include anaplasmosis, babesiosis, bacillary hemoglobinuria, hepatitis, leptospirosis, and postparturient hemoglobinemia, as well as poisoning by rape (brassica), onion, phenothiazine, or nitrates. Poisoning by metals such as arsenic, mercury, lead, and thallium may mimic the gastrointestinal effect of acute massive copper poisoning.

Treatment

The maintenance of a proper copper:molybdenum ratio in the diet is imperative for the prevention of feed-related chronic copper toxicosis. This requires the analysis of both copper and molybdenum in the complete diet. Most forages and total diets contain 0.5 to 1.5 ppm molybdenum, and sodium molybdate can be added to obtain a proper copper:molybdenum ratio. Molybdenum addition should always be under 5 ppm in the total diet. Molybdenum-containing licks or mineral mixtures may also be used for preventive purposes (86 kg salt, 64 kg gypsum, and 0.45 kg sodium molybdate). Molybdenum incorporated into phosphate fertilizer (114 g/acre) can be used to increase the molybdenum content of pasture. Sheep diets can be supplemented with 100 ppm zinc to help reduce liver copper storage. Swine diets containing excess copper should be fortified with zinc and iron.

Animals suffering from the acute hemolytic crisis of copper toxicosis have a poor prognosis. Fluid replacement therapy is suggested, using a balanced electrolyte solution unless a blood transfusion is indicated due to blood loss. Daily oral administration of 200 mg ammonium or sodium molybdate plus 500 mg sodium thiosulfate for up to 3 weeks will help decrease the body burden of copper. Daily oral administration of the copper chelating agent *d*-penicillamine at 50 mg/kg for 6 days will greatly enhance copper excretion.

Ammonium tetrathiomolybdate has been used experimentally as a treatment for copper toxicosis in sheep. Intravenous or subcutaneous administration of 1.7 to 3.4 mg/kg ammonium tetrathiomolybdate on alternate days for three treatments decreased the mortality rate in animals that had developed a hemolytic episode. Currently, however, there is no licensed product in the United States.

BIBLIOGRAPHY

Howell JM Gawthorne JM (eds): Copper in Animals and Man, Volumes I and II. Boca Raton, FL, CRC Press, 1987.
Humphries WR, Morrice PC, Bremner I: A convenient method for the treatment of chronic copper poisoning in sheep using subcutaneous ammonium tetrathiomolybdate. Vet Rec 123:51–53, 1988.
Osweiler GD, Carson TL, Buck WB, Van Gelder GA (eds): Clinical and Diagnostic Veterinary Toxicology, 3rd ed. Dubuque, Kendall/Hunt, 1985.
Smith RM, Thompson LJ: Causes and treatment of copper toxicosis in sheep. Proc Fall Conf Vet Univ Ill 69:1–8, 1988.

Fluoride Toxicosis

J. L. SHUPE, DVM
C. V. BAGLEY, DVM
A. E. OLSON, MS
H. B. PETERSON, PhD

Fluoride toxicosis, often called fluorosis, results from the intake of excessive amounts of fluorides. Animals are exposed to various forms and concentrations of fluorides when they ingest certain feeds and waters, but they absorb only minimal amounts from the atmosphere. Gaseous or particulate fluorides in the air inhaled by animals are generally of little consequence to their health. Livestock normally consume variable low-level amounts of fluoride with no known adverse effects. Ingestion of fluorides in proper amounts has been shown to exert beneficial effects on some tissues and physiologic processes in humans and animals.

DISEASE FORMS

Acute Fluoride Toxicosis

Fluoride toxicosis may be either acute or chronic. Acute fluoride toxicosis is relatively rare, and it most often results from ingestion of organic and inorganic fluoride compounds such as sodium fluorosilicate, sodium fluoride, sodium fluoroacetate, and methyl fluoroacetate. Some plants metabolize inorganic fluoride into various organic fluoride compounds, especially fluoroacetate. Fluoroacetate may accumulate in such plants to concentrations that are extremely toxic to herbivorous animals.

The rapidity with which signs of fluoride toxicosis appear and the exact nature of the signs depend on the amount and type of fluoride ingested. Clinical signs may include restlessness, stiffness, anorexia, excessive salivation, nausea, vomiting, incontinence of urine and feces, reduced milk production in lactating animals, clonic convulsions, weakness, severe depression, and cardiac failure. Chemical analyses of blood and urine from affected animals characteristically reveal high fluoride contents. Necropsy findings vary, but there is most often severe gastric and intestinal inflammation, degenerative changes in kidney tubular epithelium, epicardial and endocardial petechiae and ecchymoses, myocardial lesions, and pulmonary congestion and edema.

Published with the approval of the Utah State University Agricultural Experiment Station, Logan, Utah, as Journal Paper No. 3988.

Chronic Fluoride Toxicosis

The much more common chronic fluoride toxicosis develops gradually and insidiously. The following topics all relate to the chronic form of fluorosis. Months or even years may intervene between the beginning of excess fluoride ingestion and the development of readily observable clinical signs. Some manifestations of chronic fluoride toxicosis may be confused with other toxicoses or certain debilitating or degenerative diseases. It may be characterized by dental fluorosis, osteofluorosis, or both.

SOURCES

Forage crops are usually the most widespread source of excessive fluorides for livestock. These crops may be contaminated by fluoride-laden industrial effluents, by wind-blown or rain-splashed soil of high fluoride content, or by sprinkler irrigation water high in fluoride. In addition, some drinking water supplies contain appreciable amounts of fluorides and contribute to the total fluoride intake. Improperly defluorinated inorganic phosphates, when used to provide supplementary dietary phosphorus, may be a major fluoride source in the diets of many domestic animals. The Association of American Feed Control Officials recommends a phosphorus:fluoride ratio of at least 100:1 for defluorinated phosphate. Properly used, such phosphates are safe for livestock supplementation.

All possible sources of fluoride should be analyzed to ascertain their contribution to the total intake of the animals in question.

INFLUENCING FACTORS

The expression or severity of fluoride toxicosis may be altered or influenced by the following factors: (1) amount of fluoride ingested, (2) duration of fluoride ingestion, (3) bioavailability of ingested fluorides, (4) variations in fluoride ingestion levels (intermittent exposure), (5) species of animal, (6) age at time of ingestion, (7) nutritional status, (8) exposure to other substances (with synergistic or alleviating effects), (9) general state of health of the animal, (10) stress, and (11) individual biologic response.

SPECIES TOLERANCES

Tolerance levels for various livestock species have been determined. Where applicable, different levels have been calculated for the long-term (production and reproduction animals) and the short-term (fattening and slaughter animals). The recommended levels are listed in Table 1. The values are for sodium fluoride or for compounds of similar bioavailability (toxicity) in the total dietary intake. Less-soluble fluoride compounds, such as calcium fluoride, are less toxic. Fluorides in water are more bioavailable and thus more toxic than those ingested in dietary dry matter. The variations in relative toxicities of the different fluoride forms or sources must also be considered when evaluating fluoride toxicosis.

CLINICAL SIGNS

Dental Fluorosis

Fluorides have a great affinity for developing and mineralizing teeth. Such teeth are extremely sensitive to excessive fluoride. Some of the primary and most distinctive lesions induced by excessive fluoride ingestion are found in teeth. Because of the nature and complexity of the disease, however, such dental lesions should not be the sole criterion for diagnosis. Once the teeth have formed, mineralized, and erupted into the oral cavity, fluoride ingestion will have little or no effect on them. Thus young animals are most susceptible to dental fluorosis.

Fluoride-induced dental lesions are influenced by the 11 factors previously mentioned. The gross lesions may best be described by one or more of the following terms:

Mottling. White, chalk-like opaque areas or horizontal striations in the enamel.
Chalkiness. Dull white to pale yellow chalk-like appearance.
Hypoplasia. Defective formation and structure.
Hypomineralization. Defective mineralization.
Discoloration. Pale white, creamy yellow, brown or black.
Attrition. Excessive abnormal wear.

Severely affected teeth are discolored (chalky white or creamy yellow to brownish black), usually subject to increased attrition, and may also have lost enamel, with exposure of the dentine.

Clinical dental fluorosis is usually classified using numerical values (Fig. 1). The incisor teeth are evaluated for enamel quality, defects, and abrasion pattern (Fig. 2). The usual classification system ranges from 0 (normal) to 5 (severe fluoride effects). The more difficult to examine cheek (premolar and molar) teeth are classified 0 to 5 based on attrition patterns only.

Osteofluorosis

Fluorides have great affinity for bone as well as for developing and mineralizing teeth. Excessive fluoride may affect bones at any time during an animal's life, but bones of young animals are more responsive to excessive fluoride levels than bones of mature animals. Osteofluorosis has been seen in animals with normal teeth, which illustrates the effect of age.

The amount of fluoride stored in bone normally increases over time without inducing any demonstrable changes in bone structure and function. There will be structural changes in

Table 1. RECOMMENDED FLUORIDE TOLERANCE LEVELS IN FEED AND WATER FOR DOMESTIC ANIMALS BASED ON CLINICAL SIGNS AND LESIONS*

Species	Feed† mg/kg (ppm)	Water‡ (mg/L)
Heifers, dairy and beef	30	2.5–4
Dairy cattle, mature	40	3–6
Beef cattle, mature	50	4–8
Finishing cattle	100	12–15
Breeding ewes	60	5–8
Feeder lambs	150	12–15
Horses	60	4–8
Swine, growing	70	5–8
Turkeys, growing	100	10–12
Chickens, growing	150	10–13
Dogs	50	3–8
Mink	45	3–8

*Biologic availability depends on chemical composition. Dissolved fluoride in water appears to be more readily assimilated. The values must be reduced proportionally when both water and feed contain appreciable amounts of fluorides.
†This is a suggested guide when fluoride in the feed is the principal source of fluoride.
‡The average ambient air temperature and the physical and biologic activity of the animals influence the amount of water consumed and hence the wide range of tolerance levels suggested. For active animals in a warm climate, the lower values should be used as critical level indicators.

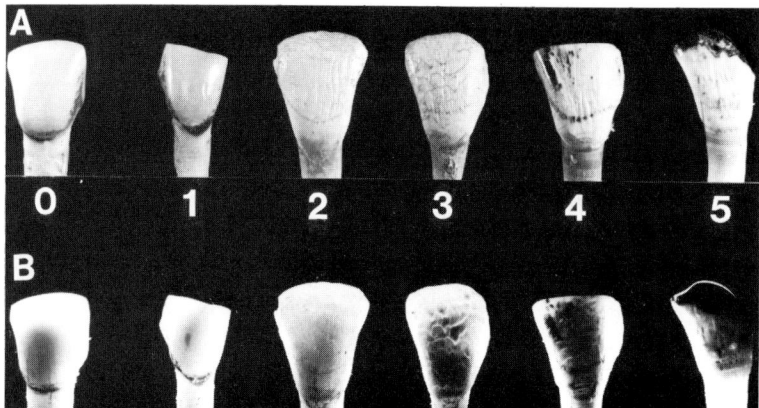

Figure 1. Classification of representative incisor teeth from cattle is from 0 to 5, reading from left to right in both *A* and *B*. *A* is with direct light; *B* is with transmitted light. (From Shupe JL, Minor ML, Greenwood DA, et al: Am J Vet Res 24:964–984, 1963.)

bone if significantly higher than normal amounts of fluoride are ingested over an extended length of time.

In livestock, clinically palpable bone lesions usually first appear on the mandible, ribs, and medial portions of the metatarsal and metacarpal bones. The lesions are generally bilateral and somewhat symmetric. Characteristic histologic changes are associated with the various degrees of osteofluorosis. The type of bone changes seen depends on the factors that influence fluoride toxicosis.

Animals with moderate to severe osteofluorosis sometimes exhibit an intermittent nonspecific stiffness that may be associated with periods of stress, periosteal overgrowths, and calcification of periarticular structures and tendon insertions. While this stiffness or "lameness" is often transitory and intermittent, it limits grazing or feeding and impairs animal performance. The type of stiffness is not definitive for fluoride toxicosis.

Other generalized but nonspecific clinical signs sometimes associated with chronic fluoride toxicosis are unthriftiness; thickened, dry, unpliable skin; and other signs of poor performance.

In addition to noting clinical signs, analyses should be made of blood, urine, and of water and all dietary components ingested by animals suspected of having fluoride toxicosis so that the cause may be elucidated.

Infertility, Carcinogenicity, and Teratogenicity

Well-controlled, long-term studies of chronic fluoride toxicity in domestic animals and detailed necropsy findings from clinical studies of animals that ingested different levels of fluoride showed no evidence that fluoride was carcinogenic or teratogenic or that it directly decreased fertility. Lameness and poor body condition resulting from chronic fluoride toxicity could predispose an animal to decreased fertility.

The placenta usually serves as a barrier to transfer of circulating fluorides from the dam's blood to the developing fetus. Therefore offspring of even severely affected females have only slightly elevated fluoride levels in tissues and no demonstrable lesions.

NECROPSY FINDINGS

If warranted by clinical examinations and chemical analyses, necropsies should be performed on selected, representative animals. For economic reasons, some animals may be sacrificed at a commercial abattoir and, after appropriate tissues are taken for detailed study and evaluation, the carcasses can be used for meat. There is no significant accumulation of fluorides in soft tissue. Ninety-six per cent or more of the fluoride in an animal's body is contained in the bones and teeth.

Dental Lesions

All permanent teeth should be carefully examined for evidence of fluoride-induced dental lesions. If lesions are present in the incisor teeth, they should be correlated with lesions in the cheek teeth, which developed during the same period of the animal's life.

Skeletal Lesions

Grossly, bones that are severely affected by fluoride appear chalky white, have a roughened irregular periosteal surface, and are larger in diameter and heavier than normal (Fig. 3). The major bone changes are located on the periosteal surface. Secondary peri- and intra-articular changes may be associated with severe or persistent lesions. The nature of the bone changes varies with the level and duration of fluoride intake and the other factors listed above. One or more of the following conditions may occur: osteosclerosis, osteoporosis, hyperostosis, osteophytosis, or osteomalacia.

Radiology

The changes (e.g., increased density, porosity, hyperostosis, and osteophytosis) may be demonstrated radiographically as well as grossly. The usefulness of the radiographic evidence will depend on the degree and severity of osteofluorosis.

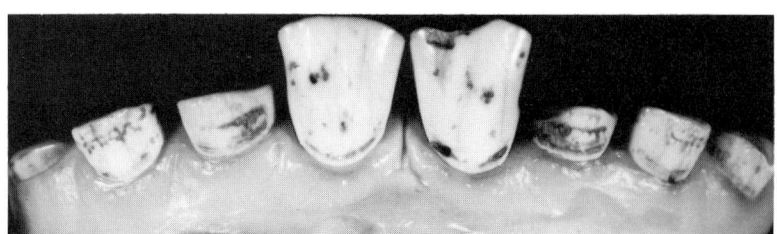

Figure 2. Permanent bovine incisor teeth. Note the chalkiness and discoloration of the enamel, hypoplasia, and excessive bilateral abrasion.

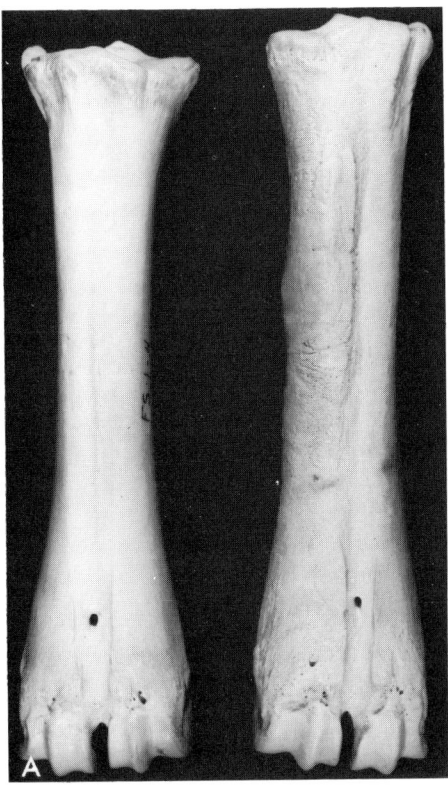
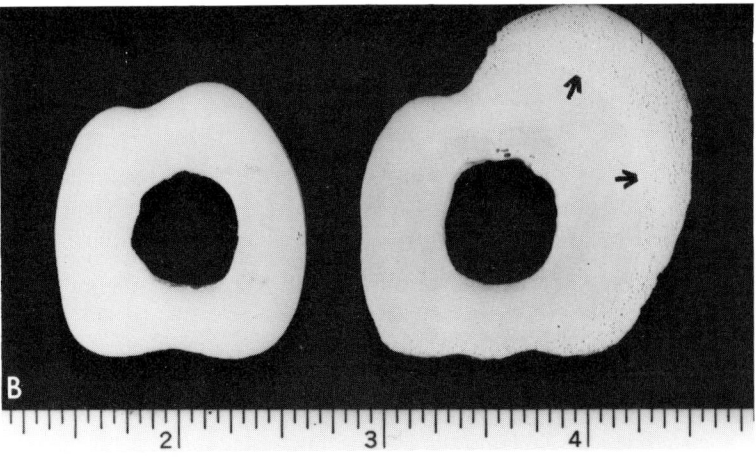

Figure 3. *A*, Metatarsal bones from two cows of the same breed, size, and age. The bone on the left is normal, while the bone on the right shows severe osteofluorosis. *B*, Cross-section of the two metatarsal bones shown in *A*. The section of bone from *arrows* outward is fluoride-induced abnormal bone.

Histopathology

Microscopic evaluation of fluoride-affected bones provides additional information on the described changes. Excessive periosteal, and at times endosteal, bone formation occurs. Porous areas, with excessive bone resorption or accelerated remodeling, appear when the proper balance between bone removal and bone replacement is disrupted. Osteones formed under the influence of excessive fluorides often vary in size and shape, and the osteocytes are often clumped or irregularly located near the periphery of the osteone rather than evenly distributed throughout the osteone. Abnormal canaliculi are associated with the clumped abnormal cells.

Pathogenesis of Osteofluorosis

The precise pathogenesis of osteofluorosis is not fully understood but appears to involve three phases: (1) elevated fluoride levels in the bone without detectable structural changes, (2) microscopic and radiographic bone changes with alterations of function, and (3) sequential and progressive structural bone changes that result in abnormal bone structure and function with resultant alterations of mechanical properties. The abnormal bone appears to result from an acceleration of the remodeling rate in existing bone accompanied by compensatory periosteal and, at times, endosteal proliferation. The osteoblasts are adversely affected and produce a defective organic matrix that is irregularly and defectively mineralized.

Chemical Analyses

Other valuable information may be provided by chemical analyses of bone for fluoride content, especially if certain precautions are taken in sampling. Sampling sites should be consistent so that test results will be representative and can be properly interpreted. Medial or lateral aspects of some long bones (even at the same proximal or distal levels) may vary in degree of change and amount of fluoride. Fluoride content of bones normally increases with age, even in animals on a lifelong low-fluoride intake.

Fluorides do not accumulate in soft tissues or in visceral organs in sufficient quantities to provide reliable, accurate, and consistent diagnostic information. Nor have fluorides been shown to induce characteristic, consistent, demonstrable changes in the visceral organs or soft tissues.

It is best to use a laboratory that routinely tests for fluoride, preferably one that is certified nationally for fluoride analyses.

DIAGNOSIS

Information from the examinations and procedures discussed should be carefully evaluated and correlated before making a definitive diagnosis of chronic fluoride toxicosis. Compare results of clinical examinations with necropsy findings. Chemical analyses, especially of bone, reflect past exposure to fluoride. The following signs and lesions are of particular importance: (1) mottling and abrasion of permanent teeth, (2) degree of osteofluorosis, (3) intermittent lameness, and (4) amount of fluorine in the urine. The first three signs were discussed previously.

Urine samples, if properly collected, analyzed, and interpreted, can assist in the diagnosis and evaluation of fluoride toxicosis. Individual random samples may be too variable to provide reliable information. Collect adequate numbers of uncontaminated samples at various intervals to provide accurate, representative values. The time of day that samples are taken and total urinary output also affect results. Counteract, insofar as possible, variations in volume of urine output by correcting specific gravity to 1.040.

Urine is a major means of fluoride elimination from the body. On a low-level fluoride diet the urinary fluoride content from animals rises slightly as the animals age, as does the fluoride content of their bones. Urinary fluoride levels may remain high for some time after animals are changed from a high- to low-fluoride diet; that is, urine values may not reflect current levels of fluoride intake. Under most circumstances specific gravity corrected urine values of less than 6 ppm fluoride are considered normal.

Analyze all sources of feed, including mineral supplements, and all sources of drinking water for fluoride content. Standardize sampling and analytic techniques to insure reliable data.

Intensive efforts should be made in regard to forage crop sampling to sample accurately what the animals have actually been ingesting. Fluorides accumulate on, as well as in, the plant structure, so do not wash samples before analysis. In areas of infrequent rainfall, results of samples taken just after a rainfall will differ significantly from samples taken just before. Mature vegetation will have a higher fluoride content than lush vegetation that has grown rapidly.

There is considerable experimental information on the fluoride tolerances of animals to fluoride in feed when animals are housed and managed under ideal experimental conditions. There is a paucity of information, however, on tolerances of animals under field conditions when they may not be properly sheltered and managed. Data are also lacking on tolerances of some animals to waterborne fluoride. Responses of animals to waterborne fluoride vary, as ambient air temperature influences the amount of water consumed.

Husbandry or management practices may also affect the expression of fluoride toxicosis. Obtain a complete clinical history of each animal, which should include information such as changes in rangeland grazing patterns and variable feed sources. These may produce intermittent excessive fluoride exposure in animals.

Other trace element toxicoses or deficiencies may alter or mimic aspects of chronic fluoride toxicosis. Some debilitating diseases, such as degenerative joint disease (osteoarthritis), may also mimic aspects of clinical fluoride toxicosis.

All available clinical and analytic data, coupled with a complete and knowledgeable understanding of the complexity of chronic fluoride toxicosis, should be utilized in diagnosing the condition. No single criterion is sufficient for a definitive diagnosis. Correlate clinical signs with laboratory analyses and with necropsy findings, when required. In making a definite diagnosis and final evaluation of fluoride toxicosis, the signs and lesions that the animals show should take precedence over fluoride analyses of current feed and water supplies.

TREATMENT

There is no known specific, successful treatment for chronic fluoride toxicosis. Supportive and symptomatic treatment based on the degree and extent of signs and lesions may be given. Lesions induced by excessive fluoride ingestion are not completely reversible. Dental lesions are irreversible, and lesions severe enough to hasten dental abrasion will accelerate wear, especially with rough, abrasive feeds.

Osteofluorotic lesions may be prevented by reducing the total fluoride intake to normal levels. Animals with extensive bone lesions do not live long enough for the bone to remodel to normal. After animals stop ingesting excessive fluoride levels, normal bone is laid down over previously induced osteofluorotic bones.

Animals adversely affected by fluoride toxicosis may be assisted by providing adequate nutrition and by avoiding physiologic stresses. Feed enough of a nutritionally well balanced diet to promote desirable performance and growth. Feed herbivorous animals as much good quality roughage as possible, and reduce or eliminate poor quality abrasive roughage. Succulent grains may be advisable in some cases.

If it is not possible to remove animals from toxic sources of fluorides, some preventive relief may be obtained by feeding alleviating compounds. Beneficial effects have been observed after feeding adequate mineral supplements and after adding calcium carbonate, magnesium, or aluminum compounds to the diet. Cattle fed aluminum sulfate as 1 per cent of their total dry matter intake for 4 years deposited 30 to 42 per cent less fluoride in their ribs than did control animals that consumed equally high dietary levels of fluoride. Including some aluminum (most often aluminum sulfate) or calcium (calcium carbonate) compounds in the diet has lessened the effects of fluoride. Some researchers have reported reduced dental lesions or reduced bone storage of fluorides or both when calcium or aluminum compounds were included in the diet. A nutritionally correct balance of other minerals, particularly phosphorus, should be maintained to obtain maximum benefits from aluminum and calcium additions. This may necessitate utilization of phosphate supplements.

PREVENTION

Livestock owners, animal feed processors, and industrialists can act to prevent fluoride toxicosis. The total amount of fluoride in feed, including mineral supplements, should not exceed normal recommended levels. Analyze all sources of drinking water. Naturally warm spring waters frequently contain excessive amounts of fluorides. Soils high in fluoride may also be a problem. The high-fluoride soils are primarily involved when they are naturally carried by wind or rain onto forage plants, not by translocation from the roots into the leaves and stems. Avoid overgrazing on high-fluoride soils to reduce the chance that livestock will ingest soil during close grazing.

Be aware of potential pollution from new industries or changes in industrial procedures. Fluoride toxicosis has been observed near some long-established operations that had no history of excessive fluoride pollution. Such companies may have utilized a new source of raw materials or altered their processing procedures, and only then started releasing excessive amounts of fluorides. Historically, phosphate smelters; aluminum, steel, and brick plants; and some coal-fired electricity generating plants have been emitters of fluorides. Another area of concern is the rapid expansion of sprinkler irrigation using geothermal or other high-fluoride-content waters. Some of these waters are safe for use in flood irrigation, but unpublished data indicate a high fluoride content in forage sprinkled with water containing high levels of fluoride (5 to 10 mg/L).

Livestock owners should routinely monitor all phases of animal health and should be aware of problems that may occur with infectious agents, nutritional imbalances, and toxicoses of all kinds, including fluoride toxicosis. Fluoride toxicosis in animals can be prevented and controlled when the complexity of the disease is realized, it is properly diagnosed, and the source of excessive fluorides is eliminated.

BIBLIOGRAPHY

Roholm K: Fluorine Intoxication: A Clinical-Hygienic Study with a Review of the Literature and Some Experimental Investigations. London, HK Lewis, 1937.

Shupe JL, Ammerman CB, Peeler HT, et al: Effects of Fluorides in Animals. Washington, DC, National Academy of Sciences/National Research Council, 1974, pp 1–70.

Shupe JL, Peterson HB, Leone NC (eds): Fluorides: Effects on Vegetation, Animals and Humans. Proceedings of International Symposium on Fluorides, Utah State University. Salt Lake City, Paragon Press, 1983.

Miscellaneous Toxicoses

Polybrominated Biphenyls (PBBs)

STEPHEN F. SUNDLOF, DVM, PhD, Diplomate, ABVT

The polybrominated biphenyls (PBBs) are manmade industrial chemicals that are no longer manufactured or marketed in the United States. Like many other halogenated hydrocarbon compounds, including the polychlorinated biphenyls (PCBs) and DDT, the PBBs are extremely persistent within the environment and they accumulate in animal tissues. The largest mass contamination of livestock in the United States occurred in 1973, when more than 6000 swine, 30,000 cattle, and 1.5 million chickens were destroyed after it was discovered that animal feed had been accidentally contaminated with PBBs, resulting in adulteration of animal carcasses.

SOURCE

Approximately 5 million pounds of PBBs were manufactured by the Michigan Chemical Corporation from 1970 until 1974, when production was discontinued. PBBs were produced as flame retardants for use in a wide variety of commercial products. In 1973 a nationwide paper shortage severely reduced the availability of paper bags. As a result, the Michigan Chemical Corporation, which produced mineral supplements as well as PBBs, was forced to use plain brown bags to package their products. PBBs and magnesium oxide were packaged in identical bags, with only a small label attached to the bags on which was stenciled the name "FireMaster" for the PBBs or "NutriMaster" for the magnesium oxide. A major feed mill in Michigan ordered magnesium oxide for incorporation into animal feeds, but at least part of the shipment of magnesium oxide turned out to be PBBs. It was later estimated that 650 lb of PBBs were incorporated into livestock rations, most of which occurred between August and December 1973.[9] As a result of this mistake, losses in addition to the numbers of condemned livestock included 5 million eggs, 34,000 lb of dry milk, 18,000 lb of cheese, 300 lb of butter, and 788 tons of feed. More than 30 dairy herds were quarantined. In 1974 the cost to the state of Michigan and responsible private companies was estimated to range from $26 million to $45 million.[4]

TOXIC PRINCIPLE AND MECHANISM OF ACTION

PBBs are the bromine analogues of PCBs, and like PCBs they are produced as mixtures containing a variety of isomers. The isomer 2,2'4,4',5,5'-hexabromobiphenyl represents about 60 per cent of the specific PBB mixture that caused the problems in Michigan.

The acute oral dose LD_{50} in the rat is 21.5 g/kg,[9] but lower total doses are lethal when divided and given daily for longer periods, such that a total dose of 3.3 g/kg administered over a 30-day period was lethal to rats.[10] The lethal total dose of PBBs in most mammalian and avian species is generally considered to be greater than 1 g/kg body weight, or greater than 500 ppm in the diet.[9] Total doses of 0.15 mg/kg of PBBs have no effect on the health or performance of lactating cattle.[8]

The clinical signs and lesions associated with PBB toxicosis are very similar to those produced by chlorinated dibenzodioxins, especially 2,3,7,8-tetrachlorodibenzo-p-dioxin (TCDD). It is not surprising, therefore, that all of the highly toxic PBB isomers approximate 2,3,7,8-TCDD in size and shape. Currently it is thought that both the dioxins and the toxic PBB isomers interact with a cytoplasmic receptor that in turn activates RNA synthesis in the nucleus and ultimately leads to the production of specific mono-oxygenase enzymes.[17] How this process of enzyme induction relates to specific pathologic changes is not known.

CLINICAL SIGNS

Because of the limited total production of PBBs (which amounted to only a small fraction of the PCBs produced), the probability of accidental poisoning in livestock must today be considered extremely remote. The following discussion of clinical signs and postmortem lesions should be read from a historical perspective, as incidents of PBB contamination and poisoning are not expected to recur.

In the Michigan incident, dairy cattle were affected to a greater extent than were other livestock species. The onset of clinical signs was slow and subtle, developing over a period of several months. Cattle showing clinical signs were estimated to have received rations containing from 4000 to 13,000 ppm of PBBs. Weight loss and decreased milk production were the first signs noticed by dairy workers. A few weeks after parturition, the body weight of cattle fell rapidly and average milk production dropped to 15 to 30 lb/day. After 2 months of lactation, many cows ceased to produce milk. Following the drop in weight and milk production, cattle often developed any of a wide number of infectious and noninfectious diseases, listed in Table 1.

General clinical signs in cattle exposed to PBBs either by accident or under experimental conditions include anorexia, emaciation, dehydration, excessive lacrimation, hyperkeratosis, and fetal deaths.[5, 11] Clinical signs that were reported following the Michigan incident but not in controlled feeding studies include hematomas, abscesses, abnormal hoof growth, hair loss, liver abscesses and necrosis, and metritis.[11] There are no consistent hematologic changes, but increased blood urea nitrogen, serum glutamic oxaloacetic transaminase, and serum cholesterol have been reported.[6, 7] Cows receiving daily doses of 250 mg/cow for 60 days or more experienced repro-

Table 1. CLINICAL DISORDERS REPORTED IN CATTLE FOLLOWING ACCIDENTAL EXPOSURE TO PBBs

Infectious Disorders	Reproductive Disorders
Pneumonia	Decreased fertility
Gastrointestinal disorders	Increased incidence of abortion
Hepatic disorders	Lowered survival rate of offspring
Mastitis	Decreased hatchability of eggs in poultry
Metritis	
Pyelonephritis	**Skin Disorders**
Inflammatory joint disease	Hyperkeratosis
Subcutaneous abscesses	Matting of the hair on the thorax
Chronic nasal discharge	Alopecia
Ocular mucopurulent discharge	Abnormal hoof growth

ductive disorders, particularly related to and following a high incidence of dystocia due to larger than normal birth weights.[20]

Behavioral changes also were noted by dairy workers. Cows that were usually familiar with milking and handling became unable to master these routines. The affected cows ceased to function in the social routine of the herd and stood apart from the herd. Even today it remains unclear as to which of the many abnormal clinical signs were the result of PBB exposure and which were due to poor nutrition and management or to other disease processes unrelated to PBBs.

Egg production in laying hens decreases in response to a PBB-induced decreased feed consumption, and there is a dose-related reduction in hatchability that occurs independently of feed intake.[1] Significant reductions in hatchability occur when hens are maintained on diets containing 30 to 40 ppm of PBBs, and offspring from PBB-fed hens experience higher mortality and lower growth rates than chicks from unexposed hens.[14]

PATHOLOGY

Most of the postmortem changes seen in Michigan cattle were the result of infectious diseases and not the direct result of PBB exposure. The pathologic lesions, in the order in which they were most frequently observed, are listed in Table 2.

Unlike most other species studied, liver lesions in cattle are relatively minor and consist of diffuse areas of centrilobular fatty degeneration, dilation of sinusoids, and depletion of glycogen.[12] The most pronounced lesions occur in the kidneys of cattle moribund from the toxic effects of PBBs. Kidneys may be doubled in size, distended with fluid, and pale tan to gray in color. Perirenal lymph nodes may be enlarged and edematous. Microscopic lesions include dilation of the convoluted tubules and collecting ducts and degenerative changes in the tubular epithelial cells.[12] Hyperkeratosis, especially of the eyelids, was a common lesion in cattle poisoned by PBBs in the Michigan incident.[12, 13, 16] Atrophy of the thymus occurs when cattle are exposed to high doses of PBBs,[12] but enlargement of the thymus has also been reported.

In avian species there is an increase in liver weight[15] with swelling of mitochondria and vacuolation of hepatocytes.[3] Reduction in the size of the bursa of Fabricius was observed in cockerels fed diets containing 10 ppm of PBBs.[3]

Hepatic lesions in swine consist of swollen hepatocytes, fatty changes, and centrilobular necrosis. In addition, thyroid hyperplasia has been reported in neonates born to sows that were fed diets containing PBBs during gestation.[18]

Table 2. POST-MORTEM LESIONS REPORTED IN CATTLE FOLLOWING ACCIDENTAL EXPOSURE TO PBBs IN DESCENDING ORDER OF FREQUENCY

Generalized lymph node enlargement
Lung changes typical of pneumonia
Small overall size of the animal
Enlarged thymus
Splenomegaly
Liver lesions: abscesses, adhesions, inflammation, degeneration
Renal lesions: inflammation, hydronephrosis, cysts, calculi
Peritonitis
Hyperkeratosis
Uterine lesions
Myocardial lesions and endocardial lesions
Serous atrophy of adipose tissue
Joint lesions
Intestinal hyperemia and serosal lesions due to peritonitis

DIAGNOSIS

Because PBBs are no longer manufactured in the United States, the probability of encountering a PBB-poisoned animal is remote. Clinical signs and postmortem lesions associated with high exposure to PBBs are not sufficiently distinctive to support a definitive diagnosis of poisoning.

The problem of PBB residues in animal carcasses, milk, or eggs is of primary concern to the veterinarian. If there is any question that a residue problem may exist, the veterinarian should submit samples of feed, mineral mix, rumen or stomach contents, milk, eggs, liver, and adipose tissue to a qualified laboratory for chemical analysis of PBBs. Because the present-day threat of PBB adulteration of animal-derived foods is considered to be minimal, in 1987 the U.S. Food and Drug Administration revoked all action levels in milk and dairy products, meat, eggs, and animal feeds.

TREATMENT

As with PCBs there is no treatment for PBB exposure, and because of the residue hazard to the human population, slaughter and disposal of animal carcasses may be the best alternative. Once absorbed, PBBs eventually distribute to adipose tissue, where they can accumulate to concentrations far exceeding the concentration in the diet. Because metabolism and excretion from adipose tissue are virtually nonexistent, elimination can occur only if the lipids themselves are mobilized into the circulation. Lipids may be mobilized under conditions of negative energy intake, lactation, or egg production. These three conditions lead to enhanced elimination of PCBs, but in the latter two cases result in residues in milk and eggs, respectively. The half-life of PBBs in lactating cows is estimated to be as long as 6 months,[19] whereas half-lives in nonlactating animals are thought to be considerably longer.[9]

Methods for enhancing the elimination of PBBs in livestock have been uniformly unsuccessful. Feeding phenobarbital to cows in an attempt to increase hepatic metabolism of PBBs did not affect excretion in milk and feces or the apparent half-life of residues in milk fat or body fat. Similarly, oral administration of activated charcoal did not increase excretion of PBBs in the milk or feces.[2]

REFERENCES

1. Cecil HC, Bitman J: Toxicity of polybrominated biphenyl and its effects on reproduction of white leghorn hens. Poultry Sci 57:1027–1036, 1978.
2. Cook RM, Prewitt LR, Fries GF: Effects of activated carbon, phenobarbital, and vitamins A, D, and E on polybrominated biphenyl excretion in cows. J Dairy Sci 61:414–419, 1978.
3. Dharma DN, Sleight SD, Ringer RK, Aust SD: Pathologic effects of 2,2′,4,4′,5,5′- and 2,3′,4,4′,5,5′-hexabromobiphenyl in white leghorn cockerels. Avian Dis 26:542–552, 1982.
4. Dunkel AE: An updating on the polybrominated biphenyl disaster in Michigan. J Am Vet Med Assoc 167:838–841, 1975.
5. Durst HI, Willett LB, Brumm CJ, Mercer HD: Effects of polybrominated biphenyls on health and performance of pregnant Holstein heifers. J Dairy Sci 60:1294–1300, 1977.
6. Durst HI, Willett LB, Brumm CJ, Schanbacher FL: Changes in blood and urine composition from feeding polybrominated biphenyls to pregnant Holstein heifers. J Dairy Sci 61:197–205, 1978.
7. Durst HI, Willett LB, Schanbacher FL, Moorehead PD: Effects of PBBs on cattle. I. Clinical evaluations and clinical chemistry. Environ Health Perspect 23:83–89, 1978.
8. Fries GF: Effect of low exposure to polybrominated biphenyl on production and other indicators of dairy herd performance. J Dairy Sci 66:1303–1311, 1983.
9. Fries GF: The PBB episode in Michigan: an overall appraisal. CRC Critical Reviews in Toxicology 64:105–156, 1985.

10. Gupta BN, Moore JA: Toxicologic assessments of a commercial polybrominated biphenyl mixture in the rat. Am J Vet Res 40:1458–1468, 1979.
11. Jackson TF, Halbert FL: A toxic syndrome associated with the feeding of polybrominated biphenyl-contaminated protein concentrate to dairy cattle. J Am Vet Med Assoc 165:437–439, 1974.
12. Moorehead PD, Willett LB, Brumm CJ, Mercer HD: Pathology of experimentally induced polybrominated biphenyl toxicosis in pregnant heifers. J Am Vet Med Assoc 170:307–313, 1977.
13. Moorehead PD, Willet LB, Schanbacher FL: Effects of PBB on cattle. II. Gross pathology and histopathology. Environ Health Perspect 23:111–118, 1978.
14. Polin D, Ringer RK: PBB fed to adult female chickens: its effect on egg production, viability of offspring, and residues in tissues and eggs. Environ Health Perspect 23:283–290, 1978.
15. Ringer RK, Polin D: The biological effects of polybrominated biphenyls in avian species. Fed Proc 36:1894–1898, 1977.
16. Robl MG, Jenkins DH, Wingender RJ, Gordon DE: Toxicity and residue studies in dairy animals with FireMaster FF-1 (polybrominated biphenyls). Environ Health Perspect 23:91–97, 1978.
17. Safe S: Polychlorinated biphenyls (PCBs) and polybrominated biphenyls (PBBs): biochemistry, toxicology, and mechanism of action. CRC Critical Reviews in Toxicology 13:319–395, 1984.
18. Werner PR, Sleight SD: Toxicosis in sows and their pigs caused by feeding rations containing polybrominated biphenyls during pregnancy and lactation. Am J Vet Res 42:183–188, 1981.
19. Willett LB, Durst HI: Effects of PBBs on cattle. IV. Distribution and clearance of components of Firemaster BP-6. Environ Health Perspect 23:67–74, 1978.
20. Willett LB, Schanbacher FL, Durst HI, Moorehead PD: Long-term performance and health of cows experimentally exposed to polybrominated biphenyls. J Dairy Sci 63:2090–2102, 1980.

Polychlorinated Biphenyl (PCB) Toxicosis

STEPHEN F. SUNDLOF, DVM, PhD, Diplomate, ABVT

The polychlorinated biphenyls (PCBs) are manmade chemical compounds often characterized as environmental contaminants. Despite their notoricty and the widely held perception that they are potent toxicants, PCB poisoning episodes in livestock are relatively rare and occur only following massive exposure to these compounds. Nevertheless, when overt poisoning in animals occurs, it generally indicates a much greater problem in the form of large-scale contamination of the food supply and the environment.

SOURCES

PCBs were first manufactured for commercial use in 1929. The name PCBs refers to a mixture of 209 theoretically possible isomers consisting of a biphenyl nucleus to which are attached chlorine atoms varying in number from 1 to 10. The degree of chlorination in commercial formulations of PCBs is determined according to the intended use of the final product. In the United States, PCBs were manufactured by the Monsanto Corporation under the trade name Aroclors. The per cent of chlorine in the formulation is reflected in the naming of the products, so that Aroclor 1242, Aroclor 1248, Aroclor 1254, and Aroclor 1260 contain 42, 48, 54, and 60 per cent chlorine by weight, respectively. Prior to their withdrawal from the marketplace, PCBs were incorporated into a wide variety of products, including waterproofing agents, flame retardants, protective coatings, oil varnishes, adhesives, molding compounds, plasticizers, carbonless copy paper, hydraulic fluid, heat exchanger fluid, dielectric fluid in capacitors and transformers, microscope immersion oil, expoxy resins, and several others. In 1971 the sale of PCBs was restricted to closed systems only. These included hydraulic fluids, heat exchanger fluids, and dielectric fluids. In 1979 the production and sale of PCBs in the United States were discontinued.

Although PCBs have not been sold for more than a decade, they remain a threat to livestock and other animals, including humans. PCBs are very stable, even under conditions of extreme heat and pressure. In addition, PCBs are relatively inert and do not react with other chemicals. These properties render PCBs ideal compounds for their intended industrial purposes, but it is these same properties that result in their accumulation in the environment and in living organisms.[14]

Because of their lipophilic nature and resistance to metabolic degradation, the half-life of PCBs may vary from a few hours to several hundred years depending on the specific isomer in question.[9] PCBs with long half-lives accumulate in food chains such that organisms occupying the highest trophic levels will attain the highest concentrations of PCBs. In aquatic ecosystems, predatory fish can concentrate PCBs 75,000-fold over the concentration in the water.[3] This biomagnification process has caused devastating effects in predatory birds and mink and represents a health threat to humans.

Most incidents of PCB poisoning or contamination of livestock have resulted from the leakage of PCBs from electrical transformers, heat exchangers, and other closed systems; from silo sealants and epoxy paints containing PCBs; or from the topical application of insecticides formulated in waste oils containing PCBs. The largest single incident of PCB contamination occurred in 1971, when 70,000 tons of fish meal were found to be contaminated with PCBs, resulting in the mandatory slaughter of 77,000 chickens that had consumed the contaminated feed. The U.S. Food and Drug Administration also called for 75,000 eggs to be destroyed, although an additional 60,000 eggs had already been consumed by the general public. PCBs had entered the fish meal through a leaky heat exchanger used in the pasteurization process to eliminate *Salmonella* organisms from the feed.[11] In Maine, where PCB residues in feeds were very high, an estimated 1.4 million broilers were destroyed in early 1972 because PCB residues in excess of 5 ppm were found in visceral fat.[2] Similar incidents on a smaller scale have occurred at various times. Silage from silos sealed with PCB-containing sealants has resulted in milk being discarded due to PCB concentrations in excess of action levels.[15] Poultry exhibit overt signs of intoxication when housed in cages painted with PCB-containing epoxy paints. The clinical syndrome has been termed chick edema disease.[4]

TOXIC PRINCIPLE AND MECHANISM OF ACTION

Most PCB isomers are of low toxicity, and field cases of acute PCB poisoning are rare. Certain PCB isomers, however, appear to be fairly potent toxicants. Furthermore, trace impurities in the form of toxic dibenzofurans may be present in some commercial PCBs.

The LD_{50} values for commercial PCBs in rats vary from 1000 to 10,000 mg/kg. The more highly chlorinated PCBs are generally considered more toxic than the lower chlorinated compounds, but toxicity appears to be more closely correlated with the positions rather than the number of chlorine atoms on the phenyl groups.[13] The clinical signs and lesions associated with PCB toxicosis are very similar to those produced by chlorinated dibenzodioxins, especially 2,3,7,8-tetrachlorodibenzo-*p*-dioxin (TCDD). It is not surprising, therefore, that all of the highly toxic PCB isomers approximate 2,3,7,8-TCDD in size and shape. Currently it is thought that both the dioxins and the toxic PCB isomers interact with a cytoplasmic receptor that in turn activates RNA synthesis in the nucleus and ultimately leads to the production of specific mono-oxygenase enzymes.[13] How this process of enzyme induction relates to specific pathologic changes is not known.

CLINICAL SIGNS

Acute or even chronic PCB intoxication is rare, and most problems confronting the veterinarian will be limited to residues. The clinical signs associated with PCB poisoning are similar to those in animals poisoned with 2,3,7,8-TCDD. General clinical signs in all livestock species include depressed weight gains and production performance, suppression of the immune system, and impaired reproductive performance.

Following dermal exposure to oil from back rubbers containing 60 to 70 per cent PCBs, cattle developed anorexia, shortness of breath, frothing at the mouth, increased thirst, diarrhea, evidence of abdominal pain, recumbency, and depression.[13]

Clinical signs of PCB poisoning in chickens and turkeys consist of edema, listlessness,[8] depressed growth rates, anemia, and decreased egg hatchability without affecting shell quality.[2,15]

Swine develop an increased susceptibility to respiratory infections and gastric disorders when maintained from weaning to market weight on diets containing PCBs at 20 ppm.[7] Sows fed diets containing 20 ppm of commercial PCB mixture (Aroclor 1242) during lactation farrowed significantly fewer pigs than control sows.[6]

Mink are the most sensitive of the domestic animals to the toxic effects of PCBs. Commercial mink ranches located around the Great Lakes provide approximately one third of the mink's diet from salmon caught from the lakes. Over the years that PCBs were marketed, the salmon accumulated these compounds to concentrations of 5 ppm. Mink that were exposed to PCBs at these concentrations in the diet were unable to reproduce or suffered a high incidence of kit mortality.[1]

PATHOLOGY

Gross lesions in cattle include hemorrhages on the serosa of the duodenum, ileum, and large intestine, and hyperemia of the mucosa of the gastrointestinal tract. Microscopic lesions include hemorrhages in the interstitial tissue of the renal medulla, moderate fatty changes of the liver, hemorrhages in muscular layers of the intestine, and inflammation of the mucosa of the intestine.[13]

Swine fed diets containing 20 ppm of PCBs from weaning to market weight developed erosions of the gastric mucosa and an increased incidence of pneumonia compared with control animals.[7] Germ-free pigs fed 12.5 to 100 ppm PCB (Aroclor 1254) in the diet developed enlarged, mottled livers, erosions of the gastric mucosa, hemorrhages through the mesentery and intestinal wall, fibrinous pericarditis, and thymic hypoplasia. Microscopic lesions included hepatic centrilobular necrosis, interstitial myocarditis, endocarditis, gastric erosions, and colitis.[10]

Sheep fed diets containing 20 ppm of PCBs from weaning to market weight were more susceptible to pneumonia than undosed control animals.[7]

Lesions in poultry include generalized edema, swollen hemorrhagic kidneys, hydropericardium, pericarditis, hepatic centrilobular necrosis, and marked tubular dilation and numerous casts in kidneys.[4,8]

RESIDUES

Residues are a far more serious consequence of PCB exposure than are the toxic effects. In the vast majority of exposure incidents, violative residues will be present without any signs of overt poisoning. In lactating cows fed up to 1000 mg PCBs/day (Aroclor 1254) for 60 days, no adverse health effects or effects on production were observed even though residues in milk fat approached 100 ppm, a value 67 times the official tolerance of 1.5 ppm.[17,18] Feeding young pigs a diet containing 250 ppm PCBs resulted in an increased rate of weight gain and produced no gross or microscopic lesions, yet PCB concentrations in adipose tissue reached values ranging from 100 to 200 ppm.[12]

Once exposure has occurred, the elimination of PCBs from the animal proceeds at a very slow rate. Continued exposure leads to accumulation of PCBs in body tissues, with the highest concentrations in adipose tissue. Once PCBs have distributed to fat, there are no mechanisms for their excretion unless the lipids themselves are mobilized into the circulation. Lipids may be mobilized under conditions of negative energy intake, lactation, or egg production. These three conditions lead to enhanced elimination of PCBs, but in the latter two cases result in residues in milk and eggs, respectively. Because adulterated feed is the most common source of PCBs, residue contamination may often extend throughout the entire herd or flock.

DIAGNOSIS

Exposure to PCBs rarely results in clinical toxicosis. Even when clinical signs are present, they are not sufficiently distinctive to allow a definitive diagnosis of PCB poisoning. More often PCB exposure is detected through routine food safety monitoring programs conducted by state or federal regulatory agencies.

If PCB exposure is suspected, samples of feed, silage, silo paint, stomach or rumen contents, liver, and adipose tissue should be sent to a laboratory for chemical analysis. If laboratory results confirm the presence of PCBs, it is important that the source of contamination be identified to prevent further exposure and to ascertain the extent of contamination to other animals. This may require assistance from federal, state, or local health officials.

TREATMENT

There is no specific treatment for PCB intoxication. Animals exhibiting clinical signs should receive supportive therapy, and efforts should be directed toward identifying and eliminating sources of PCBs.

Methods for enhancing the elimination of PCBs have focused on three separate pathways. These include preventing intestinal reabsorption by administration of oral adsorbents such as activated charcoal, enhancing the metabolism of absorbed PCBs by administering hepatic microsomal inducing agents such as phenobarbital, and mobilizing PCBs from adipose tissue reservoirs by restricting dietary intake. To date these methods have been largely unsuccessful. Feeding cows activated charcoal, phenobarbital, or both had little if any effect on the elimination of PCBs.[5] PCB depletion in laying hens was not affected by feeding a low-energy diet designed to mobilize body fat.[14] In most instances if residues are much above the tolerance level, it may be economically sound to destroy contaminated animals and dispose adulterated carcasses in a manner that will prevent environmental contamination.

REFERENCES

1. Aulerich RJ Ringer RK Seagran HL, Youatt WG: Effects of feeding Coho salmon and other Great Lakes fish on mink reproduction. Can J Zool 49:611–616, 1971.
2. Combs GF, Scott ML: The effects of polychlorinated biphenyls on birds. World's Poultry Science Journal 33:31–46, 1977.
3. Cordle F, Corneliussen P, Jelinek C, et al: Human exposure to polychlorinated biphenyls and polybrominated biphenyls. Environ Health Perspect 24:157–172, 1978.
4. Flick DF, O'Dell RG, Childs VA: Studies of chick edema disease 3. Similar symptoms produced by feeding chlorinated biphenyl. Poult Sci 44:1460, 1965.
5. Fries GF: Polychlorinated biphenyl residues in milk of environmentally and experimentally contaminated cows. Environ Health Perspect 1:55, 1972.
6. Hansen LG, Byerly CS, Metcalf RL, Bevill RF: Effect of a polychlorinated biphenyl mixture on swine reproduction and tissue residues. Am J Vet Res 36:23–26, 1975.
7. Hansen LG, Wilson DW, Teske RH: Effects on growing swine and sheep of two polychlorinated biphenyls. Am J Vet Res 37:1021–1024, 1976.
8. Holleman KA, Barnett BD, Wicker GW: Response of chicks and turkey poults to Aroclor 1242. Poult Sci 55:2354–2356, 1976.
9. Matthews HB, Anderson MW: Effect of chlorination on the distribution and excretion of polychlorinated biphenyls. Drug Metab Dispos 3:371–380, 1975.
10. Miniats OP, Platonow NS, Geissinger HD: Experimental polychlorinated biphenyl toxicosis in germfree pigs. Can J Comp Med 42:192–199, 1978.
11. Pichirallo J: PCB's: leaks of toxic substances raises issue of effects, regulation. Science 173:899–892, 1971.
12. Platonow NS, Meads EB, Liptrap RM, Lotz F: Effects of some commercial preparations of polychlorinated biphenyls in growing piglets. Can J Comp Med 40:421–428, 1976.
13. Robens J, Anthony HD: Polychlorinated biphenyl contamination of feeder cattle. J Am Vet Med Assoc 177:613, 1980.
14. Safe S: Polychlorinated biphenyls (PCBs) and polybrominated biphenyls (PBBs): biochemistry, toxicology, and mechanism of action. CRC Critical Reviews in Toxicology 13:319–395, 1984.
15. Scott ML, Zimmerman JR, Marinsky S, Mullenhoff PA: Effects of PCBs, DDT, and mercury compounds on egg production, hatchability and shell quality in chickens and Japanese quail. Poult Sci 54:350–368, 1975.
16. Skrentny RF, Hemken RW, Dorough HW: Silo sealants as a source of polychlorinated biphenyl (PCB) contamination of animal feed. Bull Environ Contam Toxicol 6:409–416, 1971.
17. Willett LB, Liu T-TY, Durst HI, et al: Productivity and health of Dairy cows fed polychlorinated biphenyls. J Anim Sci 61(Suppl 1):360, 1985.
18. Willett LB, Liu T-TY, Durst HI, et al: Health and productivity of Dairy cows fed polychlorinated biphenyls. Fundam Appl Toxicol 9:60–67, 1987.

Petroleum and Petroleum Products

LOYD D. ROWE, DVM
WILLIAM C. EDWARDS, DVM

The ingestion of crude oil or petroleum distillates occasionally causes illness or death in domestic ruminants. Cattle are involved more frequently than are sheep or goats. Carelessness in allowing ruminants free access to open containers of gasoline, kerosene, tractor fuel, or waste crankcase oil has resulted in incidents of poisoning. In certain areas of the United States, pollution of rangeland with petroleum hydrocarbons or other oil field wastes has commonly been associated with oil exploration, drilling, production, and transportation activities. Cases of petroleum hydrocarbon poisoning related to oil field activities commonly result from leaks in oil gathering or transporting systems. Ruptured pipelines can release large quantities of crude oil in a short period, causing significant pollution of pastures and water supplies. Similar incidents can result from accidents involving railroad or truck tank cars.

Cattle have been known to consume up to several gallons of crude oil at one time. The circumstances under which these animals ingest crude oil or other petroleum products are varied. It appears that ruminants ingest these materials when they are thirsty and water is not readily available, when petroleum or petroleum products contaminate normal sources of food or water, when seeking salt, or when grazing poor quality pasture. Ruminants are curious; feeder calves seemingly ingest petroleum to provide variety to their diet. Intoxication occurs most frequently and mortality is highest when accustomed water sources are contaminated.

Crude oil is a mixture of over 6000 different hydrocarbons and metals, and the composition varies with the reserve from which it is produced. Certain crude oils, the so-called "sour crudes," are high in sulfur and consequently have a telltale odor. In this parlance, crude oils low in sulfur are termed "sweet crudes." The toxicity of a crude oil or other petroleum hydrocarbon mixture appears to be related to its content of volatile hydrocarbon components and not to its content of sulfur. Upon exposure to the environment, the composition of crude oil undergoes rapid change by means of a process called "weathering." Weathering includes loss of volatile hydrocarbons through evaporation, leaching of water-soluble components, photochemical reactions, and microbial degradation. Since weathering reduces the concentration of volatile components, it appears to be an important factor in reducing the toxicity of crude oils.

The acute toxicity of a particular hydrocarbon mixture is determined primarily by its aspiration hazard and its irritant activity on pulmonary tissue. For crude oils, this correlates with the content of volatile components such as gasoline, naphtha, and kerosene. Hydrocarbon mixtures of high volatility and low viscosity appear to be more readily aspirated than their less volatile, more viscous counterparts. Aspiration may occur during ingestion, or abnormal eructation may introduce oil into an open glottis. The ability of an oil to induce bloat or vomiting may contribute to the likelihood that oil from the rumen will be aspirated. When aspirated, gasoline, naphtha, and kerosene produce tracheitis, bronchitis, and acute bronchopneumonia that is often fatal. Heavier petroleum hydrocarbons are less irritating and produce a more subacute lipoid pneumonia. Microorganisms carried into the lungs by the aspirated oil may be important to the final outcome. Animals aspirating relatively small amounts of oil may develop pulmonary abscesses, with death occurring after several weeks or months. The more volatile straight chain and aromatic hydrocarbons have an anesthetic-like action if absorbed systemically. The lighter petroleum distillates applied to the skin may cause irritation, thickening, and fissuring. Gasoline, naphtha, and kerosene are moderate dermal irritants. The irritant properties of gas oil, diesel oil, and fuel oil fractions are intermediate, while those of lubricating oils are slight.

CLINICAL SIGNS

Petroleum hydrocarbon poisoning in ruminants can involve the digestive, respiratory, and central nervous systems. In fatal cases, pneumonia due to the aspiration of liquid hydrocarbons into the lungs is the usual cause of death. Acute bloat may cause sudden death in some animals immediately following consumption of fresh, highly volatile crudes, gasoline, or naphtha. The production of bloat appears to be due, at least in part, to the rapid expansion of highly volatile hydrocarbons upon warming in the rumen. When aspiration does not occur, anorexia, decreased rumen motility, mild depression, and weight loss over a period of 1 to 2 weeks may be the only adverse effects observed despite the ingestion of large quantities (up to 40 ml/kg) of crude oil. Single oral doses of 200 ml of odorless kerosene or light petroleum solvent given to cattle caused no harm other than a reduction (40 to 90 per cent) in food intake over a 3- to 4-day period. In cases where cattle ingest substantial amounts of oil, regurgitation is common and oil may be seen on the lips and muzzle. Oily ingesta may be vomited after consumption of crude oils high in volatile components but is less likely with heavier fractions such as kerosene. Gross evidence of oil in the feces may not appear for several days after ingestion of oil. At this time the feces may become somewhat dry and formed if light fractions such as gasoline, naphtha, or kerosene are predominant. In contrast, consumption of a crude oil in which heavier lubricating distillates are predominant may result in catharsis. Clinical signs of pneumonia and possibly pleuritis may be seen in cattle that aspirate fresh, highly volatile crudes or volatile distillates. Signs in affected animals may include coughing; rapid, shallow respiration; increased heart rate; reluctance to move; holding the head in a low attitude; weakness; an oil-stained mucous nasal discharge; and a dehydrated appearance. Death usually occurs several days after ingestion. Respiratory signs following aspiration of heavier, less volatile crude oils may be limited to dyspnea shortly before death. Animals that survive the acute effects of aspiration may develop pulmonary abscesses. Such animals may gradually lose condition, walk stiffly with an arched back, and die after periods of up to several months.

Signs of central nervous system derangement have occurred in some cattle intoxicated with crude oil, condensate, diesel fuel, or kerosene. These signs included excitability, depression, shivering, head tremors, confusion, apparent visual disturbances, incoordination, mydriasis, prostration, and clonic-tonic convulsions. In experimental work, the appearance of abnormal nervous system signs was generally associated with the development of pneumonia, suggesting that systemic absorption of low molecular weight hydrocarbons took place from the lungs rather than directly from the digestive tract.

CLINICAL BIOCHEMISTRY AND HEMATOLOGY

Cattle may develop hypoglycemia 4 days or more after ingestion of crude oil or other petroleum distillates. Hypoglycemia may be due to prolonged anorexia, disruption of normal rumen function, or both. Hematologic changes are usually associated with the development of pneumonia and are indicative of mild to moderate hemoconcentration. These changes include increased packed cell volume and hemoglobin concentration. Blood urea nitrogen levels may also increase. The leukocyte response may be characterized by initial leukopenia (neutropenia, lymphopenia, and eosinopenia) followed over the next 2 to 3 days by a relative increase in neutrophils. The total leukocyte count may remain depressed, return to normal, or become moderately elevated.

PATHOLOGY

Lesions of foreign-body pneumonia are the most common finding at necropsy. These may be accompanied by localized pleuritis and even hydrothorax if light hydrocarbon materials such as gasoline, naphtha, or crude oil with a high content of these components has been aspirated. The distribution of pulmonary lesions is usually bilateral and includes the caudoventral apical, cardiac, cranioventral diaphragmatic, and intermediate lobes. The affected portions are usually dark red, consolidated, and, in animals surviving several days after aspiration, may contain multiple abscesses. Oil may not be visible in pulmonary tissue. Large encapsulated pulmonary abscesses may be found in cattle surviving up to several months following aspiration of oil. Reflux esophagitis characterized by linear ulcerations along the length of the organ and severe dermatitis below the anus were found in a fatally affected calf given kerosene (8 ml/kg/day) for 10 days. Oil may not be visible in the rumen of cattle that die more than 4 days after ingestion. Hepatopathy and renal tubular nephrosis have been reported in some cases of crude oil and refined petroleum hydrocarbon exposure.

DIAGNOSIS

The diagnosis of poisoning from oil field wastes can be one of the more difficult problems facing the veterinarian. A diagnosis cannot be made on circumstantial evidence alone. This is particularly true in cases involving generally poor performance. A potential for litigation exists whenever cattle in close proximity to drilling or production sites become ill or die. Such incidents may or may not be related to oil field operations. Many cases of suspected poisoning by oil field wastes turn out to be other disease or management problems. This emphasizes the need for thoroughness in the diagnostic investigation. The importance of a thorough clinical examination of exposed animals and a careful postmortem examination is obvious. When possible, sick, moribund, or recently deceased animals should be submitted to a veterinary diagnostic laboratory for pathologic examination and appropriate toxicologic tests.

In recently exposed animals, the presence of oil in lung, rumen contents, or fecal material may be suggested by its odor, or oil can sometimes be visualized by placing these materials in warm water, causing the oil to separate and collect at the surface. Specimens may be examined under ultraviolet light, as some petroleum hydrocarbons produce a yellow to yellow-green fluorescence under these conditions. Other compounds, including some drugs, also produce such fluorescence. Regardless of the perceived presence of petroleum odor or fluorescence, it is recommended that affected lung tissue, gastrointestinal contents, liver, kidney, and samples of the suspected source of exposure be submitted for more specific laboratory tests. Samples for laboratory analysis should be carefully protected from cross-contamination during necropsy as well as during transportation to the laboratory. Laboratory analysis should include an attempt to identify and quantify any petroleum hydrocarbon residues present and match them to the suspected source.

The finding of oil in the gastrointestinal tract does not necessarily justify a diagnosis of oil poisoning. Most oils are of low toxicity if not aspirated into the lungs. Positive chemical findings accompanied by appropriate clinical signs and lesions confirm a diagnosis of petroleum intoxication with a reasonable degree of diagnostic certainty. When investigating animal health problems in an oil field environment, one should keep in mind that poisonous materials other than petroleum hydrocarbons may be present, and that traumatic injury and electrocution are sometimes possible. Hazardous materials include explosives, lead-containing "pipe dope," lithium-containing lubricants, arsenicals, chromium compounds, organophosphate esters, and caustic acids and alkali. A wide variety of toxic and caustic chemicals are used in drilling muds. These potentially toxic compounds may become available to livestock when reserve or "sludge" pits overflow or are inadequately fenced. Salt water is a potential cause of poisoning in the oil field. Salt poisoning should be suspected when cattle are thought to have consumed brine from reserve pits or accidental salt-water spills. Cattle with an adequate supply of fresh water will usually not consume enough brine to induce salt toxicosis. Petroleum and salt-water ingestion seem to be more frequent in the winter months. This may be related to freezing of normal water supplies or accidental opening of valves to petroleum or salt-water storage tanks by cattle congregated around unfenced tank batteries for protection from cold winds. Death by drowning or exhaustion has occasionally occurred in livestock that have fallen into reserve pits.

Waste oils, such as used crankcase oil, may be hazardous to livestock owing more to the presence of toxic contaminants than to natural petroleum hydrocarbons. Waste oil may contain toxic combustion products, heavy metals, and various other toxic substances. Waste oils have, on occasion, been found to contain such highly toxic materials as tetrachlorodibenzodioxin (TCDD).

Diagnosis of illness in livestock exposed to petroleum hydrocarbons, salt water, or other oil field wastes that do not die acutely or from aspiration pneumonia can be problematic. Debilitating diseases such as parasitism or poor nutrition must be considered. Currently available experimental evidence indicates that ingestion of petroleum hydrocarbons once or daily for several days can cause short-term anorexia and weight loss, but generally does not induce chronic poor performance in cattle in the absence of lung damage due to aspiration of oil.

Prognosis hinges primarily on whether aspiration has occurred or will occur. Aspiration pneumonia does not usually respond well to treatment, and if it occurs prognosis is grave. Signs of aspiration may not appear for several days; therefore prognosis based on initial clinical findings may be misleading. Exposed animals should not be sent to market until the possibility of chemical residues in tissues that might constitute a public health hazard has passed.

TREATMENT

Recommendations for treatment of petroleum hydrocarbon ingestion in livestock based on controlled research are not available. Approaches to treatment presented in the following discussion are based on current knowledge of the pathogenesis of experimental crude oil and kerosene poisoning in cattle.

Animals developing potentially lethal bloat should be treated by passing a stomach tube and allowing the hydrocarbon vapors to escape. Use of a trocar should be avoided, if possible, because of the danger of peritonitis caused by seepage of liquid hydrocarbons into the peritoneal cavity.

In the absence of serious bloating, the primary objective of treatment should be to prevent aspiration of oil into the lungs. Subordinate objectives are to mitigate gastrointestinal dysfunction and limit systemic absorption. Rumen lavage via stomach tube is contraindicated because of the increased danger of aspiration of oil. Although not practical or economical in cases involving many animals, the most efficient means of reducing the danger of aspiration is removal of rumen contents via rumenotomy and replacement with rumen material from healthy animals. Cases involving prolonged anorexia may also respond to this procedure. Hypoglycemic animals should be treated with glucose intravenously, and dehydrated animals should be given appropriate fluid therapy.

When rumenotomy is not feasible, the careful administration of an activated charcoal slurry or vegetable oil (500 to 1000 ml) by nasogastric tube may reduce the hazard of aspiration by absorbing or increasing the viscosity, respectively, of the oil mixture in the rumen. A saline cathartic should be given to hasten evacuation of the gastrointestinal tract. Animals that consume only a small amount of petroleum hydrocarbons may respond to removal from the source of exposure and feeding of a good quality roughage such as alfalfa. Such animals should be monitored for several days for signs of respiratory involvement or rumen dysfunction.

Treatment of aspiration pneumonia is rarely effective. The administration of a broad-spectrum antibiotic for 7 to 10 days after aspiration may prevent or reduce the severity of infection in the lung. The use of anti-inflammatory agents such as dexamethasone in reducing chemical irritation to lung tissue is controversial. Steroid therapy in hydrocarbon aspiration pneumonia did not improve outcome in a double-blind controlled human study.

Prevention of oil poisoning can be accomplished only by assuring that animals do not gain access to petroleum hydrocarbons. Most cases involve human error or poor management decisions. Livestock should never be given free access to open containers holding petroleum products. Adequate fencing of animals away from oil field operations or other sources of oil should always be provided.

BIBLIOGRAPHY

Edwards WC: Toxicology of oil field wastes. Vet Clin North Am: Food Anim Pract 5:363–374, 1989.
Ellenhorn MJ, Barceloux DG: Medical Toxicology: Diagnosis and Treatment of Human Poisoning. New York, Elsevier, 1988, pp 940–947.
Gleason MN, Gosselin RE, Hodge HC, Smith RP: Clinical Toxicology of Commercial Products, Acute Poisoning. Baltimore, Williams & Wilkins, 1969, pp 132–137.
Ranger SF: A case of diesel oil poisoning in a ewe. Vet Rec 99:508–509, 1976.
Rowe LD, Dollahite JW, Camp BJ: Toxicity of two crude oils and kerosene to cattle. J Am Vet Med Assoc 162:61–66, 1973.

Coal Tar and Phenols

WILSON K. RUMBEIHA, BVM, PhD
FREDERICK W. OEHME, DVM, PhD

Cresols (phenolic compounds), crude creosote (composed of cresols, heavy oils, and anthracene), and pitch are the three classes of coal tar derivatives. These compounds are widely used for their antiseptic, herbicidal, or physical characteristics in lumber, agricultural, construction, and other industries. Because of their wide applications and their strong antiseptic properties, these compounds have been responsible for severe losses in the food animal industry, especially in swine and through residues in food products.

PHENOLS AND DERIVATIVES

Phenol is a highly reactive compound that has been widely used in the past as a disinfectant and antiseptic. Because of its high toxicity in humans and animals, however, it has been replaced by *phenolic derivatives*, which have retained the strong antiseptic properties but have reduced animal and human toxicity. Phenol and its congeners have broad-spectrum insecticidal, bactericidal, and herbicidal properties. In veterinary medicine, for example, they are being used as surgical scrubs (hexachlorophene, o-phenylphenol, and cresol). In the agricultural sector, dinitrophenol and dinitrocresol are used as herbicides. Pentachlorophenol (Penta) is widely used as a wood preservative, but other chlorophenols are also used for the same purpose.

Dinitrophenol and dinitrocresol are highly toxic to all classes of livestock. They are rapidly absorbed through the skin and lungs, and toxicity can occur if animals are accidentally sprayed or have immediate access to herbage that has recently been sprayed. These compounds markedly increase oxygen consumption and cause depletion of glycogen reserves. Clinically the affected animals have fever, dyspnea, acidosis, jaundice, tachycardia, and convulsions, followed by coma and death with a rapid onset of rigor mortis.

Pentachlorophenol-treated lumber used in farm construction, as well as sawdust and wood shavings from lumber treated with Penta, are sources of poisoning in food animals, including swine. Another possible source of exposure is the consumption of concentrates of these disinfectants. Besides the direct effects of Penta itself, Penta has been found to be contaminated with dieldrin, polychlorinated dibenzo-p-dioxins (PCDDs), and polychlorinated dibenzofurans, which have also been incriminated as toxicants.

Clinical Signs of Poisoning

Phenol is a highly corrosive contact poison. The oral median lethal dose (LD_{50}) in most domestic animals is between 100 and 500 mg/kg of body weight (BW). The fatal chronic dose for swine is between 27 and 55 mg/kg BW. Poisoning by phenol and Penta has been reported in swine, foals, and young cattle. In swine small doses stimulate the central nervous system and depress the heart, leading to vascular collapse. Stillbirths and early piglet mortality have been reported in sows kept in farrowing crates painted with Penta. Extensive necrosis of the skin around the abdomen and mammary glands have also been observed in sows kept in similarly treated farrowing pens. The baby pigs born of affected sows are dehydrated and exhibit burns on nostrils and tongues, and watery diarrhea is frequently observed. Experimental oral drenching with a Penta preservative in swine causes abdominal pain, retching and vomiting, central nervous system depression, and posterior paralysis. The phenolic compounds are rapidly absorbed by dermal contact, ingestion, or inhalation. Fetal death in utero presumably is caused by phenol absorbed through the skin of the dam. Piglets younger than 1 week of age are the most sensitive. Death in piglets born in farrowing houses painted with Penta appears to be caused by direct toxicity of Penta absorbed through the skin and also by the failure of the dam to nurse because of mammary irritation and wounds.

Necropsy lesions are consistent with the protein coagulative properties of phenolic compounds. There is extensive coagulative necrosis of the skin if exposure has been cutaneous. In case of oral exposure, there is catarrhal inflammation of the digestive tract. The carcass is icteric. Histopathologically, there is centrilobular necrosis of the liver. Subcapsular edema occurs in the kidney, and petechial to ecchymotic hemorrhages occur in the renal parenchyma.

COAL TAR AND PINE-TAR PITCH

These are polynuclear hydrocarbon residues left over after the coal tar distillation process. Clay pigeons, tar paper, creosote-treated wood, and bitumen-based flooring are typical sources of exposure, and animals are affected by directly chewing on these items. Swine are the most susceptible to creosote poisoning. For example, whereas only 3 brush applications of creosote to farrowing pens caused stillbirths in pigs, the LD_{50} of creosote in calves is 4 g/kg BW. Swine consuming 15 g of clay pigeons over a 5-day period will die. Floor slabs containing one third lignite pitch reduced growth rate in pigs by approximately 25%.

Clinical Signs of Poisoning

The first sign of pitch poisoning in swine is the finding of dead pigs. Other pigs are depressed, weak, ataxic, and icteric. Severely affected pigs progress to sternal recumbency, become comatose, and die. The acute nature of pitch poisoning results from the progressive destructive properties of the coal tar–pitch compounds on the liver, which results in an increase in fluids in the thoracic and abdominal cavities. Sudden death is often triggered by exertion. Rarely, a chronic illness characterized by anorexia, depression, weakness, rough hair coat, anemia, and icterus may affect several animals in the herd for several days before death. Affected animals have increased respiratory rates and incoordination and eventually experience sternal recumbency, dyspnea, coma, and death. Hyperkeratosis, stillbirths, and abortions are observed in sows and are partly induced by malabsorption of vitamin A and reduced storage of vitamin A in the liver because of liver injury. The prognosis of swine showing clinical signs is poor.

At necropsy, coal tar poisoning is characterized by a markedly swollen liver with a mottled appearance. The carcass is icteric with large quantities of fluid present in the peritoneal, pleural, and pericardial cavities. Histologically, there is centrilobular necrosis in the liver. In chronic cases the liver is fibrotic.

DIAGNOSIS OF COAL TAR AND PHENOL POISONING

The clinical signs attendant to poisoning by coal tar and phenolic derivatives are not pathognomonic. Therefore, a history of exposure to these compounds is an important part of the diagnosis. Animals that exhibit acute illness and death following exercise or those that are found dead, with others exhibiting muscular fasciculations and icterus with a history of exposure to phenolic compounds are highly indicative of poisoning by coal tar or phenolic compounds. Because of the corrosive nature of these compounds, coagulative necrosis of the skin or gastrointestinal tract is evident. Oral lesions induce hypersalivation and, in the case of the pig, vomiting. Animals are apprehensive, hyperactive, and ataxic, and panting is common. Advanced cases of poisoning are characterized by muscle fasciculations and cardiac arrhythmias, and some animals may be in shock. Histopathologic examination of the liver reveals centrilobular necrosis. Renal tubular degeneration and necrosis are apparent in the kidney. Confirmation of poisoning can be made by performing one of two simple tests available, as follows:

1. To 10.0 ml of urine add 1.0 ml of a 20% aqueous solution of ferric chloride. A purple color is positive.
2. To 10.0 ml of urine add 1–2 ml of Millon's reagent (10 g of mercury in 20.0 ml nitric acid). A red color is positive.

TREATMENT AND PREVENTION

Poisoning by phenolic compounds should be considered an emergency. There is no specific treatment for phenolic intoxications. In case of topical exposure, wash the skin with liquid dish-washing detergent and rinse thoroughly with copious amounts of water. Alternatively, dilute and remove topical phenols using polyethylene glycol or glycerol, if available. In case of oral exposure, give activated charcoal to bind unabsorbed toxicants. Follow up 2 hours later with a saline cathartic, such as magnesium sulfate, 0.2 to 2 g/kg BW. Avoid gastric lavage and emesis if severe upper gastrointestinal tract damage is present. Protect the liver and the kidney by giving N-acetylcysteine, 140 mg/kg BW loading dose, followed by 50 mg/kg BW intravenously every 12 hours for 5 doses. Vitamin A therapy is also recommended. Supportive treatment is vital and should include maintenance of normal body temperature and respiration and correction of acid-base and electrolyte imbalances. Treat any external wounds according to standard procedures.

BIBLIOGRAPHY

Cappock RW, Mouston MS, Lillie LE: The toxicology of detergents, bleaches, antiseptics and disinfectants in small animals. Vet Hum Toxicol 30:463–473, 1988.
Humphreys DJ: Tar derivatives. In Veterinary Toxicology, 3rd ed. London, Bailliere Tindall, 1988, pp 205–207.
Kore AM, Kiesche-Nesselrodt A: Toxicology of household cleaning products and disinfectants. Vet Clin North Am 20:525–538, 1990.
Liao JTF, Oehme FW: Literature reviews on phenolic compounds. 1. Phenol Vet Hum Toxicol 22:160–164, 1980.
Oehme FW: New information on the toxicity of phenolic compounds in small animals. Gaines Newer Knowledge About Dogs 21:8–15, 1971.

Zootoxins

MURRAY E. FOWLER, DVM

Zootoxicosis is a disease condition caused by the bite, sting, or ingestion of a venomous animal. Many species of snakes, arachnids, and insects have venomous bites or stings. Most lack sufficient potency to cause more than transient discomfort to livestock. Generally the incidence of toxicity is very low in food animals, although in certain local geographic areas the density of venomous snakes or insects may result in considerable loss.

The species listed in Tables 1 and 2 are capable of causing disease, death, or both in livestock animals in the United States.

Venoms are complex organic substances composed of a wide variety of chemicals, including enzymes, peptides, polypeptides, amines, glycoside anticoagulants, and, in the case of some ants, formic acid. Venoms may act locally, causing tissue necrosis, vascular thrombosis, and hemorrhage, or may be transported to other sites throughout the body, causing neurotoxicity and hemolysis. Venoms are also allergenic, making previously sensitized animals susceptible to anaphylactic shock.

Table 1. VENOMOUS ANIMALS CAUSING ZOOTOXICOSIS OF FOOD ANIMALS IN NORTH AMERICA

Snakes
Rattlesnake (Crotalus sp.)
Copperhead (Agkistrodon contortrix)
Cottonmouth (Agkistrodon piscivorus)

Arachnids
Black widow spider (Lactrodectus mactans)
Scorpion (Centuroides sp.)

SNAKES

It is impossible to describe precise clinical signs of poisonings from all the myriad types of venomous snakes found worldwide. The reader is directed to the literature for specific information on exotic species in a particular area of the world.[1, 4] Unfortunately it is not outside the realm of possibility for an animal to suffer a bite from an exotic species, such as the cobra in the United States, as such snakes have escaped from captivity or have been deliberately released into the wild.

Bites from copperheads and water moccasins are usually innocuous in livestock. Therefore this discussion is confined to the effects of rattlesnake bites.

Clinical Signs

Bites on the limbs cause erythema and marked edema at the injection site. Necrosis may result from the cytotoxic effects of venom, particularly that of the larger rattlesnakes. Based on reports of similar bites in humans, intense pain is associated with the swelling. Animals wince on palpation or manipulation of a swollen limb, which is a good clue that enables differentiation between snake bite and edema caused by venous stasis. Locomotion may be stiff and painful.

The exact site of envenomation is rarely visible. Shortly after the time of the bite, pronounced swelling will obliterate the marks of penetration. Bites on the head produce similar signs, with the added hazard of impaired breathing if swelling closes the nostrils. Death can result from occlusion of the airways. A bloodstained frothy discharge from the nostrils is common in bites on the muzzle. One or both eyes may be swollen shut, resulting in temporary blindness and inability to locate food.

Most North American rattlesnake venoms produce minimal neural signs. The Mojave green rattlesnake, Crotalus scutulatus, is an exception, injecting a potent neurotoxic venom. Cattle and sheep are grazed in the deserts inhabited by this snake, and bites may occur. Paralysis, convulsions, and death may ensue before local reactions become prominent. Diagnosis of such a bite would be extremely difficult without a satisfactory history.

Swine are not totally resistant to snake bite, but injection of the venom into subcutaneous fat diminishes absorption and severity of toxicity.[5]

Diagnosis

Differential diagnosis must include contusions and fractures of the head or limbs. Radiographs may be required. Abscess of the pharyngeal or parotid regions may cause venous stasis and edema of the head. Cellulitis from clostridial infections may mimic limb bites. Rattlesnakes are active only during warm seasons, so bites would likely be precluded during cold winter months.

Treatment

Rattlesnake bite in livestock is treated symptomatically. Immediate cool hydrotherapy minimizes edema of an affected limb. Once the swelling has formed, warm hydrotherapy may effectively stimulate circulation and removal of tissue fluids. Bites on the head and neck require more intensive therapy. A tracheotomy is necessary if airways become obstructed.

Antihistamines are contraindicated because their hypotensive action may be additive with that of the venom. Corticosteroids may be beneficial in reducing inflammation but are not required for successful management of a bite.

Table 2. POISONOUS INSECTS

Common Name	Scientific Name	Geographic Location
California harvester ant	Pogonomyrmex californicus	TX to UT and CA
Western harvester ant	P. occidentalis	KS, CO, WY, AZ, NV
Red harvester ant	P. barbatus	KS, LA to UT, CA
Red imported fire ant	Solenopsis invicta	Southeast, Southwest
Black imported fire ant	S. richteri	MS
Common fire ant	S. geminata	TX to SC, FL
Southern fire ant	S. xyloni	CA to SC, FL
Honey bee	Apis mellifera	Ubiquitous
African honey bee	A. mellifera adansonii	Mexico, South America
Hornets	Vespula sp.	Ubiquitous
Wasps	Polistes sp.	Ubiquitous
Striped blister beetle	Epicauta vittata	Midwest south to TX

Antivenin administration to livestock victims of snake bite in the western and northern sections of the United States is rarely warranted except for calves, lambs, or piglets. In most cases specific diagnosis is rarely made early enough for antivenin administration to be beneficial.

Bites of the large eastern diamondback rattlesnake, C. adamanteus, may be lethal to cattle, sheep, and goats. If an animal is observed being bitten by such a snake, it is advisable to administer specific antivenin* intravenously within 2 hours. From two to four vials should be given, and the patient should be monitored for 8 to 10 hours to determine if additional antivenin is needed.

If necrosis and sloughing of tissue begins, the necrotic tissue should be debrided followed by routine wound care. Parenteral antibiotics may be indicated if vital tissues, joints, tendons, or nerves are exposed.

SPIDERS AND SCORPIONS

Although animals are susceptible to the effects of spider and scorpion venoms, documented bites in livestock are rare.

INSECTS

Damage to livestock from poisonous insect bites is uncommon, but the hazard should be recognized. Stings from bees, wasps, hornets, and ants cause the same discomfort in animals as in humans.[7]

Insect venoms are allergenic, so multiple stings can be serious, especially if days or weeks elapse between envenomations. Sensitized animals may suffer anaphylaxis. Diagnosis is difficult if not impossible unless the sting and subsequent clinical signs are observed.

Occasionally an animal will become entrapped in an area where bees, wasps, or ants become enraged and descend upon the victim in large numbers, inflicting hundreds or thousands of stings. Such massive injections of venom may elicit a shock response, and death within minutes to hours may ensue, or a delayed response with signs similar to those of serum sickness may develop in 2 to 12 days.

In India, giant Indian bees, Apis dorsata, have killed water buffalo and even an elephant.[1] In the United States, individuals of all livestock species are potential victims of colonial wasp and bee attacks if an animal harasses the colony.

The African honey bee, A. mellifera adansonii, has spread to South America, where it is called the killer bee.[1–3, 7] In Brazil, 300 to 400 human deaths a year have been attributed to stinging by masses of this bee. Numerous livestock also have been killed. Killer bees have spread from South America northward through Central America and Mexico and are now within 150 miles of Texas. All control methods attempted have been ineffectual. Veterinarians may expect to see an increased prevalence of bee stings in livestock operations wherever this species appears.

The venom of killer bees is similar to that of the honey bee, A. mellifera. However, killer bees are much more aggressive than honey bees, making the hazard of serious envenomation greater.

STINGING ANTS

There are hundreds of species of ants. Some only bite, others only sting, and a third group both bites and stings.[2, 3] Livestock losses from multiple stings from the third group are recorded for a number of species (Table 2). The red imported fire ant, Solenopsis invicta (S. salvissima richteri), is indigenous to central Brazil but entered the United States in the 1940s and is now a serious pest throughout the southeastern states and west as far as Texas.[2, 3] Control methods have been unsuccessful in halting the spread of this pest, and suitable habitat for the species exists across the southern tier of states to California and northward into Nevada, Utah, Oklahoma, Arkansas, and Tennessee, and into New Jersey and New York on the East Coast.[2] The black imported fire ant, S. richteri, was identified in Alabama in 1918. It still exists in a limited pocket in northern Mississippi.

Species of fire ants native to the United States include the common fire ant, S. geminata, and the Southern fire ant, S. xyloni. These ants are local pests and may cause illness in debilitated or neonate animals.[2, 3]

Another group of ants, called harvester ants (Pogonomyrmex sp.) are pugnacious, vicious stingers and may cause mild envenomation.

Biology of the Ant

The red imported fire ant is the most important of the ants as far as livestock envenomation is concerned. Worker ants vary from 1.6 to 5.8 mm in length. Body color is red to reddish brown. The nonworking males and females are slightly larger.

There may be as many as 30 colonies per acre. The colonies are hard encrusted mounds between 25 and 65 cm in diameter and may contain 30,000 to 100,000 workers. Fire ants colonize pastures, corrals, and farmyards. Red imported fire ants eat roots, stems, buds, and fruits of plants. Seedling trees may be girdled. These ants are also predators of insects and debilitated or immobile mammals, birds, and reptiles. Healthy adult livestock are minimally affected, but neonates, juveniles, and

---

*Antivenin (Crotalidae) Polyvalent, available from Wyeth Laboratories, Marietta, PA 17547.

animals that are disabled and recumbent may be attacked and killed if in the vicinity of multiple colonies.

Fire ants bite and while grasping the victim arch the back and thrust the stinger into the skin, sometimes in multiple locations. The sting elicits an immediate sharp, painful sensation. Within a few minutes an urticarial wheal forms, which then transforms into a pustule.

The venom of the imported fire ant is unique among venoms in that it contains among other chemicals an alkaloid,[2] soltenopsin A. The venom produces a necrotoxic and hemolytic action. Though the venom of other species of fire ants is also potent, these species are less aggressive than the red ants.

Diagnosis

Single insect bites or stings produce local transient erythema, swelling, and pain. Without an adequate history, differential diagnosis must include contusions, foreign-body penetration, localized cellulitis, and urticaria. Differentiation of systemic effects include drug reactions and other shock-inducing conditions.

Treatment

Local treatment of single insect bites or stings is similar to that used for snake bites.

With multiple envenomation or severe reaction, injections of corticosteroids are indicated. Dexamethasone, 2 mg/kg every 4 hours intramuscularly or intravenously, will aid in diminishing inflammatory and allergic response. If shock or anaphylaxis occurs, quick administration of epinephrine 1:1000 in doses of 1 ml/50 kg body weight is indicated.

BLISTER BEETLES

The bodies of beetles of the genus *Epicauta* sp. contains variable amounts of cantharidin, a potent vesicating agent.[6,8] A change in agricultural practices now may result in the incorporation of dried beetles in hay in sufficient quantity to cause lethal poisoning if ingested. Blister beetles develop massive colonies in growing hay crops on which they feed (primarily alfalfa). In the past, mowing, drying, and baling techniques allowed the beetles to move out of the drying hay. Now the hay is cut, crimped, and swathed in a single operation to facilitate quick drying. A colony of beetles may be crushed and left to dry in a section of the hay, which is then incorporated into the bale. As little as 4 g of dried beetles may be lethal. Horses are most commonly poisoned, but in livestock, poisoning should be considered as well.[8]

Clinical signs vary with the dose ingested. Massive doses may cause shock and death within a few hours.[8] Lesser doses cause gastroenteritis and nephritis. Cantharidin produces an intense, direct irritation of the mucous membranes of the esophagus, stomach, and intestines. Excretion is via the kidneys, resulting in transfer of the irritant effect to the urinary tract.[8]

Altered clinical pathologic parameters include hypocalcemia, leukocytosis, elevated serum protein, blood urea nitrogen, and packed cell volume.[8] Other signs that may be observed include colic, dysuria, hematuria, diarrhea, incoordination, pulmonary edema, and dyspnea. The body temperature may elevate to 41.1°C (106°F).[8]

Lesions include vesication, erosions, and ulceration of the gastrointestinal tract. There is inflammation of the renal pelvis, urethra, and bladder mucosa.[8] Myocarditis is frequently observed, as are pulmonary edema, petechial hemorrhages of serosal surfaces, hepatomegaly, and splenomegaly.[8]

There is no specific treatment. General shock therapy is indicated, accompanied by correction of the hypocalcemia. Activated charcoal and mineral oil aid in protecting the intestinal mucosis if administered early in the onset of the disease.

REFERENCES

1. Caras R: Venomous Animals of the World. Englewood Cliffs, NJ, Prentice-Hall, 1974.
2. Ebeling W: Urban Entomology. Los Angeles, University of California, Division of Agricultural Sciences, 1975, pp 346–353.
3. Harwood RF, James MT: Entomology in Human and Animal Health, 7th ed. New York, Macmillan, 1979, pp 430–433.
4. Moore GM: Poisonous Snakes of the World. Washington, DC, United States Government Printing Office, NAVMED P-5099, 1966.
5. Oehme FW, Brown JF, Fowler ME: Toxins of animal origin. *In* Casarett LJ, Doull J (eds): Toxicology. New York, Macmillan, 1975.
6. Panciera RJ: Cantharidin (blister beetle) poisoning. *In* Mausmann RA, McAllister ES (eds): Equine Medicine and Surgery, Vol. 1, 3rd ed. Santa Barbara, CA, 1982, pp 203–204.
7. Rathmayer W: Hymenoptera: the aculeate wasps, ants and bees. *In* Grzimek B (ed): Grzimek's Animal Life Encyclopedia, Vol. 2: Insects. New York, Van Nostrand-Reinhold, 1975.
8. Schoeb TR, Panciera RJ: Pathology of blister beetle (*Epicauta*) poisoning in horses. Vet Pathol 16:18, 1979.

SECTION 7 ☐ ☐ ☐ ☐ ☐ ☐
Viruses, Chlamydiae, and Mycoplasmas

A. KONRAD EUGSTER, DVM, PhD, Consulting Editor

Diagnosis of Viral Diseases

ROBERT A. CRANDELL, DVM, BS, MPH

A laboratory diagnosis of a viral disease may not influence the course of treatment. However, an accurate diagnosis of disease is important for reasons other than therapeutic purposes. The demonstration of a virus as the etiologic agent may provide the necessary information to introduce control measures for preventing the recurrence or spread of the disease. This is especially true for those virus diseases for which specific vaccines are available. The discovery of new viral entities and the early recognition of foreign animal diseases are 2 very important reasons for establishing a definitive diagnosis. It is true that a diagnosis is in retrospect. The diagnostic report often reaches the clinician after the animal has either died or recovered; however, the constant vigil in the search for causes of new disease entities is paramount to the livestock industry. This fact was most vividly demonstrated recently with the introduction of African swine fever virus into the Western Hemisphere. It is essential that the clinician notify the appropriate veterinary authorities whenever a reportable or exotic disease is suspected.

Modern biotechnology is providing techniques for the development of more rapid and sensitive diagnostic tests. New immunodiagnostic tests are now available for detecting viral antigen in tissue and antibody in serum. Two of the more commonly used techniques are immunofluorescence and the enzyme-linked immunosorbent assay (ELISA). Although DNA/RNA probes have been developed as diagnostic aids for the detection of molecular subunits of the infecting viruses in body fluids and tissues, the conventional laboratory methods of virus isolation prevail in the diagnostic laboratory. Immunohistochemical techniques, such as the avidin biotin complex (ABC) method, are useful for demonstrating viral antigens in formalin-fixed paraffin-embedded tissues.

There are 3 basic approaches for obtaining a laboratory diagnosis of a viral infection. They are (1) examination of animal tissues for pathologic changes, (2) detection of viral antigen in tissues and body fluids, and (3) demonstration of the appearance of or rise in serum titer to a specific antigen during a recent disease.

Pathologic examinations include the examination of impression smears and histologic sections. In these procedures, the tissues are examined for pathologic changes.

The observation of characteristic pathologic lesions or the demonstration of typical inclusion bodies is of diagnostic value in some viral diseases. Some examples in which inclusion bodies are helpful in arriving at a diagnosis are canine distemper, rabies, herpesvirus, and animal and fowl pox infections. In conditions such as cytomegalic inclusion disease (inclusion body rhinitis) of swine, the diagnosis is generally dependent on the finding of large intranuclear inclusions. Bovine abortions due to infectious bovine rhinotracheitis are often recognized by their characteristic histopathologic lesions in the fetal tissues.

The technique of "smear diagnosis" is sometimes helpful in virus diseases associated with inclusion bodies. It has been advocated for diseases such as canine hepatitis (adenovirus) and avian laryngotracheitis. However, it has limited usefulness and is not routinely used. Because many inclusion bodies are transient in nature, they are either absent or sparse during the later stages of illness and will not be found. The recognition of specific viral inclusions in tissue smears is difficult and requires experience.

In certain virus diseases in which these methods are applied, it is desirable to confirm the findings by some other procedure. It is always advisable in doubtful cases to freeze some tissue at the time of necropsy for further study. If inclusions or lesions suggestive of a virus infection are found on histologic examination, the frozen tissue may be used for isolation or fluorescent antibody studies. On the other hand, if the diagnosis is obviously of nonviral origin, the material can be discarded.

The demonstration of rabies antigen in tissues by fluorescent staining has become widely used in veterinary diagnostic medicine. The fluorescent antibody test for rabies diagnosis is more sensitive than is the smear technique and compares very well with the results obtained by mouse inoculation. The antigen-antibody reaction is highly specific. The test is a visual observation of the localization of virus antigen in the tissues by its combination (reaction) with specific serum antibody labeled (conjugated) with fluorescein isothiocyanate.

Specific examples of other viral diseases in which the fluorescent antibody test is useful for detection of virus in clinical and necropsy material are calf rotavirus, infectious bovine rhinotracheitis, bovine respiratory syncytial virus, pseudorabies, and transmissible gastroenteritis.

The application of the electron microscope to the diagnosis of virus infections has advanced the art of diagnostic medicine. The visualization of virus particles in clinical and necropsy specimens has contributed greatly to the recognition of new disease entities and to the identification of many of the old ones. A diagnosis of pox infections can be made within an hour by electron microscopic examination of preparations of crusts from the lesions, whereas days are required by cell culture methods.

The isolation and identification of viruses is the most costly approach to diagnosis in terms of resources and time. However, it is the method of choice under the following circumstances: (1) in undescribed disease conditions in which the etiologic agent has not been demonstrated and grown in the laboratory, (2) in highly acute illness with early death, (3) in those diseases involving viruses of multiple antigenic subtypes, and (4) in all suspect cases of an exotic or foreign disease.

In the first situation, the initial isolation and propagation of the viral agent from a new disease entity is necessary before any serologic test is possible. Without the antigen (causative agent) and efficient means of producing it, a serologic procedure cannot be developed. In those illnesses resulting in an early death, there may be insufficient time for the development of a demonstrable specific antibody response. Therefore, the recovery of the agent from tissue or body fluids is the only means in making a diagnosis. Picornaviruses have been shown to exist in a multiplicity of antigenic types or subtypes in some species of animals (bovine and porcine). In these species, it is desirable at times to attempt virus isolation rather than to perform serologic tests against so many viruses. Also, it must be remembered that there is a limit to the number of serologic procedures that can be performed on 1 serum sample. This is particularly true in cases of the smaller animals, in which the quantity of serum is sometimes limited.

It is also advisable periodically to isolate viruses from animals with the more common known diseases. This offers an opportunity to conduct laboratory studies on the viruses in search of any biologic or antigenic alteration in current field strains. This knowledge is important, and particularly so, if vaccines are used in their control.

When clinical material is submitted for virus isolation, it is recommended that paired (acute and convalescent) sera be included if available. If a virus is recovered, the sera can then be tested for specific antibodies against the isolate. This is important in determining the role that the virus played in the disease. Animals, like humans, harbor many viruses that at times do not cause illness. The mere isolation of a virus from a clinical or pathologic specimen does not always constitute a definitive diagnosis.

Serologic procedures offer far greater usefulness in diagnostic medicine than do the other 2 approaches. Generally, serologic methods provide laboratory information faster and they are less expensive. However, serologic methods do not give the same degree of assurance of etiologic involvement. As stated earlier, serologic tests are limited to those diseases in which the causative agent has been isolated and can be successfully propagated. Serologic methods are not applicable in fatal infections in which there has been insufficient time for the development of specific antibody. Isolation of the etiologic agent is then the only means of obtaining a diagnosis.

Serum specimens must be paired because only a rise in specific antibody titer is positive evidence of current infection. The first sample should be collected as early as possible in the illness and the second from 2 to 4 weeks later during convalescence. Serologic tests now employed routinely for the diagnosis of common virus diseases are the serum neutralization, complement fixation, hemagglutination inhibition, latex agglutination, immunodiffusion, and indirect fluorescent antibody test. More recently, the enzyme-linked immunosorbent assay (ELISA) has become available for detecting antibody in animal serum. The companion tests for some pseudorabies vaccines are playing an important role in the eradication of pseudorabies.

The demonstration of antibodies in a single serum specimen is of little diagnostic value. It may be only an expression of the vaccination status of the animal or prior experience with the virus at an undetermined time. The occurrence of infectious bovine rhinotracheitis antibody in many bovine populations is reported to be very common. With a high prevalence of positive animals, it is mandatory that paired sera be required if meaningful laboratory results are to be obtained. Serologic data on single serum specimens are useful in providing information on disease incidence, herd infections, and distribution if they are interpreted with caution.

COLLECTION AND PREPARATION OF SPECIMENS

Specimens for Virus Isolation

Materials for isolation should be obtained in the early acute, febrile stage of illness. The choice of specimen is obviously the material that is most likely to contain the virus. Therefore, the source of material will depend on the nature of the clinical disease. For example, if the disease syndrome involves the respiratory system, nasal secretions would be the clinical specimen of choice. Because many animal viruses manifest themselves by producing diseases with varied clinical signs, it is necessary to obtain material according to the type of illness. This is particularly true with some enteroviruses and the viruses belonging to the herpesvirus group. Clinical and necropsy specimens should be collected with aseptic precautions, and sterile containers should be used. The usual clinical materials submitted include nasal, ocular, and vaginal swabs; blood; skin lesions; and feces.

A diagnosis for some virus diseases is best achieved by performing several diagnostic procedures. The recommended clinical and necropsy specimens for virus isolation, electron microscopy, and immunofluorescent staining are listed in Table 1. The table is intended to serve as a guide for the selection of specimens for virus diagnosis. The clinician should consult the diagnostic laboratory for more detailed information. It is also recommended that more than one animal be examined from an outbreak.

Swabs are obtained by using a sterile dry cotton swab to absorb the secretions from the conjunctival, nasal, oropharyngeal, or vaginal mucosa. Preferably, swabs should be immersed immediately into a tube containing about 1 to 2 ml of transport medium. The swab is rinsed in the medium, and the fluid is pressed out against the side of the collecting vessel. The fluid should be a balanced salt solution buffered near neutral pH and contain a protein that helps preserve the stability of the virus. Suggested transport fluid is Hanks' balanced salt solution with either 0.5 per cent gelatin, bovine serum albumin, or skim milk. If a transport medium is unavailable, place the cotton swab into a sterile blood-collecting tube and close with the rubber stopper. Material from skin lesions is also collected in a similar manner.

Feces (10 to 15 g) and necropsy specimens should be placed in a small wide-mouth hard glass jar or in a carton made of plastic or heavy waxed paper (Dixie cup) with a tight sealing lid. Although rectal swabs are not as effective as feces, they may be collected with a moist cotton swab and handled like the nasal swabs.

All specimens for virus isolation should be frozen if it takes more than a few hours to transport them to the laboratory. When delivered immediately, they should be kept on wet ice.

Table 1. RECOMMENDED SPECIMENS FOR VIRUS ISOLATION, ELECTRON MICROSCOPY, AND FLUORESCENT ANTIBODY TEST*

Anatomic Site or Type of Illness	Associated Virus	Clinical Specimen	Necropsy Specimen
Respiratory infections	Adenovirus	Nasal and ocular secretions, feces	Lung, feces
	Bovine virus diarrhea	Nasal secretions, whole blood	Lung, spleen
	Bovine respiratory syncytial virus	Nasal secretions	Lung
	Infectious bovine rhinotracheitis	Nasal and ocular secretions	Lung, tracheal swab
	Influenza	Nasal and ocular secretions	Lung, tracheal swab
	Parainfluenza	Nasal and ocular secretions	Lung, tracheal swab
	Pseudorabies (Aujeszky's)	Nasal secretions	Tonsil, lung, brain
Infections of mucous membranes and skin	Poxviruses	Lesion scrapings, biopsy	Lesions
	Mammillitis (herpesvirus)	Lesion scrapings, biopsy	Lesions
	Foot-and-mouth disease		
	Vesicular stomatitis	Vesicular fluid, epithelial covering of lesion	Vesicular fluid, epithelial covering of lesion
	Vesicular exanthema		
	Swine vesicular disease		
Infections of central nervous system	Enteroviruses	Nasal swab, feces	Tonsil, brain (swine); feces (cattle and swine)
	Infectious bovine rhinotracheitis	Nasal secretions	Brain, lung, tracheal swab
	Cache Valley virus	Blood	Heart blood of fetus or lamb (serology)
	Pseudorabies (Aujeszky's)	Nasal secretions, tonsillar swab	Brain, spinal cord (sheep and cattle); brain, tonsil (swine); liver, spleen
	Rabies	Skin biopsy of muzzle	Brain
Enteric infections	Bovine virus diarrhea	Blood, oral lesions, feces	Spleen, mesenteric nodes, intestinal mucosa, feces
	Enterovirus	Feces, oral-pharyngeal swab	Feces, tonsils
	Rinderpest	Blood	Spleen, mesenteric lymph nodes
	Transmissible gastroenteritis (TGE)	Feces, nasal secretions	Tonsils, jejunum, ileum, feces
	Rotaviruses	Feces	Feces
	Parvovirus	Feces	Feces
	Coronavirus	Feces	Feces
Hemorrhagic syndrome (viremia)	African swine fever	Blood	Spleen, liver, tonsil, lymph nodes, blood
	Hog cholera	Tonsil biopsy	Tonsil, spleen, liver, brain
	Bluetongue	Blood (heparinized)	Heart blood, spleen
Genital infections and abortions	Infectious bovine rhinotracheitis		Tissue from aborted fetus: liver, spleen, lung, brain, kidney
	Cache Valley virus		
	Enteroviruses	Vaginal secretions, serum from dam or sow	Body fluids for serology
	Bovine virus diarrhea		
	Pseudorabies (Aujeszky's)		Lung (mummified fetus)
	Parvovirus (swine)		Fetal heart blood, spleen, bone marrow
	Bluetongue		

*Serum should be collected at the same time clinical specimens are obtained and again in 2 to 3 weeks for serologic testing.

For longer periods of time, dry ice is recommended. The specimens must be in an airtight container because dry ice releases carbon dioxide gas, which is deleterious to most viruses.

Leak-proof stoppers or caps should be used on all jars and tubes. Cork stoppers should not be used unless they are paraffin-treated. Always secure the tops in place with several turns of a high-quality adhesive tape.

No preservatives or fixatives should be added to specimens for virus isolation.

Serum for Serologic Tests

Blood should be collected in a clean, sterile, dry tube or syringe without an anticoagulant. An adequate amount of serum can be obtained from 10 to 15 ml of whole blood. The larger quantity of serum is desirable to allow multiple tests, confirmation, or repetition of equivocal results. If bleeding is accomplished with a syringe, the needle should be removed before the blood is transferred to a sterile, dry tube. This precaution will reduce hemolysis. Rubber-stoppered Vacutainer tubes without an anticoagulant are recommended for large animals. The tube should stand at room temperature for at least 30 minutes (longer time may be desired) to allow time for the clot to form. The specimen is then refrigerated at 4° C (household refrigerator) to accelerate the contraction of the clot. The clot is separated by centrifugation at 1500 rpm for 10 minutes. The serum is carefully withdrawn from the clot with a sterile pipette. A rubber bulb attached to a Pasteur pipette is a very convenient means of removing the serum. The serum is transferred preferably to a sterile, rubber-stoppered tube. Screw-capped tubes are not recommended because leakage frequently occurs. If screw-capped tubes are used, the cap should be secured in place with adhesive tape. When a centrifuge and pipettes are not available, the clear serum can be removed from the clot by pouring into another sterile tube. It is recommended that the serum be separated from the clot before the serum is shipped to the laboratory.

The sterility and condition of serum for a serodiagnosis cannot be overemphasized. Serum specimens with a microbial contamination or hemolysis are unsatisfactory for testing. Because living cell cultures or animals are used in serum neutralization tests, any contamination of the serum will result in death of the host employed. Hemolysis of red blood cells in serum interferes with the complement fixation tests and should be avoided. Preservatives such as phenol or merthiolate should not be added because they are toxic to cell cultures. Whole blood intended for serologic testing should never be frozen.

PACKAGING AND SHIPPING OF SPECIMENS

Identification of Specimens

Each individual specimen tube or jar should be clearly identified with the animal's number, date of collection, and type of specimen. It is recommended that adhesive tape be used to label each container. All information should be either typewritten or printed with a lead pencil. Fountain pens, ballpoint pens, wax, or indelible pencils and markers should not be used to identify specimens. Markings made by these items become illegible through handling.

Packaging

Proper packaging not only ensures the safety of the specimens but also protects the mails and the personnel handling them.

Frozen specimens for virus isolation should be individually wrapped with an absorbent material such as cotton or paper towels. The wrapped specimens are then packed in a small cylindric shipping container, can, or any sturdy carton. The specimen package is then placed in the center of a larger insulated box next to dry ice. The specimen and dry ice are surrounded with about 15 cm of shock-resistant material (cotton, crumpled newspaper). It is important to have sufficient packing material to compensate for the loss of dry ice by evaporation. This will prevent the specimen from rattling freely in the package. Never ship dry ice in an airtight container.

It is recommended that serum samples for serologic tests be shipped under refrigeration. The tubes must be packed adequately to protect them against leakage or breakage. The specimens should be shipped by the most rapid means.

Shipping

If long distances are involved, the specimens should be sent by air mail. In cases of virus isolation specimens, it is recommended that the diagnostic laboratory be notified by telephone of the contents, carrier, and estimated time of arrival. Frozen specimens should never be shipped over weekends or holidays. It is desirable to have specimens arrive at the laboratory during the working day.

All specimens should be accompanied with the standard laboratory submission form. The history should be as complete as possible. Additional information such as the vaccination status of an animal is necessary in interpreting serologic results.

Consultation by telephone should be made to the laboratory, if any doubt exists in the type of specimen to collect or method of shipment.

Shipments should be identified as being "Perishable," "Biologic Material," "Packed in Dry Ice," "Protect from Extreme Heat," "Fragile," or any other suitable designation to help safeguard the contents and exposed persons.

When in doubt as to the mailability of any material, consult your local postmaster.

In addition to the mails, specimens may be shipped by United Parcel Service or bus transportation. If air transportation is used, the shipper must follow appropriate regulations.

BIBLIOGRAPHY

Acceptance of hazards, restricted, or perishable matter. Publication 51, January 1989, United States Postal Service, Washington, DC 20260–5361.

Viral Diseases of Cattle

Infectious Bovine Rhinotracheitis

ROBERT A. CRANDELL, DVM, BS, MPH

Infectious bovine rhinotracheitis was first recognized in the United States as an acute, febrile, highly contagious respiratory illness of cattle. The causative agent is a virus that is now known to be the cause of a variety of clinical syndromes. The respiratory disease produced by this virus is often called necrotic rhinitis and red nose. The genital infections are referred to as coital vesicular exanthema, infectious pustular vulvovaginitis, and infectious pustular balanoposthitis. The virus is responsible for severe economic losses to the cattle industry, and it has worldwide distribution.

ETIOLOGY

Infectious bovine rhinotracheitis (IBR) is caused by bovine herpesvirus 1 (BHV-1). Because the virus is also the cause of infectious pustular vulvovaginitis (IPV), it is sometimes referred to as IBR/IPV. All isolated IBR viruses belong to 1 serotype. Although they are serologically indistinguishable, the viruses produce a variety of clinical manifestations. Molecular studies on IBR isolates from various anatomic sites have shown that some differ in their DNA fingerprints. IBR virus is sensitive to lipid solvents, heat, and acid but persists for several days at 4° C and remains viable for years when it is frozen. The virus grows well in a large number of cell cultures, and with the exception of rabbits, it does not produce illness in the common laboratory animals and embryonating eggs.

EPIZOOTIOLOGY

IBR is recognized as the cause of 2 different diseases within 2 population groups of cattle. In areas where there is a high concentration of cattle, the most important disease involves the respiratory system, whereas in the less populated areas, the diseases of the reproductive system are more common.

IBR was first recognized in the United States as a respiratory disease of cattle in 1950. The disease occurred sporadically in feedlots, where it became known as red nose, dust pneumonia, and necrotic rhinotracheitis. The upper respiratory disease also occurred in dairy herds in epizootic proportions. Infections of the respiratory tract continue to be prevalent where large concentrations of dairy and beef cattle are assembled.

Clinical signs usually appear in feeder cattle 7 days to 2 weeks after they enter the feedlot. Virus shed from the ocular and nasal secretions is transmitted to susceptible cattle by direct contact. Feeder calves usually enter the feedlot at an age after they have lost their maternal (passive) antibody and are susceptible to infection. Additional insults from shipment, exposure to multiple infectious agents, and other stresses reduce their resistance to infection.

The reproductive form of the disease is transmitted primarily by coitus. Genital infections are more common in the conventionally managed European dairy and beef herds. The virus is shed in secretions of the reproductive organs.

After introduction into the Western feedlots, the virus adapted to the new host-environmental relationship by acquiring an affinity for the respiratory tract. Because the animal population of the feedlots is mostly steers and heifers that are reproductively inactive, the virus was probably unable to maintain itself as a genital type infection. Explosive outbreaks of infections of the genitalia have occurred by use of IBR virus–contaminated semen for artificial insemination.

Although cattle are considered to be the major reservoir of IBR infection, BHV-1–related herpesviruses have been isolated from goats, water buffalo, antelope, red deer, and wildebeest. Antibodies have been demonstrated in several wildlife species. BHV-1 has been isolated from pigs with clinical genital infections.

The virus can persist in the animal for years after an infection. These latent infections are potential sources for new outbreaks. Latent virus is reactivated with injections of corticosteroids that result in active shedding of infectious virus.

It is believed that stress from a number of causes may induce reactivation of the virus. New outbreaks in feedlots and closed herds may result from excretion of virus from a latent carrier. All seropositive animals should be considered potential carriers. The feature of latency in IBR infections presents a problem with the shipment and export of cattle to IBR-free areas.

CLINICAL FORMS AND SIGNS

IBR infections are manifested in a variety of clinical forms. The clinical diseases caused by the IBR virus can be grouped as (1) respiratory tract infections, (2) conjunctivitis, (3) genital tract infections and abortions, (4) central nervous system infection, (5) fatal generalized disease of neonatal calves, and (6) miscellaneous.

Respiratory Tract Infections

The respiratory disease was the first clinical manifestation of the IBR infection recognized in the United States and is the most common form of the disease. The respiratory illness has a sudden onset and is characterized by fever of 40° C to 41.5° C, salivation, rhinitis, loss of appetite, rapid and shallow respiration, and dyspnea. Dairy cattle experience an abrupt drop in milk production.

The nasal secretions are serous at first, and the nasal mucosa is hyperemic. In severe cases, the exudate becomes copious and fibrinopurulent and is loosely attached to the mucosal surface. Beneath the exudate, the mucosa is reddened and may contain necrotic foci. In advanced cases, the airways become blocked, which results in respiratory distress with open-mouth breathing.

Generally, auscultation reveals nothing more than the sounds due to obstruction of upper air passages. In field cases, pneumonia is a common complication, and rales become audible.

Conjunctivitis is not a consistent sign in the respiratory disease. When present, the ocular discharges become copious and purulent as the disease progresses.

The acute stage of illness lasts from 5 to 10 days, and most animals will recover between 10 and 14 days. The mortality rate is higher in the more stressed animal, and death is usually the result of a bacterial bronchopneumonia.

Conjunctivitis

Although a severe conjunctivitis with profuse lacrimation is common in the typical respiratory form of IBR infection, it may also occur as the primary clinical feature in some infections. The conjunctiva is inflamed and edematous, and the condition is usually bilateral. The ocular discharge is clear initially but becomes mucopurulent after bacterial involvement. The hair on the side of the face below the eyes becomes wet and soiled. Corneal opacities may occur and are often confused with other conditions, such as infectious keratitis.

Genital Tract Infections and Abortions

Infectious pustular vulvovaginitis is the name given to the infection of the vaginal and vulvar mucosa. This disease has been known in Europe since the mid-19th century as Blaschenausschlag. The infection in bulls is called balanoposthitis. Genital infection has occurred concurrently in herds with the respiratory form of the disease.

The acute infection develops within 1 to 3 days after coitus. The disease may be mild and unnoticed; however, in severe infections, animals exhibit pain, dysuria, and frequent urination, and tail swishing is common. The vulva is edematous and hyperemic, and the mucosal surface is covered with small pustules. These coalesce, forming white necrotic plaques that leave ulcers on removal from the mucosal surface. These changes extend into the vagina and are accompanied by a mucopurulent exudate. The lesions may heal in 10 to 14 days, but a vaginal discharge may persist in some animals for several weeks.

Lesions similar to those described for pustular vulvovaginitis develop on the mucosa of the penis and prepuce of infected bulls. Secondary infections are common with a mucopurulent discharge present at the preputial orifice. Semen becomes contaminated with virus from these lesions. In severe cases, extensive adhesions and penile distortion may occur.

Central Nervous System Infection

IBR virus has been isolated from the brains of fatal cases of nonpurulent meningoencephalitis in young calves. The disease has been described in both dairy and beef calves. The animals refuse to eat and exhibit intermittent generalized tremors with periods of excitement characterized by incoordinated movements, running, circling, and stumbling. These are followed by depression, recumbency, coma, and death.

Generalized Disease of Neonatal Calves

A fatal generalized infection occurs in neonatal calves that become infected in utero or early after birth. The temperature may exceed 40° C and is accompanied by complete anorexia, depression, and respiratory distress. A serous ocular discharge and diarrhea may be present. The condition is often associated with a herd experiencing abortions.

Miscellaneous

Infections of the udder and intestinal tract have been reported but seldom appear as a distinct clinical entity.

DIAGNOSIS

The clinical and pathologic features of the disease are helpful in obtaining a presumptive diagnosis. IBR should be considered in any sudden outbreak of an upper respiratory infection and in cases of vaginitis and abortions. The presence of white plaques on the mucosal surface of the nasal cavity and vagina is suggestive of IBR infection. A typical finding at necropsy is an inflamed trachea with a fibropurulent exudate loosely attached to the mucosal surface. Although intranuclear inclusion bodies are a characteristic feature of the herpesvirus infections, they are not a common histologic finding.

A definitive diagnosis can be obtained by laboratory procedures. The virus is easily isolated from a number of infected tissues by cell culture techniques. Clinical specimens selected for virus isolation should be collected during the febrile stage of illness. The type of specimen to collect is determined by the form of disease. Swabs containing ocular and nasal secretions are recommended in cases of conjunctivitis and respiratory forms of the disease. Vaginal and preputial swabs are the specimens of choice for diagnosing genital infections.

The fluorescent antibody technique is used to detect IBR virus in tissue from aborted fetuses and neonatal calves succumbing to a generalized infection. The liver, spleen, kidney, lung, and adrenals are the preferred tissues and are also used for virus isolation. Histopathologic examination of the fetal liver often reveals intranuclear inclusion bodies in epithelial cells surrounding areas of necrosis.

The central nervous system infections must be differentiated from lead poisoning and other infectious diseases such as pseudo-rabies, rabies, *Haemophilus somnus* septicemia, and listeriosis.

The serum neutralization test is the most commonly used serologic procedure to measure the specific IBR antibodies in the serum. Because a rise in the antibody titer is evidence of a recent infection, it is necessary to test paired serum samples. The first sample should be obtained during the acute stage of illness, and the second is collected 2 to 3 weeks later. Titers on single serum specimens are of no diagnostic significance.

A complete history is necessary for a meaningful interpretation of laboratory results.

TREATMENT

Because IBR is a virus infection, the therapy is directed toward controlling the secondary bacterial complications. The early administration of antibiotics with supportive therapy is recommended. Institute good husbandry practices to reduce and minimize stress. Isolate sick animals and provide shelter, food, and water. Results of recent studies indicate that the use of corticosteroids is contraindicated in the treatment of bronchopneumonia in cattle. *The administration of corticosteroids will reactivate latent IBR virus infections in cattle.*

PREVENTION AND CONTROL

Vaccines have played a major role in the prevention and control of IBR infections. Good management practices without vaccination have been relatively ineffective in preventing the spread of the virus to susceptible herds. The development of latent infections in recovered animals with virus shedding has contributed to the difficulty in preventing the introduction of the virus into clean herds. The isolation of severely infected cattle during an outbreak will, however, tend to limit the spread and severity of the disease within a herd.

Several types of effective vaccines are marketed. The parenteral modified live virus (MLV) is not recommended for use in pregnant animals. The intranasal MLV vaccines are reported to be safe for use in pregnant animals. Parenteral vaccines are considered by some to be easier to administer than the intranasal vaccines are because less animal restraint is required. The parenteral vaccines are available in combination with bovine virus diarrhea (BVD) and parainfluenza-3 (PI_3) viruses. Some IBR intranasal vaccines contain PI_3 virus.

An inactivated IBR vaccine is available as a single virus vaccine or in combination with other agents.

There are no licensed genetic engineered vaccines.

The vaccination program, selection of vaccine, and frequency of vaccination are usually determined by the local circumstances and the practitioner's experience. Although a few general recommendations concerning vaccinations have been made, the recommendation of the manufacturer on the package insert should be followed. It has been suggested that all breeding females be vaccinated between 5 and 6 months of age. If calves are vaccinated earlier, they should be revaccinated after 5 months but at least 1 month before breeding. Colostral acquired antibodies persist for about 5 months and will interfere with the effectiveness of the vaccine. Some preconditioning programs recommend that feeder calves be vaccinated at the time of weaning and at least 1 month before shipment. Unconditioned feeder calves are often vaccinated at the time of arrival at the feedlot. Although the practice of vaccinating cattle in the face of an outbreak is common, it can be hazardous. Vaccines are recommended for use in healthy animals. Vaccination of sick animals against IBR is an additional stress on the animals, particularly if the present illness is caused by another agent or is in combination with the IBR virus.

PUBLIC HEALTH CONSIDERATIONS

There is no known direct health hazard of IBR virus to humans.

BIBLIOGRAPHY

Kahrs RF: Infectious bovine rhinotracheitis: a review and update. J Am Vet Med Assoc 171:1055, 1977.
Kahrs RF: Infectious bovine rhinotracheitis. *In* Viral Disease of Cattle, 1st ed. Ames, IA, Iowa State University Press, 1981, p 135.
Pastoret PP, Thiry E, Brochier B, Derboven G: Bovid herpesvirus 1 infection of cattle: pathogenesis, latency, consequences of latency. Ann Rech Vet 13:211, 1982.

Bovine Mammillitis

W. B. MARTIN, PhD, DVSM, CIBiol, FIBiol, FRSE, MRCVS

Bovine mammillitis (bovine herpes or ulcerative mammillitis) is a disease of lactating cows caused by bovine herpesvirus 2 (BHV-2). The virus causes two distinct syndromes: ulcers on the teats and udders of lactating cows (mammillitis), and widespread nodules in the skin of cattle (pseudo–lumpy skin disease). In calves, ulcers occur on the nose and in the mouth.

EPIZOOTIOLOGY

Infection with BHV-2 has been recognized in Europe, Africa, Australia, New Zealand, and the United States. In temperate regions, bovine mammillitis is seen only in the autumn and early winter, generally in milking cows. The disease is not seen every year in any area, although occasionally severe outbreaks can occur locally on several farms. The method of spread between farms is not known, but it is possible that biting flies carry the virus mechanically between herds. Latent infection occurs, and it may be that susceptible pregnant cows get infected but only develop recognizable disease shortly after parturition. It has been postulated that changes in the hormonal and immune mechanisms at calving and reduced skin temperature may allow the virus to replicate with the development of overt disease.

Useful reference and review articles on this disease are available.[1-3]

CLINICAL SIGNS AND LESIONS

Primiparous heifers are often first affected. These develop lesions within a few days of calving. A succession of such cases can occur within the herd, and subsequently infection can spread to other cows.

Signs of general illness are usually absent. One or more teats develop lesions suddenly. The initial lesion is usually a firm, raised, oval plaque 1 to 2 cm in diameter in the wall of the teat. In another type of lesion, the skin over a large part of the teats and udder becomes discolored, hard, and inflexible. Vesicles, which are generally large and single, are seen infrequently.

Plaques on the teats rapidly break down to leave deep, ragged, painful ulcers (Fig. 1), whereas infected areas on the udder and perineum are more extensive but the ulceration is more superficial. Dark brown or black crusts, composed of serous exudate, blood, and necrotic skin, then cover the ulcers, beneath which healing occurs by granulation, with eventual regrowth of epithelium. Damage caused during milking slows down the healing process so that raw ulcers may be evident on the teats of individual cows for several weeks. Some cows may develop mastitis, which can result in the loss of one or more of the quarters.

In pseudo–lumpy skin disease, hard nodules (2 to 3 cm diameter) develop in the skin, particularly over the neck, thorax, and perineum. As on the teats, the skin covering the nodules becomes necrotic and, together with exudate, forms into hard, oval crusts that gradually separate from the skin as healing takes place. Regrowth of the hair takes time, so that hairless patches may be evident for months.

The main histologic changes produced by infection with BHV-2 are inflammation, hydropic degeneration, edema, and necrosis of the epidermis. Acidophilic or lightly basophilic intranuclear inclusion bodies and syncytia are present in the early lesions.

DIAGNOSIS

Herpetic lesions on the teats may be mistaken for traumatic injury or other infections such as foot-and-mouth disease or cowpox. The association with recent calving in those that are affected first and the seasonal incidence are helpful diagnostic factors. For laboratory confirmation of the viral cause, the fluid that exudes or can be expressed from the lesions should be collected into transport medium. Fragments of skin picked from the edge of the ulcers are also a useful source of virus. The dried scab material is generally unsatisfactory for virus isolation. Tissue for histologic examination is not readily obtained from teat lesions but is readily available from skin nodules in cases of pseudo–lumpy skin disease.

TREATMENT, PREVENTION, AND CONTROL

Treatment is generally palliative. Some antiviral substances have been shown to inhibit the replication of BHV-2 in cell cultures, of which the purine nucleoside 9-β-D-arabinofuranosyladenine (ara-A) would seem to be most active. Confirmed reports of their effectiveness in treating outbreaks of disease are awaited, however. No commercial vaccine is available for the control of herpes mammillitis.

Extra hygienic measures should be adopted to reduce the risk of spreading infection between cows or to the calves. If possible, affected cows should be milked last; milking machine teat clusters should be immersed in a halogen disinfectant between milking each cow; and after milking, teats should be dipped in an iodophore solution because this will inactivate any free herpesvirus and reduce secondary infection. Calves should not be fed milk from affected cows, nor should they be allowed to suck these cows.

Because the epidemiology of BHV-2 infection is not completely understood, no method of prevention can be recommended with certainty. Flies possibly transport the virus; therefore dry cows and heifers should be kept away from wooded areas, if possible, and treated periodically with insecticidal preparations.

PUBLIC HEALTH CONSIDERATIONS

There is no convincing evidence that BHV-2 will cause disease in humans.

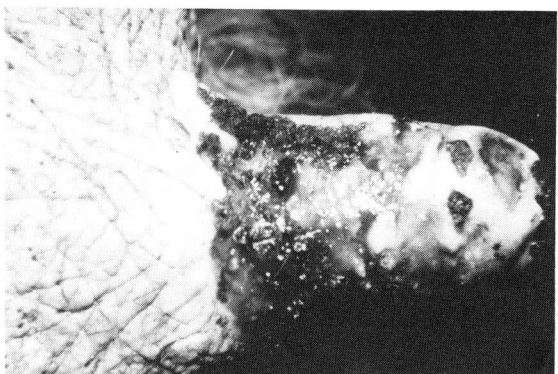

Figure 1. Severe teat lesions caused by bovine mammillitis virus.

REFERENCES

1. Cilli V, Castrucci G: Infection of cattle with bovine herpesvirus 2. Folia Vet Latina 6:1–44, 1976.
2. Gibbs EPJ, Rweyemamu MM: Bovine herpesvirus. Part II. Bovine herpesvirus 2 and 3. Vet Bull 47:411–425, 1977.
3. Martin WB: Bovine mammillitis virus. In Dinter Z, Morein B (eds): Virus Infections of Ruminants. Amsterdam, Elsevier Science Publishers B.V., 1990, pp 109–116.

Malignant Catarrhal Fever

ANTHONY E. CASTRO, DVM, PHD

Malignant catarrhal fever (MCF) has been described as a sporadic but highly fatal clinicopathologic condition of cattle. This viral disease of domesticated and exotic ruminant species has been characterized as a sheep-associated (European or American) form and as a wildebeest-derived (African) form. Recognition of the sheep-associated form of MCF has occurred worldwide, although the wildebeest-derived MCF is no longer limited to the African continent.

ETIOLOGY

The wildebeest-derived MCF is caused by a lymphotropic herpesvirus (Bovid herpesvirus, type 3), which is classified as a gamma herpesvirinae. This herpesvirus was initially isolated from a blue wildebeest in Africa by Plowright and associates. The herpesvirus of MCF has cubic symmetry (icosahedral) and is 100 to 240 nm in diameter, and the nucleocapsid is contained within an envelope. The herpesvirus is highly cell-associated and induces syncytia (i.e., multinucleated giant cells) with intranuclear (Cowdry type A) inclusion bodies. This virus has been classified as alcelaphine herpesvirus (AHV) 1 and 2, which are antigenically related but genetically distinct. Only 1 serotype is known. The prototype strain of AHV (WC11) and other known strains (16) are different from other bovine herpesviruses as determined by restriction endonuclease fingerprinting of their DNA. The alcelaphine herpesvirus is extremely susceptible to freezing, although it can remain viable within cells placed at 4° to 5° C for periods ranging to 30 days. Cell-free AHV is infectious; however, it is known to be shed in this form only by newborn wildebeest calves for a 3-month period. AHV can be propagated in cells of other nonruminant species after adaptation. An etiologic agent has not yet been identified for the sheep-associated form of MCF. Nevertheless, there is serologic evidence that sheep, goats, and individual cattle contain antibodies that react with AHV.

EPIZOOTIOLOGY

Worldwide, domestic cattle, buffaloes, bison, gaurs, greater kudus, deer, and antelope species have been reported to be affected by MCF. The incidence is generally sporadic, although epizootics of MCF, especially in cattle and red deer, have occurred. Mortality is usually 95 to 100 per cent after onset of clinical signs. In clinically ill animals, death usually occurs between 2 and 12 days after onset of pyrexia. The disease has no reference to age, sex, or breeds of cattle. The AHV has been experimentally adapted to rabbits. Wildebeest are carriers of AHV-1, and hartebeest and topi are known inapparent carriers of the AHV-2. In these alcelaphine species, induction of virus excretion has occurred after betamethasone injections. Sheep inoculated with the AHV have developed tumor-like masses, and malignant transformation of cells in vivo and in vitro may occur because MCF is a lymphoproliferative disease.

The AHV occurs in nasal and ocular secretions of young wildebeest in a cell-free state. Cattle, however, have cell-associated virus, but not cell-free virus, in secretions, and this may explain the noncontagious nature of MCF when contact occurs with MCF-affected cattle. The association of virus with whole blood has led to the experimental reproduction of MCF in cattle by intravenous inoculation of blood obtained from clinically ill ruminants. However, the means by which AHV is transmitted in nature is not completely understood. The method of transmission of sheep-associated MCF has yet to be determined but appears to occur during lambing. The etiologic agent of sheep-associated MCF is suspected to be a herpesvirus based on serologic finding, but the putative virus has not yet been isolated. However, there is a recent European report of an AHV isolation directly from a cow in contact with sheep which may prove to be the elusive herpesvirus of sheep-associated MCF.

CLINICAL SIGNS

Of the herpesviruses of cattle, only AHV is known to persist in a viremic stage for prolonged intervals. Clinical forms of MCF have been characterized as (1) peracute with generalized disease, (2) intestinal, (3) head and eye (most common), and (4) a catarrhal form with mild symptoms of catarrh (Figs. 1 to 3). The clinical signs of MCF include a high fever spike of 41° to 41.6° C at 16 to 18 days, an encrusted muzzle, a mucopurulent catarrh, inflammatory and degenerative lesions or erosions of the alimentary tract and also the respiratory tract with associated bronchopneumonia, ophthalmia with corneal opacity commencing at the limbus with eventual blindness, enlargement of lymph nodes, and diarrhea. The incubation period for wildebeest-derived MCF is between 2 and 8 weeks; however, the sheep-associated form may extend to 200 days.

DIAGNOSIS

The diagnosis of MCF is based on characteristic pathologic findings, ability to transmit disease by inoculation of blood into susceptible species, serologic conversion, and histopathologic evidence of a necrotizing vasculitis. The basic pathologic process includes a lymphoreticular cell proliferation in blood vessels of brain, kidney, and liver; angiitis and cell infiltration;

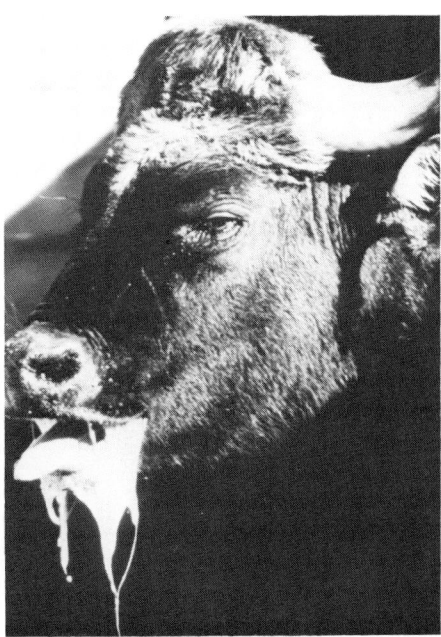

Figure 1. Mucopurulent catarrh associated with clinical malignant catarrhal fever in an Indian gaur (*Bos gaurus*). (Photographed by Dr. P. McCoy at the Oklahoma City Zoo.)

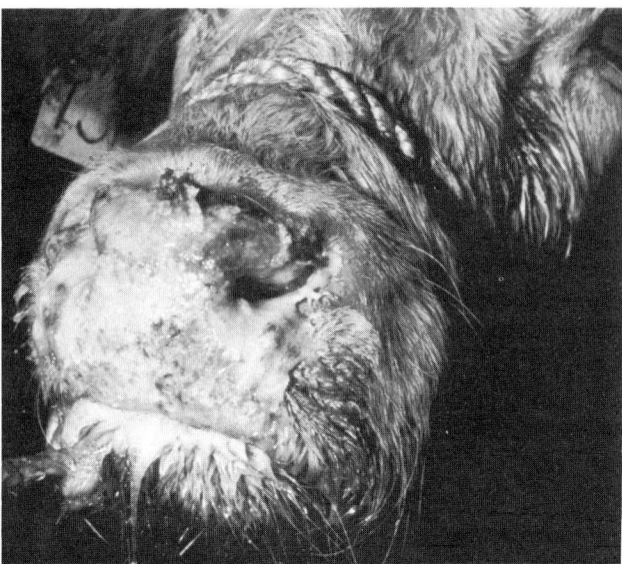

Figure 2. Mucopurulent catarrh and encrusted muzzle of a steer inoculated with alcepaphine herpesvirus (Oklahoma strain). (Courtesy of Dr. J. A. House, PIADC, New York.)

necrosis in paracortical areas of the lymph nodes; and a progressive destruction and associated dysfunction of thymic T cells.

Virus isolation can be accomplished from fresh buffy coat cells collected in heparinized blood and co-cultivated with cell cultures of fetal bovine kidney or thyroid cells. Identification of isolates of AHV can be made by immunofluorescent procedures or by serum-virus neutralization (SVN). By SVN, a serum titer of 1:4 or greater is indicative of exposure to AHV.

Differential diagnoses should include the mucosal disease complex, BVD-IBR, bluetongue, rinderpest, vesicular diseases (foot-and-mouth disease, vesicular stomatitis), Borna disease, salmonellosis, certain toxicoses (mycotoxins), and a wide variety of encephalitides of cattle. Because of the atypical cases that have been reported, laboratory diagnosis should be used for confirmation. An enzyme-linked immunosorbent assay (ELISA) for MCF that identified seropositive ruminants has been reported. Recently, several virus strains have been typed by restriction endonuclease analysis, and a cloned DNA probe to AHV has been developed that may prove useful in the examination of lymphocytes of clinically affected or carrier animals.

TREATMENT

An effective treatment for MCF has not been developed. Treatment with corticosteroids, although palliative, is contraindicated because of exacerbation of the clinical disease and possible abortion. Antibiotics and fluid therapy may prevent secondary clinical problems but will not prolong the life of a clinically ill animal. The AHV appears sensitive to bovine-derived interferons and, although costly, may be indicated in treatment of valuable breeding stock. Herpesvirus-inhibiting drugs (i.e., acyclovir, ganciclovir, or DHPG) have not yet been tested in animal hosts.

PREVENTION AND CONTROL

Presently, control procedures are not available except for the isolation of clinical cases (usually these are fatal). Although arthropod vectors could provide a mechanical transfer, there is no evidence that this is a mode of transmission. However, virus can be transmitted by common needles or during dehorning procedures. If sheep that are lambing are present, segregation from cattle should be considered. An experimental vaccine for MCF has had limited success. The cloned DNA probe described, which detects specific DNA sequences of AHV, offers the promise of detecting viral DNA sequences in AHV-infected cells of carrier species that can first be amplified by application of the polymerase chain reaction. Reports of tumor-like lesions in experimentally infected sheep, the fulminating septicemia-like disease, and the highly cell-associated nature of AHV indicate that clinically ill animals are unsuited for human or animal consumption. The known strains of AHV have not been shown to infect humans.

BIBLIOGRAPHY

Castro AE, Daley GG, Zimmer MA, et al: Malignant catarrhal fever in an Indian gaur and greater kudu: experimental transmission, isolation and identification of a herpesvirus. Am J Vet Res 43:5–11, 1982.
Heuschele WP, Castro AE: Malignant catarrhal fever. In Olsen RG, Krakowka S, Blakeslee JR (eds): Comparative Pathobiology of Viral Disease, vol 1. Boca Raton, FL, CRC Press, 1985, pp 115–125.
Plowright W: Malignant catarrhal fever. Rev Sci Tech Off Int Epiz 5:897–918, 1986.
Schuller W, Cerny-Reoterer S, Silber R: Evidence that the sheep associated form of malignant catarrhal fever is caused by a herpes virus. J Vet Med 337:447, 1990.
Shih LM, Zee YC, Castro AE: Comparison of genomes of malignant catarrhal fever–associated herpesviruses by restriction endonuclease analysis. Arch Virol 109:145–151, 1989.

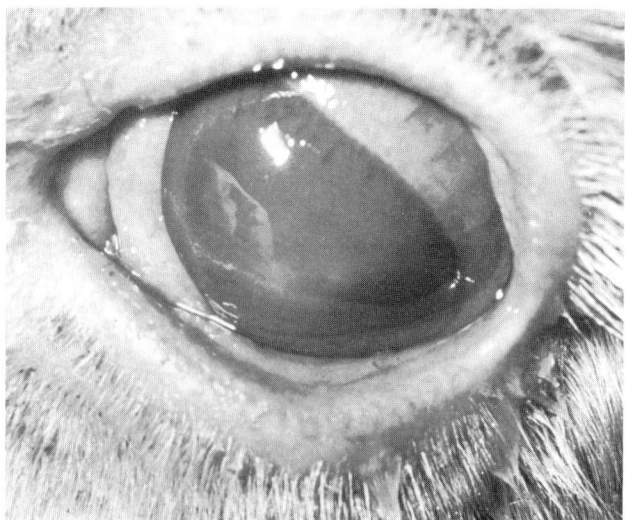

Figure 3. Characteristic corneal opacity in a steer inoculated with alcepaphine herpesvirus (Oklahoma strain). (Courtesy of Dr. J. A. House, PIADC, New York.)

Pseudorabies (Aujeszky's Disease, "Mad Itch")

ROBERT A. CRANDELL, DVM, BS, MPH

Pseudorabies is an infectious disease affecting many animal species including the domestic ruminants. In cattle, sheep, and goats, the disease is acute and is characterized by a severe local pruritus with a high mortality. The infected pig is the source of infection for ruminants.

ETIOLOGY

Pseudorabies is caused by a virus belonging to the herpesvirus group. The virus is relatively stable but is inactivated by 5 per cent phenol, sodium hypochlorite, 2 per cent sodium hydroxide, and quaternary ammonia.

EPIZOOTIOLOGY

The virus is transmitted to cattle through the nasal secretions and saliva of infected pigs. In the past, it was thought that infections in cattle and sheep were the result of direct contact with the pigs; however, results of investigations of natural infections indicate that these species can also become infected through the respiratory tract. The virus has been recovered from the nasal mucosa, lungs, brain, and spinal cord of cattle. Infections in cattle and other species have always been considered fatal. However, there is serologic evidence suggesting that some cattle have survived a pseudorabies infection.

CLINICAL SIGNS

Intense pruritus is the characteristic sign of illness in cattle. Recent observations indicate that not all cattle exposed by the respiratory route may exhibit pruritus. Some cattle will bloat and die acutely. Body temperatures of 40.5° to 41.5° C have been recorded. The duration of illness is usually short, lasting only 1 to 2 days. Infected animals will lick, bite, or rub the site of intense pruritus. Localized areas are frequently found on the head, chest, flank, perineum, and hindlegs. The animal often rubs the affected part so that an open wound is inflicted (Fig. 1). Infected cattle may not eat and often bellow and stomp their feet. The animals may show aggressiveness, a staggering gait, and partial paralysis of the hindquarters. Cattle, sheep, and goats of both sexes and of all ages and breeds are susceptible to infection. With a few exceptions, most infections in cattle are fatal.

The clinical syndrome in sheep and goats is similar to that observed in the disease of cattle.

DIAGNOSIS

Clinical pseudorabies infection in cattle is usually recognized by the intense localized pruritus. However, in some cattle infected by the oral and nasal route, pruritus was not a major clinical feature. If pruritus is present in the anterior portion of the animal, brain stem and spinal cord from the thoracic area should be collected for virus isolation. Brain and spinal cord from the lumbar region are preferred when pruritus and paralysis occur in the posterior part of the body. Lung and brain stem should also be submitted from those acute fatal cases without pruritus.

TREATMENT

There is no treatment that will reverse the course of illness after clinical signs appear.

PREVENTION AND CONTROL

Vaccination of cattle against pseudorabies has been reported from Europe; however, there are no vaccines available for cattle in the United States. For preventing the spread of pseudorabies infection to domestic ruminants, they should be removed from all contact with swine. Bovine pseudorabies has been associated with feral pigs; therefore, feral pigs should not be allowed to mingle with cattle or domestic pigs.

BIBLIOGRAPHY

Baker JC, Esser MB, Larson VL: Pseudorabies in a goat. J Am Vet Med Assoc 181:607, 1982.
Beasley VR, Crandell RA, Buck WB, et al: A clinical episode demonstrating variable characteristics of pseudorabies infection in cattle. Vet Res Commun 4:125–129, 1980.
Bitsch V: A study of outbreaks of Aujeszky's disease in cattle. 1. Virological and epidemiological findings. Acta Vet Scand 16:420–433, 1975.

Cowpox and Bovine Vaccinia Mammillitis

E. PAUL J. GIBBS, BVSc, PhD, FRCVS

Whereas cowpox was once regarded as an etiologic entity, a clinically indistinguishable teat infection can be caused by both cowpox and vaccinia viruses. Whether vaccinia virus developed from cowpox virus after Jenner's use of the virus as described in 1798 to protect people against smallpox has long been a source of controversy. Whatever the provenance of vaccinia virus, the 2 viruses can be easily differentiated by laboratory techniques. Although the mammillitis caused by these 2 viruses is identical, the different epidemiology of the 2 infections has necessitated a more exact taxonomy. The term *cowpox* is now used to denote an infection of the bovine teat skin by cowpox virus, and *bovine vaccinia mammillitis* refers to an infection with vaccinia virus.

EPIZOOTIOLOGY

Cowpox is only infrequently recorded and then only in Western Europe.[1] The epidemiology of the disease is unknown. Cowpox virus is occasionally isolated from skin infections in humans and carnivores, including domestic cats, when no direct contact with cattle can be established. In view of

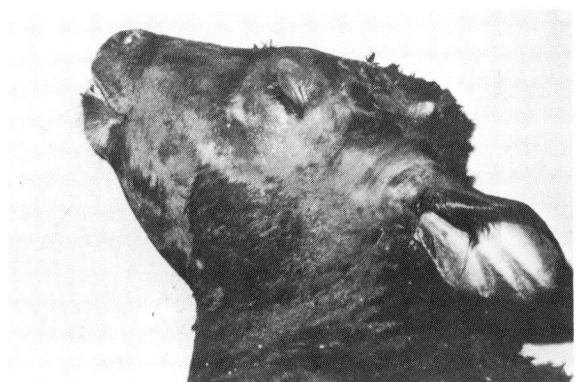

Figure 1. Pseudorabies in a calf. Note swelling and loss of hair about the left orbital region and base of ear.

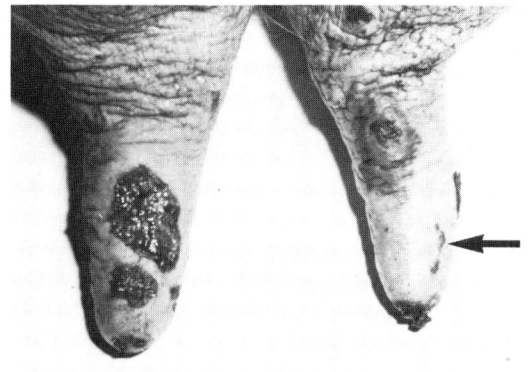

Figure 1. Ulcerated and scabbed lesions of cowpox approximately 1 week after onset of clinical signs. The arrow indicates a pseudocowpox lesion present as a second infection.

these observations, it has been suggested that a rodent or similar animal reservoir exists in which cowpox infection is probably subclinical.[2] Outbreaks of mammillitis associated with vaccinia virus have occurred throughout the world.[1] The source of infection of these outbreaks has invariably been the smallpox vaccination site of the farmer or a member of his family.* Because most countries have now discontinued vaccination against smallpox (as a result of the global eradication of this disease), outbreaks of bovine vaccinia mammillitis are unlikely to occur from this source. If recombinant vaccines based on vaccinia virus as a vector are ever licensed for human and veterinary use, it is possible, despite the reduced virulence of these recombinant vaccines, that clinical cases of bovine vaccinia mammillitis could reappear.

The method of transmission of vaccinia and cowpox viruses among cows has not been studied. The skin of the teats is normally resistant to infection unless abrasions or small wounds exist. These are, however, common in most herds, and the viruses are probably spread by the milking machine and the hands of attendants. Mechanical transmission of virus by biting insects has also been suggested.

CLINICAL SIGNS AND LESIONS

The incubation period is approximately 5 days, after which tenderness of the affected teats is noticed. Erythema with localized edema occurs at the site of future pock development, leading within 48 hours to the formation of a multiloculated vesicle. The vesicle rapidly progresses to a pustule that subsequently ruptures and suppurates. A thick red scab classically follows, but in milking cows, ulceration is common (Fig. 1). Healing is complete within 4 weeks. Lesions often affect all 4 teats and may extend to the skin of the udder.

DIAGNOSIS

The following points should be remembered (Table 1).[3]

1. Examine the whole herd, not only severely affected stock presented by the farmer. A comparison of the developmental stages helps considerably in the differentiation of the condition, and mature lesions are often similar regardless of cause. A close examination of herds obviously affected with bovine herpes mammillitis or cowpox often reveals pseudocowpox as a second viral infection. Teat warts are also present in most herds.

2. If vesicles are noticed on the teats, consider foot-and-mouth disease, vesicular stomatitis, and other reportable diseases.

3. Calves sucking cows affected with bovine herpes mammillitis, pseudocowpox, or cowpox may show similar muzzle or oral lesions. The infection associated with pseudocowpox is indistinguishable from bovine papular stomatitis. Note that a generalized skin disease can be caused by the virus of bovine herpes mammillitis.

4. A history of recent smallpox vaccination in the farmer's family may support the diagnosis of bovine vaccinia mammillitis. This is now unlikely because most countries do not allow vaccination. In the United States and Russia, however, military personnel are vaccinated against smallpox.

Laboratory confirmation of the clinical diagnosis is advised for cowpox and bovine vaccinia mammillitis because these infections constitute a danger to public health.

The collection and examination of samples for the laboratory diagnosis is discussed in the literature.[3]

In susceptible herds infected with cowpox or bovine vaccinia mammillitis, it may be up to 3 months before the herd is free of disease. Several animals may need to be slaughtered because of the subsequent bacterial mastitis.

TREATMENT

There are no specific antiviral drugs readily available for treating skin infections of the teat. Topical corticosteroids—

---

*Readers will note the subtle irony; they should also remember that the root for "vaccination" and "vaccinia" is *vacca*, Latin for cow.

Table 1. A SUMMARY OF THE DIFFERENTIAL DIAGNOSES OF COWPOX/BOVINE VACCINIA MAMMILLITIS, PSEUDOCOWPOX, AND BOVINE HERPES MAMMILLITIS

Feature	Cowpox/Bovine Vaccinia Mammillitis	Pseudocowpox	Bovine Herpes Mammillitis
Geographic distribution	Western Europe/worldwide	Worldwide	Worldwide
Seasonal incidence	None	None, but outbreaks more common in fall and spring	Summer and fall
Characteristic clinical appearance	Moderate edema; vesicles soon form pustules that subsequently rupture and scab or remain as large ulcers; lesions are essentially proliferative	No vesication; papules progress to scabs that are shed, leaving the pathognomonic lesions; lesions are essentially proliferative	Extensive edema and vesication giving rise to extensive ulcers that later scab; lesions are essentially ulcerative
Course of infection in the individual animal (uncomplicated)	3 to 4 weeks	6 weeks	3 to 4 weeks
Immunity	Probably lifelong	3 to 4 months, although some cows may be chronically infected	Probably lifelong; cattle may become virus carriers
Human infection	May give severe localized or generalized skin lesions	Localized skin lesions (milker's nodule)	Not recognized

in some cases combined with a local anesthetic and antibiotics—have been used to alleviate the pain associated with the early lesions of mammillitis, but their effectiveness has not been evaluated.

Once a teat lesion has become established, it is very difficult to avoid secondary bacterial infection. Response to treatment is often slow owing to repeated infection and the trauma of milking or suckling a calf.

Antibiotic creams often prove too expensive for herd use. Teat dipping as discussed later is simpler and probably as effective.

PREVENTION AND CONTROL

1. Quarantine and examine newly purchased cattle for 14 days before introduction to the milking herd.
2. Isolate infected cows or, if not possible, milk last.
3. Minimize risk of disease transmission by flies. Reduce fly population by improved husbandry and use of insecticides. Apply insect repellents to cattle, and incorporate teat dipping (after milking) into milking regimen. (Note that most teat dips are viricidal, particularly those that have a low pH; they are also repellant to insects.)
4. Minimize risk of infection by ensuring cattle have teats free of minor abrasions. Improve husbandry (e.g., avoid gateways that are excessively muddy; use teat dips that incorporate an emollient such as lanolin or glycerol to promote a supple teat skin).
5. Minimize transmission of virus by fomites. Disinfect the teat cups of the milking machine between cows. Make attendants wear rubber gloves, which should be disinfected regularly. Do not allow attendants to visit other herds.
6. Although vaccinia virus could be used for protection of cattle against cowpox and bovine vaccinia mammillitis, the infrequency of these infections precludes prophylactic use.

REFERENCES

1. Gibbs EPJ, Johnson RH, Collings DF: Cowpox in a dairy herd in the United Kingdom. Vet Rec 92:56–64, 1973.
2. Baxby D, Gaskell RM, Gaskell CJ, Bennet M: Ecology of orthopoxviruses and use of recombinant vaccinia vaccines. Lancet 2: 850–851, 1986.
3. Gibbs EPJ, Johnson RH, Osborne AD: The differential diagnosis of viral skin infections of the bovine teat. Vet Rec 87:602–609, 1970.

Pseudocowpox

E. PAUL J. GIBBS, BVSc, PhD, FRCVS

Pseudocowpox is caused by a poxvirus that is morphologically and serologically different from cowpox and vaccinia viruses. The virus is classified in the genus *Parapox* with the viruses of contagious pustular dermatitis (synonyms are "orf" and "contagious ecthyma") and bovine papular stomatitis.

EPIZOOTIOLOGY

The disease, which has in the past been referred to as false or spurious cowpox, varicella, waterpox, udderpox, and natural cowpox, occurs commonly in most countries of the world.[1]

Jenner[2] recognized the disease, but it was not until the 1960s that it was demonstrated to be distinct from cowpox.[3]

Lesions of pseudocowpox may be seen in herds at any time of the year, and there seems to be only a temporary immunity to reinfection (approximately 4 to 6 months).[1] In many herds, pseudocowpox is a chronic problem, and lesions are usually seen as relatively mild scabbing that causes little inconvenience. Cyclic waves of reinfection occur in these herds, often coinciding with inclement weather or calving of the majority of the herd. In completely susceptible herds, initial introduction of the virus may result in an acute infection that rapidly involves the majority of the herd. Severe lesions can also occur in susceptible stock introduced into chronically infected herds. Pseudocowpox also occurs in beef herds.

CLINICAL SIGNS AND LESIONS

The clinical appearance of pseudocowpox is extremely variable, possibly owing to the generally mild nature of the infection, the susceptibility of cattle to reinfection, and the influence of the environment. Initial acute lesions in a susceptible animal are associated with a painful localized edema and erythema with a thin film of exudate over the edematous area; vesicle formation is uncommon. Within 48 hours of onset of signs, a small papule develops, shortly followed by the formation of an elevated, small, dark red scab. The edges of the lesion then extend, and the center becomes umbilicated; at 1 week, the lesion measures approximately 1 cm in diameter. By 10 days, the central scab tends to desquamate, leaving a slightly raised scab commonly termed a ring or horseshoe scab that is pathognomonic for the disease (Fig. 1). One teat may have several such lesions that coalesce to form linear scabs. The majority of lesions desquamate by 6 weeks without leaving scars, although occasionally cattle develop chronic infection. Only rarely is ulceration noted.

DIAGNOSIS

The differentiation of pseudocowpox from other diseases of the skin of the teat has been discussed in the preceding article on cowpox. Pseudocowpox causes a mild skin lesion in humans commonly called milker's nodule.[4]

Pseudocowpox is a chronic problem in most herds, as

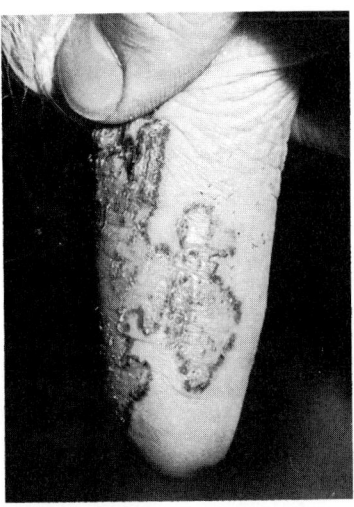

Figure 1. Extensive confluent "ring" scabs of pseudocowpox approximately 10 days after onset of clinical signs. This type of lesion appears to be pathognomonic for pseudocowpox.

mentioned previously. Good management will reduce the severity of the problem but will rarely eliminate it.

TREATMENT, PREVENTION, AND CONTROL

Treatment, prevention, and control of pseudocowpox are as discussed for cowpox in the preceding article.

REFERENCES

1. Gibbs EPJ, Osborne AD: Observations on the epidemiology of pseudocowpox in South West England and South Wales. Br Vet J 130:150–159, 1974.
2. Jenner E: An enquiry into the causes and effects of *Variolae vaccinae*, a disease discovered in some of the western counties of England particularly Gloucestershire and known by the name of cowpox. London, Sampson Low, 1798.
3. Moscovici C, Cohen EP, Sanders J, Delong SS: Isolation of a viral agent from pseudocowpox disease. Science 141:915–916, 1963.
4. Nagington J, Lauder IM, Smith JS: Bovine papular stomatitis, pseudocowpox and milker's nodules. Vet Rec 81:306–313, 1967.

Bovine Papular Stomatitis
ROBERT A. CRANDELL, DVM, BS, MPH

The disease bovine papular stomatitis (BPS) has been described throughout the world. It is caused by a virus that affects cattle of all ages and both sexes. Although this virus has been considered to be of little economic importance, significant economic losses have occurred in individual outbreaks. The disease is important in the differential diagnosis of any bovine disease causing oral lesions.

ETIOLOGY

The virus belongs to the genus *Parapoxvirus*, a large DNA-containing virus that is inactivated by lipid solvents. Although its relationship to other bovine poxviruses is not clear, some evidence suggests antigenic similarity. The virus has a limited host range. The common laboratory animals such as mice, rabbits, and embryonating eggs are resistant to infection.

EPIZOOTIOLOGY

Bovine papular stomatitis is a ubiquitous disease. It is believed that the natural host is limited to the bovine species; however, human infections do occur. The virus is shed in the nasal secretions and saliva, and it spreads from animal to animal by contact. The lesions contain infective virus; on inoculation into susceptible calves, the disease is produced.

Generally, this is a disease of high morbidity and low mortality. The severity of the illness and mortality is influenced by the presence of certain predisposing factors. Chemical toxicity, parasitism, nutritional deficiencies, and other infectious agents in combination with BPS have been associated with animal losses. The stress associated with movement of animals is also a predisposing factor. Clinical outbreaks of BPS have occurred in feeder animals after shipment to feedlots and in young animals after importation by air. In well-managed herds without predisposing factors, the disease may go unnoticed. Mild infections are often found only by careful examination of the animals.

The incidence of lesions in young cattle in infected herds ranges from 10 to 100 per cent. The disease occurs throughout the year without any particular relationship to seasons. Both dairy and beef cattle are affected, and there are no known differences in breed susceptibility. However, most reported cases have involved beef cattle. The disease occurs in all ages of cattle but is more severe in the very young calf.

The occurrence of clinical BPS after stress from shipment or other factors suggests that latent infections may exist. Because the disease is seen predominantly in younger animals, the cows are probably the source of infection.

CLINICAL FEATURES

BPS generally occurs as a mild disease without systemic signs. The disease may go undetected in many cases if the mouth is not examined. In the very young and in old, debilitated animals with complications, there may be a loss of appetite and excessive salivation. Clinical signs caused by other agents often confuse the clinical diagnosis of BPS.

The number and location of lesions vary considerably. The number of lesions in an animal may range from a single focus in one area to multiple lesions in different anatomic sites. The lesions are found chiefly on the muzzle, nostrils, lip, buccal papillae, dental pad, hard palate, soft palate, and lateral and ventral surface of the tongue. Although not common, lesions described as "wart-like" have occurred on the side, abdomen, rear legs, and scrotum and prepuce of bulls. The pox lesions become infected with bacteria and have an offensive odor. At necropsy, lesions may be found on the mucosa of the esophagus (Fig. 1) and in the omasum, rumen, and reticulum, particularly in young animals. The most common lesion appears as a reddened focus that develops rapidly into a raised papule. The papule is either circular or oblong and hyperemic. The papule increases in size, and central necrosis occurs (Fig. 2). The center becomes white and roughened, and the lesion is surrounded by a hyperemic border. The lesions persist from a few days to several weeks. The lesions finally regress, leaving a red-brown discoloration of the tissue. The lesions of the

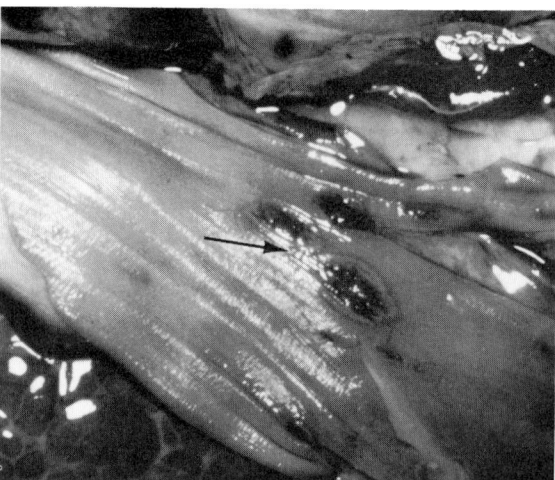

Figure 1. Erosions (*arrow*) on the mucosal surface of the esophagus of a calf with bovine papular stomatitis. (From Crandell RA, Gosser HS: J Am Vet Med Assoc 165:282, 1974. Courtesy of the Journal of the American Veterinary Medical Association.)

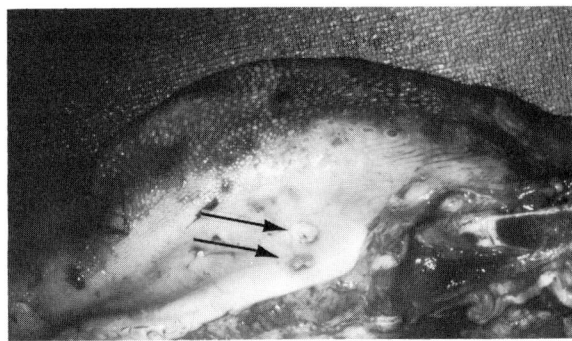

Figure 2. Lesions (*arrows*) on the tongue of a cow with bovine papular stomatitis.

hard palate follow the palatine ridges. Large circular lesions characterized by raised edges and necrotic centers surrounded by concentric colored rings are common on the soft palate. Vesiculation is not a feature of the lesion.

The course of the disease runs from a few days to several months, and the outcome varies. Recurrence of lesions is a common feature of this disease. The immune response measured by the serum neutralization test is low and of short duration.

DIAGNOSIS

Virus isolation, histopathology, and electron microscopy are useful laboratory procedures for diagnosis of this disease. The virus has been isolated in cell culture from oral secretions and biopsy and necropsy specimens. The virus has been demonstrated in skin scrapings of bovine lesions and from necropsy material by electron microscopy techniques. The characteristic feature observed during histopathologic examination is the presence of cytoplasmic inclusion bodies in the cytoplasm in areas of hydropic degeneration.

The presence of systemic lesions with oral lesions may confuse the clinical diagnosis. Several infectious diseases that exhibit oral lesions need to be considered in the differential diagnosis. They are malignant catarrhal fever, bovine virus diarrhea, foot-and-mouth disease, rinderpest, vesicular stomatitis, and mycotic stomatitis.

PREVENTION AND CONTROL

There are no vaccines available for preventive measures. Although the disease occurs in well-managed herds, the losses are minimal. Good nutrition and freedom from parasites and unnecessary stress factors are recommended.

TREATMENT

The lesions in calves with mild infections will regress spontaneously without treatment. In the more severe cases in which mixed infections are common, good husbandry is important. Antibiotic therapy is recommended to reduce secondary infections.

PUBLIC HEALTH CONSIDERATIONS

Humans acquire the infection by handling infected cattle. The virus from the oral lesions contaminates the nasal and oral secretions. The most common sites of infection for humans are on the arms and hands. The virus enters the exposed skin through a cut, bite, or scratch. Lesions appear at the site of entrance within 3 to 6 days after exposure. The lesion in humans follows a course similar to that in cattle, and on histologic examination the lesions are identical. Regression is complete within 3 to 4 weeks without treatment.

BIBLIOGRAPHY

Carson CA, Kerr KM: Bovine papular stomatitis with apparent transmission to man. J Am Vet Med Assoc 151:183, 1967.
Crandell RA, Gosser HS: Ulcerative esophagitis associated with poxvirus infection in a calf. J Am Vet Med Assoc 165:282, 1974.
Griesemer RA, Cole CR: Bovine papular stomatitis. 1. Recognition in the United States. J Am Vet Med Assoc 137:404, 1960.

Lumpy Skin Disease
CELESTINE O. NJOKU, DVM, PhD, FRVCS

Lumpy skin disease (LSD), a highly infectious viral disease of cattle and buffalo, is characterized by poxlike intracutaneous firm nodules varying in size from 0.5 to 5 cm in diameter, edema of the limbs, superficial lymph node swelling, and lymphangitis.

ETIOLOGY

LSD is caused by a virus immunologically related to sheep and goat poxviruses (capripox). By means of tissue culture techniques, 3 distinct groups of cytopathic agents associated with LSD have been isolated.

Group I (BZD) viruses or "orphan viruses," isolated from the skin of some clinically normal cattle and from the suspensions of skin nodules or lymph nodules of LSD cattle, apparently produce no signs of the disease.

Group II (Allerton) virus, recovered from skin nodules, saliva, nasal secretions, and semen of affected cattle, produces a mild form of LSD. The virus is pathogenic for cattle by the intradermal, intravenous, and subcutaneous routes of inoculation of lesion suspensions or infected tissue culture fluids.

Group III (Neethling) virus, isolated from the blood, saliva, semen, and nasal mucus (but not from the urine or feces) of infected cattle, is the cause of LSD in cattle. It persists in the skin nodules for about 33 days and has been isolated and propagated in lamb testis and lamb kidney cell cultures.

EPIZOOTIOLOGY

LSD is mainly a disease of cattle and buffalo and seems to be restricted to the African continent, although a similar disease was observed in herds of cattle in Iowa. Since LSD was reported in Northern Rhodesia (now Zambia) in 1929, it has spread to many other African countries including Botswana (1943); Republic of South Africa (1944); Southern Rhodesia, now Zimbabwe (1945); Swaziland, Basutoland, and Mozambique (1946); Malagasy Republic (1954); Zaire (1955); Kenya (1957); Uganda (1958); Rwanda, Burundi, Angola, South West Africa (now Namibia), and Cameroun (1960); Sudan (1971); Niger (1973); and Nigeria (1974).

The mode of transmission is still controversial because the disease had been reported to spread where direct or indirect contact between the infected and susceptible animals could be excluded. Even quarantine measures have failed to prevent the disease. Its rapid spread and the ease with which it traverses long distances suggest insect vectors, such as mosquitoes, arthropods, birds, and fomites. The concept of insect transmission has been buttressed by the isolation of the virus from *Biomyia fasciata* and *Stomoxys calcitrans* caught on cattle with LSD. Other suggested means of transmission are by ingestion of feed contaminated with saliva from LSD cattle and by suckling of milk from infected cows.

The disease has been experimentally transmitted by injection of infective blood (collected before the eruption of nodules) or emulsified nodules into susceptible cattle.

CLINICAL SIGNS AND LESIONS

The appearance of nodules in the skin and other body systems like the digestive, respiratory, and reproductive tracts occurs after an initial viremia and fever.

The incubation period is 2 to 5 weeks in natural infection and 4 to 14 days in experimentally induced infection. Morbidity rates range between 80 and 90 per cent, and mortality rates are usually due to secondary bacterial infection.

The first clinical sign observed is a diphasic fever reaching 41 °C. The cutaneous eruption follows the second phase in about 7 to 10 days. These nodules measure about 0.5 to 5 cm and rarely 10 cm in diameter and may affect the entire surface or any part of the body, especially the neck, brisket, back, thighs, legs, perineum, udder, and scrotum. In long-haired animals or in hairy parts of the body, the smaller nodules may not be very obvious. On the other hand, the hair over the large nodules stands erect, thereby exaggerating their size and appearance. Nodules on the muzzle, vulva, prepuce, nostrils, eyes, and mouth tend to be softer and rupture easily, leaving erosions and ulcers. Oral lesions cause increased salivation, those in the respiratory tract cause dyspnea due to occlusion, and those in the reproductive tract cause pain during copulation. Conjunctivitis and keratitis are observed at times.

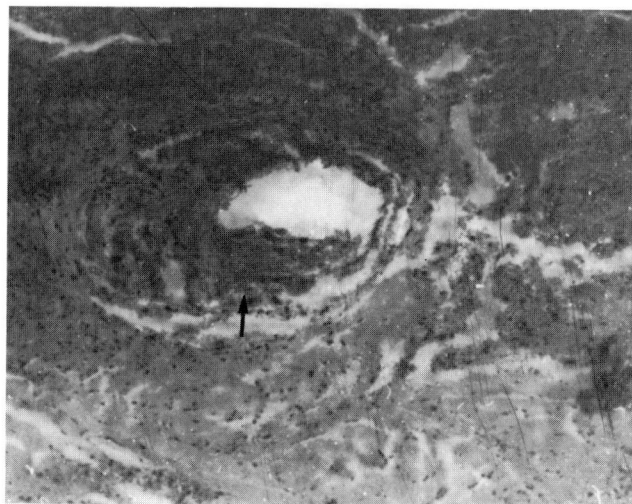

Figure 2. Blood vessel with thrombus (*arrow*).

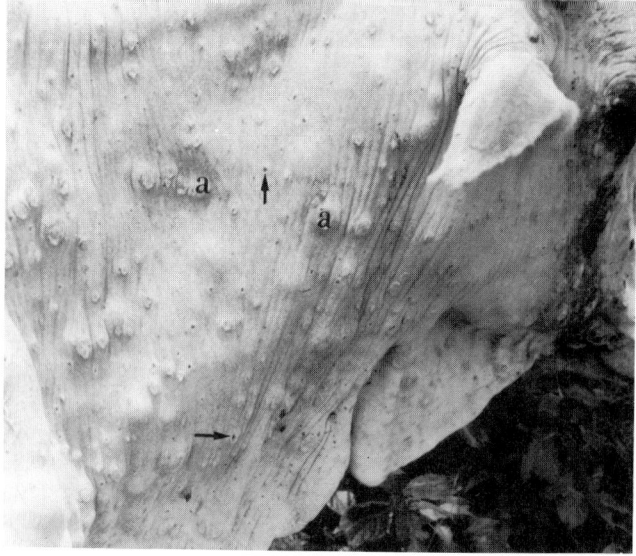

Figure 1. Lumpy skin disease. Cow with skin nodules of varying sizes and necrotic surfaces or "sit fasts" (*a*) resulting in craters (*arrows*) after shedding.

Induration of the skin nodules, which may persist for months, can occur, but usually these lesions undergo necrosis. A narrow (2 to 4 mm wide) groove or "moat" forms around the upper part of the lesion, separating it from the fairly normal skin. This forms a "sit fast" that is eventually shed, leaving behind craters of varying depths and sizes (Fig. 1). These craters could serve as portals for secondary bacterial infection, with resultant metastatic abscesses in the regional lymph nodes, lungs, and other organs. In other cases, scar formation is evident.

Palpable swelling of the superficial lymph nodes (especially the prescapular, precrural, and parotid) and thickening of the lymphatics may occur. In some cases, slight or marked edematous swellings of the limbs, dewlap, udder, vulva, scrotum, and prepuce may occur.

Apart from the cutaneous lesions already described, those of the alimentary and respiratory systems are usually covered by necrotic or ulcerated epithelium. The pulmonary lesions lead to edema and purulent pneumonia. Extensive granulation and cicatrization follow the development of the lesions in the trachea. A generalized lymphadenitis characterized by swelling and edema of the glands is a constant feature.

The microscopic changes in the disease involve the mesodermal tissues of the stratum papillaris, reticularis, and subcutis and then the surface epithelia, hair follicles, and associated glands. Below the epithelium, the early lesions include varying degrees of edema, fibroplasia, and perivascular cuffing with mononuclear cells (macrophages, lymphocytes, plasma cells) and some neutrophils and eosinophils. The macrophages contain intracytoplasmic inclusion bodies. These cuffed vessels are usually thrombosed (Fig. 2), possibly resulting in the overlying necrotic "sit fast" (Fig. 3).

The epidermal cells and sebaceous gland epithelial cells develop increased acidophilia, and many contain large cytoplasmic vacuoles with inclusion bodies. The vacuoles may coalesce to form microvesiculation.

DIAGNOSIS

Diagnosis of LSD can be made on the basis of the appearance of characteristic skin lesions. However, it may be confused with urticaria, dermatophilosis, besnoitiosis, severe tick and insect bites, demodectic mange, and pseudo–lumpy skin disease. LSD may coexist with any of these diseases.

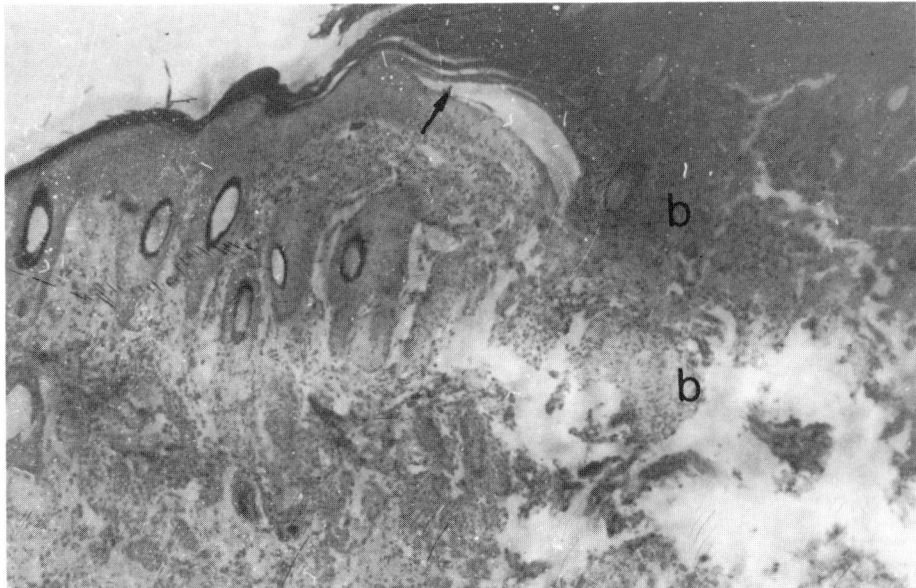

Figure 3. "Sit fast" or sequestrum. Notice line of separation (*arrow*) of necrotic tissue (*b*). (Phloxine tartrazine sulfate stain ×56.)

For definitive diagnosis, histopathologic examination of the skin nodule biopsies for characteristic features of the disease, animal (cattle) inoculation, and viral isolation and identification (by tissue culture) are imperative. Fluorescent antibody and ferritin tagging techniques can be used in identification of the virus particles in infected skin specimens and cell cultures. Electron microscopy and serology may be used too.

TREATMENT

Specific treatment for LSD is not available, but prevention and control of secondary infections are necessary and helpful.

PREVENTION

Efforts to confine the disease by quarantine measures have failed, whereas slaughter of animals with very active cases, restriction of stock movement, and insect eradication have helped in checking the disease.

In enzootic areas, prophylactic immunization with sheep poxvirus propagated in tissue culture and the egg-adapted, attenuated vaccine developed in South Africa have proved satisfactory and effective.

Recovery from natural infection confers a short-lived immunity of about 11 months.

BIBLIOGRAPHY

Bida SA: Confirmation by histopathology of the probable wide spread of lumpy skin disease (LSD) in Nigeria. Bull Anim Health Prod 25:317–324, 1977.

Emerging Diseases of Animals. FAO Agriculture Studies No. 61. Rome, FAO/UN, 1963, pp 177–201.

Henning MW: Knopvelsiekte, lumpy skin disease. *In* Animal Diseases in South Africa. Pretoria, Central News Agency, 1956, pp 1023–1036.

Jubb KVF, Kennedy PC: Pathology of Domestic Animals, 3rd ed. New York, Academic Press, 1970, pp 596–600.

Bovine Adenoviruses

DONALD MATTSON, DVM, PhD

Bovine adenoviruses (BAV) possess certain physicochemical properties in common with adenoviruses of other animal species; however, they also possess some uniquely different characteristics. Nine antigenic types of BAV are recognized, but several additional isolates have been described and are awaiting official classification. Bovine adenoviruses are classified into 2 subgroups, subgroup 1 (types 1 to 3 and 9) and subgroup 2 (types 4 to 8). Major criteria for this division are based on replicative ability in designated cell cultures and antigenic characteristics as well as other properties. Selected BAV types have been shown to be resistant to inactivation by common disinfectants (70 per cent alcohol, alkyl benzyldimethylammonium chloride, chlorhexidine, dilute solution of sodium hypochlorite, and synthetic detergents with iodine).

EPIZOOTIOLOGY

All BAV types are believed to be distributed worldwide. These viruses are very infectious, and 70 to 80 per cent of adult cattle possess serum-virus neutralizing (SN) antibodies to those viruses present within a herd.

BAV type 3 has been studied more extensively in the United States and serves as a model for other subgroup 1 members. BAV type 3 is usually present in most large dairy and beef cattle herds. Calves frequently become infected between 2 and 4 months of age. Infection is usually expressed in an enzootic fashion in dairy calves, or the virus may spread in an epizootic fashion when large numbers of susceptible beef or dairy calves are first placed in close confinement. By the time calves are 6 to 8 months of age, 40 to 60 per cent are serologically positive. If young calves are placed in large feeding establishments, seroconversion rates during the succeeding 4 weeks may vary from 20 to 40 per cent.

Epizootiologic studies with members of the subgroup 2 BAV have not been conducted in the United States. Three members of this subgroup (types 4, 6, and 7) have been isolated in this country. Studies conducted in Europe indicate that all types are widely distributed. Infection rate is highest when calves are 2 to 6 months old.

All BAV types are probably transmitted by direct animal contact or by aerosol transmission. The viruses are shed in lacrimal and nasal secretions as well as feces.

CLINICAL SIGNS AND LESIONS

Most infections with BAV are not clinically apparent. When clinical signs of disease are present, they are similar to those caused by other agents. The expression of clinical disease is believed to be determined by a variety of factors related to the virulence of the virus strain, concurrent infection with other microorganisms, stress, environmental conditions, and management practices. Expression of acute respiratory disease in calves is particularly intensified during concurrent infection with bovine viral diarrhea virus.

Calves infected naturally or experimentally with BAV may show signs of an upper and lower respiratory tract disease with concurrent enteritis. BAV type 3 is believed to be a more important respiratory tract pathogen than are other members of the subgroup 1 viruses. Clinical signs of BAV type 3 infection include conjunctivitis, pyrexia, cough, hyperpnea, and dyspnea. Pathologic changes are characterized by areas of lung collapse, emphysema, and edema. Histologic features include evidence of bronchitis, bronchiolitis, and alveolar wall infiltration. Intranuclear inclusions may be detected in infected cells.

Pneumoenteritis and enteritis have been associated more frequently with infection by the subgroup 2 BAV. Clinical signs of disease consist of an excessive conjunctival and nasal discharge, pyrexia, hyperpnea, dyspnea, cough, and diarrhea. Infection with the subgroup 2 viruses may result in a viremia, which allows the virus to localize in a number of organs. Intranuclear inclusions may be detected in endothelial cells of the blood vascular system for a brief period of time during the viremic phase.

Bovine adenovirus type 7 has been isolated from cases of the so-called weak calf syndrome. This disease is characterized by birth of calves that are listless and that have polyarthritis, subcutaneous hemorrhage over the joints, and fibrinosanguineous synovial fluid. Areas most often affected include the hock, metatarsal, and metacarpal joints.

BAV has been isolated from cattle with conjunctivitis and keratoconjunctivitis in Australia. Invasion of the bacteria *Neisseria catarrhalis* and *Moraxella bovis* was sometimes associated with the production of keratoconjunctivitis. The specific virus strains that were recovered in Australia from cases of this disease have not been isolated in the United States. However, BAV type 3 and other types have been isolated from cases of conjunctivitis in the United States.

DIAGNOSIS

Diagnosis of BAV infection is complicated by several factors. Frequently, these viruses are not detected by routine electron microscopy examination of feces because they are shed in too low a concentration. Members of the subgroup 1 group will replicate in a variety of cell cultures, but samples must be blind passaged 2 to 3 times for successful isolation. Subgroup 2 adenoviruses must be blind passaged 3 to 4 times in primary calf testicular or embryonic spleen or thyroid cell cultures. Samples for virus isolation must be taken early in the disease. Fluorescent antibody (FA) examination of tissue is the best way to detect viral antigen. This test is subgroup-specific and will confirm the diagnosis of adenovirus infection without delineating individual antigenic types of virus.

Serologic diagnosis of infection is complicated by the fact that SN tests are type-specific and there are numerous types of these viruses. Most diagnostic laboratories do not perform SN tests for bovine adenoviruses. Enzyme-linked immunosorbent assay has been described and, like the FA test, is subgroup-specific. This technique is an excellent way to provide evidence of infection with unspecified adenovirus types, and its use is expected to gain popularity as laboratories attempt to provide improved diagnostic services for respiratory and enteric diseases of cattle.

TREATMENT

There is no specific treatment for adenoviral infection in cattle.

PREVENTION AND CONTROL

There are no vaccines currently available in the United States for prevention of bovine adenoviral infection.

BIBLIOGRAPHY

Kahrs RF: Adenoviruses. *In* Viral Diseases of Cattle. Ames, IA, Iowa State University Press, 1981, pp 61–70.
Mattson DE, Norman BB, Dunbar JR: Bovine adenovirus type 3 infection in feedlot calves. Am J Vet Res 49:67–69, 1988.
Richer L, Lamontagne L: Association of bovine viral diarrhea virus with multiple viral infections in bovine respiratory disease outbreaks. Can Vet J 29:713–717, 1988.

Papillomatosis in Cattle
CARL OLSON, DVM, PhD

Cutaneous papillomatosis occurs in cattle, sheep, goats, horses, rabbits, fish, and humans. An oral papillomatosis occurs in dogs and rabbits. These warts, infectious verrucae, or papillomas are usually regarded as benign epithelial tumors. Viruses causing these tumors are similar in morphologic appearance but different in their other characteristics. The bovine papillomavirus (BPV), the ovine papillomavirus, and the deer fibroma virus will cause a fibroblastic tumor in the hamster. Otherwise, the known papillomaviruses are oncogenic only for their own species of origin. In addition, BPV will cause a fibroblastic tumor in horses, and evidence of the BPV genome is found in naturally occurring equine sarcoids.

EPIZOOTIOLOGY

Bovine papillomatosis is worldwide in distribution and is more common in cattle younger than 2 years of age that are housed in close contact with each other. The skin surfaces of the neck, legs, back, and abdomen are the more usual sites, because these locations are probably more subject to abrasions and wounds through which the virus may infect the tissues. Cutaneous papillomas in cattle can be of various size, depending on the area infected, and have a cauliflower-like appearance and a fibroma base in the dermis. Fibropapillomas of the penis and vulvovaginal mucosa have a smooth surface with less epithelial proliferation. The infective virus is concentrated in the outer keratinized epithelium of the papilloma and, when shed, can readily contaminate fomites such as fences, stanchions, and boards of the stable. These fomites with virus readily transmit the disease to susceptible cattle by causing skin wounds. Immunity develops in a few weeks after exposure to the virus, and older animals are more resistant than are very young animals, probably because of prior inapparent exposure. The incubation period for cutaneous warts produced by BPV is approximately 30 days, and the duration of both naturally and experimentally produced fibropapillomas ranges from 1 to 12 months before regression.

CLINICAL SIGNS AND LESIONS

BPV causes fibroplasia or fibroblastic tumors of the dermis in addition to the epithelial hyperplasia. These are more properly called fibropapillomas. Progressively growing fibroblastic tumors of the brain can be experimentally produced in cattle and hamsters. Polypoid tumors of the urinary bladder can be produced with BPV in calves. In certain areas of the world, such as northern Japan, parts of Brazil, Scotland, Colombia, and Turkey, enzootic bovine hematuria is associated with the bracken fern grown in certain soils as well as with BPV. A plant carcinogen seems to operate together with the BPV in causing these tumors. On bracken farms of the west coast of Scotland, papillomas and carcinomas are found on the tongue, pharynx, esophagus, esophageal groove, rumen, and intestine. A virus morphologically similar to BPV exists in these lesions, and extracts of the tumor have produced typical papillomas in the esophagus, palate, and skin. BPV is a DNA virus, and by molecular hybridization there are 9 distinct types and indications of more types. Although 2 of these types (types 1 and 2) can be differentiated, they do have partial immunologic relationships.

BPV and the other papillomaviruses multiply only in epithelial cells. Morphologic evidence of infectious BPV cannot be found in the fibroblast that has been stimulated to neoplasia, but genome DNA sequences of BPV can be demonstrated by molecular hybridization.

The potential for BPV to produce tumors of the intestinal tract or the urinary bladder in concert with a carcinogen from bracken fern and its ability to transform fibroblasts into a neoplastic state may mean that BPV has a broader and more serious potential for neoplasia than thus far has been recognized. Therefore, other types of tumors could be considered as possibly involved with the virus.

Troublesome papilloma-like lesions not infrequently develop on teats and at the teat meatus of milking cows. This is a proliferation of epithelium as in a papilloma, but it lacks the fibroplasia of the underlying dermis as seen in the typical fibropapilloma of BPV. The etiologic agent of this condition is a papillomavirus.

An atypical wart problem in cattle lacks the dermal fibroma component of the typical BPV-induced cutaneous fibropapilloma. The atypical tumors tend to persist rather than regress and involve adult animals as well as young stock. The atypical papillomas contain a virus morphologically identical to the typical BPV. Experimental transmission of the atypical wart virus has been partially successful. A 3-year herd vaccination program using atypical wart homogenates failed to influence the natural incidence of the disease.

PREVENTION AND CONTROL

Antibodies (precipitin, complement fixing, or hemagglutination inhibiting) can readily be found after exposure to BPV or commercial bovine wart vaccines. Formalized suspension of bovine warts with inactivated virus provides a vaccine for prophylactic immunization when cutaneous warts are a problem in a herd of cattle. Such problems can exist in cattle used for show; in those being sent to slaughter, in which antemortem inspection may cause a reduced price; and, particularly, in bull studs, because young bulls can develop fibropapilloma of the penis, which may render them of no value as a bull stud. Such penile lesions tend to recur after surgery with eventual deformation. Therapeutic use of vaccine has been rather extensive in the past with variable but usually poor results. A controlled test of vaccine in an experimental trial of its therapeutic effect indicated that it was of no value.

Cryosurgery with liquid nitrogen has recently come into use and should be very effective when the cutaneous papillomas are not too large. In the absence of liquid nitrogen with its instrumentation, it should be possible, with care to protect the operator, to freeze the fibropapilloma in a similar manner with dry ice.

BIBLIOGRAPHY

Barthold SW, Koller LD, Olson C, et al: Atypical warts in cattle. J Am Vet Med Assoc 165:276, 1974.
Barthold SW, Olson C, Larson LL: Precipitin response of cattle to commercial wart vaccine. Am J Vet Res 37:449, 1976.
Jarrett WFH, McNeil PE, Grimshaw WTR, et al: High incidence area of cattle cancer with a possible interaction between an environmental carcinogen and a papilloma virus. Nature 274:215, 1978.
Koller LD, Olson C: Attempted transmission of warts from man, cattle, and horses and of deer fibroma, to selected hosts. J Invest Dermatol 58:366, 1972.
Lancaster WD, Olson C: Animal papilloma viruses. Microbiol Rev 46:191, 1982.
Olson C, Gordon DE, Robl MG, Lee KP: Oncogenicity of bovine papilloma virus. Arch Environ Health 19:827, 1969.
Olson RO, Olson C, Easterday BC: Papillomatosis of the bovine teat. Am J Vet Res 43:2250, 1982.
Spradbrow P: Papilloma viruses, papillomas, and ocular cutaneous carcinomas in ruminant animals. Cold Spring Harbor Conference, Papilloma Viruses, 1982, p 73.

Bovine Parvoviruses
J. STORZ, DVM, PhD

Bovine parvoviruses (BPV) are icosahedral viruses with a diameter of 20 to 22 nm. Four structural polypeptides with approximate molecular weights of 80,000, 72,000, 62,000, and 60,000 daltons compose the capsid, which surrounds a single-stranded DNA genome of about 5550 nucleotides. Parvoviruses are extremely resistant to chemical and physical inactivating factors. The most reliable disinfection is achieved with 0.5 per cent sodium hypochlorite or ethylene oxide in the form of a nonexplosive mixture of 10 per cent ethylene oxide and 90 per cent carbon dioxide. All bovine parvoviral isolates agglutinate guinea pig and human type O erythrocytes. The isolates from cattle are antigenically related or identical to BPV-1. One BPV strain isolated in Japan appears to differ and is separated as BPV-2. Bovine parvoviruses differ antigenically from parvoviruses isolated from humans, pigs, cats, dogs, rats, and rabbits.[1,2]

BPV replicate to similar titers in bovine fetal testicle, spleen (BFS), and adrenal cells, but replication is less efficient in bovine fetal kidney cells and several cell lines. The host-cell range is virtually restricted to bovine cells. The cytopathic effect resulting from bovine parvovirus replication in actively dividing BFS cells is distinctive and reproducible. Intranuclear inclusions with unique morphologic appearance are formed in infected cells and can be detected after Giemsa or acridine orange staining.[2]

EPIZOOTIOLOGY

Evidence for parvovirus infection of cattle through detection of antibodies was found in the United States, Algiers, Japan, England, and Austria. The incidence of cattle with antibodies ranged from 46 to 86 per cent. The majority of the serum samples involved newborn calves and cattle to 12 months of age. The highest percentage of positive calves was found in February in Austria, where the only attempt was made to analyze seasonal distribution. The infectious chain consisting of intestinal shedding and oral or oropharyngeal exposure is maintained within the cattle population.[1,2] Vertical transmission of BPV was proved through detection of significant antibody titers in fetal serum and through isolation of parvovirus from tissues of fetuses from naturally occurring abortions. This pathogenic potential of BPV was confirmed through experimental inoculations of pregnant cows or direct fetal inoculations.[3]

CLINICAL SIGNS

Most parvoviral isolates described were made from fecal specimens of calves suffering from enteritis, combined occasionally with febrile respiratory illness and conjunctivitis. In several instances, parvoviruses were isolated from feces of young cattle that were clinically normal. The diarrhea was mild to moderately severe in orally inoculated calves. Calves given the inoculum intravenously developed a more severe, watery diarrhea and became prostrate. The body temperatures reached 41° C 2 days after exposure.[2]

Pregnant cows did not develop adverse clinical signs immediately after inoculation. Their temperature and behavior remained normal. Abortions occurred in the first and early second trimesters. The aborted fetuses were edematous, and the placentas were edematous and had necrotic cotyledons.[3] A serologic survey in 12 commercial dairy herds indicated that BPV may be involved in other reproductive problems. The BPV seroreactor cows experienced higher rates of embryonic mortality and required more services per conception than did nonreactor cattle.[4]

LABORATORY DIAGNOSIS

Considering the high incidence of cattle with antibody titers, it is apparent that isolation of parvovirus from natural infections was relatively sporadic and inefficient with the various methods used. A cell-associated virus technique employing parasynchronous BFS cells was most reliable and recovered parvovirus from 82.5 per cent of fluorescent antibody–positive tissue specimens. Serum free of antibodies against BPV or inhibitors of their hemagglutination must be used for successful isolation attempts and virus propagation.[2]

An efficient method to detect antibodies against BPV is the hemagglutination inhibition (HI) test employing guinea pig or human type O red blood cells. The HI antibody titers corresponded well with results obtained through infectivity neutralization tests and other methods for the detection of antibodies.[1,2]

PREVENTION AND VACCINATION

A high percentage of cattle in the United States and other parts of the world have antibodies resulting from natural infections. There are herds of cattle that do not have antibodies, and they are thus without experience with this infection. Attempts to vaccinate cattle have not been described. As we learn more about the nature of this infection in cattle and the pathogenic potential of BPV, efforts to develop means of vaccination may be warranted, particularly for the prevention of reproductive disease problems.

REFERENCES

1. Abinanti FR, Warfield MS: Recovery of a hemadsorbing virus (HADEN) from the gastrointestinal tract of calves. Virology 14:288–289, 1961.
2. Storz J, Leary JJ, Carlson JH, Bates RC: Parvoviruses associated with diarrhea in calves. Proceedings, Colloquium on Selected Diarrheal Diseases of Young Animals and Humans. J Am Vet Med Assoc 173:624–627, 1978.
3. Storz J, Young S, Carroll EJ, et al: Parvovirus infection of the bovine fetus: distribution of infection, antibody response and age-related susceptibility. Am J Vet Res 39:1099–1102, 1978.
4. Barnes MA, Wright RE, Bodine AB, Alberty CF: Frequency of bluetongue and bovine parvovirus infection in cattle in South Carolina dairy herds. Am J Vet Res 43:1078–1080, 1982.

Bovine Viral Diarrhea–Mucosal Disease

WERNER P. HEUSCHELE, DVM, PhD

Bovine viral diarrhea–mucosal disease (BVD) is a contagious viral disease of cattle and other ruminants first seen in 1946 in New York as a gastroenteritis with severe diarrhea, ulcerations of the muzzle and nasal and oral cavities, fever, leukopenia, reduction in milk secretion, cessation of rumination, and abortions. A similar disease exhibiting the same signs and lesions (only more severe, resembling rinderpest) occurred in Iowa in 1953. This disease was named mucosal disease. It is now recognized that both disease entities were caused by the same virus. Mucosal disease appears to be the consequence of fetal infection with noncytopathic BVD virus between 58 and 128 days' gestation. In many, this leads to persistent infection and specific immunotolerance. In some calves there is stunting and early deaths, whereas others may remain healthy and develop to maturity. Subsequent infection of such persistently infected animals by a cytopathic strain of BVD virus usually leads to the severe, highly fatal mucosal disease.

ETIOLOGY

The causative RNA virus is a member of the family Togaviridae and the genus *Pestivirus*, which also includes hog cholera virus and the virus of Border disease of sheep. The 3 viruses are antigenically closely related and cross-react serologically by virus neutralization, immunoprecipitation, and immunofluorescence. All are enveloped, ranging in size from 20 to 65 nm.

There is minor antigenic variation among BVD virus strains or isolates, but all cross-neutralize.

The virus is readily inactivated by heat, low and high pH, and most disinfectants but is stable at low temperatures. It grows readily in cell cultures of bovine, ovine, or porcine origin. Although several cytopathogenic strains have been isolated, a larger proportion of BVD virus field isolates are noncytopathogenic in cell cultures.

EPIZOOTIOLOGY

Cattle are commonly infected with BVD virus throughout the world. In the United States, infection prevalence ranges between 60 and 80 per cent as revealed by serologic surveys. Natural infection with BVD virus also occurs in sheep, goats, swine, and many wild ruminant species including deer, antelope, buffaloes, and so on in which clinical disease of varying severity is occasionally seen.

Domestic cattle are considered the principal reservoir of BVD virus. It is believed that latent persistent infections are common in cattle. Clinical BVD occurs most frequently in cattle 6 months to 2 years of age.

The virus of BVD is shed in feces and nasopharyngeal secretions. It is readily transmitted by aerosol droplets and direct and indirect contact. Fecal contamination of food and water sources is undoubtedly an important means of infection spread, with the oral route being the most probable route of entry. Entry via the respiratory tract by inhalation of infectious aerosols may also occur. It is possible that flies and other flying arthropods may serve as vectors of BVD virus from one premise to another. Mechanical transmission on contaminated clothing, footwear, equipment, utensils, and vehicles is also possible. Vertical transmission is considered common.

CLINICAL SIGNS AND LESIONS

A majority of BVD infections are subclinical, involving only a biphasic fever and leukopenia followed by an immune response if they are uncomplicated by a concurrent infection. The wide range of clinical responses to BVD virus infection is very likely due to several factors: difference in the pathogenicity of virus strains, susceptibility of exposed herds, concurrent infections, stress conditions, and management factors. BVD virus is associated with many episodes of bovine respiratory disease (BRD) and is therefore a major component of the BRD complex. Usually other infectious agents are concurrently involved with BRD. The BVD virus may increase the pathogenicity of other infectious agents because of its suppressive effects on the host cellular and humoral defense mechanisms. Clinical signs and lesions may therefore often be referable to the coinfecting agents.

A typical outbreak of acute BVD will usually have the following features: a gradual build-up of cases beginning 1 to 3 weeks after the introduction of new animals, onset of fever, depression, anorexia, tachypnea, tachycardia, nasal discharge progressing from serous to mucopurulent, cough, hyperemia of nasal and sometimes oral mucosa, and encrustation around the nares and on the muzzle. Diarrhea is observed 2 to 3 days after the initial onset of fever, progressing from loose watery stools to bloody stools with considerable mucus. Oral erosions appear in the mouth accompanied by hypersalivation from 3 to 7 days after the first fever. Laminitis may be observed in some animals. Pregnant cows may abort during or after the clinical episode or may produce calves with congenital abnormalities, especially cerebellar hypoplasia and ocular dysgenesis.

In some cases or herd outbreaks, diarrhea and typical erosive lesions may be minimal or absent, and respiratory signs are the only manifestations of BVD infection.

Chronic BVD may occur as a sequela to acute BVD or subclinical infections and is often manifested by intermittent diarrhea and nasal discharge and persistent ocular discharge. Chronic lameness due to laminitis and interdigital necrosis may be seen. Chronic patients often fail to develop circulating BVD antibodies and may have persistent viral infection. Areas of alopecia and reddening or hyperkeratosis of the skin, especially on the neck, may occur. Chronically infected animals usually appear unthrifty, often emaciated.

Although BVD virus primarily attacks the digestive tract, it also has a strong affinity for the lymphoreticular tissues, causing necrosis of lymphocytes and macrophages. Phagocytic functions of macrophages and neutrophils are impaired, and both B and T lymphocytes are suppressed. The result is immunosuppression and diminution of nonspecific cellular defense mechanisms as well. This can result in enhanced pathogenicity of other coinfecting organisms such as *Pasteurella* spp., coronavirus, rotavirus, *Cryptosporidium* spp., and so on.

In addition to erosions of the muzzle and all surfaces of the oral cavity, lesions of BVD may include linear esophageal erosions and erosions on the ruminal pillars, omasum, and abomasum. The pyloric portion of the abomasum may be edematous and hemorrhagic. Catarrhal enteritis may progress to include hemorrhage, erosions, and ulcers of the intestinal mucosa. There is swelling of Peyer's patches, often accompanied by necrosis and hemorrhage.

On histologic examination, there are varying degrees of necrosis of the germinal centers in lymph nodes and the spleen. In younger animals, there may be marked atrophy of the thymus. Edema and inflammatory cell infiltration of the intestinal mucosa occur in varying degrees of severity throughout the digestive tract.

When BVD infection is associated with BRD complex, lesions are usually related to associated organisms such as *Pasteurella* spp. and the major respiratory viruses.

DIAGNOSIS

Clinical diagnosis of BVD in a herd must be based on examination of several animals. A combination of clinical signs, lesions, and epizootiologic features of an outbreak is usually a reasonable basis for a provisional diagnosis of BVD. When fever, leukopenia (a total leukocyte count of 4000/mm^3 or less), respiratory signs, diarrhea, depression, and oral erosions are present, BVD should be strongly suspected.

BVD resembles several other diseases that cause erosive and ulcerative lesions in the digestive tract. Rinderpest produces clinical signs and lesions very similar to the severe acute mucosal disease form of BVD. In general, rinderpest has a higher morbidity and mortality than does BVD. Malignant catarrhal fever (MCF) also strongly resembles BVD, presenting pronounced respiratory signs, erosions in the digestive tract, leukopenia, and occasionally diarrhea. Ocular involvement (ophthalmitis) is common in MCF and less so in BVD, and MCF episodes usually involve a lower morbidity (i.e., sporadic cases).

The differential diagnosis should also include bluetongue, vesicular diseases, infectious bovine rhinotracheitis, papular and ulcerative stomatitis, ingestion of caustic substances, and other causes of diarrhea such as salmonellosis, coccidiosis, and enteric viruses.

Definitive diagnosis requires laboratory procedures such as virus isolation, identification of viral antigens in tissue sections by immunofluorescence or enzyme immunoassay, and demonstration of rising antibody titers between acute and convalescent serum samples. Serologic methods used to demonstrate BVD serum antibodies include complement fixation, indirect immunofluorescence, enzyme immunoassay, immunodiffusion precipitation, and virus neutralization, the last-named being preferred by most laboratories. The demonstration of a 4-fold or greater rise in virus neutralizing antibody titers between acute and convalescent serum samples provides a sound basis for the diagnosis of BVD infection. Isolation of BVD virus or demonstration of BVD antigens from specimens adds further confirmation.

Appropriate specimens for laboratory examination should include (1) paired sera, that is, an acute-phase sample and a sample collected 2 to 4 weeks later; (2) nasal swabs in Stewart's transport medium, which are available commercially; (3) feces or rectal swabs; and (4) unclotted blood with anticoagulants such as heparin or EDTA from clinically ill animals. Tissues from fresh necropsy cases for virus examination and histopathology should include tonsil, spleen, maxillary and mesenteric lymph nodes, lung, kidney, and a section of ileum containing Peyer's patches (tied off and unopened).

The recent development of molecular probes from cloned C-DNA complementary to viral RNA segments has provided a highly sensitive means of detecting BVD virus in various materials such as feces, blood, lymphocytes, and tissues by nucleic acid hybridization. Although still experimental and technically complex, this has promise as a useful tool for detecting adventitious BVD in biologics and for epidemiologic studies.

Because of the relatively high incidence of BVD infection in bovine fetuses, the isolation of BVD viruses or the demonstration of BVD antibodies in serum from an aborted late-term fetus may not necessarily be diagnostic; that is, BVD should not be considered the cause of the abortion unless BVD lesions are present or cases of BVD have recently occurred in the herd.

TREATMENT

Treatment of animals with clinical BVD is largely symptomatic and aimed at controlling diarrhea, respiratory signs, and secondary bacterial invaders. Antidiarrheals, antimicrobials such as antibiotics and sulfonamides, expectorants, and fluid and electrolyte therapy are used but in cases of severe acute mucosal disease are seldom of much benefit. Corticosteroids are contraindicated because they produce immunosuppression, which is additive to that produced by the BVD viral infection.

Sick animals should be separated from the rest of the herd.

PREVENTION AND CONTROL

Vaccination of susceptible cattle has been the principal approach to the prevention and control of BVD. The use of modified live virus BVD vaccines has been a subject of controversy. Some modified live virus (MLV) vaccines appear to be less attenuated than others and have been associated with postvaccinal disease complications, especially when they have been used in stressed, recently shipped cattle. Recent reports suggest that some MLV BVD vaccines cause some immunosuppression. However, post-vaccinal BVD disease can also be attributed to circumstances in which animals were in incubative stages of BVD at the time of vaccination. Contamination of MLV vaccines with adventitious virulent BVD virus also may occur occasionally. Mucosal disease may also occur in animals with persistent noncytopathic BVD viral infections after their vaccination with some MLV BVD vaccines. It would therefore appear that killed virus vaccines would be preferable to live ones. It is doubtful that current killed virus BVD vaccines confer immunity of as high a degree, quality, or duration as do the MLV vaccines. They have the advantage of being safe in pregnant cows and carry no risk of inducing postvaccinal disease.

Immunity conferred by BVD vaccines has also been a controversial topic. It is questionable whether vaccine prepared with a single BVD virus strain will provide lifelong protection against all BVD viral strains as was once believed. Field experience suggests that immunity against heterologous BVD strains may be of relatively short duration (i.e., 8 to 12 months). It is therefore recommended that animals be revaccinated annually in dairy or breeder stock. Beef cattle destined for feedlots should be vaccinated at 4 to 6 months of age, preferably before weaning stress.

In areas of high BVD endemicity, earlier vaccination at 2 to 4 weeks of age is advised, but this should be followed by a booster vaccination at 6 to 8 months of age, because persisting maternal passive antibodies may reduce the magnitude of the immune response to vaccine in the young animal.

Although current vaccines for BVD have their limitations, they have proved to be of considerable value in reducing the impact of this costly disease. Undoubtedly, newer technologies of genetically engineered subunit vaccines for BVD will provide safer, more efficacious vaccines in the near future.

BIBLIOGRAPHY

Baker JC: Bovine viral diarrhea virus: a review. J Am Vet Med Assoc 190:1449–1458, 1987.
Bolin SR, McClurkin AW, Cutlip RC, Coria MF: Severe clinical disease induced in cattle persistently infected with non-cytopathic bovine viral diarrhea virus by superinfection with cytopathic bovine viral diarrhea virus. Am J Vet Res 46:573–576, 1985.
Potgieter LND: Immunosuppression in cattle as a result of bovine viral diarrhea virus infection. Agri-Pract 9:7–14, 1988.
Potgieter LND, Brock KV: Detection of bovine viral diarrhea virus by spot hybridization with probes prepared from cloned C-DNA sequences. J Vet Diagn Invest 1:29–33, 1988.
Radostits OM, Littlejohns IR: New concepts in the pathogenesis, diagnosis and control of diseases caused by bovine viral diarrhea virus. Can Vet J 29:513–528, 1988.

Bovine Reoviruses

SASHI B. MOHANTY, BVSc, PhD

Reoviruses are of special interest in comparative virology because the agents of animal origin are indistinguishable from those of human origin. Antibodies against these viruses have been found in a wide range of domestic and wild animals. They have been isolated from both the respiratory and intestinal tracts of apparently healthy cattle and are antigenically identical to human serotypes. Three mammalian serotypes are recognized, and the existence of 4 subtypes of type 2 has been reported. Reoviruses, members of the genus *Reovirus* in the virus family Reoviridae, are 60 to 80 nm in diameter with icosahedral symmetry and a double protein shell. They have a double-stranded segmented RNA genome and are resistant to pH 3, ether, and chloroform, and they agglutinate human O red blood cells. Type 3 also agglutinates bovine red blood cells.

Reoviruses do not grow well in cell cultures of bovine origin, and they produce little or no cytopathic effects in bovine kidney cells. However, they produce good cytopathic effects and eosinophilic intracytoplasmic inclusions in monkey kidney, in mouse fibroblast (L-929) cells, and in various human cell lines.

EPIZOOTIOLOGY

Antibodies to all 3 types of reoviruses are widespread in cattle populations. The virus enters via the fecal-oral and respiratory routes. Infected cattle shed reoviruses in the feces and nasal and conjunctival discharges for up to 1 month. Susceptible cattle may become infected through contact with these sources. Although interspecies infection can occur, it does not appear to be significant under natural conditions. Cattle could harbor reoviruses and transmit them to humans or vice versa.

CLINICAL SIGNS AND LESIONS

The role of bovine reoviruses in the respiratory syndrome is not clear, and it appears that they cause an inapparent infection in nature. These viruses are considered less important in the etiology of bovine respiratory and enteric diseases than are other primary viral agents. In one study, calves experimentally infected with reovirus type 1 had mild clinical signs characterized by a mild fever, anorexia, hyperpnea, nasal discharge, and coughing. Young calves were more susceptible than were older ones. In other studies, types 1 and 2 induced no clinical illness in colostrum-deprived calves, but these calves had pneumonia at necropsy. *Pasteurella* spp. may not enhance reovirus infection, and maternal antibodies do not protect calves from these viral infections.

Gross lesions are confined to the lungs particularly at the roots. Histologic changes are similar to those found in other virus infections of the bovine respiratory tract and are mainly exudative. Interstitial pneumonia and epithelialization of alveoli are common features.

DIAGNOSIS

Bovine reoviral infection may not be detected clinically. Pneumonia at necropsy has been found in cattle infected with bovine parainfluenza-3 and rhinoviruses that had no clinical signs. This possibility should be considered in the diagnosis of reovirus infections. Virus isolation from clinical specimens and seroconversion are considered adequate for diagnosis. Virus neutralization or the hemagglutination inhibition test can be used for demonstrating a rising antibody titer (4-fold or greater) in acute and convalescent serum samples.

TREATMENT, PREVENTION, AND CONTROL

Antibiotics are given only for secondary bacterial infections. There is no vaccine available.

BIBLIOGRAPHY

Darbyshire JH: Acute respiratory/enteric disease in calves. *In* Dinter Z, Morein B (eds): Virus Infections of Ruminants, vol 3. Amsterdam, Elsevier Science Publishers, B. V., 1990, pp 217–225.
Lamont PH: Reoviruses. J Am Vet Med Assoc 152:870, 1968.
Mohanty SB, Dutta SK: Veterinary Virology. Philadelphia, Lea & Febiger, 1981, pp 129–131.
Trainor PD, et al: Experimental infection of calves with reovirus type 1. Am J Epidemiol 83:217, 1966.

Bluetongue in Cattle*
THOMAS E. WALTON, DVM, PhD

Bluetongue is an infectious, noncontagious, arthropod-borne virus disease of domestic and wild ruminants. At least 24 distinct serotypes of bluetongue virus (BTV) have been identified worldwide. In the United States, 5 serotypes have been identified: 2, 10, 11, 13, and 17; serotype 17 is unique to North America. In adult cattle, the disease is generally mild or inapparent with clinical signs being reported only occasionally. Some researchers believe that BTV-infected cattle are important reservoirs of the virus in the epizootiology of the disease. In the United States, BTV serotypes have been isolated from cattle, sheep, wild ruminants, and hematophagous insects in 32 states; serologic evidence of BTV activity has been reported in 48 states, but livestock in the northern (Great Lakes and New England) states are generally considered to be free of BTV. Occasional incursions with BTV serotype 11 have been documented virologically and serologically in the Okanagan Valley of British Columbia, but Canada normally is considered to be BTV-free. In Mexico, BTV serotypes 10, 11, 13, and 17, identical to those identified in the United States, have been isolated. Bluetongue disease is seasonal in areas in which the vector activity is interrupted by inclement weather (e.g., freezing temperatures). Epizootic activity generally has been reported in areas with temperate climates. In tropical or subtropical areas with yearlong vector activity, BTV is enzootic, and reports of clinical disease are only occasionally received. In cattle, the most significant economic losses are associated with governmental restrictions on the importation or international movement of cattle, bull semen, and fertilized bovine ova. Reproductive losses in cattle, similar to those described in pregnant cows and the bovine fetus after bovine viral diarrhea (BVD) virus infection, have been associated with the isolation of BTV. Whether BTV is coincidentally present or related to the pathogenesis of the abortions, congenital deformities, and weak or stillborn calves is controversial and unproven.

The principal biologic vector of BTV in the United States is the biting midge, *Culicoides variipennis*. Although other species of *Culicoides* occur in the United States, only *C. insignis*, which is found from central Florida and to the south into the Caribbean islands and Central America, is considered another possible vector. *C. variipennis* was used experimentally to transmit BTV to and from infected sheep and cattle. Although *Culicoides* spp. will feed on many animal species and on humans, many species appear to be preferentially attracted to cattle, compared with other ruminants; this may be a factor of significance in the epizootiology of bluetongue. After ingestion of a BTV-infected blood meal, the vector is believed to remain infected for life. Cattle and horses may become allergic to the salivary antigens in the bites of female

---

*All material in this article is in the public domain, with the exception of any borrowed figures or tables.

C. variipennis and develop a condition known as allergic dermatitis or "sweet itch."

Cattle may have prolonged viremias lasting from months to more than a year. This prolonged viremia appears to perpetuate the disease in temperate areas where the adult vector is active only seasonally. Several investigators have shown that BTV can be isolated from the semen of infected bulls during the acute phase of the infection. This excretion is ascribed by some investigators to contamination of semen with viremic blood. Reports of longer duration seminal excretion, infection of the dam by insemination with infected semen, infection of the fetus in utero, and fetal lesions or abortions due to BTV have not been independently substantiated. Experimentally, BTV infection of preimplantation embryos from cattle was shown to cause rapid cytolysis of the developing embryos; this suggested that early in utero exposure was unlikely to produce persistently infected calves, deformed fetuses, or late abortions. If the embryo is encased in the intact zona pellucida, BTV infection is prevented.

Concerns about BTV have been expressed by importers and users of bull semen for artificial insemination. As a result, restrictions have been applied to the importation of semen by certain countries. It has been documented and is generally accepted by the scientific community and the artificial insemination industry that there is no realistic danger of BTV infection from the use of commercially collected, prepared, extended, and tested semen. It is also generally accepted that there is no danger of BTV infection from the use of embryo transfer if ova are properly washed and handled.

CLINICAL SIGNS AND LESIONS

Bluetongue virus infection in cattle is unlike the typical field cases observed in sheep. Bluetongue in cattle is generally a subclinical infection, and only a small number of cattle show acute clinical signs. Inoculation of susceptible cattle with BTV isolated from acutely ill cattle has failed to reproduce the acute signs most often associated with field cases. The morbidity is variable but involves fewer than 10 per cent of infected cattle; mortality rarely occurs. On serologic examination, most cattle develop serum antibodies without showing clinical signs. Serologic surveys have shown antibody prevalence of cattle in the western and southwestern states to be more than 50 per cent.

In naturally infected cattle, fevers are transient and range from 40° to 41° C. Rapid, shallow respiration often accompanies the fever. Early in the course of infection, the animal may be stiff or lame, but from which it tends to "warm out." This may be the most frequent complaint identified by the owner. Increased salivation and lacrimation may precede the inflammatory and ulcerative lesions of the oral mucosa. Drooling is often associated with swelling of the lips, gums, and tongue. Ulcers develop on the dental pad, lips, gums, and anterior part of the tongue; in severe cases, there may be extensive necrosis of the dental pad. The skin of the muzzle may have a burned or necrotic appearance and may be dry, cracked, and peeling. The skin on the neck, back, flanks, and perineal area may be infected in severe cases, and large patches of skin may slough. Skin lesions are accompanied by alopecia and an overall loss of condition. The udder and teats of dairy cows and nursing beef cows may be swollen and ulcerated. Coronitis, lameness, and sloughing of the horny laminae may occur as the disease progresses.

Whereas congenital dysfunctions and lesions including hydrocephaly, blindness, cataracts, ataxia, arthrogryposis, gingival hyperplasia, agnathia, and prognathia have been reported in calves naturally and experimentally infected in utero with BTV, confirmation of an unequivocal relationship between BTV infection and the congenital syndrome has not been provided. Many of the lesions ascribed to BTV infection are similar to those documented after in utero infection of the bovine fetus with BVD virus. Confirmation of the involvement of BTV in the pathogenesis of the clinical fetal syndrome described or association as a dual infection with BVD or other viruses must await the rigorous application of modern technology in well-designed and controlled experimental studies.

DIAGNOSIS

Clinical signs of bluetongue in cattle are similar to those caused by photosensitization, poisonous plant intoxications, and infectious diseases such as epizootic hemorrhagic disease (caused by a virus morphologically and antigenically related to BTV), vesicular stomatitis, BVD infection, infectious rhinotracheitis, and mycotic stomatitis (etiology unknown) and such exotic diseases as foot-and-mouth disease and rinderpest. The accurate diagnosis of bluetongue in cattle must be made by virus isolation. Isolation of BTV can be made from infected blood or tissues by the inoculation of embryonating chicken eggs; of cell cultures such as baby hamster kidney (BHK-21), African green monkey kidney (Vero), bovine endothelial (CPAE), and *C. variipennis* cell lines; or of susceptible sheep. Confirmation of BTV is made by using indirect immunofluorescence, immunoperoxidase staining, enzyme-linked immunosorbent assay (ELISA), and virus neutralization techniques. Serotyping of BTV isolates is done by using plaque inhibition or plaque reduction procedures in cell culture monolayers and by polyacrylamide gel electrophoretic techniques. Although not yet available for routine use in diagnostic laboratories, modern molecular biologic procedures such as nucleic acid hybridizations, immunoassays, polymerase chain reactions, and monoclonal antibodies with various markers may soon become available for more sensitive BTV diagnoses. Antibody in cattle can be serologically detected by use of the modified direct complement fixation, agar gel immunodiffusion, hemolysis-in-gel, ELISA, and serum neutralization tests. The serum neutralization test can be used to identify serotype-specific antibodies in previously infected cattle.

TREATMENT AND PREVENTION

Antibiotics are frequently used to treat cattle with lesions from BTV infection in an effort to control secondary bacterial infections. Localized lesions on the muzzle and teats can be treated topically to minimize infection and promote healing. If pityriasis and alopecia are extensive, animals should be protected from the sun. When oral lesions are present, good management is necessary for maintenance of body weight. Infected animals should be separated from the herd and fed less rough forage for minimizing trauma to the oral mucosa.

There are no federally licensed or approved BTV vaccines available in the United States for use in cattle. Whereas some work has been done with traditional attenuated and inactivated vaccines and with modern subunit or "genetically engineered" vaccines, there is no documented need for a vaccine, and there are few expressions of interest by the industry in such vaccines for cattle.

The control of bluetongue within an infected cattle herd is difficult because of subclinical infections and persistently viremic cattle. The single most important measure for cattle is vector control. Careful water management is essential to the control of *C. variipennis*; the larvae are found in the soft, silty, polluted mud in overflow areas around stock tanks or leaking septic systems and along the edges of ponds, ditches, and streams in which there is a high organic content from manure. Improving drainage and eliminating sources of animal and human pollution or sewage effluent will reduce the numbers of potential virus vectors.

Good herd management may help control the spread of the disease. Moving animals from low-lying areas in which larval development sites are located to a higher elevation may be useful. Treatment of larval developmental sites can include physical disruption of the site or the use of approved larvicides such as a granular formula of temephos. Animals can be protected by the use of topical or parenteral pesticides such as fenvalerate or permethrin in ear tags or tapes and ivermectin, or by the use of insect repellents. Premise treatment with residual fenvalerate or permethrin spray and housing of exceptionally valuable individual cattle at dusk and dawn, when *Culicoides* feed, may protect them from infection because *Culicoides* normally do not enter structures.

BIBLIOGRAPHY

Barber TL, Jochim MM, Osburn BI: Bluetongue and related orbiviruses. Prog Clin Biol Res 178, 1985.
Gibbs EPJ, Greiner EC: Bluetongue and epizootic hemorrhagic disease. *In* Monath TP (ed): The Arboviruses: Epidemiology and Ecology, vol 2. Boca Raton, FL, CRC Press, 1988, pp 39–70.
Jones RH, Luedke AJ, Walton TE, Metcalf HE: Bluetongue in the United States: an entomological perspective toward control. World Anim Rev 38:2–8, 1981.

Bovine Rhinoviruses

BRUCE D. ROSENQUIST, DVM, PHD

Although human rhinoviruses (RV) currently number 100 distinct antigenic serotypes, only 2 serotypes of bovine RV are officially recognized. Most isolates have been characterized as bovine RV type 1. A third serotype or serologic variant, distinguishable by serum neutralization tests from types 1 and 2, has been proposed and described in Japan and the United States (Missouri). These serotypes are members of the Picornaviridae family.

EPIZOOTIOLOGY

Human RV do not cause infection in cattle, and bovine RV do not cause infection in humans. Infection is no doubt worldwide and has been documented in England, Europe, Japan, Africa, and the United States. Exposure of calves is widespread. Infection with type 1 or proposed type 3 appears to be more common than with type 2. Approximately 95 per cent of Missouri beef and dairy calves less than 1 year of age that have been tested are seropositive to type 1 RV; virtually 100 per cent of those tested are seropositive by 10 to 12 months.

CLINICAL SIGNS AND LESIONS

Rhinoviruses, the most common cause of human colds, also cause respiratory infections in cattle. Opinions vary as to pathogenicity of bovine RV. The author's personal prejudice, based on human RV literature and personal bovine RV experience, is that these viruses are important agents in the multifactorial etiology of bovine respiratory disease. In some cases, these have been the only viruses demonstrable in calves with respiratory disease. This does not rule out other agents or complicating factors. Clinical signs ascribed to RV infection include fever, lacrimation, nasal discharge, coughing, and increased respiratory rate. There may be no clinical signs observed.

DIAGNOSIS

Diagnosis requires laboratory confirmation of clinical suspicions by virus isolation in appropriate cell cultures or demonstration of a significant rise in neutralizing antibody titer between acute and convalescent phase sera. The type of rhinovirus can be determined with the use of serotype-specific antisera. At present, laboratory diagnosis is primarily confined to specialized laboratories.

TREATMENT

There is no specific treatment for RV infections. Treatment consists of supportive therapy and control of secondary infections. Endogenous and exogenous interferon may aid in protection against bovine RV infection.

PREVENTION AND CONTROL

Vaccines are not available.

Foot-and-Mouth Disease in Cattle

JERRY CALLIS, DVM, MS, DSc
DOUGLAS GREGG, DVM, MEd, PhD

Foot-and-mouth disease (FMD) is an acute, highly communicable disease caused by a virus of the *Aphthovirus* genus of the family Picornaviridae. There are 7 distinct immunologic types, and immunity to 1 serotype does not confer protection against the other 6. The virus is antigenically labile, which results in numerous subtypes within each serotype. Subtypes may complicate control. Vaccination with some subtypes will not necessarily protect animals against other strains of the virus within the same serotype.

Infectivity of FMD virus may be destroyed by chemicals such as acids, alkalis, formalin, and aziridines and by physical means such as high temperature, ultraviolet light, and x-rays. Under natural conditions, the virus has been shown to survive for 14 days in a stall and for as long as 20 weeks on sacks and hay. A shift in the pH in either direction below 6 and above 9 makes conditions for survival less favorable. The most commonly used disinfectants are 2 per cent caustic soda, 4 per cent soda ash, and 2 per cent acetic acid.

EPIZOOTIOLOGY

Foot-and-mouth disease virus infects domesticated and wild cloven-hoofed animals, armadillos, rats, nutria, grizzly bears, and elephants. Dogs, cats, rabbits, chinchilla, mice, guinea pigs, and chickens are susceptible to experimental infection. Humans can also be infected but only rarely; thus, FMD is not a public health problem. The disease occurs in livestock in all of the large land masses of the world where livestock are raised except Australia, New Zealand, North and Central America, and Greenland. The European Community has been free of FMD since 1989. The incidence in Western Europe is low because of systematic application of well-produced and tested vaccines, control of movement of animals, and eradication efforts including decontamination when the disease occurs. The virus is spread by contact between infected and susceptible animals, by contaminated animal products such as meat and milk, by the airborne route, and by mechanical transfer. The virus in muscle is inactivated within 48 hours of slaughter but survives for longer periods in bones, lymph nodes, and clots of blood. Cattle, sheep, goats, and cape buffalo have become carriers after recovery and are thought to serve as reservoirs between outbreaks. Contaminated products also serve to transmit the virus from one continent to another. However, removal of the bone has been shown to remove most of the virus. For example, Great Britain and other European countries have limited imports from FMD-infected countries to boneless beef for the last 20 years, and such shipments have not been demonstrated to be responsible for introduction of the virus into Europe.

CLINICAL SIGNS AND LESIONS

FMD virus causes blisters or vesicles in the mouth (including the tongue, lips, gums, pharynx, teats, and palate) and on the feet. There is also a sharp rise in body temperature of 1° to 3° C. Infected animals salivate, smack their lips, and are reluctant to move because of the pain caused by the blisters. These blisters rupture and leave eroded areas (Figs. 1 and 2).

DIAGNOSIS

There are other infections of the bovine that can be confused with FMD. Some of these are vesicular stomatitis, bovine papular stomatitis, infectious bovine rhinotracheitis, rinderpest, bluetongue, and malignant catarrhal fever. For this reason, a diagnosis of FMD based on clinical signs should be avoided, especially when it is the first occurrence of such a disease in the area. Specimens from the infected animal should be referred to an official laboratory with experienced staff and biocontainment facilities for containing the virus. There it can be diagnosed by isolation of the virus and identification by complement fixation, virus neutralization, enzyme-linked immunosorbent assay, and inoculation tests in livestock including the horse, which is not susceptible to FMD but is susceptible to vesicular stomatitis.

PREVENTION AND CONTROL

In countries that are free from the disease, there are strict prohibitions on importation of animals or animal products from infected countries. Products that have been processed so that their freedom from the virus is ensured, such as by cooking or drying, may be permitted entry. Some FMD-free

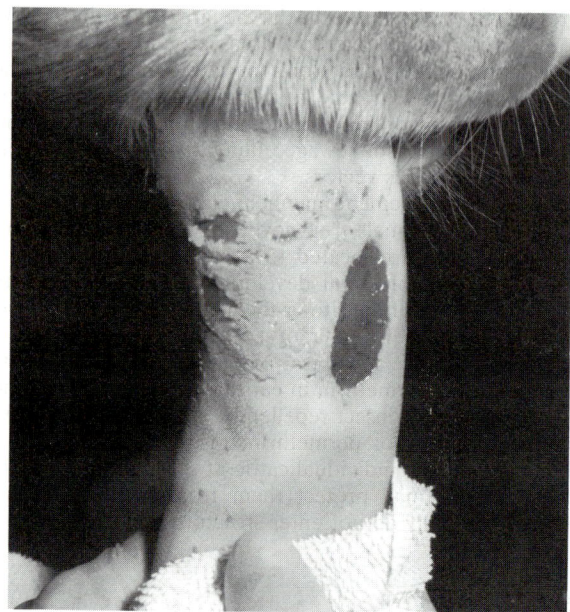

Figure 1. An eroded vesicular lesion and adjacent friable epithelium on a bovine tongue infected with foot-and-mouth disease virus.

countries accept deboned beef from infected countries. When FMD occurs, the disease-free countries eradicate it by slaughtering the infected animals, destroying the carcass by burning or burying, and decontaminating the premises. These procedures are practiced in several countries in Europe and North America.

Vaccines have been available since the 1930s and are used to control the incidence of infection in countries where FMD is enzootic or where eradication is impractical because of costs. In Western Europe, the judicious application of well-produced

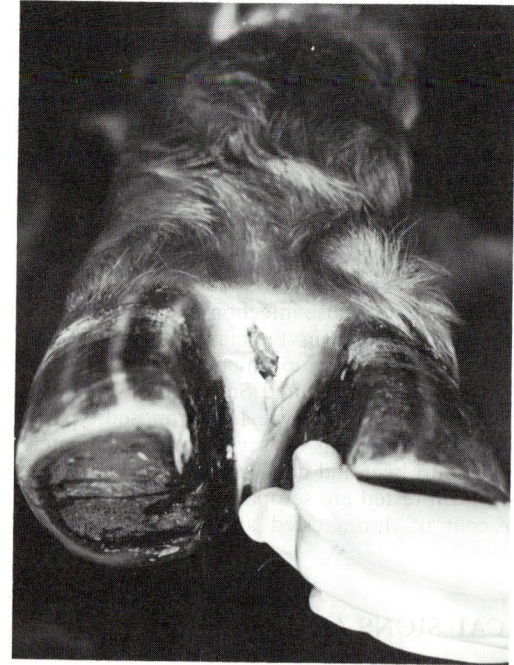

Figure 2. Ruptured vesicle on the foot of a bovine caused by foot-and-mouth disease virus.

and tested vaccines is generally considered to be responsible for the low incidence of the disease. Vaccination alone has never been responsible for eradication of the disease. In endemic areas, vaccination is used to control the incidence of infection, and it has been used to lower the incidence to such levels that slaughter is economically feasible in eradication campaigns. There are expectations that better and less risky vaccines may become available through biotechnology, but none have been commercialized since protection of livestock was first demonstrated with such a product in 1981.

Bovine Rotavirus
THOMAS L. LESTER, DVM, PhD, ACVM

Rotavirus is a genus of viruses belonging to the family Reoviridae. They have been separated into 4 groups, A to D, by enzyme-linked immunosorbent assay (ELISA), complement fixation test, immunoelectron microscopy, and RNA genome sizing. All rotaviruses share a common group-specific antigen (VP6) associated with the inner capsid. Species specificity or serotypes are determined by antigens (VP3 and 7) located on the outer capsid. Most bovine isolates are from group A. Group B and group C have been isolated rarely from cattle but form an increasing proportion of isolates from sheep and pigs.

EPIZOOTIOLOGY

Rotavirus infections have been reported in a wide variety of animals including humans, cattle, horses, dogs, sheep, goats, swine, antelope, monkeys, mice, rabbits, deer, chicken, turkeys, and ducks. Zoonosis is not considered a problem; however, cross-species infections can be experimentally induced. Disease is generally associated with the young but can occur at all ages and has been demonstrated in adult cattle. Exposure is widespread, and most cows have antibodies. The virus can survive for several days in feces, which is the main source of infection. Infected adults can excrete sufficient virus to serve as initiators of infection in calves, which then excrete large quantities of virus to infect others. Disease outbreaks occur most commonly in herds in which sick animals are not separated and orofecal transmission is allowed to occur. Infection can be initiated by almost any infectious fecal contamination. Sources have included contaminated teats, feed, bedding, equipment, people, and the introduction or mixing of animals from infected herds.

CLINICAL SIGNS AND LESIONS

Clinical signs occur in calves 1 day to 3 weeks of age with 5 to 10 days being the most frequent. The incubation period is 18 to 96 hours. The virus replicates in absorptive columnar epithelial cells of the jejunum and ileum. These are replaced by flattened squamous to cuboid epithelial cells deficient in digestive enzymes and absorptive capacity. This leads to malabsorption as well as alteration of electrolyte transport systems, which causes a profuse diarrhea. The onset of clinical signs is generally rapid, within 2 to 3 hours, but the severity can vary among calves. Signs include mild anorexia, depression, and diarrhea. The feces may be watery, brown, or green and may contain blood and mucus. Weight loss of 10 to 25 per cent may occur, and mortality may be high. Duration and mortality appear to be related to other factors such as secondary infections (bacterial or viral), stress, and the quality and type of passively acquired antibodies. Mortality is generally recognized to result from loss of electrolytes and water with resulting dehydration, acidosis, and systemic shock.

Necropsy findings are generally rather nondescript. The stomach may contain some milk or mucoid fluid. The intestinal contents are generally watery and can vary in color. The intestinal mucosa may be normal to reddened or hemorrhagic, depending on the type of severity of secondary infections.

DIAGNOSIS

Diagnosis of rotavirus infection depends on the demonstration of virus or virus-specific antigens in the feces or intestinal mucus. Methods used to detect rotavirus include the following.

1. Electron microscopy by negative staining. This procedure is rather insensitive and requires a large number of particles in the feces. Detection can be enhanced by the use of antiserum to form immunoaggregates (immunoelectron microscopy).
2. Sandwich ELISA. "Rotazyme" type tests, based on human kits, detect group A antigens in feces and compare well with electron microscopic techniques. However, owing to their specificity, they will not detect groups B to D or other virus that might be present.
3. Isolation can be accomplished but is difficult and time-consuming.
4. Fluorescent antibody technique can be used on fecal smear and intestinal mucosa impressions or frozen sections.

TREATMENT

Diarrhea in very young calves with secondary bacterial complication will require immediate and careful treatment, but 3-week-old calves with no secondary complications may recover rapidly with no treatment. When practical, milk feeding should be stopped. Calves with 5 per cent or less loss of body weight due to dehydration should be given fluids orally. Calves with 5 to 10 per cent dehydration should be given fluids orally and parenterally. Calves with greater than 10 per cent dehydration should be given fluids intravenously. For combating secondary bacterial infection, antibiotics should be given parenterally. In some cases, orally administered antibiotics are beneficial.

After treatment, recovery will be slow. Repair of the absorptive epithelium and return to function may require several weeks with resultant persistent diarrhea and poor-growing calves.

PREVENTION

Reducing exposure is the most effective method of preventing rotavirus infection. Management practices such as care in not introducing the virus by addition of infected or contaminated animals or materials, reducing stocking density, removing animals with diarrhea, and the like are recommended.

Local antibodies on the mucosal surface of the intestine appear to be important in the protection against rotavirus infections. Vaccines for oral administration to calves are available. Efficacy, however, can be varied, depending on serotypes present, maternal antibody concentrations, exposure levels, and vaccine administration. Vaccination of the cows has also been reported to reduce the incidence of infection in calves. The rationale in cow vaccination is both to reduce excretion of the virus by infected or carrier animals and to increase the concentration of maternal antibodies to the neonate's intestine (lactogenic immunity).

BIBLIOGRAPHY

Lewis LD: Calf diarrhea. Part III. Management, prevention and treatment of diarrhea. Norden News 53:22, 1978.
Mebus CA, Newman LE: Scanning electron, light and fluorescent microscopy of intestine of gnotobiotic calf infected with reovirus-like agent. Am J Vet Res 38:533, 1977.
Saif LJ, Theil KW: Viral Diarrheas of Man and Animals. Boca Raton, FL, CRC Press, 1989.

Calf Coronavirus Diarrhea

THOMAS L. LESTER, DVM, PhD, ACVM

Also known as calf neonatal diarrhea virus, calf coronavirus diarrhea is caused by a virus in genus *Coronavirus* of the family Coronaviridae. Coronaviruses have been isolated from a wide range of animals, and although there is considerable serologic cross-reactivity, isolates are generally considered host-specific. There is only 1 bovine serotype recognized, and it is not known to cross-react with any other coronavirus isolate. Coronaviruses are moderately labile and may survive for 1 to 2 days at room temperature. They are stable across a wide pH range (3 to 8) and will survive passage through the alimentary tract. Coronaviruses are difficult to isolate and grow in in vitro systems. Many strains have yet to be artificially propagated.

EPIZOOTIOLOGY

Calf coronavirus infections are host-specific for the bovine. The disease is probably worldwide in distribution. Difficulty in propagating the virus has delayed the recognition and study of this disease. Route of infection is orofecal through contact with contaminated teats, feed, equipment, and the like. The viral titer in feces can be as high as 10^{10} particles per gram of feces. Coronaviruses can also establish long-term infections in their natural hosts, thus producing inapparent persistent carriers.

CLINICAL SIGNS

Of the viruses that cause diarrhea in neonatal calves, coronavirus induces the most severe disease. The incubation period in experimentally infected calves is 20 to 36 hours. The disease is most prevalent in calves 1 day to 3 or more weeks of age. Initially the calves are only moderately depressed, eat slowly, and have a liquid yellowish diarrhea that may contain curds and mucus. The major difference between coronaviral and rotaviral disease is the lack of anorexia; coronavirus-infected calves will appear hungry and continue to eat. If fed milk, these calves will continue to have diarrhea for 5 to 6 days. The volume of feces will vary with the amount of milk or fluid ingested. Calves fed normal amounts of milk can die of severe dehydration 48 to 72 hours after onset of signs. Persistent diarrhea is believed to be due to the destruction of the absorptive epithelium of the intestinal villi primarily in the large intestine. Severely shortened villi and occasionally fusion of adjacent villi are also seen in the small intestine.

Gross necropsy lesions are not remarkable in uncomplicated natural infections. There is generally milk in the abomasum with normal feces in the small intestine. Colon contents are watery. Mucosal changes are generally due to secondary infections.

DIAGNOSIS

The most definitive diagnosis of coronaviral infection is by demonstration of viral antigens in the spiral colon by fluorescent antibody techniques. Electron microscopy can be used to demonstrate virus in intestine and feces. Recognition of coronavirus can be difficult owing to pleomorphism of the particles and debris in the sample. Immunoelectron microscopy for antibody-induced viral aggregates can be helpful. Viral isolation may be attempted, but all strains are difficult to recover, and many have not been successfully grown in in vitro systems.

TREATMENT

Treatment as described for rotavirus infection in ruminants is also applicable to bovine coronavirus infection. However, therapy may have to be continued for a longer period because of the more prolonged alteration of the small intestinal mucosa in coronavirus infection.

PREVENTION

As with rotavirus infection, management practices to reduce exposure are important. Serum antibodies have been detected in calves but do not appear to be protective. The coproantibody system is important in protection of the calf from coronavirus infection. Both locally induced and lactogenic antibodies are important. To develop maximal resistance, a calf should become infected in the presence of some antibodies developing during a subclinical infection. Coronavirus oral vaccines can induce resistance to challenge within 72 hours of administration. Efficacy, however, is influenced by timing of vaccination relative to first nursing and exposure to field virus as well as levels of maternal antibody. Cow vaccinations have also been reported to reduce the incidence of clinical disease in neonatal calves.

BIBLIOGRAPHY

Lewis LD, Phillips RW: Pathophysiologic changes due to coronavirus-induced diarrhea in the calf. J Am Vet Med Assoc 173:636, 1978.
Mebus CA, Newman LE, Stair EL Jr: Scanning electron, light and immunofluorescent microscopy of intestine of gnotobiotic calf infected with diarrhea coronavirus. Am J Vet Res 36:1, 1975.
Mebus CA, Torres-Medina A, Twiehaus MJ, Bass E: Immune response to orally administered calf reovirus-like agent and coronavirus-vaccine. Dev Biol Stand 33:393, 1976.
Saif LJ, Theil RW: Viral Diarrheas of Man and Animals. Boca Raton, FL, CRC Press, 1989.

Rift Valley Fever in Cattle*

JOHN C. MORRILL, DVM, PHD

Rift Valley fever (RVF) is an acute, arthropod-borne, viral disease primarily affecting sheep, cattle, goats, and humans. The etiologic agent is an RNA virus of the family Bunyaviridae, genus *Phlebovirus*. A number of virus strains including Entebbe, Smithburn, Lunyo, Zinga, and ZH–501 have been identified; but all isolates examined are indistinguishable by routine serologic tests. Like most enveloped virions, RVF virus is sensitive to lipid solvents, detergents, and low pH (<6.2). At neutral or alkaline pH and in the presence of protein, such as in blood or serum, the virus is extraordinarily stable and may retain its infectivity for up to 4 months at 4° C. Virus-infected specimens held at 0° C have remained infective for 8 years, and in serum, infectivity is retained for up to 3 hours at 56° C. Formalin, betapropiolactone (0.4 per cent final concentration), and acetic acid (2.0 per cent) are effective chemical inactivants.

EPIZOOTIOLOGY

Rift Valley fever or enzootic hepatitis was first described in detail in 1931 after an investigation of a disease in sheep in the Rift Valley of Kenya. In 1951, an outbreak in South Africa demonstrated that the disease was not confined to that limited geographic region, and since that time, several outbreaks have occurred in East and South Africa. Subsequent serosurveys and virus-isolation studies have shown RVF to be present throughout Africa. The 1977 RVF outbreak in Egypt was the first reported occurrence of the virus outside sub-Saharan Africa. That outbreak caused extensive livestock losses and human disease. Since then, there has been no recurrence of RVF, and serosurveys throughout Egypt have failed to show evidence of active RVF transmission. The first documented RVF epidemic in West Africa occurred in the Senegal River flood plain in 1987 and resulted in high morbidity and mortality in the human population within the affected area. Recent clinical and serologic evidence suggests RVF is active in Madagascar.

The natural host range for RVF virus includes mosquitoes, sheep, cattle, buffalo, camels, goats, other ruminants, and humans. Several species of laboratory and wild rodents are susceptible to RVF; reductions in local rodent populations have been noted during outbreaks, but their role in virus maintenance and transmission is unlikely to be of epidemiologic significance. Various avian and reptilian species have been tested for susceptibility and are refractory to RVF. Outbreaks among cattle and sheep are characterized by widespread abortion and rapidly fatal neonatal disease. Fulminant neonatal disease may be the first indication of RVF in areas where abortion rates are high owing to other abortogenic agents. Disease progression and severity of disease are generally inversely proportional to age (Table 1). Adult cattle and sheep may suffer mortality rates of 10 to 30 per cent or higher, depending on the nutritional state of the animal; but in animals less than 7 days old, fatality rates may approach 100 per cent. The disease in humans is usually a temporarily incapacitating illness, although complications of hemorrhagic fever, encephalitis, and retinal disease occur in fewer than 2 per cent of human infections.

---

*All material in this article is in the public domain, with the exception of any borrowed figures or tables.

The views of the author do not purport to reflect the position of the Department of the Army or the Department of Defense.

Table 1. SUSCEPTIBILITY OF VARIOUS ANIMAL HOSTS FOR RIFT VALLEY FEVER VIRUS

4+	3+	2+	1+	−
Lamb*	Humans	Goat	Cat	Swine
Kid*	Sheep	Camel	Dog	Chicken
Calf*	Calf (>1-week-old)	Cattle	Horse	Guinea pig
Puppies*		Buffalo		Rabbit
Kittens*				
Mouse				
Hamster				

4+ = 100 per cent fatal, high viremia; 3+ = severe illness with some mortality, abortion, and viremia; 2+ = illness, abortion, and viremia; 1+ = abortion, viremia, some illness to no overt signs of disease; − = refractory to natural disease and in those species tested to laboratory infection.
*Less than 1-week-old.
Note: It is likely that with extensive laboratory testing, the very young of several species noted above would fall into the 4+ classification. Also, on the basis of data from recent epizootics, humans are placed under the 3+ column.

Epidemics of RVF typically center around large concentrations of sheep and cattle. In the absence of epidemics, a cycle of enzootic circulation exists in many regions of Africa. Livestock infections, probably acquired by the bite of infected mosquitoes, result in low rates of disease and abortion that are undiagnosed because of confusion with other livestock diseases and a lack of diagnostic capabilities. Reservoirs for RVF virus are unidentified, although there is now evidence to support the hypothesis of interepidemic maintenance via transovarial transmission in certain *Aedes* mosquitoes. Mosquitoes of many species of the genera *Aedes*, *Anopheles*, *Culex*, *Eretmapodites*, and *Mansonia* can transmit RVF virus under field conditions. During the Egyptian epizootic in 1977, *Culex pipiens* was an important mosquito vector.

Humans may be infected by aerosol in the laboratory and during slaughter of viremic animals, but aerosol transmission between infected and susceptible animals appears less important than is mosquito transmission. Blood and serum from RVF virus–infected animals are sources for aerosol infection of humans. Abattoir workers, farmers, veterinarians, and laboratory technicians have the principal at-risk occupations for this route of transmission. The major natural means of RVF transmission is by bite of infected mosquitoes, although mechanical transmission by arthropods is possible. Consumption of milk or meat from infected animals does not appear to be a common means of transmission.

CLINICAL SIGNS

Clinical signs vary considerably and are related to the species and age of the animal involved. Abortions and infertility have been the principal signs of RVF in adult cattle. Other overt signs are infrequent but include fever of 40° to 42° C, congestion of mucous membranes, salivation, anorexia, general weakness, fetid diarrhea, and a rapid decrease in milk production. Leukopenia and elevated serum aspartate aminotransferase, γ-glutamyltransferase, and lactic dehydrogenase values are common. Experimentally infected cattle are viremic for 2 to 5 days. No long-term carrier state in animals has been identified. Infection of calves results in a febrile response, labored breathing, and death.

The most consistent pathologic changes in all species affected involve the liver. In infected calves, less than 7 days old, lesions are similar to those of newborn lambs. The liver is enlarged with necrotic foci scattered throughout the parenchyma. As these necrotic areas enlarge, extensive destruction of normal hepatic architecture occurs. Hemorrhages are seen infrequently in the abomasum and intestinal tract.

DIAGNOSIS

An epidemiologic pattern suggestive of RVF includes short incubation period; high mortality in lambs, calves, and kids that are less than 1 week of age; illness in adult sheep and cattle; high abortion rate among cows and ewes; liver lesions at necropsy; an acute febrile disease in humans; and the presence of dense populations of arthropod vectors. A differential diagnosis should include bluetongue, ephemeral fever, Wesselsbron virus infection, and Middleburg virus infection. Potentially confusing diseases are brucellosis, vibriosis, trichomoniasis, and bracken or arsenic poisoning.

In the laboratory, a characteristic histopathologic finding of liver necrosis in all susceptible animals often provides the first clue that the disease is RVF. A definitive diagnosis of RVF is accomplished only by isolating and identifying the virus or by observing a 4-fold rise in specific, neutralizing antibody titer between acute and convalescent sera. During past epizootics, the most common material used for virus isolation included whole blood or serum collected at the peak of pyrexia and specimens of liver, placenta, and fetus. Samples from liver, spleen, brain, kidney, and heart should be collected in 10 per cent buffered formalin for histologic examination. Infected humans are also a source of diagnostic material; and, if possible, suspected mosquito vectors should be collected for virus-isolation studies. Samples should be transported on wet ice, but if they are frozen and dry ice is used, the specimens must be protected from exposure to carbon dioxide.

Virus can be isolated in a number of common cell-culture systems. Laboratory animals of choice for isolation are suckling mice, adult mice, and hamsters. RVF virus is one of the few viruses that will kill adult mice and hamsters within 1 to 4 days after intraperitoneal inoculation. Serologic techniques used to demonstrate RVF virus antibody in domestic animals and humans include hemagglutination inhibition, complement fixation, indirect fluorescent antibody, agar gel diffusion, plaque-reduction neutralization, and enzyme-linked immunosorbent assay (ELISA) tests. ELISA techniques have provided a rapid, specific, and reliable means of demonstrating viral antigen and IgM and IgG antibodies in suspect tissue and serum. The ELISA can be readily adapted to rapidly test large numbers of samples to monitor the progress of epidemic disease. Nucleic acid hybridization and enzyme immunochemistry techniques for detection of viral antigen have been useful but are less sensitive than is virus isolation; nonetheless, in epidemic situations, they readily identify the presence of antigen in the infected population.

TREATMENT

No specific treatments are currently available. Rift Valley fever virus is sensitive to several antiviral agents and interferon in vitro. Experimental studies in RVF virus–infected rhesus macaques show that ribavirin and recombinant interferon-α are effective prophylactic drugs and have chemotherapeutic efficacy when given early in the course of infection.

PREVENTION AND CONTROL

Passive antibody therapy, by administration of immune plasma or serum, may be effective, provided the neutralizing antibody titer of the plasma or serum is known and sufficient quantity is given; however, it is not practical in an epizootic. Under experimental conditions, neonatal calves obtained complete protection through ingestion of colostrum from immune dams. Removal of animals to an altitude at which mosquitoes are absent or application of residual insecticides to animals and their pens and barns has been suggested, although movement of animals during an epizootic is undesirable and rarely practical, and effectiveness of residual insecticides in animal holding areas is dependent on vector habits. Limiting amplification of virus in domestic animals will probably block extensive human disease, and mass vaccination is the method of choice in controlling RVF during an epizootic. Effective live-attenuated and killed veterinary vaccines for RVF are in use in many African countries. The live-attenuated Smithburn strain provides long-lasting immunity but is abortogenic in pregnant ewes. The World Health Organization (WHO) recommends that the current live-virus vaccines be used only in enzootic areas of Africa.

Killed vaccines are recommended by WHO for use outside enzootic areas of Africa. A formalin-inactivated vaccine is safe for pregnant ewes but provides only short-term immunity and requires stringent production controls to ensure the absence of residual live virus.

Recently, a mutagen-attenuated vaccine was developed and is being tested. Under experimental conditions, this vaccine was nonpathogenic, nonabortogenic, and immunogenic for pregnant cows and ewes. Susceptible neonatal calves and lambs have been inoculated with the vaccine at 1 day of age and have withstood experimental infection with virulent virus with no untoward effects. More extensive field studies are anticipated in the future.

BIBLIOGRAPHY

Lupton HW, Peters CJ: Rift Valley fever. Proc US Anim Health Assoc 87:279–290, 1984.
Shope RE, Peters CJ, Davies FG: The spread of Rift Valley fever and approaches to its control. Bull WHO 60:229–304, 1982.
Swartz TA, Klingberg MA, Goldman N (eds): Rift Valley Fever. Contributions to Epidemiology and Biostatistics, vol 3. Basel, S. Karger, 1981, pp 1–196.
Walker JS: Rift Valley Fever. Foreign Animal Diseases. Richmond, VA, U.S. Animal Health Association, 1975, pp 209–221.

Akabane Disease in Cattle
A. J. DELLA-PORTA, BSc, PhD

Akabane disease is a congenital disease of cattle, sheep, and goats characterized by hydranencephaly (HE), arthrogryposis (AG), micrencephaly, and porencephaly. It usually occurs as localized epizootics and less frequently as sporadic cases. There may also be an increased incidence of abortion and stillbirth in the months preceding the epizootic of congenital AG/HE.

The disease is caused by Akabane virus, an insect-transmitted virus (arbovirus) belonging to the family Bunyaviridae, which occurs as an inapparent infection in nonimmune animals. If infection occurs during early pregnancy (principally during the early stages of brain development in the fetus), the virus may cross the placenta and the resulting infection of the fetus may cause deformities. The disease has been reported in Australia, Japan, Israel, and Turkey, and the virus has also been isolated in Kenya and South Africa. Akabane disease has occurred every few years as localized epizootics in Australia for at least the last 40 years and in Japan for at least 30 years.

In an area where the suspect insect vector is endemic, most animals become infected early in their life and only isolated, sporadic cases of Akabane disease are seen. Epizootics are thought to occur when extended, warm, humid summers favor the extension of virus-infected insects beyond their normal geographic distribution to areas populated by susceptible pregnant animals.

CLINICAL SIGNS

Infection in the pregnant animal is inapparent. In some instances the first sign of disease is an increase in abortions. In calves the apparent sequence of principal clinical signs appears to be mild incoordination followed by AG ("curly calves," fixed flexion, and sometimes extension of one or more limbs) and then HE ("dummy calves," blindness, with large portions of the brain replaced by fluid). These syndromes can overlap in sequence, and animals can be seen exhibiting more than one of the clinical signs.

The central nervous system lesions can vary from mild to very severe, with absence of most of the cerebrum. When AG is present, the gross appearance of the brain and spinal cord is often normal, but microscopically there is a severe, diffuse loss of myelinated fibers from the lateral and ventral horn neurons and a loss of nerve fibers from ventral spinal nerves. There is also severe atrophy of the skeletal muscles. In the HE seen toward the end of the epizootic, both cerebral hemispheres of the majority of affected animals are almost completely replaced by fluid. Several of the pathologic changes can occur simultaneously and should not be considered as clearly defined, separate stages in Akabane disease.

DIAGNOSIS

As Akabane virus has not been isolated from congenitally affected offspring born at term and only occasionally from aborted fetuses, proof of infection must be based on serologic and pathologic evidence. In an outbreak the most important specimens for diagnosis are a sample of serum from the mother and a precolostrum sample from its affected offspring. Samples of brain and cervical, thoracic, and lumbar regions of the spinal cord should be preserved in 10 per cent neutral formalin for histologic examination.

Serologic diagnosis of infection is based on a neutralization test in African green monkey kidney Vero cells. If both the serum from the dam and the precolostrum serum from the offspring contain neutralizing antibodies against Akabane virus, this virus probably caused the in utero damage to the fetus.

Similar congenital deformities in calves may be caused by bluetongue virus infection, may be of genetic or environmental origin, or may be associated with teratogenic chemicals. The deformities may also be of some unknown origin. The detection of elevated levels of specific immunoglobulin (IgG_1) in precolostrum serum samples from the affected calf would indicate whether an infectious agent was involved.

PREVENTION

As only susceptible pregnant animals can be involved in Akabane disease, prevention involves ensuring either that immunity to Akabane virus infection is developed early in life or in a nonbreeding period, or that animals are not pregnant when virus-infected insects are likely to be present in the area. An inactivated vaccine is available in Japan and may prove useful in preventing Akabane disease.

BIBLIOGRAPHY

Hartley WJ, De Sarum WG, Della-Porta AJ, et al: Pathology of congenital bovine epizootic arthrogryposis and hydranencephaly and its relationship to Akabane virus. Aust Vet J 53:319–325, 1977.
Kurogi H, Inaba Y, Takahashi E, et al: Congenital abnormalities in newborn calves after inoculation of pregnant cows with Akabane virus. Infect Immunol 17:338–343, 1977.
McPhee, DA, Della-Porta AJ: Biochemical and serological comparisons of Australian bunyaviruses belonging to the Simbu serogroup. J Gen Virol 69:1007–1017, 1988.
Porterfield JS, Della-Porta AJ: Bunyaviridae: infections and diagnosis. In Kurstak E, Kurstak C (eds): Comparative Diagnosis of Viral Diseases, Vol. 4, Part B. New York, Academic Press, 1981, pp 479–508.

Parainfluenza-3 Virus*

GLYNN H. FRANK, DVM, MS, PHD

Parainfluenza-3 (PI-3) virus is a paramyxovirus, and thus far all bovine and ovine isolates compose one serologic group. The virus hemagglutinates the red blood cells and grows on primary cells and established cell lines of a number of species. The cytopathic effect (CPE) usually includes syncytium formation and intracytoplasmic and sometimes intranuclear inclusions. Markers to differentiate strains have included hemagglutination patterns, neuraminidase content, and CPE type, but the stability of the markers is in question.

EPIZOOTIOLOGY

PI-3 virus has been associated with respiratory disease in cattle and sheep and has been isolated from aborted fetuses. It is one of the most common viruses involved in the "shipping fever complex" of cattle. The virus is found worldwide, and from numerous serologic surveys appears to be ubiquitous in cattle and sheep. Seronegative cattle are relatively rare and are highly susceptible to the virus.

CLINICAL SIGNS

Uncomplicated PI-3 viral infections are mild, and the majority are asymptomatic. Young calves often seroconvert with no history of respiratory disease. The economic importance of the virus lies in its ability to predispose cattle to *Pasteurella haemolytica* pneumonia, the most common form of acute respiratory disease in feedlot cattle.

P. haemolytica is most likely to occur in calves that have been subjected to the stresses of the marketing procedure and transportation. It most commonly occurs within 1 to 2 weeks after arrival at the feedyard. Lung lesions of experimental uncomplicated PI-3 viral infections are quickly resolved, but

---
*All material in this article is in the public domain, with the exception of any borrowed figures or tables.

the virus can persist in the alveolar macrophages, and the natural clearance of *P. haemolytica* from the lungs is impaired. Naturally occurring PI-3 virus infections that become severe are part of a respiratory disease complex that involves other etiologic agents. Viral lesions will usually be overshadowed by those of bacterial pneumonia. The role of PI-3 virus in respiratory disease of sheep is much the same as in cattle.

DIAGNOSIS

PI-3 virus is readily isolated from nasal mucus during the acute phase of respiratory disease but is usually not isolated during recovery. At necropsy the virus can be isolated from several tissues of the respiratory tract but persists in the lungs for a longer time than in other tissues. In addition to detection by virus isolation and identification, the involvement of PI-3 virus in a respiratory disease outbreak is detected by serologic evidence. In the diagnostic laboratory the virus is easily identified by standard procedures.

TREATMENT

Treatment is necessary only in complicated infections. These are evident as acute cases of respiratory disease, and treatment consists of treating for bacterial pneumonia.

PREVENTION

A wide variety of vaccines, both killed and attenuated, are available. Currently they all consist of PI-3 virus in combination with other agents. Vaccines have been shown to lessen the severity of experimental PI-3 virus infection in cattle and sheep. The use of modified live vaccines that include infectious bovine rhinotracheitis (IBR) virus for respiratory disease in sheep is questionable because of the introduction of IBR virus into sheep. The efficacy of vaccines in cattle under field conditions is difficult to determine because of the large variety of etiologic agents involved in the bovine respiratory disease complex.

BIBLIOGRAPHY

Frank GH: Paramyxovirus and pneumovirus diseases of animals and birds: comparative aspects and diagnosis. In Kurstak E, Kurstak C (eds): Comparative Diagnosis of Viral Diseases, Vol. IV. New York, Academic Press, 1981, pp 187–233.
Frank GH, Marshall RG: Parainfluenza-3 virus infection of cattle. J Am Vet Med Assoc 163:858, 1973.
Khars RF: Parainfluenza-3. In Khars RF (ed): Viral Diseases of Cattle, 1st ed. Ames, IA, Iowa State University Press, 1981, pp 171–181.

Rinderpest
FAROUK M. HAMDY, DVM, PHD

Rinderpest (RP), or cattle plague, is a highly contagious, usually fatal, acute or subacute disease of ruminants characterized by fever, lacrimation, nasal discharge, profuse diarrhea, and necrotic erosions of the epithelium of the mouth and other mucosa of the digestive tract.

ETIOLOGY

The cause is a member of the genus *Morbillivirus* of the family Paramyxoviridae. Other members of the genus *Morbillivirus* are those causing human measles, canine distemper, and pest of small ruminants (peste des petits ruminants). Other possible candidates for this genus are PMV 107, isolated from cattle with encephalomyelitis; the 72-p-535 viral isolate, isolated from a clinical case of malignant catarrhal fever in Colorado; and Hhl, isolated from apparently normal as well as sick hedgehogs in the United Kingdom.

PHYSICOCHEMICAL PROPERTIES

The RP virion is enveloped and is therefore sensitive to lipid solvents. It shares antigens with other members of the genus. Although RP virus does not have a hemagglutin property like that of the measles virus, RP convalescent or immune bovine serum inhibits agglutination of monkey erythrocytes by the measles virus.

Morphologically RP virus is pleomorphic; the most common shape is spheroid with a diameter of 100 to 300 nm. Less common virions are enveloped filaments up to 1 μm long. Thin sections of infected cells reveal nucleocapsids, usually in the cytoplasm and viral particles exiting the plasma membranes of infected cells. As in all members of the *Morbillivirus* genus, there are seven major proteins and two minor polypeptides.

The viral RNA is single-stranded with an approximate sedimentation constant of 495.

Molecular weight is $4.8 \times 10 - 6.0 \times 10$.

STABILITY

Outside its host, the virus survives best at either low or high relative humidities. Relative humidity between 50 and 60 per cent is lethal to the virus. It is sensitive to heat, light, and both high and low pH. The optimal pH is 7.2 to 7.8.

Virus stability is enhanced in a 1-M solution of magnesium sulfate. This phenomenon has been utilized advantageously in the preparation of vaccine diluents.

RP-infected carcasses are rendered noninfectious following autolysis and putrefaction.

SUSCEPTIBILITY

A list of the natural hosts of RP virus was updated by Scott in 1981 (see Bibliography). Cattle and buffalo are the most important natural hosts. Wild strains of RP virus vary in their host affinities and virulence. Generally members of the order Artiodactyla are susceptible to infection with RP virus; however, RP virus may not attack all the susceptible species at risk.

Goat and sheep have been reported to suffer from lethal RP infection in India. There are some doubts, however, as to the validity of such reports. It appears that many of these outbreaks in sheep and goats in India may well have been caused by peste des petits ruminants virus. Outside India the disease has been observed in goats and sheep only sporadically. Asian pigs are susceptible to lethal RP, while European pigs are infected only subclinically.

CLINICAL SIGNS

The incubation period ranges from 3 to 9 days. A short, sharp rise in body temperature then occurs, and the following signs develop: erosine stomatitis, lacrimation, serous nasal discharge that quickly turns mucopurulent, fetid odor, diarrhea, dehydration, terminal hypothermia, and death. The disease in enzootic regions is usually much less dramatic and is often modified and more difficult to recognize.

Clinical reactions in cattle and buffalo are similar and vary from peracute to acute and from subacute to inapparent. The acute reaction is the typical form in fully susceptible cattle and is manifested by inappetence, fever, and depression. Other signs are shallow and rapid respiration, retarded rumination, and a drop in milk yield in lactating cows. Congestion of the buccal, nasal, conjunctival, and vulvar mucosa is evident. Elevated pinheads of white necrotic epithelium become visible in the mouth and nasal passages. These erode, enlarge, and coalesce. As body temperature falls, diarrhea develops that is characterized by watery, mucoid feces containing perhaps shreds of epithelium and necrotic debris streaked with blood.

GROSS LESIONS

Whitish, punched-out erosions appear at the mucosal surfaces of the lower lip, gums, soft palate, and, less frequently, in the anterior portion of the esophagus and the ventral surface of the free portion of the tongue. Mucosa of the abomasum is congested or hemorrhagic and may reveal erosions. Natural contractions cause the necrotic tissue to lift off and produce shallow erosions. This occurs so readily that erosions are usually the first lesions observed; their margins are sharp, and the bases are reddened by the underlying congested capillaries. The initial minute erosions enlarge and coalesce to form extensive defects. Ulceration may supervene.

Lesions of the small intestine are less severe but are of the same general character. One may see streaks of congestions and white points, with erosions developing in the margins of mucosal folds. These usually are best developed in the upper duodenum and in the ileum. The ileocecal valve and surrounding cecal mucosa are congested and eroded.

There is often edema and hemorrhagic enteritis, especially in the cecum, cecocolic junction, and rectum. This is often described as zebra striping because of hemorrhages of the longitudinal folds of the mucosa. Lymph nodes are usually edematous. Peyer's patches are inflamed and may be hemorrhagic or necrotic.

Petechiae are common in the upper respiratory mucosa, and small erosions may develop on the larynx. Slight erosive lesions may be exhibited in the mucosa of the bladder and vagina.

The mucosa becomes necrotic and grayish in affected foci and then sloughs, leaving sharply marginated, irregular erosions, the bases of which are intensely hyperemic and ooze blood.

Acute congestion and edema of the conjuntiva may be followed by purulent conjunctivitis and corneal ulceration. Skin lesions have been reported, especially in buffalo, but are considered rare.

PATHOGENESIS

RP virus has a special affinity for epithelial cells of the upper respiratory tract, the gastrointestinal tract, and both T and B lymphocytes.

In natural disease the upper respiratory tract is the principal route of infection. The virus localizes in the palatine tonsils and the regional lymph nodes.

The virus replicates in the lymphoid tissues with formation of polykaryocytes or syncytia.

The lesions of stratified squamous epithelium originate in the basal layer. A few and then many epithelial cells undergo necrosis; the nuclei become pyknotic and fragmented.

MICROSCOPIC FINDINGS

The cryptal epithelium in the small intestine may become necrotic, and syncytia may form in crypts. Associated villi may be somewhat atrophic. Small hemorrhages occur from the intensely congested blood vessels. There is diffuse edema of the submucosa, but little leukocytic infiltration.

Necrosis of lymphocytes is extreme. It begins in the germinal centers and proceeds until virtually all mature lymphocytes are lost in individual follicles, leaving only a reticular mesh. Polykaryocytes form in the lymph and hemolymph nodes. There is often an increase in the number of other leukocytes in the sinuses. Similar lesions occur in the spleen, tonsils, and Peyer's patches.

Cellular syncytia and intracytoplasmic as well as intranuclear inclusion bodies may help to differentiate RP from BVD histologically.

TRANSMISSION

RP virus is naturally transmitted to susceptible animals through infected droplets from sick animals via aerosols, secretions, or excretions. Virgin-soil epizootics have been consistently traced to importation of live animals. Very rarely transmission has occurred through fomites, that is, contact with contaminated bedding, fodder, or water. Controlled experiments have shown that pigs could be infected when fed uncooked contaminated meat scraps.

IMMUNOLOGIC PROPERTIES

All strains of RP virus are immunologically homogeneous, and only minute differences can be demonstrated by modern technology.

RP virus is highly immunogenic; cattle that survive natural infection or are adequately vaccinated develop solid, lifelong immunity.

DIAGNOSIS

RP can be provisionally diagnosed on the basis of history, clinical signs, and pathologic lesions. Confirmation of a presumptive field diagnosis is easily achieved by serologic detection of RP viral-specific antigens in tissues of affected animals. Many serologic tests are employed in this task, including agar gel immunodiffusion, counter immunoelectrophoresis, complement fixation, immunofluorescence, and immunoperoxidase staining. Virus isolation in cell culture and its identification by virus neutralization test are also conducted but take longer.

Detection of antibodies, to determine rising titers in paired serum samples, is also used in enzootic regions to diagnose RP infection by employing serum neutralization or complement fixation tests.

Histopathologic examination for characteristic tissue alterations, including necrotic lesions with syncytia and cytoplasmic and nuclear inclusion bodies, can also be used.

DIFFERENTIAL DIAGNOSIS

Infection with RP virus activates latent pathogens and may confuse diagnosis. Bovine virus diarrhea is clinically similar to RP, but the causal viruses are serologically distinct. Therefore laboratory diagnosis can be easily achieved. Infectious bovine rhinotracheitis, malignant catarrhal fever, hemorrhagic septicemia, and other conditions such as arsenic poisoning, salmonellosis, theileriasis, and trypanosomiasis could be confused with RP. RP in sheep and goats must be differentiated from peste des petits ruminants through virus isolation and identification confirmed by virus neutralization test.

COLLECTION OF SPECIMENS FOR DIAGNOSIS

Specimens for diagnosis should be collected from several sick or sacrificed animals at the onset of fever through the erosive mucosal phase, but before the onset of diarrhea. Clear lacrimal secretions, uncoagulated blood, lymph nodes, tonsils, and gum debris are adequate samples for virus isolation or detection of viral antigens. Paired serum samples are also useful for detection of specific antibodies.

Specimens should be chilled until they reach the laboratory. No transport medium is required; particularly glycerol should not be used, as it is virucidal for RP virus.

A set of specimens fixed in buffered formalin can be dispatched at ambient temperature, but it should be protected from overheating or freezing.

PREVENTION AND CONTROL

To maintain their status, RP-free countries should not take risks by importing live cattle or other susceptible animals from enzootic regions. If this embargo is not practical, that is, in zoologic ruminants, these animals should be tested twice for antibody 30 days apart with negative results. Upon arrival in an RP-free country, imported animals should be kept in quarantine and retested negative for antibody before their release.

Cell culture RP vaccines are currently the most widely used for cattle and buffalo immunization. Usually vaccination is practiced as a prophylactic measure in enzootic regions or in RP-free areas adjacent to enzootic regions. If properly produced and administered, vaccine is safe and induces solid, permanent immunity.

If the disease should manage to reach an RP-free country, it can be successfully eradicated by quarantine and vaccination or by quarantine and slaughter.

RP is still prevalent in Africa, South Asia, and the Middle East. The United Nations Food and Agriculture Organization has been coordinating activities to launch massive vaccination campaigns at these three frontiers. The hope is to eradicate RP virus from the globe as the World Health Organization has achieved with smallpox. This is technically feasible, but it will take quality animal health management, commitment, and persistence on the part of interested governments.

The most recent developments in the production of RP vaccines are a thermostable vaccine virus mutant and the subviral vaccine; these two products are important improvements to the already efficient RP cell culture vaccines.

Proper disposal of carcasses, decontamination of infected premises, and strict quarantine are the sanitary measures necessary for control, containment, and eventual eradication of RP.

EPIZOOTIOLOGY

RP is one of the most fatal diseases of cloven-hooved animals and has caused tremendous catastrophes by decimating cattle populations during the last 100 years. It is highly contagious; the morbidity rate may reach 100 per cent, and the mortality rate may exceed 90 per cent in a susceptible cattle population. In areas previously free of the disease, epizootic RP affects all ages of susceptible animals.

On many occasions, especially in times of war, RP has been spread from Asia to Europe, where it has caused tremendous losses in the cattle population. RP has never occurred in North America and only once in the Western Hemisphere, where it occurred in Brazil after the importation of Zebu cattle from India. The disease was recognized relatively early, and the death toll was only 1000 cattle, with another 2000 sacrificed.

With the development of speedy modes of transportation for people and animals, the threat of introduction of RP has increased. Veterinarians should be aware of the status of animal diseases throughout the world and should be able to recognize RP quickly if measures for prevention of its introduction ever fail. The Soviet Union experienced a small outbreak of RP early in 1990 after 63 years of freedom from this disease.

Being enzootic in parts of Africa, South Asia, and the Middle East, RP remains one of the foremost causes of mortality in these regions. Although RP appears to attach ungulates of the order Artiodactyla, not all species in this order are affected. Wild RP viral strains vary widely in their infectivity, and this infectivity seems to vary with time. While cattle and buffalo are the most important victims, sheep and goats, especially in India, have been reported to suffer from fatal RP. The Asian domestic pig succumbs to RP infection, while the European variety of domestic pig appears to be infected only subclinically.

Many species of wildlife in Africa, for example, buffalo, eland, kudu, bongo, bushbuck, hushpig, giraffe, warthog, impala, and Thomson's gazelle, are susceptible.

In enzootic areas, calves of susceptible dams and those of immune dams whose maternal antibodies have waned before they receive vaccinations are the principal victims.

BIBLIOGRAPHY

DeBoer CJ, Barber TL: pH and thermal stability of rinderpest virus. Arch Ges Virusforsh 15:98–108, 1964.

Fenner F: Classification and nomenclature of viruses. Second report of international committee on taxomony of viruses. Intervirology 7:59, 1976.

Maurer FD, et al: The pathology of rinderpest. Proc 92nd Ann Mtg Am Vet Med Assoc, Minneapolis, 1955, pp 201–211.

Nakamura J, MacLeod AJ: The complement fixation test and its adaptation to the diagnosis of rinderpest. J Comp Pathol 69:11–69, 1959.

Plowright W: Rinderpest virus. Ann NY Acad Sci 101:327–382, 1962.

Plowright W, Cruickshank JG, Waterson AP: The morphology of rinderpest virus. Virology 17:118–122, 1962.

Plowright W, Ferris RD: Studies with rinderpest virus in tissue culture: the use of attenuated vaccine for cattle. Res Vet Sci 3:172–182, 1962.

Plowright W, Ferris RD: Studies with rinderpest virus in tissue culture. III. The stability of cultured virus and its use in virus neutralization tests. Arch Ges Virusforsch 11:516–533, 1962.

Scott GR: The incidence of rinderpest in sheep and goats. Bull Epiz Dis Afr 3:117–118, 1955.

Scott GR: Rinderpest. Adv Vet Sci 9:113–224, 1964.

Scott GR: Rinderpest. In Davies JW, Karstad LH, Trainer DD (eds): Infectious Diseases of Wild Mammals, 2nd ed. Ames, IA, Iowa State University Press, 1981, pp 18–30.

Scott GR, Taylor WP, Rossiter PB: Manual on the Diagnosis of Rinderpest. FAO Animal Production and Health Series No. 23. Rome, United Nations Food and Agriculture Organization, 1986.

White G: A specific diffusable antigen of rinderpest virus demonstrated by the agar double diffusion precipitation reaction. Nature 181:1409, 1958.

Bovine Respiratory Syncytial Virus

MALCOLM H. SMITH, DVM, PHD

Bovine respiratory syncytial virus (BRSV) was first recognized as causing disease in cattle in 1970. The human counterpart virus, RSV, has been recognized since the late 1950s and is the major cause of severe, life-threatening lower respiratory disease in infants and young children.

Since 1970 BRSV has been recognized worldwide as being associated with bovine respiratory disease of varying severity. BRSV will infect cattle of all ages, types, and breeds. It is now apparent that BRSV plays a major role in respiratory disease of all cattle.

BRSV is a member of the family Paramyxoviridae and is classified a pneumovirus. It is a fragile, pleomorphic, easily inactivated virus that derives its name from the formation of characteristic masses of fused cells, or syncytia, in cell culture and in the infected animal. BRSV and respiratory syncytial viruses from other species, including sheep, goats, and humans, are similar but distinct antigenically.

CLINICAL SIGNS AND LESIONS

The spectrum of clinical signs extends from subclinical to mild to life-threatening. The high incidence of antibody in cattle populations is indicative of widespread subclinical infection.

Clinical signs include elevated temperature, hyperpnea, increased harshness in respiratory sounds, and spontaneous coughing that can vary from dry and nonproductive to moist. Coughing can often be easily induced. Nasal discharge in varying degrees is often present. Conjunctivitis may be seen but is not a common feature. Most cases recover spontaneously. Severe cases often progress to death in spite of treatment.

Most efforts to infect calves experimentally have resulted in only mild or subclinical manifestation of disease, whereas others have succeeded in producing severe disease. It would appear that there are differences in pathogenicity among virus isolates. In both naturally and experimentally infected calves, temperatures may be elevated to 41 to 43°C (107 to 109°F), often without clinical signs of disease.

The pathogenesis of BRSV-induced respiratory disease is far from clear. A biphasic disease pattern has been described, with an initial, mild infection followed by a severe, often fatal episode with extensive emphysema evident. Immune-mediated disease is a likely explanation for some of these cases. The involvement of immunoglobulin E (IgE) in the pathogenesis of severe disease has been described. The association of BRSV with atypical interstitial pneumonia of feedlot cattle would support the hypothesis that immune mechanisms may be involved with severe disease.

Postmortem examination of fatal BRSV pneumonia presents a variety of lesions, including consolidation of anteroventral lobes with varying degrees of emphysema and edema. Secondary bacterial infection is often evident, usually *Pasteurella haemolytica* with associated fibrinous pleuritis. Fatal pneumonia can occur with only BRSV and with no secondary bacterial involvement.

Microscopic features of respiratory tract lesions in fatal cases include necrotizing bronchiolitis, bronchiolitis obliterans, interstitial pneumonia, and edema with hyaline membrane formation. Syncytia with or without inclusions are frequently observed.

DIAGNOSIS

Serologic studies indicate that 40 to 50 per cent of respiratory disease outbreaks in feeder calves involve BRSV. However, there are few salient features that would assist a clinician in making a presumptive diagnosis of BRSV-induced disease. A diagnosis is often made only by virus isolation, a demonstration of a rise in antibody to the virus, or both. BRSV is difficult to isolate because of its lability and because nasal swab material is usually taken too late. Samples taken early in the clinical course, when high temperatures exist and before signs of severe respiratory disease appear, are most likely to be successful in yielding the virus. Many cell types support replication of BRSV.

Immunofluorescent techniques, both direct and indirect, and serum neutralization tests are used to detect antibody to BRSV. Recently a hemagglutination inhibition test has been described. Enzyme-linked immunosorbent assay tests have been used with varying degrees of success. By the time severe signs of respiratory disease are noted, the antibody titer may already be quite elevated and the acute and convalescent serum titers may be inverted. A number of animals in an outbreak should be sampled for meaningful serologic studies.

TREATMENT, PREVENTION, AND CONTROL

Conventional treatment with antibiotics and supportive therapy to combat secondary infections is usually successful. Where severe clinical manifestations exist with emphysema, and death occurs within the infected herd, more vigorous therapy with antihistamines and corticosteroids in addition to antibiotics and supportive therapy may be necessary.

Conventional management practices, such as preconditioning to lessen the stress coincident with weaning, are often helpful in disease prevention. Vaccines have become available and are currently widely used. Good efficacy has been observed, especially when the vaccine is a part of a total herd health program. Recent evidence of severe disease resulting from use of vaccine concurrent with natural infection signals caution to indiscriminate vaccine use.

BIBLIOGRAPHY

Baker JC: Bovine respiratory syncytial virus: pathogenesis, clinical signs, diagnosis, treatment and prevention. Compendium on Continuing Education for the Practicing Veterinarian, 8:F31–F38, 1986.
Collins JK, Jensen R, Smith GH, et al: Association of bovine respiratory syncytial virus with atypical interstitial pneumonia in feedlot cattle. Am J Vet Res 49:1045–1049, 1988.
Kimman TG, Sol J, Westenbrink F, Straver PJ: A severe outbreak of respiratory tract disease associated with bovine respiratory syncytial virus probably enhanced by vaccination with modified live vaccine. Vet Q 11:250–253, 1989.
Stewart RS, Gershwin L: Role of IgE in the pathogenesis of bovine respiratory syncytial virus in sequential infections in vaccinated and nonvaccinated calves. Am J Vet Res 50:349–355, 1989.

Vesicular Stomatitis Virus in Cattle

ALVIN W. SMITH, DVM, PHD

Vesicular stomatitis (VS) viruses belong to the family Rhabdoviridae and the genus *Vesiculovirus*. They are bullet-shaped, 65 × 185 nm in size, with a helically arranged single-stranded RNA genome, and their surface envelope is covered with spikes 10 nm long.

They are inactivated by lipid solvents and heat (58°C for 30 minutes) but will survive for several weeks in soils at 4 to 6°C and are resistant within a pH range of 2 to 11.

The first VS virus was isolated in 1925 from vesicles of cattle in Indiana and is the prototype virus. Subsequent isolates have been grouped into three serotypes: (1) Indiana with three strains as follows: Indiana 1 (Indiana strain), Indiana 2 (Cocal and Argentina strains), and Indiana 3 (Alagoas and Brazil strains); (2) New Jersey, represented by a single strain; and (3) Isfahan with three strains as follows: Isfahan (*Phlebotomus* strain from Iran), Chandipura (human strain from India), and Piry (opossum strain from Brazil).

VS virus is inactivated in 10 minutes by 1 per cent formalin; 1:200 Wescodyne[1]; benzalkonium chloride (Roccal) (10 per cent at 1:200); 1:1000 Roccal[2]; and 1:50 hexachlorophene (Septisol[3]). Lye (2 per cent sodium hydroxide) has been used but will not deactivate the virus in 2 hours.

EPIZOOTIOLOGY

Vesicular stomatitis virus will cause clinical infection in naturally exposed cattle, swine, horses, deer, and humans. Sheep can be experimentally infected, and although there have been occasional reports of field infections, sheep are considered quite resistant. Other species having shown serologic conversion under conditions of natural exposure are javelinas, turkeys, raccoons, bobcats, skunks, opossums, squirrels, antelopes, monkeys, sloths, porcupines, bats, and some rodents. Experimentally the virus will infect all the common laboratory rodents and chinchillas, ferrets, and chickens. Dogs are refractive. The virus will replicate in mosquitoes, leaf hoppers, and sand flies, and transovarian passage has been demonstrated in *Phlebotomus* flies. Mechanical transmission by nonbiting insect pests has also been suggested.

The virus is confined to the New World, primarily the United States, Mexico, Central America, Venezuela, Colombia, Ecuador, and Peru. The disease stays endemic in the more tropical zones, which include the Gulf Coast, Georgia, and the Carolinas, then extends into Veracruz, Mexico, and into Colombia. During the spring and summer under favorable conditions, every 10 years or so, VS will spread in epizootic fashion into the temperate zones of the United States, Brazil, and Argentina. Alaska, western Canada, New England, and eastern Canada have not experienced epizootics of VS. When epizootics do occur in the United States, they move northward up the river valleys of the Appalachian chain, upper Mississippi, and Rocky Mountains as the summer progresses and occasionally extend north into central Canada. Epizootic spread is favored when environmental temperatures are above 20°C, lush vegetation occurs in river valleys, and some shade is present. Deserts, high mountains, and open plains act as barriers to spread. The epizootic form of the disease primarily affects cattle and horses, and the movement of infected animals can readily spread the disease.

The precise mechanisms of transmission and reasons for occasional epizootic spread out of endemic areas are not understood. Two important aspects of past epizootics have been that the incubation period is less than 7 days and the disease dies out with the first killing frost in the autumn. The extensive and costly epizootic of 1982 did not follow this pattern: one dairy broke with the disease in a way that suggested a 30-day incubation period, and other outbreaks in dairies of the central valley of California occurred through the winter on into March of the following year.

CLINICAL SIGNS

The most important aspect of this disease is that the clinical disease in cattle mimics that in swine and must be rapidly differentiated from foot-and-mouth disease. Once animals become infected, vesicular lesions will occur on the tongue, lips, gums, teats, and coronary bands. If there are oral lesions, these will be accompanied by profuse salivation and a reluctance to eat. The incubation period is usually 2 to 4 days, and older animals will be more frequently affected. Economic losses in dairy and swine herds can be considerable, especially if there is secondary mycotic or bacterial invasion of lesions. Uncomplicated cases will fully recover in 2 weeks.

DIAGNOSIS

If horses have lesions, a presumptive diagnosis of VS can be made on clinical evidence because there are no other virus diseases that mimic the signs and lesions seen in horses. Laboratory diagnosis in cattle and swine is absolutely essential for differentiation from foot-and-mouth disease and must be made on the basis of virus isolation and the presence of specific antibodies. Appropriate laboratory specimens are epithelial tissues covering the vesicle and the vesicular fluid. These should be placed in buffered glycerol or frozen for shipment. Paired acute and convalescent serum samples are useful for complement fixation and serum neutralization tests. One of the newer, rapid diagnostic tests is a tissue microtitration complement fixation (TMCF) test, which can be performed in 3 hours at any time of the day or night. Although it has not been described for field cases, direct electron microscopic examination of lesion material could, in appropriate samples, rapidly and easily differentiate the rhabdovirus of VS from the enterovirus of foot-and-mouth disease and the calicivirus of vesicular exanthema of swine.

TREATMENT

There is no specific treatment except supportive therapy, for example, feeding soft foods, providing rest and an abundance of water, and ensuring early treatment of secondary infections.

PREVENTION AND CONTROL

During epizootics, livestock movements and other common mechanisms for contact transmission should be avoided; however, severely restrictive control measures within epizootic areas may not be warranted because of the sporadic nature of the disease. A vaccine has been developed and approved for use in the United States but has not been field tested during one of the periodic epizootics that occur in United States cattle. Newer vaccines incorporating novel methods of viral inactivation and genetic manipulation are currently being developed for a variety of rhabdoviruses, but most have not been licensed yet.

BIBLIOGRAPHY

Callis J, Dardiri J, Ferris AH, et al: Illustrated Manual for the Recognition and Diagnosis of Certain Animal Diseases. Mexico–United States Commission

---

[1]Wescodyne, West Chemical Co.
[2]Winthrop Laboratories.
[3]Calgon.

for the Prevention of Foot and Mouth Disease, Plum Island Animal Disease Center, 1982, pp 17–19.

Jenney EW: Vesicular stomatitis in the United States during the last 5 years (1963–1967). Proc 71st Ann Mtg US Livestock Sanit Assoc, 1967, pp 371–385.

Snyder ML, Jenney EW, Erickson GA, Carbrey EA: The 1982 resurgence of vesicular stomatitis in the United States: a summary of laboratory diagnostic findings. Am Assoc Vet Lab Diagnosticians, 25th Ann Proc, 1983, pp 221–228.

Bovine Ephemeral Fever

P. B. SPRADBROW, BVSc, PhD, DVSc

Bovine ephemeral fever (BEF) virus is a vector-transmitted rhabdovirus. The insect vectors have not been specifically identified, but they are believed to include species of *Culicoides* and possibly mosquitoes. Only a single serologic type of BEF virus is known. However, in Australia other rhabdoviruses with a distant serologic relationship to BEF virus have been isolated. The presence of these viruses complicates the interpretation of serologic surveys.

EPIZOOTIOLOGY

BEF is a viral disease of cattle and possibly water buffalo. Other species of domestic animals are apparently insusceptible, and reservoirs of infection among feral animals or birds have not been identified. BEF occurs in Australia, Asia, and Africa. Sporadic cases occur in endemic areas, and there are occasional extensive epizootics. The mortality rate is usually low, possibly less than 1 per cent.

BEF virus does not spread between cattle by contact. There is a brief period of viremia at the time when the animal is clinically ill, and blood-sucking vectors are presumably infected at this time. Some infected animals develop viremia but show no obvious clinical signs. Recovered carriers are not recognized. The seasonal incidence of the disease is related to periods of vector activity.

BEF is not a killing disease. It is serious because it results in a great reduction in milk yield and because it immobilizes animals, making normal husbandry and marketing procedures impossible.

CLINICAL SIGNS

The early clinical signs of BEF are inappetence and pyrexia. The fever is biphasic, and the temperature is normal or nearly normal between the two peaks. Stiffness or lameness is the most obvious sign in cattle in the field. This symptom usually develops a little after the febrile response begins, but it does not occur in all animals. Lameness usually affects more than one leg, and animals often become recumbent. There is a sudden and severe drop in milk production in lactating cows. Many animals experience difficulty swallowing and salivate excessively.

Other inconstant clinical signs are shivering, nasal and ocular discharge, edema affecting the area around joints, and subcutaneous emphysema. Fever and lameness usually abate after 3 or 4 days. A few animals remain recumbent for long periods after the temperature returns to normal. Pregnant animals do not abort, but a reduction in semen quality occurs in some bulls.

The blood picture is one of leukocytosis and neutrophilia, returning to normal within a few days of recovery. Necropsy changes are usually slight and include edema of lymph nodes, congestion of abomasal mucous membranes, and variable inflammatory changes on serosal surfaces.

The pathogenesis of BEF has not been fully explained. The basic gross lesion appears to be a serofibrinous polyserositis, presumably resulting from capillary damage to serosal surfaces in the body cavity and joints. The virus appears to be noncytolytic in bovine cells. Both interferons and interleukin-1 have been proposed as mediators of the inflammatory changes in BEF.

DIAGNOSIS

BEF is usually diagnosed on clinical grounds, especially during an epizootic. Isolated cases need to be differentiated from bovine chlamydiosis.

The laboratory diagnosis depends on the demonstration of viremia or of rising levels of neutralizing antibody. BEF virus can be isolated by serial, intracerebral passage in suckling mice or in Vero or baby hamster kidney cell cultures. An insect cell line derived from *Aedes albopictus* has greater sensitivity. Diagnosis is also possible by fluorescent antibody staining of blood smears prepared during viremia. Neutralizing antibodies are most conveniently detected in cell cultures.

The prognosis is usually favorable unless recumbency has been prolonged. Animals that have been down for long periods may die or may be permanently ataxic.

TREATMENT

There is no specific treatment for BEF. Recumbent animals should be provided with shade and water. Nonspecific therapy aims at reducing fever and alleviating joint pain. Oral medication with liquids should be avoided because many animals have difficulty swallowing.

Acetylsalicylic acid (Acetobols[1]) is given orally as a bolus or in a gelatin capsule to control fever. The dose for mature cattle is 60 to 120 g every 12 hours. Phenylbutazone, which has antipyretic action similar to that of acetylsalicylic acid, has additional anti-inflammatory action. In artificially infected cattle, repeated treatment with phenylbutazone initiated before or shortly after the start of pyrexia suppressed the development of clinical signs. However, viremia and development of immunity were not affected. This drug can be given intravenously, which is an advantage in animals that will not readily take oral medication. Phenylbutazone is obtainable in combination with isopyrin (Tomanol[2]). Tomanol contains 120 mg phenylbutazone and 240 mg isopyrin per milliliter and is given by slow intravenous drip or by intramuscular injection. The dose for a mature animal is 20 to 30 ml.

PREVENTION

Vector control is not usually a practical remedy. BEF virus vaccines are used in South Africa, Australia, and Japan. The vaccine widely used in Australia uses living virus grown in cultures of Vero cells and mixed with the saponin-based adjuvant Quil A[3] immediately before administration. Immunity following natural infection is long-lasting.

---

[1]Available from Parnell Laboratories Pty. Ltd., Peakhurst, N.S.W., 2210, Australia.
[2]Available from Intervet Pty. Ltd., Artarmon, N.S.W. 2064, Australia.
[3]Available from Arthur Webster Pty. Ltd., Castle Hill, N.S.W. 2154, Australia.

BIBLIOGRAPHY

Bryden DI: Ephemeral fever. *In* The Post Graduate Committee in Veterinary Science: The Therapeutic Jungle. Proceedings No. 39. Sydney, Austrl, University of Sydney, 1978, pp 312–314.

Spradbrow PB: Vaccines against bovine ephemeral fever. Aust Vet J 53:351, 1977.

Uren MF: Bovine ephemeral fever. Aust Vet J 66:233, 1989.

Uren MF, St. George TD, Zakrzewski H: The effect of anti-inflammatory agents on the clinical expression of bovine ephemeral fever. Vet Microbiol 19:99, 1989.

Young PL, Spradbrow PB: The clinical response of cattle to experimental infection with bovine ephemeral fever virus. Vet Record 126:86, 1990.

Bovine Leukemia Virus*

JANICE M. MILLER, DVM, PHD, MS, BS

Lymphatic cancer in cattle is known by several terms, including leukemia, leukosis, lymphosarcoma, and malignant lymphoma. The disease was first described in eastern Europe in about 1900. As case reports accumulated, it became clear that there were four different clinicopathologic forms of lymphoid neoplasia, which were designated calf, thymic, skin, and adult. Epidemiologic studies indicated that the adult form was contagious, and it was called enzootic bovine leukosis (EBL). The other three forms were called sporadic because there was no evidence that they were infectious. The accuracy of this classification was finally proven in the 1970s, when it was shown that a retrovirus, bovine leukemia virus (BLV), causes adult-type leukosis but is not involved in pathogenesis of sporadic forms. No etiology has been identified for calf, thymic, or skin leukosis.

ETIOLOGY

BLV is an antigenically unique, horizontally transmitted oncogenic retrovirus. The mode of replication in infected cells is characteristic of viruses belonging to the retrovirus family. Genetic information, which exists as RNA, is copied with the aid of a specific viral enzyme into a "mirror image" DNA molecule. This DNA, called the provirus, is then integrated into chromosomal DNA and becomes part of the infected cell's genetic information. Thereafter the provirus is perpetuated at each subsequent cell division, even in the absence of further virus replication and in the presence of viral-specific antibody.

Because BLV-infected cattle do not produce significant amounts of cell-free virus, environmental or chemical inactivation of the agent is not a pertinent consideration. Infection is apparently transmitted by introduction of viable lymphocytes from an infected to a susceptible animal. After this transfer occurs, lymphocytes become activated and produce complete virus particles that are infectious for the new host. BLV transmission can be prevented only if infected lymphocytes are destroyed. Freezing, drying, and temperatures above 50° C are lethal to lymphocytes, but the cells can survive in blood at 4°C for at least 2 weeks and in serum even longer. Chemical inactivation of infective lymphocytes has not been studied, but any solvent or nonisotonic liquid would be expected to cause lysis.

---

*All material in this article is in the public domain, with the exception of any borrowed figures or tables.

EPIZOOTIOLOGY

Cattle are the primary natural host of BLV. Sheep can be infected experimentally; there are a few reports of natural infections in sheep, but the source and mode of transmission were not determined. The distribution of BLV is worldwide, although prevalence of infection varies greatly from one geographic region to another. Many countries in Europe, through long-standing efforts to control the spread of leukosis, have succeeded in reducing virus prevalence to very low levels, and in some regions infection has been totally eliminated. In the United States, BLV prevalence in dairy cattle ranges from 10 to 50 per cent in various parts of the country. In the same areas, infection in beef cattle is less common, ranging from 1 to 20 per cent. Regardless of production type, BLV prevalence in an individual herd can be very high, sometimes involving virtually all adult animals. Transmission of BLV apparently requires close, prolonged contact, and it is believed that most infections result from blood transfer into the skin of a susceptible animal. The most likely mechanisms for this type of transfer appear to be insects (over short distances) and traumatic, surgical, or other similar events that lead to blood contamination. There seems to be little or no risk of transmission by semen from infected bulls if artificial insemination is used; however, the close contact involved in natural service presents a greater potential for spreading virus. Calves can carry BLV at birth as a result of in utero exposure, but in most herds this involves less than 10 per cent of the calves from infected dams. Although milk from infected cows contains cells with provirus, oral transmission to nursing calves is a rare event, probably because most of them receive enough colostral antibody to neutralize virus particles produced in the gut.

CLINICAL SIGNS AND LESIONS

The lymphosarcoma produced by BLV occurs in adult cattle, usually between 4 and 8 years of age. The location of tumors is unpredictable, but frequent sites are lymph nodes, heart, abomasum, kidney, spleen, uterus, lumbar spinal cord, and retrobulbar lymphatic tissue. Symptoms vary depending on the organ or tissues affected, but weight loss and decreased milk production are frequent nonspecific signs that accompany tumor development. The most obvious clinical signs of lymphosarcoma are enlargement of peripheral lymph nodes or exopthalmos due to tumor in the posterior orbit. When there is heart involvement, a marked jugular pulse and ventral edema in the neck may be present. Abomasal tumors often lead to ulcers, which are detected by the appearance of dark blood in the feces. Splenic lesions generally are not recognized clinically unless the organ becomes so large that it ruptures. Uterine and pelvic lymph node tumors may cause breeding problems and are often detected by rectal palpation. Posterior paresis or paralysis is the typical symptom associated with tumor in the spinal canal.

Cattle with EBL may have elevated lymphocyte counts in peripheral blood, but leukemia is not a typical manifestation of lymphosarcoma. Infection with BLV causes some animals (approximately one third) to develop persistent lymphocytosis, and this condition can be present for many years in the absence of other clinical signs. Although a few lymphocytotic cattle develop tumor, it is unwise to use the blood profile for prognosis or diagnosis.

For comparison to EBL, a brief summary of clinical findings in sporadic (non-BLV related) bovine leukosis is presented here.

The *calf* form usually appears when animals are less than 6 months old and has been seen in fetuses. The hallmark of this form is tumor involvement of virtually all hematopoietic tissues and other organ systems as well. High blood lymphocyte counts are common.

An animal with *thymic* form is typically between 6 months and 2 years of age. The common clinical presentation is diffuse, firm swelling in the ventral neck, sometimes accompanied by enlargement of prescapular lymph nodes. Leukocyte counts are usually within normal limits.

Skin leukosis, the rarest form, is most frequently seen in young adults. Tumors occur only in the skin and usually regress after a few weeks. There may be a subsequent recurrence of generalized lymphosarcoma, which is fatal.

DIAGNOSIS

In considering the diagnosis of EBL, it is important to recognize that there are two different problems. One is diagnosis of *disease* (tumor), and the other is diagnosis of BLV *infection*. Only a few infected cattle (usually less than 1 per cent annually) develop lymphosarcoma. Environmental, immunologic, genetic, or other factors probably play an important role in determining which animals become clinically affected.

A conclusive diagnosis of lymphosarcoma requires histopathologic examination of affected tissue. A presumptive diagnosis is usually accurate, however, if clinical history and physical examination suggest a noninflammatory proliferation of lymphatic tissue. Histopathologic confirmation is needed to rule out granulomatous disease or some other type of neoplasm that would produce similar gross tissue changes. Specimens for study should be submitted to the diagnostic laboratory in 10 per cent formalin.

Establishment of etiologic diagnosis requires identification of BLV infection. Because the virus persists, there is constant production of antigen and consequently a marked antibody response. Infected cattle can be detected by a number of serologic tests. The most sensitive test is radioimmunoassay (RIA), but application of the technique has been limited due to relatively high cost and requirement for sophisticated technology. Enzyme-linked immunosorbent assays (ELISA) are easier to perform and almost as sensitive as RIA. Because it is simple and inexpensive, the agar gel immunodiffusion (AGID) test is widely used. BLV infection can be detected by AGID within 2 to 3 months after virus exposure; thereafter the antibody titer rarely falls below a detectable level. The only time a positive AGID test is inconclusive is in the case of calves less than 6 months old. Because colostral antibody may persist for that length of time, a serologic test cannot determine if calves have active infection or just passive antibody. In this situation virus isolation is the only diagnostic test possible, and because it is technically very difficult, few laboratories provide the service.

TREATMENT

There is no treatment for animals with tumor. BLV infection is always persistent and cannot be eliminated by any drug currently available.

PREVENTION AND CONTROL

The only way to prevent EBL (lymphosarcoma) is to prevent BLV infection. Because the virus spreads primarily by contact, control must be instituted at the herd level unless animal(s) to be protected can be isolated. BLV can be eradicated from a herd by repeated serologic testing of animals over 6 months of age, followed by rapid removal of infected cattle. If testing is conducted at 3-month intervals, the herd is usually BLV free after the second or third test. A few European countries have used such procedures to eradicate BLV, and several others have instituted programs designed to reduce spread of infection. For this reason serologic testing is now frequently incorporated into regulations for international trade. The resulting economic impact on sales of cattle, semen, and embryos has been the most serious national problem associated with BLV. Vaccination against infection may be feasible, but the protective antigen would seroconvert animals and make them ineligible for export certification. In some herds tumor incidence is high enough to create substantial economic loss; however, demand for a vaccine has not been sufficient to stimulate commercial interest in the research and development necessary to prove safety and efficacy.

BIBLIOGRAPHY

Miller JM, Van Der Maaten MJ: Bovine leukosis—its importance to the dairy industry in the United States. J Dairy Sci 65:2194–2203, 1982.
Stober M: The clinical picture of the enzootic and sporadic forms of bovine leukosis. Bov Pract 16:119–129, 1981.
Thurmond MC, Burridge MJ: Application of research to control of bovine leukemia virus infection and to exportation of bovine leukemia virus-free cattle and semen. J Am Vet Med Assoc 181:1531–1534, 1982.

Bovine Breda Virus (Torovirus)

GERALD N. WOODE, BVetMed, DVetMed

Two viruses that have been isolated from the diarrheic feces of either horses (Berne virus) or calves (Breda virus) are related and have been placed in the proposed Toroviridae family. Similar viruses have been demonstrated in the diarrheic feces of children, and from serologic evidence the presence of similar viruses in swine, sheep, goats, rabbits, and wild mice is probable. Although toroviruses do not share antigens with coronaviruses, superficially the morphology of the two virus families is similar, causing confusion in the viral diagnosis of diarrheic samples by electron microscopy.

ETIOLOGY

The Berne virus, Breda virus, and human viruses share antigens when tested by enzyme-linked immunosorbent assays (ELISA) or by immunoelectron microscopy. Breda virus isolates have been subdivided into two serotype groups by hemagglutination inhibition reactions, although both serotypes cross-react by immunofluorescence with infected intestinal sections and by ELISA. Breda virus serotype 1 is represented by Iowa isolate 1, and Breda virus serotype 2 by Iowa isolate 2 and the Ohio isolate. Apart from one report that has not been confirmed, Breda viruses have not been adapted to cell culture, and all studies on the morphology, replication, and biochemical properties of the virions have been obtained by the infection of gnotobiotic calves. Berne virus, in contrast, is adapted to cell culture, and the taxonomic properties of the group have been determined with this virus and then compared with the in vivo cultured Breda virus.

In negatively stained preparations the virus particles are either elongated or curved into a kidney shape (105 to 140 × 12 to 40 nm) or spherical (mean diameter of 82 nm). Peplomers are present in the envelope, measuring approximately 7 to 9 nm (Breda virus serotype 1) or 20 nm (Berne virus and Breda virus serotype 2). The presence of short, stubby peplomers on many particles aids in the differentiation from coronavirus, as does the rather characteristic kidney shape, if these particles predominate in the preparation being examined. The virions contain ssRNA of positive polarity and four major proteins. Replication occurs in the cytoplasm with the budding of preformed tubular capsids through Golgi membranes and endoplasmic reticulum, and host-cell nuclear function is required.

EPIZOOTIOLOGY

From serologic evidence, Breda virus infections are common in cattle in the United States, the Netherlands, France, and Germany. Breda virus has been isolated from calves in the United States, France, and Germany. Approximately 90 per cent of cattle sera are positive for Breda virus antibody. In contrast to these data, the presence of the virus is infrequently demonstrated in diarrheic samples. This may be due to a combination of two problems. First, few laboratories possess the diagnostic expertise to identify Breda virus. Second, the excretion of the virus at detectable levels in many calves is restricted to 1 to 2 days during the postinfection period.

Little is known about the survival and spread of the virus under farm conditions. Experimentally the fecal-oral route of transmission is successful, and the viruses probably have the same survivability outside the host as do the coronaviruses. For long-term (more than 6 months) the virus probably survives by continual reinfection of adults or through the agency of carrier cows, as has been suggested for coronaviruses. Under acute epizootic conditions of housed animals, viral infections spread rapidly from calf to calf.

CLINICAL SIGNS AND LESIONS

Calves develop diarrhea within 48 to 72 hours postinfection. The color of the diarrheic feces is largely dependent on the diet, varying from white to yellow scours for the wholly milk-fed animal to brown or green for older calves. The clinical signs are not distinguishable from diarrheas induced by rotavirus, coronavirus, *Escherichia coli*, and *Cryptosporidium*. Both the small and the large intestines are infected; thus the diarrhea is usually more watery than that seen in uncomplicated rotavirus diarrhea. As for most enteric infections, the severity of the disease varies considerably between outbreaks. Calves may show mild to severe diarrhea of 1 to 4 days' duration followed by rapid recovery or death after severe loss of weight and dehydration. Cold stress appears to predispose calves to a higher mortality rate, although experimental studies by the author and colleagues in gnotobiotic and conventionally reared calves suggest that animal-to-animal variation is more important in determining the outcome of the infection than is the role of environmental factors or mixed infections. Lesions occur in the epithelium of the small intestine from midjejunum through the ileum and also in the epithelial cells of all parts of the large intestine. Both crypt and villous epithelial cells are infected, including the dome epithelial cells covering Peyer's patches. Infected cells slough off, the villi collapse in atrophy, and maldigestion and malabsorption develop. There is an acute inflammatory response with cellular infiltration. Tubular structures, similar in size to the inner tubular structure of the virion, are observed in both the nucleus and the cytoplasm. Breda virus has been isolated recently from the larynx, trachea, and lungs of calves that died after severe respiratory disease.

DIAGNOSIS

Fecal samples are taken during the first 3 days of diarrhea. The diagnostic method of choice at present is immunoelectron microscopy (IEM), although hemagglutination and hemagglutination inhibition (HAI) tests and ELISA for antigen identification in feces have proved useful. IEM and HAI are largely serotype-specific tests, and thus unrecognized serotypes may appear as false negatives. In ELISA tests and immunofluorescence, antibodies react with the torovirus-group antigens.

TREATMENT

The treatment as described for rotavirus and coronavirus infections in calves is applicable to Breda virus infections.

PREVENTION

As little is known concerning the epidemiology of the infection, prevention is based on a common sense approach. Both direct and indirect transmission between calves can be controlled to a limited extent by good management practices, and isolation of all sick calves is recommended as soon as possible. Adding colostrum to the daily diet of calves for the first 7 to 14 days will probably reduce the incidence of infection. There is no vaccine for Breda virus.

SUPPLEMENTAL READING

Horzinek MC, Flewett TH, Saif LJ, et al: A new family of vertebrate viruses: Toroviridae. Intervirol 27:17–24, 1987.
Koopmans M, Van Den Boom U, Woode GN, Horzinek MC: Seroepidemiology of Breda virus in cattle using ELISA. Vet Microbiol 19:233–243, 1989.
Pohlenz JFL, Cheville NF, Woode GN, Mokresh AH: Cellular lesions in intestinal mucosa of gnotobiotic calves experimentally infected with a new unclassified bovine virus (Breda virus). Vet Pathol 21:407–417, 1984.
Vanopdenbosch E, Wellemans G, Petroff K: Breda virus associated with respiratory disease in calves. Vet Rec 129:203, 1991.
Weiss M, Steck F, Kaderli R: Antibodies to Berne virus in horses and other animals. Vet Microbiol 9:523–531, 1984.
Woode GN, Reed DE, Runnels PL, et al: Studies with an unclassified virus isolated from diarrheic calves. Vet Microbiol 7:221–240, 1982.
Woode GN, Saif LJ, Quesada M, et al: Comparative studies on three isolates of Breda virus of calves. Amer J Vet Res 46:1003–1010, 1985.

Bovine Astroviruses

JANICE C. BRIDGER, BSc, PhD

In the electron microscope, bovine astroviruses are characterized by the presence of a five- or six-pointed star on a proportion of the smooth-edged, 28-nm particles. British and American bovine astroviruses were strongly related by immunofluorescence but did not cross-react with astroviruses from other animal species. Antigenic differences were detected between American bovine astroviruses by cross-neutralization tests; at least two serotypes were identified. There is insufficient knowledge to allow astroviruses to be assigned to a particular virus group.

EPIZOOTIOLOGY

Bovine astroviruses have often been identified in the United Kingdom and the United States in association with established gut pathogens. Eleven of 22 herds examined in the United Kingdom and 30 per cent of cattle sera from the United States possessed antibody. The virus is found in the feces of both normal and diarrheic calves. On three farms in southern England, 60 to 100 per cent of calves excreted astroviruses in the first 5 weeks of life, although in the United States only 2.6 per cent of 1060 samples from diarrheic calves aged 3 days to 3 weeks were astrovirus positive.

It is likely that astroviruses are species specific, as human and bovine astroviruses failed to infect experimental piglets and cross-immunofluorescence between astroviruses from humans, cattle, and lambs does not occur.

CLINICAL SIGNS

Diarrhea was not produced after inoculation of gnotobiotic calves aged 0 to 49 days with uncultured astroviruses obtained from British or American cattle. Mild villus atrophy was found in the mid–small intestine with the one British isolate studied, however, and feces became yellow and slightly soft at the time of excretion of the American astrovirus. Infection was found in the epithelium of the dome villi of the jejunal and ileal Peyer's patches.

DIAGNOSIS

Bovine astroviruses can be identified by electron microscopy after concentration by ultracentrifugation or by inoculation of primary calf kidney or testicular cells with fecal preparations. After 24 to 72 hours' incubation, individual cells are detected by immunofluorescence with bovine astrovirus-specific antisera. To date, only one bovine astrovirus has been passaged serially in cell cultures after incorporation of trypsin in the medium. Solid-phase immunoassays are still to be developed.

TREATMENT, PREVENTION, AND CONTROL

As there is little evidence that bovine astroviruses are pathogens, no control is indicated.

BIBLIOGRAPHY

Aroonprasert D, Fagerland JA, Kelso NE, et al: Cultivation and partial characterisation of bovine astrovirus. Vet Microbiol 19:113–125, 1989.
Bridger JC, Hall GA, Brown JF: Characterisation of a calici-like virus (Newbury agent) found in association with astrovirus in bovine diarrhoea. Infect Immun 43:133–138, 1984.
Bridger JC: Small viruses associated with gastroenteritis in animals. *In* Saif LJ, Theil KW (eds): Viral Diarrheas of Man and Animals. Boca Raton, FL, CRC Press, 1990, pp 161–182.

Bovine Calici-like Viruses
JANICE C. BRIDGER, BSc, PhD

Calici-like viruses resemble accepted caliciviruses in their size (diameter approximately 33 nm) and in the surface morphology of their particles, although the strains studied to date have not shown the clear "one-plus-six" pattern characteristic of caliciviruses and have not been propagated in cell culture. At least two, and possibly three, "types" occur that are not cross-protective.

EPIZOOTIOLOGY

Calici-like viruses have been seen in the feces of calves in the United Kingdom, Germany, the United States, and Canada. They were identified in 26 per cent of outbreaks of calf diarrhea investigated in southern Britain from 1981 to 1983 in the feces of calves aged 2 to 21 days. They have been found either in association with other known enteric pathogens or alone. Little is known about interspecies infectivity; similar viruses occur in gastroenteritis of humans, but their relationship, if any, to the bovine viruses remains to be elucidated.

CLINICAL SIGNS

Oral inoculation of gnotobiotic calves up to 8 weeks of age with inocula consisting of uncultured viruses produces anorexia, diarrhea, and xylose malabsorption, although anorexia may not always occur. Feces become lighter in color, often yellow, and the volume excreted increases two- to tenfold. With the SRV-1 strain, small-intestinal damage is restricted to the anterior half of the small intestine, where desquamation of degenerate enterocytes results in stunted villi.

DIAGNOSIS

The only available method of diagnosis is electron microscopic examination of feces after differential centrifugation and negative staining. The number of particles tends to be lower than that usually found with rotaviruses and enteric coronaviruses. Solid-phase immunoassays are still to be developed.

TREATMENT, PREVENTION, AND CONTROL

No specific therapeutic studies have been performed, and there are no available vaccines, but oral rehydration therapy is likely to be of value. If calici-like viruses are widespread in the cattle population, colostrum and early milk are likely to contain protective levels of antibody.

BIBLIOGRAPHY

Bridger JC: Small viruses associated with gastroenteritis in animals. *In* Saif LJ, Theil KW (eds): Viral Diarrheas of Man and Animals. Boca Raton, FL, CRC Press, 1990, pp 161–182.

Bovine Spongiform Encephalopathy (Cow Madness, Raging Cow Disease, Mad Cow Disease)

HOWARD W. WHITFORD, DVM, PhD

Bovine spongiform encephalopathy (BSE) is a recently recognized disease of cattle that thus far is confined to cattle originating from Great Britain. It is a sporadic, slowly progressive neurologic disorder of adult cattle. No cases have been diagnosed in the United States as of January 1992.

ETIOLOGY

Although not firmly established, the cause of BSE is believed to be the scrapie agent of sheep or a cattle-adapted strain of scrapie.

EPIZOOTIOLOGY

The first clinical case of BSE was seen in 1985 in Friesian cattle from widely separated geographic locations in England, the highest incidence being in southern England. Cases have also been reported from Scotland, Wales, France, Switzerland, and Ireland. Two cases have been reported from the Sultanate of Oman in Jersey cows imported from England. A similar condition has also been reported in captive eland, nyala, oryx, kudu, and gemsbock in England.

In 1986 only sporadic cases were seen. In 1987, 100 cases were reported. By mid-1988, 500 cases had been reported, and by the end of 1988 a cumulative total of 2160 cases had been seen. By mid-1990 there were over 14,700 confirmed cases, with about 1200 new cases being recognized each month. Except as noted earlier, all cases have been confined to Great Britain, and almost 90 per cent are in Holstein-Friesian cattle.

By means of computer modeling, exposure was retrospectively determined to have occurred about 1981 or 1982, with an incubation period ranging from 2.5 to 8 years. In the early 1980s the rendering industry largely discontinued a solvent extraction procedure, which is further evidence of the time of exposure and route of transmission of BSE. This process normally would remove fats and lipids that make up the bulk of brain tissue, and it also used live steam. Additionally there was a marked increase in the sheep population in Great Britain since 1980, which in turn increased the amount of sheep by-products to be rendered. Taken together there appear to be enough data to support the hypothesis that BSE in cattle was due to scrapie-infected ovine tissue inadequately decontaminated in the rendering process and incorporated into commercial bovine dairy rations.

CLINICAL SIGNS

Clinical signs are observed only in adult cattle, and initially these are apprehension, hyperesthesia, and mild incoordination. With time the neurologic signs progress to include kicking, aggressive behavior, difficult handling, hypermetria (goose-stepping), and increasing incoordination with falling and difficulty in rising. No pruritus (itching) has been reported.

In the final stages of the disease, head tremors, hypersensitivity to touch or sound, recumbency, or frenzied behavior usually necessitates slaughter. Once seen, the signs become progressively more apparent and death is inevitable. The course of the disease varies from 2 weeks to 14 months; however, most affected animals die within 4 months of onset.

DIAGNOSIS

Since there are no clinical pathology or gross necropsy lesions to aid diagnosis, confirmation of the disease in cattle showing typical antemortem signs is only by histologic examination of certain brain stem gray matter locations. The changes are bilaterally symmetrical and degenerative, consisting of vacuolation of the gray matter neutropil and neurons. Although minimal neuronal vacuolation is found in healthy cattle, it is not found in the gray matter neutropil.

In addition to the abnormal neuronal and neutropil vacuolation, the presence of fibrils that closely resemble those found in sheep with scrapie (scrapie-associated fibrils) is demonstrated by electron microscopy in brain tissue of cattle having BSE.

Mice inoculated with brain tissue from affected cattle develop typical neurologic signs and histologic changes in their brain tissue.

TREATMENT

No treatment is available for BSE.

PUBLIC HEALTH CONSIDERATIONS

The BSE outbreak in Great Britain has resulted in much negative press coverage and political rhetoric concerning the safety of human consumption of beef and dairy products. The only human diseases attributed to the unconventional viral agents (slow viruses) are Creutzfeldt-Jakob (CJ) and kuru. Scrapie-infected sheep (preclinical) have obviously been in the human food chain for many years, and some areas such as New Zealand, Australia, and New Guinea are free of scrapie. Epidemiologic evidence shows that CJ disease and kuru occur at about the same rate in people from scrapie-free regions as in those from scrapie-infected areas.

Since extraneural bovine tissues have very low titers of the disease-causing agent, and since historically the transmissible degenerative encephalopathies require relatively large doses of infectious agent orally to establish infection, it would appear that the risk of foodborne transmission of BSE to the human population is quite minimal. No information could be found as to whether cooking alters the viability of the agent of BSE.

PREVENTION AND CONTROL

In 1988 Great Britain banned the inclusion of all ruminant-derived protein, including meat and bone meal, in ruminant rations. On the assumption that cattle are dead-end hosts with no lateral or vertical transmission, the disease should reach its peak of approximately one case/1000 cattle/year until the late 1990s, when it should disappear.

However, if cattle-to-cattle transmission does occur, the incidence of disease should decrease as a result of the 1988 ban but then increase at an unknown rate to an unknown magnitude well into the next century. If, on the other hand, transmission is only in utero (vertical) and not horizontal, the disease should run its course naturally and not be sustained.

In the United States, brains of cattle dying from undiagnosed neurologic disease are being submitted to the National Veterinary Services Laboratory for BSE screening.

BIBLIOGRAPHY

Bolis CL, Gibbs CJ, Wilesmith JW, et al: Proceedings of an international roundtable on bovine spongiform encephalopathy. J Am Vet Med Assoc 196:1673–1690, 1990.
Gibbs CJ, Bolis CL, Asher DM, et al: Recommendations of the International Round Table Workshop on bovine spongiform encephalopathy. J Am Vet Med Assoc 200:164–167, 1992.
Scott PR, Aldridge BM, Clarke M, et al: Bovine spongiform encephalopathy in a cow in the United Kingdom. J Am Vet Med Assoc 195:1745–1747, 1989.
Taylor DM: Bovine spongiform encephalopathy and human health. Vet Rec 125:413–415, 1989.
Wells GAH, Scott AC, Johnson CT, et al: A novel progressive spongiform encephalopathy in cattle. Vet Rec 121:419–420, 1987.

Chlamydial Disease in Cattle

Bovine Chlamydiosis

A. KONRAD EUGSTER, DVM, PhD

Chlamydial agents are obligate intracellular bacteria with a unique biphasic development cycle; they are susceptible to certain antibiotics, particularly tetracyclines. The genus *Chlamydia* consists of two well-defined species, *C. trachomatis* and *C. psittaci*. Two major serotypes have been identified in cattle: type one includes all isolates from abortion and enteric infections, and type two includes isolates recovered from cases of polyarthritis and encephalomyelitis.

ABORTION AND GENITAL INFECTIONS

Chlamydial Abortion

Chlamydiae have been identified as a cause of abortion in cattle in North America, Europe, Africa, and certain Asian countries. Generally no clinical signs are evident in cows prior to abortion. Cows of all ages are susceptible, and abortion can occur as early as the fifth month of gestation; however, most abortions occur during the last trimester of pregnancy. Stillborn and weak calves can also be born. Placentas are frequently retained, and rebreeding problems are encountered. Chlamydial abortions are usually sporadic, but as many as 20 per cent of the cows have been reported to abort in a given herd.

A separate disease entity known as epizootic bovine abortion, or "foothill" abortion, exists in California. Although chlamydiae were isolated from some of these aborted fetuses, it now appears that this disease is vector-transmitted (*Ornithodoros coriaceus*, Koch ticks); however, the infective principle within these ticks has not yet been positively identified. Chlamydiae were not isolated from these ticks, although they have been recovered from other ticks, and involvement of vectors in transmission of chlamydiae requires further studies.

The pathogenic events leading to abortion are not clearly understood. A likely route is the intestinal tract. Intestinal infections (clinically inapparent or overt) are relatively common, and abortions have been induced experimentally with enteric isolates. A venereal transmission may also be possible, inasmuch as heifers inseminated with *Chlamydia*-containing semen did not conceive.

Clinical Signs

Abortions usually occur without any prior clinical signs. Reduction of milk production, retained placentas, metritis, and rebreeding problems can be present postpartum. Placentitis is a consistent lesion. The trophoblastic epithelium is necrotic, especially in the inter- and periplacentomal areas. Fibrinopurulent exudate may be present between the endometrium and the chorion. The intercotyledonary chorion may be of gelatinous (edematous) or leathery consistency.

Lesions in the fetus vary considerably depending on the stage of infection. Fetal lesions may be minimal in cases in which the infection remained localized in the placenta and the abortion occurred prior to a fetal chlamydemia. Fetuses may show petechiae in the subcutis, thymus, and mucous/serosal surfaces; ascites; swollen livers with a mottled surface; and enlarged lymph nodes. Necrotic foci, vasculitis, and other inflammatory reactions may be seen in various somatic organs of the fetus, including the brain.

Diagnosis

None of the fetal or placental lesions are characteristic enough for a positive diagnosis without laboratory confirmation. Intracytoplasmic chlamydial inclusions are most abundant in the chorionic placental epithelial cells. Gimenez stain is preferred over Giemsa and hematoxylin-eosin (H & E) stains. *Chlamydia* can also be isolated in chick embryos or tissue culture from the placenta or various fetal tissues. The complement fixation test is a group-specific test, and a positive serologic diagnosis for chlamydial abortion is difficult to achieve. A rise in antibody titer between the time of abortion and 14 days postpartum would be a good indicator for a causative chlamydial involvement in the abortion.

Treatment and Prevention

Since cows do not show any signs prior to abortions, they are difficult to prevent. Two to 5 g chlortetracycline day/cow incorporated in pelleted alfalfa or protein molasses blocks reduced the abortion rate in a field trial. However, this is an expensive prophylactic regimen and is not practical except in special circumstances in which a severe, confirmed chlamydial abortion problem exists in a given herd. No chlamydial vaccines are available for use in cattle.

Seminal Vesiculitis Syndrome

This condition of primarily young bulls is characterized by a chronic inflammation of the epididymis, testicles, and accessory sex glands. The ejaculate usually contains large numbers of leukocytes and low numbers of spermatozoa with poor motility and primary and secondary sperm abnormalities. There are several causes for this syndrome; chlamydiae have been isolated from some affected bulls. Infertility is obviously a problem in herds with affected bulls; however, chlamydial abortions have not been reported in such herds. Seminal vesiculitis syndrome is diagnosed clinically during breeding soundness examinations. An etiologic diagnosis can be made only by isolation of chlamydiae or other pathogens from the ejaculate.

Chlamydial Endometritis

A report from Europe attributes *Chlamydia* as a cause of sterility. Chlamydial elementary bodies were demonstrated in the vaginal discharge. Endometritis has also been experimentally induced by directly placing chlamydiae into the uterus.

A similar condition has so far not been reported in the Americas.

ENTERIC CHLAMYDIAL INFECTIONS

Chlamydial infections of the intestine, particularly of the ileum, are not uncommon; they are clinically inapparent in adult cattle but can cause diarrhea in young calves. The most severe signs are observed in newborn calves, especially in those that do not receive colostrum or receive inadequate amounts.

In experimentally inoculated, colostrum-deprived calves, *Chlamydia* caused severe diarrhea as well as pneumonia, polyarthritis, and, in some cases, death.

Diagnosis

A laboratory diagnosis (isolation of *Chlamydia* in tissue culture or chick embryos) is essential to differentiate this condition from the many causes of neonatal diarrhea.

Treatment

Fluid therapy and chlortetracycline (2.2 to 4.4 mg/kg body weight for 7 days) are indicated if a positive diagnosis has been established.

RESPIRATORY CHLAMYDIAL INFECTION

Cattle affected by an uncomplicated chlamydial pneumonia have fever, serous or mucopurulent nasal discharge, cough, and dyspnea. All ages of cattle are susceptible. Infections with *Mycoplasma*, *Pasteurella*, *Corynebacterium*, and *Streptococcus* can occur simultaneously or secondarily, obviously adding to the severity of the disease.

Affected parts of the lung are well demarcated, firm, and located in the ventral parts of the anterior lobes. Bronchitis, bronchiolitis, peribronchitis with lymphocytic cuffing, and alveolitis are observed on histologic examination.

Diagnosis

Neither clinical signs nor lesions are characteristic enough to allow a diagnosis of *Chlamydia*-induced pneumonia. Isolation of the organism from lung, nasal secretions, or mediastinal lymph nodes has been used successfully to substantiate a diagnosis.

Treatment

Sick animals should be treated daily with either 11 mg/kg tetracycline or 135 to 200 mg/kg sulfamethazine until they recover.

Prevention

No vaccine is available. Sulfamethazine or sulfathiazole (135 mg/kg) in the drinking water may be indicated as a preventative.

CHLAMYDIAL POLYARTHRITIS

This condition occurs only in young calves. It follows a systemic chlamydial infection and other signs such as inappetence, fever, and diarrhea. The infection in some cases may also start in utero, as calves may be born weak and are reluctant to move.

Clinical Signs and Lesions

The joints are usually enlarged and painful on palpation. Calves frequently die despite various antibiotic treatments. Radiologic examinations are generally unrevealing. All joints can be affected, but usually weight-bearing joints of the extremities and the atlanto-occipital joint are more severely involved. There is excessive turbid yellow synovial fluid present, frequently containing fibrin plaques. The articular cartilage usually does not show any lesions. The periarticular area and especially the tendon sheaths are edematous, hyperemic, and hemorrhagic (petechiae as well as ecchymoses). The reactive changes in the synovial membranes and periarticular tissues are inflammatory and proliferative.

Diagnosis

Synovial cells and inflammatory cells may contain chlamydial inclusions when stained with Giemsa or Gimenez. Isolation of *Chlamydia* from synovial fluid is achieved early in the disease course. A rise in antibody titer (complement fixation test) to *Chlamydia* between acute and convalescent samples is also of diagnostic aid.

Treatment and Prevention

Treatment of affected calves with tetracyclines or penicillin has generally not been beneficial.

CHLAMYDIAL CONJUNCTIVITIS

Chlamydial conjunctivitis is a well-recognized disease entity in guinea pigs, sheep, goats, and humans. In cattle only one report from Czechoslovakia describes the isolation of *Chlamydia* from animals with keratoconjunctivitis and the experimental reproduction of the disease in calves. Conjunctivitis has also been observed concurrently with polyarthritis in experimentally inoculated calves.

CHLAMYDIAL ENCEPHALOMYELITIS

This disease, also known as sporadic bovine encephalomyelitis (SBE), has been confirmed in various parts of the world in predominantly 6-month- to 3-year-old calves. This disease is not to be confused with SBE of viral origin (possibly a morbillivirus), which is extremely rare and has only been reported sporadically in Switzerland and southern Germany.

Clinical Signs

A marked fever is observed about 14 days after exposure. Inappetence, excessive salivation, and diarrhea are also frequent early signs. Some cattle recover at this stage, whereas some develop nervous signs leading to stiff gait, circling, staggering, and paralysis. All parts of the brain and cord may show perivascular cuffs consisting of mononuclear cells.

Diagnosis

Isolation of *Chlamydia* from the brain along with the histologic changes is diagnostic.

Treatment and Prevention

Tetracyclines at therapeutic levels are effective if given early in the disease course, before extensive chlamydial replication in the brain occurs.

BIBLIOGRAPHY

Pienaar JG, Schutte AP: The occurrence and pathology of chlamydiosis in domestic and laboratory animals: a review. Onderstepoort J Vet Res 42:77–90, 1975.

Storz J: Chlamydia and Chlamydia-Induced Diseases. Springfield, IL, Charles C Thomas, 1971.

Storz J, Whiteman CE: Bovine chlamydial abortions. Bovine Pract 16:71–75, 1981.

Mycoplasmosis in Cattle

Bovine Mycoplasmosis

MERWIN L. FREY, DVM, PhD

Within the class Mollicutes, over 20 species of the genera *Mycoplasma*, *Ureaplasma*, and *Acholeplasma* have been isolated from disease conditions in cattle. A number of these species are known to be important pathogens. Organisms within the three genera are all commonly called "mycoplasmas." Mycoplasmas possess the primary characteristics of bacteria and are genetically similar to a few of them. They differ from other bacteria most notably in lacking a rigid cell wall and in being much smaller than most. Because of these two properties they are as filterable as the larger viruses. Mycoplasmas have a proportionately small genome and limited metabolic capabilities and thus require complex media for their isolation and culture. They are very susceptible to chemical and physical environmental factors, yet they flourish in target tissues of susceptible hosts.

EPIZOOTIOLOGY

Mycoplasmas generally cause insidious diseases that spread relatively slowly from animal to animal. The usual means of primary infection is by direct, droplet, or fomite contact between nasal, oral, ocular, teat, and genital orifices and mucous membranes, but infection by aerosols also occurs. Infective aerosols are created when mycoplasmas are present in splattered urine or milk or in coughed bronchial secretions, and they may be long-lived because of the small organism size. Once the infection is established, hematogenous spread to other organs is possible with some species. Many infections become chronic or latent, and thus are a source of later spread to new susceptible animals.

CLINICAL SIGNS

Bovine Respiratory Mycoplasmosis

Mycoplasma mycoides subspecies *mycoides* causes contagious bovine pleuropneumonia (CBPP), a severe fibrinous pneumonia that was eradicated from the United States about a century ago. Mycoplasmas currently endemic to North America cause less severe cuffing pneumonias and alveolitis rather than fibrinous pneumonia. Mycoplasmas infection in bovine respiratory disease (BRD) is not often diagnosed, but serologic studies and observed efficacy of antimycoplasmal antibiotics in many BRD outbreaks have led to a presumption of widespread infection. *M. bovis* is the species most often associated with BRD in North America. It can cause or complicate respiratory disease directly, but it is also important in its potential for hematogenous spread elsewhere to cause arthritis, mastitis, and possibly a generalized immunosuppression. *M. dispar* and *Ureaplasma* spp. are probably associated with respiratory disease of calves at least as frequently as is *M. bovis*, but being harder to isolate are less well recognized as respiratory pathogens. As with *M. bovis*, they are present in a large percentage of properly tested pneumonic calf lungs.

Mycoplasmal Mastitis

Many of the mycoplasma species that infect cattle can cause mastitis in lactating animals, but *M. bovis* is the one most frequently isolated from severe outbreaks. The first sign of mastitis caused by *M. bovis* is a sudden drop in milk flow, usually affecting more than one quarter of the mammary gland. A painless mammary swelling often signals the onset of mastitis, although occasionally there is simply a cessation of lactation. The milk may at first be thicker than normal and frequently goes through several changes in appearance to an increasingly yellow or tan color and then becomes purulent, watery, and fibrin-filled. Recovery of normal appearance usually occurs within about 2 weeks, although milk flow may remain well below normal for the duration of the lactation. Less frequent clinical signs include febrile response, arthritis, anorexia, and respiratory disease. There is usually a marked eosinophilic response in the mycoplasma-infected udder. Other species not infrequently causing mastitis are *M. californicum*, *M. canadense*, *M. alkalescens*, *M. bovigenitalium*, and *Ureaplasma diversum*. Mycoplasmal mastitis is more of a problem in herds in which large groups of cows may be treated at one time, for example, antibiotic prophylaxis of a group of cows at drying-off time. Without urgent sanitary precautions and testing with isolation or culling of affected cows, widespread infection and a precipitous drop in herd milk production may result.

Mycoplasmal Arthritis

Arthritis is a fairly common clinical sign in mycoplasma-infected cattle. It may be the only sign in young calves affected with CBPP. Among calves infected with mycoplasmas indigenous to North America, it usually appears secondary to respiratory disease or in milk-fed dairy calves following ingestion of milk from a herd affected with mycoplasmal mastitis. Although isolations of a number of species have been made from arthritic joints, the two species most often isolated are *M. bovis* and *M. bovigenitalium*. Bovine serogroup 7 and *M. alkalescens* also have been isolated from severe outbreaks of arthritis and have caused arthritis in experimentally infected calves.

In natural infections, one or two joints in one limb may be affected or more than one limb may be involved. Sometimes the lameness may shift from one limb to another. There is mild or no febrile response, but severely affected joints themselves feel quite warm to the touch. Mycoplasmal arthritis following a respiratory disease outbreak typically affects up to 5 or 10 per cent of the animals showing signs of BRD, but occasionally a considerably higher percentage is lame. Swelling usually becomes marked in affected joints after a day or two. A considerable increase in joint fluid is present, and it is frequently somewhat cloudy. Pure cultures of the causative mycoplasma can be cultured from the fluid early in untreated cases. After a week or two it becomes much harder to isolate the organisms, as there is a high concentration of specific antibodies in the synovia. Experimentally *M. bovis* has been shown to cause severe arthritis in the cervical spine. Such lesions may contribute to the severe depression sometimes seen in calves with respiratory disease.

Genital Tract Mycoplasmosis

Many bovine mycoplasmas have been isolated from various parts of normal and diseased male and female genital tracts. *M. bovis* is the mycoplasma most often associated causally with genital tract disease in cattle, and it causes endometritis, salpingitis, salpingoperitonitis, and infertility in experimental infections in cows. It causes seminal vesiculitis, epididymitis, and orchitis in bulls, and it is frequently isolated from semen, where it seems to cause decreased motility of spermatozoa. Other species, especially *M. bovigenitalium*, are thought to cause occasional abortions. *Ureaplasma* spp. are known to cause granular vulvovaginitis. They and *M. canadense* are also frequently present in bull semen.

Keratoconjunctivitis

M. bovoculi, *Acholeplasma oculi*, and *Ureaplasma* spp. are frequently isolated from infectious bovine keratoconjunctivitis (IBK) but from normal eyes as well. Experimentally *M. bovoculi* may cause a mild keratitis by itself, and, more important, it has been shown to be one of several predisposing insults leading to development of IBK when there is concomitant infection with *Moraxella bovis*.

DIAGNOSIS

Methods of diagnosis of mycoplasma infections are difficult, costly, and frequently unavailable. Consequently clinicians and pathologists must usually make presumptive diagnoses on the basis of clinical signs, lesions, and histopathology, and treatment must be empirical. Some diagnostic laboratories that work with large numbers of milk samples are able to provide isolation and identification services for the common mastitis-causing mycoplasmas. Reports indicate that testing of bulk tank samples for pathogenic mycoplasmas is an effective way of detecting a very low percentage of infected cows. Routine checks would be very desirable in those areas of intensive milk production where mycoplasmal mastitis is known to be common.

TREATMENT AND CONTROL

Tetracyclines, tylosin, lincomycin, and spectinomycin (or preferably the last two combined) are the antibiotics most frequently used successfully against the mycoplasmas. Based on their effectiveness in vitro and in experimental infections, mitomycin, tiamulin, and two tetracycline derivatives, doxycycline and minocycline, would appear to be viable choices where approved for use. High-side dosages are recommended for mycoplasmal infections, as the organisms are sequestered where antibiotics do not penetrate readily. Oral antibiotic therapy started early against respiratory mycoplasmosis may prevent further progression of the disease. Oxytetracycline or chlortetracycline at about 16.5 mg/kg body weight has been suggested as an effective daily oral dose rate.

The control of mycoplasmal mastitis is difficult, at best, and antibiotics are of little help. Early diagnosis is essential in preventing spread of infection to additional cows, as segregation or culling of infected animals is necessary. Unfortunately shedding of mycoplasmas begins one to several days before onset of clinical signs. The best control is containment by bulk tank or string sampling, stringent milking hygiene, and avoidance of aerosolization during stripping and other milking procedures.

Effective CBPP vaccines are available in areas where the disease is endemic. Vaccines for mycoplasma infections in swine and chickens have recently become available in the United States, giving hope for eventual development of vaccines for some of the more important mycoplasma infections of cattle.

BIBLIOGRAPHY

Bushnell RB: *Mycoplasma* mastitis. *In* Jarrett JA (ed): Symposium on Bovine Mastitis; Vet Clin North Am: Lg Anim Prac 6:301–312, 1984.
Gourlay RN, Howard CJ: Respiratory mycoplasmosis. Adv Vet Sci Comp Med 26:289–332, 1982.
Jasper DE: The role of *Mycoplasma* in bovine mastitis. J Am Vet Med Assoc 181:158–162, 1982.
Stalheim OHV: Mycoplasmal respiratory diseases of ruminants: a review and update. J Am Vet Med Assoc 182:403–406, 1983.

Viral Diseases of Sheep and Goats

Caprine and Ovine Herpesviruses

A. KONRAD EUGSTER, DVM, PHD

A herpesvirus serologically distinct from bovine herpesvirus I (IBR virus) was originally isolated in California in 1972 from seven kids suffering from a severe systemic infection. Abortions also occurred in this affected herd, but virus isolation was not performed on tissues from aborted fetuses. Since then, herpesviruses have been isolated from aborted sheep and goat fetuses and from goats with vulvovaginitis, chronic pneumonia, wart-like lesions, and proliferative lesions around the mouth and hard palate. A herpesvirus was also isolated from sheep affected with pulmonary adenomatosis; however, current consensus is that herpesviruses do not play a role in the etiology of pulmonary adenomatosis.

With the exception of the original isolates from goats in the early 1970s in California, New Zealand, and Switzerland and an isolate obtained in 1984 from goats with vulvovaginitis, herpesviruses isolated from sheep and goats are serologically closely related or indistinguishable from IBR virus. The vulvovaginitis isolate is closely related to Bovid herpesvirus type 6, the original caprine herpesvirus isolate.

Experimental inoculation of goats with IBR virus has resulted in respiratory disease of varying severity in one experiment and has failed to induce any clinical disease in other experiments.

The fact that herpesviruses serologically indistinguishable from IBR have been isolated from sheep and goats points to these species as a potential source of IBR for cattle and to a possible interspecies transmission of IBR virus between cattle, sheep, and goats.

No vaccine against herpesviruses in sheep and goats is available, and the effectiveness of IBR vaccines in sheep and goats on an experimental basis has not been ascertained.

BIBLIOGRAPHY

Rosadio RH, Evermann JF, Mueller GM: Spectrum of naturally occurring disease associated with herpesvirus infections of goats and sheep. Agri-Practice 5:20–25, 1984.
Saito JK, Gribble DH, Berrios PE, et al: A new herpesvirus isolate from goats: preliminary report. Am J Vet Res 35:845–848, 1974.

Sheep and Goat Pox

E. PAUL J. GIBBS, BVSC, PHD, FRCVS

Sheep and goat pox virus are classified in the genus *Capripox*, which includes the virus of lumpy skin disease of cattle.[1] Sheep or goat pox virus protects cattle from infection with lumpy skin disease in geographic areas where sheep and goat pox are absent. Sheep and goat pox are often considered host-specific; however, in those areas of the world, particularly Africa, where sheep and goats are herded together, nonhost-dependent strains exist. For the present it should be accepted that sheep and goat pox are caused by the same virus.

The virus is transmitted by aerosol and by direct contact with sick animals or fomites.

Sheep or goat pox is the most important pox disease of domesticated animals and can cause extensive epidemics in which a large number of sheep and goats may die. The disease is common in the Middle East, the Indian subcontinent, and Africa, mostly north of the equator; it has been eradicated from most of Europe and has not been reported from the Americas or Australia.

CLINICAL SIGNS (Figs. 1 and 2)

Sheep and goats of all ages can be affected. However, the disease is more severe in young animals. The first signs of disease are rhinitis, conjunctivitis, and pyrexia. Animals tend to stand with an arched back, have a poor coat, and lose their appetite. Cutaneous nodules (0.5 to 1.5 cm diameter) develop 1 to 2 days later, often accompanied by lesions on the external nares, on the lips, and within the mouth. The extent of nodule

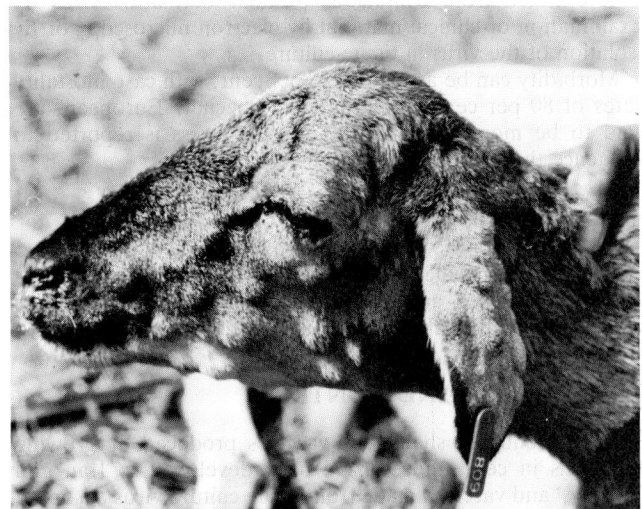

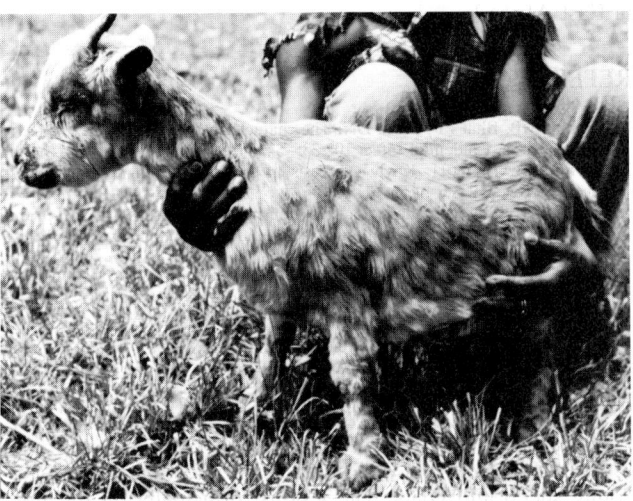

Figures 1 and 2. Sheep and goat pox. (Courtesy of M. A. Bonniwell.)

formation is variable; they are most obvious in the areas of skin where the wool/hair is shortest, such as the head, neck, ears, axillae, groin, perineum, and under the tail. The nodules mostly scab—although some regress without scab development—and these persist for 3 to 4 weeks.

Lesions within the mouth may be present on the tongue and gums; they tend to ulcerate. High mortality rates occur when lesions develop in the respiratory and alimentary tracts. Postmortem observations show these lesions in the lungs as multiple consolidated areas (0.5 to 2.0 cm diameter) beneath the pleural surface. Secondary bacterial pneumonia is the common cause of death. Similar lesions may be seen in the liver, kidneys, abomasum, and other organs.

DIAGNOSIS

Sheep and goat pox are reportable diseases in most countries of the world, and any clinical suspicion of disease should be reported to the appropriate authorities. Classic sheep and goat pox present little difficulty in diagnosis, but on occasion disease may be mild and may be complicated by the presence of contagious pustular dermatitis (synonyms are orf and contagious ecthyma) and dermatophilosis in the affected flock. In such cases laboratory confirmation is advised.

In the laboratory, sheep and goat pox virus can easily be differentiated from contagious pustular dermatitis virus by examination of clinical material by electron microscopy or by isolation of the virus in tissue culture.

Morbidity can be as high as 75 per cent, with case mortality rates of 80 per cent. Some breeds, especially European, are said to be more susceptible, and heat stress is reported to influence the severity of disease.

TREATMENT

There is no specific treatment, but severely affected animals should be housed and given antibiotics. In some countries affected animals or flocks must be slaughtered.

PREVENTION AND CONTROL

Live attenuated sheep pox vaccines produced by growing the virus in cell cultures have been developed in Iran and Turkey,[2] and vaccines made from tissue culture virus adsorbed onto aluminum hydroxide and treated with formalin are in use in East Africa.[3]

REFERENCES

1. Kitching RP, Bhat PP, Black DN: The characterization of African strains of capripoxvirus. Epidemiol Infect 102:335–343, 1989.
2. Martin WB, Ergin H, Koylu A: Tests in sheep of attenuated sheep pox vaccines. Res Vet Sci 14:53–61, 1973.
3. Davies FG: Characteristics of a virus causing a pox disease in sheep and goats in Kenya, with observations on the epidemiology and control. J Hyg 76:163–171, 1976.

Contagious Ecthyma
ROBERT A. CRANDELL, DVM, BS, MPH

Contagious ecthyma (CE) is an acute infection primarily of young sheep and goats. The lesions, principally on the lips, are characterized by vesiculopapular eruptions followed by development of pustules and scabs. Economic loss is usually in the reduction of weight gains and death of feedlot lambs. The disease in animals is commonly known as sore mouth, scabby mouth, lip and leg ulceration, and contagious pustular dermatitis, and the human disease is referred to as orf.

ETIOLOGY

The virus causing CE belongs to the genus *Parapoxvirus* and is inactivated by chloroform. There is only one serotype, but biologic differences exist among strains. The virus survives for long periods outside the body in dried scabs. Exposure to heat at 60° C for 30 minutes destroys the infectivity of the virus. CE virus propagates in a variety of cell cultures of caprine, ovine, and bovine tissues.

EPIZOOTIOLOGY

Sheep and goats are the natural hosts. CE infections have been reported in musk-oxen (*Ovibos moschatus*), Dall sheep (*O. dalli*), Rocky Mountain bighorn sheep (*O. e. canadensis*), mountain goats (*Oreamnus moschatus*), chamois (*Rupicapra rupicapra*), tahr (*Hemitragus jemlahicus*), steinbok (*Raphicerus campestris*), and reindeer (*Rangifer tarandus*). Human infections are occupation related.

CE is found worldwide wherever sheep are raised. There is a seasonal incidence, with most cases occurring during the lambing season and within 2 weeks after lambs enter feedlots. The disease is more prevalent in young animals, and both sexes and all breeds are susceptible. Morbidity is high in infected flocks, but mortality is low. Cases complicated by bacterial infections may result in death.

Infection is spread among animals by direct and indirect methods. The disease is perpetuated under crowded conditions by animal-to-animal contact. Lambs become infected by nursing ewes with active lesions on their teats and udder. The virus is transmitted by fomites contaminated by virus containing scabs and saliva.

CLINICAL SIGNS AND LESIONS

The characteristic feature of this disease is the occurrence of epidermal lesions, particularly on the lips and face of the infected animal. Naturally infected young animals usually develop lesions within 4 to 7 days after exposure to the virus. The lesion begins as a red raised macule and progresses through papule, vesicle, and pustule stages. The vesicles increase in size, advance to the pustular stage, and rupture and release a yellowish exudate. Yellow-brown crusts or scabs form, covering the affected area. The epithelial cells proliferate, forming nodules that may coalesce into larger masses. The lesions may extend to the mucous membrane of the buccal cavity and spread to other parts of the body. Usually they occur at the commissure of the lips and extend along the lip, affecting the gum (Fig. 1), and may involve both sides of the mouth. In the southwestern United States, gum lesions are not a feature of the disease in sheep and goats. Occasionally lesions develop on the eyelids, nares, feet, and teats and udder of ewes. Infections also occur at the site of docking, forming dark, crusty scabs along the incision. Extensive lesions on the face and in the mouth are painful to the animal and may lead to anorexia and weight loss. The course of the illness varies between 1 and 4 weeks. In severe cases the animals are overcome by secondary bacterial infections.

Recovery from clinical disease does not result in lifelong

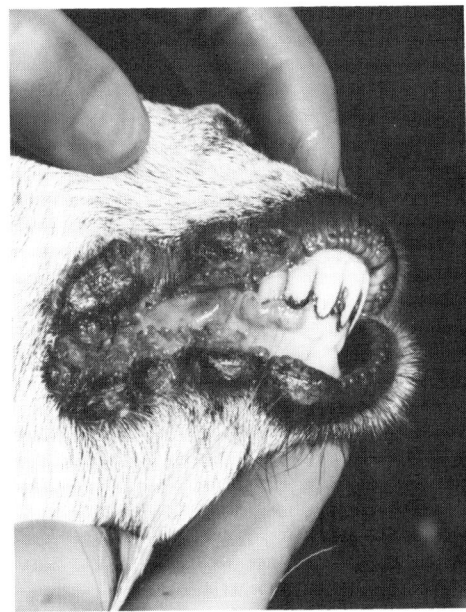

Figure 1. Lesions of contagious ecthyma on the lips and gum of doe. (Courtesy of Dr. R. S. Ott and J Am Vet Med Assoc 173:81–82, 1978.)

immunity, and animals may become reinfected within a year. In older, partially immune sheep, small, dark, hard epithelial tags may occur at the commissure of the lips and go unnoticed. These are a source of infection to handlers. It is because of this short-lived immunity and the addition of susceptible animals to flocks that sporadic outbreaks recur within the same flocks. The persistence of the virus in flocks suggests that latent infections occur.

DIAGNOSIS

A diagnosis is most often made on the clinical appearance of the lesions. A history of previous outbreaks in the flock should be considered in the diagnosis-making process. The presence of oral and foot lesions may confuse the clinical diagnosis with other diseases. Several infectious diseases that should be considered in a differential diagnosis are bluetongue, sheep pox, ulcerative dermatosis, and foot-and-mouth disease. Scabs, scrapings, and lesion biopsies should be submitted to the diagnostic laboratory.

Virus isolation, histopathology, and fluorescent and electron microscopy are useful laboratory procedures in making a definitive diagnosis of this disease. The virus can be isolated in cell culture from scabs and scrapings of the lesion. Specific antigen is demonstrable in frozen sections of the lesion by fluorescent microscopy. CE virus is readily detected in affected tissue by electron microscopy. The characteristic feature of the histopathology is the ballooning degeneration of the epithelial cells. Eosinophilic intracytoplasmic inclusion bodies have been described, but they are not a consistent finding.

CONTROL AND TREATMENT

There are licensed live, dried ecthyma virus vaccines available to prevent this disease in sheep and goats. Vaccination is recommended for each lamb and kid crop in infected flocks because the virus is resistant to environmental conditions. Range lambs should be vaccinated at least 10 days before shipment to the feedlot. The vaccine is administered to scarified skin of wool-free areas such as the inside surface of the thigh and flank or the underside of the tail. Although the vaccine is recommended only for healthy animals, the course of illness has been shortened in some outbreaks after vaccination.

The live virus vaccines should not be used within 24 hours of dipping or spraying. People vaccinating the animals should take the proper precaution against infecting themselves with the vaccine virus. All vaccination instruments should be properly disposed.

Lesions may be softened with an antibiotic-containing ointment. Removal of scabs causes bleeding and delays healing.

PUBLIC HEALTH CONSIDERATIONS

Veterinarians, veterinary students, ranchers, and sheep shearers acquire the infection by handling infected animals. The virus from the mouth lesions contaminates the saliva and wool and enters open lesions on the skin and arms of the handler. The disease in man is generally benign and self-limiting.

Occasionally human infections become generalized.

BIBLIOGRAPHY

Dieterich RA, Spencer GR, Burger D, et al: Contagious ecthyma in Alaska musk-oxen and Dall sheep. J Am Vet Med Assoc 179:1140–1143, 1981.
Jensen R, Swift BL: Contagious ecthyma. In Diseases of Sheep. Philadelphia, Lea & Febiger, 1982, pp 109–111.
Moore RM Jr: Human orf in the United States, 1972. J Infect Dis 127:731–732, 1973.

Ovine and Caprine Adenoviruses

DONALD MATTSON, DVM, PhD

Currently six antigenic types of ovine adenoviruses (OAV) are recognized. While only two types of caprine adenoviruses (CAV) have been described, the number of both OAV and CAV is expected to increase as research continues. In addition, adenovirus strains previously classified as bovine adenoviruses (BAV) have been recovered from sheep.

EPIZOOTIOLOGY

There have been comparatively few reports concerning the distribution and prevalence of various types of OAV. In one serologic survey conducted in Scotland, the prevalence of infection with selected types of OAV varied from 21 to 68 per cent. In a survey conducted in Oregon, the prevalence of antibodies in serum of adult sheep varied from 21 to 60 per cent with OAV type 6 and an unclassified isolate. In addition, antibodies were found in 24 and 57 per cent, respectively, of normal adult goats.

These data do not provide sufficient information to make an accurate conclusion concerning the distribution and prevalence of OAV and CAV infection. These viruses are probably widespread. The possible role of interspecies transmission of virus between sheep, goats, and cattle has not been investigated.

OAV are believed to be transmitted by direct contact or by aerosol droplet. In experimentally infected lambs, virus is shed in lacrimal and nasal secretions, feces, and, with some isolates, urine.

CLINICAL SIGNS

Most isolations of OAV have been from normal lambs. Other isolations have been made from normal lambs in flocks that had a past history of respiratory or enteric disease or both. There have been some reports that have directly implicated these viruses as etiologic agents of enteric and respiratory disease in neonatal lambs. Lambs experimentally infected with various OAV or BAV isolates usually show mild clinical signs of disease and pathologic changes. Clinical signs of disease include pyrexia, anorexia, hyperpnea, dyspnea, conjunctivitis, cough, and diarrhea. Lungs have variable degrees of atelectasis and edema. Microscopic lesions include swelling, proliferation and necrosis of the bronchiolar epithelial cells, and an increased proliferation of cells in the alveolar septa. Infection may localize in the alimentary tract and produce a catarrhal enteritis. Virus may also replicate in the kidneys and produce swelling and proliferation of endothelial cells.

Lambs infected with selected OAV isolates followed by *Pasteurella haemolytica* develop more severe clinical signs of disease and pathologic changes than when infected by either microorganism individually.

DIAGNOSIS

For viral isolation, samples should be taken early in the disease from the conjunctiva, nasal cavity, and/or feces. Samples at necropsy should be taken from the affected portions of the respiratory or enteric tract and their regional lymphatic tissue. Virus can be isolated using traditional procedures in lamb kidney cell cultures. In early stages of infection, virus-infected cells can be detected by the fluorescent antibody (FA) technique. While the FA technique is not conducted by most diagnostic laboratories in the United States, the procedure will detect the group-specific viral antigen and should be a useful tool in diagnosing infection caused by unspecified strains of OAV, CAV, or BAV.

TREATMENT

Treatment should be symptomatic and directed toward controlling infection by secondary microorganisms.

PREVENTION AND CONTROL

There are no vaccines available in the United States for the prevention of ovine or caprine adenoviral infection.

BIBLIOGRAPHY

Lehmkuhl HD, Cutlip RC: Characterization of two serotypes of adenovirus isolated from sheep in the central United States. Am J Vet Res 45:562–566, 1984.
Lehmkuhl HD, Contreras JA, Cutlip RC, Brogden KA: Clinical and microbiological findings in lambs inoculated with *Pasteurella haemolytica* after infection with ovine adenovirus type 6. Am J Vet Res 50:671–675, 1989.

Papillomatosis in Sheep and Goats
CARL OLSON, DVM, PhD

Naturally occurring warts with virus were found on the legs and muzzle of sheep in two different outbreaks. The ovine papilloma virus produced warts in experimental sheep and fibromas in hamsters, but no lesions were produced in cattle or goats. Cutaneous papillomas have been reported in goats, and in one instance these apparently progressed to carcinoma. The infrequent observation or reports of papillomas in sheep and goats may be due to the masking of such lesions by wool and hair or to the fact that the condition is rare in these animals. Papilloma virus and carcinoma have been associated in cattle and sheep of Australia. Sunlight and longevity of animals seem to be additional factors.

For further information on papilloma viruses see Papillomatosis in Cattle.

BIBLIOGRAPHY

Gibbs EPJ, Smale CJ, Lawman MJP: Warts in sheep. J Comp Path 85:327, 1975.
Moulton JE: Cutaneous papillomas on the udders of milk goats. North Am Vet 35:29, 1954.
Theilen GH, Wheeldon EB, East N, et al: Goat papillomatosis. Cold Spring Harbor Conference—Papilloma Viruses. 1982, p 73.

Border Disease
BENNIE I. OSBURN, DVM, PhD

Border disease (BD) is a congenital infectious disease of sheep. Infection of embryos and fetuses results in embryonic death with resorption, fetal death, and birth of lambs with developmental abnormalities of the skin, nervous and endocrine systems, and bones. BD was first reported in sheep along the Welsh border of the United Kingdom; since then it has been observed in New Zealand, Australia, Europe, the United States, and Canada. In New Zealand affected lambs are called "hairy shakers," whereas in the western United States they are known as "fuzzies." The disease has been observed in most of the sheep-raising areas of the United States.

ETIOLOGY

The etiologic agent of BD is a pestivirus of the Togaviridae family. The noncytopathogenic agent is closely related to bovine viral diarrhea (BVD) virus and to hog cholera virus.

BD virus readily passes through the placenta of ewes infected between 16 and 80 days' gestation. Embryos and fetuses infected from 20 to 45 days after conception undergo embryonic or fetal death with resorption or abortion. Infection of the fetus between 45 and 80 days' gestation causes abnormalities of those organs undergoing major development, including the skin, nervous, lymphoid, thyroid, and skeletal systems and possibly others. Lambs infected through 80 days' gestation become persistently infected and immunologically compromised. The persistent infection lasts for the duration of the animal's life, serving as a reservoir of infection for others. There is no evidence that the virus infection is associated with clinical disease in the postnatal period other than abortion in susceptible ewes.

INCIDENCE

Clinical evidence of BD is most apparent at lambing time, when as many as 50 per cent of the flock may be affected. Ewes are nonpregnant, abort, or deliver weak and/or malformed lambs. Serologic studies reveal that close to 90 per cent or more of the ewes in a flock may be affected; however, clinical expression of disease occurs only in those lambs whose ewes were infected between 16 and 80 days' gestation.

TRANSMISSION

Natural transmission apparently occurs through contact with secretions and excretions of body fluids and tissues from infected animals. Urine, saliva, and placental fluids and tissues contain infective virus, and these serve as an important source for susceptible sheep. Appearance of the disease in a flock is usually associated with introduction of persistently infected animals that have minimal or no clinical evidence of disease. Persistently infected animals have been known to be viremic for over 2 years.

CLINICAL SYNDROME

BD is a disease of the embryo and fetus. The various forms of disease expression are related to the particular time during embryonic and fetal development that infection occurs. There are three major effects of infection:

1. *Embryonic and fetal death.* Infection during the embryonic and early fetal period (16 to 45 days' gestation) often leads to death and resorption of the embryo or fetus. The principal manifestation in flocks where this occurs is a small lamb crop because of many open ewes.
2. *Abnormal lambs.* The classic picture of BD is the birth of small, weak lambs with hairy fleece and congenital tremors. Infection of fetal lambs between 45 and 80 days' gestation leads to dysplastic development of the hair follicles and nervous system and dysfunction of the thyroid gland. This is associated with hypothyroidism characterized by low T_3 and T_4 levels. Lambs are usually small in stature with a preponderance of hairy fleece rather than wool. Often there is a dark pigmented area on the dorsal aspect of the neck. Tonic-clonic tremors may be so severe in some cases that lambs are unable to stand or suckle. Most of these lambs die within the first few days of birth.
3. *Weak lambs.* Birth of small, weak lambs with minimal neurologic and fleece abnormalities occurs in a small per cent of outbreaks. These lambs may survive with appropriate husbandry; however, they become the principal carriers of infection because they are persistently infected with BD virus.

The usual clinical history includes all three of these syndromes. The percentage of affected lambs with typical signs of hairy fleece and congenital tremors will vary and depends on the gestation period when infection occurred. The birth of these abnormal lambs usually prompts the livestock worker to seek veterinary service. A critical review of past breeding records and of the current lamb crop will reveal a number of open, dry ewes and an unusually large number of neonatal deaths leading to a reduced lamb crop. If infection occurs in 1 year, the ewes appear to recover from infection and develop sufficient immunity so that cases of BD are minimal the following year.

PATHOLOGY

The principal gross findings consist of hairy fleece in place of wool, hyperpigmentation over the dorsal cervical area, and a small, undernourished lamb. Radiographs of long bones reveal dense bands around growth plates, suggesting arrested growth during fetal development. The cranium is domed in severely affected individuals. Microscopic changes are in the nervous system and consist of dysmyelinogenesis and hypercellularity of the white matter. Special myelin stains are required to detect the lack of myelin in the cerebellum and spinal cord.

IMMUNOLOGY

The increased susceptibility to other infections and the poor viability due to intercurrent infections have been attributed to immune deficits. There is evidence of depressed cell-mediated immune responsiveness. Antibody responses to BD virus are negligible, further suggesting that affected lambs are immunocompromised. The failure of the immune system to overcome BD virus and eliminate the virus from the system is probably the result of immunomodulation resulting from the fetal viral infection.

DIAGNOSIS

An impression of BD can be gained by obtaining a flock history consisting of a combination of reduced lamb crop, abortions, weak lambs with poor viability, and lambs with hairy fleece and congenital tremors. Submission of a single specimen does not allow a definitive diagnosis unless BD virus is isolated. A definitive diagnosis can be made upon isolation of virus from heparinized peripheral blood or brain, spinal cord, spleen, and bone marrow from affected lambs. Frozen tissues can be examined for evidence of BD viral antigens with fluorescent-tagged hyperimmune BVD antiserum. The thyroid gland contains considerable BD viral antigen. Nervous tissue fixed in formalin can be examined for hypercellularity and decreased myelin staining of white matter.

Serologic evaluation of ewe and affected lamb sera for evidence of antibodies to pestiviruses such as BD and BVD may assist diagnosis.

PREVENTION

The usual history associated with outbreaks of BD is that if it occurs one year, it is an insignificant cause of losses in the succeeding year. Infection usually spreads through a flock, resulting in subclinical viral infection and recovery with good immunity. Precautions need to be taken in flocks where BD carriers are introduced to susceptible populations with no previous history of BD infection. This must be considered as well in ewes and flocks where flock immunity to BD has declined.

Recently there have been reports suggesting that BVD vaccines prescribed for cattle when given to sheep may provide sufficient immunity for sheep flocks at risk. Inactivated or killed BVD vaccines should be used on sheep until an appropriate licensed product for sheep immunity is available.

BIBLIOGRAPHY

Anderson CA, Higgins RJ, Smith ME, Osburn BI: Border disease virus–induced decrease in thyroid hormone levels with associated hypomyelination. Lab Invest 57:168, 1987.

Anderson CA, Sawyer MA, Higgins RJ, et al: Experimentally induced ovine border disease: extensive hypomyelination with minimal viral antigen in neonatal spinal cord. Am Vet Res 48:499–503, 1987.

Barlow RM, Gardiner AC: Experiments in border disease. 1. Transmission, pathology and some serological aspects of the experimental disease. J Comp Path 79:397–405, 1969.

Osburn BI, Crenshaw GL, Jackson TA: Unthriftiness, hairy fleece, and tremors in newborn lambs. J Am Vet Med Assoc 160:442–445, 1972.

Terlecki S: Border disease: a viral teratogen of farm animals. Vet Ann 17:74–79, 1977.

Foot-and-Mouth Disease in Sheep and Goats

JERRY CALLIS, DVMS, DSc
DOUGLAS GREGG, DVM MEd, PhD

Foot-and-mouth disease (FMD) is caused by a picornavirus. There are seven distinct immunologic types and numerous subtypes within each. The virus is antigenically labile, and to protect by vaccination it is necessary to produce vaccines homologous with the virus in the field.

EPIZOOTIOLOGY

Foot-and-mouth disease occurs in all species of cloven-hoofed animals. The disease is generally less severe in sheep and goats than in cattle and swine. The virus has a tendency to become species adapted, and in such instances the infection in sheep and goats may be severe. Such an outbreak occurred in 1990 in Israel, killing only young lambs; no sheep or lambs developed vesicles. FMD virus occurs worldwide except in Australia, New Zealand, North and Central America, and Greenland; the European Community has been free of FMD since 1989. The virus is transmitted by infected animals and animal products. It can also be airborne. Recovered sheep and goats become carriers of the virus; although it has not been proven, they are thought to be responsible for spreading the virus to susceptible animals.

CLINICAL SIGNS

Sheep and goats suffer less than cattle and swine. In some instances clinical signs are not readily evident. The most pronounced sign is lameness. Careful examination is necessary to notice the usually small vesicles or erosions on the dental pad and tongue and between the claws (Fig. 1). In severe infections, pregnant sheep and goats may abort.

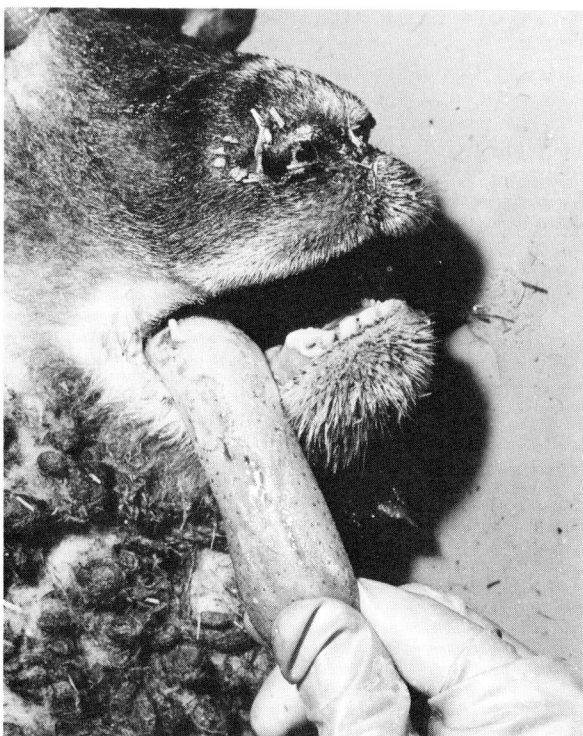

Figure 1. Ruptured vesicles on tongue of sheep infected with FMD virus.

DIAGNOSIS

Sheep and goats are also susceptible to vesicular stomatitis, bluetongue, and contagious ecthyma. The lesions of FMD and these diseases show common features; therefore laboratory tests are essential for differential diagnosis. FMD is diagnosed by isolation of the virus or by tests for virus or antibody by complement fixation, virus neutralization, agar gel precipitin, and enzyme-linked immunosorbent assays.

TREATMENT

There is no specific cure for FMD. Palliative treatment may make the animal more comfortable.

PREVENTION AND CONTROL

Prevention is the best policy. Susceptible animals should be isolated from infected animals or animal products. In FMD-free countries when the disease appears, infected animals are slaughtered, the carcasses are destroyed by burial or burning, and the premises are decontaminated. Vaccines have been available since the 1930s but are not widely used in sheep and goats because these species are less susceptible than cattle. The insidious nature of the infection in these species makes them particularly dangerous during outbreaks, and signs of infection may go unnoticed.

BIBLIOGRAPHY

Bachrach HL: Foot-and-mouth disease. Ann Rev Microbiol 22:201, 1968.
Callis JJ, McKercher PD: Foot-and-mouth disease. In Dunne HW, Leman AD

(eds): Diseases of Swine, 5th ed. Ames, IA, Iowa State University Press, 1981, pp 278–287.

McVicar JW, Sutmoller P: Sheep and goats as foot-and-mouth disease carriers. Proc Ann Mtg US Livestock Sanit Assoc 72:400, 1969.

St. George N: The epizootiology and epidemiology of foot-and-mouth disease carriers. Adv Vet Sci Comp Med 14:261, 307, 1970.

Ovine and Caprine Reoviruses

SASHI B. MOHANTY, BVSc, PhD

All three types of reoviruses, similar to those found in humans, have been isolated from sheep. They have been isolated from nasal and rectal swabs of lambs with respiratory signs and diarrhea and from the nasal secretions and feces of clinically normal lambs. These viruses replicate in embryonic lamb kidney cells and produce cytopathic effects. Seroepidemiologic surveys indicate that antibodies to reoviruses are widespread in sheep populations. There is no report of caprine reoviral isolation.

CLINICAL SIGNS

It appears that reovirus type 1 is capable of producing respiratory and enteric diseases in sheep. Mild signs of these diseases attributed to reovirus type 1 have been observed in natural outbreaks. An ovine reovirus type 1 isolate induced respiratory illness and diarrhea in 2- to 4-week-old lambs. Reovirus types 2 and 3, however, induced no clinical signs in experimentally infected sheep. Focal consolidation of lungs, interstitial pneumonia, and catarrh of the mucous membranes of the upper respiratory and intestinal tracts were seen with type 1 reoviral infection.

DIAGNOSIS, PREVENTION, AND CONTROL

Virus isolation and seroconversion are considered adequate for diagnosis. There is no vaccine available.

BIBLIOGRAPHY

Belak S, Palfi V: Isolation of reovirus type 1 from lambs showing respiratory and intestinal symptoms. Arch Ges Virusforsch 44:177, 1974.

McFerran JB, Nelson R, Clarke JK: Isolation and characterization of reoviruses isolated from sheep. Arch Ges Virusforsch 40:72, 1973.

Snodgrass DR, Burrols DR, Wells PN: Isolation of reovirus type 2 from respiratory tract of sheep. Arch Virol 52:143, 1976.

Bluetongue in Sheep*

THOMAS E. WALTON, DVM, PhD

Bluetongue (BT) is an infectious, noncontagious, arthropodborne virus disease of domestic and wild ruminants. At least 24 distinct serotypes of BT virus (BTV) have been identified worldwide. In the United States, five serotypes have been identified: 2, 10, 11, 13, and 17, the latter of which is unique to North America. In sheep, the disease may be inapparent to very severe, with marked clinical signs and substantial death losses reported. Goats can be infected but rarely show viremia or clinical signs of the disease. Some researchers believe that sheep are the primary indicators of BTV activity. The severity of clinical BT in sheep appears to be related to age, breed, individual animal susceptibility, environmental conditions, stress, vector competence, occurrence of dual infections with multiple serotypes, virus serotype, and virus pathogenicity.

In the United States, BTV serotypes have been isolated from cattle, sheep, wild ruminants, and/or hematophagous insects in 32 states; serologic evidence of BTV activity has been reported in 48 states, but livestock in the northern (Great Lakes and New England) states are considered to be free of BTV. Occasional incursions of BTV serotype 11 have been documented virologically and serologically into the Okanagan Valley of British Columbia, but Canada normally is considered to be BTV free. In Mexico, BTV serotypes 10, 11, 13, and 17, identical to those identified in the United States, have been isolated. BT disease is seasonal in areas in which the vector activity is interrupted by inclement weather, for example, freezing temperatures. Epizootic activity has been reported generally in areas with temperate climates; in tropical or subtropical areas with yearlong vector activity, BTV is enzootic and reports of clinical disease are only occasionally received. In sheep the most significant economic impact is associated with deaths, loss of condition and wool, and therapeutic expenses.

ETIOLOGY

BTV and the antigenically related epizootic hemorrhagic disease (EHD) virus of deer are morphologically classified as Orbiviruses in the family Reoviridae. The virus has a segmented, double-stranded ribonucleic acid (RNA) genome in a core particle with 32 capsomeres arranged in icosahedral symmetry. The 10 genomic segments code for 10 structural and nonstructural proteins. The core particle is surrounded by an outer capsid layer containing two major virus-specific polypeptides; VP (virus protein) 7 is the major antigen associated with the group-specific reactivity detected by complement fixation, immunofluorescence, and agar gel immunodiffusion tests, while VP 2 is the major antigen associated with the serotype-specific reactivity detected by the neutralization and hemagglutination inhibition tests. Genome segment reassortment between serotypes has been reported in mixed serotypic infections of cells, insects, and ruminants. While BTV does not have an essential lipid membrane, the virion is membranophilic and generally found in association with host-cell membranes unless it has been treated with a lipid solvent. For this reason, BTV in blood is most closely associated with the erythrocytic fraction rather than with the plasma.

EPIZOOTIOLOGY

The host range of BTV includes sheep, cattle, goats, and other species of Artiodactyla. Clinical disease commonly occurs in sheep and wild ruminants but rarely occurs in cattle and goats.

The principal biologic vector of BTV in the United States is the biting midge *Culicoides variipennis*. Although other species of *Culicoides* occur in the United States, only *C. insignis*, which is found from Central Florida and to the south into the Caribbean islands and Central America, is considered

---

*All material in this article is in the public domain, with the exception of any borrowed figures or tables.

another possible vector in the Northern Hemisphere. *C. variipennis* was used experimentally to transmit BTV to and from infected sheep and cattle. Although *Culicoides* spp. will feed on many animal species and on humans, many species appear to be preferentially attracted to cattle rather than to sheep; this may be related to the size of cattle. After ingestion of a BTV-infected blood meal, the female vector is believed to remain infected for life. *C. variipennis* females feed at dawn and dusk and require a blood meal to produce eggs. Epizootics are seen when the midge populations reach peak numbers, generally in the late summer or early fall before the first frost.

In sheep, in utero infections of the fetus have been reported from infections with attenuated vaccine virus strains of BTV during pregnancy. In rams BTV has been isolated from the semen, but the significance is not known.

CLINICAL SIGNS AND LESIONS

BTV infection in sheep produces a subclinical, mild, or severe infection with morbidity of 50 per cent in some flocks. In breeding ewes and feeder lambs, mortality may reach 30 to 50 per cent of clinically affected animals. Serologic surveys have shown high antibody prevalence in sheep in the western and southwestern United States.

Clinical signs are more pronounced in naturally infected than in experimentally infected sheep. Inoculation of susceptible sheep with BTV isolates from acutely ill cattle has failed to reproduce the acute signs most often associated with field cases. In naturally and experimentally infected sheep, the incubation period is 6 to 14 days. Signs of illness include fever to 41.5°C within 4 to 8 days after infection; excessive salivation; catarrhal nasal discharge; and edema and congestion of the lips, ears, and oral mucosa. Rapid, shallow respiration often accompanies the fever. Increased salivation and lacrimation may precede the inflammatory and ulcerative lesions of the oral mucosa. Drooling is often associated with swelling of the lips, gums, and tongue. Ulcers develop on the dental pad, lips, gums, and anterior part of the tongue; in severe cases there may be extensive necrosis of the dental pad. The skin of the muzzle may have a burned or necrotic appearance and may be dry, cracked, and peeling. Anorexia and loss of condition frequently occur. The high fever may produce weak wool of low quality or the fleece may be dropped.

Bacterial bronchopneumonia secondary to aspiration of vomitus is observed in severely infected sheep. The bluish-colored, cyanotic, congested tongue, from which the disease was named, occurs after natural infections but is rarely observed after experimental infections. Coronitis, lameness, and sloughing of the horny laminae may occur as the disease progresses. Although it has been reported in South Africa, necrosis of skeletal muscle manifested as scoliosis has not been reported with the five United States serotypes.

Abortion and congenital deformities such as hydranencephaly may occur in fetuses of ewes naturally infected or vaccinated with BTV. Viremia persisting for up to 2 months has been reported in blood and tissues of newborn lambs from ewes experimentally infected in midgestation. Newborn lambs have an effective passively acquired immunity that may last up to 6 months. Spring lambs lose this immunity at the peak summer activity of BTV, resulting in severe economic losses.

DIAGNOSIS

A presumptive diagnosis of BT in sheep can be made on the basis of the clinical signs, which occur during mid- to late summer or early fall. Signs of BT in sheep are similar to those caused by photosensitization; poisonous plant intoxications; infectious diseases such as contagious ecthyma (soremouth), mycotic stomatitis, and infestation with nose bots; and such exotic diseases as foot-and-mouth disease, sheep pox, and peste des petits ruminants. The closely related EHD virus will infect sheep and produce a detectable viremia, but clinical signs have not been reported. A confirmed diagnosis of BTV in sheep requires the isolation and identification of the virus or a demonstrable rise in serum antibody titer in paired acute and convalescent serum samples.

Isolation of BTV can be made from infected blood or tissues by the inoculation of embryonating chicken eggs; of cell cultures such as baby hamster kidney (BHK-21), African green monkey kidney (Vero), bovine endothelial (CPAE), and *C. variipennis* cell lines; or of susceptible sheep. Confirmation of BTV is made by using indirect immunofluorescence, immunoperoxidase staining, enzyme-linked immunosorbent assay (ELISA), and virus neutralization techniques. Serotyping of BTV isolates is done by using plaque inhibition or reduction procedures in cell culture monolayers and by polyacrylamide gel electrophoretic techniques. While not yet available for routine use in diagnostic laboratories, modern molecular biologic procedures such as nucleic acid hybridizations, radioimmunoassays, polymerase chain reactions, and monoclonal antibodies with various markers may soon become available for more sensitive BTV diagnoses.

Antibody in sheep can be serologically detected by using the modified direct complement fixation, agar gel immunodiffusion (AGID), hemolysis-in-gel, ELISA, and serum neutralization tests. Currently the serologic test of choice by importing countries is the AGID or bluetongue immunodiffusion (BTID) test.

TREATMENT AND PREVENTION

There is only one federally licensed and approved BTV vaccine available in the United States for use in sheep. This commercially available attenuated vaccine was produced against BTV serotype 10 in bovine kidney cell cultures. Unfortunately most clinical BTV activity that occurs in the United States is caused by serotypes 11 and 17. Cross-protection among BTV serotypes has been reported to be limited and variable. In spite of the lack of specific immunity to other BTV serotypes, many ranchers choose to use the serotype 10 vaccine early in an outbreak because the identity of the infecting serotype is frequently unavailable for several weeks after an outbreak begins. In addition, BTV has been reported to be a potent interferon inducer, and some believe the available vaccine may provide some antiviral protection. While work has been done to produce traditional attenuated vaccine virus candidates to the other United States serotypes, and to develop inactivation methods for BTV, commercialization of this technology has not been pursued. Modern subunit or "genetically engineered" vaccines may become an economically viable reality in the future as advances in molecular biology are made.

Antibiotics are frequently used to treat sheep with lesions from BTV infection in an effort to control secondary bacterial infections. Localized lesions on the muzzle and teats can be treated topically to minimize infection and promote healing. When oral lesions are present, good flock management is necessary to increase survivability of infected sheep and to maintain their body weight. Infected animals should be separated from the flock and fed less rough forage to minimize trauma to the oral mucosa.

The control of BT within an infected sheep flock is difficult because of the large numbers of infected *Culicoides* females attacking sheep at the same time. The most important therapeutic measures for sheep are vector control and administration of vaccine. Careful water management is essential to the control of *C. variipennis*; the larvae are found in the soft, silty, polluted mud in overflow areas around stock tanks or leaking septic systems and along the edges of ponds, ditches, and streams in which there is a high organic content from manure. Improving drainage and eliminating sources of animal and human pollution or sewage effluent will reduce the number of potential virus vectors. Treatment of larval developmental sites can include physical disruption of the site or the use of approved larvicides such as a granular formulation of temephos at the label rate for polluted waters.

Good flock management may help to control the spread of the disease. Moving animals from low-lying areas in which larval developmental sites are located to higher elevations may be useful. In the western United States, BT outbreaks in sheep generally do not occur until sheep are returned to lower elevations from summer pasture in the mountains.

Animals can be protected by the use of topical pesticides such as fenvalerate or permethrin in ear tags or tapes, parenteral pesticides such as ivermectin, or insect repellents. Premise treatment with residual fenvalerate or permethrin spray and housing of sheep at dusk and dawn, when *Culicoides* feed, may protect them from infection because *Culicoides* normally do not enter structures.

BIBLIOGRAPHY

Barber TL, Jochim MM, Osburn BI (eds.): Bluetongue and related orbiviruses. *In* Progress in Clinical and Biologic Research, Vol. 178. New York, Alan R. Liss, 1985.
Gibbs EPJ, Greiner EC: Bluetongue and epizootic hemorrhagic disease. *In* Monath TP (ed): The Arboviruses: Epidemiology and Ecology. Boca Raton, FL, CRC Press, 1988, pp 39–70.
Jones RH, Luedke AJ, Walton TE, Metcalf HE: Bluetongue in the United States—an entomological perspective toward control. World Anim Rev 38:2–8, 1981.

Ovine Rotavirus

THOMAS L. LESTER, DVM, PhD, ACVM

Rotavirus is a genus of viruses belonging to the family Reoviridae. They have been separated into four groups, A to D, by enzyme-linked immunosorbent assay (ELISA), complement fixation test, immunoelectron microscopy, and RNA genome sizing. All rotavirus share a common group-specific antigen (VP6) associated with the inner capsid. Species specificity or serotypes are determined by antigens (VP3 and 7) located on the outer capsid. Most ovine isolates are from group A; however, groups B and C are forming an increasing proportion of isolates from sheep and pigs.

EPIZOOTIOLOGY

Rotavirus infections have been reported in a wide variety of animals, including humans, cattle, horses, dogs, sheep, goats, swine, antelope, monkeys, mice, rabbits, deer, chickens, turkeys, and ducks. Zoonosis is not considered a problem; however, cross-species infections can be experimentally induced. Disease is generally associated with the young but can occur at all ages and has been demonstrated in adult sheep. Exposure is widespread, and many ewes have antibodies. The virus can survive for several days in feces, which is the main source of infection. Infected adults can excrete sufficient virus to serve as initiators of infection in lambs, which then excrete large quantities of virus to infect others. Disease outbreaks occur most commonly in herds where sick animals are not separated and orofecal transmission is allowed to occur. Infection can be initiated by almost any infectious fecal contamination. Sources have included contaminated teats, feed, bedding, equipment, and people and the introduction or mixing of animals from infected herds.

CLINICAL SIGNS AND LESIONS

Clinical signs occur in lambs 1 day to 3 weeks of age. The incubation period has been reported as short as 10 to 20 hours. The virus replicates in absorptive columnar epithelial cells of the jejunum and ileum. These are replaced by flattened squamous to cuboidal epithelial cells deficient in digestive enzymes and absorptive capacity. This leads to malabsorption as well as alteration of electrolyte transport systems, causing profuse diarrhea. The onset of clinical signs is generally rapid, within 2 to 3 hours, but the severity can vary among lambs. Signs include mild anorexia, depression, and diarrhea. Duration and mortality appear to be related to other factors such as secondary infections (bacterial or viral) and stress and to the quality and type of passively acquired antibodies. Mortality is generally recognized to result from loss of electrolytes and water with resulting dehydration, acidosis, and systemic shock.

Necropsy findings are generally rather nondescript. The stomach may contain some milk or mucoid fluid. The intestinal contents are generally watery and can vary in color. The intestinal mucosa may be normal, hyperemic, or hemorrhagic, depending on the type and severity of secondary infections.

DIAGNOSIS

Diagnosis of rotavirus infection depends on demonstrating virus or virus-specific antigens in the feces or intestinal mucosa. Methods used to detect rotaviruses include

1. Electron microscopy by negative staining. This procedure is rather insensitive and requires a large number of particles in the feces. Detection can be enhanced by the use of antiserum to form immunoaggregates (immunoelectron microscopy).
2. Sandwich ELISA-"rotazyme" type tests, based on human tests, detect group A antigens in feces and compare well with electron microscopy techniques. However, owing to their specificity, they will not detect groups B to D or other viruses that might be present.
3. Isolation can be accomplished but is difficult and time-consuming.
4. Fluorescent antibody techniques can be used on fecal smears and intestinal mucosa impressions or frozen sections of the intestinal mucosa.

TREATMENT

Neonatal diarrheas should be treated similarly in most species. Procedures described for bovine rotavirus infections also apply for ovine rotavirus infections.

PREVENTION

Reducing exposure is the most effective method of preventing rotavirus infection. Management practices such as care in not introducing the virus by addition of infected or contaminated animals or materials, reducing stocking density, and removing animals with diarrhea are recommended.

Local antibodies on the mucosal surface of the intestine appear to be important in the protection against rotavirus infections. Vaccination of ewes has been reported to reduce the incidence of infection in lambs.

BIBLIOGRAPHY

Saif LJ, Theil KW: Viral Diarrheas of Man and Animals. Boca Raton, FL, CRC Press, 1989.
Snodgrass DR, Anguss KW, Gray EW: Rotavirus infection in lambs: pathogenesis and pathology. Arch Virol 55:263–274, 1977.
Snodgrass DR, Wells RP: The immunoprophylaxis of rotavirus infections in lambs. Vet Rec 102:146–148, 1978.

Nairobi Sheep Disease

HUGH W. REID, BVM&S, DTVM, PhD, MRCVS

Nairobi sheep disease (NSD) is an arthropod-transmitted virus infection of sheep and goats characterized by a marked febrile response followed by profuse watery diarrhea that frequently becomes hemorrhagic. The course of disease may be peracute, acute, mild, or inapparent, with a case mortality frequently over 80 per cent.

The virus of NSD belongs to the *Nairovirus* genus within the family of arthropod-transmitted viruses known as the Bunyaviridae. Nairoviruses have distinct structural and antigenic characteristics and can be subdivided into six serogroups. The serogroup to which NSD virus belongs also contains Dugbe and Ganjam viruses isolated from ticks in Nigeria and India, respectively. The virus measures 90 to 100 nm in diameter and contains RNA; all isolates appear to be antigenically identical. In the laboratory the virus may be propagated by intracerebral inoculation of mice or in baby hamster kidney cell line (BHK-21) cultures, in which it produces characteristic perinuclear inclusion bodies and forms plaques under an overlay of carboxy-methylcellulose. Detection of viral antigen by immunoperoxidase in a cell line derived from *Rhipicephalus appendiculatus* has also been reported and may be superior for quantitative assays of viral infectivity.

EPIZOOTIOLOGY

NSD was first described in 1910 as a fatal gastroenteritis of trade sheep in Kenya. The subsequent studies of Montgomery in 1917 established that the disease was caused by a virus transmitted by *R. appendicalatus* ticks that had previously engorged on sheep reacting to infection. Thus NSD virus became the first identified tickborne virus.

Following the recognition of NSD in the area around Nairobi, its distribution within Kenya was found to correspond generally to that of *R. appendiculatus*. The disease has subsequently been identified in Uganda, northern Somalia, and probably Zaire and Ruanda. There is serologic evidence that it is present in Botswana, Ethiopia, Tanzania, and South Africa.

Natural transmission between sheep occurs only by tick bite. Both transtadial and transovarial transmissions have been demonstrated in the tick vector.

Experimentally, *R. appendiculatus* is an efficient vector of the virus, and the distribution of the disease in Kenya corresponds to that of this tick. However, other ticks can transmit the virus, which has been isolated on a number of occasions from field collections of *Amblyomma variegatum*, suggesting that the epidemiology of NSD may be complex. Furthermore, in Somalia it is evident that *R. pulchellus* effectively transmits virus and appears to be the main vector in this region. Thus the suggestion by earlier workers that *R. appendiculatus* is the sole vector of NSD can no longer be accepted.

Naturally occurring infection of the native fauna of Africa has not been identified, and domestic animals other than sheep and goats are refractory to infection. Antibody detected in wild ruminants is probably due to infection with serologically related viruses. Thus it has been concluded that NSD is maintained in a sheep-tick-sheep cycle, and as Ganjam and NSD viruses appear to be identical, it is currently suggested that NSD may be a strain of Ganjam introduced into Africa from India.

CLINICAL SIGNS

All breeds of sheep and goats are susceptible. The mortality rate of African sheep tends to be high, even up to 80 per cent, whereas that of European breeds is seldom more than 50 per cent. Goats appear to be less susceptible, with a mortality rate of 10 per cent, but losses in the field have been reported to reach 88 per cent.

Following exposure to infected ticks, the incubation period is 4 to 6 days. Pyrexia of sudden onset is the first sign, with temperature rising rapidly to 40 to 42° C. Affected animals are dull and anorexic, and there may be a mucous nasal discharge. Shortly thereafter, watery green feces are voided and may become hemorrhagic. Distress and constant straining are evident, and the nasal discharge often becomes blood-tinged. The external genitalia of ewes swell, and pregnant animals frequently abort. Death may follow within 24 hours of the onset of signs but can be delayed for as long as 6 days. It is generally considered that the prognosis is poor if diarrhea develops.

At postmortem examination the hindquarters are usually soiled with feces and the nostrils caked with blood-tinged nasal discharge. The principal lesions are seen in the gastrointestinal tract, extending from the abomasum to the rectum. The mucosa of the abomasum and small intestine is edematous and hyperemic and may be hemorrhagic, particularly in the region of the pylorus and ileocecal valve. The most severe lesions are found in the large intestine, extending from the cecum sometimes as far as the rectum. The lumen may be filled with blood, and longitudinal hemorrhages extend along the tops of the folds that are edematous. Serosal hemorrhages may also be present.

In addition, the trachea is frequently hyperemic and may contain blood-tinged froth, whereas in a proportion of cases the lungs have lesions associated with secondary pasteurella pneumonia. Frequently ecchymoses are present on the endocardium and petechial hemorrhages on the epicardium. The genital tract, particularly of pregnant ewes, is edematous and hyperemic, and the mucous membranes are catarrhal. Lymph nodes are enlarged and moist, and the malpighian corpuscles of the spleen are prominent.

The only histologic changes that are consistently present and considered to be of diagnostic value are a severe glomerulotubular nephritis associated with hyaline and epithelial casts and a generalized vascular congestion of the kidney that is most marked around the glomeruli.

DIAGNOSIS

The clinical and postmortem picture cannot be relied on to provide a specific diagnosis, and confirmation depends on laboratory tests. From dead animals the isolation of virus from plasma, spleen, and mesenteric lymph node homogenates by intracerebral inoculation of suckling mice should be attempted. Tissue culture is less sensitive for primary isolation of virus, as generally isolates must be serially passaged two to five times before cytopathic effects can be detected. In recovered animals the detection of serum antibody will indicate previous infection with NSD virus. Animals that recover are immune for life, and though neutralizing antibody is not readily detected, high titers of antibody may be detected by fluorescent or indirect hemagglutination tests and are maintained for at least 15 months. Among the conditions that must be considered in the differential diagnosis are Rift Valley fever, rinderpest, peste des petits ruminants, salmonellosis, pasteurellosis, babesiosis, coccidiosis, helminthiasis, heartwater, and poisoning.

PREVENTION

Viruses serially passaged by intracerebral inoculation of mice or in tissue culture lose pathogenicity for sheep and have been used as attenuated live virus vaccines. However, the degree of attenuation is accompanied by a loss of immunogenicity. Thus, owing to the variability in susceptibility of different breeds of sheep, none of these vaccines has proved generally acceptable. An inactivated vaccine prepared from virus propagated in baby hamster kidney cells and then formalinized and precipitated with methanol produced a high level of resistance to laboratory challenge but has not yet been assessed in the field.

BIBLIOGRAPHY

Clerx JPM, Casals J, Bishop DHL: Structural characteristics of Nairoviruses (genus *Nairovirus*, Bunyaviridae). J Gen Virol 55:165–178, 1981.
Daubney R, Hudson JR: Nairobi sheep disease. Parasitology 23:507–524, 1931.
Davies GF: Nairobi sheep disease in Kenya. The isolation of virus from sheep and goats, ticks and possible maintenance hosts. J Hyg 81:259–265, 1978.
Munz E, Reimann M, Jager H: Qualitative and quantitative detection of Nairobi sheep disease virus antigen by immunoperoxidase in BHK-sheep kidney and tick cell cultures. Zbl Vet Med B 31:231–239, 1919.

Rift Valley Fever in Sheep and Goats*

JOHN C. MORRILL, DVM, PhD

Rift Valley fever (RVF) is caused by an arthropodborne virus of the family Bunyaviridae genus *Phlebovirus*. RVF has been described through serosurveys and virus-isolation studies in most countries of sub-Saharan Africa and Madagascar. The exportation of RVF to Egypt and the resultant devastating epidemic in 1977 emphasize the necessity for continual vigilance anywhere mosquitoes, sheep, and cattle are found. To date, no outbreaks have been reported outside Africa, although modern transportation provides a means for global transmission. The possibility of infected humans carrying the virus from country to country is very real. Consequently international travelers should be made aware of the clinical symptoms of the disease and of the importance of the disease to other humans and to domestic animals. The disease is characterized by a short incubation period, fever, hepatitis, abortion, and death, with newborn lambs, calves, and puppies being highly susceptible.

For additional information see Rift Valley Fever in Cattle.

EPIZOOTIOLOGY

Domestic ruminants and humans are natural vertebrate hosts for RVF. Mice, lambs less than 7 days old, and baby hamsters are the most susceptible experimental animals. Explosive epidemics occur periodically and are associated with periods of heavy rainfall and dense or expanding vector populations. Transovarial transmission in certain *Aedes* mosquitoes provides a probable mechanism for maintenance of the virus during interepidemic periods. The eggs may remain dormant in depressions, called "dambos" in East Africa or "pans" in South Africa, that are subject to inundation. When flooding occurs, the eggs hatch and infected larvae emerge and develop into infected adults. Through monitoring of changes in vegetation, satellite remote sensing is being used to identify areas of flooding that may trigger hatching of floodwater *Aedes* and provide breeding sites for secondary vectors. These secondary vectors are primarily mosquitoes, especially *Culex* species, although culicoides and sandflies may play limited roles in biologic transmission and, along with other arthropods, mechanical transmission.

In Africa, disease seems to be limited to domestic ruminants, with imported European animals being more severely affected than native African breeds. Sheep and cattle are the primary domestic ruminant species affected by RVF virus, with goats being involved to a lesser extent.

CLINICAL SIGNS

Widespread abortion and rapidly fatal neonatal disease characterize RVF outbreaks among sheep and cattle. Newborn lambs and kids are highly susceptible to infection with RVF virus and may suffer 90 to 100 per cent mortality rates. Experimentally infected lambs experience an acute febrile response, often exceeding 42°C, followed by collapse and death within 24 to 48 hours. Experimentally infected pregnant ewes experience a fever of up to 42°C for 1 to 4 days, followed by prostration and death or recovery; abortion occurs 5 to 20 days later in survivors. A definite leukopenia, most severe in younger animals, which corresponds to maximal viremia and temperature response, is seen, often followed by leukocytosis in later stages of the disease. Mortality ranges from 10 to 30 per cent in adult animals.

Other clinical signs in adults are inconsistent but may include an unsteady gait, vomiting, mucopurulent nasal discharge, injected conjunctiva, and hyperemia of the oral mucosa. Febrile animals have been observed submerging their muzzles in water, presumably seeking relief from the fever. The disease in goats is less severe, although abortions are reported, and the incidence of seroconversion after an epizootic is much lower than in sheep.

The liver is the primary site of virus replication, and initial mild hepatocellular changes rapidly progress to final massive

---
*All material in this article is in the public domain, with the exception of any borrowed figures or tables.

necrosis. As the disease progresses in newborn lambs, the necrotic foci may enlarge to 2 mm in diameter and the liver becomes friable, irregularly congested, and may become mottled brown or yellow in color. Hepatic lesions in adult sheep and goats are not as severe as those found in lambs, but multiple necrotic areas may be present. In some animals only small, microscopic necrotic areas with varying degrees of visceral and serosal hemorrhages are seen. Coagulated blood may be found in the lumen of the gallbladder in those cases with marked hemorrhage in the liver.

DIAGNOSIS

The same diagnostic procedures used for RVF in cattle can be used for the disease in sheep and goats. Diseases that may confound a diagnosis include enterotoxemia of sheep, Nairobi sheep disease, and ovine enzootic abortion, as well as many of the diseases listed in the article Rift Valley Fever in Cattle. Amnionic fluid and the serosanguinous fluid in the thorax of aborted lamb fetuses may have virus titers in excess of 10^8 plaque-forming units per milliliter, providing a source of environmental contamination as well as diagnostic material.

TREATMENT

No specific treatments are currently available.

PREVENTION AND CONTROL

Immunization of susceptible animals is the most effective means of controlling RVF. Vector control in enzootic areas is expensive and may be only moderately successful. If control of mosquitoes and biting flies is implemented, larvacides should be incorporated into the program to increase effectiveness. Movement of livestock during an epizootic should be regulated to prevent extension of the disease to RVF-free areas. To reduce the risk of aerosol transmission, sick animals should not be slaughtered. Two types of RVF vaccines are currently in use: a live attenuated vaccine for use in sheep and cattle and formalin-inactivated vaccines for animals and humans. Both have limitations that affect their usefulness. A recently developed mutagen-attenuated RVF vaccine has potential as an effective immunogen for human and veterinary use. This vaccine is nonpathogenic in neonatal lambs and calves and is nonpathogenic and nonabortogenic in pregnant ewes and cows. Vaccinated dams and their fetuses, as well as vaccinated neonates, were protected against experimental challenge with virulent virus.

BIBLIOGRAPHY

Assad F, Davies FG, Eddy GA, et al: The use of veterinary vaccines for prevention and control of Rift Valley fever: memorandum from a WHO/FAO meeting. Bull WHO, 61:261–268, 1983.
Meegan JM, Shope RE: Emerging concepts on Rift Valley fever. In Pollard M (ed): Perspectives in Virology, XI. New York, Alan R. Liss, 1981, pp 267–287.
Peters CJ, Meegan JM: Rift Valley fever. In Steele JN (ed): Handbook Series in Zoonoses, Section B, Viral Zoonoses, Vol. 1. Boca Raton FL, CRC Press, 1981, pp 403–420.
Weiss KE: Rift Valley fever—a review. Bull Epizoot Dis Afr 5:431–458, 1957.

Akabane Disease in Sheep and Goats

A. J. DELLA-PORTA, BSc, PhD

Akabane disease is a congenital disease of cattle, sheep, and goats characterized by hydranencephaly (HE), arthrogryposis (AG), micrencephaly, and porencephaly. It usually occurs as localized epizootics and less frequently as sporadic cases. This disease is caused by Akabane virus, an insect-transmitted virus (arbovirus) belonging to the family Bunyaviridae, that occurs as an inapparent infection of nonimmune pregnant animals during the first trimester of pregnancy. The disease has been seen in lambs in Australia, Israel, and Turkey and in goats in Israel. Akabane virus is probably present throughout much of Africa and Asia. A similar disease syndrome has been reported in sheep in Texas and has been associated with infection by the Bunyavirus Cache Valley virus.

CLINICAL SIGNS

Infection in the pregnant animal is inapparent. There may be an increase observed in the number of abortions or an apparent decrease in the number of ewes and goats reaching parturition. At birth, many of the lambs and kids may be suffering from HE, AG, micrencephaly, and other skeletal and nervous system impairments. These syndromes can overlap in sequence, and animals can be seen exhibiting more than one of the clinical signs.

The central nervous lesions are similar to those seen in calves (see Akabane Disease in Cattle).

DIAGNOSIS

As Akabane virus has not been isolated from congenitally affected offspring born at term, proof of infection must be based on serologic and pathologic evidence. Serologic evidence is based on the presence of virus-neutralizing antibodies against Akabane virus in the precolostrum serum sample from the affected offspring.

BIBLIOGRAPHY

Chung SI, Livingstone CW Jr, Edwards JF, et al: Evidence that Cache Valley viruses induce congenital malformations in sheep. Vet Microbiol 21:297–307, 1990.
Kurogi H, Inaba Y, Takahashi E, et al: Experimental infection of pregnant goats with Akabane virus. Natl Inst Anim Health Q 17:1–9, 1977.
Parsonson IM, Della-Porta AJ, O'Halloran ML, et al: Akabane virus infection in the pregnant ewe. 1. Growth of virus in the foetus and the development of the foetal immune response. Vet Microbiol 6:197–207, 1981.
Porterfield JS, Della-Porta AJ: Bunyaviridae: infections and diagnosis. In Kurstak E, Kurstak C (eds): Comparative Diagnosis of Viral Diseases, Vol. 4, Part B. New York, Academic Press, 1981, pp 479–508.

Maedi-Visna (Ovine Progressive Pneumonia, Zwoegerziekte)*

RANDALL C. CUTLIP, DVM, PhD

Maedi and visna are Icelandic terms for a chronic progressive viral disease of adult sheep, known also as ovine progressive pneumonia (OPP) in the United States and zwoegerziekte in Holland. In Iceland the disease was initially described as two

---

*All material in this article is in the public domain, with the exception of any borrowed figures or tables.

separate entities: a chronic pneumonitis called maedi, meaning dyspnea, and a chronic encephalitis called visna, meaning wasting.

ETIOLOGY

The maedi-visna virus is an exogenous RNA retrovirus of the lentivirus group that is closely related to the virus of caprine arthritis-encephalitis. Structurally the virus contains a dense 40-nm core surrounded by a single envelope with 8-nm spikes. The core is formed in the peripheral cytoplasm of the infected cell and is enveloped in host-cell membrane by a budding process. The mature virus is 80 to 120 nm in diameter. Major detectable antigenic components are polypeptides of the core and glycoproteins of the envelope. The core proteins are stable, but the glycoproteins, important in serum neutralization, are subject to antigenic drift. Thus multiple minor variants are detected by serum neutralization. The virus is readily inactivated by heat, drying, and disinfectants but is stable at refrigeration temperature (4°C) or less.

EPIZOOTIOLOGY AND PATHOGENESIS

Infection with maedi-visna virus is common in most sheep-raising areas of the world, but clinical disease is uncommon. Australia and New Zealand are reported to be free of the virus. Based on serologic testing, about 26 per cent of sheep in the United States are persistently infected. However, infection may reach 100 per cent in some flocks. There is rarely more than a 5 per cent annual loss in a flock, and clinical signs are not seen in some flocks. Some breeds (Icelandic, Texel, Border Leicester, Finnish) and their crosses appear to be more susceptible than other breeds to clinical disease. Recent studies indicate that some breeds are also more susceptible to infection. Goats are the only species other than sheep known to be susceptible to persistent infection by the maedi-visna virus. A transient infection can be induced experimentally in rabbits. Transmission of virus is primarily through the milk to young lambs, but can occur at any time by close contact but rarely before birth.

Infection with maedi-visna virus is unconventional in that a carrier state persists in the presence of circulating homologous antibodies. Thus a positive serologic test indicates persistent infection. The virus is carried in a nonproductive state as DNA copies (provirus) that are integrated into the chromosomal nucleic acid of infected cells, mainly circulating monocytes. Disease is induced when the infected monocytes mature into tissue macrophages in the lungs or elsewhere and a productive infection is established. Lesions are believed to be immune mediated through prolonged stimulation by viral antigen on the surface of infected macrophages. It is not known why some sheep are clinically affected while others are not affected, but pathogenicity probably relates to the capacity of infected macrophages to produce viral antigen and the immune response to that antigen. Most sheep seroconvert 2 to 3 weeks after infection with the virus; however, it is theoretically possible for the provirus to be carried in a nonproductive state for years or for the life of the sheep without causing seroconversion or clinical effect. Most sheep infected with maedi-visna virus die as the result of a secondary bacterial pneumonia.

CLINICAL SIGNS AND LESIONS

The cardinal clinical feature of maedi-visna is a continuous weight loss that leads to death after several weeks or months. Respiration becomes progressively labored. Mastitis, seen as a swollen, firm udder with poor milk production for 2 to 3 weeks following lambing, is a common feature. Rarely there is a central nervous system disturbance characterized by listlessness and an advancing hindquarter paralysis. Severe lameness, because of chronic degenerative arthritis of the carpal and tarsal joints, is occasionally seen. All or any combination of clinical signs may be seen in individual sheep. The incubation period is more than 1 year, and death is inevitable once signs appear. Affected sheep are afebrile and continue to eat. Signs may be exacerbated during times of stress, such as lambing, nursing, or inclement weather.

At necropsy the lungs fail to deflate fully and weigh two to three times normal. They are diffusely involved, grayish pink with gray patches, of a firm, spongy consistency, and dry. The anterioventral areas are frequently dark red and consolidated because of secondary bacterial infection. Thoracic lymph nodes are enlarged three to four times normal. Affected joints have focal necrosis of the articular cartilage and subchondral bone, fibroplasia of the synovium and capsule, and, in advanced cases, may contain a dry chalky material.

The characteristic histologic feature of maedi-visna is lymphoproliferative inflammation in the interstitium of affected tissues. Alveolar septa of the lungs are thickened by accumulation of mononuclear cells and, in many cases, by excessive fibromuscular tissue. Pulmonary epithelial hyperplasia is usually minimal but may become extensive, resulting in an adenomatous appearance that has been confused with pulmonary adenomatosis (jaagsiekte). The mastitis is characterized by accumulation of lymphocytes in the interstitium and formation of lymphoid nodules around collecting ducts. Ductal epithelium may be degenerate or sloughed. Neural lesions vary from a simple cuffing of blood vessels with lymphocytes to necrosis of the ependyma and subependymal neuropil. Articular lesions are those of a chronic nonsuppurative lymphocytic inflammation with degeneration of cartilage and subchondral bone.

DIAGNOSIS

Infection can be diagnosed by serologic testing or by isolating virus from buffy coats or other tissues. Diagnosis of disease is dependent on finding typical signs and lesions.

TREATMENT

No treatment is effective. Supportive therapy to control secondary infections and appropriate husbandry will usually prolong life for a few weeks to months.

PREVENTION AND CONTROL

The only known method of preventing infection is to avoid exposure to the virus. Once a flock is infected, the disease can be controlled by removing serologically positive animals from the flock or by isolating lambs from the flock at birth. Serologic monitoring of the flock for several years is necessary to assure elimination of the virus. Maedi-visna was eradicated from Iceland by slaughtering all sheep on infected and contiguous farms.

BIBLIOGRAPHY

Cutlip RC, Lehmkuhl HD, Brogden KA, Bolin SR: Mastitis associated with ovine progressive pneumonia virus infection in sheep. Am J Vet Res 46:326–328, 1985.

Cutlip RC, Lehmkuhl HD, Wood RL, Brogden KA: Arthritis associated with ovine progressive pneumonia. Am J Vet Res 46:65–68, 1985.
Dawson M: Maedi/visna. A review. Vet Rec 106:212–216, 1980.
Gendelman HE, Narayan O, Kennedy-Stoskopf S, et al: Tropism of sheep lentiviruses for monocytes: susceptibility to infection and virus gene expression increases during maturation of monocytes to macrophages. J Virol 58:67–74, 1986.
Opendra N, Clements JE: Biology and pathogenesis of lentiviruses. J Gen Virol 70:1617–1639, 1989.

Caprine Arthritis-Encephalitis Virus

DONALD P. KNOWLES, JR., DVM, PhD
WILLIAM P. CHEEVERS, PhD

The lentivirus caprine arthritis-encephalitis virus (CAEV) causes inflammation in synovial spaces, mammary gland, brain, and lung. Arthritis, the form seen most often clinically, is characterized by bilateral or unilateral swelling of carpal joints (Fig. 1). Mastitis is clinically recognized as diffuse swelling of the mammary gland with associated firmness. Encephalitis, which occurs most often in goats 1 to 5 months of age, presents as an ascending paralysis. An interstitial pneumonia, similar to that described for sheep infected with ovine progressive pneumonia virus, has been found in goats infected with CAEV.

INCIDENCE

CAEV occurs worldwide, with the highest prevalence of infected goats occurring in industrialized countries. A 1981 serologic survey of 1160 goats from 24 states within the United States revealed that 81 per cent of the goats tested were seropositive. Other industrialized countries such as Canada, France, Norway, and Switzerland have CAEV prevalence levels of 65 per cent or greater, and within individual infected herds, up to 100 per cent of the goats may have CAEV antibody. In contrast, Australia, New Zealand, and England have prevalence levels of 10 per cent or less. Developing countries with no or low levels of CAEV-positive goats include Kenya, Mexico, Peru, Somalia, Sudan, South Africa, and Fiji.

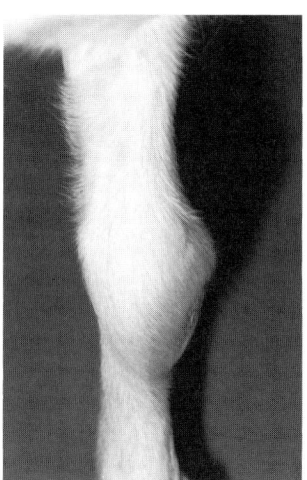

Figure 1. Carpus from a 5-year-old goat experimentally infected with CAEV as a kid. Notice the marked periarticular swelling.

Clinical disease as measured by swelling of the carpal joints varies among herds and occurs in approximately 9 to 38 per cent of seropositive animals. The incidence of clinical mastitis, encephalitis, and pneumonia caused by CAEV is not documented; however, the encephalitic form appears to be rare in the United States.

ETIOLOGY

CAEV is a retrovirus in the subfamily Lentivirinae. Other members of Lentivirinae are the causative viruses of equine infectious anemia, ovine progressive pneumonia, and the acquired immunodeficiency syndromes of humans and nonhuman primates. Recent additions to Lentivirinae are the feline immunodeficiency and bovine immunodeficiency viruses. Primary cultures of caprine synovial membrane, choroid plexus, and blood monocytes support CAEV replication.

TRANSMISSION

Transmission occurs most efficiently to kids during nursing via colostrum and milk. Horizontal transmission of CAEV is usually not efficient; however, an exception to this is contact between lactating does, which may lead to rapid transmission. Intrauterine infection is rare, if it occurs at all, and transmission by aerosol has not been demonstrated.

PATHOGENESIS

Of the multiorgan systems that CAEV affects, the pathogenesis of the arthritis is best understood. Carpal swelling can be detected as early as 6 months after experimental oral infection of newborn kids. In approximately 25 to 40 per cent of experimentally infected kids, the course of the carpal swelling is progressive and characterized by recurrent episodes of active arthritis interspersed with periods of quiescence. It appears that the goats which eventually develop the most severe carpal arthritis have recurrent episodes of periarticular swelling early in the disease course.

The cell type infected by CAEV, both in vitro and in vivo, appears to be macrophages. Synovial membrane cells have characteristics of macrophages and may serve as an additional cell for CAEV replication in vivo. Evaluation of synovial fluid from arthritic joints indicates that (1) there is a high concentration of immune reactants including cells and immunoglobulin in the synovial fluid, (2) a large amount of the synovial fluid antibody is specific for CAEV, (3) virus can often be isolated from synovial fluid, (4) the isolation of virus from the synovial fluid correlates with the severity of arthritis as measured by joint swelling, and (5) virus expressing antigenically variable neutralization-sensitive epitopes arises in joint fluid during chronic CAEV arthritis. Additionally, goats challenged with CAEV during persistent CAEV infection or after vaccination with inactivated virus develop more severe arthritis than do uninfected or nonvaccinated goats.

These observations support the hypothesis that CAEV arthritis is an immunopathologic process in which specific antibody and sensitized lymphocytes react with CAEV antigen in the synovial cavity. Furthermore, virus isolates expressing antigenically variable neutralization-sensitive epitopes and the immune response to these variants may contribute to periods of inflammation and progression of the arthritis.

CLINICAL SIGNS

Clinically, the arthritis caused by CAEV is characterized by bilateral or unilateral swelling of carpal joints (Fig. 1). Clinical features of advanced disease are emaciation, rough and long hair coat, gait abnormalities, and carpal hygroma.

The encephalitic form of CAEV infection is recognized most often in goats 1 to 5 months of age. Clinically, an ascending paralysis leads to recumbency. Even though recumbent, the goats are afebrile, are alert, and maintain a good appetite. More severe signs include upward deviation of the head, twisting of the neck, and paddling movements of the feet. Regardless of the stage of progression, signs rarely if ever regress owing to the irreversible central nervous system damage.

The mastitis caused by CAEV presents as a diffuse swelling of the mammary gland with associated firmness. In some does, there is a marked acute swelling of the mammary gland that decreases with time; however, the mammary gland never completely returns to its original size or consistency. Experience with experimentally infected herds indicates that the udder of nonpregnant does is susceptible to CAEV-induced mastitis. As is the case with the arthritis caused by CAEV, there is wide variation in the eventual clinical severity of the mastitis.

An interstitial pneumonia, similar to that described for sheep infected with ovine progressive pneumonia virus, is found in goats infected with CAEV. The pneumonia is usually found in herds with a high prevalence of goats serologically positive for CAEV. Clinically, the pneumonia primarily affects adults, is insidious in onset, and is progressive. The goats have histories of gradual weight loss and respiratory distress.

NECROPSY FINDINGS

Although the carpal joints are often the only joints with clinically apparent periarticular swelling, on histologic examination, the atlanto-occipital, fetlock (metacarpal), and stifle joints and atlantal and supraspinous bursae are also commonly affected. In joints with advanced disease, there is often discolored synovial fluid, marked thickening of the joint capsule, and periarticular mineralization. Articular cartilage usually remains intact. On histologic examination, the arthritis is characterized by a proliferative synovitis. There is synovial membrane hyperplasia, villous hypertrophy, and infiltration by lymphocytes, macrophages, and plasma cells (Fig. 2). In goats that develop severe disease, there is often fibrosis, necrosis, and mineralization of synovial membranes and periarticular collagenous structures.

In the encephalitic form of CAEV infection, gross lesions of the brain and spinal cord are sometimes visible as brown areas of softening; however, the lesions are often discernible only microscopically. On histologic examination, the inflammation involves primarily the white matter and meninges and is characterized by infiltrations of lymphocytes and demyelination.

The mastitis caused by CAEV is characterized histologically by multifocal to diffuse periductal accumulations of lymphocytes, macrophages, and plasma cells. In the more severe cases, affected parts of the mammary gland resemble lymphoid tissue.

Lungs affected by CAEV infection are swollen, are firm on palpation, and have 1 to 2 mm gray foci on the cut surface. On histologic examination, the alveolar septa are irregularly thickened with lymphocytes and macrophages. Lymphoid aggregates are present in some septa, usually adjacent to small

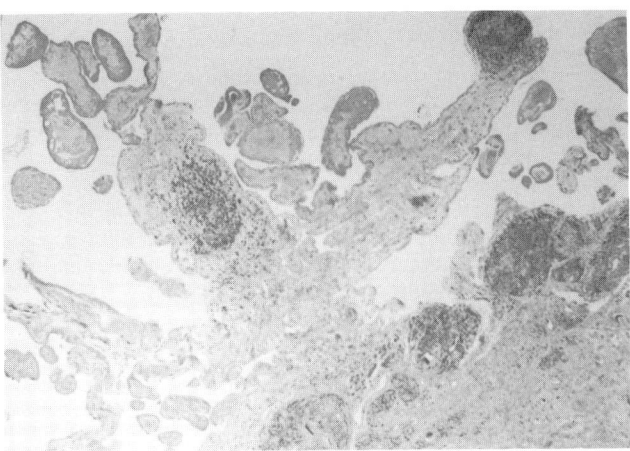

Figure 2. Radiocarpal synovium of CAEV-infected goat. Notice the synovial membrane hyperplasia, ischemic necrosis, and synovial and subsynovial cellular infiltrates. (Hematoxylin and eosin.)

vessels and bronchioles. Bronchial lymph nodes are often hyperplastic.

DIAGNOSIS

The most practical approach to confirming a diagnosis of CAEV infection is a combination of serology and clinical evaluation. A widely used serologic test is the agar-gel immunodiffusion test. This test measures primarily antibodies against the viral surface glycoprotein gp135 and core protein p28. An enzyme-linked immunosorbent assay (ELISA) that measures anti-CAEV antibodies has been described but is not currently in wide use. Interpretation of a positive serologic test to CAEV in regard to predicting potential herd impact requires an understanding of the dynamics of a lentiviral infection. Persistence of virus in the individual animal is a consequence of the ability of lentiviruses to establish a latent infection of monocytes. The result of persistence is that a positive serologic test to CAEV indicates the goat is infected for life and is a continual potential source for virus transmission.

CONTROL

The important aspects of CAEV infection that must be considered in designing a prevention program are the following: (1) CAEV persists for life in the infected host. (2) A major route of transmission is to kids via colostrum and milk during nursing. (3) Contact transmission among adults can occur. (4) There can be marked variability among individual goats in the time from infection to a positive serologic test. With consideration of these aspects of CAEV pathogenesis, a practical approach to preventing CAEV infection of newborn goats and reducing the prevalence of CAEV within a herd was devised. First, all kids must be immediately removed from the dam at birth, and there should be no contact of the newborn kids with secretions of the dam. The kids should be isolated from infected goats and provided colostrum from known virus-free does. Colostrum from CAEV-positive does can be used if it is treated at 56° C for 1 hour. Further nutrition consisting of goat milk must be from does free of virus, pasteurized cow milk, or pasteurized goat milk from infected does. Goats raised in this manner should be serologically tested for CAEV every 6 months, and those testing positive must be removed.

TREATMENT

With the current absence of a vaccine to prevent infection or a method to clear individual goats of CAEV, any treatment of clinical disease is only palliative. Management of caprine arthritis-encephalitis must be at the level of preventing transmission and reducing the prevalence of infected goats within a herd. Any attempt to decrease CAEV infection in a goat herd must take into account that a positive serologic result indicates a goat is infected for life and a potential, continual source for transmission of CAEV.

BIBLIOGRAPHY

Adams DS, Klevjer-Anderson P, Carlson JL, et al: Transmission and control of caprine arthritis-encephalitis virus. Am J Vet Res 44:1670–1676, 1983.
Adams DS, Oliver RE, Ameghino E, et al: Global survey of serological evidence of caprine arthritis-encephalitis virus infection. Vet Rec 115:493–495, 1984.
Crawford TB, Adams DS: Caprine arthritis-encephalitis: clinical features and presence of antibody in selected goat populations. J Am Vet Med Assoc 178:713–719, 1981.
Crawford TB, Adams DS, Cheevers WP, Cork LC: Chronic arthritis in goats caused by a retrovirus. Science 207:997–999, 1980.
Robinson WF, Ellis TM: Caprine arthritis-encephalitis virus infection: from recognition to eradication. Aust Vet J 63:237–241, 1986.

Ovine Astroviruses
JANICE C. BRIDGER, BSc, PhD

By negative-stain electron microscopy, the 30-nm particles appear circular in outline with a 5- or 6-pointed stellate configuration on the surface. Although morphologically indistinguishable from astroviruses of other species, ovine astroviruses do not cross-react by immunofluorescence with convalescent antisera. Particles contain single-stranded RNA. To date, only 1 strain has been studied.

EPIZOOTIOLOGY

No information is available on the significance of astroviruses in ovine enteritis or on the prevalence of infection. The virus is recognized only in the United Kingdom, where it was identified in an outbreak of diarrhea in lambs 4 to 6 weeks old. Experimental infection can be produced by oral inoculation of bacteria-free fecal filtrates in gnotobiotic lambs 1 to 3 days old.

CLINICAL SIGNS

The single strain studied produced a mild diarrhea in gnotobiotic lambs 1 to 3 days old. Histologic damage was confined to the middle and posterior small intestine, where villus height–crypt depth ratios were reduced and epithelial cells on the distal parts of villi immunofluoresced. Crystalline arrays of virus particles were seen in the cytoplasm of infected cells.

DIAGNOSIS

Electron microscopy, particularly with ammonium molybdate as the negative stain, is used to identify astroviruses in feces; a simple preparative procedure without centrifugation is adequate to demonstrate particles. Alternatively, immunofluorescent staining of cryostat sections of small intestine may be used, but the highest rate of cell infection was found to be during the incubation period. Unlike human and bovine astroviruses, ovine astroviruses are not detectable by cell culture inoculation; they have not been shown to infect cell cultures, even on primary passage.

TREATMENT, PREVENTION, AND CONTROL

No specific therapeutic studies have been conducted, but the pathogenesis suggests that oral rehydration would be beneficial. No vaccines are available. Passive protection by maternal antibody may be possible, but natural levels in the ovine population are unknown.

BIBLIOGRAPHY

Bridger JC: Small viruses associated with gastroenteritis in animals. In Saif LJ, Theil KW (eds): Viral Diarrheas of Man and Animals. Boca Raton, FL, CRC Press, 1990, pp 161–182.
Kurtz JB, Lee TW: Astroviruses: human and animal. In Bock G, Whelan J (eds): Ciba Foundation Symposium 128: Novel Diarrhoea Viruses. Chichester, UK, John Wiley & Sons Ltd, 1987, pp 92–107.
Snodgrass DR: Astroviruses in diarrhea of young animals and children. In Kurstak E, Kurstak C (eds): Comparative Diagnosis of Viral Disease IVB. New York, Academic Press, 1981, pp 659–669.

Arthrogryposis-Hydranencephaly in Sheep: Cache Valley Virus Infection
ROBERT A. CRANDELL, BS, DVM, MPH

Cache Valley virus (CVV) infection is a recently reported virus disease of sheep in the United States. The virus has been isolated from mosquitoes and large vertebrates. The disease mimics Akabane virus infection of sheep and goats and is characterized by congenital arthrogryposis and central nervous system (CNS) malformations. Both diseases are vector-borne and are caused by viruses belonging to the same family. They have similar pathologic changes without clinical disease in the ewe, and both occur as epizootics. CVV was isolated from a sheep and cow in Texas in 1981, but it was not until 1987 that the virus was associated with disease in sheep.

ETIOLOGY

CVV is an arthropod-borne virus belonging to the Bunyamwera serogroup, family Bunyaviridae, genus *Bunyavirus*. The virus was first isolated from the mosquito (*Culiseta inornata*) in the Cache Valley of Utah in 1956. The virus is chloroform-sensitive and replicates in cell culture and in suckling and weanling mice.

EPIZOOTIOLOGY

The virus is widely distributed in North America. The virus or specific antibody has been demonstrated in arthropods and vertebrates in at least 25 states within the United States, 4 provinces of Canada, northern Mexico, and Jamaica. CVV first isolated from *Culiseta inornata* in 1956 has since been isolated from a wide range of mosquito vectors. The virus has recently been isolated from the blood of a horse, cow, and sheep. Transmission cycles and reservoirs are not known. However, during the breeding season before the Texas epizootic, there was an unusual amount of rainfall and a high density of flying insects. These conditions have also been observed in other recognized outbreaks.

CLINICAL DISEASE

After the bite of an infected mosquito, an asymptomatic viremia develops in the ewe with production of neutralizing antibodies. It has been shown that when the fetus is inoculated with the virus between 27 and 54 days of gestation, an infection occurs and congenital abnormalities develop. Infections during this time may result in arthrogryposis, CNS malformations, readsorption, and mummification. When fetuses are infected with Akabane virus at 76 days' gestation, they develop specific antibodies, and it is believed that the same response occurs in CVV infection. No clinical illness has been observed in naturally affected rams.

Most affected lambs are delivered at term and are stillborn. Those alive at birth are weak and unable to walk. In multiple births, all lambs may be affected; however, normal lambs do occur with mummified fetuses or affected lambs. Dystocia may be a complication when severe malformations are present, and the ewe may require assistance in delivery.

Severe to mild arthrogryposis with skeletal muscle hypoplasia occurs in the affected lambs (Fig. 1). All joints may be involved, with multiple joints being immobilized and fixed in flexion. Torticollis, scoliosis, and kyphosis are present in the more severely affected lambs. Gross lesions in the CNS consist of microencephaly, cerebellar hypoplasia, micromyelia, hydrocephalus, hydranencephaly, and porencephaly.

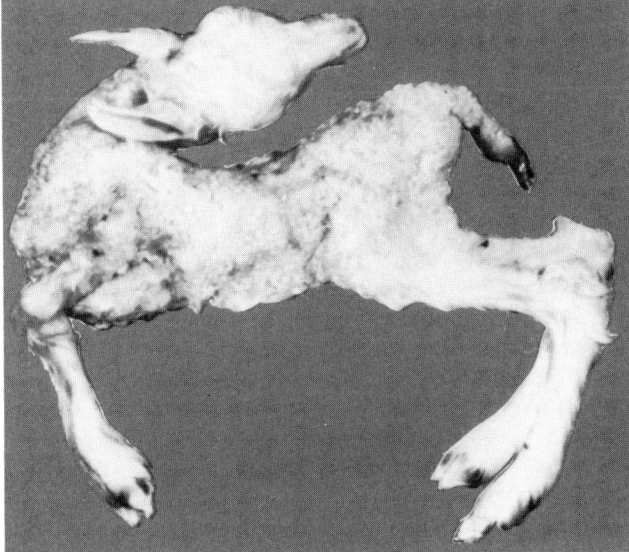

Figure 1. Lamb with severe arthrogryposis from a natural outbreak of CVV. (From Crandell RA, Livingston CW Jr, Shelton MJ: J Vet Diagn Invest 1:62–65, 1989. Courtesy of the American Association of Veterinary Laboratory Diagnosticians.)

DIAGNOSIS

The clinical, pathologic, and epizootiologic features of the disease are helpful in determining a presumptive diagnosis. CVV infection should be considered whenever a high incidence of severe arthrogryposis occurs during the lambing season. The diagnosis of CVV infection is based on the demonstration of specific CVV antibodies in precolostral serum collected from heart blood of affected lambs.

The virus has not been isolated from the tissues or fluids of term lambs. It is believed that the virus is neutralized by the antibody that develops after the 76th day of gestation. Positive serologic reaction in the ewes is evidence that they have been exposed to the virus at some time.

Other conditions causing fetal malformations in which CVV must be differentiated are bovine viral diarrhea (BVD), bluetongue (BT), border disease (BD), Akabane infection, spider lamb syndrome, and toxicosis by teratogenic plants. Although BVD, BT, and BD viruses induce CNS lesions in ruminants, musculoskeletal deformities are not a feature of the infections. The clinical, pathologic, immunologic, and epizootiologic characteristics of CVV infections are similar to Akabane virus infection. The two virus infections can be differentiated by serologic means. Spider lamb syndrome, a genetic defect observed in the Suffolk breed, differs from arthrogryposishydranencephaly in that lambs are born weak and have abnormalities of the musculoskeletal system without CNS lesions. The involvement of a plant toxicosis is determined by searching the pastures for the presence of poisonous plants.

PREVENTION AND CONTROL

There is no vaccine available for the immunization of sheep against CVV infection. Because of the relationship between the time of infection of the fetus and the period of gestation in the development of lesions, anything that will prevent or reduce exposure to the vectors during the breeding season is recommended. Good water and herd management may help reduce the spread of the infection. There should be good drainage around the stock tanks, and other mosquito breeding areas should be eliminated. The breeding stock may be sprayed for insects and moved from lower lands to higher elevations for avoiding exposure to vectors. Neutralization tests on the serum from the older breeding stock will provide evidence of the existence of CVV in the area and indicate the immunologic status of the herd.

BIBLIOGRAPHY

Chung SI, Livingston CW Jr, Edwards JF, et al: Congenital malformations in sheep resulting from in utero inoculation of Cache Valley virus. Am J Vet Res 51:1645–1648, 1990.

Crandell RA, Livingston CW Jr, Shelton MJ: Laboratory investigation of a naturally occurring outbreak of arthrogryposis-hydranencephaly in Texas sheep. J Vet Diagn Invest 1:62–65, 1989.

Edwards JF, Livingston CW Jr, Chung SI, Collisson EW: Ovine arthrogryposis and central nervous system malformations associated with in utero Cache Valley virus infection: spontaneous disease. Vet Pathol 26:33–39, 1989.

Scrapie

HOWARD W. WHITFORD, DVM, PhD

Scrapie is a neurodegenerative disease of sheep caused by a subviral agent thought to be a prion. A prion in its broadest sense is a strand of nucleic acid having no outer protein coat. Virino, slow virus, and unconventional virus are other terms used to describe the scrapie agent. This agent has some very extraordinary properties. It has never been visualized with the electron microscope, but filtration studies indicate that it is 50 to 60 nm in diameter. The scrapie agent is extremely resistant to heat and chemical disinfectants. Infected brain tissue heated to 100° C for 8 hours is capable of causing disease when it is injected into sheep. Likewise, infected mouse brain stored in 10 per cent formalin for up to 4 months remains infective for mice and goats.

EPIZOOTIOLOGY

Sheep are the natural host for scrapie. Mink encephalopathy and kuru in humans are closely related, if not host-adapted scrapie agent. The recent (1985) outbreak of bovine spongiform encephalopathy in cattle in Great Britain is also thought to be bovine-adapted scrapie transmitted to cattle by the feeding of rendered sheep by-products infected with scrapie. Scrapie has been experimentally reproduced in goats, mink, laboratory primates, and a variety of laboratory rodents.

Geographically, scrapie is widespread. The disease occurs in sheep in Great Britain, Belgium, France, Germany, Spain, India, Iceland, Canada, and the United States. The disease was also recognized in South Africa, Australia, and New Zealand after importation of infected sheep from Great Britain. Prompt quarantine and slaughter resulted in the eradication of the disease in these countries.

In the United States, the number of flocks with scrapie has increased dramatically during the 1980s, compared with the 1970s. No more than 6 scrapie-infected flocks in any 1 year were reported during 1974 to 1979. In 1980, 11 flocks were reported; these have increased each year to 52 flocks in 1988. The number of states having infected flocks has increased from 9 in 1984 to 20 in 1988.

The most commonly affected breed of sheep is the Suffolk. In the United States, this breed accounts for about 74 per cent of the infected flocks. Cheviot, Hampshire, and Swaledale have higher incidence of natural scrapie than do other breeds, although no breed of sheep or goats has been found to be resistant. Most natural outbreaks can be traced to Suffolks.

There is an apparent genetic link with susceptibility to scrapie. This was firmly established with the discovery of the Sip (short incubation period) gene having two alleles sA and pA. Those sheep having sAsA or sApA die much sooner from intracerebral inoculation than do pApA sheep. If the agent is given subcutaneously, the pApA sheep survive a natural life span, whereas the sAsA and sApA sheep develop clinical scrapie.

Transmission of scrapie occurs only horizontally. There is no evidence that the disease agent is transmitted in utero, although the agent has been found in the female reproductive organs. Research in this area is ongoing, but thus far it appears that embryos collected from scrapie-infected ewes and implanted in scrapie-free ewes produce scrapie-free offspring and vice versa. Likewise, the agent has never been demonstrated in lacteal secretions. It is believed that lambs are exposed at an early age via nasal and fecal shedding from infected dams. Resistance to the infection increases with age.

The pathogenesis of scrapie has been laboriously worked out by Hadlow and Eklund. In experimentally infected animals, the agent is initially in the lymphoreticular system, namely, the retropharyngeal lymph nodes and spleen. Next it is detected in the intestine, where it replicates slowly for months or years. Although a blood phase has never been demonstrated, it is probably carried to the central nervous system by the blood. The agent reaches the brain stem most likely via the cranial nerves and replicates in those parts of the brain that result in the clinical signs (incoordination, pruritus, and so on). The agent is not cleared from the extraneural tissue and continues to be shed throughout the course of the disease.

CLINICAL SIGNS

In natural outbreaks of scrapie, clinical signs may occur in sheep between the ages of 18 months and 6 years, most commonly in animals 30 to 60 months of age. Neurologic manifestations are the only ante-mortem signs noted. These develop very slowly and insidiously. Initially the animals appear apprehensive. They then become excitable and overreact to routine stimuli. As the disease progresses, tremors of the head and neck with the head held high may be noted. Muscle tremors of the flanks and thighs may also develop. Pruritus, usually beginning at the tail head and progressing anteriorly over the flanks and ribs, develops with resultant scratching and loss of wool (Fig. 1). Serpentine tongue movements accompany the scratching. Licking and wool biting affected areas are common. Incoordination that becomes progressively pronounced develops until the animal becomes recumbent and invariably dies. The clinical disease may occur over a period as short as a few weeks or as long as a year, but most cases last between 6 weeks and 6 months. During the clinical course, the animal remains alert with a good appetite, but weight loss will occur.

Post-mortem examination of animals dying of scrapie shows no gross abnormalities with the exception of localized skin trauma due to scratching. On microscopic examination, the lesions are confined to the central nervous system, where degenerative changes are seen. These changes are confined to the cerebellar cortex, medulla oblongata, pons, midbrain, diencephalon, and corpus striatum and consist of pyknotic and shrunken neurons, cytoplasmic vacuoles, and astrocytosis. Few, if any, changes are noted in the spinal cord or cerebral cortex.

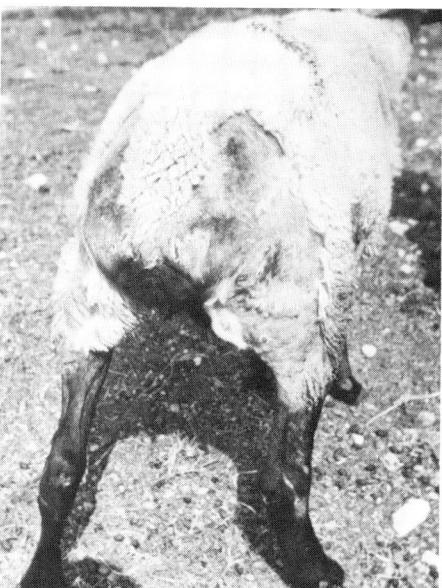

Figure 1. Scrapie-infected sheep showing wool loss due to pruritus and scratching. (Courtesy of Dr. Wilbur Clark, Scrapie Field Trial, Mission, TX.)

DIAGNOSIS

At the present time, scrapie in a live animal cannot be definitively diagnosed by use of current laboratory procedures. This is because the infectious agent has never been isolated, purified, or propagated outside the animal host. The scrapie agent produces no detectable humoral or cellular antibody and has never been demonstrated in blood. The agent incorporates with host glycoprotein to become PrP (prion protein), which accumulates as aggregates to form scrapie-associated fibrils in brain, spleen, and lymph nodes during the development of the disease. Work is currently under way to isolate and purify these structures so that antibodies can be raised that are specific for the scrapie-associated fibrils and become a useful rapid diagnostic tool.

A tentative diagnosis is based on history of exposure, long incubation period, age of the animal, and clinical signs (some animals may not have pruritus) progressing to death. Histopathologic lesions in the brain and transmission of the disease to mice by inoculation with infected tissue confirm the diagnosis.

Differential diagnosis includes encephalopathies due to other infectious agents (such as *Listeria*, louping ill, visna, maedi, caprine arthritis-encephalitis), polioencephalomalacia, and pruritic dermatitis caused by bacteria or fungi. The age of the animal and response to specific therapy should rule out other disease conditions.

Scrapie is a reportable disease, and the appropriate state and federal animal health officials should be contacted if scrapie is suspected.

TREATMENT

No treatment has been found to be effective, and none should be attempted.

PREVENTION AND CONTROL

The historical approach to prevention and control of scrapie has been to slaughter herds that have experienced the disease, tracing back to herds of origin and destroying them also. This method proved successful in eradicating the disease in New Zealand and Australia, probably owing to the early recognition and prompt action more than to the method itself.

In the United States, an official eradication program was begun in 1952 in which affected sheep as well as the whole flock were killed; in 1957, the source flocks were included in the slaughter program. This program reduced the prevalence of scrapie to very few flocks.

However, in 1983, a critical change in the eradication program was put into effect. Because of shortage of indemnity money and concern over eliminating certain valuable blood lines, whole flocks were no longer slaughtered, and only blood kin parents and progeny were killed. This change ignored the horizontal transmission of the disease and resulted in a dramatic increase in infected flocks.

In 1989, this program was abandoned, and at the present time there is no official eradication program for scrapie. There is, however, a voluntary program being developed by producer groups, animal health officials, veterinarians, renderers, and the federal government through a negotiated rule-making process. In 1991, The Negotiated Rulemaking Committee adopted the following control measures for scrapie: (1) a one-time indemnification program for infection and source flocks; (2) a voluntary flock certification program; and (3) permanent, highly visible identification for the interstate movement of sheep from infected or source flocks.

BIBLIOGRAPHY

Eklund CM, Hadlow WJ: The slow virus diseases. *In* Steele JH (ed): CRC Handbook Series in Zoonoses. Boca Raton, FL, CRC Press, 1981.
Fact Sheet: Scrapie—Background, Negotiated Rulemaking, Proposed Voluntary Scrapie Flock Certification Program. USDA, APHIS, February, 1991.
Gadjusek DC, Gibbs CJ Jr, Alpers M: Slow, Latent, and Temperate Virus Infections. United States Department of Health, Education and Welfare, Public Health Service, National Institutes of Health, National Institute of Neurological Diseases and Blindness, 1965.
Hadlow WJ, Eklund CM: Scrapie: A Virus-Induced Chronic Encephalopathy of Sheep. Infections of the Nervous System. Research Publication of The Association for Research in Nervous and Mental Disease, vol XLIV, 1968.
Jensen F, Swift BL: Scrapie. *In* Kimberling CV (ed): Diseases of Sheep, 3rd ed. Philadelphia, Lea & Febiger, 1988, pp 334–341.

Sheep Pulmonary Adenomatosis (Sheep Pulmonary Carcinoma, Jaagsiekte)*

RANDALL C. CUTLIP, DVM, PhD

Sheep pulmonary adenomatosis, sheep pulmonary carcinoma, or jaagsiekte, an Afrikaans term meaning "driving sickness," is an infectious bronchoalveolar carcinoma of the lungs of sheep that occasionally metastasizes to regional lymph nodes and rarely to other nodes and organs.

ETIOLOGIC AGENT

A type D retrovirus with a 25,000 molecular weight protein antigenically related to the Mason-Pfizer monkey virus has been shown by several laboratories to be associated with experimental production of the disease. This virus has been shown to replicate in cell cultures derived from the tumor and is presumed to be the sole etiologic agent. The virus has limited genetic and antigenic relatedness to ovine and caprine lentiviruses (ovine progressive pneumonia and caprine arthritis-encephalitis viruses). A herpesvirus is frequently associated with the disease and may be involved in a secondary role but more likely is a latent virus that is activated by the neoplasm. Ovine progressive pneumonia (maedi-visna) virus is also frequently found with the type D retrovirus, and a combination of these 2 diseases is common.

EPIZOOTIOLOGY

Sheep pulmonary adenomatosis was first described in South Africa in 1891 and was thought to have been present since 1850. The disease is common in Europe, Africa, Asia, and South America but is rare in the United States. There are no known differences in susceptibility among different breeds of sheep. Sheep appear to be the primary natural host, although the disease also occurs naturally in goats. The disease can be transmitted experimentally to sheep and goats by intratracheal administration of lung homogenate or pulmonary lavage fluid

---

*All material in this article is in the public domain, with the exception of any borrowed figures or tables.

from affected sheep. Natural transmission occurs by aerosol and probably by contact with food or water contaminated by secretions from the respiratory tract of affected sheep. Death rates in a flock usually are less than 2 per cent annually, but death rates as high as 50 per cent have been reported.

CLINICAL SIGNS AND LESIONS

The disease is characterized clinically by a long and variable incubation period of 2 months to 2 years, an insidious onset, and a slow progression to death after several weeks. The incubation period is shortened to as little as 2 weeks when neonatal lambs are inoculated intratracheally with infectious fluid or tumor tissue. Signs are progressive dyspnea, tachypnea, and loss of weight. Late in the disease, excess secretions produced in the lungs by neoplastic cells cause moist rales, and fluid may run from the nostrils when the rear of an affected sheep is elevated. In uncomplicated cases, body temperature and appetite are normal and coughing is rare. Death from bacterial pneumonia is a common sequel to the neoplasm.

Macroscopic lesions are unevenly distributed in the lungs, with the ventral parts most severely affected. Lesions are usually bilateral and vary within the same lung from small discrete areas of less then 1 cm in diameter to large confluent areas that are several centimeters in diameter. Affected areas of the lungs are reddish-gray to bluish-gray in color, firm in consistency, and wet on cut surface. The lungs may be 2 to 3 times normal weight. On microscopic examination, the lesion is a papillary adenocarcinoma with variable amounts of fibrous and myxomatous stroma. Discrete nodules of myxomatous stroma are present in some tumors. Alveoli surrounding tumor foci are usually filled with macrophages. The neoplastic epithelial cells arise from type II alveolar epithelial cells and from nonciliated bronchiolar epithelial (Clara) cells. Metastatic lesions are usually small and mimic the primary lesion in microscopic appearance.

DIAGNOSIS

Sheep pulmonary adenomatosis may be suspected from clinical signs, but a definitive diagnosis is dependent on finding characteristic lesions in the lungs. The lesion must be differentiated from epithelial hyperplasia resulting from various bacterial and parasitic infections or caustic agents.

TREATMENT

No treatment is effective against the neoplasm, but life may be prolonged by treating with antibiotics for prevention of secondary pneumonia.

PREVENTION AND CONTROL

The lack of a simple diagnostic test limits effective control. The disease was eradicated from Iceland by slaughtering all affected sheep and their contacts. On the basis of epidemiologic data, removing affected sheep from a flock or rearing lambs in isolation would be a useful control measure.

BIBLIOGRAPHY

Cutlip RC, Young S: Sheep pulmonary adenomatosis (jaagsiekte) in the United States. Am J Vet Res 43:2108–2113, 1982.
DeMartini JC, Rosadio RH, Lairmore MD: The etiology and pathogenesis of ovine pulmonary carcinoma (sheep pulmonary adenomatosis). Vet Microbiol 17:219–236, 1988.
Querat G, Barban V, Sauze N, et al: Characteristics of a novel lentivirus derived from South African sheep with pulmonary adenocarcinoma (jaagsiekte). Virology 158:158–167, 1987.
Sharp JM: Sheep pulmonary adenomatosis: a contagious tumour and its cause. Cancer Surv 6:73–83, 1987.

Ovine and Caprine Mycoplasmoses
SØREN ROSENDAL, DVM, PhD

Mycoplasmas are significant pathogens of sheep and goats on a worldwide scale. Perhaps because of the close phylogenetic relationship between these animal species, many members of their mycoplasma flora are shared. Mycoplasma diseases tend to be enzootic or epizootic in nature and are most serious in large and crowded herds subjected to various stress factors. Mycoplasma diseases in sheep and goats fall into the following categories: pneumonia, mastitis, conjunctivitis, genitourinary tract diseases, and septicemia.

PNEUMONIA

Mycoplasma ovipneumoniae is a cause of both acute and chronic pneumonia in sheep and goats. In sheep, at least, it contributes together with *Pasteurella haemolytica* to exudative and proliferative pneumonia. The role of viruses promoting virulence of *M. ovipneumoniae* is not clear. Disease is most frequent in lambs and kids raised under crowded conditions. Wet and cold conditions seem to predispose as much as dry and dusty conditions do to the aggravation of mycoplasma pneumonia. The animals develop a dry hacking cough and nasal discharge that may progress and become more productive with time. The respiratory distress may be easily visible and audible by auscultation of the cranial thorax. Mortality, even when the pneumonia is untreated, is low, but the affected animals thrive poorly.

Specific diagnosis rests on isolating *M. ovipneumoniae* from bronchoalveolar lavage samples or from lung tissue at post mortem. *M. ovipneumoniae* is a fragile organism, and samples should be brought frozen to the diagnostic laboratory for culture. *M. ovipneumoniae* is fastidious and requires special media but is easily identified on the basis of growth characteristics and antigens. Diagnosis by serologic methods is less reliable owing to the ubiquitous nature of *M. ovipneumoniae* in the upper airways of sheep and goats.

Treatment should be aimed at maintaining antimicrobial drug levels in the lung tissue with effect against both mycoplasmas and bacteria. Drugs such as spectinomycin, tylosin, quinolones, oxytetracycline, tiamulin, and gentamicin may be effective.

No vaccines are currently available to protect lambs and goat kids against *M. ovipneumoniae*. The best preventive measures are those directed toward reducing infection pressures, social and environmental stress burdens.

The classic form of contagious caprine pleuropneumonia (CCPP) is caused by mycoplasmas tentatively labeled the F-38 group, which is closely related to *M. capricolum*, *M. mycoides* subsp. *mycoides*, and *M. mycoides* subsp. *capri*. Classic CCPP has so far been diagnosed in Africa and Asia.

Control and prevention of CCPP is based on diagnosis of cases and carriers by clinical, post-mortem, and serologic procedures followed by slaughter and restriction of movement of potential carrier animals into areas free of infection. A vaccine developed in Kenya is showing promise.

MASTITIS

Contagious agalactia caused by *Mycoplasma agalactiae* is an important disease of sheep and goats in Africa, Asia, and Mediterranean countries of Europe. Infections spread by carriers, and outbreaks with high morbidity and some mortality may occur upon introduction into susceptible herds. The mammary infection leads to agalactia and involution of the gland and therefore lost milk production. The infection will occasionally progress to septicemia and death or occasionally to arthritis or keratoconjunctivitis. Diagnosis of infection requires culture of milk samples on suitable media and proper identification of the *Mycoplasma* isolate. *M. agalactiae* infections in sheep or goat populations outside the countries with endemic problems should be reported and appropriate measures taken for elimination.

Mastitis in goats in countries with no evidence of contagious agalactia may occasionally be caused by the caprine variant of *M. mycoides* subsp. *mycoides*, *M. putrefaciens*, or *M. capricolum*. Suspicion should be raised when bacterial cultures of milk or secretions from mastitic does are negative or give pinpoint colonies with slight α-hemolysis. Milk from infected does may cause severe septicemia and high mortality in nursing kids or bucket-fed animals. This can be prevented by pasteurizing the milk before use. Sporadic cases of mycoplasma mastitis should be culled. Long-term treatment with tylosin or similar drugs may be attempted in very valuable or pregnant animals. The specific diagnosis is based on isolation and identification of the mycoplasma in question, a task normally accomplished only by highly specialized laboratories.

CONJUNCTIVITIS

Infectious keratoconjunctivitis of sheep and goats occurs worldwide. *Mycoplasma conjunctivae* is introduced into herds by carrier animals and may spread rapidly among all the animals. The initial signs include conjunctivitis ("pinkeye") with hyperemia, edema, and increased lacrimation. The tears flow over the lower eyelid and wet the hair on the face. Later in the course, the cornea becomes cloudy and opaque, which leads to temporary blindness. The corneal and conjunctival inflammation usually subsides after 1 to 2 weeks as immunity increases. Corneal ulceration and permanent scarring is rare and more likely due to secondary bacterial infections. The animals do not seem to be affected in terms of productivity or feed intake. The diagnosis is based on culture of lacrimal fluid or eye swabs in appropriate medium followed by identification of isolates.

Treatment includes tetracycline ointments instilled into the eye and elimination of dust, ammonia, insects, or other external factors that may impede spontaneous recovery or aggravate the problem.

GENITOURINARY TRACT INFECTIONS

Mycoplasmas are commonly isolated from the genital tract of sheep and goats. The role in specific diseases is not clear at this point but should be carefully evaluated, with consideration of the numbers of mycoplasmas isolated, species isolated, and other possible intercurrent pathogenic microorganisms. Mycoplasma taxon 2D has been associated with vulvovaginitis and reproductive failure. Ureaplasmas may cause a mild vulvovaginitis and have been incriminated in cases of urinary calculi in goats on a low-calcium diet. Because of the sporadic nature of mycoplasma diseases of the genitourinary tract, treatment is rarely considered.

SEPTICEMIA

Mycoplasmas of the caprine variant of *M. mycoides* subsp. *mycoides* may cause septicemia in addition to local infections of the lungs, mammary gland, tonsils, or outer ear. Outbreaks of septicemia are observed in goat kids exposed to contaminated milk. The animals show signs of prostration, increased respiratory rate, increased body temperature, and often swollen joints. Mortality is usually high. Diagnosis is secured by isolation of the organism. Experienced bacteriologists suspect mycoplasmas when blood agar plates grow pinpoint α-hemolytic colonies that do not stain with Gram's stains. Transfer of colonies from blood agar plates or primary isolation on mycoplasma agar results in rapid growth of relatively large colonies, which usually reach 1 to 2 mm in diameter in 2 to 3 days. The caprine variant of *M. mycoides* subsp. *mycoides* is therefore often referred to as the "large colony type." In contrast to the caprine variant, the bovine variant grows slowly and produces small colonies on mycoplasma agar. The bovine variant (or "small colony type") of *M. mycoides* subsp. *mycoides* is the cause of contagious bovine pleuropneumonia, a disease confined to Africa, Asia, and limited areas of Spain and Portugal. The caprine variant occurs in most countries of the world including the United States and Canada. In addition to isolating the caprine variant of *M. mycoides* subsp. *mycoides*, it may be possible to diagnose chronic infections with serologic tests, such as the complement fixation test or an indirect hemagglutination test.

Treatment may be attempted with use of macrolide, quinolone, tetracycline, or aminoglycoside antibiotics but seldom leads to complete recovery. Preventive measures such as control of stressors and intercurrent diseases and elimination of milk shedders should prove effective. Experimental vaccines developed to prevent mastitis outbreaks have shown promise.

BIBLIOGRAPHY

Cotten GS: Caprine-ovine mycoplasmas. *In* Tully JG, Whitcomb RF (eds): The Mycoplasmas, vol 2, New York, Academic Press, 1979, pp 105–132.
Rosendal S: Ovine and caprine mycoplasmas. *In* Whitford E (ed): Diagnosis of Mycoplasmoses in Domestic Animals. Ames, Iowa State University Press, in press.

Viral Diseases of Swine

Porcine Pseudorabies (Aujeszky's Disease)

ROBERT A. CRANDELL, DVM, BS, MPH

Pseudorabies is an infectious, naturally occurring virus disease affecting many animal species. The disease is known as Aujeszky's disease, mad itch, and infectious bulbar paralysis. In cattle, sheep, dogs, and cats, the disease is characterized by a severe local pruritus with a high mortality. The clinical disease in pigs varies with the age of the animals. There is a worldwide interest in the control of this economically important virus disease.

ETIOLOGY

Pseudorabies (PR) is caused by a herpesvirus, a large DNA virus measuring 150 to 180 nm in diameter. All PR viruses studied belong to 1 serotype. Although the virus strains are indistinguishable serologically, there are variations in virulence and biologic characteristics among strains. Molecular differences (DNA fingerprints) can be demonstrated between field and vaccine strains by restriction endonuclease analysis. Like other herpesviruses, PR virus has the ability to persist in the host as a latent infection. The virus is relatively stable, and the survival time outside of the animal's body is dependent on the environmental conditions. The virus is readily inactivated with chloroform, ether, 1 per cent sodium hydroxide, and 5 per cent phenol. The virus replicates with cytopathic changes in a wide variety of cell cultures derived from different animal species. The rabbit is most sensitive of the laboratory animals to infection.

EPIZOOTIOLOGY

Pseudorabies-infected swine are believed to be the primary source of infection for other animals and the host reservoir for the perpetuation of the virus in nature. The communicability of the virus from swine to other species, and particularly to other swine, is the most important single factor known in the transmission of PR virus. Infected swine transmit the virus through the nasal secretions, saliva, milk, and placenta; the virus is transmitted by boars during service.

Survivors of an outbreak develop a long-lasting antibody. The virus persists in recovered animals as a latent infection. These animals become carriers, and under certain stresses, the virus is reactivated and serves as a source of infection to susceptible animals.

The reservoirs of the virus and the nature of spread from farm to farm are not understood. Although the virus has been isolated from a number of wildlife species, their importance as a reservoir and their role in the spread of the virus are not conclusive. Badgers, raccoons, skunks, rats, foxes, coyotes, and opposums have been found to be naturally infected. The source of infection is believed to be from feeding on infected swine carcasses.

Dogs and cats are highly susceptible to infection by the oral route. It is common to have a sudden illness and death in these animals on swine farms before the disease is recognized in the swine.

CLINICAL SIGNS

Porcine PR occurs both as a clinical and a subclinical infection; however, the morbidity and mortality is highest in the newborn pig. In the older pig, the disease generally occurs as a milder clinical disease or an inapparent infection.

The illness in the very young and weaning-age pig has a sudden onset and progresses rapidly, with resultant high death losses. Newborn pigs from infected sows die as early as 1 day of age, with the average age of death being about 1 week; however, deaths may extend over a period of 1 month after farrowing. Temperature may exceed 40.5° C. Depression, tremors, incoordination, and convulsions are observed before death. Respiratory signs are the most predominant clinical feature with some strains of virus. Diarrhea and vomition may be present but are not a constant feature of the disease.

Disorientation is common, and if the pigs are not confined, they will wander off and die. Pigs have been observed to rub their heads against walls and run into objects with their snouts to the ground. Death losses in litters of very young pigs may approach 100 per cent, whereas death losses may reach 40 to 60 per cent in the 3- to 4-week-old pigs.

Outbreaks in feeder operations have occurred as late as 1 month after the addition of new animals. In the 3- to 5-month-old pig, the clinical signs may persist as long as 7 or 8 days after onset. The death losses are less than in the younger pigs. Temperatures may reach 41.5° C, and the animals usually stop eating and may vomit. Head and body tremors, circling, and paddling movements of varying degrees are characteristic. Some infected pigs weighing 45 to 68 kg have been described as having a "wobbly motion." Death is preceded by convulsions and prostration.

A respiratory form of the disease has also been observed in sows and gilts. The animals have fever, may cough or sneeze, and go off feed. Abortions may occur during the early or late stages of gestation. In the later stages of pregnancy, the fetus may be retained and become mummified. Some sows will absorb the fetuses, whereas others will farrow stillborn pigs. Many sows will have a fever, go off feed, and may vomit for several days at the time of farrowing or immediately thereafter. Occasionally a sow or gilt will die. A few animals may rub their noses or heads; however, the "mad itch" syndrome seen in other species is generally absent in swine. Some herds experience breeding problems with sows and gilts after an outbreak.

DIAGNOSIS

A clinical diagnosis of PR should always be confirmed by laboratory methods because the clinical signs mimic other diseases, and PR may also occur concurrently with another condition.

The disease is confirmed by the isolation and identification of the virus and by the fluorescent antibody test. The recommended specimens for virus isolation from suspect pigs are the tonsils and portions of the olfactory lobes, pons, and medulla. The tonsil is the choice tissue for the fluorescent antibody test. The virus may be present in other tissues such as the lung, liver, and spleen of some animals. It is important that tissue from more than 1 animal from a suspect herd be submitted to the laboratory because the virus is not recovered from all animals, and not all tonsils are positive by the fluorescent antibody test.

Some of the swine diseases from which PR must be differentiated are enterovirus infections, water deprivation (salt poisoning), and hog cholera. Rabies is of special concern with cattle and in peculiar-acting wild animals.

Serologic methods (serum neutralization, enzyme-linked immunosorbent assay, latex agglutination) are useful in surveys and for monitoring herds but are not recommended for the identification of an outbreak. Demonstrable antibodies are not present in the serum of animals during the acute stage of illness.

TREATMENT

There is no treatment that will reverse the course of illness after clinical signs appear. Although the administration of hyperimmune serum to baby pigs is effective in reducing death losses during an outbreak, there is no commercial source for the serum. Vaccines are used as preventive measures; in some infected herds, vaccination has helped reduce the economic loss.

CONTROL AND ERADICATION

Serologic testing and restricting the movement of positive animals are important features of a control program. It is recommended that animals have a negative test before entering exhibitions and herds as replacement breeding stock. Replacement gilts and boars should be tested within 30 days of movement, held in isolation for 30 days, and retested negative before being added to the new herd.

Early recognition of the disease is important in controlling the spread of the virus. When PR is suspected in a herd, the sick animals should be isolated until a laboratory diagnosis can be made. When PR is confirmed, the herd should be quarantined, and traffic to and from the premises should be controlled. All dead animals should be buried or burned. Dogs and cats should not be allowed to comingle with swine or eat dead pigs. Although it is difficult, every effort should be made to control wildlife. Feral swine are known to be carriers of PR virus and should not have access to premises where domestic swine are raised.

There are 3 recommended methods for the elimination of PR virus from an infected herd: depopulation and repopulation; test and removal; and offspring segregation, which has several options. It is also advisable to determine the status of virus circulation in the herd before a method of virus elimination is selected. Herd vaccination may be useful in combination with the control program. Advantages and disadvantages and other considerations of the various programs are discussed in detail in the bibliography. Many European countries, New Zealand (North Island), and the United States are committed to eradication of the disease. The United States has a 5-stage state-federal industry PR eradication program. The goal is to eradicate the disease in domestic swine by the year 2000. The recent advances in biotechnology have made a major impact on the eradication of this disease. Marker vaccines (gene deletions) produced by genetic engineering are playing a major role in the programs. With specially designed diagnostic kits, vaccinated animals can be distinguished from field-infected animals. The serologic test kits are referred to as a companion test for the vaccine. At the present time, 3 tests that can differentiate between infection titers and those induced by vaccine have been licensed by the United States Department of Agriculture.

PUBLIC HEALTH CONSIDERATIONS

There are no known public health concerns associated with PR virus–infected animals.

BIBLIOGRAPHY

Crandell RA: Pseudorabies (Aujeszky's disease). Vet Clin North Am [Large Anim Pract] 4:321–331, 1982.
McConnell S, Kit M, Sit S: Pseudorabies virus gene-deleted vaccines. In 62nd Annual Western Veterinary Conference, Biotechnology and Applications in Veterinary Practice. USDA, APHIS, 1990, pp 16–24.
Mock RE, Crandell RA, Mesfin GM: Induced latency in pseudorabies vaccinated pigs. Can J Comp Med 45:56–59, 1981.
Morrison RB, Thawley DG: Elimination of PRV from large swine herds. Report of the Pseudorabies Committee, Appendix 3. In Proceedings, 93rd Annual Meeting, U.S. Animal Health Association, 1989, pp 479–485.
Pseudorabies. 9CFT Part 85. Federal Register, vol 55, no 90, 1990, pp 19245–19253.
Thawley DG, Gustafson DP, Beran GW: Procedures for the elimination of pseudorabies virus from herds of swine. J Am Vet Med Assoc 181:1513–1518, 1982.

Porcine Cytomegalovirus (Inclusion Body Rhinitis)
ROBERT ASSAF, AGR, MScV

Porcine cytomegalovirus (PCMV) is associated with pig inclusion body rhinitis and death in very young piglets and fetuses. Occasionally, the virus causes a systemic disease in susceptible older pigs.

ETIOLOGY

PCMV is a DNA virus belonging to the herpesvirus family and is sensitive to ether and chloroform. Only 1 serotype has been reported. The virus grows in lung macrophages, porcine fallopian tube cell line, and primary pig testis cells.

EPIZOOTIOLOGY

PCVM is host-specific and probably occurs worldwide. The disease is most commonly propagated via the nasal route. The economic importance of the disease is not well known; however, it seems that the virus is emerging as an economically significant pathogen for some swine herds with minimal disease status.

CLINICAL SIGNS AND LESIONS

Natural outbreaks include symptoms of shivering, sneezing, respiratory distress, and death in piglets. Usually, pigs older than 3 weeks are asymptomatic. Early postnatal or congenital infection also occurs and is associated with mummification, stillbirths, neonatal death, and runt pigs. Moreover, infection with PCMV immediately after coitus can lead to infection of the embryo, depending on the kinetics of virus-host interaction.

In piglets, the infection produces widespread petechiae and edema involving most commonly the thoracic cavity and subcutaneous tissues. In older animals, no macroscopic lesions are found. Basophilic intranuclear inclusion bodies and cytomegaly are seen in numerous cells.

DIAGNOSIS

Serologic diagnosis is based on the indirect immunofluorescence test (IIF) or enzyme-linked immunosorbent assay (ELISA). Virus may be isolated from nasal mucosa, lung, and kidney. Viral antigen can be detected by the IIF test on frozen sections of infected tissue.

TREATMENT AND PREVENTION

There is no specific treatment for PCMV infection. Good management and abstention from introducing new stock during the mating period and the first month of pregnancy should be practiced.

BIBLIOGRAPHY

Assaf R, Bouillant AMP, Di Franco E: Enzyme-linked immunosorbent assay for the detection of antibodies to porcine cytomegalovirus. Can J Comp Med 46:183–185, 1982.
Edington N: Porcine cytomegalovirus infection. In Disease of Swine, 5th ed. Ames, IA, Iowa State University Press, 1981, pp 271–277.
Edington N, Wrathall AE, Done JT: Porcine cytomegalovirus (PCMV) in early gestation. J Vet Microbiol 17:117–128, 1988.
Orr JP, Althouse E, Dulac GC, Durham JK: Epizootic infection of a minimal disease swine herd with herpesvirus. Can Vet J 20:45–50, 1988.

Swine Pox

DEOKI N. TRIPATHY, BVSC & AH, PHD, MS

ETIOLOGY

Swine pox is caused by swine poxvirus, which belongs to the genus *Suipoxvirus* of the Poxviridae family. This virus is highly host-specific, and the disease is characterized by development of cutaneous lesions in susceptible young pigs.

EPIZOOTIOLOGY

Swine pox is worldwide in distribution and affects primarily the susceptible population of young pigs. Once introduced in a large herd, the disease is maintained for a long time owing to constant availability of susceptible young pigs as replacement stock and the resistance of the virus to environmental conditions. The virus can survive in the dried crusts for at least 1 year.

TRANSMISSION

Swine pox is transmitted by direct contact associated with skin injury. The louse *Hematopinus suis*, under natural conditions, acts as a mechanical vector of the virus and may carry the virus for weeks or months. The lice puncture the skin and provide necessary injury for permitting entry of the virus. The severity of the disease is influenced by louse infestation and the degree of injury. Injuries from mechanical irritations or other blood-sucking external parasites can bring results similar to those of lice injuries. Skin lesions of poxvirus infection in a newborn piglet suggesting transplacental infection have been reported.

CLINICAL SIGNS

The incubation period varies from 4 to 6 days and sometimes 12 to 14 days. The onset may be marked by a mild transient fever and inappetence. The initial skin lesions are small, round, erythematous spots that increase in size and thickness to form reddish papules of about 2 mm in diameter. These papules enlarge to 2 to 5 mm in diameter and become vesicles and then form umbilicated pustules. The vesicular stage is of short duration and is often missed. With rapid drying of the exudate, scabs are formed with depressed centers. Desquamation of the scabs or crusts leaves a small, white, discolored spot. The course of the disease is 1½ to 3½ weeks. The lesions occur primarily on the abdomen and inner aspects of the thighs but may occur on other areas (Fig. 1A). Udder and teat lesions may occur in some sows that nurse infected piglets. In such cases, loss of piglets may occur because of low milk consumption resulting from painfully infected teats. Regional lymphadenopathy has been observed.

DIAGNOSIS

Swine pox may be suspected when characteristic cutaneous pox lesions are observed. Swine are also susceptible to vaccinia virus (genus *Orthopoxvirus* of the Poxviridae family), which has a wide host range and causes similar lesions. Restriction endonuclease analysis of DNA from swine poxvirus and vaccinia virus reveals marked differences in the genome of these viruses. However, because of discontinuation of human vaccination, chances of animal infections by vaccinia virus in the future are unlikely. Swine pox should be clinically differentiated from other cutaneous infections (e.g., vesicular exanthema, vesicular stomatitis, foot and mouth disease, erysipelas), parasitic skin diseases, and allergic skin conditions.

Virions of typical poxvirus morphology can be detected under the electron microscope in negatively stained preparations or in ultrathin sections of cutaneous lesions. Swine poxvirus has a restricted host range; it affects swine only, can be isolated in cell cultures of swine origin only, and does not grow in embryonated eggs or other laboratory animals.

Swine poxvirus has an affinity for epidermal cells. Histopathologic examination of a cutaneous biopsy may be helpful in diagnosis. Swine poxvirus causes hydropic degeneration and hyperplasia of epidermal cells. Infected cells contain eosinophilic cytoplasmic inclusion bodies and nuclear vacuolation that is characteristic of swine poxvirus infection (Fig. 1B). Swine poxvirus–infected cells reveal cytoplasmic fluorescence when they are reacted with fluorescent antibody against swine poxvirus. Cloned genomic fragments of swine poxvirus, e.g., thymidine kinase gene, can be used as a diagnostic probe to detect specific viral DNA in the skin lesions.

Pigs recovered from swine poxvirus are refactory to challenge with swine poxvirus, which indicates development of active immunity.

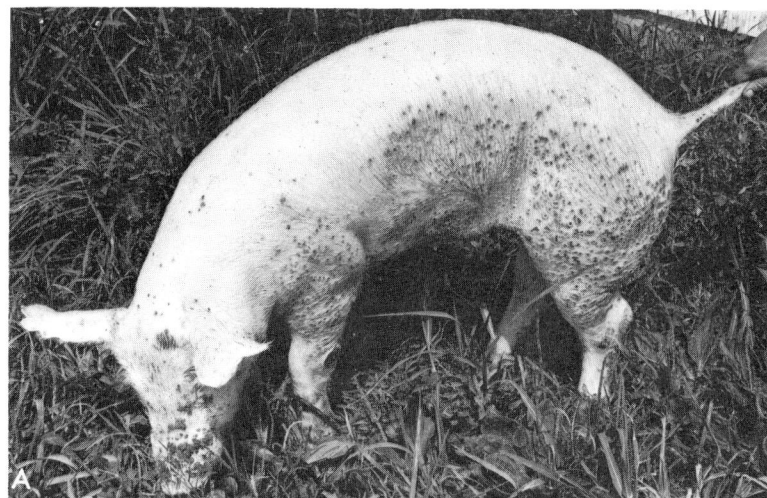
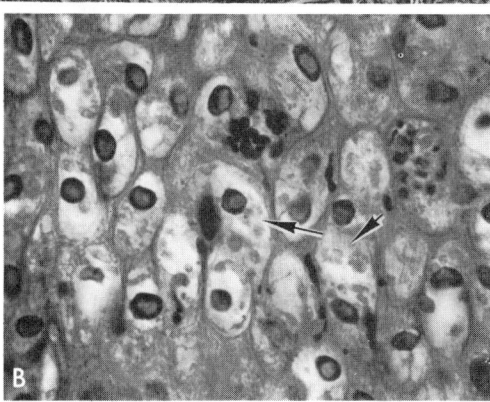

Figure 1. Swine pox. *A,* Cutaneous lesions in a pig 14 days after intravenous inoculation with swine poxvirus. (From Miller RB, Olsen LD: Am J Vet Res 41:341–347, 1980. Courtesy of the American Veterinary Medical Association.) *B,* Microscopic epidermal changes characterized by hydropic degeneration, cytoplasmic inclusions *(arrows),* and nuclear vacuolations. (Hematoxylin and eosin, × 450. Courtesy of Dr. Robert A. Crandell.)

TREATMENT

There is no specific therapy for swine pox. If the disease is associated with lice infestation, primary attempts should be aimed at the elimination of the lice. Insecticides are applied by dipping or spraying of animals or by dusting of the bedding. Only those insecticides should be used that are approved for use on swine to control lice.

BIBLIOGRAPHY

Kasza L: Swinepox. *In* Leman AD, Straw B, Glock RD, et al (eds): Diseases of Swine, 6th ed. Ames, Iowa State University Press, 1986, pp 315–320.
Neufeld JL: Spontaneous pustular dermatitis in a newborn piglet associated with a poxvirus. Can Vet J 22:156–158, 1981.
Schnitzlein WM, Tripathy DN: Identification and nucleotide sequence of the thymidine kinase gene of swinepox virus. Virology 181:727–732, 1991.
Tripathy DN, Hanson LE, Crandell RA: Poxviruses of veterinary importance: diagnosis of infections. *In* Kurstak E, Kurstak C (eds): Comparative Diagnosis of Viral Diseases, vol III. New York, Academic Press, 1981, pp 267–346.

Porcine Adenoviruses

DONALD MATTSON, DVM, PhD

There are 4 recognized types of porcine adenoviruses (PAV). However, additional isolates have been described that have been shown to vary antigenically from the prototype strains, so the number of officially recognized strains is expected to increase.

There have been no reports regarding the resistance of PAV to disinfectants. If PAV are like other members of the Adenoviridae family, they should be very resistant to most common disinfectants. One PAV isolate has been shown to withstand inactivation for 10 days or more at 25° C.

EPIZOOTIOLOGY

Porcine adenoviruses are widely distributed and appear to be present in most countries. There may be some regional predominance of individual types. Few serologic survey studies have been undertaken, and an accurate figure concerning prevalence of infection cannot be given. One study showed that the main period of infectivity in young pigs was immediately after weaning. PAVs replicate extensively in the nasal cavity, tonsils, and alimentary tract. The method of viral transmission is probably by direct contact. Chronic infection takes place in the intestinal tract and kidney. The role of virus shedding in the urine and transmission of infection has not been investigated.

CLINICAL SIGNS AND LESIONS

Infection is usually not associated with clinical signs of disease, and most investigators consider PAV to be of little pathogenic significance with the possible exception of PAV type 4.

Some PAVs have been recovered from neonatal pigs with diarrhea. Experimental infectivity studies with gnotobiotic pigs have usually failed to reproduce the disease. In 1 study in which enteritis was reproduced, the severity of disease was mild.

Some strains of PAV have been shown to have an affinity for the respiratory tract. In disease transmission studies, there was no clinical evidence of disease, and minimal lesions were observed in the lungs. A synergistic effect between PAV type 4 and *Mycoplasma hyopneumoniae* has been proposed.

PAV type 4 was originally isolated from a 10-week-old pig with encephalitis. Several investigators have attempted to transmit the disease in gnotobiotic colostrum-deprived pigs. The virus was shown to replicate extensively in the intestinal tract during the first week of infection, but neurologic signs did not develop. Histopathologic changes consistent with meningoencephalitis were produced 2 to 3 weeks after infection; a complex pathogenesis for central nervous system infection was proposed.

DIAGNOSIS

For viral isolation, samples should be taken from tissue or organs showing pathologic changes. In the early stages of the disease, virus-infected cells can be detected by the fluorescent antibody technique.

Paired serum samples should be submitted for serologic diagnosis. An agar-gel precipitation test has been used to detect antibody titer increase to the group-specific antigen. For type-specific testing, the serum-virus neutralization test must be used. Many diagnostic laboratories do not provide serologic or fluorescent antibody testing for PAV.

TREATMENT

There is no specific treatment for adenoviral infection.

PREVENTION AND CONTROL

There are no vaccines available for prevention of PAV infection.

BIBLIOGRAPHY

Coussement W, Ducatelle R, Charlier G, Hoorens J: Adenovirus enteritis in pigs. Am J Vet Res 42:1905–1911, 1981.
Sanford SE, Hoover DM: Enteric adenovirus infection in pigs. Can J Comp Med 47:396–400, 1983.

Porcine Parvovirus–Induced Reproductive Failure of Swine*

WILLIAM L. MENGELING, DVM, PhD

Porcine parvovirus (PPV)–induced reproductive failure is characterized by prenatal infections and death, usually without accompanying maternal clinical signs. Dams are most often exposed oronasally, and embryos and fetuses are subsequently

*All material in this article is in the public domain, with the exception of any borrowed figures or tables.

infected transplacentally. A venereal route of exposure is also possible because PPV has been isolated from boar semen. The virus is distributed among swine throughout the world, and all strains that have been compared are antigenically similar or identical. In the United States, PPV is ubiquitous and the disease is common. However, on the basis of an as yet unpublished study completed in 1989, it appears that the extensive use of vaccines during recent years has markedly reduced the incidence of the disease from that suggested by a similar study completed in 1978.

Reproductive failure is the probable consequence of exposure of nonimmune females to PPV any time during the first half (8 weeks) of gestation. Later exposure is often innocuous for fetuses because they may not be infected transplacentally for 2 or more weeks; and by 10 weeks of gestational age, fetuses are usually immunocompetent and relatively resistant. However, the effect of late fetal infection on neonatal survival has not been determined.

When an entire litter is infected at about the same time, the effects on both dam and litter can be considered according to the stage of gestation as follows.

1. Embryo (≤30 days): Embryos die and are resorbed, and the dam returns to estrus. Subsequent copulation and conception are followed by an uneventful pregnancy. However, on the basis of observations of naturally occurring cases, older embryos may not always be completely resorbed. The result is that females return to estrus and accept the boar but do not conceive. The latter possibility is speculative and has not been confirmed experimentally.

2. Early fetus (~30 days to ~70 days): Fetuses die and become relatively dehydrated (mummified). The dam does not return to estrus, and farrowing is often delayed. Many affected dams are marketed when they fail to farrow at the expected time, and they appear nonpregnant as a result of resorption of fetal and associated extrafetal fluids.

3. Late fetus (~70 days to term): Most infected fetuses survive in utero and produce antibody to PPV. Nevertheless, the virus persists, and it can be disseminated at farrowing in extrafetal fluids and by neonates.

When only part of a litter is infected transplacentally, then some or all littermates can be infected by intrauterine spread of virus. Because intrauterine spread is often relatively slow, particularly when fetuses are able to produce antibody, a litter may become infected progressively over almost the entire interval of gestation. Therefore, all of the effects on embryos and fetuses that were described in the preceding paragraph can be represented in a single litter. Additionally, 1 or more pigs of a litter may be stillborn when dead littermates cause a prolonged gestation or farrowing interval or both. Note, however, that in such cases, one would expect to find mummified fetuses as well as stillborn pigs.

CLINICAL SIGNS

Maternal infection is usually subclinical. A mild, transient fever and leukopenia have been shown under experimental conditions. The possibility of PPV-induced reproductive failure can be considered when an unusually large number of bred females return to estrus, fail to farrow despite being anestrous, farrow small litters, or farrow a large proportion of mummified fetuses. When maternal exposure is near midgestation, the abdominal girth of pregnant females will often decrease noticeably as fetuses die and associated fluids are resorbed. There is no evidence that abortion is a significant feature of the naturally occurring disease. The virus has not been associated unequivocally with any other disease syndrome, and boars seem clinically unaffected.

NECROPSY LESIONS

Most fetuses that die as a direct result of PPV infection are in an advanced stage of autolysis and mummification when they are farrowed. Consequently, a thorough necropsy examination is limited to the relatively few infected fetuses that die near term or are stillborn. Macroscopic lesions have not been reported for such fetuses, but microscopic lesions of meningoencephalitis have been suggested as pathognomonic for PPV infection. These lesions consist of perivascular cuffing with proliferating adventitial cells, histiocytes, and plasma cells in the leptomeninges and parenchymatous tissue of the brain, excluding the cerebellum.

DIAGNOSIS

A tentative diagnosis of PPV-induced reproductive failure is based on a high incidence of embryonic or fetal death or both, an absence of concurrent or previous maternal illness, and an absence or low incidence of abortion. Although numerous other agents have been associated with the same or a similar syndrome, recent studies suggest that PPV is the most common infectious cause.

For a confirmed diagnosis, tissue from affected fetuses must be submitted to a laboratory, where it can be tested for viral antigen, viral hemagglutinin, and infectious virus. The tissue of choice is lung collected from mummified fetuses. Tissues from live and stillborn pigs are much less suitable because they are more likely to either be noninfected or contain antibody that would interfere with testing. Several whole mummified fetuses or their lungs should be sent refrigerated or frozen to the laboratory. The fastest and most definitive diagnostic method is to examine cryostat-microtome sections of tissue by immunofluorescence microscopy. Viral antigen is extremely stable and remains reactive for months after fetal death. The usual finding is masses of viral antigen throughout the tissue. Tissue can also be triturated and tested for viral hemagglutinin or infectious virus or both. Infectivity is less stable than is either antigenicity or hemagglutinating activity, however, and isolation of virus from mummified tissues is sometimes unsuccessful.

Results of testing maternal sera for hemagglutination inhibiting antibody are significant when serum samples collected at about the time of farrowing are free of antibody—and thus preclude the involvement of PPV—and when 2 or more serum samples collected at different times during gestation reveal seroconversion. When infection is early in gestation and embryos are resorbed, maternal seroconversion is the only means by which a probable diagnosis can be made. Because PPV is ubiquitous, the presence of antibody in maternal serum collected only at about the time of farrowing is of no diagnostic significance.

Sera collected from neonates before they ingest colostrum can also be tested by hemagglutination inhibiting antibody, and often titers are as high as those of adults. Although the presence of antibody in serum of neonates of small litters or of litters with dead and mummified fetuses is reasonable evidence for a causal role for PPV, it obviously is less definitive than is demonstrating viral antigen in tissue of dead fetuses.

TREATMENT

There is no treatment.

PREVENTION

Porcine parvovirus–induced reproductive failure can be prevented by vaccination or by exposing females to virulent virus several weeks before breeding to establish immunity. Boars should also be immune so that the chance of their disseminating the virus by various routes, including semen, is minimized. Exposure to virulent virus can sometimes be accomplished by commingling gilts and boars with other swine that may be shedding PPV (e.g., older breeding stock) or by placing them in potentially contaminated quarters. However, neither procedure is dependable or selective. Vaccines are available commercially. To be effective, vaccines should be administered only after passively acquired (colostral) antibody has disappeared.

BIBLIOGRAPHY

Cartwright SF, Huck RA: Viruses isolated in association with herd infertility, abortions and stillbirths in pigs. Vet Rec 81:196–197, 1967.
Joo HS, Donaldson-Wood CR, Johnson RH: Observations on the pathogenesis of porcine parvovirus infection. Arch Virol 51:123–129, 1976.
Mengeling WL: Prevalence of porcine parvovirus-induced reproductive failure: an abattoir study. J Am Vet Med Assoc 172:1291–1294, 1978.
Mengeling WL, Cutlip RC, Wilson RA, et al: Fetal mummification associated with porcine parvovirus infection. J Am Vet Med Assoc 166:993–995, 1975.
Mengeling WL, Paul PS, Brown TT: Transplacental infection and embryonic death following maternal exposure to porcine parvovirus near the time of conception. Arch Virol 65:55–62, 1980.

Mystery Pig Disease*
WILLIAM L. MENGELING, DVM, PhD

Mystery pig disease (MPD) is the name most commonly used to refer to a reproductive syndrome of swine first recognized and described in Wabash County, Indiana, in 1989. It has since been reported in most of the major swine-producing areas of the United States and in several countries of Western Europe. The disease is characterized clinically by maternal signs of fever, anorexia, and minor respiratory distress followed by reproductive losses that include aborted, stillborn, and weak pigs and a higher than usual preweaning mortality. In addition, pigs affected before weaning sometimes develop severe dyspnea. Microscopic lesions in affected pigs include those of interstitial pneumonia, myocarditis, and encephalitis. During the course of some epizootics, there has been a temporal progression from aborted litters, to litters containing many stillborn pigs, to litters that appear normal at birth but have a poor rate of preweaning survival.

Most of the case histories and epizootiologic studies associated with MPD have been consistent with an infectious etiologic agent. However, identity of the putative agent remained highly controversial until scientists at the Central Veterinary Institute in Lelystad, the Netherlands, reported their isolation of a virus from affected pigs and experimental reproduction of the disease. They suggested that because the cause of the disease is no longer a mystery, it might be more appropriately named porcine epidemic abortion and respiratory syndrome (PEARS). On the basis of recent serologic and virologic studies in the United States, it now appears that the same virus, or a virus very similar to the Lelystad virus, is the cause of MPD in this country. Confirmation of this likelihood awaits further characterization of the virus and the disease.

---

*All material in this article is in the public domain, with the exception of any borrowed figures or tables.

African Swine Fever

H. A. McDANIEL, DVM, PhD

African swine fever (ASF) is a highly contagious viral disease that affects only swine. Acute, subacute, chronic, and inapparent forms occur in domestic swine, and an inapparent form occurs in truly wild swine such as wart hogs, bush pigs, and giant forest hogs.

ETIOLOGY

ASF is caused by a relatively large DNA virus that is resistant to some of the traditional disinfectants and environmental conditions that inactivate many other viruses. This virus may remain viable in soil, blood, bone marrow, or pork at room temperature for several months.

There are 4 types and numerous strains of ASF virus. Recovered pigs usually resist challenge with homologous strains of virus but appear to be fully susceptible to heterologous strains. Antibodies often reach a very high titer in recovered pigs, but classic virus neutralizing antibodies have not been demonstrated.

Two commercially available disinfectants that have been found to be effective against ASF virus are One-Stroke-Environ* and Vanodyne-FAM.† Both products are also sold under other trade names.

EPIZOOTIOLOGY

The first reports of ASF were from East Africa in 1909. Outbreaks have occurred in several European countries, the Dominican Republic, Haiti, Cuba, and Brazil. It remains enzootic only in Africa, the western portion of Spain, Portugal, and Sardinia.

In 1971, ASF first occurred in the Western Hemisphere in Cuba. A stamping out program was quickly implemented. Within a few months, over 400,000 swine died or were slaughtered because they were considered to be infected or exposed. No more cases occurred in Cuba during this outbreak.

In 1978, ASF was found in 4 widely separated areas: Sardinia, Malta, the Dominican Republic, and Brazil. During the previous year, a marked increase in the incidence of ASF occurred in Spain and Portugal, and this may have been the source of virus for the new outbreaks found in 1978. From the Dominican Republic, it spread to Haiti and finally in 1980 to Cuba before the outbreak was finally stamped out. There is no reason to believe the ASF found in Cuba in 1980 was due to virus that remained from the 1971 outbreak.

There is much still to be learned about ASF before an adequate explanation can be provided for the cyclic nature of the incidence in enzootic areas and the factors that cause this disease to change from being highly lethal for most pigs that become infected during the first few months of an outbreak to a chronic or inapparent form after the disease has been present in the area a year or more.

TRANSMISSION

Transmission is by direct or indirect contact. Soft ticks, *Ornithodoros moubata* and *O. erraticus*, serve as biologic reservoirs and vectors of ASF virus in Africa and on the Iberian Peninsula.

O. puertoricensis and *O. turicata* found on several Caribbean islands and in Florida, respectively, have been shown experimentally to be capable of transmitting ASF virus in a biologically secure laboratory. However, similar ticks collected in the Dominican Republic and Haiti were thoroughly examined and found not to contain ASF virus. During the repopulation of large areas where ASF had been prevalent 1 or 2 years earlier, there was no recurrence of this disease when noninfected pigs were brought onto the farm.

CLINICAL SIGNS AND LESIONS

The first signs of ASF are often depression and fever, but 1 or 2 pigs may be found dead without apparent prior illness. In totally white pigs, the most obvious change is often red to reddish-blue hyperemia and congestion of the skin over the snout, ears, and fetlock, under the belly, up the sides, and over the hindquarters. However, this discoloration is not usually apparent on swine with pigmented skin. The skin of yellow, almost white, or white spotted hogs usually remains normal in color. As soon as illness becomes apparent, ASF-infected pigs will usually become febrile and have a body temperature of 41° to 42° C. Fever is an important differential diagnostic criterion and will indicate the illness or sudden death is not due to poisoning, as is often suspected by the owner. Pigs with ASF do not usually huddle together as tightly as those with hog cholera do (Fig. 1).

Pregnant animals often abort soon after the onset of illness regardless of the stage of pregnancy. Sows that abort often die in 3 to 6 days. Petechia and ecchymotic hemorrhage may be found on the fetal membranes or skin of aborted fetuses.

Infected swine usually continue to eat and drink until near death. They are more alert than might be expected with fever and such a high body temperature. Incoordination, trembling convulsions, and muscular twitching are not usually seen, and when present, they are not as marked as in hog cholera. However, coughing and dyspnea are more severe than in uncomplicated hog cholera. Diarrhea is seldom seen in uncomplicated ASF.

Ascites may be the first abnormality seen when the carcass is opened. Excessive straw-colored or blood-tinged fluid may be found in the pleural or peritoneal cavities and pericardial sac. If ascites has been present long enough for fibrin to have formed and fluids to have been reabsorbed, fibrin tags may be present on any internal organ surface similar to the fibrin deposits seen in mycoplasmal and certain bacterial infections.

The vascular system is severely damaged. Impaired blood coagulation, thrombocytopenia, and probably other tissue damages allow edema and hemorrhage to be found in any tissue. Hemorrhage is more often seen in visceral organs, especially lymph nodes, lungs, heart, and kidneys; on the serosal surface of intestine and diaphragm; and on the serosal and mucosal surface of the stomach. The hemorrhage is usually petechia but also often ecchymotic.

The spleen may be normal, but in about 50 per cent of affected animals, it will be swollen to 2 or 3 times the normal size, very friable with the splenic pulp having the consistency of currant jelly. Occasionally it will be normal in size but with infarcts indistinguishable from those seen in hog cholera.

The liver is usually swollen, congested, and dark red or clay-colored. The surface may have a fine granular or slightly rough appearance due to the parenchymatous tissue swelling more than the interlobular connective tissue. Occasionally, well-demarcated focal blotchy areas will be seen on the surface

---

*Vestal Laboratories, St. Louis, MO 63166.
†Vanodyne International Ltd., Eccles, Manchester, England; and Pfizer International, New York, NY 10017.

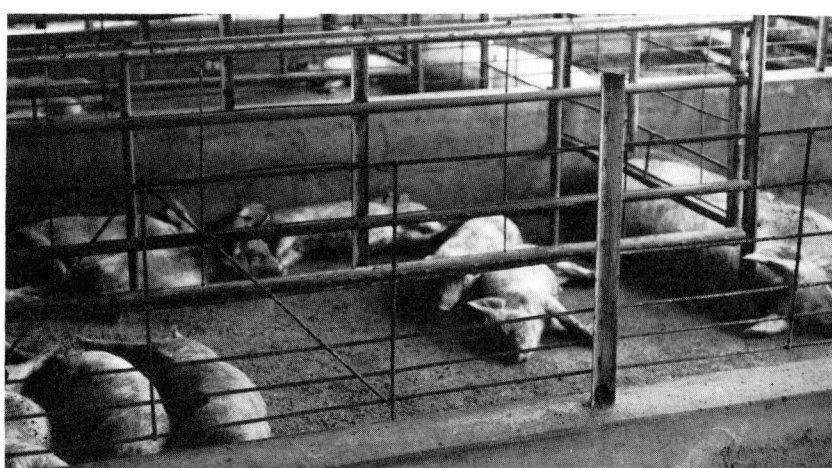

Figure 1. Swine infected with ASF in Dominican Republic. Note that they do not pile together as in hog cholera.

and extending into the parenchyma. They may be lighter or darker than the surrounding liver tissue.

The gallbladder is often edematous and may be over 0.5 cm thick and opaque. The blood vessels are often so engorged they appear to be ready to rupture. The bile may contain sufficient blood to cause coagulation of the blood-bile mixture, and fibrin from the clot may be adhered to the mucosa of the gallbladder.

Lymph nodes throughout the body are usually edematous and hemorrhagic. The hemorrhage may be subcapsular as in hog cholera or diffuse. When lymph node hemorrhage is diffuse and extensive, the nodes have the appearance of a shiny blood clot and are 2 to 4 times larger than normal. The gastrohepatic and renal nodes are the ones most frequently and most severely affected. Usually the lymph nodes in the pleural and peritoneal cavities are more hemorrhagic and swollen than are the body nodes, but those in the head and neck region may also be severely affected.

In a small percentage of infected pigs, the mucosa of the stomach, especially the fundic portion, will appear bright blood-red. Close examination will reveal that the mucosa is coated with a mixture of mucus and blood. Free blood in the stomach or intestine is rarely seen.

Peyer's patches throughout the small intestine may be edematous and occasionally necrotic. The intestinal contents are usually normal, but when bloody dysentery occurs, the colon will usually contain large amounts of blood.

Tonsillar abscesses and button ulcers near the cecal orifice are usually absent. Petechiae on the epiglottis and mucosa of the urinary bladder are not seen as frequently as in hog cholera.

Kidney involvement is variable, even within the same herd. In approximately 10 per cent of pigs dying of ASF, the kidney will appear normal, and in about 20 per cent, the kidney will be extensively hemorrhagic (Fig. 2). In these pigs, the kidneys appear to be contained within a transparent sac filled with clotted blood. Apparently, when hemorrhage is extensive within the kidney, blood seeps through the renal capsule, forming a clot 6 to 7 mm thick around the kidney. In these cases, free blood will usually be found in the pelvis, and the cortex will be severely congested and hemorrhagic (Fig. 3). In other cases, only a few petechiae will be seen on the surface as is typically seen in pigs with hog cholera.

The lungs are usually severely affected. Petechiae and ecchymotic hemorrhage are often present on the surface and throughout the lungs. Pulmonary edema may be especially prominent in the interlobular connective tissue of the anterior dorsal quarter of the lung. There may be so much blood in the edematous fluids that the cut surface of the lung resembles severely congested liver.

PREVENTION AND TREATMENT

There is no effective therapy. A satisfactory vaccine has not been developed, and there is little hope of one in the near

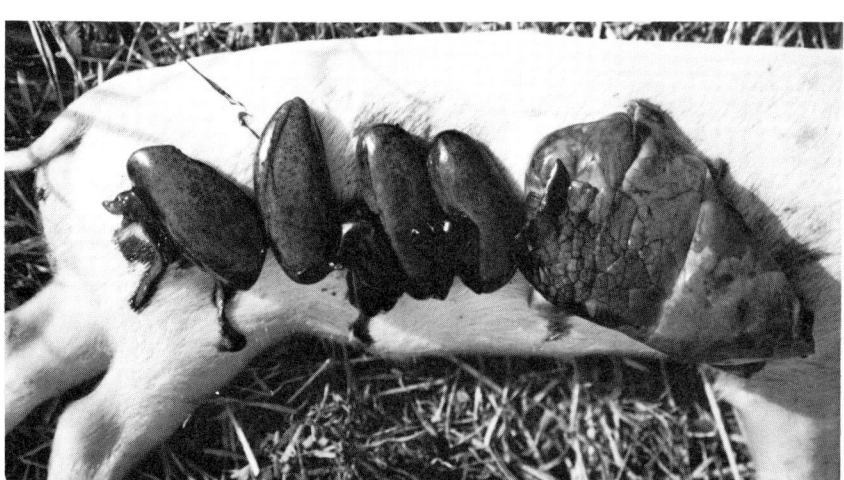

Figure 2. Kidneys and lungs from swine dying from ASF. Note the petechial and ecchymotic hemorrhage on the surface of the kidneys and the clotted blood adhering to the reflected renal capsules. In the lung, marked interlobular edema and hemorrhage are present in the dorsal anterior part of the lung, and pale blotchy areas can be seen on the surface of the diaphragmatic lobe.

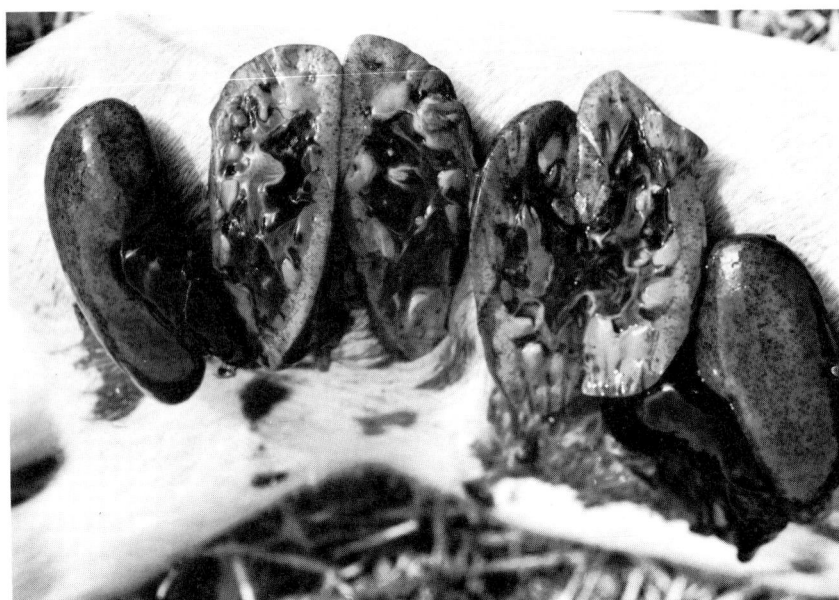

Figure 3. These are the same kidneys illustrated in Figure 2. Two have been opened to illustrate hemorrhage on the cut surface and clotted blood in the pelvis.

future because ASF antibodies are not of the typical virus neutralizing type. Many recovered swine remain carriers of ASF virus for prolonged periods and probably as long as they live. Recovered pigs may appear perfectly normal and resume normal gains or they may be unthrifty and runty with chronic pneumonia, arthritis, nephritis, and ulcerative and necrotic dermatitis.

CONTROL

Destruction of all infected and exposed swine, together with sound sanitary practices, has been effective in rapidly eradicating ASF outbreaks from several countries in Europe and the Western Hemisphere. Countries free of this disease should not allow the entry of pigs or garbage containing fresh pork scraps that originate from areas where ASF is enzootic. This includes all countries of Africa, Portugal, the western part of Spain, and Sardinia.

Early diagnosis of new ASF outbreaks is critical for stopping the spread and holding losses to a minimum. ASF should be considered during all field and laboratory diagnostic examination of sick swine. The acute form with the typical signs and lesions is almost always prevalent during the first few months of a new outbreak in previously free areas.

Quarantines applied to areas where new outbreaks are occurring plus a surrounding buffer zone are usually effective for reducing spread. This prevents swine free of ASF from being directly or indirectly exposed to infected swine. Pigs in the incubation period of ASF are extremely hazardous. Veterinarians, feedmen, and other service personnel who might visit infected farms must be extremely careful to avoid further transmission of this disease.

The first pigs that become ill in new ASF outbreaks have been erroneously diagnosed as having hog cholera. Massive hog cholera vaccination campaigns were totally ineffective, and epidemiologic studies indicate they actually contributed to further spread.

Spread of ASF to distant locations such as free countries or areas has most often occurred as a result of feeding uncooked pork scraps contained in garbage from enzootic areas. Garbage from international carriers such as airlines and ships is especially hazardous.

Government officials responsible for animal health should be immediately notified when ASF is suspected or when any unfamiliar disease of swine is encountered. They must quickly take appropriate measures to confirm the diagnosis, to institute quarantines, and to eliminate infected and exposed pigs plus other reservoirs of the virus.

BIBLIOGRAPHY

Edwards JF, Dodds WJ, Slauson DO: Coagulation changes in African swine fever virus infection. Am J Vet Res 45:2414–2420, 1984.
Hamdy FM, Dardiri AH: Clinical and immunologic responses of pigs to African swine fever virus isolated from the Western Hemisphere. Am J Vet Res 45:711–714, 1984.
Hess WR: African swine fever. In Foreign Animal Diseases: Their Prevention, Diagnosis and Control. Richmond, VA, Committee on Foreign Animal Diseases of The United States Animal Health Association, 1985.
McDaniel HA: African swine fever. In Diseases of Swine, 6th ed. Ames, IA, Iowa State University Press, 1986, pp 300–309.
Mebus CA, Dardari AH: Additional characterization of disease caused by African swine fever virus isolated from Brazil and the Dominican Republic. Proceedings, 83rd Annual Meeting of USAHA, 1979, pp 227–239.
Schlafer DH, McVicar JW, Mebus CA: African swine fever convalescent sows: subsequent pregnancy and the effect of colostral antibody on challenge inoculation of their pigs. Am J Vet Res 45:1361–1366, 1984.
Schlafer DH, Mebus CA, McVicar JW: African swine fever in neonatal pigs: passively acquired protection from colostrum or serum of recovered pigs. Am J Vet Res 45:1367–1372, 1984.

Calicivirus (Vesicular Exanthema of Swine Virus)
ALVIN W. SMITH, DVM, PhD

Vesicular exanthema of swine virus (VESV) belongs to the family Caliciviridae, of which VESV-A_{48} (isolated in California from pigs with vesicular exanthema in 1948) is the prototype species. Caliciviruses are single-stranded RNA viruses about 34 to 36 nm in diameter. They are lipid solvent–resistant but are unstable at pH 3 and at 50° C. Divalent cations (Mg^{2+}) further degrade them in the presence of heat. They can survive for long periods at 4° C and will survive for 14 days in 15° C sea water. Although they are deactivated by a variety of antiseptics, 2 per cent lye has been the disinfectant of choice.

There were 13 known serotypes of VESV isolated from swine between 1934 and 1956. Since that time, there have been 20 more serotypes of caliciviruses indistinguishable from VESV isolated from marine mammals, marine fish, and other sources. Ten of these that have been tested do infect swine, and some are more virulent for swine than are many of the original 13 VESV types. Other caliciviruses have been isolated from mink, dogs, reptiles, chimpanzees, and calves. Of these, only the calf isolate has been tested in swine, and it does produce clinical vesicular lesions in experimentally inoculated swine. There are now a total of 32 known serotypes of calicivirus worldwide, including the single serotype infecting cats. Of these, only the feline type is known not to infect swine.

EPIZOOTIOLOGY

Vesicular exanthema was said to be a new disease of pigs after its first documented appearance in 1932 in Orange County, California. That outbreak was treated as foot-and-mouth disease and eradicated; however, the disease reappeared on an annual basis through 1936. Each outbreak was controlled, and no more occurrences were reported between 1936 and 1939. From 1939 until it was eradicated in the mid-1950s, the disease was endemic in California. In 1952, VES escaped California and spread throughout all the major swine-producing areas of the United States. The last outbreak occurred in 1956. The disease was declared eradicated and was classed as a foreign animal disease in 1959. Vesicular exanthema has never been reported outside the continental United States except for single occurrences in Hawaii and Iceland, which were each traceable to shipments of pork from the United States.

Before 1972, swine were the only known naturally occurring hosts for VESV. Now the more recent calicivirus isolates of marine origin can in some cases be shown to be antigenically closer to the VES viruses than some of the VES virus serotypes are to each other. This finding, plus the reports that caliciviruses from seals and fish will infect swine and the discovery that many unrelated species of feral mammals along the coastal zones have type-specific antibodies to both the recent isolates of marine origin and the original virus types isolated from swine, leaves little doubt that these agents have broad host spectrums. In 1 series of studies, 1 calicivirus serotype was shown to infect fish, seals, swine, and monkeys.

The original outbreaks of disease were associated with feeding raw garbage, and it is now widely accepted that the virus-contaminated components in the garbage were marine products. Both marine mammals and fish are proven reservoirs for a calicivirus that causes typical vesicular lesions in experimentally exposed swine. In addition, the infection will spread horizontally and cause vesicular lesions in pen contact swine.

Although VESV has been reported only in the United States, marine mammals carrying caliciviruses infectious for swine are known to migrate along the Mexican, United States, Canadian, Alaskan, and Russian coasts. Northern fur seals harvested in Russia have type-specific antibodies for certain of these viruses. There has been no report of these agents in marine species outside the Pacific Basin and the Bering and Chukchi Seas.

CLINICAL SIGNS AND LESIONS

Vesicular exanthema of swine is indistinguishable clinically from foot-and-mouth disease, vesicular stomatitis, and swine vesicular disease. Vesicular lesions will be seen around the coronary bands of the feet and on the snout and oral tissues. Swine will show lameness with reluctance to move and will not maintain a full level of food intake. In addition to these manifestations that occur as a result of the vesicular lesions, agalactia, abortion, myocarditis, and mild encephalitis have been reported. Consequently, runting and unthriftiness are common sequelae, even though the epidermal lesions usually heal rather quickly. Morbidity is variable but can approach 100 per cent; however, mortality is low. In the past, VESV has been most often introduced into swine herds by feeding raw contaminated garbage, but infected pigs shedding virus in their body excretions can spread the disease.

DIAGNOSIS

Diagnosis is on the basis of virus isolation and serologic testing. Epithelial coverings of lesions and vesicular fluid frozen or placed in buffered glycerol are the laboratory samples of choice. Acute and convalescent sera are useful. Virus isolation can be accomplished in vero cells or pig kidney cells. Direct electron microscopic examination could be rapid and useful in differentiating this virus from those causing foot-and-mouth disease, vesicular stomatitis, and swine vesicular disease. Serum neutralization tests are necessary to identify VESV serotypes; however, complement fixation has been used for group testing, and monoclonal antibody techniques are now being developed for screening tests.

TREATMENT

Treatment should be directed toward the relief of signs and prevention of secondary infection. There are no specific chemotherapeutic agents for calicivirus infections. Should secondary infections become severe, administration of parenteral antibiotics could be indicated.

PREVENTION AND CONTROL

Vesicular exanthema of swine is classed as a foreign animal disease. Prompt reporting of all vesicular disease outbreaks is essential. Should VES be diagnosed, eradication procedures, which include slaughter, quarantine of premises, and restricted animal movements, are mandated. Recent findings confirm that these viruses are not host-specific, and they may infect a variety of species. Additional strong evidence suggests that humans may also become infected, and this should call for strong safeguards to minimize human exposure to infected materials and animals. These newly emerging concepts on the biology of caliciviruses suggest that their character is rapidly changing. As more new host species emerge and additional overviews of transmission develop, the probabilities increase that this virus could once again be introduced into domestic swine populations.

BIBLIOGRAPHY

Bankowski RA: Vesicular exanthema. Adv Vet Sci 10:23–64, 1965.
Smith AW: Focus on caliciviral disease. Foreign Animal Disease Report, USDA–APHIS 11-3:8–16, 1983.
Smith AW, Akers TG: Vesicular exanthema of swine. J Am Vet Med Assoc 169:700–703, 1976.
Smith AW, Boyt PM: Caliciviruses of ocean origin. J Zoo Wildl Med 21:3–23, 1990.

Enteroviral Encephalomyelitis of Pigs (Teschen Disease)

TALMAGE T. BROWN, JR., DVM, PHD

Enteroviral encephalomyelitis was originally described in 1929 as a severe, devastating neurologic disease of pigs in the Teschen district of Czechoslovakia. During World War II, Teschen disease spread in Eastern and central Europe and later was reported in the island republic of Madagascar, located off the southeast coast of Africa. With one possible exception, Teschen disease has not been reported in Western Europe since 1980. In 1984, an outbreak of polioencephalomyelitis, caused by a serotype 2 porcine enterovirus and clinically similar to Teschen disease, was reported in a herd of fattening pigs in West Germany. Teschen disease continues to be a clinically important disease in Madagascar and a less common but threatening disease in the Ukraine. Disease control by vaccination is practiced in these 2 areas. A milder form of enteroviral encephalomyelitis, most commonly referred to as Talfan disease but also called poliomyelitis suum, benign epizootic paresis, and polioencephalomyelitis, has been reported in Europe, North America, South America, and Australia. The milder disease occurs sporadically and, when recognized, is viewed more as a nuisance than as a serious disease problem. Teschen/Talfan disease has not been recognized in China or Taiwan. Viruses antigenically related to Teschen disease virus have been isolated in Japan from nondiseased pigs, but clinical disease has not been observed. Serologic evidence suggests that subclinical infections of swine with strains of porcine enterovirus, indistinguishable from those that cause Teschen/Talfan disease, are common in some parts of Europe.

ETIOLOGY

Porcine enteroviruses are subdivided into 11 serogroups with strains of serotype 1 being the most common cause of Teschen or Talfan disease. Serotypes 2, 3, and 5 may also cause neurologic disease, although usually of milder degree. Other diseases associated with porcine enterovirus infection include diarrhea, pneumonia, myocarditis, and reproductive failure.

The small, RNA-containing, nonenveloped enteroviruses are resistant to many chemicals and are capable of surviving in the environment for many months. Sodium hypochlorite, caustic soda, and 70 per cent alcohol are the most effective chemicals for inactivating enteroviruses. Because of the highly resistant nature of enteroviruses, they are often difficult to eliminate from contaminated premises, which probably contributes to continual enteroviral infections in some swine herds. Transmission can occur directly by the fecal-oral route, indirectly by housing susceptible pigs in contaminated premises, or by feeding uncooked contaminated pork products.

EPIZOOTIOLOGY

Even though most porcine enterovirus infections are subclinical, infections by virulent strains of serotype 1 may cause neurologic disease that involves up to 50 per cent of a herd. High morbidity usually occurs in herds infected for the first time, especially if there are a large number of young, susceptible pigs in the herd. Swine of all ages are susceptible to enterovirus infection when a herd is first infected, but once infection is established, clinical disease is usually limited to pigs less than 12 weeks of age. Pigs infected with virulent enterovirus, at less than 2 weeks of age, are the most severely affected. Typically, clinical disease is not seen in all litters of a herd, and of the litters affected, often less than half of the pigs will become clinically ill. In small to moderate-sized herds (50 to 150 animals), clinical disease may continue to appear for several months and then disappear unless susceptible animals are brought into the herd. In large herds of 400 to 500 or more animals, disease may persist with a few clinical cases appearing each year. Herd mortality depends on the virulence of the infecting strain of enterovirus and previous herd experience with enterovirus infections. Susceptible herds infected with a highly virulent neurogenic strain of enterovirus may have death losses approaching 100 per cent. More commonly, clinical disease is mild to moderate, and death losses are few to absent.

CLINICAL SIGNS AND LESIONS

Pigs infected with a virulent strain of enterovirus may show general signs of illness, including anorexia, lethargy, and fever (40° to 41° C) before the onset of neurologic signs, or remain bright and alert with good appetites and normal temperatures. Signs of illness usually appear 14 to 21 days after exposure to enterovirus, often simultaneously in a number of pigs in the same litter or in different litters. Some degree of rear limb ataxia and weakness are typically the first signs of neurologic disease and are usually seen in pigs over 2 weeks and less than 12 weeks of age. During the early stages of disease, affected pigs may huddle or respond to noise, touch, or sudden movement by developing generalized muscle tremors, tonic-clonic muscle spasms in the rear legs, or convulsive seizures. Paresis may worsen for 2 to 3 days, extending from the rear to the front legs, and then gradually improve with recovery in 1 or 2 weeks. Occasionally, recovery may take 3 or more weeks or be incomplete with some muscle wasting and residual paralysis. Infection by a highly virulent, neurogenic strain may result in paresis, paralysis, recumbency, and death, usually by the third or fourth day and nearly always within 2 weeks.

Significant gross lesions are not seen at necropsy. Specific microscopic lesions are limited to the central nervous system; there is nonsuppurative inflammation focused primarily on the gray matter of the brain stem, cerebellum, and spinal cord that is characterized by neuronal necrosis, neuronophagia, glia nodules, and perivascular lymphocytic cuffs.

DIAGNOSIS

Enteroviral encephalomyelitis must be differentiated from a variety of neurologic disorders affecting swine, including pseudorabies, hog cholera, African swine fever, rabies, edema disease, and salt poisoning. The clinical signs of these disorders overlap; therefore diagnosis should be based on a complete history, observation of the full spectrum of symptoms, postmortem examination of affected animals, and, if possible, isolation and identification of the causative agent. Neurologic signs suggesting spinal cord injury are more suggestive of enteroviral infection than are signs of cerebral dysfunction such as blindness, aimless walking, or convulsions. Tissues for virus isolation should be collected fresh and submitted immediately to an appropriate diagnostic laboratory. If immediate submission is not possible, fresh tissues should be refrigerated (4° C) for submission later. Paired serum samples, taken at least 14 days apart, may be of value in, retrospectively, establishing the cause of the disease.

TREATMENT AND PREVENTION

There is no treatment for enteroviral encephalomyelitis, but supportive therapy for prevention of secondary infections may be considered if the value of the animal warrants it.

Vaccination is practiced in those areas where Teschen disease is a substantial problem and vaccination is economically feasible. Both inactivated and attenuated live virus vaccines have been used effectively. If a virulent strain of enterovirus is introduced into a herd, sick pigs should be isolated from clinically normal animals, especially those 12 weeks old or younger. If it is economically feasible, sick pigs should be removed from the herd. In endemic areas, new breeding stock should be introduced into the herd long enough before breeding so that ample opportunity is given for exposure to and infection with indigenous agents, thereby enhancing the chances of colostral antibody protection of the offspring. Depopulation of infected herds and repopulation with specific pathogen-free stock has not been an effective approach to eliminating porcine enteroviruses because of the highly resistant nature of enteroviruses. Spread of Teschen disease has been effectively controlled by restrictions on the importations of swine and pork products from countries in which Teschen disease is endemic.

BIBLIOGRAPHY

Derbyshire JB: Porcine enterovirus (polioencephalomyelitis). *In* Pensaert MB (ed): Virus infections of Porcines. Amsterdam, Elsevier Science Publishers BV, 1989, pp 225–233.
Kaplan MM, Meranze DR: Porcine virus encephalomyelitis and its possible biological relationship to human poliomyelitis. Vet Med 43:330–341, 1948.
Mills JHL, Nielsen SW: Porcine polioencephalomyelitides. Adv Vet Sci 12:33–104, 1968.

Swine Vesicular Disease

ALVIN W. SMITH, DVM, PhD

Swine vesicular disease (SVD) is classed as a foreign animal disease, and the causal agent is one of the picornaviruses (small RNA viruses) grouped as an enterovirus. It has icosahedral symmetry and appears generally round with a diameter of 28 nm. SVD virus is serologically and biologically closely related to the human enterovirus coxsackie B-5 but not other porcine enteroviruses. However, there are strain differences between isolates of SVD virus. It is stable for many months in the environment and has been isolated from earthworms collected above the infected carcasses of buried pigs. Restocking of premises after depopulation has been difficult because of viral persistence in the environment. Hams taken from infected pigs and processed in the Parma tradition have been shown to consistently harbor viable virus for 6 months but not 1 year after slaughter. Salami and pepperoni containing dried contaminated pork retained residual infective virus for at least 200 days. The virus is acid-resistant and heat-stabilized in the presence of divalent cations (50° C and 1 M Mg^{2+}).

EPIZOOTIOLOGY

Swine and humans are the only known hosts to be naturally infected. Newborn mice are susceptible by intracerebral and intraperitoneal inoculations but become refractory to infection by 7 days of age. SVD is a new disease of pigs that was first recognized in 1966 in Lombardy, Italy, and initially was indistinguishable from foot-and-mouth disease. In 1971, the disease was diagnosed in Hong Kong, then the following year in Staffordshire, England. By 1974, SVD had been discovered in France, Poland, Austria, Germany, Switzerland, Japan, and Taiwan. Indirect evidence suggests that the People's Republic of China has also experienced occurrences of SVD. At this time, it should be considered endemic in parts of Asia and Europe. Efforts in England to eradicate the disease appear to have succeeded.

The international spread of SVD virus has occurred primarily by the trans-shipment of exposed pigs and infected pork products. Once SVD becomes established, direct contact with infected swine, contaminated garbage, swine-holding facilities, or swine-handling equipment appears to be the major source of continuing exposure. There are no known reservoirs in nature other than swine. Although humans are susceptible to SVD viral infection and this agent may have arisen as a variant of a human coxsackievirus, there is no evidence of a human reservoir for SVD.

CLINICAL SIGNS AND LESIONS

The incubation period for SVD is 2 to 6 days, and seroconversion can be shown by day 4. Clinically the disease is indistinguishable from foot-and-mouth disease, vesicular stomatitis, and vesicular exanthema of swine. Lameness of sudden onset is usually the first sign and is more obvious in larger and heavier animals. Temperatures may be elevated 2° to 4° C, and there is a reluctance to eat. Vesicles appear on the coronary band, dew claws, interdigital space, and heel of the foot. In natural infections, the snout, tongue, and lips are more frequently involved, and fluid-filled vesicles, tags of epidermis, or erosions will be seen. Lesions other than vesicles on epithelial surfaces have not been described grossly. Recovery is usually rapid, and barring secondary involvement, swine will usually return to normal within 3 weeks. Morbidity is high and mortality is low, except in newborn pigs, in which mortality is also high.

DIAGNOSIS

Although the condition cannot be clinically differentiated from foot-and-mouth disease, vesicular exanthema of swine, or vesicular stomatitis, the presence of lesions in contact cattle would tend to eliminate SVD, and the absence of lesions in exposed cattle would suggest SVD. Laboratory diagnosis is essential, and both lesion material and serum should be submitted. The epithelial coverings of the vesicles and vesicular fluid are samples of choice. These should be placed in buffered glycerol or frozen for shipment. Virus isolation, complement fixation, and virus neutralization are the tests of choice. Direct electron microscopic examination may easily differentiate this virus from the bullet-shaped virus of vesicular stomatitis or the typical caliciviruses of vesicular exanthema of swine but not the enterovirus of foot-and-mouth disease. Immunoelectron microscopy should rapidly differentiate SVD and foot-and-mouth disease viruses if adequate quantities of antigen are available from processed laboratory specimens. An enzyme-linked immunosorbent assay (ELISA) test has been developed for detection and quantification of SVD antibodies.

TREATMENT

Specific therapy is not available; however, the disease is self-limiting, and recovery is usually complete within 3 weeks, except for newborn pigs. Symptomatic treatment and good sanitation for reducing secondary infections are useful. If secondary infection does occur, parenteral antimicrobials may be useful.

PREVENTION AND CONTROL

This is a foreign animal disease that has not been reported in the United States. All outbreaks of vesicular disease should be reported immediately to a regulatory veterinarian. If a diagnosed outbreak of SVD does occur, eradication measures would be instituted and would include slaughter of infected animals, quarantine of infected premises, and restriction of swine movements. Because of the resistance of this agent to environmental effects and to many of the accepted food processing procedures, the threat of this disease being introduced into the United States is very real.

BIBLIOGRAPHY

Armstrong RM, Barnett IT: An enzyme-linked immunosorbent assay (ELISA) against swine vesicular disease virus (SVDV). J Virol Methods 25:71–80, 1989.

Callis JJ, Dardiri AH, Ferris DH, et al: Illustrated Manual for the Recognition and Diagnosis of Certain Animal Diseases. Mexico–United States Commission for the Prevention of Foot and Mouth Disease. Plum Island Animal Disease Center, 1982, pp 19–21.

Graves JH, McKercher PD: Swine vesicular disease. Proceedings, 77th Annual Meeting, U.S. Animal Health Association, 1973, pp 155–159.

Encephalitis–Vomiting and Wasting Disease Complex of Swine*

WILLIAM L. MENGELING, DVM, PhD

The term "encephalitis–vomiting and wasting disease complex" is used to encompass the variety of clinical manifestations of infection of swine with a neurotropic porcine coronavirus. The virus is named hemagglutinating encephalomyelitis virus (HEV) in reference to its ability to agglutinate erythrocytes of several species of animals and to its neuropathogenicity.

There are 2 primary clinical forms of the disease complex. One form is peracute to acute. It is characterized clinically by nervous signs and histopathologically by lesions of nonsuppurative encephalomyelitis. This form does not have a specific name, but it is probably the same as a condition first reported in Canada in 1959 and referred to as Ontario encephalomyelitis. The second primary form of the disease complex is subacute to chronic. It is characterized clinically by vomition and progressive emaciation and is called vomiting and wasting disease (VWD). Lesions of mild nonsuppurative encephalomyelitis have been found in pigs killed early in the course of VWD. Some European scientists have referred to isolates from pigs affected with VWD as VWD virus, but there is no evidence that such isolates differ from HEV either structurally or antigenically.

EPIZOOTIOLOGY AND PATHOGENESIS

Infection with HEV is common, particularly in areas of concentrated swine production. Conversely, clinical disease is rare and confined almost exclusively to pigs within their first few weeks of life. Although epizootiology and pathogenesis have not been completely defined, the following events seem most probable on the basis of information currently available. Virus is disseminated through aerosols and by direct contact of infected and noninfected pigs. In most pigs, infection is subclinical and limited mainly to the initial sites of viral replication in the upper respiratory tract and tonsil. Occasionally, virus invades the central nervous system by extension through peripheral nerves to cause disease. The extent of central nervous system damage apparently determines the type and severity of clinical signs. In at least some cases, HEV can also infect neurons of the digestive tract.

CLINICAL SIGNS

Under experimental conditions, clinical signs appear 4 to 8 days after oronasal exposure. A somewhat shorter incubation for some naturally occurring cases is suggested by case histories. Although signs are variable, they can be grouped according to the 2 main forms of clinical illness. Signs of the peracute to acute form are hyperesthesia, muscle tremors, incoordination, collapse, nystagmus, and paddling movements. Many affected pigs also vomit. Some pigs die within 24 hours after the initial appearance of signs. Signs of the subacute to chronic form are vomition and either progressive emaciation or failure to gain weight at a normal rate. Inappetence and listlessness are common to both forms, and occasionally these are the only signs that are observed. In such cases, pigs may recover completely. Sometimes there are marked differences in the susceptibility of pigs even within the same litter. Although morbidity and mortality are variable, they may reach 100 per cent of the baby pigs in some herds.

NECROPSY LESIONS

There are no consistent macroscopic lesions of pigs infected with HEV. In pigs affected with VWD, the gastrointestinal tract is usually relatively empty because of inappetence and vomition. The sparse stomach contents may be bile-stained. Areas of pulmonary consolidation have been observed in experimentally infected pigs.

Microscopic lesions of nonsuppurative encephalomyelitis are often extensive in pigs with nervous signs, and viral infection of neurons has been demonstrated by immunofluorescence microscopy. Lesions consist of perivascular cuffing with mononuclear cells, glial nodules, and neuronophagia. Most are in the gray matter of the brain stem and anterior spinal cord. Similar but less extensive lesions are found in pigs killed early in the course of VWD. This observation, plus the fact that HEV is seldom isolated from the gastrointestinal tract, has led to the hypothesis that VWD is due to limited but irreparable neuronal damage. Microscopic, inflammatory lesions of the respiratory tract have been observed with both forms of the disease. The association of HEV with such lesions has been confirmed by virus isolation and immunofluorescence microscopy.

---

*All material in this article is in the public domain, with the exception of any borrowed figures or tables.

DIAGNOSIS

A tentative diagnosis of the encephalitis–vomiting and wasting disease complex is based on the occurrence of characteristic clinical signs mainly or entirely among pigs within the first few weeks of their life. Although pseudorabies virus and porcine enteroviruses can cause similar nervous signs and vomition, they more often affect older pigs as well. Transmissible gastroenteritis virus also causes baby pigs to vomit, but the absence of nervous signs and the presence of diarrhea with transmissible gastroenteritis are distinguishing features.

A definitive diagnosis depends on isolation of HEV from nervous tissue or demonstration of HEV-infected neurons by immunofluorescence microscopy. Because HEV is ubiquitous among swine, neither the detection of antibody nor the isolation of the virus from non-nervous tissue can be considered probable diagnostic evidence. The tissue of choice for diagnostic purposes is brain stem collected from a pig that has had clinical signs for no more than 48 hours and preferably less than 24 hours. The brain stem is cut symmetrically in halves, and one half is fixed in 10 per cent formalin for histologic examination. The other half is further divided into 2 parts. One part is used for attempted virus isolation, and the other is cut into thin sections with a cryostat-microtome for examination by direct immunofluorescence microscopy. Several studies have confirmed that virus isolation is usually unsuccessful after 1 or 2 days of clinical signs. One possible contributing factor is that because of the relatively long incubation period (perhaps reflecting the time required for the virus to reach the central nervous system), humoral antibody is present at or soon after the appearance of clinical signs.

TREATMENT

Treatment to reduce dehydration and electrolyte imbalance in cases of persistent vomition and to control secondary pathogens with antibiotics depends on the value of the affected pigs.

PREVENTION

Clinical disease is usually self-limiting. Most or all litters born over a period of 1 to 2 weeks may be affected, but eventually, through exposure of dams before farrowing, neonates are protected by colostral antibody. Passively acquired immunity may explain, in part, why the disease is so rare despite the probability that many pigs are initially exposed to HEV during the first few weeks of their life. Although the development of a vaccine is technically feasible, the sporadic nature of the disease makes vaccination economically unlikely.

BIBLIOGRAPHY

Andries K, Pensaert MB: Virus isolation and immunofluorescence in different organs of pigs infected with hemagglutinating encephalomyelitis virus. Am J Vet Res 41:215–218, 1980.

Mengeling WL, Cutlip RC: Pathogenicity of field isolates of hemagglutinating encephalomyelitis virus for neonatal pigs. J Am Vet Med Assoc 168:236–239, 1976.

Pensaert MB, Andries K: Hemagglutinating encephalomyelitis virus infection. In Leman AD, Straw B, Glock RD, et al (eds): Diseases of Swine, 6th ed. Ames, IA, Iowa State University Press, 1986, pp 310–315.

SMEDI and Other Porcine Enteroviruses*

WILLIAM L. MENGELING, DVM, PhD

The acronym SMEDI was introduced into the veterinary literature in 1965 to designate porcine enteroviruses (SMEDI viruses) that caused a syndrome of reproductive failure of swine characterized by stillbirth, mummification, embryonic death, and infertility (SMEDI syndrome). Subsequent reports that several other viruses cause the same, or a similar, syndrome have resulted in the ambiguous usage and interpretation of SMEDI when the term is used as an adjective to describe viruses associated with reproductive failure. Whereas some veterinary scientists and practitioners still adhere to the original definition of a SMEDI virus, perhaps the more common usage of the term is for any virus that causes embryonic or fetal death, or both, in the absence of maternal clinical signs and without ensuing abortion. Viruses in addition to porcine enteroviruses that have been reported to meet the aforementioned criteria are porcine parvovirus, reovirus, adenovirus, Japanese B encephalitis virus, porcine cytomegalovirus, and, most recently, encephalomyocarditis virus. All but Japanese B encephalitis virus are present and common among swine in the United States; however, there is substantial evidence to indicate that porcine parvovirus is the cause of most such cases.

Porcine enteroviruses have also been reported to be associated with other clinical diseases, namely, enteritis, pneumonitis, pericarditis, myocarditis, and polioencephalomyelitis. With the exception of polioencephalomyelitis, however, their role in these conditions is unclear. The most severe form of polioencephalitis caused by porcine enterovirus (i.e., Teschen disease) is discussed in a previous article.

BIBLIOGRAPHY

Huang J, Gentry RF, Zarkower A: Experimental infection of pregnant sows with porcine enteroviruses. Am J Vet Res 41:469–473, 1980.

Kim HS, Joo HS, Bergeland ME: Serologic, virologic, and histopathologic observations of encephalomyocarditis virus infection in mummified and stillborn pigs. J Vet Diagn Invest 1:101–104, 1989.

Encephalomyocarditis Virus*

JOSEPH H. GAINER, DVM

The encephalomyocarditis virus (EMCV) is a small picornavirus (of the genus *Cardiovirus*) that survives well outside the host. It is inactivated by hypochlorites and by iodinated compounds.

EPIZOOTIOLOGY

EMCV has been isolated sporadically in natural infections from a wide variety of species from around the world since 1940: human beings and the subhuman primates baboons, chimpanzees, and monkeys; the domesticated animals calves, African elephants, and pigs; the *Taeniorhynchus* mosquitoes; and small wild rodents including cotton rats, mongoose, rats,

---

*All material in this article is in the public domain, with the exception of any borrowed figures or tables.

squirrels, and water rats. The pig is the domestic animal most often infected, and many infections with deaths of the pigs occurred in Florida in the 1960s. Isolations of EMCV and the presence of positive antibodies suggesting EMCV infections have been reported from Minnesota and Canada from 1985 to 1990. In the late 1980s, infections have been reported from swine in Italy and Cuba; devastating infections have occurred in several swine herds in Australia in the mid-1970s.

Mortality in swine, although usually low, has been 100 per cent in young piglets. The rat likely serves as a reservoir of this enterovirus, contaminating the food and drinking water with infected feces. Immunotoxic chemicals may aggravate the infection in pigs as they do in experimental EMCV infections in mice.

Reproductive failure and neonatal losses in sows and their pigs associated with possible EMCV infection have been reported from Minnesota and Australia from 1985 to 1990.

CLINICAL SIGNS AND LESIONS

Sudden death, suggesting myocardial failure, in young 2- to 4-month-old pigs, subhuman primates, and elephants is the principal sign. Pathognomonic lesions are small (1 to 2 × 5 to 10 mm) grayish-white foci in the right myocardium. The foci consist microscopically of calcification and lymphocytic, monocytic infiltration. Infected hearts contain high levels of virus; altered electrocardiographic patterns have been seen in pigs experimentally infected with the virus. Stillborn and mummified porcine fetuses from swine farms experiencing reproductive problems have been associated with EMCV antibody, EMCV isolation, and nonsuppurative myocarditis and encephalitis in the dead fetuses.

DIAGNOSIS

Suspect EMCV infections are confirmed by virus isolation and identification of suspect virus with specific antiserum. Sudden death of animals with characteristic heart lesions is strongly presumptive.

TREATMENT

There is no treatment available at present.

PREVENTION AND CONTROL

Rat control should help prevent the spread of the virus. Outbreaks usually run short courses with immunity occurring in surviving animals. No commercial vaccines have been developed.

BIBLIOGRAPHY

Acland HM, Littlejohns IR: Encephalomyocarditis virus infection of pigs. 1. An outbreak in New South Wales. Aust Vet J 51:409–415, 1975.
Christianson WT, Kim HS, Joo HS, Barnes DM: Reproductive and neonatal losses associated with possible encephalomyocarditis virus infection in pigs. Vet Rec 126:54–57, 1990.
Gainer JH: Effects of viruses on the heart. In Bourne GH (ed): Hearts and Heart-like Organs, vol 3. Pathology and Surgery of the Heart. New York, Academic Press, 1980, pp 189–237.

Foot-and-Mouth Disease in Pigs

JERRY CALLIS, DVM, MS, DSc
DOUGLAS GREGG, DVM, MEd, PhD

Foot-and-mouth disease (FMD) is caused by a picornavirus. There are 7 distinct serotypes and many subtypes within each owing to the antigenic lability of the virus. A shift in the pH to 6 and below or to 9 and above creates a less favorable environment for infectivity. Two per cent caustic soda, 4 per cent soda ash, and 2 per cent acetic acid are good disinfectants.

EPIZOOTIOLOGY

FMD virus infects all species of animals, domestic and wild, that have cloven hoofs. Other naturally infected species include armadillos, hedgehogs, rats, nutria, grizzly bears, and elephants. Dogs, cats, rabbits, guinea pigs, chickens, mice, and chinchilla may be experimentally infected. Swine, in contrast to cattle, sheep, and goats, have not been shown to become carriers after infection and recovery.

CLINICAL SIGNS AND LESIONS

The clinical signs of FMD infection in swine are vesicles or erosions on the snout, lips, and tongue, on the coronary band, and between the claws on the feet. Infected animals have an elevated temperature and are reluctant to stand or move because of pain caused by blisters on their feet (Figs. 1 and 2). During infection, the milk from infected sows may contain 10^5 plaque-forming units of virus per milliliter. Piglets nursing such animals are readily infected, and the mortality is high as a result of viral necrosis of the heart muscle.

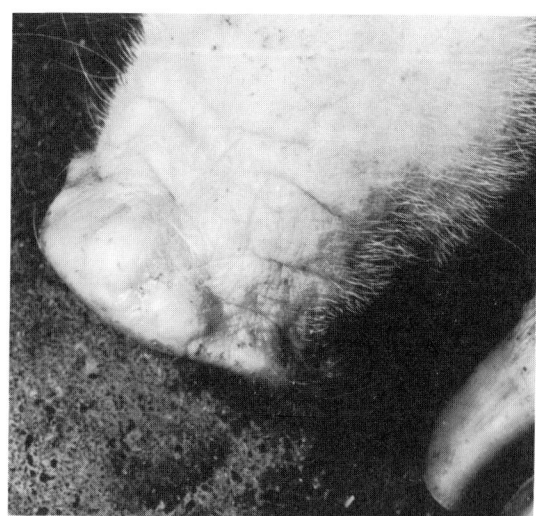

Figure 1. Two unruptured vesicles on the snout of a pig infected with foot-and-mouth disease virus.

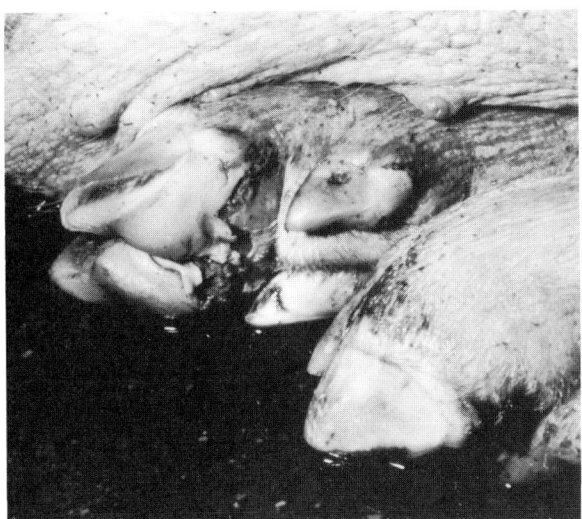

Figure 2. Broken vesicles on the foot pads and the coronary band of one dewclaw of a pig infected with foot-and-mouth disease virus.

DIAGNOSIS

Blisters or vesicles in the mouth, in the dorsal snout, or on the feet and an elevated temperature are characteristic of FMD in swine; however, these same lesions occur in 3 other vesicular infections in swine, including vesicular stomatitis, vesicular exanthema of swine, and swine vesicular disease. For this reason, a laboratory diagnosis is essential. Diagnosis can be made by isolation of the virus and identification by complement fixation, virus neutralization, agar-gel precipitin tests, and enzyme-linked immunosorbent assay.

TREATMENT

There is no specific cure for the disease. Palliative treatment may make the animals more comfortable.

PREVENTION AND CONTROL

The best way to prevent infection is to avoid contact with infected or recovered animals and their products. In the FMD-free countries, the disease is eradicated by slaughter of the infected animals, destruction of the carcasses, and disinfection of the premises. Vaccines have been available since the 1930s but are generally more effective for cattle than for swine. In recent years, vaccines containing oil adjuvants have been used with more success in swine. In control programs, it is also essential to control movement of infected animals and products for preventing aerosols of the viruses and transmission by air.

BIBLIOGRAPHY

Bachrach HL: Foot-and-mouth disease. Ann Rev Microbiol 22:201, 1968.
Callis JJ, McKercher PD: Foot-and-mouth disease. *In* Leman AD, et al (eds): Diseases of Swine, 5th ed. Ames, IA, Iowa State University Press, 1981, pp 278–287.
Cottral GE: Diagnosis of bovine vesicular disease. J Am Vet Med Assoc 161:1293, 1972.

Hog Cholera*

JAMES E. PEARSON, DVM, MS

Hog cholera is a highly contagious disease of swine caused by a small, 40 to 50 nm, enveloped RNA virus with cubic capsid symmetry. The hog cholera virus (HCV) belongs to the family Togaviridae and genus *Pestivirus* and is antigenically related to bovine viral diarrhea virus and border disease virus. There is no major antigenic difference between HCV isolates, but different strains will vary considerably in their virulence and pathogenicity. Hog cholera virus is inactivated by heat (60 minutes at 56° C), lipolytic chemicals (detergents), and the common disinfectants including hypochlorite, cresol, sodium orthophenylphenate, and 2 per cent sodium hydroxide. Its survival in blood, feces, or saliva is dependent on the environment. HCV has been recovered from processed hams and bacon after 85 days. Natural freeze-drying in temperate zones during winter will permit long survival. Synonyms are classical swine fever, virus-schweinepest, and peste du porc.

EPIZOOTIOLOGY

Hog cholera is found worldwide except in countries from which it has been eradicated or was never present (e.g., Australia, Canada, Denmark, Great Britain, Iceland, Ireland, New Zealand, the Scandinavian countries, and the United States). Although other animal species may be infected experimentally, the pig is the only natural host and reservoir. The virus is transmitted by lacrimal and nasal discharges, saliva, urine, feces, and tissues of infected pigs. Sources of infection include pig movement, garbage feeding, live virus vaccines, in utero infection in pregnant sows, insect transmission by mechanical means, contaminated instruments, and persistently infected piglets. Continuous farrowing may ensure persistence of virus of low virulence with continuing infection and losses in baby pigs. Transport of pork or pork products from infected pigs is the usual method of movement over long distances.

CLINICAL SIGNS AND LESIONS

Pigs affected with acute hog cholera look and act sick; the disease usually progresses rapidly to death, and remissions are rare. Initially, only a few pigs are affected. They appear drowsy and stand with arched backs, drooping heads, and straight tails. The sick pigs huddle together as though they were cold. Although pigs will continue to drink water, anorexia soon becomes complete. There is also a fever with temperatures as high as 42.2° C (most in the range of 41° to 42° C). There is a leukopenia with leukocyte counts as low as 3000/mm^3 of blood. Marked lacrimal discharge is observed with conjunctivitis so severe that the eyes may be pasted shut. Constipation develops during the febrile period and is followed by severe diarrhea. Eventually the pigs become gaunt and have a weak, staggering gait. Purple discoloration of the skin and convulsions may be observed just before death. In chronic hog cholera, clinical signs are less severe, pigs survive longer, and remissions occur. Pigs will resume eating but do not finish their ration so that weight is not gained, and some pigs become runts that can survive more than 100 days. Many of the pigs that survive will no longer be viremic. If secondary bacterial invaders become involved, other clinical signs may be observed.

Inapparent or unnoticed hog cholera is caused by low-

---

*All material in this article is in the public domain, with the exception of any borrowed figures or tables.

virulence strains that fail to produce typical clinical signs. In affected herds, the only clinical signs observed are baby pig deaths, stillbirths, abortions, and mummified fetuses. The administration of modified live virus vaccine to pregnant sows may cause this syndrome. Newborn pigs may show tremors or trembling (shakers) related to cerebellar hypoplasia and hypomyelinogenesis. A sequel of congenital HCV infection is "late onset" disease, which occurs 2 to 11 months after birth. Pigs develop mild anorexia and depression, conjunctivitis, dermatitis, diarrhea, and central nervous system disturbance. Pigs usually survive 6 months but eventually die; all have a persistent viremia.

The pathogenesis and lesions of HCV infection are due to the affinity of the virus for epithelium and the reticuloendothelial system. Primary invasion is through the oronasal epithelium, and severe impairment of metabolism is caused by damage to the vascular endothelium. Entry of the virus is by ingestion or inhalation, with the tonsil as the primary site of viral replication. Virus is transferred to regional lymph nodes and then by blood to the other lymph nodes, spleen, bone marrow, and lymphoid structure of the small intestines. The parenchymatous organs are invaded after 3 to 4 days. Edema and swelling of the infected vascular endothelium result in thrombosis, infarction, and hemorrhage. Common lesions are infarcts of the spleen, button ulcers in the large intestine, and petechial hemorrhages in the lungs, epiglottis, bladder, and kidney. Other frequent lesions are edema and peripheral hemorrhage of the lymph nodes and hemorrhage and necrosis of the tonsil. In chronic hog cholera, lesions are less severe, and bronchopneumonia may be seen.

DIAGNOSIS

The diagnosis may be confirmed by laboratory examinations that detect viral antigen and isolate the virus or detect antibody titers in sera from convalescent pigs. Tonsil, spleen, and mandibular lymph nodes should be submitted. Thin sections of tonsil can be cut in a cryostat, and virus-infected cells in the tonsillar crypts may be detected by immunofluorescence. Splenic suspensions may be inoculated into pig kidney cell cultures. After overnight incubation of the cultures, infected cells can be detected by immunofluorescence. Inapparent hog cholera can be confirmed in nonvaccinated pigs by detecting hog cholera antibody with the neutralization test, enzyme-linked immunosorbent assay, or peroxidase-linked assay.

PREVENTION AND CONTROL

There is no effective treatment for hog cholera. Upon confirmation of the diagnosis, some pigs may be saved by prompt vaccination of the herd with a live attenuated vaccine. The commonly used vaccines are attenuated by passage in rabbits (C strain) or cell culture (Japanese GPE strain or French Thiveral strain). If pregnant sows are present, they also should be vaccinated but sent to slaughter before they farrow.

In a country where hog cholera is enzootic, a regular vaccination program is the safest method of preventing the disease. Young pigs can be vaccinated at 4 weeks of age. If vaccinated at less than 8 weeks, breeding animals should be revaccinated at 5 to 6 months of age. The breeding herd should be revaccinated at least once a year before breeding.

Clinical hog cholera can be controlled with an adequate vaccination program. However, ultimate hog cholera control in a country or state must involve eradication of the disease. This requires the cooperation of the government, veterinary profession, and swine industry. An initial phase of intensive vaccination, followed by detection and quarantine of infected herds, and finally slaughter and disposal of infected pigs has successfully eradicated hog cholera.

BIBLIOGRAPHY

Liess B: Classical Swine Fever and Related Viral Diseases. Boston, Martinus Nijhoff, 1988.
Van Oirschot JT: Hog cholera. In Leman AD, et al (eds): Disease of Swine, 6th ed. Ames, IA, Iowa State University Press, 1986, pp 289–300.

Japanese Encephalitis (Flavivirus)*

JAMES E. PEARSON, DVM, MS

Japanese encephalitis is caused by a 40 to 50 nm single-stranded RNA virus, genus *Flavivirus*, family Flaviviridae.

EPIZOOTIOLOGY

The virus is mosquito-borne and infects humans, other animals, and birds. Swine develop high concentrations of virus in their blood and serve as the primary amplifying hosts. Japanese encephalitis virus is inactivated by heat (30 minutes at 56° C), lipid solvents, and sodium hypochlorite. Japanese encephalitis is enzootic in Southeast Asia, including Russia, China, Nepal, Kampuchea, Sri Lanka, Philippines, Indonesia, India, Korea, Vietnam, Laos, Burma, and Japan. Synonyms are Japanese B encephalitis, Japanese equine encephalitis, Russian autumnal encephalitis, and summer encephalitis.

CLINICAL SIGNS AND LESIONS

Japanese encephalitis virus infection in humans is often subclinical, but there may be systemic diseases, especially in children under 12 years, with fever, headache, prostration, stiff neck, and encephalitis. Mortality after clinical disease is approximately 25 per cent, and 50 per cent develop neuropsychiatric sequelae. Cattle, sheep, and goats have inapparent infections. In horses, the disease is generally inapparent, but fatal encephalitis has been recognized. When pregnant sows are infected, severe economic losses occur. The virus spreads to the fetuses, causing stillbirths, mummified hydrocephalic fetuses, and weak pigs in approximately half of the infected sows. Some of the weak piglets have nervous signs. Japanese encephalitis virus infection of boars can cause infertility and reduced sexual drive. The virus may be isolated from the semen. Clinical signs are usually observed only in very young pigs.

DIAGNOSIS

Japanese encephalitis may be isolated from the tissues of infected animals by use of suckling mice, chick embryos, or cell cultures. A serologic diagnosis may be made by detecting IgM in serum with the enzyme-linked immunosorbent assay

---

*All material in this article is in the public domain, with the exception of any borrowed figures or tables.

test or a rise in antibody titer with virus neutralization, hemagglutination inhibition, or complement-fixation tests performed on paired (acute and convalescent) sera.

PREVENTION AND CONTROL

Both attenuated live virus and inactivated vaccines are used to prevent baby pig losses and to protect horses. Young gilts and boars should be vaccinated before breeding. When inactivated vaccines are used, at least 2 doses should be given at an interval of 2 to 3 weeks. In temperate climates, the vaccination should be done before the mosquito season.

BIBLIOGRAPHY

Acha PN, Szyfres B: Zoonoses and Communicable Diseases Common to Man and Animals. Washington, DC, World Health Organization, 1989, pp 376–380.
Burke DS, Leake CJ: Japanese encephalitis. In Monath TP (ed): The Arboviruses: Epidemiology and Ecology, vol 3. Boca Raton, FL, CRC Press, 1988, pp 63–92.
Joo HS: Japanese B encephalitis infection. In Leman AD, et al (eds): Disease of Swine, 6th ed. Ames, IA, Iowa State University Press, 1986, pp 407–411.
Rosen L: The natural history of Japanese encephalitis virus. Ann Rev Microbiol 40:395–414, 1986.

Porcine Reoviruses
SASHI B. MOHANTY, BVSc, PhD

Reovirus types 1 and 3, isolated from apparently normal pigs and pigs with clinical disease, are serologically identical to human reoviruses. Antibodies to these agents are highly prevalent in swine populations. Porcine reoviruses grow and produce cytopathic effects in cell cultures of porcine origin and a variety of other mammalian cells. They may produce initial cytopathic effects in HEP-2 and PK-15 cell lines, but they cannot be maintained by serial passage in these cells. Reovirus type 1 was isolated from healthy pigs, from pigs with respiratory illness, and from aborted fetuses. Type 3 was isolated from pigs with dyspnea.

CLINICAL SIGNS AND LESIONS

The pathogenic role of porcine reoviruses is not fully understood, and further investigations are required for elucidation of their role. Pigs experimentally infected with reovirus type 1 of human origin and with types 1 and 3 of porcine origin had only a mild, transient febrile reaction. Older pigs, however, had no reaction to type 3 reovirus. Experimental infection of sows between 40 and 80 days of gestation resulted in stillbirths, mummified fetuses, and small weak pigs.

No gross lesions have been described. Histologic changes confined to the lungs are mild and focal. Lobular alveolar emphysema, peribronchiolar lymphocytic infiltration, and thickened alveolar walls are seen in type 3 reoviral infection.

DIAGNOSIS, PREVENTION, AND CONTROL

Virus isolation and seroconversion are adequate for a diagnosis. Histopathologic changes may also be helpful. There is no vaccine.

BIBLIOGRAPHY

McAdaragh JP, Robl MG: Experimental reovirus infection of pregnant sows. Proceedings, 4th International Congress, Pig Veterinary Society, Iowa State University, 1976, pp DDI.
McFerran JB: Reovirus infection. In Leman AD, et al (eds): Diseases of Swine, 5th ed. Ames, IA, Iowa State University Press, 1981, pp 330–334.

Porcine Rotavirus
LINDA J. SAIF, PhD, MS

Rotaviruses are so named because of their wheel-like appearance when they are viewed by electron microscopy. Like other members of the Reoviridae family, these viruses have segmented double-stranded RNA genomes and are very resistant to environmental conditions and many disinfectants. Early studies revealed that porcine rotaviruses share a common antigen and cross-react serologically with rotaviruses from other mammalian hosts. Some isolates with other distinct antigens were recently recovered from pigs. Porcine rotaviruses are now separated into at least 4 groups, designated A, B, C, and E, with members of each group sharing their own distinctive common antigen. The original rotaviruses belong to group A and are the most frequently diagnosed in pigs. Little information is available about the prevalence of infections with nongroup A rotaviruses in pigs, largely owing to a lack of diagnostic tests for their routine detection. Consequently, group A rotaviruses are the focus of this report. At present, at least 3 serotypes of group A porcine rotaviruses occur; infection with 1 serotype may not protect pigs against challenge with an unrelated serotype.

EPIZOOTIOLOGY

Rotaviruses are spread by the fecal-oral route and are a common cause of diarrhea in many young animals including pigs. Because of excretion of the virus in large numbers in feces of infected pigs and the stability of the virus in the environment, rotavirus infections are common and widespread in pigs, and enzootic infections probably occur in all herds. Pigs generally become infected between 1 and 3 weeks of age and again 1 week after weaning. The clinical syndrome is often referred to as milk scours, white scours, or 3-week scours. The age of peak incidence and severity of the disease vary under different management conditions and are highly influenced by the degree of passive immunity and viral exposure.

CLINICAL SIGNS AND LESIONS

Rotavirus infects the villous enterocytes of the small intestine, which leads to their destruction and villous atrophy. Consequently, the normal digestive-absorptive processes are impaired, and an acute, transitory malabsorptive diarrhea results.

Most rotavirus infections occur in nursing pigs at 1 to 5 weeks of age, coincident with the presence of passively transferred milk antibodies in the gut. These antibodies moderate the severity of rotavirus infections such that most pigs develop only subclinical infections or transient diarrhea. However, in environments heavily contaminated with virus, such as continuous farrowing operations, more severe rotaviral diarrhea with dehydration and increased mortality may occur in pigs of progressively younger ages. Thorough cleaning and disinfection of the farrowing or nursery units is needed to interrupt this cycle of increasingly severe diarrhea. In addition, the severity of the disease and mortality rate may be increased by concurrent infections with other pathogens (*Escherichia coli*, coccidia, transmissible gastroenteritis and other enteric viruses), inadequate intake of immune milk, or stress, especially chilling.

DIAGNOSIS

An etiologic diagnosis is necessary for distinguishing diarrhea caused by rotavirus from that caused by enzootic transmissible gastroenteritis virus, coccidia, and enteropathogenic *E. coli*. Specimens to submit for laboratory diagnosis include feces or gut segments or contents from pigs in the early stages of diarrhea. Diagnosis consists of the demonstration of virus in feces by immune electron microscopy or enzyme-linked immunosorbent assay (ELISA) or detection of infected enterocytes by fluorescent antibody staining of gut sections or smears. Specific antiserum is needed in each assay to distinguish group A from nongroup A rotaviruses. Serology is of little aid in diagnosis because most swine are seropositive for rotavirus antibodies.

Newer molecular methods based on detection of viral nucleic acids have been developed for diagnosis and differentiation of rotaviruses. These include RNA electropherotyping (analysis of the migration patterns of rotaviral RNA genome segments in polyacrylamide gels) and use of nucleic acid hybridization probes. The latter method or use of monoclonal antibodies in ELISA can also be used to identify rotavirus groups and differentiate serotypes. All of these methods can be performed with use of feces or gut contents collected in the early stages of diarrhea and stored frozen.

TREATMENT, PREVENTION, AND CONTROL

Because rotaviruses are ubiquitous and highly stable in the environment, methods for their eradication or prevention of infection are unlikely. Therefore emphasis must be on reducing exposure of neonatal or recently weaned highly susceptible pigs to virus and enhancing active and passive immunity to prevent clinical disease. The following management procedures may be useful in reducing the severity of rotaviral infections: good sanitation and use of disinfectants (phenol derivatives and formaldehydes are the most effective) to reduce the level of viral exposure; provision of optimal environmental conditions to pigs (especially adequate heat); control of other concurrent infections; and use of "all-in, all-out" systems in farrowing and nursery units. A licensed vaccine is available for vaccinating pregnant swine and suckling pigs. In theory, the vaccine should boost rotavirus antibody titers in the colostrum and milk of the mother and provide enhanced lactogenic immunity to the nursing pigs. However, no independent studies of vaccine efficacy for protection of nursing pigs against rotavirus diarrhea have been reported. In one study, maternal antibodies were postulated to interfere with active immunization of pigs with the vaccine, with resultant failure of the vaccine to prevent rotavirus diarrhea in weaned pigs. Antibiotics and other drugs are ineffective against rotaviral infections and are indicated only in cases of concurrent or secondary bacterial infections.

BIBLIOGRAPHY

Hoblet KH, Saif LJ, Kohler EM, et al: Efficacy of an orally administered modified live porcine origin rotavirus vaccine against postweaning diarrhea in pigs. Am J Vet Res 47:1697–1703, 1986.
Saif LJ, Theil KW (eds): Viral Diarrheas of Man and Animals. Boca Raton, FL, CRC Press, 1990.
Saif LJ, Rosen BI: Porcine rotavirus. In Castro AE, Heuschele WP (eds): Diagnostic Veterinary Virology: A Practitioner's Guide. Baltimore, Williams & Wilkins, 1992, pp 239–243.
Woode GN: Rotavirus. In Leman AD, et al (eds): Diseases of Swine, 6th ed. Ames, IA, Iowa State University Press, 1986, pp 368–382.

Transmissible Gastroenteritis Virus

LINDA J. SAIF, PhD, MS

Transmissible gastroenteritis (TGE) is a contagious enteric viral disease affecting swine of all ages, with diarrhea and vomiting the prominent clinical signs. When disease outbreaks occur in seronegative herds, TGE virus (TGEV) often causes 100 per cent mortality in pigs under 2 weeks of age. Because there is no effective practical treatment and commercially available vaccines are of limited efficacy, TGE infections represent a major cause of loss to the swine industry.

TGEV is a porcine coronavirus, with only 1 known serotype. The virus has an envelope and is inactivated by high temperature ($>32°$ C), sunlight, and a variety of disinfectants. TGEV is antigenically related to coronaviruses of cats and dogs. More recently, outbreaks of mild respiratory disease without diarrhea, caused by TGEV variants, have been reported in swine in Europe and the United States. These TGEV variants, referred to as porcine respiratory coronaviruses (PRCV), are indistinguishable from TGEV by conventional serologic methods. Both TGEV and PRCV infections induce neutralizing antibodies in pigs that are qualitatively and quantitatively similar. The PRCV is now enzootic in the swine population in Europe, and in recent surveys, nearly 100 per cent of the swine farms in Belgium tested positive for antibodies to PRCV (and consequently TGEV).

EPIZOOTIOLOGY

TGE occurs primarily during the winter months. This may relate to greater survival of the virus and its more efficient spread at cold temperatures. Although the disease is restricted to swine, dogs and cats can become infected with TGEV and shed virus in their stools for up to 2 weeks. Thus dogs and cats as well as starlings, which tend to flock into feedlots during winter, may be involved in the herd-to-herd spread of TGEV during epizootics. Other possible modes of transmission from herd to herd include newly introduced infected animals, especially feeder pigs, and mechanical spread of virus via fecal contamination of footwear, clothes, vehicles, feed, and equipment. The aerogenic route of spread has been suggested as the major means of transmission of PRCV throughout European swine herds.

Within a herd, the natural route of infection may be by fecal-oral or aerosol transmission of virus in densely populated herds. The PRCV is readily transmitted by the aerosol or oronasal route of inoculation. The PRCV appears to spread aerogenically over long distances, even into swine herds that use strict sanitary measures. Fecal or nasal shedding of TGEV persists for up to 2 weeks. Although TGEV has been recovered from respiratory and intestinal tissues at 104 days after infection, it is unknown whether such persistently infected animals can shed viable virus for longer than 2 weeks after the initial infection. Sentinel pigs placed in a herd at 3 to 5 months after a TGE outbreak remained free of infection. The duration of nasal shedding of virus in pigs infected with PRCV has not been well documented, but in these disease outbreaks or in artificially challenged pigs, fecal shedding of PRCV has not been demonstrated.

Two distinct forms of TGE occur in swine herds: epizootic and enzootic. Epizootic TGE occurs after introduction of the virus into a susceptible (seronegative) herd. The virus spreads rapidly within a herd, affecting swine of all ages. Unless there is a continual source of susceptible animals, the disease usually runs its course in 2 to 4 weeks. Clinical signs may include inappetence, lethargy, diarrhea, and vomiting. Pigs under 2 weeks of age are the most severely affected, and mortality may approach 100 per cent. Lactating sows often develop anorexia and agalactia. Such severe clinical signs aid in diagnosis of epizootic TGE in the United States but may be difficult to differentiate from those due to porcine epidemic diarrhea virus, an unrelated enteric coronavirus that occurs in swine herds in Europe.

Enzootic TGE persists in partially immune herds with frequent or continuous farrowings or frequent addition of susceptible swine, such as feeder pig operations. It is characterized by high morbidity but lower mortality (10 to 20 per cent), both rates being influenced by the pig's age when it is infected. It is also influenced by the level of immunity in the herd, with previously infected sows transmitting a variable degree of passive immunity via colostrum and milk to their suckling piglets. Diarrhea usually occurs in pigs from 1 to 3 weeks of age, when the level of viral exposure exceeds the level of passive immunity. In some herds, the disease occurs primarily postweaning after the abrupt curtailment of lactogenic immunity; or it is first established in older swine, eventually spreading to younger piglets. An etiologic diagnosis is necessary for distinguishing TGE from other enzootic diarrheal infections. Serologic surveys indicated about 30 to 50 per cent of swine herds in the United States were positive for TGEV antibodies. This contrasts with the situation in Europe, where PRCV infections are widespread and the number of swine herds seropositive for antibodies to TGEV approaches 100 per cent.

The PRCV also causes enzootic infections in swine herds, having spread extensively throughout Western Europe and in countries such as Denmark, which was previously free of TGEV. PRCV infections persist on closed breeding farms with cyclic episodes most common during winter and spring. Respiratory infections with PRCV generally occur after weaning, in pigs between 5 and 10 weeks of age, in the presence of passive serum antibodies. Infections are usually subclinical but may be accompanied by mild signs of respiratory disease; no diarrhea or fecal shedding of virus is observed. In the United States to date, isolates of PRCV have been recovered only from swine herds in Indiana, North Carolina, and Arkansas.

CLINICAL SIGNS AND LESIONS

As noted previously, clinical signs vary in herds experiencing enzootic or epizootic outbreaks of TGE. TGEV infects and destroys the villous enterocytes of the small intestine, which results in villous atrophy. This causes impaired digestion, accumulation of fluids in the intestine, diarrhea, dehydration and weight loss, and death in severe cases. The severity of clinical signs, duration of the disease, and mortality are inversely related to age. Clinical signs, particularly diarrhea and dehydration, are most pronounced in seronegative piglets infected under 2 weeks of age in which mortality approaches 100 per cent. Clinical signs in adult swine are usually limited to inappetence and mild diarrhea, although lactating sows may show more severe disease.

The PRCV replicates in nasal mucosa, trachea, and lung and may cause variable degrees of interstitial pneumonia. Little or no viral replication is observed in the intestine. Clinical signs were not seen in pigs artificially inoculated with PRCV; in field outbreaks, only subclinical or mild respiratory infections were usually observed.

DIAGNOSIS

A presumptive diagnosis of epizootic TGE can be made in the United States and Canada on the basis of clinical signs and herd history, particularly if piglets are affected. Porcine epidemic diarrhea virus infection, which occurs in Europe, resembles TGE, but it has not been diagnosed in North America. Enzootic TGE requires an etiologic diagnosis for differentiating it from enteric diseases with similar clinical signs such as *Escherichia coli* infection, coccidiosis, and rotaviral diarrhea. Like TGEV, the last two pathogens may also induce villous atrophy. TGE may be diagnosed by one or more of the following laboratory tests: detection of virus or viral antigen by immunofluorescence (IF), enzyme-linked immunosorbent assay (ELISA), or immune electron microscopy (IEM); isolation of virus in cell culture; and detection of rising antibody titers in serum. The IF, ELISA, and IEM tests are rapid with results available within 48 hours, whereas the last 2 tests usually require at least 1 week for final results. Immunofluorescence tests on mucosal smears or sections of the small intestine collected from pigs near the onset of diarrhea are most often employed for the detection of TGEV. For diagnosis of the infection in live animals, stools collected near the onset of diarrhea can be tested in ELISA or by IEM, or paired sera may be examined for antibodies in virus neutralization tests. However, the virus neutralization test provides only retrospective evidence of infection and will not differentiate between infections with TGEV and PRCV.

Currently, none of these tests allow differentiation of TGEV from PRCV. However, evaluation of clinical signs, histologic lesions, and tissue distribution of viral antigen may provide useful information because PRCV does not cause diarrhea or villous atrophy and replicates almost exclusively in respiratory tissues. PRCV has been detected in live animals by IF staining of nasal epithelial cells or isolation of virus from nasal secretions. More recently, a competition blocking ELISA test based on use of monoclonal antibodies that react with TGEV but fail to recognize PRCV has been developed in Europe for serologic differentiation of TGEV- from PRCV-infected animals. Presently, only this test provides the differential information required for export of TGE-free swine, for animals testing seropositive to TGEV in countries where PRCV infections also occur. Preliminary data also suggest cDNA probes specific for TGEV but nonreactive with PRCV may distinguish between the 2 viruses in nucleic acid hybridization tests.

TREATMENT, PREVENTION, AND CONTROL

Although sows naturally infected with TGEV previously transmit effective passive immunity against TGE to their offspring, commercial vaccines are of limited efficacy in providing the level of lactogenic immunity necessary for preventing the epizootic form of TGE. Moreover, there is no specific treatment for the disease. Therefore, management factors play an important role in preventing spread of the infection within a herd or to other herds and reducing losses in a TGE-infected herd. For control of the spread of TGE within or between herds, dead pigs should be incinerated and sows due to farrow within about 10 days of the outbreak should be removed from the contaminated facility. The transport of virus via contaminated feces should be avoided by careful disinfection of boots, shoes, and clothing; controlled access of vehicles or people; and control of starlings and flies around swine premises. Cats, dogs, foxes, and possibly other wildlife may also disseminate the virus to other farms, so their access to swine herds should be controlled. Because carrier swine may introduce TGEV into a herd, newly acquired or previously infected pigs should be isolated for at least 1 month before being added to a TGE-free herd; alternatively, only TGEV seronegative pigs might be added to such a herd.

Possible methods for control of enzootic TGE include administration of the commercial vaccines to seropositive sows (previously naturally infected) to boost the level of passive immunity transferred to suckling pigs. This approach should decrease infection of younger pigs with TGEV, thereby reducing mortality. Secondly, an "all-in, all-out" management system to prevent the continual influx of susceptible pigs into the herd or facility and permit thorough cleaning and disinfection of the premises between groups is important in breaking the cycle of infection.

In the face of a TGE epizootic, death losses may be decreased by keeping pigs warm (>32° C) and dry and providing free access to water. If possible, cross-suckling of infected or susceptible young pigs on TGE-immune sows may also reduce losses. If concurrent or secondary bacterial infections occur, antibacterial therapy may be indicated, but this will not affect the course of a TGEV infection.

During an outbreak, deliberate infection of sows due to farrow more than 2 weeks hence with the autogenous virulent virus may be useful. This is accomplished by feeding the guts (minced and diluted in water) from newly infected pigs as a slurry to the sows. If adequately exposed to infectious virus, sows should develop immunity in approximately 2 weeks and passively transmit such immunity to their newborn piglets. In such situations, deliberate exposure of all older pigs on the same farm may be warranted in order to shorten the total time the disease progresses through the herd and ensure more uniform exposure levels in all animals. Hazards associated with planned infections include possible spread of other pathogens or dissemination of the virus to other herds.

Preliminary studies in Europe of cross-protection between PRCV and TGEV indicate that prior infection of pigs with PRCV does not prevent infection or diarrhea after challenge with TGEV. However, some reduction in clinical signs and virus shedding was reported, which suggests that prior infection with PRCV moderates the severity of TGEV infections. Furthermore, sows primed by a PRCV infection undergo a rapid secondary immune response upon exposure to TGEV, with increased antibody levels in milk. This enhanced passive immunity apparently moderates the severity of TGE outbreaks such that piglet mortality is decreased and the disease course is shortened relative to that seen previously during typical outbreaks of epizootic TGE.

BIBLIOGRAPHY

Bohl EH: Transmissible gastroenteritis (classical enteric variant). In Pensaert MB (ed): Virus Infections of Porcines. Amsterdam, Elsevier Science, 1989, pp 139–153.

Hill H, Biwer J, Wood R, Wesley R: Porcine respiratory coronavirus isolated from two U.S. swine herds. Denver, CO, Proceedings, American Association of Swine Practitioners, 1990, pp 333–335.

Pensaert MB: Transmissible gastroenteritis virus (respiratory variant). In Pensaert MB (ed): Virus Infections of Porcines. Amsterdam, Elsevier Science, 1989, pp 154–165.

Pensaert MB: Porcine respiratory coronavirus related to transmissible gastroenteritis virus. Agri-Practice 10:17–21, 1989.

Saif LJ, Bohl EH: Transmissible gastroenteritis virus. In Leman AD, et al (eds): Diseases of Swine, 6th ed. Ames, IA, Iowa State University Press, 1986, pp 225–274.

Saif LJ, Heckert RA: Enteric coronaviruses. In Saif LJ, Theil KW (eds): Viral Diarrheas of Man and Animals. Boca Raton, FL, CRC Press, 1990, pp 185–252.

Porcine Epidemic Diarrhea Virus

LINDA J. SAIF, PhD, MS

The porcine epidemic diarrhea virus (PEDV) was first identified as a coronavirus in England and Belgium in 1978 in association with transmissible gastroenteritis (TGE)–like outbreaks of acute diarrhea in swine of all ages. It was subsequently shown to be antigenically unrelated to transmissible gastroenteritis virus (TGEV) or other known coronaviruses. PEDV or antibodies to PEDV have been identified in swine from Europe, Taiwan, and China but not from the United States. A recent survey of swine sera from midwestern states in the United States again failed to detect antibodies to PEDV, confirming the earlier findings.

At present, there is only 1 known serotype of PEDV. On the basis of serologic testing, the virus first appeared in Belgium swine about 1971, coincident with the first reported clinical outbreaks. No antibodies were detected in swine sera collected before this date. The origin of PEDV is unknown.

EPIZOOTIOLOGY

PEDV is a cause of diarrhea, most commonly in weaned pigs, feeder pigs, and finishing swine. Recent serosurveys in Belgium and Germany have indicated 19 to 33 per cent of swine farms tested positive for antibodies to PEDV. PEDV is transmitted by the fecal-oral route. Disease outbreaks often occur on farms within a few days after sale or purchase of pigs.

Similar to TGE, PED outbreaks occur primarily during the winter months in breeding herds. Much clinical variation may occur among outbreaks. On some farms, piglets under 1 week of age are the most severely affected, developing watery diarrhea with variable vomiting and mortality rates (50 to 90 per cent). This form resembles TGE, except PEDV spreads more slowly through the herd (4 to 5 weeks), and mortality rates are lower in baby pigs. In other outbreaks, weaned and adult pigs are more severely affected than are suckling pigs, which develop only mild diarrhea and low mortality. Among finishing swine, 100 per cent morbidity is common, with a 1 to 3 per cent mortality rate; these animals may die acutely, with acute back muscle necrosis frequently observed.

PEDV is probably spread mechanically among farms by personnel and equipment. In addition, weaned and feeder pigs may become carrier animals, providing a reservoir for spread of virus both within a herd and among herds.

CLINICAL SIGNS AND LESIONS

As noted, infection of swine with PEDV may cause a variety of clinical signs, most of which resemble TGE. Like TGEV, PEDV infects villous enterocytes, which leads to villous atrophy and ensuing diarrhea. Differences observed between TGEV and PEDV in their pathogenesis include the following: TGEV infection progresses more rapidly and induces more severe villous atrophy; PEDV, but not TGEV, infects small intestinal crypt and also colonic epithelial cells.

DIAGNOSIS

Clinical signs and histopathologic lesions are not sufficient for diagnosis of PED because such findings are similar to ones seen in TGE outbreaks. Specific tests are available in Europe for identification of PEDV or viral antigen in feces or gut sections. These include immunofluorescent staining of gut sections or smears and enzyme-linked immunosorbent assay (ELISA) or immune electron microscopy for detection of virus from feces or gut contents. An indirect immunofluorescent test or blocking ELISA can be used for detection and titration of antibodies to PEDV.

TREATMENT, PREVENTION, AND CONTROL

Because of the recent emergence of this disease, there is little information on its prevention and control. A key emphasis, as for many other enteric viral infections, must be on proper management for prevention or control of disease outbreaks. Spread of PEDV by animal and human movement necessitates proper disinfection and security procedures on and around swine premises. During an outbreak of PED, measures similar to ones used in TGE outbreaks may help reduce piglet mortality. These include free access of infected pigs to water to reduce dehydration, provision of supplemental heat to piglets, short-term withholding of feed in finishing units, and isolation of farrowing units containing newborn piglets. The feeding of gut contents from recently infected piglets to pregnant sows at least 2 weeks before farrowing may stimulate lactogenic immunity and provide some protection to suckling piglets, although this has not been definitively proved for PED. Antibiotics are of no value unless secondary bacterial infections are a contributing factor to the disease syndrome.

BIBLIOGRAPHY

Pensaert MB: Porcine epidemic diarrhea virus. *In* Leman AD, et al (eds): Diseases of Swine, 6th ed. Ames, IA, Iowa State University Press, 1986, pp 402–406.

Pensaert MB: Porcine epidemic diarrhea virus. *In* Pensaert MB (ed): Virus Infections of Porcines. Amsterdam, Elsevier Science, 1989, pp 167–176.

Saif LJ, Heckert RA: Enteric coronaviruses. *In* Saif LJ, Theil KW (eds): Viral Diarrheas of Man and Animals. Boca Raton, FL, CRC Press, 1990, pp 185–252.

Swine Influenza

B. C. EASTERDAY, DVM, PhD

Swine influenza (SI), also known as swine flu, hog flu, and pig flu, is a specific, acute, infectious, respiratory disease of swine caused by a type A influenza virus. The disease is characterized by sudden onset, coughing, dyspnea, fever, prostration, and rapid recovery. The mortality rate is low except in very young piglets and cases complicated by other infections or conditions.

ETIOLOGY

The cause of SI is a type A influenza virus. It is one of many such viruses of diverse antigenic characteristics found in humans, horses, and many domestic and wild avian species. The influenza viruses belong to the family Orthomyxoviridae. They have enveloped virions 80 to 120 nm in diameter that may be spherical, elongated, or pleomorphic. The structural proteins on the surface of the virion, hemagglutinin (H) and neuraminidase (N), are the significant surface antigens. Antibodies to the hemagglutinin are protective against viruses containing the same hemagglutinin. Antibodies are also formed against the neuraminidase antigen, but they are less important in providing protection from infection.

Swine influenza virus (SIV) has been remarkably stable in its antigenic characteristics over 60 years. However, there has been definite antigenic drifting, and the contemporary strains are clearly distinguishable from the older ones. Coexisting subpopulations with antigenically and biologically distinguishable hemagglutinins may be found in SIVs isolated from swine and humans. Influenza viruses with swine characteristics, but clearly distinguishable antigenically from classic swine strains, have been recovered from avian species.

It is clear that swine have become infected with at least 4 distinct type A influenza viruses. These include the "classic" SIV, with the antigenic characteristics H1N1 (formerly Hsw1N1); the Hong Kong influenza virus H3N2 and its antigenic variants; the "Russian" influenza virus, an H1N1 virus; and, more recently, an H1N1 virus with some of the classic SIV antigenic characteristics but generally considered to be of avian origin.

EPIZOOTIOLOGY

The first appearance of SI in a swine population is generally associated with the movement of animals (e.g., the introduction of breeding stock, introduction of feeder pigs, or return of show stock to the farm). Once the infection has appeared in a swine-breeding operation or any environment in which there is no complete depopulation, it is likely to be maintained in the herd with at least annual episodes of acute disease. It is generally reported that outbreaks are explosive, with all of the pigs in the herd becoming ill at the same time. However, owners who observe their herds closely are often aware of 1 or a few pigs with signs of the disease 2 to 5 days before the whole herd is involved. Although the precise method of transmission is not known, it is presumed to be direct pig-to-pig transmission by the nasopharyngeal route. Nasal secretions are laden with virus during the acute febrile stages of infection, which provides an abundant source of infectious materials for susceptible animals.

It is quite clear that although outbreaks of SI are generally seasonal, especially in the north central United States, the infection and disease are present throughout the year.

It has been clear since 1976 that SIV may be transmitted from pigs to humans and may cause acute respiratory disease. Most of the documented cases of transmission of SIV resulting in acute respiratory disease in humans in contact with swine have been in young men under 30 years of age. In the United States there is a plentiful source of virus in the pig populations, and there are thousands of contacts between human beings and pigs every day. Such exposure constitutes an occupational hazard and a potential public health problem of undetermined magnitude and significance. In 1988, a pregnant woman contracted a fatal swine influenza virus infection while visiting a swine show area at a county fair in Wisconsin.

CLINICAL SIGNS AND LESIONS

Classic SI, as it occurs in nature, is a herd disease. It is most frequently described as a disease of autumn, winter, and early spring. There is a sudden onset of signs, most of which are referable to the respiratory tract. Coughing, inactivity, and inappetence are generally the first signs noticed. This proceeds to labored and jerky breathing and prolonged paroxysmal coughing. Great prostration and complete anorexia along with conjunctivitis, nasal discharge, and loss of weight are common. Body temperature is commonly elevated to 42.2° C (106° F) or greater. This state of severe illness remains practically unchanged for 5 to 7 days, after which there is remarkably fast recovery. The morbidity rate will approach 100 per cent. The mortality rate in uncomplicated cases is usually less than 1 per cent. Most death losses are in suckling pigs.

The lesions observed in acute swine influenza are those of a viral pneumonia. The mucosa of the pharynx, larynx, trachea, and large bronchi is hyperemic and covered with mucus. The small bronchi and bronchioles are completely filled with exudate. There is a sharp line of demarcation between normal and pneumonic lung. Cervical and mediastinal lymph nodes are enlarged and edematous and may be congested.

In fatal cases with the more severe lesions, there is more fibrin in the bronchial exudate and accumulation of fibrin on the pleural surfaces of the lung and thoracic wall. In natural fatal cases, there may be a lobular pneumonia involving about 60 per cent of all lobes. The involved areas were plum-colored and slightly firm.

DIAGNOSIS

SI may be suspected when there is an outbreak of acute respiratory disease involving most or all of the pigs in a herd. Although signs of the classic disease may be present, a clinical diagnosis is presumptive. There are conditions that are clinically identical to classic SI that are not caused by the SIV. Furthermore, the SIV has been recovered from cases of poorly defined respiratory disease that have no similarity to the classic disease. SI must be differentiated from enzootic pneumonia of pigs and other acute and chronic respiratory diseases.

A definitive diagnosis of SI can be made only by the isolation and identification of SIV or by demonstration of specific antibodies. The most common method for isolation of virus is by intra-amniotic or intra-allantoic inoculation of embryonated (10 to 12 days) chicken eggs. Nasal mucus is obtained by swabbing and is then suspended in a suitable transport medium such as glycerol-saline and injected into the embryonated eggs. Pharyngeal mucus may be obtained by swabbing in very small pigs, in which it is difficult to swab the nasal passages. Virus is more likely to be found in nasal secretion during the febrile period than after the fever has subsided.

Serologic diagnosis of SI requires the testing of paired serum samples, one obtained during the acute phase of the disease and the other 3 to 4 weeks after the first sample, to demonstrate an increase in amount of antibody. The hemagglutination inhibition test is most commonly employed for serologic diagnosis of SI.

Positive diagnosis of the disease by serologic and virologic means among suckling or weanling pigs from dams with antibody to the virus may be complicated. Maternal antibody persists 2 to 4 months, depending on the initial level. It has been shown that weanling pigs with maternal antibody may be infected and may shed virus.

TREATMENT

There is no specific therapy for SI. Careful nursing is important, with the provision of a comfortable, draft-free shelter. Clean, dry, dust-free bedding should be provided. Pigs should not be moved or transported during the acute stages of the disease to avoid additional stress to the respiratory system.

Expectorants are commonly used as a herd treatment and are administered in the drinking water. Antimicrobial agents have been used on a herd basis to control concurrent or secondary bacterial infections.

PREVENTION

There are no licensed vaccines available in the United States for the prevention of SI.

BIBLIOGRAPHY

Easterday BC: Swine influenza. In Leman AD, et al (eds): Diseases of Swine, 5th ed. Ames, IA, Iowa State University Press, 1981, p 184.
Gillespie JH, Timoney JF: Swine influenza. In Gillespie JH, Timoney JF (eds): Hagan and Bruner's Infectious Diseases of Domestic Animals, 7th ed. Ithaca, NY, Cornell University Press, 1981, p 711.
Kaplan MM, Webster RG: The epidemiology of influenza. Sci Am 237:88–105, 1977.

Paramyxovirus (Blue Eye Disease of Swine)

ALBERTO STEPHANO, DVM, MC

The blue eye is a disease of pigs associated with a paramyxovirus infection and characterized by central nervous system disorders, reproductive failure, and corneal opacity.

This new disease emerged in 1980 in central Mexico with numerous outbreaks of encephalitis and corneal opacity in piglets, from which a hemagglutinating virus was isolated. This virus was identified as a member of the Paramyxoviridae group and was shown not to be serologically related to previously described paramyxoviruses; it was named the blue eye paramyxovirus (BEP). The blue eye has become an economically important disease of pigs because it produces mortality with nervous system disorders in piglets and, in some outbreaks in older pigs, causes reproductive failure in the sow and infertility with orchitis and epididymitis in boars.

This disease has not been reported elsewhere, nor have clinical signs similar to those described in blue eye been observed in other species.

ETIOLOGY

The BEP, a member of the family Paramyxoviridae, is more or less spherical, measuring from 135×148 nm to 257×360 nm; the particle has a surface covered with a layer of closely spaced projections or spikes and contains a nucleocapsid. It easily replicates in a great variety of primary cultures and cell line monolayer cultures as well as in chick embryos; in the primary pig kidney and in the PK-15 monolayer cultures, syncytium formation and intracytoplasmic inclusion bodies occur. It hemagglutinates erythrocytes from domestic and laboratory animals as well as human cells. Spontaneous elution at 37° C is observed. Infected PK-15 cells were also positive to hemadsorption with chicken erythrocytes. Antisera prepared against paramyxovirus serotypes 1, 2, 3, 4, 6, and 7 as well as parainfluenza serotypes 1, 2, 3, 4a, 4b, and 5 were not able to affect the BEP infectivity. The BEP is inactivated with ether, chloroform, formalin, β-propiolactone, and heat treatment.

EPIZOOTIOLOGY

The blue eye has been confirmed only in pigs in Mexico. It first appeared in La Piedad, Michoacan, in 1980, and spread to 12 different states. The northwest and the Yucatan Peninsula, which are swine-producing areas, remain free of the disease. Blue eye is more common from March to July, which are the driest and hottest months of the year in the affected area, but outbreaks are observed throughout the year.

In commercial breeding units, the problem may start in any area; usually it is first observed in the farrowing house, with central nervous system signs and high piglet mortality. At about the same time, the farmer may observe corneal opacity.

Of the litters farrowed during an outbreak, 20 to 65 per cent are affected. In these litters, the piglet morbidity is between 20 and 50 per cent; the mortality of the affected pigs is between 87 and 90 per cent. The piglet mortality lasts 2 to 9 weeks, depending mainly on the system of management.

Transmission has been confirmed to occur by direct contact with infected pigs. Pigs subclinically infected are the main source of the disease; the virus may also be disseminated by people and vehicles. Other sources of infection have not been demonstrated, but wind and possibly birds could be incriminated.

It has been proved that the disease is self-limiting in close herds. The mortality rate rises rapidly and falls within a short time. Once the initial outbreak is over, no new clinical cases appear unless susceptible pigs are introduced to an infected farm, as has been observed on farms that operate on a continuous-flow pattern. Some farms after an outbreak may have occasional cases of corneal opacity without mortality or other manifestations.

Naturally infected animals develop antibodies that usually persist throughout their life. Infected farms within an enzootic area have become affected 3 years later.

Experimentally, the BEP affects mice and chick embryos; rabbits, dogs, and cats do not show clinical signs, but the rabbit produced antibodies.

CLINICAL SIGNS AND LESIONS

The clinical signs are variable and depend mainly on the age of the pig. Piglets 2 to 15 days old are most susceptible. The first clinical signs are fever, a staring hair coat, and an arched back followed by progressive nervous signs: ataxia, weakness, rigidity mainly of the hind legs, muscle tremor, abnormal posture, and prostration generally in lateral recumbency. Some piglets suffer from conjunctivitis with swollen eyelids and lacrimation. Often the eyelids are closed and adherent with exudate. In 1 to 10 per cent of the affected piglets, either unilateral or bilateral corneal opacity is present. Corneal opacity can frequently be seen in piglets without other signs and is commonly observed to resolve spontaneously. Some piglets may be found dead without prior illness.

After weaning, pigs more than 30 days old usually remain asymptomatic, but some show moderate and transient clinical signs such as anorexia, fever, sneezing, and coughing. Nervous system signs are rare. Only 1 to 4 per cent of pigs older than 30 days have corneal opacity, and the mortality is low. Badly managed farms have usually had central nervous system manifestations and mortality in pigs up to 45 kg.

Most of the adult animals are clinically normal. Some of them show moderate anorexia, and a few corneal opacity. Central nervous system manifestations have been observed. In pregnant sows, an increase in the number of animals returning to estrus is observed. This sign lasts 6 to 8 months. Abortion has been observed in some dams. During outbreaks, there is also an increase in stillbirths and mummified fetuses up to 24 per cent and 5 per cent, respectively. In boars, there is a reduction in fertility associated with an increase in the size of the testicle and epididymis, usually unilateral, and later there is testicular atrophy with hardness of the epididymis; 14 to 40 per cent of the boars in the farm are so affected.

There are no specific gross changes. A mild pneumonia is frequently observed at the ventral tips of the cranial lung lobes. Mild gastric distention with milk (in piglets), distention of the urinary bladder with urine, and small accumulation of fluid with fibrin in the peritoneal cavity were observed. Brain congestion was also a feature. Conjunctivitis, chemosis, and varied degrees of corneal opacity have been confirmed; vesicle formation, ulcers, and keratoconus in the cornea as well as exudate in the anterior chamber have been observed. Recently, pericardiac and kidney hemorrhages have been observed.

In boars, there are orchitis, epididymitis, and, later, testicular atrophy with or without granulomatous formations in the epididymis.

The main histologic changes are located in the brain and spinal cord. There is a nonsuppurative encephalomyelitis affecting mainly the gray matter of the thalamus, midbrain, and cerebral cortex. This is characterized by multifocal and diffuse gliosis; perivascular cuffing with lymphocytes, plasma cells, and reticular cells; neuronal necrosis; neuronophagia; meningitis; and choroiditis. Intracytoplasmic inclusion bodies are found in neurons. There are variations in the severity and extent of these lesions.

The lungs have localized, scattered areas of interstitial pneumonia characterized by thickened septa with mononuclear cell infiltration.

Changes in the eye are mainly observed in those animals with corneal opacity and consist of corneal edema and anterior uveitis with neutrophils, macrophages, and mononuclear cells infiltrating mainly the iridocorneal endothelium. The external epithelium of the cornea is often with cytoplasmic vesicles, and in some, intracytoplasmic inclusions are observed in the epithelial cells near the corneoscleral angle.

DIAGNOSIS

The diagnosis of blue eye is based on the clinical signs and the pathologic findings. Encephalitis, corneal opacity, and reproductive failure in the sow or orchitis and epididymitis in the boar give the basis for a diagnosis. The nonsuppurative encephalitis, anterior uveitis, and keratitis also contribute.

Serologic tests such as hemagglutination inhibiting antibodies, neutralizing antibodies, and enzyme-linked immunosorbent assay (ELISA) have been developed to identify positive animals. Until now, hemagglutination inhibition has been the most reliable. Also, a direct immunofluorescence test has been performed in tissue section and monolayers by use of a conjugate prepared with rabbit or pig serum.

Virus isolation is easily performed in monolayers of PK-15 cells with brain and tonsil samples. A cytopathic effect characterized by syncytium formation occurs.

Differential diagnosis from other encephalitides and causes

of reproductive failure needs to be performed, especially against Aujeszky's disease. Only the BEP produces corneal opacity in up to 30 per cent of pigs.

PREVENTION AND CONTROL

Elimination of the blue eye paramyxovirus from infected herds has been performed by management practices such as closing the herd; cleaning and disinfecting; all-in, all-out; and elimination of clinically affected animals (nervous signs or infertile boars). This is followed by serologic testing, herd performance analyses, and sentinel BEP-seronegative pigs for confirming the elimination of the BEP.

A vaccine of killed virus, elaborated in cell monolayer cultures, is being developed; preliminary trials are encouraging.

BIBLIOGRAPHY

Stephano HA, Gay GM, Ramirez TC, Maqueda AJJ: Estudio de un brote de Encefalitis en lechones por un virus hemoaglutinante. Mexico, Memorias del XVII Congreso de la Sociacion Mexicana de Veterinarios Especialistas en Cerdos, 1981, p 43.
Stephano HA, Gay GM: Experimental studies of a new viral syndrome in pigs called "blue eye" characterized by encephalitis and corneal opacity. Ghent, Belgium, Proceedings, 8th International Pig Veterinary Society Congress, 1984, p 71.
Stephano HA, Gay GM: El sindrome del ojo azul en cerdos I. Sintesis Porcina 4:42–49, 1985.
Stephano HA, Gay M, Kresse J: Properties of a paramyxovirus associated to a new syndrome (blue eye) characterized by encephalitis, reproductive failure and corneal opacity. Barcelona, Spain, Proceedings, 9th International Pig Veterinary Society Congress, 1986, p 455.
Stephano HA, Gay GM: Encefalitis, trastornos reproductivos y opacidad de la cornea en cerdos (sindrome del ojo azul) asociados a un paramyxovirus. Estudio cronologico. Med Vet 3:359–362, 1986.
Stephano HA, Gay GM: Encefalitis, falla reproductiva y opacidad de la cornea, ojo azul. Sintesis Porcina 5:26–39, 1986.
Stephano HA, Gay GM: El sindrome del ojo azul. Una nueva enfermedad en cerdos asociada a un paramyxovirus. Vet Mexico 17:120–122, 1986.
Stephano HA, Gay GM, Ramirez TC: Encephalomyelitis, reproductive failure and corneal opacity in pigs, associated with a new paramyxovirus infection (blue eye). Vet Rec 122:6–10, 1988.

Vesicular Stomatitis Virus in Swine

ALVIN W. SMITH, DVM, PhD

The etiologic agent, a Rhabdoviridae of the genus *Vesiculovirus*, has been discussed in detail in Vesicular Stomatitis Virus in Cattle. Also included in that article is additional information on epizootiology, clinical signs and lesions, diagnosis, treatment, prevention, and control.

There are some differences, however, between the virus in cattle and that in swine. During the periodic epizootics that occur, pigs have not been involved to the same extent as cattle and horses have been. Swine that ingest the virus will develop antibodies but not clinical disease, and garbage feeding has not been a means of transmission or a concern in the control of the disease in pigs. Intravenous injections of virus will cause foot and snout lesions. Fighting and abrading mucous membranes may be other primary means of spread in pigs. Pigs that contract the disease through natural exposure are seen to have foot lesions more often than snout lesions, and lameness may be the only sign noted on initial examination.

The diagnosis of vesicular stomatitis in swine is more complicated than it is in cattle because the disease must be differentiated from swine vesicular disease (an enterovirus) and vesicular exanthema of swine (a calicivirus) in addition to foot-and-mouth disease. All 4 of these virus diseases of swine occur with mouth and foot lesions that are clinically identical. Virus isolation or visualization and serologic examinations are essential for rapid and definitive diagnosis of this disease in pigs.

BIBLIOGRAPHY

Redelman D, Nichol S, Klieform R, et al: Experimental vesicular stomatitis virus infection of swine: extent of infection and immunological response. Vet Immunol Immunopathol 20:345–361, 1989.

Mycoplasmosis of Swine

Swine Mycoplasmosis

C. H. ARMSTRONG, DVM, PhD
RICHARD F. ROSS, DVM, PhD

PNEUMONIA CAUSED BY *Mycoplasma hyopneumoniae*

Mycoplasmal pneumonia of swine (MPS; also called enzootic pneumonia of pigs) is a chronic disease that occurs in all of the major swine-producing regions of the world. A high proportion of all conventional herds are affected. The disease also occurs in some minimal disease or SPF herds. Annual losses in the United States have been estimated to be $200 million.

The causative agent of MPS is *Mycoplasma* (M.) *hyopneumoniae* (*suipneumoniae*). The only known host of *M. hyopneumoniae* is the pig. Transmission is from infected pig to susceptible pig via infective aerosols or contact. Swine of all ages are susceptible to MPS; however, in affected herds, young pigs may be resistant to infection as a result of maternal antibodies. These pigs become infected at two to four months of age when they are commingled with older swine in the growing and finishing units.

The typical lesion is purple in color and lobular in distribution and is most apt to be seen in the ventral aspects of the apical and cardiac lobes of the lungs. During the active phase of infection, lobules are slightly swollen and have a lymphoid texture when cut. The airways of such lungs contain a sticky white exudate that is laden with *M. hyopneumoniae* organisms. Later, the lobules are contracted slightly, and the airways contain little or no exudate. Eventually, lesions in uncomplicated cases resolve completely, with only slight fibrosis.

MPS is characterized by high morbidity and zero mortality. Clinical signs include a chronic, dry, nonproductive cough;

rough hair coat; retarded growth rate; and inefficient utilization of feed. The severity of these signs is influenced directly by the quality of the environment and by concurrent diseases such as bacterial pneumonias and ascarid migration.

Many laboratories diagnose MPS entirely on the basis of gross and microscopic lesions. The lesions associated with MPS are characteristic but not pathognomonic. Consequently, the use of lesions as the sole criterion of MPS can result in false-positive diagnoses. It should also be emphasized that the absence of gross lesions does not prove freedom from infection. A definitive diagnosis requires that *M. hyopneumoniae* be visualized in immunofluorescence (IF)–stained lung sections or that it be recovered culturally. The preferred specimen is a lung in the active stage of infection. The IF test should be performed first because it is rapid and relatively inexpensive. The IF test is specific, and positive results are reliable; however, negative results do not prove absence of infection. Therefore, IF-negative lungs should be examined culturally. Unfortunately, few diagnostic laboratories are capable of isolating and identifying *M. hyopneumoniae* owing to its fastidious nature. The complement fixation test and indirect hemagglutination test have been used to diagnose MPS ante mortem. These tests are useful when they are applied on a herd basis but lack the sensitivity and the specificity for reliably identifying infected swine on an individual basis. The enzyme-linked immunosorbent assay (ELISA) with Tween 20 extract of *M. hyopneumoniae* holds promise of being a highly sensitive and specific serodiagnostic test for MPS.

Control of MPS is best accomplished by providing good ventilation and optimal temperature, avoiding overcrowding, and controlling associated diseases such as bacterial pneumonias, atrophic rhinitis, and ascariasis. Tetracyclines, lincomycin, tylosin, and tiamulin have been reported to reduce the incidence and severity of lesions and improve growth rate and feed utilization efficiency of MPS-affected swine. Tetracyclines have been shown to control MPS, if medication is begun before exposure. Conclusive evidence that any available antibiotic is highly effective in controlling the mycoplasma component of naturally occurring swine pneumonia has not been presented. Antibiotics are useful for controlling the bacterial component of swine pneumonia.

POLYSEROSITIS AND ARTHRITIS CAUSED BY *Mycoplasma hyorhinis*

Mycoplasma hyorhinis is a common inhabitant of the nasal cavity of pigs in all parts of the world. Piglets acquire the infection early in life via aerosols from or contact with older pigs and infected littermates. *M. hyorhinis* remains localized in the nasal cavity in most pigs and causes no perceptible illness. Some sort of stress appears to be a prerequisite to clinical disease; that is, stress leads to septicemia with a resulting localization of the organism in joints and on serosal membranes.

The disease occurs most commonly in pigs 3 to 10 weeks of age and occasionally in young adult swine. First evidence of illness appears 3 to 10 days after stress. Clinical signs include fever, restlessness, dull hair coat, reluctance to move, abdominal tenderness, labored breathing, swollen joints, and lameness. Acute-phase lesions consist of serofibrinous pleuritis, pericarditis, peritonitis, synovitis, and arthritis. There is regression of the signs associated with polyserositis in 10 to 14 days. The most severe signs of arthritis are seen after the acute phase of illness has passed. Arthritis generally persists for 2 to 3 months, and some swine may be lame for as long as 6 months.

Diagnosis depends on isolating *M. hyorhinis* from affected tissues. *M. hyorhinis* grows well on a variety of mycoplasmal media and is relatively easy to isolate and identify. Swine in the acute phase of the disease are preferred diagnostic specimens, especially for the polyserositis phase of infection. However, the organism can be recovered from joints for several weeks after the acute phase of the disease. Diseases that must be differentiated include Glasser's disease (a polyserositis caused by *Haemophilus parasuis*); polyserositis caused by agents such as *Streptococcus suis*, *Pasteurella multocida*, or *Salmonella* spp.; and erysipelas arthritis.

M. hyorhinis is susceptible in vitro to a variety of antibiotics, but the use of such compounds clinically is disappointing. The best way to control the disease is to reduce stress, that is, to control respiratory and intestinal infections and to provide a good environment.

ARTHRITIS CAUSED BY *Mycoplasma hyosynoviae*

A high percentage of sows in the United States harbor *M. hyosynoviae* in their nasopharynx. Pigs acquire the infection from adult carriers or from infected penmates via nasopharyngeal secretions. Most pigs are at least 6 to 8 weeks of age before they become infected. Intranasal exposure is followed in 2 to 4 days by septicemia. The septicemia persists for 8 to 10 days and may lead to joint infection. The factors leading to joint disease have not been defined. Age may be important. It has been suggested that exposure before 10 weeks of age results in inapparent disease and resistance to arthritis later in life. Arthritis reportedly is more severe in certain genetic strains of heavily muscled swine with straight legs. It has also been suggested that swine with osteochondrosis may experience more severe arthritis when they are infected with *M. hyosynoviae*.

M. hyosynoviae induces a nonsuppurative polyarthritis with little or no fever. There is no polyserositis. The disease is most common in swine 10 to 20 weeks of age. It is characterized by an acute lameness of sudden onset that persists 3 to 10 days. The acute phase is usually followed by gradual recovery. Synovial fluid is increased in volume and at first is serosanguineous and later yellowish-brown.

A definitive diagnosis depends on isolation of the causative agent. *M. hyosynoviae* is readily recovered from affected joints during the acute phase of illness but disappears rapidly thereafter. Synovial fluids should be collected from several untreated swine and examined by a microbiologist familiar with the mycoplasmas.

Swine in the acute phase of the disease respond well to intramuscular tylosin, lincomycin, or tiamulin. Prevention includes use of breeding stock with good leg conformation and avoidance of stress during the period of greatest susceptibility. Early weaning and subsequent rearing in the absence of carrier swine may also be effective.

BIBLIOGRAPHY

Ross RF: Mycoplasmal diseases. *In* Leman AD, et al (eds): Diseases of Swine, 5th ed. Ames, IA, Iowa State University Press, 1981, pp 535–549.

Whittlestone P: Porcine mycoplasmas. *In* Tully JG, Whitcomb RF (eds): The Mycoplasmas, vol II. New York, Academic Press, 1979, pp 133–176.

SECTION 8
Bacterial and Fungal Diseases

SØREN ROSENDAL, DVM, PhD, Consulting Editor
JOHN F. PRESCOTT, Vet MB, PhD, Consulting Editor

Haemophilus parasuis Infection (Glasser's Disease)

NONIE L. SMART, BSc, DVM, MSc

Haemophilus parasuis causes polyserositis and polyarthritis in susceptible pigs. This syndrome was named Glasser's disease in 1910, at the time when K. Glasser first described the sporadic occurrence of this disease in young weaned pigs. More recently, outbreaks of Glasser's disease associated with high morbidity and high mortality have occurred in groups of SPF pigs of all ages. For this reason, Glasser's disease has taken on new importance in modern swine practice.

ETIOLOGIC AGENT

H. parasuis is a gram-negative coccobacillus that is normally found in the nasal passages of apparently healthy conventionally raised swine. There is some evidence that *H. parasuis* is associated with the development of enzootic pneumonia and atrophic rhinitis, but a large proportion of *H. parasuis* culture-positive pigs show no clinical signs as a result of infection.

H. parasuis requires V factor (NAD) for cultivation on blood agar, but unlike some other *Haemophilus* organisms, it does not require the X factor (heme) for growth. There is a great deal of genetic heterogeneity between isolates of *H. parasuis*; however, a classification system based on phenotypic, genotypic, or virulence differences between strains has not yet been fully worked out.

PATHOGENESIS

In conventional pig herds, Glasser's disease usually occurs sporadically in young weaned pigs. Affected animals may die, but more often they exhibit unthriftiness as a result of chronic sequelae. Because *H. parasuis* is widespread in conventional swine environments, young pigs are exposed to the organism at birth or shortly thereafter. Piglets are passively protected from Glasser's disease by maternal antibodies and develop active immunity at about 8 weeks of age. Piglets that receive inadequate or poor-quality colostrum or those that are stressed at the time when maternal antibody begins to wane are at risk of developing Glasser's disease. In rare instances, large numbers of young pigs may become affected with Glasser's disease. These outbreaks are usually traced to extreme environmental conditions at or after weaning, such as chilling, mixing, or transit.

Glasser's disease in SPF pigs can be quite different. In situations in which SPF pigs have been exposed to conventional pigs (after the sale of breeding stock or the mixing of fattening pigs), outbreaks of Glasser's disease with high morbidity and mortality have occurred in the SPF pigs, whereas the conventional pigs remained unaffected. Specific pathogen-free pigs do not develop immunity to Glasser's disease because *H. parasuis* is often absent from the SPF environment. Thus clinical disease in this group of pigs correlates with their first exposure to *H. parasuis* regardless of age. There are some SPF herds infected with organisms identified as *H. parasuis*, but these organisms do not appear to stimulate serum antibodies that are protective against other field strains of *H. parasuis*. For this reason, culture-positive pigs may be quite susceptible to Glasser's disease when they are moved from SPF or minimal disease facilities.

CLINICAL SIGNS

Clinical signs usually begin 2 to 7 days after infection. The clinical course of Glasser's disease may range from peracute to chronic, and thus the clinical signs will vary accordingly. In peracute cases, apparently healthy animals may die within 12 to 24 hours. This syndrome is most common to SPF pigs. Less acute disease is characterized by an initial inappetence, depression, and pyrexia that may be accompanied by lameness involving one or more limbs. Joints may be hot and swollen, and as a result of the pain, pigs may squeal and assume a dog-sitting position. As the disease progresses, neurologic signs such as incoordination, recumbency, and convulsions may become apparent. Death soon follows the initiation of these signs. Animals that recover from infection are often chronically lame or unthrifty. Other clinical signs of Glasser's disease that have been reported are dyspnea, coughing, purple discoloration of the skin of extremities, and swelling of eyelids and ears.

NECROPSY

Lesions seen at post-mortem examination may vary depending on the length of the clinical course of infection and immune response of the pig. When pigs die acutely, the gross post-mortem lesions are often negligible. When pigs have shown a clinical course of several days, fibrinous serositis and serous effusion may be found in association with meninges, pleura, pericardium, peritoneum, and synovia. The extent of the lesions may range from mild to severe and occur singly or in combination. The latter necropsy picture is most common to conventional pigs, whereas SPF pigs are much more likely to die quickly with minimal post-mortem lesions. Other lesions reported include swollen liver, spleen, and lymph nodes; pulmonary edema; and renal glomerular necrosis. Pleural adhesions are often found at slaughter in recovered or subclinical cases.

DIAGNOSIS

A diagnosis of Glasser's disease is based on a history of exposure of SPF pigs to conventional swine, post-mortem findings, or isolation of *H. parasuis* from body fluids or tissues other than the respiratory tract. Gram-stained smears of fibrinous exudate may also be used to confirm the presence of bacteria. Seroconversion of *H. parasuis*–negative SPF pigs has been used to confirm exposure of pigs to *H. parasuis*; however, serologic surveys are not performed under routine circumstances.

Unfortunately, *H. parasuis* may be difficult to isolate under usual laboratory conditions even if fresh tissue specimens are cultured. Small opaque colonies appear in 24 to 36 hours, and isolates that satellite *Staphylococcus aureus* colonies or NAD-impregnated disks can tentatively be identified as *Haemophilus* organisms on the basis of their requirement for V factor. The use of a selective medium incorporating lincomycin, bacitracin, and crystal violet in a chocolate agar will reduce the overgrowth of more vigorous organisms and increase the chance of recovery of this fastidious bacterium.

DIFFERENTIAL DIAGNOSIS

Infectious and noninfectious conditions that present similarly to Glasser's disease include sudden death, septicemia, lameness, and diseases of neurologic dysfunction. Sudden death due to nutritional myopathy, exsanguination due to gastric ulceration, salt toxicosis, and fibrinous pleuropneumonia caused by *Actinobacillus pleuropneumoniae* can usually be differentiated at post mortem. Bacterial causes of septicemia such as β-hemolytic streptococci, *Escherichia coli*, or *Salmonella* can be cultured under routine laboratory conditions, as can the other infectious agents *(Streptococcus suis* and *E. rhusiopathiae)* that might mimic Glasser's disease. *Mycoplasma hyorhinis* causes a disease similar to Glasser's disease but in younger pigs, and the clinical signs are usually milder with lower mortality and with lameness as the predominant sign. Viral agents that cause nervous disease can usually be ruled out on the basis of clinical and histopathologic considerations.

TREATMENT

Antibiotic treatment of pigs affected with Glasser's disease is often unrewarding. Affected animals may not respond to therapy unless they are treated very early in the clinical course of the disease, and those that do survive may develop chronic sequelae. Administration of antibiotics via water is usually less effective than is parenteral therapy because sick pigs are usually anorectic. Antibiotics recommended for use include chloramphenicol (not permitted for use in food animals in North America), ampicillin, penicillin, tetracycline, and trimethoprim-sulfamethoxazole; penicillin is the drug of choice.

In outbreaks involving large numbers of SPF pigs, the spread of clinical infection within the herd may be controlled by vaccination of all susceptible animals including pregnant sows and weaned piglets.

PREVENTION

In conventional pigs, in which Glasser's disease is enzootic, attention should be given to management practices that affect the quality of the environment for young pigs. It is particularly important that transfer of passive immunity to piglets be optimized. The effectiveness of vaccination in controlling enzootic Glasser's disease has not been determined.

Specific pathogen-free pigs, of all ages, should be vaccinated at least 2 to 3 weeks before anticipated exposure to conventional swine. All vaccinates should receive a booster dose 2 to 3 weeks after the initial inoculation. Animals must be closely monitored upon arrival at the new facility, preferably isolated from the main herd and integrated in a stepwise fashion. Prophylactic antibiotics given parenterally or in feed or water have not been shown to be effective in preventing Glasser's disease outbreaks in SPF pigs introduced to conventional facilities. In order to prevent the entry of *H. parasuis* into an SPF facility, it is essential that these animals be maintained in strict isolation from conventional swine.

BIBLIOGRAPHY

Leman AD, Straw B, Glock RD, et al: Diseases of Swine, 6th ed. Ames, IA, Iowa State University Press, 1986, pp 426–428.
Nielsen R, Danielson V: An outbreak of Glasser's disease. Studies on etiology, serology, and effect of vaccination. Nord Vet Med 27:20–25, 1975.

Nonvenereal Campylobacteriosis

ROGER MARSHALL, BVSc, MS, PhD

The diseases covered under this heading are those resulting from infection with *Campylobacter* spp. Diarrhea is the sign generally associated with *C. jejuni* and *C. coli* infection, whereas abortions and infertility are associated with *C. fetus* subsp. *fetus*, *C. fetus* subsp. *venerealis*, and *C. cryaerophilia*. Bovine abortions and infertility, however, are dealt with in a separate section. The significance of *Campylobacter* spp. as diarrhea producers has been debated over the years, and the widespread distribution of these organisms among animals has not made their etiologic role any easier to establish. The association of these bacteria with healthy animals does not mean that they do not contribute to disease, either on their own or in partnership with other microorganisms. The more recent definition of *C. cryaerophilia*, an aerotolerant campylobacter, has made us realize that there may be more organisms in this genus whose role has yet to be elucidated. An attempt has been made in this section to indicate the extent of knowledge about the contribution of the various campylobacter to production animal disease.

CATTLE

Etiology

Campylobacter jejuni and *C. coli* are associated with disease in cattle but have also been isolated from normal animals. Pure cultures of *C. jejuni* have been used to reproduce enteric disease in both milk-fed and ruminating calves as well as in adult cattle. Infection with *C. fetus* subsp. *fetus* can initiate clinical changes resembling those produced by *C. jejuni*.

Distribution is worldwide but uncommon when animals are kept at pasture or in feedlots. Clinical disease is still not common but is more likely if the animals are housed and under a high standard of hygiene. This is presumed to be because housed animals are less likely to have acquired an immunity as a result of low-level challenge. The infection may occur in neonatal calves from the ingestion of milk that has become contaminated with feces containing *Campylobacter* or as a result of *Campylobacter* mastitis. In older animals, ingestion of contaminated feed is the most likely source.

Clinical Signs

Enteric disease due to *Campylobacter* spp. is generally regarded as mild and of minor clinical significance. Animals may be depressed and sometimes have an elevated temperature. The incubation period is 1 to 4 days; the animals remain clinically affected for up to 16 days. Dark feces with blood flecks are also sometimes seen. In experimental infections, calves produced thick mucoid feces sometimes with flecks of blood in the mucus within 72 hours. In a number of clinical cases as well as in experimental studies, an associated mild pneumonia with coughing has been reported, and *C. jejuni* has been isolated from lung lesions.

Diagnostic Features

Campylobacter may not be easily isolated from the feces owing to the intermittent nature of the excretion and depending on the efficiency of the isolation medium used. A rise in antibody titer against homologous organisms is consistently found in experimental infections, and it is assumed that this also occurs with natural infections. *C. jejuni* and *C. fetus* subsp. *fetus* are isolated from the mucosa of ileum, cecum, and colon and sometimes gallbladder, jejunum, abomasum, and mesenteric lymph nodes of domestic animals. The ubiquitous nature of *C. jejuni* makes it difficult to determine the relevance of its isolation from the environment, from other animal sources, and even on occasions from pathologic samples. There is a great need for a technique to differentiate pathogenic from nonpathogenic strains. DNA studies have shown that there are a large number of genotypes within the species that can be differentiated by DNA fingerprinting methods. The degree to which these strains are animal species–specific in their ability to colonize, let alone produce disease, is not yet defined.

Necropsy Findings

The ileum is the most frequently affected section of the intestine with excess clear mucus present and dark contents. The serosal surface of the ileum is pale, the walls are thickened and fleshy, and the mucosa is rough, granular, and slightly red. The jejunum may also be affected to a greater or lesser extent. The cecum and colon are usually grossly normal. Stunted villi, dilated crypts often filled with inflammatory cells, dilated capillaries, and mononuclear cell infiltration in small intestinal mucosa are all signs of enteric disease, but these are not specific to *Campylobacter* infection.

Treatment and Control

Owing to the poorly understood nature of this infection, it is usually not necessary to do anything other than treat cases symptomatically; but should antibiotics be deemed necessary, neomycin, erythromycin, or tetracyclines have been found to be useful. No control program is usually necessary; diarrheic illness is mild and self-limiting. Prognosis is generally good. Clinical signs disappear in time, and the number of organisms that can be found in the feces gradually reduces.

Public Health Aspects

C. jejuni causes diarrhea in human beings, and epidemiologic links between bovine and human infection have been made. Most of these infections have been due to the consumption of unpasteurized milk and have resulted in large outbreaks. *C. fetus* subsp. *fetus* is also capable of producing an enteric syndrome in human subjects that is similar to that caused by *C. jejuni* but is generally less severe. *Campylobacter*-like organisms can initiate lesions with features of those of *C. jejuni*. This organism may act in concert with other enteric disease agents and result in a disease more severe than either agent alone is capable of producing.

SHEEP

Etiology

Two species of *Campylobacter* have been isolated from the feces or enteric tracts of sheep. They are *C. fetus* subsp. *fetus* and *C. jejuni*. *Campylobacter*-like organisms and *C. jejuni* are commonly isolated from healthy grazing sheep and appear to be normal inhabitants of the gut. Distribution is worldwide, but disease is not common. Infection with all these types of *Campylobacter* is probably acquired by ingestion of feed or water contaminated with feces. An animal infected with *C. fetus* subsp. *fetus* may suffer a bacteremia; if the animal is pregnant, this may be followed by a fetal septicemia with hepatitis and death and expulsion of the fetus. The consequences of *C. fetus* subsp. *fetus* infection are much less equivocal than are those that follow *C. jejuni* infection. There is little information on the degree of immunity that may develop as a result of natural infection to either species. The large number of serotypes present in the environment in some countries makes it likely that immunity resulting from infection with one serotype will be of limited protective value because of the presence of many other serotypes. Little is known about the pathogenesis of campylobacter enteritis in sheep; more is known about the abortion aspects of the disease. *C. fetus* subsp. *fetus* is a well-recognized cause of abortion and stillbirth in ewes in late pregnancy. During interepidemic times, the abortion-producing organisms are carried in the gallbladder and intestine of sheep and are spread by fecal contamination of food and water. After ingestion of the *Campylobacter* organisms, ewes may experience a bacteremia for up to 1 to 2 weeks, during which time, if the ewe is in the latter part of pregnancy, the placenta and the fetus become infected.

Clinical Signs

In some field outbreaks of colitis with its associated diarrhea, *Campylobacter*-like organisms have been isolated that may play a role, but this has yet to be substantiated. Blood-flecked mucoid feces, but not diarrhea, have been induced experimentally in ewes by giving *C. jejuni* orally. Abortion and stillbirth occur in late pregnancy.

Diagnostic Features

Campylobacter spp. are found in the intestines, feces, and gallbladder. All clinical specimens should be kept at 4° C and cultured within 6 hours. In outbreaks of abortion, the etiologic agent must be distinguished from other possible causes such as *Toxoplasma gondii*, *Chlamydia psittaci*, and *Listeria monocytogenes*. The number of ewes aborting and the necropsy appearance of the liver and cotyledons will help. *Campylobacter* can be readily demonstrated in a stained smear made directly from the fetal abomasal contents or from a cotyledon. The abortions usually affect only 1 or 2 ewes at the start of the outbreak, but this is followed by an abortion storm in which up to 20 per cent of the flock or even higher may be affected, if the flock has a large proportion of maiden (2-tooth) ewes. The outbreak results in widespread contamination of pasture with the products of abortion, which leads to heavy contamination of the farm with *C. fetus* subsp. *fetus*. There is no venereal spread of the infection. Lambs are sometimes born alive but are weak and usually die within a few days. A convalescent immunity may occur in the ewes that will prevent subsequent infections for 2 to 3 years. Ewes that abort usually produce normal lambs in subsequent years.

Necropsy Findings

In cases of enteritis, an increased fluidity of the colonic contents may be all that is seen. In severe cases, ascites, subcutaneous edema, and loss of adipose tissue may be seen. A necropsy appearance seen in a high proportion of abortion cases is pale areas of focal necrosis in liver, up to 25 mm in size, often with reddened margins. The cotyledon appears edematous, a general feature of abortions. Erosion of the cecal and colonic superficial epithelium and infiltration of the lamina propria by neutrophils occur, with flattened epithelium and dilated glands containing necrotic debris. Some severe cases show deeper ulceration of the mucosa. The microscopic appearance of the cotyledon is sufficiently characteristic that it should always, when possible, be submitted to the diagnostic laboratory.

Treatment and Control

Treatment is usually not necessary for enteritis cases, but with outbreaks of abortions, streptomycin at the rate of 70 mg/kg body weight has been used. The success of such treatment depends on the stage of the epidemic, the earlier the better. The value of the sheep will determine if such an expense is warranted. The enteric form of the disease is usually self-limiting and therefore requires no specific control program. A vaccine produced from a killed suspension of *C. fetus* subsp. *fetus* is available in some countries for control of abortion outbreaks, but to be effective it must be given before animals are exposed to infection. The success of the vaccine will depend on how well the field strains are represented in the vaccine. If a diagnosis is made early enough, vaccination may be used to protect those ewes not yet exposed. Because of the sporadic nature of this disease and the low unit value of the animals, it is seldom justified to maintain this vaccination program beyond the year of the outbreak. However, annual vaccination is recommended if abortions are known to occur each year. As an alternative to this regimen, only replacement ewes, especially young ewes, need be vaccinated. The first dose is given before the rams are put out and the second dose at the time the rams are withdrawn. By the end of an outbreak, most of the ewes are likely to have been exposed to infection and will have developed an immunity. In these cases, vaccination is usually reserved for any new ewes that are to be added to the flock.

Public Health Aspects

The role of sheep meat as a source of *C. jejuni* infections in humans has not been seriously investigated and so far no epidemiologic linkage has been established. Mouth-to-mouth resuscitation of weak lambs, however, can present a hazard, and a condition known as shepherd's scours has been recognized.

GOATS

Occasional reports of abortion due to *C. fetus* subsp. *fetus* or *C. jejuni* have been documented.

PIGS

Etiology

The significance of *C. coli* and *C. jejuni* infections in pigs has been the subject of debate, and the discovery of *Serpula (Treponema) hyodysenteriae* as the causal organism of swine dysentery relegated *C. coli* to the status of nonpathogen. However, large numbers of *C. coli* have been recovered from the inflamed intestinal mucosa of young pigs without there being any evidence of *Treponema* spp. infection. Therefore, the possibility that *C. coli* can, on occasions, act alone or in concert with other potential pathogens to produce disease cannot be ruled out. Surveys have shown that 60 to 100 per cent of postweaning pigs are infected with *C. coli*. Infected sows are the major source of infection for piglets. *C. jejuni* is rarely isolated from pigs. Experimental oral inoculation of 7-day-old colostrum-deprived pigs, conventional suckling pigs, and conventional weaned pigs has been undertaken. Within 4 days of inoculation, both the preweaned groups developed elevated temperatures and mucoid yellow diarrhea containing occasional flecks of blood in the feces; the mucosa was hyperemic, and the mesenteric lymph nodes were enlarged. No clinical signs were seen in the weaned animals.

Distribution is worldwide; young pigs become colonized within the first few days of life with the same strains colonizing either their dam or the pig that they are suckling. Infection is by ingestion.

Clinical Signs

Diarrhea supposedly resulting from *C. coli* infection is of varying severity but usually mild. The significance of this infection is negligible or unclear.

Diagnostic Features

Culturing the organism can be meaningless because its recovery is so common. A demonstrable serologic titer is likely to be more significant.

Necropsy Findings

Mild to moderate inflammation of the small intestinal mucosa is seen with possible enlargement of the draining lymph nodes. Nonspecific signs of enteric disease may occur such as stunted villi, dilated crypts containing inflammatory cells, dilated capillaries, and mononuclear cell infiltration.

Treatment and Control

The diarrhea is usually self-limiting; therefore control measures are usually not needed. Symptomatic treatment should be given; when necessary, neomycin, erythromycin, and tetracyclines can be used. Prognosis is generally good, especially if body fluid loss is controlled.

Public Health Aspects

Pig meat is considered a likely source of *C. coli* infection in humans, although extensive biotyping, serotyping, or DNA fingerprinting of pig isolates for comparison with human strains has not yet been reported.

Bovine Venereal Campylobacteriosis

JOHN DUFTY, BVSc, RDA
JILL VAUGHAN, BAppSc, FAIMLS, MASM

During the last few years, there has been an upsurge of interest in the campylobacters of medical and veterinary importance. As a consequence, substantial advances have been made in both the definition of this group of bacteria and the conditions they cause. In fact, these organisms have emerged as a common cause of gastrointestinal upsets in humans and in some instances are being isolated as frequently as are *Salmonella* sp. and *Shigella* sp. In the veterinary field, however, most attention still centers around *Campylobacter fetus* (formerly known as *Vibrio fetus*), which has long been recognized as a cause of infertility and abortion in cattle.

ETIOLOGY

There are 2 subspecies of *C. fetus*, both of which cause reproductive disorders in cattle. One of these, *C. fetus* subsp. *fetus*, is responsible for sporadic abortions in sheep and cattle. It cannot live in the nongravid uterus for long but is found in the gut and gallbladder of a wide range of animals, including birds, and spreads from one host to another by the ingestion of contaminated material. The organism is able to invade the body and can reach the gravid uterus via the blood stream.

Bovine venereal campylobacteriosis, on the other hand, is caused by *C. fetus* subsp. *venerealis*. This is a gram-negative, non-sporing, motile, spirally curved thin rod that possesses a single polar flagellum. In young cultures, microscopic cell morphology varies from comma-shaped single cells to double cells joined end to end to give a gull-winged or S-shaped outline. Longer spiral forms are more numerous after prolonged incubation; in old cultures or samples exposed to oxygen, coccoid forms or spheroplasts predominate.

C. fetus is strictly microaerophilic, growing at 25° and 37° C. It does not ferment carbohydrates, nor does it produce acid as a metabolic end-product. It is relatively slow-growing, and the typical domed, light gray or pearly-white colonies are not readily visible until after at least 3 days' incubation in a reduced atmosphere at 37° C. It will not grow at 43° C, and its resistance to both heat and desiccation is low.

Other important characteristics that differentiate *C. fetus*, the type species, from other members of the genus are the presence of catalase, an inability both to produce hydrogen sulfide on triple sugar iron medium and to hydrolyze hippurate, its sensitivity to cephalothin (30 μg), and resistance to nalidixic acid (30 μg). Overall, the subdivision of this genus into species and subspecies can be made on the basis of relatively few biochemical criteria.

C. fetus subsp. *venerealis* can also be separated on the basis of hydrogen sulfide production into 2 biotypes, *venerealis* and *intermedius*, the latter giving a positive test result when lead acetate is used as the indicator and the medium contains 0.02 per cent cystine. Both biotypes are, however, unable to grow on media containing 1 per cent glycine, a feature that distinguishes them from *C. fetus* subsp. *fetus*.

OCCURRENCE

Bovine venereal campylobacteriosis is widely distributed and endemic throughout most countries of the world. It is found only in cattle but is present in both dairy and beef herds held under a wide range of environmental and management conditions. The disease is one of the most important infectious causes of reduced breeding efficiency, economic losses arising through shortened lactation periods and reduced milk yields in seasonally calving dairy herds (fewer calves being available for sale or as potential herd replacements), and an increased culling rate due to more infertile or sterile cattle.

The distribution of each of the 2 biotypes of *C. fetus* subsp. *venerealis* appears to be somewhat variable; whereas biotype *venerealis* is generally more widespread, biotype *intermedius* is commonly isolated in Argentina, some parts of the United States, and the northern half of Australia.

EPIZOOTIOLOGY

Bovine venereal campylobacteriosis is a true venereal disease of cattle; the causal organism is confined to the female reproductive tract and the preputial cavity of bulls. Under normal circumstances, transmission of *C. fetus* subsp. *venerealis* occurs during the mating of a carrier bull with susceptible females. Spread can also occur through the artificial insemination of cattle with non–antibiotic-treated semen obtained from an infected bull. Transmission from one female to another by direct contact and contamination of the vulval lips is highly unlikely, whereas it can occur among communally held bulls during mounting or in artificial insemination centers through inadequately cleansed and disinfected collection equipment.

There is considerable variation (38 to 78 per cent) in the ability of carrier bulls to transmit the organism to susceptible females. This is probably due to differences in the number of *Campylobacter* organisms carried in the prepuce and ultimately deposited in the vagina at the time of service.

Heifers and cows that have had no prior contact with *C. fetus* subsp. *venerealis* are, for all practical purposes, highly and equally susceptible to infection. However, it is not unusual for a few individuals (up to 5 per cent) to resist infection despite repeated exposure to carrier bulls or the deposition of large numbers of viable organisms into the reproductive tract.

After transmission to susceptible females, the organism can be found initially in the vagina, cervix, uterus, and oviducts. Infection of the uterus and oviducts persists for up to 2 months, but thereafter it is progressively eliminated and by the end of the third month is usually confined to the cervix and vagina. In 10 to 20 per cent of animals, infection is confined to the vagina and does not appear to have any adverse effects on fertility. There is a marked decline in the number of infected animals around the time of conception, but up to 10 per cent may continue to harbor the organism until after calving, when most become free within the ensuing 3 months.

Females that fail to conceive often remain infected for over 6 months, and possibly half of these may still carry *C. fetus* subsp. *venerealis* in the vagina for up to 10 months after initial infection.

Although between 30 and 70 per cent of animals that have recovered from genital campylobacteriosis may become reinfected during the next breeding season, they possess a well-developed resistance to the effects of the disease, and their fertility is only slightly impaired. However, this resistance declines with time and in the majority of cases has largely vanished within 3 to 4 years of initial infection.

In bulls, *C. fetus* subsp. *venerealis* can be demonstrated on the mucosal surfaces of the prepuce, glans penis, anterior urethral opening, and distal portion of the urethra. In general, the prevalence of infection increases with the age group of the bulls; this is attributed to a greater opportunity for contact with infected females. Experience has shown, however, that bulls less than 3 years old either are difficult to infect or tend to recover within a few weeks after exposure. Older bulls, especially those over 5 years, are much easier to infect, and because a protective immunity is not induced, they can remain carriers for long periods of time if not permanently. The greater susceptibility of older bulls has been attributed to greater folding of the preputial mucosa and an increase in the size and number of epithelial crypts on the penis, which provides a favorable environment for the organism.

CLINICAL SIGNS

Female cattle suffering from venereal campylobacteriosis exhibit various signs of infertility, the most common being repeated returns to service. The interestral periods are often prolonged, and there is an increased proportion of cycles with a duration of 25 to 35 days or longer. Anestrus is not often encountered, and abnormal genital discharges are only occasionally seen.

In the absence of any other condition, the time required to mate all cattle once is normal, but the conception rate to first service is reduced considerably and may be as low as 20 to 30 per cent. As the breeding season advances, the general level of fertility improves, with most animals finally conceiving by the third to fifth month. By this time, the overall conception rate is 85 to 95 per cent, and the average number of services per conception is between 2.5 and 3.5. A small number (5 to 10 per cent) of cattle fail to conceive despite repeated returns to service, whereas a similar proportion abort between the fourth and sixth months of pregnancy. The incidence of abortions, however, appears to depend on the number or nature of organisms present in the uterus. Large numbers of campylobacters are commonly associated with early embryonic death and infertility; smaller numbers may permit pregnancy to last for 4 to 6 months. Organisms of the biotype *intermedius* seem to be more often associated with abortions, possibly because of a lower pathogenicity.

In herds that have not previously been exposed to *C. fetus* subsp. *venerealis*, the average time taken from the first infective service to conception is usually over 40 days and in particular instances may exceed 60 days. As a result, both the subsequent calving period and the intercalving interval are extended by a similar amount. Thus the number of cattle calving within a year of their previous parturition is reduced by between one third and one half.

In areas where the disease is endemic and herds are chronically infected, only the heifers and newly introduced cattle are susceptible and suffer from infertility. Previously exposed cattle, on the other hand, either resist infection or show near-normal breeding pattern despite becoming reinfected. Under these circumstances, the actual degree of infertility observed will depend on the age structure of the herd and the prior exposure status of each animal in it.

The presence of *C. fetus* subsp. *venerealis* in the preputial cavity of the bull is not associated with any clinical signs, nor is there any change in semen quality. Essentially, the bull acts as a normal carrier of the organism.

HISTOPATHOLOGY

Venereal campylobacteriosis causes an endometritis, cervicitis, and salpingitis, all of which are relatively mild and superficial. Lesions are first seen 2 to 3 weeks after the animal becomes infected, reach a peak at 2 to 3 months, and are generally completely resolved by 4 to 5 months. The changes are not pathognomonic for the disease, but the duration of infertility is directly referable to the presence of endometritis. It is presumed the inflammatory response creates an environment hostile to the developing embryo, but other views have suggested a direct microbial effect on the viability of the egg or conceptus or a functional disturbance of the cervix causing the termination of pregnancy.

The most typical lesion is a focal or occasionally diffuse plasmacytosis. This is sometimes accompanied by a neutrophilic reaction that is also usually focal. Lymphocytic infiltration is less frequent but sometimes extensive in nature. Inflammation is most marked around the endometrial glands, which become filled with debris and leukocytes and are then destroyed and replaced by epithelial cells. Salpingitis may lead to sterility due to thickening of the oviduct wall, loss or fusion of villi, and narrowing or occlusion of the lumen, which prevents the egg from passing into the uterus.

In the case of recognizable abortions, there is a placentitis and extensive edema of the fetal membranes, which limits the interchange of gases and nutrients between the dam and fetus. It has also been suggested abortion may be due to an allergic response to heat-stable endotoxin, which has been shown to be an abortifacient in cattle.

DIAGNOSIS

If the herd history indicates the possible presence of venereal campylobacteriosis, confirmatory evidence can be obtained by demonstrating the organism itself in mucus, preputial secretions, semen, or aborted fetuses or by testing for specific antibody to *C. fetus* subsp. *venerealis* in vaginal mucus.

Owing to the slow growth of *C. fetus* subsp. *venerealis* and its susceptibility to oxygen, the detection of carrier bulls by cultural examination of semen or preputial secretions presents some problems, particularly when there is a delay between the collection of samples and their processing in the laboratory. However, the development of transport enrichment media in which samples can be kept for several days before culturing on solid selective medium has been shown to improve isolation rates from 59 to 85 per cent. The method used to obtain preputial secretions also influences efficiency; suction pipettes or instruments that can swab or scrape the mucosal surface are better than is the washing technique, which inherently reduces the concentration of organism in the sample.

Bacteriologic examination of vaginal mucus from recently infected cattle is diagnostically valuable when samples can be cultured on selective solid medium within 6 to 8 hours of collection. If this is not possible, enriched transport medium can be used to ensure the samples reach the laboratory in good condition. Under these circumstances, up to 60 per cent of infected animals can be detected; the isolation rates are higher during the early phase of an outbreak and lower after 2 months, when immunity is stimulated and animals start conceiving. Recovery rates of *C. fetus* subsp. *venerealis* are also higher in samples of estrus mucus than in those collected during diestrus.

The selective isolation of *C. fetus* enables a provisional diagnosis to be made within 3 days of culture; confirmation of subspecies and biotype requires up to another week. The direct fluorescent antibody test is a valuable alternative in permitting the rapid demonstration of *C. fetus* and its differentiation from other campylobacters. The technique does not enable the differentiation of the *venerealis* and *fetus* subspecies, but this is of lesser significance when the herd history points to infertility as the main clinical condition. *C. fetus* subsp. *fetus* can occasionally be found in the prepuce of bulls, especially those subject to prolapse and fecal contamination, and this possibility should also be borne in mind in deciding on the test to be used. There is also an occasional problem with overgrowth by contaminating organisms and a high background of nonspecific fluorescent staining, but this can be minimized by the addition of formalin to samples. The immunofluorescent test can also be applied to aborted fetuses, but in these cases it is best used an an adjunct to the cultural examination of abomasal liquid, liver, and spleen to enable differentiation of the subspecies.

The vaginal mucus agglutination (VMA) test can be used as a herd test for previous infection provided sufficient samples are obtained. It can also indicate a current infection through rising antibody titers being found in sequential samples, taken by pipette or tampon, a few weeks apart.

The VMA test has a relatively low degree of sensitivity in that only about 50 per cent of females develop agglutinins, and these do not appear until the second month after initial infection or even later. The persistence of antibody is also quite variable; up to one half of animals become negative within 6 months, whereas others may be positive for years. Samples of vaginal mucus obtained around the time of estrus tend to give more false-negative reactions; this is probably due to a simple dilution effect. False-positive results, on the other hand, are more frequent in samples obtained at metestrus or in those containing blood due to an inflammatory condition of the posterior genital tract or to trauma when mucus is collected. In these instances, the lowered specificity is due to the presence in the contaminating blood of cross-reactive antibody directed against *C. fetus* subsp. *fetus*.

False-positive reactions can be overcome to some extent by use of a comparative VMA test in which samples are examined against agglutinating antigens derived from both subspecies of *C. fetus*. The problem can also be reduced by employing the indirect hemagglutination or complement fixation test, but false-positive reactions still occur in at least 1 per cent of mucus samples from non-infected cattle. The use of serum as the test sample is of little value owing to high background antibody titers to *C. fetus* subsp. *fetus* and the poor serologic response to *C. fetus* subsp. *venerealis*.

Tests should also be carried out to exclude trichomoniasis as a cause of infertility or early abortion and *Brucella abortus* as a possible cause of late abortions.

CONTROL

The best method of controlling and eventually eradicating venereal campylobacteriosis from infected herds of cattle is the use of artificial insemination for several years. The method, however, relies on the availability of semen from noninfected bulls, and strict control measures are needed in artificial insemination centers for ensuring freedom from disease. Ideally, all bulls should be tested for and found free of *C. fetus* subsp. *venerealis* before use. When valuable sires are identified as carriers, a course of antibiotic treatment should be instituted and further retesting carried out.

The most efficient method of treatment involves the deposition into the preputial cavity of 10 ml of a 50 per cent solution of dihydrostreptomycin. The preputial opening is then held closed while the exterior of the sheath is massaged for at least 5 minutes. The procedure is repeated twice more at 24-hour intervals; and at the first and last treatments, the bull is also given a subcutaneous injection of dihydrostreptomycin at a rate of 22 mg/kg body weight (10 mg/lb). Preputial massage can induce urination, and if this occurs at an early stage, the procedure will need to be repeated. This should be avoided whenever possible because antibiotic treatment can cause ulceration and sloughing of the penile mucosa. There is also the possibility of resistant strains of *C. fetus* emerging or *Escherichia coli* developing with enzymes that can inactivate the antibiotic, rendering treatment ineffective. The problem can be minimized in some individuals by deliberately inducing urination before the introduction of antibiotic into the prepuce.

Because antibiotic treatment does not alter a bull's susceptibility to reinfection, strict management procedures must also be adopted at artificial insemination centers, especially those providing a custom collection service, for preventing the spread of disease if it is introduced. Such measures should include (1) separate accommodation for all bulls; (2) strict control over animal movement and thorough cleaning and disinfection of pens before different animals are moved into them; (3) ensuring all teaser animals are free of disease and that hair over the hindquarters is kept short and disinfected between mounts by different bulls; (4) use of separate collection equipment for each bull; and (5) addition of antibiotics at the correct concentration to extended semen.

In those areas where an artificial insemination service is not available, a split- or 2-herd system of management can be adopted. With this procedure, suspect or known infected cattle are kept separate from unexposed and susceptible animals, which form the nucleus of a new breeding herd. This procedure, however, is difficult to maintain for long periods especially when holdings are large, subdivision and fencing are inadequate, and bull control is poor.

Under these circumstances, vaccination provides a valuable alternative means of control. All animals initially require 2 doses of vaccine; these are given 4 weeks apart, and the second dose is given a month before mating is due to commence. Revaccination can be undertaken either annually or biennially, using a single dose, which is given a month before joining.

If female cattle are vaccinated in this manner, between two thirds and three quarters of all animals will be protected from venereal campylobacteriosis. The immunity conferred by vaccination is largely directed against the establishment of infection and not the effects of the disease, which under experimental conditions is equally severe in both infected vaccinated and control animals. Thus, in an outbreak, vaccination may not be of immediate benefit to those animals already infected or those that will contract the disease during the next month or so. However, some studies suggest vaccination may shorten the duration of a pre-existing infection or reduce the level of reinfection during the next breeding season.

Antibiotics are of little value in infected females unless treatment is undertaken during the early stage of an outbreak. When treatment is adopted, it normally involves the infusion into the uterus of an oily preparation containing 1 to 2 g streptomycin and 1 million units of penicillin. Although this procedure will temporarily reduce the overall level of infection in the herd, it is not very useful after the third or fourth month, when conception can be expected to occur owing to a developing natural immunity.

Whereas the treatment or vaccination of female cattle will help maintain a reasonable level of fertility, the disease will not be contained unless control procedures also involve the bull. Treatment of infected bulls or their culling and replacement by less susceptible young bulls can reduce the carrier rate considerably. However, this approach can only be regarded as a temporary measure, and in order to prevent reinfection, vaccination should also be carried out. This has the dual function of curing an existing infection and preventing the establishment of the carrier state in previously unexposed animals. It should be emphasized that 2 doses of vaccine must be given initially. A single dose can cause a substantial reduction in the number of organisms isolated from the prepuce of carrier bulls, but the complete elimination or the prevention of infection can be achieved only by a second dose of vaccine a month later.

It has also been demonstrated that the vaccination of bulls reduces their ability to mechanically transmit *C. fetus* subsp. *venerealis* from one female to another. The experimental evidence available suggests that passive spread of the organism is low when the interval between mating of an infected and a susceptible female by a vaccinated bull exceeds 24 hours. Any management practice, including the synchronization of estrus, that increases the sexual activity of the bull and reduces the interval between matings is therefore likely to result in a much higher transmission rate.

The eradication of bovine venereal campylobacteriosis from infected herds is not likely to be achieved by vaccination alone. Efforts must also be made to minimize mechanical or passive spread by treating or culling exposed or known infected females or segregating them from noninfected susceptible animals. If spread is prevented, the disease should disappear within 2 breeding seasons, but it would be prudent to ensure that during this time all female replacements are also vaccinated before entry into the breeding herd.

BIBLIOGRAPHY

Clark BL: Review of bovine vibriosis. Aust Vet J 47:103–107, 1971.
Corbeil LB, Schurig GG, Duncan JR, et al: Immunity in the female bovine reproductive tract based on the response to *"Campylobacter fetus."* Adv Exp Med Biol 137:729–743, 1981.
Garcia MM, Eaglesome MD, Rigby C: Campylobacters important in veterinary medicine. Vet Bull 53:793–818, 1983.
Hoffer MA: Bovine campylobacteriosis: a review. Can Vet J 22:327–330, 1981.

Campylobacter Proliferative Enteropathies of Pigs

G. H. K. LAWSON, BVM & SC, PhD, MRCVS
A. C. ROWLAND, BSc, MRCVS

The term "proliferative enteropathy" is a pathologic description of a group of diseases with common underlying characteristic histologic changes of the intestine. The important microscopic features are the presence of proliferating immature enterocytes and that these altered cells contain bacteria within the apical cytoplasm. There is considerable support for the opinion that these intracellular bacteria are important in the etiology of the condition, but at this time the disease is largely defined by its pathologic lesions.

The abnormal crypt cells that characterize the condition continue to divide, which leads to a thickened mucosa made up of elongated, branched crypts. The histologic change can generally be appreciated grossly as a thickening of the mucous membrane. Lesions that comprise such a thickened proliferating mucosa without other significant intestinal change are described as adenomatous or porcine intestinal adenomatosis. In certain circumstances, the proliferative mucosa undergoes necrosis, which may vary from superficial destruction to a deep coagulative necrosis; in the latter case, the affected mucosa is replaced by a yellow cheesy exudate that retains the original form of the intestine. This pathologic presentation, when severe, is described as necrotic enteritis.

In survivors of such changes, the mucosa may be ulcerated, and compensatory muscle hypertrophy may result in a thickened or "hosepipe" gut. These changes are identified as regional ileitis.

Some proliferative lesions culminate in blood leakage. These intestines show the characteristic mucosal thickening together with a formed blood clot or free blood in the intestinal lumen. They are known as proliferative hemorrhagic enteropathy (PHE). The lesions of all these conditions are most common in the lower ileum. PHE tends to be confined to the small intestines, whereas the other conditions may occur in the large bowel either in association with or sometimes without small intestinal involvement.

OCCURRENCE

The disease is worldwide in its occurrence and has been present in pigs for many decades; however, it has only been since the commercial exploitation of high health production methods that the disease has made a dramatic and important impact on pig production. Many minimal disease or equivalent status herds have suffered from the clinical effects, which have the characteristics of a highly contagious disease. Signs are those attributable to PHE in this acute disease form, with 12 to 50 per cent of the adult herd showing clinical signs and a mortality of half those clinically affected. Whereas the hemorrhagic form of the disease may spread clinically from animal to animal, the disease can also affect single or small numbers of pigs with adjoining animals remaining unaffected. In certain countries, PHE can be a repeated problem in animals involved in growth trials.

Most other manifestations of the disease are less dramatic than is the hemorrhagic form, and therefore it is less easy to evaluate their effect. Mortality in herds experiencing clinical porcine intestinal adenomatosis/necrotic enteritis may reach 1 per cent, with some 0.89 to 2.5 per cent of animals being detectably affected. Lesions can be present in animals presented for slaughter; the incidence of such lesion is generally low (0.7 to 1.63 per cent), but occasionally a high proportion (40 per cent) of the pigs killed are affected.

ETIOLOGY

Experiments confirm that the disease is infectious and that all the pathologic conditions described as proliferative enteropathy are the result of infection by similar or closely related agents. A variety of *Campylobacter* spp. but principally *C.*

mucosalis and *C. hyointestinalis* can often be recovered from the intestinal lesions; this, along with the curved or S-shaped morphologic features of the intracellular organism, has led to the concept of proliferative enteropathy as a campylobacter-associated enteropathy. Recent work, however, has clearly identified the intracellular organism or *Campylobacter*-like organism as distinct and antigenically largely unrelated to the campylobacters that can be isolated in culture from the lesions of proliferative enteropathy. It would appear, therefore, that at the present time, the intracellular organism has not been grown in conventional bacteriologic media. Although the potential importance of other agents has been promoted, current evidence suggests that the intracellular organism plays a crucial role in the pathogenesis of the disease.

CLINICAL SIGNS

Symptoms of PHE are generally those of acute-onset intestinal blood loss with concomitant profound anemia in adult pigs. The hemorrhagic form of the disease mainly affects mature animals (more than 4½ to 5 months of age), although on occasion all ages including sucklers may be involved. Unlike other forms of proliferative enteropathy, the clinical condition is not preceded by a period of wasting. Initial anemia is often sufficiently severe to cause sudden death without premonitory symptoms. Feces in affected animals contain blood either altered or fresh and may be diarrheic or formed but without free excess mucus. Vomiting may be present along with anorexia, but fever is not present other than as a slight or transient feature. Recovery takes place progressively over a period of about a week. Pregnant animals may abort, the majority within days of the onset of symptoms.

Adenomatosis or associated conditions (necrotic enteritis or regional ileitis) can occur at any time in the fattening period and may commence as early as 6 weeks of age. The most prominent signs are those of loss of appetite and failure to gain weight. Affected animals become hairy, are poorly fleshed, and show intermittent episodes of diarrhea. Such symptoms remain in evidence for up to 6 weeks, but most animals thereafter regain appetite and subsequently make satisfactory progress to slaughter. Necrotic enteritis or regional ileitis is most commonly manifested as sudden death in previously unthrifty pigs; regional ileitis may terminate in intestinal rupture and peritonitis. Although adenomatosis may be apparent clinically, it may also be present as a subclinical entity with the only manifestation that of depressed weight gains.

DIAGNOSIS

PHE has to be differentiated from other enteric diseases demonstrating blood in the feces, notably swine dysentery, gastric ulceration, intestinal anthrax, warfarin toxicosis, salmonellosis, and certain mycotoxicoses. Only in gastric ulceration, warfarin poisoning, and mycotoxicosis is the anemia comparable in severity to that seen in PHE. Confirmation of diagnosis in the living animal can be achieved by demonstrating the intracellular organism in the feces by use of indirect fluorescent antibody techniques with specific monoclonal antibody or by serum assay in which the antibody response is short-lived and involves principally IgM. In the absence of such tests, confirmation depends on demonstration of typical lesions and the intracellular organism; a useful simple diagnostic aid is the staining by modified Ziehl-Neelsen technique of mucosal smears, which, with care in preparation, can demonstrate the intracellular organism. PHE cases found dead must be differentiated from an occasional but frequent intestinal catastrophy described as intestinal torsion or colonic bloat, in which, however, the intestinal wall remains thin, the lumen is distended by gas, and the hemorrhagic contents are never clotted.

Diagnosis of the wasting syndrome is more difficult, although both sero-techniques for antigen and antibody are applicable but not generally available. A wide variety of specific and nonspecific conditions can cause failure to gain weight, and as with PHE, the diagnosis will usually rest on necropsy, microscopy of stained smears, and histology.

The principal conditions that may cause confusion in diagnosis are weaner colitis; nutritional deficiencies, notably niacin and vitamin E (in young piglets); other intestinal aberrations; and chronic respiratory disease.

TREATMENT

Most current therapy is aimed at ameliorating the clinical effects of the disease; controlled studies on the effects of therapy are not available, and most clinical observations are confined to visual assessment and a cessation of mortality. In dealing with a disease syndrome expressed as a complex of pathologic lesions, some with superimposed secondary infection, it is often not clear whether the proliferative lesion or the secondary infection is being modified by treatment.

Our knowledge of the epidemiology of infection is poor. Clinical cases often occur after movement of animals; it is uncertain whether this is clinical expression of a previously subclinical infection or whether infection has been acquired at the new location. The decision as to which is most likely is important, even if it is impossible to assess accurately. One decision requires isolation and treatment of incoming pigs, the other, exposure to infection with a period of prophylactic treatment to prevent clinical disease and allow immunity to develop. The period of exposure to potential infection is critical and should not exceed 3 weeks; otherwise there is risk of the occurrence of clinical cases. The method is empiric, and there is no certainty that exposure has taken place and consequent immunity has developed. Procedures such as these have been adopted and are considered to minimize losses and signs in both PHE and porcine intestinal adenomatosis. Deliberate exposure to infection generally merely involves introducing animals into a unit or environment in which infection is believed to be present.

A wide variety of antibacterials have been used to treat clinical proliferative enteropathy, but field or experimental evidence of the efficacy of any on the primary lesion is lacking. Preventive therapy after exposure often utilizes in-feed tetracycline (100 ppm) for 2 to 3 weeks, sometimes in combination with other drugs (penicillin G, 50 ppm; sulfamethazine, 100 ppm). Other antimicrobials, especially tylosin, sometimes in combination with sulfonamides, are employed, but their use has not been well evaluated. The mortality associated with necrotic enteritis may on occasion be controlled by dimetridazole (500 ppm), although other evidence suggests that this drug may have limited activity against the intracellular organism.

A variety of drugs have been used on farms in an effort to control the disease, the effects being monitored by the presence of lesions at slaughter. Such reports have not been controlled but may be an indication of efficacy; halquinol and oliquindox, 60 to 120 and 25 to 50 ppm respectively, appeared useful, but both on occasion failed to control the presence of lesions for reasons that were not investigated. This drug failure may merely indicate either that on-farm usage was not correctly carried out or that susceptibility of the intracellular organism may vary. Drug withdrawal periods before slaughter are of crucial importance, and withdrawal periods of more than 21 days may allow clinical cases to occur before slaughter. Circumstantial evidence suggests that continuous in-feed tetracycline to growers leaves animals susceptible to infection on withdrawal of the drug. Such treatment therefore may lead to an adult population vulnerable to the effects of infection. Not all drugs mentioned may be approved for use by certain national authorities.

CONTROL

Animals may be infected and be asymptomatic. There is no known test that reliably detects all infections and no certainty that infection is absent from a herd whatever the status, although cesarian-derived or similar herds that have never shown symptoms may be free from infection. Other animal species are affected by a similar disease associated with closely related bacteria, and hamsters and mice are susceptible to infectious material of swine origin. It is possible, therefore, that infection may be introduced into free herds by either infected pigs or rodents. Maintenance of a closed herd with elimination of rodents is at the moment the only advice that can be offered to exclude infection.

BIBLIOGRAPHY

Lawson GHK, Rowland AC: *Campylobacter sputorum* subsp *mucosalis*. In Butzler JP (ed): Infections in Man and Animals. Boca Raton, FL, CRC Press, 1984, pp 207–225.
Lomax LG, Glock RD, Hogan J: Porcine proliferative enteritis: field studies. Vet Med 77:1777–1786, 1982.
Rowland AC, Lawson GHK: Porcine proliferative enteropathies. In Leman AD, et al (eds): Diseases of Swine, 7th ed. Ames, IA, Iowa State University Press, 1991.

Borreliosis in Cattle

ELIZABETH C. BURGESS, DVM, PhD

Borreliosis is defined as disease caused by infection with a spirochete belonging to the genus *Borrelia*. In this article, 2 different spirochetal infections are addressed, Lyme borreliosis caused by *B. burgdorferi*, and epizootic bovine abortion caused by *B. coriacae*.

LYME BORRELIOSIS

Lyme borreliosis is an important infectious disease that affects domestic animals as well as wildlife and humans. Human infections can vary from a mild skin rash to arthritis and neurologic and cardiac manifestations. The disease in humans has been recognized in the United States since 1969, and the number of cases has increased annually since that time. In 1989, 7402 human cases were reported in the United States. The disease in cattle is still poorly understood. There has been 1 reported case of Lyme borreliosis in cattle and several reports of cattle with antibodies to the organism. The information presented in this article represents information obtained from these limited sources and by extrapolation from other species.

Etiology

Lyme borreliosis is caused by a spirochete, *Borrelia burgdorferi*, which belongs to the genus *Borrelia*. They are flexible helical cells with dimensions of 0.18 to 0.25 μm by 4 to 30 μm. The spirochete is motile and has regular coiling. The cells are gram-negative and stain with Giemsa and Warthin-Starry stains. They are visible by phase-contrast or darkfield but not by brightfield microscopy. *B. burgdorferi* is microaerophilic and grows best at 33° to 34° C.

Occurrence

The incidence of Lyme borreliosis in cattle is not known.

Pathogenesis

The exact mechanisms of the pathogenesis of borreliosis are not completely known. It is postulated that both direct and indirect effects of the spirochete are involved. Direct effects include the production of a spirochetal lipopolysaccharide that produces a pyrogenic reaction and production of cell-wall peptidoglycan that may induce persistent joint inflammation. Indirect effects include the production of immune complexes that may be present in the serum and synovial fluid of infected humans in abnormal amounts, which suggests an immune-mediated inflammatory reaction. When these complexes localize in the joints, they may produce inflammatory joint disease. Interleukin-1 production by macrophages may produce increases in collagenase and prostaglandin E2 secreted by synovial cells. Collagenase may play a role in the digestion of articular cartilage. Spirochetes may cause mast cell degranulation and the release of inflammatory mediators.

Transmission

The main route of transmission of *B. burgdorferi* is by the bite of an infected tick of the ixodid family *(Ixodes dammini* or *Ixodes pacificus)*. *I. dammini* is a 3-host tick. The juvenile stages feed on mice, whereas the adults feed primarily on deer. The principal vertebrate maintenance hosts for *B. burgdorferi* are *Peromyscus leucopus* (white-footed mouse) and *Odocoileus virginianus* (white-tailed deer). *I. dammini* lives in grassy and wooded areas and feeds on small and large animals, including small rodents, birds, raccoons, opossums, deer, horses, dogs, cats, and humans. The adults will feed on cattle. Adult ticks are abundant in the spring and fall. The adult ticks are small, about two thirds the size of *Dermacentor variabilis*, and the females have an orange body. Transmission has been shown by direct contact in dogs and *Peromyscus* spp. in the absence of an arthropod vector, possibly by direct contact with infected urine. The spirochete has been isolated from the urine of dogs, *Peromyscus* spp., and cows. It is postulated that contact transmission occurs by exposure to infected urine.

Organs Involved

There has been only 1 reported case of Lyme borreliosis in cattle that describes the organs involved and the lesions. Organs involved in that case include joint synovia, joint cartilage, kidneys, lymph nodes, heart, liver, lung, and mammary gland. It is not known whether other organs may also be involved.

Clinical Signs

In acute cases, the most common sign is a sudden onset of lameness in 1 or more legs. The lameness may or may not be accompanied by a fever (up to 41° C, or 105° F) and swollen joints. In chronic cases, there may be weight loss and arthritis may develop. In one report, 13 lactating dairy cows had erythema, warmth, swelling, and hypersensitivity of the skin of the ventral udder and lower rear legs. There was mild lameness with swollen pastern and fetlock joints. Milk production was diminished.

Clinical Pathology and Necropsy Lesions

The clinical pathologic presentation varies from a normal hemogram to leukocytosis with neutrophilia and anemia. Necropsy lesions may include thickened joint capsules with a proliferation of the synovial membranes with lymphoplasmacytic infiltrates. Myocarditis, membranoproliferative glomerulopathy and tubular epithelial degeneration of the kidney, interstitial pneumonitis, and plasmacytic proliferation of lymph nodes have been reported. Not all cases will have all lesions.

Diagnosis

A combination of clinical signs with serologic tests provides the most effective diagnostic procedure. There are several diagnostic tests for detecting antibodies to *B. burgdorferi*. The most frequently used are the indirect immunofluorescent antibody test (IFA), the enzyme-linked immunosorbent assay (ELISA), and the Western blot. The IFA and ELISA are specific for antibodies to the genus *Borrelia* but not for *B. burgdorferi*. Cross-reactions may occur with other *Borrelia* species. The only other known *Borrelia* species in cattle in the United States are *B. coriacae* and the nonpathogenic spirochete *B. theileri*. The Western blot technique can distinguish *B. burgdorferi* if the animal has antibodies to the species-specific 31 kd or 34 kd proteins of *B. burgdorferi*. Diagnosis cannot be made on the presence of antibodies alone because there can be asymptomatic infections. If serum is collected early in the acute stage of the disease, when serologic tests are usually negative, a second sample should be submitted 2 to 3 weeks later when a measurable antibody titer should have developed. Antibiotic treatment can block the immune response early in the disease. Isolation of spirochetes may take as long as 4 months, which makes it of little value for diagnosis. The development of a new technique (polymerase chain reaction) for detection of specific spirochetal nucleic acid sequences in blood, urine, or tissues may prove to be of significant aid in diagnosis in the future.

Treatment

No controlled studies have been done on antibiotic treatment of Lyme borreliosis in cattle.

Prevention

No vaccine is presently available for use in cattle. Prevention is based on tick control and sanitary measures for preventing exposure of feed to rodents and birds, because birds and rodents can bring infected ticks into barns, and rodents may shed spirochetes in their urine.

EPIZOOTIC BOVINE ABORTION

Epizootic bovine abortion (EBA) is generally an asymptomatic infection of adult cattle that may result in abortion during late pregnancy and the birth of weak calves. The disease has been reported from the far West of the United States for 60 years and has been associated with the bite of a soft tick *(Ornithodoros coriaceus)*. A spirochete *(Borrelia coriacae)* has been isolated from this tick and has been associated with EBA. The spirochete has been seen in the blood of calves with lesions of EBA, and lesions of EBA were found in fetuses from cows superinfected with the spirochete.

Etiology

EBA has been associated with the spirochete *Borrelia coriacae*. The spirochete, a member of the genus *Borrelia*, is highly motile and helical in form. It is 8 to 10 µm in length and 0.3 to 0.4 µm in diameter. There are 11 to 15 periplasmic flagella. *B. coriacae* does not readily infect mice, whereas *B. burgdorferi* does infect mice. It is microaerophilic and can be grown in Barbour-Stoener-Kelly medium at 30° C. It is visible by darkfield or phase-contrast microscopy.

Occurrence and Transmission

The occurrence of EBA is related to the distribution of the soft tick *(O. coriaceus)*, which includes the Sierra Nevada mountain range and the coastal range mountains of California. Transmission is by the bite of an infected *Ornithodoros coriaceus*, a soft tick feeding primarily on cattle and deer. Adult cows are infected by the bite of spirochete-infected ticks, and then the organism is passed transplacentally to the developing fetus. Abortion usually occurs during the last trimester of pregnancy.

Clinical Signs

Adult animals usually show no clinical signs other than abortion late in pregnancy. Calves may be born weak and die. Generalized edema and abdominal distention may be present. Calves may have enlarged palpable superficial cervical lymph nodes and petechiae of the mucous membranes. Retention of the placenta may occur, but breeding capacity is not impaired.

Clinical Pathology and Necropsy Lesions

Lesions include proliferation of lymphocytes and macrophages. There is macrophage infiltration of the liver stroma, which may cause compression atrophy of the hepatocytes. Macrophages also infiltrate the thymus and lung. Focal granulomas and subacute perivasculitis of the lung may occur.

Diagnosis

Diagnosis is difficult and must be made on the history of abortion in the last trimester of gestation. A history of cattle recently introduced from an EBA-free region is significant. Finding spirochetes on silver stain of aborted fetal tissues and typical histologic tissues will confirm the diagnosis.

Treatment and Prevention

No clinical trials have been done on treatment. A prophylactic dose of chlortetracycline in the feed at 2 g daily per cow has been shown to reduce abortion rates. No vaccine is available for use. Tick control measures will help prevent exposure to the organism.

BIBLIOGRAPHY

LYME BORRELIOSIS

Bosler EM, Schulze TL: The prevalence and significance of *Borrelia burgdorferi* in the urine of feral reservoir animals. Zentralbl Bakteriol Mikrobiol Hyg (A) 263:40–44, 1986.

Burgess EC, Gendron-Fitzpatrick A, Wright WO: Arthritis and systemic disease caused by *Borrelia burgdorferi* in a cow. J Am Vet Med Assoc 191:1468–1470, 1987.

Burgess EC: *Borrelia burgdorferi* infection in Wisconsin horses and cows. Ann NY Acad Sci 539:235–243, 1988.

Post JE, Shaw EE, Wright SD: Suspected borreliosis in cattle. Ann NY Acad Sci 539:488, 1988.

EPIZOOTIC BOVINE ABORTION

Kennedy PC, Casaro LAP, Kimsey PB, et al: Epizootic bovine abortion: histogenesis of the fetal lesions. Am J Vet Res 44:1040–1048, 1983.

Kimsey PB, Bushnell RB, Casaro AP, et al: Studies on the pathogenesis of epizootic bovine abortion. Am J Vet Res 44:1266–1271, 1983.

Osebold JW, Osburn BI, Spezialetti R, et al: Histopathologic changes in bovine fetuses after repeated reintroduction of a spirochete-like agent into pregnant heifers: association with epizootic bovine abortion. Am J Vet Res 48:627–633, 1987.

Escherichia coli Infections in Farm Animals

JOHN M. FAIRBROTHER, BVSc, PhD

Escherichia coli is an important cause of disease in young animals. *E. coli* infection is found worldwide in most mammalian species including humans.

The most common clinical manifestations of *E. coli* infection are neonatal and postweaning diarrhea and edema disease in young pigs; neonatal diarrhea, dysentery, and septicemia in young calves and lambs; and mastitis in adult cattle.

ETIOLOGY AND PATHOGENESIS

E. coli is a gram-negative, facultative anaerobic rod found in the normal intestinal flora and grows easily on most culture media. *E. coli* is classified into 150 to 200 serotypes or serogroups on the basis of somatic (O), capsular (K), and flagellar (H) antigens. Only strains of a restricted number of serogroups are pathogenic and are classified into categories or pathotypes on the basis of the production of virulence factors. The most important categories in farm animals are enterotoxigenic or enterotoxemic *E. coli* (ETEC); verotoxigenic *E. coli* (VTEC); septicemic; and nonsepticemic extraintestinal *E. coli*. Less common categories found in farm animals are enteropathogenic *E. coli* (EPEC) and enterohemorrhagic *E. coli* (EHEC); strains of these groups are also called attaching and effacing *E. coli* (AEEC) because of the way in which they attach to the intestinal mucosa. The relationship between VTEC and AEEC strains needs to be defined, because these strains may be identical. Enteroinvasive *E. coli* (EIEC) are rarely observed in farm animals. Certain serogroups are associated with specific disease manifestations in each animal species (Table 1). Most *E. coli* causing diarrhea in farm animals are ETEC. These strains produce fimbriae (pili) that mediate bacterial attachment to the small intestinal mucosa. The most important fimbrial antigens are F4 (K88), F5 (K99), F6 (987P), and F41. These strains then produce one or more of the enterotoxins STa, STb, or LT, which stimulate the secretion of water into the intestinal lumen and subsequently cause diarrhea with few pathologic changes to the intestinal mucosa. The most important pathotypes, that is, combinations of fimbriae and enterotoxins, are listed in Table 1. F4-producing isolates occasionally proliferate rapidly in the small intestine of young pigs and produce rapid death with the typical lesions of hemorrhagic gastroenteritis, congestion, and thrombi in the mucosa of the stomach and small intestine. These lesions probably result from a rapid release of bacterial lipopolysaccharide from the intestine into the circulation.

More recently, AEEC, which attach closely to the small and large intestinal mucosa and efface the microvilli, have been associated with diarrhea in postweaning pigs and dysentery in young calves. Lesions are multifocal and range from mild and scattered through the large and small intestine to severe and involving mostly the cecum and colon. In pigs, lesions include light to moderate inflammation of the lamina propria, enterocyte desquamation and some mild ulceration, and light to moderate villous atrophy in the small intestine. In calves, lesions are often more severe and are mostly found in the colon. Calf isolates often produce verocytotoxin [VT] (synonymous with Shiga-like toxin [SLT]). These isolates tend to induce more extensive lesions of hemorrhagic colitis: edema, ulceration, and erosions in the large intestinal mucosa and consequently hemorrhage into the intestinal lumen. The pathogenesis of these lesions is not yet well understood. Edema disease in weaned piglets is caused by VTEC, mostly of serogroups 0138, 0139, and 0141. These strains proliferate in the small intestine and produce a variant of VT II, which enters the circulation and causes lesions associated with endothelial cell damage.

E. coli septicemia is mostly observed in young animals with low maternal antibody levels and is caused by strains able to resist the bactericidal effects of serum complement and grow in body fluids with low available levels of iron. These strains belong to a restricted number of serogroups and often produce the fimbrial antigens F165 and CS31A. The role of these fimbriae in the pathogenesis of the disease is not yet well understood. In contrast to enteric *E. coli* infections, *E. coli* mastitis is caused by a large variety of serotypes similar to those found in the intestinal flora of adult cattle. After fecal contamination from the immediate environment of the cow, *E. coli* enter the teat end and remain in the teat canal and lactiferous sinuses. The *E. coli* either are rapidly eliminated by infiltrating neutrophils with mild damage to the epithelial cells of the teat sinus or proliferate rapidly and cause more extensive epithelial damage in the secretory areas of the mammary gland owing to diffusion of endotoxin and possibly other cytotoxins. A wide variety of serotypes of *E. coli* may be involved in other extraintestinal and nonspecific infections such as wound or urinary tract infections.

CLINICAL SIGNS

The clinical signs of the disease depend on the virulence factors of the infecting *E. coli* and the age and immune status

Table 1. SEROGROUPS AND VIRULENCE FACTORS OF *E. coli* CAUSING DISEASE IN FARM ANIMALS

	Disease	Serogroup	Virulence Factors
Pig	Neonatal diarrhea	08, 045, 0138, 0141, 0147, 0149, 0157	F4 (K88), F5 (K99), F6 (987P), F41, LT, STa, STb
		08, 09, 020, 064, 0101	F5 (K99), F41, STa
	Postweaning diarrhea	08, 045, 0138, 0139, 0141, 0147, 0149, 0157	F4 (K88), F (?), LT, STb, VT, AEEC
	Edema disease	0138, 0139, 0141	VT II$_e$ (SLT II$_v$)
Calf, lamb	Neonatal diarrhea	08, 09, 020, 064, 0101	F5 (K99), F41, STa
	Septicemia	011, 025, 020, 035, 078, 0115	Aerobactin, Col V, F165, CS31A
Cow	Mastitis	Diverse	Endotoxin

of the animals. ETEC cause a severe watery diarrhea followed by dehydration, metabolic acidosis, and death. In certain cases, the infection may be so rapid that death occurs before the development of diarrhea. One or more animals in a group are affected. In calves, piglets, and lambs, neonatal ETEC diarrhea is mostly observed in the first few days after birth. In piglets, a less watery diarrhea is also observed in the first 1 to 2 weeks of age and also after weaning, with low mortality and often decreased weight gain. Hemorrhagic gastroenteritis occurs in unweaned and recently weaned pigs and manifests as rapid death with some cutaneous cyanosis of the extremities or less acutely with hyperthermia, diarrhea, and anorexia. In edema disease, recently weaned pigs die suddenly, sometimes with edema of the eyelids. E. coli septicemia occurs in calves in the first few days of life and in lambs at 2 to 3 weeks of age. It is characterized by an acute generalized infection, sometimes with diarrhea, with signs of shock often followed by death. In some animals, the infection becomes localized, causing polyarthritis and meningitis. E. coli mastitis affects lactating cattle and may vary from a very mild inflammation with some clotting and swelling of the gland to a very acute reaction with no early signs of inflammation in the gland, but a rapid build-up of E. coli and widespread damage to the udder, followed by signs of toxemia and possibly death.

DIAGNOSIS

In the live animal, presumptive diagnosis of enteric E. coli infection is based on clinical history and signs, determination of fecal pH, and confirmation by culture of E. coli in the feces. Diagnosis is more definitive if the E. coli belong to a pathogenic serogroup and are positive for fimbrial antigens by agglutination, enzyme-linked immunosorbent assay (ELISA), immunofluorescence, or gene probe and positive for enterotoxins by the infant mouse test, tissue culture assay, pig gut loop test, or gene probe. Fecal material may also be tested directly for the presence of these virulence factors.

On post-mortem examination, diagnosis of E. coli infection may be confirmed by demonstration of typical lesions and bacterial intestinal colonization on histopathologic, immunoperoxidase, or immunofluorescent study and by cultural identification of the appropriate E. coli. Diagnosis of E. coli septicemia can be confirmed by culture of E. coli of the appropriate serogroup.

CONTROL OF E. coli DISEASE

Treatment

Treatment of E. coli disease is mostly aimed at removal of the pathogenic E. coli and should be rapidly instituted to be as effective as possible. However, diagnosis of E. coli infection should be confirmed by culture, and antibiotic sensitivity tests should be performed; antibiotic sensitivity varies greatly between E. coli isolates. A broad-spectrum antibiotic treatment could be used initially until the results of antibiotic sensitivity are known. Antimicrobial agents against which E. coli isolates have developed the least resistance are gentamicin, trimethoprim-sulfamethoxazole, cephalothin, amikacin, and apramycin. On the other hand, isolates are becoming increasingly resistant to ampicillin, neomycin and kanamycin, spectinomycin, tetracycline, and sulfisoxazole. The route of administration would depend on the type of infection and the choice of antibiotic. In E. coli diarrhea, oral administration is often more practical. If septicemia or more generalized infection is present, parenteral administration is indicated. The main problem with the use of antibiotic therapy is the rapid development of antibiotic resistance by E. coli. Many E. coli isolates demonstrate multiple resistance to antibiotics. An alternative approach to the treatment of E. coli diarrhea is the use of bacteriophages. This approach has been successful experimentally but has not been applied in the field. In E. coli diarrhea, it is important to treat dehydration and acidosis. In less severe cases, electrolyte replacement solutions should be given orally as soon as possible. In more severe cases, intravenous fluid therapy may be required. Drugs with antisecretory properties such as chlorpromazine and berberine sulfate may be useful for the treatment of diarrhea due to ETEC isolates. However, many of these drugs have undesirable side effects.

Immunoprophylaxis

Early immunity to E. coli infection in young farm animals is provided by antibodies obtained in the colostrum. Failure to receive or absorb an adequate level of colostral antibodies through the small intestinal gut wall within the first 24 hours after birth predisposes young animals to both enteric ETEC infection and systemic E. coli infection. Immunoglobulin levels, particularly in calves, may be estimated by the zinc sulfate or sodium sulfite turbidity tests during the first 48 hours after birth. Immunodeficient animals can be treated with plasma from an adult animal originating from the same area and in contact with the same E. coli serogroups or with colostrum taken from an older cow in the herd and stored frozen until time of use. Oral administration of specific anti-F5 (K99) monoclonal antibodies to calves within the first 12 hours after birth appears to prevent intestinal colonization by F5-positive ETEC isolates.

Vaccination programs are helpful for the control of ETEC infections in young animals. Identification of virulence determinants important in the pathogenesis of ETEC diarrhea, particularly in neonates, has resulted in the production of more efficient vaccines. Vaccination of the dam before parturition is the most effective way of ensuring the transfer of specific antibody in the colostrum and in the milk for protection of newborn animals and in the first few weeks of life. Bacterins containing strains representing the most important serogroups and producing the appropriate fimbrial antigens are commercially available for vaccination of farm animals. They are usually given parenterally at about 6 weeks and 2 weeks before parturition and show a variable response in field conditions. More recently, recombinant DNA technology has enabled the production of large quantities of purified fimbrial antigens for use in parenteral vaccines for immunization of the dam. Unfortunately, however, more widespread vaccination has led to a change in the bacterial population. For example, fewer F4-positive ETEC are being isolated from neonatal piglets, and F4-negative isolates are emerging from classic F4-positive serogroups. Recombinant DNA technology is being used to produce toxoid forms of the enterotoxins LT and STa. Conjugation of nonimmunogenic STa to carrier proteins has given protection in experimental conditions but has shown less encouraging results in the field. Addition of these components to fimbrial vaccines will provide protection against the emerging ETEC with new fimbrial antigens in neonates and against ETEC negative for the known fimbrial antigens but commonly found in older pigs. Live autogenous oral vaccines, consisting of ETEC isolates from a particular herd, are commonly used in the United States. These are given to the dam 3 to 4 weeks before farrowing and offer good protection if the appropriate isolates are present. With the advent of recombinant technology, these vaccines should become less necessary. Oral or parenteral immunization of young piglets with live or killed

ETEC vaccines may reduce the incidence of postweaning diarrhea and improve growth rate of early weaned pigs.

Husbandry

A program for prevention of *E. coli* infection should be aimed at reduction of numbers of pathogenic *E. coli* in the environment by good hygiene, maintenance of suitable environmental conditions, and provision of a high level of immunity. Because most pathogenic *E. coli* in enteric infections belong to a limited number of serogroups, enteric *E. coli* infection could be eliminated from some herds.

Young farm animals should be maintained at an adequate environmental temperature in a dry area free of drafts in order to reduce the effects of chilling on intestinal motility and resistance to enteric infection and septicemia. New animals should be quarantined for avoiding introduction of different pathotypes to which existing animals have very little immunity. Calving pens should be thoroughly decontaminated between batches of calves for reducing the population of pathogenic *E. coli* in the immediate environment. It has been found that the longer calving houses are used, the greater is the incidence of *E. coli* infection. Similarly, the design of farrowing crates is important in reducing contamination of young piglets. Use of the all-in, all-out system of farrowing, with a period of rest and thorough disinfection between farrowings, will reduce the incidence of enteric infection.

Careful attention to diet after weaning can reduce the incidence of postweaning diarrhea in pigs. A highly digestible, milk-based diet, fed in liquid form at frequent intervals, reduces the incidence of postweaning diarrhea and results in improved growth rates.

Occurrence of *E. coli* mastitis is a direct reflection of poor hygienic conditions of winter housing. Thus, control measures should be aimed not only at regular teat end decontamination, but also at maintenance of clean and dry bedding and disinfection of the immediate environment of the cow.

BIBLIOGRAPHY

Fairbrother JM: Enteric colibacillosis. *In* Leman AD, Straw BE, Mengeling WL, Taylor DJ, D'Allaire S: Diseases of Swine, 7th ed. Ames, IA, Iowa State University Press, 1991.
Holland RE: Some infectious causes of diarrhea in young farm animals. Clin Microbiol Rev 3:345–375, 1990.
Wray C, Morris JA: Aspects of colibacillosis in farm animals. J Hyg Camb 95:577–593, 1985.
Zeman DH, Thomson JU, Francis DH: Diagnosis, treatment, and management of enteric colibacillosis. Vet Med 84:794–802, 1989.

Eubacterium suis Infection

SCOTT A. DEE, DVM, MS

In 1957, an anaerobic diphtheroid bacterium was isolated from cases of cystitis and pyelonephritis in swine herds in the United Kingdom and classified as *Corynebacterium suis*. It has since been reclassified into the genus *Eubacterium* and isolated in many European countries as well as in North and South America, Australia, and China.

The prevalence of urinary tract infections induced by *Eubacterium suis* has increased as intensive management practices have changed the pigs' environment. It has been isolated from the pen floor of 10-week-old pigs and is a normal inhabitant of the boar prepuce. Transmission to the sow is believed to occur at breeding, but the factors that allow *E. suis* to survive in the vaginal tract and subsequently migrate to the bladder are unknown. The vagina is naturally acidic, and *E. suis* requires an alkaline environment; however, elevated estrogen levels in the sow are capable of causing an increase in urinary pH that may enhance survivability. The organism is piliated, which may allow improved adhesion in the vagina, whereas the short, wide urethra of the sow may enhance accessibility to the urinary tract.

The problem is much more prominent in older sows (6+ parity) housed in gestation stalls because of the higher incidence of fecal contamination of the perineal region as well as lack of exercise, reduced water consumption, and infrequent urination. Urine stagnation leads to increased urinary pH, which enhances the growth of *E. suis*. The organism produces urease, which splits urea-releasing ammonium ions that damage bladder epithelial cells. The elevated pH also initiates the precipitation of calcium, magnesium, and phosphate salts, which results in calculi formation. These changes predispose the kidney to pyelonephritis similar to *Corynebacterium renale* infection in the bovine.

CLINICAL SIGNS

E. suis infection affects the kidneys, ureters, and bladder, producing acute or chronic renal failure. In the acute phase of infection, the animal is anorexic and unwilling to rise. It may urinate pus or blood. Mortality is high (up to 100 per cent) if the infection is not treated immediately. If the animal survives the initial infection, it can suffer severe weight loss and becomes polyuric and polydipsic. It may continue to discharge pus or blood, and a white precipitate may form on the lips of the vulva. Typically, the sow becomes a repeat breeder with subsequent poor reproductive performance and is culled. It is hypothesized that the infection ascends into the uterus at breeding, damaging the endometrial lining, which results in reduced conception rates.

DIAGNOSIS

The presence of an acutely sick sow with hematuria should place *E. suis*–induced cystitis-pyelonephritis at the top of the differential list. Other causes of acute illness or sudden death include mesenteric torsion, bacterial septicemia, endometritis, and coliform mastitis; however, hematuria is not commonly found with these conditions. Chronic weight loss secondary to renal disease can result from leptospirosis, *Stephanurus dentatus* infection, and a variety of toxicoses such as long-term gentamicin usage as well as cadmium, citrinin, ochratoxin, and pigweed poisoning. The practitioner must not forget to investigate other potential causes of chronic weight loss such as malnutrition, locomotor problems, parasitism, ulcers, pneumonia, or intestinal diseases such as ileitis or dysentery. Finally, diseases such as African swine fever and hog cholera are capable of inducing glomerulonephritis and subsequent renal failure.

PATHOLOGY

Pathologic changes associated with *E. suis* infection are striking. Inflammatory reactions on the mucosal surface of the bladder may be hemorrhagic, purulent, or necrotic. The bladder wall is thickened, and deposits of granular material may be present in the lumen. The urine is usually red-brown in color, with a foul odor. The ureters may increase in size up to 1 to 1.5 cm in diameter. Unilateral or bilateral pyelonephritis may occur with the cortical, medullary, and pelvic regions distended with pus, blood, or foul-smelling urine.

MICROBIOLOGY

Isolation of *E. suis* to support the initial diagnosis and establish a therapeutic protocol is important. For enhancement of growth, strict anaerobiosis is required. If cultures are to be taken in the field, a small opening (½ inch in length) in the bladder should be made; the culture is taken and placed immediately into anaerobic transport medium (Cary-Blair). In order to attempt the highest possible isolation rate, portable incubators, culture media, and anaerobic jars can be carried to the necropsy site. If tissues are to be taken to the laboratory, the neck of the bladder should be tied off with umbilical tape, and 1 kidney should remain unopened.

The preferred medium is colistin–nalidixic acid (CNA) agar, which consists of Columbia agar with 5 per cent sheep red blood cells as well as colistin sulfate (10 mg/L), nalidixic acid (15 mg/L), and metronidazole (50 mg/L). It is commercially available and does an excellent job of reducing gram-negative contaminants of the urinary tract. The anaerobic environment is maintained with use of gas pack jars; incubation is 37° C for 5 to 7 days.

Morphologic features on blood agar are unique. Gray, pinpoint, smooth-edged colonies, 1 mm in diameter, can be seen after 48 to 72 hours of incubation. Over the next 24 to 48 hours, the morphologic character changes to flat, dry, opaque colonies 4 to 5 mm in diameter with serrated edges. There is no hemolysis. Gram staining reveals gram-positive rods with typical corynebacterial morphology. The organism is urease-positive, catalase-negative and ferments maltose, xylose, arabinose, and starch. Glucose and sucrose fermentation is variable. Gelatin hydrolysis, Voges-Proskauer, and methyl red tests are negative, as are nitrate reduction and esculin hydrolysis. Urinalysis indicates a severe bacteriuria ($\geq 10^5$/ml), proteinuria, hematuria, and pyuria. The pH can rise to 8 to 8.5, and the primary calculi produced are struvite, calcium oxalate, apatite, calcium phosphate, and urate. Analysis of these "bladder stones" indicates the majority are of struvite composition.

TREATMENT

If acute *E. suis* infection is recognized early, treatment can be very successful. It is important to choose an antibiotic that not only is effective against the organism and nontoxic to the already impaired renal system but will be active at the urinary pH produced by *E. suis*. Antibiotics known to be effective are ampicillin, penicillin, tetracycline, and the cephalosporins. Because of their safety, efficacy, and primary route of excretion being the urinary tract, the drugs of choice are ampicillin and penicillin. Both are active at an alkaline pH; ampicillin has the greater spectrum of activity. A veterinary-client-patient relationship is necessary for the use of this drug in swine in the United States. Acutely sick animals have been effectively treated with 5 mg/lb of ampicillin twice daily or penicillin once a day (s.i.d.) intramuscularly for 3 to 5 days. The withdrawal times are 21 days and 7 days, respectively. Other antibiotics such as the tetracyclines have been reported to be effective but are known to be nephrotoxic, and their activity is reduced at an alkaline pH. Cephalosporins are expensive, and first-generation compounds are contraindicated in cases of renal disease.

With the chronic form, the prognosis for full recovery is poor. Sows often develop into repeat breeders, and culling is the most cost-effective measure rather than long-term therapy. If the affected females are of significant value, proper therapeutic measures should be taken and the sows rested for an entire estrous cycle. One boar should be designated to breed these infected animals, and this "dirty boar" should not be allowed to service a noninfected sow in order to reduce the spread of infection throughout the breeding herd.

Large-scale outbreaks of urinary tract disease are rare; however, water-soluble ampicillin is approved for use in swine, and water consumption is not usually a problem. The withdrawal time is 24 hours, and free-choice water should be available at all times. Feed-grade antibiotics are rarely cost-effective. Affected animals are anorexic, and the bioavailability of certain antibiotics such as penicillin is reduced owing to degradation in the gastrointestinal tract.

Infusion of boar sheaths with penicillin or tetracycline has been reported to be effective in some instances. This may be helpful in reducing bacterial numbers in the short term, but it is questionable whether long-term "flushing" programs are cost-effective. With the high prevalence of *E. suis* on today's modern hog farm, it is better to control bacterial build-up and prevent the problem from occurring.

PREVENTION

Eradication of *E. suis* is not practical; therefore, one must recognize the factors that increase the animal's susceptibility to the problem. As mentioned earlier, good hygiene in breeding and gestation is critical. Manure should be removed regularly from behind the sow stalls, and gestation stalls should be washed and disinfected as groups are moved to farrowing. Breeding pens should be washed and disinfected as needed. For ensuring proper disinfection against *E. suis*, disinfectant sensitivities can be run. Sterile cotton swabs dipped into vials of diluted disinfectant are placed on agar inoculated with the bacteria, similar to a Kirby-Bauer antibiotic sensitivity test. Zones of inhibition will be seen if the organism is sensitive to that disinfectant. The phenols, formaldehyde-based or quaternary ammonium compounds, have been shown to be effective against *E. suis*; the quaternary ammonium compounds are preferred because of the minimal skin irritation produced.

When hand mating, the producer should wear plastic gloves for reducing contamination. Fecal material on the vulva or prepuce should be wiped off with a paper towel before mating. Walking behind sow stalls daily looking for discharges, examining the level of fecal contamination on sows, and watching urination for pus or blood are good diagnostic tools for monitoring the level of urinary tract infection on the farm.

Proper hygiene during farrowing is important as well. Regular manure removal and cleanliness reduce the incidence of urogenital infections. When assisting farrowings, producers should wear plastic sleeves that are well lubricated and wash the sow's perineal region before entering the reproductive tract. Sows should be treated with benzathine penicillin after such measures have been taken.

Proper design of gestation stalls is also important. The 7-foot-long stall should include *at least* 3 feet and preferably 3½ to 4 feet of slats under the sow. Gang slats of 4 inches in width with 1-inch gaps improve manure removal. New slat designs look promising, particularly those slats that run perpendicular to the sow with the gap space increasing in width toward the back of the stall. The solid portion of the floor should be gently sloped to allow ease of water and urine run-off. The trough should be inlaid, *not raised*, in order to prevent excessive wetness in the stall after drinking. New gestation stall designs that allow animals to turn around may prove beneficial in reduction of urinary tract infections in stalled sows.

Maximizing water consumption is necessary to induce frequent urination and flushing of the bladder. Frequent watering and twice-a-day feedings will help the sows spend more time on their feet. Reducing feet and leg injuries will also help promote frequent activity in the stall.

Nutritional modifications may also help water consumption, particularly by increasing salt content in the ration. Gestation diets should run 0.35 to 0.5 per cent salt. Acidifying the urine through addition of vitamin C, ammonium chloride, or DL-methionine has been discussed, but the practitioner must work closely with a nutritionist for ensuring that changes in the rations do not impair their nutritional value or reduce feed consumption in any way.

Vaccination against *E. suis* is not common but has been used in conjunction with Parvo-Lepto prebreeding vaccines. However, revised United States Department of Agriculture rules involving biologics may limit the accessibility of such products unless the antigens are federally licensed.

In conclusion, good management and proper building design for ensuring a high level of hygiene and a comfortable living environment still remain the best defense against *E. suis*–induced urinary tract infection in swine.

BIBLIOGRAPHY

Walker RL, MacLachlan NJ: Isolation of *Eubacterium suis* from sows with cystitis. J Am Vet Med Assoc 195:1104–1107, 1989.
Jones JET: Corynebacterial infections. *In* Leman AD, Straw B, Glock RD, et al (eds): Diseases of Swine, 6th ed. Ames, IA, Iowa State University Press, 1986, pp 617–621.
Jones JET: Urinary system. *In* Leman AD, Straw B, Glock RD, et al (eds): Diseases of Swine, 6th ed. Ames, IA, Iowa State University Press, 1986, pp 162–167.

Nocardioses

JOHN A. LYNCH, DVM, MSc, DVSc, Diplomate, ACVM

DEFINITION

Nocardioses are noncontagious, pyogranulomatous infections caused by exogenous, nocardioform bacteria. Numerous genera, species, and subtypes are now included in this group. *Nocardia asteroides* and *Nocardia farcinica* are the most frequently reported veterinary isolates, but other species are being increasingly implicated as sporadic pathogens of humans and other animals. Nocardioses may occur as isolated cases or in epizootic proportions. Infection follows traumatic or iatrogenic implantation of foreign material, inhalation, or wound contamination. The pathogenic nocardioforms are globally distributed soil organisms that are found in higher prevalence in African and North American soils than in those of other continents that have been studied. Nocardioses are recognized worldwide, although the form called bovine farcy is largely restricted to Africa, Asia, and the Middle East. Nocardial mastitis can cause economically significant losses in cattle and goat herds from repeated ineffective therapy, lost production, and lost genetic potential from culling. Human infection is not a zoonosis.

CLINICAL SIGNS

Typically, nocardiosis occurs as a localized infection; however, fever and other systemic signs may be present. The site of infection is dependent on the route of entry of the organisms. Response to antimicrobial drugs is consistently poor, despite in vitro tests, when advanced necrosis and fibrosis are present.

MYCETOMA (INCLUDING BOVINE FARCY). Mycetoma is characterized by tumefaction, draining sinuses, and granule formation as a result of traumatic inoculation of soil organisms, usually at a distal site in a single limb. Bovine farcy is a specific, severe form involving subcutaneous lymphatic spread of *Nocardia farcinica* to local lymph nodes, with or without *Mycobacterium farcinogenes*.

PNEUMONIA. This rare form of chronic pneumonia occurs in calves under 6 months of age or in goats. Laboratory assistance is required for diagnosis. Inhalation is the presumed route of entry.

ABORTION. Nocardial abortion, which is also rare, has been described in cattle and swine. It can originate from contamination of the genital tract during prior obstetric manipulations. Fetal death follows either placental necrosis or fetal septicemia.

MASTITIS. This is the most frequent clinical form of disease in food-producing animals, predominantly affecting mature cattle and goats. Major epizootics have occurred for incompletely understood reasons in France, Switzerland, and Canada in the past decade, as have occasional regional outbreaks in the United States. This ascending infection may occur as acute mastitis with fever and malaise, a chronic nonresponsive form, or a subclinical or preclinical infection. Heifers that have not received intramammary infusions are rarely affected.

SEPTICEMIA. Septicemic disease is infrequent but has been described and histologically confirmed. It usually follows prolonged localized disease. Sudden death after chronic nocardial mastitis is sporadically reported, but histologic confirmation of postulated nocardial septicemia is seldom documented.

CLINICAL PATHOLOGY AND NECROPSY LESIONS

In all forms of this disease, a chronic granulomatous tissue reaction with intermittent drainage through sinuses or natural orifices is typical. Mycetomas have a distal limb distribution, affecting skin and subcutaneous tissues. Bovine farcy is a nodular, suppurative dermatitis with granulomatous involvement of lymphatics and regional lymph nodes. In nocardial mastitis, multiple, caseating granulomas with a lobular distribution can be found. These are often large and involve the dorsal portions of affected glands and supramammary lymph nodes. Only 1 gland is usually involved. Initial glandular secretions may be watery with flakes, granules, or clumps. Thick, flocculent pus exudes in advanced cases. Leukopenia with a left shift may be present. Somatic cell counts for clinically infected quarters reach 1 to 8×10^6 cells/ml, and California Mastitis Test scores are routinely 3+. Branching, filamentous, modified acid-fast bacilli can be observed in secretions or tissues.

DIAGNOSIS

Diagnosis of nocardial mycetoma or farcy requires microscopic examination or culture for differentiation of the condition from eumycotic mycetoma, sporotrichosis, or bacterial cellulitis due to other agents. Index cases of nocardial mastitis in herds require similar laboratory assistance for etiologic differentiation from infection due to *Staphylococcus aureus, Actinomyces pyogenes*, atypical mycobacteria, or fungi. Because of sporadic shedding of the organism, subsequent cases of nocardial mastitis may be more accurately diagnosed in herds on the basis of clinical findings, persistently high somatic cell counts, and abnormalities of the milk, unless serial cultures are performed. Accurate identification of the isolated nocardioform to the species and even the genus level is difficult. Initial growth takes 48 to 72 hours, producing a small, chalky colony that develops a waxy, orange pigment and embeds in the agar. On microscopic examination, a mixture of gram-positive cocci, bacilli, and branching forms are observed. *Nocardia* retains the modified acid-fast stain. In vitro susceptibility testing is of marginal value in directing therapy. It can be a useful adjunct in the identification of nocardioforms to the level of both genus (*Nocardia*: kanamycin resistant, rifampicin resistant, sulfadimethoxine susceptible) and species (cefamandole, carbenicillin, gentamicin results vary with the species). Catalase demonstration, growth on Sabouraud's agar, production of aerial hyphae on slide culture, esculin hydrolysis, urease production, and lysozyme resistance are additional simple but beneficial tests.

TREATMENT

Potentiated sulfonamides are most commonly recommended for treatment, and they have proved effective in treating nocardial pneumonia. The prognosis for all nocardioses should be guarded to poor.

Treatment of nocardial mastitis rarely results in complete elimination of the organism, although temporary remissions in late lactation and intermittent negative cultures are common. Once the infection is confirmed, the animal should be shipped to slaughter at the earliest convenience. Most isolates are susceptible to tetracyclines, erythromycin, and potentiated sulfonamides as well as some of the new cephalosporins, fluoroquinolones, and potentiated aminopenicillins. The use of these drugs by the recommended route and dosage may alleviate systemic or more severe local reactions sufficiently to maintain a cow until parturition. Repeated intermittent therapy, cessation of secretion with sclerosing agents such as 500 ml of 2 per cent formalin, or even mastectomy may be considered for exceptionally valuable cows. Whereas early diagnosis might allow a more satisfactory response to treatment, most cows appear to become infected during dry-treatment infusion, and clinical infection is not recognized until 1 to 2 months into lactation. Thus, the infection is generally in an advanced, chronic stage when initial therapy is instituted. Only rigorous attention to hygiene and relentless culling of all clinically affected or culture-positive animals appear to be effective in achieving long-term elimination of the problem from infected herds. At the time of diagnosis of the index case, producers should be advised of the frustrating nature of the disease, the insidious and persistent character of the infection in herds, and the potential for substantial economic loss if an aggressive control program is not strictly maintained.

PREVENTION

Considerations relative to prevention are largely restricted to nocardial mastitis. *Nocardia* is an environmental cause of mastitis, rather than a contagious cause. However, it is common to find multiple cases in herds. This may be a result of simultaneous or sequential exposure to the same contaminated source, rather than true cow-to-cow transmission. Infected cows do provide a nidus of infection in herds. Contaminated multidose intramammary products or teat dips have been incriminated or suspected as sources. Isolation of the organism from such products retrospectively is difficult owing to a variety of biologic factors, and incrimination of a specific product may require the application of carefully controlled epidemiologic studies. Blanket dry-cow therapy and the use of neomycin-based dry-cow infusions have been identified as significant risk factors in infected herds. Selective dry-cow therapy and the exclusive use of individually packaged, sterile, nonirritant intramammary infusions are advisable in known-infected herds. Strict attention to aseptic infusion techniques must be reinforced. The activity of disinfectants against nocardioforms is variable, but chlorine at 100 to 400 ppm for 5 to 60 minutes is reported bactericidal for mastitis isolates. Infected, suspected, or recently introduced cows should be milked last and isolated if possible.

This is an extremely disconcerting problem for producers because of the significant economic impact on individual affected herds, the lack of response to therapy, and the need to take control measures that contradict those advocated for control of contagious mastitis pathogens. An empathetic, patient, and informative approach is required to assist producers in the management of this disease.

BIBLIOGRAPHY

Beaman BL, Sugar AM: *Nocardia* in naturally acquired and experimental infections in animals. J Hyg Camb 91:393–419, 1983.
Collins CH, Yates MD, Uttley AHC: Presumptive identification of nocardias in a clinical laboratory. J Appl Bacteriol 65:55–59, 1988.
Sears PM: Nocardial mastitis in cattle: diagnosis, treatment and prevention. Compend Contin Educ Pract Vet 8:F41–F46, 1986.

Dermatophilosis
D. H. LLOYD, B Vet Med, PhD, FRCVS

DEFINITION

Dermatophilosis is a seasonal proliferative and exudative skin disease, principally affecting mammals, that occurs throughout the world. The disease is also known as streptothricosis and, in sheep, as lumpy wool or mycotic dermatitis. The term "strawberry foot rot" is used to describe an ovine syndrome involving the distal limbs in which concurrent infection with orf occurs. Oral dermatophilosis has been described in cattle, buffaloes, cats, and humans. Subcutaneous lesions have been reported in cattle, lizards, and humans.

INCIDENCE

Subclinical skin infection is common in endemic areas, particularly in sheep. Clinical disease is usually associated with wet weather, and morbidity may be 100 per cent. In African cattle, a higher incidence has been demonstrated in mature animals and males; however, in South America, infection is more prevalent in young animals. There is considerable breed variation in susceptibility. Zebu cattle are generally more resistant than is *Bos taurus*, but West African N'dama and Muturu breeds are highly resistant. In sheep, the disease is more prevalent in the fine-wooled breeds; lambs under 5 weeks old are particularly susceptible.

ETIOLOGY AND PATHOGENESIS

The causative organism, *Dermatophilus congolensis*, is an aerobic, gram-positive, filamentous bacterium normally found only in the epidermis. Its infective stage is a motile coccoid zoospore that is attracted toward breaks in the stratum corneum and germinates to form a mycelium that proliferates within the living epidermis. The mature mycelium becomes divided into packets of zoospores, which remain in the scabs formed by epidermal hyperkeratosis and can survive for long periods. On wetting, they are released and may initiate new infections. During dry weather, spontaneous recovery occurs in most animals, but the disease may persist in small chronic lesions, commonly on the ears. Scabs remaining attached to the coat also act as reservoirs of infection. Transmission of the disease may be by contact or through the agency of ticks and flies, which may also abrade the skin surface and inoculate the causative organism. Skin susceptibility is increased by trauma, the effects of prolonged or heavy rainfall, exposure of unpigmented skin to the sun, malnutrition, and intercurrent disease. The immunosuppressive effects of infestation with the tick *Amblyomma variegatum* are associated with severe infections in cattle and goats.

Dermatophilus infection at sites other than the skin has generally been seen in young or debilitated animals. In pigs, tonsillar infection with a *Dermatophilus*-like organism has been described, but this appears to be a different bacterial species.

IMPORTANCE

Hides and skins from diseased animals are unsuitable for use as leather; fleeces containing scabs are downgraded. The disease may cause decreased milk production and reduced fertility in dairy cattle. Performance of draft cattle may be greatly impaired. More severely affected animals suffer from cachexia and death.

CLINICAL SIGNS

The disease is first recognized when exudation and incipient scab formation mat the hairs, forming the characteristic "paintbrush" lesions. As the lesions develop, thick, dense scabs are formed, adjacent affected sites coalesce, and 50 per cent or more of the body may be affected. Acute, generalized infection may occur in as little as 2 weeks, or the disease may extend progressively over periods of months or years. Mild infections may heal within 2 weeks in dry conditions and often pass unnoticed. Moist lesions in the fleeces of sheep are predisposed to fleece-rot and fly-strike.

The lesions can vary greatly in appearance and may be found on any part of the body. On haired skin, the scabs form flat plaques or hornlike projections; but on relatively hairless areas such as the perineum where wetting occurs, the scabs tend to be lost and the skin may become thickened, convoluted, and secondarily infected with other bacteria. In early lesions, hairs are found protruding from the scabs, but these subsequently disappear. The undersides of the scabs are typically concave and covered with a yellowish exudate when removed. The underlying skin has a red, coarsely granular, and often hemorrhagic appearance. On healing, the scabs separate from the skin but remain attached to the hairs.

Oral lesions in buffaloes and bulls appear as erosions or raised granulomatous lesions affecting the palate, lips, and dorsal surface of the tongue. Subcutaneous and lymph node abscesses infected with *D. congolensis* have been reported in cattle, sheep, and a goat.

CLINICAL PATHOLOGY AND NECROPSY LESIONS

D. congolensis is seen as branching filaments composed of multiple rows of gram-positive cocci in stained smears obtained from freshly removed scabs; motile zoospores may be observed in emulsified preparations from such scabs. In chronic or secondarily infected lesions, the organism may not be readily found. In granulomatous oral, subcutaneous, and lymph node lesions, club-forming granulomas very similar to those in actinomycosis may be seen.

The disease may be associated with a decrease in the serum albumin-globulin ratio; enlargement of lymph nodes and toxic changes in the liver and spleen may be found. Intercurrent disease, leading to other pathologic signs, may be present. Serum antibodies are produced in response to infection. They are not protective, but serologic tests may be used to identify subclinical infection.

DIAGNOSIS

Diagnosis is based on the characteristic appearance of the skin lesions and demonstration of the causative organism in scabs or skin specimens. The seasonal nature of the disease and its association with humid conditions may assist in diagnosis. It should be differentiated from other skin conditions leading to scab formation on the skin. Bovine sarcoptic mange may produce a similar clinical condition, and fleece-rot may be confused with the disease although the typical scabs of dermatophilosis are not present. Infections of the muzzle may be confused with orf and "peste des petits ruminants" in sheep and malignant catarrh or mucosal disease in cattle. Concurrent infection with these diseases may occur. Lesions at sites other than the skin are usually seen in association with skin infection and in young or debilitated individuals.

TREATMENT

The objectives are to halt invasion and reinfection of the epidermis. Invasion can be stopped by intramuscular injection of penicillin and streptomycin (or dihydrostreptomycin) either as a single dose (70,000 IU penicillin and 70 mg streptomycin per kilogram body weight) or in 5 daily injections (5000 IU penicillin and 5 mg streptomycin per kilogram). Long-acting oxytetracycline (20 mg/kg) given as a single injection is also effective in most cases in cattle. Alternatively, 5-day treatment with tetracyclines, chloramphenicol,* or spiramycin at normal therapeutic levels can be substituted. Successful treatment leads to separation of scabs from the skin surface; however,

---

*An unapproved drug in food animals in the United States.

under wet conditions, reinfection may occur. Cases already advanced before treatment may fail to respond.

Topical therapy is less effective but may succeed in mild or early cases. Sprays containing 0.3 to 1 per cent copper or zinc sulfate or cresols have been used. An aluminum sulfate–insecticide dip (M.D. Dip*) may control the disease in sheep.

Changes in management including bringing animals into dry conditions and elimination of *A. variegatum* (see Prevention) will promote spontaneous recovery in many cases.

PREVENTION

In sheep, the disease can be prevented by dusting the fleece with potash alum or aluminum sulfate during the wet periods of the year (M.D. Dusting Powder*). These substances may also be used in dips, as in M.D. Dip, which contains an insecticide and reduces the hazard of fly-strike. The disease may be minimized by changes in management. Shearing should not be carried out during wet weather, and dipping or jetting should be avoided when fleeces are long. Cuts and abrasions after shearing may be disinfected by dipping in 0.5 per cent zinc sulfate solution. Outbreaks in young lambs may be avoided by lambing during dry weather.

In cattle, control depends on the identification and elimination of predisposing factors such as ectoparasitic attack (ticks, flies, midges), abrasions due to thorny vegetation, intercurrent disease, malnutrition, and other stress factors. Where *A. variegatum* infestation occurs, this should be eliminated. In endemic areas, breeding for resistance and the introduction of less susceptible breeds should be considered. Intradermal vaccination with live cultures of *Dermatophilus* reduces the incidence and severity of the disease, but effective preparations for field use are not yet available.

Eradication of the infection is generally impracticable owing to the widespread nature of the disease and the difficulty in identifying subclinical infections.

PUBLIC HEALTH SIGNIFICANCE

Dermatophilosis is a zoonotic disease, and care should be taken in handling infected animals.

BIBLIOGRAPHY

Ilemobade AA: Clinical experience in the use of chemotherapy for bovine dermatophilosis in Nigeria. Prev Vet Med 2:83, 1984.
Lloyd DH, Sellers KC: *Dermatophilus* Infection in Animals and Man. New York, Academic Press, 1976.
Lloyd DH: Dermatophilosis: a review of the epidemiology, diagnosis and control. Proceedings of the CTA/CARDI Agricultural Seminar, Improving Health and Nutrition, Antigua, 1990. Trinidad, Caribbean Agricultural Research and Development Institute.

---

*Coopers/Pitman-Moore Ltd., Harefield, Middlesex, U.K.

Systemic Mycoses
JOHN PRESCOTT, VET MB, PhD

This discussion considers fungal infections of food-producing mammals that affect any organ except the superficial layers of the skin. The agents that cause systemic mycoses are part of the microbial flora of the external or internal environment. Those inhabiting the external environment, which constitute most of the organisms to be considered, are of low virulence. Animals are constantly exposed via the respiratory or intestinal route without adverse effects. Whether the agents assume a pathogenic role depends on developments that change the host-environmental equilibrium, such as (1) a derangement in the physiology of the animal, for example, hormonal changes caused by advanced pregnancy, certain pituitary tumors, or other immunosuppressive event; (2) an abnormal increase in the abundance of the fungi in the immediate environment, such as moldy feed and bedding, or through antibacterial therapy that removes competition with bacteria; and (3) the introduction of fungal cells by routes other than the respiratory or alimentary tract, such as mammary glands, wounds, or uterus. The bulk of systemic mycoses are therefore sporadic, most often in individual animals or in groups of animals subjected to comparable predisposition or exposure. Confirmation of these diseases involves pathologic (including histopathologic) and cultural diagnosis. Special fungal stains include Wright's, Giemsa's, silver, and periodic acid–Schiff (PAS) stains; in addition, yeasts but not molds stain with Gram's stain. Fungal hyphae and large yeasts may be readily seen on wet mount examination.

Treatment is rarely attempted or successful in food animals, and antimycotic drugs have had limited use. The proven means of dealing with systemic mycoses in food-producing mammals are largely confined to preventive measures instituted when the cause has been established by diagnostic tests.

ETIOLOGY

The most important mycotic syndromes recognized in food animals, primarily bovine abortion and mastitis, can be caused by a variety of fungal agents. With the exception of some of the *Candida* spp. (especially *Candida albicans*) and, possibly, *Rhinosporidium seeberi*, all the fungi involved are free-living saprophytes of dead or decaying organic matter.

Aspergillus

Aspergillus spp. are common molds found in virtually every habitat. They grow as branching filaments (hyphae) with frequent subdivisions (septa). They develop pigmented fruiting bodies at their free ends, with chains of spores (conidia). The color and structure of the fruiting bodies are characteristic for each species. The most common species that affects animals is *A. fumigatus*. Septated hyphae can be demonstrated in unstained wet mounts, in Giemsa's- or Wright's-stained fixed smears, and in stained sections of pathologic material. Their presence in lesions justifies a provisional diagnosis of aspergillosis.

Zygomycetes or Phycomycetes

The Zygomycetes or Phycomycetes, also called mucoraceous fungi, are as abundant and cosmopolitan as *Aspergillus* is. They differ in possessing few or no subdivisions in their usually broader hyphae, the only structures found in tissue. The fruiting bodies, which develop in culture, are spherical or oblong vesicles (sporangia). The shape of the sporangia, their support stalks (sporangiophores), and their relation to other hyphal features are important in determining genus and species. The genera important in animal diseases are *Mucor*, *Rhizopus*, *Absidia*, and *Mortierella*. A zygomycotic infection is suggested by the presence of broad, readily collapsing and twisting, nonseptate hyphae in smears or sections.

Histoplasma

Histoplasma capsulatum is a saprophytic fungus concentrated in the eastern central United States, but endemic foci are known in many parts of the world. *H. capsulatum* is dimorphic, that is, fungi occurring as molds in their saprophytic phase and as yeasts in their tissue phase. The yeasts can be demonstrated in Giemsa's-, Wright's-, PAS-, or silver-stained smears or sections within phagocytic cells of infected hosts. At room temperature, these yeasts grow into the mold phase again, producing characteristic thick-walled spores called tuberculate because of their studded exterior. At 37° C they grow as yeasts. Demonstration of the 2 phases is required for definitive identification.

Coccidioides

Coccidioides immitis, the agent of coccidioidomycosis, is another dimorphic fungus confined to certain parts of the Western Hemisphere, where soil and climate favor its growth. All authentic instances of diseases in all humans and animals are traceable to these areas. In the United States, they are in parts of California, Arizona, New Mexico, and Texas. The saprophytic phase of *C. immitis* is mycelial, which is also the form in which the fungus grows on agar plates at either room temperature or 37° C. In the parasitic phase, after inhalation or, rarely, traumatic introduction, the arthrospore is transformed into a spherical structure (spherule, sporangium) in which nonbudding endospores develop. These, upon liberation from the mature spherule, may be disseminated to other tissues, in which another cycle of sporangium and endospore formation can be initiated. Culturing the sporangial phase on the usual media results in reversion to the filamentous mold form. The spherules can be demonstrated in wet mounts of bronchial washes or exudate and in stained sections of tissue.

Cryptococcus

Cryptococcus neoformans is encountered only in the yeast form. The organism lives in soil, its growth being enhanced by bird feces. On morphologic examination, *C. neoformans* is a spherical cell that reproduces by budding. The most striking feature is the presence of a mucoid capsule of varying thickness.

Candida

Candida spp., of which *C. albicans* is most prevalent in infections, is normally present on the mucous membranes, especially of the alimentary tract. Infections are most commonly endogenous.

Candida spp. are basically yeasts that propagate by budding. The predominant cell shape is oval, and buds may be single or multiple. Under altered nutritional and atmospheric conditions, *Candida* spp. form mycelium by spore germination or pseudomycelium by cellular elongation and filament formation. This is also characteristic of *Candida* in its invasive phase, when it is actively growing in tissue rather than on mucus-containing membranes.

Candida in its yeast, mycelial, and pseudomycelial forms is readily demonstrable in Gram's-stained smears of infected material.

Rhinosporidium seeberi

Most cases of infection are in tropical or subtropical climates. The pathogen has never been convincingly cultured on artificial media. In the parasitic state, it forms large vesicles, up to several hundred micrometers in diameter, in which endospores are generated. Their large size and anatomic predilection for the nasal mucosa differentiate them from the spherules (sporangia) of *C. immitis*. The natural reservoir of the agent is unknown.

Prototheca

Prototheca spp. are algae devoid of chlorophyll. They resemble yeasts superficially in being basically unicellular nucleated organisms enclosed by rigid cell walls. They undergo endosporulation, forming a sporangium from which, through internal cleavage, a new crop of organisms is produced and eventually liberated. Sporangia are readily demonstrated in unstained exudates and in culture suspensions as spherical to oval bodies, about 20 μm in diameter, containing a variable number of endospores. They stain with special fungal stains. They grow readily on common isolation media. Colonies resemble those of yeasts, being white to off-white in color and creamy in consistency. Microscopic examination will reveal the characteristic pattern of spherical to oval cells at varying stages of endosporulation.

All the agents mentioned are potentially pathogenic to humans under much the same conditions as for animals. The noncontagious nature of the diseases makes transmission from infected animals to humans a rather minor concern.

GENITAL INFECTIONS AND ABORTIONS

Incidence

The most prominent mycotic problem in food animals is abortion. Whereas less than 40 per cent of all abortions in cattle can be associated with an infectious agent, fungal agents are blamed for about 2 to 30 per cent of this total. The rate varies from year to year and from place to place. Fungal agents rank among the leading causes of bovine abortion, competing in the United States with viral abortion due to IBR virus and in Europe with various bacteria, including *Brucella abortus* and *Leptospira*. Mycotic abortion in other food animal species is rare.

Etiology

A wide variety of fungal species have been implicated. *Aspergillus fumigatus* accounts for about two thirds or more of all mycotic abortions. It is followed in frequency by the zygomycotic fungi (*Mucor, Rhizopus, Mortierella,* and *Absidia*).

Epidemiology

The source of infection in most cases is external. Fungal spores are present in varying amounts in the feed and air, and the alimentary and respiratory tracts are portals of infection.

Genital infections may develop from commensal flora of the vagina or from contaminated semen. Breeding problems due to this type of infection involve yeasts more often than molds and are manifested in failures to conceive. Semen used for artificial insemination has repeatedly been shown to contain yeasts. In occasional instances, such contamination has been related to breeding problems, metritis, and even early abortion. Although various fungi of preputial origin have been demonstrated in semen, an important source of the fungi is semen extenders and other additives.

Mycotic abortions may occur at any time of gestation beginning in the third month, but they are most common in later pregnancy. The seasonal incidence shows a peak during winter. The circumstances responsible are (1) confinement in stables with greater likelihood of prolonged respiratory exposure to suspended spores in high concentration, (2) the use of harvested feeds in which there has been fungal growth, and, often, (3) the prevalence of animals in the advanced stages of pregnancy. Other predisposing factors may include steroid use, antibacterial drugs in feed, and increased feeding of stored rather than fresh feeds. For example, in some studies, moisture and pH of hay and of silage have been related to mold infestation. High-moisture hay or moldy or rotten silage commonly contains common saprophytic fungi. In the outcome of exposure, quantitative aspects are of great importance, because abortions in cattle have frequently been related to the use of obviously moldy feed.

Pathogenesis

Most bovine mycotic abortions are the result of generalized infections via the respiratory and alimentary routes. Manifestations in these systems (e.g., granulomas in the lung and ulcers in the stomach) are usually subclinical but lead to blood-borne dissemination. Localization in the placenta results in placentitis, necrosis, and hemorrhage, with eventual separation of the chorion from the maternal placental tissue by an exudate in which fungal hyphae abound. Penetration of tissue and blood vessels is thought to be aided, at least in the case of certain fungi, by necrotizing enzymes. Attempts to account for the placental localization of fungi have revealed substances in tissue extracts of cattle that stimulate germination of fungal spores and growth of fungi. The chemical nature of such substances has not been adequately defined, nor is it necessarily the total explanation of the abortion process.

Clinical Signs and Pathology

Clinically, there are few features that differentiate mycotic from other abortions at the same stage of pregnancy. In the majority of cases, no general illness is present in the aborting cow, although fatal, fulminating pneumonia after *Mortierella wolfii* infection has been reported in New Zealand, which was followed within 1 to 5 days by fulminating and ultimately fatal pneumonia in the majority of affected animals. Such systemic complications by *M. wolfii* abortions have not been common elsewhere.

The aborted fetuses may be grossly normal. A variable percentage (2 to 25 per cent) have ringworm-like skin lesions in which fungal elements can be demonstrated. They are concentrated in the head and neck region. Such lesions are observed with *Aspergillus*- and zygomycete-induced abortions. Internal lesions of the fetus may include general lymphadenitis, dehydration, and emaciation. Mycotic colonization of lungs, liver, spleen, and brain may occur. Grossly recognizable mold colonies may be floating in the abomasal or amniotic fluid.

The most significant lesions of mycotic abortion are necrotizing hemorrhagic placentitis, manifested grossly by brownish discoloration, and swollen necrotic placentomes with thickened edges distorting the structure into a cup-like shape. There is much adventitious placentation and thickening of intercotyledonary areas. The cotyledons adhere firmly to the maternal caruncles, so that retention of the placenta is very common.

On microscopic examination, the basic lesion is one of vasculitis, with hyphal invasion of the vessel walls, especially when zygomycotic agents are involved. Thrombosis, hemorrhage, necrosis, and inflammation with neutrophilic components predominating follow. Microscopic fetal lesions include bronchopneumonia and, where skin lesions are present, necrotizing epidermitis.

Extragenital lesions in the cows consist of pyogranulomatous nodules in various internal organs, particularly lung and kidneys. In cases of fatal pneumonia described as an abortion sequela due to *M. wolfii*, a fibrinohemorrhagic process is evident.

Diagnosis

The diagnosis of mycotic abortion rests on the demonstration of fungi in association with significant lesions. The mere demonstration or, even less conclusively, culture of fungi from specimens obtained after abortions or from genital tracts does not constitute adequate evidence of a causative role for the fungi. The ubiquity of fungi and the almost invariable contamination of placenta and fetus before examination render the presence of fungi in such material very likely. Fungi must be demonstrated as integral parts of the lesions before their etiologic significance can be fully established.

For pathologic examination, placental tissues, especially cotyledons, should be submitted. If the entire fetus cannot be promptly forwarded to a laboratory, skin lesions, lymph nodes, lung, and stomach with its contents securely tied off should be forwarded. Duplicate tissue samples can be placed into 10 per cent formalin. The stomach contents may be preserved for microscopic examination by addition of 1 part formalin to 9 parts fluid. Fungi do not tolerate putrefactive tissue changes well, nor do they benefit from freezing.

Treatment and Control

To date, no specific control measures are available. A reasonable preventive step is the elimination of moldy feeds and, as far as possible, removal from moldy environments. Most cows that survive an episode of fungal abortion return to breed normally, without special treatment.

MYCOTIC MASTITIS

Incidence

The incidence of mycotic mastitis ranges from about 1 to 10 per cent of total mastitis of infectious origin. These figures may have little relevance to individual herds, in which outbreaks, usually triggered by some management factor, may involve the majority of milking cows. A large variety of fungal agents have been implicated. The most frequent are the yeastlike fungi, particularly *Candida* spp. and *Cryptococcus* spp. Rare genera are *Hansenula, Pichia, Rhodotorula, Torulopsis, Trichosporon,* and *Saccharomyces*. Mold mastitis is rarely encountered, but there have been incriminations of *A. fumigatus* in a greater number of instances in recent years, particularly in Europe. *Pseudallescheria (Petriellidium) boydii* has been implicated on occasion, and there is growing awareness of the alga *Prototheca* sp. (usually *P. zopfii*) causing mastitis.

Epidemiology

Like all mastitis, mycotic mastitis is decisively influenced by management factors. Two aspects of dairy routine are particularly pertinent, milking hygiene and the use of antimicrobial drugs, especially by intramammary infusion. Inadequate milking hygiene may permit the passage of mastitis-producing agents from one mammary gland to another, converting a basically fortuitous, sporadic infection into a transmissible disease of potentially epidemic proportions. Mycotic mastitis as a herd problem is related to machine milking and other practices involving rapid successive contact of udders with persons or equipment capable of acting as vehicles of transmission.

The use of antibacterial drugs can play a part in the production of mastitis in 2 possible ways. First, it can provide the mechanical means of introducing fungal spores into the gland, because these are abundant in the environment, including the skin of the udder. Yeasts have also been found in freshly opened antibiotic preparations, which suggests contamination during manufacture. Second, some antimicrobials are suspected of stimulating fungal growth and depressing certain host defense factors. Tetracycline has been described as having both these effects with regard to *C. albicans*. Circumstances surrounding mycotic mastitis outbreaks frequently include preceding or ongoing antibacterial intramammary therapy.

Clinical Signs, Pathogenesis, and Pathology

Fungal mastitis has no consistent peculiarities to differentiate it from bacterial mastitis. Reduced milk flow, swelling, and greater firmness of the affected gland are observed along with varying abnormalities in the appearance of the milk and positive results of the California Mastitis Test. Fevers with "spiking" temperatures may occur but have not been correlated with demonstrable fungemia. The duration and course of the disease are highly variable, depending on the infecting agent and on the size of the infecting dose. The most severe fungal mastitis is caused by *C. neoformans*, which can extend over weeks and months, lead to complete suppression of milk flow, and leave glands with diminished or lost milk-secreting ability. By contrast, infection with other yeasts (*Candida* spp., *Trichosporon* spp.) takes a more benign and frequently self-limiting course. Whenever herds undergoing outbreaks of fungal mastitis have been investigated, a large proportion of infected but clinically normal animals were identified, even when *C. neoformans* was present.

The pathologic changes evoked by yeasts are pyogranulomatous reactions. The acute phase is characterized by neutrophilic and eosinophilic exudates. Histiocytic infiltration and granuloma formation follow. In gross appearance, edema predominates early, with granulomatous foci and fibrotic changes occurring in advanced lesions.

In *A. fumigatus* mastitis, a chronic progressive course is usually observed with suppurative lesions predominating at necropsy. Protothecal mastitis, although varying from acute to chronic to inapparent, also appears to follow a progressive, irreversible course ending eventually in the destruction of the infected gland.

Diagnosis

In the absence of specific clinical criteria, the demonstration of the causative agent by direct microscopic findings and culture is a requirement for establishing a diagnosis of fungal mastitis. The manner of collection, promptness of handling, and method of processing determine results. The presence of fungi (e.g., *Candida* spp.) in the environment, on the skin, and even in the teat canal and sinus would render the isolation of small numbers of the organisms of doubtful significance. However, finding yeast cells in fresh milk by direct microscopic examinations of fixed stained smears indicates the presence of considerable numbers and points to infection. *Candida* cells are readily stained by Gram's stain and appear as predominantly purple, often budding ovoids. Cryptococcal cells do not show any consistent staining patterns with Gram's stain and are apt to be overlooked.

Both *Candida* and *Cryptococcus* will grow on most common culture media, including blood and Sabouraud's agar at either room temperature or 37° C. Several days should be allowed for colonial growth to develop. The specific identification of the yeast is based on morphologic and physiologic tests. Several simple commercially available systems of yeast identification exist for clinically prominent species. Hyphal fragments can be demonstrated in centrifuged mammary secretions by wet mounts in 15 per cent potassium hydroxide. *A. fumigatus* grows well on blood agar and most other common media and is identified on the basis of fruiting structure morphology. Demonstration and culture of *Prototheca* spp. have been described earlier.

Treatment and Control

There is at present no established treatment for fungal mastitis, and many cases may resolve spontaneously in 2 to 4 weeks. In fact, no intramammary antimycotic drug has been approved to date for use in the United States. Recommendations followed in Europe include intramammary nystatin ointment at the rate of 3 g on 3 successive days, or nystatin solution at the rate of 250,000 units in 2.5 ml on at least 2 successive days but to no more than 2 quarters at one time because of the toxic local and systemic effects that the aqueous solution may elicit. Clotrimazole is also suggested and can be used as ointment or as aqueous solution at the rate of 100 to 200 mg/quarter in 10 to 20 ml, 2 to 4 times at 24-hour intervals. Another drug that has been suggested for treatment of *Candida* mastitis is intramammary natamycin (Pimaricin) given as 2.5 or 5 per cent solution in 20 or 10 ml, respectively, on 3 successive days.

In vitro test results showed yeasts isolated from bovine mastitis most susceptible to clotrimazole. Results varied with regard to other antimycotics, including miconazole, nystatin, and 5-fluorocytosine. One study rated ketoconazole next best to clotrimazole.

Treatment of *Prototheca* mastitis with most antibacterial antibiotics is ineffective. Strains are, however, sensitive to myxin and nystatin, with a proportion sensitive to polymyxin B, amphotericin B, and gentamicin. There is no published experience on their use in treatment. Approaches to control have usually involved repeated cultural examination for identifying infected cows, which are then immediately culled. This approach is combined with environmental, especially water, hygiene.

There are no recommendations, based on adequate field or experimental studies, concerning the treatment of mastitis due to molds.

OTHER MYCOSES

Aspergillosis

Sporadic clinical aspergillosis in cattle, sheep, and swine as either isolated cases or limited outbreaks has been reported from all parts of the world. Primarily young animals or debilitated animals are involved. Either the respiratory or alimentary tract is affected and constitutes the likely portal of infection. General cases with lesions in kidney, liver, and lungs are also sometimes observed.

Massive exposure to moldy feed and bedding, dietary acidosis, and extended administration of antimicrobial drugs have been found associated with infection. Subclinical infections have been shown to be widespread in cattle, with both pulmonary and intestinal localizations reported. Several instances of fatal infections in newborn animals, especially lambs, point to the likelihood of prenatal exposure.

Acute cases exhibit hemorrhagic, necrotic lesions associated with vasculitis and thrombosis. More chronic cases are characterized by granuloma formation and fibrosis. Eosinophils may be prominent in association with the lesions and in the circulating blood. The agent will appear as septate filaments, 2 to 3 μm in diameter, fairly regular in outline, and generally branching at acute angles. In progressive pulmonary aspergillosis, cavitation may occur, with the fungus growing freely in the lumen of the cavities, producing cottony, aerial mycelia, complete with pigmented fruiting bodies. A frequent feature of chronic and subclinical aspergillosis is the presence of "asteroid" bodies, that is, hyphal nests surrounded by radiating acidophilic projections.

Zygomycoses

Systemic infection with Zygomycetes occurs primarily in cattle but also in swine. Reports of infections in sheep are extremely rare. The genera involved are mainly *Mucor*, *Absidia*, and *Rhizopus*. Many cases are based on histopathologic findings only, so that no genus, let alone species, identification is possible. A noteworthy incidence of *Mortierella* infections has been reported mainly from New Zealand.

The epidemiology of these infections, like that of aspergillosis, is related to acidosis, inappropriate diet, and concurrent infection due to other fungi, bacteria, or viruses. Unusually concentrated exposure to the agents is also thought to play a part. Gastrointestinal tract involvement predominates, especially in pigs. Several cases of neonatal encephalitis have been observed in cattle.

Reports of zygomycotic infections, especially in young animals, describe acute signs and lesions more often than is the case with aspergillosis. Gastrointestinal tract disturbances are frequently the first sign, including anorexia and mucosanguineous diarrhea. Ruminal atony, bloat, and colic have been observed in affected cattle. Other forms affect mainly the lymph nodes of the intestinal tract or thorax.

The gross lesions in the gastrointestinal tract are ulcerations of stomach and intestine. Any part of the stomach can be involved. In ruminants, the rumen and abomasum are the usual sites. Depending on the acuteness of the condition, hemorrhagic, necrotic, suppurative, or nodular granulomatous features will predominate in that order. The basic lesion is vasculitis, affecting either arteries or veins and initiated by hyphal invasion of the vessel wall. Thrombosis and vascular disintegration follow, causing hemorrhage, necrosis, and suppuration that are grossly observable. In the lymphadenitic form, the only lesions may be granulomas in the nodes that range from a few millimeters in diameter to those that have replaced all recognizable lymph node tissue. Hyphae will be apparent and distinguishable from those of *Aspergillus* spp. by their larger size (up to 7 μm), their irregular outline, their relative lack of septa, and their greater tendency to branch to right angles.

In swine, gastric zygomycosis has been reported infrequently as a cause of mucosal or transmural hemorrhagic ulcers, sometimes in pigs as young as 1 week old. Predisposing factors may include liberal use of antibiotics in piglets or their dams. In older pigs, zygomycosis is sometimes associated with minor mesenteric lymph node granulomas.

No successful treatment has been established.

Candidiasis

Most *Candida* infections have been encountered in cattle and swine. The localization, other than in bovine mastitis, has been predominantly in the alimentary tract from the mouth to the intestine. Septicemic and pneumonic infections are seen rarely.

The source of the causative agents may be the mucous membranes of the animals themselves containing *C. albicans*, as well as the skin and external environment containing other *Candida* spp. The prolonged use of broad-spectrum antibacterial drugs is frequently a factor in initiating clinical candidiasis. The disruption of the normal microbial balance in the digestive tract produces the overgrowth by the yeasts. In some cases, massive prolonged exposure to contaminated feed has been implicated in the absence of, or in addition to, antibiotics.

The common clinical form of candidiasis is thrush and enteritis in calves and young pigs. Thrush is an ulcerative pseudomembranous inflammation of the mucous membranes of the mouth, esophagus, and stomach (rumen). The process in the intestine is similar but not usually referred to as thrush. Clinical signs will reflect the location of the process; inappetence, excessive salivation, and vomiting occur in oral and upper digestive tract infections. Intestinal infections are also characterized by diarrhea.

Lesions are those of ulcerative inflammation with varying amounts of overlying fibrinous exudate. As long as the process is relatively superficial, the yeast forms of *Candida* predominate. With invasion of deeper tissue, pseudomycelial and mycelial structures replace the yeasts.

Confirmation of candidiasis requires demonstration of *Candida* spp. in significant numbers in association with compatible lesions. The recovery of *Candida* from oral or rectal swabs and even from tracheobronchial washes does not establish the diagnosis. Overgrowth without significant pathogenic activity is a distinct possibility with these fungi. Finding a preponderance of filamentous forms would be much more suggestive of a disease. Microbiologic observations must be evaluated in the light of pathologic and clinical evidence.

The agents of candidiasis are readily cultured on common media over a wide range of temperatures. There are few reports of successful treatment of clinical candidiasis, especially from this country. Experience in Europe showed favorable results with oral nystatin and amphotericin B in isolated instances. Control measures should be directed at removing underlying causes.

Histoplasmosis and Coccidioidomycosis

Instances of clinical histoplasmosis in livestock are extremely rare. Existing reports concern cattle and pigs. Respiratory lesions were present in all 6 cases but 1, in which the lesions were in the liver.

Among food-producing mammals, only cattle are infected with *C. immitis* to any significant extent. The infection is quite common in endemic areas but invariably subclinical and evident only at post-mortem examination, when thoracic lymphadenitis and small lung lesions may be noted. Coccidioidomycosis in sheep has been reported. The infection is of no economic importance in livestock.

Mycotic Nasal Infections

A variety of fungi have been implicated in nasal infections. Among food-producing animals, only cattle have been involved. The lesions are nasal granulomas and polyps, which lead to respiratory distress of varying severity. Best known among the polyp-forming infections is rhinosporidiosis, a disease mostly seen in tropical and subtropical climates but occasionally seen in the United States. Polyps, pedunculated or not, form in 1 nostril. They are soft and pink and bleed readily. The whitish specks they contain are the spherules (sporangia) previously mentioned. Treatment is through surgical excision. A report from Argentina refers to cures in 9 cases after treatment with calcium, isoniazid (isonicotinic acid hydrazide), and 60 per cent sodium iodide.

Bovine granulomas with and without polyp formations have been found associated with infections by pigmented saprophytic fungi (pheohyphomycosis). Some of these infections were accompanied by fairly widespread involvement of skin and lymph nodes. The agents included among other black (dematiaceous) fungi mainly *Drechslera rostrata* and *D. spicifera*. The lesions have been described as mycetomas, and allergy is assumed by many workers to be involved. No medical treatment is known.

ANTIFUNGAL DRUGS

Medical treatment of deep mycosis in food animals is a virtually unexplored field, in part because antifungal drugs suitable for such treatment are relatively new and have not been adequately tested in food-producing mammals. It is to be expected that this situation will change and that drugs presently in use on humans and companion animals will be utilized on meat and dairy stock. A brief characterization of the types of drugs used on fungal infections is therefore appropriate. Present antifungal drugs fall into 3 chemical categories.

1. The polyenes are represented by nystatin (Mycostatin*) and amphotericin B (Fungizone*). They are characterized by limited solubility in water and poor absorbability from the gastrointestinal tract. They are also quite toxic. Nystatin is useful only for topical application or intestinal infection, mostly of yeasts. Amphotericin B, which is at present the mainstay of antifungal therapy in humans, is given by intravenous injection. Systemic amphotericin B has not been used in food animals. Natamycin is effective against a wide range of filamentous fungi and yeasts. It is poorly absorbed and is therefore not useful in systemic infections but has been used effectively in the treatment of mycotic mastitis.

2. A more recently introduced antimycotic is 5-fluorocytosine (flucytosine, e.g., Ancobon†), which is readily absorbed from the gastrointestinal tract and is generally well tolerated. Its usefulness so far has been confined largely to the treatment of infections due to yeastlike fungi, particularly candidiasis and cryptococcosis. A further limitation to the use of 5-fluorocytosine is the existence of resistant strains of these yeasts in nature and the common emergence of resistance in the course of treatment. Susceptibility tests are advisable for establishing the appropriateness of this drug in each instance its use is considered.

3. The most recent additions to the antimycotic armamentarium are the various imidazole derivatives, for example, miconazole (Monistat‡), clotrimazole (Lotrimin§), and ketoconazole (Nizoral‡). Some of these drugs (e.g., miconazole), can be used both topically and systemically, whereas others are for topical use only (e.g., clotrimazole). The imidazole derivatives have a rather broad spectrum of activity and affect both yeasts and mycelial fungi. They are effective when administered orally. Resistance has so far not been a major problem. The drugs even have some antibacterial activity and inhibit dermatophytes as well. Their toxicity is much less than that of amphotericin B.

Acknowledgment

This article is based on the section Systemic Mycoses written by Dr. E. L. Biberstein for the second edition of Current Veterinary Therapy: Food Animal Practice.

BIBLIOGRAPHY

Ainsworth GC, Austwick PKC: Fungal Diseases of Animals, 2nd ed. England, Commonwealth Agricultural Bureaux, Farnham Royal, 1973.
Jungerman PF, Schwartzman RM: Veterinary Medical Mycology. Philadelphia, Lea & Febiger, 1973.
McDonald JS, Richard JL, Anderson AJ, Fichter RE: In vitro antimycotic sensitivity of yeasts isolated from infected bovine mammary glands. Am J Vet Res 41:1987–1990, 1980.
Pepin GA: Bovine mycotic abortion. Vet Annu 23:79–90, 1983.
Rippon JW: Medical Mycology, 2nd ed. Philadelphia, WB Saunders, 1982.
Weigt V, Ahlers D: Zur Atiologie, Symptomatologie und Therapie der Hefemastitis bein Rind. Dtsch Tieraerztl Wochenschr 89:234–238, 1982.

Swine Mycobacterial Disease

J. GLENN SONGER, PhD

ETIOLOGY

In the early 1900s, human and bovine tuberculosis were much more prevalent than they are today, and the organisms found as etiologic agents of tuberculosis in swine were often of either bovine (*Mycobacterium bovis*) or human (*M. tuberculosis*) type. However, *M. avium* began to appear more frequently during the second quarter of the century and has gradually overtaken *M. bovis* and *M. tuberculosis* in importance as a cause of mycobacterial disease in swine. During the past 15 years, isolation from swine of mycobacteria other than *M. avium* has been uncommon, and this is an increasing trend worldwide. Reports of extensive involvement of *M. bovis* in tuberculosis of swine have usually addressed animals produced outside the United States or those fed improperly cooked wastes from cattle slaughtering plants.

Tuberculosis in chickens or other fowl remains a periodic source of infection for swine. Pig-to-pig transmission of tuberculosis may also be a problem, apparently owing to shedding in feces of *M. avium* from lesions in the intestinal wall. The major sources of infection are chickens or other birds and contaminated woodshavings. Pig-to-pig transmission is not significant because infection is not maintained in a herd once the external source has been eliminated. Infections of other tissues, such as lungs, mammary glands, and uterus, also occur and may represent a means of dissemination. Feeding of improperly processed contaminated, mainly chicken, food waste is another possible means for the spread of swine tuberculosis.

The environment may also be a reservoir of *M. avium*. The organism has been reported to survive more than 4 years in soil and other materials contaminated by chickens with tuberculosis. A new facet of swine tuberculosis, especially in large confined herds, is its association with woodshavings used for bedding. Outbreaks usually involve 30 to 60 per cent of slaughter swine. Serovars of *M. avium* recovered from swine can often be recovered by bacteriologic culture of sawdust and

---

*E. R. Squibb & Sons, Princeton, NJ 08540.
†Hoffmann–La Roche, Inc., Nutley, NJ 07110.
‡Janssen Pharmaceutical, Inc., New Brunswick, NJ 08903.
§Schering Corporation, Kenilworth, NJ 07033.

woodshavings from the same premises. The organism survives in these materials for long periods of time (up to 160 days at 18° to 22° C under experimental conditions and at least 4 years under natural conditions) and may multiply if provided with proper conditions of moisture and temperature. Seasonal variation in these conditions correlates with seasonal occurrence of tuberculosis in some herds.

Mention should also be made of other mycobacteria occasionally isolated from granulomatous lesions in lymph nodes of swine. Isolation of the human opportunist pathogens *M. kansasii*, *M. xenopi*, and *M. fortuitum* has been described, but the greatest usefulness of these findings may be in determining if swine and humans are infected from a similar source. *M. chelonei* has been isolated from pigs and is of potential significance to human health, because the same organism has been found in prosthetic heart valves prepared from swine. *M. paratuberculosis*, the cause of paratuberculosis (Johne's disease), and *M. microti*, the vole bacillus, have also been isolated from pigs, but the significance of these findings is unknown.

SIGNIFICANCE

Mycobacterium avium–induced infections in pigs bear little resemblance to what is commonly called tuberculosis in cattle or humans. In contrast to the progressive nature of disease caused by *M. tuberculosis* or *M. bovis*, *M. avium* infection in pigs rarely produces clinical signs. Some have, in fact, suggested that it be called swine mycobacteriosis rather than tuberculosis.

There is no evidence for transmission of the infection from pigs to humans, either by direct contact or by consuming pork products, but the possibility of such transmission is the basis for current meat inspection regulations. Up until about 20 years ago, swine tissues with lesions determined by gross inspection to be tuberculous were trimmed and discarded. This is a reasonable step. However, a regulation adopted in 1972 in the United States calls for cooking (170° F, 30 minutes) all of the carcasses found to have at least 2 isolated tuberculous lesions; these carcasses are designated "passed for cooking" or PFC. Carcasses processed in this manner lose most of their economic worth, and the additional labor required at slaughter exacerbates the situation. The absence of cooking facilities in many processing plants requires that PFC carcasses be condemned.

Estimates of the prevalence of swine tuberculosis have usually been based on the rate of detection of lesions by federal meat inspectors. On the basis of this methodology, the annual prevalence of mycobacterial disease in swine is about 5 per 1000 in all hogs slaughtered under federal inspection, which costs the pork industry an estimated $2.5 to $3 million annually. It is likely that this figure is influenced by both false-positives (due to infection by organisms such as *Rhodococcus equi* and the occurrence of culturally negative, "healed" lesions) and false-negatives (due to the presence of *M. avium* in lymph nodes in the absence of gross and even microscopic lesions).

The public health significance of *M. avium* infections may be increasing. Of specific interest are reports on the involvement of serovars of *M. avium* in disease in patients with acquired immune deficiency syndrome.

PATHOGENESIS

Pigs usually develop tuberculous lesions after ingestion of feed contaminated with *M. avium*, as determined by the high percentage of pigs developing lesions in lymph nodes associated with the digestive tract, compared with lymph nodes draining other organ systems. When swallowed, *M. avium* attaches to epithelial cells and eventually penetrates the wall of the gastrointestinal tract. Macrophages engulf organisms that infiltrate the subepithelial space and then carry them to the regional lymph nodes, usually the cervical or mesenteric nodes. Lesion development occurs in these nodes, and as noted, progressive disease is rare. Pigs may be most susceptible to this infectious process during the first few days of life. Rarely, miliary tubercular lesions may develop in the liver after spread by the portal vein from the intestine.

DIAGNOSIS

Because of the absence of significant effects of *M. avium* infection in the pig, clinical diagnosis is usually not possible. Thus diagnosis requires detection of typical gross and microscopic lesions and isolation and identification of *M. avium* or other mycobacteria. The tuberculin skin test, in which intradermal administration of 0.1 ml tuberculin or PPD into the dorsal surface of the ear produces a zone of erythema and possibly necrosis in 24 to 48 hours, may be beneficial as a herd test. However, it must be used with circumspection, because it displays high false-positive and false-negative rates. No other diagnostic test is in common use, but development of such tests should be encouraged. An efficacious blood test, such as the enzyme-linked immunosorbent assay (ELISA), could eliminate the double handling of animals required by use of the skin test, and blood samples submitted for other tests, such as pseudorabies and brucellosis, could likewise be used to test for tuberculosis.

As noted, lesions produced by *M. avium* infection in swine are typically confined to the lymph nodes associated with the digestive tract. In gross appearance, lesions are nodular and are white to yellow in color, sometimes exhibiting a slightly greenish cast. They vary in size from barely visible to 10 mm in diameter. Although active lesions are rarely calcified, lesions that are several months of age (such as those found in slaughter pigs that were exposed to the infection soon after birth) may be calcified, as suggested by their gritty texture on cutting. Caseous exudate is usually seen, and diffuse fibrosis and proliferation of epithelioid and giant cells is a distinctive characteristic of lesions. The mycobacterial etiologic agent of the lesions cannot be determined by examination of gross and microscopic lesions but requires bacteriologic examination for determining whether the causative agent is *M. avium* or another organism such as *M. bovis* or *M. tuberculosis*.

THERAPY

No vaccine is available at present. No antimicrobial agents have been shown to be effective in preventing or treating the infection.

PREVENTION AND CONTROL

Swine mycobacterial disease is better prevented than controlled. Contact between pigs and birds should be strictly controlled, including keeping wild birds away from feed storage areas. A common practice is to refrain from mixing swine and poultry production on the same farm. Hogs should not be housed in old poultry buildings unless they are constructed in such a way as to allow thorough cleaning and disinfection with a phenol-based disinfectant (such as Amphyl) or a 2 to 3 per cent cresylic acid solution. Quaternary ammonium disinfectants are not effective against mycobacteria. Concrete surfaces and equipment such as farrowing crates and feeders must also be disinfected. Because little is known about effective decontamination of infected soil, concrete lots should be used whenever possible.

Use of woodshavings for bedding (especially in farrowing buildings) should be eliminated, if possible. Whereas many producers have used woodshavings as swine bedding without significant problems, others have been forced out of business because of the economic strain of dealing with tuberculosis in their animals. If woodshavings are used as bedding, they should be kept dry, both at the sawmill and on the farm, and anecdotal information suggests that shavings from kiln-dried lumber are less likely to contain *M. avium* than are shavings from green lumber. Improperly cooked garbage or other material that might contain viable pathogenic mycobacteria must not be fed to pigs. When possible, breeding stock should be purchased from tuberculosis-free herds.

Once the source of the infection is found and eliminated (e.g., infected bedding), the producer may be able to wait the approximate 6-month period until all exposed pigs have been slaughtered and the disease disappears. The infection will not be maintained in the herd by pigs. Alternatively, infected herds may be depopulated and then repopulated with stock from tuberculosis-free herds, but the important point is to find and remove the source. Another strategy for managing an outbreak of disease after removal of the source is based on the fact that lesions caused by *M. avium* often regress and disappear with age. Infected gilts can be kept, for adding to the herd size or replacing retired breeders, and when these animals are sold at the end of their usefulness as breeding stock, the lesions may have disappeared.

BIBLIOGRAPHY

Grange JM, Yates MD, Broughton E: The avian tubercle bacillus and its relatives. J Appl Bacteriol 68:411–431, 1990.
Thoen CO, Karlson AG: Tuberculosis. *In* Leman AD, et al (eds): Diseases of Swine, 6th ed. Ames, IA, Iowa State University Press, 1986, pp 484–493.

Tuberculosis
L. D. KONYHA, DVM, MS

Tuberculosis is an infectious disease caused by certain pathogenic acid-fast organisms of the genus *Mycobacterium* and is usually characterized by the formation of nodular granulomas known as tubercles. Although commonly a chronic, debilitating disease, tuberculosis can occasionally assume an acute, rapidly progressive course.

ETIOLOGY

Three main types of tubercle bacilli are recognized: human, bovine, and avian. Their causative organisms are classified in *Bergey's Manual of Systematic Bacteriology* as *Mycobacterium tuberculosis*, *M. bovis*, and *M. avium*, respectively. Because tubercle bacilli do not multiply except in infected animals, their principal reservoirs in nature are the 3 groups of animals mentioned. Although certain morphologic and cultural differences are described, these can vary considerably and cannot be depended on for accurate identification. Many biochemical tests have been devised that are extremely useful in classifying mycobacteria. The most common are the niacin, catalase, arylsulfatase, and growth inhibition tests. The mycobacterial tube agglutination test described by Schaefer has provided a useful procedure for the classification of *M. avium* complex organisms. Cattle are susceptible to human tuberculosis, but lesions of this infection are seldom reported. Although there are cases on record of generalized bovine tuberculosis caused by the avian strain, they are unusual. If avian infection becomes established in bovines, gross lesions generally are limited to the mesenteric lymph nodes. During the 7-year period from October 1, 1982, to September 30, 1989, *M. bovis* accounted for 64.2 per cent of the total isolations of mycobacteria from specimens submitted to the National Veterinary Services Laboratories for examination for tuberculosis.

EPIDEMIOLOGY

Bovine tuberculosis is known to exist in all parts of the world. Of the 176 countries reporting in the 1988 Animal Health Yearbook, 4 indicated bovine tuberculosis to be an exceptional occurrence, 62 reported a low sporadic occurrence, 21 reported it as enzootic, 3 reported a high occurrence, and 7 stated the disease exists but the occurrence is unknown. Even though tuberculosis in cattle in the United States has been reduced to a low sporadic occurrence, there were still 3 new *M. bovis*–infected herds in fiscal year 1989, and 13 in fiscal year 1990, so reports of epizootics of the disease continue.

PATHOGENESIS

The disease commences with the formation of the primary focus, which is in the lungs in about 90 per cent of the cases. Lymphatic drainage from the primary focus leads to the formation of a caseous lesion in the corresponding lymph node, and this lesion, together with the primary focus, is known as the primary complex.

Whenever the organisms localize, their activity stimulates the formation of tumor-like masses called tubercles. Any body tissue can be affected, but lesions are most frequently observed in lymph nodes (bronchial, mediastinal, portal, and cervical), lungs, liver, spleen, and surfaces of the body cavities. The bacilli spread throughout tissues by extension onto surfaces in contact with a lesion, or they may be transported in body cavity fluids. Bacilli may also be disseminated in the vascular system subsequent to vessel erosion at a lesion site.

GENERAL MODE OF SPREAD

The tuberculous cow is the greatest source of danger to healthy cattle, and an infected animal not promptly removed from the herd is a potential source of reinfection. Active lesions contain myriad bacilli, capable of wide dissemination through the natural body openings. In diseased cattle, this is most frequently by way of the respiratory tract. Bronchial exudates teeming with organisms may be expelled into the manger or watering trough by coughing, or exudates may be swallowed and expelled in the feces. Animals that ingest contaminated feed or water may contract the disease. Inhalation of contaminated aerosols is an important mode by which the disease is disseminated in closed barns with poor ventilation. Contaminated dust, droplets, or dried secretions can enter the respiratory tract and cause infection in susceptible animals.

Viable organisms can also be eliminated in milk, even in the absence of udder lesions. Calves sometimes are infected during the first few hours or days of life by nursing an infected dam. Many calves in the past were infected by ingestion of unpasteurized skimmed milk from diseased cows. Calves may infrequently be infected as a result of intrauterine exposure.

CLINICAL SIGNS

Clinical signs of tuberculosis in cattle in the United States are seldom encountered today because the intradermal tuberculin test results facilitate presumptive diagnosis and elimination of infected animals before signs appear. Before the national bovine tuberculosis eradication program, however, the signs associated with this disease were commonly observed.

The evidence of tuberculosis exhibited by any animal depends on the extent and location of lesions. Characteristic signs are often lacking even in advanced stages of the disease in which many organs may be involved. Lung involvement may be manifested by a cough that can be induced by changes in temperature or by manual pressure on the trachea. Dyspnea and other signs of low-grade pneumonia are also evidence of lung involvement. In advanced cases, lymph nodes are frequently greatly enlarged and may obstruct air passages, the alimentary tract, or blood vessels. Lymph nodes of the head and neck may become visibly affected and sometimes rupture and drain to the outside. Involvement of the digestive tract is characterized by intermittent diarrhea and by constipation in some instances. Extreme emaciation and acute respiratory distress may occur during the terminal stages. Lesions involving the female genitalia are possible. Primary uterine infection may rarely occur after service by an infected bull. However, tuberculosis is efficiently transmitted by artificial insemination with contaminated semen. The male genitalia are seldom involved; however, when penile lesions are present, they appear to be limited to the submucosa of the glans, sheath, and adjacent lymphatics.

PATHOLOGIC PICTURE

On necropsy, tuberculous granulomas usually have a yellowish appearance and are caseous, caseocalcareous, or calcified in consistency. The appearance may sometimes be purulent. The caseous center is usually dry and firm and covered by a fibrous connective capsule of varying thickness. In recent years, calcification has been seen less commonly. The lesions may be so small that they are missed by the unaided eye or so large as to involve the greater part of the organ. Bronchopneumonia may be observed grossly in instances of lung lesions, and there may be some microscopic evidence of fluid accumulations. Lesions may be situated in any one of the lung lobes, causing a productive bronchopneumonia that, in turn, gives rise to lesions in the bronchotracheal tree and regional lymph nodes.

Tubercle bacilli entering the body are phagocytized by neutrophils almost immediately. The neutrophils are destroyed by the multiplying mycobacteria, and as dead cells they stimulate the accumulation of epithelioid cells that engulf the neutrophils and mycobacteria. The bacilli are not destroyed, but multiply within the epithelioid cells and apparently stimulate a strong cytotoxic T-cell response that destroys adjoining cells. This causes an area of caseous necrosis and the beginning of a tubercle. As epithelioid cells encircle the necrotic area, the cellular nuclei disappear from the center of the tubercle, and structural detail is lost. A number of epithelioid cells coalesce, forming multinucleated giant cells (Langhans' cells). These cells are characteristic but not pathognomonic of tubercles. They are also found in granulomatous lesions seen in other chronic inflammatory diseases. Acid-fast bacilli may be demonstrated throughout a lesion in epithelioid cells, in giant cells, and in necrotic debris. Granulation tissue forms and is usually surrounded by a zone of lymphocytes and fibroblasts, frequently near a blood vessel.

DIAGNOSIS

Clinical evidence of tuberculosis is usually lacking; therefore, its diagnosis in individual animals and an eradication program were not possible before the discovery of tuberculin by Koch in 1890. Tuberculin, a concentrated sterile culture filtrate of tubercle bacilli grown on glycerinated beef broth, and more recently on synthetic media, provides a means of detecting the diseased animal. Animals affected with tuberculosis are allergic to the proteins contained in the tuberculin and give characteristic delayed reactions when exposed to them. If tuberculin is deposited in the deep layers of the skin (intradermally), a local reaction characterized by swelling and inflammation is induced in infected animals. In the United States, the caudal fold is the preferred injection site for the intradermal tuberculin test. The injection site is examined by observation and palpation 72 hours after injection.

Nearly all countries of the world are now using a strain of *Mycobacterium bovis* for the preparation of mammalian tuberculin. Heat-concentrated synthetic media tuberculin (OT) is still used in some countries, but a majority (including the United States) are now using a purified protein derivative (PPD) tuberculin at a protein concentration of 1 mg/ml (3 mg/ml in Australia). PPD tuberculins are preferable because they are easier to standardize, more stable, and more specific.

Although remarkably effective, the intradermal test has certain limitations, as do all diagnostic tests. No antigen (tuberculin) is entirely specific. Significant intradermal responses are induced not only by infection with the homologous organism (*M. bovis*) but also to varying degrees by several heterologous organisms, primarily other mycobacteria. All caudal fold–responding animals in herds that are not known to be infected with *M. bovis* in areas of the world where bovine tuberculosis has been nearly eradicated (such as the United States) should be retested by the comparative-cervical (c-c) test. In the United States, only specifically approved state or federal regulatory veterinarians are permitted to conduct the c-c test using PPD tuberculins of equal biologic potency as determined in sensitized guinea pigs. The c-c test is contraindicated in cattle in known *M. bovis*–infected herds.

TREATMENT

Until the discovery of the antituberculosis drug isonicotinic acid hydrazine, or isoniazid (INH), there was no practical therapeutic agent available for the treatment of bovine tuberculosis. Reports from South Africa indicate that it is economically feasible to treat cattle with INH. See Table 1 for the protocol for treatment in South Africa.

Isoniazid therapy may have potential value in countries where the incidence of bovine tuberculosis is high and "test and slaughter" methods are not yet feasible. However, the disadvantages of treatment with INH are so great (up to 25

Table 1. ISONIAZID (INH) TREATMENT OF BOVINE TUBERCULOSIS

Choice of Herds for Treatment
Large herds (≥200), high producers, and herds with infection rate over 30 per cent; or
Positively reacting herds of valuable stud animals or when special blood lines are involved

Doses of INH
Infected cattle and cattle with suspicious reactions:
 20 mg/kg daily (maximum 12 g/day for bulls and 10 g/day for cows) for 2 months
 Then same dose 3 times weekly for another 5 months
Cattle with negative reactions:
 10 mg/kg daily (maximum 4.5 g/day for adults; 2.2 g/day for calves) for 2 months

---

per cent refractory cases, emergence of drug-resistant strains, elimination of INH in the milk, and the danger of relapse when the drug is withdrawn) that the treatment of bovine tuberculosis is not permitted in the United States.

PREVENTION AND CONTROL

Eradication of bovine tuberculosis is a major objective that has nearly been achieved in many countries of Europe, North America (including the United States), Japan, New Zealand, and Australia. The basis of these eradication programs has been the systematic application of the tuberculin test and the slaughter of the reactors.

The best preventive measure against the introduction of bovine tuberculosis is a negative tuberculin test before exchange of ownership, whether movements are international, interstate, or local in nature. A complete epidemiologic investigation, with testing when indicated, should be conducted on every regular-kill animal found to have lesions of tuberculosis on routine post-mortem examination.

Since 1890, various types of vaccines have been advocated for cattle, but none has produced effective immunity to bovine tuberculosis. Recent investigations in Malawi confirm that whereas bacille Calmette-Guérin (BCG) vaccine (the most successful immunizing agent in humans) reduces the severity of the initial disease in cattle, it does not completely prevent infection. Besides affording no practical protection to cattle, vaccination induces hypersensitivity to tuberculin and, thus, interferes with diagnostic test results. Countries that have attempted to use vaccination as the basis of a control program ultimately abandon the procedure in favor of the "test and slaughter" method.

BIBLIOGRAPHY

Animal Health Yearbook, FAO-WHO-OIE, 1988.
Francis J: Tuberculosis in Animals and Man. London, Cassel & Co, Ltd, 1958.
Rich AR: The Pathogenesis of Tuberculosis, 2nd ed. Springfield, IL, Charles C Thomas, 1950, pp 3–118.
Schaefer WB: Serologic identification and classification of the atypical mycobacteria by agglutination. Am Rev Respir Dis 96:115, 1965.
Smith HA, Jones TC, Hunt RD: Veterinary Pathology, 5th ed. Philadelphia, Lea & Febiger, 1983.
Wayne LG, Kubica GP: Family Mycobacteriaceae. In Sneath PHA (ed): Bergey's Manual of Systematic Bacteriology, vol 2. Baltimore, Williams & Wilkins, 1986, pp 1436–1457.

Paratuberculosis (Johne's Disease)
DANIEL G. BUTLER, DVM, MSc, PhD

Paratuberculosis or Johne's disease is an infectious, chronic granulomatous, enteric disease of domestic and wild ruminants caused by *Mycobacterium paratuberculosis* that occurs worldwide.[1]

Surveys in North America confirm the presence of the disease in cattle in the majority of states in the United States with a prevalence in ileocecal lymph nodes ranging from 1 to 19 per cent. The economic loss in the state of Wisconsin alone was estimated to be over $52 million per year.[2] The causative agent is a small, acid-fast organism, 1 to 2 by 0.5 μm, that inhabits the intestinal mucosa of the ileal and cecal area and adjacent mesenteric lymph nodes. The pathognomonic histologic finding is the presence of acid-fast organisms in clumps in these tissues.

The organism, which grows very slowly in the host and in specific culture media, can cross-infect sheep and cattle. To date, it is difficult to differentiate *M. paratuberculosis* from related species such as *M. avium*, although absolute dependence on exogenous mycobactin for in vitro growth is the common criterion. *M. paratuberculosis* survives outside the host in buildings for up to a year and in moist feces on pasture for 3 to 9 months. Although vertical transmission has been reported, infection is most commonly transmitted horizontally by the ingestion of food and water contaminated with feces from an infected animal shedding the organism.[3]

Spontaneous and experimental infection in cattle is characterized by chronic diarrhea and severe muscle wasting. However, the disease in sheep and goats is more typically a chronic wasting condition without diarrhea.

Because resistance to the organism increases with age, it is thought that clinical cases have been infected as neonates by repeated ingestion of the organism while nursing an infected dam. Depending on the age of the neonate, the number of ingested organisms, the degree of exposure, the status of natural resistance, the breed of the animal (Channel Island cattle are most susceptible), and the development of acquired immunity, the organisms may be eliminated or the animal may develop chronic infection of the intestinal mucosa and associated mesenteric lymph nodes. The chronically infected animals intermittently shed the organism in their feces and thus become a reservoir for infection in the herd. A proportion of these animals may go on to develop clinical disease as adults. Tonsillar and intestinal lymph tissue[4] as well as direct invasion of the intestinal mucosa have been suggested as portals of entry of the organism with subsequent dissemination within macrophages. The organism has been isolated from semen and the genital organs of bulls with Johne's disease, but the importance of venereal transmission in spreading infection is not established. Spontaneous and experimental infection of horses and pigs has periodically been reported. To date, no good laboratory animal model to facilitate experimental investigation has been described.

The isolation of a mycobactin-dependent *M. paratuberculosis*-like organism from humans with chronic inflammatory bowel disease begs the question of the zoonotic potential of *M. paratuberculosis*.

CLINICAL SIGNS

Cattle

After an incubation period of 1 or more years, those animals that fail to clear the organism become subclinically infected with intestinal lesions. Experimental intravenous inoculation of calves with *M. paratuberculosis* reduces this incubation period by 50 per cent. Infected animals carry the organism throughout their lives and shed it intermittently in their feces, with or without overt clinical signs of weight loss and chronic diarrhea. Commonly, these clinical signs become apparent in cattle at 2 to 6 years of age. Although terminally the diarrhea is severe and is associated with extreme muscle wasting and decreased milk production, acidosis is not a feature of the disease. Further, feed intake remains normal until it is compromised in the terminal stages of the disease by the severe debilitated state of the animal. The characteristic gross necropsy lesion is a corrugated appearance of the distal small intestine primarily associated with mucosal infiltration by inflammatory cells. Prominent mesenteric, submucosal, and serosal lymphatics and mesenteric lymph nodes have also been described.

Sheep and Goats

Clinical signs in small ruminants mimic those seen in cattle except that the progressive weight loss usually continues without evidence of diarrhea. Because affected animals also maintain a normal appetite, they are easily overlooked until they are severely emaciated. Gross and histologic necropsy findings are similar to those described for cattle, although the organism may often be found in the intestine proximal to the ileum.

DIAGNOSIS

In known infected herds and flocks, the astute manager can readily recognize the problem once unthriftiness becomes apparent. However, Johne's disease in cattle must be differentiated from chronic local peritonitis; liver abscessation; helminth parasitism in the early stages; and winter dysentery, pyelonephritis, and chronic salmonellosis in the later stages. In small ruminants, the disease must be differentiated from other causes of chronic wasting such as helminth parasitism and undernutrition associated with poor or abnormal dentition and inadequate energy intake because of a poor-quality ration or starvation.

To date, the gold standard for confirmation of the diagnosis in an individual animal has been histologic examination of tissue collected at surgery or at necropsy for ascertaining the presence of clumps of acid-fast organisms in the intestinal submucosa or cecal or mesenteric lymph nodes. Recently, rectal biopsy, as opposed to rectal scraping, has been recommended as a useful, expedient, and cheap clinical diagnostic procedure. Obviously, false-positive results are not possible, but negative results in this procedure do not rule out the infection. Likewise, although fecal culture is 100 per cent specific, it is estimated to detect only about 30 per cent of individual infected animals. As a herd test, however, fecal culture is considered to be both 100 per cent specific and 100 per cent sensitive in identifying infected herds of 25 animals or more and an essential component of any Johne's disease control program.

Agar-gel immunodiffusion (AGID), complement fixation test (CFT), and enzyme-linked immunosorbent assay (ELISA) are available for serologic diagnosis. The reliability of these tests improves as the disease progresses, so that they are usually positive in animals with marked clinical disease. They are unreliable in detecting subclinically affected carrier animals.

Unfortunately, even fecal culture combined with a variety of immunologic tests (CFT, AGID, ELISA, IV Johnin) cannot detect all animals infected with *M. paratuberculosis* because of the variability of fecal shedding and the unpredictable humoral and cell-mediated immune response relative to the spectrum of subclinical, clinical, and terminal disease. It is anticipated that the commercial production of DNA probes of high sensitivity and specificity for *M. paratuberculosis* in feces will greatly facilitate the diagnosis and control of this disease.

TREATMENT AND CONTROL

Prolonged antibiotic therapy with a variety of drugs including antituberculosis drugs has not been successful and is therefore not recommended.

Unattenuated, attenuated, heat killed, or disrupted vacuum-dried fragments of MPTB have been injected subcutaneously, usually in the brisket area, to boost immunity. Although a single dose of vaccine at 1 to 35 days of age before exposure to infection reduces and delays the onset of clinical signs and reduces mortality, it does not prevent Johne's disease in cattle, sheep, or goats. Vaccination reduces the extent of intestinal lesions and fecal shedding but does not eliminate infection from the herd or flock. For this reason, and because vaccination may cause animals to react to tuberculin, federal and state agencies that permit the use of vaccine require that a supervised Johne's disease control program that involves fecal culture of the entire herd twice yearly, culling of all positive animals and their offspring, and institution of hygienic precautions for limiting the spread of infection be rigidly followed. Relative to the last measure, fecal contamination of feed and drinking water, strip grazing, and low-lying wet pasture areas should be avoided. In the absence of vaccination and culture, additional approaches to control include rearing young away from their mothers for 12 months before reintroduction to the farm; feeding these animals pasteurized colostrum in the first 24 hours of life; provision of piped, non–fecally contaminated water to the herd; culling of any of the offspring of animals that develop clinical disease; and early recognition and removal of animals with clinical illness.

REFERENCES

1. Chiodini RJ, Van Kruiningen HJ, Merkal RS: Ruminant paratuberculosis (Johne's disease). the current status and future prospects. Cornell Vet 74:218–262, 1984.
2. Merkal RS, Whipple DL, Sacks JM, Snyder GR: Prevalence of *Mycobacterium paratuberculosis* in ileocecal lymph nodes of cattle culled in the United States. J Am Vet Med Assoc 190:676–680, 1987.
3. Thomas GW: Johne's disease (paratuberculosis) in goats. In Gruncell CSG, Hill FWG, Raw MZ (eds): Veterinary Annual, vol 25. Bristol, Scientechnica, 1985, pp 231–235.
4. Payne JM, Rankin JD: The pathogenesis of experimental Johne's disease in calves. Res Vet Sci 2:167–174, 1961.

Actinobacillosis and Actinomycosis

R. D. WALKER, PhD, MS

ACTINOBACILLOSIS

Actinobacillosis is caused by bacteria belonging to the genus *Actinobacillus*. These organisms are pleomorphic gram-negative rods that may appear as coccobacilli to long filamentous rods when they are Gram-stained. Most bacteria belonging to this genus are part of the normal flora of the respiratory, alimentary, or genital tracts of healthy animals. Disease develops when these organisms are allowed to spread beyond the confines of colonized mucosal barriers. Whereas capsules have not been demonstrated on most species of *Actinobacillus*, *A. actinomycetemcomitans*, *A. equuli*, and *A. suis* do produce an extracellular slime. The capsular material from *A. actinomycetemcomitans* may play an active role in tissue destruction. This organism also produces bacteriocin, which is inhibitory to other bacteria. It is not known whether other species of *Actinobacillus*, associated with disease in food animals, possess this same virulence factor, but it is not uncommon, on properly collected specimens, to isolate the *Actinobacillus* pathogen in pure culture. It has recently been reported that several species of *Actinobacillus* produce a toxin that is similar genetically to the leukotoxin produced by *Pasteurella haemolytica* and the α-hemolysins produced by *Escherichia coli*, *Proteus vulgaris*, *P. mirabilis*, and *Morganella morganii*. Except for the leukotoxin produced by *A. actinomycetemcomitans*, the role this toxin plays in disease production has not been elucidated. Pathogens associated with disease in food animals include *A. lignieresii*, *A. equuli*, *A. pleuropneumoniae*, *A. suis*, *A. actinoides*, and *A. seminis*. Infections caused by *A. pleuropneumoniae* are described in a separate section. *Actinobacillus actinoides*, because of the possibility that it is the same organism as *Haemophilus somnus*, is not discussed here.

Habitat

These organisms are normal inhabitants of mucous membranes of the respiratory, alimentary, and genital tracts of numerous animal species throughout the world. When they cause disease, it is usually sporadic and due to a break in the integrity of the protective barriers on which they have colonized. Outbreaks may occasionally occur but are usually a result of some underlying cause that has traumatized the mucous membranes of the animals affected, thus allowing the *Actinobacillus* sp. to invade otherwise sterile tissue.

Actinobacillus lignieresii

This organism has a worldwide distribution and has been isolated from disease processes in sheep, pigs, chickens, horses, dogs, and humans. It is part of the normal flora of the alimentary canal of cattle and sheep.

The most frequently seen lesions are in cattle and consist of multiple, hard, granulomatous abscesses in soft tissues of the head and upper alimentary canal and associated lymph nodes. The frequent involvement of the tongue has led to the term "wooden tongue." Other tissues that may be infected by this organism include the pleura, lungs, liver, udder, lymph nodes, and subcutaneous tissues. Abscesses usually begin as firm nodules that eventually ulcerate and discharge a viscous, white to faintly green exudate. This exudate may contain small (≤1 mm) grayish-white granules. In sheep, lesions are seen in the skin (especially around the head), lungs, testes, and mammary glands but not the tongue. In pigs, an *A. lignieresii*–like organism may occasionally be isolated from abscesses in the udder.

A. lignieresii relies on a break in the integrity of the epithelial cell lining of the alimentary canal to cause disease. Such breaks can occur with the feeding of coarse feeds such as dry haylage. Once the bacterium has been introduced into these otherwise sterile tissues, local abscesses develop. From these abscesses the organism may, on rare occasions, spread to other body sites through the lymphatics (most common route), by hematogenous spread, by injection, or by aspiration into the lungs, in which a similar type of lesion develops.

Diagnosis of actinobacillosis is usually made from the isolation of the causative bacteria from granulomatous lesions in conjunction with clinical signs and physical examination. Specimens for culture should be collected by aspiration from closed lesions, transferred to a sterile container, and transported to the laboratory on ice. Purulent material from the abscesses may contain small (≤1 mm) grayish-white, sulfur-like granules. Gram staining of the granules, after they are crushed in 10 per cent sodium hydroxide, will reveal small, gram-negative rods and coccobacilli with examination under oil immersion.

TREATMENT. Traditionally, topical or systemic iodine has been used and shown to be effective in the treatment of this disease. More recently, with increased concerns over food safety, the use of these products in dairy cows has been discouraged. *A. lignieresii* has also been shown to be susceptible to streptomycin, sulfonamides, ampicillin, and tetracyclines in vitro. When these drugs are used, they should be administered at high doses for several weeks.

Actinobacillus suis

Actinobacillus suis was first isolated from diseased pigs in 1962 and placed in the genus *Actinobacillus* on the basis of biochemical similarities and DNA homologies. *A. suis* has a worldwide distribution, with disease caused by this bacterium being largely restricted to the swine population. A genetically similar organism, *Actinobacillus equuli*, produces similar lesions in pigs. However, *A. suis* is hemolytic, which helps distinguish it from the nonhemolytic *A. equuli*.

A. suis is most frequently associated with acute septicemia in pigs from 3 days up to 6 weeks of age. The septicemic illness may involve up to a third of a litter and has a rapid onset with piglets dying anywhere from 15 hours to 3 days after the onset of infection. This organism has also been associated with arthritis, pneumonia, pericarditis, nephritis, subcutaneous abscesses, meningitis, and metritis in older pigs. Outbreaks of septicemic illness in specific pathogen free (SPF) sows has resulted in elevated temperatures and "diamond skin lesions" similar to those seen with erysipelas.

It is believed that the organism gains access to the vascular system through the upper respiratory tract. *A. suis* has been isolated from the vagina and tonsils of healthy pigs, and these sources may serve as the means of transmission from adult to baby pigs. Once the bacterium has gained access to the neonatal animal, its route of infection is probably through the mucous membranes or umbilicus, enhanced partly by the immunologic immaturity of the host defenses. Infections in adult animals are rare, probably because of widespread infection in the neonate.

Because of the infrequency of the disease as a whole, and its sporadic nature, it has been difficult to justify the development of preventive measures. When the disease entity has been diagnosed, *A. suis* has been shown to be susceptible to ampicillin, cephalothin, trimethoprim-sulfadiazine, streptomycin, and the tetracyclines.

Actinobacillus seminis

The taxonomic placement of this organism is unknown. Recent studies have shown that it is genetically unrelated to *Actinobacillus* or *Haemophilus*. It occurs primarily as a pathogen of sheep, in which it has been associated with epididymitis and seminal vesiculitis in rams, mastitis in ewes, and purulent polyarthritis in lambs.

ACTINOMYCOSIS

Actinomycosis is a subacute or chronic disease caused by any of several closely related species of *Actinomyces*, all of which are members of the normal flora of the mouth and gastrointestinal tract of the animals in which they cause disease. In cattle, the predominant lesion associated with actinomycosis involves bony tissues of the head and is caused by *A. bovis*, although *A. israeli* has also been isolated from some lesions. Actinomycosis is often associated with a mixed bacterial flora involving pyogenic aerobic and anaerobic bacteria. Bacteria belonging to this genus are gram-positive, pleomorphic rods that may appear as coccobacillary forms (primarily *A. pyogenes*), straight or slightly curved rods, or filaments that exhibit true branching. Most species grow best under anaerobic conditions at 35° to 37° C, with carbon dioxide being required for maximal growth. In food animals, *A. bovis* and *A. pyogenes* account for most of the cases of actinomycosis, although *A. suis* may be a frequent isolate from chronic granulomatous and suppurative mastitis in sows. *A. bovis* is the etiologic agent of lumpy jaw in cattle and has occasionally been associated with primary lung infections in cattle. There are also reports of its isolation from mastitic udders in pigs. *A. pyogenes* has been isolated from numerous soft tissue infections in cattle and other animal species including pneumonia, mastitis, abscesses, and polyarthritis.

Actinomyces are not highly virulent pathogens. Rather they are endogenous oral commensals that, on introduction into soft tissues as a result of traumatic or surgical injuries, produce chronic infections that spread unimpeded along anatomic barriers. These infections are characterized by suppurative granulomas, which in the case of *A. bovis* form external sinuses that discharge characteristic sulfur-like granules.

Habitat

Except for *A. suis*, the species of *Actinomyces* that have been associated with infectious disease in domestic animals are considered to be part of the normal flora, primarily of the oral cavity, of the animal species in which they cause disease. Attempts to demonstrate these organisms in the gastrointestinal tract have been unsuccessful. The habitat of *A. suis* is unknown, although it is suspected that trauma due to the action of the teeth of the suckling pigs is thought to provide both the inoculum and the tissue injury necessary for actinomycosis of the mammary gland of pigs.

Actinomyces bovis

Actinomycosis (lumpy jaw) caused by *A. bovis*, or sometimes *A. israeli*, is a chronic, suppurative, and granulomatous infection. It is characterized by pyogenic lesions, with interconnecting sinus tracts containing granules (usually 1 to 3 mm in diameter) composed of microcolonies of the bacteria embedded in tissue elements. Infections by this organism in other animals are rare but may include lumpy jaw in sheep and goats and fistula withers and poll evil, associated with *Brucella abortus*, in horses. This organism is part of the normal flora of the oral cavity of the animal species in which it causes disease. Thus, most of these infections originate from an endogenous source.

Perhaps the best known actinomycete infection occurring in animals is bovine actinomycosis (lumpy jaw). The infection occurs after an abrasion or penetrating wound to the oral mucosal surface, on which this organism has colonized, that allows it to gain access into deeper tissues. Once the organism has penetrated into these tissues, it spreads to contiguous areas along tissue planes, with resultant nodules and abscesses. Whereas the organism often infects bony tissues of the head (primarily mandible and maxilla), it may sometimes cause suppurative granulomatous disease in adjacent soft tissue. As the infectious process continues, it becomes a chronic progressive infection with hard, tumor-like masses. Nodules may coalesce, forming sinuses, many of which may open at the skin to discharge pus that contains sulfur-like granules. Depending on the severity of the infection, organisms may be ingested or aspirated with resultant visceral or pulmonary actinomycosis, respectively. Infection may also spread hematogenously with resultant abscesses at other body sites including mammary tissue.

The mechanism of pathogenesis of *A. bovis* infections has not been clearly elucidated. It is suspected that pathogenesis may be related to the inability of the host to remove organisms and the toxicity of their metabolic products once they have been introduced into deeper tissues, thus stimulating a granulomatous reaction. Many infections caused by *A. bovis* are polymicrobial in nature, and the other organisms present may also contribute to the pathogenesis of the disease process.

Diagnosis of lumpy jaw and related diseases may be made clinically in conjunction with a microscopic examination of the pus from the nodules or discharge from the draining tracts. Sulfur-like granules in the exudate may be examined by transferring them to a glass slide. The addition of 10 per cent sodium hydroxide digests the purulent material around the granules, which may then be gently crushed under a cover slip. A Gram stain of the crushed granule will reveal pleomorphic gram-positive club-shaped rods and filaments radiating from the center of the granule with examination under oil immersion. Confirmation may be made by isolation of *A. bovis* from granules or infected tissues by routine culture techniques.

Treatment of lumpy jaw and related diseases in other animal species is generally unsuccessful unless it is initiated early in the disease process and aggressively. For successful therapy, treatment should include surgical debridement and prolonged (weeks to months) antimicrobial chemotherapy. The drug of choice for the treatment of actinomycosis is penicillin, administered parenterally, although tetracyclines have also been used successfully. Because of the potential for mixed infections, some investigators feel that ampicillin and amoxicillin have an advantage over penicillin because of their broader spectrum. Sodium iodide solution administered intravenously or injected locally into the tumorous masses has also been used successfully, and potassium iodide administered orally has been recommended. However, the use of these products in animals whose milk will enter the human food chain is discouraged.

Actinomyces pyogenes

Actinomyces (Corynebacterium) pyogenes is a commensal of cutaneous and mucosal surfaces of cattle and other animal species and has been associated with many pyogenic disease conditions in many animal species, including cattle, sheep, goats, and pigs. These include pneumonia and mastitis in cattle, peritonitis and pleuritis in pigs, and various forms of suppurative lesions in other animal species including sheep and horses. It has also been reported in rabbits. It is most commonly isolated from pyogenic infections in cattle, sheep, and pigs.

The mechanism by which *A. pyogenes* gains access to infected body sites has not yet been elucidated. However, on the basis of its slow rate of growth and lack of potent virulence factors, one might assume that it is introduced into tissues along with foreign material, introduced into tissue with reproved. The implantation is repeated every 3 months as long as the diet remains high in protein.

BIBLIOGRAPHY

Doherty M: Outbreak of posthitis in grazing wethers in Scotland. Vet Rec 116:372–373, 1985.

C. bovis UDDER INFECTION OF DAIRY CATTLE

Corynebacterium bovis has been regarded as both a harmless commensal of the bovine udder and a minor mastitis pathogen, because its presence in the teat canal and cistern results in only a mild increase in somatic cell count and does not adversely affect milk yield or composition. *C. bovis* is frequently isolated from bovine milk samples in herds in which routine teat disinfection and antibiotic dry-cow treatment are not practiced. Results from a multiple-herd survey in Ontario found an infection rate with *C. bovis* of 20, 36, and 86 per cent at the quarter, cow, and herd level, respectively. Not using routine teat disinfection and no or selected dry-cow therapy were associated with a high *C. bovis* quarter infection rate. *C. bovis* is extremely contagious during lactation, and colonization has been shown to persist during the nonlactating and peripartum periods. In one study, dry-cow therapy eliminated 67 per cent of *C. bovis* infections.

There has been interest in *C. bovis* as a natural biologic control mechanism against infection by important mastitis pathogens. Some but not all studies have shown a protective effect of *C. bovis* colonization on new infection rates by certain major pathogens. Overall, the results indicate that colonization of quarters by *C. bovis* may reduce the risk of infection by other bacteria, but that this effect is small and easily overcome. The mechanisms of enhanced resistance to new intramammary infections may be due to inhibited penetration of other pathogens by the competitive adherence of *C. bovis* to the squamous epithelium of the teat end area or the pre-existing leukocytosis in *C. bovis*–colonized udders.

C. bovis grows slowly on blood agar, forming small, white to cream colonies by 48 hours' incubation. The colonies are usually found in areas where milk fat is concentrated. In contrast to *Actinomyces pyogenes*, *C. bovis* is nonhemolytic and catalase-positive.

BIBLIOGRAPHY

Brooks BW, Barnum DA, Meek AH: An observational study of *Corynebacterium bovis* in selected Ontario dairy herds. Can J Comp Med 47:73–78, 1983.
Sordillo LM, Oliver SP, Doane RM, et al: Duration of experimentally induced *Corynebacterium bovis* colonization of bovine mammary glands during the lactating, nonlactating, and peripartum periods. Am J Vet Res 50:267–270, 1989.

Leptospirosis
JOHN F. PRESCOTT, VET MB, PHD

Leptospirosis is a fascinating, complex, and important bacterial infection of animals responsible for significant economic loss in livestock, particularly through abortion and stillbirth, and for zoonotic infection of humans. Many aspects of leptospirosis in farm animals are poorly understood, in part because of difficulties with diagnostic methods, the complexities of the host-leptospire relationship, the changing pattern of infection as a result of vaccination, and other reasons. Leptospirosis in livestock is largely a hidden disease that may cause considerable frustration in diagnosis and control. It should be considered a series of separate infections caused by individual serovars within a particular host, rather than a single disease with a common epidemiology, host response, and means of control.

ETIOLOGY

Leptospirosis is caused by any of the individual serovars of *Leptospira interrogans*, of which there are over 180, grouped within 19 serogroups on the basis of shared antigens. *L. interrogans* is a slender spirochete that does not stain with usual bacterial stains and is difficult to isolate in the laboratory. Serotyping to distinguish isolates into serovars is increasingly being replaced by the simpler and more informative technique of genotyping. For example, serovar *hardjo* can be distinguished into 2 genotypes, hardjoprajitno (a virulent genotype found in cattle in Europe) and hardjo-bovis (a less virulent genotype isolated from cattle in many parts of the world). Isolates once identified in the United States as serovars *szwajizak* and *balcanica* in cattle have been reidentified by genotyping as the more mundane serovar *hardjo*. Isolates previously identified as serovar *pomona* in North America have recently mostly been identified by genotyping as being truly serovar *kennewicki* and have been further subdivided into pig-associated and cattle-associated subtypes. It is referred to as *pomona* in this discussion.

Although many serovars are recognized internationally, only a limited number are endemic to any particular region. The endemic serovars in North America are shown in Table 1.

Each serovar is adapted to particular maintenance ("reservoir") hosts (Table 1), although they may cause disease in any mammalian species. The serovar behaves differently within its maintenance host species than it does in other, incidental ("accidental"), host species. A maintenance host relationship is characterized by high susceptibility to infection; endemic transmission within the host species; relatively low pathogenicity of the serovar for its host; a tendency to cause chronic rather than acute disease, producing insidious economic loss through reproductive losses; persistence of the serovar in the kidney and sometimes the genital tract; a low antibody (microscopic agglutination test, MAT) response to infection, and therefore difficulties in diagnosis; and, suspected in some cases, low efficacy of vaccination in prevention of infection. Examples of this relationship are serovar *bratislava* in swine and serovar

Table 1. COMMON LEPTOSPIRAL SEROVARS AND THEIR MAINTENANCE HOSTS IN NORTH AMERICA

Serovar	Maintenance Host	Serovar	Maintenance Host
autumnalis	Rodents	*hardjo*	Cattle
Australis serogroup (*bratislava*)	Swine, horses	*icterohaemorrhagiae*	Rats
canicola	Dogs	*pomona**	Pig, skunk, raccoon, opossum, and others
grippotyphosa	Raccoon, opossum, squirrels, and others		

*Pomona (kennewicki) does not occur in Britain.

hardjo type hardjo-bovis in cattle. By contrast, an incidental host relationship is characterized by relatively low susceptibility to infection but high pathogenicity for the host, with a tendency to cause acute, severe rather than chronic disease; sporadic transmission within the host species and acquisition of infection from other species, sometimes in epizootic form; a short kidney phase; marked antibody response to infection, making for ease of diagnosis; and the efficacy of vaccination in preventing infection. An example of this relationship is serovar *pomona (kennewicki)* infection in cattle.

These distinctions in behavior between animal species as either maintenance or incidental hosts are not absolute. One exception is infection of swine by serovar *pomona*, in which swine behave as an intermediate between the 2 forms, with the organism persisting in the kidney but the host showing a marked antibody response to infection and responding well to vaccination.

TRANSMISSION

Transmission may be direct, particularly in a maintenance host, for example, through urine splashing, through placental or uterine discharges after abortion, venereally, through milk, or across the placenta in the case of congenitally infected animals. Infection of incidental hosts is more commonly indirect, through environmental contamination by the urine of carrier animals. Environmental conditions are critical in determining the success of indirect transmission, survival of the leptospires being favored by moisture, moderately warm temperatures (optimal around 28° C), and neutral or mildly alkaline soil and water pH. Under ideal conditions, leptospires may survive weeks or months in water-saturated soil or in stagnant water; survival may be a matter of minutes in dry soil at temperatures under 10° C or over 34° C. In temperate climates, leptospirosis thus occurs particularly in the autumn and early winter, when optimal environmental conditions occur, which may also coincide with high populations of wildlife carriers.

PATHOGENESIS

Leptospires penetrate exposed mucous membranes and water-softened skin and, after a 4- to 10-day incubation, disseminate to many organs (especially liver, kidneys, lungs, the reproductive tract such as the udder and placenta, cerebrospinal fluid) in a leptospiremic phase lasting up to 7 days. Agglutinating antibody production, which can first be detected about 6 days after leptospiremia, stops the bacteremic phase, so that the organism persists only in sites of poor antibody penetration (proximal convoluted tubules of the kidney, sometimes cerebrospinal fluid, rarely vitreous humor of the eye) and, for certain serovars, in the genital tract of maintenance hosts. Acute clinical disease may be seen in the leptospiremic phase, particularly in young animals.

Chronic infection is associated with persistence of leptospires in the sites described and in the reproductive tract. Leptospires persist in the kidneys and are shed in the urine for several weeks in incidental hosts but for 6 months or longer, even perhaps for life in some cases, in maintenance hosts. Localization and persistence in the uterus of pregnant animals may result in fetal infection, with subsequent abortion, stillbirth, the birth of live animals of poor viability, or occasionally the birth of healthy but infected offspring. An animal usually aborts only once. In maintenance hosts, such as serovar *bratislava* infection in swine or *hardjo* infection in cattle, infection may persist in the oviduct and uterus, and occasionally the udder, as well as in the male genital tract (testes, seminal vesicles, prostate). Leptospires have been demonstrated in bull semen and may be spread by mating but probably not by artificial insemination when semen is treated with antibiotics. Venereal transmission seems to be common in Australis serogroup *(bratislava)* infection in swine.

CLINICAL SIGNS

Most leptospiral infections are largely subclinical, particularly in nonpregnant and nonlactating animals, detected only by the presence of antibody in sampled animals or minor lesions of interstitial nephritis in the kidneys at slaughter. Disease may be acute or subacute, associated with the leptospiremic phase of the infection, or chronic, occurring later and associated with reproductive loss through abortion and stillbirth and, in *bratislava* infection in swine, probably also infertility. *Hardjo* infection in cattle may also be associated with infertility, but this is less clear.

Cattle

Serovars of major importance are *hardjo* and *pomona* type kennewicki in North America and *hardjo* in Europe. Illness due to other serovars are relatively unimportant. Seroprevalence (MAT titers ≥100) in cattle in the United States is approximately *hardjo*, 25 per cent; *pomona*, 17 per cent; *icterohaemorrhagiae*, 16 per cent; and *canicola*, 9.5 per cent. In recent years, infection with serovar *hardjo* has become increasingly recognized along with the apparent decline in importance of serovar *pomona*.

ACUTE INFECTION. The most severe but uncommon manifestation of acute infection occurs in calves infected with incidental serovars, particularly *pomona*. Clinical signs are high fever, hemolytic anemia, hemoglobinuria, jaundice, pulmonary congestion, occasionally meningitis, and high mortality. In cows, additionally, agalactia with small quantities of blood-tinged milk is also typical. Recovery is prolonged.

The most common form of acute disease occurs in dairy cows as a marked (2- to 10-day) drop in milk production with transient pyrexia. In this acute "milk drop syndrome" or "flabby udder mastitis" form, the milk has the consistency of colostrum, with thick clots, yellow staining, and high somatic cell count, and the udder has a uniformly soft texture. This form most commonly occurs with serovar *hardjo* type hardjoprajitno but may be caused by other serovars. Leptospiral "milk drop syndrome" varies from an epizootic infection in a previously unexposed herd, involving over half the herd over a period of 1 or 2 months, to a more common endemic infection affecting cows in their first or second lactation. Recovery is usually in 10 days, without treatment, although cows in late lactation may dry off. A subclinical form of this "milk drop syndrome" may occur in *hardjo*-infected lactating cows in the absence of clinical evidence of infection.

CHRONIC INFECTION. The chronic form of disease, most commonly associated with serovars *hardjo* and *pomona*, is fetal infection in pregnant cows presenting as abortion, stillbirth, or the birth of premature and weak infected calves. Infected but apparently healthy calves may also be born. Retention of fetal membranes may follow *hardjo* abortion. Abortion or stillbirth is commonly the only manifestation of infection but may sometimes be related to an episode of illness up to 6 weeks *(pomona)* or 12 weeks *(hardjo)* earlier. Serovar *hardjo* type hardjoprajitno appears to be more virulent than, and to cause more abortion than, type hardjo-bovis.

Accurate data for the frequency of abortion due to *hardjo* and *pomona* are not readily available in North America. Abortion due to *pomona* has decreased in importance over the last decades, probably because of vaccination. Abortion and stillbirth due to *hardjo* are recognized more commonly. *Hardjo* is more important than is *pomona* because it causes endemic rather than more incidental and usually sporadic infection. In Northern Ireland, where the more virulent type hardjoprajitno occurs, *hardjo* was recognized as responsible for nearly half of all bovine abortions in one study. Type hardjoprajitno was isolated from the majority of aborted fetuses, whereas type hardjo-bovis was isolated mainly from the kidney and genital tract of carrier cows. In one large study in Ontario, where the less virulent type hardjo-bovis occurs, serovar *hardjo* caused about 6 per cent of abortions; no *pomona* abortions were recognized.

The pattern of *hardjo* infection in a herd varies with the husbandry conditions and possibly with the type of *hardjo* present. Much of our understanding comes from Britain, where the more virulent hardjoprajitno is present, and therefore may not be fully applicable to North America. In Britain, where heifers are often reared separately from the main herd, abortion and stillbirth commonly occur in a proportion of these susceptible animals after their introduction into an endemically infected herd. In such herds, between 3 and 10 per cent of cows in the herd may abort or produce stillborn or weak calves. Hathaway and others (1986) described 4 patterns of *hardjo* infection in cattle in Britain, based on herd serology and history. These patterns were endemic infection, described in the preceding; active infection in yearlings, in which subsequent abortion was rare; frequent and high titers in cows of all ages indicating recent infection in a susceptible herd; and a "fading herd infection" in which titers were confined largely to older cows but their significance was unclear. A recent detailed study in Ontario showed that *hardjo* infection and abortion was largely a problem in beef rather than in dairy cattle, and that the serologic pattern conformed most to the pattern of "fading herd infection." More details on the patterns of infection in herds in North America are needed.

Infertility, which has apparently responded to vaccination, has been suggested in *hardjo*-infected herds. Such infertility, which has not been well documented, may follow localization of leptospires in the uterus and oviduct of *hardjo* carriers, an event that does not occur with incidental serovars.

Swine

Whereas any leptospire may infect and cause disease in swine, until recently the most common and important serovar recognized in swine in North America was *pomona* (type kennewicki), a subtype of which is host-adapted to swine. In Australia and some European countries, *tarassovi* (formerly *hyos*), another swine-adapted pathogen, causes losses as serious as those of *pomona*. Serovars such as *canicola* and *grippotyphosa* have been locally important. Antibody to *icterohaemorrhagiae* is widespread, but the serovar is of no disease significance. Understanding of leptospirosis in swine is rapidly changing with the recognition of the widespread and dominant prevalence of antibodies to the Australis serogroup (serovars *bratislava*, *lora*, *muenchen*) and the isolation particularly of *bratislava* and *muenchen* from aborted and stillborn pigs. In contrast to other serovars, the role and importance of Australis serogroup in swine is not fully understood, in part because of the difficulty of isolating these leptospires.

ACUTE INFECTION. Only a small proportion of infected animals develop clinical illness, a transient and mild episode of fever, anorexia, and depression that is generally unrecognized. Hemoglobinuria and jaundice occur rarely in piglets.

CHRONIC INFECTION

Serovars Other than Australis Serogroup. Abortion in the last trimester of pregnancy and the birth of stillborn or of weak and unthrifty piglets are results of chronic infection. In nonpregnant swine, variable lesions of interstitial nephritis are commonly observed grossly at slaughter. Infection with *pomona* or *tarassovi* may result in a "storm" of abortion when it is first introduced into a susceptible herd but diminishes once herd immunity develops, to affect mainly the gilts.

Australis Serogroup Infection. Evidence for the role of serovars *bratislava* and *muenchen* in abortion includes their recovery from 30 per cent of aborted and stillborn swine over an 8-year period by Ellis and colleagues in Northern Ireland, their isolation from the kidneys and genital tracts of recently aborting sows, the significant improvement in fertility and number of piglets born in sows vaccinated with *bratislava* reported in Italy and the United States, and serologic studies showing significant relationship of titers to infertility in sows. The complexity of the situation is illustrated, however, by one study, which found that sows with antibodies were significantly more likely to produce live pigs than were sows without antibodies.

In Northern Ireland, W. A. Ellis (1989) has described late-term abortion and stillbirth caused by Australis serogroup leptospires as being characterized by the birth of live, dying, and dead piglets. Infection in herds in Ireland often had a 2-year cyclicity. There was marked annual variation in infection in Northern Ireland, from 6 to 40 per cent in different years.

A distinct syndrome also associated with Australis serogroup is a repeat breeder syndrome, described by Ellis as endemic in most breeding herds in Northern Ireland. Disease is most noticeable in sows in certain age groups, particularly those bred for the first time to infected boars. Disease is at its worst when susceptible animals are introduced into an endemically infected herd, for example, when sows from SPF herds are brought into the herd. Serovars *bratislava* and *muenchen* have been commonly isolated from the genital tracts of sows and boars in infected herds; venereal transmission is thought to be a major means of transmission. In Britain, *bratislava* type B2b is almost exclusively isolated from swine and from aborted fetuses; type B2a is widespread in several hosts, including swine, but is rarely isolated from aborted piglets. This pattern is not so apparent in the United States, where B2a and B2b, and an additional type B1, have been isolated from cases of reproductive failure as well as from the kidneys of swine at slaughter. All 3 types have even been isolated from piglets in the same litter. One genotype of serovar *muenchen* is isolated mainly from aborted piglets.

The fascinating and important findings of Ellis and his colleagues in Ireland have not yet been fully confirmed in the United States. Recently, serovar *bratislava* was isolated from stillborn and weak pigs in Iowa by Bolin and Cassells. This same group has associated *bratislava* infection with stillborn pigs, with weak neonatal pigs, and less commonly with abortion. The importance of this infection in swine in North America will emerge with further work, including experimental inoculations, and as diagnostic methods improve.

Sheep and Goats

Sheep appear less susceptible than are cattle to clinical leptospirosis. The major serovar of sheep is *hardjo*, which is maintained in a maintenance cycle independent of cattle. Other serovars may also cause disease. Acute disease in lambs is characterized by fever, hemolytic anemia, hemoglobinuria, and jaundice. *Hardjo* infection of ewes may cause late-term abortion, stillbirth, weak lambs, and agalactia in recently lambed ewes. Other serovars occasionally cause abortion. Leptospirosis in goats has attracted little attention.

PATHOLOGY AND NECROPSY FINDINGS

In acute infection, calves and piglets show pathologic changes of subserosal and submucosal hemorrhage, hemolytic anemia, hemoglobinuria, and jaundice, with histologic changes of interstitial nephritis and centrilobular hepatic necrosis.

In chronic infection, pathologic findings in most aborted bovine fetuses are often negligible. Mild focal tubular necrosis and interstitial nephritis may be present in the kidneys. Jaundice is recognized rarely. In swine, non-mummified fetuses often show excess serosal effusions and quite commonly scattered 1- to 4-mm necrotic foci in the liver. Jaundice is rare. Adult swine, especially those infected by serovar *pomona*, and cattle infected with *hardjo* commonly show 1- to 3-mm gray foci of chronic lymphocytic interstitial nephritis scattered over the kidney cortex.

DIAGNOSIS

The diagnosis of leptospirosis depends on good laboratory facilities combined with clinical history.

Demonstration of Leptospires

Darkfield microscopy of fetal fluids and silver staining of tissue sections are insensitive methods for the demonstration of leptospires that may give false-positive results. Immunofluorescence of urine, of homogenates of fetal lung and kidney, or of placenta is an excellent technique for demonstration of leptospires in experienced laboratories. Difficulties may be experienced with serovar *bratislava*. Leptospires die rapidly in tissues or body fluids unless they are kept at 4° C. As well as by examination of fresh material, results may also be improved if samples are submitted to laboratories in leptospiral transport medium. Isolation of leptospires is generally expensive, time-consuming, and unavailable. It is especially difficult for serovar *bratislava* and *hardjo* type hardjoprajitno. Immunofluorescence is more readily available and often as sensitive. Recognition of leptospires in the urine of cows that have recently aborted does not distinguish these animals from renal carriers. The use of DNA hybridization techniques for leptospiral diagnosis promises to revolutionize understanding and control of leptospirosis in maintenance hosts.

Serologic Studies

Serologic diagnosis with use of the microscopic agglutination test (MAT) is the approach commonly used to diagnose leptospirosis in animals. It is particularly useful in diagnosis of disease caused by incidental, non–host-adapted serovars or acute disease caused by host-adapted serovars. It is less useful in diagnosis of chronic disease in maintenance hosts because antibody response to infection may be negligible in chronic infections or may persist from subclinical infections. The herd serologic response to infection is often more helpful than is the individual's response in chronic infections in maintenance hosts. In abortion or stillbirth, it is often useful to do serologic testing on fetal fluids, but dilutions should start at 1:10, in contrast to adult studies, in which the usual starting dilution is 1:100.

In the MAT, a titer ≥100 is regarded as "significant." There are several considerations in evaluating the MAT response. The MAT is a serogroup (and especially serovar) specific test, so serovars representative of all suspected serogroups should be tested. It detects IgM better than IgG antibody. The MAT has low sensitivity in chronic leptospirosis in maintenance hosts. The MAT is not adequate for detection of the carrier state in maintenance hosts, because titers ≥100 against host-adapted serovars have low sensitivity but high specificity. The MAT is not a measure of immunity to infection; vaccination produces a largely IgG response, with low (100 to 400) and transient (1- to 4-month) titers, but immunity commonly persists in vaccinated animals long after MAT titers are negative. Paradoxic reactions may occur with the MAT early in the course of an acute infection, with a marked MAT response to a serovar other than the infecting serovar. Vaccination may mask the MAT response to natural and experimental infection. Poor interlaboratory reproducibility in the MAT has been described and is particularly a problem with fetal serology because titers are often so low.

Cattle

Titers ≥100 are considered significant, and a 4-fold rise in titer on a paired sample taken 2 weeks apart (acute, convalescent) tested at the same time is diagnostic. Paired samples in an individual animal are particularly useful for acute and subacute infections. Titers in these animals are often considerably greater than 100. In abortion caused by incidental serovars, MAT titers against *pomona* and other incidental serovars are high, often ≥3000.

Paired sera are of no value in chronic infections because abortion occurs weeks after infection, so that titers are static or declining. For chronic *hardjo* infections, a recently aborting cow with a titer ≥300 has about a 60 per cent, of ≥1000 an 80 per cent, and ≥3000 a 90 per cent chance of fetal infection. If several aborting cows show high titers (≥300), this is usually sufficient evidence for the diagnosis of leptospirosis in unvaccinated herds. However, one quarter of cows with *hardjo*-infected fetuses may have no detectable MAT titer.

Because of these serodiagnostic difficulties in chronic disease, herd rather than individual serology may be useful for determining the presence of active infection, especially due to *hardjo*. The herd should be divided for sampling into different management and age groups for representative testing. Hathaway and others suggested testing 10 animals each from the groups yearlings, first calvers, second calvers, and older cows. For *hardjo* infection, titers ≥300 indicate active infection, and for incidental serovars, titers are often higher (≥1000 to 3000). The herd serologic pictures will show seasonal and individual variation over time. Diagnosis of chronic infections is thus best made by combination of direct detection of leptospires with individual and herd serology.

Swine

Several fetuses in each litter must be examined for leptospires, for example, by pooling kidneys and lungs from 4 piglets for immunofluorescence. Serosal effusions or the vitreous humor of the eye may show viable leptospires, especially in *pomona* or *tarossavi* infections, which can be identified by darkfield or immunofluorescence microscopy. Serologic testing on several piglets (aborted, stillborn, or weak piglets that have not sucked) in the litter is a particularly useful way for identifying *bratislava* or *muenchen* infection (using *bratislava* as the Australis serogroup antigen). Titers may be as low as 1:10, and are rarely over 1:100, and reactions with other serovars (especially *icterohaemorrhagiae*) may occur, but these usually have a lower titer than that to *bratislava*. Several litters should be so examined before it is concluded that Australis serogroup leptospires are not involved.

Sows that have recently aborted because of *pomona, tarassovi*, or incidental serovars often have high MAT titers (1000 to 30,000). A paired titer does not usually rise. Because individual sows may show low titers, testing a dozen herdmates is often valuable. MAT titers in sows aborting because of Australis serogroup leptospires are unhelpful; whereas many have low but non-rising titers (100 to 400), many will be MAT-negative, even at 1:10 dilution. Seroconversion may, however, occasionally be demonstrated. Herdmates may show titers ≥100, but these cannot be readily distinguished from those often found in swine.

TREATMENT AND CONTROL

Animals with acute leptospirosis can be treated with streptomycin (12.5 mg/kg twice daily for 3 days) or tetracycline (10 to 15 mg/kg twice daily for 3 to 5 days). Streptomycin treatment can be combined with ampicillin or large doses of penicillin G. Leptospires are also highly susceptible to erythromycin, tiamulin, and tylosin, although these antibiotics cannot be relied on to remove the renal carrier state. A single dose of streptomycin will usually remove the chronic renal carrier state caused by *pomona* or serovars other than *bratislava* or *hardjo*.

Control is based on prevention, vaccination, and treatment. In all cases, there should be limitation of direct and indirect transmission by carriers of incidental infections (for example, by rodent control around buildings, fencing of swampy ground or streams). Immunity is serovar (often serogroup) specific. Polyvalent vaccines containing common serovars endemic to the host and region are generally available. These may contain unnecessary serovars (for example, *canicola* and *icterohaemorrhagiae*). Different vaccines vary in efficacy, and vaccine failures may occur.

There are 2 basic approaches to control: eradication by a combination of progressive identification of carriers and antibiotic treatment; or control by annual herd vaccination and judicious injection of streptomycin. The disadvantage of eradication is that it leaves the herd open to infection by leptospires introduced by livestock carriers, which may not be detected because of the poor sensitivity of the MAT, or by carriers of other species, such as wildlife. The disadvantage of control by vaccination is that it may be an unnecessary routine procedure, although it is usually combined with other antigens. Many farmers, however, vaccinate as an inexpensive form of insurance. The decision on which approach to use depends on the purpose of the herd, its history, and its seroprevalence of leptospirosis; most people will favor control over eradication.

Cattle

Annual vaccination with appropriate bacterins of all cattle in a closed herd, or twice yearly vaccination in an open herd, is the most effective approach to control. Newly introduced cattle should be treated once, and preferably several times, with dihydrostreptomycin (25 mg/kg intramuscularly, once daily [s.i.d.]) for removal of most renal carriage and vaccinated before they enter the herd. Streptomycin treatment will not remove all carriers of *hardjo* but is usually effective for *pomona*. Vaccination can be combined with streptomycin treatment in the face of an outbreak. Calves should be 6 months or older before vaccination, which should be done twice with a month interval; younger animals respond poorly. Vaccination thereafter is with a single dose annually. Because of the short-lasting low-titer MAT response, annual vaccination with most available vaccines will progressively reduce and eventually abolish the herd seroprevalence of leptospirosis. In an infected animal, such as one with an MAT titer, vaccination will not reduce urinary shedding but often considerably increases and prolongs the titer. Persistent low-titer reactions, which may last for years, may prevent bulls from entering studs or cattle from being exported. Treatment often does not abolish these titers. Because of the low sensitivity of the MAT test in detecting serovar *hardjo* carriers, international recommendations (International Zoo-Sanitary Code, Office International des Epizooties) for importation of livestock suggest reliance on antibiotic treatment before movement, rather than on serologic testing. Regulations generally should be changed for bull studs or export requirements to allow control by a combination of vaccination and streptomycin treatment rather than the use of the insensitive MAT test to "detect" *hardjo* carrier animals.

Field evidence has shown that *hardjo* vaccination reduces reproductive losses due to *hardjo* infection as well as leptospiruria. Disturbingly, some well-designed experimental studies have shown that *hardjo* vaccination does not prevent kidney establishment, urinary shedding, or fetal infection after conjunctival infection with type *hardjo-bovis*. Such vaccination, however, prevents an MAT response to infection and may hinder the ability to isolate leptospires present in the urine. More information on the efficacy of vaccination of cattle against *hardjo* is required. Vaccination with incidental serovars usually gives excellent protection against challenge.

Swine

A single streptomycin injection (25 mg/kg intramuscularly) stops leptospiruria in the majority of swine infected with *pomona*, although administration for 3 days may be slightly more effective. The value of streptomycin in the treatment of Australis serogroup infections has not been investigated but would be likely to be less effective than for *pomona*. Penicillin is ineffective against the carrier state. Administration of tetracycline in feed (800 to 1000 g/ton) has in some, but not all, cases eliminated renal infections with *pomona*. Herd administration of tetracyclines at 4000 g/ton on a month-on, month-off pattern has been used to control Australis serogroup infection, but infection usually recurs within 4 or 5 months of cessation of treatment (Ellis, 1989).

Vaccines will markedly reduce abortion and stillbirth rates, and they will reduce but may not fully eliminate renal colonization and leptospiruria. They have, however, been used to eradicate infection in combination with hygienic measures. Double vaccination of gilts just before mating, and of vaccinated sows at each weaning, is a useful approach to control on endemically affected farms. Field studies of *bratislava* vaccines have shown that their use has been followed by increased litter sizes and farrowing rates. Their efficacy under controlled experimental infections has not been determined. Eradication of *pomona* and *tarassovi* has been done by a combination of serologic testing, isolation, vaccination, and treatment of positive animals. Control can be achieved by a combination of twice-yearly vaccination, with antibiotic treatment and double vaccination of all introduced pigs. Careful design of effluent channels and pen and pig separation can reduce transmission.

BIBLIOGRAPHY

Bolin CA, Cassells JA: Isolation of *Leptospira interrogans* serovar *bratislava* from stillborn and weak pigs in Iowa. J Am Vet Med Assoc 196:1601–1603, 1990.

Bolin CA, Thiermann AB, Handsaker AL, Foley JW: Effect of vaccination with a pentavalent leptospiral vaccine on *Leptospira interrogans* serovar *hardjo* type hardjo-bovis infection of pregnant cattle. Am J Vet Res 50:161–165, 1989.
Ellis WA: The diagnosis of leptospirosis in farm animals. *In* Ellis WA, Little TWA (eds): The Present State of Leptospirosis Diagnosis and Control. Dordrecht, Martinus Nijhoff, pp 13–24.
Ellis WA: Effects of leptospirosis on bovine reproduction. *In* Morrow DA (ed): Current Therapy in Theriogenology, 2nd ed. Philadelphia, WB Saunders, 1986, pp 267–271.
Ellis WA: *Leptospira australis* infection in pigs. Pig Vet J 22:83–92, 1989.
Ellis WA, Michna SW: Bovine leptospirosis: infection by the Hebdomadis serogroup and abortion—a herd study. Vet Rec 99:409–412, 1976.
Frantz JC, Hanson LE, Brown AL: Effect of vaccination with a bacterin containing *Leptospira interrogans* serovar *bratislava* on the breeding performance of swine herds. Am J Vet Res 50:1044–1047, 1989.
Hanson LE, Tripathy DN: Leptospirosis. *In* Leman AD, et al (eds): Diseases of Swine, 5th ed. Ames, IA, Iowa State University Press, 1986, pp 591–599.
Hanson LE, Tripathy DN, Killinger AH: Current status of leptospirosis immunization in swine and cattle. J Am Vet Med Assoc 161:1235–1243, 1972.
Hathaway SC, Little TW, Pritchard DG: Problems associated with the serological diagnosis of *Leptospira interrogans* serovar *hardjo* infection in bovine populations. Vet Rec 119:84–86, 1986.
Prescott JF, Miller RB, Nicholson VM, et al: Seroprevalence and association with abortion of leptospirosis in cattle in Ontario. Can J Vet Res 52:210–215, 1988.

The *Haemophilus somnus* Complex

PETER B. LITTLE, DVM, PhD

Haemophilus somnus was first recognized as the cause of a fatal septicemic disease of feedlot cattle with severe neurologic complications (thromboembolic meningoencephalitis [TME], sleeper syndrome). The organism is now known to be involved in bovine pneumonia, mastitis, arthritis, tendonitis, vaginitis, endometritis, abortion, and recently has been isolated from conjunctivitis and myocardial abscessation.

ETIOLOGY

H. somnus is a gram-negative non–spore-forming coccobacillary organism that requires 10 per cent carbon dioxide in air for optimal growth. It does not need an X or V factor for growth, a traditional requirement for placement in the genus *Haemophilus*. Recent DNA homology studies show that it belongs in the family Pasteurellaceae but in a unique, as yet unnamed, genus. Therefore the organism will soon be renamed. *H. somnus* can be isolated on brain-heart infusion agar supplemented with 10 per cent bovine blood and 0.5 per cent yeast extract. Growth occurs as 1- to 2-mm regularly convex, slightly yellow, glistening colonies in 2 or 3 days. Thiamine monophosphate, cysteine hydrochloride, and soluble starch potentiate growth of *H. somnus*.

OCCURRENCE

Infectious TME was first recognized in Colorado in 1956, and *H. somnus* was connected with it in California in 1960. Over the last two decades the disease has moved northerly and westerly across the continent, probably in association with feeder cattle movement. There appears to be little doubt that similar, or even identical, organisms were isolated from bovine disease as early as 1927 in the United States and 1950 in Canada. *H. somnus* syndromes have been reported from many countries (the United States, Canada, Switzerland, Belgium, France, Italy, Germany, Australia, New Zealand, Poland, Japan, Brazil, Argentina, Romania, and Russia), and it is likely present in most countries with a cattle industry. A sheep pathogen related to *H. somnus* called *Histophilus ovis* has been identified in New Zealand, Australia, and Canada. *H. ovis* experimentally produces lesions of TME in cattle.

PREVALENCE

The total prevalence of TME in its various forms is not known. However, when TME occurs in a feedlot, from 0.1 to 1 per cent of the cattle are affected with the acute and often fatal disease. In a 2-year Canadian study, only 11 per cent of feedlots had the disease in both years, and the average overall population mortality rate for 3 years was 0.1 per cent. Serologic studies suggest that 20 to 50 per cent of cattle are seropositive to *H. somnus*, although cross-reactivity induced by *H. agni*, *Actinobacillus lignieresii*, *Listeria monocytogenes*, *Campylobacter fetus*, and other bacteria may account for some positive test results. As many as 20 per cent of pneumonia cases in calves are associated with *H. somnus* as pure or mixed infections. There is an 80 to 90 per cent genital carrier rate in bulls, but it is considerably lower in cows. It is now known that pathogenic TME strains are carried in the genital tract of cows. The organism is seldom isolated from the upper respiratory tract of healthy cattle. Although deaths caused by myocardial abscessation in western Canadian feedlot cattle is high, incidence figures are not yet available.

PATHOGENESIS

Experimental work has clarified some aspects of the pathogenesis of *H. somnus* septicemic disease. The mode of entry is unresolved, although the nasopharyngeal and pulmonary routes are the most likely. Intratracheal instillation or intravenous administration of *H. somnus* is capable of reproducing the pulmonary and acute septicemic disease and TME lesions. Serum antibody levels give no indication of an animal's vulnerability to infection, suggesting that a complex host-bacterial relationship exists that produces the fatal effects. Fc receptors have been identified on the surface of *H. somnus*, and these may protect it from bactericidal activity. Neutrophils but not macrophages are able to kill *H. somnus*, so the type and rapidity of host cellular response to infection may influence the severity of disease. The organism has a cell-associated cytotoxic effect that contracts endothelial cells and activates clotting. This appears to be responsible for the widespread thrombotic phenomena in the organs of affected animals. Little is known of the pathogenesis of the pulmonary lesions; however, the response is typical of other acute and chronic bacterial pneumonic processes. Myocardial abscessation appears to be the result of nonfatal bacteremic infection in partially immune cattle or infections with *H. somnus* strains of lower pathogenicity. The organisms form septic foci in the myocardium, and over several weeks or months abscesses form that eventually cause sudden death or signs of heart failure. In abortion, thrombotic phenomena in the fetus and necrosis of the placenta lead to death of the fetus.

CLINICAL SIGNS

TME is found in cattle 4 months to 3 years of age but most frequently in 7- to 9-month-old feedlot calves. The onset of disease in a group of calves is usually within 4 weeks of commencement of the feeder period, sometimes in association with respiratory disease. Animals affected with TME are found dead or are separated from the group. They are depressed and walk reluctantly, often with a stiff, knuckling gait. Fever of 41°C (106°F), muscle tremor, weakness, and recumbency rapidly supervene in untreated cases. The severe septicemic shock often obscures neurologic signs, but ataxia, stiff neck, blindness, nystagmus, and circling are reported. Premortal endotoxemic coma accounts for the sleeper syndrome. At this stage the temperature is subnormal and respiration has an interrupted expiratory phase. Pathognomonic multifocal hemorrhagic retinal infarcts are observed in 20 per cent of cases. Cerebrospinal fluid (CSF) of a comatose animal is cloudy. Smear or culture results help confirm the presence of the coccobacillus.

In calves the signs of the bronchopneumonic respiratory syndrome due to *H. somnus* are poor condition, fever, and hacking cough. Bilateral consolidation of the anteroventral lung lobes occurs, and moist rales may be auscultated. An acute respiratory form has a shorter course with fever, rapid weight loss, dyspnea, and extensive consolidation of the lungs. Pleuritic rubs may be auscultated.

Arthritis, an uncommon chronic form of the disease, is seen in animals that have averted the fatal septicemic form. It is characterized by swollen joints and tendon sheaths. The joint fluid is serosanguineous with fibrin flecks; purulent exudate is not seen. Affected cattle are in poor condition. With myocardial abscessation the animal is found dead 5 to 6 weeks into the feeder period or has a syndrome of recurrent fevers and eventual respiratory distress and depression from left heart failure.

The endometritis syndrome (described principally in Australia and Europe) is characterized by a purulent vaginal discharge and, frequently, red granular vaginitis and cervicitis after breeding. The period between calving and conception may be significantly prolonged. *Ureaplasma* and *H. somnus* may coexist. Abortion with retained placenta occurs at 7 to 9 months of gestation but is rare. Diagnosis is confirmed by microscopic demonstration of fetal and placental lesions and by bacterial culture.

PATHOLOGY AND NECROPSY FINDINGS

Septicemic *H. somnus* produces lesions in many organs but particularly in the nervous system. Lesions are found in the brain, eye, spinal cord, skeletal muscles, urinary bladder, heart, kidney, joints, tendon sheaths, lungs, and retropharyngeal lymph nodes. In genital carriers the organism may be isolated from the prepuce and from the region of the cervix or Bartholin's glands in the vagina.

The hematologic pattern of septicemic *H. somnus* is that of endotoxic shock with pronounced neutropenia and the presence of fibrin split products. Neutrophilic pleocytosis is present in the CSF with counts as high as 500/µl. Pándy's test for CSF globulin is positive, and the creatine phosphokinase levels in the CSF may be elevated.

Petechial and ecchymotic hemorrhages are found in the subcutaneous tissues, fascial planes, and muscle of cattle with TME. Endocardial and epicardial ecchymotic hemorrhages may be severe. Joints and tendon sheaths frequently contain excess fluid and fibrin strands. This is often very noticeable in the atlanto-occipital joint when the head is removed. The retropharyngeal lymph nodes are enlarged and red. Focal 0.5- to 2-cm hemorrhagic lesions are often found in the larynx, heart, retina, intestines, kidneys, and mucosal surface of the bladder. Pathognomonic lesions are seen in the brain in 75 to 80 per cent of cases. Grossly these lesions are multifocal hemorrhagic infarcts, generally 2 mm to 2 cm in diameter, bright red, and found over the cortex as well as on cut sections (Fig. 1). Focal red lesions of the spinal cord are best observed on cut surface. A slight to moderate cloudiness of the meninges and CSF indicates the prominent acute meningitis that is always present.

The acute fibrinous pneumonic and pleuritic lesions of *H. somnus* infection in feedlot cattle are comparable to the usually more common *Pasteurella haemolytica* lesions. Microscopically, fibrinous pneumonia and necrotic bronchiolitis are evident. In younger calves the respiratory lesions of *H. somnus* are those of chronic, suppurative bronchopneumonia. There are anteroventral consolidation, prominent pus-filled bronchioles, and frequently gray necrotic foci (2 to 4 mm). Tissue from the junction between normal and affected lung gives the best yield of the organism in culture. Myocardial abscessation should be suspected in sudden deaths and in those with severe pulmonary edema similar in severity to that seen in anaphylactic shock. Multiple slices of the ventricular walls and papillary muscles are necessary to observe the multiple small miliary abscesses or the larger ragged-walled abscesses (Fig. 2).

Aborted fetuses may have gross petechial hemorrhages in tissues with focal necrotic placentitis. Microscopic and bacteriologic analyses of placenta and fetus are usually necessary for diagnosis, however. Little is known about the uterine lesions in the endometrial form of the disease.

DIAGNOSIS

H. somnus septicemia should be suspected in feedlot cattle when sudden death occurs or when they are afflicted with pyrexia, depression, and stiffness. Ophthalmoscopic examination can help confirm the diagnosis in the 20 per cent of live animals affected with retinal infarcts in this disease. The presence of acute meningitis can be confirmed with a cisternal CSF tap. Multifocal hemorrhagic infarcts in the brain at necropsy are characteristic. Culture on brain-heart infusion agar with 5 per cent bovine blood and 0.5 per cent yeast extract (Difco[1]) in 10 per cent carbon dioxide will assist the

---
[1]Baxter Lab, Mississauga, Ontario, Canada.

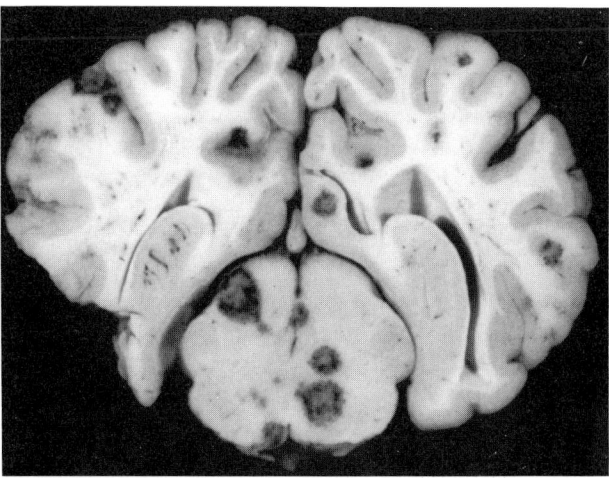

Figure 1. Feedlot steer with multiple focal septic infarcts in the parietal cortex caused by *H. somnus* (TME).

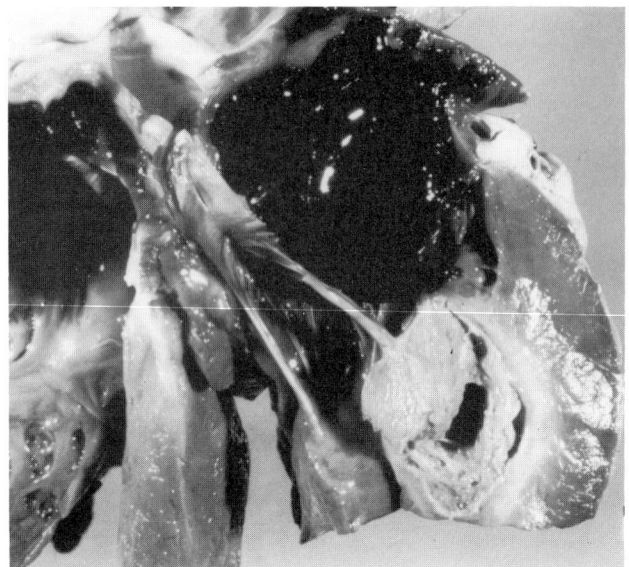

Figure 2. *H. somnus* myocardial abscess in the papillary muscle of a 700-lb feedlot steer. (Photo courtesy of M. Savic, DVM, DVSc, Guelph, Ontario.)

veterinarian in confirming the diagnosis. Commonly the organism cannot be isolated from animals treated with antibiotics before death.

TME is frequently confused with other feedlot cattle disease involving the CNS. Cattle with polioencephalomalacia (PE) separate from the group in a manner similar to those with TME, but fever is usually absent. In PE there are consistent neurologic signs of bilateral blindness and preserved pupillary light reflexes, with moderate to severe opisthotonos, hyperesthesia, and clonic convulsions in later stages. Bilateral medial dorsal strabismus is a valuable but inconsistent feature of PE. A CSF analysis may show some macrophages, but the suppurative meningitic exudate typical of TME is not found. Listeriosis is characterized by fever and depression, but in most cases the cranial nerve signs indicative of focal medullary lesions will assist in separating listeriosis from TME. In listeriosis, the CSF analysis indicates mild to moderate lymphocytic meningitis.

TME cases that are treated early and that have predominantly spinal infarctive lesions are a special problem in regard to differential diagnosis of rabies, spinal abscess, and vertebral fractures associated with calcium and phosphorus dietary imbalances. The history of acute febrile diseases that rapidly resolved with antibiotic treatment, leaving residual paralysis without progressively abnormal neurologic signs, separates TME spinal disease from rabies, vertebral fracture, and abscesses. Treated animals are bright and alert and eat well. They become star boarders until the owner recognizes the futility of continuous special care.

Respiratory disease caused by *H. somnus* must be differentiated from respiratory disease caused by *P. haemolytica, P. multocida, Actinomyces pyogenes,* and *Mycoplasma* sp. Necropsy with microbiologic confirmation is usually necessary for diagnosis, although *H. somnus* can often be isolated from the noses of animals with *H. somnus* pneumonia. The myocardial abscessation syndrome may be confused with any other cause of sudden death in feeder cattle. The intermittent fever and left heart failure may be confused clinically with right ventricular vegetative endocarditis caused by *A. pyogenes* or *Fusiformis necrophorum*. The accompanying severe pulmonary edema seen at necropsy is often mistaken for anaphylactic shock.

H. somnus should be suspected as a cause of infertility in beef and dairy cows if the disease is associated with postbreeding endometritis, vaginitis, and purulent discharge. The disease must be differentiated from trichomoniasis, *Ureaplasma* infection, campylobacteriosis, and infectious pustular vulvovaginitis. Microbiologic studies of the vaginal exudate are required to identify accurately each of these conditions. Special cultural procedures may be required since *H. somnus* is often overgrown with aerobic bacteria such as *Proteus, Coryneform, Escherichia coli,* and *Streptococcus* in these cases.

A clinical diagnosis on the basis of signs and lesions is not usually possible in cases of pneumonia, abortion, conjunctivitis, and mastitis caused by *H. somnus*. Cultural confirmation is required in order to make a diagnosis. Host resistance to *H. somnus* does not correlate with most antibody tests; however, the IgG_2 immunoglobulin subtype has a role in preparing *H. somnus* for phagocytosis, and it may also be used to assist in identifying vaccinated or naturally infected animals. *H. somnus* IgG_2 titers measured in acute and convalescent sera may prove useful in identifying herd infections.

PROGNOSIS

Early treatment of TME while the animal is still ambulatory generally results in dramatic recovery since the organism is highly sensitive to most systemic antibiotics. Recumbent animals having advanced septicemia and the attendant brain and spinal cord infarcts are poor candidates for treatment and should be destroyed.

PREVENTION AND THERAPY

H. somnus will survive for long periods on fomites contaminated with infected exudate and blood; therefore pressure spraying of watering areas, feedbunks, and yards, with a period of drying and sunlight, will reduce bacterial contamination when yards are quickly restocked. More important is the recognition that many cattle are carriers of genital infections. Intermingling of cattle groups heightens the opportunity for cross-infection of susceptible cattle. Overcrowding of cattle similarly increases the chances of infection of susceptible cattle from the respiratory droplets and urinary or genital secretions of infected cattle.

Rational treatment, in addition to intravenous antibiotic infusion (see later), should include treatment for endotoxic shock such as intravenous isotonic fluid therapy and corticosteroids (1 mg/kg body weight dexamethasone). The endothelial damage that coexists in this disease might be addressed by heparin therapy, but its use, while preventing incipient thrombosis, may potentiate hemorrhage in more advanced lesions; such therapy has not yet been evaluated in *H. somnus* disease and would be considered experimental. Neutrophil phagocytosis and killing of *H. somnus* might be enhanced by the parenteral use of granulocyte-macrophage colony stimulating factor (GM-CSF). Its use in cattle just prior to or on entry into the feedlot might raise an animal's resistance to *H. somnus* and other bacterial diseases. Bovine GM-CSF is not yet available commercially, and current material has a short biologic half-life. Further research is necessary before this potentially valuable therapy can be recommended as prophylactic treatment.

Several bacterins are currently available for use against *H. somnus*. All require two doses, and many contain antigens to other common bacterial diseases. The economic value of vaccination to prevent TME has been questioned because of the sporadic nature of the disease. Under good management conditions and reliable surveillance, early antibiotic therapy is probably the most economical. However, if cattle surveillance is less than optimal, vaccination may be indicated to prevent TME. The efficacy of vaccination to prevent many forms of the disease has not been demonstrated.

ANTIBIOTICS

Early intravenous therapy with antibiotic is essential in *H. somnus* disease. The organism fortunately is sensitive to a wide variety of antibiotics, and a recent in vitro study of 25 *H. somnus* isolates from differing forms of the disease indicated that the following were effective for all: sulfamethoxazole-trimethoprim, cefoxitin, cefotaxime, ciprofloxacin, erythromycin, amoxicillin, gentamicin, sulbactam/ampicillin, penicillin, tetracycline, amakacin, and chloramphenicol. Chloramphenicol is not approved for food animal use in the United States or Canada. Neomycin, sulfonamide, lincomycin, and spectinomycin are often ineffective. Intravenous tetracycline (10 mg/kg body weight) is probably the economical treatment of choice.

BIBLIOGRAPHY

Davidson JN, Carpenter TE, Hjerpe CA: An example of an economic decision analysis approach to the problem of thromboembolic meningoencephalitis (TME) in feedlot cattle. Cornell Vet 71:383–390, 1981.

Humphrey JD, Stephens LR: *Haemophilus somnus*: a review. Vet Bull 53:987–1004, 1983.

Silva SVPS, Little PB: The protective effect of vaccination against experimental pneumonia in cattle with *Haemophilus somnus* outer membrane antigens and interference by lipopolysaccharide. Can J Vet Res 54:326–330, 1990.

Porcine *Actinobacillus* Pleuropneumonia

SØREN ROSENDAL, DVM, PHD

Pleuropneumonia in pigs is the disease caused by *Actinobacillus pleuropneumoniae*. The organism was originally classified within the genus *Hemophilus* because it was shown to require the growth factor nicotinamide adenine dinucleotide (NAD). Comparative genetic studies have clearly determined, however, that the pathogen belongs to the genus *Actinobacillus*.

Pleuropneumonia is a disease of worldwide distribution. There are 12 capsular serotypes, of which serotype 5 is further subdivided into 5a and 5b. The distribution of these serotypes varies from continent to continent. In North America, serotypes 1, 5, and 7 are currently the most prevalent, with serotypes 2, 3, 4, and 6 of sporadic occurrence only.

Infection with *A. pleuropneumoniae* may result in peracute, acute, or chronic pleuropneumonia or in inapparent infection. From the earliest outbreaks, described in the 1960s, this disease has been sweeping through most major pork-producing countries in the world, where the incidence of peracute and acute pleuropneumonia reached epizootic levels but declined to sporadic incidence after a few years. The reasons for this decline are most likely increased acquired and innate resistance and adjustment of managerial procedures to alleviate environmental stress factors. Currently many herds are infected, but they have only sporadic cases of acute pleuropneumonia and a certain prevalence of chronic disease, depending on the quality of husbandry. Losses due to pleuropneumonia are substantial and are incurred from mortality, lost marketability, cost of medication and veterinary service, reduced feed conversion efficiency, and cost of trimming carcasses for pleurisy lesions at slaughter. During the epizootics of acute pleuropneumonia in North America in the late 1970s and early 1980s, losses to individual producers often led to bankruptcy.

AGENT AND PATHOGENESIS

A. pleuropneumoniae is a gram-negative coccobacillus that is apparently specifically adapted to parasitize the porcine host. The organism is fragile in the environment and seems to transmit only between pigs having contact or in close proximity of each other. The bacterium colonizes the nasal epithelium and tonsils. Invasion of the lower airways in susceptible pigs leads to an acute inflammatory response. The virulent bacteria possess a large, protective polysaccharide capsule, enabling them to evade phagocytosis by the neutrophils attracted to the lung by the lipopolysaccharide (endotoxin). Lipopolysaccharide and protein cytotoxins released from the bacterium are responsible for dramatic vascular breakdown, neutrophil and macrophage cytotoxicity leading to generation of inflammatory mediators, tissue active enzymes, and oxygen radicals. In highly susceptible pigs the acute inflammation involves the entire lung within hours, and leads to death due to pulmonary edema, hemorrhage, and shock. In less susceptible pigs the inflammation is confined to parts of the lung, which undergo necrosis and eventually turn into sequestra or abscesses. Because of the dramatic exudation during the acute phase of the inflammation abscesses, sequestra or scars are invariably associated with pleuritic adhesions.

Whether pigs become only subclinically infected, develop localized pleuropneumonia leading to lung necrosis and pleurisy, or develop the acute lethal form depends on exposure dose and specific and nonspecific host resistance. The latter is determined by previous exposure, vaccination, and stress factors. Although laboratory studies suggest that serotype 1 strains are the most virulent, all serotypes have been isolated from field cases of acute lethal pleuropneumonia.

CLINICAL SIGNS

The clinical course of pleuropneumonia varies from peracute, acute, to chronic. New outbreaks often occur a few days after carrier pigs have been introduced into a herd lacking immunity. The period of incubation can be very short, for example, only 10 to 18 hours. Animals observed to be perfectly normal in the evening may be found dead in the morning, or animals loaded on a truck for shipment to packing plants via stockyards may develop disease as a result of exposure on the truck and be found dead on arrival. Froth and blood around the mouth and nostrils of pigs found dead with no preceding signs of pneumonia are strong indications of pleuropneumonia. Pigs with acute signs of pleuropneumonia are prostrated, lying singly and often in sternal recumbency or in a "sitting dog" position. They are severely dyspneic with a rapid, thumping breathing pattern. They are very reluctant to move and will soon sit or lie down if stirred up. The body temperature is elevated and often between 41 and 42°C. The respiration is labored and audible owing to the fluid accumulation in the airways. When the animals approach the moribund stage, hemorrhagic froth can often be observed around the nostrils;

in some animals cyanotic changes occur at the ears and other extreme parts of the body.

Chronic pleuropneumonia–suffering pigs may have had a previous bout of acute pleuropneumonia that went unrecognized or was treated. Pigs with chronic pleuropneumonia have reduced feed intake and are much less active than their healthy counterparts. Coughing may be observed occasionally but is by no means characteristic. Chronic pleuropneumonia is one of the primary reasons for increased days to market.

NECROPSY LESIONS

The changes observed in the respiratory tract are quite characteristic of pleuropneumonia and very helpful for arriving at a specific diagnosis. In pigs with peracute or acute pleuropneumonia the airways are filled with hemorrhagic froth. The lungs are heavy and fail to collapse when removed from the thorax. The interlobular septa are very conspicuous owing to distention with edema and hemorrhage. The lymph nodes are enlarged, wet, and hemorrhagic. The pleural cavity has abundant serohemorrhagic fluid, particularly in the peracute phase, whereas in the more protracted cases the fluid may not be present because the animal is often dehydrated. The lungs are covered with a layer of fibrin, which in peracute cases resembles ground glass and in protracted cases forms a layer that can easily be peeled away. Hemorrhagic fluid drains in abundance from fresh cut surfaces. There is often pericarditis, but there are no lesions in organs outside the thoracic cavity.

Histologically the lung tissue has lost the natural honeycombed structure and is replaced by fibrin, hemorrhage, and inflammatory cells primarily of the mononuclear type. There is marked vascular inflammation with thrombosis. In acute to subacute cases the lung has an abundance of basophilic spindle-shaped cells forming swirly patterns. Except in peracute cases there are very few neutrophils present in the lung.

Chronic pleuropneumonia is macroscopically characterized by necrosis, sequestration, and abscessation. If the areas of necrosis are sufficiently small, healing may leave only scar tissue. The lung lesions are invariably associated with pleuritic fibrous adhesions. Histologically the areas with chronic pleuropneumonia have coagulation necrosis surrounded by layers of basophilic spindle-shaped cells and fibrous tissue.

DIAGNOSIS

Outbreaks of acute pleuropneumonia can often be related to a recent introduction of new stock of carrier pigs or, in the case of latently infected herds, to social or environmental stress such as a break in climate control, management faults, or intercurrent diseases. The clinical signs and the course of disease as described should lead to a tentative diagnosis of pleuropneumonia. Definitive diagnosis of pleuropneumonia is easily made at necropsy on the basis of the characteristic lesions and isolation of *A. pleuropneumoniae* from the lung tissue. With the exception of very young pigs the pathogen is rarely isolated from organs outside the thoracic cavity. *A. pleuropneumoniae* grows on blood agar supplemented with NAD or as a satellite around nurser bacteria such as *Staphylococcus aureus* or *Escherichia coli*. The organism is a gram-negative coccobacillus, hemolytic, and urease positive and ferments sucrose and mannitol. Serotyping is most conveniently done using coagglutination reaction. It is possible to demonstrate the organism in lung tissue using fluorescent antibody tests or coagglutination with tissue fluid as antigen. Isolation of the organism, however, affords the opportunity to determine the antimicrobial susceptibility.

Chronic pleuropneumonia is difficult to diagnose clinically without a history of preceding acute cases in the herd. In the laboratory the organism is readily isolated from the center of lung abscesses or sequestra. In the living animal it may be possible to isolate *A. pleuropneumoniae* from nasal or tonsilar swabs, in which case advantage should be taken of a selective medium containing blood, NAD, crystal violet, bacitracin, and lincomycin. Chronically infected pigs develop antibodies to a number of antigens of *A. pleuropneumoniae*. For serotype-specific diagnosis of infection, serologic tests using capsular antigen appear to be most reliable.

Swine erysipelas should be kept in mind as a possible differential diagnosis in herds unvaccinated for erysipelas, and hog cholera may be considered in countries where both diseases occur. Acute pleuropneumonia may also be confused with swine influenza, but the latter would not have the mortality of the former or the chronic sequelae.

TREATMENT

Prompt antimicrobial treatment is required in the face of acute outbreaks of pleuropneumonia in order to curb morbidity and mortality and further spread of disease. Unfortunately no one antimicrobial drug is universally effective because of antimicrobial resistance among strains of *A. pleuropneumoniae*. Until antimicrobial susceptibility profiles have been obtained on isolates from an outbreak, injectable drugs with good and sustained levels in the lung tissue should be used. Recommended drugs are listed in Table 1. Plasmid-mediated antimicrobial resistance has been recognized in the cases of penicillin, ampicillin, streptomycin, tetracycline, and chloramphenicol. Chloramphenicol is no longer permitted for use in food animals in many countries, including the United States and Canada. Initial treatment may require several injections, and it is important to inspect the herd several times around the clock in order to treat new cases at the earliest possible stage. Treatment of pleuropneumonia may also be administered in the drinking water or feed but would benefit only those animals with normal feed and water intake. Chronic pleuropneumonia is not curable owing to the inability to reach the bacteria in the center of lung necroses or abscesses, but part of the growth-depressing effect may be alleviated by medication. Sick pigs should be isolated in order to secure optimal opportunity for uptake of medicated feed or water and to reduce the challenge for the healthy penmates.

PREVENTION

The fact that *A. pleuropneumoniae* is a pathogen restricted to pigs and only transmits by contact makes pleuropneumonia

Table 1. ANTIMICROBIAL DRUGS FOR TREATMENT OR CONTROL OF *ACTINOBACILLUS* PLEUROPNEUMONIA

Drug	Injectable Dose	Feed, Water Medication (ppm)
Penicillin	10–20,000 IU/kg	
Ampicillin	10 mg/kg	
Trimethoprim/ sulfamethoxazole	2.5/12.5 mg/kg	
Oxytetracycline	10 mg/kg	1600
Gentamicin	10 mg/kg	
Ceftiofur	3 mg/kg	
Danofloxacin	1.25 mg/kg	25
Enrofloxacin	10 mg/kg	100–200
Tiamulin	10–15 mg/kg	200

a preventable disease by use of simple management strategies. Practicing closed-herd management virtually eliminates the risk of introducing the agent. Supplemental stock entering a closed herd must come from other closed herds that have been ascertained to be free of pleuropneumonia on the basis of serologic surveillance in addition to clinical and postmortem evidence of disease-free status. Pigs of unknown status entering a herd with *A. pleuropneumoniae* may be conditioned by 2 to 3 weeks of feed or water medication. Producers buying weaners for fattening should secure supply known to be free of pleuropneumonia from a single supplier. If this arrangement is not possible it may be advisable to use the all-in–all-out production system, involving either the entire barn or well-separated sections.

Outbreaks of disease in chronically infected herds is related to environmental stress factors. Prevention therefore must be based on maintaining conditions that assure optimal resistance among the pigs and lowest possible infection pressure. In herds in which losses are substantial and incorrectable by management procedures, it may be advisable to depopulate and restock with specific pathogen-free (SPF) pigs or pigs from herds ascertained to be free of pleuropneumonia by serology and other clinical or laboratory diagnostic approaches. An eradication program based on medicated early weaning may be implemented in herds with appropriate facilities and labor resources.

Vaccination against pleuropneumonia using bacterins has been shown to protect against mortality but not always against chronic lung lesions. Newer vaccines incorporating extracellular antigens may be more efficacious. Certainly vaccination should be considered in chronically infected herds with recurring acute flare-ups of disease and also when pigs are moved from disease-free herds into herds with pleuropneumonia or of unknown status. Commercial vaccines are protective primarily against homologous serotypes. Therefore isolates from the herd in which vaccination is performed should be serotyped to ascertain whether the vaccine will work. Alternatively autogenous vaccines may be used.

BIBLIOGRAPHY

Devenish J, Rosendal S, Basse JT: Humoral antibody response and protective immunity in swine following immunization with the 104 Kilodalton hemolysin of *Actinobacillus pleuropneumoniae*. Infect Immun 58:3829–3832, 1990.

Huether MJ, Fedorka-Cray PJ, Pfannenstiel MA, Anderson GA: Plasmid profiles and antibiotic susceptibility of *Haemophilus pleuropneumoniae* serotypes 1, 2, 3, 5 and 7. FEMS Microbiology Letters 48:179–182, 1987.

Rosendal S, Mitchell WR. Epidemiology of *Haemophilus pleuropneumoniae* infection in pigs: a survey of Ontario pork producers, 1981. Can J Comp Med 47:1–5, 1983.

Willson PJ, Osborne AD: Comparison of common antibiotic therapies for *Haemophilus pleuropneumonia* in pigs. Can Vet J 26:312–316, 1985.

Brucellosis

PAUL NICOLETTI, DVM, MS

Brucellosis in food-producing animals is caused by four of the six members of the genus *Brucella*. Infections in cattle are caused primarily by *B. abortus*, in swine by *B. suis*, in goats and sheep by *B. melitensis*, and also in sheep by *B. ovis*. Cross-species infections are uncommon, and clinical symptoms are rare.

HISTORY

In 1886 a micrococcus was isolated from the spleen of human patients, and the disease it caused was called undulant fever in 1897. In 1904 a young British physician, Bruce, was commissioned to determine the cause of the human malady on the Isle of Malta. In the meantime a Danish veterinarian, Bang, had isolated a microorganism from an aborting heifer that was later to be called *B. abortus*. Traum, in California in 1914, isolated *B. suis* from a sow. In 1953 Buddle and Boyes, in Australia and New Zealand, identified *B. ovis* as a cause of epididymitis in sheep.

Brucellosis is the term now used for infections by any member of the genus *Brucella*. In humans it is occasionally referred to as undulant fever or Malta fever and in cattle as Bang's disease. All species infect humans except *B. ovis* and *B. neotomae*. There are no residual *B. melitensis* infections in the United States. Sporadic cases occur in goats and humans when introduced from and contracted in other countries, respectively.

The incidence of cattle brucellosis in the United States was reduced from 5 per cent in 1957 to approximately 0.2 per cent in 1989, according to the US Department of Agriculture (USDA) statistics. Twenty-seven states were classified free of cattle brucellosis. The actual losses due to the disease are difficult to estimate but are given as approximately $35 million annually from abortions, decreased milk yield (especially due to early calving), temporary or occasional permanent sterility, and sale and replacement of diseased cattle. Estimates of losses are not available for human, swine, or sheep infections. The incidence of swine brucellosis has declined to approximately 0.04 per cent among marketed swine. Approximately two thirds of the states of the United States are validated brucellosis free.

ETIOLOGY

Brucellae are gram-negative coccobacilli that are nonmotile and nonencapsulated. They are aerobic, but some species require carbon dioxide for cultivation. The colonies appear in approximately 4 to 5 days and are round and convex, displaying a somewhat characteristic bluish color when examined with light transmitted at a 45-degree angle.

Differentiation of species and biovars in the genus *Brucella* is based on various growth requirements, sensitivity to dyes in media, oxidation of metabolic substrates, serologic reactions, and bacteriophage susceptibility (Table 1).

CLINICAL SIGNS

Cattle

After ingestion of the coccobacilli there is temporary septicemia with phagocytosis by neutrophils and fixed macrophages of local lymph nodes. The predilection sites are the endometrium and fetal placenta in the pregnant cow and the supramammary lymph nodes and the udder. Uterine infection is probably related to the presence of a natural compound, erythritol, which stimulates the growth of *B. abortus*. The severity of uterine infection varies, but the numbers of organisms are greatest at the time of abortion or parturition. Genital infection usually disappears within 30 days after calving but may recur at subsequent pregnancies. Inflammation of the allantochorion may interfere with circulation to the fetus and cause subsequent death and expulsion. Abortions frequently

Table 1. SOME GENERAL CHARACTERISTICS OF FOUR SPECIES OF *BRUCELLA**

Species	Number of Biovars	Growth Requirements			
		CO_2	H_2S	Basic Fuchsin	Thionin
B. melitensis	3	−	−	+	+
B. abortus	8	+	+	+	−
B. suis	4	−	+	−	+
B. ovis	1	+	−	+	+

*Variations occur among some biovars.

occur after the fifth month of pregnancy, and a retained placenta may follow. Not all infections result in abortion, and few cattle abort more than once. A small percentage of cattle spontaneously recover. A high percentage of cattle have permanent udder infection with shedding of organisms in the milk.

In the bull, *B. abortus* may produce orchitis with abscesses, epididymitis (Fig. 1), and inflammation of accessory reproductive organs. Orchitis is usually unilateral and results in reduced libido and impaired fertility. Brucellae may be discharged in the semen.

Swine

Clinical evidence of *B. suis* infections varies and is influenced by many factors. The typical syndrome is that of abortion or birth of stillborn or weak pigs, infertility, orchitis (Fig. 2), and sometimes posterior paralysis or lameness due to spondylitis. Genital infection is more permanent in boars than in sows. The semen usually contains large numbers of organisms, and sows may become infected during breeding.

Sheep and Goats

B. melitensis infections occur in both sheep and goats and produce abortions in late pregnancy (Fig. 3). The abortion rate varies considerably, and susceptibility also varies among breeds of sheep. Infected ewes and goats excrete organisms in the milk and in vaginal discharges. Sheep may recover from the disease.

B. ovis infections in sheep are usually demonstrated by epididymitis and orchitis. There may be abortions even though the ewe appears to be more resistant than the ram, and the

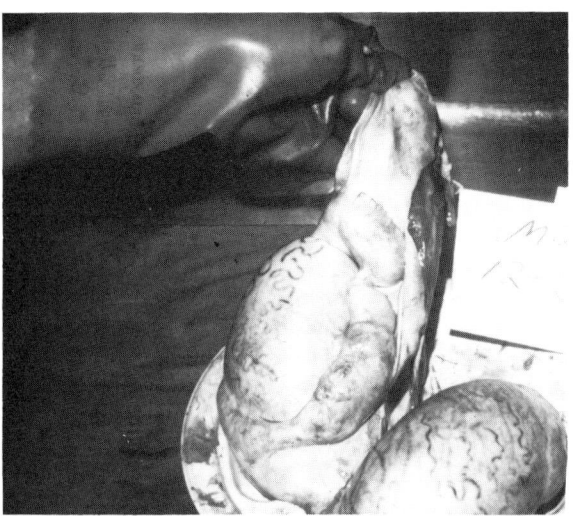

Figure 1. Epididymitis in a bull with *B. abortus* infection.

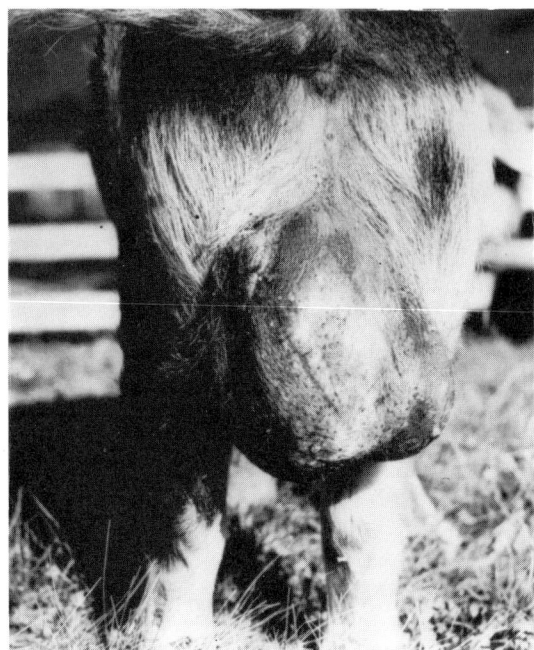

Figure 2. Unilateral orchitis from *B. suis*. (Courtesy of Dr. B. Deyoe, Retired, Nevada, IA.)

disease may not persist. Gross lesions of scrotal edema, fibrosis, and adhesions are observed. There may be aspermia and abnormalities in motility or morphology of spermatozoa. Transmission is from ram to ram during preputial or rectal contact and from ram to ewe during mating, although this appears to be uncommon.

DIAGNOSIS

A correct diagnosis depends on herd or flock history along with information concerning the individual. Serologic, bacteriologic, or pathologic examinations may be necessary.

Antibodies to *Brucella* are found in a number of fluids, but most tests are performed on serum or milk. Herd surveillance methods include milk-ring and blood tests on marketed cattle. The milk-ring test is much more efficient, as it surveys nearly all of the population at one time. Identification of infected herds is also through blood tests for cattle marketed for breeding or slaughter. This method depends on the sale of an

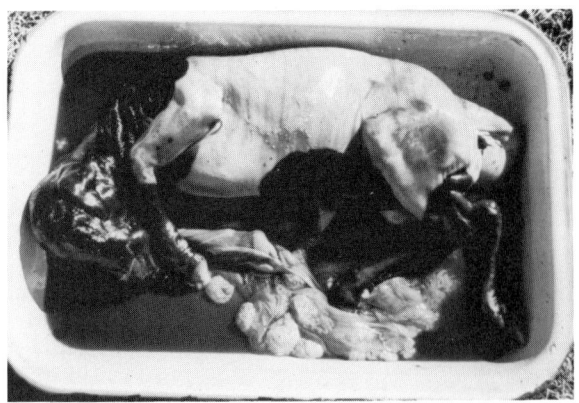

Figure 3. Abortus from sheep with brucellosis.

animal with positive results, and it may be slow to identify infected herds.

SEROLOGY

Positive results from serologic tests indicate present or past exposure to an antigenic stimulus and cannot always be equated with infection. They also do not measure immunity.

The only international standard for the diagnosis of brucellosis in individual cattle is the tube agglutination test (Fig. 4), which measures antibodies in international units. The test methods and interpretation of results vary in both veterinary and human medicine and from country to country. In the United States, tests on cattle are considered positive if the serum reacts in the 1:100 or greater dilution and is from a nonvaccinate and in the 1:200 dilution and is from a vaccinate. Test results from cattle with lower titers are classified as suspect or negative, depending on vaccination status. The tube agglutination test is influenced by many factors, and there are many false-positive and false-negative results. Causes of false results are early or chronic infections, vaccination, and heterospecific antigens. The difficulties in performing the test and in interpreting results have led to the development and use of several other procedures. The tube agglutination test is mostly performed in the United States and several other countries when required for international commerce of cattle.

Plate Agglutination Test

This rapid test is comparable to the tube agglutination test in sensitivity and is subject to most of the same factors that influence the results. Other tests have largely replaced the plate agglutination test.

Card Test or Rose Bengal Test

This test (Fig. 5) is performed on a card, a white tile, or a machine. It is simple and can be completed at the farm, ranch, market facility, or laboratory. The test is a good screening procedure (there are few false-negative results) and should generally be supported by other tests (there may be many false-positive results, especially in vaccinated populations) and information on herd and individual history.

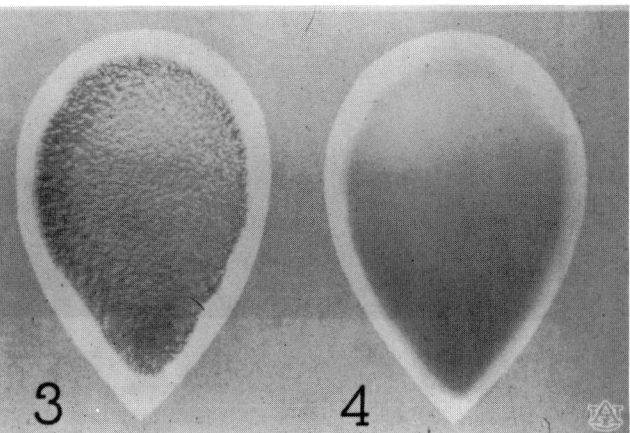
Figure 5. Card test showing agglutination (left).

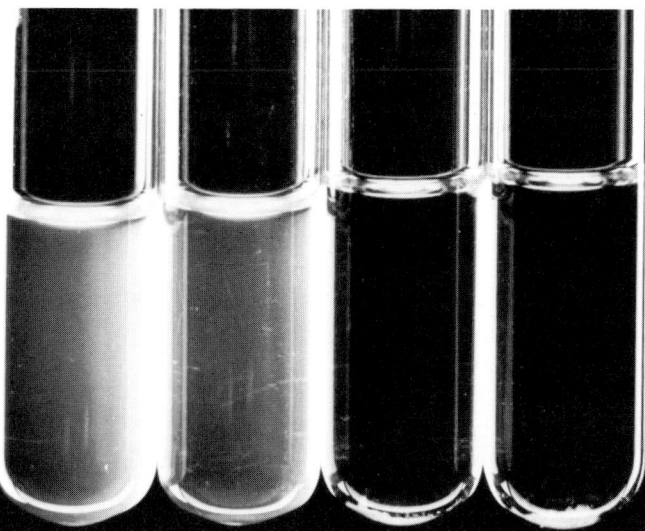
Figure 4. Tube agglutination test with negative (left) and positive (right) results.

Rivanol Precipitation Test

This procedure depends on the precipitation of high molecular weight agglutinins and examination of the supernatant with a special antigen. It is less sensitive than the tube or plate agglutination test or the card test and is more simple than the complement fixation test.

Complement Fixation Test

Many studies have shown the superiority of this test in specificity and sensitivity, especially for chronically infected or vaccinated cattle.

The Particle Concentration Fluorescence Immunoassay (PCFIA) has been developed by a commercial company (IDEXX Corp., Portland, ME) and utilizes submicron polystyrene particles to which soluble antigens and a fluorescence marker are attached. The system is automated and used as a screening test. Other test methods that have been used are enzyme-linked immunosorbent assay (ELISA), buffered acid antigen, heat inactivation, mercaptoethanol, Coombs' antiglobulin, hemagglutination, milk-ring, and whey tests, and vaginal mucus and semen plasma agglutination.

Regardless of the test used, the results should be properly evaluated. Emphasis should be placed on kinds of antibodies (qualitative) instead of numbers of antibodies (quantitative) and on bacteriologic studies of appropriate specimens.

BACTERIOLOGY

The milk and other udder secretions are good sources of organisms. The supramammary lymph nodes are the preferential site at necropsy, but other lymph nodes are also useful. Abomasal fluids should be cultured from the fetus.

Swine

There is an agreement that individual animal test results are less accurate in swine than in cattle. There may be false-negative or false-positive results. A herd test result profile is best. The card test is very useful, and supplemental procedures can be used. Sites for cultures should include the lymph nodes, especially those in the cervical region, and the seminal vesicles.

Sheep and Goats

There is no international standard for the selection of a test or interpretations of results for *B. melitensis* infections. The tube agglutination test or the rose bengal test is generally used, but complement fixation and dermal hypersensitivity tests are preferred by many workers. Bacteriologic examinations are of vaginal discharges, milk, lymph nodes, placentae, and aborted fetuses.

The diagnosis of *B. ovis* infection requires a clinical examination, semen evaluation, and interpretation of results of the complement fixation test on blood sera and cultures if indicated. A gel diffusion test has also given good results. Recent research studies have found that an indirect ELISA is superior in sensitivity to other procedures.

EPIDEMIOLOGY

The infected cow is the source of most infections through discharges and products associated with parturition (Fig. 6). She is generally not infectious to other cattle by 2 to 4 weeks after parturition. Hygienic measures are important but may not be effective in controlling the disease owing to seronegative infected cattle that abort or calve normally. The variable incubation period of a few weeks to several months is related to the gestation period and severity of exposure.

Brucellae are intracellular parasites and, in this environment, are not antigenic and are protected from host defenses and chemotherapy.

Calves born to infected cows and those ingesting contaminated milk are temporarily infected. The permanency of this infection has been disputed. However, it is now certain that latent infections occur, but the frequency and contributing factors are unknown. An additional problem is that the heifer becomes seronegative during most of prepuberty and prior to calving. There have been many reports of latent infections that have resulted in new herd infections or in reinfections of herds considered free of brucellosis.

Under normal conditions the bull appears to play a minor, if any, role in the transmission of brucellosis. However, contaminated semen used in artificial insemination may result in infections.

Brucellosis in wildlife species has rarely proven to be a problem in transmission to domesticated livestock except under special circumstances. The disease exists in certain bison and elk populations in the United States and in caribou and reindeer populations in the Arctic.

Brucella organisms may survive within protected environments for several weeks, but sunlight kills them within a few hours. The virulence of strains varies, but no satisfactory in vitro method for its measurement has been developed.

TREATMENT

Development of a satisfactory treatment for brucellosis in domestic animals has been difficult. Spontaneous recoveries occur among all species, and the percentages vary.

There has been success in treating *B. ovis* infections in sheep and *B. abortus* in cattle with tetracyclines and streptomycin, but use of these regimens has been limited owing to costs and regulatory aspects of cattle brucellosis.

PUBLIC HEALTH CONSIDERATIONS

Brucellosis is a true zoonosis, and control in humans is directly related to its prevalence among animals. Occupationally related infections predominate, with slaughterhouse workers being the highest risk group.

B. melitensis is considered the most virulent species for humans, followed by *B. suis* and *B. abortus* in that order.

Direct contact with contaminated fluids and tissues is the chief source of infection. Outbreaks in slaughterhouses have been reported due to inhalation of *B. suis*. Accidental inoculation of strain 19 among veterinarians and laboratory workers is not uncommon. Ingestion of contaminated and unpasteurized dairy products is a very serious public health problem where *B. melitensis* is prevalent.

The symptoms in humans vary in severity from acute to chronic, and many infections are undiagnosed. The classic symptoms are headache, undulating fever, joint pains, chills, and weakness. Relapses after apparent successful treatment are not uncommon. The serum agglutination test is most often used to aid in the diagnosis, but methods of performing the test and interpretations of results may vary. The card test is

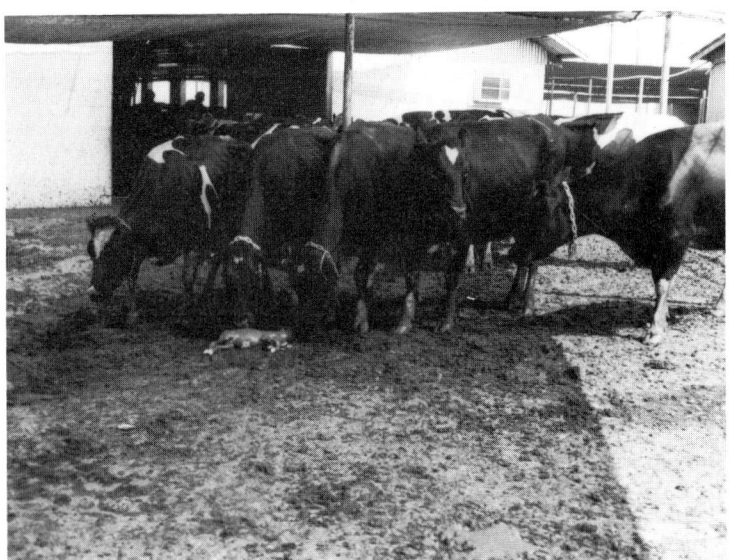

Figure 6. Ingestion is the most common source of *Brucella* infection, such as an aborted fetus.

very useful for acute infections. Intradermic tests should be avoided.

Acute infections respond well to oral tetracycline and intramuscular streptomycin. An early diagnosis combined with proper and prolonged treatment is important.

CONTROL

The control of brucellosis is both a herd owner's and a regulatory agency's responsibility. The major phases are identification and slaughter of diseased livestock, vaccination, herd management, and control of livestock movements.

Strain 19 is the only approved vaccine in the United States to prevent *B. abortus* infections. Other vaccines such as 45/20 and H38 have been studied by many investigators, often with conflicting findings. An attenuated strain of *B. melitensis*, Rev 1, is used in other countries for control of *B. melitensis* and sometimes *B. ovis* and is very effective. Adjuvant vaccines have been used to prevent *B. ovis* infections.

Currently strain 19 is recommended for vaccination of calves 4 to 12 months of age. It is also used for adult cattle in a lowered dose and under restricted conditions. High rates of vaccination in herds are important to reduction of infection rates.

The immunity produced by *Brucella* vaccines is cell mediated and related to dose and virulence of the challenge strain. The effectiveness of vaccination is best when a high percentage of the herd is immunized so that exposure potential is minimized. Individual effectiveness is often quoted to be about 65 to 70 per cent, but herd effectiveness is much greater. Vaccinated animals are much more likely to resist the disease or to have less severe disease, so fewer organisms are excreted.

The herd size is very important in brucellosis control, especially if there is close confinement. Introduction of replacement animals increases the risk of herd infection. The status of the herd of origin is very important. Negative test results on purchased animals are not satisfactory means of preventing introduction of cattle that are incubating the disease. Isolation and retests are recommended.

A cooperative program for control and eradication of bovine brucellosis began in 1934 largely as a drought relief effort. It received special emphasis in the early 1950s, and the current federal budget in the United States is about $65 million annually. The Uniform Methods and Rules are administered by the USDA. Strain 19 vaccination has been an integral part of the program, with peak usage in 1988, when approximately 10 million calves were vaccinated. The program emphasizes surveillance methods, prompt herd tests, slaughter of seropositive animals, vaccination, and owner cooperation.

Swine

Purchase of swine from *Brucella*-free herds or rearing replacements is the best prevention. If brucellosis exists it is best to depopulate the herd. A second proposal is to retain young pigs and test them prior to breeding and farrowing. A third but inferior approach is to test and remove reactors until the last two herd tests reveal no more infected swine. The criteria for validating herds and areas are given in the Uniform Methods and Rules.

Sheep and Goats

Where *B. melitensis* exists, consideration is given to slaughter of the entire flock or herd. Use of Rev 1 vaccine, with or without identification, along with slaughter of infected animals is another form of control. Rev 1 vaccine has been recommended for young female sheep and goats. Recent studies have found successful and more practical control using a reduced dose of Rev 1 in sexually mature animals.

The control of *B. ovis* is accomplished by maintaining young rams separate from mature rams. In addition, mature sheep are examined, and those with clinical and serologic evidence of infection are slaughtered. In some countries Rev 1 vaccine is also used.

BIBLIOGRAPHY

Alton GG, Jones LM, Angus RD, Verger JM: Techniques for the Brucellosis Laboratory. Paris, Institut National de la Recherche Agronomique, 1988.
Deyoe BL: Brucellosis. *In* Leman AD, Straw B, Glock RO, et al (eds): Diseases of Swine, 6th ed. Ames, IA, Iowa State University Press, 1986, pp 599–607.
Kimberling CV: Jensen and Swift's Diseases of Sheep, 3rd ed. Philadelphia, Lea & Febiger, 1988.
Nicoletti P: The Epidemiology of Bovine Brucellosis. *In* Brandly CA, Carnelius CE (eds): Advances in Veterinary Science and Comparative Medicine, Vol. 24. New York, Academic Press, 1980.
Nielson K, Duncan JR (eds): Animal Brucellosis. Boca Raton, FL, CRC Press, 1990.

Pasteurellosis in Cattle
PATRICIA E. SHEWEN, BSc, DVM, MSc, PhD
KENNETH G. BATEMAN, DVM, MSc

Pasteurella multocida and *P. haemolytica* are commensals of the ruminant nasopharynx. Pneumonia is the most common form of bovine pasteurellosis, and its onset is typically related to environmental stress. Pneumonic pasteurellosis is the major cause of death due to undifferentiated bovine respiratory disease, or shipping fever, in feedlot cattle, which is estimated to cause losses in excess of $800 million annually in North America. The usual isolates from this fibrinous bronchopneumonia are *P. haemolytica* A1 (biotype A serotype 1) and/or *P. multocida* serotype A. While viruses, mycoplasma, and other organisms may contribute with environmental stress to the initiation of disease, the pneumonic lesions and death can be attributed to the pasteurellae. Young dairy and veal calves housed in crowded or poorly ventilated conditions also develop pneumonic pasteurellosis, recognized as one form of enzootic pneumonia. Pasteurellae have also been isolated from cases of sporadic pneumonia in adult dairy cattle, localized infections, abortion, mastitis, meningitis, and rarely acute fatal septicemia.

SEPTICEMIA

P. multocida types B2 and E2 cause hemorrhagic septicemia, which is an important disease of cattle and water buffalo in Southeast Asia, Africa, and the Middle East. Disease is transmitted by contact with latent carriers, which harbor organisms in the tonsil and shed intermittently when stressed. Outbreaks occur most often in the rainy season both because infectious organisms may survive in moist soil and because waterways disseminate organisms from infected carcasses. There is a strong association between nomadic husbandry and disease. Morbidity rates vary from 5 per cent in areas where disease is endemic to 100 per cent among naive animals. In North America sporadic outbreaks in bison have been reported, but in domestic cattle disease is so rare as to be considered nonexistent.

Clinical signs appear within 2 to 5 days after inhalation or ingestion. First reports may be of sudden death without other signs. Peracute and acute cases must be differentiated from other causes of sudden death, such as snakebite, lightning, anthrax, rinderpest, and blackleg. Typically, initial fever and inappetence are followed by respiratory distress with profuse salivation and nasal discharge. There is characteristic swelling of the head, throat, and brisket, swollen hemorrhagic lymph nodes, and numerous mucosal and subserosal petechial hemorrhages. Untreated septicemia results in death.

At necropsy, subcutaneous infiltration of serogelatinous fluid in the upper body is readily apparent. Petechial and ecchymotic hemorrhages are seen in the subcutis, connective tissues, lymph nodes, gastrointestinal tract, and heart. There may be marked serofibrinous pericarditis, pleuritis, and peritonitis with adhesions. Pneumonia, if present, resembles typical pneumonic pasteurellosis.

Treatment

The acute course of disease generally makes treatment of clinically sick animals futile. Once disease is recognized, all in-contact animals with fever should be isolated and treated. Sulphadimidine (33 per cent solution) intravenously is commonly used in Southeast Asia. Intramuscularly administered oxytetracycline or penicillin-streptomycin combinations are also effective. There are no reports of antibiotic resistance among strains of *P. multocida* isolated from hemorrhagic septicemia. Hyperimmune serum, although effective, is rarely used.

Prevention

In countries where hemorrhagic septicemia occurs, vaccination with indigenous strains, recently passaged in animals, is the principal means of control. Several vaccines are available. All are formalinized bacterins of similar efficacy. Endotoxin-induced anaphylactic shock following vaccination may occur. In well-managed herds, calves are vaccinated at 3 to 6 months of age, boosted 3 months later, and then boosted annually. Calves less than 3 months of age do not respond to vaccination, but disease is rare in animals less than 6 months old. In free-range or nomadic animals, annual vaccination prior to the rainy season is recommended.

RESPIRATORY DISEASE

While both *P. multocida* and *P. haemolytica* are normal inhabitants of the upper respiratory tract of cattle, only *P. multocida* is readily recovered from nasal swabs of clinically healthy animals. *P. haemolytica* is cultured infrequently and sporadically, and type A2 predominates. When cattle are stressed by weaning, shipment, or intensive rearing conditions, the rate of isolation increases and serotype 1 predominates. It is now thought that *P. haemolytica* A1 is carried in the tonsillar area of the pharynx. Under stressful conditions, for unknown reasons, the bacterium replicates rapidly and large numbers of organisms ascend into the nasal passages coincidentally with their descent in aerosol droplets into the lung. Clearance of *P. haemolytica* is ineffective because of depressed mucociliary function and alveolar macrophage activity brought about by stress, concurrent infection with respiratory viruses, or the bacterium itself. In the lung, rapidly growing *P. haemolytica* produces a polysaccharide capsule, which inhibits phagocytosis; fimbriae, which permit adherence and colonization; and a leukotoxin/hemolysin, which inhibits the function of and also destroys alveolar macrophages, neutrophils, and other white cells. The resultant release of proteolytic enzymes and fibrinogenic factors from dying phagocytes induces the severe fibrinous pneumonia typical of shipping fever. Endotoxin released into the lung probably contributes to lesions, if only by inducing neutrophil influx. Death is due to respiratory failure.

Lesions are typically anteroventral, although in severe cases the entire lung may be involved. In acute pneumonia there is an accumulation of serofibrinous exudate on pleural surfaces and within the thorax. Later, fibrinous adhesions develop between lung lobes and between the lungs, thorax, and pericardium. The normal architecture of the lung may be indistinguishable, and affected lobes are consolidated, hemorrhagic, or necrotic. Airways are filled with blood-stained fibrinous exudate. Histologically, in early stages there is atelectasis, bronchiolitis, fibrinous exudate, neutrophils, and cell debris in alveolar spaces. Macrophages may have engulfed pasteurellae—many are oat-shaped "streaming" macrophages. Later there is distension of lymphatic vessels with fibrin and areas of coagulation necrosis surrounded by zones of inflammatory cells and fibrinous tissue.

P. multocida type A is occasionally isolated with *P. haemolytica* from fibrinous bronchopneumonia at necropsy, and it may participate in development of the lesions typical of shipping fever. However, the pathogenic role of *P. multocida* is less well studied. The organism is encapsulated, and some strains of type A produce the dermonecrotic toxin implicated in atrophic rhinitis, although most pneumonic isolates have not been characterized for toxin production. Occasionally *P. multocida* is the only bacterium isolated. Typically these pneumonias lack the fibrinous characteristics described above.

The cardinal signs of pneumonic pasteurellosis include depression (recognized by hanging head, standing alone), loss of appetite, and fever. Fever alone is not sufficient for diagnosis, since many febrile animals never develop respiratory signs or go off feed. Animals that exhibit fever with no other clinical signs cannot be shown to have poorer weight gains when compared with treated (sick) calves. In fact, fever by itself may be a positive indicator of effective clearance/immune mechanisms at work. Research has shown that the incidence of fever may be well over twice that of the incidence of treatment for pneumonia. Respiratory signs are apparent as pneumonia develops and are initially observed as increased respiratory rate and shallow respiration. Mucoid or purulent nasal discharge is an inconsistent feature probably dependent on the degree of concurrent viral infection. A serous discharge may result from failure of a depressed calf to lick its nose. As pneumonia progresses there is audible breathing, and often an expiratory grunt and friction sounds can be heard on auscultation, especially anteroventrally. Terminally the temperature may be subnormal and the respiratory rate may be normal or very low.

Treatment

Successful treatment of pneumonic pasteurellosis is dependent on early application of the correct antimicrobial at adequate dosage, at correct frequency, and for an adequate duration. The concurrent nursing care (housing, nutrition, and handling) of the cattle can be as important as the particular antimicrobial therapy that is administered.

Antimicrobial sensitivity testing in combination with knowledge of the pharmacokinetics of the various antimicrobials remains the preliminary means upon which therapeutic decisions must be based. Undoubtedly the in vivo results of therapy become an important adjunct when available. *P. multocida* isolates exhibit little antimicrobial resistance and remain sensitive to the commonly used antimicrobials even after prolonged exposure. On the other hand, evidence is emerging that *P. haemolytica* seems to have, at least in the "wild" strains isolated pretreatment, two distinct patterns of antimicrobial resistance that are serotype related and plasmid encoded. Approximately half of the A1 and A2 isolates are resistant to sulfonamides. *P. haemolytica* A2 is generally sensitive to the other commonly used antimicrobials (Table 1), while A1 demonstrates a consistent, plasmid-encoded resistance to ampicillin, penicillin, and tetracycline. Despite this, most isolates of *P. haemolytica* obtained pretreatment are not antimicrobial resistant and therefore are probably A2. Once antimicrobial therapy has been administered, the isolates obtained from either the live or the dead animal are almost invariably resistant to ampicillin, penicillin, and tetracycline. There would therefore seem to be a shift in the predominant population of *P. haemolytica* in the animal after antimicrobial exposure.

There are well-substantiated but unpublished cases in which prolonged use of a given antimicrobial in a therapeutic protocol has led to the selection of *P. haemolytica* with resistance patterns substantially different from those generally described. For example, with continued use of penicillin in a treatment protocol of a closed herd, *P. haemolytica* isolates resistant to penicillin but sensitive to ampicillin and tetracycline were obtained from a number of case fatalities. Recent work has shown a strong correlation between the antimicrobial sensitivity patterns of *Pasteurella* spp. obtained from the culture of nasopharyngeal swabs and bronchoalveolar lavage culture. Although this correlation is not always accurate at the individual animal level, the relationship is strong enough at the group level to recommend that pretreatment nasopharyngeal swabs be obtained from a sample of calves in which resistance to the currently employed antimicrobial is suspected as the cause of treatment failure.

Table 1. SUITABLE ANTIMICROBIALS FOR THE TREATMENT OF PNEUMONIC PASTEURELLOSIS IN CATTLE

Antimicrobial	Dosage and Route
Individual Therapy	
Procaine penicillin G	45,000 IU/kg body weight[a] intramuscularly or subcutaneously[b] once a day
Oxytetracycline	10 mg/kg body weight[a] intramuscularly once a day
Long-acting oxytetracycline[c]	20 mg/kg body weight intramuscularly once *every 72 hours*
Trimethoprim-sulfadoxine[d]	3 ml/45 kg body weight intramuscularly once a day
Sulbactam-ampicillin[c, e]	2.5 ml/45 kg body weight intramuscularly once a day
Ceftiofur sodium[f]	1.0 mg/kg body weight intramuscularly once a day
Tilmicosin[c, g]	10 mg/kg body weight subcutaneously once *every 72 hours*
Mass Prophylactic Medication	
Long-acting oxytetracycline[c]	20 mg/kg body weight intramuscularly once *every 72 hours*
Tilmicosin[c, g]	10 mg/kg body weight subcutaneously once *every 72 hours*

[a]Extralabel dosage.
[b]Extralabel route.
[c]Not approved for use in lactating dairy cows.
[d]40 mg/ml trimethoprim; 200 mg/ml sulfadoxine.
[e]Synergistin (60 mg/ml sulbactam; 120 mg/ml ampicillin), rogar/STB, London, Ontario.
[f]Excenel (50 mg/ml ceftiofur), Upjohn, Orangeville, Ontario.
[g]Micotil (300 mg/ml tilmicosin), Provel, London, Ontario.

There is an amazing lack of published information from clinical field trials of antimicrobial therapy. Two published clinical trials compared procaine penicillin, oxytetracycline, and trimethoprim-sulfadoxine as first-line antimicrobials under two different types of management conditions. Different (both extralabel) dosages of penicillin and oxytetracycline were used in each trial. There were no differences in the response, relapse, or case fatality rates among the three antimicrobials, although differing definitions of these rates were used in each trial. Both authors found that the likelihood of relapse was greater in calves treated in the first few days postarrival in the feedlot.

Suggested treatment protocols are often based on treatment of depressed, anorexic, febrile (>40°C) animals for 2 days with the first-line antimicrobial, evaluation of response on the third day, and, if favorable, continued therapy for an additional 1 or 2 days for a total of 3 or 4 days of therapy. If a case is nonresponsive on the third day, based on a failure of the temperature to drop below 40°C, a second-line antimicrobial should be employed for 3 or 4 days. Relapses should be treated with the second-line antimicrobial for 3 to 6 days depending on the response (temperature decline). Inexpensive, narrow-spectrum antimicrobials such as penicillin or oxytetracycline are often employed as first-line therapy, with the more expensive, broader-spectrum drugs employed as second- and occasionally third-line therapy. In light of the presence of plasmid-encoded resistance to penicillin, ampicillin, and tetracycline, it is not advisable to use penicillin and oxytetracycline in a protocol as first- and second-line drugs. Because of growing concerns over extralabel dosages, some veterinarians and managers choose to avoid penicillin and oxytetracycline owing to the high dosages and subsequently increased withdrawal times that are necessary.

Long-acting oxytetracycline (20 mg/kg body weight) and tilmicosin (10 mg/kg body weight) are both effective antibiotics that maintain therapeutic blood levels for 3 days and inhibitory pulmonary tissue levels for still longer. These products can be used in place of three daily injections of other conventional products with resultant savings in labor and stress associated with daily therapy. One of the most important advantages may be that their use allows the cattle to leave the relatively contaminated environment of the hospital earlier. However, if the animal is not hospitalized, there is the risk that nonresponsive cases will not be identified and changed to second-line therapy or at least have the original therapy extended for a few days. Very experienced pen checkers may be able to evaluate response subjectively and avoid high case fatality rates, but this aspect deserves close monitoring and assessment.

Ancillary therapy, such as corticosteroid and nonsteroidal anti-inflammatories, is considered unproven and potentially harmful when used in a broad manner. While they may have the benefits of reducing inflammation and sequestering neutrophils away from the lung, it is felt that because the febrile response is suppressed, therapy may be prematurely terminated.

The response, relapse, and case fatality rates will vary with the quality of cattle, time of year, age of calf, and feedlot management practices. Generally a favorable response to therapy is considered to be a drop in the rectal temperature to below 40°C by the third day of therapy (48 hours after first treatment). Response rates (by this definition) of greater than 80 per cent are quite acceptable. Relapse rates of greater than 20 per cent should be cause for concern and warrant investigation of potential contributing factors. If cattle arrive at the feedlot in reasonably good condition, case fatality rates can be maintained at 3 to 4 per cent. Yearling cattle, while not generally suffering from morbidity rates as high as calves, often seem to have higher case fatality rates. This may result from detection relatively late in the course of disease compared with calves or from inadequate treatment of previous pulmonary damage.

When response, relapse, or case fatality rates are unacceptable, there is a tendency to blame the antimicrobial. This should be investigated via culture and sensitivity of pretreatment nasal swabs from new cases of pneumonia. All too often, however, the investigation ends here rather than focusing on the epidemiologic characteristics of the problem animals. For example, is the problem high relapse rates in fresh pulls (first-time cases) or relapses that go on to die? Higher relapse rates are an expected phenomenon in cattle treated during the first few days postarrival, possibly as a result of more advanced pneumonia. On the other hand, overcrowded hospital pens can pose a high risk of dissemination of various infectious organisms, including resistant pasteurellae. Even under the best of management there will be occasional deaths due to pneumonic pasteurellosis of untreated cattle or animals in the feeding pen with no recent history of therapy. Such cases should generally constitute less than 20 per cent of fibrinous pneumonia mortality.

Prevention

Available methods of prophylactic antimicrobial therapy include feed and water medication as well as injectable medication of in-contact animals. Despite anecdotal evidence in support of water medication, there are no clinical trials to document its efficacy, and evidence from an observational study showed the use of sulfonamides in the water to be associated with decreased treatment rates but increased mortality rates.

The addition of chlortetracycline to the feed at levels from 1 to 4 g/head/day during the first 2 weeks postarrival or the combination of 350 mg sulfamethazine and 350 mg chlortetracycline/head/day for the first 3 to 4 weeks has been shown to be useful in reducing the morbidity and improving weight gains. A crucial factor in the success of feed medication is early, adequate dry matter consumption to ensure intake of sufficient amounts of the antimicrobial before pneumonic pasteurellosis occurs. It remains to be proven whether initial increased weight gain is maintained through the remainder of the feeding period or whether in fact unmedicated calves exhibit compensatory gains after the first month on feed. The effectiveness of the antimicrobial if used as a subsequent therapeutic agent in these groups is unknown. The expected cost:benefit ratio in each situation should be closely examined.

The greatest danger associated with feed or water medication is the false sense of security that it can create in some managers. If this occurs, cases are more advanced when detected, resulting in poor response, high relapse, and high case fatality rates.

One of the most promising but sometimes frustrating methods of antimicrobial prophylaxis is the mass individual medication of cattle prior to the expected or during the early onset of pneumonic pasteurellosis in the group. It can be difficult to anticipate that the outbreak will be severe enough to warrant mass medication and to time it accurately. Where cattle always originate from similar sources (e.g., auction marts) and data available from previous epidemic curves indicate early and substantial (greater than 30 per cent treatment rates) outbreaks of pneumonia, injection upon arrival or at a fixed time (e.g., 3 days) postarrival with long-acting oxytetracycline or tilmicosin can be a very effective strategy. Such application of antimicrobials does not necessarily lead to greater total amounts being used. In situations in which sources and morbidity rates may not be consistent, decisions may be made on a group-to-group basis by deciding to medicate when, for example, greater than 8 to 10 per cent of the cattle in a pen have been treated over a 3-day period. Some practitioners suggest that mass medication be carried out whenever a pen death (untreated mortality) due to fibrinous pneumonia occurs, since lack of adequate observation of the group on the part of the manager is likely to be associated with the presence of other advanced cases in that pen.

Although *P. multocida* or *P. haemolytica* are necessary causes of pneumonic pasteurellosis, the simple presence of either organism alone is not a sufficient cause of the disease. Prior or simultaneous exposure of the animal to other infectious agents and/or management stressors are necessary for the development of this disease. It is also prudent to remember that when evaluating the effectiveness of a preventive procedure directed against *Pasteurella* spp. that there are numerous other sufficient causes of bacterial pneumonia and still many more causes of undifferentiated bovine respiratory disease. Since pneumonic pasteurellosis can be produced experimentally following challenge of the respiratory tract with either infectious bovine rhinotracheitis (IBR) virus or parainfluenza-3 virus, vaccination against these viruses has been recommended as part of preconditioning and prevaccination programs prior to shipment of calves. Minimal success has been attained, however, and recent evidence suggests that, despite being susceptible to IBR, infection with this virus during the first 4 weeks postarrival is not common. Calves vaccinated both experimentally and in the field with formalin-killed pasteurella bacterins are at best not better off than controls. At worst, evidence suggests that killed bacterins may be harmful. Commercially produced live *P. haemolytica* vaccines have had relatively little effect in field situations despite promising results in laboratory trials.

Over the last 10 years various researchers have isolated a leukotoxin produced by actively growing cultures of *P. haemolytica*. This leukotoxin is immunogenic, and a cell-free vaccine containing high levels of the toxin (Presponse[1]) has been produced and available commercially since 1988.

The results of two large clinical trials to evaluate the efficacy of Presponse under commercial feedlot conditions have been published. In the first trial, auction-mart calves were vaccinated twice: at arrival and again 1 to 5 days later. In this feedlot (with controls experiencing treatment rates of 60 per cent and mortality due to fibrinous pneumonia over 2 per cent) there were significant reductions in relapse, mortality, and case fatality rates attributable to vaccination. A second trial examined the effect of vaccination with Presponse 3 weeks prior to shipment and upon arrival at the feedlot. Morbidity, relapse, and mortality rates due to fibrinous pneumonia were unaffected by vaccination. Weight gains to 90 days were almost identical in the four groups. An examination of the effect of a single vaccination of auction-mart calves upon arrival showed a 20 per cent reduction in the relapse rate of vaccinated calves as the only significant difference. In conclusion, it would appear that the greatest benefits to be realized with this product may be in high-risk auction-mart calves fed in lots that have relatively high case fatality rates owing to fibrinous pneumonia. Careful cost:benefit analysis of each situation would therefore be preferable to blanket statements on efficacy.

BIBLIOGRAPHY

Bateman KG, Martin SW, Shewen PE, Menzies PI: An evaluation of antimicrobial therapy for undifferentiated bovine respiratory disease. Can Vet J 31:689–696, 1990.

---

[1]Available from Langford, Inc., Guelph, Ontario, Canada, and Langford Labs, Kansas City.

Mechor GD, Jim GK, Janzen ED: Comparison of penicillin, oxytetracycline, and trimethoprim-sulfadoxine in the treatment of acute undifferentiated bovine respiratory disease. Can Vet J 29:438–443, 1988.
Schumann FJ, Janzen ED, McKinnon JJ: Prophylactic tilmicosin medication of feedlot calves at arrival. Can Vet J 31:285–288, 1990.
Thorlakson B, Martin W, Peters D: A field trial to evaluate the efficacy of a commercial *Pasteurella haemolytica* bacterial extract in preventing bovine respiratory disease. Can Vet J 31:573–579, 1990.

Pasteurellosis in Swine

JENS PETER NIELSEN, DVM, PhD
POUL BÆKBO, DVM, PhD

Pasteurella multocida infections cause some of the most prevalent and economically important respiratory diseases in pigs: progressive atrophic rhinitis and purulent bronchopneumonia as part of the enzootic pneumonia complex. Septicemia caused by *P. multocida* strains may be seen sporadically in young piglets. In order for disease to develop, predisposing factors are necessary. Healthy pigs can withstand a massive experimental dose of *P. multocida* without developing disease, and the organism can be recovered from the nose, tonsils, and lungs of most pigs in the field. A chromosomally encoded protein toxin, known as the *P. multocida* toxin (PMT), is now recognized as an important virulence factor produced by some *P. multocida* strains. The toxin is highly active and causes turbinate bone atrophy, liver and kidney damage, and growth retardation.

PROGRESSIVE ATROPHIC RHINITIS

Epidemiology

Progressive atrophic rhinitis (PAR) is common in most pig-producing countries. The occurrence of clinical atrophic rhinitis and the presence of toxigenic *P. multocida* in herds is closely related. The economically important part of the atrophic rhinitis complex is caused by infection with toxigenic *P. multocida* and is named PAR because of the progressive character of the resulting turbinate atrophy.[1] However, pigs may remain subclinically infected for years in herds in which predisposing factors are under control. In a Danish survey, toxigenic *P. multocida* was demonstrated in 84 per cent of herds with clinical PAR and in 12 per cent of herds without clinical PAR. Daily weight gain may be reduced as much as 10 to 15 per cent in pigs with severe turbinate atrophy, leading to economic losses. The nonprogressive form of atrophic rhinitis is generally subclinical and is caused by *Bordetella bronchiseptica* and nontoxigenic *P. multocida*.

Toxigenic and nontoxigenic *P. multocida* is found in a variety of host species, including birds, mammalian carnivores, and herbivores, as well as humans, which may have implications for the spread of the infection.

Etiology

Toxigenic *P. multocida* strains from pigs belong to capsular type A or D and are now classified as *P. multocida* spp. *multocida*. Infection with toxigenic *P. multocida* usually takes place before the age of 4 weeks, but infection and subsequent turbinate atrophy may occur in pigs several months old. The turbinate atrophy and growth-retarding effect seen in clinical cases of PAR can be produced in piglets by intraperitoneal injection of purified PMT, thus confirming the central role of PMT in PAR.[2]

Predisposing Factors

Concurrent infections, substandard management, and poor environment are factors predisposing to PAR. *B. bronchiseptica* infection is widespread in pig herds and increases the prevalence of clinical atrophic rhinitis in herds infected with toxigenic *P. multocida*. Other microorganisms that may predispose to PAR include *Mycoplasma hyorhinis* and inclusion body rhinitis virus. Herds with large farrowing units, or preweaned and weaned piglets sharing the same airspace, tend to have a higher prevalence of PAR. Toxigenic *P. multocida* is present in the air in buildings with infected pigs. Transmission of the infection may take place through the ventilation system. The influence of other environmental factors is poorly documented, but high levels of ammonia, dust, or other noxious substances are considered to be important.

Clinical Signs and Diagnosis

The most characteristic clinical signs of atrophic rhinitis are deviation and shortening of the snout, typically seen in pigs older than 8 weeks. Less characteristic signs include wrinkling of the skin covering the snout and broadening of the snout. Serous or purulent nasal discharge or epistaxis is often observed, as is tear staining. A short, sharp sneeze is often heard in weaners suffering from atrophic rhinitis, but sneezing is not in itself indicative of PAR since it may be caused by a variety of infections. The clinical diagnosis is easy in fulminant outbreaks even though clinical inspection usually reveals a spectrum from typical rhinitis to borderline cases. Turbinate atrophy may be present in pigs without clinical snout changes.

The postmortem diagnosis is made on snout transversal sections at the level of the upper jaw second premolar tooth. Atrophy is most easily detected in the ventral turbinate. Since the *B. bronchiseptica* infection may induce a reversible turbinate atrophy in piglets 6 to 12 weeks old, atrophy seen in this age group is inconclusive with regard to PAR. Microbiologic or serologic examination can identify carrier animals in which no bone deformation is present. Pigs from subclinically infected herds may develop clinical disease under adverse conditions or transmit the infection to other herds. Toxigenic *P. multocida* is isolated from nasal swabs of live animals or tissue from the respiratory system at necropsy. Detection of PMT antibodies is not yet used routinely.

Control and Treatment

Antibiotic therapy may be used in combination with other procedures to control and prevent the disease. Prophylactic medication of piglets one to three times before weaning may be given as intramuscular injections of either oxytetracycline (20 mg/kg) or ampicillin (25 mg/kg) at days 7, 14, and 21. Resistance of *P. multocida* to these drugs is rare, while resistance towards sulfonamides has been observed. Feed medication postweaning has been used at a dose of 400 ppm of oxytetracycline, but attainable serum levels are far below minimal inhibitory concentrations for *P. multocida*. Vaccines containing *P. multocida* toxoid, *P. multocida* whole cells, and *B. bronchiseptica* antigens have been employed successfully for the control of atrophic rhinitis. A new generation of single-component vaccines, consisting of either purified *P. multocida* toxoid or nontoxic PMT derivatives, have proved very efficient against the combined infection with *B. bronchiseptica* and *P. multocida*. The PMT antigen in atrophic rhinitis vaccines is probably required since the toxin is the key virulence factor in the pathogenesis of PAR. Vaccination of sows gives high immunity to the suckling piglets while they are at the greatest risk for infection with toxigenic *P. multocida*. Gilts are normally vaccinated twice before first farrowing, followed by booster vaccination before each consecutive farrowing. Vaccination of pigs at 5 and 8 weeks has been proposed by some workers. The reduced prevalence of PAR following vaccination with *B. bronchiseptica* antigens may be due to protection against this predisposing infection.

Control measures should include correction of management and environment, as well as vaccination and medication in severe outbreaks. The infection pressure should be lowered by segregation of clinically affected animals. Dividing the farrowing facility into smaller units and constructing separate weaner units will usually help to control the disease. Cold drafts and wet corners in farrowing crates should be avoided. Special attention should be given to the early winter period in cold-climate regions since the disease is known to accelerate during this season.

Successful eradication of PAR requires depopulation and then repopulation with specific pathogen-free (SPF) pigs free of infection with toxigenic *P. multocida*. Long-term studies in the Danish SPF system indicate that introduction of toxigenic *P. multocida* in SPF herds is relatively uncommon compared with other respiratory pathogens.

PNEUMONIA

Epidemiology

Worldwide, *P. multocida* is by far the most common bacterium isolated from pneumonic lesions in pigs. It is typically isolated from 30 to 80 per cent of lungs concomitantly infected with *Mycoplasma hyopneumoniae*. Approximately 20 to 50 per cent of all isolates are toxigenic. The most important predisposing condition for the *P. multocida* pulmonary infection is *M. hyopneumoniae*. Other predisposing infections are swine influenza, pseudorabies, hog cholera, and migrating *Ascaris suum* larvae. *P. multocida* may be seen as a secondary invader in lesions caused by *Actinobacillus pleuropneumoniae*. Excess ammonia, dust, or airborne bacteria may also predispose to lung infection. In contrast to what has been shown for PAR, the *P. multocida* toxin does not seem to determine the severity of the pulmonary lesions. Thus the effect of PMT in pulmonary infections may be exerted in the liver or kidney. Growth retardation following infection with toxigenic *P. multocida* has been observed. It has been shown that pigs with primary *M. hyopneumoniae* infection and subsequent toxigenic *P. multocida* infection had a reduced daily weight gain of about 100 g compared with pigs infected with nontoxigenic *P. multocida*.[3]

Clinical Signs and Pathology

The aggravation of an existing *M. hyopneumoniae* infection with *P. multocida* results in moist cough, dyspnea (thumping), depression, anorexia, and fever (40 to 42°C). Depending on the severity of the pneumonia, some pigs will recover in 5 to 10 days without treatment, but others will become chronically ill with reduced feed intake and weight loss. The mortality rate is usually low (<5 per cent). The purulent bronchopneumonia caused by *P. multocida* is usually located in the cranial and ventral parts of the lungs. The lesions are reddish gray, and the lung tissue is firm and rich in fluid. The pleura is usually normal, although some strains of *P. multocida* have been reported to cause pleuritis with or without an underlying pneumonia. Abscess formation seems to occur only in combined infections with *Actinomyces pyogenes*.

Diagnosis

The diagnosis of *P. multocida* infection must be based on the clinical signs described above, the necropsy lesions, and isolation of the bacterium. An important differential diagnosis is chronic pleuropneumonia caused by *A. pleuropneumoniae*, which is often indistinguishable clinically from *P. multocida* pneumonia. In these cases the diagnosis must be based on serologic evaluation, necropsy lesions, and bacteriologic examination.

Prevention and Control

The aim is elimination of the predisposing factors. *M. hyopneumoniae* infection might be eradicated by depopulation and restocking with SPF animals. However, the costs and the risk of reinfection by airborne spread must be considered when using this approach. Efficient vaccines against pulmonary *P. multocida* infections are not available. Whether the *P. multocida* toxoid vaccines against PAR can prevent the growth-retarding effect of the *P. multocida* toxin in pulmonary infections remains to be determined.

Antibiotic treatment together with management improvement might lower the infection pressure and increase the resistance of the pigs. The most efficient antibiotics against *P. multocida* are ampicillin (25 mg/kg), oxytetracycline (10 to 20 mg/kg), and tiamulin (10 to 20 mg/kg). A rather high proportion of lung isolates are resistant to sulfonamides. Individual parenteral treatment for 3 days is preferable. In outbreaks with high morbidity or in outbreaks when sudden rise in morbidity occurs, herd treatment for 5 to 7 days in the feed or drinking water must be considered, together with individual treatment of the most severely affected pigs. Ampicillin and tetracycline are not very suitable for oral use because of a low bioavailability when in contact with feed. For oral treatment, tiamulin is a reasonable choice because of its high absorption from the gastrointestinal tract.

Beneficial management strategies include operation of closed herds, all-in–all-out production of fatteners, low stocking density, small fattening sections, closed pens, and an optimal air quality (the indicator carbon dioxide <1.000 to 1.500 ppm). Medication of all piglets during the first week after weaning together with all-in-all-out production benefits productivity.

BIBLIOGRAPHY

1. Pedersen KB, Nielsen JP, Foged NT, et al: Atrophic rhinitis in pigs: proposal for a revised definition. Vet Rec 122:190–191, 1988.
2. Chanter N, Rutter JM: Pasteurellosis in pigs: the determinants of virulence of toxigenic *Pasteurella multocida*. In Adlam C, Rutter JM (eds): Pasteurella and Pasteurellosis. London, Academic Press, 1989, pp 161–195.
3. Bækbo P: Pathogenic properties of *Pasteurella multocida* in the lungs of pigs. The significance of toxin production. Proc 10th Int Pig Vet Soc Cong, 1988, p 58.

Swine Dysentery
ROBERT D. GLOCK, DVM, PhD

Swine dysentery (bloody scours) is a common diarrheal disease in swine throughout the world. It is feared by swine producers because it is easily transmitted and tends to cause long-term economic losses. Exact prevalence is not known because of a lack of reliable methods for determining whether there may be carrier animals in a particular herd. However, some estimates place the infection rate at up to 40 per cent of the swine herds in the United States.

The term swine dysentery refers to a specific disease. The primary causative agent, and the key to transmission of the disease, is an anaerobic spirochete, *Serpula (Treponema) hyodysenteriae*. Other gram-negative bacteria, which are normally present in swine intestines, may play a synergistic role in the pathogenesis.

Mechanisms of pathogenesis in swine dysentery have not been clearly defined, but *S. hyodysenteriae* are located deep in crypts and often invade the epithelial layer of the large intestine. Dissemination is not characteristic, and the effects on the host are the result of the severe inflammation diffusely affecting the large intestine.

CLINICAL SIGNS

All ages of swine are susceptible to swine dysentery, but pigs in the postweaning and early fattening periods are most frequently affected. The disease is rarely seen in suckling pigs. Peracute deaths, before onset of diarrhea, are infrequently encountered. These pigs usually have typical enteric lesions. Clinical signs in most pigs begin as mucoid diarrhea, which often progresses to dysentery with blood, mucus, and fibrin in the feces. Initially flecks of blood may be found scattered in the mucoid feces. If the disease progresses, the blood may be thoroughly mixed in watery feces. Abdominal pain, weight loss, and dehydration cause a gaunt, arched-back appearance. The diarrhea and anorexia result in depletion of serum electrolytes, metabolic acidosis, and some deaths. However, the majority of economic losses are the result of reduced performance, cost of continuous medication, and loss of breeding-stock markets.

DIAGNOSIS

It is important to recognize that there are many causes of diarrhea or dysentery. A diagnosis of swine dysentery should include an appropriate history such as the recent movement of swine into a clean herd. Previously infected pigs may have no clinical signs until after the stress of movement, environmental change, or altered feeding routine. The incubation period of swine dysentery may range from 2 or 3 days to a number of months, depending on the amount of exposure and host resistance. Some swine carry the disease without showing any clinical signs. However, clinical signs often appear within 1 or 2 weeks after exposure.

Clinical dysentery with blood in the feces may be caused by other diseases, such as salmonellosis, trichuriasis, and proliferative enteritis (intestinal adenomatosis, ileitis). Gastric ulcers can also cause blood-stained feces, although the feces are usually darker and more firm than those of swine dysentery.

Necropsy of an acutely affected pig may be essential. Specific lesions of swine dysentery are limited to the large intestine, which is usually hyperemic and edematous. The mucosa is diffusely inflamed, swollen, and covered by variable combinations of mucus, fibrin, blood, and cellular debris, depending on the stage of the disease. Salmonellosis differs because lesions are usually also found in other parts of the intestine or in other organs. Trichuriasis is best diagnosed by carefully inspecting the cecal and colonic mucosa for the parasites. The lesions in proliferative enteritis are located in the small intestine. Histopathology may be necessary for confirmation.

Laboratory diagnosis of swine dysentery includes examination of mucosal scrapings (or dysenteric feces) by dark-field or phase microscopy to identify numerous large, motile spirochetes with tapered ends. These can also be identified in smears stained with crystal violet or Victoria blue 4-R, and they can be seen in silver-stained histologic sections of the large intestine. The intestine has diffuse edema, crypt dilation, superficial erosion, and mucosal hyperemia. The reliability of these presumptive diagnostic aids is jeopardized by the fact that very similar nonpathogenic spirochetes, *S. innocens*, may be found in large numbers in pigs without swine dysentery.

Definitive diagnosis of swine dysentery is based on isolation and identification of *S. hyodysenteriae* from colonic mucosal or rectal swabs. Trypticase soy agar with 5 per cent bovine blood and selectively inhibitory antibiotics such as 400 μg/ml spectinomycin may be streaked, incubated anaerobically at 42°C, and examined for the presence of typical complete hemolysis. Specimens submitted for culture should be kept cool and moist but not frozen. It is also important to culture for *Salmonella* spp. Combinations of infections with swine dysentery, salmonellosis, and trichuriasis are common, so the mere presence of one organism does not exclude the presence of others.

Detection of individual carrier animals is very difficult, but rectal swab cultures and serologic tests on specimens from numerous animals have some promise as methods of determining carrier animals in the herd.

CONTROL

After establishing a diagnosis of swine dysentery, medication in the feed or water is recommended. In a very acute outbreak, medication of water is preferred because of reduced feed consumption by sick pigs. Parenteral treatment with drugs, such as tylosin or lincomycin, is also useful in some cases. Initial medication can then be followed by the use of therapeutic or control levels of medications available as feed additives. The disease is likely to persist in infected premises, so it is frequently necessary to medicate continuously or, at least, repeatedly. Table 1 lists some drugs commonly used for treatment of swine dysentery.

It is imperative that pig comfort and sanitation be given primary attention in any control program. There is a direct correlation between levels of contamination and severity of the disease.

Combinations of sanitation, medication, and isolation have been used to eliminate the infection from some herds. Success depends on a good cooperative effort between a determined herd manager and an experienced veterinarian. Possible ap-

Table 1. SOME DRUGS USED FOR TREATMENT OF SWINE DYSENTERY*

Compound	Water	Feed
Bacitracin	+	+
Carbadox	−	+
Dimetridazole†	+	+
Gentamicin	+	−
Ipronidazole†	+	+
Lincomycin	+	+
Sodium arsanilate	+	+
Tiamulin	+	+
Tylosin	+	+
Virginiamycin	+	+

*Always follow label direction for dosage and withdrawal before slaughter.
†Use of these compounds is prohibited in the United States.

proaches to eradication are described by Walter and Kinyon and by Fujioka and colleagues (see Bibliography).

PREVENTION

The most important consideration in prevention of swine dysentery is to maintain a closed herd. Any new stock should be purchased from a reliable supplier who can provide a history free of swine dysentery. Any new arrivals should be isolated and observed for several weeks before entry into the main herd. If diarrhea should occur, feces should be analyzed by culture to determine if *S. hyodysenteriae* are present. It is also imperative that animals be transported in a truck that has been thoroughly cleaned.

S. hyodysenteriae can survive for at least a few days in moist, cool feces, so infection can also be easily transmitted by fomites, such as truck tires and boots. Mice have been shown to be long-term carriers of infection, so rodent control is an important part of control programs.

It may be wise to use preventive levels of medications in situations in which animals of unknown origin are combined with the herd or previously contaminated facilities are used. Survival times of *S. hyodysenteriae* range from a few hours or less on clean, dry surfaces to a number of weeks in cool, moist feces. Survival time in anaerobically stored wastes may be quite long.

BIBLIOGRAPHY

Fujioka K, Nakamoto S, Nishida H, et al: A trial of Lincomix 44 Premix for the eradication of swine dysentery. Proc Int Pig Vet Soc 11th Cong, July 1–5, 1990, p 132.
Harris DL, Glock RD: Swine dysentery. *In* Leman AD, Straw B, Glock RD, et al (eds): Diseases of Swine. Ames, IA, Iowa State University Press, 1986, pp 494–507.
Kinyon JM, Harris DL, Glock RD: Enteropathogenicity of various isolates of *Treponema hyodysenteriae*. Infect Immunol 15:638–646, 1977.
Songer JG, Kinyon JM, Harris DL: Selective medium for isolation of *Treponema hyodysenteriae*. J Clin Microbiol 4:57–60, 1976.
Walter DH, Kinyon JM: Recent MIC determinations of six antimicrobials for *Treponema hyodysenteriae* in the United States; use of tiamulin to eliminate swine dysentery from two farrow to finish herds. Proc Int Pig Vet Soc 11th Cong, July 1–5, 1990, p 129.

Salmonellosis

GEORGE A. KENNEDY, DVM, PhD, Diplomate, ACVP
CLAIR M. HIBBS, DVM, PhD

Salmonellosis is a ubiquitous disease affecting nearly all species of vertebrates. It is caused by a large number of serovars of *Salmonella* spp. These are gram-negative, pleomorphic, generally motile, aerobic, and facultatively anaerobic rods that are tissue invasive and induce inflammation and tissue damage. Precise classification of salmonellae is controversial. The most common proposal places all salmonellae into one of three species: *S. typhi, S. choleraesuis,* and *S. enteritidis.* In this scheme all other salmonellae are serovars of *S. enteritidis* (e.g., *S. enteritidis* serovar *typhimurium*). Some serovars are further subdivided into biovars, for example, *S. choleraesuis* biovar *kunzendorf,* or *S. enteritidis* serovar *typhimurium* biovar *copenhagen.* Over 2000 serovars have been identified.

For convenience, in this discussion we will use the older species designations, for example, *S. typhimurium (copenhagen).* Knowledge of the serovar can be important in that it may influence the way a given outbreak is most effectively managed; for example, the likelihood and duration of carrier animals, the choice of a systemic antibiotic rather than an enteric antibiotic, the probable source of the infection, and the zoonotic potential.

Clinically the disease may be systemic or enteric and may be acute or chronic. The disease tends to occur in the very young, the debilitated, or the very old, although all ages may be affected.

Subclinical carriers are common in all species, which makes salmonellosis difficult to control. Carrier animals that are transported or stressed in some other way shed organisms more readily. Concentrated animal populations and poor sanitation also enhance the maintenance of this organism in the environment. Salmonellae may survive in soil or stagnant water for many months. The organisms survive freezing but are readily inactivated by heat and sunlight. Morbidity and mortality may be quite high, depending on the type of husbandry, dose, age, immune status, stability of intestinal flora, weather, other environmental circumstances, and concomitant diseases, among other factors. Cases of salmonellosis seem to be increasing, owing in part both to more concentrated husbandry and to better diagnostic capabilities. Contaminated water, feed, pasture, and carrier animals are all possible sources of the organism. Liquid slurries from manure pits are major sources of contamination for pastures and other fields.

Ingestion is the usual method of transmission. The organisms are facultative intracellular pathogens that can invade cells and localize in lymphoid tissue and in macrophages of the monocyte-phagocyte system (MPS). As salmonellae proliferate they release endotoxin, often resulting in endotoxic shock. Salmonellae are sometimes opportunistic pathogens secondary to some other primary disease.

Some *Salmonella* serovars are non–host-adapted, while others have adapted to a particular species. *S. typhimurium,* the most commonly isolated serovar from all animals, is a nonhost-adapted serovar. *S. choleraesuis (kunzendorf)* and *S. typhisuis* are pathogens of swine only, whereas *S. dublin* is relatively host specific for cattle. Host-adapted serovars tend to occur exclusively, or at least most commonly, in one species and also tend to produce inapparent, chronic shedders more commonly than nonhost-adapted serovars. The practical application of this is that, when confronted with an outbreak of a host-adapted serovar, the most likely source of the infection will have been a chronic shedder or recrudescence of an infection in a chronic carrier.

CLINICAL SIGNS

Pigs

Salmonellosis can occur in all ages of pigs but is most likely to occur in weanling or feeder pigs. The clinical signs may vary from peracute septicemia to chronic enterocolitis. Salmonellosis is not common in nursing pigs but occasionally causes diarrhea, septicemia, and even central nervous system (CNS) signs. In piglets, depression and rapid death are the main features, but enteritis, particularly necrotic enteritis, may occur. Laboratory identification methods may be necessary to differentiate salmonellosis from diseases caused by *Escherichia coli,* enteric viruses, coccidia, streptococci that cause septicemia, or *Clostridium perfringens* type C.

Septicemic salmonellosis is generally due to *S. choleraesuis (kunzendorf).* It occurs mainly in weanling or young feeder pigs and frequently follows some form of stress. Fever, depression, prostration, and sudden death are characteristic of the acute septicemic form. Pigs may huddle as if cold. Reddish or purplish skin blotches that blanch on pressure are common but nonspecific clinical signs of septicemia. CNS signs due to meningitis or encephalitis or both may occur in a variable number of pigs. Diarrhea is usually not a prominent feature of septicemic salmonellosis but may occur in animals that survive more than a couple of days. Mortality is high, but morbidity tends to be lower than with the enteric forms.

Acute enteric salmonellosis is characterized by watery to mucohemorrhagic, fetid diarrhea, along with fever, weakness, and anorexia. Shreds of fibrin, sloughing mucosa, and some fresh blood are often present in the feces. Morbidity and mortality may be high. Many survivors of the enteric form will be unthrifty and may remain carriers. A rectal stricture syndrome may also be a sequel to enteric salmonellosis. *S. typhimurium* is the most common cause of enteric salmonellosis in swine.

The chronic enteric form is less common. It may or may not follow an outbreak of the acute enteric form. Persistent watery, yellowish diarrhea, unthriftiness, and intermittent fever characterize the chronic enteric form. Recovered pigs may remain permanently stunted.

Differential diagnosis of septicemic salmonellosis includes erysipelas, streptococcal septicemia, edema disease, pseudorabies, and hog cholera. For the enteric form, swine dysentery, proliferative ileitis (campylobacteriosis) and its manifestations, and whipworms need to be diagnostically differentiated. Mixed infections are common; an example is salmonellosis superimposed on swine dysentery.

Cattle

Salmonellosis affects both dairy and beef cattle. It is more difficult to categorize the disease in cattle as strictly systemic or enteric since in any given case one form may merge into the other, particularly in calves. Prevalence of the various serovars changes with different geographic localities, but *S. typhimurium* tends to be common worldwide. *S. dublin, S. newport,* and *S. anatum* are also among important serovars in cattle but tend to have more patchy geographic distributions. *S. dublin,* once confined to the Pacific Northwest in the United States, is becoming more widespread geographically, and severe outbreaks have occurred in the Southwest and Midwest.

Acute salmonellosis is more common in dairy than beef calves. It usually does not occur in calves less than 2 weeks old. However, it has occurred in beef calves on pasture and in calves less than 1 week old. A common history includes a moderately high incidence of intractable diarrhea with some deaths and with calves continuing to develop the disease over an extended period. The initial fever may or may not have subsided by the time the calf is examined. The temperature commonly drops upon initiation of diarrhea. Extreme weakness is often a prominent sign. The most characteristic feature is brownish, watery diarrhea with shreds and flakes of fibrin and sloughing mucosa and streaks of fresh blood. Meningitis, polyarthritis, and pneumonia may occur in septicemic cases. Even in the enteric form most calves will be terminally septicemic, and those that survive may remain unthrifty. Sources of infection may be inapparent carrier animals or newly purchased calves, contaminated feed, water, or bedding. Transport, lack of colostrum, and cold or wet weather are among the predisposing factors.

Clinical signs in adult cattle are acute illness with depression, fever, cessation of milk flow, and severe diarrhea. Parturition can be a precipitating factor. The diarrheic feces tend to be fetid and watery and to contain mucus, fibrinous casts, and sometimes considerable quantities of fresh blood. Persistent diarrhea and unthriftiness characterize the more chronic syndrome. Pregnant animals may abort. Although abortion is more commonly associated with *S. dublin,* it may occur with a variety of serovars. Cows may or may not be sick at the time of abortion. The disease may become enzootic on some premises, particularly dairies.

Salmonellosis in the feedlot may occur anytime during the fattening period, but it generally appears soon after cattle arrive in the feedlot owing to the stresses and infection encountered in shipping. Feeding green chopped alfalfa and green chopped corn may aggravate the disease. A sudden onset of semifluid to mucohemorrhagic diarrhea accompanied by depression, fever, and weakness is characteristic. The diarrhea may mimic bovine viral diarrhea (BVD) or coccidiosis.

Differential diagnosis includes colibacillosis and viral diarrhea in calves, and BVD, Johne's disease, coccidiosis, parasitism, and certain poisonings, such as arsenic, in older calves and adults.

Blood studies may reveal leukopenia early in the course of the disease, but there are no consistent clinical pathologic findings.

Sheep and Goats

Salmonellosis is most frequent and economically most important in feeder lambs. It generally affects lambs soon after arrival at the lot. Affected lambs will have watery diarrhea that often contains mucus and streaks of blood. Fever and depression are less specific features. Morbidity may exceed 25 per cent, and mortality can be high. Salmonellosis in feedlot lambs must be differentiated from coccidiosis and enterotoxemia. Coccidiosis is more common, tends to appear 1 to 3 weeks after arrival, and commonly causes more blood in the feces.

Several serovars of *Salmonella* may cause abortions in ewe and lamb flocks. The ewe is usually sick at the time of abortion with *S. typhimurium* or *S. dublin* infections, whereas *S. arizona* and *S. montevideo* may cause abortions in healthy-appearing ewes. *S. abortus ovis,* a host-adapted serovar causing abortion in sheep and goats, appears to be restricted to parts of Europe.

Salmonellosis in goats is reported to be generally similar to the disease in cattle. It occurs in neonatal goats, older nursing kids, and adults. The enteric form is most common, with a watery or hemorrhagic diarrhea. Coccidiosis, parasitism, and enterotoxemia should be included in the differential diagnosis.

NECROPSY FINDINGS

No gross lesions can be considered pathognomonic, but some may be highly suggestive. Ingestion of the organism is followed by invasion of the intestinal epithelial cells and subsequent localization in the macrophages of the lymphoid follicles of the digestive tract. The high concentration of lymphoid tissue in the ileum, cecum, and colon predisposes these areas to severe lesions. The pathogenesis is not entirely understood, but cellular invasion and elaboration of an enterotoxin(s) and a cytotoxin, as well as an endotoxin, are thought to be involved in the development of the lesions. Depending on various factors, such as serovar and host resistance, the organisms may remain localized in the intestinal mucosa and mesenteric nodes or may gain entrance to the blood and become disseminated. Invasion of epithelial cells and macrophages is followed by multiplication of the organisms and an inflammatory reaction with vascular damage, thrombosis, hemorrhage, and necrosis. Pneumonia frequently occurs after systemic invasion; thus in systemic salmonellosis the lungs are often a tissue of choice for culturing salmonellae. The stomachs of monogastric animals generally have reddened mucosae, while the abomasa of ruminants may or may not have inflamed mucosae. Miliary foci of necrosis and inflammation are rarely observed grossly in the liver but frequently occur histologically. Occasionally one finds edema of the gall bladder wall.

Splenic enlargement is a common finding in swine and may occur in ruminants, but not as consistently. Generalized lymphadenopathy usually occurs in systemic cases. In enteric cases the mesenteric lymph nodes are consistently enlarged and frequently hemorrhagic. In pigs, petechial hemorrhages may be present on the cortical surface of the kidneys ("turkey egg kidney") and on the mucosal surface of the urinary bladder. Serosal hemorrhages occur on any of the visceral organs and are a common nonspecific occurrence on the epicardial surface of the heart.

Intestinal changes are generally confined to the lower jejunum, ileum, cecum, and colon. This can be an important point of differentiation, as swine dysentery due to *Serpula* (*Treponema*) *hyodysenteriae* is confined to the cecum and colon. The mucosal surface with salmonellosis may vary from an angry red to grayish yellow with adherent flakes of fibrin. The latter is associated with the more chronic form of salmonellosis. Pseudomembrane formation, ulceration, serosanguineous material, and whitish flecks of fibrin with sloughing mucosa, sometimes forming casts of the intestinal lumen, may be observed within the intestines in all species. In these cases the intestinal wall is often thickened and rigid, especially in pigs, giving rise to the term "garden hose gut." Necroproliferative ileitis thought to be caused by *Campylobacter* spp. is the main differential diagnosis. Septic polyarthritis is a less frequently observed lesion and mainly restricted to young animals.

Lung, tied-off sections of affected intestine, and mesenteric lymph nodes have been the most productive tissues for recovery of salmonellae in our laboratories, followed in frequency of successful isolations by liver, spleen, and kidney. Thinly sliced pieces of tissue should also be submitted in 10 per cent neutral buffered formalin for histologic examination. Histologic lesions are suggestive but not pathognomonic for salmonellosis. On the other hand, simply isolating a salmonella from the intestine is not proof of its involvement in the animal's illness, and distinction must be made between infection and clinical disease.

PREVENTION

Salmonellae are widespread in the environment, and clinically normal carriers occur; thus prevention is not always easy. Prevention of the disease involves considerable labor and dedication on the part of both owner and veterinarian. Common medical sense should prevail. Closed-herd operations are best when possible. Quarantine of replacement stock for 2 to 4 weeks is helpful but not fully effective because of the carrier state. Many cases occur as a result of exposure of susceptible animals to inapparent carriers; therefore purchase of replacement stock from herds with no history of salmonellosis is helpful. Identification of carriers by culture procedures is difficult because of intermittent shedding, and serologic examination for antibody titers to salmonellae is unreliable.

It is advisable to purchase feedstuffs from reputable manufacturers and dealers. Dried milk, meat scraps, bone meal, and other animal or fish products are potential sources of salmonellae unless properly processed. Forages and grains are not generally a source of salmonellae, but contaminated haylage has been a source. Hay and grain may be contaminated by rodent or bird excreta.

Effluent from human sewage is a common source of salmonellae. Some rural homes have effluent discharging directly into lots or fields. Two severe cases of salmonellosis in beef calves, investigated by one of the authors, involved household effluents running into the calving areas.

Vaccination may have preventive value in some situations, but results are not consistent. A combination *S. typhimurium*/*S. dublin* bacterin is available in the United States. Autogenous bacterins have been used with variable success. Attenuated live vaccines have reportedly been used with varying success in the United Kingdom. With some salmonella vaccines, anaphylactic reactions have occurred following a second or booster dose. Research using metabolically altered or mutant strains of salmonella are promising, and such vaccines may be available in the future.

Livestock owners with infected animals should use precautions when disposing of infected carcasses to prevent contamination of barns, pens, and equipment. Several years ago one of the authors performed a bacteriologic survey of a horse slaughter plant. Salmonellae were isolated from holding pens, sewer drains, shackle hooks used to transport carcasses, the doorway to the cooler, boning knives, and other areas and objects. This demonstrates a need for careful prevention of contamination. There are numerous reports of different ways of spreading salmonellae by contaminated equipment. Cleaning and disinfection will help to prevent spread of the organism. The common phenolic-, chlorine-, and iodine-based disinfectants are all effective.

TREATMENT

Basically therapy of animals with clinical salmonellosis involves the use of antibiotics, supportive measures, good nursing care, good hygiene, and, if possible, separation of the sick from the healthy.

The role of antibiotics is controversial, as they apparently do not eliminate the carrier state and may contribute to the development of antibiotic-resistant strains. Furthermore the results are often disappointing, particularly if not instituted early in the course of the disease. Experimental studies in swine suggest that continuous inclusion of an antibiotic in the feed to which the resident salmonellae are susceptible should reduce the prevalence and severity of the disease, although it may not affect the infection rate and may be of little benefit if initiated once clinical signs have appeared.

In clinically ill animals the usual approach is to administer antibiotics orally and, when feasible, parenterally. When dealing with the septicemic form and treating the animal with oral antibiotics, a drug that is absorbed and reaches effective blood levels should be used. The choice of antibiotics should be based on antibiotic sensitivity tests and approval for use in food animals. When sensitivity results are not available, the choice should be one of the drugs usually effective against salmonellae. This may vary in different geographic locations. In our laboratories antibacterial drugs to which currently there are the fewest resistant strains of salmonellae include gentamicin, trimethoprim-sulfadiazine, ampicillin, apramycin, enrofloxacin, and amikacin. Of these only ampicillin is cleared for treating salmonellosis in food animals at this time in the United States. The nitrofurans have been used as water and feed additives for treatment of salmonellosis but are no longer available for use in food animals in the United States. Strains resistant in vitro to neomycin, tetracyclines, spectinomycin, carbadox, ceftiofur, and the sulfonamide drugs are common.

In most herd situations individual parenteral treatment is difficult to administer, and medication via the water source is most practical. Medicated water is better than medicated feed, as ill animals will generally continue to drink but feed intake may be greatly reduced.

When conditions permit, individual treatment may be practical, and parenteral antibiotics and fluids to combat dehydration and metabolic acidosis are indicated. Management manipulations that reduce stress and fecal-oral contamination will be helpful. Strict sanitation to lower exposure is frequently the most beneficial treatment and preventive measure. With ruminants, switching to an easily digestible, higher-roughage ration is sometimes of benefit. Culling chronically unthrifty animals is a useful management procedure, as these animals often remain sources of environmental contamination.

PUBLIC HEALTH CONSIDERATIONS

Salmonellosis is reported to be the most important animal-borne bacterial infection of humans. Most serovars are potentially infective for people. The disease usually takes the form of gastroenteritis, but systemic disease with fatalities occurs. Humans may contract salmonellosis by direct or indirect contact with actively or latently infected animals, their excreta, or their food products. Human-to-human transmission is also important.

The stress of being shipped to slaughter often increases fecal shedding in latent carriers. This and constant recontamination of holding pens at slaughter facilities can result in widespread contamination of carcasses and food products. More often, food products may become contaminated by breakdown in hygienic precautions at the time of processing, display, preparation, or storage.

Poultry and poultry products are considered the most frequent animal source of human infection, but pork, beef, and dairy products are also frequently incriminated. Even some smoked and cooked meat products may harbor salmonellae. Milk is less frequently a problem, as pasteurization destroys the organism.

Although salmonellosis has not been found to be more prevalent in livestock owners or their families than in other families, the potential danger needs to be recognized by attending veterinarians when dealing with suspected or confirmed cases of salmonellosis. Cases of serious salmonellosis in veterinarians have occurred.

BIBLIOGRAPHY

Bulgin MS: Salmonella dublin: what veterinarians should know. J Am Vet Med Assoc 182:116–118, 1983.
Bulgin MS, Anderson BC: Salmonellosis in goats. J Am Vet Med Assoc 178:720–723, 1981.
Hibbs CM, Foltz VD: Bovine salmonellosis associated with contaminated creek water and human infection. Vet Med Small Anim Clin 59:1153–1155, 1964.
Morehouse LG: Salmonellosis in swine and its control. J Am Vet Med Assoc 160:593–602, 1972.
Pelzer KD: Salmonellosis (zoonosis up-date). J Am Vet Med Assoc 195:456–463, 1989.
Rings MD: Salmonellosis in calves. Vet Clin North Am: Food Anim Pract 1:529–539, 1985.
Whitlock RH: Therapeutic strategies involving antimicrobial treatment of the gastrointestinal tract in large animals. J Am Vet Med Assoc 185:1210–1213, 1984.
Wilcock BP, Armstrong CH, Olander HJ: The significance of serotype in the clinical and pathological features of naturally occurring porcine salmonellosis. Can J Comp Med 40:80–88, 1976.
Wray C, Sojka WJ: Reviews of the progress of dairy science; bovine salmonellosis. J Dairy Res 44:383–425, 1977.

Anthrax
ARNOLD F. KAUFMANN, DVM, MS

Anthrax is an acute infectious disease of food animals caused by *Bacillus anthracis*. The disease has a worldwide distribution and can affect a wide range of mammalian species, including humans.

B. anthracis is a member of the normal bacterial flora of numerous soil types sharing a pH higher than 6. Although naturally contaminated soil is the primary reservoir of infection, outbreaks have been traced to a variety of other sources, such as animal-origin feed and fertilizer, river water contaminated by wastes from animal-product processing, and even crops raised on contaminated soil.

Within the United States anthrax tends to be restricted to certain regions, such as the lower Mississippi River Valley. Outbreaks, however, have occurred in virtually every state. Even in recognized areas of endemic disease, anthrax occurs very irregularly. Many years may elapse between sporadic cases and epizootics in a high-risk area. Multiple small sporadic outbreaks are reported each year in the United States, but epizootics are uncommon.

Outbreaks in grazing animals occur primarily in warm seasons of the year when the minimum daily temperature is above 16°C, but documented cases have occurred even in midwinter in northern states. Epizootics tend to follow periods of marked climatic or ecologic change, such as heavy rainfall, flooding, or drought.

In food animals, infection usually results from ingestion of contaminated feed. Anthrax is not communicable directly between animals except in instances such as swine feeding on carcasses. Transmission by biting flies can take place, but recent studies indicate that biting insects have an insignificant role in anthrax epizootics.

The attack rate in an outbreak is variable, but the case:fatality ratio is high, usually exceeding 90 per cent. Compared with cattle, sheep and goats are highly susceptible to experimental infection, whereas swine are much more resistant. Under field conditions, however, the attack rate by species on the same pasture does not necessarily correlate with relative species susceptibility, presumably because of differences in grazing patterns. Relative risk also varies with age (lambs and calves are seldom affected) and sex (bulls are much more susceptible to infection than cows).

CLINICAL SIGNS

The incubation period of natural anthrax is typically 3 to 7 days, but it may range from 1 to 14 days or more. The clinical course is from peracute to chronic. Sudden death in animals that appeared normal a few hours earlier is common.

In ruminant livestock the acute illness is characterized by abrupt onset of fever (temperature may rise to 42°C), variably followed by anorexia, ruminal stasis, signs of abdominal pain, hematuria, and blood-tinged diarrhea. Pregnant animals may abort, and milk production in lactating animals often abruptly declines, with milk being abnormal or blood tinged. Subcutaneous edematous swellings may be present, particularly on the ventral aspect of the neck. Death usually occurs within 1 to 3 days after onset, with severe depression, respiratory distress, muscular tremors, and convulsions being common terminal events. Occasionally animals survive the infection without treatment, but this is uncommon. Chronic infection is rarely found in cattle. When found, however, it is characterized by localized edematous swelling on the ventral neck, thorax, and shoulders.

In swine the disease is similar to that in ruminants, except edematous swelling of the head and neck is much more common. The swelling may be so extensive as to interfere with breathing and swallowing. Chronic infection localized to the tonsils and cervical lymph nodes is common.

NECROPSY FINDINGS

The carcasses of animals that died of anthrax tend to putrify rapidly and develop incomplete rigor mortis. Blood may exude from the nose, mouth, and anus. The blood is dark, clots poorly, and flows freely from cut surfaces.

The lesions of anthrax result from widespread damage to the reticuloendothelial system and vasculature. In ruminants the spleen is almost always greatly enlarged, dark, and soft. The necrotic and engorged red pulp will readily exude from incisions in the splenic capsule.

The lymph nodes, particularly in the region of the initial infection site, will be hemorrhagic and edematous. Hemorrhages of various sizes are common on the serosal surfaces of the abdomen and thorax, as well as the epicardium and endocardium. A localized to diffuse gelatinous edema is commonly present under the serosa of the various organs, between skeletal muscle groups, and in the subcutis. A small amount of serous to blood-tinged fluid is usually present in the body cavities. Hemorrhages frequently occur along the gastrointestinal tract mucosa. Ulcers, particularly over Peyer's patches, may also be noted.

In swine the lesions tend to be restricted to the tonsils, cervical lymph nodes, and surrounding tissues. The lymphatic tissues of the head and neck will be enlarged and appear a mottled salmon to a brick-red color on cut surface. Diphtheritic membranes or ulcers may develop over the pharyngeal surface of the tonsils. A thick layer of gelatinous edema generally surrounds the involved lymphatic tissues.

DIAGNOSIS

Anthrax may be confused with a wide range of diseases causing sudden death. Definitive diagnosis through isolation of *B. anthracis* from affected tissues, however, is generally not difficult.

If anthrax is suspected, complete necropsy of affected animals should be avoided to reduce environmental contamination and health risks to personnel. A small amount of blood collected aseptically from a superficial vessel such as the jugular vein is the preferred diagnostic specimen. For shipment to the laboratory, the blood can be left in the syringe, which in turn should be enclosed in a leak-proof container. The blood can also be submitted to the laboratory as a dried specimen on a sterile swab or small piece of sterile cotton umbilical tape, or, if necessary, as thin smears on microscopic slides. An ear from the carcass is not a desirable specimen. In swine with localized disease, a small piece of affected lymphatic tissue that has been collected aseptically should be submitted. Tissue specimens other than dried blood should be shipped refrigerated or frozen.

Examination of blood smears from recently dead animals is used for field diagnosis but may be misleading. On Wright- or Giemsa-stained blood smears, *B. anthracis* will appear as single to short-chained bacilli with blunted ends. The presence of a capsule about the bacilli is the important distinguishing feature of the anthrax organism in such preparations. Fluorescent antibody procedures are also used in the diagnosis of anthrax.

TREATMENT

The anthrax bacillus is highly susceptible to a number of antimicrobial agents, including penicillin, amoxicillin, erythromycin, chloramphenicol, gentamicin, streptomycin, and ciprofloxacin. Under field conditions penicillin and oxytetracycline have been reported most consistently as being therapeutically effective. The common recommended daily dose of penicillin for swine, sheep, and goats is 22,000 IU/kg; the daily dose for cattle is 5 to 10 million units. Therapy should be continued for at least 5 days, and the daily dose should be administered in two equal parts at 12-hour intervals for the first 2 days. In severely ill animals, the initial dose should be administered intravenously.

The daily oxytetracycline dose, administered intravenously or intramuscularly, is 4.4 mg/kg for all species. The daily dose should be divided into two equal parts for the initial period of therapy, as with penicillin.

Antibiotics should not be administered to healthy animals recently vaccinated against anthrax. The only anthrax vaccines in common use are live spore products, which must germinate and grow in the vaccinated animal's body to provide protection. Experimental evidence indicates that concurrent administration of antibiotics and anthrax vaccine negates the protective effect of the vaccine.

Hyperimmune anthrax serum has been recommended for use in conjunction with antibiotic therapy. Such serum, however, is not available in the United States.

PREVENTION

Annual vaccination of livestock in areas of endemic anthrax is recommended. The nonencapsulated Sterne strain vaccine is almost universally used for this purpose. Vaccination should be done 2 to 4 weeks prior to the season that outbreaks are expected. Animals should not be vaccinated within 60 days of anticipated slaughter. Antibiotics should not be administered within 7 days of vaccination.

The Sterne strain anthrax vaccine (Anthrax Spore Vaccine and Thraxol-2; see Table 1) is administered subcutaneously. The dose recommended by the manufacturers varies from 1 to 2 ml. A second dose administered 2 to 4 weeks after the first dose is commonly recommended. Field experience indicates that equal protection is given by either one or two doses. Immunity develops about 7 days after vaccination. Localized subcutaneous edema commonly develops within 24 hours at the injection site and lasts several days. This edema is rarely severe. Localized anthrax at the site of injection with the Sterne strain anthrax vaccine has been reported in llama calves.

Table 1. ANTHRAX VACCINES

Name	Supplier	Species	Dose
Anthrax Spore Vaccine	Colorado Serum Co., Denver, CO	Cattle, goats, sheep, swine	1 ml
Thraxol-2	Mobay Animal Health, Shawnee Mission, KS	Cattle	2 ml
		Sheep, swine	1 ml

Progressive edema at the site of inoculation may occur in goats.

All outbreaks should be reported to local regulatory and public health officials. Quarantine should be placed on affected premises to prevent infected animals from being marketed. All susceptible livestock on affected and surrounding premises should be vaccinated. Prior to vaccination of dairy cattle at the time of an outbreak, the procedures required by state health authorities should be determined. If the outbreak is associated with a discrete source, such as contaminated bone meal, antibiotic treatment of exposed animals and removal of the source may be more effective than vaccination in reducing losses.

Carcasses of animals that die of anthrax should be either burned completely or buried deeply (2 m of soil) to reduce environmental contamination. Covering the carcasses with a layer of quicklime (calcium oxide) at burial is often recommended; the benefit of this procedure is unknown. Bedding and other contaminated material should also be burned or buried.

BIBLIOGRAPHY

Cartwright ME, McChesney AE, Jones RL: Vaccination-related anthrax in three llamas. J Am Vet Med Assoc 191:715–716, 1987.
Kaufmann AF, Fox MD, Kolb RC: Anthrax in Louisiana, 1971: an evaluation of the Sterne strain anthrax vaccine. J Am Vet Med Assoc 163:442–368, 1973.
Turnbull PCB: Proceeding of the international workshop on anthrax. Salisbury Med Bull 68:1–105, 1990.
Van Ness GB: Ecology of anthrax. Science 172:1303–1307, 1971.

Diseases Caused by *Clostridium* Species
Tetanus; Botulism; and Clostridial Myositis, Cellulitis, Hemoglobinuria, Abomasitis, and Hepatitis

HENRY STAEMPFLI, DVM, DR MED VET,
 DIPLOMATE, ACVIM
OLIMPO OLIVER, DVM, MSC

Diseases caused by *Clostridium* spp. are still of considerable economic importance in farm animals. The ubiquitous presence of the organisms in soil and intestinal contents of animals makes eradication of diseases impossible. In almost all instances diseases caused by *Clostridium* may be prevented by vaccination. Polyvalent vaccines with up to seven antigens are commercially available and highly effective.

TETANUS

Definition, Occurrence, and Incidence

In food animals tetanus causes a generalized, or occasionally localized, hypertonia of the skeletal muscles, frequently accompanied by clonic paroxysmal muscular spasms. The disease occurs throughout the world and is more prevalent in tropical countries. The incidence decreases in order from cattle and buffalo to camels, sheep, goats, and pigs. This variation is due to difference in susceptibility and to the ecology of *C. tetani*. The organisms are commonly present in feces and are continuously shed into the environment, where they sporulate and persist for long periods. Tetanus is usually seen in sporadic individual cases, but occasionally outbreaks occur in cattle, young pigs, and lambs. Mortality is high in younger ruminants. Adult cattle have a higher recovery rate, possibly because of a greater concentration of circulating naturally acquired antitoxin antibodies. In adult dairy cattle tetanus occurs most commonly as a postparturient complication following retention of placenta.

Etiology and Pathogenesis

C. tetani is a strictly anaerobic, gram-positive bacterium. Infection most often results from contamination of a wound. Upon entrance into devitalized tissue with an anaerobic environment, *C. tetani* will convert into the vegetative form and produce toxin within 4 to 8 hours. The tetanus bacteria remain localized and do not commonly invade surrounding tissue. Tetanus toxin (tetanospasmin) is locally produced, diffuses to surrounding tissue, enters the lymphatics and blood, and ascends retrogradely along axons to the spinal cord. It acts by irreversibly blocking the inhibitory synapses of the spinal cord motoneuron, resulting in overactivity of extensor muscles (extensor rigidity) and in uncontrolled stimulation of voluntary muscles. Death most often occurs by asphyxiation. In outbreaks the tetanus bacteria may proliferate in the forestomachs of normal cattle to produce sufficient concentrations of toxin to result in clinical signs. The toxin may also be ingested in the feed and enter via wounds in the mouth.

Clinical Signs

The first signs usually occur after an incubation period of 1 to 3 weeks and include stiff gait, prolapse of the third eyelid, and trismus (lockjaw). The prolapse of the third eyelid can be accentuated by sudden lifting of the muzzle. With progression of signs the stiffness becomes more obvious and involves the head, neck, all four extremities, and the tail. Other signs observed include an exaggerated response to external stimuli, erect ear carriage, and drooling of saliva. Regurgitation of food and water may be present owing to laryngeal and pharyngeal spasm, preventing normal deglutition. Secondary aspiration pneumonia is a potential sequel. At a later stage the animals become dehydrated owing to decreased water intake, hypersalivation, and profuse sweating. Temperature and heart rate are normal early in the course of the disease but rise when muscular tone is increased. Cattle may be mildly bloated as an early sign (esophagus: striated muscle) but maintain normal rumen motility (rumen: smooth muscle). As disease progresses there is great difficulty in walking, and the animal may adopt the "sawhorse" posture. Tetanic convulsions, accompanied by opisthotonos, often occur following external stimuli.

Clinical Pathology and Necropsy

Serum muscle enzymes (AST, CK, and LDH) are likely to be elevated. Stress hyperglycemia may occur. Dehydrated cattle may become acidotic (loss of saliva) and may have elevated serum urea and creatinine (prerenal). No gross or histologic lesions are seen on postmortem examination of uncomplicated cases. Aspiration pneumonia, prolonged recumbency, and severe dehydration may lead to lesions in lungs, extremities, and kidneys.

Diagnosis

Clinical signs in well-advanced disease are related to spasms of voluntary muscles and are usually not confused with other diseases. Early cases should be differentiated from hypomagnesemic tetany, polioencephalomalacia, rabies, other cerebrospinal meningitides, lead poisoning, and enterotoxemia in lambs. In cattle the stiff gait in polyarthritis may be confused with tetanus. In enzootic muscular dystrophy there is usually no tetany. Attempts at measuring blood levels of tetanospasmin for confirmation of tetanus are often unsatisfactory. Tetanus can be confirmed bacteriologically by demonstrating *C. tetani* in an infected wound, if present.

Treatment

The goals of therapy include elimination of the local infection (wound débridement); parenteral and local procaine penicillin G (25,000 IU/kg b.i.d. for 3 to 5 days followed by s.i.d. for another 5 days; or long-acting penicillin); neutralization of circulating toxin (1500 IU tetanus antitoxin subcutaneously s.i.d. for 3 to 5 days); and relaxation of muscle tetany (acetyl promazine 0.05 mg/kg intramuscularly b.i.d.; xylazine dose 0.05 to 0.1 mg/kg intramuscularly or 0.016 to 0.034 mg/kg intravenously b.i.d.) until severe signs subside (10 to 12 days). Supportive treatment by keeping the animals in a dark, quiet, well-bedded stall is important. If recurrent bloat occurs, a rumen fistula may be indicated. This allows the animal to receive feed and water temporarily through the fistula. Recovery is a slow process (weeks to months).

Prevention

Proper skin and instrument disinfection at the time of castration, docking, and shearing could prevent many tetanus cases. Passive immunization with 1500 to 2000 IU tetanus antitoxin in calves and 200 IU in lambs has reduced the incidence of disease after these procedures on tetanus-prone farms. The protection lasts only 10 to 14 days, and the toxoid, an aluminium-precipitated formalin-treated toxin given intramuscularly at the same time but at a different site, gives immunity after 2 weeks and lasts at least 12 months. Prevention of tetanus in lambs is achieved by vaccinating ewes in the last 2 to 3 weeks of gestation and the lambs at 2 to 3 months of age. Vaccination of cattle is usually not indicated unless an outbreak of disease has occurred.

BOTULISM

Definition, Occurrence, and Incidence

Botulism is a fatal, progressive, flaccid paralysis of all voluntary muscles caused by the ingestion of botulinum toxin in contaminated food or water. Cattle, sheep, goats, and horses are more susceptible than pigs, dogs, and cats. The organisms are common inhabitants of the gastrointestinal tract of herbivores and other animals and may persist in the environment in its sporulated form for long periods. The source of toxin for animals is usually a dead animal (carrion), which may include decaying rodents, birds including dead chickens in poultry manure, or other animals. Proliferation of *C. botulinum* is also possible in decaying plant material (rotten hay and silage). Sporadic epizootics have been reported from many countries and in recent years have been associated with the feeding of poultry litter or its use on pasture, as well as with the use of "big-bale" silage. The disease is seasonal in range animals, occurring mainly during drought periods, when feed is sparse and animals have a depraved appetite owing to phosphorus deficiency. Mortality in cattle is usually 90 to 95 per cent.

Etiology and Pathogenesis

C. botulinum is a spore-forming, anaerobic, gram-positive rod, mainly proliferating in decaying animal and plant material. It is commonly found in soil samples and aquatic sediments. Different types (A to G) have been identified, and different types predominate in different soils. The derivative toxins produced by the different serologic types are physically and chemically very similar to each other and closely resemble tetanospasmin. Following ingestion, clinical signs appear after 24 to 48 hours. The toxin is absorbed as a protoxin and converted by endogenous gastrointestinal proteases into the active form. The paralysis follows a three-step event: (1) recognition of a receptor on the nerve ending and irreversible binding at that site; (2) internalization of a portion of the molecule into the nerve cell; and (3) action of this internalized fragment to prevent acetylcholine release at the motoneuronal junction. Only peripheral cholinergic synapses are affected. The animals die of respiratory paralysis.

Clinical Signs

Incubation period varies with amount of ingested toxin, with individual susceptibility, and may last from days to weeks. Peracute cases may die without prior clinical signs. In most cases the disease is subacute and death ensues within 2 to 6 days.

Cattle

The first clinical signs are decreased tongue tone and problems with deglutition and prehension of food, followed by progressive muscular weakness until animals become recumbent in a parturient paresis-like posture. The tongue may be protruding. Early weakness is usually manifested by ataxia and a stumbling gait affecting the hind legs first. Oral examination can be performed without resistance (decreased jaw tone), and there is ptosis and occasionally a delayed pupillary light reflex. Skin sensation is retained. In some cases there is no obvious impairment of deglutition, and animals continue to eat until they die.

Sheep

Flaccid paralysis does not occur in sheep until late in the disease. There is stiffness in the gait. Salivation and serous nasal discharge are common.

Clinical Pathology and Necropsy

Marked indicanuria, glycosuria, and albuminuria have been observed in cattle but are not consistent findings. In peracute cases toxin can be demonstrated in serum by mouse inoculation. Toxin is often not detected in the serum of subacute cases. Nonspecific changes in the serum biochemical profile may be seen in dehydrated recumbent animals.

There are no specific changes at necropsy. Cattle that died often have a very dry omasum and a mild enteritis with congestion of intestinal mucosa. There may be nonspecific hemorrhages in the subendocardium and subepicardium. Perivascular hemorrhages have been reported in the corpus striatum and cerebrocortex.

Diagnosis

Diagnosis by demonstration of toxin is often impossible and therefore relies on the clinical manifestation and epidemiologic pattern of the cases. The veterinarian should look for a potential source of toxin, such as the presence of a carrion-contaminating hay, silage, or water. Filtrates of the stomach and intestinal contents can be tested for presence of toxins but are frequently negative. In epizootics, suspected feed material may be fed to susceptible animals to establish a diagnosis.

Recumbent animals and findings at necropsy resemble cows with parturient paresis. Other differential diagnoses should include diseases of the central nervous system and spinal cord, such as the paralytic form of rabies; Aujeszky's disease; sporadic bovine encephalomyelitis (Buss disease); listeriosis; polioencephalomalacia; lead poisoning; miscellaneous plant poisonings; and bovine spongiform encephalopathy. In sheep, louping-ill and some cases of scrapie and plant poisoning may be misdiagnosed as botulism.

Treatment

Treatment should only be attempted in subacute cases. Therapy is mainly symptomatic and should include fluid and nutritional support and general nursing care. Feeding potentially contaminated feeds should cease until the source of the toxin is established, the type of toxin identified, and the rest of the herd vaccinated. Ruminal lavage, administration of lactic acid (50 to 80 ml lactic acid in 5 to 10 L water per stomach tube in adult cattle), or purgatives have been suggested to remove or inactivate toxin in the intestinal tract. Polyvalent serum containing antibotulinum toxin antibodies (anti-C and -D mostly) may be tried in very early cases and in animals believed to be at risk, but once toxin is bound at the synapses it cannot be neutralized. Anticholinesterases such as neostigmine have been used with contradictory results. The type of toxoid for vaccination depends on results of mouse protection testing or historical experience with a specific type in an endemic area.

Prevention

Control measures consist mainly of good husbandry: proper disposal of carcasses (especially in range cattle areas); avoiding the use of contaminated and spoiled feed (hay, silage); and supplementing phosphorus in deficient regions to prevent pica. In areas with enzootic disease, vaccination with a type-specific or bivalent vaccine (cattle: types C and D toxoid) is recommended. A single dose of vaccine gives good immunity after 2 weeks and lasts for about 24 months.

BLACKLEG (EMPHYSEMATOUS GANGRENE)

Definition, Occurrence, and Incidence

Blackleg is a peracute, noncontagious, highly fatal infection of skeletal muscle with *C. chauvoei (C. feseri)* characterized by gaseous edema of muscles and severe toxemia. Less common causes of infection include *C. septicum, C. novyi,* and *C. sordellii.* Blackleg is common in cattle and rarely seen in sheep. The infection is soilborne, but the portal of entrance into the body is still in dispute. The disease affects mainly young cattle (6 months to 2 years) on pastures in blackleg-prone regions. Most cases occur during the hot months of the year. Blackleg may cause enormous economic loss in endemic areas, with mortality approaching 100 per cent, especially where there is frequent flooding.

Etiology and Pathogenesis

C. chauvoei and other agents of blackleg are anaerobic, motile, spore-forming organisms. The spores may survive for many years in the soil. Mixed infections are common. It is assumed that the port of entry is through the mucosa of the alimentary tract. The bacteria can be found in the spleen, liver, and alimentary tract of normal animals. The stimulus causing postulated "latent" spores to proliferate in muscle tissues is often unknown, but muscle trauma associated with transporting, herding, and handling has been incriminated as creating suitable conditions in the muscle to allow bacterial multiplication and myonecrosis. Several toxic compounds (cytolysins, necrotizing enzymes) are produced by *C. chauvoei,* causing severe local damage and widespread organ dysfunction.

Clinical Signs

Cattle

Peracute cases are often found dead. The incubation period is 1 to 3 days. Prior to local signs there is depression, anorexia, rumen stasis, high fever (41 to 42°C), and tachycardia (>100/min). These early signs are usually followed by marked lameness with pronounced muscle swelling of the upper part of the affected leg. Lesions can also occasionally be found on the base of the tongue, the brisket, and the udder. There is regional lymphadenopathy. The developing edema shows crepitus on palpation and tympanic sounds on percussion. The skin is often discolored in affected areas. On cut section a serosanguineous rancid fluid appears and gas escapes.

Sheep

Subcutaneous edema is uncommon, and crepitation is often absent. There is high fever, anorexia, and depression followed by rapid death. The first clinical signs observed are lameness, often involving multiple limbs.

Clinical Pathology and Necropsy

Culture, cytology, and Gram's stain may be attempted on fine-needle aspirates of affected tissues. Serum enzymes derived from skeletal muscle (CK, AST, and LDH) are significantly elevated. Terminally sick animals have secondary complications, such as toxemia and hypovolemia. Clotting of blood occurs rapidly. For necropsy, cadavers must be fresh to avoid the rapid local infiltration of other clostridial organisms, which might confuse the bacteriologic diagnosis. On necropsy, affected areas (connective tissues and muscles) are filled with rancid serosanguineous fluid and gas pockets, which crepitate when squeezed. The affected muscles appear dry, showing red and black areas with islands of necrosis. Toward the periphery of the lesion the muscle is dark red and moist with edema fluid. There is lymphadenopathy. Spleen and liver often look normal but may show gaseous distention. Secondary findings include pulmonary edema, degenerated heart muscle, and some degree of degeneration in the other solid organs. To detect localized lesions it is important to examine all skeletal muscles of the carcass, including tongue and diaphragm.

Diagnosis

Isolation and identification of *C. chauvoei* and related clostridia are quite demanding, whereas detection by immunofluorescence is relatively simple using commercially available conjugated antisera. Clinically and on gross necropsy, malignant edema should be ruled out. The epidemiology (local incidence, season, age group, pasture environment) and bacterial confirmation are therefore crucial. Anthrax and lightning strike do not show the typical gaseous edemas. Necropsy findings in bacillary hemoglobinuria are very similar.

Treatment

Treatment is often too late. Large doses of penicillin (20,000 IU/kg b.i.d.) are given to animals that are not moribund. Local antibiotic treatment in affected areas has been attempted. Drainage and slashing of affected tissue to allow oxygen into the tissue may be tried to save individual animals. Supportive treatment (parenteral fluids, analgesics, etc.) is crucial.

Prevention

On farms and in regions where the disease is endemic, annual vaccination of cattle between 6 months and 2 years should be performed shortly before expected epizootics (spring, summer). The formalin-killed, aluminium-precipitated bacterin from a local strain of *C. chauvoei* is best. Early vaccination (3 weeks of age) with subsequent revaccination has been recommended on disease-prone farms. Immunity develops after 2 weeks, but morbidity and mortality may continue for some time in outbreak situations. The incidence may be reduced by prophylactic antibiotic treatments (procaine penicillin 10,000 IU/kg intramuscularly once daily [s.i.d.]) for up to 2 weeks. Movement from affected pastures is recommended. In sheep less than 1 year of age, good immunity does not develop postvaccination, and vaccination of young first-lambing ewes 3 weeks before parturition is suggested. This will give permanent protection of the adult animals and passive protection of lambs up to 3 weeks of age. In sheep, multivalent clostridial vaccines are preferred.

Carcasses of animals should be destroyed by burning or deep burial in safe, nonpasture areas to limit soil contamination.

MALIGNANT EDEMA

Definition, Occurrence, and Incidence

Malignant edema is an often fatal wound (castration, injections, dystocia) infection caused by one of several *Clostridium* spp. It is characterized by signs of acute inflammation at the site of infection and by systemic toxemia. All ages and species of food animals may be affected. The disease occurs sporadically, mostly in individual animals, and only rarely in outbreaks (e.g., contaminated dip in sheep having shearing or docking wounds).

Etiology and Pathogenesis

Clostridia causing malignant edema are common inhabitants of the intestinal tract and the environment as spore-forming soil organisms. The species isolated from malignant edema cases include mainly *C. septicum* but also *C. chauvoei, C. perfringens, C. sordelli,* and *C. novyi.* Toxigenic clostridia, which are either locally present in tissue or, more often, deposited there by wound contamination, multiply in traumatized tissue. Several different toxins and enzymes produced by the bacteria create a local lesion but are also absorbed systemically to produce toxemia. Bacteremia may develop terminally. The target tissues of the different toxins produced are mainly capillary endothelial cells, platelets, and red blood cells, which are destroyed. Local tissue necrosis may also be produced by increased pressure owing to gas production, resulting in reduced venous return.

Clinical Signs

Shortly after infection (12 to 48 hours) there is local inflammation and painful warm edema of cutis, subcutis, and muscle. There may or may not be crepitation on palpation and percussion indicating presence of gas. Regional lymphadenopathy is present, and the patients are febrile (40 to 42°C), depressed, anorexic, weak, and tachycardic. Complications may include pulmonary edema and diarrhea. If not treated early, animals usually succumb to the infection within 2 to 5 days. When infection occurs after parturition, there is cushion-like swelling of the vulvar region with a foul-smelling, reddish discharge. The swelling extends into the pelvic tissues, perineum, and down between the hind legs. In "swelled head" of rams, which may follow fighting, the edema is initially restricted to the head. Pigs usually have very little evidence of emphysema.

Clinical Pathology and Necropsy

Generally similar to those described under blackleg. There may be some variations in the gross appearance of the lesions depending on the principal pathogen involved. The distinctive characteristics are severe edema and the formation of gas bubbles in connective tissues and muscles associated with a wound or other sites of entry.

Diagnosis

Often there is history of surgery, obstetric complications, injection, or wounds preceding onset of malignant edema. It is very difficult to differentiate from blackleg, and the causative organism can be identified only by laboratory methods such as fine-needle aspirates and fluorescent antibody staining of affected tissues.

Treatment

Cases should be considered emergencies because of the peracute nature of the disease and the poor prognosis. Antitoxin (multivalent serum) may be given early in the disease but is difficult to obtain. Penicillin (20,000 IU/kg intramuscularly b.i.d.) systemically and/or locally is specifically indicated because of its high activity and bactericidal action. Surgical incision to provide drainage and local irrigation with 3 per cent hydrogen peroxide should be attempted.

Prevention

Hygiene is essential to prevent the infection. In enzootic areas vaccination with multivalent or specific formalinized bacterin has given satisfactory results. All wounds should be properly débrided and treated to prevent contamination, especially with fecal material. In areas where there is anecdotal evidence of increased incidence of injection-related malignant edema (mostly after prostaglandin injections), practitioners have successfully prevented the disease by injecting penicillin locally with the product used. The carcasses of affected animals should be disposed of as for blackleg cases. Stalls should be cleaned and disinfected.

BACILLARY HEMOGLOBINURIA

Definition, Occurrence, and Incidence

Bacillary hemoglobinuria (BHU) is an acute, toxemic, and highly fatal clostridial disease, with the liver being the main target organ. The disease occurs worldwide, is sporadic, and most commonly affects cattle and occasionally sheep and pigs. In North America it is seen more commonly during the summer and early fall. BHU occurs more frequently in areas where fascioliasis is a problem and is spread from infected areas to noninfected areas by flooding, natural drainage, contaminated feed, or carrier animals. In the United States BHU occurs predominantly in poorly drained pastures, particularly where the soil is alkaline (pH 8.0 or higher). Bacillary hemoglobinuria is rare in calves less than 1 year old and cattle with poor body condition. On endemic farms the mortality averages 5 per cent, but mortality rates up to 25 per cent have been observed in outbreaks among feedlot cattle.

Etiology and Pathogenesis

BHU is caused by *C. haemolyticum*. It is a soilborne anaerobe. The organism has been successfully isolated from the bone of dead animals up to 1 year after death. *C. haemolyticum* produces several exotoxins. Beta toxin is mainly responsible for the tissue damage. The infection results from ingestion, and in some instances from inhalation, of the clostridial spores, which are then absorbed and transported via blood to the liver. Once in the liver, the spores may remain latent for an indefinite time and may be isolated from healthy cattle. It has been difficult to determine the natural incubation period of the disease, but, from experimental and observational evidence, it seems that local hepatic injury is necessary to trigger the onset. It has been suggested that either telangiectasis, necrobacillosis, fascioliasis, or *Cysticercus tenuicollis* is the triggering factor causing local anaerobic conditions for germination of dormant spores. Once spore germination occurs there is local production of exotoxins. These exotoxins cause severe hepatic necrosis and local thrombosis. With the increasing concentrations of exotoxin in the blood, erythrolysis ensues, producing acute hemolytic anemia and hemoglobinuria. Beta toxin also causes endothelial damage of arterioles throughout the body with extravasation of blood into the tissue and body cavities.

Clinical Signs

Animals with peracute disease die before any signs have been noted. In acute cases the animals stand separated from the rest of the herd and appear very ill. The back is arched, and the abdomen is "tucked up." Appetite, lactation, rumination, and defecation suddenly cease. Animals are reluctant to move and have to be forced to walk. Grunting occurs when walking. Tachycardia, tachypnea, and weak pulse are present. Fever (40 to 41°C) is prominent throughout the clinical disease, with subnormal temperature being observed terminally. Initially there is frequent passage of small amounts of bile-stained feces, later often progressing to diarrhea. The urine is dark red with no erythrocytes present; jaundice may be observed, and anemia may be severe. The duration of the clinical syndrome is 18 to 36 hours. Death occurs as a consequence of the severe hemolytic anemia and toxemia. Mortality in untreated animals reaches 95 per cent.

Clinical Pathology and Necropsy

Anemia with a hematocrit as low as 0.10 L/L (10 per cent) is frequently observed, and the red cell count is low and may reach values as low as one million cells per microliter. Hemoglobin can also drop to 35 g/L. The white blood cell count is highly variable; the urine is red in color and contains hemoglobin. Blood culture may be positive. Necropsy findings are characterized by subcutaneous edema, petechiae, and diffuse hemorrhages throughout the body. The pleural and peritoneal cavities contain large quantities of hemoglobin-stained transudate. Hemorrhagic abomasitis and enteritis may be present. Red urine is found in the bladder; the lungs are edematous, and bronchi are filled with a blood-tinged foam. Large hepatic infarcts are always present and are pathognomonic. They vary from 5 to 25 cm in diameter, are pale and conical in shape on cut surface, and are often surrounded by a reddish zone of congestion. Histologically the necrotic liver tissue is sharply demarcated from the unaffected tissue by a wide band of bacteria and a mild leukocytic infiltrate. *C. haemolyticum* can be consistently isolated from heart blood, the liver infarct, and sometimes from other organs of fresh carcasses. Postmortem invaders may obscure its presence.

Diagnosis

Clinical diagnosis of BHU is mainly done by excluding other causes of hemoglobinuria. Peracute disease is difficult to diagnose. Appropriate specimens from dead animals should be collected, especially those tissues showing pathologic lesions. BHU can be confused with acute leptospirosis, postparturient hemoglobinuria, and hemolytic anemia caused by cruciferous plants, including rape or kale. The plant-induced hemoglobinurias are usually not accompanied by severe febrile reactions.

Babesiosis and anaplasmosis are geographically limited, and protozoal parasites can be detected in peripheral blood smears. Pyelonephritis, enzootic hematuria, and cystitis have intact red cells in urine. Chronic copper poisoning, especially in sheep, is differentiated at postmortem by the absence of the liver infarcts.

Causes of sudden death in cattle and sheep, such as in anthrax, blackleg, and infectious necrotic hepatitis, have to be differentiated from BHU, especially when terminal hematuria occurs.

Treatment

If treatment is attempted, 500 to 1000 ml *C. haemolyticum* antitoxin should be administered along with specific antibiotics: procaine penicillin (20,000 IU/kg intramuscularly b.i.d.) or tetracycline (10 mg/kg intravenously or intramuscularly s.i.d.) to control the infection. The response to the antibiotic treatment without the antitoxin is poor. Supportive treatments with blood transfusions, parenteral fluid, and electrolytes may help to control the hemolytic anemia and the dehydration. Animals should be kept in a quiet environment to avoid additional stress. Bulls should not be used for service up to 3 weeks after recovery because of the danger of liver rupture and hemorrhage. Vitamins and iron should be administered to recovering animals.

Prevention

BHU can be prevented by the use of vaccination. The vaccine can be administered at any age but is recommended to be used at 6 months of age and again within 3 to 4 weeks, with boosters annually in low-exposure areas and every 6 months in high-exposure areas. Multiway clostridial vaccines include *C. haemolyticum* and are efficacious. In low-prevalence areas vaccination may not be economically reasonable.

BRAXY

Definition, Occurrence, and Incidence

Braxy is a rare, acute, hemorrhagic abomasitis of sheep caused by *C. septicum* and is associated with toxemia and high mortality (about 50 per cent). The disease is mostly seen in the winter in animals eating frozen silage or hay. The age groups most commonly affected are weaned to yearling sheep. The disease occurs worldwide but appears to be rare in North America. A similar syndrome has been reported in a beef calf.

Etiology and Pathogenesis

C. septicum, a soilborne organism and probably a normal commensal in the gastrointestinal tract of sheep, invades the abomasal wall under favorable conditions, causing severe abomasitis and toxemia.

Clinical Signs

The course of braxy is peracute. There is sudden onset of depression, segregation from the group, high fever, and death ensuing within hours. There may be signs of colic and abdominal distention.

Clinical Pathology and Necropsy

Antemortem laboratory tests are of little value. Major changes are observed in the abomasal wall and include congestion of the mucosa with areas of necrosis, gas accumulation, and ulceration. Histologically there is acute, severe, transmural abomasitis. Besides changes associated with toxemia, no other histologic lesions are present.

Diagnosis

Because of the acute nature of the disease, clinical diagnosis is very difficult. Grain overload may produce similar signs, but there are no lesions in the abomasum at necropsy. The syndrome resembles infectious necrotic hepatitis but lacks the liver lesions. Diagnosis is established by direct isolation of *C. septicum* from abomasal tissue or by demonstrating the organism by immunofluorescence of frozen abomasal sections of smears.

Treatment

No treatment of value has been reported.

Prevention

In areas where the problem is prevalent, prophylactic vaccination with formalin-killed whole culture of *C. septicum* given 2 weeks apart has proven to be very effective.

BLACK DISEASE (INFECTIOUS NECROTIC HEPATITIS)

Definition, Occurrence, and Incidence

Black disease (infectious necrotic hepatitis) is a peracute, highly fatal clostridial disease occurring in sheep and cattle and occasionally in pigs. Horses and goats may also be affected.

Black disease has a worldwide distribution. A close association between black disease and fascioliasis has been established. There is a marked seasonal occurrence in the summer, and the disease occurs in well-nourished adult sheep between 2 and 4 years of age. Fecal contamination of pasture, infected carcasses, and flooding are the main sources of infection. The infection is also spread by birds and wild animals. In sheep the morbidity is about 5 per cent, with up to 50 per cent being reported.

Etiology and Pathogenesis

Black disease is caused by *C. novyi* type B and a concurrent hepatic insult, most commonly due to *Fasciola hepatica*. The disease has been reproduced in sheep by administration of spores to animals previously infected with fluke metacercariae. *C. tenuicollis* has also been implicated as a possible way of precipitating hepatic insult.

The spores of *C. novyi* are ingested and transported to the liver, where they may remain dormant or proliferate in injured anoxic liver tissue. *C. novyi* type B usually produces alpha and beta exotoxin, causing hepatic necrosis, toxemia (mostly alpha toxin), and often death.

Clinical Signs

Sheep or cattle with black disease are frequently found dead without preceding signs of disease. Clinically affected animals tend to separate from the flock, are unwilling to move, and may fall if driven. Early in the disease body temperature is increased (40 to 42°C) but tends to fall to normal or subnormal levels in moribund animals. There is tachypnea, and sheep usually remain in sternal recumbency and may even die in this posture. The course of the clinical disease is very short (hours). The clinical findings in cattle are similar to sheep, but the course is usually longer (1 to 2 days). New cases may occur up to 9 weeks after removal from fluke-infested pastures or up to 14 days after vaccination is initiated.

Clinical Pathology and Necropsy

Antemortem laboratory tests are rarely possible because of the peracute course. The carcass undergoes very rapid putrefaction. Subcutaneous blood vessels are engorged and cause the carcass to blacken (black disease). Varying amounts of fluid are present in the pericardial sac and pleural and peritoneal cavities. Hemorrhages of the endocardium are a consistent finding.

There is a generalized engorgement of the liver, with areas of necrosis, 1 to 2 cm in diameter, surrounded by a zone of hyperemia. Hepatic necrosis is most frequently subcapsular in the diaphragmatic lobe and consists of a central zone of necrosis surrounded by leukocytes and large numbers of clostridia.

Diagnosis

The diagnosis is based on the history and postmortem findings. The lesions are often unremarkable, and, if there is considerable damage by *Fasciola* spp., diagnosis may be very difficult. Definitive diagnosis is reached by demonstration of the organism in the lesion or presence of preformed mouse lethal toxin. Bacteria are easily identified in smears of hepatic tissue by immunofluorescence.

Other causes of sudden death, such as clostridial infections (enterotoxemia, bacillary hemoglobinuria, and blackleg) and anthrax, should be considered. In sheep, acute fascioliasis can cause heavy mortalities, with a postmortem finding similar to that in black disease. Therefore laboratory diagnosis is necessary for a definite diagnosis.

Treatment

There is no effective treatment available. The longer course in cattle may allow the use of broad-spectrum antibiotics or penicillin.

Prevention

Based on epidemiology of black disease, the control can be effected by eliminating fascioliasis. Vaccination with aluminium-precipitated toxoid is highly effective even in the face of an outbreak. It is recommended that the initial vaccination be repeated 3 to 4 weeks later, with annual boosters on problem farms.

BIBLIOGRAPHY

TETANUS

Wallis AS: Some observations of the epidemiology of tetanus in cattle. Vet Rec 75:188–191, 1963.

BOTULISM

Hariharan H, Mitchell WR: Type C botulism: the agent host spectrum and environment. Vet Bull 47:95–100, 1977.
Rings DM: Bacterial meningitis and diseases caused by bacterial toxins. Vet Clin North Am: Food Anim Pract 3:85–98, 1987.

BACILLARY HEMOGLOBINURIA

Stogdale L, Booth AJ: Bacillary hemoglobinuria in cattle. Comp Cont Ed 6:S284–S290, 1984.

BLACK DISEASE

Bagadi HO: Infectious necrotic hepatitis (black disease) of sheep. Vet Bull 44:385–388, 1974.

Clostridial Enterotoxemia (*Clostridium perfringens*)
DONNA M. GATEWOOD, DVM, MS
M. M. CHENGAPPA, BVSc, PhD

Clostridial enteric disease in domestic animals is most frequently caused by *Clostridium perfringens*. There are five types of *C. perfringens* that can cause variable lesions in a variety of organ systems; the syndromes are known collectively as enterotoxemia, which is an acute, infectious, noncontagious disease that originates in the gut of affected animals. Characteristic lesions are the result of toxins produced by the specific type of *C. perfringens* present in the gut.

C. perfringens is nearly ubiquitous in nature and can be isolated from the alimentary tract of healthy animals. Conditions that favor multiplication of the organism and promote toxin production may result in disease in susceptible animals. Abrupt switching of animals from a high-roughage to a high-concentrate diet frequently precedes an outbreak.

C. perfringens types C and D are the most prevalent causes of enterotoxemia in the United States, while types A and E occur with less frequency. Type B is not known to be a problem in the United States. All five types have antigenic similarities and produce toxins in common. Since the clinical disease syndromes produced by the five types differ, each syndrome will be discussed separately. Diagnosis, treatment, and prevention are the same for all types, however, and will therefore be discussed together.

TYPE A ENTEROTOXEMIA

Type A *C. perfringens* is distributed worldwide and is the only one of the five types that is well adapted to survival in soil as well as in the alimentary tract of animals and humans. Although type A is frequently isolated, it is infrequently associated with disease outbreaks. Type A is responsible for "yellow lamb" disease, which is seen sporadically in California and Oregon in the spring, when lambs are nursing heavily. The primary feature of this disease appears to be intravascular hemolysis and capillary damage caused by large quantities of alpha toxin absorbed through the small intestine. Morbidity may reach 30 per cent or more, and mortality may be close to 100 per cent.

In calves the disease is suspected of taking one of two forms. The first is similar to that seen in lambs but occurs with less frequency and decreased severity in calves. The second form is associated with acute abdominal syndrome. This syndrome is sporadic, although some midwestern herds have experienced a prevalence of up to 40 per cent.

Clinical Signs

Affected lambs are acutely depressed, icteric, anemic and hemoglobinuric, dyspneic, and have pale mucous membranes. Icterus is the predominant feature of the syndrome and is evident on all mucosal surfaces. Although abdominal discomfort may be the initial sign of disease, diarrhea is seldom a feature of this disease in sheep. Most affected animals die of acute hemolytic crisis within 6 to 12 hours after the onset of clinical signs. The clinical signs, lesions, and mortality are much less severe in calves.

Acute abdominal syndrome in calves is characterized by acute onset of abdominal tympany or bloat, colic, anorexia, lassitude, and depression with or without diarrhea or sudden death. In some cases affected calves have a history of diarrhea in the first week of life followed by recovery and development of acute abdominal syndrome 1 to 2 weeks later.

There is evidence that *C. perfringens* type A may cause enterotoxigenic diarrhea in neonatal pigs, but the disease has not been fully characterized.

Necropsy Findings

Postmortem lesions in lambs include dark kidneys, a swollen spleen, and an enlarged, pale, friable liver. Excessive fluid may be present in the pericardial and peritoneal cavities. Lesions are less severe in calves. Postmortem lesions in calves with acute abdominal syndrome include abomasitis, abomasal erosions, varying degrees of abomasal ulcerations, and grayish to black fluid in the rumen and abomasum.

TYPE B ENTEROTOXEMIA

Type B enterotoxemia is not observed in North America, Australia, or New Zealand but has been reported in Europe, South Africa, and the Middle East. It causes dysentery in newborn lambs and calves up to 2 weeks of age.

C. perfringens type B elaborates three of the major *C.*

perfringens toxins (alpha, beta, epsilon) and can therefore resemble other *C. perfringens* infections. A definitive diagnosis can be made only through culture and identification of the organism.

Clinical Signs

In lambs sudden death may occur, but more frequently the onset is characterized by listlessness, unwillingness to suckle, and abdominal pain followed by fetid diarrhea. Mortality is close to 100 per cent, with death occurring within a few hours after the onset of clinical signs. The disease in calves is similar to that seen in lambs but is generally less severe and runs a course of 2 to 4 days. Older calves up to 10 weeks of age may be affected.

Necropsy Findings

The most prominent lesion is an extensive hemorrhagic enteritis. The intestinal mucosa is congested, and ulcerations and necrosis are present on the intestinal walls. Free blood may be seen in the intestinal lumen, and the peritoneal cavity often contains hemorrhagic fluid. The liver is usually enlarged and friable, and the mediastinal lymph nodes are enlarged and edematous.

TYPE C ENTEROTOXEMIA

C. perfringens type C is the cause of hemorrhagic enteritis in adult sheep and in lambs, calves, kids, and piglets less than 2 weeks of age. It is the most widespread cause of hemorrhagic enterotoxemia in domestic livestock in North America and is the result of the beta toxin that characterizes this type. In adult sheep the disease is referred to as "struck" or "Romney Marsh disease," and is seen primarily in Great Britain. Mortality is 5 to 15 per cent in adult animals but may approach 100 per cent in young animals.

Clinical Signs

In calves and lambs the disease is most frequently observed within the first few days of life. The beta toxin associated with the disease is destroyed by trypsin, and it is thought that low levels of trypsin in the immature digestive tract may play a role in the pathogenesis. Clinical signs include diarrhea, dysentery, and colic, although sudden death is frequently a feature of this syndrome. In some individuals opisthotonos and tetany may be observed just prior to death. Those few affected animals that survive are usually unthrifty and stunted.

In piglets the disease most frequently occurs as epizootics, which may remain as enzootics. Whole litters may be affected, and the mortality rate is high. Clinical signs are similar to those seen in calves and lambs.

In adult sheep there is no diarrhea, but affected animals may show signs of acute abdominal pain. Frequently the infection is peracute, and death occurs suddenly with convulsions.

Necropsy Findings

In young animals extensive hemorrhagic inflammation of the jejunum and ileum is the most striking feature of the disease. The peritoneal cavity may contain serohemorrhagic fluid, and there may be peritonitis. Ecchymotic and petechial hemorrhages are usually present on serosal surfaces, as well as in the spleen, thymus, heart, meninges, and brain.

In adults the peritoneum contains a large volume (up to 3 L) of serous fluid. The peritoneal vessels are intensely congested, and peritoneal hemorrhages may be present. The small intestine has areas of superficial mucosal necrosis, and ulcers are usually present, particularly in the jejunum. Other organs show evidence of acute toxemia, including copious pleural and pericardial transudate. The causative agent is usually distributed throughout the tissues, and if necropsy is delayed the disease may be confused with blackleg.

TYPE D ENTEROTOXEMIA

Type D enterotoxemia ("overeating disease," "pulpy kidney disease," "braxy-like disease") is the most common form of enterotoxemia in sheep and goats and has worldwide distribution. It is also seen in feedlot cattle, although cattle are less frequently affected than sheep. In all species, affected animals are usually well nourished and are on a high plane of nutrition. Single lambs less than 12 weeks old that are nursing high-producing ewes are most frequently affected; affected calves are usually 1 to 3 months of age. Adult sheep are occasionally affected.

The epsilon toxin responsible for type D disease requires trypsin activation to be fully potent. The mechanism of action of epsilon toxin is not well understood, but it is believed to act on the liver, causing altered metabolism of glycogen, which results in hyperglycemia and subsequent glycosuria. In addition, it appears to cause vascular damage in the brain and kidney, where there is an abundance of toxin receptor sites.

Clinical Signs

In most lambs and calves the disease is peracute and the animal is found dead. Some individuals may exhibit neurologic signs, such as ataxia, blindness, or convulsions, just prior to death. There is usually no evidence of intestinal involvement unless the disease runs a course of several days. These individuals may produce dark, semifluid feces; this is most frequently seen in goats or adult sheep. Goats are likely to develop a more chronic form of the disease, characterized by severe, persistent diarrhea lasting for several days.

Necropsy Findings

Gross lesions are variable and in peracute cases may be absent. These individuals often have a rumen and abomasum filled with concentrated feed.

Epsilon toxin is absorbed by the small intestine and causes increased vascular permeability in many tissues. Observable lesions include petechial and ecchymotic hemorrhage on the serosal surfaces of the rumen, abomasum and duodenum, diaphragm, and abdominal muscles. There is an excess of pericardial fluid, and the epicardium and endocardium may have hemorrhages. Animals that die after a more chronic course of the disease may have fluid in the lungs and focal necrosis and edema of the brain. The effects of epsilon toxin on renal vasculature may contribute to more rapid autolysis of the kidneys, causing them to appear hyperemic, soft, and friable. This is most prominent in affected sheep but is not evident if carcasses are examined immediately after death.

TYPE E ENTEROTOXEMIA

This is a rare disease that has been reported in calves and lambs. The syndrome appears to be similar to type C enterotoxemia. Calves die acutely, and necropsy examination reveals hemorrhagic enteritis and enlarged mesenteric lymph nodes.

DIAGNOSIS OF ENTEROTOXEMIA

Enterotoxemia should be suspected if sudden death occurs in apparently healthy young calves, lambs, piglets, or older animals on full feed. A presumptive diagnosis can be made if stained smears of fresh intestinal contents reveal large numbers of gram-positive rods.

Laboratory confirmation is necessary for a definitive diagnosis and to determine which *C. perfringens* type is involved. In addition to isolation and identification, many workers feel it is necessary to demonstrate the specific toxins in order to reach a definitive diagnosis. Samples of intestinal contents collected from several places along the digestive tract should be obtained as quickly as possible after death. The toxins are unstable, so samples should be refrigerated and sent to the appropriate laboratory in refrigerated packs. The addition of one drop of chloroform per 10 ml of sample helps to stabilize the toxins. There is no established concentration of toxin that is indicative of disease; the presence of toxin together with characteristic lesions and history is sufficient for definitive diagnosis.

A diagnosis of type D enterotoxemia requires demonstration of epsilon toxin in the intestine. Lambs usually also show glucosuria.

Type A enterotoxemia may resemble copper poisoning, leptospirosis, or bacillary hemoglobinuria. The other enterotoxemias may appear similar to acute bloat, thromboembolic meningoencephalitis (TEME), polioencephalomalacia (PEM), or acute poisoning. Copper levels in liver tissues of below 150 ppm on a wet-weight basis will eliminate copper poisoning as a possible diagnosis. Serologic surveys of individuals in the herd and histopathologic studies of affected tissues will differentiate leptospirosis. The absence of characteristic liver infarction will eliminate bacillary hemoglobinuria as a cause. Animals suffering from bloat usually have frothy material in the rumen and engorgement of superficial blood vessels. Animals with TEME and PEM generally do not die as acutely; characteristic gross and histopathologic lesions associated with these diseases should differentiate them from enterotoxemia.

TREATMENT AND PREVENTION

Treatment is generally of little benefit in those animals showing clinical signs of enterotoxemia. Once the toxin is present in sufficient quantity to cause acute clinical signs, its effects are generally irreversible. Treatment of the chronic form of type D enterotoxemia in goats may be more successful.

During a herd or flock outbreak, antitoxins and oral sulfonamides should be administered to all potentially susceptible individuals. The antitoxin will provide passive immunity for up to 3 weeks and should be given as quickly as possible after a presumptive diagnosis is made to minimize losses. Vaccines should also be given to both susceptible animals and dams, and a vaccination program should be instituted to prevent future outbreaks.

Prevention is the most effective means of controlling clostridial enterotoxemia. Losses due to type D infection in lamb feedlots are best controlled by increasing the roughage in the diet and decreasing the concentrates. However, this may not be economically feasible. Administration of type C and D toxoids is usually effective in controlling the disease. All individuals entering the feedlot should be given two injections administered 2 weeks apart.

Newborns can be protected by vaccinating the dam 2 to 3 months prior to parturition and again 3 to 5 weeks later with type B, C, and D toxoids. Annual booster injections given 1 month prior to parturition will provide protection to subsequent offspring through ingestion of colostrum. This practice should be routine in sheep flocks.

Offspring delivered to nonimmunized dams can be given antitoxin or hyperimmune serum to provide passive immunity. This will last about 3 weeks, after which time the toxoid should be effective in preventing disease.

Type A *C. perfringens* is a relatively poor antigen, and there are currently no biologics available for preventive use. Control of type A infections may be achieved only through management practices.

Streptococcal Disease
E. DENIS ERICKSON, DVM, PhD

Streptococcal infections were some of the earliest diseases studied, and they continue to be major causes of economic loss to the livestock industries. Infections caused by these organisms form a long list involving most livestock species and virtually all body systems. Emphasis will be placed on those streptococcal diseases of food animals that are of particular veterinary and economic importance. Current methods have allowed a more precise classification of the streptococci, resulting in new names for some; however, the earlier, more familiar names will be used in this article. Serologic grouping and typing of pathogenic streptococci continue to be useful classification tools.

STREPTOCOCCAL INFECTIONS OF RUMINANTS

Streptococcal infections of sheep and goats are not common. Does may develop streptococcal mastitis, while streptococcal septicemia and localized infections occur sporadically in the young. Meningoencephalitis, septic arthritis, and otitis media may occur. Bovine streptococcal infections other than mastitis are also of relatively minor importance. Incidental and opportunistic infections of various organ systems may occur but do not represent well-defined syndromes with consistent streptococcal etiology. Respiratory and genital infections as well as abscesses have been described. Various streptococcal species, including *Streptococcus equisimilis, S. zooepidemicus, S. pneumoniae*, and various alpha and nonhemolytic streptococci, may be involved. Streptococcal infections of the udder, however, are a significant veterinary problem and cause of economic loss.

STREPTOCOCCAL MASTITIS OF CATTLE

Streptococcal mastitis is commonly divided into two groups based on the etiology: those infections caused by *S. agalactiae* and those caused by other streptococci (nonagalactiae mastitis). *S. agalactiae* is highly contagious and resides almost exclusively in the udder, while other streptococci may be found in the environment. These differences influence the strategies and outcomes of control programs.

Etiology

Bovine mastitis may be caused by several species of streptococci, *S. agalactiae*, *S. dysgalactiae*, and *S. uberis* being the most common. Other streptococci, including *S. pyogenes*, group G streptococci, and *S. pneumoniae*, have been implicated in sporadic cases. Various alpha hemolytic streptococci are readily isolated from the skin and teat canal of cows, but their pathogenicity is uncertain.

S. agalactiae, in spite of its susceptibility to several common antibiotics, still exists in herds in which mastitis control procedures have not been adopted. The infected udder is the usual reservoir for transmission of infections to healthy animals. *S. agalactiae* can be carried by some adult human beings and may cause serious disease in infants. Human isolates have been shown under experimental conditions to produce bovine mastitis, but *S. agalactiae* from cows is not regarded as a source for human infection.

Mastitis results when organisms reach sufficient numbers at the teat end, cross the teat canal, adhere to host epithelial cells, and multiply in the gland. Streptococcal cells reach the acinar level of the ductular system, and some penetrate below the secretory epithelium, causing an acute exudative neutrophilic reaction. In later stages a mononuclear cell infiltration develops in areas of chronic inflammation. Fibrosis and scar tissue develop, which, in addition to the cellular debris, cause obstruction of the ductular system and progressive loss in milk production, particularly for *S. agalactiae* infections.

Clinical Signs

Streptococcal mastitis may be seen as an acute local inflammatory disease of the udder with abnormal milk and a systemic reaction. However, chronic subclinical infections are more frequent and may be detectable only by special cow-side tests, such as the California Mastitis Test (CMT), or by laboratory analysis of the milk. *S. agalactiae* infections are more common in herds in which mastitis control procedures are not being used. In these herds both acute and chronic infections may be found. In those herds in which mastitis control procedures are being used, *S. dysgalactiae* and *S. uberis* infections are more common.

Diagnosis

While mastitis must be viewed as a herd problem, the careful clinical examination of individual animals is necessary. In addition to the obvious signs of acute mammary inflammation and abnormal milk, examination of the udder may reveal damaged teat ends associated with improper milking equipment, freezing, or trauma. Resolution of the mastitis problem will occur only following remedy of these predisposing problems or risk factors.

The herd evaluation should include a thorough laboratory analysis of the milk, including determination of the herd somatic cell count and microbiologic analysis of bulk tank milk. Further analysis should include regular testing of all lactating quarters with the CMT or a similar system for detection of elevated leukocyte numbers. While microbiologic analysis of all quarters is ideal, much information on the infections within a herd can be obtained by sampling a proportion of the quarters that score greater than trace on the CMT.

Treatment

The treatment of mastitis should have at least three components: good nursing care of the cow and udder, provision of antibiotic and other supportive treatments, and prevention of reinfection or superinfection. While many dairy workers abhor the chore, nursing care, particularly frequent stripping of affected quarters, is a first step to recovery. The goal for *S. agalactiae*-infected herds is eradication of the infection. *S. dysgalactiae* and *S. uberis* are present in the environment and are less amenable to eradication from the herd. While *S. agalactiae* is usually sensitive to penicillin, the susceptibility patterns of other streptococcal udder pathogens are much less predictable; therefore it is valuable to monitor these patterns by antibiotic susceptibility testing of herd isolates. For intramammary infusion, only sterile, properly formulated products prepared by licensed commercial drug manufacturers should be used. Too often hand-mixed preparations in multidose containers are found in dairies. These preparations and the method in which they are used are often the source of new udder infections. Intramammary infusions deliver high concentrations of antibiotic into the ductular system. Depending on lipid solubility, degree of ionization, and protein binding, parenterally administered antibiotics may achieve high levels in both tissues and milk. Dosages must be those indicated by the manufacturer, with the upper limits being used for parenteral administration.

Prevention

Preventive measures for the control of bovine streptococcal mastitis have received exhaustive description and review in the veterinary and dairy science literature. The cornerstone of most programs includes a properly functioning milking system, single-use towels to clean and dry the udder before attaching milkers, and teat dipping using an approved germicide after each milking. Early detection and treatment of clinical cases of mastitis and infusion of appropriate antibiotics at the time of drying off are important. The objective is to reduce both the duration and the number of infections.

An equally important objective is to reduce the use of antibiotics for cost and public health reasons. Both systemic and local immunizations have been studied to increase natural defenses. An enhanced level of antibodies in milk to *S. agalactiae* has been produced, but the duration of effective protection is limited using currently available strategies.

STREPTOCOCCAL DISEASES OF SWINE

Streptococcal infections are associated with several important and specific disease syndromes of pigs.

Streptococcus suis

Etiology

S. suis is a Lancefield group D streptococcus. There are at least 29 serotypes based on capsular antigens, and there is some relationship between serotype and the clinical disease syndrome. Serotypes 2, 1/2, 3, and 8 appear to be the most prevalent, but patterns of occurrence may vary geographically. *S. suis* has its greatest impact on large, intensively managed herds in which other major diseases are controlled. Overcrowding and poor air quality are predisposing factors. Disease episodes have been reported from virtually all swine-raising areas of the world. All ages of pigs may be affected, but the typical case of septicemia and meningoencephalitis occurs in nursing pigs and in weaned pigs, particularly in the 8- to 12-week age group. The incidence varies greatly within an infected herd and among herds under differing environmental and management conditions.

S. suis has been isolated from other animals, including cattle and horses. Infection in human beings, particularly meningitis, is well documented. People associated with swine production and the handling of pork are at greatest risk.

In pigs the organism gains entry by the mouth and nose and colonizes the palatine tonsils. Following colonization, *S. suis* can be transported to distant sites, including the central nervous system, using mononuclear cells as vehicles. As many as 100 per cent of a herd may harbor *S. suis* in their tonsils, and these pigs are a constant source of infection for susceptible penmates.

Clinical Signs

Pigs with overwhelming infection die suddenly. Preweaned pigs will stop nursing and become lethargic and recumbent. With meningitis, signs of central nervous system (CNS) disorder may be seen, including incoordination, paddling, and opisthotonos. This disease may resemble pseudorabies, from which it must be differentiated. In more chronic stages, pigs may be left with residual CNS signs and lameness following septicemia of polyarthritis. Weaned pigs develop bronchopneumonia. This may be a pure infection or may involve other agents such as *Actinobacillus pleuropneumoniae*, *Pasteurella multocida*, or *Salmonella* species. *S. suis* has been recovered from aborted fetuses and the postpartum genital tract of sows.

Pathology

No gross lesions are seen in pigs dying peracutely; in those which survive longer, the common finding is a fibrinopurulent exudative polyserositis. Different strains and serotypes of the organism vary in pathogenicity and tissue tropism. Meningoencephalitis is a common finding but may not be noticed except on histopathologic examination. Polyarthritis, meningitis, bronchopneumonia, and polyserositis may occur individually or concurrently. Less common lesions of young pigs include pericarditis, myocarditis, and valvular endocarditis.

Diagnosis

Confirmation of *S. suis* infection must rely on postmortem and microbiologic examinations. As mentioned, the spectrum of clinical signs allows this infection to be confused with other viremic and septicemic diseases causing meningitis, polyserositis, pneumonia, and arthritis. *S. equisimilis*, *Hemophilus parasuis*, *A. pleuropneumoniae*, and pseudorabies virus are possible alternate or concurrent diagnoses. *S. suis* may be confused with closely related streptococci. Accurate identification should include serologic, morphologic, and biochemical criteria.

Tissue sections from a variety of organs, including the brain and meninges, tonsil, lung, parenchymatous organs, and synovial membranes should be fixed in buffered formalin for histopathologic study. Large blocks of the same tissues should be transported to the laboratory at 4°C for microbiologic analysis.

Treatment

Treatment includes good nursing care and specific antibiotic therapy. Weaned pigs with clinical signs should be moved to a hospital pen with clean and dry bedding, adequate heat, and ventilation. Severely affected pigs should be given more intensive nursing, including hand feeding, or be euthanized for necropsy.

While most reports indicate *S. suis* isolates are susceptible to penicillin, ampicillin, and trimethoprim-sulfonamide, their susceptibility to other antibiotics is much more variable. In a recent study, 43 per cent of 122 *S. suis* isolates were only moderately sensitive (minimum inhibitory concentration [MIC] 0.25 to 2.0 μg/mL) and 6 per cent were resistant (MIC 4.0 μg/mL) to penicillin. Therefore it is important to have susceptibility tests done to ensure appropriate antibiotic selection. Because *S. suis* is widely distributed in various tissues, the higher end of the dosage range should be used. Procaine penicillin at 10 to 20,000 IU/kg intramuscularly once a day (s.i.d.) or b.i.d. or ampicillin at 10 mg/kg body weight intramuscularly t.i.d. have been used.

Prevention

There are at least three avenues for the control of *S. suis* infection: management techniques, antibiotics, and vaccines. However, because of its sporadic nature, the disease can be frustrating to control. The use of management practices that reduce stress and exposure to *S. suis* must precede and accompany any other control measures. Problems with overcrowding and air quality must be corrected. Pigs from different age groups or sources should not be mixed, and an all-in–all-out management system should be used. *S. suis* may survive for several days, even weeks, in feces and dust at cool temperatures. It is readily killed by most commercial disinfectants. Pest control, particularly flies, must be an integral part of a hygiene program.

Feed-mixed antimicrobials have been used as a means of controlling infection during peak risk times, such as the moving and commingling of pigs, or to control the spread of an enzootic. Once again, selection of antimicrobials must be based on susceptibility testing. Neither antibiotics nor immunization can be expected to eliminate the infection of carrier pigs.

Commercial and autogenous vaccines are now in use. Since protection is serotype specific, vaccine components must correlate with on-farm strains. Some practitioners find autogenous vaccines to be more effective than commercial vaccines. This suggests that there may be antigens, in addition to those associated with type specificity, that are significant in protection.

Eradication of the infection on a premises may be attempted by depopulation and thorough cleaning and disinfection followed by a rest period of at least 6 weeks. The problem arises with repopulation, as most herds have carrier animals, and methods for detection of infected pigs are unreliable.

Streptococcus porcinus

Cervical lymphadenitis (jowl abscess) has been a major cause of carcass trim or condemnation in the North American swine industry. The cause of this disease is a group E, beta-hemolytic streptococcus now called *S. porcinus*. Interestingly, this disease is not of economic importance in other countries in spite of its presence in those swine herds. These same streptococci may be found in a variety of other lesions such as arthritis, pericarditis, and encephalitis, but the frequency and economic significance of these infections are low.

The development of abscesses may be accompanied by pyrexia, inappetance, and a neutrophilia, but the systemic effects are minimal. Palpable thick-walled abscesses develop in the throat region and may rupture.

Abscesses in pigs may be caused by a variety of streptococcal and nonstreptococcal agents. Aspirates, carefully collected to avoid contamination, are inoculated on selective media. Identification of *S. porcinus* requires biochemical and serologic procedures.

Well-formed abscesses and the infection in carrier pigs are unlikely to respond to antibiotic therapy. Group E streptococcal infections have been controlled in young pigs by adding antibiotics to starter feed. The tetracyclines have been suggested, but antibiotic selection should be based on susceptibility testing. An avirulent oral vaccine given to postweaned pigs protected more than 90 per cent of those challenged.

OTHER STREPTOCOCCAL INFECTIONS

A variety of other streptococci may cause sporadic infections of pigs. *S. equisimilis* and group L streptococci are commonly associated with a wide variety of pyogenic infections of pigs, including meningitis, otitis, pneumonia, arthritis, endocarditis, abscesses, septicemia, and pyoderma. These infections are most commonly seen in young pigs. A syndrome of ear necrosis is also seen in young pigs from which streptococci are isolated, often in combination with staphylococci. Endometritis and abortion is yet another syndrome attributable to these streptococci.

Antibiotics, particularly penicillin or ampicillin, are used in treatment as previously described. Multivalent bacterins containing *S. equisimilis* are available but may provide limited protection.

S. durans has been associated with enteritis in dogs, foals, and pigs. The organism is isolated in essentially pure culture from the intestine of affected animals. In these infections numerous gram-positive cocci are seen closely adherent to the brush border of villus enterocytes on histologic examination. The significance and prevalence of this infection are not known.

BIBLIOGRAPHY

Clifton-Hadley FA: The epidemiology, diagnosis, treatment and control of *Streptococcus suis* type 2 infection. Proc Ann Mtg Am Assoc Swine Pract 471–491, 1986.
Higgins R, Gottschalk M: An update on *Streptococcus suis* identification. J Vet Diagn Invest 2:249–252, 1990.
Soback S: Mastitis therapy—past, present and future. *In* International Symposium on Bovine Mastitis, Indianapolis. Arlington, VA, National Mastitis Council, 1990, pp 244–251.
Watts JL: Etiological agents of bovine mastitis. Vet Microbiol 16:41–66, 1988.

Staphylococcal Diseases

LUC A. DEVRIESE, DVM

Staphylococcal infections in animals are of a very diverse nature, and different staphylococcal species may act as etiologic agents. In food animals *S. aureus* is involved most often. *S. hyicus* is a cause of certain skin infections in pigs and cattle, and several other staphylococcal species, such as *S. chromogenes, S. simulans, S. epidermidis, S. warneri*, and *S. caprae*, cause subclinical mastitis in cattle and goats. These bacteria have more limited disease-causing abilities than *S. aureus*. The pathogenicity of staphylococci and especially of *S. aureus* is based on a complex and poorly understood array of virulence factors rather than on a single or dominant toxin.

EPIZOOTIOLOGY

Most *S. aureus* strains belong to biotypes or ecovars that usually colonize and infect distinct host species. Strains can be assigned to a human, a bovine, an ovine, a poultry, or a hare or rabbit biotype. Some animal hosts, such as chickens, turkeys, and sheep, are colonized almost exclusively by a single biotype, while others, such as cattle and pigs, are colonized by several biotypes. Human biotype strains rarely infect animals, and animal strains rarely infect humans.

Staphylococci are closely associated with their animal and human hosts, but they may survive to some extent away from body surfaces. They commonly do not act as infectious agents that enter and spread through a group or herd. Most probably they are transmitted from parent to young and persist in the nares or other body orifices of all or many individuals of a group. The possibility that certain epidemic strains occur in animal herds as they do in human hospitals cannot be excluded, however. In ruminants the teat skin is a common carrier site. The intact hairy skin appears to be devoid of *S. aureus*. The bacteria are seeded from their usual carrier sites on body surfaces and may gain entry and proliferate in superficial wounds, abrasions, or insect bites. They are the most common starting points of staphylococcal disease.

S. hyicus apparently does not infect humans, and many other coagulase-negative species are also confined to animals.

CLINICAL SIGNS AND PATHOGENESIS

S. aureus and other staphylococci are commonly associated with infections of the skin and related tissues such as the udder. Hematogenous dissemination may result in acute septicemia and toxemia or in chronic abscesses in kidneys, joints, or other internal organs. The most important specific diseases will be discussed.

Staphylococcal Mastitis

Staphylococcal mastitis in ruminants is more often chronic and subclinical than clinical. Infections caused by the coagulase-negative species cause less severe lesions than *S. aureus* and are often self-curing. Infections caused by *S. aureus* may be peracute and gangrenous, but this is a rare form of disease that usually occurs in the postparturient period. The more common form of clinical *S. aureus* infection develops mostly without systemic symptoms except for a slight elevation of body temperature in the first stages of the disease.

Mastitis of sows is rarely caused by staphylococci. These bacteria do not seem to play a role in the mastitis-metritis-agalactia (MMA) syndrome of sows.

Exudative Epidermitis of Pigs and Cattle

Exudative epidermitis caused by *S. hyicus* affects mainly young pigs from a few days of age to a few months. The disease is characterized in its early stages by epidermolysis without purulent inflammation characteristic of most staphylococcal lesions. Other bacteria, often gram-negatives, gain entry into the lesions and complicate the picture. Skin function may become heavily affected, resulting in growth impairment. Internal lesions, typically urethral edema and arthritis, may also occur.

S. hyicus exudative epidermitis is clearly infectious, but the factors that favor the spread of this condition are unknown. The organism is present in virtually all pig herds, and differences in virulence between strains are not clear. The maternal immune status of the pigs may be of importance, as well as the more or less frequent occurrence of insect bites and small skin wounds.

S. hyicus is also involved in exudative skin conditions and much more rarely in joint infections of cattle. In moderate climates the bovine skin condition is secondary to mange.

Staphylococcosis in Sheep

The *S. aureus* subspecies *anaerobius* is the etiologic agent of Morel's abscess disease, a chronic condition involving abscedation of ganglia in the anterior part of the body and subcutaneous and intramuscular abscesses. The disease occurs in European Mediterranean countries, in Africa, and in Asia.

The common type of facultatively anaerobic *S. aureus* causes neonatal infections with focal suppurative myocarditis as the most consistent lesion. In mature sheep, periorbital eczema, a severe ulcerative pyoderma, can be seen, and in lambs staphylococcal folliculitis and "tick pyemia," an infection transmitted by tick bites resulting in septicemia, can occur.

DIAGNOSIS

Certain conditions, such as exudative epidermitis, are clinically very typical, but most others require laboratory examinations and culture for diagnosis. Gram's or fast hematologic stains can be helpful, but negative results do not exclude staphylococcal infection.

TREATMENT

Staphylococcal mastitis is notoriously difficult to treat. Results decrease with increasing number of lactations, duration of infection before treatment, and length of lactation period. These factors are more important than the type of antibiotic treatment given and the in vitro susceptibility of the infecting strain. Better results are obtained with dry cow treatment and development of strategies that aim to minimize the proliferation of *S. aureus* in a herd: general hygiene, including washing and disinfecting, teat dipping or spraying to reduce teat-end colonization, and maintenance and control of the milking equipment to avoid teat injury. Culling of chronic shedders and relapsing older cows is especially important.

Antibiotic treatment is most often by intramammary infusion. Systemic treatment with weakly basic antibiotics, such as spiramycin and lincomycin, may be useful in the first stages of the disease and, according to some investigators, also in chronic cases. In most countries a majority of bovine *S. aureus* produce exopenicillinases (β-lactamases), which affect penicillin G and the broad-spectrum penicillins ampicillin and amoxicillin. A slightly lowered response to systemic penicillin G therapy has been observed in mastitis caused by penicillinase producers, however. Similar comparative data on local treatment are not available, but cephalosporins, penicillinase-stable penicillins, and also amoxicillin combined with clavulanic acid, which counteracts penicillinase, are generally recommended. Rare human ecovar strains resistant to penicillinase-stable penicillins and cephalosporins, a special resistance type important in human nosocomial infections, have been observed in bovine mastitis, but these infections were self-limiting. Antibiotic treatment is further discussed in the article on mastitis.

Also in other types of staphylococcal infection, efficacy of antibiotic treatments is often impeded by antibiotic resistance. This is notably the case in porcine exudative epidermitis. Systemic macrolide or lincosamide treatments, which may give excellent results in uncomplicated cases, are totally ineffective in infections caused by in vitro resistant strains. Antibiotic susceptibility testing is indicated in these cases.

In skin as in mammary infections, all measures that decrease opportunities for staphylococcal proliferation outside carrier sites are important. Superficial skin damage caused by trauma or exoparasites should be controlled. Staphylococci are susceptible to the commonly used disinfectants, and their use can be helpful in the prevention of skin infections. Systemic and local antibiotic treatments used in veterinary medicine are unable to eliminate in vitro susceptible staphylococci from carrier sites. They may suppress the staphylococcal flora temporarily.

The incidence of surgical staphylococcal infections is strongly influenced by surgical techniques. Low numbers of bacteria may cause infection when foreign bodies, such as inert particles, prostheses, or catheters, are present, but relatively high numbers are needed to cause infection in clean wounds or incisions. Also, occlusion favors superficial staphylococcal skin infection.

BIBLIOGRAPHY

Anderson EC: Veterinary aspects of staphylococci. *In* Easmon CSF, Adlam C (eds): Staphylococci and Staphylococcal Infections. London and New York, Academic Press, 1983, pp 193–241.

Devriese LA: Staphylococci in healthy and diseased animals. J Appl Bacteriol 69(Suppl):71S–80S, 1990.

Swine Erysipelas
JERRY P. KUNESH, DVM, MS, PhD

Erysipelas of swine is a contagious disease caused by *Erysipelothrix rhusiopathiae*, a bacterium that also infects many other species that may be a source of infection to swine. The most common of these are mice, pigeons, sparrows, and blackbirds. Turkeys, cattle, sheep, goats, horses, and many others may also be infected. Distribution of the disease is worldwide, but regional differences are recognized. The factors that predispose swine to infection are not well understood.

CLINICAL SIGNS

Acute erysipelas is characterized by elevated temperature of 41°C or higher and depression. When disturbed, affected animals are irritable and noticeably lame. Abortions may be observed. Occasionally, individual pigs may be found dead without observed illness. Generally, inappetence and other symptoms of illness will be observed. As the disease process progresses, raised rhomboid erythematous skin lesions may be observed.

Subacute forms of this disease present the same clinical signs in a mild form, while chronic forms are characterized by lameness and varying degrees of arthritis.

PATHOLOGIC CHANGES

Rhomboid skin lesions are generally considered to be pathognomonic, but similar lesions have been reported in pigs with septicemia caused by *Actinobacillus suis*. All other lesions, that is, enlarged spleen, hemostasis, and hemorrhagic lymph nodes, are associated with septicemia and are not specific for swine erysipelas. In the chronic forms, vegetative endocarditis and lesions of arthritis are suggestive of swine erysipelas.

DIAGNOSIS

The arthritic form of the disease must be differentiated from streptococcal, staphylococcal, and mycoplasmal infections. In rare cases *Actinomyces pyogenes* or *Brucella* may present a similar clinical picture. In the absence of rhomboid skin lesions, bacterial cultures are necessary to differentiate erysipelas from other septicemic conditions. Although possibly rare, *A. suis* should be considered, even in the presence of typical skin lesions.

TREATMENT

Penicillin is considered to be the drug of choice. Recommended dosage is 10,000 to 20,000 IU/kg body weight. Other antibiotics that are effective include ceftiofur, 3.0 mg/kg; lincomycin, 10.0 mg/kg; tylosin, 4.5 to 9 mg/kg; and oxytetracycline, 10 to 20 mg/kg, depending on product used.

The foregoing should be injected intramuscularly so that therapeutic levels are sustained for 4 to 5 days. Any of the tetracyclines or lincomycin may be used for herd treatment by incorporation into the feed or water, in accordance with label directions, as an adjunct to individual treatment. In all cases the preslaughter withdrawal period must be observed to avoid tissue residues.

Antiserum is available and may be used for herd treatment. More commonly antiserum use is restricted to suckling or recently weaned piglets and is according to label directions in conjunction with injectable penicillin.

PREVENTION AND CONTROL

Prevention of erysipelas on farms or in areas where the disease is a problem is best accomplished by using either bacterins or attenuated live immunizing agents. Breeding stock should be immunized twice annually. Market animals immunized before 4 weeks of age should be revaccinated after 6 weeks of age if protection is to last until the animals are marketed.

Erysipelas can be avoided by following a systematic immunization program, purchasing replacement stock from herds where the disease has not occurred, using good sanitation and disinfecting procedures, and protecting feed supplies from contamination by soil or feces.

BIBLIOGRAPHY

Wood RL: Erysipelas. *In* Leman AD, Straw BE, Glock RD, et al (eds): Diseases of Swine, 6th ed. Ames, IA, University of Iowa Press, 1986, pp 571–583.

Listeriosis (Circling Disease, Silage Sickness)
STANLEY M. DENNIS, BVSc, PhD, FRCVS, FRCPath

Listeriosis is an infectious disease caused by *Listeria monocytogenes*. In ruminants it is characterized primarily by encephalitis or abortion in adults and by septicemia in fetuses and neonates. In monogastric animals it is usually characterized by septicemia with focal hepatic necrosis. In ruminants, especially sheep, listeriosis has been called "circling disease" and, in Iceland, "silage sickness."

Listeriosis is worldwide in distribution and affects a wide variety of mammalian and avian species, including humans. It is more prevalent in temperate and colder climates.

ETIOLOGICAL AGENT

Two pathogenic species of *Listeria* are recognized. *L. monocytogenes* is the principal pathogen of animals and humans, and *L. ivanovii* is an occasional pathogen of animals and humans. Sixteen serovars have been identified in the genus *Listeria*. Common serovars in animals in the United States are 1 and 4b.

L. ivanovii (previously *L. monocytogenes* serovar 5) is pathogenic especially for pregnant sheep. It has been isolated from healthy animals, human carriers, the environment, and, very occasionally, ill people. It is characterized by wide zones of hemolysis on blood agar in contrast to the narrow zone of *L. monocytogenes*.

Listeria are small, motile, pleomorphic, gram-positive, nonsporing coccobacilli. *Listeria* strains grow well on usual bacterial media. Primary isolation of *Listeria* is better under microaerophilic conditions. *Listeria* grow under a wide temperature range, with the optimum temperature between 30 and 37°C. Its ability to grow at 4°C is important diagnostically and is the basis for the "cold enrichment" method for primary isolation of *Listeria* from suspected cases of listeric encephalitis. Brain suspensions are held at 4°C and cultured weekly. This procedure is not required for fetal or placental tissues in which *L. monocytogenes* or *L. ivanovii* are present in large numbers.

EPIZOOTIOLOGY

The natural habitat of *Listeria* is soil and the mammalian intestinal tract. Vegetation and silage become contaminated with soil and/or feces. Grazing animals, domestic and feral, ingest *Listeria* and further contaminate soil and vegetation, thereby establishing an ecologic listeric cycle. Animal-to-animal transmission by fecal-to-oral route occurs (Fig. 1). The most important transmitters are silage, grass, surface water, and dust. Animal-to-human transmission may occur directly or indirectly via milk, cheese, meat, eggs, vegetables, etc. Listeriosis is more of a geonosis or anthroponosis than a zoonosis. Animal and human infections go their own way, and cross-infection, such as an occupational infection, is probably accidental.

L. monocytogenes has been isolated from feces of healthy animals and humans. The majority of listeric infections are too mild to be recognized clinically and are inapparent or

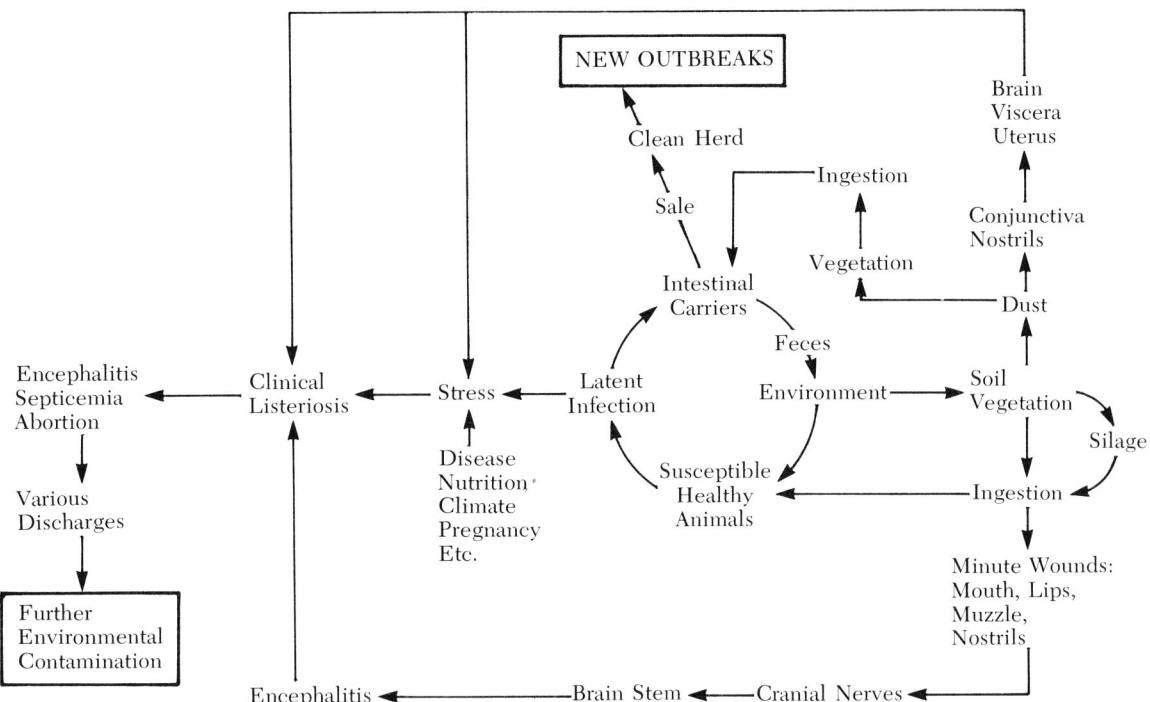

Figure 1. Animal-environment cycle of listerial infection in domestic animals.

latent. Asymptomatic intestinal carriers are common in all species.

Sporadic cases of listeric encephalitis are common. Over a period of months, up to 5 per cent of a cattle herd or 10 per cent of a sheep flock may become infected. Listeriosis is primarily a winter-spring disease. Confined sheep and cattle, especially those being fed silage, have a higher incidence than range animals. Listeriosis affects animals of all breeds, sexes, and ages.

Recovery of *Listeria* from milk of both mastitic and normal cows emphasizes the potential danger of milkborne listeriosis in animal and human populations. Excretion of *Listeria* in milk is usually intermittent but may persist for periods exceeding a single lactation. *Listeria* have also been isolated from the milk of sheep, goats, and women.

The distal intestinal tract is regarded as a reservoir from which *Listeria* are able to invade tissues when the body's defenses are impaired. The most important single source of both clinical and asymptomatic listeric infections is gross environmental contamination. *Listeria* can multiply in soil at 18 to 20°C. As a result it is present on many types of grass, hay, and other crops. In a cool, damp environment *Listeria* can survive in organic matter for years. Its survival is good in grass, soil, and silage of near-neutral pH but is poor in acid soil and good silage.

Listeria are saprophytes living in a plant-soil environment and can be contracted by animals and humans practically anywhere, especially in temperate climates. Outbreaks of listeriosis in sheep and cattle have been attributed to silage. Poor quality or poorly cured silage (pH 5.6 or greater) provides a favorable substrate for *Listeria* present on grass or crops to grow. Pit silage appears to be involved more than that in tower-type silos, possibly by greater soil and fecal matter being introduced by tractors during filling and packing. Frequency of listeriosis tends to increase as the lower and damper layers of silage are consumed, shortly before animals are turned out to graze in spring. It is postulated that listeric-contaminated silage results in a large number of latent infections, often approaching 100 per cent of the herd or flock, but clinical listeriosis develops in only a few animals.

L. monocytogenes has high infectivity but low pathogenicity, and clinical *Listeria* infection is usually not manifested unless the host's resistance is reduced by various stress factors, intercurrent disease, or pregnancy. Asymptomatic intestinal carriers from infected herds or flocks disseminate listeric infection to clean herds or flocks upon their introduction.

PATHOGENESIS

The initial route of exposure is ingestion of *Listeria*-contaminated soil, vegetation, or silage. The prevalence of encephalitis or septicemia in a group of animals during an outbreak of listeriosis under different environmental conditions suggests that *Listeria* gain entry by several routes: encephalitis via minute wounds in buccal mucosa, inhalation, or conjunctival contamination; or septicemia and latent infection by ingestion and inhalation. *L. monocytogenes* has a predilection to localize in the intestinal wall, placenta, and medulla oblongata.

Listeria encephalitis is essentially a local infection of the brain stem resulting from *L. monocytogenes* ascending via cranial nerves. Susceptible animals are exposed to *L. monocytogenes* in contaminated feed, especially silage. Grass and grain awns can result in abrasions and small puncture wounds in the buccal mucosa, lips, muzzle, and nostrils. *Listeria* penetrate these tissues innervated by cranial nerves, especially the trigeminal, and migrate along one or more branches to the medulla oblongata and pons. The lesions are confined to the brain, and the clinical signs vary according to the functions of the damaged neurons. The selective localization of *L. monocytogenes* in the brain stem is often unilateral and accounts for the signs of facial paralysis and circling.

Septicemic or visceral listeriosis affects organs other than the brain, and the principal manifestations are visceral lesions, especially hepatic, and placentitis with abortion. *Listeria* invading the body orally tend to localize in the intestinal wall, especially in Peyer's patches, and result in inapparent listeric infection and prolonged fecal excretion; in some cases bacteremia with localization in various organs or even a fatal septicemia may develop. *Listeria* may be excreted to the external environment in feces, milk, tears, nasal secretion, urine, and uterine discharge and perpetuate the listeric infection cycle.

The placenta of all pregnant domestic animals is highly susceptible to listeric infection and results in placentitis, fetal death, abortion, stillbirths, neonatal deaths, and possibly viable carriers. The uterus is extensively involved only when fetal and placental tissues are retained. Although *Listeria* metritis is constant, it has little or no lasting effect on reproductive function, but *Listeria* may be shed for a month or more. Sporadic abortions resulting from some stress during pregnancy and from development of listeric congenital infection in individual animals are more likely than a herd or flock pathogen spreading horizontally and causing abortion epizootics.

Listeria encephalitis and *Listeria* abortion rarely occur together.

CLINICAL SIGNS

Clinical *Listeria* infection is generally associated with characteristic syndromes in various groups of susceptible animals: encephalitis in adult ruminants, septicemia in swine and neonatal ruminants, and abortion and perinatal mortality in all species, especially ruminants. Infection is more common in ruminants fed silage.

Ruminants

Encephalitis is the most frequently recognized form of listeric infection and is of economic importance. It affects sheep, cattle, goats, and occasionally pigs and generally occurs in winter and early spring. Although both sexes and all ages are affected, it is more common during the first 3 years of life. The morbidity rate is low, but mortality is high.

Listeria encephalitis in sheep and goats is acute, with death occurring as early as 4 to 48 hours after onset of clinical signs, and recovery is rare. In cattle the disease is more chronic, with most surviving for 4 to 14 days. Spontaneous recovery is frequent, but recovered animals often have long-lasting brain damage.

Clinical signs of *Listeria* encephalitis in ruminants are similar but may differ in severity. The incubation period is unknown, probably 2 to 3 weeks. Affected animals become depressed, disoriented, febrile, indifferent to their surroundings, and usually separate themselves from the rest of the flock or herd. In the early stages, affected animals tend to crowd into corners and lean or push their heads against stationary objects, such as mangers and fences, as if unable to stand. Facial paralysis with dropping ear, dilated nostril, and lowered eyelid on the affected side often develop, more commonly in cattle than sheep. Torticollis may develop. Often, intermittent twitching and paralysis of facial and throat muscles and tongue, which usually protrudes, interfere with swallowing, resulting in profuse salivation. Marked nasal discharge and anorexia are common. Strabismus and conjunctivitis are also common, and an animal may appear blind. If it walks, it stumbles and moves in circles, always in the same direction. Paralysis of limbs is progressive. In the terminal stages the animal falls and is unable to rise without assistance. Prostration followed by coma and death may develop rapidly. During recumbency and even in coma, the affected animal lies constantly on the same side despite attempts to change it to the other side. Deaths cease suddenly when sheep are turned out to pasture.

Primary *Listeria* septicemia in adult ruminants, usually sheep, is reported in Europe and is relatively rare in the United States. The affected animals have general weakness, inappetence, and respiratory distress. The mortality is not as high as that resulting from listeric encephalitis. *L. monocytogenes* has been isolated from the conjunctival sac of cows and calves with keratoconjunctivitis and from mastitic milk. Listeriosis has been incriminated in diarrhea in dairy cows.

Listeria encephalitis is rarely observed in neonatal lambs and calves before the rumen becomes functional. In these neonates listeric infection is manifested by septicemia similar to that in monogastric animals.

Swine

Listeria infection in swine is uncommon. It results in septicemia, encephalitis, localized internal abscesses, and pox-like skin lesions. Mixed infections with hog cholera, erysipelas, and influenza are reported.

Listeriosis in swine is usually septicemic, with sudden anorexia, coughing, and respiratory distress. In piglets the main signs are depression, fever, prostration, and death. Encephalitis has been reported in older pigs. Signs of central nervous system (CNS) disturbances include trembling, incoordination, caudal paralysis, stilted gait of the forelegs, and progressive weakness followed by death. Infection during pregnancy may be followed by abortion.

Listeriosis in swine, either septicemic or encephalitic, usually runs a rapid and fatal course of 3 to 4 days. The majority of swine listeric infections, however, apparently do not manifest clinical signs, and outbreaks are usually self-limiting.

Pregnant Animals

Regardless of animal species, stage of gestation, or route of infection, the uterine contents quickly become infected with *L. monocytogenes*. Most listeric abortions occur in the last trimester but may occur at any stage of gestation. Near term, the fetus may be stillborn, born alive and die in a few hours or days, or survive. No premonitory signs of abortion are observed, and most dams exhibit little or no signs of general infection and spontaneously recover. The abortion rate in sheep is reported to range from 1 to 20 per cent, with the average being about 10 per cent. Abortion in sheep occurs within 3 to 11 days after exposure, depending on the route of infection.

NECROPSY FINDINGS

There are no gross lesions in animals dying from *Listeria* encephalitis apart from some congestion of meningeal vessels and an increase in cerebrospinal fluid. Microscopic lesions are confined primarily to the pons, medulla, and anterior spinal cord. Marked perivascular cuffing of mononuclear cells and varying degrees of focal necrosis develop. In sheep and goats, neutrophils predominate in the necrotic foci, resulting in microabscesses. There is edema, hemorrhage, neuron degeneration, neuronophagia, congestion, and some thrombi. In cattle the perivascular cuffs are smaller and the focal lesions are usually limited to edema and small accumulations of microglial cells and lymphocytes. Rarely are lesions as extensive as those in sheep—an observation in keeping with the more chronic nature of bovine encephalitis.

In septicemic listeriosis, small necrotic foci may be found in any viscera, especially liver.

L. monocytogenes has been recovered from acute or chronic cases of bovine mastitis and keratoconjunctivitis.

Fetuses aborting from listeric placentitis may be slightly to markedly autolytic. There is excess fluid in the serous cavities, clear to blood tinged; some fibrin in the abdominal cavity; and numerous small necrotic foci, up to 2 mm in diameter, in the liver, especially the right half. These lesions are usually not masked by autolysis, grossly or microscopically. Necrotic foci may also be found in other organs, such as lungs and spleen. Shallow erosions, 1 to 3 mm in diameter, may be present in the abomasal mucosa. Gram-stained smears of abomasal contents revealed numerous gram-positive, pleomorphic coccobacilli.

DIAGNOSIS

Listeria encephalitis is diagnosed by typical CNS signs and laboratory findings: circling, lateral inclination of the head, and facial paralysis. These signs, especially in sheep and cattle fed silage, suggest listeriosis. When encephalitis occurs in cattle and results in death, prompt examination should be made for both listeriosis and rabies. In sheep, not cattle, listeric encephalitis is confirmed by finding the characteristic microabscesses in the midbrain.

Listeria encephalitis must be differentiated from other diseases, such as those listed in Table 1.

Listeria abortion must be differentiated from other causes of abortion, such as brucellosis, campylobacteriosis, salmonellosis, infectious bovine rhinotracheitis, enzootic ovine abortion, leptospirosis, and parvovirus, depending on species affected.

Listeria infection is confirmed by isolating and identifying *L. monocytogenes*. Difficulties are often encountered in isolating *Listeria* from fresh tissues, especially brain. Direct-stained smears, especially of fetal or placental tissues, may reveal large numbers of pleomorphic, gram-positive, small rods suggestive of listeriosis. Fluorescent antibody techniques are effective for rapidly diagnosing and identifying *L. monocytogenes* in smears from animals dead or aborted from listeriosis, and from milk and meat.

Serologic procedures are being used more for diagnosing listeriosis, but their value in animals has not been established.

Hematologic examination is of little value in ruminants.

TREATMENT

Listeria are sensitive to many antibiotics, especially ampicillin, erythromycin, and rifampicin. Ampicillin has low toxicity and provides an effective level in cerebrospinal fluid. Penicillin in high doses is the most economic antibiotic for food animals.

Early treatment is important, before onset of severe CNS signs. Prognosis for *Listeria* encephalitis depends on duration and severity of clinical signs before treatment; if the animal is recumbent, treatment is of little use. Penicillin in high doses intramuscularly (44,000 units/kg, b.i.d.) for 7 to 14 days and then half dosage for another 7 to 14 days is effective in cattle. Dehydration, acid-base imbalances, and electrolyte disturbances must be corrected. Supportive therapy such as nursing, analgesics, vitamin E–selenium, and ruminal content transfer may be required.

Treatment is less effective in sheep, as *Listeria* encephalitis progresses more rapidly in this species and is usually advanced before detection. Initially penicillin (44,000 units/kg) should be administered intravenously and then intramuscularly b.i.d. for 7 to 10 days. With *Listeria* abortion, long-acting penicillin intramuscularly may be effective prophylactically. Penicillin or chloramphenicol and penicillin have been reported to be successful in septicemic listeriosis.

Corticosteroids are contraindicated in the treatment of listeriosis.

IMMUNITY

Immunologic protection against listeriosis is primarily cell mediated. A recent study suggested humoral immunity was also a factor in the clinical course of infection in goats and in the elimination of *Listeria* from the gastrointestinal tract.

Formol and heat-killed *Listeria* vaccines give poor protection. Good results with live attenuated vaccines in sheep have been reported from Bulgaria, Germany, Norway, and Russia. The Bulgarian vaccine contains two attenuated strains of *L. monocytogenes*, serovars 1/2 and 4b. Healthy sheep over 3 months of age, including pregnant ewes, are given 2 ml (approximately 4×10^9 organisms) subcutaneously, and protective immunity results within 2 weeks and lasts for at least 10 months. Annual revaccination is recommended in those countries where the vaccine is cost-effective.

CONTROL

Institution of general principles for controlling infectious diseases and good hygiene are the only control measures available in North America at present. When listeriosis has broken out, affected animals should be isolated and treated and dead animals disposed of as quickly as possible by a rendering plant or preferably by burning or burying deeply under quicklime. Buildings housing affected or in-contact animals should be thoroughly cleaned and disinfected, and all contaminated or suspected bedding and feed burned.

Reduce silage feeding and avoid feeding any spoiled silage. In affected feedlots, constant feeding of low-level tetracyclines may be beneficial.

Animals with nonfatal *Listeria* infection or those recovering following antibiotic therapy may be carriers for long periods and should therefore probably be eliminated. Some lactating cows with listeriosis may excrete *Listeria* via their milk for long periods and are a public health hazard.

Table 1. DIFFERENTIAL DIAGNOSIS OF *LISTERIA* ENCEPHALITIS

Cattle	Sheep	Swine
Rabies	Rabies	Rabies
Lead poisoning	Polioencephalomalacia	Aujeszky's disease
Ketosis	Pregnancy toxemia	Hog cholera
Acute gastroenteritis	Brain abscess	Erysipelas
Aujeszky's disease	Gid	Intoxications
Viral encephalitis		Influenza
		Nutritional disturbances

BIBLIOGRAPHY

Gray ML, Killinger AH: *Listeria monocytogenes* and listeric infections. Bacteriol Rev 30:309, 1966.
Gudding R, Nesse LL, Gronstol H: Immunization against infections caused by *Listeria monocytogenes* in sheep. Vet Rec 125:111, 1989.
Miettinen A, Husu J, Tuomi J: Serum antibody response to *Listeria monocytogenes*, listerial excretion, and clinical characteristics in experimentally infected goats. J Clin Microbiol 28:340, 1990.
Rebhun WC, deLahunta A: Diagnosis and treatment of bovine listeriosis. J Am Vet Med Assoc 180:395, 1982.
Scarratt WK: Ovine listeric encephalitis. Comp Cont Educ Pract Vet 9:F28, 1987.

SECTION 9
Protozoal and Rickettsial Diseases

SAREL R. VAN AMSTEL, BVSc, MMed Vet (Med), Consulting Editor

Babesiosis

DANIËL THEODORUS DE WAAL, BVSc

DEFINITION

Babesiosis, also known as piroplasmosis, tick fever, redwater, Texas fever, splenic fever, and tristeza, is a tick-borne disease of cattle, sheep, goats, and swine caused by intra-erythrocytic protozoan parasites of the genus *Babesia*. The disease is characterized by fever, erythrocyte destruction resulting in anemia, anorexia, hemoglobinuria in certain instances, icterus, occasionally central nervous system involvement, and death in severe cases.

EPIDEMIOLOGY

Babesiosis has a worldwide distribution that corresponds to the distribution of the vector ticks. The prevalence of ticks responsible for the transmission of babesiosis and anaplasmosis in cattle is one of the most important factors hindering the introduction of more productive livestock and the upgrading of existing livestock in the developing countries. Babesiosis in cattle is of major economic importance and is discussed mainly, with brief reference to babesiosis in other species.

Etiologic Agents, Vectors, and Distribution

Babesiosis in cattle is primarily caused by 4 *Babesia* spp. The most important are *Babesia bovis* and *Babesia bigemina*; both have a worldwide distribution including large parts of Africa, southern Europe, southern Asia, Australia, and Central and South America as well as many islands in the Caribbean and South Pacific. Their distribution corresponds to the occurrence of their 1-host tick vectors *Boophilus microplus*, *Boophilus decoloratus*, and *Boophilus annulatus*.

Babesia divergens, transmitted by the 3-host tick *Ixodes ricinus*, has been reported throughout northern Europe including Ireland, Scotland, and western England.

Babesia major, usually less pathogenic than the other bovine *Babesia*, occurs in essentially the same temperate zones in which *Babesia divergens* is found and is transmitted by the 3-host tick *Haemaphysalis punctata*. It has, however, also been reported from Africa, Israel, South America, and the Soviet Union.

Transmission

Babesia organisms are transmitted by ticks only, and mechanical transmission does not occur. Non–vector-borne transmission, such as intrauterine or iatrogenic infection, is epidemiologically insignificant.

Babesia follow a highly specific pathway of infection in certain tick stages, depending on the species involved. Engorging female ticks usually acquire the infection, after which the *Babesia* erythrocytic stages undergo transformation into sexual stages and finally into sporokinetes in the gut of the replete female tick. This is followed by transovarial transmission. Depending on the *Babesia* and tick species, larvae, nymphae, or adults of the next generation can then transmit the infection.

The Host

European *(Bos taurus)*, Sanga, and Zebu *(Bos indicus)* breeds are all susceptible to babesiosis, but *Bos indicus* and their crosses with *Bos taurus* often possess appreciable resistance. After recovery, a latent infection usually develops, which may persist for variable periods.

Calves under 2 months of age from previously unexposed cows are highly susceptible to the infection and its effects, whereas the offspring of immune mothers are resistant. This is presumably because of a passive transfer of immunity via the colostrum. After the age of 2 months, all calves develop a natural, nonspecific, innate resistance that persists for at least a further 4 to 6 months and is not dependent on the immune status of the cow.

Endemic (enzootic) stability is achieved in areas where all calves are frequently exposed to the parasite while they are still protected by colostral and innate immunity (i.e., first 6 to 9 months of age). Under such conditions, clinical babesiosis is minimal. However, endemic instability occurs if some animals fail to become infected for prolonged periods after birth. Such animals remain susceptible, and when they are infected as adults, severe clinical reactions can occur. Various factors, such as changes in climatic conditions and frequency of acaricidal treatment, can influence the tick populations and therefore the enzootic stability in a region.

Mortality among imported susceptible cattle can be as high as 50 per cent. Other indirect losses can occur through weight loss, loss in milk production, abortions, and temporary infertility in animals surviving acute babesiosis.

Babesia Infection in Other Animal Species

Babesia infections in sheep, goats, and swine are of lesser importance as a cause of clinical disease and have a limited distribution.

In sheep, 2 species occur, *Babesia mortasi* (large) and *Babesia ovis* (small). These are transmitted by tick species of the genera *Haemaphysalis, Rhipicephalus, Ixodes,* and *Dermacentor*. These parasites have been recorded from Europe, the Middle East, the Soviet Union, Asia, and parts of Africa. *Babesia ovis* has been incriminated as the cause of severe disease in sheep in southern Europe, Turkey, and Iran.

Babesia trautmanni (large) may be a severe pathogen of pigs and has been recorded from the Soviet Union, southern Europe, and Africa. *Babesia perroncitoi* is a small *Babesia* with a distribution limited to the Sudan, Italy, and North Africa. The vector of *B. trautmanni* has been identified as being *Rhipicephalus simus* (D. T. de Waal and L. M. López Rebollar, unpublished observations, 1990). The vectors of *B. perroncitoi* are still unknown.

CLINICAL SIGNS

Clinical signs associated with *Babesia* infections are influenced by the susceptibility of the host. This, in turn, is influenced by factors such as age, breed, and environmental stress as well as the species or strain of *Babesia* involved. The incubation period varies from 2 to 3 weeks after tick infestation.

Clinical signs include fever ($\geq 40°$ C), which is usually present for several days before other signs develop such as anorexia, depression, weakness, dehydration, and sometimes icterus. Hemoglobinuria occurs earlier and more consistently during the course of infections with *B. bigemina* than with *B. bovis*. Cerebral babesiosis develops in some *B. bovis* infections and is characterized by a variety of signs related to the central nervous system, which include hyperesthesia, nystagmus, circling, head pressing, aggression, convulsions, and coma. The outcome is almost invariably fatal.

In subacute infection, the symptoms are less pronounced and are often difficult to detect. Calves infected before 9 months of age often develop an inapparent form of the disease.

CLINICAL PATHOLOGY AND GENERAL PATHOLOGY

The pathogenesis of *Babesia* infection is highly complex, as evidenced by multisystemic involvement. Two events that occur in the host appear to play a central role in the pathogenesis of babesiosis, namely, the release of pharmacologically active substances and erythrocyte destruction.

In the case of *B. bovis* infections, proteases released by the parasites cause fibrinogen hydrolysis resulting in soluble fibrin complexes that adhere to infected erythrocyte membranes, with subsequent aggregation of these cells in the vasculature. This leads to circulatory stasis with anoxic degenerative changes particularly in the brain, kidney, and skeletal musculature.

Activation of plasma kallikrein coincides with multiplication of *B. bovis* parasites in the blood. Kallikrein produces increased vascular permeability and vasodilation, which can result in circulatory stasis and shock. Activation of the kinin system, coagulation, and the other vascular changes are not a feature in *B. bigemina* infections.

A macrocytic, hypochromic anemia resulting from intravascular hemolysis is a feature of *Babesia* infections. This results in a drop in the packed cell volume, which may fall to less than 10 per cent. In *B. bovis* infections, the initial fall in the packed cell volume is largely a result of the associated circulatory disturbances. The red blood cell count may decrease to less than $3 \times 10^6/mm^3$ and the total hemoglobin level to less than 50 g/L. Microscopic evidence of an anemic response is evident within a few days.

Damage to internal organs resulting from hypoxia is further complicated by the release of host protein, for example, hemoglobin and other tissue breakdown products that damage the kidneys and liver. This may be evident by an increase in the blood urea nitrogen, creatinine, aspartate transaminase, alanine transaminase, and lactic dehydrogenase. Proteinuria develops during the acute phase of the infection, and a metabolic and respiratory alkalosis develops as evidenced by increased bicarbonate levels and a lowered arterial blood carbon dioxide tension.

Death in acute cases frequently occurs within 5 to 7 days of the onset of clinical signs and is usually associated with the vascular and multiorgan changes described. Post-mortem changes associated with babesiosis include watery blood, a pale carcass, icterus, splenomegaly, hepatomegaly (yellow-brown in color), swollen dark-colored kidneys, partly congested lungs, lung edema (more common in *B. bigemina* infection), and dark red urine due to hemoglobinuria (more pronounced in *B. bigemina* infection). In the case of cerebral babesiosis, the gray matter of the cerebrum and cerebellum is congested and has a characteristically cherry-pink color.

Microscopic sludging of parasitized red blood cells in the peripheral circulation and evidence of vascular stasis are striking in acute *B. bovis* infections. Other lesions seen are hyaline casts in kidney tubular lumens with tubular epithelial necrosis, centrilobular hydropic or fatty degeneration of the liver, congestion of the sinusoids of the spleen, and a reduced ratio of white to red pulp. Lung edema and myocardial hemorrhages may also be evident.

In subacute cases, the carcass is pale and icteric with varying degrees of swelling and congestion of the internal organs.

DIAGNOSIS

The clinical signs, the history, and the geographic region are often suggestive of babesiosis but are not absolutely characteristic of the disease. Therefore microscopic demonstration of the parasite is necessary to confirm the diagnosis. It is also important for identifying the *Babesia* sp. involved because this can influence the control measures, treatment regimen, and prognosis. It can also provide data on the incidence of *Babesia* spp. for epidemiologic studies.

Peripheral blood collected from the tip of the tail is used to make both thick and thin blood smears. On post-mortem examination, blood or organ as well as brain smears should be made. Blood smears are allowed to air dry, the thin smears are fixed in methanol, and both thick and thin smears are then stained with use of the Romanovsky-type dyes, such as Giemsa, which usually gives the best results. In the interpretation of smears, recognition of the particular *Babesia* sp. is of primary importance because it is often necessary for determining whether the organism is associated with clinical disease. Low-level parasitemias are significant only if they are accompanied by clinical signs such as anemia.

Identification of the particular *Babesia* sp. involved is more difficult on post-mortem specimens because the organisms tend to assume a rounded-off appearance within a few hours after death. However, accumulations of parasites in organ smears or big differences in the parasitemias in the general and peripheral circulation are indicative of *B. bovis* infection.

The morphologic diversity of *Babesia* parasites can make it difficult to differentiate between them. *B. bovis* is a "small" *Babesia* measuring up to 2 μm in diameter. Single organisms are round, oval, or irregular in shape; paired forms are piriform or club-shaped with an obtuse angle between the paired merozoites. Large forms of *B. bovis* are, however, not uncommon.

B. bigemina is larger, around 4 to 5 × 2 to 3 μm, and can extend the full width of an erythrocyte. Single forms of *B. bigemina* are enlongated or ameboid in shape. Paired forms are piriform with an acute angle between the merozoites.

B. divergens is a piriform, paired, or club-shaped organism, smaller than *B. bovis*, and is around 1.5 to 2.0 × 0.4 μm. It frequently occurs on the margin of red blood cells.

B. major is very similar to but slightly smaller than *B. bigemina*.

A variety of serologic tests have been used to demonstrate the presence of antibodies to *Babesia* spp. The most commonly used include the complement fixation, indirect fluorescent antibody, indirect hemagglutination, radioimmunoassay, and enzyme-linked immunosorbent assay (ELISA) tests. Of these, the indirect fluorescent antibody test is the most popular. Some cross-reactions between *B. bovis* and *B. bigemina* have been observed, however, which makes accurate serologic differentiation difficult.

DIFFERENTIAL DIAGNOSIS

Babesiosis should be differentiated from anaplasmosis in animals showing anemia and icterus. Hemolysis, hemoglobinuria, and icterus may also occur in cattle suffering from leptospirosis as well as noninfectious conditions such as chronic copper poisoning and intoxicatious with *Brassica* and *Allium* spp. In Africa, cerebral babesiosis caused by *B. bovis* must be differentiated from nervous conditions of cattle, including heartwater, cerebral theileriosis, plant poisonings, chlorinated hydrocarbon, pesticide poisoning, and others.

PROGNOSIS

If the infection is treated early, the prognosis is good; however, when the pathologic changes are more advanced, the prognosis is guarded. Cerebral babesiosis is invariably fatal.

TREATMENT

In some areas, such as the United States, a successful *Boophilus* tick eradication program has led to the disappearance of cattle babesiosis. However, in vast areas of the world, including Africa, Asia, and Australia, ticks have not been eradicated and the disease persists and is controlled by a variety of measures including chemotherapy, chemoprophylaxis, vaccination, and tick control.

If specific treatment is given early in the course of bovine babesiosis, recovery usually takes place, but often animals are first seen when anemia, weakness, and neurologic signs are advanced. In these cases, supportive treatment is most important. If at all possible, animals should be made comfortable in a cool, shaded area with ready access to feed and water. Other supportive measures may include blood transfusions, fluid therapy, hematinics, and other symptomatic treatment as indicated. The animal's temperament, the location, and the stage of infection must also be taken into account. Fractious animals may best be left alone because exertion and excitement associated with restraint may contribute to death.

Treatment of babesiosis is usually directed toward moderating the clinical signs of fever and anemia associated with the infection. Some babesiacides are so specific and effective that one injection will eliminate the parasite from the host, which will then also eliminate the source of infection for ticks. This could be advantageous in cases in which total eradication of the disease is desired, but it is not recommended in endemic areas where re-exposure is likely. These drugs induce a sterile immunity that will persist for a variable period of time depending on the antigenic stimulus, which in turn is correlated with the level of parasitemia at the time of treatment. Animals exposed during this period of sterile immunity will become infected and may show varying degrees of illness.

The availability of babesiacides varies from country to country, depending on registration and import restrictions. The majority of drugs used in the treatment of babesiosis in cattle are listed in Table 1. The exact mode of action for most of the compounds is not as yet clear.

In acute *B. bovis* infections, large doses of corticosteroids and heparin may help offset the hypotensive and hypercoagulable state of the animal. In cases of cerebral babesiosis, intravenous use of osmotic diuretics such as mannitol and glucose may provide temporary relief.

PREVENTION

Eradication of tick vectors is probably the most desirable solution for the prevention of tick-borne diseases. For this approach to be successful, a good infrastructure is needed with the necessary funding, as well as support from local cattle producers. Tick eradication has been successful only in a very few countries in which ticks have made temporary incursions into environments ecologically unsuitable for their long-term survival, or in the case of a newly introduced species (e.g., *B. microplus* in Florida). In other regions, such as South America, Africa, Australia, Asia, and Europe, where ticks are well established, their eradication as a method of preventing babesiosis is economically unjustifiable. The development of acaricidal resistance with intensive chemical tick control also remains a problem, whereas the presence of alternative hosts (such as game) inordinately complicates tick eradication. The alternative approach of allowing natural endemic stability to develop by limiting the degree of tick control is the more practical one. It is now recognized by livestock industries in many of these areas that the long-term approach should be to integrate control measures with the strategic use of acaricides, the administration of vaccines in endemically unstable areas, and the use of tick-resistant cattle breeds.

Vaccines

The necessity to control other tick species inevitably affects the vectors of babesiosis and therefore the epidemiology of the disease.

With an effective vaccine, endemic stability can be created artificially by inoculating all the cattle in a herd. The most commonly used method for vaccination against babesiosis in cattle is inoculation with bovine blood containing live attenuated *Babesia* organisms. This method of vaccination has been successfully applied in areas such as Australia, South Africa, and Israel. These vaccines, however, have certain disadvantages that prohibit their wide use in many countries:

Table 1. DRUGS SUCCESSFULLY USED IN THE TREATMENT OF BABESIOSIS IN CATTLE

Drug	Dosage	Route of Administration	Uses	Disadvantages (Side Effects)
Trypan blue	2–3 mg/kg	IV	B. bigemina	Not effective against small babesias; discoloration of animal's flesh; can cause severe tissue sloughing if not given IV
Acridine derivatives Euflavine[1]	4–8 ml/100 kg as 5% solution	IV	B. bigemina B. bovis B. divergens	Highly irritant if not given IV
Diamidine derivatives Amicarbalide Diampron[1]	5–10 mg/kg	IM	B. bigemina B. divergens B. bovis	
Diminazene Berenil[2]	3–5 mg/kg	IM	B. bigemina B. bovis B. divergens	
Imidocarb Imizol[3]	1–3 mg/kg	SC or IM	B. bigemina B. bovis B. divergens	Prophylactic activity up to 8 weeks depending on dose and Babesia spp. involved; nephrotoxic; cholinesterase inhibitor; slowly metabolized and eliminated—tissue residues
Phenamidine Lomadine[1]	8–13.5 mg/kg	SC or IM	B. bigemina B. bovis	Cholinesterase inhibition
Quinoline derivatives Quinuronium Babesan[4]	1 mg/kg	SC	B. bigemina B. bovis B. divergens	Low therapeutic index Slow effect against B. bovis Side effects associated with the stimulation of the parasympathetic nervous system

IM = intramuscular; IV = intravenous; SC = subcutaneous.
[1]May & Baker Ltd., Dagenham, England.
[2]Hoechst, Frankfurt, Germany.
[3]Burroughs Wellcome & Co., London, England.
[4]ICI, Macclesfield, Cheshire, England.
Many of these preparations are sold under a variety of trade names. Consult publications such as Veterinary Pharmaceuticals and Biologicals, 6th ed. Lenexa, KS, Veterinary Medicine Publishing Co, 1989/1990.

- Elaborate facilities and skilled personnel are required to maintain donor cattle in tick-free conditions.
- The transmission of other pathogens to cattle is possible.
- The vaccines have a very short shelf life.
- The vaccines contain normal bovine proteins that could lead to hemolytic anemia (neonatal isoerythrolysis) in the suckling calf owing to the presence of antibodies in the colostrum of dams vaccinated with blood vaccines.

Continued efforts are therefore being made to develop other vaccines, including the following:

- The irradiation of B. bovis, B. divergens, and B. bigemina parasites at between 200 and 300 Gy resulted in some attenuation of the parasites. In most cases, a mild parasitemia developed with various degrees of immunity to challenge.
- A killed B. bigemina and B. bovis vaccine. Plasma from cattle infected with B. bigemina, B. bovis, and B. divergens engendered variable protection against homologous species challenge.
- Most research on babesial vaccines is now concentrated on the isolation of specific parasitic antigens for the development of a vaccine with recombinant technology.

Tick-Resistant Cattle

Tick resistance in cattle may be defined as the ability of cattle to limit the survival of the number of ticks feeding on them. This has been reported by many observers. Such resistance results in limited tick infestation, failure to complete their development (i.e., failure to engorge and produce fertile eggs), and an extended life cycle. On the whole, therefore, tick-resistant cattle appear to offer an effective means of controlling tick-borne diseases, in combination with other tick management systems.

Chemoprophylaxis

Imidocarb and diminazene are the only two babesiacides with useful prophylactic properties in the short-term control and prevention of babesiosis. Treatment with imidocarb (3 mg/kg) will prevent overt B. bovis infections for at least 4 weeks, B. bigemina infections for 8 weeks, and infections with B. divergens for about 2 weeks. Diminazene (3.5 mg/kg) will protect cattle against B. bovis and B. bigemina for 2 and 4 weeks, respectively. Because drugs cannot be administered periodically to cattle for their entire lifetime, chemoprophylaxis in endemic areas is realistic only if a protective asymptomatic infection can be induced when the rate of transmission of Babesia by ticks is of such a level as to ensure infection of all or most of the cattle while they are still protected by a suitable level of babesiacide.

BIBLIOGRAPHY

Callow LL: Animal Health in Australia, vol 5. Protozoal and Rickettsial Diseases. Canberra, Australian Bureau of Animal Health, 1984.
Joyner LP, Donnelly J: The epidemiology of babesial infections. Adv Parasitol 17:115–140, 1979.
Levine ND: Veterinary Protozoology. Ames, IA, Iowa State University Press, 1985.
Mahoney DF: Babesia of domestic animals. In Kreier JP (ed): Parasitic Protozoa, vol 4. New York, Academic Press, 1977, pp 1–51.
Ristic M, Ambroise-Thomas P, Kreier JP (eds): Malaria and Babesiosis. Research Findings and Control Measures. Dordrecht, Martinus Nijhoff Publishers, 1984.
Ristic M, Kreier JP (eds): Babesiosis. New York, Academic Press, 1981.
Ristic M (ed): Babesiosis of Domestic Animals and Man. Boca Raton, FL, CRC Press, 1988.
Zwart D, Brocklesby DW: Babesiosis: non-specific resistance, immunological factors and pathogenesis. Adv Parasitol 17:50–114, 1979.

Bovine Anaplasmosis

WILHELM HEINRICH STOLTSZ, BVSc

Bovine anaplasmosis is an infectious vector-borne disease of cattle caused by obligate intraerythrocytic rickettsia-like organisms of the genus *Anaplasma*. The disease is generally characterized by fever, inappetence, a drop in milk yield, progressive anemia, icterus, and constipation.

Three species of the causative organism occur in cattle, *A. marginale*, *A. centrale* and *A. caudatum*.[1] *A. marginale*, by far the most widely distributed *Anaplasma* sp., is the most pathogenic of the three, and infection in susceptible animals often leads to severe disease symptoms and mortality. *A. centrale*, which enjoys a far more limited natural distribution than does *A. marginale*, is less pathogenic and responsible for a relatively mild form of the disease in cattle. However, *A. centrale* may cause severe clinical reactions in susceptible adult cattle and should not be disregarded.

EPIDEMIOLOGY

Occurrence

Anaplasmosis caused by *A. marginale* has been reported from most tropical and subtropical parts of the world. It occurs in Europe bordering on the Mediterranean, the Middle and Far East, South America, the Caribbean, the Soviet Union, Australia, North America, and large parts of the African continent. *A. centrale* was isolated from a naturally infected bovine heifer in South Africa early in this century (1911) and has since been widely used in the form of a live blood vaccine for the protection of cattle against *A. marginale* infection. Because it has been demonstrated that the *A. centrale* vaccine strain remains tick-transmissible despite several decades of needle passage in cattle, this species may occur naturally in countries in which it has been used as a vaccine.

Susceptible Hosts

Although anaplasmosis is essentially a disease of cattle, potentially affecting animals of any age, breed, or sex, *Anaplasma* spp. are known to also infect a wide range of North American and African wild ruminant species. Infections in these hosts are usually inapparent. The importance of free-living wild ruminants as reservoir hosts of *Anaplasma* spp. pathogenic to cattle has not been fully investigated, yet it would appear that at least in Africa and North America, infections can be maintained indefinitely in these hosts in the absence of cattle. Sheep and goats, as well as certain wild ruminants, can be latently infected with *A. marginale* and the organism can be maintained in these animals by serial passage for lengthy periods, after which time some degree of attenuation apparently occurs.

Calves born to immune or nonimmune dams possess an innate resistance protecting them from severe clinical disease. This nonspecific resistance is probably greatest at the age of 6 months and tends to diminish with increasing age of the animal. Calves up to the age of 9 months or even 1 year usually show no clinical signs or develop only a mild form of the disease, whereas animals between 1 year and 2 years of age may develop acute, but rarely fatal, disease symptoms. Acute and occasionally fatal infections occur in cattle up to 3 years of age; in cattle older than 3 years, the disease is often peracute and frequently fatal. In endemic areas, without strict vector control, the majority of animals should become infected during the first year of their lives. This would lead to their developing long-term specific immunity, which should result in disease stability with minimal incidence of clinical disease in a herd.

Transmission

At least 20 tick species have been shown experimentally to be capable of transmitting anaplasmosis. These include argasid ticks (*Ornithodorus* spp. and *Argas persicus*) and a number of 1-host, 2-host, and 3-host ixodid tick species, of which *Boophilus* spp., *Dermacentor* spp., and *Rhipicephalus* spp. are regarded as the most important. Trans-stadial (larva to nymph or nymph to adult) and intrastadial transmission (e.g., transfer of male ticks between hosts) appear to be the usual modes of transmission employed by both 1-host and multihost ticks. The occasional reports of transovarial transmission are considered to be exceptional.

Mechanical transmission of anaplasmosis by hematophagous arthropods, particularly blood-sucking flies such as horseflies (*Tabanus* spp.), stable flies (*Stomoxys* spp.), and mosquitoes (*Psorophora* spp. and *Anopheles* spp.), is considered important in the maintenance of infection, even in the absence of tick vectors. Flies of the genera *Musca*, *Chrysops*, and *Siphora*, and eye gnats (*Hippelates* spp.) have also been incriminated as potential vectors. However, transmission is accomplished only if flies feeding on an infected host are transferred to a susceptible host with a delay of no more than a few minutes. Therefore, the risk of mechanical transmission by blood-sucking flies is greatest where cattle are maintained in close association with one another, such as in dairy herds and feedlots. However, ticks, which act as biologic vectors, are generally regarded as more important vectors than flies. It should be borne in mind that mechanical transmission can also take place by iatrogenic means, through the unsanitary use of instruments employed for vaccination, dehorning, castration, and tattooing that become contaminated with fresh infected blood.

There seems to be some disagreement among authors regarding the importance of transplacental transmission of anaplasmosis. Although many consider it to be an insignificant mode of transmission, intrauterine infection of calves was found under controlled experimental conditions to occur in up to 30.8 per cent of calves born to cows undergoing acute primary reactions during pregnancy and in 12.8 per cent of calves from carrier dams. Intrauterine infection may lead to fetal death and abortion, but most calves infected in utero never develop any detectable signs of anaplasmosis and can only be identified by serologic testing or biologically by the subinoculation of blood. It should therefore be considered an important factor in anaplasmosis eradication schemes directed at vector control only.

Incidence

Considering the fact that anaplasmosis can be transmitted by such a variety of means, it is not surprising that the disease is widespread in so many parts of the world. Since the advent of rapid serologic screening tests, these have been applied to accurately determine the prevalence in particular areas or herds, greatly facilitating the choice of appropriate control measures.

The incidence of clinical disease varies greatly within en-

---

[1] Syn. *Paranaplasma caudatum/Paranaplasma discoides*, which has only been isolated from mixed infections with *A. marginale* and by the use of special techniques, can be demonstrated to have appendages in the form of a tapering tail, a loop, or a ring.

demic areas and is influenced by management factors such as the control measures employed, if any, and stock movement in and out of such areas. The boundaries of these endemic areas may vary with climatic changes, which influence the prevalence of arthropod vector populations. Anaplasmosis generally shows a strong seasonal incidence; clinical cases and outbreaks occur more frequently during the warmer summer and autumn months, coinciding with periods of greater arthropod vector activity.

Ecologic factors of terrain, climate, and vegetation may also favor the propagation of large numbers of wild ruminants that could potentially act as reservoirs of infection and support large vector populations. Outbreaks have also been known to occur after mass vaccination programs, when a few carrier animals were present among the vaccinates and blood-contaminated hypodermic needles were used to inoculate several animals.

Importance

Anaplasmosis has for many years been recognized as a disease of major economic importance to the cattle industry in most tropical and subtropical regions. The development of modern transport systems with the subsequent movement of carrier animals into previously uninfected (non-endemic) areas has also led to the gradual spread of the disease into temperate zones. In many countries, it is considered the most important tick-borne disease of cattle. In the United States, anaplasmosis is considered the second most important disease affecting the cattle industry, and annual economic losses are estimated to be in excess of $100 million.

Mortality rates due to anaplasmosis may vary from very low to high (50 to 60 per cent or more). No absolute control method has yet been developed, and losses from anaplasmosis may be high even in areas with sophisticated veterinary services. In Canada and parts of the United States, isolated pockets of infection were successfully eradicated, but usually only at the high cost of slaughtering all serologically positive animals.

Apart from mortality, anaplasmosis also results in other economic losses. These include lower productivity due to loss of body mass of diseased animals, drop in milk production, and reproductive disorders (abortion and temporary infertility) as well as high costs incurred by the implementation of costly preventive and curative measures.

PATHOGENESIS

The incubation or prepatent period is usually defined as the interval between the time of exposure and the time when the first *Anaplasma* bodies are detected in stained blood films. Under experimental conditions in which a blood inoculum is used to infect animals, this period varies from 15 to 45 days depending on the size of the inoculum of infected blood, with the length of the former increasing inversely proportional to the latter. The incubation period after natural infection usually varies from 3 to 5 weeks. During the incubation period, the organisms multiply in the blood, infecting only erythrocytes, without causing host-cell lysis.

During the patent period, organisms are removed from circulation by erythrophagocytosis, which may result in a rapidly developing anemia. The anemia is usually more severe than can be accounted for by simple destruction of parasitized erythrocytes alone and is probably largely the result of an autoimmune response due to alteration of the erythrocyte membrane by the parasite. The presence of opsonizing and hemagglutinating antibodies to erythrocytes probably results in the phagocytosis of infected as well as uninfected cells by the reticuloendothelial system.

Anemia increases over a period of 4 to 15 days, during which time animals may lose up to 70 per cent of their circulating erythrocytes. Because destruction of erythrocytes occurs by phagocytosis rather than by intravascular hemolysis, icterus develops but not hemoglobinemia and hemoglobinuria. Secondary effects include damage to various organs due to hypoxia.

In adult cattle, it would seem that the competence of the reticuloendothelial system and immunologic responsiveness of individual animals, to a large extent, determine the outcome of anaplasmosis. Convalescence after patent infection and anemia is usually slow and may last several months, particularly in older animals. It starts with increased hematopoiesis, which is characterized by reticulocytosis, anisocytosis, polychromatophilia, basophilic stippling, and Howell-Jolly bodies. The animal gradually recovers, with hematologic and clinical signs returning to normal, but small numbers of *Anaplasma* bodies persist in circulation, rendering the animal a premune carrier. Splenectomy of carrier animals often results in severe relapse parasitemias, which indicates the importance of the spleen in controlling infection.

CLINICAL SIGNS

Most clinical signs of anaplasmosis are related to an acute anemia and a febrile response. If infected animals are not thoroughly examined, clinical signs are only consistently observed when 40 to 50 per cent of erythrocytes have been destroyed. Peracute, acute, chronic, and mild forms of anaplasmosis are recognized in cattle.

Acute anaplasmosis is the most frequently encountered form and is usually characterized initially by fever, anemia, increased heart and respiration rates, inappetence, muscle weakness, and depression. Inspection of the mucous membranes should reveal them to be pale, and the blood appears watery and thin on examination. A drop in milk yield may be noticed early in dairy cows and become more pronounced as the disease progresses. Icterus, muscle tremors, gastrointestinal atony, constipation, and dehydration only become apparent a few days after the onset of symptoms. Upon exertion, animals often show signs of severe respiratory distress, and myocardial hypoxia together with such additional stress as herding, restraint, treatment, and obesity predisposes to cardiac arrest.

Diarrhea has been reported to occur during the early stages of the disease, but usually the feces are dry, partly covered in mucus, and bile-stained. Loss of condition and body mass may vary from slight to marked. Nervous symptoms that may occur include signs of restlessness or aggressiveness and are probably due to cerebral hypoxia. In severe cases, pregnant animals (especially in late pregnancy) may abort, and temporary infertility has also been observed in bulls.

Although a febrile response is often considered to be an early symptom of anaplasmosis, it would appear that this is not consistent. In some fatal cases, the body temperature remains below 40° C throughout the course of the disease, and in others the febrile response is only noticeable at the peak of the anemic crisis. The fever may be continuous or intermittent, dropping to normal or subnormal levels before death.

Blood smears made during the time when clinical signs are most pronounced may require careful examination for demonstration of the organisms. The percentage of infected cells drops as infected cells are removed and immature erythrocytes are added to the circulation. *Anaplasma* apparently do not infect immature erythrocytes, but the presence of a regenerative anemia complicates the differention of parasites from basophilic inclusions in erythrocytes.

Peracute anaplasmosis is occasionally seen in highly susceptible purebred adult animals or high-producing dairy cows. It constitutes the most severe form of the disease and is frequently fatal. Animals succumb to infection within hours of the onset of clinical symptoms. In addition to anemia, the milk flow in cows is suspended; extensive salivation and rapid heart and respiration rates are noted, and animals may exhibit irrational behavior and signs of nervousness. Animals so affected usually die before icterus develops; on examination of blood smears, a very high parasitemia is observed (60 to 80 per cent of erythrocytes may be parasitized).

Chronic disease may follow the acute stage and is manifested by a slow recovery that may last from a few weeks to 3 months or longer. During this period, the animal may not produce optimally and appears to be in a less than satisfactory condition.

Calves up to the age of 1 year show few if any clinical signs of disease, and when these are present, they are usually of a mild nature. However, splenectomized calves are as susceptible to disease as are adult cattle.

Prognosis

Because the anemia results mainly from the destruction of infected erythrocytes, the severity of the disease is usually proportional to the number of infected erythrocytes at the peak of infection. Some strains of *A. marginale* also appear to be more virulent than others, resulting in higher peak parasitemias and a greater autoimmune response followed subsequently by lower packed cell volumes (hematocrit values). In the absence of specific treatment, recovery is dependent on the rate of destruction of erythrocytes and the responsiveness of the bone marrow. Therefore, with slower multiplication of the organism and lower peak parasitemia, followed by a rather gradual onset of anemia, the development of an adequate bone marrow response and recovery are more likely. Similarly, if specific treatment is implemented before severe anemia and icterus develop (hematocrit values above 15 per cent), the prognosis is fairly good. The prognosis is less favorable in animals that develop severe anemia and icterus, owing mainly to the hypoxic effect on the heart muscle, which in turn could result in cardiac failure. Hematocrit values below 11 per cent usually indicate a poor prognosis.

Because of the autoimmune nature of the disease, severe anemia may still develop in animals after relatively early treatment. Advanced age, pregnancy, lactation, and stress during the period of peak anemia adversely influence the prognosis. Water intake, return of appetite, and hematologic evidence of increased bone marrow activity are favorable prognostic signs.

CLINICAL PATHOLOGY

Clinical pathologic tests are seldom used to confirm a diagnosis of anaplasmosis. Very little change, except a decrease in hemoglobin and concomitant decrease in oxygen content, is noticed in the blood profile before the onset of the anemic crisis. This is indicative of the onset of anemia. The most important finding during the anemic crisis is, however, that of a low packed cell volume, the extent of which influences the prognosis. Leukocytosis is often detected. Other changes include increases in the levels of blood urea nitrogen, total bilirubin (mostly unconjugated), aspartate aminotransferase, and alkaline phosphatase as well as a decrease in blood pH and bicarbonate concentrations. Increased osmotic fragility of erythrocytes, preceded by a decrease in erythrocytic acetylcholinesterase, has also been reported.

PATHOLOGY

Gross Pathology

Gross pathologic lesions can be correlated with the clinical signs and are typical of an acute anemia brought about by massive erythrophagocytosis. The tissues generally appear pale and anemic, or icteric in advanced cases, and the blood appears thin and watery. The color of the mucous membranes may range from pale to dark yellow. Emaciation, dehydration, and serous atrophy of fatty tissues may also be apparent.

Owing to the involvement of the reticuloendothelial system in erythrophagocytosis, splenomegaly is almost invariably present. On cut surface, the spleen bulges and the pulp is reddish-brown with prominent follicles. The liver is enlarged and appears yellowish-brown in color. The gallbladder appears enlarged and is distended with thick yellow-green bile. The colon and rectum usually contain dry hard feces covered in a variable amount of thick mucus. Occasionally a mild catarrhal enteritis is noted. If severe anemia is present, degenerative changes may be seen in the liver and kidneys. A variable amount of straw-colored fluid may be present in the pleural cavity, and petechial hemorrhages are occasionally seen on the epicardium and pericardium. The lungs are usually pale and edematous, and a variable amount of froth may be present in the trachea and bronchi. The heart is often pale and flabby.

Histopathology

Histologic findings can similarly be correlated to the events occurring during the pathogenesis of the disease. Evidence of a regenerative anemia, characterized by the presence of anisocytosis, polychromatophilia, basophilic stippling, and Howell-Jolly bodies, is found. Phagocytosed erythrocytes and parasites or their remnants may be seen in macrophages. Degenerative changes associated with anemia and hypoxia are noted in various organs, including the liver, kidneys, and myocardium. Hemosiderin accumulation occurs in many organs but is most extensive in the spleen, liver, and kidneys. Canaliculi in the liver are often distended as a result of bile stasis, and this further contributes to the hepatic disease. Usually the bone marrow is hyperplastic, but in chronic cases there may be evidence of depletion.

DIAGNOSIS

When the many epidemiologic factors involved in the disease are taken into consideration, a tentative diagnosis of anaplasmosis can usually be made on the basis of geographic region, history, clinical signs, and post-mortem lesions.

During the acute stage of the disease, a diagnosis in the individual animal is usually made on the basis of clinical signs, hematologic changes, and microscopic examination of stained blood smears. A definitive diagnosis of anaplasmosis depends on the demonstration of *Anaplasma* bodies in erythrocytes of clinically affected animals. In Giemsa-stained blood smears, the organisms appear as homogeneous, dense, deep purple, more or less round bodies 0.3 to 1.0 μm in diameter. In *A. marginale* infections, approximately 80 to 90 per cent of parasites are situated at or near the periphery of erythrocytes, whereas in *A. centrale* infections, approximately 80 per cent of parasites occupy a more central position in the cells. Occasionally, mixed infections of both parasites may be encountered in the same animal, which may preclude species differentiation.

Detection of the chronic or carrier stage of infection is, however, more difficult. Although carrier animals serve as reservoirs of infection, they cannot be clinically differentiated from uninfected cattle, and the low numbers of parasites present in their blood often defy detection by microscopic means. Serologic methods are thus required to detect latent infections. The direct and indirect fluorescent antibody tests, complement fixation test, capillary tube agglutination test, enzyme-linked immunosorbent assay (ELISA), simple latex agglutination test, radioimmunoassay, and rapid card agglutination test have been applied successfully to the detection of subclinical forms of anaplasmosis. The complement fixation test and capillary tube agglutination test have been found to be more than 90 per cent accurate. The rapid card agglutination test, which was developed later and shows comparable accuracy, has advantages in its relative simplicity and rapidity with which results are obtained. The complement fixation and rapid card agglutination tests are the most widely used and recognized diagnostic tests. The high degree of serologic cross-reactivity between *A. marginale* and *A. centrale* generally precludes species-specific diagnosis and should be taken into consideration in areas where *A. centrale* is endemic.

Infection in a carrier animal can also be confirmed by subinoculation of blood into a susceptible splenectomized calf, but this is usually too expensive and impractical for routine use under field conditions.

More recently, specific DNA probes that detect *Anaplasma* DNA in infected animals have been developed. These probes do not suffer from the same limitations of serologic techniques with regard to cross-reactions (some probes even allow differentiation of *A. marginale* and *A. centrale*) and persistent positive reactions following elimination of the parasite. However, because of the high cost of reagents, DNA probes have thus far mainly been used experimentally and are unlikely to completely replace serologic techniques in large-scale epidemiologic surveys.

Differential Diagnosis

None of the clinical signs of anaplasmosis is pathognomonic; therefore, differentiation from infectious and noninfectious causes of similar nonspecific clinical symptoms, such as fever, anemia, icterus, depression, inappetence, drop in milk yield, abortion, and nervous signs, is necessary. Similarly, on postmortem examination, conditions that primarily cause lesions attributable to anemia resulting from erythrophagocytosis or icterus should be considered.

Confirmation of a diagnosis of anaplasmosis ultimately depends on the microscopic demonstration of *Anaplasma* bodies in erythrocytes of an affected animal. It should, however, be borne in mind that at the time when clinical signs are most pronounced, and examination of blood smears is most likely to be performed, very often the parasitemia might be low. This is due to the fact that at the height of the anemic crisis, most of the infected erythrocytes have already been removed from the circulation. In addition, the presence of a regenerative anemia at this stage requires careful examination to distinguish *Anaplasma* bodies from basophilic stippling in reticulocytes, Howell-Jolly bodies, and possibly other stained particulate matter in erythrocytes.

In countries in which bovine babesiosis occurs, it is the disease with which anaplasmosis is most likely to be confused. The clinical signs of babesiosis closely resemble those of anaplasmosis, and many of the epidemiologic factors show marked similarities. One of the main distinguishing clinical features in anaplasmosis is the absence of hemoglobinuria in an anemic or icteric animal. However, hemoglobinuria is not a constant feature in all *Babesia* infections. In addition, the course of anaplasmosis in cattle is usually of longer duration than babesiosis. Although a diarrhea, which commonly occurs in babesiosis, may be present in acute anaplasmosis, constipation and ruminal stasis (leading to chronic weight loss) are most frequently observed. The possibility of concurrent infections of *Babesia* spp. and *Anaplasma* spp. in an animal should also not be excluded.

Anemia and progressive weight loss are also clinical signs often associated with *Trypanosoma* spp. infections. Trypanosomiasis, however, usually occurs within well-defined tsetse-infested areas. Within these areas, particular attention should be paid to the microscopic examination of wet films and thick blood smears for the detection of trypanosomes. *Theileria* spp. infective to cattle may, to a greater or lesser extent, also cause symptoms reminiscent of anaplasmosis (e.g., *Theileria mutans*, which may cause severe anemia). Theileriosis, however, affects cattle of all age groups equally and can usually be distinguished by the presence of enlarged lymph nodes and the microscopic demonstration of schizonts in lymph node biopsy smears or large numbers of piroplasms in blood smears. Anemia or icterus may also occur in cattle suffering from leptospirosis, post-parturient hemoglobinuria, bacillary hemoglobinuria, chronic copper poisoning, and intoxications with a variety of toxic plants (e.g., *Brassica* spp., *Senecio* spp., and *Allium* spp.) In these conditions, hemoglobinemia and hemoglobinuria are usually also present. Intoxication with plants causing hepatotoxicity (e.g., *Lantana* spp. and *Microcystis aeruginosa*) and in which icterus is often one of the principal signs, should also be considered.

Behavioral changes (such as aggression) and nervous symptoms, occasionally observed in cattle suffering from anaplasmosis, may also be encountered in animals suffering from heartwater, cerebral babesiosis, cerebral theileriosis, rabies, sporadic bovine encephalomyelitis (where these diseases occur), and bacterial meningitis and meningoencephalitis as well as noninfectious conditions such as chlorinated hydrocarbon pesticide poisoning, lead poisoning, vitamin B_1 deficiency (resulting in cerebrocortical necrosis), and plant poisonings (*Albizia* spp., *Cynanchum* spp., *Sarcostemma viminale*, and others).

TREATMENT

When individual cattle are treated for anaplasmosis, both the parasite (specific chemotherapy) and the resulting anemia (supportive therapy) require consideration. Once a large number of erythrocytes are invaded by *Anaplasma*, infected as well as uninfected erythrocytes are rapidly phagocytosed, followed by anemia and concomitant secondary complications due to tissue hypoxia. Therefore chemotherapy before the development of a high parasitemia is considered essential for a favorable prognosis. Very often, however, by the time an animal with clinical anaplasmosis is noticed, the parasitemia is already declining and the animal is suffering from anemia.

Reacting cattle are a major source of infection to uninfected animals and should be separated from healthy cattle. Discretion should be applied in deciding whether to remove the infected animals or the diseased ones, because severely affected animals could succumb from exertion. The provision of adequate protection against the elements, easy access to good feed and water, continued close observation, and the administration of any additional chemotherapy with minimal exertion of the animal also require consideration and are recommended.

The tetracycline drugs (tetracycline hydrochloride,[1] chlortetracycline,[2] oxytetracycline,[3] and doxycycline[4]) are the most widely used chemotherapeutic drugs for the treatment of anaplasmosis. Chlortetracycline is usually administered via the oral route, whereas the others are administered intramuscularly or intravenously. Gloxazone[5] (an experimental drug) and imidocarb[6] also have specific chemotherapeutic effects on *Anaplasma* but have not been approved for commercial distribution in all countries in which anaplasmosis occurs. Both gloxazone and imidocarb occasionally cause toxic side effects. Imidocarb should be administered intramuscularly or subcutaneously, for the intravenous route can be hazardous and is not recommended. The recommended therapeutic dose of imidocarb is 2 to 5 mg/kg. Gloxazone can be administered intravenously, intramuscularly, or subcutaneously, but side effects appear less severe and the efficacy of the drug is not affected when the last 2 routes are used. The recommended therapeutic dose of gloxazone is 5 mg/kg. Imidocarb has the advantage of being highly effective against *Babesia* spp.; thus, the necessity of making a differential diagnosis is avoided where anaplasmosis and babesiosis occur in the same area. However, this practice is not recommended, because a specific diagnosis is essential for the implementation of appropriate control measures.

A single dosage of a long-acting tetracycline formulation[7] (200 mg/ml) at the rate of 20 mg/kg administered intramuscularly, or 1 or more (preferably 2 to 3) injections of a standard oxytetracycline formulation of lower concentration (50 to 150 mg/ml) administered intravenously or intramuscularly at the rate of 11 mg/kg (at 24- to 48-hour intervals), is recommended for the treatment of clinical anaplasmosis. The recommended therapeutic dose of doxycycline (100 mg/ml) is 4 to 10 mg/kg administered intramuscularly or slowly intravenously. The dose may be repeated after 24 to 48 hours, and a total of 2 to 3 injections is recommended.

The use of blood transfusion in cattle with acute anemia seems logical, yet results are often disappointing. To be effective, large volumes of blood (2 to 4 L, depending on the size of the animal) need to be transfused, but even 4 L of blood has on occasion been transfused to adult cattle without apparent benefit. Blood should be administered slowly, with the risks of increased blood pressure and the possibility of anaphylactic shock reactions due to incompatible blood types kept in mind. Owing to accelerated removal of erythrocytes in cattle with anaplasmosis, the benefits derived from blood transfusion are of short duration (24 to 48 hours), and transfusions should therefore be repeated. Blood transfusion is not recommended in animals that are restless and difficult to restrain, or in cases with apparent icterus. Together with hypoxic liver degeneration, icterus also suggests myocardial damage, in which case transfusion may cause additional cardiac stress and lead to heart failure.

In addition to specific treatment and attempting to limit stress factors, the use of supportive therapy may be beneficial and is usually recommended. Although hematinic drugs probably do not have adequate time to stimulate erythropoiesis sufficiently to influence mortality, these and liver supportive drugs may reduce the time required for convalescence. Gastrointestinal disturbances such as ruminal stasis, constipation, and lack of appetite often complicate recovery; when indicated, attempts should be made to correct these disorders with rumenotorics, mild laxatives, and appetite stimulants.

CONTROL

Control of anaplasmosis can be achieved by a variety of methods, which generally include 1 or more of the following:

- Eliminating the source of infection by chemotherapy of carrier cattle (chemosterilization).
- Protecting susceptible cattle against clinical disease by prolonged chemotherapy during exposure (chemoprophylaxis).
- Controlling the vectors.
- Establishing widespread immunity in the cattle population by vaccination.

The method of choice and its efficacy will depend largely on epidemiologic and economic considerations. Control in most endemic areas is, however, difficult and expensive because of the complex involvement of a variety of arthropod vectors and the presence of large numbers of domestic and wild ruminant reservoirs.

Eliminating the Carrier Stage

With the advent of sensitive serologic tests, a control method was developed whereby the source of infection (carriers) in a herd could be eliminated. It consists of testing the herd, identifying the carriers, and removing them by slaughter, segregation and isolation from the rest of the herd, or sterilizing the infection by chemotherapy (see Tables 1 and 2). This approach has successfully been used in parts of the United States but is usually only feasible in areas of low incidence. Cattle cleared of infection are susceptible to reinfection but show resistance to clinical anaplasmosis (sterile immunity) for variable periods of up to 30 months.

Treatment for eliminating *Anaplasma* infections in most endemic areas is considered to be contraindicated because of the high risk of reinfection and the relative susceptibility of the cattle population in the absence of any long-term immunity that accompanies low-level persistent infections (premunity). Animals eventually become susceptible and reinfection may result in clinical disease, depending on the degree and duration of sterile immunity. Thus the alternative of controlling clinical disease is the more realistic and economically feasible method adopted in most tropical and subtropical regions.

Where indicated, *Anaplasma* infections in cattle can be eliminated by a number of treatment regimens with use of tetracycline drugs. These are summarized in Table 1. Intravenous injections of tetracycline should be administered slowly. With intramuscular administration, large doses should preferably be divided between 2 or more injection sites. Oral administration has advantages in the ease of treatment on a herd basis and the availability of economical feed premixes. Consistent elimination of infections by oral application is often difficult to obtain owing to differences in the consumption of medicated feed or salt-mineral mixes by individual animals. It is therefore important to mix the drug with a highly palatable feed supplement so that adequate medication by free-choice feeding is ensured. Feeding of the higher levels of chlortetracycline may cause transient diarrhea, anorexia, and weight

---

[1]Polyotic. Lederle Laboratories, American Cyanamid Co., Pearl River, NY.
[2]Aureomycin. Lederle Laboratories, American Cyanamid Co., Pearl River, NY.
[3]Liquamycin, Terramycin. Charles Pfizer & Co., Inc., New York, NY.
[4]Charles Pfizer & Co., New York, NY.
[5]356-C-61, α-ethoxyethylglyoxal dithiosemicarbazone. Burroughs Wellcome Co., Research Triangle Park, NC.
[6]4A65, imizol, 3,3′bis-(2-imidazolin-2-yl)-carbanilide dihydrochloride (or dipropionate). Burroughs Wellcome Co., Research Triangle Park, NC.
[7]L-200, Liquamycin/LA, Terramycin/LA (long-acting 200 mg oxytetracycline/ml). Charles Pfizer & Co., Inc., New York, NY.

Table 1. TREATMENT REGIMENS FOR THE ELIMINATION OF *ANAPLASMA* INFECTION WITH THE TETRACYCLINE DRUGS

Drug	Rate of Administration	Route	Number of Treatments	Interval
Tetracycline	11 mg/kg	IV or IM	5–10	Daily
Oxytetracycline	11 mg/kg	IV or IM	10–14	Daily
Chlortetracycline	33 mg/kg	IV	16	Daily
Chlortetracycline	2.2 mg/kg	Orally	41	Daily
Chlortetracycline	5.5 mg/kg	Orally	45	Daily
Chlortetracycline	1.1 mg/kg	Orally	120	Daily[1]
Chlortetracycline	11 mg/kg	Orally	30–60	Daily
Chlortetracycline	11 mg/kg	Orally	60	Daily
Chlortetracycline	5.5 mg/kg	Orally	60	Daily
Chlortetracycline	3.3 mg/kg	Orally	60	Daily
Chlortetracycline	11 mg/kg	Orally	45–60	Daily
Oxytetracycline	22 mg/kg	IV or IM	5	Daily
Oxytetracycline (LA)	20 mg/kg	IM	2–4	7 days
Oxytetracycline (LA)	20 mg/kg	IM	4	3 days

IV = intravenous; IM = intramuscular; LA = long-acting formulation.
[1]Negative status determined by serologic procedures.
Source: Modified from Kuttler KL: Current anaplasmosis control techniques in the United States. J S Afr Vet Assoc 50:314–320, 1979.

loss during the first week, but medicated feed should not be withdrawn during this period.

Alternative treatment regimens involving the use of gloxazone, imidocarb, or both that have been reported to be effective in eliminating *Anaplasma* infections in cattle are summarized in Table 2. Although imidocarb has very few toxic side effects at normal recommended therapeutic doses, when doses are repeated or increased to eliminate infections, the toxic range is approached and transient symptoms of toxicity frequently occur. The severity is dose-related, and symptoms include salivation, serous nasal discharge, diarrhea, and dyspnea. Mortality may occur at doses of 20 mg/kg or above, even with administration in divided doses.

However, neither of the treatment regimens listed in Tables 1 and 2 consistently eliminates infections in all treated animals. Therefore, all control programs aimed at eliminating the parasite by chemotherapy should include serologic screening of the herd after treatment. The disappearance of specific antibodies from the serum of treated cattle is used to indicate successful sterilization of infection. However, serum from animals in which the infection has been cleared may still react positively to these tests for several months. Testing should thus only be conducted 6 months or longer after treatment is completed. Any animals subsequently found to be serologically positive should be regarded as treatment failures and either retreated or separated from the rest of the herd.

The possibility of transplacental infection of calves should not be underestimated in such eradication programs. However, serum from uninfected calves born from infected dams may also react positively in serologic tests for variable periods of up to 3 months owing to the presence of colostral antibodies.

Re-exposure of carrier animals to infection during the period of treatment may result in reinfection and failure to eliminate the infections. Programs aimed at the elimination of the carrier state are thus best conducted during the period of lowest vector activity.

Temporary or Prolonged Protection by Chemotherapy (Chemoprophylaxis)

Intramuscular administrations of oxytetracycline at 21- to 28-day intervals to all susceptible cattle throughout the vector season, and continued for a further 1 to 2 months after the end thereof, will prevent clinical disease in animals that become infected but will not sterilize the infections. Thus, infected animals would become carriers and subsequently develop premunity. The recommended dose of oxytetracycline is 6.6 to 11 mg/kg (50 to 150 mg/ml formulations) or 20 mg/kg (200 mg/ml long-acting formulations). For doxycycline (100 mg/ml), the dose is 4 to 10 mg/kg.

Similar protection is afforded by the continuous daily oral administration of chlortetracycline at a rate of 1.1 mg/kg throughout the vector season, or 0.22 to 0.55 mg/kg throughout the year. It is essential that all animals consume sufficient quantities of the medicated feed or feed supplement for ensuring an adequate intake of chlortetracycline. The use of sustained-release oxytetracycline boluses, which provide therapeutic drug levels for up to 60 days, should impose fewer management and labor constraints.

In all cases in which tetracyclines are used to prevent clinical anaplasmosis, animals should be observed closely for any clinical signs of disease after withdrawal of medication.

Control of Vectors

For preventing mechanical transmission by the use of blood-contaminated instruments, all contaminated instruments should be washed in clean water or disinfectant before use on the next animal. Clean hypodermic needles and syringes should preferably be used for each animal.

The fact that anaplasmosis can be transmitted both biologically and mechanically by a variety of arthropod vectors, which are difficult to control effectively, has led many to believe that alternative approaches to intensive vector control (such as chemoprophylaxis, chemosterilization, or vaccination) are more desirable. This is true for most endemic areas, in which it may be desirable that all animals be exposed to infection at a young age for ensuring that they develop premunity while they are least susceptible to clinical disease. However, the importance of vector control has clearly been demonstrated in incidents in which, after successful elimination of carriers by chemotherapy, the prevalence of anaplasmosis

Table 2. TREATMENT REGIMENS USING OXYTETRACYCLINE PLUS GLOXAZONE, OXYTETRACYCLINE PLUS IMIDOCARB, IMIDOCARB, AND IMIDOCARB PLUS GLOXAZONE FOR THE ELIMINATION OF *ANAPLASMA* INFECTION

Drug	Rate of Administration	Route	Number of Treatments	Interval
Oxytetracycline[1]	11 mg/kg	IV	3	1 or 2 days
+ Gloxazone	5–10 mg/kg	IV	3	1 or 2 days
Oxytetracycline	20 mg/kg	IM	4	7 days
+ Imidocarb	5 mg/kg	IM or SC	2	14 days
Oxytetracycline (LA)	20 mg/kg	IM	4	7 days
+ Imidocarb	5 mg/kg	IM or SC	2	7, 14, or 21 days
Imidocarb	4–6 mg/kg	IM or SC	3	Daily
Imidocarb	2 mg/kg	IM or SC	3	Daily
+ Gloxazone	5 mg/kg	IV	3	Daily
Imidocarb[2]	4–5 mg/kg	IM or SC	2	14 days

IV = intravenous; IM = intramuscular; SC = subcutaneous; LA = long-acting formulation.
[1]Splenectomized calves tested.
[2]Adult cattle tested.
Source: Modified from Kuttler KL: Current anaplasmosis control techniques in the United States. J S Afr Vet Assoc 50:314–320, 1979.

in cattle herds returned to pretreatment levels in the absence of vector control.

Control of vector ticks is more readily achieved than that of biting flies. However, because of a variety of epidemiologic and management factors (e.g., the potential role of wild ruminants as hosts of vector ticks and of *Anaplasma*, as well as the development of acaricide resistance in vector tick populations), vector control alone cannot be considered a practical and reliable method of preventing transmission of anaplasmosis. Intensive vector control will, however, reduce the dissemination of anaplasmosis in a susceptible herd and can substantially reduce the number of clinical cases occurring during an outbreak.

In most anaplasmosis endemic areas, vector control is generally only practiced to reduce tick and fly worry, or as part of a general vector-borne disease control strategy. If too vigorous, vector control could result in an unstable disease situation (an increase in incidence of clinical anaplasmosis as well as other tick-borne diseases, e.g., babesiosis and heartwater) due to unreliable exposure of animals at a young age to natural infection, especially in areas marginal for survival of vectors. Therefore, a vaccination program is usually recommended to ensure widespread immunity in the cattle population.

Vaccination

Vaccination is employed either as a routine preventive measure or to provide long-term protection in the face of or following an outbreak of anaplasmosis. A single administration of a live vaccine generally induces a strong cell-mediated response of long duration, affording greater protection against clinical disease than killed vaccines, which require multiple injections.

As a preventive measure, live vaccines are often used as an adjunct to natural infection in endemic areas for ensuring that all animals are exposed to infection at a young age when they are least susceptible to clinical disease. Therefore, it is generally recommended that calves be vaccinated at approximately 6 months of age and limited vector control be applied to young animals, allowing maximal exposure to field challenge, which should result in the development of a lifelong immunity in these animals.

The administration of any live vaccine involves a certain amount of risk, particularly in older, debilitated, or pregnant animals. Because older cattle are more susceptible, vaccination is indicated only when such susceptible animals are to be introduced into anaplasmosis endemic areas or after an outbreak. Adult cattle should be vaccinated only under strict supervision and treated with recommended therapeutic drugs at the first sign of development of clinical disease. Pregnant cows should preferably be vaccinated only after calving.

Both *A. marginale* and *A. centrale* produce persistent low-level infections (carrier infections) in cattle that are accompanied by lifelong immunity in the animal. Premunition, as these carrier infections are referred to, has been widely used as the basis for immunization against anaplasmosis. However, carrier cattle are considered undesirable in some epidemiologic situations, such as in areas of low incidence where control may be directed at total eradication of the disease.

A vaccine containing killed *A. marginale*[1] has been developed that is not infective but provides a transient low level of resistance to anaplasmosis and is the only vaccine presently approved for use in the United States. Whichever vaccine is used, all recommendations of the manufacturer regarding storage, handling, and administration should be closely followed.

A. marginale *Vaccines*

The relative resistance of young calves to anaplasmosis has in the past led to the practice of inoculating calves with blood from *A. marginale* carrier cattle. Mild infections are induced that are usually followed by spontaneous recovery and the development of a carrier state with solid immunity.

More recently, quality-controlled frozen stabilates of virulent *A. marginale* have been prepared, which, when used to appropriate dilution, produce moderate infections that may or may not require chemotherapy, depending on the age and natural resistance of the animals. However, severe reactions and mortality have occurred even after inoculation of very small doses of *A. marginale*.

An attenuated, sheep-adapted, live *A. marginale* vaccine[1] has been developed that is commercially available in South America. It produces mild, almost inapparent infection in calves but induces substantial long-lasting immunity against virulent *A. marginale* challenge. There have, however, been reports of reversion to virulence. This attenuated vaccine is produced as a frozen vaccine and dispensed in liquid nitrogen. It is administered intramuscularly in 1 to 2 ml doses.

Anaplaz vaccine is a lyophilized blood-based antigen of bovine origin that is reconstituted with an oil adjuvant. Vaccination does not prevent infection with *A. marginale* but does aid in the prevention of severe clinical disease. Exposed animals subsequently become carriers, which renders them premune and resistant to reinfection. For initial vaccination, it is recommended that 2 doses of the vaccine be administered subcutaneously at an interval of 4 to 6 weeks. Protection from clinical disease is reportedly provided approximately 2 weeks after the second dose. Therefore, vaccination should be scheduled so that the second injection is given at least 2 weeks before the start of the vector season. Protection afforded by the killed vaccine is of relatively short duration; an annual booster injection is recommended, administered approximately 2 weeks before each subsequent vector season. A major drawback of the vaccine is its induction of neonatal isohemolytic anemia in some calves after ingestion of colostrum from vaccinated dams. The use of a similar vaccine prepared from *A. marginale*–infected sheep blood or chemical modification of the antigen should overcome the problem of neonatal isohemolytic anemia.

A. centrale *Vaccines*

Premunizing cattle with *A. centrale*–infected bovine blood has for many decades been the most widely used method of vaccination in many countries. The vaccine has been distributed either as a refrigerated fresh blood vaccine or in frozen stabilate form, the dose being 1 to 2 ml administered subcutaneously or intramuscularly, and occasionally intravenously.

A. centrale usually causes mild or inapparent infections in cattle, but vaccination neither prevents infection with *A. marginale* nor provides complete protection against virulent *A. marginale* challenge. It does, however, reduce the severity of a subsequent *A. marginale* infection, which results in the development of a solid resistance to further field challenge in infected animals. Although generally considered a mild pathogen, *A. centrale* may occasionally cause serious disease symptoms in highly susceptible animals.

The various immunization procedures are summarized in

---

[1]Anaplaz. Fort Dodge Laboratories, Fort Dodge, IA.

[1]VIVAN. Anchor Laboratories, Guadalajara, Mexico.

tabular form in Table 3 together with an evaluation of their use in cattle of different age groups and relative efficacy of the vaccines as immunizing antigens.

HANDLING AN OUTBREAK OF ANAPLASMOSIS

Usually only adult cattle are affected. Exposure of all animals to natural infection at a young age will lead to widespread immunity within a cattle population and ensure a stable disease situation (i.e., no or very low incidence of clinical disease in an anaplasmosis endemic area). However, low or fluctuating vector populations, especially in areas marginally suitable for their survival, as well as a low incidence of carriers may result in varying proportions of the animals in different age groups being susceptible, leading to an unstable disease situation (i.e., high incidence of clinical disease in an endemic area). Disease instability due to low rate of transmission may also result from overzealous vector control measures.

In most endemic areas, clinical cases of anaplasmosis occur only sporadically during periods of increased vector activity. Outbreaks in which several animals are affected within a short period of time may involve one or more managemental or epidemiologic factors that lead to an unstable disease situation, including the introduction of carrier animals into a previously uninfected herd. These factors should be assessed to determine whether eradication is feasible, because this will in turn influence the decision on the method of choice to be implemented to control losses and prevent further outbreaks. The following should serve as general guidelines:

1. Separate clinically affected animals from the rest of the herd and implement appropriate specific and supportive therapy. Handle diseased animals with care to prevent losses due to overexertion.
2. Treat reacting cattle with a suitable insecticide-acaricide (pour-on or spraying), for they are a major source of infection to the rest of the herd, through both tick transmission and mechanical transmission by biting flies.
3. Some protection against infection should also be provided to the rest of the herd through periodic application of a suitable insecticide-acaricide by spraying, dipping, or pour-on. In endemic areas where the establishment of low-level infection is relied on for immunization (vaccination with live vaccines and natural exposure), calves under the age of 9 months need not be treated with acaricides.
4. Several animals in the herd may be in the incubation stage of the disease and show no clinical signs. Therefore, close supervision is required to identify such animals at the first signs of illness for implementing early treatment.
5. No prophylactic drugs are available, but temporary protection can be provided to animals incubating the disease by parenteral administration of oxytetracycline at a rate of 6.6 to 11 mg/kg. A single injection may not have the desired effect, merely prolonging the incubation period and delaying the onset of clinical disease. Longer-term protection can be achieved by repeating the oxytetracycline treatments at 21- to 28-day intervals. At the time of the outbreak, it will not be possible to determine which animals have not been exposed, and which have been exposed and are incubating the disease. Therefore, all animals have to be regarded as having been exposed, which requires the treatment of all susceptible animals. Depending on the number of susceptible animals in a herd, this may be a very costly undertaking and in most instances should probably be reserved for valuable, high-risk animals such as pregnant cows, older animals, and bulls.
6. Prolonged oral administration of chlortetracycline at a rate of 1.1 mg/kg will suppress clinical anaplasmosis in animals already incubating the disease and prevent clinical disease in those animals subsequently exposed. If there is a delay before oral medication can be initiated, temporary protection can be provided by the parenteral administration of oxytetracycline. Regardless of whether parenteral or oral administration is decided upon to provide temporary or prolonged protection, animals should be closely observed for any signs of anaplasmosis when the treatment is discontinued.
7. As soon as the temporary measures for preventing clinical disease have been employed, measures for providing long-term protection should be implemented. All epidemiologic factors involved in the outbreak need to be carefully evaluated, with various economic considerations also being taken into

Table 3. PROCEDURES FOR ANAPLASMOSIS IMMUNIZATION

	Calves <8 Months Old	Cattle 8 Months to 2 Years Old	Cattle >2 Years Old	Relative Efficacy
Virulent field *Anaplasma marginale*	Safe NR	Not safe NR	Not safe NR	+ + + +
Virulent field *A. marginale* with therapy	Safe NR	Safe NR	Not safe NR	+ + + +
Dilute stabilate of *A. marginale*	Safe R	Safe NR	Not safe NR	+ + + +
Dilute stabilate (*A. marginale*)	Safe R	Safe R	Safe R	+ + + +
Attenuated *A. marginale*	Safe NR[1]	Safe R	Safe R[2]	+ + +
A. centrale	Safe R	Safe R	Safe R[2]	+ +
Killed vaccine (Anaplaz)	Safe NR	Safe NR	Safe R	+

R = recommended; NR = not recommended.
[1]The mildness of the organism is such that a satisfactory replicating infection that results in premunity is not always produced in calves of this age.
[2]Not recommended for lactating dairy cattle or pregnant cows.
   + + + +   Maximum protection against needle and field challenge.
   + + +   Solid protection against needle challenge. Variable response against some field challenges.
   + +   Partial protection against both needle and field challenge. Prevents death losses by either challenge.
   +   Partial protection against needle challenge. Will usually prevent death losses against a moderate challenge. Imposes neonatal isohemolytic anemia hazards in producing cows.
Source: Modified from Kuttler KL: Current anaplasmosis control techniques in the United States. J S Afr Vet Assoc 50:314–320, 1979.

account. Once a decision has been reached on the most suitable control program, it should be implemented as soon as possible to prevent further outbreaks. The most frequently used programs for long-term protection in endemic areas include the vaccination of all animals to achieve a stable disease situation.

8. In endemic areas in which vaccination with live vaccines is opted for, calves between the ages of 3 and 9 months can be vaccinated immediately without the risk of their developing severe vaccine reactions. Animals receiving tetracycline drug therapy should be vaccinated only after withdrawal of treatment. (Where vaccination with Anaplaz is indicated, it can be carried out concurrently with tetracycline treatment to provide temporary protection until adequate immunity has developed after vaccination.) While the possible risks involved in vaccinating adult cattle with live vaccines are borne in mind, all adult animals should be vaccinated in numbers not too large to make handling and proper supervision impossible. Pregnant cows should preferably be temporarily protected by chemotherapy or vector control and vaccinated after calving. Strict vector control measures should be maintained for at least 2 months after vaccination so that adequate time is provided for the development of protective immunity before exposure to natural challenge.

BIBLIOGRAPHY

Carson CA, Buening GM: The immune response of cattle to live and inactivated *Anaplasma* vaccines and response to challenge. J S Afr Vet Assoc 50:330–331, 1979.

Jones EW, Brock WE: Bovine anaplasmosis: its diagnosis, treatment, and control. J Am Vet Med Assoc 149:1624–1633, 1966.

Kuttler KL: Current anaplasmosis control techniques in the United States. J S Afr Vet Assoc 50:314–320, 1979.

Kuttler KL: *Anaplasma* infections in wild and domestic ruminants: a review. J Wildl Dis 20:12–20, 1984.

Losos GJ: Anaplasmosis. In Losos GJ (ed): Infectious Tropical Diseases of Domestic Animals. Harlow, UK, Longman Scientific and Technical, 1986, pp 741–795.

Potgieter FT: Epizootiology and control of anaplasmosis in South Africa. J S Afr Vet Assoc 50:367–372, 1979.

Potgieter FT, Van Rensburg L: The persistence of colostral *Anaplasma* antibodies and incidence of *in utero* transmission of *Anaplasma* infections in calves under laboratory conditions. Onderstepoort J Vet Res 54:557–560, 1987.

Ristic M: Anaplasmosis. Adv Vet Sci 6:111–192, 1960.

Ristic M: Anaplasmosis. In Weinman D, Ristic M (eds): Infectious Blood Diseases of Man and Animals, vol 2. New York, Academic Press, 1968, pp 473–542.

Ristic M: Anaplasmosis. In Amstutz HE (ed): Bovine Medicine and Surgery, vol 4. Santa Barbara, CA, American Veterinary Publications, 1980, pp 324–348.

Ristic M: Anaplasmosis. In Ristic M, McIntyre I (eds): Current Topics in Veterinary Medicine and Animal Science, vol 6. Diseases of Cattle in the Tropics. The Hague, Martinus Nijhoff, 1981, pp 327–344.

Rogers RJ, Shiels IA: Epidemiology and control of anaplasmosis in Australia. J S Afr Vet Assoc 50:363–366, 1979.

Wilson AJ: Observations on the pathogenesis of anaplasmosis in cattle with particular reference to nutrition, breed and age. J S Afr Vet Assoc 50:293–295, 1979.

Wilson AJ, Ronohardjo P: Some factors affecting the control of bovine anaplasmosis with special reference to Australia and Indonesia. In Riemann HP, Burridge MP (eds): Developments in Animal and Veterinary Sciences, vol 15. Impact of Diseases on Livestock Production in the Tropics. New York, Elsevier Science Publishing Company, 1984, pp 121–134.

Besnoitiosis
(Elephant Skin Disease, Olifantsvelsiekte [Afrikaans], Anasarque des Bovidés)

RUDOLPH D. BIGALKE, BVSc, DVSc

Bovine besnoitiosis is a disease of cattle caused by the protozoan parasite *Besnoitia besnoiti*. It is characterized by typical skin lesions, particularly in the chronic stage of the disease. The way in which bovine besnoitiosis is transmitted has not been definitely determined, but it is assumed that a carnivorous host features in the life cycle, as is the case with some other *Besnoitia* spp. The disease has a relatively widespread distribution in Africa, but its occurrence is sporadic. It has also been recorded in Israel, France (where it was originally described), southwestern Russia (Kazakhstan), South Korea, Portugal, and Venezuela.

Besnoitiosis has also been recognized as a clinical entity in goats in Kenya, but the *Besnoitia* sp. responsible for the disease has not been identified, and the epizootiology of caprine besnoitiosis requires further investigation.

EPIZOOTIOLOGY

The distribution of bovine besnoitiosis suggests a preference for a less temperate, even subtropical to tropical climate. Although the incidence of the disease in South Africa appears to have declined over the last 2 decades, it still seems to be more prevalent there than in any other country; the majority of fresh cases are observed during the warmer, moister months of the year. In South Africa, it is mainly a disease of beef cattle farmed extensively under ranching conditions.

All breeds of cattle and all sexes seem to be susceptible, but for unknown reasons the disease is rarely encountered in calves under 6 months of age. Relatively few animals, however, develop the typical clinical form of the disease. A survey conducted in South Africa by examination of the scleral conjunctiva of 5018 animals for the presence of cysts of *B. besnoiti* revealed an infection rate of 8.5 per cent, but typical skin lesions were observed in only 1.5 per cent of the cattle studied. Serologic surveys suggested the existence of an even higher incidence of clinically inapparent infections than was found in the aforementioned survey.

Experimental and circumstantial field evidence suggests that chronically infected cattle harboring large numbers of cysts possibly serve as carriers of the disease. No naturally infected hosts other than cattle have hitherto been found. *Besnoitia* strains isolated from 2 species of antelope (blue wildebeest and impala), although antigenically closely related to bovine strains of *B. besnoiti*, were virtually apathogenic for cattle and revealed viscerotropic rather than dermatotropic tissue affinities in artificially infected bovine and rabbit hosts. Consequently, it seems most unlikely that naturally infected antelope harboring these strains would serve as carriers for the typical bovine disease.

Experimental and circumstantial field evidence also indicates that bovine besnoitiosis can be transmitted mechanically by blood-sucking insects from chronically infected to susceptible cattle. This method of transmission probably plays some role in the epizootiology of the disease. It does not, however, solve the transmission riddle because mechanical transmission did not produce typical clinical cases, as are seen in the field.

It seems logical to surmise that a carnivorous final host also exists for *B. besnoiti*, as is the case for some other *Besnoitia* spp. *Felis lybica* has been incriminated in Russia (Kazakhstan), but hitherto it has not been possible to confirm these findings. It also seems unlikely that cattle could serve as a source of infection for such a small wild cat under natural conditions. An unknown cycle involving a carnivorous host therefore probably occurs in nature.

ETIOLOGY AND PATHOGENESIS

The etiologic agent of bovine besnoitiosis, *B. besnoiti*, is morphologically similar to *Toxoplasma* and *Sarcocystis*, indicating its coccidian nature and justifying its classification in the phylum Apicomplexa, family Sarcocystidae, and subfamily Toxoplasmatinae.

It is currently assumed that cattle, which serve as intermediate hosts, contract besnoitiosis by ingestion of mature isosporan-type oocysts ($\pm 15 \times 13$ μm in size, according to unconfirmed Russian (Kazakhstan) studies) shed in the feces of a presumed feline final host.

If this assumption is correct, sporozoites escaping from the oocyst presumably enter the bovine circulation and then multiply by endodyogeny in endothelial cells of blood vessels, particularly in the dermis, subcutis, fascia, upper respiratory tract, and testes. Merozoite-like endozoites, $\pm 5.9 \times 2.3$ μm in size, reinvade adjacent and other cells to produce further endozoites. This portion of the developmental cycle is associated with the acute anasarca stage of the disease.

The initial developmental cycle is superseded by cyst formation when activated hypertrophic cystozoite-containing histiocytic cells become detectable in the same sites in which the endozoites were formed. Characteristic thick-walled cysts (Fig. 1), filled with cystozoites $\pm 8.4 \times 1.9$ μm in size, are formed and grow to reach a diameter of 400 μm. The formation and persistence of large numbers of cysts is associated with the chronic scleroderma stage of the disease. Cyst production is finite, however, all cysts apparently arising from the endozoitic proliferation cycle referred to previously.

CLINICAL SIGNS

An incubation period of 4 days was recorded after infection of cattle, in the unconfirmed study cited before, with sporu-

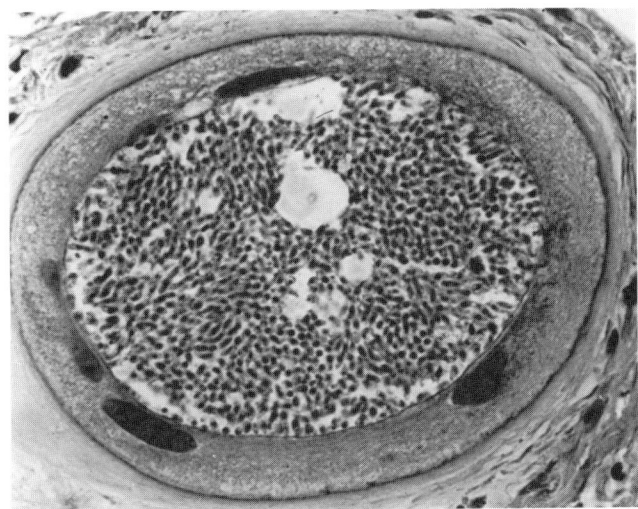

Figure 1. Developing cyst of *Besnoitia besnoiti* in hypertrophic histiocyte. Extracellular homogeneous layer of cyst wall, compressed cytoplasm of histiocyte containing several nuclei, and vacuole containing numerous cystozoites are clearly distinguishable.

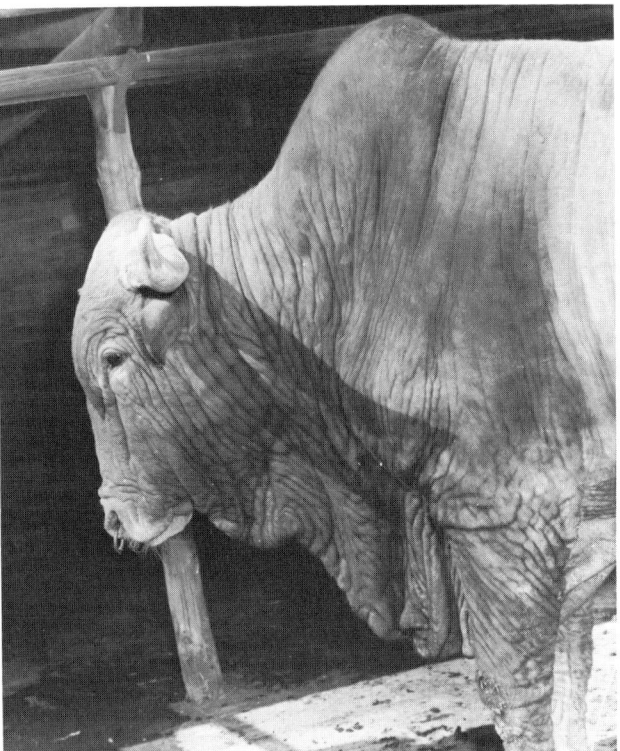

Figure 2. Clinical signs of a typical chronic case in the scleroderma stage of the disease. Note thickening and excessive wrinkling of skin of forelimbs, head, and neck.

lated oocysts of feline origin, whereas it was approximately 14 days after mechanical transmission of the disease.

Clinically affected cattle initially develop a pronounced, sustained febrile reaction; morning temperatures reach 40° to 41° C and even higher. Pyrexia is accompanied by progressive inappetence and loss of weight. Animals are listless, are inclined to seek the shade, walk with a slow gait, and prefer the recumbent position. Hyperemia of the muzzle, periorbital skin, and scrotum and a variable degree of anasarca may be evident. The testes are swollen and painful, indicative of a severe orchitis. The anasarca stage may go entirely unnoticed in the field.

Animals rarely succumb in the anasarca stage. Autopsy of such animals reveals, in addition to the lesions already described, widespread petechiae and ecchymoses in the subcutis, edema of the lymph nodes and testicular parenchyma, and a mucous to mucopurulent rhinitis. On histopathologic examination, parasitized vessels show endothelial necrosis, intimal fibrinoid degeneration, and necrosis with consequent edema, thrombosis, hemorrhage, and necrosis in surrounding tissues.

The anasarca stage is followed by the chronic scleroderma stage of the disease characterized by a progressive thickening, hardening, and prominent folding and puckering of the skin, which may be extensive or more localized (Fig. 2). Pronounced thickening of the limbs accompanied by slow, apparently painful movement—if the very listless and usually recumbent animals are forced to move—may be seen in severe cases. A mucopurulent nasal discharge, which forms crusts and may clog the nostrils, and stridor may occur.

Microscopic examination reveals the presence of numerous cysts in the dermis, subcutis, and intermuscular fascia (Fig. 3). The muscles and tendons of the limbs, synovial sheaths, periosteum of the metatarsal and metacarpal bones, testicular

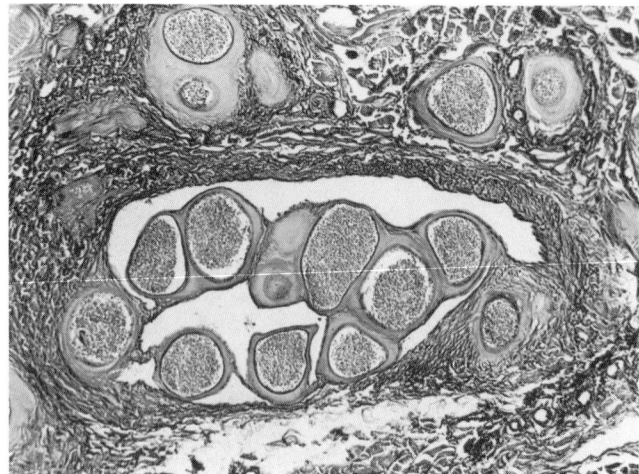

Figure 3. Cluster of cysts of *Besnoitia besnoiti* in dermis. Note homogeneous cyst walls.

parenchyma, mucosa of the nose and upper respiratory tract, superficial veins, and scleral conjunctiva are often heavily parasitized. Most of the cysts are enclosed by a thin layer of collagen. When the organisms die off, they elicit a granulomatous reaction. Very large numbers of rapidly growing cysts in the dermal papillae and other parts of the stratum papillare, the accompanying fibrosis and granulomatous reactions, and hyperkeratosis and acanthosis account for development of the typical scleroderma.

These symptoms are usually accompanied by an undulant, low-level febrile reaction that persists for several weeks as well as a poor appetite and emaciation. More pronounced fever and anorexia occur in the very severe, often fatal cases. Bulls are usually rendered permanently infertile in severe cases owing to the development of atrophic and indurated testes. Downgrading, due to trimming, or even condemnation of carcasses with large numbers of cysts in the fasciae and intermuscular connective tissue also contributes to the economic importance of the disease.

Most cattle that are not too severely affected survive, but convalescence is slow. The characteristic scleroderma and alopecia are, however, lifelong features despite a gradual improvement in the appearance of such animals, which seems to be associated with a decrease in the numbers of cysts due to their degeneration.

Surveys conducted by scrutiny of the scleral conjunctiva, in which cysts become visible to the naked eye, and serologic tests indicate that most animals that become infected in the field contract a clinically inapparent form of the disease.

In Kenya, besnoitiosis in goats is characterized by alopecia and the presence of large numbers of cysts in the dermis and other sites similar to those observed in cattle.

DIAGNOSIS

Bovine besnoitiosis can be diagnosed quite readily in the scleroderma stage on its clinical manifestations. If necessary, the diagnosis can be confirmed by histopathologic demonstration of large numbers of cysts in the dermis of affected skin taken by biopsy or at necropsy.

Diagnosis in the anasarca stage of the disease is difficult, however. Free or intracellular endozoites of *B. besnoiti* in monocytic cells may be demonstrated for several days in peripheral blood smears at the height of the febrile reaction, but they are scarce and hence difficult to find. On the other hand, cystozoites originating from punctured cysts are often quite plentiful in blood smears made from chronic scleroderma cases. Both endozoites and cystozoites are merozoite-like in appearance and therefore not diagnostic for besnoitiosis.

Visible cysts are often quite plentiful in the scleral conjunctiva of chronic scleroderma cases. They can even be detected in small numbers in clinically inapparent cases. Their identity may be confirmed by biopsy and further processing of the material for microscopic examination.

Serologic tests are useful aids for studies on the epizootiology of the disease and the efficacy of vaccination but not, as yet, for diagnostic purposes.

TREATMENT

No specific remedy has hitherto been found for the treatment of natural cases. Oxytetracycline has been shown to have a delaying effect on the course of the disease in artificially infected rabbits if the antibiotic is administered concurrently with infection. It has no noticeable curative effect on natural bovine cases.

Tetracyclines, wound dressings, myiasis control, and provision of shade and nutritious feed and water ad libitum are advocated as supportive treatment.

PREVENTION

A live cell-culture vaccine, which was developed from a strain of *B. besnoiti* isolated from blue wildebeest, is used to a limited extent in South Africa. It is recommended for use in weaners and older animals. Vaccination has been shown to protect cattle against the clinical form of the disease for several years but not to prevent clinically inapparent infections from taking place entirely. Indirect fluorescent antibody tests have, however, revealed that antibody levels to a homologous antigen start declining at 180 days after vaccination. Annual revaccination for 2 to 3 years is therefore advocated.

Systematic annual elimination of all chronically infected cattle, detected by examination of the scleral conjunctiva for cysts, in a closed herd on a farm in the enzootic area over a period of several years appeared to result in a decrease of fresh infections. It will not be possible, however, to determine with any measure of certainty whether measures based on the elimination of presumed carriers have any chance to succeed until the epizootiology of the disease is better understood.

BIBLIOGRAPHY

Basson PA, McCully RM, Bigalke RD: Observations on the pathogenesis of bovine and antelope strains of *Besnoitia besnoiti* (Marotel, 1912) infection in cattle and rabbits. Onderstepoort J Vet Res 37:105–126, 1970.

Bigalke RD: New concepts on the epidemiological features of bovine besnoitiosis as determined by laboratory and field investigations. Onderstepoort J Vet Res 35:3–138, 1968.

Bigalke RD: Besnoitiosis and globidiosis. *In* Ristic M, Kreier JP (eds): Diseases of Cattle in the Tropics. New York, Academic Press, 1981, pp 429–442.

Bwangamoi O, Carles AB, Wandera JG: An epidemic of besnoitiosis in goats in Kenya. Vet Rec 125:46, 1989.

McCully RM, Basson PA, Van Niekerk JW, Bigalke RD: Observations on *Besnoitia* cysts in the cardiovascular systems of some wild antelopes and domestic cattle. Onderstepoort J Vet Res 33:245–275, 1966.

Pols JW: Studies on bovine besnoitiosis with special reference to the aetiology. Onderstepoort J Vet Res 28:265–356, 1960.

Shkap V, Pipano E, Greenblatt C: Enzyme-linked immunosorbent assay for detection of antibodies against *Besnoitia besnoiti* in cattle. Trop Anim Health Prod 16:233–238, 1984.

Shkap V, Pipano E, Greenblatt C: Cultivation of *Besnoitia besnoiti* and evaluation of susceptibility of laboratory animals to cultured parasites. Vet Parasitol 23:169–178, 1987.

Coccidiosis

B. L. PENZHORN, DSc, BVSc
G. E. SWAN, BVSc, MMed Vet (Pharm et Tox)

Coccidiosis has been termed a manmade disease; it is generally a problem not of extensive ranching, but of feedlots and other intensive husbandry systems. Low-level infections occur in most wild or domestic animals under extensive conditions. Intensification favors reproduction of coccidia, and the well-balanced host-parasite relationship is disturbed. Intestinal coccidiosis of food animals is caused by obligatory, monoxenous, intracellular protozoan parasites of the genera *Eimeria* and *Isospora*. Oocysts of *Eimeria* spp. have 4 sporocysts, each with 2 sporozoites; oocysts of *Isospora* spp. have 2 sporocysts, each with 4 sporozoites.

Coccidia are very host-specific. Nearly all animals are infected with 1 or more species of coccidia, but clinical symptoms are usually observed in young or stressed animals only; infection therefore does not necessarily result in disease. Coccidiosis is considered the fifth most important bovine disease in the United States; *Isospora suis* is incriminated in up to 20 per cent of piglet diarrhea cases.

LIFE CYCLE

The life cycles of all coccidia are basically similar (Fig. 1). Sporulated oocysts are ingested by the host; after exposure to bile and trypsin in the small intestine, sporozoites are released. These penetrate the gut epithelium and round off to form meronts (schizonts), which undergo multiple fission, the first merogony (schizogony). Merozoites are released into the gut lumen, penetrate epithelial cells, and repeat the process (the second merogony). Second-stage merozoites are released into the gut lumen, penetrate epithelial cells, and initiate the sexual stage of the cycle. (A third merogony occurs in some species.) Some merozoites round off and form macrogamonts, which give rise directly to macrogametes that remain in situ; others form microgamonts, which undergo merogony to form large numbers of flagellated microgametes that are released into the gut lumen and reach the macrogametes. Syngamy (fertilization) takes place, and a diploid zygote is formed. Eosinophilic granules in the cytoplasm migrate to the periphery of the zygote, where they fuse to form a protective layer. The unsporulated oocyst, which contains a single cell, the sporont, enters the gut lumen and is passed with the feces. The infection is therefore self-limiting in the host. Animals are continually exposed to reinfection, however.

Sporulation occurs outside the body and can be completed within 48 hours but may take longer, depending on the species. In the presence of oxygen, the sporont undergoes meiosis, with the formation of a polar body. Now haploid, the sporont divides into 4 sporoblasts (*Eimeria*), each turning into a sporocyst containing 2 sporozoites, or 2 sporoblasts (*Isospora*), each forming a sporocyst containing 4 sporozoites.

Optimal conditions for sporulation are high humidity and an environmental temperature of 28° to 30° C. Oocysts are sensitive to desiccation and to high temperatures: they are destroyed immediately by boiling water or steam and within

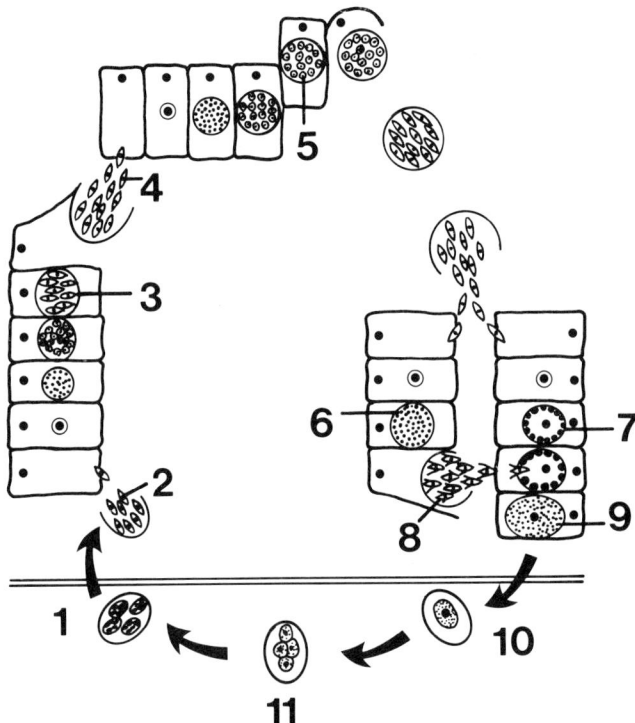

Figure 1. Generalized life cycle of coccidia. *1*, Ingestion of sporulated oocyst by host. *2*, Release of sporozoites and penetration of gut epithelium, followed by first merogony. *3*, First-generation meront with merozoites. *4*, Release of merozoites into gut lumen and penetration of gut epithelium, followed by second merogony. *5*, Second-generation meront. *6*, Microgamont. *7*, Macrogamont, giving rise to a single macrogamete. *8*, Release of flagellated microgametes into gut lumen, followed by syngamy with macrogamete *in situ*. *9*, Zygote. *10*, Unsporulated oocyst shed in feces. *11*, Sporulation outside host. (Redrawn after Urquhart GM, et al: Veterinary Parasitology (Veterinary Series). Harlow, UK, Longman Group UK, Ltd., 1987, p 218.

10 minutes at 50° C. They can be stored for years at 4° to 5° C but are destroyed by freezing. Oocysts are fairly resistant to chemical disinfectant and detergents.

SPECIES INVOLVED

Coccidian species may be identified by morphologic differences, especially of sporulated oocysts, and biologic differences (i.e., sporulation time and location, shape and size of endogenous stages). Size of the oocyst is an important criterion; shape, number of layers forming the wall, nature of the wall (smooth, rough, patterned), and presence or absence of a small pore at one end (micropyle) that may be covered by a cap are other differentiating features. The recognized coccidian species recovered from production animals are listed in Table 1. The most important coccidia of the various hosts are the following.[20]

Cattle (Fig. 2)

E. bovis is the most common cause of bovine coccidiosis. Oocysts are ovoid, smooth, and about 27 to 29 × 20 to 21 μm. First-generation meronts are large (about 303 × 281 μm) and found in endothelial cells of lacteals within villi of the small intestine. Second-generation meronts (about 10 × 19 μm) occur in epithelial cells of villi of the cecum and colon.

Table 1. LIST OF *EIMERIA* AND *ISOSPORA* SPECIES RECOVERED FROM PRODUCTION ANIMALS

Cattle	Goats
Eimeria alabamensis	*Eimeria alijevi*
Eimeria auburnensis	*Eimeria apsheronica*
Eimeria bovis	*Eimeria arloingi*
Eimeria brasiliensis	*Eimeria caprina*
Eimeria bukidnonensis	*Eimeria caprovina*
Eimeria canadensis	*Eimeria christenseni*
Eimeria cylindrica	*Eimeria gilruthi*
Eimeria ellipsoidalis	*Eimeria hirci*
Eimeria illinoisensis	*Eimeria jolchijevi*
Eimeria pellita	*Eimeria kocharii*
Eimeria subspherica	*Eimeria ninakohlyakimovae*
Eimeria wyomingensis	*Eimeria pallida*
Eimeria zuernii	*Eimeria punctata*
Sheep	**Pigs**
Eimeria ahsata	*Eimeria betica*
Eimeria crandallis	*Eimeria debliecki*
Eimeria faurei	*Eimeria guevarai*
Eimeria gonzalezi	*Eimeria neodebliecki*
Eimeria granulosa	*Eimeria perminuta*
Eimeria intricata	*Eimeria polita*
Eimeria marsica	*Eimeria porci*
Eimeria ovina	*Eimeria residualis*
Eimeria ovinoidalis	*Eimeria scabra*
Eimeria pallida	*Eimeria spinosa*
Eimeria parva	*Eimeria suis*
Eimeria punctata	
Eimeria weybridgensis	*Isospora suis*
Eimeria gilruthi	

Source: Data from Levine ND: Veterinary Protozoology. Ames, IA, Iowa State University Press, 1985.

Gamonts occur in villi of the cecum and colon, extending into the terminal ileum in heavy infections.

E. zuernii is highly pathogenic, causing bloody diarrhea. Oocysts are subspherical or ovoid, smooth, and about 18 × 15 μm. Merents (about 13 × 10 μm) occur in epithelial cells of villi of the small and large intestine; gamonts also occur there.

Sheep

E. ahsata is markedly pathogenic. Oocysts are ellipsoid to somewhat ovoid, are smooth, have a micropyle and micropylar cap, and are about 29 to 44 × 17 to 30 μm. There is a single asexual generation; merents (about 184 × 165 μm) occur in the mucosa of the central part of the small intestine. Gamonts are mostly in the epithelial cells lining the intestinal glands.

E. ovinoidalis is markedly pathogenic. Oocysts are ellipsoid or subspherical to somewhat ovoid, smooth, and about 16 to 28 × 14 to 23 μm and have neither micropyle nor micropylar cap. The life cycle is uncertain; it parasitizes especially the posterior part of the small intestine and also the cecum and colon.

E. ovina is not very pathogenic but is extremely common. Oocysts resemble those of *E. ahsata,* but are smaller, about 23 to 36 × 16 to 24 μm. A single asexual generation is known: in endothelial cells of central lacteals of villi of the small intestine, about 122 to 146 μm. Gamonts occur in epithelial cells of the villi.

Goats

E. ninakohlyakimovae is probably the most pathogenic species.[4] Oocysts are ellipsoid to ovoid, about 23 × 18 μm, and lack a micropyle. Developmental stages occur in the lower small intestine and large intestine.

E. arloingi has ellipsoid to slightly ovoid, smooth oocysts, with micropyle and micropylar cap, 22 to 36 × 16 to 26 μm.

It presumably forms giant merents 280 × 150 μm in the endothelial cells of the lacteals of the jejunum, and other merents about 10 to 14 × 9 to 10 μm in the epithelial cells of some glands of the jejunum. Gamonts are in the mucosa of the small intestine and upper colon.

E. christenseni can be fatal to Angora kids.[4] Oocysts are ovoid, about 38 × 25 μm, with a dome-shaped micropylar cap. Developmental stages occur in the jejunum, ileum, and mesenteric lymph nodes.

Pigs

Isospora suis has spherical to subspherical smooth oocysts, 17 to 25 × 16 to 21 μm, without a micropyle.[17] Asexual stages occur in the epithelium of the small intestine and sometimes of the colon.

IMMUNITY

Coccidiosis is mainly a problem in young animals, which indicates that immunity may play a protective role in older individuals. Immunity against coccidia is species-specific; animals exposed to recurrent low-grade infection over a long period and those that recover from the disease develop an immunity to the species by which they were infected. The strength and duration of immunity differs for the various species. Unfortunately, the most pathogenic species seem to be the least immunogenic. Because immunity is not absolute and recovered animals often are continually reinfected, they serve as sources of infection for other animals. Stress may also reduce immunity and allow recurrent clinical signs.

Different stages of the coccidian life cycle seem to differ in their ability to induce protective immune responses; the sexual stage seems to have little, if any, immunizing potential, even against homologous stages. The sporozoite itself is probably not very immunogenic.

The duration of immunity in the absence of reinfection is difficult to ascertain because of the ubiquity of the organism and the difficulty in eliminating extraneous infection. It has been claimed, however, that calves experimentally infected with *E. bovis* became resistant to reinfection within 14 days and showed marked resistance by 3 months and moderate resistance at 7 months. Very young lambs experimentally infected were found to be resistant to the pathogenic effects of some coccidia but were able to respond to them immunologically when challenged.[14]

PATHOGENESIS[19]

Coccidia are intracellular parasites restricted, with a few exceptions, to the epithelial cells of the host's intestine. Coccidiosis involves extensive destruction of the host's intestinal epithelium. Different species usually prefer specific parts of the intestine for their various developmental stages. Many species of coccidia are pathogenic, but others are not. Pathogenicity depends on a multitude of factors, such as size of the infecting dose, size of endogenous stages, number of host cells destroyed, depth of penetration of the host's tissues, and degree of immunity of the host.

First-generation merents are often found in the epithelial cells of the crypts of Lieberkühn; subsequent generations and gamonts usually develop along the sides and near the tips of the villi. In *E. bovis,* the large first-generation merents containing up to 120,000 merozoites occur in the endothelial cells of the lacteals in the villi of the small intestine and can cause

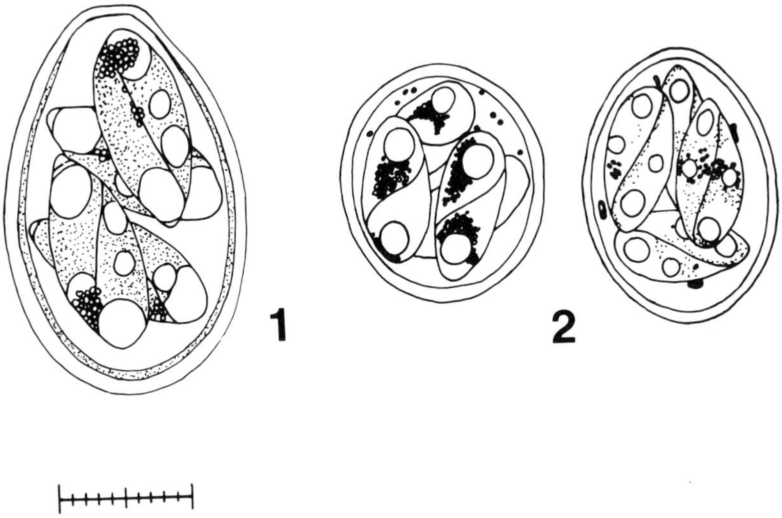

Figure 2. Sporulated oocysts of pathogenic bovine coccidia. *1, Eimeria bovis. 2, E. zuernii* (bar: 10 μm). (Redrawn after Levine ND: Veterinary Protozoology. Ames, IA, Iowa State University Press, 1985.)

disruption of blood vessels, with resultant hemorrhage into the gut lumen. Species in which large endogenous stages develop below the host-cell nucleus close to the basement membrane appear to cause greater inflammatory responses.

An increase in the infective dose of sporulated oocysts results in an increase in pathogenic effects. Large numbers of developing asexual stages may result in disruption of the villous epithelium. The effects of coccidiosis are most severe when the parasites develop in the absorptive areas of the small intestine. Villous atrophy, which often occurs in coccidiosis, results in a reduction of the surface area available for absorption of nutrients and water. Histologic changes may lead to reduced enzyme activity, especially of those enzymes concerned with absorption and transport mechanisms of the cells; alkaline phosphatases are reduced when villous atrophy is marked. Changes in permeability occur in the intestinal wall, which interfere with the uptake of nutrients and water. These changes allow nutrients, including serum proteins, to escape into the intestinal lumen. Coccidiosis may be regarded as a protein-losing enteropathy; the strongly acidic intestinal contents that accompany protein loss impair the absorption of nutrients.

Concurrent infections may enhance the effect of coccidia. In dairy calves, the presence of the nematode *Trichostrongylus colubriformis*, affecting the same general region of the intestine as *Eimeria* spp., was thought to have had a synergistic effect on the development of *Eimeria*.[6]

Experimental *Isospora suis* infection in gnotobiotic piglets resulted in a biphasic disease course with villous atrophy and necrosis of the intestinal epithelium at 4 to 6 and 8 to 10 days after inoculation. The presence of normal bacterial flora markedly influenced the survival rate of piglets but did not appear to affect the histopathologic changes. Mild limited focal necrosis and bile stasis were present in the liver at 8 to 10 days after inoculation, as was ectasia of lymph vessels in the intestinal lymph nodes.[16]

CLINICAL SIGNS

Cattle

In mild cases, cattle show diarrhea and may be listless and anorexic for a few days. Severe cases show hemorrhagic diarrhea; feces may contain mucus and strands of sloughed intestinal mucosa. Fresh, unclotted blood may dribble from the anus. The animal has a rough, staring hair coat. Tenesmus may lead to protrusion of the anus. The tail and hindquarters may be soiled with liquid feces, often leading to myiasis. The animal is anorexic and listless and becomes emaciated, dehydrated, and weak. Animals that do not die recover very slowly. In one trial, feed consumption of affected calves was reduced for 13 weeks and water consumption for 4 to 5 weeks after infection; 10 months later, the calves still weighed appreciably less than did the control group.[11]

"Nervous coccidiosis" of idiopathic origin associated with high mortality may occur, especially with *E. zuernii* infections. In addition to acute diarrhea, the animals show muscle tremors, convulsions, opisthotonos, nystagmus, and occasionally blindness. The symptoms resemble those of hypomagnesemia. Could malabsorption play a role in the pathogenesis?

Sheep

Profuse, watery diarrhea is the most conspicuous sign, associated with emaciation, dehydration, tenesmus, and rectal prolapse. Soiling of the wool often leads to myiasis.

Goats

Depending on the *Eimeria* sp. involved, there may be catarrhal enteritis to hemorrhagic diarrhea. The kid may die of blood loss, dehydration, or secondary bacterial septicemia.

Pigs

Piglets aged 5 to 14 days are usually affected. Clinical disease is characterized by a severe, yellow to gray, frothy to pasty, rancid-smelling diarrhea. No blood is seen in the feces. Piglets may vomit and become dehydrated but generally continue to suckle. Mortality may reach 20 per cent, and survivors suffer reduced weight gains.

DIAGNOSIS

Clinical coccidiosis is associated with late asexual or early sexual stages of the life cycle; passage of oocysts lags behind onset of clinical signs. A diagnosis is confirmed by demonstrating the parasite in clinically affected animals. However, mere presence of coccidia does not necessarily indicate clinical coccidiosis, because some species are apathogenic; partial immunity to pathogenic species may result in low-grade infections that are not harmful to the host. On the other hand, asexual stages of *E. zuernii* in cattle, for instance, may cause such severe symptoms that the animal may die before oocysts have been produced; absence of oocysts in feces may therefore not necessarily rule out coccidiosis.

Merozoites may be seen in smears made of the hemorrhagic stools of severely affected cattle. A simple and fast method for demonstrating oocysts is to place a small amount of feces on a microscope slide, mixing it with a drop of water; place a cover slip over the mixture and examine microscopically. (Oocysts may not be found owing to the small amount of feces examined.)

Flotation techniques are generally used to concentrate oocysts in the feces. Sheather's sugar solution is a good flotation medium because it evaporates rather slowly and does not distort the oocysts. It is prepared by adding 500 g sucrose to 320 ml water; boil gently, stirring frequently, until the solution is clear; allow to cool and add 6.5 g melted phenol as a preservative. For counting oocysts, a modification of the McMaster technique is used.[8]

Oocysts can be sporulated by mixing feces with several volumes of 2.5 per cent potassium dichromate solution (to prevent bacterial growth), placing the mixture in a thin layer in a Petri dish, and allowing it to stand for 1 day to 2 weeks, depending on species.

Microscopic examination of scrapings or stained sections of intestinal tissues showing gross lesions may be used to diagnose coccidiosis at necropsy. Scrapings of lesions are mixed on a slide with a little physiologic saline solution.

TREATMENT

Many drugs have been used for the control of coccidiosis.[15] The development of anticoccidial agents for use in ruminants and swine has largely resulted from an extension of development of anticoccidials in poultry. However, not all of the anticoccidials available for use in poultry have been tested or have been found to be effective in ruminants and swine.

The recommended label use, dosage, dosage form, and withdrawal period of the most important drugs used in cattle, goats, sheep, and swine are given in Table 2.

Anticoccidial drugs are used both therapeutically and prophylactically. Drugs that are traditionally used to treat clinically affected ruminants include sulfonamides, nitrofurazone, amprolium, monensin, and lasalocid.[15] Amprolium is currently still the drug of choice for the treatment of a coccidial infection in ruminants. In some countries, amprolium is used in combination with ethopabate. However, this combination has not been shown to have additive anticoccidial effects in ruminants relative to amprolium given alone.

Sulfonamides are also commonly used for the treatment of coccidiosis in ruminants but are only partially effective.[21] Sulfaguanidine, sulfamethazine, sulfadimidine, and sulfaquinoxaline are the major compounds that have been used. Their concurrent antibacterial activity may contribute to their efficacy by controlling secondary bacterial invaders.[5] Longer-acting sulfonamides such as sulfachlorpyrazine and sulfadimethoxine are the most active sulfonamides for use in poultry,[5] but very little information is available on their use in ruminants. Cruthers and Szanto[5] used sulfachlorpyrazine orally at 50 mg/kg for 3 to 5 consecutive days successfully in a few naturally infected cases of bovine coccidiosis. Potentiated sulfonamide mixtures such as sulfonamides with either trimethoprim (sulfadiazine and trimethoprim: Tribrissen) or ormethoprim (sulfadimethoxine and ormethoprim: Rofenaid) have been found to have synergistic activity against coccidia in poultry[21] but have also not been evaluated in ruminants. The gut-active sulfonamides, succinylsulfathiazole and phthalylsulfathiazole, should not be used for the treatment of coccidiosis because these products become active only in the large intestine.[1]

The carboxylic ionophores monensin and lasalocid are not registered for use as anticoccidial agents in ruminants in the United States but are commercially available as feed additives for use in cattle for improving feed efficiency and increasing rate of weight gain.[9] These drugs are less effective for curative purposes and are best used for preventive measures.[15]

Nitrofurazone is not approved for use in animals in the United States.

Toltrazuril belongs to a novel chemical class of anticoccidials, the symmetric triazinetriones, and is registered for use in poultry in some countries. It has recently been used at a single dose of 20 mg/kg in sheep against natural coccidial infections with excellent results.[13, 25] Diclazuril (Vecoxan), from this group, has recently been registered for use in sheep and goats in South Africa.

In pigs, anticoccidial treatment is normally limited to the treatment of *Isopora suis*. Sulfonamides, amprolium, and nitrofurazone have been used with variable success.[7]

Clinical coccidiosis is difficult to treat, and success is normally limited. By the time the disease has progressed to the sexual stage of the life cycle and oocysts are appearing, substantial destruction of the epithelium of the intestine has taken place and recovery is slow. In addition, in many of these cases, the parasites have already passed through the stages against which the anticoccidial drugs are effective, and treatment is less effective.[9] Treatment of clinically affected animals should therefore include supportive therapy to aid in the repair of damaged gut and to limit secondary infection. Specific treatment of concurrent infestations with helminths may also be indicated.[2] Where animals are penned, clinically infected animals should be removed and housed separately. Other animals in the pen not showing signs should also be treated because they have potentially been exposed and may harbor early developmental stages that are susceptible to treatment.[9]

Prophylactic treatment is designed to prevent the occurrence of coccidiosis on a herd or flock basis. Treatment is coupled to certain management procedures or given under conditions where the potential exists for outbreaks. Drugs available for prophylactic medication include amprolium and decoquinate as well as the ionophores monensin and lasalocid (see Table 2). Preventive medication is usually given continually in the feed over extended periods. In ruminants, with the exception of animals accustomed to a concentrate ration, administration of such prophylactic drugs is not always practical and may be difficult to implement. An anticoccidial compound capable of controlling the severity of or preventing coccidiosis after a single application, as in the case of toltrazuril in sheep,[13] or intraruminal delivery devices like those used by Parker and associates[22] to deliver monensin to weaner calves may facilitate administration of these compounds in the future. In swine, the same drugs are used as for the prevention of coccidiosis in ruminants.[26] For treatment to be successful, important management procedures must be instituted concurrently as discussed under control.

Ionophores have a relatively narrow margin of safety, and errors in dosage and feed mixing procedures may result in toxicity. Potentiation of toxicosis by the concurrent administration of tiamulin and monensin may occur.[27] High levels of amprolium incorporated into feed may cause a thiamine deficiency, but it is reversible by addition of thiamine to the diet.[21] Anticoccidial activity of the drug may be reversed with excess dietary thiamine.

Table 2. RECOMMENDED USE, DOSAGE, DOSAGE FORM, AND WITHDRAWAL PERIOD OF ANTICOCCIDIAL DRUGS USED IN CATTLE, GOATS, SHEEP, AND SWINE

Drug	Trade Names	Use	Animal	Dosage	Dosage Forms	Withdrawal Time (days)
Amprolium	Amprol Corid	Therapeutic	Cattle	10 mg/kg daily for 5 days	20% soluble powder	1
			Sheep	50 mg/kg daily for 5 days	9.6% solution	
			Goats	100 mg/kg daily for 5 days	25% feed additive	
					1.25% crumbles	
			Swine	25–65 mg/kg once or twice daily for 3–4 days		
		Prophylactic	Cattle, sheep, and goats	5–10 mg/kg daily for 21 days		
			Swine	25 mg/kg in piglets for first 3–4 days of life		
Sulfonamides[1]						
Sulfamethazine		Therapeutic	Cattle, sheep, and goats	50–100 mg/kg daily for 4 days	Soluble powder or bolus	15
Sulfaquinoxaline					9.6% liquid soluble powder, and feed additive	10
Sulfaguanidine		Prophylactic	Sheep	0.5–3 g per lamb per day for 20 days		15
			Swine	1 g/15 kg for 7–10 days		
Ionophores[2]						
Monensin	Rumensin	Prophylactic	Cattle, sheep, and goats	1 mg/kg for 30 days	Feed additive	
Lasalocid	Avatec	Prophylactic	Cattle, sheep, and goats	0.5–1 mg/kg per day for up to 6 weeks	Feed additive	
Nitrofurazone[3]	Furacin	Therapeutic	All	10–20 mg/kg daily for 5 days	88.9% m/m	5/swine
Decoquinate	Deccox	Prophylactic	Cattle	0.5 mg/kg in feed for at least 28 days	6% premix for addition to feed	0
Toltrazuril[3]	Baycox	Therapeutic	Sheep	Single treatment at 20 mg/kg	25% liquid	Unknown
Diclazuril[3]	Vecoxan	Therapeutic	Sheep and goats	1 mg/kg orally	2.5% suspension	1

[1]Several trade names.
[2]Licensed as growth promoter but not as anticoccidial.
[3]Not licensed for use in the United States.

CONTROL

Coccidiosis usually occurs in young animals or in stressed older animals. Severity of the disease is directly related to the number of sporulated oocysts ingested by the animal. Control should therefore be based on (1) reduction of the number of sporulated oocysts available and (2) reduction of stress factors.

Reduction of oocyst numbers depends on good hygiene. In penned animals, feces should be removed daily. Pens should be kept dry; leaking water troughs should be repaired. Penned animals should preferably be of the same age, because older animals may serve as sources of infection. Feed should not be placed on the floor, but in elevated troughs, to prevent fecal contamination; troughs should be constructed in such a manner that sheep and goats cannot get onto them.

Before sows enter farrowing pens, the pens should be cleaned thoroughly with water under pressure for removal of fecal material, treated with a phenol-containing compound, and then steam-cleaned.[10] Anticoccidials in the sow's feed will also reduce the number of oocysts shed.

General sound management policies should be applied in order to reduce stress factors. Overcrowding should be prevented. Adequate shelter should be provided. High-energy feed should be provided during and after stressful periods such as transport, cold spells, shearing, and weaning. Anticoccidials may be added to the feed, especially before and during stressful periods.

There is as yet no vaccine available. Controlled exposure may be achieved by gradually withdrawing the anticoccidials from the feed of susceptible animals, especially young ones. This will allow the animals to acquire a controlled parasite burden and develop immunity, while being protected against clinical disease.

REFERENCES

1. Bevill RF: Sulphonamides. *In* Booth NH, McDonald LE (eds): Veterinary Pharmacology and Therapeutics. Ames, IA, Iowa State University Press, 1988, pp 785–795.
2. Catchpole J, Harris TJ: Interaction between coccidia and *Nematodirus battus* on lambs on pasture. Vet Rec 124:603–605, 1989.
3. Catchpole J, Nolan A, Gregory MW, Arthur MJ: Observations on the effects of monensin on the production of antibodies to coccidia in lambs. Vet Rec 118:75–76, 1986.
4. Craig TM: Epidemiology and control of coccidia in goats. Vet Clin North Am [Food Anim Pract] 2:389–395, 1986.
5. Cruthers LR, Szanto J: The pharmacotherapeutics of gastrointestinal protozoans. *In* Phillipson AT, Hall LW, Pritchard WR (ed): Scientific Foundations of Veterinary Medicine. London, William Heinemann Medical Books, 1980, pp 186–200.
6. Davis LR, Herlich H, Bowman GW: Studies on experimental concurrent infections of dairy calves with coccidia and nematodes. IV. *Eimeria* spp. and the small hairworm, *Trichostrongylus colubriformis*. Am J Vet Res 21:188–194, 1960.
7. Doré M, Morin M: Porcine neonatal coccidiosis: evaluation of monensin as preventive therapy. Can Vet J 28:663–666, 1987.
8. Ernst JV, Benz GW: Coccidiosis. *In* Ristic M, McIntyre I (eds): Current Topics in Veterinary Medicine and Animal Science, vol 6. Diseases of Cattle in the Tropics. The Hague, Martinus Nijhoff, 1981, pp 377–392.
9. Ernst JV, Benz GW: Intestinal coccidiosis in cattle. Vet Clin North Am [Food Anim Pract] 2:283–291, 1986.
10. Ernst JV, Lindsay DS, Current WL: Control of *Isospora suis*–induced coccidiosis on a swine farm. Am J Vet Res 46:643–645, 1985.
11. Fitzgerald PR, Mansfield ME: Effects of bovine coccidiosis on certain blood components, feed consumption, and body weight changes of calves. Am J Vet Res 33:1391–1397, 1972.
12. Foreyt WJ: Epidemiology and control of coccidia in sheep. Vet Clin North Am [Food Anim Pract] 2:383–388, 1986.

13. Gjerde B, Helle O: Efficacy of Toltrazuril in the prevention of coccidiosis in naturally infected lambs on pasture. Acta Vet Scand 27:124–137, 1986.
14. Gregory MW, Catchpole J: Ovine coccidiosis: heavy infection in young lambs increases resistance without causing disease. Vet Rec 124:458–461, 1989.
15. Gregory MW, Joyner LP, Catchpole J: Medication against ovine coccidiosis: a review. Vet Rec Commun 5:307–325, 1981/1982.
16. Harleman JH, Meyer RC: Pathogenicity of *Isospora suis* in gnotobiotic and conventionalised piglets. Vet Rec 116:561–565, 1985.
17. Levine ND: Veterinary Protozoology. Ames, IA, Iowa State University Press, 1985.
18. Lindsay DS, Current WL, Taylor JR: Effects of experimentally induced *Isospora suis* infection on morbidity, mortality, and weight gains in nursing pigs. Am J Vet Res 46:1511–1512, 1985.
19. Long PL: Pathogenicity of enteric protozoa. *In* Phillipson AT, Hall LW, Pritchard WR (eds): Scientific Foundations of Veterinary Medicine. London, William Heinemann Medical Books, 1980, pp 215–220.
20. Long PL (ed): The Biology of the Coccidia. London, Edward Arnold, 1982.
21. McDougald LR, Roberson EL: Antiprotozoal drugs. *In* Booth NH, McDonald LE (eds): Veterinary Pharmacology and Therapeutics. Ames, IA, Iowa State University Press, 1988, pp 950–968.
22. Parker RJ, Jones GW, Ellis KJ, et al: Post weaning coccidiosis in beef calves in the dry tropics: experimental control with continuous monensin supplementation via intra-ruminal devices and concurrent epidemiological observations. Trop Anim Health Prod 18:198–208, 1986.
23. Schillhorn Van Veen TW: Coccidiosis in ruminants. Compend Contin Educ Pract Vet 8:F52–F58, 1986.
24. Stuart BP, Lindsay DS: Coccidiosis in swine. Vet Clin North Am [Food Anim Pract] 2:455–468, 1986.
25. Taylor SM, Kenny J: Coccidiocidal efficacy of a single treatment of Toltrazuril in naturally infected lambs. Vet Rec 123:573, 1988.
26. Tubbs RC: Controlling coccidiosis in neonatal pigs. VM/Food Anim Pract June:646–650, 1987.
27. Van Vleet JF, Runnels LJ, Cook JR, Scheidt AB: Monensin toxicosis in swine: potentiation by tiamulin administration and ameliorative effect of treatment with selenium and/or vitamin E. Am J Vet Res 48:1520–1524, 1987.

Trypanosomiasis
(Surra; Nagana, Samore, or Tsetse Fly Disease)

ROBERT J. CONNOR, MVSc, D Vet Med, MRCVS

Trypanosomiases are diseases of people and domestic animals resulting from infection with parasitic protozoa of the genus *Trypanosoma*. Trypanosomes parasitize all classes of vertebrates and are transmitted from host to host by hematophagous vectors. Usually trypanosomal infections are not pathogenic; however, several species of trypanosomes that parasitize mammals are less well adapted and commonly cause disease.

The trypanosomiases form a group of diseases; each species of pathogenic trypanosome causes the disease trypanosomiasis. The course of a trypanosomal infection varies considerably, depending on the species of trypanosome and the host species involved. Trypanosomiasis is generally characterized by intermittent presence of parasites in the blood and intermittent fever. Most infections are chronic. Affected animals become anemic and weak; they lose weight and body condition, their productivity is reduced, and, often, mortality rates are high.

Animal trypanosomiasis occurs widely in the tropics and subtropics and is well recognized, having various local names such as mal de caderas in equines of Central and South America; surra in equines and camels in India; and nagana, samore, or tsetse fly disease in sub-Saharan Africa. Human trypanosomiasis occurs as Chagas' disease in Central and South America and as sleeping sickness in Africa.

Animal trypanosomiasis causes huge economic losses that are greatest in the vast tsetse-infested tracts of sub-Saharan Africa. Tsetse flies transmit trypanosomes to natural wild animal hosts; several species of these trypanosomes are pathogenic to domestic animals (Table 1). Beyond the limits of tsetse infestation, *T. evansi* and *T. vivax* are transmitted by other hematophagous flies. *T. evansi* is a serious pathogen of camels in northern Africa; it also occurs in southern Russia, the Indian subcontinent, and the Near and Far East and affects mainly equines, buffaloes, and pigs. In Central and South America, *T. evansi* affects mainly equines, whereas *T. vivax* is the cause of bovine trypanosomiasis in this region.

ETIOLOGY AND LIFE CYCLE

Trypanosomes are kinetoplastid protozoa and typically require 2 hosts for completion of their life cycle. Pathogenic trypanosomes of livestock are "salivarian"; they multiply in the blood, tissues, or body fluids of the vertebrate host and are transmitted between vertebrate hosts with the saliva of blood-sucking flies as they feed. In the tsetse fly, trypanosomes undergo a cycle of development and maturation before infective metacyclic trypanosomes are transmitted to the next host. In contrast, *T. evansi* has no cycle of development in the vectors and is transmitted mechanically on the contaminated mouthparts of biting flies as they complete interrupted blood meals. Although *T. vivax* is an important tsetse-transmitted pathogen of livestock, it has become established outside tsetse habitats; in these areas, it is transmitted mechanically.

From the site of inoculation in the skin, trypanosomes reach

Table 1. PATHOGENICITY[1] OF SALIVARIAN TRYPANOSOMES IN LIVESTOCK

Trypanosome Subgenus	Trypanosome Species	Cattle	Goats and Sheep	Pigs	Camels	Equines
Trypanozoon	*T. brucei*[2]	+	+ +	+	+ + +	+ + +
	T. evansi[3]	+ +	+	+ +	+ + +	+ + +
	T. equiperdum[4]	−	−	−	−	+ + +
Nannomonas	*T. congolense*	+ + +	+ +	+	+ +	+ +
	T. simiae	−	+	+ + +	+ + +	−
Duttonella	*T. vivax*	+ + +	+ +	−	+ +	+ +
Pycnomonas	*T. suis*[5]	−	−	+ +	−	−

− not pathogenic; + mildly pathogenic; + + moderately pathogenic; + + + severely pathogenic.
[1]Under usual field conditions, but which is modified by many factors.
[2]*T. brucei gambiense* and *T. brucei rhodesiense* cause human sleeping sickness in West and East Africa, respectively, and have animal reservoirs, in which pathogenicity is low. *T. brucei brucei* is not infective to humans.
[3]Mechanical transmission by biting flies other than tsetse.
[4]Transmission is venereal.
[5]Rarely encountered.

the blood stream via the lymphatics. The parasites then multiply by longitudinal binary fission; parasitemia becomes patent some 10 to 14 days after the infective blood meal. Infection is characterized by alternate parasitemia and aparasitemia, which is attributable to the phenomenon of antigenic variation. Each trypanosome has a dense glycoprotein (and thus antigenic) surface coat. Antibodies specific to one type of antigenic coat cause complement-mediated lysis of the parasites. The ability of trypanosomes to vary the antigenic nature of the coat enables the parasite population to evade the full effects of the host's immune response. The large antigenic repertoire results in prolonged infections and chronic disease. Trypanosomes, especially of the subgenus *Trypanozoon* (Table 1), tend to invade extravascular spaces, such as the aqueous humor of the eye and cerebrospinal fluid. Such infections are often aparasitemic.

The pathogenicity of trypanosomes varies with the different species of host; for example, *T. simiae* is a serious pathogen of pigs to which cattle are refractory. The converse is true with *T. vivax*.

EPIZOOTIOLOGY

Management is central to the epizootiology of animal trypanosomiasis. It frequently determines the extent to which livestock are exposed to challenge and also governs their general health and nutritional status. The other key aspects of the epizootiology of trypanosomiasis involve interactions of parasites, vectors, and livestock. Climate affects vector activity and abundance and frequently influences husbandry practices; these factors result in seasonal changes in disease incidence.

Important variations also occur in the virulence of trypanosomes within a single species; the susceptibility of different species and breeds of livestock to infection and disease; and the efficiency with which the different vectors transmit infection.

Sylvatic cycles of trypanosome transmission occur in tsetseinfested areas, in which both the tsetse flies and the wild animal hosts constitute reservoirs of infection. The entry of domestic animals into these areas is quickly followed by the emergence of trypanosomiasis. The wild animal hosts are tolerant of trypanosomal infection, a trait shared by some breeds of livestock such as the N'Dama and Muturu breeds of cattle. Even within breeds of trypanosusceptible cattle, some individuals are more tolerant than others. However, tolerance is not synonymous with absolute resistance, and when infected trypanotolerant animals are stressed, parasitemia flares up, often precipitating disease.

In common with other vector-borne diseases, trypanosomiasis occurs as a herd problem that becomes increasingly serious as fly numbers increase.

PATHOGENESIS

Metacyclic trypanosomes may produce a transient inflammatory lesion—a chancre—at the site of inoculation in the skin. The subsequent onset of parasitemia is accompanied by fever, which subsides in aparasitemic periods. The interval between peaks of parasitemia ranges from 4 to 12 days initially, with the first peak usually lasting several days. In long-standing infections, parasites may be undetectable for many weeks; when parasitemia does occur, it is often low-grade and afebrile.

The successive antibody responses to the different antigenic populations of trypanosomes lead to the destruction of large numbers of parasites. This is accompanied by the release of parasite-derived enzymes and host-derived cytokines into the circulation. Cellular debris and complexed antigen and antibody are removed by the cells of the mononuclear phagocyte system, which becomes enlarged as infection progresses. Erythrocytes, damaged after the onset of parasitemia, are also phagocytosed, and the onset of anemia occurs early in infection. Although it appears that the ability of an animal to control parasitemia is linked to less severe anemia, in chronic infections, in which parasitemias are scanty, anemia persists as a result of dyshematopoiesis.

Damage to the microvasculature, induced by immune complexes and vasoactive substances, contributes to tissue damage and organ dysfunction. *Trypanozoon* spp. are more tissue invasive than are the other species and produce marked cellular infiltration and more severe lesions. Trypanosomiasis also induces immunosuppression, which renders affected animals more susceptible to secondary infections.

CLINICAL SIGNS

Clinical signs of trypanosomiasis are variable. They depend on the rapidity of onset of anemia and the degree of impairment of organ function. Disease may be acute, subacute, or chronic. *T. simiae* usually causes peracute disease and sudden death in pigs, and acute cases of *T. vivax* infections in cattle also occur; however, generally, trypanosomiasis runs a chronic course.

Acute disease often causes abortion; in dairy cattle, a suddenly reduced milk yield is a common presenting sign. Acutely affected animals are dejected, often have a stiff gait, and are inappetent. On examination, pulse rate and respiratory rate are raised, and rectal temperature may reach 41° C. In early acute cases, mucous membranes are congested and there may be bilateral excessive lacrimation. Some acutely affected animals become recumbent and anorexic and die within 1 to 3 weeks of the onset of signs.

Other cases survive and may enter a subacute phase in which the predominant signs are listlessness, loss of weight and condition, enlargement of superficial lymph nodes, and a dry, lackluster coat. A marked jugular pulse develops; it is associated with pale mucous membranes and raised pulse and respiratory rates. In febrile periods, rectal temperatures of cattle range from 39° to 39.5° C. Although animals continue to eat, they gradually lose weight. Death may occur after several weeks or even months, but many animals survive the subacute infection and enter the chronic phase.

Chronic trypanosomiasis is very common and may result from partial recovery from more acute infection or from an initial subclinical infection. Typically, animals are pitiably emaciated and lethargic and have dry, inelastic scaly skin and sparse, poor-quality coats. Enlarged prefemoral lymph nodes and hemal lymph nodes and pronounced jugular pulse are readily visible. Mucous membranes are very pale, but animals are afebrile; they may collapse from the exertion of resisting restraint. Death may occur many months or even years after infection, and it is usually due to congestive heart failure.

In subclinically infected animals, acute clinical episodes are precipitated by such stresses as lowered nutritional plane, increased production demands (lactation, work, or pregnancy), or intercurrent disease. This applies equally to trypanotolerant and trypanosusceptible breeds.

Trypanosomiasis is a herd problem and reduces all aspects of production: fertility, birth weights, lactation, weaning weights, growth, work output, and survival. Trypanosomiasis predisposes animals to other diseases, which may mask the underlying trypanosomal infection.

PATHOLOGY

There are no pathognomonic features of trypanosomiasis. The most consistent findings are associated with anemia. With the onset of parasitemia and fever, the hematocrit begins to fall: in cattle, from a value of 32 per cent, it may be reduced to 20 per cent or less in a few weeks. Anemia is initially normochromic and normocytic but becomes microcytic in chronic infections. Leukocytosis, thrombocytopenia, and hypocomplementemia also occur. Endocrine disturbances have been described in experimental infections, and altered plasma levels of several hormones, including cortisol and thyroxine, have been demonstrated.

The gross pathologic changes in acute cases differ from those of chronic cases. In acute cases, carcasses may be in reasonably good condition although mucous membranes may be pale. Petechial and ecchymotic hemorrhages are usually present on serosal surfaces; lymph nodes are enlarged and have a watery appearance when incised. In chronic cases, carcasses are severely emaciated and have a pale and watery appearance. Residual fat around the heart and kidneys is gelatinous, and excessive straw-colored fluid is present in the pericardial sac and in pleural and peritoneal cavities. Lymph nodes and spleen are usually enlarged, but hemorrhages are not a feature of chronic trypanosomiasis.

Extensive microscopic lesions occur in trypanosomiasis and are prominent in the vascular and lymphoid systems.

DIAGNOSIS

Diagnosis of trypanosomiasis is notoriously difficult: there are no specific clinical signs, parasitemia is intermittent, and infection is not synonymous with disease—especially in tolerant breeds. A history of trypanocide use in a herd, combined with the presence of vectors and the presenting clinical signs, enables a tentative diagnosis to be made. Response to therapy may provide a presumptive diagnosis, but the only way of confirming a diagnosis in a clinically affected animal is to demonstrate and identify trypanosomes in body fluids.

Direct parasitologic methods commonly used are the microscopic examination of fresh wet blood smears or of Giemsa-stained thick and thin blood or lymph smears. The examination of fresh wet preparations of the buffy coat of centrifuged blood with dark-field phase-contrast illumination is the most sensitive direct diagnostic method. It has an added advantage because the hematocrit can be measured before the buffy coat is examined for the presence of live, motile trypanosomes. On a herd basis, the hematocrit profile and the detection of trypanosomal infections in a proportion of the animals are sufficient for a herd diagnosis to be reached. Repeated sampling of an individual animal is often necessary to confirm a diagnosis.

The subinoculation of blood into laboratory rodents or other animals has limited diagnostic value in clinical practice. Many indirect methods have been used as adjuncts to the diagnosis of trypanosomiasis. Of these, the most useful are the indirect fluorescent antibody test and the enzyme-linked immunosorbent assay (ELISA). These methods are indicated for epizootiologic rather than clinical use. However, the recent development of antitrypanosomal, species-specific, monoclonal antibodies gives hope for more sensitive diagnosis, and methods using these reagents are being evaluated.

Intercurrent disease frequently masks trypanosomiasis and often results in quite serious underestimation of its true extent. In its chronic form, trypanosomiasis can be easily mistaken for malnutrition or helminthiasis; indeed, these conditions are often concurrent. Acute trypanosomiasis must be differentiated from anthrax, anaplasmosis, babesiosis, theileriosis, and hemorrhagic septicemia. Pathogenic trypanosomes of cattle must also be distinguished from the usually nonpathogenic, ubiquitous *Trypanosoma theileri*, which is a much larger trypanosome, being up to 100 μm long compared with 10 to 30 μm.

TREATMENT

The satisfactory treatment of trypanosomiasis requires correctly administered trypanocidal therapy and supportive measures. Recovery is more rapid when treated animals are well rested and well fed. However, chronic trypanosomiasis often fails to respond to therapy owing to irreversible dyshematopoiesis. Conversely, treatment early in infection produces a quick improvement. Few trypanocidal drugs are marketed (Table 2). The last compound, isometamidium, was marketed in 1961, since which time several trypanocides have been withdrawn because of the widespread emergence of drug-resistant strains of trypanosomes. Cross-resistance between diminazene (also a babesiacide) and isometamidium has not often been found, and these 2 trypanocides are referred to as a "sanative pair." Their alternate use in herds in trypanosomiasis-enzootic areas is widely practiced to control the risk of drug resistance arising.

The therapeutic indices of trypanocides are low and vary with the host species. Diminazene, for example, is highly toxic to camels and equines, and quinapyramine must be used with care in all species: animals must be rested before and after treatment. Trypanocides are usually supplied in dry form as powder, granules, or tablets, which have to be dissolved in sterile water for injection. Careful attention to the preparation of solutions of trypanocides, to body weight estimation and to injection techniques, is essential for ensuring that curative dosages are actually administered. Trypanocides, especially isometamidium, are irritant substances and may cause severe inflammation at the injection site.

In areas where the incidence of infection is too high to be contained by a therapeutic approach, herd prophylaxis is practiced. In order for the retreatment interval needed to maintain systemic trypanocidal drug levels to be reliably determined, constant parasitologic and clinical surveillance is essential. The duration of protection is affected by many factors, the main one being the dosage rate used. Protection usually lasts from 2 to 4 months, depending on the season.

The trypanocides are not equally effective against all trypanosomal species. In cattle, the main pathogenic species are *T. congolense* and *T. vivax*, both of which may be treated with diminazene, homidium, or isometamidium. However, diminazene has been associated more often with resistance in *T. vivax*, and homidium more often with resistance in *T. congolense*. Isometamidium has prophylactic properties and is usually reserved for that purpose. When prophylaxis with isometamidium is practiced, herd sanative treatments with diminazene are given in low-risk periods to remove residual, potentially isometamidium-resistant infections. Homidium is chemically related to isometamidium, and cross-resistance between these compounds does occur.

The use of trypanocides in goats and sheep is similar in principle to that in cattle. However, *T. brucei*, whereas generally not being pathogenic in cattle, is a significant pathogen of small ruminants. Diminazene is the drug of choice for the treatment of *T. brucei* infections and should be used at a higher dosage rate (7 mg/kg) for treatment of infections with this species. Caution is needed to avoid damage to the sciatic

Table 2. GENERIC AND TRADE NAMES OF TRYPANOCIDES FOR THE TREATMENT AND PREVENTION OF ANIMAL TRYPANOSOMIASIS

Compound						
Generic Name	Trade Name	Manufacturer	Action	Range of Dosage Rates (mg/kg)	Route of Administration	Remarks
Diminazene aceturate	Berenil	Hoechst AG, Germany	T	3.5–7.0	IM SC	Also babesiacidal; toxic to horses, donkeys, dogs, and camels
	Ganasag	Squibb, US	T	3.5–7.0	IM or SC	
Homidium bromide	Ethidium	CAMCO Animal Health, UK	T(P)	1.0	IM	
Homidium chloride	Novidium	Rhône-Merieux, France	T(P)	1.0	IM	
Isometamidium	Samorin	Rhône-Merieux, France	P/T	0.25–1.0	IM, IV[3]	Toxic above 2 mg/kg; highly irritant; avoid SC administration
	Trypamidium	Rhône-Poulenc Sante, France	P/T	0.25–1.0	IM, IV[3]	
Quinapyramine sulfate[1]	Antrycide	Coopers Animal Health Ltd, UK	T	3.0–5.0	SC	Rest animals before and after treatment
Quinapyramine prosalt[1]	Antrycide Prosalt[2] R.F.	Coopers Animal Health Ltd, UK	PT	3.0–5.0	SC	Dosage calculated as sulfate
Suramin	Naganol Antrypol	Bayer, Germany	T	10.0	IV	Severe local reactions by other routes

Update: Recently, the new trypanocide mel cy has been introduced to treat *T. evansi* and *T. brucei* infections. It is marketed as Cymelarsan by Rhône-Merieux, France, and is used at a dosage rate of 0.25 to 0.5 mg/kg by IM or SC injection. The IM route is preferred in equines.

Many of these preparations are sold under a variety of trade names. Consult publications such as Veterinary Pharmaceuticals and Biologicals, 6th ed. Lenexa, KS, Veterinary Medicine Publishing Co, 1989/1990.

[1]Reintroduced in 1985 to treat mainly *T. evansi* infections.
[2]Prosalt is a mixture of sulfate and chloride salts of quinapyramine.
[3]Given by very slow injection of 1 per cent W/V solution at 0.5 mg/kg.

T = therapeutic action; P = prophylactic action; (P) = short prophylactic activity; IM = intramuscular; IV = intravenous; SC = subcutaneous.

nerve of small stock during intramuscular injections, particularly when isometamidium is given repeatedly.

T. simiae is the main pathogenic trypanosome of pigs. Treatment of infections is not usually successful because of the rapidity of onset of disease, its short duration, and the invariably fatal outcome. In the face of outbreaks, herd prophylaxis has been attempted with variable results. Treatment with quinapyramine sulfate at 5 mg/kg given at the same time as diminazene at 10 mg/kg can effect a cure, but relapses are common. Prophylaxis may be achieved with isometamidium at high dosage rates: up to 25 mg/kg has been used. Quinapyramine-suramin complexes have also been used prophylactically, but they are not commercially available.

For the treatment of *T. evansi* infections, quinapyramine sulfate or suramin is indicated. Relapses are common because the parasite invades extravascular spaces in which trypanocidal drug levels may not be achieved. Resistance to these 2 compounds has been reported. The subcutaneous injection of quinapyramine is generally well tolerated in camels if they are rested for 2 hours after treatment. Little information is available on the treatment of *T. evansi* infections in buffaloes or pigs.

CONTROL

The contribution made by good management to the control of trypanosomiasis is frequently overlooked. It often determines the level of exposure to trypanosome challenge, the plane of nutrition, the general health status, and the production demands on livestock. Furthermore, selection of trypanotolerant breeds will control the extent of the disease problem, although animals will probably still become infected.

No vaccine is available for the control of trypanosomiasis because of the antigenic complexity of the causal organisms. Nevertheless, under certain circumstances, judicious therapeutic measures promote drug-assisted acquired immunity. Immunity in such circumstances is limited to the locally prevalent serodemes. Chemotherapy and chemoprophylaxis are extensively practiced, the former more so, and these measures permit livestock production in trypanosomiasis-enzootic areas. An understanding of local epizootiology and constant surveillance are necessary so that necessary modifications are able to be made to drug regimens for improving trypanosomiasis control.

Vector control has been highly effective in some parts of Africa. Control measures directed against the tsetse fly currently include aerial application of the nonresidual insecticide endosulfan; selective application of DDT to tsetse resting sites, by ground spraying teams; tsetse attractant odor-baited, insecticide-treated cloth targets (or screens) and odor-baited traps; and complementary sterile male release in control areas. More recently, cattle have been treated with pyrethroids for control of the tsetse. These insecticides, which also have acaricidal properties, are applied by dipping, by spraying, or by means of topical pour-on formulations. The wider use of this "live bait" method on a seasonal basis could produce good control of mechanically transmitted trypanosomiasis, the vectors of which often have pronounced seasonal activity.

For obtaining the best control of animal trypanosomiasis, several methods should be combined, all of which require close supervision and surveillance.

BIBLIOGRAPHY

Hoare CA: The Trypanosomes of Mammals: A Zoological Monograph. Oxford, Blackwell Scientific Publications, 1972.
Jordan AM: Trypanosomiasis Control and African Rural Development. London, Longman, 1986.
Leach TM, Roberts CJ: Present status of chemotherapy and chemoprophylaxis of animal trypanosomiasis in the eastern hemisphere. Pharmacol Ther 13:91–147, 1981.
Losos GJ: Infectious Tropical Diseases of Domestic Animals. Canada, Longman Scientific and Technical, 1986, pp 182–318.
Mulligan HW, Potts WH: The African Trypanosomiases. London, George Allen and Unwin/Ministry of Overseas Development, 1970.
Stephen LE: Trypanosomiasis. A Veterinary Perspective. Oxford, Pergamon Press, 1986.

Trichomoniasis in Cattle

STAN HERR, BVSc, BVSc(Hons), MMed Vet (Gyn),
Diplomate, Agric

DEFINITION OF CONDITION

Bovine trichomoniasis is a venereal disease of cattle caused by a protozoan and characterized by irregular estrous cycles and infertility due to the early death of the embryo and resorption of the conceptus. A low percentage of discernible early abortions (between 3 and 5 months' gestation) and pyometra are also seen. The disease is common wherever natural breeding of cattle is practiced and has been found under these circumstances whenever serious attempts to demonstrate the organism have been applied. It is especially prevalent where communal grazing is practiced and where old bulls (over 4 years of age) are used.[1]

The causative organism is *Trichomonas foetus*,[2] which is a trichomonad with 3 anterior and 1 posterior flagella and a characteristic undulating membrane. Three serotypes are described, namely, *brisbane*, *belfast*, and *manley*,[3] but no differences in pathogenicity have been found. The organism is found as a parasite of the genital tract of both sexes in cattle. In the male, it is confined mainly to the fornix of the prepuce and the mucosa of the penis.[2] Its presence in other parts of the male genital tract is considered incidental.[2] In the female, it is found in the vagina, cervix, uterus, and oviducts.[2] In practice, the most important means of transmission of infection is by coitus.[4]

There is a distinct possibility that *T. foetus* may survive the process of deep freezing semen.[2,5] The artificial insemination industry usually goes to great lengths to ensure that all bulls used for collection of semen are proved to be clear of *T. foetus* infection[1] by 3 preputial wash examinations spaced 1 week apart on acquisition of the bull and annual examinations thereafter.

Sexually active females of all ages are equally susceptible but tend to rid themselves of the infection if they are allowed to cycle normally for a period of 2 to 6 months.[6-9] When pyometra develops after infection, the animal will usually not cycle and will remain infected for much longer periods. A few females will retain the infection throughout a normal gestation and only clear themselves after 2 to 3 normal cycles postpartum.[6,9] A partial immunity has been shown to develop in infected females[10] but occurs in the presence of superinfection. No such immunity has been seen in bulls of any age.

Infection between bulls may be possible if a susceptible bull mounts another that has recently been contaminated by an infected bull.[6] Iatrogenic transfer between bulls is possible if basic sterile techniques are not followed in the preputial washing of a number of bulls. Artificial insemination is also capable of spreading infection if hygiene of a poor standard is applied.[8] Transmission by contact or carry-over by flies between females is improbable.[11] Mechanical transfer of infection by a nonsusceptible young bull from an infected to a susceptible female has been demonstrated only when the 2 services occurred within a short time span of less than 30 minutes.[11]

In the area served by the Veterinary Research Institute, Onderstepoort, *T. foetus* was isolated from 156 (35 per cent) of 446 herds where the bulls were examined by preputial washes in the years 1980 to 1985. In these same specimens, 457 (14 per cent) of 3195 bulls proved to be infected. Similar results were found in the 1988–1989 period. This must not be construed as a survey result because many of the specimens were submitted because of infertility problems in the herds.

All breeds of bulls were found to be infected, and it could not be proved that some breeds were more or less prone to infection than were others. Experience has shown that young bulls (1 to 3 years) are resistant to infection,[12] but *T. foetus* was isolated from bulls younger than 2 years in the author's laboratory and has also been reported by Ball and colleagues.[1] There was no indication that this phenomenon was coupled to any specific breed or to either *Bos indicus* or *Bos taurus* types. The development of deeper epithelial crypts in the mucosa of the sheath is the theory advanced for the greater susceptibility of bulls older than 4 years.[2]

The percentage of cows that will be infected by an infected bull may vary greatly. Work done by Clark and associates[10] showed this rate of infection to be 31 (42 per cent) of 73 cows in the first year, whereas 40 previously uninfected cows all became infected in the second year. In the same work, it was found that cows were reinfected in subsequent years but retained the infection for shorter periods.

An economic analysis of losses due to trichomoniasis in a 940-cow Californian dairy herd was $66,538 or $665 per infected cow.[8]

CLINICAL SIGNS

In the female, a mild vaginitis, cervicitis, or endometritis may occur with a primary infection, but usually no external symptoms can be perceived[2] (Fig. 1). A watery discharge with flakes of pus may be seen in samples from vaginal aspiration.[13] A pyometra, which may occur in 5 per cent of cases,[2] often yields only small quantities of a watery, odorless, grayish-white pus[9] that often goes unnoticed. The pyometra fluid contains large numbers of trichomonads.[2,9] Abortion, which occurs up to 5 months' gestation, may often go unnoticed, but the amniotic and allantoic fluids as well as the fetal stomach content yield large numbers of *T. foetus*.[9]

The breeding record of the herd will show a lower than normal conception rate of between 40 and 70 per cent.[2,3,12] During the breeding season, a large percentage of recently infected cows and heifers will show irregular returns to service.[7] The subsequent calving season will have few early calvers and

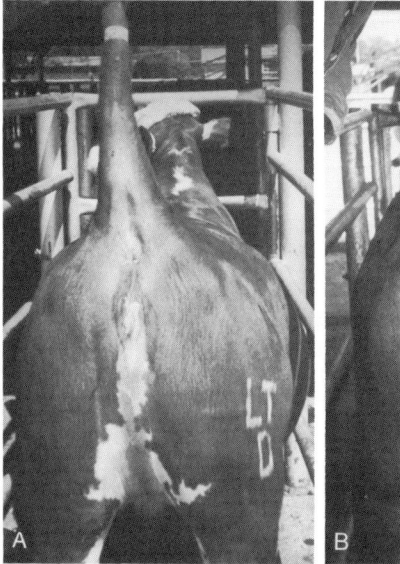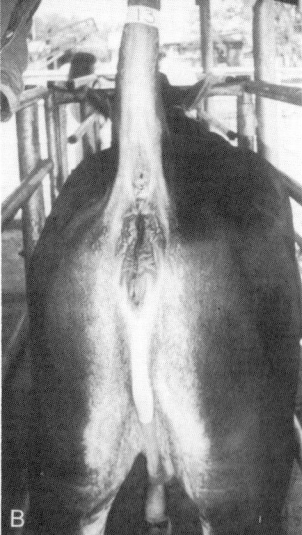

Figure 1. No pus on the tails of heifers infected with *Trichomonas foetus* for 5 (*A*) and 2 weeks (*B*).

many late calvers. These patterns may be obscured by factors such as not all bulls being infected, the presence of immune cows, the recent introduction of infection,[6] and the fact that not all females served by an infected bull become infected.[10]

The young bull (1 to 3 years of age) that comes into contact with *T. foetus* does not develop any signs of infection, and colonization of the prepuce seldom occurs.[2, 12, 14, 15] In the older bull, *T. foetus* readily colonizes the mucosa of the prepuce and penis,[16] presumably because of the deeper crypts in the mucosa.[2] With primary infection, swelling of the prepuce with a mucopurulent discharge may occur but does not last beyond 2 weeks and usually goes unnoticed.[9] *T. foetus* infection is limited to the preputial secretions and does not invade the mucosa.[16] Older bulls remain chronically infected, although spontaneous recovery occurs in a few cases.[5]

In the female, the infection occurs in the vagina at the time of coitus. From here, the trichomonads migrate through the cervix to the uterus and oviducts. They cause a vaginitis, endometritis, or salpingitis where they have colonized the mucosa, but no lesions are seen up to 50 days after infection.[17] If salpingitis occurs, fertilization may be affected. The endometritis may cause death of the embryo by interference with either nutrition or nidation. The embryo or fetus may be affected until the fifth month of gestation, but not more than 5 per cent of cases will abort this late.[2] Most affected females will either abort or resorb the dead embryo 14 to 18 days after infection,[9] which results in irregular returns to service. Jubb and coworkers[18] describe a slight opacity of the normally clear estral mucus in infection, but this effect is often a normal occurrence brought about by the migration of leukocytes at the end of estrus.[19] Some, not more than 5 per cent,[2] of the dead embryos will be retained, with the development of a pyometra that may not be resolved for many months. Except for these cases, females will spontaneously clear themselves of the infection within 2 to 6 months[6-8] and will show a convalescent immunity to reinfection.[2] Rarely, a female conceives despite infection and will then carry the infection throughout the gestation.[6, 8] Females encountering the infection again during the second season show a measure of immunity and become pregnant more readily than in the first encounter with *T. foetus*.[10] A few females will become permanently sterile after the development of endometritis or salpingitis, as will animals that have developed pyometra.[9]

NECROPSY

No gross lesions are seen in bulls infected with *T. foetus*[16] unless they are observed within 2 weeks of infection, when swelling of the prepuce and a mucopurulent discharge may occur.[9] On histologic examination, mixed cellular infiltration and debris may be seen in the crypts, but the causative organism is not demonstrable.[16, 18]

No gross or microscopic lesions of the female genital tract are seen before 50 days after infection.[17] The same investigators reported varying degrees of vaginitis, cervicitis, endometritis, salpingitis, and pyometra as well as the absence of some or all of these lesions between 50 and 100 days after infection, in some instances. The organism was demonstrated by them on the surface and in the lumen of endometrial glands by use of a silver stain.

In cases of pyometra after *T. foetus* infection, the uterine contents are usually voluminous, fluid, nonodorous, and grayish-white and contain trichomonads in great numbers.[2, 9] In a study carried out in the author's laboratory on experimental infection with *T. foetus*, a single heifer in a group of 17 retained a pyometra of several liters for a period of 8 months after infection, and a cow that produced a 4- to 5-month *Trichomonas*-positive abortion had an accumulation of floccular, yellowish, nonodorous pus in the pregnant horn of the uterus. On microscopic examination, the fluid from the pyometra case resembled a pure culture of *T. foetus*.

DIAGNOSIS

The diagnosis depends on the finding of the organism in at least 1 animal in the herd. Preputial douches from bulls are the favored diagnostic medium where laboratory facilities are available.[20] Recently a diagnostic pouch has become commercially available for use in bulls.* When direct examination of smegma is relied on, suction through a plastic insemination pipette or scraping (with suitable instruments) of the mucosa in the region of the fornix is applied.[21, 22] For preputial douching, the bull is restrained in a race or chute. The bull's tail is raised straight up so that kicking is discouraged, and a coarse brush is used to brush his back. Alternatively, a rectal probe from an ejaculator may be inserted with the voltage turned up slightly to produce mild stimulation. In both cases, the procedure described apparently dissuades the bull from urinating while the preputial wash is done. A rope is placed in a noose around the hindleg, above the hock, on the same side from which the douche is to be done. The end of this rope is wrapped around a pole and held (Fig. 2). This prevents the bull from kicking forward with any force but allows quick release should the bull go down. The preputial hairs are clipped down to 1 cm long. The opening of the prepuce is not washed because this promotes urination. Fifty milliliters of phosphate buffered saline (pH 7.2) is run into the bull's prepuce with the use of a sterile funnel and 1.5 m rubber tube of 10 mm outside and 5 mm inside diameter, while the opening of the prepuce is clamped closed around the tube with a gloved hand. The funnel is held in the raised position while the prepuce is massaged vigorously 100 times. The funnel is then lowered until the fluid drains back into it, at which point the tip of the tube is clamped shut and then passed into the collecting bottle. A good preputial wash specimen is slightly

---

*InPouch-TF. BioMed Diagnostics, Santa Clara, CA 95050.

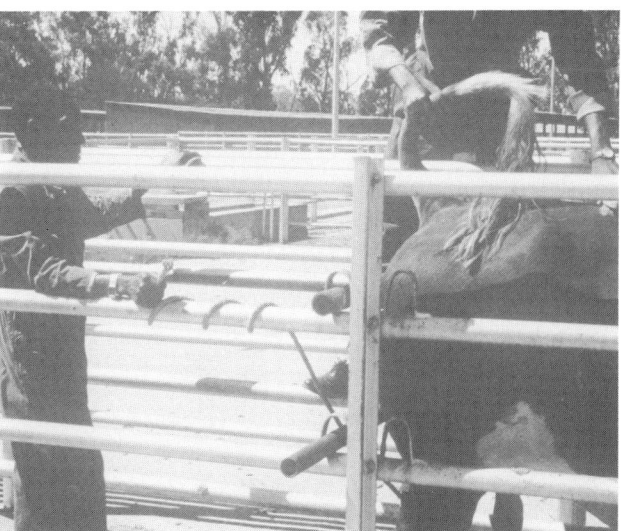

Figure 2. Bull in crush for preputial wash. Note tail held straight up, loose loop of rope above hock on right hindleg.

opaque and whitish in color. Should the bull urinate into the preputial wash, it can nevertheless still be processed because *T. foetus* survives well in urine.[16] A fresh funnel, tube, and pair of gloves are used for each bull to obviate the chances of carrying the infection over. The collected preputial wash is placed in a polystyrene box with bottles of ice to keep it cool and away from sunlight. Although *T. foetus* survives well in buffered salt solution (Ringer's lactate) for 24 hours at 4° C,[23] the preputial wash must arrive at the laboratory within 6 to 8 hours for ensuring the survival of any *Campylobacter* species that may be present. Reece and colleagues[23] describe a transport medium of milk with or without antibiotics in which *T. foetus* survives for up to 96 hours. In the author's experience, however, this medium does not support the survival of *C. foetus*.

The preputial wash is centrifuged at 1200 g for 10 minutes and the supernatant fluid decanted as soon as the centrifuge has stopped, allowing no time for the trichomonads to move back into the fluid. The pellet is resuspended in 1 ml of phosphate buffered saline, examined directly with phase-contrast or darkfield microscopy (1 drop under a cover slip) and also inoculated (4 drops) into 2 of 3 semisolid media (Table 1). One is a modification of Plastridge's medium,[24] the second a modification of Stenton's medium,[25] and the third a modified commercial medium (Table 1).

T. foetus has a characteristic undulating membrane that is seen as a wave motion on one side of the organism when it is viewed under phase-contrast or darkfield microscopy.[2, 9, 25] It is identified and differentiated from other protozoa that may be present in the preputial wash by this characteristic and the presence of 3 anterior and 1 posterior flagella.[26] In the author's experience, the organism tends to be piriform and elongated when a fresh specimen is viewed (Fig. 3), but it shows pleomorphism and a tendency to become spherical (Fig. 4) on in vitro culture. The overall approximate size is 8 to 18 μm × 4 to 9 μm.[20] *T. foetus* can be recognized by its jerky, rolling motion at magnifications of 100× and 250× under phase-contrast and dark-field microscopy. The ancillary structures are better seen with magnifications of 400× and 500×.

In the author's laboratory, it has been found that with direct examination of the centrifuged specimen, only 38 per cent of the herds and bulls were diagnosed as positive, as opposed to the culture of the organism. Other workers have diagnosed 73 per cent of known positive bulls using direct examination only.[20] Nevertheless, many infected herds and bulls would be missed if direct examination alone were relied on.

Serologic tests on either serum or vaginal mucus are possible. They cannot be used to identify individual infected animals but are useful as herd tests.[20] Direct examination and culture of pyometra fluid, fetal stomach content, and vaginal mucus may also be used to demonstrate the infection. Where the fetus has been mutilated, a deep swab of the external auditory meatus often yields a pure culture of the organism, easily identified by direct examination. Vaginal mucus is aspirated from the fornix of the vagina by guiding a plastic insemination pipette with a hand in the rectum and applying suction through a rubber tube connected to a 20-ml syringe. Because the probability of isolating *T. foetus* from vaginal mucus depends

Table 1. MEDIA FOR THE SUCCESSFUL ISOLATION OF *TRICHOMONAS FOETUS*

Ingredient	Modified Plastridge	Modified Stenton	Oxoid CM 161
Trichomonas medium CM 161[1]	—	—	37.5 g
Nutrient broth[2]	16 g	16 g	—
Ascorbic acid[2]	—	0.75 g	—
Agar[3]	0.7 g	1 g	—
Sterile distilled water[4]	750 ml	900 ml	900 ml
D (+) Glucose[5]	10 g	—	—
Sterile distilled water for glucose[6]	50 ml	—	—
Sterile horse or cattle serum[7]	200 ml	100 ml	100 ml

1. The media are dispensed in 12-ml aliquots in 20-ml screw-capped McCartney bottles.
2. Sterile liquid paraffin (0.5 ml) is added to each bottle of modified Stenton's medium to create an anaerobic condition in the medium.
3. The media may be stored at 4°C for up to 1 month before use.
4. On the day that the media are to be inoculated, an antibiotic mixture as outlined below is added to each 12 ml of medium to control bacterial and fungal contaminants.

Antibiotics		
Sodium benzylpenicillin[8]	(1,000,000 IU)	0.6 g
Streptomycin sulfate[9]		1.0 g
Amphotericin B[10]		5.0 mg
Sterile distilled water[11]		100.0 ml

5. Inoculated media are intubated at 32 to 37°C and examined at 48, 96, and 144 hours before being discarded as negative. A drop from the bottom of the culture is taken because more trichomonads congregate at this level.

[1]Oxoid Ltd., Basingstoke, Hampshire, England.
[2]Biolab Chemicals, 2 Bernard St., Colbyn 0083, Pretoria, South Africa.
[3]Biolab Diagnostics, P.O. Box 1998, Halfway House 1685, South Africa.
[4]The ingredients are dissolved in the stated quantity of water and autoclaved at 121°C for 15 minutes, then cooled at 50°C before the other ingredients are added.
[5]E. Merck, Darmstadt, West Germany.
[6]The glucose is dissolved in this amount of water and autoclaved at 109°C for 20 minutes, cooled at 50°C, and then added to the rest of the medium.
[7]The sterile horse or cattle serum is inactivated at 60°C for 30 minutes and then added to the rest of the medium.
[8]Novopen, Novo Industries, P.O. Box 783155, Sandton 2146, South Africa.
[9]Novo-strep, Novo Industries, as above.
[10]Fungizone for tissue culture, E.R. Squibb & Sons, Princeton, NJ 08540.
[11]After the antibiotics are dissolved in the water, 1 ml of the solution is added to each 12-ml aliquot of medium, giving a final concentration per milliliter of 769 IU or 462 μg penicillin, 769 μg streptomycin sulfate, and 3.8 μg amphotericin B.
Many of these preparations are sold under a variety of trade names.
Consult publications such as Veterinary Pharmaceuticals and Biologicals, 6th ed. Lenexa, KS, Veterinary Medicine Publishing Co, 1989/1990.

on the quality of the fluid aspirated,[13] it is suggested that only nonodorous samples be submitted for isolation of the organism. Low-volume and more mucoid samples are poor specimens for the isolation of *T. foetus*.[13] In addition, the percentage of positive samples will depend on the time elapsed since infection, the phase of the estrous cycle, and the percentage of the herd tested. The sensitivity of direct examination as a means of testing can be as low as 56 per cent.[20]

The syndrome of infertility and irregular cycles with a few early abortions caused by *T. foetus* is indistinguishable from that caused by *Campylobacter fetus*.[2,6] The 2 diseases can be diagnosed only by laboratory investigation. *T. foetus* must be distinguished on morphologic grounds from other protozoal contaminants of preputial washes or smegma. Pyometra may be caused primarily or secondarily by a variety of infectious agents. Early abortion may be caused by a number of factors other than infectious agents. Infertility, likewise, may be due to a variety of causes mainly managerial and nutritional.

TREATMENT

No effective methods of treatment are available that are approved for use in cattle, and control of the disease is presently dependent on managerial control and the development of an efficacious vaccine.[2]

Earlier treatments depended on topical application of flavine ointments and other trichomonicides, all of which proved both too labor-intensive and not very efficacious. More recent treatments with imidazole compounds proved efficacious, but all these substances are either no longer marketed or not approved for use in cattle.[2]

PREVENTION

An essential component of any control program is the establishment of a closed herd. Spending $10,000 on fencing

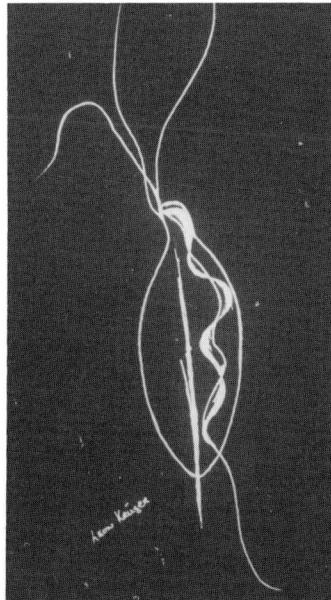

Figure 3. *Trichomonas foetus* sketched by Leon Kruger from direct dark-field microscopy examination of a preputial wash. Note that the central protruding rod (axostyle) is not visible microscopically under these conditions.

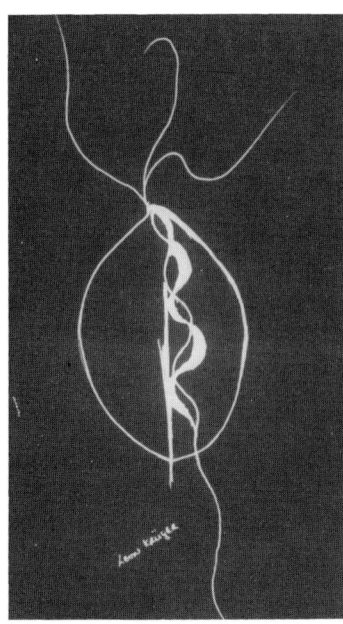

Figure 4. *Trichomonas foetus* more spherical as seen on culture.

is a good investment when there is a potential calf crop loss of $60,000 involved. In addition, all introductions to the herd must be carefully examined. Virgin heifers and bulls may be freely introduced. Older bulls should not be introduced unless they have been bought from a known clean source and have tested negative on 3 preputial washes at weekly intervals.[5,6] Older cows should be introduced only if they come from a certified clean herd, because it is well nigh impossible to test a nonpregnant cow and certify it clean of infection[9] unless she has calved normally and is 90 days postpartum, with regular cycles, and has not been served. Besides keeping a closed herd with strict examination of all introductions, a plan for controlling the disease must be designed for each individual property. This entails employing the methods described below to fit viable management skills and economic design.

Methods for prevention include building up a separate clean herd using virgin bulls on virgin heifers, while the older infected herd is removed by normal attrition. This demands good management to ensure that the herds do not mix.

Cull all bulls older than 4 years and use bulls as young as possible, preferably 1 to 3 years of age.[12] In some herds, it may be possible to use bulls of 1 to 2 years of age which have been bred on the property, for a season, and then sell them to slaughter. When such bulls have to be purchased, this is seldom an economical proposition.

The principle of culling cows in infected herds that are not pregnant 5 months after the end of the breeding season should be applied wherever feasible because nonpregnant females at this time are likely to be infected,[15] and all abortions due to *T. foetus* should have occurred before 5 months' gestation.[2] Special care must be taken to identify all cows with pyometra, because these should also be culled.

The use of artificial insemination, with attention to normal hygienic practice, will prevent the spread of the disease, provided that the semen comes from certified *Trichomonas*-free bulls. If females to be inseminated have had contact with the infection, they must first be allowed 2 to 6 months of sexual rest because they can remain infected for this period.[6-8] The same must be done if clean bulls are to be used on a group of females previously exposed to infection.

Although the chances for the isolation of *T. foetus* from

bulls during the breeding season are lower than normal (60 per cent instead of 90 per cent),[2] the advantage of monitoring bulls during the breeding season is the detection of infection early enough for corrective measures to be taken, thus saving a threatened calf crop.

In an affected herd, a small percentage of cows may calve normally yet retain the infection throughout the gestation period and up to 3 normal cycles thereafter.[9] These circumstances make it imperative that all bulls be tested after the breeding season or at least before the next breeding season.

Wherever possible, a short breeding season (60 to 90 days) should be introduced, and the bulls should be isolated from the breeding herd outside the breeding season.[2,3,6] Test all bulls 3 times at weekly intervals before and after the breeding season and cull all positives.

Encouraging results have been reported on experimental vaccines.[4,27] A *T. foetus* killed vaccine* is conditionally licensed in the United States, but no reports on its efficacy in the field have been published to date.

I would like to acknowledge the contributions of all my coworkers and predecessors and the technicians of the section of the Veterinary Research Institute, Onderstepoort, who over the years have built up the knowledge and technology of our present system. In this regard and in no particular order they are Drs. A. P. Schutte, G. P. Retief, L. A. Te Brugge, S. M. Pefanis, and L. M. M. Ribeiro and Messrs. D. Roux, P. M. Pieterson, C. G. Venter, L. Kruger, A. G. S. Gous, and E. Claassen.

REFERENCES

1. Ball L, Dargatz DA, Cheney JM, Mortimer RG: Control of venereal disease in infected herds. Vet Clin North Am [Food Anim Pract] 3:561–574, 1987.
2. BonDurant RH: Diagnosis, treatment and control of bovine trichomoniasis. Compend Contin Educ 7:S178–S188, 1985.
3. Dennet DP, Reece RL, Barasa JO, Johnson RH: Observations on the incidence and distribution of serotypes of *Tritrichomonas foetus* in beef cattle in north-eastern Australia. Aust Vet J 50:427–431, 1974.
4. Clark BL, Dufty JH, Parsonson IM: Immunisation of bulls against trichomoniasis. Aust Vet J 60:178–179, 1983.
5. Clark BL, White MB, Banfield JC: Diagnosis of *Trichomonas foetus* infection in bulls. Aust Vet J 47:181–183, 1971.
6. Abbitt B: Trichomoniasis in cattle. In Morrow DA (ed): Current Therapy in Theriogenology. Philadelphia, WB Saunders, 1980, pp 482–488.
7. Fitzgerald PR: Bovine trichomoniasis. Vet Clin North Am [Food Anim Pract] 2:277–282, 1986.
8. Goodger WJ, Skirrow SZ: Epidemiology and economic analyses of an unusually long epizootic of trichomoniasis in a large California dairy herd. J Am Vet Med Assoc 189:772–776, 1986.
9. Riedmuller L: *Tritrichomonas foetus*. In Kreier JP (ed): Parasitic Protozoa. New York, Academic Press, 1978.
10. Clark BL, Dufty JH, Parsonson IM: The effect of *Tritrichomonas foetus* infection on calving rates in beef cattle. Aust Vet J 60:71–74, 1983.
11. Clark BL, Dufty JH, Parsonson IM: Studies on the transmission of *Tritrichomonas foetus*. Aust Vet J 53:170–172, 1977.
12. Clark BL, Parsonson IM, White MB, et al: Control of trichomoniasis in a large herd of beef cattle. Aust Vet J 50:424–426, 1974.
13. Pierce AE: The mucus agglutination test for the diagnosis of bovine trichomoniasis. Vet Rec 61:347–349, 1949.
14. Christensen HR, Clark BL: Spread of *Tritrichomonas foetus* in beef bulls in an infected herd. Aust Vet J 55:205, 1979.
15. Christensen HR, Clark BL, Parsonson IM: Incidence of *Tritrichomonas foetus* in young replacement bulls following introduction into an infected herd. Aust Vet J 53:132–134, 1977.
16. Parsonson IM, Clark BL, Dufty J: The pathogenesis of *Tritrichomonas foetus* infection in the bull. Aust Vet J 50:421–423, 1974.
17. Parsonson IM, Clark BL, Dufty JH: Early pathogenesis and pathology of *Tritrichomonas foetus* infection in virgin heifers. J Comp Pathol 86:59–66, 1976.
18. Jubb KVF, Kennedy PC, Palmer N: Pathology of Domestic Animals, 3rd ed, vol 3. New York, Academic Press, 1985.
19. Paisley LG, Mickelson WD, Anderson PB: Mechanisms and therapy for retained fetal membranes and uterine infections of cows: a review. Theriogenology 25:353–381, 1986.
20. Skirrow SZ, BonDurant RH: Bovine trichomoniasis. Vet Bull 58:591–603, 1988.
21. Tedesco LF, Errico F, Del Baglivi LP: Comparison of three sampling methods for the diagnosis of genital vibriosis in the bull. Aust Vet J 53:470–472, 1977.
22. Tedesco LF, Errico F, Del Baglivi LP: Diagnosis of *Tritrichomonas foetus* infection in bulls using two sampling methods and a transport medium. Aust Vet J 55:322–324, 1979.
23. Reece RL, Dennett DP, Johnson RH: Some observations on cultural and transport conditions for *Tritrichomonas foetus* var. *brisbane*. Aust Vet J 60:62–63, 1983.
24. Plastridge WN: Cultivation of a bacteria-free strain of *Trichomonas foetus*. J Bacteriol 45:196–197, 1943.
25. Lowe GH: The Trichomonads. Public Health Laboratory Service, Monograph Series 9. London, Her Majesty's Stationery Office, 1978.
26. Morgan BB, Noland LE: Laboratory methods for differentiating *Trichomonas foetus* from other protozoa in the diagnosis of trichomoniasis in cattle. J Am Vet Med Assoc 102:11–15, 1943.
27. Clark BL, Emery DL, Dufty JH: Therapeutic immunisation of bulls with membranes and glycoproteins of *Trichomonas foetus* var. *brisbane*. Aust Vet J 61:65–66, 1984.

---

*American Home Products, Fort Dodge Laboratories Inc., Fort Dodge, IA 50501.

Cryptosporidiosis
COLIN G. STEWART, BVMS, BVSc(Hons), MSc

Cryptosporidium spp. are coccidia of the family Cryptosporidiidae. They are protozoan parasites that can cause diarrhea in neonatal calves, lambs, kids, and piglets. The disease is common in North America, Europe, and Australia; however, cases have been reported from many parts of the world. Infections have been reported in a variety of animal species including birds, reptiles, mammals, and humans.

ETIOLOGY AND LIFE CYCLE

Four valid species of *Cryptosporidium* are recognized. The most common species infecting mammals is *C. parvum*, whereas *C. muris* is less common in food animals. *C. baileyi* and *C. meleagridis* infect birds. The life cycle is similar to that of other intestinal coccidia but differs in that they develop just under the surface membrane of the host cell. Transmission is by ingestion of oocysts present in fecal material. After ingestion, sporozoites are released and penetrate the brush border and develop into meronts within a parasitophorous vacuole in the microvillous region of the host cells. The meronts are small and contain merozoites, which are released and produce a second generation of meronts. Merozoites released from these second-generation meronts enter further cells, producing macrogamonts and microgamonts. Fertilization follows with the production of oocysts, which sporulate within the host cell. The oocysts then develop a resistant thick wall and are passed out in the feces. They are round or ellipsoid and contain 4 sporozoites. These oocysts, which are infective, then contaminate food and water supplies, resulting in spread to other animals. The life cycle is shorter than that of other coccidia. Infected animals shed oocysts within 3 to 5 days of infection and continue to shed oocysts for about 10 days.

EPIDEMIOLOGY AND PATHOGENESIS

The oocysts are resistant to environmental conditions and can survive for months if they are maintained in a cool moist environment. In many cases, *Cryptosporidium* is reported in conjunction with other pathogens; however, in some cases, *Cryptosporidium* has been reported as the only cause of diarrhea. In calves, a high morbidity and low mortality occur.

In foals, infection has been associated with the combined immunodeficiency syndrome. As sporulation occurs within the host, autoinfection is possible. This results in persistent infection and has been recorded in immunologically compromised humans. This may also explain why ingestion of a small number of oocysts can cause a severe infection.

Cryptosporidiosis is an important zoonosis. Fecal material from infected animals may contaminate water or food supplies intended for human consumption. This results in diarrhea in normal persons, which can be life-threatening in immunodeficient individuals.

The exact mechanism by which *Cryptosporidium* causes diarrhea is not known. Maldigestion due to reduced activity of membrane-bound digestive enzymes and malabsorption as a result of villous atrophy are probably important mechanisms.

CLINICAL SIGNS AND LESIONS

In many cases, infections are subclinical. In natural outbreaks, clinical disease is most common in animals between 1 and 3 weeks of age. Most cases reported have been in calves; however, lambs, kids, and piglets may also be affected. Acute diarrhea is seen in calves between 1 and 3 weeks of age that lasts for about 1 to 2 weeks. The diarrhea is similar to that of other enteric disease. Depression and anorexia is followed by the development of a profuse, often yellow, watery nonhemorrhagic diarrhea accompanied by dehydration, weight loss, and sometimes death. After a few days, the feces become pasty and the diarrhea becomes intermittent. Relapses may occur after apparent recovery. Vomiting may occur in piglets. *C. parvum* is usually associated with a profuse watery diarrhea in calves under 21 days of age, whereas *C. muris* causes milder diarrhea in older animals.

The lesions vary from mild to moderate enteritis with a progression in the severity of lesions toward the terminal portion of the ileum. In general, there is a good correlation between mucosal injury and the severity of the disease. The carcass is emaciated and dehydrated. On histologic examination, most cases of diarrhea show disarrangement and exfoliation of enterocytes. The villi are fused and become covered with cuboid enterocytes. This feature is particularly prevalent in cryptosporidiosis. The organisms can be seen as small basophilic dots in the microvilli. Ring or crescent-shaped forms may also occur.

DIAGNOSIS

Diagnosis depends on the demonstration of oocysts in the feces of young animals with clinical signs of enteritis, or organisms can be seen in histologic sections. Endogenous development stages are located within the brush border or microvillous layer of the epithelial cell of the intestine. Parasites are more easily demonstrated in tissues stained with Giemsa. In the feces, oocysts can be concentrated by flotation methods and stained with Giemsa or safranine–methylene blue. *C. parvum* oocysts can be differentiated from *C. muris* because they are smaller. *C. parvum* measures 5×4.5 µm (4.5 to 5.4×4.2 to 5) and *C. muris* 7.4×5.6 µm (6.6 to 7.9 $\times$ 5.3 to 6.5). In many cases, more than 1 pathogen causing enteritis may be present although *Cryptosporidium* may be the only cause of diarrhea. Other pathogens often associated with *Cryptosporidium* infection are rotavirus, coronavirus, enterotoxigenic *Escherichia coli*, and *Salmonella* spp. In these cases, the various enteropathogens act synergistically to increase mortality. Environmental stress, such as exposure to cold temperatures, may also increase the mortality. Because many cases of cryptosporidiosis infection are subclinical, it is important to associate the presence of clinical signs and/or histologic lesions with the presence of the parasite before a definitive diagnosis is made.

TREATMENT AND PREVENTION

No specific therapeutic agent has been described for *Cryptosporidium*. Symptomatic treatment should be given. The animals should be kept warm, dry, and well fed. Fluid therapy should be given in cases of dehydration. If managed in this way, most animals will recover unless other pathogens are also involved.

Prevention should be aimed at a reduction of the number of oocysts ingested. Calves and other young animals should be raised in a clean, dry environment and obtain adequate colostrum from their dams at birth. Sick animals should be removed and kept in separate pens. Emphasis should be on regular removal of all fecal material rather than on chemical disinfection because oocysts are resistant to many disinfectants. If disinfectants are used, the most effective are 10 per cent formalin or 5 per cent ammonia.

BIBLIOGRAPHY

Angus KW: Cryptosporidiosis in domestic animals and humans. In Pract 9:47–49, 1987.
Kirkpatrick CE, Farrel JP: Cryptosporidiosis. Compend Contin Educ Vet 6:154–162, 1984.
Tzipori S: The relative importance of enteric pathogens affecting neonates of domestic animals. Adv Vet Sci Comp Med 29:103–206, 1985.

Ovine Eperythrozoonosis
COLIN G. STEWART, BVMS, BVSc(Hons), MSc

Eperythrozoon spp. are members of the family Bartonellaceae in the order Rickettsiales. *E. ovis* infects the red blood cells of sheep. It has been isolated from many countries and usually produces mild clinical signs in experimentally inoculated animals. In certain circumstances, it is associated with a severe disease in young sheep known as ill-thrift. This condition is restricted to certain geographic situations and has been reported from Australia, New Zealand, France, Norway, and South Africa. Ill-thrift is characterized by a failure of young sheep to thrive when sheep of all other ages appear to be in good health.

ETIOLOGY AND EPIDEMIOLOGY

E. ovis appears as a delicate pleomorphic organism, 0.55 to 1.0 µm in diameter, which stains pale purple to pinkish with May-Grünwald-Giemsa stain. Rings, triangles, rods, commas, ovoid bodies, and bell- and rocket-shaped forms may be seen in stained blood smears. Parasites are found both on erythrocytes and lying free between the cellular elements in blood smears. A single organism may be present, or the entire surface may be covered with parasites with a tendency to cluster on the margin of the erythrocyte.

In sheep experimentally infected with *E. ovis*, a febrile

reaction occurs for several days. Parasites appear in the blood at about the same time and multiply rapidly so that they may be up to 100 times more numerous than the erythrocytes. With the development of anemia, the parasitemia declines rapidly until very few organisms are seen. Recovery then occurs. Relapses may occur in some animals. Only those animals with prolonged parasitemias show signs of ill health. The typical ill-thrift syndrome does not occur.

The role of *E. ovis* as the causative agent of ill-thrift is still controversial. Many outbreaks of ill-thrift are associated with the presence of *E. ovis*; however, the parasite can also be isolated from properties where the disease does not occur. The persistence of both ill-thrift and *E. ovis* on properties where other causes of failure to gain weight have been eliminated, such as mineral and nutritional deficiencies and helminth infestations, suggests that ill-thrift may be caused primarily by *E. ovis*. At present, there is no proof that *E. ovis* is the sole causative agent.

In South Africa, *Anaplasma ovis*, *Cytoecetes phagocytophila*, *Theileria ovis*, *Borrelia theileri*, and *Ehrlichia ovina* have also been isolated on properties where ill-thrift occurs. Mixed infections of these parasites with *E. ovis* appear to have a synergistic effect resulting in more severe disease. In other countries where ill-thrift occurs, these additional parasites have not been reported.

New infections of *E. ovis* appear to be prevalent when large populations of mosquitoes are present. *Culex annulirostris* has been shown to be a vector. The sheep ked *Melophagus ovinus* and certain tick species can also transmit the parasite. Mechanical transmission appears to be important with infective material remaining on the mosquitoes' mouthparts during interrupted feeding.

Ill-thrift occurs mainly from areas of high rainfall. In some properties, there appears to be a gradual build-up of the disease, which takes several years to reach maximal severity. At first lambs are normal; however, as time passes, more and more lambs are affected until, after several years, virtually the entire crop may be infected.

CLINICAL SIGNS AND LESIONS

The clinical signs vary from subclinical infection to an ill-thrift syndrome associated with severe clinical disease with high morbidity and mortality. On properties with ill-thrift, lambs usually grow normally for the first 2 to 3 months of age. After this, their growth becomes retarded. Lambs are listless, anorexic, anemic, and pot-bellied and lag behind the flock, stagger, breathe rapidly, and, in severe cases, may collapse and die when exercised. A small proportion of animals may develop diarrhea and hemoglobinuria. Mild icterus is seen in some lambs, which is easier seen at slaughter. The characteristic finding is a decreased growth rate resulting in generalized stunting of affected lambs. The condition may persist up to 15 months of age. The morbidity may be as high as 100 per cent and the mortality up to 50 per cent.

Lesions consist of anemia sometimes accompanied by icterus, splenomegaly, and emaciation with excess peritoneal and pericardial fluids in the body cavities. The anemia is macrocytic and normochromic, although in less severe cases it is normocytic and normochromic.

DIAGNOSIS AND DIFFERENTIAL DIAGNOSIS

Diagnosis depends on the demonstration of severe anemia and failure to gain normal body weight together with the demonstration of *E. ovis* in the affected flock. The geographic situation is also an important consideration because ill-thrift appears to be restricted to certain areas. In many cases, by the time severe anemia has developed, the parasitemia has declined, making demonstration of *E. ovis* difficult. At least 50 blood smears from normal and sick animals may have to be examined to demonstrate *E. ovis*. The presence of a macrocytic or normocytic and normochromic anemia also has diagnostic value. As autoantibodies are produced during the development of the parasite, a positive antiglobulin test is an additional diagnostic aid. This test is particularly useful in differential diagnosis because autoantibodies do not occur in anemia of sheep due to other causes.

It is important to eliminate all other causes of anemia and loss in weight before a diagnosis of ill-thrift is made. These include mineral deficiencies, helminth infestation, and malnutrition. The response of animals to dietary supplementation with cobalt, selenium, and other elements should be carried out to eliminate the possibility of these conditions. Parasitic diseases should be excluded on necropsy findings and response to anthelmintic treatment.

TREATMENT AND CONTROL

Although experimental infections of *E. ovis* are susceptible to treatment with tetracyclines, spirotrypan, and imidocarb, in cases of ill-thrift treatment is often disappointing. The use of drugs during outbreaks of disease is controversial. Some people have claimed beneficial results, whereas others suggest that the extra stress of handling during treatment is more hazardous than allowing the infection to run its course. Affected animals should be given nutritious feed, sheltered from the elements, and disturbed as little as possible.

In affected flocks, supplementary feeding should be given to lambs from about 2 months of age. This will help the lambs to overcome the critical period during which ill-thrift is likely to occur. Pregnant and nursing ewes should also be given supplementary feed so that the lambs produced are in good condition.

BIBLIOGRAPHY

Burroughs GW: The significance of *Eperythrozoon ovis* in ill-thrift in sheep in the Eastern Cape coastal areas of South Africa. J S Afr Vet Assoc 59:195–199, 1989.
Callow LL: Animal Health in Australia, vol 5. Protozoal and Rickettsial Diseases. Canberra, Australian Government Public Service, 1984.
Sheriff D, Clapp KH, Reid MA: *Eperythrozoon ovis* infection in South Australia. Aust Vet J 42:169–177, 1966.

Porcine Eperythrozoonosis
R. K. LOVEDAY, BVSc, Diplomate, Med Vet

Eperythrozoonosis of swine is an infectious disease characterized by anemia resulting from red blood cell infection with the rickettsial organism *Eperythrozoon suis*. This parasite occurs epicellularly on erythrocytes and occasionally free in the plasma of infected pigs. Infection is generally followed by a lifelong subclinical carrier state that may become activated to overt disease under stress conditions. Stress-induced relapse is principally found in sows at farrowing as an acute self-limiting, febrile reaction over a few days. Litters of such sows may become infected in utero or shortly after birth via arthropod transmission.

This disease is well known in the United States and has also been reported from Europe, Taiwan, and parts of Africa. The examination of 1500 pig sera in the United States by means of the indirect hemagglutination test showed 7 per cent to be suspect at a titer of 40 and 8 per cent positive at a titer of 80 or higher. Examination of blood films from 570 apparently healthy German pigs found 5.7 per cent of them to be harboring *E. suis*. It is probable that a pure *Eperythrozoon* parasitemia alone is a rare occurrence, and generally the infection is associated with intercurrent disease caused by other agents. This concept, plus the existence of subclinical carriers, has precluded an accurate assessment of the actual economic significance of eperythrozoonosis to the swine industry. It is reasonably certain, however, that this condition in infected herds that are poorly managed and suffering from the stresses of mange or other conditions can become an unsuspected but costly problem.

ETIOLOGY

The parasite may be visualized in Giemsa-stained thin blood films prepared from acute, febrile clinical cases and especially from infected piglets up to 7 days of age, usually as ring forms, sometimes coccoid or budding forms, 0.8 to 1 μm in size, lying on the red blood cell surface. The organisms may be difficult to find once the height of the anemia has subsided, and they must also be carefully distinguished from artifacts caused by stain deposit. For diagnostic purposes, blood collected in EDTA is stated to be superior to heparinized or citrated samples submitted to a laboratory. A smaller (0.5 to 0.8 μm) organism, *E. parvum*, has also been described, is serologically distinct from *E. suis*, and is regarded as nonpathogenic.

EPIDEMIOLOGY

Eperythrozoonosis spreads rapidly within a newly exposed herd, but the methods of transmission under natural conditions are not clear. Apart from transplacental transmission, arthropod vectors are believed to be important, and the hog louse (*Haematopinus suis*) has been shown to transmit *E. parvum*. A role for biting flies and mosquitoes is suspected but not yet finally substantiated. Mechanical transmission could readily occur in most pig herds from contaminated hypodermic needles and instruments used in tail docking, castration, and ear notching unless hygienic precautions are observed.

Eperythrozoon infection may complicate other diseases as already mentioned and may increase problems where immunosuppressive stresses such as overcrowding, poor ventilation, and heat stress are already present. The anemia that develops has been ascribed to autoimmune hemolysis caused by cold autoantibodies attaching to red blood cells, which are then removed from circulation by phagocytosis in the spleen and lymph nodes. These IgM cold agglutinins are correlated with the serum antibody measured by the indirect hemagglutination test.

CLINICAL SIGNS

Cases of eperythrozoonosis are mostly suspected in newly farrowed sows or in young litters up to about 10 days old. In both cases, confirmation of the diagnosis should be made from blood films, and care is required in excluding other possible aggravating conditions. The sow may present with a high fever, up to 41.5° C, which returns to normal within 2 to 4 days. Other signs during this period are depression, loss of appetite, reduced milk production, and constipation. Recovery without treatment is the rule provided no serious puerperal complication has arisen, such as endometritis or mastitis. After weaning, a chronic form of the disease occurs in some sows showing signs of serious debility and anemia, often accompanied by anestrus or nonpregnancy. Such animals often fail to gain condition with extra feeding and may well be suffering from pyelonephritis or gastric ulceration. When the animal is not responding to treatment (usually the injection of a broad-spectrum long-acting antibacterial drug), consideration should be given to culling before further loss of condition renders the sow unmarketable.

In suckling pigs, the clinician is confronted with a litter some of which are showing skin pallor, weakness, and occasionally mild icterus. The visible mucosae of the colored breeds will be paler than usual. Navel bleeding at birth is ascribed by some to this infection, but this is unproved as yet. The disease occurs on a litter basis and is often noticeable when affected and contemporary unaffected litters are compared in the farrowing house. Infected pigs grow slowly at first but spontaneous resolution is the rule, although unevenness of size may become evident at weaning. When chronic pneumonia is present in the herd, severe "runting" may be seen at weaning as a further complication to previous Eperythrozoon infection. Whereas mortality is not high in this area, economic losses resulting from poor growth of weaners and reduced sow productivity should be carefully assessed in known infected herds.

CLINICAL PATHOLOGY AND NECROPSY LESIONS

Acute cases take up to a week from onset of infection to develop a clinically apparent anemia characterized by a reduced hematocrit and increased erythrocyte sedimentation rate. Blood films become positive in these early stages. Artificial infection of 10- to 17-week-old splenectomized pigs with 1 ml of infected blood produced a febrile response about 1 week after injection.

Necropsy findings include a thin, watery blood that clots on exposure, a varying degree of icterus, yellowish-brown swollen liver, and splenomegaly. Serous effusion into thoracic, pericardial, and peritoneal cavities may occur and be bile-stained. Microscopic lesions include red bone marrow hyperplasia, hemosiderosis in liver and spleen, and centrilobular degeneration and necrosis of liver lobules.

DIAGNOSIS

The clinical evidence of anemia and icterus in sows or suckling pigs may suggest the possibility of eperythrozoonosis, and blood smear confirmation should be sought. The herd status can be investigated by a number of serologic techniques, including indirect hemagglutination, direct or indirect immunofluorescence, complement fixation, and enzyme-liked immunosorbent assay (ELISA). Blood test some 10 to 20 sows who have recently farrowed or weaned a litter for a herd diagnosis.

Differential diagnosis must include consideration of iron and copper deficiency anemia in sucklers and leptospirosis or babesiosis in older pigs in countries where these diseases occur.

Acute copper poisoning in pigs receiving excessive amounts of copper as a growth stimulant (generally more than 500 ppm in the feed) produces gastric ulceration, severe hemolytic icteroanemia, and melena.

The prognosis for acute cases of eperythrozoonosis is reasonably good provided no complicating conditions are present. Specific treatment plus the elimination of any concomitant parasitic disease should be instituted and accompanied by improved husbandry, hygiene, and nutrition.

TREATMENT

The objective with treatment is to reduce the level of parasitemia in acute cases, usually by injection of a tetracycline. Treatment of farrowing breakdowns in infected breeding herds should be accompanied by preventive measures involving in-feed use of organic arsenicals or tetracyclines during gestation and lactation. In spite of their usefulness, however, these drugs cannot be relied upon to sterilize the infection in the majority of cases.

Confirmed cases in sucklers are treated with a single injection of 25 mg of a long-acting tetracycline and with 200 mg of iron dextran injected in the neck muscle and not in the ham. Preparations containing 20 per cent iron are preferred, but leakage from the injection site must be prevented. Some practitioners repeat the iron injection 2 weeks later if it is considered necessary. Unthrifty, underweight weaners should be given a repeat tetracycline injection and be kept in special "hospital" pens in the nursery. Feed intake in these pigs is insufficient for successful in-feed medication. Treatment for mange is also recommended at this time, and ivermectin by injection is regarded as very efficacious and economically cost-beneficial.

An alternative treatment for poor doers is the use of water medication, with either sodium arsanilate or a water-soluble tetracycline, for at least 10 days. Sows with the acute syndrome, and also sows debilitated at weaning, generally benefit from tetracycline injections.

PREVENTION

A variety of medical programs have been described for the prevention of Eperythrozoon problems, and these are briefly indicated.

1. The gestation diet may contain 90 g/ton of arsanilic acid from day 21 to day 105 of gestation. Arsanilic acid may or may not be continued thereafter in the lactation diet at a level of 45 g/ton. When 3-Nitro-4 hydroxyphenylarsanic acid (3-Nitro) is used instead of arsanilic acid, the recommended level is half that stated for arsanilic acid.
2. The lactation diet only may be medicated at a maximal level of 90 g/ton arsanilic acid.
3. Replacement gilts purchased from known or suspected Eperythrozoon-infected suppliers should be fed arsanilic acid at 90 g/ton for a month before breeding.

Because the organic arsenicals are excreted via the kidneys, it is important to warn farmers regarding the absolute necessity for an adequate water supply at all times when this medication is used. Careful control of the farm feed mixing is also a legal responsibility of the prescribing veterinarian when in-feed arsenicals are used.

As mentioned earlier, the parasite is easily transmitted from pig to pig via blood-contaminated needles or instruments used in castrating, tail docking, or ear notching. Advice should be given on the proper cleansing and disinfection of such equipment. Finally, it has been amply demonstrated by field experience that Eperythrozoon cannot be brought under control in herds in which mange and lice problems are not eliminated by appropriate action.

BIBLIOGRAPHY

Smith AR: Eperythrozoonosis. *In* Leman AD, Straw B, Glock RD, et al (eds): Diseases of Swine, 6th ed. Ames, IA, Iowa State University Press, 1986.

Bovine Ehrlichiosis and Nofel
GORDON R. SCOTT, BSc, PhD, MS, FRCVS

Bovine ehrlichiosis is a tropical, tick-borne rickettsiosis of cattle that is seldom recognized or reported. Although primary infections in the sucking young are subclinical, in older animals they cause fever, lymphadenosis, depression, loss of condition, and abortion. Nofel is a fatal stress syndrome in cachectic carriers, which terminates in an encephalosis resembling that seen in heartwater.

ETIOLOGY

The causative rickettsia, *Ehrlichia bovis*, multiplies in tissue macrophages and, rarely, in circulating monocytes, forming dense intracytoplasmic clusters of small cocci. Their colors range from lilac to deep purple on staining with Giemsa. On morphologic examination, *E. bovis* and *Ehrlichia ovina*, the causative rickettsia of ovine ehrlichiosis, are identical. Both may share antigens with *Cowdria ruminantium*, the etiologic agent of heartwater. Experimentally, *E. bovis* has been propagated in bovine leukocyte cultures.

EPIZOOTIOLOGY

The natural hosts are cattle and, perhaps, pigs. Infections in healthy calves reared in tick-infested areas are of low pathogenicity, whereas primary infections in older naive cattle reared in areas free of the vector ticks and, subsequently, exposed to infected ticks are highly pathogenic with a case mortality rate that ranges from 10 to 50 per cent. Recovered animals become carriers and, when stressed by intercurrent disease, malnutrition, water deprivation, fatigue, or adverse weather conditions, develop the severe clinical signs of nofel, which kills 5 to 25 per cent of affected animals if it is left untreated.

Bovine ehrlichiosis is not a contagious disease, being primarily transmitted by ixodid ticks: *Amblyomma variegatum* in West Africa, *Rhipicephalus appendiculatus* in southern Africa, *Hyalomma excavatum* in Iran, and *A. cajennense* in South America. In ticks, there is transstadial but not, apparently, transovarian transmission.

CLINICAL SIGNS

Infections in neonatal calves are subclinical; their presence is discovered fortuitously, for example, after splenectomy.

Older naive cattle exposed to infected ticks become ill 1 to 6 weeks after developing fevers that fluctuate widely for 7 to 10 days, during which time many of them exhibit signs of nervous derangement. Some have a transient paralysis of the larynx that disappears on recovery. Others undergo bouts of depression interspersed with periods of hyperexcitability and galloping convulsions. While depressed, they stand somnolent with lowered heads and neither eat nor ruminate but usually develop diarrhea. Pregnant cows abort. Fatally affected animals die during a convulsion.

The nofel syndrome is an exacerbation of the persistent *E. bovis* infection and occurs in stressed cachectic carrier animals. They develop fevers, grossly enlarged superficial lymph nodes, swollen drooping ears, and suppurative otitis. Many collapse and die if they are not treated immediately. Some have a subacute nonfatal relapse in which the only signs are lymphadenosis and inappetence.

HEMATOLOGY

Intracytoplasmic clusters of *E. bovis* are rarely seen in circulating monocytes. Nevertheless, the hematologic changes are diagnostically significant. There is usually a monocytosis, neutropenia, eosinopenia, and thrombocytopenia. Many immature leukocytes enter the circulation, and mitotic cells are common. The monocytes present a bizarre foamy appearance, being filled with vacuoles, a few of which may contain *E. bovis* organisms.

NECROPSY LESIONS

The gross changes mimic those seen in bovine cases of heartwater, namely, hydropericardium, lung edema, hydrothorax, and ascites. The lymph nodes are hypertrophied, edematous, and congested. The spleen is reactive, and the kidneys are congested.

On microscopic examination, *E. bovis* is most readily identified in impression smears of liver and lungs; it is never found in vascular endothelial cells, the primary site of *Cowdria ruminantium*, the etiologic rickettsia of heartwater. Spectacular microscopic changes occur in the kidneys, in which the convoluted tubules are virtually obliterated.

DIAGNOSIS

The history, clinical signs, and post-mortem lesions in primary infections in naive weaned animals are easily confused with heartwater, particularly in areas where amblyomma ticks reside. Differentiation in the live animal depends on the recognition of the bizarre monocytosis in bovine ehrlichiosis. In the dead animal, differentiation is accomplished by examining liver and lung smears and brain squash preparations. Intracytoplasmic inclusions in the smears indicate bovine ehrlichiosis; the detection of large intracytoplasmic clusters in the endothelial cells of the brain capillaries confirms the presence of heartwater.

The history and clinical signs of nofel are considered diagnostic.

IMMUNITY

Recovered cattle remain persistently infected; relapses, both subclinical and clinical, may occur and can be induced by splenectomy. However, recovered animals resist reinfection with homologous isolates of *E. bovis*.

TREATMENT AND PREVENTION (Table 1)

Infections in sucking calves are seldom recognized and, therefore, are not treated. Before older naive animals are imported into areas infested with vector ticks, steps should be taken to lessen the tick burden by frequent dipping of indigenous animals. After importation, the temperature of naive animals should be monitored regularly; when animals are found to be febrile, they are treated with tetracycline intravenously (5 mg/kg/day for 4 to 5 days).

Cases of nofel warrant immediate treatment with tetracycline without waiting for confirmation.

BIBLIOGRAPHY

Rioche M: La rickettsiose generale bovine au Senegal. Rev Elev Med Vet Pays Trop 19:485–594, 1966.

Rioche M: Lesions microscopique de la rickettsiose generale bovine a *Rickettsia (Ehrlichia) bovis* (Donatien et Lestoquard 1936). Rev Elev Med Vet Pays Trop 20:415–427, 1987.

Ovine Ehrlichiosis
GORDON R. SCOTT, BSc, PhD, MS, FRCVS

Ovine ehrlichiosis is a noncontagious, persistent rickettsial infection of sheep in Africa and Asia believed to be tick-borne and usually detected accidentally in the course of other disease investigations. Recovered sheep are carriers, and if they are severely stressed, a fatal exacerbation that mimics heartwater may result. The causative rickettsia, *Ehrlichia ovina*, was the first hemorickettsia of domestic animals to be discovered. It parasitizes circulating monocytes and tissue macrophages, multiplying in intracytoplasmic vacuoles and forming dense clusters of minute cocci. Its relationship to other ehrlichias is unknown.

EPIZOOTIOLOGY

E. ovina has been detected in sheep only on rare occasions. The known geographic distribution is north, west, and southern Africa, the Near East, and Sri Lanka. Fatal epizootics in severely malnourished and heavily tick-infested carrier sheep concurrently debilitated by severe helminthiasis are even rarer, being limited to single reports from Turkey and north and

Table 1. DRUGS USED IN BOVINE ERHLICHIOSIS

Name of Drug	Company Name and Address	Species	Dose
Terramycin Q-100 injectable solution (100 mg/ml)	Pfizer Ltd. Sandwich Kent CT13 9NJ UK	Cattle	5 mg/kg daily for 4–5 days

This preparation is sold under a variety of trade names. Consult publications such as Veterinary Pharmaceuticals and Biologicals, 6th ed. Lenexa, KS, Veterinary Medicine Publishing Co, 1989/1990.

southwest Africa. The disease is not contagious. Tick transmission is suspected, but it has been demonstrated only experimentally with *Rhipicephalus evertsi*.

CLINICAL SIGNS

Natural primary infections in young lambs are subclinical. Experimental primary infections in older sheep become evident 10 to 15 days after intravenous inoculation of infected tissue suspensions. The onset of fever is abrupt and is accompanied by depression and inappetence for 3 to 4 days, although the fever itself persists for several days longer. Recovery is rapid.

Exacerbations occur suddenly in cachectic carrier animals. Ataxia is rapidly followed by paraplegia, recumbency, and death.

HEMATOLOGY

Intracytoplasmic clusters of cocci are present in circulating monocytes and tissue macrophages 2 to 3 days after the onset of illness. Differential leukocyte counts reveal a monocytosis and a concurrent eosinopenia.

NECROPSY LESIONS

Primary infections are seldom fatal, whereas exacerbations are usually fatal. The post-mortem changes mimic those seen in heartwater with effusion into all body cavities, lung and brain edema, splenomegaly, and cardiac hemorrhages.

DIAGNOSIS

Diagnosis is difficult and depends on the detection of clusters of *E. ovina* in monocytes, macrophages, or both. Suspicions should be aroused if sheep are apparently dying of heartwater in areas where there are no amblyomma ticks. Differentiation from heartwater, however, is impossible in heartwater areas without a microscopic search; *E. ovina* occurs exclusively in monocytes and macrophages, whereas *Cowdria ruminantium* is restricted to vascular endothelial cells and neutrophils.

TREATMENT AND PREVENTION

Successful treatment of clinically obvious ovine ehrlichiosis has yet to be reported; the theoretical treatment is a course of tetracycline. Similarly, control strategies have not been formulated in the absence of concrete data on the mode of transmission. Nevertheless, avoidance of stress and control of ticks would be prudent.

BIBLIOGRAPHY

Neitz WO: *Ehrlichia ovina* infection. Bull Off Int Epiz 70:337–340, 1968.
Schulz K: A rickettsiosis new to South Africa. Onderstepoort J Vet Sci Anim Industry 13:287–289, 1939.

Swine Ehrlichiosis
GORDON R. SCOTT, BSc, PhD, MS, FRCVS

In an investigation into a suspect outbreak of hog cholera in Algeria, blood from a sick pig was subinoculated into a healthy pig, which developed an irregular fever and died 12 days later. The necropsy findings were likened to those seen in sheep affected with heartwater. In the course of a second passage, clusters of cocci were observed in monocytes and, at death, were also detected, with difficulty, in vascular endothelial cells. Drs. Donatien and Gayot named the agent *Ehrlichia suis* in 1942; their findings still await confirmation.

In 1968, Drs. Rioche and Bourdin described a virulent epidemic disease in pigs in Senegal that was associated with *Ehrlichia*-like cocci in monocytes. They emphasized that their rickettsias were not *E. suis* because vascular endothelial cells were not affected. The pigs shared the same premises as cattle, and they concluded that the pigs had been infected by ticks that had fed on cattle infected with *E. bovis*.

BIBLIOGRAPHY

Donatien A, Gayot G: Rickettsiose generale de porc. Bull Soc Pathol Exot 35:324–325, 1942.
Rioche M, Bourdin P: Rickettsiose des monocytes observee chez le porc au Senegal. Rev Elev Med Vet Pays Trop 21:455–461, 1968.

Bovine Petechial Fever
GORDON R. SCOTT, BSc, PhD, MS, FRCVS

Bovine petechial fever, or Ondiri disease, is a rickettsiosis of the bushbuck (*Tragelaphus scriptus*) endemic in the highlands of eastern Africa. Infections in imported and crossbred cattle are aberrant and dramatic, being characterized by high fluctuating fevers, agalactia, petechiation of visible mucous membranes, lymphadenosis, abortions, and high fatality rates.

ETIOLOGY

Ehrlichia (Cytoecetes) ondiri, the causative rickettsia, parasitizes the cytoplasms of circulating granulocytes and, less often, monocytes and tissue macrophages, forming open morular inclusions and dense clusters of tiny cocci (Fig. 1). It closely resembles *Ehrlichia (Cytoecetes) phagocytophila*, with which it shares common antigens.

EPIZOOTIOLOGY

Bovine petechial fever is noncontagious and is believed to be vector-borne. Although the vector has not yet been identified, its distribution is strictly limited to forest edges and patches of thick scrub inhabited by bushbuck, the normal natural host. Cattle vary markedly in their response to infection such that indigenous East Africa cattle undergo subclinical or mild reactions, whereas cattle imported from other continents react severely. Sheep and goats can be infected experimentally, and it is likely that both species are infected natu-

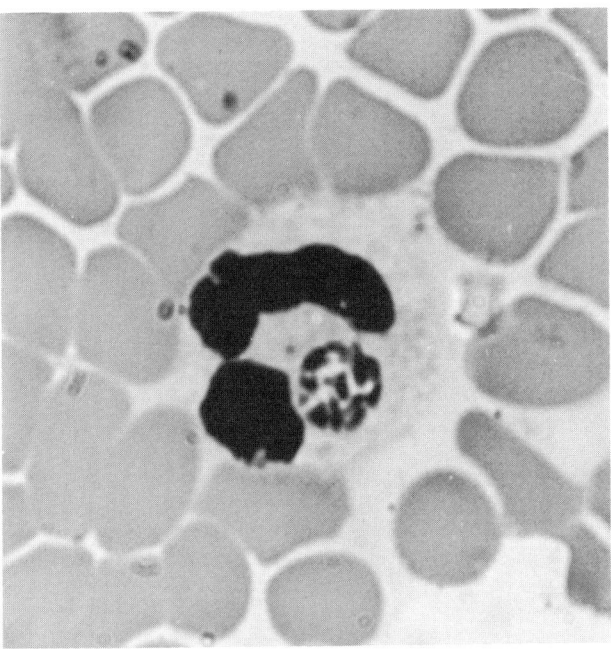

Figure 1. Morular inclusion of *Ehrlichia (Cytoecetes) ondiri* in a neutrophil of a cow affected with bovine petechial fever. (Courtesy of D. Danskin.)

rally. Infections have also been induced experimentally in impala, Thomson's gazelles, and wildebeest.

There is a spurious seasonal prevalence because cattle are at most risk when grazing is scarce and farmers are forced to herd their animals in forests and scrubland. Today, however, clinical cases are rarer than in the past because land pressure from the expanding human population in the highlands of eastern Africa has eliminated most of the pockets of bush and scrub on farmland.

CLINICAL SIGNS

Incubation periods in all species range from 5 to 14 days. Clinical signs in indigenous East African domestic and wild ruminants are usually subclinical and occasionally subacute, but in recently imported cattle they are peracute, being manifested by the sudden onset of high fever, abrupt agalactia, emerging petechiae on all visible mucous membranes, and pulmonary edema. Peracutely affected cows collapse and die within 3 days.

Reactions in naturally infected crossbred cattle and experimentally infected Thomson's gazelles are less dramatic but, nevertheless, acute. A high fluctuating fever persists for more than 1 week, but the attendant clinical signs are not marked, and affected animals continue to eat. Mucous membranes are congested within 24 hours of the onset of fever and are flecked with petechiae that are transient and fade rapidly but are continuously replaced. Epistaxis is not uncommon. Meantime, in some animals, superficial lymph nodes enlarge. A few cattle develop a unilateral conjunctivitis described as a "poached-egg eye" in which the conjunctival sacs are swollen and everted around a tense protuberant eyeball often containing a visible pool of blood in the lower part of the aqueous humor. Pregnant cows are liable to abort. The fatality rate is about 50 per cent. The experimentally infected Thomson's gazelles died after 1 to 2 weeks of illness. Recovering animals have pallid mucous membranes when the petechiae finally fade, and some may develop brisket edema.

HEMATOLOGY

All blood cells are affected. At the onset of fever, a leukopenia is already evident and is due to a disappearance of eosinophils and a severe but transient fall in lymphocytes. Thereafter, a neutropenia that persists into convalescence maintains the leukopenia. Erythrocyte numbers, packed cell volumes, and hemoglobin values are all depressed throughout the fever. In addition, a severe thrombocytopenia increases bleeding times and the risk of epistaxis. Patent parasitemias, evident at the onset of fever, persist only for a few days.

NECROPSY LESIONS

The carcass is usually in good condition. Hemorrhages involve all organs and range from numerous petechiae to ecchymoses; the subcutaneous tissues and fat are particularly involved. Ecchymoses also involve both the epicardium and endocardium. The mucosal surfaces of the alimentary, respiratory, and urogenital tracts have hemorrhages throughout their length. Carcass and visceral lymph nodes are moderately enlarged and edematous with hemorrhages in the cortex and beneath the capsule. Splenomegaly is common and is usually associated with capsular hemorrhages. Hydropericardium has been observed, but only occasionally.

The major microscopic changes are hyperplasia of cells of the lymphoid series and capillary thrombosis. Morulas and clusters of *E. ondiri* are present in the cytoplasms of sinusoidal cells in the liver. They occur also, but less commonly, in other tissue macrophages.

DIAGNOSIS

A presumptive diagnosis is relatively easy on farms where pockets of infected scrub are known to exist. Elsewhere it is difficult to differentiate bovine petechial fever from other hemorrhagic syndromes such as bracken poisoning, arsenic poisoning, hemorrhagic septicemia, peracute trypanosomiasis, peracute theileriosis, and heartwater. Confirmation of bovine petechial fever requires the demonstration of *E. ondiri* in granulocytes either in blood films prepared at the onset of illness or in impression smears of spleen, lung, and liver of a fresh carcass.

Table 1. DRUGS USED IN BOVINE PETECHIAL FEVER

Name of Drug	Company Name and Address	Species	Dose
Terramycin Q-100 injectable solution (100 mg/ml)	Pfizer Ltd. Sandwich Kent CT13 9NJ UK	Cattle	5 mg/kg intravenously for 4–5 days
Terramycin/LA injectable solution (200 mg/ml)	Pfizer Ltd. Sandwich Kent CT13 9NJ UK	Cattle	20 mg/kg intramuscularly

These preparations are sold under a variety of trade names. Consult publications such as Veterinary Pharmaceuticals and Biologicals, 6th ed. Lenexa, KS, Veterinary Medicine Publishing Co, 1989/1990.

IMMUNITY

Recovered animals resist reinfection for up to 2 years. Many, however, are carriers, and relapses occur.

TREATMENT AND PREVENTION (Table 1)

The preferred treatment is the immediate intravenous administration of a full course of tetracycline (5 mg/kg for 4 to 5 days). Alternatively, a long-acting formulation of tetracycline may be given intramuscularly (20 mg/kg). Both formulations have been used prophylactically when cattle have been put at risk by being herded in bushbuck habitats.

In recent years, extensive development of farmland has dramatically lowered the prevalence of bovine petechial fever in the highlands of East Africa. Nevertheless, clearance of scrubland and forests for grazing poses a risk of new foci emerging.

BIBLIOGRAPHY

Danskin D, Burdin ML: Bovine petechial fever. Vet Rec 75:391–394, 1963.

Tick-Borne Fever and Pasture Fever

GORDON R. SCOTT, BSc, PhD, MS, FRCVS

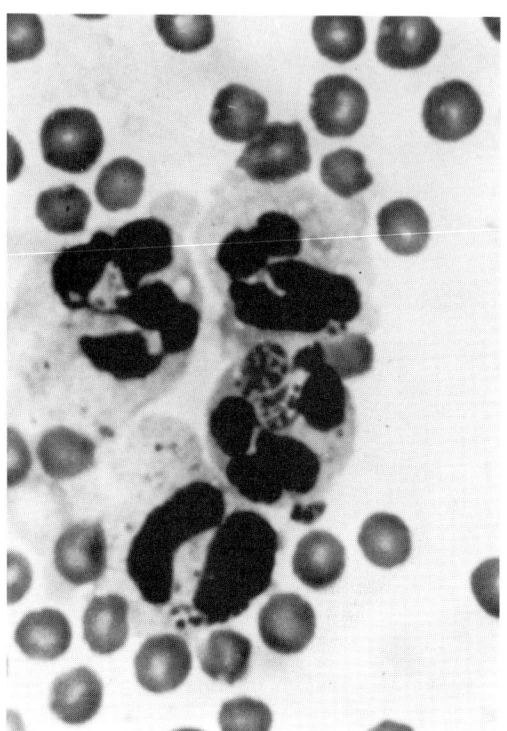

Figure 1. Ovine neutrophils parasitized by *Ehrlichia (Cytoecetes) phagocytophila*.

Tick-borne fever and pasture fever are noncontagious rickettsioses of domestic and wild ruminants. The diseases in the sucking young are characterized by minimal constitutional disturbances despite the presence of prolonged parasitemias and high fevers. In contrast, febrile adult animals pant, eat and drink less, and lose weight. Lactating animals stop secreting milk, and pregnant animals abort. Death in uncomplicated cases is rare. Defense mechanisms, however, are compromised, and a common sequel is potentiation of other pathogens; for example, affected lambs are prone to develop a crippling staphylococcal polyarthritis known as tick pyemia, and aborting ewes and cows often die from a purulent metritis.

ETIOLOGY

The responsible rickettsia, *Ehrlichia (Cytoecetes) phagocytophila,* parasitizes granulocytes and occasionally monocytes, multiplying in their cytoplasms; it is recognizable in Giemsa-stained blood films as slate-blue–colored single coccobacilli, open morulas, or dense clusters of minute cocci (Fig. 1). It appears to be identical to *Ehrlichia (Cytoecetes) ovis,* a rickettsia observed infecting granulocytes of sheep grazing the Deccan Plateau of India. It also shares antigens with *Ehrlichia (Cytoecetes) ondiri,* the causative rickettsia of bovine petechial fever in East Africa, and *Ehrlichia (Cytoecetes) equi,* rickettsiosis of horses in North America and Europe.

EPIZOOTIOLOGY

The distribution of tick-borne fever and pasture fever is defined by the distribution of ixodid vector ticks in the temperate areas of Europe, Africa, and Asia. The vector in Europe is *Ixodes ricinus* and in Asia *Rhipicephalus haemophysaloides.* The natural vector in Africa is not known. *E. phagocytophila* multiplies in ticks and is transmitted to ruminant hosts when they feed. There is no transovarian transmission. Multiplication in the tick is not an essential stage in the life cycle of the organisms, and iatrogenic transmission of a drop of blood from a parasitemic to a susceptible ruminant readily occurs. Both tick-borne fever and pasture fever have a clear-cut seasonal prevalence linked to the time of questing tick activity, which in Europe coincides with lambing out-of-doors and with the turning out of cattle from their winter quarters onto tick-infested pastures in the late spring and early summer. The infection rate in ticks is so high that most lambs born on tick-infested pastures are parasitemic before they are 2 weeks old. Abortion storms follow the exposure of naive pregnant animals to infected ticks.

Many affected animals become carriers, and several relapses of up 2 days' duration may occur. The relapses are spontaneous and are characterized by patent parasitemias with or without transient fever.

CLINICAL SIGNS

The incubation period ranges from 3 to 13 days. Sucking ruminants possess a high innate resistance that masks primary infections. In older animals, the onset of tick-borne fever is an abrupt high fever that fluctuates between 40° and 42° C for 4 to 22 days. The systemic disturbance otherwise in nonpregnant and nonlactating animals is mild, being manifested as a rapid faint pulse, rapid shallow respiration, partial inappetence, low water intake, and slight weight loss. The milk yield is transiently depressed, and most naive pregnant animals abort while they are still parasitemic 2 to 8 days after the onset of fever. The fetus is not infected, but occasionally it mummifies and is expelled several weeks later. The prolonged fevers are said to impair spermatogenesis, but the claim has been disputed.

Pasture fever occurs in lactating heifers turned out to grass. Abrupt high fevers are associated with plummeting milk yields. Appetites are depressed, coughing is frequent, and the ears droop. Homebred heifers infected originally as calves undergo milder reinfection reactions that last 1 or 2 days only.

HEMATOLOGY

Unlike the vague clinical signs seen in most animals, the hematologic changes are dramatic and diagnostic. At the onset of fever, the total leukocyte count is unaffected but the relative proportions of the neutrophils and lymphocytes are changed. Within 24 hours, leukopenia and thrombocytopenia are pronounced. The leukopenia is caused at first by a transient B-cell lymphocytopenia and an eosinopenia that is often total, and then 2 to 3 days later by a severe neutropenia. A slight monocytosis develops toward the end of the clinical response.

Patent parasitemias are restricted to granulocytes and monocytes, are evident at the onset of fever, and persist throughout the fever. Relapse parasitemias are common.

NECROPSY LESIONS

Uncomplicated deaths are rare and appear to be limited to malnourished, unthrifty animals. The lesions are reminiscent of heartwater, consisting of effusion into the body cavities, petechiae in the intestinal mucosa, frank hemorrhage into the colon, serosal and subendocardial hemorrhages, and splenomegaly. The usual lesion in an animal slaughtered during a primary reaction is splenomegaly, but often visible macroscopic lesions are absent.

Microscopic examination of impression smears of cut surfaces of the spleen, liver, and lung will reveal the presence of cytoplasmic clusters in neutrophils and tissue macrophages.

DIAGNOSIS

Fever, agalactia, and abortion are the dominant syndromes. A presumptive diagnosis is based on the clinical signs and a knowledge of the area, flock, or herd, the age of the affected animals, and the season. A history of a recent movement of naive animals to or births on tick-infested grazings is crucial. Suspicions should be confirmed by the demonstration of E. phagocytophila in blood films or impression smears.

Tick-borne fever should be considered a predisposing condition in other diseases because of its ability to exacerbate latent infections and to suppress the defense mounted against fresh infections.

IMMUNITY

Recovered animals develop antibodies, but they are not protective, and the sucking young remain fully susceptible despite the ingestion of antibodies from their dams. Carrier animals usually resist homologous reinfection, but the duration of the carrier state is very variable and appears to be related to the level of humoral antibodies at the time of reinfection. Carrier animals rarely resist heterologous reinfections even if they have patent parasitemias when they are reinfected. Reinfection reactions are clinically and parasitologically less severe and do not persist as long as primary reactions do. Reinfected pregnant animals do not abort. Frequent reinfections with either homologous or heterologous isolates eventually result in a solid immunity.

TREATMENT AND PREVENTION (Table 1)

Infected sucking young are usually not treated. Older animals respond quickly to a single dose of tetracycline (5 to 7 mg/kg) administered intravenously at the onset of fever. The single dose breaks the fever and temporarily clears the parasitemia. One week later there is a mild relapse, which ensures resistance to homologous reinfection. A full course of tetracycline, on the other hand, eliminates the rickettsias, which leaves the animal fully susceptible.

In Europe, farmers purchasing farms that are tick-infested traditionally limit their losses by buying the livestock on the farm at the same time. Thereafter, only nonpregnant new stock are brought in. Newborn animals should be exposed to infected ticks as soon as possible. In areas where tick pyemia is prevalent, early treatment of newborn lambs with a long-acting tetracycline (2 ml intramuscularly) together with the application of a "spot-on" formulation of an acaricide is justified because it protects the lambs over the first 3 weeks of age when the risk of a staphylococcal septicemia is greatest.

The recognition of tick-borne fever in countries outside Europe suggests that there is a real risk of introducing the disease to previously clean areas with purchases of carrier animals if potential ixodid tick vectors are present.

Table 1. DRUGS USED IN TICK-BORNE FEVER AND PASTURE FEVER

Name of Drug	Company Name and Address	Species	Dose
Terramycin Q-100 injectable solution (100 mg/ml)	Pfizer Ltd. Sandwich Kent CT13 9NJ UK	Cattle Sheep	5 mg/kg 7 mg/kg
Terramycin/LA injectable solution (200 mg/ml)	Pfizer Ltd. Sandwich Kent CT 13 9NJ UK	Lambs	2 ml
Spot-On Insecticide, Coopers	Coopers Pitman-Moore Crewe Hill Crewe Cheshire CW1 1UB UK	Lambs	5 ml

These preparations are sold under a variety of trade names. Consult publications such as Veterinary Pharmaceuticals and Biologicals, 6th ed. Lenexa, KS, Veterinary Medicine Publishing Co, 1989/1990.

BIBLIOGRAPHY

Paxton EA, Scott GR: Detection of antibodies to the agent of tick-borne fever by indirect immunofluorescence. Vet Microbiol 21:133–138, 1989.
Van Miert ASJPAM, Van Duin CTM, Schotman AJH, Franssen FF: Clinical, haematological and blood biochemical changes in goats after experimental infection with tick-borne fever. Vet Parasitol 16:225–233, 1984.
Woldehiwet Z: Tick-borne fever: a review. Vet Res Commun 6:163–175, 1983.

Q Fever

I. D. AITKEN, BVMS, PhD, MRCVS

Q (query) fever is an infectious human disease first recorded in Australian abattoir workers as a pyrexic illness of unknown etiology. The causative microorganism, *Coxiella burnetii*, has a broad host spectrum that includes ticks, various free-living vertebrates, and domestic animals. Infected animals constitute the natural reservoir for this worldwide and probably underreported zoonosis.

ETIOLOGY

C. burnetii is a small gram-negative obligate intracellular bacterium of the order Rickettsiales, which, although pleomorphic, most commonly has ovoid to rodlike forms (0.4 to 1 µm) that stain red with modified Ziehl-Neelsen and Macchiavello procedures and purple with Giemsa. Laboratory culture requires a living medium—embryonated hen eggs or cell culture—but because of the attendant zoonotic risk, the procedure is restricted to specialized laboratories.

On adaptation to laboratory culture, *C. burnetii* undergoes modification of antigenicity and virulence from the phase I (analogous to smooth gram-negative bacteria) found in animals to phase II (rough form). The process is reversed on reinoculating cultured organisms into animals. This antigenic variation has relevance for vaccine formulation and diagnostic serology.

Outside the host cell, *C. burnetii* is remarkably stable, resisting desiccation, putrefaction, standard concentrations of most disinfectants, and climatic extremes. This robustness, probably stemming from an ability to form endospore-like structures, accounts for persistence of environmental and fomite infection for long periods (months) after shedding by infected animals. Heat inactivation (e.g., of infected raw milk) is accomplished by high-temperature short-time exposure (74° C for 15 seconds), but lower temperatures are less efficient.

EPIDEMIOLOGY

Q fever has been found in almost all regions of the world, the Antarctic being an exception. *C. burnetii* has been identified in various species of tick, diverse wild birds, and free-living small mammals as well as in a range of domesticated animals that includes cattle, sheep, goats, buffaloes, camels, pigs, horses, dogs, and cats.

Two cycles of animal infection occur. In one, infection is maintained by ticks and free-living vertebrates, particularly rodents. *C. burnetii* can infect many species of tick and in some (e.g., *Dermacentor marginatus*, *Rhipicephalus sanguineus*) can replicate so profusely that up to 10^{10} organisms per gram of tick feces are recoverable. Dried tick feces can remain infective for up to 1 year. It is from this primary cycle that *C. burnetii* may be transmitted to domestic pets or livestock through bites from infected ticks or contact with their heavily contaminated excreta. Some cases of human infection may originate from this source.

Once it has been introduced into a herd or flock of farmed ruminants, infection with *C. burnetii* can be perpetuated without tick involvement, thus creating a cycle of infection. In large measure, establishment of enzootic infection can be attributed to the predilection of the organism for placental tissue, where its florid growth results in parturient excretion of vast numbers of infectious coxiellae that contaminate the immediate environment and spread infection to susceptible in-contact animals. Coxiellae are also present in milk and may be shed continuously or intermittently by infected cattle and goats even into the subsequent lactation. In sheep, milk excretion is much briefer. Infectious organisms are also shed in urine, feces, and oculonasal secretions. The highly resistant nature of *C. burnetii* favors its persistence in the environment, and its small size encourages wind-borne spread of infectious dust. In tick-independent enzootic cycles of infection, the virulence of the organism may be reduced.

Farmed ruminants are important reservoirs of *C. burnetii*, and serologic surveys have suggested prevalences of infection ranging from rare to 50 per cent or higher. The infection rate is highly variable from place to place with a tendency to be greater in warm, dry areas where dusty environments are common. In dogs and cats, seroprevalences of up to 45 per cent and 26 per cent have been recorded.

CLINICAL SIGNS AND LESIONS

Animal infection with *C. burnetii* is commonly asymptomatic, and it is more apt to refer to coxiellosis than to animal Q fever. However, experimental studies have demonstrated that the organism has pathogenic potential. Infection of sheep and calves by various routes has resulted in transient pyrexia and, in some cases, mild respiratory disease; intramammary inoculation induced a mastitis and systemic reaction of short duration. In a proportion of breeding and pregnant females, infection resulted in abortion, stillbirths, or the delivery of weak offspring.

The extent to which natural infections cause or contribute to clinical disease is uncertain, but sporadic cases of bovine abortion have been attributed to *C. burnetii*, as have some flock outbreaks of ovine and caprine abortion in which no other abortifacient agents could be detected. These may represent incidents arising from initial exposure of susceptible flocks to a heavy weight of infection because abortions are not associated with enzootic infections. In cattle, *C. burnetii* has been incriminated as a contributor to complex infertility problems.

In cases of abortion, the placenta may exhibit visible thickening with a superficial creamy pink exudate, but the lesions are neither consistent nor pathognomonic. On histologic examination, there is evidence of infection, sloughing of chorionic epithelial cells, and inflammatory change in intercotyledonary areas.

DIAGNOSIS

Because of the organism's affinity for the placenta, large numbers of *C. burnetii* can be seen as coccobacillary particles in stained smears, although the morphologic resemblance to *Chlamydia psittaci* must be borne in mind. If culture is required, a sample of placenta, uterine discharge, mammary secretion, or fetal liver should be referred to a specialist laboratory. Serologic tests for the detection of antibodies to coxiellae can provide confirmation of infection. The complement fixation test is still widely used but is relatively insensitive and is being replaced by immunofluorescence procedures and enzyme-linked immunosorbent assays. Rising titers indicate recent infection, and antibody may persist for many months.

TREATMENT AND CONTROL

Although *C. burnetii* is susceptible to a number of antibiotics, with oxytetracycline the preferred choice, animal treatment is not a routine procedure but may assist in control of clinical problems in which *C. burnetii* is implicated. Treatment with oxytetracycline has been used in conjunction with vaccination in dealing, apparently successfully, with an infectious chronic infertility problem in cattle.

Experimental vaccines developed for use in animals have incorporated inactivated whole cells or extracts of *C. burnetii*. Usually organisms in phase II are used because they are safer to handle during bulk culture, but some vaccines have been based on phase I organisms, which antigenically are more closely related to those occurring in natural infections. Both types of vaccine have conferred relative protection against challenge exhibited as lower infection rate, avoidance of abortion, and reduced postpartum shedding of the challenge organism. However, vaccination in calfhood or before exposure to natural infection is necessary for optimal results. A commercial inactivated vaccine incorporating both *C. burnetii* and *C. psittaci* has been marketed in some European countries.

PUBLIC HEALTH ASPECTS

With occasional exceptions, animal coxiellosis has not been regarded as an important animal health problem. However, with increasing attention now being paid to agricultural zoonoses, the role of livestock as reservoirs of *C. burnetii* will come under closer scrutiny. By no means all cases of human Q fever are traceable to livestock, and there is growing evidence that other sources, such as parturient cats, are implicated in some instances.

BIBLIOGRAPHY

Aitken ID: Clinical aspects and prevention of Q fever in animals. Eur J Epidemiol 5:420–424, 1989.
Babudieri B: Q fever: a zoonosis. Adv Vet Sci 5:81–182, 1959.
Little TWA: Q fever: an enigma. Br Vet J 139:277–283, 1983.

Toxoplasmosis*

J. P. DUBEY, MVSc, PhD

ETIOLOGIC AGENT

Toxoplasmosis is caused by the protozoan parasite *Toxoplasma gondii*. It is an intracellular coccidian parasite that is classified in the phylum Apicomplexa, class Sporozoasida, order Eucoccidiorida, suborder Eimeriorina, and family Toxoplasmatidae. Felids including the domestic cat *(Felis catus)* and the wild Felidae are the definitive hosts, and warm-blooded animals are intermediate hosts (Fig. 1).

Like all coccidian parasites, oocysts are excreted only by the definitive hosts, cats. Unsporulated, noninfective oocysts (10×11 μm) are shed in feces of infected cats. Oocysts sporulate outside in cat feces within 1 or more days, depending on the environmental conditions. Sporulated oocysts can survive in soil and the environment for many months, and they are resistant to freezing and drying. Each sporulated oocyst contains 2 sporocysts, and each sporocyst has 4 banana-shaped sporozoites (8×2 μm). Sporulated oocysts are infectious to all warm-blooded hosts, including humans.

Intermediate hosts can become infected by ingesting sporulated oocysts in food or water. Sporozoites are released from oocysts in the gut lumen and become tachyzoites (Greek *tachy*, speed; *zoite*, organism) within a few hours of penetration in host cells. Tachyzoites (6×2 μm) multiply in virtually all cells of the body by division into 2 zoites. Within 3 to 4 days, tachyzoites may become encysted in tissues and are called bradyzoites (*brady*, slow). Bradyzoites (7×2 μm) are enclosed in a thin, elastic wall, and the entire structure is called a tissue cyst. Tissue cysts are formed in many tissues, but particularly in the central nervous system and muscles. They are often elongated (up to 100 μm) in muscles and round (up to 50 μm) in the central nervous system. Tissue cysts may persist for the life of the host.

All hosts, including the definitive host, can become infected by ingesting tissue cysts. In the intermediate host, the bradyzoites become tachyzoites within a few hours of infection, and the tachyzoite-bradyzoite cycle is repeated. However, in the definitive host, the cat, bradyzoites give rise to a coccidian cycle in the small intestinal epithelium. The coccidian cycle consists of an asexual cycle (schizonts) followed by the sexual cycle (gamonts). The male parasite (microgamete) fertilizes the female (macrogamont) parasite and gives rise to an oocyst. The entire asexual and sexual cycle can be completed in the feline intestine within 3 days of ingestion of tissue cysts. The extraintestinal cycle of *Toxoplasma* in the cat is the same as in the intermediate hosts.

During pregnancy, the ingestion of tissue cysts or oocysts can cause parasitemia in the mother and lead to infection of the fetus. Congenital *T. gondii* infections are frequent in humans, sheep, and goats.

CLINICAL SIGNS AND LESIONS

Clinical signs and symptoms vary with hosts, mode of infection, immune status, and the organ parasitized. Congenitally acquired toxoplasmosis is generally more severe than is postnatally acquired toxoplasmosis.

Chorioretinitis, hydrocephalus, mental retardation, and jaundice may all be seen together in severely affected children, but chorioretinitis is the most common sequela of congenital infection in children. Hydrocephalus does not occur in sheep, goats, and other animals.

In ewes infected during pregnancy, lambs may be mummified, macerated, aborted, or stillborn or may be born weak and die within a week of birth. Lambs that survive the first week generally grow normally to adulthood and produce *T. gondii*–free lambs. Although infected adult sheep have no clinical signs, adult goats can die from toxoplasmosis. Severe congenital toxoplasmosis has been reported in cats, dogs, and pigs but not in cattle or horses.

Clinical toxoplasmosis in dogs is generally seen concurrently with canine distemper virus infection and often involves lungs, liver, and the central nervous system. Pneumonia is the most common entity in clinical toxoplasmosis in cats. Clinical toxoplasmosis has never been documented in cattle and horses.

Whereas most infections in immunocompetent humans are asymptomatic, toxoplasmosis can be fatal in immunocompromised hosts, particularly in patients with acquired immunodeficiency syndrome (AIDS) and those receiving immunotherapy for tumors and organ transplants. Whereas lymphadenopathy is the most common symptom in immunocompetent humans, encephalitis predominates in immunosuppressed patients.

---

*All material in this article is in the public domain, with the exception of any borrowed figures or tables.

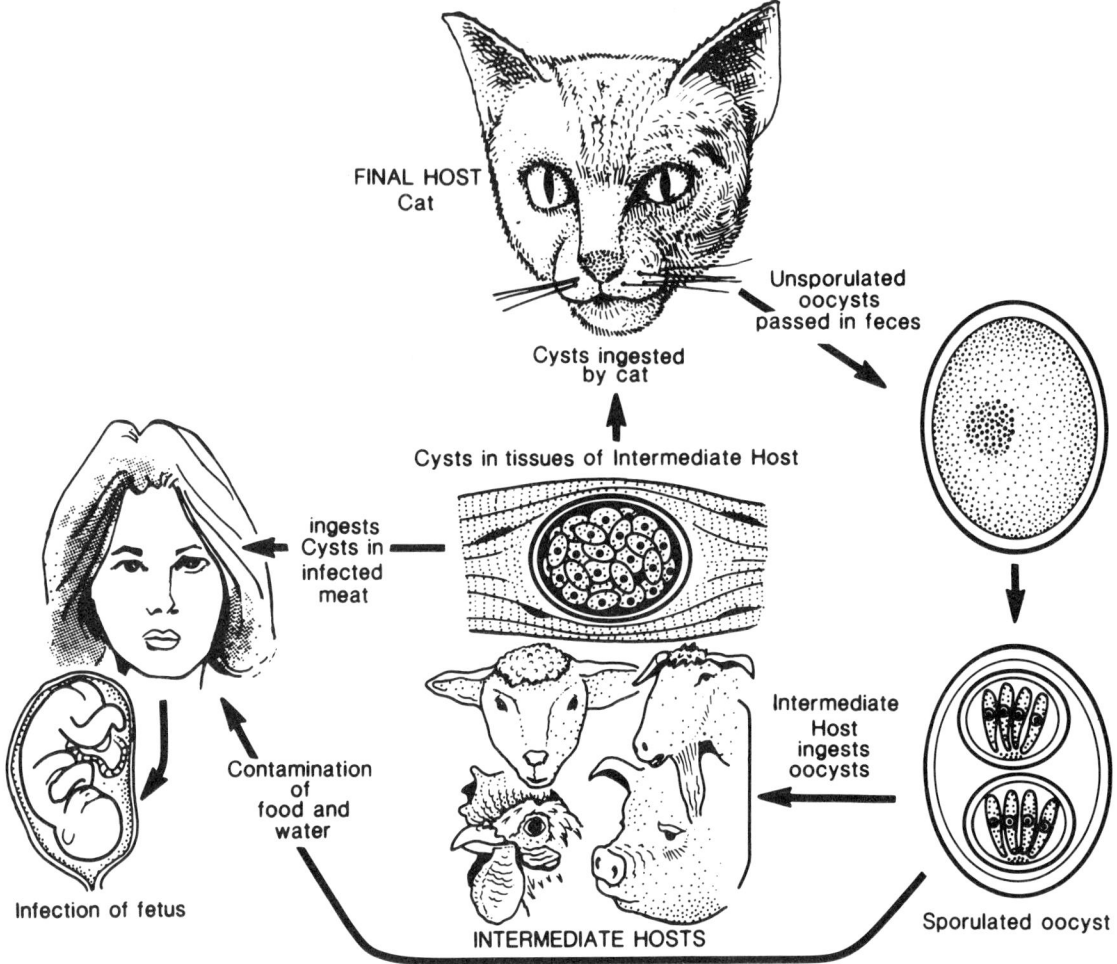

Figure 1. Life cycle of *Toxoplasma gondii*.

T. gondii causes necrosis by active multiplication in cells; it does not produce a toxin. The extent of lesions and associated clinical signs vary depending on the organ parasitized. For example, even small lesions in eyes are important. Early in the infection, *T. gondii* produces enteritis and mesenteric lymph node necrosis before lesions develop in other organs. Some hosts may die of enteritis. Pneumonia and nonsuppurative encephalitis are other important lesions. In sheep and goats, *T. gondii* causes small (1 to 5 mm) chalky-white areas of necrosis in cotyledonary villi of the placenta.

Clinical signs of toxoplasmosis are nonspecific and cannot be depended upon for definitive diagnosis. Diagnosis is aided by biologic, serologic, or histologic methods or by combinations of them. *T. gondii* can be isolated from patients by inoculation of laboratory animals (generally mice) and tissue cultures. Secretions, excretions, body fluids, and tissues taken ante mortem or tissues taken at necropsy are all possible specimens from which to attempt to isolate *T. gondii*. However, these procedures are too complicated for a routine diagnostic laboratory and can be performed only in specialized laboratories.

Finding of *T. gondii* antibodies aids diagnosis. There are numerous serologic tests for detecting humoral antibodies, and their details can be found in Dubey and Beattie (1988). A number of agglutination tests and an enzyme-linked immunosorbent assay (ELISA) are commercially available, and they have been modified to detect both IgG and IgM antibodies. The IgM antibodies appear and disappear generally sooner than do the IgG antibodies, and the difference in IgM and IgG antibody titers is helpful in determining recency of infection. IgG antibody titers may persist for life. Therefore, their presence establishes only that a host has been exposed to *T. gondii*. A 16-fold higher antibody titer in a serum taken 2 to 4 weeks after the first serum was collected more certainly indicates an acute acquired infection. In veterinary practice, this rise in antibody titer is difficult to document because acute and convalescent samples must be run at the same time. Moreover, antibodies may have already peaked by the time patients are seen in the clinic. For example, by the time goats and sheep abort owing to toxoplasmosis, the antibodies have already peaked and are of marginal help in diagnosis. However, finding antibodies in goat, sheep, and pig fetuses is indicative of congenital toxoplasmosis in the fetus because there is no maternal transplacental transfer of antibodies in ruminants and pigs.

Diagnosis can be made by finding *T. gondii* in host tissue removed by biopsy or at necropsy. A rapid diagnosis may be made by making impression smears of lesions on glass slides. After drying for 10 to 30 minutes, the smears are fixed in methyl alcohol and stained with Giemsa or any of the other stains used to stain blood smears. *T. gondii* tachyzoites are crescent-shaped, are about 6 × 2 μm, have a well-defined nucleus, and are often found in macrophages.

TREATMENT

Little is known of the efficacy of various drugs in treating naturally occurring toxoplasmosis in animals because antemortem diagnosis is rarely made. Sulfadiazine and pyrimethamine (Daraprim) are 2 drugs widely used in treatment of human toxoplasmosis. Monensin (30 mg total/day/ewe) has been advocated in some countries as a prophylactic for preventing abortion in sheep. However, the drug is not approved for this use in the United States.

PUBLIC HEALTH SIGNIFICANCE

Cats are the key in the epidemiology of toxoplasmosis. They can excrete millions of oocysts in a gram of feces without showing any clinical signs. The oocysts are very hardy and can survive in the environment for many months. Cats generally become infected by eating tissue cysts of *T. gondii* from birds and mammals. Cats excrete oocysts for only 1- to 2-week periods in their life.

Food animals become infected by ingesting food and water contaminated with *T. gondii* oocysts. Tissue cysts can persist in tissues of live animals for many months (probably for life). *T. gondii* infections are more common in sheep, goats, and pigs than in horses and cattle, which are resistant to it. Therefore, ingestion of beef is less important in the epidemiology of toxoplasmosis. Humans become infected by ingesting tissue cysts in undercooked meat or oocysts in food and water contaminated with cat feces. Approximately 40 per cent of the adult humans in the United States have antibodies to *T. gondii*, and estimates are twice that of the United States in Central and South America and in France. In approximately 1 in 1000 pregnancies, a child is born infected with *T. gondii*. Therefore, it is essential to prevent infections in humans during pregnancy.

PREVENTION AND CONTROL

For prevention of human infection, hands should be washed thoroughly with soap and water after handling meat. All cutting boards, sink tops, knives, and other materials that come in contact with uncooked meat should be washed with soap and water because the stages of *T. gondii* in meat are killed by water. The meat of any animal should be cooked to 70° C before human or animal consumption, and tasting meat while cooking it or while seasoning homemade sausages should be avoided. Pregnant women especially should avoid contact with cat feces or litter, soil, and raw meat. Pet cats should be fed only dry, canned, or cooked food. Cat litter should be emptied every day, preferably not by a pregnant woman. Gloves should be worn while gardening. Vegetables should be washed thoroughly before eating because they may have been contaminated with cat feces. Expectant mothers should be aware of the dangers of toxoplasmosis.

Because most cats become infected by eating infected tissues, cats should never be fed uncooked meat, viscera, or bones, and efforts should be made to keep cats indoors to prevent hunting. Trash cans should be covered to prevent scavenging. Although freezing can kill most *T. gondii* tissue cysts, it cannot be relied on to kill them all. Cats should be spayed to control the feline population on the farm. Dead animals should be removed promptly to prevent scavenging by cats. A vaccine for prevention of toxoplasmosis in humans or animals is not yet available.

BIBLIOGRAPHY

Dubey JP, Beattie CP: Toxoplasmosis of Animals and Man. Boca Raton, FL, CRC Press, 1988, pp 1–220.
Roberts T, Frenkel JK: Estimating economic losses and other preventable costs caused by congenital toxoplasmosis in people in the United States. J Am Vet Med Assoc 196:249–256, 1990.

Sarcocystosis*

J. P. DUBEY, MVSc, PhD

ETIOLOGIC AGENT

Sarcocystis spp. are coccidian parasites that belong to phylum Apicomplexa, class Sporozoasida, subclass Coccidiasina, order Eucoccidiorida, and family Sarcocystidae.

The name *Sarcocystis* (Greek *sarkos*, flesh; *kystis*, bladder) implies parasites in muscle and refers to sarcocysts found in striated muscles of mammals, birds, and poikilothermic animals.

Sarcocystis has an obligatory prey-predator 2-host cycle (Fig. 1). Unlike most other coccidian parasites, the asexual and sexual cycles occur in different hosts. The asexual cycle develops only in the intermediate host, which in nature is often a prey animal. Sexual stages develop only in a carnivorous definitive host. A host may have more than 1 species of *Sarcocystis*, and intermediate and definitive hosts may vary for each species of *Sarcocystis* (Table 1). The definitive host becomes infected by eating sarcocysts containing infective zoites (bradyzoites). The bradyzoites transform into male and female gamonts in the small intestine, and after fertilization, oocysts are produced. The oocysts sporulate in the lamina propria and contain 2 sporocysts, each with 4 sporozoites. The oocyst wall is thin and often breaks so that both sporocysts and oocysts are excreted in feces, usually 1 week after ingestion of sarcocysts. The asexual cycle occurs initially in vascular endothelia, later in cells in the blood stream, and finally in muscles. Two or more asexual cycles (schizonts) are produced in blood vessels. After a brief multiplication in leukocytes, merozoites enter muscles and produce sarcocysts.

Sarcocysts mature in about 1 to 2 months and become infectious for the carnivore host. Sarcocysts of some species of *Sarcocystis* may become grossly visible, for example, *S. gigantea*, *S. hirsuta*, and *S. moulei*.

CLINICAL SIGNS AND LESIONS

Sarcocysts are generally nonpathogenic for the definitive host, and not all species of *Sarcocystis* are pathogenic for intermediate hosts (Table 1). Generally, species transmitted by canids are pathogenic, whereas those transmitted by felids are nonpathogenic. *Sarcocystis cruzi*, *S. capracanis*, and *S. tenella* are the most pathogenic species for cattle, goats, and sheep, respectively. Clinical signs generally are seen during the second schizogonic cycle in blood vessels (acute phase). Three to 4 weeks after infection with a large dose of sporocysts (50,000 or more), animals develop fever, anorexia, anemia, emaciation, and hair loss (particularly on rump and tail in cattle), and some die. Pregnant animals may abort, and growth is slowed or arrested. By the time sarcocysts begin to mature, animals recover.

Dramatic gross lesions are seen in animals that die during

---

*All material in this article is in the public domain, with the exception of any borrowed figures or tables.

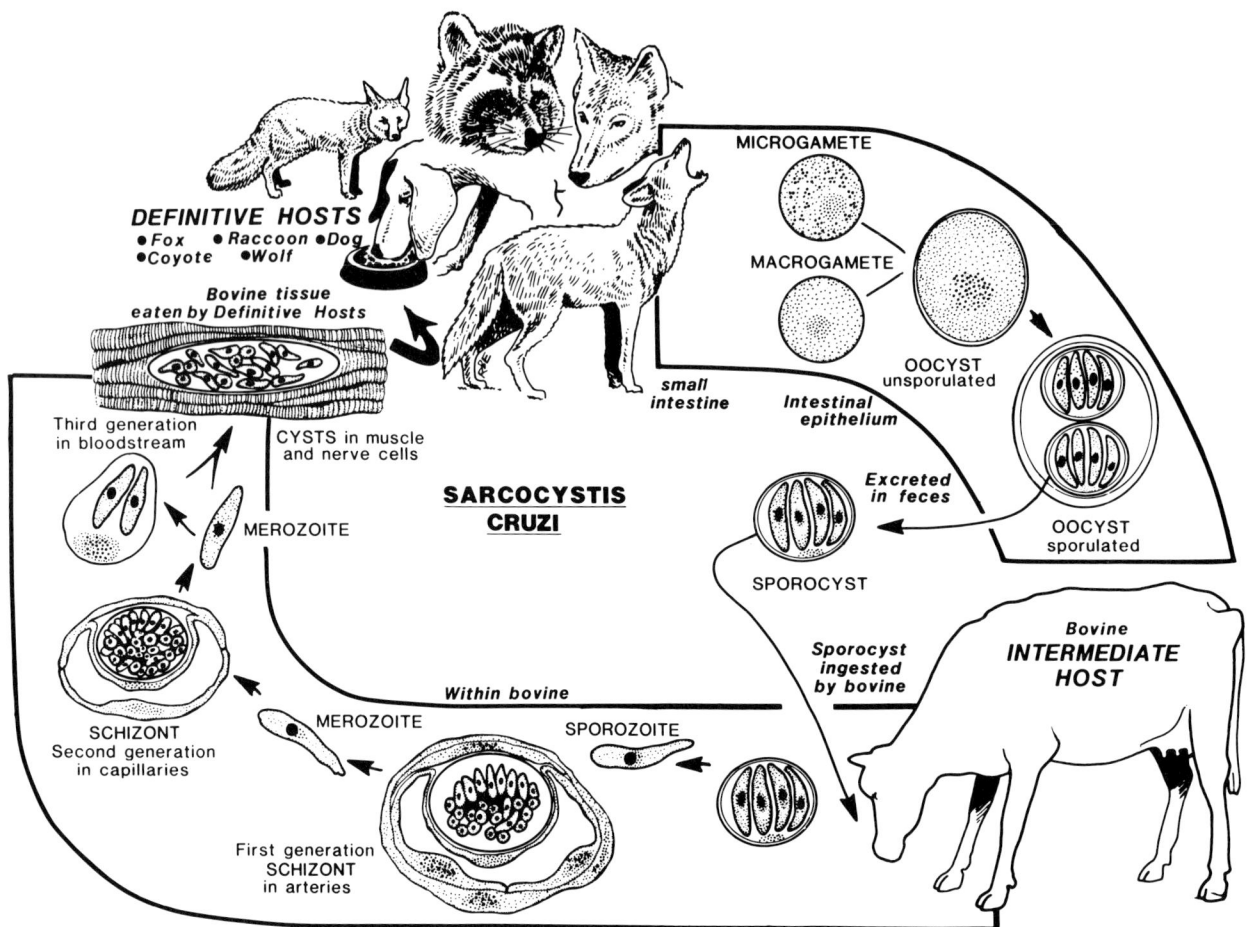

Figure 1. Life cycle of *Sarcocystis cruzi*. (From Dubey JP, Speer CA, Fayer R: Sarcocystosis of Animals and Man. Boca Raton, FL, CRC Press, 1989 pp 1–215.)

the acute phase and consist of edema, hemorrhage, and atrophy of fat. The hemorrhages are most evident on the serosa of viscera, in cardiac and skeletal muscles, and in the sclera of the eyes. Hemorrhages vary from petechia to ecchymosis several centimeters in diameter. Microscopic lesions may be seen in many organs and consist of necrosis, edema, and infiltrations of mononuclear cells. During the chronic phase, lesions are restricted to muscles and consist of nonsuppurative myositis and degeneration of sarcocysts.

DIAGNOSIS

Diagnosis of acute sarcocystosis is difficult. Naturally occurring clinical acute sarcocystosis has been observed only in cattle. The disease in cattle is generalized in nature with no specific signs. Anemia, hair loss, excessive salivation, abortion, and history of contamination of feed or water by canine feces should arouse suspicion of acute sarcocystosis. Laboratory examination should include hematology, serum enzyme chem-

Table 1. INTERMEDIATE AND DEFINITIVE HOSTS FOR SPECIES OF *SARCOCYSTIS* IN CATTLE, SHEEP, GOATS, AND PIGS

Intermediate Host	*Sarcocystis* Species	Definitive Hosts	Pathogenicity for Intermediate Host
Cattle	S. cruzi	Dog, coyote, fox, wolf, jackal, raccoon	+ +
	S. hirsuta	Cat	±
	S. hominis	Primates, humans	±
Sheep	S. tenella	Dog, coyote, fox	+ +
	S. arieticanis	Dog	+
	S. gigantea	Cat	−
	S. medsuiformis	Cat	−
Goat	S. capracanis	Dog, coyote, fox	+ +
	S. hircicanis	Dog	+
	S. moulei	Cat	−
Pig	S. miescheriana	Dog, fox, raccoon, jackal	+
	S. porcifelis	Cat	?
	S. suihominis	Humans, primates	+

+ + highly pathogenic; + pathogenic; ± mildly pathogenic; − nonpathogenic; ? unknown.

istry, and serologic examination for anti-*Sarcocystis* antibody. Serum sorbitol dehydrogenase, creatine phosphokinase, and lactic dehydrogenase levels are elevated; packed cell volume is lowered to less than 20 per cent; and levels of anti-*Sarcocystis* antibodies are elevated. Because nearly all cattle and sheep are subclinically infected with *Sarcocystis*, serologic examination alone is not diagnostic.

TREATMENT

Although prophylaxis with certain anticoccidials (monensin, lasalocid, decoquinate, salinomycin, amprolium) can reduce clinical sarcocystosis in animals treatment is not effective once clinical signs are noted. Because diagnosis is difficult, the efficacy of chemotherapy in natural outbreaks of clinical sarcocystosis is unknown.

Carnivores should be excluded from animal houses and from feed, water, and bedding for livestock. Uncooked meat should never be fed to carnivores. Freezing kills sarcocysts in meat. Dead livestock should be buried or incinerated. There is no vaccine to protect livestock from acute sarcocystosis.

BIBLIOGRAPHY

Dubey JP, Speer CA, Fayer R: Sarcocystosis of Animals and Man. Boca Raton, FL, CRC Press, 1989, pp 1–215.

Theileriosis

J. A. LAWRENCE, DPHIL, BSC, MRCVS, DTVM

Theileriosis is caused by protozoan parasites of the genus *Theileria* (synonyms: *Gonderia*, *Cytauxzoon*, *Haematoxenus*). Among food animals, the disease occurs only in ruminants. Several species of *Theileria* are recognized; their taxonomic relationship has been very confused until recent years.

In cattle, there are 2 highly pathogenic species. *Theileria parva* is the cause of East Coast fever in East and Central Africa. A variant regarded as either a subspecies, *T. parva lawrencei*, or a type, *T. parva (lawrencei)* type), is a common benign parasite of the African buffalo (*Syncerus caffer*), which, when transmitted to cattle, causes Corridor disease. *Theileria annulata* causes tropical theileriosis, which is widespread through the Mediterranean basin, the Middle East, and Asia. Other species that infect cattle in Africa are *T. mutans*, *T. taurotragi*, and *T. velifera*. They are usually benign, although *T. mutans* may be pathogenic in some circumstances. *Theileria mutans* is also thought to occur in the Caribbean region. *Theileria orientalis* (*T. buffeli*, *T. sergenti*) is a generally benign species found in the Mediterranean basin, the Middle East, Asia, and Australia which may cause disease in imported cattle.

In small ruminants, *T. lestoquardi* (*T. hirci*) causes malignant theileriosis of sheep and goats in the Mediterranean basin and the Middle East. A number of benign species that infect sheep and goats have been described in the Mediterranean basin, Africa, and Asia, but their identities are confused.

LIFE CYCLE

All species of *Theileria* are transmitted by multihost ticks. The principal vectors are as follows:

T. parva/T. taurotragi	*Rhipicephalus* spp., especially *R. appendiculatus*
T. annulata	*Hyalomma* spp., especially *H. d. detritum* (Mediterranean basin) and *H. a. anatolicum* (Asia and North Africa)
T. mutans/T. velifera	*Amblyomma* spp., especially *A. hebraeum* (southern Africa) and *A. variegatum* (remainder of Africa and Caribbean)
T. orientalis	*Haemaphysalis* spp., especially *H. longicornis* (eastern Asia and Australia) and *H. punctata* (western Asia and Mediterranean basin)
T. lestoquardi	*Hyalomma a. anatolicum*

Transmission by the tick in all species occurs from one stage to the next and not transovarially from one generation to the next, as with *Babesia*. When a larval or nymphal tick feeds on an infected animal, it ingests parasitized erythrocytes. During the period after detachment of the engorged tick from its host and its molt to the next stage, the parasites undergo a cycle of sexual development in the tick gut and then migrate through the body cavity to the salivary glands, where they undergo sporogony to produce large numbers of sporozoites. When the fully developed nymph or adult tick feeds on a susceptible host, sporozoites injected with the saliva invade lymphocytes and undergo schizogony to form schizonts. The schizonts stimulate the lymphocytes to divide and transform into lymphoblasts, and thereafter the schizonts divide synchronously with the host cells as they undergo mitosis. After a period of schizogony, merozoites are liberated from the schizonts and invade erythrocytes; thus, the life cycle is completed. The merozoites themselves divide within the erythrocytes and are liberated to invade further erythrocytes. There are differences between species of *Theileria* in the relative frequency of intralymphocytic and intraerythrocytic multiplication.

EPIDEMIOLOGY

Within an enzootic area, theileriosis is primarily a problem in introduced, nonadapted animals, in which it may cause heavy mortality. In local, adapted animals, infection is widespread in young stock, but a degree of innate resistance usually limits mortality to a low level, although infection may be a contributory factor to reduced growth rates and increased mortality under suboptimal management conditions. When theileriosis is introduced into a previously disease-free area in which the vector occurs, the disease assumes epizootic status in all types of animal and may result in devastating outbreaks, with morbidity and mortality both in excess of 90 per cent.

CLINICAL SIGNS AND LESIONS

The incubation period after attachment of an infected tick may range from 8 to 25 days, with a mean of 13 to 15 days. The first clinical signs are fever, together with increased pulse and respiration rates, followed after a few days by depression and inappetence. East Coast fever in fully susceptible animals usually follows a course of 15 days (range, 5 to 25 days) and is characterized by enlargement of superficial lymph nodes, lacrimation, photophobia and corneal opacity, constipation followed by diarrhea, petechiation of visible mucous membranes, variable anemia and icterus, progressive loss of condition, weakness and recumbency, and terminally by severe respiratory distress with a moist cough and discharge of frothy fluid from the nostrils. In the few animals that recover, convalescence is protracted, and the animals may be persistent carriers. An atypical cerebral form, "turning sickness," is seen occasionally. Corridor disease shows similar signs, but the course is usually shorter. Tropical theileriosis is clinically similar to East Coast fever, but severe anemia and icterus are constant features, with occasional hemoglobinuria. When *T. mutans* or *T. orientalis* causes clinical disease, the main features are fever and severe anemia. Malignant theileriosis of sheep and goats is clinically similar to tropical theileriosis of cattle.

Characteristic lesions in all forms of theileriosis include enlargement of peripheral and visceral lymph nodes, splenomegaly, red or white lymphoid nodules in the renal cortex, abomasal ulcers, severe pulmonary edema, and possible hydrothorax and hydropericardium. Lymphoid infiltration may be recognized microscopically in the gastrointestinal mucosa and most parenchymatous organs.

DIAGNOSIS

Schizonts ("Koch's bodies") in lymphoblasts and piroplasms in erythrocytes are easily identified in Giemsa-stained smears of blood, spleen, and lymph node; their presence in large numbers in conjunction with appropriate clinical signs and lesions is pathognomonic. It is difficult and often impossible to distinguish the species of *Theileria* microscopically; in enzootic areas, the possibility that parasites seen in smears may represent a coincidental infection with a benign species may complicate diagnosis.

Retrospective serologic diagnosis in recovered animals is possible by use of indirect immunofluorescence with schizont or piroplasm antigens.

TREATMENT

Several drugs have been developed recently that are effective against *Theileria*. Parvaquone, administered intramuscularly at a rate of 10 mg/kg on 2 occasions at 48-hour intervals, has resulted in 90 per cent recovery or better from East Coast fever in field trials. Buparvaquone at 2.5 mg/kg on a single occasion, repeated if necessary, is equally effective against East Coast fever and is also very effective against tropical theileriosis. Halofuginone lactate, administered orally at 1 mg/kg and repeated after 48 hours, is effective against both diseases but has a relatively low therapeutic index; overdosing may cause severe diarrhea. Tetracyclines appear to have some therapeutic effect in mild or early infections. None of these drugs will sterilize infection, and recovered animals may be carriers.

PREVENTION

Prevention of theileriosis is usually dependent on control of tick vectors. Susceptible animals in enzootic areas must be maintained free from ticks, if infection is to be avoided, by regular treatment with an effective acaricide or confinement to pastures, yards, or buildings that can be kept proof against accidental introduction of infected ticks. In an epizootic situation, control depends on quarantine and intensive acaricide treatment of all animals at risk.

Immunization against *T. annulata* by use of an attenuated live schizont vaccine grown in lymphoblast culture has proved effective in many countries. For *T. parva*, immunization can be achieved by an infection and treatment method using a suspension of sporozoites originating from ground-up infected ticks and simultaneous treatment with a long-acting tetracycline preparation. Because of the antigenic diversity of the parasite, a mixture of isolates is used, or a local isolate may be used within a specific area. The method has given encouraging results in trials and is being introduced on an increasing scale in the field.

BIBLIOGRAPHY

Brown CGD, Hunter AG, Luckins AG: Diseases caused by protozoa. *In* Senell MMH, Brocklesby DW (eds): Handbook on Animal Diseases in the Tropics, 4th ed. London, Baillière Tindall, 1990, pp 183–199.

Losos GJ: Infectious Tropical Diseases of Domestic Animals. Harlow, England, Longman Scientific and Technical/International Development Research Centre, 1986, pp 97–181.

Morel PC: Manual of Tropical Veterinary Parasitology. Wallingford, England, C.A.B. International, 1989, pp 390–413.

Heartwater
(Cowdriose, Kaboa, Daji, Enguruti, Khadar, Modikulogo)
PETER T. OBEREM, BSc, BVSc (Hons)

DEFINITION OF THE CONDITION

Heartwater is an infectious, virulent, inoculable, and noncontagious disease affecting domestic and wild ruminants. It is characterized in domestic ruminants by a high fever, lung edema, and hydropericardium followed in acute and peracute forms by severe nervous symptoms. The causative agent is a rickettsia, *Cowdria ruminantium*, which is borne by ticks of the *Amblyomma* genus.

GEOGRAPHIC DISTRIBUTION

It is an African disease occurring south of the Sahara and in Malagasy. The disease was also discovered on 3 islands in the Caribbean (Antigua, Guadeloupe, and Marie-Galante) in the early and late 1980s with the resultant threat of possible introduction to the American mainland, where 2 of the ticks of the genus *Amblyomma* have been found to be able to transmit the disease in the laboratory.

Despite the fact that *Amblyomma* spp. occur on the Asian continent, there is no evidence that heartwater occurs in that part of the world.

The occurrence of heartwater is limited by the distribution and occurrence of the ixodid ticks that are its vectors.

PREVALENCE

Most of the reports on the prevalence of the disease are either broad statements or estimated mortalities, or at best describe the importance of the disease in extremely localized areas.

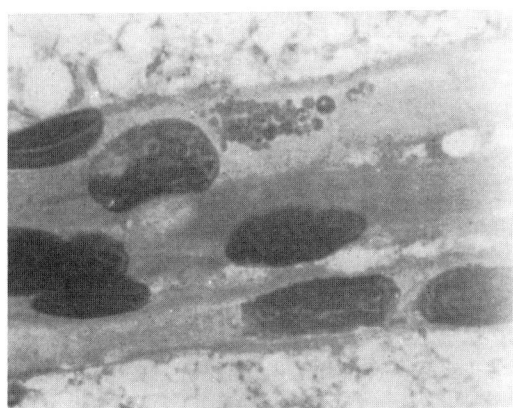

Figure 1. Etiozootiologic agent of heartwater, *Cowdria ruminantium*.

Factors such as animal breeds farmed within a particular area, the tick challenge, the infection rate within the tick population, the use of acaricides, vaccination, and enzootic stability all influence the prevalence of the disease. Nevertheless, heartwater is a severe hindrance to the importation of stock and the upgrading of indigenous breeds in Africa.

ETIOLOGIC AGENT

Heartwater in ruminants is caused by an infection with *Cowdria ruminantium*, which is currently classified as one of the rickettsiae in a large group of vector-borne parasites that can survive and grow only within living cells. On morphologic examination, the microorganism is pleomorphic, resembling a gram-negative coccus, and stains lilac-purple to blue with Giemsa.

Cowdria initially parasitizes macrophages and subsequently endothelial cells, which become distended without appearing injured (Fig. 1). In endothelial cells, the organism is usually found in colonies of tens to hundreds of organisms surrounded by a halo in the cytoplasm of the cell they parasitize, and situated to one side of the nucleus. In bovines, the endothelial cells of renal glomeruli and the superficial gray matter seem mainly to be involved. However, colonies occur in the endothelial cells of most tissues.

PATHOGENESIS

Although little or no damage to the endothelial cells can be detected microscopically, the pathophysiologic changes seem to result from an increased capillary permeability. There is some evidence to suggest that endotoxins could play a role in causing this.

There is a marked drop in cardiac output and a drop in diastolic blood pressure in the advanced stage of the disease. This probably is the result of fluid loss from the circulatory system and of pressure on the heart caused by the progressively severe hydropericardium.

Fluid accumulation in the lungs leads to pulmonary dysfunction, which results initially in a respiratory alkalosis during the early febrile stage. This changes to respiratory acidosis in more advanced cases.

Brain edema explains the nervous symptoms seen during the terminal stages of the disease.

TRANSMISSION

Twelve species of *Amblyomma* ticks are presently known to be capable of transmitting *Cowdria ruminantium*, 5 of which, although proven to be capable in the laboratory, have not been implicated in field outbreaks. *A. variegatum* is the most important and widely distributed vector in Africa; *A. hebraeum* is the only important field vector in most of southern Africa.

Cowdria is not transmitted transovarially from one generation of vector to the next. Larval or nymphal ticks must feed on hosts with rickettsemia in order to become infected before the next stage can transmit the disease.

EPIDEMIOLOGY

Ruminants may remain carriers for 60 days in cases of spontaneous recovery, and adult *Amblyomma* ticks can retain their infectivity for over 15 months. This, however, does not adequately explain where the immature ticks pick up the infection, because their peaks of seasonal abundance do not coincide with those of the adult ticks or with the peak of disease incidence, which is usually during the rainy season. Crowned guinea fowl (*Numida meleagris*), the leopard tortoise (*Geochelone pardalis*), and the spring hare (*Pedetes capensis*) have recently been shown to be subclinically susceptible to *Cowdria* infection in the laboratory. This could explain the source of infection of the immature vector ticks, of which these species are preferred hosts.

CLINICAL SIGNS

The incubation period of heartwater varies according to the species of animal infected, the route of infection, and the virulence of the isolate of infective material (Table 1). Depending on age, immune status, individual or breed susceptibility of the animal, and virulence of the isolate, the course of the disease may range from peracute to mild.

Cattle

The peracute form is usually seen in cattle of the *Bos taurus* breeds. Pyrexia develops suddenly (>41° C), and the animals die within a few hours without overt clinical signs.

Acute heartwater is the most common form of the disease in endemic areas and affects mainly cattle 3 to 18 months of age. Temperatures of 40° C and higher followed by a drop to subnormal levels shortly before death are common. Animals initially appear clinically normal before they gradually show inappetence and eventually stop feeding. Cessation of rumination and difficult breathing follow. Petechiae are visible on the mucous membrane of the conjunctiva of most animals (Fig. 2 A).

Nervous symptoms ranging from a mild incoordination to pronounced convulsions occur in the majority of acutely af-

Table 1. INCUBATION PERIOD AS AFFECTED BY SPECIES AND ROUTE OF INFECTION

Species	Natural Infection (days)		Intravenous Inoculation (days)	
	Range	Average	Range	Average
Sheep and goats	7–35	14	5–35	10
Cattle	9–29	18	7–21	12

fected animals. They are hypersensitive when handled or startled. Tapping on the head often evokes an exaggerated blinking reflex. The gait of affected animals becomes progressively more unsteady, whereas some animals show a hypermetria especially in the forelegs. Lateral recumbency follows. They then show chewing movements and opisthotonos. Extensor rigidity of the legs with bouts of pedaling movements are seen at the same time (Fig. 2 B). Large amounts of froth usually escape from the nostrils and mouth.

Diarrhea, which is often hemorrhagic, particularly in Jersey and Afrikaner cattle, is infrequently seen in animals with heartwater.

The course of the acute form of the disease runs between 2 and 6 days, and recovery is rare.

Less severe cases (subacute and mild) occur with clinical signs ranging from slightly less intense than the acute form to little or no signs at all.

Sheep and Goats

The peracute form of heartwater is most common in exotic breeds of goats; the acute form is seen most frequently in sheep.

Complications

In a low percentage of nonfatal cases of heartwater, complications such as hypostatic pneumonia and rumen stasis may occur. Permanent blindness, torticollis, and a break in the wool of sheep have also been described.

Morbidity and Mortality

Morbidity and mortality vary greatly, especially according to breed and age. Calves less than 3 weeks of age have a high degree of natural resistance (not related to the immune status of the dam), a factor important in the immunization process. This appears to be stronger in Zebu calves than in calves of European breeds.

Sheep of the Persian breed and crosses thereof have a strong natural resistance; the Angora goat is thought to be the most susceptible domestic ruminant.

CLINICAL PATHOLOGY

The main clinical pathologic changes are a progressive anemia and fluctuations in total and differential white blood cell counts, of which an eosinopenia and a lymphocytosis are most marked. A marked loss of albumins results in a drop in total serum proteins; a darkening of plasma color is explained by increases in total bilirubin.

NECROPSY LESIONS

The macroscopic lesions seen in cattle, sheep, and goats are fairly similar although quite variable in extent.

Effusion of the body cavities (ascites and hydrothorax) is a very common finding in most cases of heartwater (Fig. 3). The transparent or slightly turbid light-yellow fluid often coagulates on exposure to air. Hydropericardium, from whence the name heartwater, is seen in most cases but is generally more pronounced in the smaller domestic ruminants. In most peracute cases, edema of the lungs is seen, as is congestion of the trachea and bronchi. As expected, brain edema occurs but is sometimes difficult to detect macroscopically. Although in small stock it may not be very marked, splenomegaly is a constant finding.

Epicardial and endocardial hemorrhages, congestion of the kidneys, congestion or edema of the abomasum, enterorrhagia, and edema of the lymph nodes of the mesentery are inconsistent findings sometimes seen in carcasses at post-mortem examination. Histopathologic studies are very rarely utilized and add little to the picture, merely substantiating the macroscopic changes. Microscopic detection of the organisms in the endothelial cells by brain smear examination is, however, essential for confirmation of a diagnosis of heartwater.

DIAGNOSIS

Ante-mortem diagnosis of heartwater is extremely difficult because there are no pathognomonic signs and the course of the disease is short. Diagnosis is thus based on the classic criteria of history or epidemiology (including the presence of *Amblyomma* ticks) and clinical signs. Despite the difficulties experienced, veterinarians in areas where the disease occurs

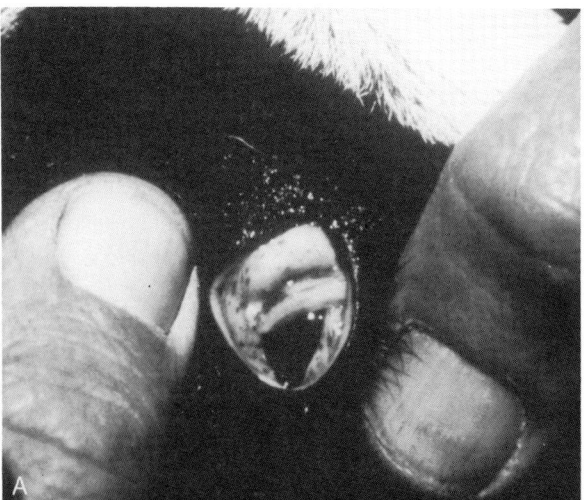 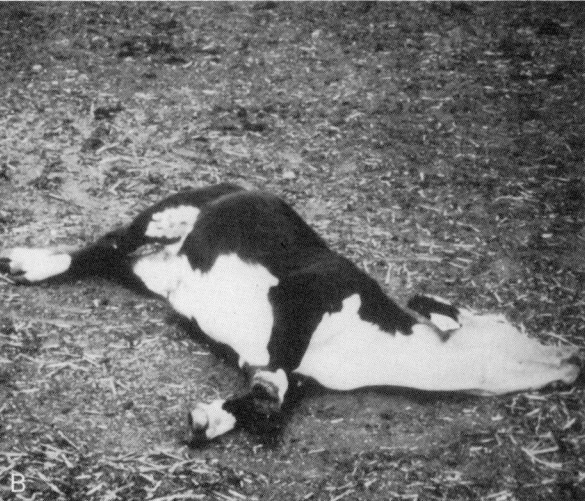

Figure 2. Clinical signs. *A*, Petechiae on the conjunctiva. *B*, Opisthotonos and rigidity of the legs.

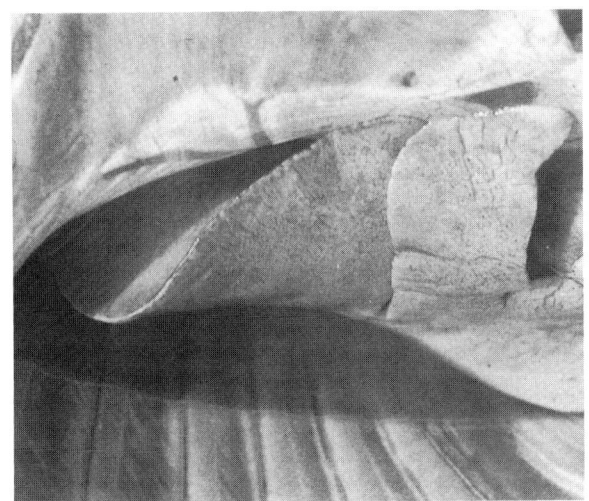

Figure 3. Effusion of body cavities is the main macroscopic pathologic change seen.

are usually quite successful in diagnosing cases that are presented in a timely manner. It has been reported that brain biopsy, although not widely used, is a reliable technique for the confirmation of the disease and that the technique, if properly performed, holds little risk for the animal.

The diagnosis of heartwater at necropsy is far simpler, although gross lesions may be inconspicuous or absent in animals dying peracutely or in animals that have been unsuccessfully specifically treated.

The history taken before commencement of the necropsy with special attention placed on clinical signs (acute death), vaccination and ectoparasite (tick) control programs, and details of the animals involved is essential.

On macroscopic examination, most ruminants dying of heartwater show effusion of body cavities, hydropericardium, edema of the lungs, splenomegaly, and widespread petechiation.

Generally, histopathologic examination is of limited value, but confirmation requires the demonstration of the causative organism in either brains smears or histopathologic sections.

The preparation of brain smears by crushing a small piece of hippocampus or cerebral gray matter between 2 glass slides has greatly simplified the confirmation of a diagnosis of heartwater (Fig. 4). Various staining methods can be used, but 30 minutes in 10 per cent Giemsa solution or 2 to 3 minutes in CAM's Quick-Stain[1] are the most useful. With both methods, the colonies of *C. ruminantium* appear lilac-purple to blue in the endothelial cells.

DIFFERENTIAL DIAGNOSIS

Numerous conditions causing nervous symptoms or acute death must be differentiated from heartwater.

NERVOUS SYMPTOMS. Rabies, cerebral babesiosis, cerebral theileriosis, meningitis, encephalitis, and abscessation of the hypophysis in goats are some of the infectious conditions that need to be considered in endemic areas. Numerous plant and pesticide poisonings also need to be differentiated: *Albizia* spp., *Sarostemma viminale*, *Solanum kwebense*, *Cynanchum* spp., and *Euphorbia mauritanica* as well as strychnine, chlorinated hydrocarbons, organophosphates, and lead.

ACUTE DEATH. Acute death due to anthrax, in which splenomegaly is even more pronounced, must also be ruled out. The presence of dark, tarry blood as opposed to a white froth as seen in heartwater and the presence of *Bacillus anthracis* in the blood smear are useful distinguishing features. Blood and brain smears are useful in the diagnosis of *Babesia bovis* (cerebral) as well.

TREATMENT

The successful treatment of field cases of heartwater remains a problem owing to the short course of the disease, which results in most cases being presented for treatment in an advanced stage.

Specific Treatment (Table 2)

Although much time and effort has been spent in search of antimicrobials active against *Cowdria ruminantium*, only tetracyclines are registered for the treatment of heartwater. Sulfonamides are reported as being effective but are rarely used where the tetracyclines are available. Rifamycin, although not registered for the purpose, has recently been found to be effective. Gloxazone is also more effective than are the tetracyclines, but unfortunately its toxicity prevents general usage.

Oxytetracycline, doxycycline, and rolitetracycline are most commonly used. Short-acting (12- to 24-hour therapeutic blood levels) formulations of oxytetracycline are administered at 10 mg/kg. This needs to be repeated at 24-hour intervals until the febrile reaction is reduced. During the early febrile stage of the disease, however, a single dose of 5 mg/kg is usually sufficient.

Long-acting oxytetracycline formulations (48- to 72-hour blood levels) need to be administered only once at 20 mg/kg.

Doxycycline is more lipid soluble and, because of a longer serum half-life, need only be given at 2 mg/kg at 24-hour intervals.

Supportive Treatment

The success achieved with the treatment of more advanced cases of heartwater depends on the supportive treatment given. However, not enough is known about the pathophysiologic mechanism to make supportive treatment really effective.

The use of drugs to reduce edema (diuretics), stabilize

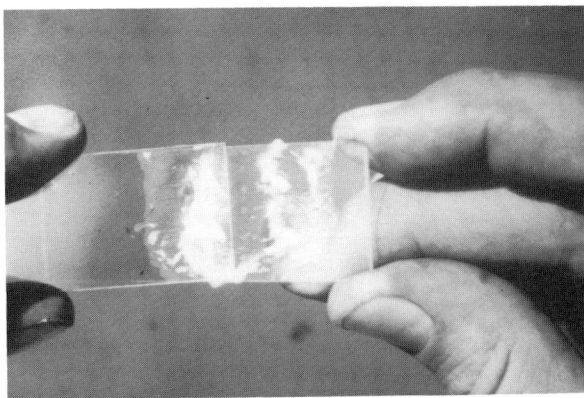

Figure 4. Brain smear used for confirmation of diagnosis at necropsy.

---

[1]CAM Quick-Stain, C. A. Milsch (Pty.) Ltd., P.O. Box 943, Krugersdorp 1740, South Africa.

Table 2. DRUGS USED FOR THE TREATMENT AND PREVENTION OF HEARTWATER

Name of Drug	Company Name and Address	Species	Dosage
Terramycin 1000	Pfizer Laboratories	Ruminants	10 mg/kg
Terramycin/LA	Pfizer Laboratories	Ruminants	20 mg/kg
Doxymycin	Milborrow Animal Health	Ruminants	2 mg/kg
Onderstepoort Heartwater Infective Blood	VRI, Onderstepoort	Ruminants	5 ml
Doximplant S	Geo Schwultz Laboratories	Sheep and goats	7.5–10 mg/kg
Doximplant B	Geo Schwultz Laboratories	Cattle	7.5–10 mg/kg

Many of these preparations are sold under a variety of trade names. Consult publications such as Veterinary Pharmaceuticals and Biologicals, 6th ed. Lenexa, KS, Veterinary Medicine Publishing Co, 1989/1990.

membranes (corticosteroids, dimethyl sulfoxide), block the effects of vasoactive compounds released with cellular death (anti-inflammatory agents), and stimulate cardiac function as well as the bleeding of animals with nervous symptoms (up to 5 L in adult cattle) have been reported as possibly reducing mortality.

Prognosis

The prognosis for recovery of cases during early febrile stages treated adequately with tetracyclines (sulfonamides or rifamycin) is good. However, once clinical signs have manifested, the response to treatment is at best erratic with a poor prognosis.

None of the 3 available drugs sterilize the treated animal of infection; fortunately, this results in a subsequent immunity that lasts about 18 months in cattle that are not reinfected and is lifelong in sheep.

CONTROL AND PREVENTION

Tick Control

Since the earliest times when the tick-borne transmission of heartwater was realized, tick control was advocated as a means of controlling the disease.

In heartwater endemic areas, treatment of the animals against ticks is essential by dipping, spraying, or, more recently, using the pour-on acaricides. There are 2 approaches:

1. "Total tick control" in which heavy reliance is placed on the ability of the acaricides to keep the susceptible stock tick-free. This is usually advocated for marginal areas where *Amblyomma* ticks are found only occasionally. Efficient management is necessary for successful implementation of this method of control.
2. The attainment of an enzootically stable situation by allowing sufficient ticks on the cattle so that young animals are infected before losing their innate age resistance.

Vaccination

A heartwater vaccine is produced commercially only in the Republic of South Africa. It consists of diluted sheep blood containing the virulent organism, which is stored frozen at less than $-77°$ C. It must be inoculated intravenously. Vaccination is thus a form of controlled exposure. There are 4 managerial regimens for this use.

1. In animals still protected by the innate age resistance, that is, calves less than 6 weeks of age, the vaccine elicits an immunity without any clinical manifestations or the necessity for treatment.
2. The standard method is used when small numbers of susceptible animals are vaccinated before being moved into a heartwater area. This entails intravenous administration of the vaccine, daily monitoring of the vaccinates' temperature, and treatment (as described earlier) as soon as they begin to show a temperature reaction (i.e., $>40°$ C).
3. The block method is used when large numbers of animals are involved (Table 3). Vaccination is done in the usual way, but instead of monitoring temperatures, the animals are all "block treated" when they are expected to start reacting.
4. The recent development of a doxycycline implant, which is placed in the subcutaneous tissue of the ear of the animal, has greatly simplified vaccination of susceptible adult animals. The slow release of doxycycline from the implant suppresses clinical signs while allowing the limited multiplication of *Cowdria*, which permits the development of immunity.

Table 3. DAY AFTER INOCULATION ON WHICH BLOCK TREATMENT IS RECOMMENDED

Ruminant Species	Breed	Day After Inoculation
Cattle	Bos taurus	14
	Bos indicus	16
Sheep	Merino	11
	Dorper	11
Goats	Angora	11
	Boergoat	12

Source: Adapted from du Plessis JL, Malan L: The block method of vaccination against heartwater. Onderstepoort J Vet Res 54:493–495, 1987.

BIBLIOGRAPHY

Camus E, Barré N: Heartwater: A Review. Paris, France, Office International des Epizooties, 1988.

Heartwater: past, present and future. International Workshop Proceedings. Onderstepoort J Vet Res 54:1–546, 1987.

SECTION 10 ☐ ☐ ☐ ☐ ☐ ☐
Diseases of the Respiratory System

JEROME G. VESTWEBER, DVM, PhD, Consulting Editor

Pathophysiology of the Respiratory Tract

JEROME G. VESTWEBER, DVM, PhD

ANATOMY AND FUNCTION OF THE RESPIRATORY TRACT

The primary function of the respiratory system is the transport of oxygen from the external environment to the body cells and delivery of carbon dioxide from the cells to the external environment. For effective respiration to take place, three interrelated mechanisms must function: (1) alveolar ventilation of the lung, (2) diffusion of gases to and from the alveoli-pulmonary capillary system, and (3) pulmonary blood flow. Respiratory disease includes any abnormality that causes disruption or failure of these mechanisms. In addition to these functions, the respiratory system is significantly involved in body temperature control, vocalization, immunity to inhaled antigens, antimicrobial action, detoxication, olfaction, and a number of important metabolic and endocrine functions.

The pulmonary system includes structures necessary for external respiration (the upper and lower airways, thoracic wall and diaphragm, pleural space, gas exchange area, and supporting structures of the lung), as well as structures necessary for internal respiration (metabolizing cells and cardiovascular system). The respiratory tract is designed so that air can be conducted easily from the nose to the peripheral alveoli; for efficient gas exchange to take place, a large alveolar surface is required. The remaining portion of the respiratory tract is made up of tubing for conducting air from the nose to the alveoli. This tubing must remain patent so that there is no obstruction to airflow.

The pulmonary system also serves the important functions of metabolic activity and lung defense. Metabolic functions include regulation of body temperature; acid-base balance; blood pressure regulation (enzymatic activation of angiotensin I to angiotensin II); and the production of histamines, prostaglandins E and F, serotonin, norepinephrine, and bradykinin.

The lungs are continuously exposed to air that contains dust, bacteria, fungi, viruses, and various noxious agents, and defense against these potentially harmful materials is controlled by a complex of protective mechanisms. The lung is normally sterile distal to the first bronchial division and is protected by numerous defense mechanisms of the upper and lower respiratory tract, which are broadly categorized as physical defenses, cellular defenses, and secretory defenses. Compromise of these defense mechanisms will result in respiratory disease.

Nasal Cavity

Smell and the conditioning of air before its passes into the trachea are important functions of the upper respiratory tract. During air movement through the turbinate area of the upper airways, inspired air is warmed to approximately body temperature and the relative humidity is raised to approximately 95 per cent. If air is not conditioned in this way, the lower respiratory mucosa becomes dry and the cilia will cease to function. The nasal cavity also functions in the aerodynamic filtration of particles larger than 10 μm by inertial impaction of these particles on the mucous membrane. Particles of 1 to 2 μm in diameter or less, which include aerosolized bacteria and viruses, will generally escape clearance by physical defenses and settle within alveoli. Humidification of incoming air is important because it increases particle size and helps particles to settle out more anteriorly in the respiratory tract. Impinged particles and secreted mucus are moved anteriorly by ciliary action to the oropharynx and swallowed. Drying of the mucous membranes is the most important cause of interference with ciliary action and hence the clearance mechanism. The temperature of the nasal cavity is lower than that of deeper parts of the respiratory tract. This phenomenon is important when temperature-sensitive mutants of viruses are employed as vaccines.

The tonsils are located strategically at the site of greatest impaction in the nasopharynx and function as immunologically active antigen-processing tissue that aids laryngopharyngeal and gastrointestinal defense. The tonsils can be a portal of entry for infectious agents into the lymphatics or adjacent tissue or can act as a source of infection to other animals.

Larynx

The laryngeal opening is relatively small and is a limiting orifice. Forceful or rapid breathing can dry and irritate the laryngeal mucosa so that bacteria become established and produce laryngeal lesions, such as necrotic laryngitis of cattle. Other irritating inhalants can result in severe laryngeal edema.

Trachea, Bronchi, and Bronchioles

The trachea gives off an accessory asymmetric bronchus to the right cranial lobe of the lung in cattle, sheep, and pigs at approximately the level of the third rib. This tracheal bronchus passes laterally and divides into the cranial and caudal bronchi, which ventilate the cranial and caudal parts of the right apical (cranial) lobe, respectively. This lobe is frequently the first to be involved in bronchopneumonia and is frequently atelectatic following birth.

The trachea bifurcates distal to the accessory bronchus into the right and left principal bronchi, which give off additional bronchi to different lobes of the lung. Further division occurs into secondary bronchi and into one terminal bronchiole that serves a primary lobule of the lung. Bronchioles are defined as airways not having cartilage in their walls; they may collapse owing to pressure from surrounding pneumonic tissue or constrict owing to smooth muscle spasm of the wall. The primary lobules are considered the basic respiratory portions of the lungs.

Inhaled particulate matter that ranges in size from 2 to 10 μm is deposited from the larynx to the terminal bronchioles on a mucociliary blanket. This is sometimes called the mucociliary transport system, and it transports mucus-particulate matter to the oropharynx, at a rate of approximately 15 mm/minute, to be swallowed. Ciliated cells are generally 250 per cell in number and beat synchronously at over 1000 strokes/minute. They extend down to the terminal bronchioles, but their numbers are few in comparison with the major bronchi and trachea. Mucus has the physical properties of viscosity and elasticity; in infection, mucus is transported poorly because of increased viscosity and reduced elasticity. Also, in bovine respiratory disease, large quantities of fibrin are likely to occur in the mucus as it is transported from the bronchi. Fibrin adds significantly to the viscosity and elasticity of mucus. The mucociliary blanket is made up of two layers: an outer gel layer derived primarily from goblet cells and an inner sol layer contributed by submucosal glands. Mucus serves to prevent epithelial dehydration and serves as a barrier to toxic agents and a vehicle for other factors important to host defense, including neutrophils, immunoglobulin A (IgA), and lactoferrin. Ninety per cent of the material deposited on the mucociliary blanket is cleared effectively within 1 hour. Factors such as dehydration, extremely cold inspired air, irritant gases such as ammonia, abnormal body electrolytes, anesthetics, general hypoxemia, or infectious agents such as viruses will impede mucociliary activity. If the presence of these factors allows pathogenic bacterial agents to colonize or remain in the upper respiratory tract for as long as 3 to 4 hours, infection probably will occur. Particles deposited on nonciliated surfaces distal to the terminal bronchioles may be cleared by slow anterior migration on a thin fluid layer normally covering nonciliated epithelium. Particles may also be phagocytized by local alveolar macrophages or neutrophils.

The cough reflex occurs in response to irritation of the respiratory tract, and the stimulus may arise anywhere between the pharynx and the secondary branches of the bronchi. The most sensitive areas are in the region of the larynx and tracheal bifurcation, whereas the smaller bronchioles are relatively insensitive. A cough may not result in expulsion of mucus from peripheral airways because of relatively low airflow rates, but compression of small airways resulting from high intrathoracic pressures can help produce a milking action that clears mucus to larger airways for subsequent removal. Difficulty in clearing secretions by this method is mainly due to increased viscosity and decreased elasticity of secretions.

Mechanical irritation of the larynx or trachea by inhalation of irritant gases, aerosols, and chemically inert dusts can produce bronchoconstriction. Reflex bronchoconstriction is a physiologic protective mechanism to prevent penetration of mechanical or chemical irritants farther into the lungs.

Lungs

The right lung is divided into the apical (cranial), middle, diaphragmatic (caudal), and accessory lobes, whereas the left lung is divided into the apical (cranial) and diaphragmatic (caudal) lobes. The right lung has 55 to 60 per cent of the total lung volume. A lobule is the functional unit of the lungs and consists of a terminal bronchiole, poorly developed respiratory bronchiole, alveolar duct, alveolar sacs, and alveoli. In comparison with other domestic animals, cattle, sheep, and pigs have very extensive interlobular connective tissue or septa around these lobules, which are continuous with a thick pleura covering the lung. This complete septum results in a lack of collateral ventilation between adjacent lobules. In addition, cattle and pigs have notably thick walled arteries and veins.

In cattle, sheep, and pigs, the terminal bronchiole is the last airway into the lobule and the respiratory bronchiole is poorly developed. This creates problems in clearing plugs of exudates from these distal terminal bronchioles because of poor collateral ventilation. Interalveolar pores (pores of Kohn) communicate between alveoli and are important in clearance mechanisms of the lung, especially if the terminal bronchioles are plugged. Normally air from unaffected alveoli will pass through the pores of Kohn and help force exudate out of the alveolus up to the mucociliary transport system. There are also bronchiolar-alveolar communications (Lambert's canals), which also permit collateral ventilation of many alveoli. If an infected mucus plug is not cleared from the terminal bronchiole, it may become organized by fibrous connective tissue and completely occlude the bronchiole, resulting in collapse of the affected lobule.

The three primary cells in the alveoli are the type I and II pneumocytes, macrophages, and a few brush cell and neuroepithelial bodies. Most of the alveolus is lined by the cytoplasm of type I pneumocytes and forms part of the blood-air barrier. At its thinnest the barrier consists of type I pneumocyte cytoplasm, fused basement membranes, and vascular endothelial cell cytoplasm. These structures can be damaged easily, resulting in exudation of edema fluid, fibrinogen, and blood cells into the alveolus. The alveolar epithelial cells are covered by an acellular duplex layer (surfactant) of highly surface-active phospholipids over a hypophase containing phospholipids, proteins, and carbohydrates.

The type II pneumocyte is regarded as a precursor of the type I cell, and, if there is lung damage, it rapidly proliferates to line the alveolus, producing what is called "alveolar epithelialization," "fetalization," or "alveolar epithelial hyperplasia." The type II pneumocytes are the cells that synthesize and secrete the surface-active phospholipids known as surfactants, which are responsible for maintaining low surface tension in the lung and preventing alveolar collapse. A lack of adequate levels of surfactant at birth can cause respiratory distress syndrome during the first days of life.

Alveolar macrophages make up 70 per cent of the free cells of the bronchoalveolar airspaces and protect the lung from bacteria in essentially two ways. First, they phagocytize and kill opsonized and nonopsonized bacteria. Second, they elaborate products that directly mediate or are responsible for attracting into the lung other inflammatory and immunologic factors essential to host defense. They have marked secretory activities, with over 50 products having been identified. When they are properly stimulated they can release neutrophil chemoattractants, an angiogenesis factor, factors that mediate B- and T-lymphocyte functions, complement, prostaglandins, platelet activating factor, leukotrienes, and a variety of lysosomal enzymes. Inflation of irritant materials will increase their numbers up to four times. The metabolic activity of macrophages has proved to require high levels of pO_2, the divalent cations (Ca^2 Mg^2), an energy source, proper pH, and isotonicity for optimum phagocytosis. Hypoxia, starvation, and acidosis will slow pulmonary clearance by alveolar macrophages.

Macrophage function also has been shown to diminish after infection with viruses. At least two bovine respiratory viruses infect alveolar macrophages. Parainfluenza-3 virus infects macrophages in vivo and in vitro, resulting in persistent infection. In vitro infection with infectious bovine rhinotracheitis virus results in reduced competence of the macrophages and subsequent cell death. *Pasteurella haemolytica* may also be able to further impair macrophage function by cytotoxicity. Thus the alveolar macrophage is the cell that provides and orchestrates the inflammatory and immune responses in the lung. These cells can become damaged, releasing enzymes that damage lung tissue and leading to conditions such as emphysema and pulmonary fibrosis.

Neutrophils account for about 2 per cent of lavage cell population in the normal bovine lung, but their numbers will increase dramatically following intrapulmonary inoculation of viruses, bacteria, and complement components. Neutrophils will enter the lung rapidly from the circulation, responding to chemotactic factors produced by alveolar macrophages, arachidonic acid products, or complement. These cells are more effective at phagocytizing and killing bacteria than alveolar macrophages because of a more intense respiratory burst, more lysosomal enzymes, and more mobility. On the negative side, they have been shown to be responsible for inducing serious lung injury themselves because of their stores of reactive products, and their function can be suppressed by challenge with infectious bovine tracheitis virus, *P. haemolytica*, and *P. multocida*.

Lymphocytes are an important cell type of the lung, both as individual cells and as aggregations known as bronchus associated lymphoid tissue (BALT). Presentation of antigen by macrophages is followed by programming of B lymphocytes for antibody production and T lymphocytes for cell-mediated immunity, with various and complex interactions between the two.

Interferon is a product of the respiratory epithelium and alveolar macrophages and is present in respiratory secretions. To induce interferon synthesis it is necessary for viruses, virus vaccines, or other synthetic polymers to penetrate respiratory cells. The affected cells release interferon, which enters unaffected cells to provide them with viral resistance by preventing viral replication. Interferon also participates in the regulation of both humoral and cellular immunity by enhancing macrophage phagocytic function and regulating B- and T-lymphocyte responses. The principle of intranasal vaccination against infectious bovine rhinotracheitis and parainfluenza-3 is that, in addition to local and systemic immunologic response, the production of interferon occurs within 1 to 2 days following administration. It has also been shown that intranasal vaccine strains of infectious bovine rhinotracheitis virus will induce nasal secretion interferon, which will help protect against bovine rhinovirus and adenovirus.

Complement components serve a beneficial role by virtue of their chemotactic and opsonization functions, mediated by the C5a and C3 peptides. Control of complement accumulation and activation is important because C5a and related peptides can also result in hypoxia, hypertension, and acute pulmonary edema and inflammation.

Lysozymes produced by neutrophils, alveolar macrophages, and glandular epithelial cells participate in bacteriolysis of gram-positive bacterial cell walls. These enzymes also participate in complement-antibody complex lysis of target cells. In addition, lactoferrin synthesized by glandular mucosal cells and polymorphonuclear leukocytes have potent bacteriostatic activity.

The contribution of the lungs to the output of immunoglobulins is frequently underestimated. Lymphoid tissue is found in the walls of conducting airways from the nasopharynx to the alveolar ducts. Nodules of lymphoid tissue are made up of about 20 per cent T cells, about 50 per cent B cells, and others that bear no detectable marker. Such nodules are probably the pulmonary analogue of gut-associated lymphoid tissue, such as Peyer's patches or the colonic lymphoid microbursa, and the term BALT is used to describe them.

Bacteria, viruses, and fungi contain a wide variety of antigens to which the immune system can respond. The four classes of immunoglobulins defined at present are immunoglobulins G, M, A, and E. IgG is the major opsonizing antibody in the respiratory tract, promoting ingestion of microbial agents by phagocytes via Fc receptors, agglutinating bacteria, neutralizing toxins, inactivating viruses, and activating complement. IgM is a large immunoglobulin and remains within the intact blood vascular system. IgE is produced by plasma cells located within the respiratory mucous membranes and, in some species, is the immunoglobulin responsible for acute allergic reactions. The respiratory tract produces local immunoglobulins, such as IgA, that play a role in neutralizing toxins, inhibiting bacterial adherence and viral binding to cell surfaces. Pulmonary capillary endothelial cells are actively responsible for removal of norepinephrine, 5-hydroxytryptamine, prostaglandin E and F, and thromboxane from the blood. Capillary endothelial cells and other lung cells may also make prostaglandins and thromboxanes under certain conditions. They may also activate angiotensin I to angiotensin II, which elevates systemic blood pressure, and inactivate bradykinin, which lowers blood pressure. They are actively antithrombogenic and control levels of other biologically active compounds that enter the systemic arterial circulation.

PATHOLOGIC REACTIONS OF THE RESPIRATORY TRACT

Major components of any disease are the structural damage caused directly by the insulting agent and the subsequent inflammatory and repair processes. Once bacteria have become established in the lung, tissue injury is mediated by several mechanisms. Toxins play a major role in tissue damage in *Pasteurella* and *Haemophilus* pneumonia. The most ubiquitous of these is the endotoxin or lipopolysaccharide (LPS) in the outer membrane of gram-negative cell walls. Endotoxins can result in the initiation of complement and coagulation cascades, which result in increased vascular permeability, coagulation, accumulations of inflammatory cells, edema, and intravascular and extravascular fibrin in the lung. Extracellular protein toxins of *P. haemolytica* have been shown to impair phagocytosis and kill macrophages and can be more cytotoxic if opsonization has taken place. This toxin is produced in log phase cultures and can be neutralized by antiserum. Other *P. haemolytica* extracellular fractions will also kill bovine neutrophils, and neutral proteases produced by the organism may cleave complement components C3 and C5.

It has been shown that immune complexes (or type III) lung injury may be involved in mycoplasma respiratory disease. Damage in these cases may involve activation of the complement cascade with the release of small vasoactive peptides C3a and C5a, which are also chemotactic for neutrophils. The migration of neutrophils to the area not only results in phagocytosis of the bacteria but also results in tissue damage owing to neutrophil products such as superoxide anion, hydrogen peroxide, and hydroxyl ions of the respiratory burst. The respiratory burst is the principal bactericidal mechanism of phagocytes.

Inflammation of the lung represents the sum of the host responses to injury and includes the complement cascade; the

Hageman factor–dependent pathways to coagulation; kinin generation; fibrinolysis; arachidonic acid metabolism; platelet activating factor; activation of mast cells and basophils; cellular recruitment; and mediator release from neutrophils, eosinophils, macrophages, and oxygen-mediated injury.

Mucous Membranes

The pathologic changes that occur with insult to the mucous membranes are similar for trauma, toxic chemical or bacterial exposure, or viral infection. The earliest changes are associated with destruction of ciliated or mucus-secretory cells, which will be sloughed into the lumen. Often in the early stages of infection, viral-infected cells will be shed before they are dead, and these cells are good specimens for viral isolation or fluorescent antibody studies. Gradually inflammation of the destroyed area develops with local intercellular edema, congestion, and leukocytic infiltration. Inferferon production, secretion of IgA, and leakage of serum immunglobulins occur with infectious agents.

The time needed for complete repair of epithelial surfaces depends on the species of animal, cause of injury, and occurrence of secondary infection. Following mechanical injury, most of the epithelium is replaced by 14 days and is fully functional by 28 days. The repair rate following viral infection varies depending on the properties of the virus. Hyperplastic changes and the presence of viral inclusion bodies are seen with viral infections.

Nasal Cavity and Larynx

Inflammatory reactions in the nasal passages are common, especially when associated with upper respiratory tract viruses, such as infectious bovine rhinotracheitis of cattle. Observation of these mucous membranes will reveal an inflamed red color. A variety of organisms, such as *P. haemolytica, P. multocida*, and *Haemophilus somnus*, are able to colonize and reside in the nasal cavity. Organisms wait for the opportunity for the defense mechanism to be compromised, which allows their establishment in the lower respiratory tract.

Inflammation of the larynx reduces the luminal size dramatically, resulting in inspiratory dyspnea. Invasion of mucous membranes and supporting cartilage by microorganisms can produce necrosis of these tissues and can result in more permanent problems, such as intraluminal granulation tissue, necrotic cartilage, and hemiplegia.

Trachea, Bronchi, and Bronchioles

Mild tracheitis, which can be detected only microscopically, is not uncommon. Severe tracheitis is most usually due to viruses, such as infectious bovine rhinotracheitis, and is also associated with upper respiratory tract diseases, such as aspiration of infected debris from oral or pharyngeal lesions or accidental administration of liquids into the trachea.

Acute bronchitis is frequently associated with many viruses or bacteria. Chronic bronchitis may be recognized clinically by a persistent cough and excessive mucus secretion because of hypertrophy of mucus-secretory glands.

The bronchiolar epithelium is very sensitive to insult from chemical agents, viruses, and parasites. Necrosis, sloughing, regeneration, hyperplasia, and organization of mucus plugs are typical responses to injury in the bronchioles. The identification of viral inclusion bodies or the finding of lungworms is the only positive indication of cause. Bronchiolitis obliterans can result from severe local injury of the bronchiolar epithelium by bacterial, viral, parasitic, or chemical agents and results in several complications in the alveoli: interference with airflow either in or out of the alveoli with resulting overinflation or collapse, reduced resistance to inhaled microorganisms and resulting pneumonia, and release of inflammatory mediators and intracellular proteases that could be involved in the pathogenesis of emphysema.

Alveolar Atelectasis or Collapse

Atelectasis is described classically as an incomplete expansion of the lungs at birth, whereas the term "collapse" is reserved for previously inflated lungs. Although complete atelectasis of the lungs is found in the stillborn animal, partial atelectasis of the anterior ventral aspect of the lungs can be found in perinatal animals following the aspiration of fluid during birth. Atelectasis is also associated with hyaline membrane disease of human infants, the cause of which is believed to be a deficiency of pulmonary surfactant. This disease is also seen in full-term neonatal pigs and cattle, but whether it is caused by a surfactant deficiency is not known.

Collapse of a lobule or lobules can be due to either bronchiolar obstruction or compression by surrounding pneumonic consolidation, abscesses, or extrapulmonary lesion such as hydrothorax, pneumothorax, or neoplasms. Collapse from bronchiolar obstruction is often encountered in cattle, sheep, and pigs because of inadequate collateral ventilation.

Emphysema

Emphysema of the lung is characterized by an increase beyond normal in the size of the air spaces distal to the terminal bronchiole and destructive changes in the alveolar walls. This distinguishes emphysema from pulmonary overinflation, in which air spaces are enlarged but destructive changes are not present in the alveolar walls. Collateral ventilation through the pores of Kohn normally allows passage of air between adjacent normal alveoli of a lobule or between functioning alveoli of adjacent lobules. If the bronchiole supplying the alveoli is obstructed, the air within the alveoli is trapped and the volume increases with inspiration, but expiratory reduction does not occur. The walls of the alveoli become overdistended and thin, vascular supply is reduced, and walls rupture to produce cystic cavities.

Interstitial emphysema is a necropsy finding of cattle and pigs owing to the entrance of air into the connective tissue of the interlobular septa. It is often a necropsy observation associated with agonal death following severe toxemia. Air may escape the lungs and travel beneath the pleura into the mediastinum, then via the thoracic inlet to the subcutaneous tissues of the neck and back. The cause of interstitial emphysema is not fully known, but increased intrapulmonary pressure due to disease may cause rupture of terminal bronchioles and result in passage of air to the interlobular septa.

Pulmonary Edema and Congestion

The barriers separating the vascular and alveolar spaces concerned with fluid balance are the capillary endothelium, basement membrane, alveolar epithelium, interstitial compartment, and pulmonary lymphatics. Movement of water into the alveolus or interstitium generally is associated with an alteration of structure and is caused by noxious agents, increased blood volume, or hydrostatic pressure. The equilibrium normally is maintained such that the alveolar surface is moist, but there is no large flux of water from the capillary bed into the alveolus. Pulmonary hypertension, heart failure, heart valve lesions, or mediastinal masses prevent the clearing of blood that comes from the lungs and may cause increased pulmonary venous pressure, with resulting congestion and edema of the lungs.

The permeability of the capillary-alveolar membranes also may be increased by infection (bacterial or viral pneumonia), endotoxins, inhaled noxious substances, uremia, allergic reactions, disseminated intravascular coagulation, and aspiration pneumonia.

Two stages of pulmonary edema are recognized. The first is interstitial edema, which is characterized by engorgement of the perivascular and peribronchial interstitial tissue. Pulmonary function is usually not affected at this stage. The second stage is alveolar edema; its development is not fully understood, but lymphatics may become overloaded so that interstitial edema increases until fluid enters the alveoli.

Pneumonia

The conventional term "pneumonia" is reserved for the pathologic condition of inflammation of the lungs. Further division of pneumonia into exudative reaction of the alveolar space and cellular infiltration or proliferation of the alveolar wall or interstitial space will cover most of the pneumonias of cattle, sheep, and swine.

The susceptibility of the bovine to pneumonia has been proposed to be due to some of the following factors: (1) a large rugose surface on the tonsil, which serves as a source of microorganisms for the lungs; (2) dependent anatomic orientation and poor oxygen perfusion of anteroventral lobes; (3) a small exchange capacity relative to body needs, minimal collateral ventilation, and anatomic compartmentalization; (4) low numbers of resident alveolar macrophages and a weak leukocytic response to infection; (5) low levels of lysozyme, an enzyme produced by neutrophils and macrophages to destroy bacteria; and (6) a relatively small endothelial mass for the clearance of toxins.

Bronchopneumonia or fibrinous pneumonia caused by *P. haemolytica* is the most common type of exudative reaction of the alveolar space. Exudation of fluid and infiltration of neutrophils into the air spaces are the major features of this disease. Experimental inoculation of *P. haemolytica* into the lungs of cattle produced the following sequence of lesions. Eighteen hours following intratracheal inoculation there were various degrees of atelectasis, infiltration of neutrophils into alveolar spaces and bronchioles, and accumulation of macrophages and fibrin in alveoli. Exudate was prominent in and around the bronchioles. By 3 days there was general distention of lymphatic vessels with fibrin and neutrophils; thrombosis of these vessels was common. A purulent exudate consisting of neutrophils and necrotic debris was present in bronchioles. Alveolar spaces contained large numbers of neutrophils, macrophages, and eosinophilic clots of fibrin. Small areas of coagulation necrosis were found in many calves. By 7 days lymphoid hyperplasia was extensive around bronchi and bronchioles; organizing obliterative bronchiolitis was observed. Small areas of necrosis were replaced by granulation tissue, and large areas of coagulation necrosis were still present. Fibrinous exudate in lymphatics and on the pleura was well organized.

As a general concept it is well to think of pneumonia passing through successive stages, and, with treatment, the response may be abbreviated or aborted at any phase. Frequently the morphologic changes do not fit the classical descriptions, but all stages represent a continuum of an inflammatory reaction.

Pulmonary adenomatosis, chronic progressive pneumonia, and atypical interstitial pneumonia are examples of cellular infiltration or proliferation of the alveolar wall or interstitial space. Chronic progressive pneumonia and pulmonary adenomatosis are important diseases in sheep. In regard to the pathogenesis of chronic progressive pneumonia, it is thought that a virus stimulates reticular and lymphocyte cells to proliferate. This results in thickening of interalveolar septa from the presence of numerous histiocytes, new fibrocytes, and collagenous fibers. As the septa thicken, the squamous epithelial cells lining the alveoli morphologically transform into cuboidal cells. In addition, the peribronchiolar and perivascular lymphoid tissues undergo hyperplasia.

Acute bovine pulmonary emphysema and edema is an important disease in certain areas of the United States. The disease is characterized by pulmonary edema and emphysema with exudation into the alveoli of a protein-rich fluid, formation of hyaline membranes, epithelialization of the alveolar lining, and fibrous thickening of the alveolar septa. The pathogenesis of acute bovine pulmonary emphysema is related to the ruminal formation of 3-methylindole from L-tryptophan, a naturally occurring amino acid and constituent of forage. Certain pasture management practices are believed to create a ruminal environment that favors the conversion of L-tryptophan to 3-methylindole. Following its production, 3-methylindole is absorbed and transported to the lung, where it is detoxified by the mixed-function oxidase system in lung Clara cells and type I pneumocytes. Metabolism of 3-methylindole by the mixed-function oxidase system results in highly reactive cytotoxic intermediates that, when present in overwhelming concentrations, are responsible for destruction of the cells in which it is produced.

BIBLIOGRAPHY

Ardan AA: Pulmonary structure, function and defense mechanisms. Proceedings of the 8th Annual Convention of the American Association of Bovine Practitioners, 1975, pp 25–28.
Breeze R: Structure, function and metabolism in the lung. Vet Clin North Am: Food Anim Pract 1:219–235, 1985.
Confer AW, Panciera RJ, Mosier DA: Bovine pneumonic pasteurellosis: immunity to *Pasteurella haemolytica*. J Am Vet Med Assoc 193:1308–1315, 1988.
Corbeil LB, Gogolewski RP: Mechanisms of bacterial injury. Vet Clin North Am: Food Anim Pract 1:367–376, 1985.
Forman AJ, Babuik LA, Baldwin F, Friend SC: Effect of infectious bovine rhinotracheitis virus infection in calves on cell populations recovered by lung lavage. Am J Vet Res 43:1174–1179, 1982.
Leid RW, Potter KA: Inflammation and mediators of lung injury. Vet Clin North Am: Food Anim Pract 1:377–400, 1985.
Liggitt HD: Defense mechanisms in the bovine lung. Vet Clin North Am: Food Anim Pract 1:347–366, 1985.
Markham RJ, Wilkie BN: Interaction between *Pasteurella haemolytica* and bovine alveolar macrophages: cytotoxic effect on macrophages and impaired phagocytosis. Am J Vet Res 41:18–22, 1980.
Osburn BI: Immunologic concepts relating to the bovine respiratory system. Proceedings of the 8th Annual Convention of the American Association of Bovine Practitioners, 1975, pp 30–32.
Sibille Y, Reynolds HY: Macrophages and polymorphonuclear neutrophils in lung defense and injury. Am Rev Respir Dis, 141:471–501, 1990.
Veit HP, Farrell RL: The anatomy and physiology of the bovine respiratory system relating to pulmonary disease. Cornell Vet 68:555–581, 1978.
Wilkie IW, Fallding MH, Shewen PE, Yager JA: The effect of *Pasteurella haemolytica* and the leukotoxin of *Pasteurella haemolytica* on bovine lung explants. Can J Vet Res 54:151–156, 1990.
Yates WG: Respiratory system. *In* Thomson RG (ed): Special Veterinary Pathology. Philadelphia, CV Mosby, 1988, pp 69–122.

Upper Respiratory System Diseases

VAUGHN L. LARSON, DVM, PhD

Diseases of the upper respiratory system, from a clinical standpoint, include those causing dysfunction from the external nares to the bifurcation of the trachea and including the paranasal sinuses. Primary diseases of this system are usually sporadic and of low incidence and therefore are misdiagnosed by practitioners as lower respiratory conditions. The lack of early diagnosis in view of the generally poor prognosis and economically nonfeasible therapeutics required often leads to needless losses of slaughter salvage value.

A systematic approach to problem solving requires careful assessment of disease history. Upper respiratory diseases are usually of a chronic progressive nature rather than of acute onset (i.e., in closely observed animals).

Clinical signs often associated with disease of the upper respiratory system are inspiratory dyspnea, mouth breathing, nasal discharge, cough and/or observed anatomic changes.

Inspiratory dyspnea is the prolongation of the inspiratory phase of respiration. This sign always indicates obstructive diseases of the upper respiratory system. Inspiratory dyspnea and airflow differentials of the nares indicate nasal cavity obstruction. Pharyngeal obstruction is often accompanied by inappetence and/or dysphagia in addition to inspiratory dyspnea. Obstructions in the larynx and trachea can usually be localized by careful auscultation.

The nasal discharge associated with upper respiratory disease often progresses from serous to mucoid to mucopurulent and may be blood tinged.

Coughing with these diseases is usually not productive. By definition productive coughing is that which causes lower tracheal rales. Coughing in severe pharyngeal or laryngeal disease may sound productive but can usually be defined by auscultation.

Open-mouth breathing may be observed with either severe upper respiratory obstructions or advanced disease of the lung.

Cases should be visually observed for evidence of swelling over the paranasal sinuses in the regions of the throat latch and trachea. All masses should be palpated. Digital examination of cervical tracheal rings is essential in cases of inspiratory dyspnea.

Endoscopy can be very helpful in localization and observation of lesions in cattle.

RHINITIS

Rhinosporidium spp. and *Helminthosporium* sp. fungi infect the nasal cavities of cattle, causing rhinitis. Allergic rhinitis is seen in pastured cattle and is called "summer snuffles." The inhalation of chemical fumes, smoke, and exhaust fumes causes an irritant rhinitis. Calves raised in confinement over pits and with inadequate ventilation often exhibit signs of rhinitis.

Clinical Signs

Nasal discharge is the most prominent sign of rhinitis. This may be serous, mucoid, or suppurative, depending on the severity and chronicity of the disease. Usually serous discharge is seen early in the clinical course and progresses to a mucoid discharge and then to a thick, suppurative exudate. Suppurative discharge is seen early in bacterial rhinitis but may not be seen in viral infections for several days or until secondary bacterial infection occurs. Nasal discharge may be blood tinged in ulcerative rhinitis. Snorting and sneezing may be observed early in the course of rhinitis. Inspiratory dyspnea is usually seen only in severe infections or allergic reactions of the mucosa. Congestion of the mucous membranes is common, and erosions or ulcers are seen in some diseases.

Clinical Pathology

The laboratory findings and pathologic lesions of rhinitis in most cases depend on the causative disease and are discussed under those headings elsewhere in the text. The nasal cavity is a convenient site for obtaining specimens for bacterial and viral isolation of causative agents.

Treatment

Bacterial rhinitis is treated with parenterally administered antimicrobials. Since rhinitis is usually part of the respiratory disease complex, the reader is referred to that section for specific therapeutic recommendations. Allergic rhinitis can be relieved by irrigation of the nasal cavities with epinephrine solutions (1 ml 1:1000 epinephrine in 100 ml water) or parenteral corticosteroids (e.g., 0.02 mg/kg body weight dexamethasone).

EPISTAXIS

Etiology

Bleeding from the nose can be due to either nasal cavity or pulmonary hemorrhage. Bleeding in the bronchial tree or hemoptysis is not always manifested as epistaxis unless it is extensive or unless the head is held low, since most blood is swallowed.

External trauma to the nasal and maxilla bones, dehorning and internal trauma from lodgment of objects in the nasal cavity, and passage of a nasogastric tube are common causes of nasal cavity hemorrhage. Usually slight hemorrhage is also observed in some cases of ulcerative rhinitis in cattle and atrophic rhinitis of swine. Nasal tumors and granulation tissue may ulcerate, causing slight recurrent epistaxis.

Severe pulmonary hemorrhage may be associated with erosion of pulmonary vessels by abscesses in chronic pneumonia. Also, severe hemorrhage may be seen following embolic showering of the lung in animals with vegetative endocarditis or thrombosis of the vena cava.

Epistaxis commonly is an early and prominent sign seen in diseases of blood coagulation. Disseminated intravascular coagulation may intervene in the course of many diseases, particularly those with endotoxemia such as gram-negative bacterial infections of the uterus and mammary gland or in enteric diseases. Liver disease and the consumption of bracken fern or moldy sweet clover are causes of epistaxis due to coagulation deficiencies.

Clinical Signs

Epistaxis may vary from slight to profuse, may be unilateral or bilateral, and may be continuous or recurrent. Some recurrent cases may present only with evidence of previous bleeding such as nasal cavity clots or blood stains on the nostrils. Unilateral epistaxis is usually due to nasal cavity or paranasal sinus hemorrhage. Epistaxis due to pulmonary hemorrhage is usually bilateral, and in severe cases the blood may run in streams from both nostrils when the head is lowered. Coughing usually accompanies hemoptysis. Blood is swallowed, with resulting melena in chronic cases. Examination of the nasal cavity, pharynx, larynx, and trachea with a flexible fiberoptic endoscope is usually helpful in determining the source of hemorrhage.

Clinical signs in animals with epistaxis vary depending on the cause of hemorrhage. Epistaxis due to trauma is often obvious. Bleeding associated with nasal cavity disease usually is accompanied by evidence of obstruction and inspiratory dyspnea. There is evidence of hemorrhage in other areas of the body in coagulopathies. Auscultation of the lungs and heart may reveal evidence of pneumonia or endocarditis if epistaxis is due to pulmonary hemorrhage.

Treatment

Epistaxis that is secondary to other diseases will resolve with successful treatment of the primary disease. Blood transfusions usually result in only transient improvement in severely anemic cases unless the primary cause of the hemorrhage is corrected. Traumatic epistaxis usually spontaneously resolves; however, bleeding time can often be reduced by repeated irrigation of the nasal cavity with epinephrine solutions (1 ml 1:1000 epinephrine in 100 ml water).

NASAL CAVITY OBSTRUCTION

Etiology

Partial obstruction of the nasal cavity commonly occurs in rhinitis because of inflammation of the mucosal lining and accumulation of exudates. Chronic obstructions are usually due to space-occupying lesions. Nasal polyps are common in cattle and sheep but rarely attain sufficient size to cause obstruction. Granulation tissue resulting from chronic infection or trauma or in reaction to foreign bodies occurs in the nasal passages. There are a few reports of nasal carcinomas and sarcomas in older food animals. Nasal adenocarcinoma of sheep and goats occurs endemically in some flocks and is thought to be due to a virus. Large obstructive growths can be caused by *Rhinosporidium* spp. and *Helminthosporium* sp. fungal infections. Nasal bots commonly cause partial obstruction in sheep. Chronic allergic rhinitis may cause eosinophilic granulomas of the nasal cavity. Actinomycosis of the maxillae may intrude into the passages.

Clinical Signs

Partial or unilateral obstruction may cause minimal signs in the nonstressed animal. Nasal discharge, inspiratory dyspnea, and stertor are usually exhibited variably depending on the degree of obstruction. Reduction or differences in airflow on expiration can be determined by placing the backs of the hands near the nostrils. Bilateral or complete occlusion of the passages causes significant distress, with the animal exhibiting mouth breathing.

The degree of obstruction and the location of the lesion can be determined by passing tubing of various sizes up the ventral meatus. Endoscopy may be used to visualize the lesion for biopsy and specific diagnosis.

Treatment

The prognosis of nasal obstruction is generally poor because of the limitations of treatment. Surgical removal of foreign bodies and polyps is possible in some cases.

SINUSITIS

Etiology

Frontal sinusitis is a common sequela of dehorning in cattle since the sinus is opened in this operation. Usually the problem spontaneously resolves. However, if the opening to the ethmoid meatus becomes occluded with exudates, the sinusitis becomes chronic. This becomes a significant problem if the dehorning incision closes prior to resolution of the sinus infection. The frontal sinuses as well as the maxillary and other paranasal sinuses can become infected as an extension of nasal cavity infections. The bones of the walls and septae can become infected by *Actinomyces bovis*. Sinus tumors of food animals rarely occur. *Oestrus ovis* larvae usually migrate to the maxillary and frontal sinuses, causing sinusitis in sheep.

Clinical Signs

A diagnosis of acute frontal sinusitis due to dehorning is usually obvious because of evidence of recent surgery. Nasal discharge is prominent, as is the spillage of exudate from the surgical opening.

Animals with acute sinusitis due to ascending infection also exhibit nasal discharge. Percussion of the sinus regions elicits a dull sound.

In chronic sinusitis there may or may not be nasal discharge, depending on the patency of the openings to the nasal cavities. Some very chronic cases will persist for months or well beyond closure of the dehorning incision. The bones over the affected sinuses may become asymmetrically elevated. Dull percussion sounds are heard over the sinuses. The swelling of the sinus cavities can cause exophthalmus and strabismus. Pressure on the brain often causes neurologic signs such as opisthotonos and ataxia. The infection may extend to the meninges with the onset of acute meningitis. Radiographs usually reveal evidence of fluid accumulation and bone lysis.

Treatment

Acute sinusitis that persists following dehorning usually resolves following irrigation via the surgical incision with disinfectants (equal parts hydrogen peroxide [3 per cent] and povidone-iodine solution [10 per cent]). The treatment of chronic sinusitis must be more intensive and is less often successful. Animals showing evidence of extension of the disease to bone due to actinomycosis should be treated with parenteral antibiotics (10 mg/kg oxytetracycline intravenously or intramuscularly s.i.d. for 10 to 14 days). Successful treatment of chronic sinusitis requires opening of the sinuses for local treatment. The sinus should be opened at the dehorning site if the condition is a dehorning sequela or by a trephine opening over the most dependent area of the affected sinus, taking care not to damage vital structures. Long-term disinfectant irrigation is required in these cases.

PHARYNGITIS, LARYNGITIS, AND TRACHEITIS

Etiology

The upper air passages are usually involved along with the whole respiratory system in diseases grouped in the respiratory disease complex. Many of the etiologic agents colonize and replicate in the upper airways early in these diseases, so early clinical signs may be restricted to these anatomic sites. The following diseases are specific to the upper respiratory tract: infectious bovine rhinotracheitis and calf diphtheria in cattle, influenza in swine, and *Corynebacterium pyogenes* laryngitis in sheep.

Clinical Signs

A nonproductive cough is the most consistent clinical sign. The cough may be painful so that the animal may extend the head and mouth breathe between coughs. The lower trachea should be auscultated during coughing, since absence of rales indicates that the origin of the cough is due to upper respiratory irritation. Manual manipulation of the throat, cold air, and dust will induce coughing. Inspiratory dyspnea and stertorous breathing are seen with severe inflammation. Extreme irritation of the pharynx occasionally causes dysphagia. The regional soft tissues and lymph nodes are uncommonly involved.

The upper respiratory system of adult cattle can be thoroughly examined with a flexible endoscope. The larynx can usually be visualized via the mouth with the aid of a bright light and a cylindric speculum.

Treatment

Infections of the upper respiratory system are treated with parenteral antibiotics at the same dosages as those recommended for the bovine respiratory disease complex. The reader is referred to that article for specific therapeutic recommendations.

TRAUMATIC PHARYNGITIS

Etiology

Food animals are often treated by forced oral administration of medicants with minimal restraint by lay workers with resulting damage to the pharynx. The injudicious administration of pills and magnets with a balling gun, liquids with a dose syringe, and fluids by esophageal feeders and the forceful passage of stiff stomach tubes cause the damage. Animals may cause similar trauma by inadvertently swallowing sharp objects. The problem with lacerations in this region is that ingesta impacts into the defects with resulting abscess or phlegmon.

Clinical Signs

The history of prior oral therapy is helpful in diagnosing this condition. Even in animals that were ill at the time of treatment there is usually a sudden deterioration in their condition. Anorexia is common, and many animals will not drink and will become dehydrated. Inspiratory dyspnea is exhibited when severe inflammation of the pharynx develops. Usually there is some soft tissue swelling or fullness noted in the throat region. In severe cases very large abscesses may form submucosally or in the regional lymph nodes. Occasionally, severe phlegmon will develop in the throat and extend to the intermandibular space or gravitate down the neck to the thoracic inlet.

In larger calves and cattle it is usually possible, via the mouth, to palpate digitally the damage in the pharyngeal mucosa. Endoscopy may be required for specific diagnosis in smaller food animals.

Treatment

In animals with extensive damage, therapy is usually unsuccessful and the best option is slaughter. Adult cattle with moderately superficial lesions can be managed by digitally removing ingesta from the defects twice a day and feeding a semifluid diet. This is done until granulation tissue fills the defect. Early in the disease a broad-spectrum antimicrobial therapy is indicated in those animals that are not to be slaughtered. Abscesses may point up later in the clinical course and can then be surgically drained.

OBSTRUCTION OF THE UPPER RESPIRATORY TRACT

Etiology

Partial and complete obstructions can occur in the pharynx, larynx, or trachea. Impediments to air movement through these structures can be due to a variety of causes. The pharynx can be impinged on by cellulitis of the throat or from abscesses or tumors in the retropharyngeal lymph nodes. In cattle and particularly calves, lymphosarcoma of these nodes often causes partial obstruction. Calf diphtheria and *C. pyogenes* laryngitis of sheep can obstruct the larynx. Edema of the larynx may occur in allergic reactions in all species, as part of edema disease in swine, and as a reaction to irritation from trauma or the inhalation of smoke or chemical fumes. Perivascular cellulitis of the jugular veins can partially collapse the trachea. The tracheal diameter is also decreased when tracheal rings are fractured, in calves with congenital malformation of the rings, or in older cattle with partial tracheal collapse, that is, "scabbard trachea."

Clinical Signs

Acute obstructions are manifested by severe dyspnea, anxiety, and cyanosis or even fatal asphyxia. Partial obstructions or those of a progressive nature are characterized by increasingly prominent thoracic movements during inspiration. Mouth breathing with extension of the head and loud stertor are prominent signs in advanced cases. Syncope or fatal asphyxia can result from agitation or forced exercise in these cases.

Calves with absent or partially developed tracheal rings usually exhibit inspiratory dyspnea and hyperpnea from birth. These malformations may be evident on tracheal palpation. Cases with less severe involvement or with partial collapse (scabbard trachea) may reach adulthood and be evident only by inspiratory dyspnea during exertion or with endoscopic examination.

Treatment

Therapy is largely dependent on the cause and therefore varies from case to case. Regardless of cause, a tracheotomy will relieve the dyspnea and facilitate examination. The prompt administration of a corticosteroid and epinephrine is indicated in animals with laryngeal edema.

BIBLIOGRAPHY

Blood DC, Henderson JA, Radostits OM, et al: Veterinary Medicine, 5th ed. Philadelphia, Lea & Febiger, 1979.
Jensen R, Swift BL: Diseases of Sheep, 2nd ed. Philadelphia, Lea & Febiger, 1982.
Leman AD, Straw B, Glock RD, et al: Diseases of Swine, 6th ed. Ames, IA, Iowa State University Press, 1991.

Pneumonia in Cattle, Sheep, and Swine

JEROME G. VESTWEBER, DVM, PhD

The term pneumonia in this article will be used for all pulmonary inflammatory lesions regardless of location or cause. This disease occurs in all food animal species (cattle, sheep, and swine) and is the main component of many respiratory syndromes, such as the respiratory disease complex, shipping fever, enzootic pneumonia, progressive pneumonia, and atypical pneumonia. Pulmonary emphysema and edema will be more fully discussed in another article in this section. Pneumonia ranks high in economic importance to the food animal industry and is extremely costly for several reasons: immunity to some of the infectious agents is generally poor, vaccination has some limitations, and antibiotic therapy must be extensively applied to control the disease. Treatment can be life-saving, but loss in production among surviving animals can also result in economic liability. A variety of factors are responsible for the development of pneumonia, but most are infectious and will be elaborated upon in individual articles on the respiratory disease complex of cattle, sheep, and swine. The most typical description of the disease when caused by a bacterial agent is a widespread, exudative, inflammatory reaction characterized by inflammatory cells as well as fluid, blood, mucus, fibrin, and necrotic debris in air passages and tissues. The location of the lesions in the lung and the components of the exudate usually allow a diagnosis of the type of pneumonia.

ETIOLOGY

Respiratory disease in food animals is due to a complex of factors that often interact to produce disease. The management and environmental stresses placed on these animals are often the deciding factors between the development of clinical diseases or the disease remaining subclinical.

Some viruses, such as parainfluenza-3, infectious bovine rhinotracheitis, and respiratory syncytial virus, may produce mild or subclinical disease if not complicated by other factors, but they are capable of inhibiting the mucociliary transport system and depressing alveolar macrophage function. The compromised respiratory tract offers the opportunity for secondary bacterial invaders, such as *Pasteurella haemolytica* and *P. multocida*, to reside and initiate the pneumonic stages. It is risky to attribute primary responsibility of an infectious agent to specific pathologic changes, but viral agents are usually associated with upper respiratory tract disease and mild pathologic changes in the lungs. The severe pathologic changes associated with pneumonia are primarily attributed to bacterial agents. Less frequently, mycotic agents and lungworms are involved in pneumonia or act in concert with viral and bacterial agents. Finally, the lung will respond to injury from chemicals, such as 3-methylindole, primarily at the alveolar level in a manner different from an infectious agent.

PATHOGENESIS

Pneumonia can be caused by inhaled irritant gases or aerosols; aspirated foreign matter; and aerogenous or hematogenous viruses, bacteria, fungi, and metazoa. In many instances the lesion is specific by virtue of its anatomic pattern or the presence of the causative agent. In many instances, however, the course is deviated beyond a specific range by secondary bacterial infections or by therapy. Even when the cause is readily ascertainable, the pathogenesis can seldom be stated with clarity except in those few infections that are consistently virulent.

The three main morphologic types of pneumonia have different pathogenesis and lesions and therefore exhibit a different appearance and texture. Bronchopneumonia commonly develops primarily in bronchi and bronchioles and spreads in a lobular fashion into the parenchyma of the anterior ventral areas. Enzootic pneumonia is an example of bronchopneumonia. Fibrinous pneumonia is an acute lobar type of pneumonia that develops in the anterior ventral areas and is characterized by exudation and fibrin in airways, between lobules, and on the pleura. Pasteurellosis, or shipping fever, is a good example of fibrinous pneumonia. Finally, interstitial pneumonia involves the lung uniformly, with alveolar walls distended and the lining cells hypertrophied or destroyed. Atypical interstitial pneumonia is a good example of this disease.

The prototype of pneumonia in most of our food animal species is fibrinous pneumonia, which is most commonly produced by *Haemophilus (Actinobacillus) pleuropneumoniae* in swine and *P. haemolytica* in cattle and sheep. Pure experimental infections with these bacterial agents without predisposing factors, such as stress, viral, mycotic, or metazoan agents, have given us a better understanding of the pathogenesis of pneumonia.

Experimental aerosol exposure of weaned pigs to 1×10^9 colony forming units of serotype 5 *H. pleuropneumoniae* resulted in the following findings. Pulmonary edema, hemorrhage, and a diffuse neutrophilic bronchiolitis and alveolitis were observed 3 and 6 hours following experimental infection. By 12 and 18 hours after infection, focal areas of coagulative necrosis had developed, which were demarcated by dense bands of inflammatory cells. A thick layer of fibrinous exudate covered the lesion. At 24 and 48 hours following infection, necrotic areas were surrounded by dense bands of degenerating leukocytes, mononuclear round cells, and mononuclear elongated or swirling cells. By 96 to 168 hours, lung abscesses and pleural adhesions had developed.

Two-week-old calves were inoculated endobronchially with 7.9×10^{10} colony-forming units of 6-hour log phase *P. haemolytica*. Twenty-four hours following infection, many of the small airways were filled with neutrophils, there was extensive edema accumulation around the small and large blood vessels, and there was hemorrhage in the alveoli. Leukocytes were seen in dilated lymph channels, and the pleura had dilated vessels, pockets of leukocytes, edema, and fibrin. At 72 hours there were extensive interstitial and alveolar edema containing fibrin, generalized distention or thrombosis of lymphatic vessels, and fibrinous pleuritis. Leukocytes and fusiform, elongate macrophages were found surrounding necrotic lung tissue.

Resolution of pneumonia by natural defense mechanisms or aided by therapy is the primary objective, but complications can occur. Pneumonia can spread to new areas of normal lung tissue. Bronchiolar epithelium that has become ulcerated or plugged with necrotic inflammatory exudate may become organized with connective tissue, resulting in a permanent bronchiole plug (bronchiolitis obliterans); this may further result in either lung collapse or emphysema.

CLINICAL SIGNS

Pneumonia can vary from the mildest syndrome, such as with enzootic pneumonia of calves or pigs, to a rapidly fatal disease, such as shipping fever. A bilateral, mucopurulent nasal discharge may or may not be present, depending on the stage or duration of the disease. With acute pneumonia, nasal discharge is usually mucopurulent, whereas if the pneumonia is more chronic, the nasal discharge may be absent.

Coughing may be exhibited and be moist and productive if there is an accumulation of loose exudate in the bronchi and bronchioles. A cough will be more dry in character if some of the following are present: the pneumonic process is in the early stages of hyperemia, there are chronic pneumonic changes in the lung, or the pneumonia is more interstitial in character.

A fever is a good indicator of acute pneumonia and can range from 40 to 41°C. With response to treatment the fever will again decrease to the normal range, but a lack of immediate fever response may suggest a viral (interstitial) pneumonia or lack of susceptibility of the causative organism. A fever that is slightly elevated (39 to 40°C) for a duration of at least 7 days suggests incomplete resolution of the pneumonic process and permanent pathologic lung changes.

Most animals will have increased depth of respiration, whereas a few will exhibit primarily shallow abdominal breathing. Most will have an inspiratory dyspnea, whereas fewer will have an expiratory dyspnea. If severe thoracic pain characterized by shallow respiratory movement and reluctance to move is present with pneumonia, it is usually indicative of a purulent pleuritis.

Extensive involvement of both lungs can result in open-mouth breathing, extension of the head, dilation of the nostrils, abduction of the elbows, and the presence of thoracic inlet movement. Animals with chronic cases of pneumonia will be depressed and exhibit inappetence and will have a gaunt appearance, fast, shallow, or labored respirations, expiratory grunt, some coughing, and usually a body temperature that is slightly elevated or within the normal range.

AUSCULTATION OF THE LUNGS

Further discussion of diagnostic auscultation can be found in the article Diagnostic Methods Applied to the Respiratory System. Sounds that are heard with a stethoscope should be interpreted with the stages of inflammation that occur with pneumonia. Bronchial sounds, which are normal over the trachea and the primary bronchi, are distinctly abnormal when they are heard over an extensive area of the lung field and usually indicate consolidation of the lungs. Crackles are always a sign of disease and are audible whenever movable exudate or edema fluid accumulates within the respiratory tract. Moist crackles are often heard in early stages of pneumonia and are generally heard throughout inspiration and expiration over affected lung tissue. If the crackles are numerous, indicate that considerable inflammatory fluid is present. When pneumonia becomes more advanced or is resolving, the crackles will become drier. A pleural friction sound is heard during both inspiration and expiration in the ventral third of the lung field and is commonly associated with primary pleuritis or fibrinous pneumonia. If pleural frictional sounds disappear, pleural adhesions may have developed or fluid (exudate) is separating the pleural surfaces.

DIAGNOSTIC METHODS

Nasal or tracheal swabs can be utilized for either bacteria or viral isolation, but caution should be used in interpreting the bacterial findings because this method may not express the true pathogenic organisms responsible for pneumonia. A transtracheal aspiration or bronchoalveolar lavage will produce more valuable information. These techniques will be discussed further in the article Diagnostic Methods Applied to the Respiratory System. Serologic testing of serum samples during the acute febrile and convalescent periods leads to viral identification but has the disadvantage of a 2-week wait to see if fourfold increase in titer occurs.

Most absolute neutrophil band cells and blood fibrinogen are elevated 24 hours following the initiation of a bacterial pneumonia. In addition, by 72 hours postinfection the total leukocyte counts are usually elevated significantly, whereas a leukopenia and lymphopenia are more common with acute viral pneumonia. With the availability of venous or arterial blood gases, a determination can also be made of pulmonary function status.

Radiographic examination will readily identify areas of abscessation, fibrosis, atelectasis, plugged bronchi and bronchioles, consolidation, and emphysema, but size of animal can limit this procedure.

PATHOLOGY

Most of the pneumonias are bilateral, with the right apical lobe being affected first because of the anterior bronchus supplying this lobe. Most of the lesions will be confined to the anterior ventral portions of the cranial, middle, and caudal lung lobes and will be dark red, gray, or red-black in color. The affected areas will be hard and heavy and possibly covered with various amounts of fibrin on the pleural surface. Interlobular connective tissue will be widened because of extensive edema, and lobulation is emphasized. Edema and hemorrhage will be evident on a cut surface. Small, irregularly shaped pale areas of coagulation necrosis may develop in the parenchyma. Extensive lesions may be accompanied by some emphysema of the remaining lung tissue.

Animals not responding to treatment may develop chronic pneumonia. Pathologic findings include collapse because of obstruction of bronchioles. These affected areas are dark red and heavy but depressed below the normal surface of the lung. The lung is variegated in color, consisting on cross sections of exaggerated lobular patterns with widened interlobular septa. Organization of pleural exudate will result in permanent pleural adhesions. If the causative organisms are pyogenic, frank abscesses may occur. Areas of emphysema can be found outside areas of pneumonia and collapse. Interstitial pneumonia usually involves both lungs and is characterized by uncollapsed, enlarged, and firm lungs. The caudal lobes are most commonly affected, and a cut surface demonstrates pleural thickening and edema. Emphysema of interlobular, subpleural, connective tissue and lymphatics is common.

Any bacterial or viral isolation taken from pathologic specimens should be accomplished in the early stages of pneumonia. If specimens are taken in the later stages, the primary pathogen may have disappeared or may be masked by changes induced by secondary agents.

TREATMENT AND PREVENTION

Antibiotic selection is usually the initial consideration in the development of a therapeutic plan for pneumonia cases. This should be based on the evidence that *Pasteurella* spp. are the principal causes of severe clinical signs, terminal lesions, and death loss to pneumonia regardless of the initial cause of respiratory disease. Other bacteria, such as *Haemophilus* spp., *Actinobacillus* spp., and *Mycoplasma* spp., may also contribute in a primary or secondary capacity. Usually *Pasteurella* spp. are sensitive to broad-spectrum antibiotics and sulfonamides. However, antibiotic sensitivity is variable because of development of resistance. Antibiotics should be administered for a minimum of 3 days, but longer if response is not complete.

Antibiotic drugs approved by the U.S. Food and Drug Administration for parenteral use in food-producing animals are aqueous procaine penicillin G, benzathine penicillin G, ampicillin trihydrate, oxytetracycline hydrochloride, tetracycline hydrochloride, dihydrostreptomycin sulfate, erythromycin, amoxicillin trihydrate, ceftiofur sodium, and tylosin. The recommended dosage, routes of administration, and withdrawal times before slaughter need to be closely observed to safeguard milk and meat supplies. Extra-label nonapproved antibiotics and sulfonamides such as gentamycin, neomycin, spectinomycin, and trimethoprim-sulfa have also been used.

Some parenteral and oral sulfonamides (sulfabromomethazine, sulfachlorpyridazine, sulfadimethoxine, and sulfamethazine) continue to be used in individual and herd medication, but they no longer appear to be as popular as antibiotics in treatment. Slow-release sulfonamides have the advantage of requiring only one episode of cattle handling, but if the pneumonia is extensive, they may not provide enough medication to resolve the infection.

Failure to get a treatment response to antibiotic or sulfonamide therapy may not always be explained by bacterial resistance but may be due to lack of early detection of the disease, advanced irreversible pathologic changes of the disease, or inadequate levels of previous therapy. Thus serious consideration of these factors should be made before using nonapproved drugs in the treatment of pneumonia. More details on the antibiotics and ancillary treatments will be found in other articles in this section.

Controversy continues over the use of corticosteroids in the treatment of pneumonia. Administration of corticosteroids early in the course of pneumonia will usually result in a clinical improvement (often a decrease in febrile response and an increase in appetite because of a euphoric effect), but these drugs at the commonly recommended dosages may increase the number of relapses and prolong the course of disease.

A highly effective method for preventing pneumonia has not been found. The bovine viral vaccines are helpful by preventing some of the predisposing effects that viral agents have on compromising the respiratory tract and allowing secondary bacterial infection. The *P. haemolytica* and *P. multocida* vaccines are questionable immunizing agents. The bacterins may actually be detrimental to the animal, whereas the modified live vaccines have demonstrated some protection. The experimental use of *P. haemolytica* bacterial-free leukotoxic culture supernatant for immunization appears to be positive. The benefit derived from preventing respiratory disease with *Haemophilus* vaccines has not been researched as well.

Avoidance of "stress" factors is sometimes unpredictable from both management and environmental standpoints, but decreasing or eliminating as many possible adverse effects to the animal will help in preventing pneumonia. The timing of management events is critical.

BIBLIOGRAPHY

Allan EM, Gibbs HA, Wiseman A, Selman IE: Sequential lesions of experimental bovine pneumonic pasteurellosis. Vet Rec 117:438–442, 1985.
Confer AW, Panciera RJ, Mosier DA: Bovine pneumonic pasteurellosis. Immunity to *Pasteurella haemolytica*. J Am Vet Med Assoc 193:1308–1316, 1988.
Groom SC, Little PB, Rosendal S: Virulence differences among three strains of *Haemophilus somnus* following intratracheal inoculation of calves. Can J Vet Res 52:349–354, 1988.
Jensen R, Pierson R, Braddy P, et al: Shipping fever pneumonia in yearling feedlot cattle. J Am Vet Med Assoc 169:500–506, 1976.
Liggett AD, Harrison LR: Sequential study of lesion development in experimental *Haemophilus* pleuropneumonia. Res Vet Sci 42:204–221, 1987.
Rehmtulla AJ, Thomson RG: A review of the lesions in shipping fever in cattle. Can Vet J 22:1–8, 1981.
Shoo MK: Experimental bovine pneumonic pasteurellosis: a review. Vet Rec 124:141–144, 1989.
Thomson RG: The pathogenesis and lesions of pneumonia in cattle. Compend Contin Educ Pract Vet 3:S403–S412, 1981.

Vestweber JG, Klemm RD, Leipold HW, et al: Experimental *Pasteurella haemolytica* pneumonia: clinical and pathological studies. Am J Vet Res 51:1792–1798, 1990.
Vestweber JG, Klemm RD, Leipold HW, Johnson DE: Pneumonic pasteurellosis induced experimentally in gnotobiotic and conventional calves inoculated with *Pasteurella haemolytica*. Am J Vet Res 51:1799–1805, 1990.
Yates WDG: A review of infectious bovine rhinotracheitis, shipping fever pneumonia and viral-bacterial synergism in respiratory disease of cattle. Can J Comp Med 46:225–263, 1982.

Acute Bovine Pulmonary Edema and Emphysema

ROGER BREEZE, BVMS, PhD, MRCVS
JAMES R. CARLSON, PhD

Acute bovine pulmonary edema and emphysema (ABPE) is an acute respiratory distress syndrome that usually occurs in the fall in adult (over 2 years old) beef cattle moved from dry, sparse grazing to lush, green pastures. The disease has been known as fog fever in Europe for at least 200 years, the word "fog" having epidemiologic connotations in that the condition is often seen in cattle on "fog" pastures (i.e., aftermath or foggage, the regrowth after a hay or silage cut). There is no association with atmospheric smog or fog. ABPE is consistently related to management practices resulting in sudden introduction of hungry adult cattle to lush grazing. In cow-calf operations in the western United States, this typically occurs when the herd is brought from dry summer range onto irrigated or fertilized aftermath pasture. The species composition of the pasture does not appear to be important, provided it is lush. ABPE has been reported on a wide variety of grasses, alfalfa, rape, kale, and turnip tops. The disease is rare in dairy cattle probably because the necessary abrupt pasture movements are unusual in a well-managed milking herd. APBE appears to be more frequent in the Hereford breed and its crosses, apparently because this is the most prevalent type of animal in cow-calf operations. No breed appears to be unaffected under the right management conditions. The available evidence supports the view that ABPE is caused by ruminal production of 3-methylindole (3MI) from ingested L-tryptophan (TRP) in herbage.[1,2] The 3MI is absorbed into the blood stream from the rumen and metabolized by a mixed-function oxidase (MFO) system in the lung to produce pneumotoxicity (Fig. 1).

CLINICAL DISEASE

The terms "ABPE" and "fog fever" have been applied to a farrago of different respiratory conditions in which interstitial emphysema has been detected clinically or at necropsy (Figs. 2 to 5). In this context ABPE and fog fever refer only to the pasture-associated syndrome, which is defined in clinical, epidemiologic, and pathologic terms.[3] Almost all outbreaks of ABPE arise within 2 weeks of pasture change, and the condition is usually limited to fat, brood cows, usually of the Hereford type. The morbidity rate is variable but often approaches 50 per cent; 30 per cent of severely affected animals die, usually within 2 days of the onset of clinical signs. In severe cases there is labored breathing with loud expiratory grunt, frothing at the mouth, and mouth breathing. On auscultation, inspiratory and expiratory sounds are usually surprisingly soft in view of the respiratory rate, and crackles

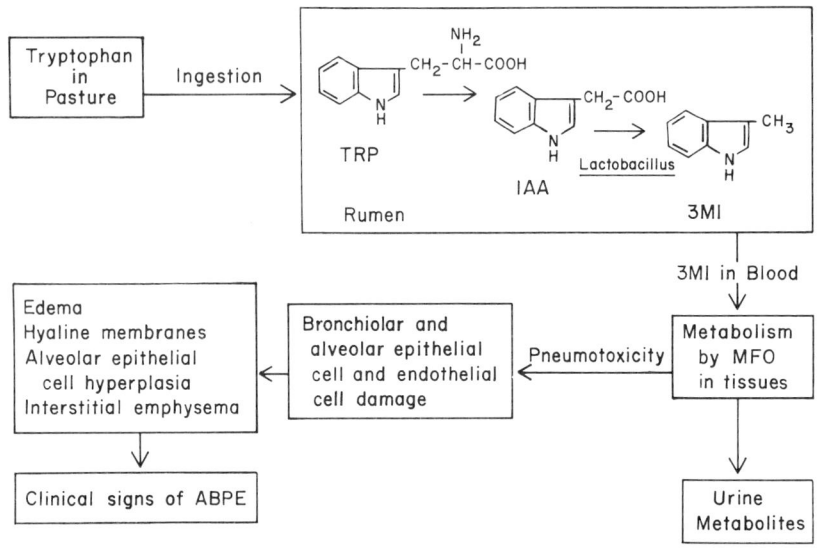

Figure 1. An outline of the pathogenesis of acute bovine pulmonary edema and emphysema (TRP = tryptophan; IAA = indoleacetic acid; 3MI = 3-methylindole; MFO = mixed function oxidase).

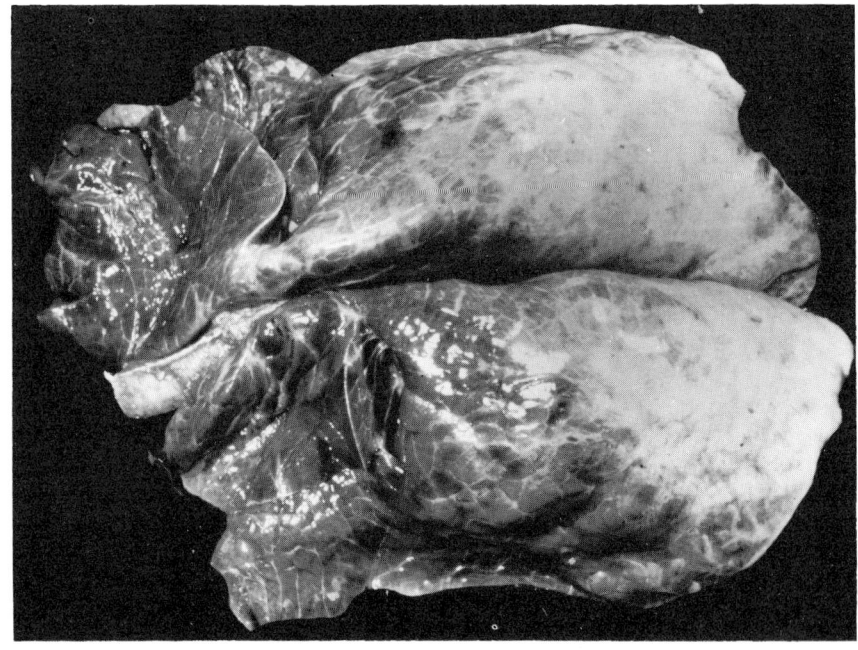

Figure 2. Fog fever: the cranial lobes are dark red and congested. There is pleural edema and interstitial emphysema in the caudal lobes, which are distended by gas bullae. The lungs are from a fatal case.

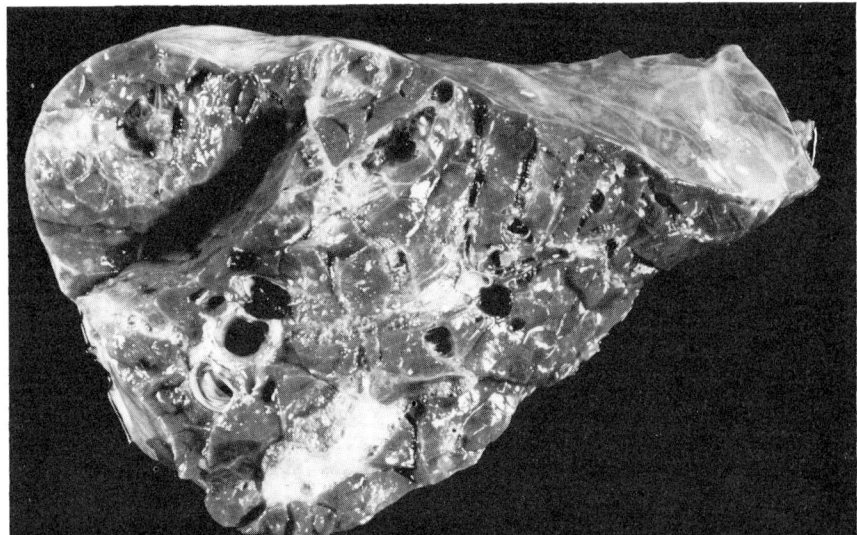

Figure 3. Fog fever: cross section of caudal lung lobe in Figure 2. Interstitial emphysema and gas bullae are evident. The lung lobes are dark red and have a smooth, shiny cut surface indicative of the presence of congestion, edema, and hyaline membranes.

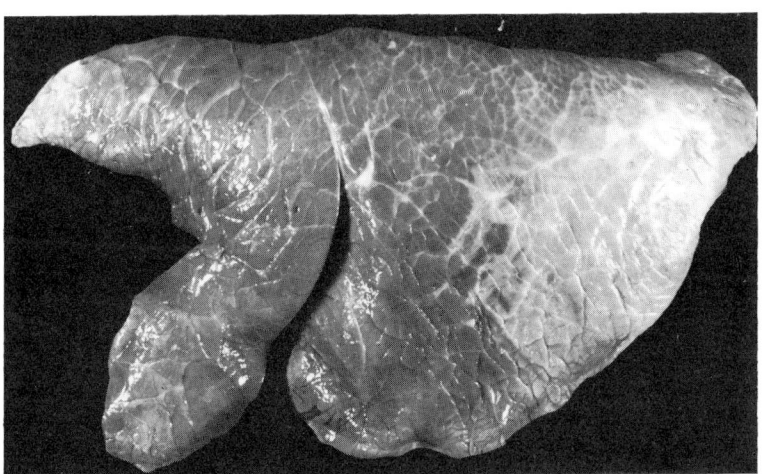

Figure 4. Fog fever: lungs of a slaughtered animal ill for 4 days. The lungs were fawn colored and very heavy.

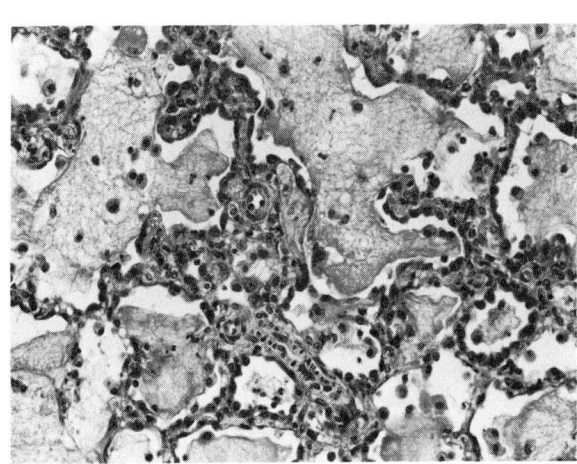

Figure 5. Histologic appearance of the lungs in fog fever. There is edema of the alveolar spaces and interalveolar septa and marked proliferation of cuboidal alveolar epithelial cells (type 2 pneumonocytes). (H & E, × 250)

(harsh or soft crackling sounds) are only occasionally detected. Severe cases improve dramatically after 3 days, and in these animals and in others that have not shown severe signs (and that may not be immediately apparent to the inexperienced observer) it is quite common to note only increased rate (50 to 80/minute) and depth of breathing. Harsh respiratory sounds are common on auscultation, and crackles and rhonchi (whistling or musical adventitious sounds) may also be noted, particularly in caudal lung fields, in this later stage. Subcutaneous emphysema may be detected in a few of these convalescing animals. In addition to these signs of respiratory disease within an affected group, there is also a tendency for the demeanor of the group to change so that the animals become more tranquil. It should be particularly noted that coughing is not a dominant feature in affected individuals nor in the group as a whole.[4,5] In animals that die there are ecchymotic and petechial hemorrhages in the larynx, trachea, and bronchi, and the airways are filled with frothy edema fluid. Cranial lung lobes are deep red or purple, and the cut surface of the lobules has a smooth, glistening, glass-like appearance, the result of severe congestion, edema, and hyaline membranes. Interstitial emphysema with large gas bullae is apparent in all parts of the lung and occasionally may also extend along the back. Pulmonary edema is very noticeable, especially in the ventral segments of the lungs, and gelatinous yellow edema fluid can be found in the interlobular septa and perivascular connective tissue. Histologically, alveoli and alveolar ducts are usually lined by eosinophilic hyaline membranes; edema fluid; a few eosinophils, neutrophils, alveolar macrophages, and multinucleated giant cells are found in the air spaces. In most animals there is some proliferation of alveolar epithelial cells. In animals that are slaughtered after at least 3 to 4 days of illness, interstitial emphysema and pulmonary edema are usually minimal. However, all the lung tissue is fawn and rubbery as a result of severe, diffuse alveolar epithelial hyperplasia, in which the alveoli in all acini are lined by a single layer of cuboidal type 2 pneumonocytes containing frequent mitotic figures. Large mononuclear cells and a mixture of alveolar macrophages and type 2 pneumonocytes are found in the alveolar spaces, together with condensed hyaline deposits and multinucleated giant cells. Interalveolar septa are edematous, and many interstitial cells and eosinophils are apparent.[6] The pulmonary lesions are obligatory for diagnosis but are not pathognomonic. This is very important diagnostically. All cases of ABPE have some combination of the lesions mentioned previously, but all animals with some combination of these lesions do not have ABPE.

TREATMENT

A distinction should be made between treatment of an animal that already shows clinical signs of disease and prevention of disease in the herd as a whole before access to lush pasture.

Many different drugs, including corticosteroids, atropine, diethylcarbamazine, epinephrine, and diuretics, are alleged to be of value in the treatment of ABPE, but none have been properly tested. Drugs acting as antagonists to postulated mediators of bovine anaphylaxis or hypersensitivity do not appear to alter the course of 3MI-induced ABPE significantly, even when given before 3MI dosage.[7] These include acetylsalicylic acid, mepyramine, sodium meclofenamate, diethylcarbamazine, and betamethasone. Experimentally the antiprostaglandin drug flunixin meglumine has proven capable of preventing or reducing lung lesions induced by 3MI. Flunixin meglumine (2.2 mg/kg body weight intramuscularly once daily for 3 days) should be given as soon as possible after clinical signs are noticed. Temporary hospital pens should be erected in the pasture to avoid driving sick animals for long distances and to facilitate handling.

Our experience is that supportive therapy is useful only if it can be given with minimal stress to the animal involved and that recovery often occurs without drug treatment. Laboratory observations of cattle given TRP or 3MI confirm that many recover spontaneously over about 10 days; relapses do not occur.

PREVENTION AND CONTROL

1. The first step in dealing with suspected ABPE is to consider the differential diagnosis and rule out other possibilities. Careful clinical or pathologic examination can distinguish a number of different disease entities frequently mistaken for ABPE.[5] Such conditions appear unlikely to cause differential diagnostic problems in typical epidemiologic situations in the western United States and elsewhere. In any event, the presence of interstitial emphysema should not be used as the sole diagnostic criterion.

2. Having established that the problem is indeed ABPE, the next step should be to remove all adult cattle and their calves from the pasture involved, taking great care to prevent unnecessary excitement or exertion in the process. In this respect it is worth noting that cows and their calves should not be separated for any reason within the first 3 weeks of a move to lush pasture. The best preventive measure thereafter is to organize grazing management so as to avoid sudden introduction of hungry adult cattle to better pastures. This is often easier said than done but can be achieved by pregrazing lush pastures with less susceptible stock, such as sheep, horses, or immature cattle; by moving cattle onto new pasture before it becomes particularly lush; or by continuous strip-grazing. Some have recommended limiting intake of pasture by offering hay or concentrates daily or by restricting grazing time during the changeover period. Others suggest that cattle should be fed only grass that has been cut and allowed to wilt during this time. All these measures may find a use under individual circumstances but are at best unreliable methods of preventing disease or limiting losses.

3. The most promising area for prevention of ABPE appears to be in the alteration of ruminal metabolism to inhibit or lower 3MI production. Oral doses of 200 mg monensin/head/day prevent TRP-induced ABPE by reducing the conversion of TRP to 3MI in the rumen of cattle subjected to abrupt change to lush pasture or given TRP experimentally.[7,8] Lasalocid at the same dosage rate also inhibits 3MI formation.[9] If current understanding of the pathogenesis of ABPE is correct, dosing with monensin or lasalocid for a few days before pasture change and for the first 7 to 10 days after introduction should prevent the disease.

These drugs can be given in custom-milled pellets as either an energy supplement (e.g., 94.85 per cent barley, 5 per cent molasses, and 0.15 per cent Rumensin 60 [monensin]) or a protein supplement (10 per cent dehydrated alfalfa, 26.6 per cent dent yellow corn, 5 per cent molasses, 58.25 per cent soybean meal, and 0.15 per cent Rumensin 60) formulated to provide 200 mg monensin (or lasalocid)/head/day when fed once daily, or as a divided dose, in a total 1-kg supplement.[8,9] Supplements should be offered in a sufficient number of tubs or troughs to allow all cattle an opportunity to feed. Care must be taken in labeling, storage, feeding, and disposal of supplements to avoid accidental ingestion by horses and other species that are more sensitive than cattle to polyether antibiotic toxicity. Such potential hazards should be fully discussed with the client.

At present, use of monensin or lasalocid to prevent ABPE in brood cows is not approved by the U.S. Food and Drug Administration, but such a claim is being pursued.

No beneficial effect of monensin or lasalocid is to be expected when the drug is given after clinical signs appear, since by this time 3MI-induced pneumotoxicity has been expressed.

4. When a clinical case of ABPE has been found in a herd, it may be beneficial to try to prevent the disease in other animals by treatment with flunixin meglumine as described above. Whether this is economically sensible will depend on the individual herd situation.

REFERENCES

1. Selman IE, Wiseman A, Breeze RG, Pirie HM: Fog fever in cattle: various theories on its aetiology. Vet Rec 99:181–184, 1976.
2. Carlson JR, Dickinson EO: Tryptophan induced pulmonary edema and emphysema in ruminants. In Keeler RF, van Kampen KR, James LF (eds): Effects of Poisonous Plants on Livestock. New York, Academic Press, 1978, pp 272–292.
3. Breeze RG, Pirie HM, Selman IE, Wiseman A: Acute respiratory distress in cattle. Vet Rec 97:226–229, 1975.
4. Selman IE, Wiseman A, Pirie HM, Breeze RG: Fog fever in cattle: clinical and epidemiological features. Vet Rec 95:139–142, 1974.
5. Selman IE, Wiseman A, Breeze RG, Pirie HM: Differential diagnosis of pulmonary disease in adult cattle in Britain. Bovine Pract 12:63–74, 1977.
6. Pirie HM, Breeze RG, Selman IE, Wiseman A: Fog fever in cattle: pathology. Vet Rec 95:479–483, 1974.
7. Hammond AC, Carlson JR, Breeze RG, Selman IE: Progress in the prevention of acute bovine pulmonary emphysema. Bovine Pract 14:9–14, 1979.
8. Potchoiba MJ, Nocerini MR, Carlson JR, Breeze RG: Effect of energy or protein supplements containing monensin on ruminal 3-methylindole formation in pastured cattle. Am J Vet Res 45:1389–1392, 1984.
9. Nocerini MR, Honeyfield DC, Carlson JR, Breeze RG: Reduction of 3-methylindole production and prevention of acute bovine pulmonary edema and emphysema with lasalocid. J Anim Sci 60:232–238, 1985.

BIBLIOGRAPHY

Breeze RG: Parasitic bronchitis and pneumonia. Vet Clin North Am 1:219–229, 1985.
Breeze RG: Respiratory disease in adult cattle. Vet Clin North Am 1:335–370, 1985.
Breeze RG, Selman IE, Pirie HM, Wiseman A: A reappraisal of atypical interstitial pneumonia in cattle. Bovine Pract 13:75–81, 1978.
Carlson JR, Yost GS: 3-Methylindole induced acute long injury resulting from ruminal fermentation of tryptophan. In Cheeke PR (ed): Toxicants of Plant Origin. Boca Raton, FL, CRC Press, 3:107–123, 1989.

Vena Caval Thrombosis

ROGER BREEZE, BVMS, PhD, MRCVS

Hemoptysis, the coughing up of blood or blood-stained sputum, can be a dramatic clinical sign in cattle. A minor degree of hemoptysis may infrequently be observed in animals with right-sided infective endocarditis, but in the author's experience massive hemoptysis is virtually indicative of one disease: thrombosis of the caudal vena cava (CVCT, caval thrombosis).

THROMBOSIS OF THE CAUDAL VENA CAVA

History, Distribution, and Epidemiology

CVCT has been known in Europe for over 80 years and is now recognized as an increasing problem in the United States.[1] CVCT is an important and common cause of cardiovascular disease in adult cattle, in the same ranks as infective endocarditis and traumatic pericarditis.[2,3] In a survey of 1998 yearling feedlot cattle, CVCT was the cause of death in 1.3 per cent. Of these, 40 per cent were affected in the first 45 days on the feedlot and a further 28 per cent during the next 45 days.[1] CVCT is associated with the rumenitis–hepatic abscess complex most prevalent in the fattening and finishing periods of feedlot management. In a Canadian survey, CVCT was present in 19.3 per cent of cattle with hepatic abscesses and was most frequent in 1- to 2-year-old cattle.[4]

Clinical Disease

CVCT may present in two forms. The most important and common is a respiratory syndrome that follows pulmonary arterial thromboembolism and the formation and rupture of pulmonary arterial aneurysms.[5] Much less frequently, cases are encountered in which the main presenting sign is gross abdominal distention due to hepatomegaly and massive ascites, but in such instances respiratory signs and pulmonary arterial lesions are also found.[6] CVCT is also reported as a cause of "sudden death" without prodromal signs. Death often occurs unexpectedly in CVCT, usually soon after an episode of severe intrapulmonary hemorrhage or hemoptysis, but this is usually preceded by other respiratory signs of at least several days' duration. It seems likely that in cases of "sudden death" these signs have passed unnoticed, the only exception being when sudden intravascular rupture of a hepatic abscess leads to rapidly fatal septicemia and septic shock.

In about half the cases there is a history of respiratory disease of only a few days' duration. These animals usually deteriorate rapidly once hemoptysis begins. Other cattle have a history of weight loss and coughing for weeks or months. Thoracic pain is often present and may be the reason for referral, but the respiratory signs are often such that the initial clinical diagnosis would appear to be chronic suppurative pneumonia—that is, until the onset of hemoptysis.

Increased rate of breathing (>30/minute at rest), increased depth of breathing, and coughing are present in every case. These signs are of little help in establishing a diagnosis, but three features are found sufficiently frequently to make this fairly straightforward, particularly when they occur together. These signs are (1) *anemia*, manifested as mucosal pallor, hemic murmur, and lowered packed cell volume (range 10 to 20 per cent; normal 28 to 35 per cent); (2) *hemoptysis*; and (3) *widespread rhonchi*. Other useful signs, which are common but not detectable in every case, are (4) *thoracic pain* at rest, while walking, or after coughing; (5) *hepatomegaly*, considered to be present if the liver projects into the right paralumbar fossa; (6) *melena*; and (7) *fever*, rectal temperature greater than 39°C. Finally, signs of congestive cardiac failure, including jugular distention and brisket edema, may be superimposed in a few animals developing chronic cor pulmonale following widespread pulmonary arterial thromboembolism.[5]

Pathogenesis (Figs. 1 to 5)

A thrombus is always present in the hepatic or intrathoracic portion of the CVC between the liver and the right atrium. Almost all thrombi are the result of thrombophlebitis, where the wall of the CVC has been infiltrated by a perivascular hepatic or postdiaphragmatic abscess from which *Fusobacterium necrophorum*, *Corynebacterium pyogenes*, or *Staphylococcus* is often recovered.[7] Most thrombi are large and often occlude the lumen of the CVC at or anterior to the openings of the hepatic veins. This gives rise to chronic venus congestion of the liver, hepatomegaly, and the development of a collateral venous circulation, which utilizes the hemiazygos, vertebral, and mammary veins to return blood to the heart. Gross abdominal enlargement due to ascites and massive hepatomegaly is uncommon and occurs only when the thrombus extends into and obstructs hepatic veins so that this collateral drainage is blocked.

Pulmonary arterial thromboembolism from the CVC thrombus is very widespread and has the following consequences: (1) there is extensive embolic occlusion of small arteries; (2) aneurysms form at sites of arterial obstruction; (3) sudden blockage of lobar or larger arteries can cause acute clinical crises or death; (4) arterial occlusion results in development of pulmonary arterial hypertension; and (5) pulmonary hypertension promotes and accelerates the formation of aneurysms and leads to cor pulmonale.[2, 3]

A peculiar feature of CVCT is the formation of multiple pulmonary arterial aneurysms at sites of thromboembolism or where the vessel wall has been weakened by arteritis, endarteritis, and thromboarteritis. Eventually the wall of the aneurysmal sac becomes so attenuated that rupture occurs and blood is ejected into the adjacent pulmonary tissue, where it passes into the bronchial system (resulting in hemoptysis) or forms large hematomata in the interstitium of the lung. Hemoptysis usually develops when an embolic abscess is located between the artery and bronchus in such a way that the bronchial and arterial walls are eroded simultaneously. Rupture of the aneurysm is immediately followed by hemoptysis since the blood is ejected directly into the bronchial system. If only the arterial wall is eroded and the bronchus remains intact, blood ejected from ruptured aneurysms cannot gain access to the bronchial system and gathers in large, lamellated interstitial hematomata that may be 20 cm or more in diameter. Such intrapulmonary hemorrhage is the cause of anemia in the absence of hemoptysis. Thoracic pain may be the result of intrapulmonary hematomata, suppurative pneumonia, and pleuritis, or dissecting aneurysms in which blood separates the tissue planes of the arterial media.

Diagnosis

Three features are of particular value in making a clinical diagnosis of CVCT: (1) anemia; (2) hemoptysis; and (3) widespread rhonchi. Thoracic pain, hepatomegaly, and melena, when present, are also useful. Hemoptysis should be distinguished from epistaxis, which might occur in infectious bovine rhinotracheitis, for example. Widespread rhonchi are detectable in many affected cattle, and the diagnostic possibilities when these sounds are scattered over a wide lung area are generally limited to CVCT, parasitic bronchitis, and fibrosing alveolitis.[8] When other findings are considered, there is little difficulty in differentiating CVCT from the latter two conditions.

Diagnosis of CVCT at necropsy presents no problem, providing the CVC is opened. This is best achieved by removing the larynx, trachea, lungs, heart, liver, and diaphragm together, then opening the vascular system; this procedure preserves the relationships of the organs and facilitates demonstration of the lesions. Hemoptysis may be wrongly attributed to the presence of primary lung abscesses if the CVC is not examined.

THROMBOSIS OF THE CRANIAL VENA CAVA

Thrombosis of the cranial vena cava is very uncommon but gives rise to venous obstruction, the development of a collateral venous circulation, embolic pneumonia, and pulmonary arterial aneurysms and thromboembolism.[9, 10]

Clinical Disease (Fig. 6)

As in CVCT, presenting signs usually suggest chronic suppurative pneumonia. The frequency of hemoptysis has not been determined. Differential diagnosis is facilitated when additional signs are present, including: (1) edema of the head; (2) jugular distention in the absence of endocarditis or traumatic pericarditis; (3) widespread rhonchi; and (4) elevated venous pressure in the head and neck.

At necropsy, significant lesions include a septic thrombus in the cranial vena cava, pulmonary arterial thromboembolism, pulmonary arteritis, aneurysm formation, and embolic pneumonia. Massive edema of the head or severe jugular distention probably develops only when the collateral circulation is inadequate.

PULMONARY THROMBOEMBOLISM

Pulmonary thromboembolism and suppurative pneumonia may be consequences of infectious processes in various areas of the body, including phlebitis of the jugular veins, endocarditis, hepatic abscess, mastitis, and metritis. Hemoptysis and aneurysm formation are not recorded in these situations. The reason for this is unclear. Pulmonary vascular hemodynamics may be unusual in vena caval thrombosis. Certainly the distribution of emboli to periarterial sites is unlike that of other diseases. It is possible that the emboli reach these unusual sites in VCT because they arrive in lymphatics or via the collateral circulation.

Treatment

Surgical removal of arterial aneurysms with ligation of the vena cava has successfully cured similar cases in humans, but this is clearly impractical for all but the most valuable cattle.

Antibiotic treatment may remove or suppress the hepatic abscess and render emboli sterile in some cases, but in the majority significant penetration and resolution of the primary lesions would appear unlikely, even supposing these could be diagnosed. Once hemoptysis and anemia are noted, prompt slaughter and salvage are the only answer. Mortality rate at present is 100 per cent.

Prevention

On the assumption that CVCT is part of the rumenitis–hepatic abscess complex, measures taken to reduce the incidence of the latter problem in the feedlot might be expected to be beneficial.

Text continued on page 653

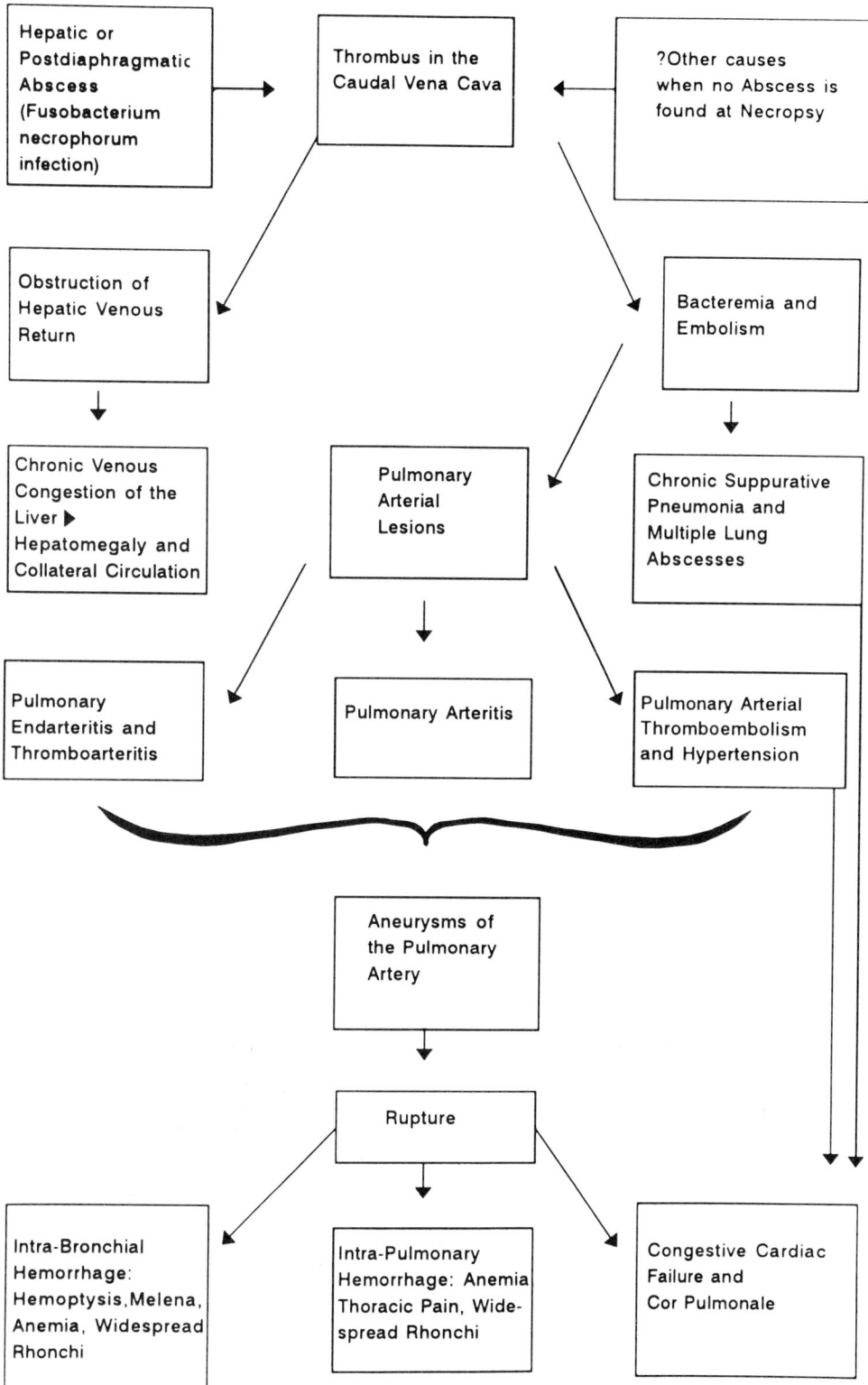

Figure 1. The pathogenesis of caudal vena caval thrombosis in cattle.

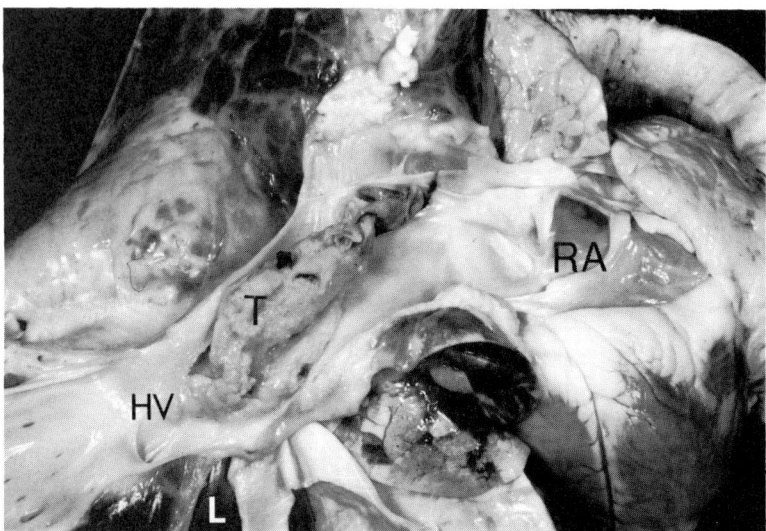

Figure 2. A rough-surfaced thrombus (T) almost occludes the lumen of the intrathoracic caudal vena cava. The liver (L), orifices of the hepatic veins (HV), and right atrium (RA) are marked.

Figure 3. Diagrammatic representation of the pathogenesis of hemoptysis and hematomata resulting from pulmonary arteritis. (i) An embolic abscess is situated adjacent to the pulmonary artery. The endothelium, intima, media, and adventitia making up the arterial wall are indicated. (ii) Extension of the abscess results in erosion of the adventitia and media of an arc of the pulmonary artery and the formation of a saccular aneurysm at the site. (iii) Erosion of vasa vasorum in the wall of the pulmonary artery results in intramural and perivascular hemorrhage between the base of the aneurysm and the surrounding abscess. (iv) There is dissection of blood between the tissue planes of the media in the vicinity of the aneurysm, and a dissecting aneurysm is formed. (v) A perivascular abscess erodes the wall of the bronchus to form a communication with the lumen. At the same time it erodes an arc of the wall of the pulmonary artery to form a saccular aneurysm surrounded by clotted blood derived from eroded vasa vasorum. (vi) Rupture of the aneurysm in (v) results in hemoptysis, and the contents of the abscess are flushed into the bronchus. (vii) A perivascular abscess that results in pulmonary arteritis and the formation of a pulmonary arterial aneurysm, but that does not erode the accompanying bronchus. (viii) Massive lamellated hematoma in the interstitium as a result of rupture of the lesion described in (vii) above. The blood cannot gain access to the bronchus (cf. vi).[3]

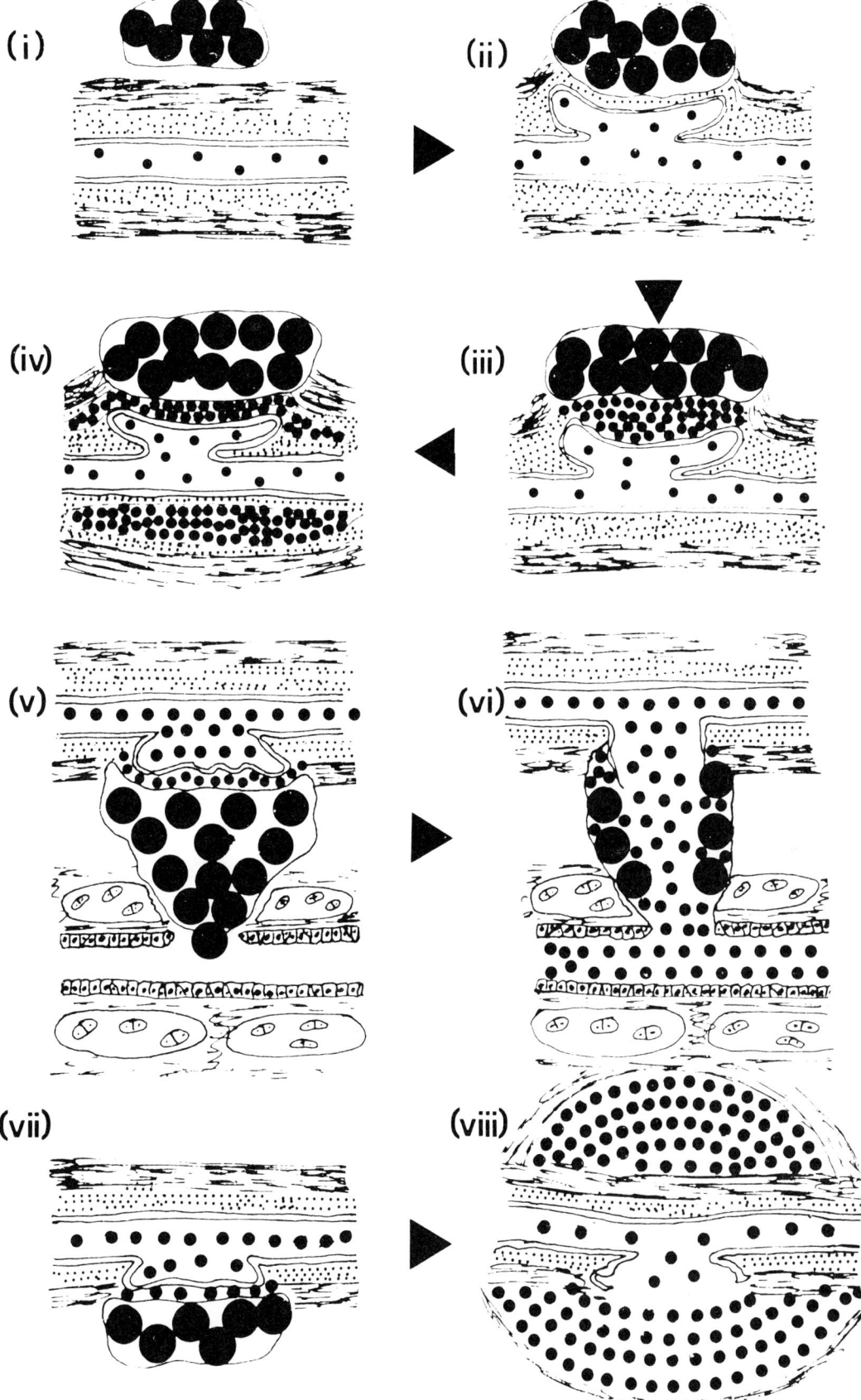

Figure 3 *See legend on opposite page*

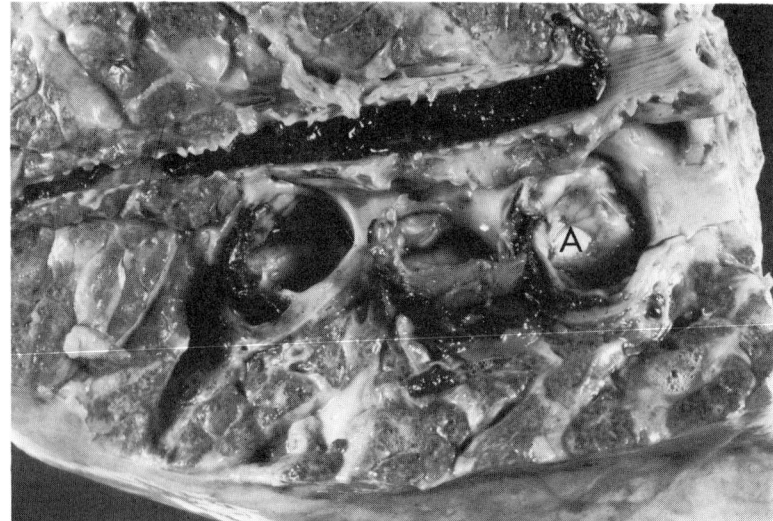

Figure 4. Three pulmonary arterial aneurysms (A) adjacent to a bronchus, which contains a cast of clotted blood. This corresponds to Figure 3 (iii).

Figure 5. Cross section through a pulmonary arterial aneurysm comparable to Figure 3 (v). A lobar artery (L) gives off a segmental branch (S) in which there is an aneurysm (A) *(solid arrows)*. Clotted blood (C) and pus surround the base of the aneurysm. The wall of the bronchus (B) is almost completely eroded *(open arrows)*.

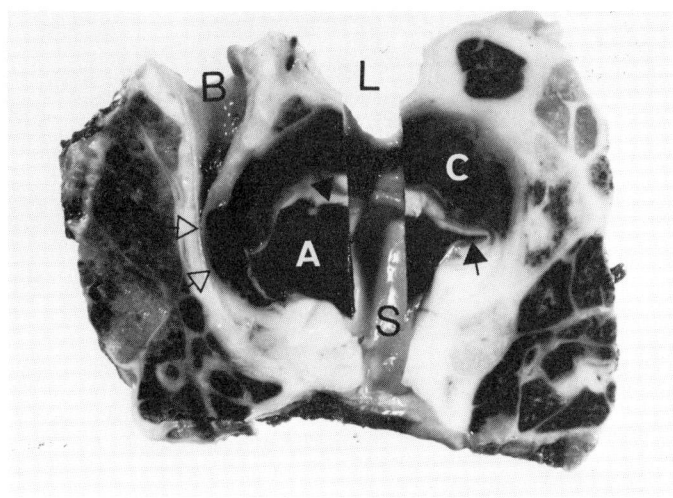

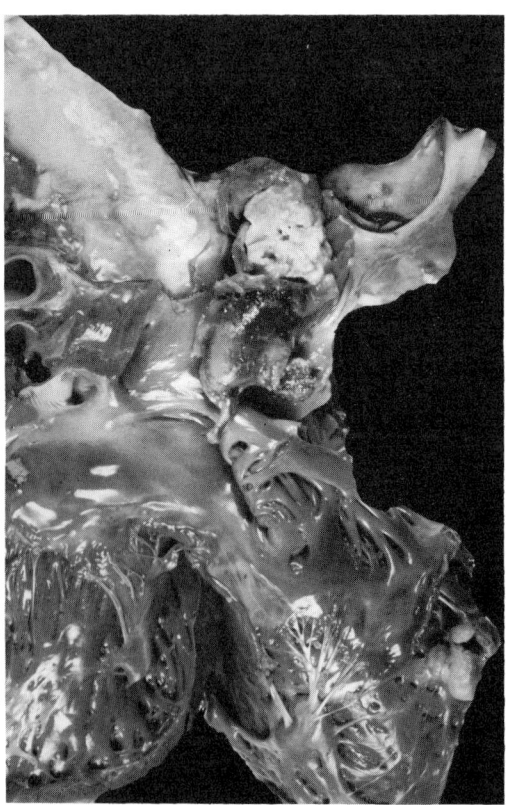

Figure 6. A septic thrombus occludes the cranial vena cava.

REFERENCES

1. Jensen R, Pierson RE, Braddy PM, et al: Embolic pulmonary aneurysms in yearling feedlot cattle. J Am Vet Med Assoc 169:518–520, 1976.
2. Breeze RG, Pirie HM, Selman IE, Wiseman A: Pulmonary arterial thromboembolism and pulmonary arterial mycotic aneurysms in cattle with vena caval thrombosis: a condition resembling the Hughes-Stovin syndrome. J Path 119:229–237, 1976.
3. Breeze RG, Pirie HM, Selman IE, Wiseman A: Hemoptysis in cattle. Bovine Pract 12:64–72, 1976.
4. Gudmundson A, Radostits OM, Doige CE: Pulmonary thromboembolism in cattle due to thrombosis of the posterior vena cava associated with hepatic abscessation. Can Vet J 19:304–309, 1978.
5. Selman IE, Wiseman A, Petrie L, et al: A respiratory syndrome in cattle resulting from thrombosis of the posterior vena cava. Vet Rec 94:459–466, 1974.
6. von Stöber M: Pyogene Thrombosen der Vena cava caudalis beim Rind. Proc IVth Int Conf Buiatrics (Zurich), 1966, pp 1–8.
7. Ikawa H, Narushima T, Kohno T: Bacteriology of caudal vena caval thrombosis in slaughter cattle. Vet Rec 120:184–186, 1987.
8. Selman IE, Wiseman A, Breeze RG, Pirie HM: Differential diagnosis of pulmonary disease in adult cattle in Britian. Bovine Pract 13:63–74, 1977.
9. Fisher EW, Pirie HM: Cardiovascular disease in domestic animals. Ann NY Acad Sci 127:606–616, 1965.
10. Breeze RG, Petrie L: Thrombosis of the cranial vena cava in a cow. Vet Rec 101:130–131, 1977.

The Bovine Respiratory Disease Complex

CHARLES A. HJERPE, DVM

DEFINITION

The etiology of the bovine respiratory disease complex is multifactorial and incompletely defined. It is believed that complex interactions between viruses, bacteria, and physical, psychologic, physiologic, and environmental stress factors are involved. When primary uncomplicated viral respiratory infections occur, the disease that results is, in most cases, subclinical or mild in nature. When severe clinical disease occurs, a bacterial bronchopneumonia and/or fibrinous pneumonia (B&FP) is nearly always present. The bacteria most frequently isolated from pneumonic bovine lungs are also commonly isolated from the oral, nasal, and oropharyngeal mucosae of normal cattle.

This definition of the bovine respiratory disease complex excludes all diseases that are limited to the upper respiratory tract (sinusitis, rhinitis, rhinosporidiosis/nasal granuloma, summer snuffles, epistaxis, pharyngitis, laryngitis, laryngeal edema, tracheitis, and tracheal edema); all sporadic diseases of the lower respiratory tract (aspiration pneumonia, metastatic pneumonia, pulmonary abscess, posterior vena caval thrombosis, hemoptysis, and milk allergy); all diseases limited to the pleural space (pleurisy, hydrothorax, hemothorax, and pneumothorax); all parasitic pneumonias; all congenital respiratory diseases; all neoplastic respiratory diseases; and all diseases included in the bovine interstitial pneumonia complex (atypical interstitial pneumonia, acute bovine pulmonary emphysema/3-methylindole toxicosis, moldy sweet potato toxicosis, perilla mint toxicosis, paraquat toxicosis, stinkwood toxicosis, extrinsic allergic alveolitis, diffuse fibrosing alveolitis, and bacteremic interstitial pneumonia).

ETIOLOGY AND PATHOGENESIS

Pulmonary Clearance Mechanisms

The lower respiratory tract is constantly exposed to bacteria, which are inhaled on dust particles and aerosolized from the nasal and oropharyngeal mucosae in droplet nuclei. Most of these particles impact on the respiratory membrane and are rapidly removed or inactivated by pulmonary clearance mechanisms. Particles larger than 2 μm in diameter are removed from the inhaled air stream by inertial impaction on the mucus layer associated with the respiratory membrane that lines the nasal passages, trachea, bronchi, and bronchioles. The nasal passages are particularly efficient in this regard. This mucus layer and the associated ciliated respiratory epithelial cells are collectively termed the "mucociliary apparatus." The mucus and associated inhaled bacteria and debris are propelled to the oropharynx by beating cilia, where they are disposed of by swallowing. Removal from the major bronchi and trachea is aided by the cough reflex.

Particles ranging in size from 0.5 to 2 μm in diameter may reach the alveoli and impact on the alveolar surface fluid film by sedimentation or Brownian movement. These particles are ordinarily rapidly phagocytized and digested primarily by pulmonary alveolar macrophages (PAM).

Because of the efficiency of these two primary pulmonary clearance mechanisms, the lower respiratory tract of the healthy, unstressed bovine is highly resistant to bacterial invasion by the aerogenous route, even with massive experimental exposure by aerosol or by intratracheal or endobronchial inoculation. However, the efficiency of the mucociliary apparatus may be adversely affected by systemic dehydration, prolonged exposure to cold air, exposure to irritant gases, and infection with certain respiratory viruses. The efficiency of the PAM may be adversely affected by starvation, exposure to cold, systemic acidosis, hypoxia, and treatment with glucocorticoids (and inferentially by stress). In vitro studies indicate that PAM function is depressed by several bovine respiratory viruses, including infectious bovine rhinotracheitis (IBR), bovine viral diarrhea (BVD), parainfluenza-3 (PI-3), and bovine respiratory syncytial virus (BRSV). Experimental infections with IBR or PI-3 viruses in cattle reduce pulmonary clearance of *Pasteurella haemolytica* and, in combination with stress, favor development of a pasteurella pneumonia. In the case of PI-3 virus, it is not known whether depressed mucociliary clearance, depressed PAM clearance, or both are involved. Although in vitro PI-3 infections in calf trachea organ cultures cause severe destruction of ciliated respiratory epithelial cells, a similar effect is not usually observed in vivo. Naturally occurring infections with IBR virus, BRSV, and bovine herpes virus type 4 are commonly associated with severe cytopathology of ciliated respiratory epithelial cells.

To summarize, bovine respiratory disease complex refers to bacterial infections of the lower respiratory tract with organisms that are normal saprophytes in the upper respiratory tract and to which the normal lower tract is constantly exposed. Clinical disease results when mucociliary and/or PAM clearance is depressed by the effects of respiratory viruses and/or stress, permitting bacterial colonization of the lower respiratory tract and initiation of a bacterial bronchopneumonia and/or fibrinous pneumonia. Of these two primary nonspecific pulmonary clearance mechanisms, PAM bactericidal activity is thought to be the most critical and important relative to the etiology of B&FP. Following initiation of respiratory viral infections, PAM function may be adversely affected for up to 2 weeks, with peak dysfunction occurring approximately 1 week postinfection. The extent of PAM suppression in experimental viral respiratory infections is directly correlated with the infectious dose of virus that has been administered.

Role of Respiratory Viruses

A large number of respiratory viruses have been isolated from cattle affected with clinical respiratory disease. These include IBR virus, African malignant catarrhal fever virus, bovine herpesvirus type 4, BVD virus, BRSV, PI-3 virus, bovine adenovirus (eight types), bovine rhinovirus (two types), reovirus (three types), bovine enterovirus (seven types), a calicivirus, bovine coronavirus, and bovine parvovirus.

IBR virus, malignant catarrhal fever virus, bovine herpesvirus type 4, BVD virus, and BRSV are capable of causing severe primary disease. Experimental infections with PI-3 virus, IBR virus, BVD virus, and bovine herpesvirus type 4 have all been shown to reduce respiratory tract resistance to pasteurella bacteria. Experimental infection of calves with IBR or PI-3 virus facilitated an explosive proliferation of *P. haemolytica A1* within the nasal passages. Rapid proliferation of *P. haemolytica A1* in the nasal passages has been shown to be a key factor in the etiology of B&FP. Large nasal bacterial populations result in increased exposure of the lower tract to aerosolized bacteria. In addition, *P. haemolytica A1* in log phase growth possesses increased virulence and pathogenicity for the bovine lung.

Experimental infections with bovine adenovirus (types 1 to 6), reovirus (type 1), bovine rhinovirus (types 1 and 2), calicivirus, and bovine coronavirus produce only a mild primary respiratory disease syndrome. Experimental BRSV infections are generally mild, but severe primary disease has been reported following simultaneous intranasal and intratracheal inoculations. Experimental infections with reovirus type 1 did not affect respiratory tract resistance to *P. multocida*.

Experimental infections with bovine adenovirus type 8, PI-3 virus, and reovirus (types 2 and 3) produce subclinical primary respiratory disease. Respiratory disease has not been produced by experimental infections with bovine enterovirus (types 1 to 7). Experimental pulmonary infections with bovine adenovirus type 7 and bovine parvovirus have not been reported.

Except for IBR virus, BVD virus, and BRSV, information concerning the relative importance of these viruses in B&FP is lacking. Serologic evidence implicating BRSV in as high as 60 per cent of field outbreaks of bovine respiratory disease has been reported from the midwestern United States. Studies in Minnesota and Iowa showed that BRSV was the viral agent most commonly identified in outbreaks of enzootic pneumonia in dairy calves and respiratory disease in weaned beef calves, respectively. Except for PI-3 and BVD, the effects of these viruses on pulmonary clearance mechanisms have not been studied in vivo. It has been found that BVD infection does not affect the clearance rate of inhaled *P. haemolytica* organisms.

Bacterial Agents

Pasteurellae, especially *P. haemolytica A1* and *P. multocida A3*, are the bacteria most frequently isolated from pneumonic bovine lungs. Less frequently isolated bacteria include *Haemophilus somnus*, *Salmonella* spp., streptococci, *Staphylococcus aureus*, *Escherichia coli*, and *Neisseria* spp. *Actinobacillus pyogenes* is frequently isolated with *Bacteroides melaninogenicus* from chronic lesions and pulmonary abscesses.

Role of Stress

Stress factors that are thought to contribute to B&FP include exhaustion, starvation, and dehydration (often resulting from transportation); weaning; ration changes; castration; dehorning; overcrowding; chilling (from confinement in cold, damp quarters or muddy pens or from exposure to drafts or inclement weather); overheating (especially when alternated with chilling); confinement in poorly ventilated quarters; exposure to stagnant air or excessive humidity; and the social adjustments associated with commingling of cattle from different sources. The occurrence of nonrespiratory diseases, such as digestive upsets from improper feeding, is an additional stress factor. Irregular consumption of high-energy rations and feeding of rations excessively high in energy prior to ruminal adaptation can result in overproduction of lactic acid in the rumen and systemic acidosis in feedlot cattle. This is a particularly serious occurrence in relation to B&FP in view of the depressing effect of systemic acidosis on PAM function. Exposure of feedlot cattle to airborne particles of pen dust in the 2.0 to 3.3 μm size range was positively correlated with the morbidity rate from B&FP. This adverse effect was compounded when cattle were also subjected to wide fluctuations in the daily temperature. Exposure of cattle to stress or abrupt climatic changes can result in explosive proliferation of nasal *P. haemolytica A1* populations, even in the absence of upper respiratory viral infections.

Role of Mycoplasmas

Mycoplasmas are frequently isolated from pneumonic bovine lungs, but their significance is unclear. Twelve species of mycoplasmas and acholeplasmas have been isolated from the bovine respiratory tract. *Mycoplasma mycoides* ssp. *mycoides* is the cause of contagious bovine pleuropneumonia. Of the remaining 11 species, only 3 (*M. bovis*, *M. dispar*, and *Ureaplasma* spp.) have been shown to be capable of causing pneumonic lesions, but clinical primary respiratory disease does not occur. Pulmonary mycoplasma infections with *M. bovis* do not affect the rate of pulmonary clearance of inhaled *P. haemolytica* organisms. Inclusion of *M. bovis* with *P. haemolytica* in intranasal inoculations has been reported to enhance the pathogenicity of *P. haemolytica* for calves. Current thinking is that pulmonary infections with *M. bovis*, *M. dispar*, or *Ureaplasma* spp. tend to be mildly synergistic with *P. haemolytica A1* and *P. multocida A3*. What is currently lacking is an effective way to make use of this information in the interest of improved prevention, control, or treatment of B&FP.

Role of Chlamydias

Chlamydia spp. are occasionally isolated from pneumonic bovine lungs but are apparently not a part of the upper respiratory microflora of normal cattle. Chlamydias are obligate intracellular bacteria. Experimental intratracheal inoculation of *Chlamydia* spp. in cattle produces a subclinical exudative bronchopneumonia. Intratracheal inoculation of a *Chlamydia* spp. isolate from a case of sporadic bovine encephalomyelitis reduced the resistance of the bovine lung to challenge by *P. haemolytica*. The relative importance of chlamydia in B&FP is unknown.

OCCURRENCE AND INCIDENCE

The potential for an outbreak of B&FP exists in virtually any population of cattle subjected to stress, in view of the ubiquity of pasteurella bacteria and many of the bovine respiratory viruses. The probability that clinical disease may result is increased by mismanagement, which increases and compounds stresses, and by commingling cattle from different sources so as to introduce new respiratory viruses for which herd immunity is lacking. Morbidity and mortality rates may rise to 100 per cent and to 30 per cent or higher, respectively, depending on the degree of mismanagement. Susceptibility to

B&FP decreases with age, although outbreaks are occasionally encountered in cattle of all ages. Transmission of respiratory viruses and bacteria occurs by direct contact, by inhalation of aerosols induced by coughing, and by ingestion of feed or water contaminated by nasal discharges and drool from infected animals.

CLINICAL SIGNS

Clinical disease does not usually occur until 6 to 10 days after cattle are stressed or new animals are introduced to the herd. The first observable signs are slight depression and inappetence manifested by gauntness. Affected animals often stand apart from the group with lowered head, drooping ears, and half-closed eyes, as if dozing. A human observer is often viewed out of the "corner" of one eye, as if discomfort results from turning the head and neck for direct, binocular viewing. In the early stages there is no dyspnea, although the respiratory rate may be elevated when there is high fever, especially when the ambient temperature is high. The muzzle may be dry and scabby in appearance. Nasal discharge may or may not be present, and it is often more indicative of the severity of the predisposing upper respiratory viral disease than of pneumonia. Coughing is never a prominent sign and is usually soft, moist, and occasional rather than paroxysmal. The rectal temperature may range from slightly above normal to 42.2°C (108°F). Diarrhea is occasionally present.

With extensive lung consolidation there is marked depression, inappetence, and dyspnea with extended head and open-mouth breathing. The rectal temperature may be elevated, normal, or subnormal. If the animal should respond to treatment at this stage, there is a marked tendency for relapse to occur within a few days to a few weeks after antimicrobial therapy is terminated. Those animals that do permanently recover may remain thin, grow slowly, and have a rough hair coat.

The distribution of the pneumonic lesion is anteroventral. Auscultation of the dorsal lung is usually normal. Rales, increased vesicular breath sounds, bronchial tones, and/or exaggerated expiratory sounds are evident upon auscultation of the anteroventral lung fields. When pleural effusion is present, there may be complete absence of respiratory sounds over the lung field below the fluid line.

PATHOLOGY

The inflammatory lesions usually develop initially in the anteroventral lung. B&FP results from tissue damage caused by release of inflammatory mediators and proteolytic enzymes from activated neutrophils, which have been attracted to the areas of bacterial colonization and lysed by the cytotoxin of *P. haemolytica*. The disease is often subclinical until more than 10 to 15 per cent of the lungs are consolidated. From 60 to 80 per cent of the lungs are usually affected in fatal cases of uncomplicated B&FP. When other diseases such as IBR, BVD, salmonellosis, mycotic rumenitis, or traumatic pharyngitis occur primarily or secondarily, only 30 to 50 per cent of the lungs may be affected. Calves younger than 4 weeks of age are an exception, in that fatal infections, which involve only 10 to 20 per cent of the lung, are often encountered. Both lungs are usually involved, although the lesions are occasionally unilateral. Healed, resolving, and inflamed areas of varying chronicity are often encountered in the same individual and can usually be correlated with a history of repeated relapses. Actively inflamed areas are swollen, firm, and engorged with blood. Inactive, resolving lesions are more nearly normal in size and are flaccid.

Pneumonic pasteurellosis usually takes the course of a bronchopneumonia, and either *P. haemolytica* or *P. multocida* may be isolated. Fibrinous pleuritis may or may not be present. In the less resistant host, or with more virulent bacteria (especially *P. haemolytica*), a more fulminating disease referred to as fibrinous (or lobar) pneumonia may occur. In the latter case a fibrinous pleuritis is invariably present, often accompanied by pleural effusion. Individual lobules are often widely separated by edematous interlobular septa. Gross evidence of airway orientation is lacking.

It is possible to determine, within limits, the approximate duration of the clinical course by a careful gross postmortem examination of the sectioned pneumonic pulmonary lobules. This determination is of value in helping to fix responsibility when it is suspected that unhealthy cattle have been purchased or that disease detection has been faulty. In fatal cases of bronchopneumonia, in which the clinical course is less than 7 days, the cut surface of the lobules is reddish-brown in color. After a 7- to 10-day course, a few tiny white foci are visible against the reddish-brown cut lobular surface. These are focal accumulations of leukocytes within and around intralobular bronchioles. After a 10- to 14-day course, increased numbers of white foci, 1 to 2 mm in diameter, are visible against the reddish-brown congested lobular parenchyma. After a 14- to 21-day course, the white foci reach maximum numbers and size (2 mm) and are packed closely together. The lobules appear yellow to white in color, as little congestion is present. Thick ribbons of yellow exudate may be expressed from the cut ends of bronchioles when the lung is compressed. After a 21- to 30-day course, beginning resolution can be noted. The sectioned lobules are yellow to white or sometimes greenish in color, and the margins of the white foci are indistinct. A thin, purulent exudate may ooze from the cut surface. Inspissated exudate may be present within necrotic foci and within some of the larger airways. Beginning abscess formation may be noted, but the capsule is poorly developed. After a 30- to 60-day course, mature abscesses may be present. The lobules are smaller than normal. The cut ends of intralobular bronchioles are dilated, and the bronchiolar walls are thickened and fibrotic. The interlobular septa are thickened by fibrosis in varying degrees. The area between bronchioles is congested and red in color. The visceral pleura may be thickened and fibrotic, and fibrous adhesions may be present between the lobes of the lung and between the visceral pleura and the chest wall.

In fatal cases of fibrinous pneumonia, in which the clinical course is less than 3 days, the cut lobular surface is reddish-black in color. After a course of 3 to 5 days, there are red as well as reddish-black areas on the lobular surface. After a 5- to 7-day course, the lobular surface is red to reddish-yellow in color. After a 7- to 14-day course, the lobular surface is yellow in color. Patients that survive for longer than 7 to 10 days will usually recover. More chronic lesions than this may be noted in cattle that die from other causes. By 14 to 30 days after the onset of signs, resolution is occurring. The majority of affected lobules are necrotic. Beginning abscess formation may be noted within some lobules. In others, the necrotic lobule may separate from the septal wall, forming an inspissated central mass. By 30 to 60 days, mature abscesses may be present. The pleura is markedly thickened and fibrotic, and the lung is adhered to the chest wall.

Pure cases of fibrinous pneumonia are seldom encountered, as some areas of bronchopneumonia are nearly always present. Sometimes fibrinous pneumonia is superimposed on lobules previously affected with bronchopneumonia. Renal infarcts are a common secondary finding with either type of process.

With either kind of pneumonia, healing is usually complete by 60 to 90 days after the onset of clinical signs, except when there is extensive pulmonary abscessation. Affected areas heal by involution of alveolar tissue, resorption of exudates, and fibrosis. Normal respiratory function is not reestablished in areas of lung in which severe bacterial infection has occurred.

TREATMENT

When effective antimicrobial therapy can be initiated on the first day that clinical signs are evident to an experienced observer and continued for 48 hours after fever, dyspnea, and toxemia have abated, and if appropriate shelter, nutrition, and nursing care are provided, mortality from acute, uncomplicated bacterial pneumonia in cattle will be negligible. Mortality is increased when disease detection is inadequate, resulting in delayed treatment; when ineffective antimicrobial drugs are utilized; when inappropriate dosages, routes of administration, or treatment intervals are selected; or when treatment is irregularly administered or prematurely terminated. Failure to promptly reinstitute treatment when relapses occur is often a factor in excessive mortality. When disease detection is adequate and a satisfactory treatment program is maintained, most fatalities from B&FP can be explained in terms of antimicrobial-resistant pasteurella bacteria. Consequently, alternative antimicrobial therapy should be considered when a satisfactory clinical response is not evident by 48 hours after initiation of primary treatment. To minimize the risk of relapse, treatment with an effective antimicrobial drug should be continued for at least 2 days after the rectal temperature has returned to the normal range (<39.5°C [103°F]) and signs of depression and dyspnea have abated. In severely affected cattle it is wise to continue treatment for 5 to 7 days after the rectal temperature has returned to the normal range.

When more than 50 to 60 per cent of a bovine animal's lungs have become consolidated, response to treatment is nearly always unsatisfactory, regardless of the treatment chosen or the antimicrobial sensitivity of the infecting organism. In those few cases that do respond, relapses are to be expected.

Relatively unsatisfactory response rates may be observed in calves shipped long distances to feedlots. These cattle may be exhausted, if not debilitated, when they finally arrive in the feedlot, and are often too tired and weak to eat for several days after arrival. If sick on arrival, or if they should become sick before recovering from the effects of shipping, response to treatment may be unsatisfactory.

B&FP in cattle is most frequently associated with *P. haemolytica*, *P. multocida*, and *A. pyogenes*. *P. haemolytica* and *P. multocida* are usually sensitive to sulfonamides, penicillin G, ampicillin, amoxicillin, tetracyclines, chloramphenicol, spectinomycin, neomycin, kanamycin, gentamicin, polymyxin B, cephalothin, cephaloridine, ceftiofur, and a combination of trimethoprim and a sulfonamide; they are usually resistant to dihydrostreptomycin and erythromycin; and they are always resistant to tylosin. *A. pyogenes* is always sensitive to penicillin G, ampicillin, amoxicillin, cephalothin, cephaloridine, and ceftiofur; it is usually sensitive to chloramphenicol, spectinomycin, neomycin, kanamycin, and a combination of trimethoprim and a sulfonamide; it is frequently resistant to erythromycin and tylosin; it is usually resistant to oxytetracycline and dihydrostreptomycin; and it is always resistant to sulfonamides and polymyxin B.

Nursing

Sick cattle should be kept dry and provided with shelter from cold winds or hot sun. Sick cattle penned together should be of similar size and should not be overcrowded. At least 12 linear inches and preferably 24 linear inches of feed bunk space and at least 40 square feet and preferably 100 square feet of pen space should be provided per animal.

Good quality long-stem pasture grass or grain hay should be available at all times. Legume hays are not recommended for sick cattle, as their use is often associated with fatal bloat. In addition to hay, a starting ration should be fed free-choice to feedlot cattle. Clean, fresh water should be available at all times. Supplementary feeding is not required for cattle on good pasture.

Use of Sulfonamides in Treatment of B&FP

All sulfonamides are bacteriostatic through competitive inhibition of bacterial para-aminobenzoic acid utilization for the synthesis of folic acid. Since bacterial cross-resistance generally occurs between all sulfonamides, selection of a specific one for treatment of B&FP in cattle should be based only on such considerations as (1) relative risk of toxicosis, (2) gastrointestinal absorption characteristics, (3) concentrations of free (active, unbound) drug achieved in blood serum, (4) cost, and (5) drug withdrawal period.

It is essential that continuously bacteriostatic blood concentrations be maintained during treatment with sulfonamides. A concentration of at least 8 to 15 mg/100 ml blood is desired, with 5 mg/100 ml being the minimum effective concentration. When using sulfonamides such as sulfadimethoxine or sulfaethoxypyridazine, in which the ratio of active drug to protein-bound drug in blood is low, even higher concentrations are probably desirable. In general, the greater the blood concentration, the better the therapeutic response (toxicosis being the limiting factor). Recommendations concerning dosages, treatment intervals, and withdrawal periods are summarized in Table 1.

From 78 to 91 per cent of *P. haemolytica* and *P. multocida* isolates recovered from nasal secretions of cattle with B&FP are sensitive to sulfonamides. *A. pyogenes* is resistant to sulfonamides. In a series of acute feedlot B&FP cases summarized by the author, 81.9 per cent responded satisfactorily when treated with sulfamethazine USP boluses as recommended (see Table 1). Sulfamethazine is suspected by the U.S. Food and Drug Administration (FDA) of being a carcinogen, and may soon be unavailable for use in food animals.

Sulfonamides are potentially toxic. Recommended dosages should not be exceeded. The treatment period should not exceed 5 to 7 days. Water should be continuously available to treated animals. Acute toxicosis, characterized by weakness, ataxia, and collapse, may occur when sulfonamides are administered by rapid intravenous injection. The problem is avoided by proper technique. In reality, sulfonamide toxicity in cattle is a relatively rare occurrence. Most toxicosis problems have involved sulfathiazole or sulfapyridine, both of which are no longer commonly used.

A combination of trimethoprim and sulfadiazine is formulated in a fixed 1:5 ratio and has been used for treatment of B&FP in preruminant calves on an extralabel basis. Marked synergistic antimicrobial activity results from sequential blockage of two successive steps in microbial synthesis of folic acid. Twice-daily oral administration in a dose of 48 mg/kg body weight or twice-daily subcutaneous administration in a dose of 30 mg/kg body weight (of combined drug) has been recommended for use in preruminant calves. This drug combination is ineffective in cattle with a functional rumen owing to rapid removal and inactivation of trimethoprim by hepatic metabolism. In the experience of the author, trimethoprim-sulfa

Table 1. SUMMARY OF LABEL DIRECTIONS FOR FDA-APPROVED SULFONAMIDE FORMULATIONS FOR TREATMENT OF BRONCHOPNEUMONIA AND FIBRINOUS PNEUMONIA IN CATTLE

Sulfonamide Product	Manufacturer/Distributor	Dosage Priming	Dosage Maintenance	Treatment Interval	Withdrawal Period Slaughter (days)	Withdrawal Period Milk (hr)
Sulfamethazine, USP	—	220 mg/kg	110 mg/kg	24 hr	10	NA[a]
Albon[b]	Hoffman-LaRoche, Inc. 340 Kingsland St. Nutley, NJ 07110	55 mg/kg	28 mg/kg	24 hr	5[c]–7[d]	60
Albon-S.R.[b,e]	Hoffman-LaRoche, Inc. 340 Kingsland St. Nutley, NJ 07110	138 mg/kg	—	7 days	12	NA
Sulfamethazine Spanbolet II[f]	SmithKline Beecham Animal Health 601 W. Cornhusker P.O. Box 80809 Lincoln, NB 68521	1 (27 g) bolus/68 kg	—	5 days	28	NA
Calf Span[f]	SmithKline Beecham Animal Health 601 W. Cornhusker P.O. Box 80809 Lincoln, NB 68521	1 (8 g) tablet/20 kg	—	3 days	18	NA
Hava-Span[f,g]	Mobay Corporation Animal Health Div. Shawnee, KS 66201	1 (22.5 g) bolus/90 kg 1 (22.5 g) bolus/45 kg	— —	3-½ days 5 days	16 16	NA NA
Sulfamethazine Sustained Bolus[f]	Fermenta Animal Health Co. 7410 N.W. Tiffany Springs Pkwy. P.O. Box 901350 Kansas City, MO 64190	1 (30 g) bolus/91 kg 1 (8.25 g) bolus/23 kg	— —	3 days 3 days	8 8	NA NA
Sustain III[f]	Quality Plus Essar Corp. 2116 8th Ave. South Fort Dodge, IA 50501	1 (32.1 g) bolus/91 kg 2 (8.02 g) bolus/45 kg	— —	3 days 3 days	12 12	NA NA

[a]NA = Not approved for use in lactating cattle.
[b]Sulfadimethoxine. Blood levels reported by the manufacturer with the recommended dose are only marginally therapeutic.
[c]After intravenous administration.
[d]After oral administration.
[e]Sustained-release bolus formulation.
[f]Sustained-release sulfamethazine bolus formulation.
[g]Therapeutic blood concentrations not obtained during the first 14 to 18 hours after administration.

therapy has not been effective in calves older than 2 weeks of age.

Use of Antibiotics in Treatment of B&FP in Cattle

Food animal drugs have been approved by the FDA for use in food-producing animals. Procaine penicillin G in aqueous suspension, benzathine penicillin G, ampicillin trihydrate, amoxicillin trihydrate, oxytetracycline hydrochloride, tetracycline hydrochloride, dihydrostreptomycin sulfate, erythromycin, tylosin, and ceftiofur are approved by the FDA for parenteral administration in cattle. Over-the-counter (OTC) food animal drugs are freely available to livestock owners through OTC sales but must be used by them according to label instructions with regard to dose, route of administration, treatment interval, maximum number of treatments administered, and withdrawal period before slaughter or marketing of milk.

Prescription legend (Rx) food animal drugs are available to livestock owners only from a licensed veterinarian or by his/her prescription and must be used according to the directions provided by the prescribing veterinarian. A veterinarian can also legally prescribe and use many nonapproved drugs in food-producing animals that are directly under his/her care or supervision. Exceptions are chloramphenicol, dimetridazole, ipronidazole, and diethylstilbestrol, which can never be legally used in food animals. In addition, it is illegal to administer sulfamethazine to female dairy cattle over 20 months of age. Use of (1) nonapproved drugs, and/or use of (2) approved OTC or Rx food animal drugs in a manner that is contrary to label instructions regarding (a) dosage, (b) route of administration, (c) treatment interval, or (d) maximum number of doses to be administered is termed extralabel use of drugs. When engaging in the extralabel use of drugs, the veterinarian assumes legal responsibility for any drug residues that are subsequently detected in meat or milk from treated animals. A veterinarian is also legally responsible when a residue is found in an animal treated with an OTC food animal drug if he/she has administered the drug without informing the owner or caretaker as to the proper withdrawal period.

The use of nonapproved drugs, or the extralabel use of approved food animal drugs, in treatment of livestock diseases should be undertaken by the veterinarian only when he/she has considered all other alternatives and is satisfied (1) that a valid veterinarian:client:patient relationship exists; (2) that a diagnosis has been made and that it has been determined that either (a) there is no approved food animal drug labeled to treat the condition or (b) drug therapy in the label dose is ineffective; and (3) that a suitably long drug withdrawal period can be enforced. In the case of aminoglycoside antibiotics (neomycin, kanamycin, gentamicin), no period of less than 4 months should be considered safe. In the absence of a recommendation from FARAD (see next paragraph), other (non-aminoglycoside) prescription antibiotics should not ordinarily be used unless a withdrawal period of at least 2 months can be ensured. Fortunately most B&FP cases can be successfully managed with one or the other of four approved antimicrobial drugs: a sulfonamide (especially sulfamethazine), procaine penicillin G, a tetracycline (especially oxytetracycline), or ceftiofur. Of the nonapproved antibiotics, only spectinomycin is sufficiently inexpensive to permit systemic use for treatment of B&FP in commercial cattle (Table 2).

Label directions concerning dosages, routes of administration, and treatment intervals have been determined empirically for nearly all existing FDA-approved antibiotics. In many instances the label recommendation does not permit the most effective use against the organisms most commonly associated with B&FP in cattle. Unfortunately the veterinarian is sometimes in the position of being forced to choose between a treatment regimen that is less than optimally effective in a substantial proportion of his/her cases and one that is effective in a greater number of cases but for which reliable drug withdrawal information is lacking. Fortunately veterinarians in the United States now have access to a computerized data bank (Food Animal Residue Avoidance Databank [FARAD]), which can assist them in developing withdrawal recommendations for a wide range of extralabel drug treatment regimens. The data bank can be accessed by phoning (916) 752–7507 (California), (217) 333–3611 (Illinois), or (904) 392–4085 (Florida).

The author has summarized recommended extralabel regimens for oxytetracycline hydrochloride, procaine penicillin G in aqueous suspension, ceftiofur, ampicillin trihydrate, amoxicillin trihydrate, spectinomycin, and tylosin (see Table 2). For comparison, a summary of label directions for antibiotics currently approved and recommended for treatment of B&FP in cattle is also provided (Table 3). The suggested extralabel regimens will, in general, maintain blood serum concentrations that are inhibitory for antibiotic-sensitive *P. haemolytica* and *P. multocida* isolates for at least two thirds of the period between treatments.

Tetracyclines

From 63 to 97 per cent of *P. haemolytica* and *P. multocida* isolates recovered from nasal secretions of cattle with B&FP and approximately 20 per cent of *A. pyogenes* isolates are sensitive to tetracyclines. Chlortetracycline and oxytetracycline are both available in forms suitable for feed or water medication, but absorption from the digestive tract of cattle is limited. Doses of 88 mg/kg body weight/day are required to achieve inhibitory (1 to 2 µg/ml) serum concentrations. Adverse effects on ruminal microflora preclude the use of large

Table 2. SUMMARY OF EXTRALABEL (PRESCRIPTION) DIRECTIONS FOR THE USE OF AUTHOR-RECOMMENDED ANTIBIOTICS FOR TREATMENT OF BRONCHOPNEUMONIA AND FIBRINOUS PNEUMONIA IN CATTLE

Antibiotic	Proprietary Name	Manufacturer/Distributor	Dosage	Route	Treatment Interval (hr)	Withdrawal Period Slaughter (days)	Withdrawal Period Milk (hr)
Oxytetracycline hydrochloride	Terramycin 100[a]	Pfizer, Inc. 235 E. 42nd Street New York, NY 10017	11 mg/kg	SC[b]	24	16[c]	84[c]
	Liquamycin LA-200	Pfizer, Inc. 235 E. 42nd Street New York, NY 10017	20 mg/kg[d]	IM[d,e]	48[d]	28[d]	—
Procaine penicillin G, aqueous suspension	Crysticillin 30 A.S. Veterinary[a]	Solvay Animal Health, Inc. PO Box 7348 Princeton, NJ 08540	66,000 U/kg	IM, SC	24	20[f]	—
Ceftiofur sodium	Naxcel[a]	The Upjohn Co. 7000 Portage Rd. Kalamazoo, MI 49001	2.2 mg/kg	IM, SC	12	Zero[c]	72[c]
Ampicillin trihydrate	Polyflex[a]	Fort Dodge Laboratories, Inc 800 5th St. Fort Dodge, IA 50501	22 mg/kg	IM, SC	24	9[c]	72[c]
Amoxicillin trihydrate	Amoxi-Inject	SmithKline Beecham Animal Health 501 5th St. Bristol, TN 37620	11 mg/kg[d]	IM, SC[d]	24[d]	25[d]	96[d]
Spectinomycin dihydrochloride pentahydrate	Spectam Injectable[g]	Sanofi Animal Health, Inc. 7101 College Blvd. Suite 610 Overland Park, KS 66210	33 mg/kg	SC	8	60[c]	120[c]
Tylosin	Tylan Injection 200[h]	Elanco Products Co. Lilly Corporate Center Indianapolis, IN 46285	44 mg/kg	IM	24	30[c]	—

[a]Dosage, treatment interval, and route of administration adjusted so as to assure an antibiotic concentration in the serum that is equal to or greater than the minimum inhibitory concentration for sensitive *P. haemolytica* and *P. multocida* isolates for no less than 67 per cent of the period between treatments.
[b]SC = Subcutaneous administration.
[c]Recommended by FARAD.
[d]Label recommendation.
[e]IM = Intramuscular administration.
[f]Recommended by the author.
[g]Dosage, treatment interval, and route of administration adjusted so as to assure an antibiotic concentration in the serum that is equal to or greater than the minimum inhibitory concentration for sensitive *P. haemolytica* and *P. multocida* isolates for no less than 50 per cent of the period between treatments.
[h]Not recommended for treatment of *Pasteurella* infections.

Table 3. SUMMARY OF LABEL DIRECTIONS FOR FDA-APPROVED AND AUTHOR-RECOMMENDED ANTIBIOTICS FOR TREATMENT OF BRONCHOPNEUMONIA AND FIBRINOUS PNEUMONIA IN CATTLE

Antibiotic	Proprietary Name	Manufacturer/ Distributor	Mode of Action	Antibacterial Spectrum	Dosage	Route	Treatment Interval (hr)	Withdrawal Period Slaughter (days)	Withdrawal Period Milk (hr)
Oxytetracycline hydrochloride	Terramycin 100	Pfizer, Inc. 235 E. 42nd Street New York, NY 10017	Bacteriostatic	Broad spectrum	11 mg/kg	IM[a], IV[b]	24	15	84[c]
	Liquamycin LA-200	Pfizer, Inc. 235 E. 42nd Street New York, NY 10017			20 mg/kg	IM	48	28	NA[d]
Procaine penicillin G, aqueous suspension	Crysticillin	Solvay Animal Health, Inc. PO Box 7348 Princeton, NJ 08540	Bactericidal	Mainly gram-positive	6600 U/kg	IM	24	4	48
Ceftiofur sodium	Naxcel	The Upjohn Co. 7000 Portage Rd. Kalamazoo, MI 49001	Bactericidal	Broad spectrum	1.1 mg/kg	IM	24	Zero	72[c]
Ampicillin trihydrate	Polyflex	Fort Dodge Laboratories, Inc. 800 5th St. Fort Dodge, IA 50501	Bactericidal	Broad spectrum	11 mg/kg	IM, SC[e]	24	6	48
Amoxicillin trihydrate	Amoxi-Inject	SmithKline Beecham Animal Health 501 5th St. Bristol, TN 37620	Bactericidal	Broad spectrum	11 mg/kg	IM, SC	24	25	96
Tylosin[f]	Tylan Injection 200	Elanco Products, Co. Lilly Corporate Center Indianapolis, IN 46285	Bacteriostatic	Mainly gram-positive	18 mg/kg	IM	24	21	NA

[a]IM = Intramuscular administration.
[b]IV = Intravenous administration.
[c]Recommended by FARAD.
[d]NA = Not approved for use in lactating dairy cattle.
[e]SC = Subcutaneous administration.
[f]Not recommended for treatment of *Pasteurella* infections.

doses of tetracyclines by the oral route for management of acute systemic bacterial infections in cattle.

Of the three major tetracyclines, only oxytetracycline hydrochloride is suitable for intramuscular or subcutaneous injection. Consequently it is the one most frequently utilized for systemic therapy. Subcutaneous administration, though not an FDA-approved procedure, is considered by the author to be the preferred method. Inhibitory serum oxytetracycline concentrations are obtained within 1 to 4 hours after subcutaneous injection. With some proprietary preparations, a substantial concentration advantage over intravenous and intramuscular administration is obtained during the last 8 to 16 hours of a 24-hour treatment interval. The frequency of postinjection abscessation is thought to be less with subcutaneous administration than with intramuscular administration. When abscessation does occur, less damage results to edible tissues. Oxytetracycline is usually injected into the dorsal midcervical muscles or the cervical subcutaneous tissues. To minimize local tissue irritation, the calculated dose is administered in multiple injection sites using a maximum volume of 10 ml/site. In a series of acute feedlot B&FP cases summarized by the author, 70.8 per cent responded satisfactorily when treated with oxytetracycline as suggested (see Table 2).

Penicillin G

From 63 to 78 per cent of *P. haemolytica* and *P. multocida* isolates recovered from nasal secretions of cattle with B&FP are sensitive to penicillin G. All *A. pyogenes* isolates are sensitive to penicillin G.

Because of rapid absorption from injection sites and rapid urinary excretion, multiple daily administration is required when treating with sodium or potassium penicillin G.

Serum concentrations of penicillin G are inhibitory for penicillin G–sensitive *P. haemolytica* and *P. multocida* isolates (0.5 to 2 µg/ml) for only 4 hours following administration of benzathine penicillin G (Bicillin Fortified[1] [benzathine penicillin G and procaine penicillin G in aqueous suspension]) in the FDA-approved regimen of 2 ml/68 kg body weight injected subcutaneously. Even at five times the approved dose, serum penicillin G concentrations are inhibitory for only 12 hours following injection.

Procaine penicillin G in aqueous suspension is the form of penicillin G best suited for treatment of B&FP in cattle. With the FDA-approved regimen of 6600 units/kg body weight injected intramuscularly (Table 3), serum penicillin G concentrations are inhibitory for penicillin G–sensitive *P. haemolytica* and *P. multocida* isolates for only 2 to 4 hours after administration. In a series of acute feedlot B&FP cases summarized by the author, 78.6 per cent responded satisfactorily when treated with procain penicillin G as suggested (see Table 2).

Ceftiofur

Ceftiofur is a third-generation cephalosporin. Ceftiofur-resistant isolates of *P. haemolytica*, *P. multocida*, and *A. pyogenes* have not yet been encountered in the clinical microbiology laboratory of the Veterinary Medical Teaching Hospital, University of California, Davis. In the opinion of the author, ceftiofur should be reserved for use in treating refrac-

---
[1]Available from Fort Dodge Laboratories, Inc., Fort Dodge, IA 50501.

tory (presumably antimicrobial-resistant bacterial) lung infections that do not respond to the less expensive standard drugs such as sulfonamides, procaine penicillin G, and oxytetracycline. More frequent routine use is likely to eventually be associated with development of ceftiofur-resistant strains of pulmonary bacterial pathogens. The label direction is for once-daily intramuscular administration in a dose of 1.1 mg/kg body weight (see Table 3). Used in this dosage regimen, serum ceftiofur concentrations are inhibitory for *P. haemolytica* and *P. multocida* isolates (0.25 μg/ml) for at least 24 hours following administration. Clinical observations indicate, however, that response rates of refractory B&FP cases are improved when ceftiofur is administered at 12-hour intervals in a dose of 2.2 mg/kg (see Table 2).

Ampicillin Trihydrate and Amoxicillin Trihydrate

Sensitivity of *P. haemolytica* and *P. multocida* isolates to ampicillin and amoxicillin closely parallels sensitivity to penicillin G. Of 390 penicillin G–resistant isolates, 82.8 per cent were also resistant to ampicillin. As with penicillin G, all *A. pyogenes* isolates are sensitive to ampicillin and amoxicillin. The suggested ampicillin treatment regimen (see Table 2) provides serum ampicillin concentrations that are continuously inhibitory for 96 per cent of ampicillin-sensitive *P. haemolytica* and *P. multocida* isolates (0.5 to 2 μg/ml).

Spectinomycin

Approximately 79 per cent of *P. haemolytica* and *P. multocida* isolates from the lungs of fatal cases of feedlot B&FP (not treated with spectinomycin) are sensitive to spectinomycin. Approximately 69 per cent of *A. pyogenes* isolates are sensitive to spectinomycin. The suggested treatment regimen (see Table 2) provides serum spectinomycin concentrations that are inhibitory for most spectinomycin-sensitive *P. haemolytica* and *P. multocida* isolates (1 to 25 μg/ml) during about 50 per cent of the interval between treatments. When used as suggested (see Table 2) in clinical cases of B&FP, the efficacy of spectinomycin therapy is comparable to that reported with sulfamethazine and procaine penicillin G.

Tylosin

The author has successfully utilized tylosin as suggested (see Table 2) as an alternative to penicillin G therapy in refractory *A. pyogenes* infections. Sensitive *A. pyogenes* isolates are inhibited by substantially lower concentrations of tylosin than of penicillin G. In addition, tylosin, being a lipophilic antimicrobial, is better able to penetrate cellular membranes (such as the capsule of abscesses) than is penicillin G, which is an ionized antimicrobial. Intramuscular administration is preferred to subcutaneous administration since absorption from subcutaneous sites is significantly retarded.

Use of tylosin in the treatment of B&FP should be limited to penicillin G–refractory *A. pyogenes* infections and infections with unusual organisms that are sensitive to tylosin and resistant to sulfonamides, penicillin G, tetracyclines, spectinomycin, and ceftiofur. In a series of acute feedlot B&FP cases treated with tylosin as suggested (see Table 2), 23 per cent responded favorably. Response rates of up to 37 per cent were obtained in chronic cases, which were more commonly associated with a *A. pyogenes* component.

Supportive Therapy

In the opinion of the author, supportive treatment (other than good husbandry as previously discussed) has little application in the treatment of uncomplicated B&FP in commercial cattle. This is especially true in production systems in which administration of treatments is delegated to lay workers. Any benefits are likely to be limited to relief of symptoms and are unlikely to influence final mortality or culling rates. Use of corticosteroids in uncomplicated cases should be discouraged since efficacy of bacteriostatic antimicrobials may be reduced. In addition, corticosteroid therapy may cause remission of fever and toxemia, resulting in premature termination of antimicrobial therapy and leading to subsequent exacerbation of clinical signs. In the hands of competent clinicians, the use of a prostaglandin antagonist such as flunixin meglumine[2] in a daily dose of 2.2 mg/kg injected intramuscularly, in combination with an appropriate antimicrobial, may be useful.

PREVENTION AND CONTROL

Recommendations for control of B&FP must consider the geographic location of the individual production unit and the production system utilized. The objective of a preventive program is to minimize economic losses from B&FP by preventing IBR, BVD, PI-3, and BRSV infections through vaccination; by eliminating, decreasing, or spacing out/separating stresses; by avoiding management practices that favor a high incidence of B&FP; and, in some cases, by immunizing against *P. haemolytica*.

Controlling B&FP in Feedlot Cattle

The B&FP problem can be reduced by utilization of "preconditioned" cattle. In a summary of seven trials performed by others, one author reported that preconditioning reduced the morbidity rate by 6 percentage points (23 per cent) and the mortality rate by 0.7 percentage points. Preconditioned cattle have been weaned and fed a milled concentrate ration on the ranch of origin for a minimum period of 30 days prior to shipment to the feedlot. Processing is performed at least 14 days prior to shipment and should include necessary vaccinations, implantation with a growth stimulant, administration of a systemic organophosphate insecticide, and treatment with an anthelmintic, if required. Horn-tipping may also be performed, but dehorning is contraindicated. B&FP losses are minimized by avoiding saleyard cattle and by buying directly from ranchers. In a feedlot serviced by the author, the mortality rate was 1.5 per cent, the culling rate was 3.2 per cent, and the medicine cost was $5.09/head in 1070 yearling saleyard steers. Corresponding values were 1.0 per cent, 1.3 per cent, and $4.20/head in 6057 yearling ranch steers fed during the same 2-year period. It was necessary to discount the saleyard cattle approximately $3.25/head to compensate for increased health problems, especially B&FP.

If cattle have not previously been vaccinated for IBR and BVD, this should be done as soon as possible after arrival at the feedlot, certainly within 48 hours. It should be understood that this is being done to prevent IBR and BVD "wrecks" and that the basic morbidity and mortality rates from B&FP will not be reduced by this practice. In fact, Canadian workers reported that vaccination of calves on arrival at the feedlot with (1) modified live virus (MLV) IBR or MLV IBR-PI-3 vaccines or (2) MLV IBR-BVD-PI-3 vaccines was associated with increases in the total mortality rate of 0.62 percentage points (significant, $P<0.05$) and 0.2 percentage points (nonsignificant), respectively (compared with nonvaccinated calves).

---

[2]Banamine Solution Veterinary, Schering Animal Health, 1011 Morris Ave., Union, NJ 07083.

Nevertheless, it is the author's opinion that IBR vaccination is absolutely essential. BVD vaccination is not as critical because most BVD infections are subclinical. Additionally, cattle arriving in feedlots are usually protected by colostral BVD antibodies or are immune from natural exposure. Susceptible groups are occasionally encountered, however, and heavy losses can be expected when B&FP and BVD occur concurrently. It is thought that the leukopenia and cellular and humoral immune system suppression resulting from BVD infection enhance the pathogenicity of pasteurella bacteria. The occurrence of postvaccinal mucosal disease has been a deterrent to widespread acceptance of BVD vaccination. This problem is associated with the use of specific commercial MLV vaccines, which should be avoided since they appear to be insufficiently attenuated. Two different groups of workers have reported adverse effects (increased morbidity rates from clinical BVD and respiratory disease) associated with the use of MLV BVD vaccines in stressed cattle. Nevertheless, the author prefers MLV IBR and BVD vaccines over inactivated vaccines when cattle cannot be immunized prior to arrival in the feedlot. Rapid achievement of immunity is paramount in an environment in which instant exposure to virulent virus is virtually assured. Intramuscular MLV IBR vaccines are favored over intranasal MLV IBR vaccines because of cost advantages, ease of administration, and negligible differences in efficacy.

Administration of either MLV or inactivated PI-3 vaccines to cattle, after arrival in the feedlot, should not be expected to provide cost-effective control of B&FP. Exposure to PI-3 virus may occur before effective immunity can develop. Additionally, a high proportion of cattle of feedlot age have significant serum antibody titers to PI-3 virus and may not benefit from immunization. Since PI-3 vaccination almost routinely fails to reduce the incidence of B&FP, it is likely that PI-3 is less important than other viruses in the etiology of B&FP. PI-3 vaccination may be desirable if it can be performed on the ranch of origin at least 2 weeks prior to transport to the feedlot. MLV PI-3 vaccines, especially intranasal vaccines, are favored over inactivated virus vaccines since nasal (local secretory) antibody production is more important in resistance than humoral antibody production.

The importance and effectiveness of BRSV vaccines for control of B&FP have yet to be fully determined under field conditions. The results of some limited field studies have shown promise, however. Both MLV and inactivated BRSV vaccines are marketed, and both are recommended for administration in two doses, 2 to 4 weeks apart. Because of the long lag period (3 to 4 weeks) between administration of the priming dose and the beginning of protection after the immunizing dose, it is unlikely that vaccination of feedlot cattle for BRSV infection, subsequent to arrival at the feedlot, will prove to be a cost-effective strategy in most situations. This is also likely to be the case for H. somnus bacterins, for the new two-dose modified live and inactivated subunit P. haemolytica vaccines, and for inactivated IBR, BVD, and PI-3 vaccines.

Upon arrival at the feedlot, cattle should be refed on hay for several days before feeding concentrate rations in order to avoid overconsumption and lactic acidosis in hungry cattle. Alternatively, cattle may be started on a milled ration containing 50 per cent roughage.

The incidence of B&FP is usually highest in groups of cattle that are least inclined to consume feedlot rations. Consequently a major effort should be undertaken to encourage feed consumption in newly received cattle by offering a palatable ration kept fresh by frequent feeding of small quantities, by promptly removing stale feed, by preventing the accumulation of "fines," and by avoiding unnecessary ration changes. Receiving pens should be wide and shallow to keep the cattle in close proximity to the feed bunks. If cattle are reluctant to feed, they can usually be coaxed to the feed bunks by frequent offerings of long-stem baled hay placed on top of the milled feed. Premature utilization of very high energy rations, before ruminal adaptation has occurred, will aggravate the B&FP problem. Once feeding of a high-energy ration has begun, it must be available free-choice at all times or lactic acidosis is likely to result. The feeding of silage during the starting period has been associated with increased rates of morbidity and mortality from B&FP.

It is especially important that cattle not be overcrowded during the first 30 days after arrival. A minimum of 40 ft^2 pen space and 12 linear inches feed-bunk space/head should be provided. An allowance of approximately 100 ft^2 pen space/head appears optimal in terms of stress reduction. The optimal group size (cattle per pen) appears to be 100 or fewer head. Groups of 500 or larger tend to be associated with higher morbidity and mortality rates.

Except for initial processing, cattle should not be handled for 30 days after arrival to minimize stress and avoid disturbing their feeding patterns. Cattle from different sources should not be commingled during the first 30 days after arrival to minimize cross-infection with respiratory viruses and to avoid stresses associated with establishing a new "pecking order." Cattle of unequal size should not be penned together since the smaller animals cannot effectively compete for feed-bunk space.

The B&FP problem is aggravated when cattle are started in an excessively dusty or muddy environment. Corral dust is controlled in starting pens with sprinkler systems. After 30 days the problem can be controlled by increasing the stocking rate, except where shade must be provided. Mud is harder to control. This is accomplished by hauling in dirt and building mounds for cattle to rest on and by reducing stocking rates to 150 to 300 ft^2 (or more) pen space/head.

Mass medication may help to reduce the incidence of B&FP. Sulfonamides are administered in full therapeutic dosages for 5 to 7 days in feed or water or individually in the form of sustained-release boluses (see Table 1). Antibiotics such as procaine penicillin G in aqueous suspension or oxytetracycline hydrochloride are administered parenterally in full therapeutic dosages, usually for 1 to 3 days. Alternatively chlortetracycline or oxytetracycline may be administered in feed or water over a 2- to 4-week period, utilizing a prophylactic dosage of 2.2 mg/kg body weight/day. Mass medication of antimicrobials in full therapeutic dosages is very effective in preventing occurrence of clinical disease during the period that a therapeutic blood antimicrobial concentration is maintained and for a few days thereafter. It is more effective in highly stressed cattle, in which the occurrence of B&FP tends to be compressed into a relatively short 7- to 10-day period. Results are maximized when initiation of treatment is delayed until significant numbers of animals begin to show clinical signs of B&FP. The occurrence of B&FP may be spread out over a 4- to 6-week period in groups of cattle that have not been significantly stressed prior to arrival in the feedlot. In such groups, short periods of mass medication may have relatively insignificant effects on final morbidity rates. A 30-day prophylactic course of feed or water medication with chlortetracycline or oxytetracycline may be of greater value. Reductions of up to 50 per cent in the morbidity rate have been commonly reported. In the experience of the author, however, this method of control has been without merit under commercial feedlot conditions. Oral administration of chlortetracycline or oxytetracycline does not produce blood serum antibiotic concentrations that are inhibitory for pasteurella bacteria, so sick cattle must be individually treated.

It should be appreciated that any mass medication scheme will suppress antimicrobial-sensitive bacteria and permit antimicrobial-resistant bacteria to increase their relative importance in the gastrointestinal and upper respiratory tract flora. An increased number of antimicrobial-resistant pasteurella pneumonia cases can be anticipated when mass medication is utilized, even though morbidity and mortality rates may be reduced by the practice. For this reason mass medication is best reserved for use in highly stressed groups, in which a high percentage would be treated anyway. Newly received cattle should be isolated, especially from cattle that have received mass medication, until the period of highest susceptibility to B&FB has passed to minimize exposure to antimicrobial-resistant pasteurella bacteria.

Conventional pasteurella bacterins, and antisera prepared against pasteurella bacteria, have been found valueless where controlled field studies have been conducted. However, preliminary results with modified live and new (inactivated) subunit *P. haemolytica* vaccines appear promising. But some (if not all) modified live *P. haemolytica* vaccines may prove to be excessively stressful for use in newly arrived feedlot cattle (as well as in other high-stress situations). Only one modified live *P. haemolytica* vaccine is specifically recommended by the manufacturer for administration to cattle arriving in feedlots (Respirvac[3]). It can be predicted that (1) effective immunization against *both P. haemolytica* and *P. multocida* will be required for effective control of B&FP, and (2) the new modified live and inactivated subunit *P. haemolytica* vaccines will be most effective when they can be administered several weeks or more before cattle are introduced to the feedlot environment.

Commercial *H. somnus* bacterins are clearly effective for prevention of thromboembolic meningoencephalitis. However, the extent to which they may be effective in reducing the incidence of B&FP is as yet undetermined. Because of the difficulty with which *H. somnus* is isolated from diseased tissues, the extent to which it may be involved in the etiology of B&FP is so far unknown. Various authors have reported its isolation from between 1.4 and 5 per cent of fatal cases of B&FP. In one large Canadian study the mortality rate (from all causes) was not significantly influenced by administration of an *H. somnus* bacterin to calves upon arrival in feedlots. In three small Indiana field trials, administration of an *H. somnus* bacterin to calves upon arrival in a feedlot did not influence the mortality rate or feedlot weight gains. In the initial trial the morbidity rate from respiratory disease was significantly reduced, from 30.8 to 19.8 per cent. In two subsequent trials, however, the morbidity rate was not reduced by vaccination. In another Canadian trial, vaccination of calves at the feedlot with an *H. somnus* bacterin was associated with a (statistically significant) 17.4 per cent reduction in steer mortality. However, the mortality rate in heifers was not reduced by vaccination. It seems clear that vaccination of cattle with an inactivated product, subsequent to arrival at the feedlot, has limited potential for effective control of a disease like B&FP (in which significant morbidity often occurs within the first 1 to 2 weeks after arrival).

Since it is not currently possible to totally prevent B&FP, effective control is highly dependent on early disease detection and prompt, rational treatment of clinical cases. It is imperative that sufficient numbers of experienced pencheckers be available for performing these tasks.

Controlling B&FP in Beef Calves on Pasture

Preweaning vaccination against both PI-3 and BRS virus infections has apparently prevented or reduced the postweaning B&FP problem on individual ranches. Vaccination should be performed (and completed by) 2 to 4 weeks prior to weaning. Intranasal MLV PI-3 vaccine is preferred. Vaccination for IBR and BVD is also desirable where there is a postweaning B&FP problem. Intranasal MLV IBR vaccine, chemically altered IBR vaccine (Cattlemaster[4]) or inactivated IBR vaccine is recommended if vaccinated calves are to be put back with unimmunized pregnant cows, to avoid the risk of IBR vaccine virus abortion.

It remains largely to be determined how useful the new modified live and inactivated subunit *P. haemolytica* vaccines may prove to be in this environment. During the last 6 years a total of six new *P. haemolytica* vaccines have been introduced in the United States. Four of these utilize modified live bacterial agents. The two new inactivated *P. haemolytica* products are subunit vaccines.

The immune mechanisms involved in resistance of the bovine lung to *P. haemolytica* infections are incompletely understood. It is clear, however, that resistance is greatly enhanced by the presence of serum and bronchoalveolar antibodies to (1) the leukotoxin of *P. haemolytica* and (2) certain surface antigens that are present in the bacterial capsule of *P. haemolytica A1*. It is believed that vaccines that produce antibodies to both (1) leukotoxin and (2) bacterial capsular antigens (in a saline extract of log phase *P. haemolytica A1*, referred to as carbohydrate protein subunit) are more effective than those that stimulate production of only one of these two types of antibodies. It has been shown that effective live *P. haemolytica* vaccines stimulate high levels of both kinds of antibodies. *P. haemolytica* bacterins in oil adjuvants stimulate high antibody titers to carbohydrate protein subunit but not to leukotoxin. Conventional aluminum hydroxide–absorbed *P. haemolytica* bacterins also do not stimulate leukotoxin antibody production and stimulate only low titers to carbohydrate protein subunit. Subunit vaccines can be produced that stimulate high levels of leukotoxin-neutralizing antibodies and/or carbohydrate protein subunit antibodies, depending on the extraction process utilized.

Vaccines that utilize modified live *P. haemolytica* bacteria will not be effective when administered within 7 days after or 3 days before systemic administration of antimicrobial agents. These same vaccines should probably not be administered simultaneously with MLV BVD vaccines, *Brucella abortus* vaccine, anthrax vaccine, or modified live anaplasmosis vaccine. Three of the new modified live *P. haemolytica* vaccines are one-dose vaccines. The new *P. haemolytica* subunit vaccines and one new modified live *P. haemolytica* vaccine are two-dose vaccines.

All six of these vaccines are relatively new products. It is still too early to predict with certainty which, if any, will stand the test of time and which will fall by the wayside. In studies performed at Oklahoma State University, vaccination of cattle with Precon-PH[5] did not stimulate production of levels of whole-cell agglutinating antibodies, which are usually associated with satisfactory immunity. Since Septimune PH-K[6] does not stimulate production of leukotoxin-neutralizing antibodies, it would not be surprising if it proved to be less efficacious than at least some others. Some (if not all) modified live *P. haemolytica* vaccines may prove to be excessively stressful for use in high-stress situations. For more information about *P. haemolytica* vaccines, the reader is referred to the author's 1990 review (see Bibliography).

To minimize stress, calves should not be handled for 2 weeks

---

[3]Available from SmithKline Beecham, Bristol, TN 37620.

[4]Available from SmithKline Beecham Animal Health, Lincoln, NB 68501-0809.
[5]Available from A. H. Robins, Richmond, VA 23220.
[6]Available from Fort Dodge Laboratories, Fort Dodge, IA 50501.

before and after weaning. Weaning stress can be reduced by avoiding corral weaning. Cows and calves are moved to a relatively small, well-fenced field with abundant forage. After 7 to 10 days weaning is accomplished by removing one third of the cows each day over a 3-day period. Two weeks after weaning, the calves can be moved to other pastures.

If corral weaning cannot be avoided, dusty or muddy conditions should be controlled. Preventive mass medication can be expected to reduce the incidence of B&FP with minimal risk of antimicrobial-resistant pasteurella pneumonia. By the time bacteria have developed resistance, the cattle are no longer under stress and are not highly susceptible to B&FP. Continuous medication of feed or water with tetracycline, chlortetracycline, or oxytetracycline, in a dose of 2.2 mg/kg body weight/day for 2 to 4 weeks after weaning, is the method of choice.

Controlling B&FP in Dairy Calves

Calves should be vaccinated against PI-3 and BRS virus infections, preferably with intranasal MLV PI-3 vaccine, approximately 2 to 4 weeks before they are weaned and placed in group pens. Vaccination for IBR and BVD is also recommended at this time.

Calves should be kept in individual crates for 2 weeks following weaning, after which time they can be placed in group pens, together with no more than 10 to 20 calves of similar age and size. Alternatively, calves can be fed milk or milk replacer for 2 to 4 weeks after grouping. Stressful procedures such as dehorning and castration should be performed at least 1 month prior to weaning and/or grouping. Ideally each group pen should be isolated from other group pens by at least 20 ft of open air space so that a respiratory disease outbreak can be confined to an affected group of calves. Each group of calves should be raised together in isolation until they are 4 to 6 months of age, after which their susceptibility to B&FP is dramatically reduced, and they can be safely mixed with larger groups of calves. It is especially important that newly weaned calves be isolated from older calves and adult cattle.

Corral dust or mud must be controlled. Calves should not be overcrowded. A minimum of 25 ft^2 pen space and 12 linear inches feed-bunk space should be provided. This should be increased to 100 ft^2 pen space/head should B&FP become a problem.

Whenever possible, housing of calves in enclosed buildings should be avoided. Adequate ventilation (in terms of the number of air changes per hour) of such structures is essential for satisfactory respiratory health and is seldom achieved. Any detectable odor of ammonia in a calf barn should be considered dangerous. Calves can tolerate very low temperatures if kept dry with adequate bedding and overhead cover and protected from drafts. Open sheds, enclosed on three sides and facing south, provide adequate shelter in severe climates with a minimum of ventilation problems. If calves must be housed, serious problems with B&FP can generally be avoided if the structure can be uniformly and continuously ventilated at a minimum rate of four air changes per hour, and draftiness, extreme temperatures, and temperature fluctuations prevented. Aerosolized bacteria rapidly die when the relative humidity within a barn can be maintained below 80 per cent by adequate ventilation.

Calves that are debilitated by parasitism, malnutrition, or viral and/or bacterial gastrointestinal infections are highly susceptible to B&FP; therefore these problems, if present, should be corrected. A sufficiently high level of nutrition should be provided to ensure average daily weight gains of from 1.5 to 1.75 lb (0.7 to 0.8 kg).

Vaccination for brucellosis with strain 19 vaccine is a stress that often triggers outbreaks of B&FP in dairy calves. Strain 19 vaccine should not be simultaneously administered with any other live vaccine. Administration of strain 19 vaccine should be timed so as to avoid periods of high susceptibility to B&FP, such as within 2 weeks of weaning, grouping, processing, vaccination with MLV vaccines, and so on.

Preventive mass medication should be avoided since problems with antimicrobial-resistant pasteurella pneumonia can be anticipated. Medication of feed or water with tetracycline, chlortetracycline, or oxytetracycline for the first 30 days after placement in group pens has not resulted in satisfactory control in the experience of the author.

Early disease detection and prompt, rational treatment of clinical cases are necessary for satisfactory control. It is possible that some of the new modified live and inactivated subunit *P. haemolytica* vaccines may prove to be helpful in the control of this problem. However, on many dairy farms the major bacterial respiratory pathogen is *P. multocida*. *P. haemolytica* vaccines do not afford cross-protection against *P. multocida* infections.

Occasionally problems with respiratory disease are encountered in young dairy calves prior to weaning. Precipitating factors usually involve inadequate ventilation within calf barns, poor colostrum management, and/or debility from uncontrolled neonatal enteric diseases. Recommendations for improved control include providing for passive neonatal immunity to IBR and BVD by way of the cow-herd vaccination program. Passive immunity is of no value for prevention of BRSV infections and is not likely to be effective in preventing many PI-3 virus infections. Vaccination of young calves (less than 3 months of age) for BRSV infections is unlikely to be of value since passively immune calves cannot be effectively immunized against BRSV and the colostrum from most cows contains BRSV antibodies. Passively immune calves *can* be actively immunized against PI-3 virus infection using MLV intranasally administered PI-3 vaccines, but not using inactivated vaccines or MLV or chemically altered intramuscularly administered PI-3 virus vaccines.

An effort should be made to reduce chilling by keeping calves dry by providing overhead shelter from rain and snow, by frequent removal and replacement of wet, soiled bedding, or by housing on slats, wire, or expanded metal. Draftiness should be controlled with appropriately constructed buildings or by windbreaks with appropriate orientation to prevailing winds. Adequate ventilation of enclosed barns is imperative and usually will require the assistance of an agricultural engineer with expertise in this area.

When respiratory disease occurs as a sequela to neonatal enteric disease, a major effort must be devoted to control of the primary problem. The following strategy is usually helpful: The calf should be born in a *dedicated* calving stall or maternity corral. The cow should not be introduced until calving is imminent and until after the stall has been cleaned out, disinfected, and rebedded. If a corral is utilized, manure and old bedding should have been removed by blading with a tractor immediately following removal of the prior occupant. Dairy calves should be removed to a disinfected individual rearing pen immediately following birth. Within 2 hours after birth, 2 to 3 L of fresh colostrum should be hand fed, and again 12 hours later. Subsequently the diet of the calf should include at least 1 L of either fresh colostrum or fresh cow's milk per (12-hour) feeding through the third week of life. Fresh cow's milk is thought to contain sufficient concentrations of specific viral neutralizing lactoglobulins to provide at least partial protection against neonatal viral enteric infections during the immediate period that the milk is being fed. Viral particles are believed to be neutralized within the gut of calves consuming milk containing protective levels of specific lactoglobulins. Passive immunity (absorbed, circulating humoral antibodies) plays only a minor role in resistance to enteric rotavirus and coronavirus infections. Colostrum usually contains very high levels of specific viral neutralizing lactoglobulins. Colostrum from cows vaccinated against rotavirus and coronavirus is highly protective, even when diluted with milk and fed in a 1:3 colostrum:milk ratio during the immediate period that it is being consumed by the calf. Since calves become relatively resistant to the clinical effects of viral enteric infections by 3 to 4 weeks of age, the practice of raising calves to that age on milk containing 25 per cent colostrum from vaccinated cows can greatly assist in the control of neonatal enteric disease and secondary respiratory disease. Rigid attention to sanitation with respect to feeding utensils and the environment of the calf is also imperative.

FIBRINOUS PLEURITIS AND PLEUROPNEUMONIA

The term fibrinous pleuritis and pleuropneumonia (FPPP) has been proposed by the author for a unique and rather uncommon disease syndrome that deserves to be included under the umbrella of the bovine respiratory disease complex. The usual bovine respiratory disease syndrome caused by *H. somnus*, which has been reported by others, presents as a subacute to chronic bronchopneumonia.

Etiology and Epidemiology

FPPP is an acute infection of the lung and/or pleura with *H. somnus*, often in conjunction with pasteurella bacteria. It is thought that stress and concurrent respiratory viral infections are prerequisites, as in B&FP. Cattle are usually affected between the fourteenth and thirtieth days after arrival in the feedlot.

FPPP usually occurs sporadically and is usually of minor economic significance. A total of 11 fatal cases were diagnosed in a total of 96,092 head of cattle received by a single feedlot over a 5-year period (a mortality rate of 0.01 per cent). Then, during the subsequent year, an outbreak of FPPP occurred and 40 fatal cases were diagnosed. Thirty-three of these occurred in a population of 8682 cattle received during a single month (a mortality rate of 0.38 per cent). Mortality rates in affected groups (lots) ranged from 0.18 to 2.03 per cent.

The precise morbidity rate of FPPP cannot be determined under commercial feedlot conditions. Because exacerbations of pleuritis and pneumonia and chronic unthriftiness would be anticipated in survivors, and because only five such cases were recognized during an 8-year period of observation, it is believed that most affected cattle die. All ages, breeds, and sexes of feedlot cattle appear to be equally susceptible to FPPP.

FPPP is sometimes associated with the occurrence *of Haemophilus* thromboembolic meningoencephalitis (TEME). In the outbreak of FPPP observed by the author, six cases of TEME occurred within 3 days of the time that sister cattle, in the same lots (groups) as the cattle with TEME, were affected with fatal FPPP.

Clinical Signs

Onset is sudden and usually characterized by high fever, anorexia, marked depression, and dyspnea. The course was 2 days or less in 42 of 55 fatalities (76 per cent). Occasionally the course was as long as 57 days.

Pathology

When the chest is opened, one or both pleural spaces are found to be completely obliterated by massive accumulations of yellow fibrin and straw-colored fluid. A 5- to 8-cm-thick sheet of fibrin is adhered to the pleura of the affected lung. In a few cases only the pleura and pleural space are affected. Usually, however, a pleuropneumonia is also present. In these instances the dependent parts of the affected lung are firm. Affected lobules are pinkish-tan and separated by enlarged, white interlobular septa. In some cases lesions of acute or subacute B&FP accompany those of pleuropneumonia.

On histopathologic examination the interlobular septa are dilated with edema fluid and fibrin, are focally necrotic, and are separated from adjacent lung parenchyma by a zone of leukocytes. Airways are normal or mildly infiltrated with leukocytes. Alveoli are congested, flooded with edema fluid, atelectatic, or mildly infiltrated with leukocytes.

Treatment

The treatment regimens recommended for B&FP are also recommended for treatment of FPPP, although most cases are probably not amenable to treatment.

Control

As with TEME (and unlike B&FP), losses from FPPP are abruptly terminated when chlortetracycline or oxytetracycline is administered in the ration to affected groups in a dosage of 2.2 mg/kg body weight/day for 10 days. New cases are prevented from the third day of the medication period and do not ordinarily begin again when treatment is terminated.

Commercial *H. somnus* bacterins would presumably afford protection if administered a sufficient period of time prior to exposure for immunity to develop. With usual and expected rates of occurrence, bacterins are not a cost-effective means of control.

BIBLIOGRAPHY

Confer AW, Panciera RJ, Mosier DA: Bovine pneumonic pasteurellosis: immunity to *Pasteurella haemolytica*. J Am Vet Med Assoc 193:1308–1316, 1988.
Hjerpe CA: Bovine vaccines and herd vaccination programs. Vet Clin North Am: Food Anim Pract 6:171–260, 1990.
Liggit HD: Defense mechanisms in the bovine lung. Vet Clin North Am: Food Anim Pract 1:347–366, 1985.

Causal Factors in Swine Pneumonia

BARBARA STRAW, DVM, PhD

GENERAL EPIDEMIOLOGIC CONSIDERATIONS

Pneumonia in swine, especially the chronic forms, must be viewed as a complex. Most cases are caused by infectious agents, but they are strongly influenced by contributing factors. Clinical disease occurs when pigs exposed to a number of microorganisms experience stress and lowered resistance owing to the influence of environmental conditions, genetics, or management practices.

Infectious Agents

Numerous infectious agents can be involved in the pneumonia complex (Table 1). Some are highly pathogenic primary agents capable of causing extensive lung lesions and severe clinical signs. Many other primary pathogens produce only faint lesions without clinical significance. Other organisms are not capable of initiating disease but act as secondary invaders, intensifying damage caused by primary pathogens.

Spread of pneumonia between herds occurs most often through infectious contacts (primarily purchase of pigs and, to a lesser extent, transport vehicles, birds, people, etc.), or sometimes through airborne transmission. Airborne transmission over several kilometers has been demonstrated for porcine respiratory coronavirus (PRCV), *Mycoplasma hyopneumoniae*, and pseudorabies. Factors increasing the risk of airborne spread include large herd size, mechanical ventilation, proximity to other herds, direction and velocity of the prevailing winds, cloud cover, minimum turbulence, level topography, and relative humidity over 90 per cent.

The infectious agents responsible for swine pneumonia are extremely common in the swine population. Various surveys have estimated the per cent of midwestern herds positive for *Actinobacillus pleuropneumoniae* as 70 to 80 per cent and for *M. hyopneumoniae* as over 90 per cent. Bacterial flora identified in live healthy 20- to 30-kg specific pathogen–free (SPF) pigs typically belonged to two or three species, most often streptococci (nonhemolytic, α-hemolytic), staphylococci, *Escherichia coli*, *Klebsiella*, and *Corynebacterium*. *Haemophilus parasuis* and *Bordetella bronchiseptica* were rarely isolated, and *Pasteurella multocida* was never isolated. By contrast, in about 40 per cent of conventionally reared pigs, *H. parasuis* and *M. hyorhinis* were also detected. These two organisms act as commensals when the respiratory defense system is competent, and a constant low level of exposure exists for all animals. Outbreaks occur when this does not happen, that is, in small herds, in herds with restricted contact between individuals (early weaning, strict age separation), and in hysterectomy-derived SPF herds. *A. pleuropneumoniae* and *M. hyopneumoniae* are common at the herd level but are seldom isolated from healthy individuals. Their presence in the herd is usually associated with clinical or more often subclinical disease, particularly during the critical period in young pigs when passive immunity is replaced by active immunity. Although pneumonia organisms are widely distributed throughout herds, the presence of pneumonia agents in the herd is not well correlated with severity or extent of infection.

Table 1. INFECTIOUS AGENTS ASSOCIATED WITH PNEUMONIA

Bacteria	Mycoplasma
Actinobacillus pleuropneumoniae	*Mycoplasma hyopneumoniae*
Pasteurella multocida	*Mycoplasma hyorhinis*
Salmonella cholerasuis	
Bordetella bronchiseptica	**Parasites**
Haemophilus parasuis	*Ascaris suum*
Streptococcus suis	*Metastrongylus* spp.
Klebsiella pneumoniae	
Corynebacterium pyogenes	
Viruses	
Swine influenza	
Pseudorabies virus	
Swine mystery disease virus (Lelystad or SIRS virus)	

Interaction Between Infectious Agents

Clinically significant disease is seldom the result of infection with only one pathogen. More typically, several microorganisms are involved. Primary pathogens reduce local and sometimes also systemic defense mechanisms of the host, allowing secondary invaders to colonize the lung. Primary pathogens are usually viruses or mycoplasmas, while secondary invaders are bacteria. For example, susceptibility to *A. pleuropneumoniae* is increased following infection with swine influenza or pseudorabies. Pigs infected with *M. hyopneumoniae* have decreased resistance to *A. pleuropneumoniae*.

There may be cases in which one organism may diminish rather than intensify the effect of another. Because of shared antigens, there may be some cross-protection between *A. pleuropneumoniae* serotypes 2 and 6, and between PRCV and transmissible gastroenteritis.

Environment and Management

As more sensitive microbiologic and serologic methods were developed, it became obvious that differences between levels of pneumonia in different herds were not primarily due to type of organisms present. Epidemiologic techniques subsequently revealed the major impact of environment and management on clinical disease. Therefore practical control of pneumonia is primarily based on modifying environment and management when possible and using medication and vaccination when physical limitations prevent their adoption.

Farm Type–Degree of Integration

Farms producing all their own animals (closed) have less pneumonia than farms that purchase feeder pigs (open). Studies find the prevalence of pneumonia to be nearly twice as great in open versus closed herds. Typically farms that purchase feeder pigs buy from multiple sources, so pigs with differing microbiologic and immunologic backgrounds are mixed together. Pigs purchased from only one source do not have a substantially greater risk of pneumonia than the closed herd. Purchase of stock from sales barns confers the greatest risk of pleuropneumonia. Obviously respiratory problems can be expected if pigs with low health status are introduced into a herd with better health. However, it is also risky to introduce high-health animals into herds with lower health status. High-health animals, insufficiently protected by specific immunity, easily develop clinical disease. As a consequence there is a sudden rise in excretion of pathogens, and the established equilibrium between infection and immunity in the lower-health herd is unbalanced.

Pneumonia control is greatly simplified in farrow-to-feeder and feeder-to-finish herds compared with that in farrow-to-finish herds owing to the "pathogen generator" effect associated with growing pigs. In farrow-to-finish herds periodic transmission of airborne pathogens from growers to the breeding herd is inevitable. In herds with an inadequate separation between pigs of different age groups there remains a continuous transmission of microbials from older to younger pigs with a subsequent continuous replication of pathogens. Dissimilar environmental needs of different age groups may be a contributing factor.

Movement of Pigs Through Facilities

Numerous studies have demonstrated the benefit of utilizing all-in–all-out movement of pigs into buildings compared with continuous addition and removal of animals. Prevalence of pneumonia in facilities with all-in–all-out flow is generally 20 to 25 per cent less than in continuous-flow facilities.

Mixing and Sorting of Pigs

Frequently when animals are moved from nursery to grower barn or grower barn to finishing barn, they are regrouped so that all animals in a pen are approximately the same size. Farms with all-in–all-out pig flow have less tendency to mix or regroup animals, but often at least a few animals are sorted out and moved back. By contrast, farms with continuous flow of animals are conspicuous for the amount of mixing and regrouping. Often pneumonia is the reason pigs fail to grow as rapidly as their contemporaries. Thus when pigs are mixed, healthy younger animals under stress of establishing a new social order are placed in contact with older diseased pigs.

Number of Animals in Herd/Room

Generally the risk of contracting respiratory disease increases with increasing herd size. However, very large herds frequently have a lower level of respiratory disease than middle-sized herds. This probably occurs because very large herd facilities are forced to subdivide and move pigs in groups, while for small and middle-sized herds it is not cost-effective to divide facilities for all-in–all-out production. Therefore the health status of middle-sized and small swine herds often is surpassed by that of large herds.

Pneumonia is spread by aerosol and direct contact. The number of possible disease transmissions increases exponentially as the number of animals increases according to the following formula:

Number of possible disease transmissions = $n^2 - n$

where n = number of animals.

Barns that contain fewer pigs have less pneumonia than barns with more animals. The ideal barn capacity is between 150 and 300 animals. The number of pigs housed in the same air space significantly affects prevalence of pneumonia even on farms with all-in–all-out production.

Floor Space per Pig

Densely crowded pigs have higher levels of pneumonia than pigs that are allowed more space. Herds that crowd pigs beyond a recommended level of 0.7 m^2/pig have increased levels of pneumonia. There is also some evidence that when the number of pigs per pen is reduced, the level of pneumonia is also lessened.

Ventilation

Forced ventilation is required in confinement facilities to remove excess moisture and waste gases. The smaller the air space allotted per pig, the higher the air exchange needed. While air exchange rates of greater than 60 m^3/hour/pig have been associated with reduced frequencies of pneumonia, it is not possible to offset an increase in stocking density with a proportional increase in ventilation rate. For example, if stocking rate is doubled in a fixed air space, ventilation rate would have to be increased by 10 times to maintain the same clearance of air contaminants. Ventilation systems often recirculate air, and this mixing of air contributes to spread of respiratory pathogens in the barn. Pneumonia is less severe in buildings with negative pressure ventilation where the polluted air is removed and exchanged for totally fresh air.

Within confinement facilities the amount of air space per animal is significantly associated with risk of pneumonia. Based on amount of pneumonia occurring at slaughter, an air space of at least 3 m^3/pig in the growing-finishing period has been recommended. This amount of space is especially critical in continuous-flow facilities.

Lack of uniform airflow through a building is associated with increased levels of pneumonia. Pigs raised in buildings with solid pen dividers, which minimize draftiness, have less severe pneumonia than pigs raised in an open environment.

Temperature

Cold environmental temperatures reduce the young pig's ability to clear bacteria from its lungs. Cold, uninsulated concrete floors, which cause heat loss from the pig's body through conduction, are associated with higher levels of pneumonia.

Ammonia

Ammonia in concentrations of 10 to 100 ppm interferes with respiratory tract function and predisposes the pig to infection. Prolonged exposure to 20 ppm ammonia caused excessive nasal, lacrimal, and oral secretions, increased coughing, and increased the number of bacteria in the lungs. Usually the ammonia concentration in pigpens is less than 20 ppm. However, ammonia concentrations as low as 11 ppm have shown clinical association with pneumonia.

Waste Disposal System

Liquid manure handling and slatted floors are associated with higher levels of pneumonia. This is possibly due to a cold environment, drafts, and high ammonia concentration, which frequently accompany slatted flooring.

Dust

While aerial hog-house dust can induce acute or chronic malfunction of the respiratory tract in humans, there is little evidence to incriminate it as a major contributor to swine pneumonia. Several investigations have failed to demonstrate any significant relation between dust and respiratory disease in pigs.

Other Diseases

Pigs from herds in which diarrhea occurs either in unweaned or weaned pigs are at a greater risk of developing pneumonia. Litters of pigs with rotavirus or transmissible gastroenteritis (TGE) have been shown to have higher rates of respiratory disease than virus-free litters.

Outbreaks of pneumonia have been reported in which control could not be achieved until pigs were treated for mange.

Within-farm studies have generally failed to demonstrate an association between the presence of atrophic rhinitis and pneumonia, while between-farm studies have shown that herds with high levels of one disease tend also to have high levels of the other. Shared predisposing factors probably account for herd associations, but within individuals, atrophic rhinitis does not predispose to pneumonia.

Migration of *Ascaris suum* enhances lesions of pneumonia in swine. Lung consolidation in mycoplasmal pneumonia may be increased 10 times if pigs undergo concomitant ascarid migration.

Castration

Slaughter surveillance of market swine shows the prevalences of pneumonia and pleuritis in castrated males to be 10 per cent higher than in females.

Nutrition

Low protein content or feed restriction exacerbates the effects of pneumonia in swine. Two studies reported that restricted access to drinking water produced higher levels of pneumonia.

Heredity

Respiratory disorders are to some extent influenced by heredity. Antibody production and phagocytic functions of pulmonary alveolar macrophages differ between breeds. Yorkshire pigs have been shown to have higher levels of pneumonia than Hampshire, Landrace, or Duroc pigs.

DIAGNOSIS OF RESPIRATORY DISEASE

Definitive diagnoses of respiratory diseases are based on a combination of history, clinical observation, laboratory tests, necropsy, and slaughter checks. A clinical diagnosis can only be tentative, as respiratory distress may result from dysfunction of other organs. Also, certain disorders of the respiratory system may be without clinical signs or signs typical for respiratory disorders. Often acute pleuropneumonia may be widespread in a herd before the disease is discovered. Clinical signs of "lazy pigs" and decreased appetite in fatteners should trigger investigation of possible pneumonia etiologies.

Table 2 lists various differentiating features of coughing, dyspnea, and pneumonia in swine.

MONITORING PNEUMONIA

Pneumonia levels are monitored to provide feedback for use in determining the appropriateness and efficacy of specific intervention. Action is taken to reduce economic loss or maintain health status of seed stock. Pneumonia has been estimated to reduce average daily gain by 37 g for every 10 per cent of the lung with lesions. Certain facilities will buy replacements only from *M. hyopneumoniae*–free or *A. pleuropneumoniae*–free herds. Monitoring diseases of the respiratory tract entails collecting data from clinical and production records, laboratory tests, and slaughter examinations.

Examinations in the Herd

Clinical observations include the amount of coughing or dyspnea and unevenness in size. Postmortem examinations of dead or euthanized animals are used to determine the character of lesions and for isolation of infectious agents. Records are reviewed for feed consumption, growth rate, number of treatments, and accumulated mortality. Weight or age of dead pigs should be noted.

Laboratory Tests

Tremendous progress in biotechnology has accelerated the development of new, highly specific laboratory tests for pneumonia. Typically sera from 20 to 30 sows are examined for antibodies to *M. hyopneumoniae* and different serotypes of *A. pleuropneumoniae*. Testing for colostral instead of serum antibodies may improve the diagnostic value of testing to monitor pleuropneumonia and mycoplasmal pneumonia.

Examinations of Slaughter Swine

Slaughter checks are used to determine the extent and character (reflection of etiology) of pneumonia. Commonly used measures include prevalence and severity of lesions such as consolidation, pneumonic abscesses, and pleuritis. Recent infections show up as darker, firm areas of the lung; fissures in lung tissue represent earlier resolved lesions. Details of various examination techniques are recorded elsewhere.

Interpretation of slaughter findings are made in light of the dynamic nature of infection and seasonal influences. Acute infection resolves in 6 to 8 weeks, so lesions at slaughter reflect only the last part of the finishing period. Fissures in lung tissue indicate earlier infection. Pneumonia is most prevalent and severe in pigs slaughtered in the spring and fall and is mildest in the summer.

CONTROL OF PNEUMONIA

Pathogenic microorganisms are involved in all respiratory disorders of importance. While it is possible to eliminate certain organisms from the herd, in practice it is impossible to protect pigs from every pathogenic microorganism, and the development of respiratory disease fundamentally depends on the balance between pressure from pathogenic microorganisms and the pigs' ability to resist them. This equilibrium is very fragile and greatly affected by the above-mentioned factors. Therefore control of pneumonia at the herd level is based on two principles: (1) elimination of certain pathogens and (2) strengthening the herd's defense mechanisms and diminishing the infection pressure in the herd.

Elimination of Pathogens from the Herd

Freedom from certain pathogens greatly simplifies pneumonia control. However, this can be accomplished only if the agent in question can be definitively identified, transmission routes can be effectively blocked, sufficient diagnostic capacity is available, and the owner is highly motivated.

Specific Pathogen–Free (SPF) Swine Production

Some herds have achieved freedom from *M. hyopneumoniae* and *A. pleuropneumoniae* by establishing the herd from caesarian-derived stock, raised in isolation from other pigs. The usual contributing factors (crowding, lack of age separation, infection with influenza or pseudorabies, enteric disorders, etc.) are tolerated to a greater extent in SPF herds than in conventional herds infected with these two organisms. Secondary SPF herds enjoy many of the same advantages.

Medicated Early Weaning (MEW)

A. pleuropneumoniae and *M. hyopneumoniae* may be eliminated from the growing-finishing section by weaning piglets before 10 days of age, giving them high doses of injectable and feed medication, and raising them in a facility far removed from the sow herd.

Culling Techniques

Heavy medication in conjunction with repeated serologic testing and removal of positive sows has been used to eradicate

Table 2. CHARACTERISTICS OF DISEASES THAT CAUSE COUGH AND DYSPNEA IN PIGS

Clinical Signs	Associated Agents	Necropsy Findings	Diagnosis
Signs primarily referable to the respiratory tract. Dyspnea, cough, anorexia, fever, abdominal respiration, varying severities of clinical signs in a group of pigs.	M. hyopneumoniae A. pleuropneumoniae S. cholerasuis B. bronchiseptica Pseudorabies virus M. hyorhinis P. multocida H. parasuis Streptococcus Klebsiella Corynebacterium	Usually cranioventral distribution of lesions. Firm areas of tissue with variable intralobular edema. Fibrinous pleuritis suggests involvement with A. pleuropneumoniae, H. parasuis, P. multocida, M. hyorhinis, or S. cholerasuis.	Culture of organism. Fluorescent antibody (FA) test for mycoplasma. Serology or FA for pseudorabies.
Rapid clinical course, high fever, anorexia, depression, severe dyspnea, open-mouth breathing, cyanosis, foamy, blood-tinged discharge from nose and mouth.	A. pleuropneumoniae	Acute hemorrhagic necrosis distributed throughout the lungs, especially dorsally in the diaphragmatic lobes. Fibrinous pleurisy; some blood-tinged fluid in the pleural cavity. Bloody foam in the trachea.	Isolation of organism. Serology. Pathology.
Coughing with minimal other signs.	A. suum	Areas of atelectasis, hemorrhage, edema, and emphysema in lung. Septal and periseptal hemorrhage and necrosis in the liver.	Fecal examination for eggs (may be negative early). Typical necropsy findings. History of access to soil (absolute requirement for Metastrongylus).
	Metastrongylus spp.	Bronchitis, bronchiolitis in caudoventral margins of the diaphragmatic lobes. Areas of atelectasis.	
Dyspnea, abdominal respiration, cyanosis, no coughing.	Diaphragmatic hernia (possibly related to selenium deficiency, genetics, trauma)	Tear in diaphragm. Abdominal organs in chest.	Necropsy.
No coughing, but dyspnea and cyanosis, depression, fever, anorexia and reluctance to move, lameness, stiff gait, swollen joints, ataxia, convulsions.	H. parasuis M. hyorhinis S. suis	Fibrinous to serofibrinous pleuritis, pericarditis, arthritis, and meningitis.	Isolation of organism.
Very acute onset, near 100% morbidity, extreme prostration, complete anorexia, labored jerky respiration, hard paroxysmal cough, fever.	Swine influenza	Often there is no opportunity to do a necropsy since death due to uncomplicated swine influenza is rare. Tenacious mucus in pharynx, larynx, trachea, and bronchi. Depressed deep-purple areas in lung.	Physical examination. Serology. Virus isolation from pharyngeal swab.
Signs of systemic disease, sneezing, coughing, dyspnea, fever, anorexia, vomiting, constipation initially then diarrhea, possibly tremors, ataxia, and convulsions.	Hog cholera African swine fever	Edematous tissue, swollen edematous lymph nodes with mottled hemorrhage, petechial or ecchymotic hemorrhage in bladder and kidneys, enlarged liver and spleen, splenic infarcts.	FA test.
	Pseudorabies	Few gross lesions, necrotic tonsillitis and pharyngitis, small white necrotic foci in liver.	Virus isolation or FA test on tonsil.
Labored respiration, minor cough.	F. moniliforme toxicity	Pulmonary edema and hydrothorax.	Necropsy, mycotoxin analysis on feed.
Rapid or abdominal respiration, moist nonproductive cough if present, pale mucous membranes.	Anemia	Pale musculature, lung edema, dilated heart, excess pericardial fluid, contracted spleen.	Packed cell volume 15–20%. Hemoglobin concentration 6–7 g/dl.
Rapid, panting respiration, no cough, open-mouth breathing, gasping, extremely high temperature.	Porcine stress syndrome Heat prostration Puffer sow syndrome	Areas of pale, soft, or exudative muscle. Edema and congestion of lungs. Rapid autolysis.	Creatine kinase. Physical examination.
Rapid or abdominal respiration, moist nonproductive cough, subcutaneous edema, enlarged abdomen.	Cardiac insufficiency	Enlarged dilated heart, valvular endocarditis, pulmonary edema, enlarged liver.	Necropsy.

A. pleuropneumoniae from smaller herds with low initial prevalence of infection.

Long-Term Control: Increasing Herd Defense Mechanisms and Reducing Infection Pressure

Long-term control of pneumonia often requires more radical and expensive changes in production systems and housing. Long-term strategies should incorporate as many of the control options as possible. Table 3 lists factors that influence pneumonia and their relative importance.

Practical application of disease control principles does not necessarily require expensive construction. Large finishing barns may be partitioned into rooms using sheets of heavy plastic to create walls. Pressure-treated plywood is placed below the floor, extending into the liquid surface of the pit to totally separate ventilation between sections. Barn sections should be designed to hold the number of animals that are introduced (weaned) in a 2-week or, more ideally, 1-week period and then operated on an all-in–all-out basis.

Ventilation and housing should be carefully assessed and deficiencies corrected. Often this requires adding additional insulation, placing solid partitions between pens, and supplying the correct amount of air exchange while maintaining incoming airflow at 600 ft/minute.

Farms that purchase feeder pigs should locate a single source of high-health pigs. Even with conventional pigs, a single source allows buyer and seller to design vaccination, worm, and mange control programs.

Table 3. DISEASE DETERMINING HERD FACTORS WITH DETRIMENTAL EFFECT ON PNEUMONIA

Factor	Degree of Effect
Production System	
Large herd size	+++
High stocking density	+++
Conventional health system (not SPF or minimal disease production system)	+++
Introduction of animals from herds with unknown/low health status	+++
Continuous flow of animals through the facilities	+++
Housing	
Badly insulated and ventilated facilities (cold or fluctuating temperature, inadequate air exchange, drafts)	+++
Poor division of facilities combined with housing of different aged animals in same air space	+++
Pen dividers without solid separations	+++
Large grower-finisher apartments (>200–300 pigs)	++
Nutrition	
Caloric intake insufficient	+
Improper content of macro-microelements in feed	+
Presence of Nonrespiratory Pathogens	
Colibacillosis	++
Dysentery	++
Mange	+
Ascarids	+
Management	
Poor control of climate	+++
Poor monitoring of signs of disease	++
Lack of or incorrect treatment	++
Lack of or incorrect preventive measures (vaccinations, strategic medications)	++
Poor care of sick animals (isolation, handling)	+
Poor hygiene	++

Source: Adapted from Christensen G, Mousing J: Respiratory system. *In* Leman AD, Straw BE, et al (eds): Diseases of Swine, 7th ed. Ames, IA, Iowa State University Press, 1992.

Short-Term Control Measures

Short-term measures against pneumonia include strategic medication procedures, vaccination, immediate treatment of sick animals, climate modification, and isolation or dispersion arrangements.

Medication

Successful control of pneumonia outbreaks requires immediate medication of diseased individuals and penmates. Pigs showing clinical signs should be treated for 2 to 3 days by injection since their consumption of water and feed is significantly decreased. Pigs in contact with clinically diseased individuals should be medicated in the feed or water for 4 to 7 days.

Strategic medication is useful when outbreaks can be anticipated. Common times for the development of clinical pneumonia include about 1 week after pigs are moved to the grower-finisher unit, and at about 50 to 75 kg, when passive immunity to *A. pleuropneumoniae* is lost. Feed or water medication should be given for 4 to 7 days just prior to when signs of disease are expected. Hopefully medication will prevent severe consequences of infection but still allow pigs to receive sufficient exposure to the current infections to develop immunity. Totally preventing exposure only delays the outbreak. Pulse medication has been used to achieve immunity while protecting pigs. Regimens used include a 5-day period of medication every 2 weeks and medication 2 days out of every week.

Vaccination

Vaccines against pseudorabies are generally efficacious. However, existing vaccines against pleuropneumonia, enzootic pneumonia, and influenza have only limited value. Some oil-adjuvanted *A. pleuropneumoniae* vaccines reduce mortality but do little to lessen prevalence or severity of lesions.

Dispersion

During an outbreak, new cases of pneumonia can be avoided by dispersing pigs over a large area. If weather conditions permit, pigs may be moved to an outside lot.

Climate Modification

Obvious deficiencies in environment should be corrected. Hovers or plastic partitions can be erected to reduce drafts. Sources of dampness should be removed. Provision of straw bedding raises the effective environmental temperature. Air exchange should not be compromised in order to increase air temperature.

BIBLIOGRAPHY

Alexander TJL, Harris DL: Methods of disease control. *In* Leman AD, Straw BE, et al (eds): Diseases of Swine, 7th ed. Ames, IA, Iowa State University Press, 1992.

Christensen G, Mousing J: Respiratory system. *In* Leman AD, Straw BE, et al (eds): Diseases of Swine, 7th ed. Ames, IA, Iowa State University Press, 1992.

Straw BE: Factors that contribute to the development of swine pneumonia. Vet Med Aug: 747–756, 1986.

Straw BE, Backstrom L, Leman AD: Evaluation of swine at slaughter. Part 1—Sample size, mechanics of examination, scoring systems and seasonal effects. Compendium of Continuing Education 8:541, 1986.

Management of Respiratory Disease in Sheep

NEIL ANDERSON, DVM, PhD

Respiratory disease in sheep is a major cause of loss to producers. Infectious agents that cause etiologically specific diseases (Table 1) are variably present in sheep flocks, serving as a reservoir for infection of weaned and feeder lambs and newly introduced or commingled sheep, as well as of in-flock sheep. Interactions between *Pasteurella haemolytica, Mycoplasma ovipneumoniae*, and parainfluenza-3 virus appear to be pivotal factors in acute and chronic (nonprogressive) pneumonia in sheep. *P. haemolytica* infects lungs previously infected with PI-3 virus, *M. ovipneumoniae*, or ovine progressive pneumonia (OPP) but is less likely to do so in the absence of these or other predisposing infections. Adenoviruses may also predispose sheep lung to *P. haemolytica* infection. Because these transmissible agents (microbes and parasites) are, for the most part, not eradicable from the sheep flock, the producer is best advised to acknowledge their potential presence and to focus on disease avoidance strategies. The veterinarian and the producer should work as a team to develop specific strategies that address each of the principles of disease control cited below.

RISK FACTORS AND PREVENTION

The overwhelming influence of environmental and management factors in minimizing or intensifying respiratory disease and the benefits to profitability of preventing rather than treating respiratory disease make a persuasive case for giving a discussion of risk factors and prevention first importance. The health status of the flock is increasingly seen as (1) a major determinant of productivity over time, (2) responsive to the use of simple, often one-time and low-cost technologies that enhance the quality of life and thus the productivity of sheep, and (3) of such importance to the long-term viability of the enterprise that reducing risk of respiratory disease becomes an integral and irreducible part of enterprise forward planning. Knowing and avoiding or minimizing the impact of the risk factors makes it possible to minimize respiratory disease and to use therapies with greater expectation of efficacy.

The following three major principles of disease control serve as guides to managing respiratory disease in sheep:

1. Prevent exposure of sheep to transmissible agents of respiratory disease when possible; minimize exposure at all times.

2. Enhance resistance to prevent or reduce the spread of respiratory diseases between sheep within the flock.

3. Manage the environment to avoid or minimize stressors that trigger respiratory disease.

Each of these strategies includes the concept of risk assessment; each bears a cost that must be factored into enterprise planning.

Step one, for veterinarian and producer, is to inventory the present respiratory health status of the flock. A critical visual assessment of the flock is essential. Sheep displaying severe respiratory disease should be isolated and examined individually, and severely affected sheep should be necropsied. Necropsy and laboratory examinations identify causative agents and provide an objective basis for production medicine strategies. Less severely ill sheep may be isolated and treated appropriately and/or culled. These data should be assessed in the light of recently documented respiratory cases in the flock and known prevalence of respiratory disease of sheep in the area. In going through step one, the veterinarian and producer will develop a mutual sense of the risk of production loss due to respiratory disease in the flock. They will also have begun to prevent exposure by removing sheep with respiratory disease from contact with clinically healthy sheep. It is useful to reiterate to the producer that the short-term goal is to identify and prevent the most prevalent respiratory disease.

A strategy to minimize exposure of clinically healthy sheep to respiratory disease agents is to quarantine (30 days minimum) all newly acquired sheep and to isolate clinically ill sheep in separate buildings or distant pens. Sheep (replacement ewes or feeder lambs) purchased from a single source, without commingling and without recourse to channels of trade, are less likely to experience severe outbreaks of respiratory disease, particularly if quarantined upon arrival and if aggressive surveillance is made daily for signs of illness (see Flock Therapy below). Bringing unacclimated sheep (not quarantined) or sheep from undocumented sources (e.g., public markets) into contact with the existing ewe flock is to place those sheep at risk for exposure to active cases of respiratory disease. Most of the transmissible agents of respiratory disease (bacteria, chlamydia, mycoplasmas, and viruses) are harbored at nasopharyngeal (including lymphoid) sites, as well as in tracheobronchial and pulmonary tissues of carrier, convalescent, or actively infected sheep. These agents are distributed into the environment and thus to susceptible sheep in aerosols, by nose-to-nose contact, or via water or feed.

A second strategy is to close the breeding flock on the female side by introducing all genetic inputs through purchased rams. Careful prepurchase examination and quarantine of rams for 30 days upon arrival reduces the risk of clinical respiratory disease in the ewe flock. Although rams carrying and shedding respiratory disease agents are not excluded by this strategy, clinical disease in ewes may be minimized or avoided because, after quarantine, rams will likely shed smaller numbers of the agent into the environment and by direct contact. If each of these actions is taken early on, the prevalence of respiratory disease among ewes may be substantially reduced.

Step two is to enhance resistance to respiratory diseases among the clinically healthy sheep. General resistance to respiratory disease should be enhanced by

Table 1. INFECTIOUS AGENTS COMMONLY CAUSING RESPIRATORY DISEASE IN SHEEP, SEGREGATED AS TO SIGNS, PRIMARY SITE OF INFECTION, AND TIME COURSE OF DISEASE

Acute Upper Respiratory	**Chronic Upper Respiratory**
Parainfluenza-3 virus	*Oestrus ovis*
Respiratory syncytial virus	Nasal adenocarcinoma
Ovine adenovirus	*Dictyocaulus filariae*
Reovirus type 1	*Muellerius capillaris*
Chlamydia psittaci	*Protostrongylus rufescens*
Mycoplasma ovipneumoniae*	
Acute Lower Respiratory	**Chronic Lower Respiratory**‡
Pasteurella haemolytica†	*Corynebacterium pseudotuberculosis* (ovis)
Haemophilus somnus	*Actinomyces pyogenes*
Pulmonary aspergillosis	Ovine progressive pneumonia (OPP virus)
	Pulmonary aspergillosis

*Pathogenicity uncertain.

†*P. haemolytica* superinfection of acute upper respiratory disease results in pasteurella pneumonia.

‡Frequently a mixed infection, particularly if OPP virus is the underlying cause.

1. Assuring that the grazing/feeding program maintains the desired body condition score of the ewe flock throughout the production cycle. Appropriate nutrient inputs are necessary for development of optimal general resistance to respiratory disease and for optimal protective responses to natural exposure or vaccination. Water, salt, and minerals are essential to good nutrition; vitamins may be needed in some situations (e.g., old forage, drought, by-product feedstuffs).

2. Identifying and reducing the internal and external parasite burden of ewes and lambs. Regular anthelmintic treatment should be instituted, coupled with periodic fecal flotation examinations for parasite eggs, so that drug efficacy is assured. By giving ivermectin in late autumn, nasal bots *(Oestrus ovis)* will also be removed.

3. Specific resistance to certain infectious respiratory diseases has been shown to reduce morbidity and mortality in sheep.

Vaccines directed against ruminant respiratory pathogens are not currently licensed for use in sheep in the United States, and their use must be accepted as extralabel by both veterinarians and producers. In the United States, vaccine costs and variable efficacy in sheep, especially in instances in which vaccine is relied on for prevention but environmental factors are not dealt with, have mitigated against the use of bovine respiratory vaccines in commercial ewe flocks. Lamb feeders often defer the use of respiratory vaccines for the same reasons.

Owners of purebred sheep flocks that have stock of considerable genetic worth may request their veterinarian to recommend a vaccination program to prevent outbreaks of clinical respiratory disease. Yearly vaccination of ewes and of lambs prior to weaning with intranasal PI-3 MLV (modified live virus) vaccine has been demonstrated to reduce losses due to *P. haemolytica* pneumonia effectively. *P. haemolytica* bacterins must contain antigenic material from the biotype and serotype present in the flock, since cross-protection does not occur among biotypes or serotypes. Costs for vaccines/bacterins and labor can exceed expected net return from the procedure, so vaccine usage must clearly contribute to profitability or not be used. Active immunity to microbial respiratory pathogens may be attained without clinical disease or loss through the acquisition of organisms by contact with other sheep in the flock if the sheep are well nourished and not stressed.

Step three is management of the environment to reduce the impact of stressors. Environmental risk factors for respiratory disease in sheep include transport, crowding, high humidity within shelters and barns, toxic gases, chilling due to low temperatures and/or drafts, lack of shade or windbreak, abrupt changes in feedstuffs or feeding schedule, and increased dust in buildings or lots. While it is not possible to control climate and weather, it is usually possible to modify the impact of heat, chilling drafts, humidity, and rainfall by placement of trees, structures, curtains, and other windbreaks. Opening the ridge of structures is a way to provide upward drainage of warm, moisture-laden air, which reduces humidity. Dampening lots by water spray provides short-term control of dust. Regular cleaning of feed bunks and proper drainage around water sources will contribute to a more healthful environment.

Adequate ventilation of structures, including opening the ridge, reduces humidity and aerosol density and removes dust and gases, which is of prime importance in preventing respiratory diseases. Sheep will find the best available comfort zone, so indoor-outdoor access should be provided.

Late autumn, winter, and early spring lambing in North America are increasingly done as some variant of "shed-lambing," in which high humidity is an important and potentially controllable risk factor for sheep production. The building environment should be characterized by low-velocity cfm air movement to affect air exchange, yet without chilling drafts (e.g., 25 cubic feet per minute [cfm]/1000 lb animal weight, continuously, in cool to cold weather). This usually calls for relatively high ceilings so as to enclose a large volume of air, such that intrusion air from doorways, ducts, and fans is tempered by dilution. Warm, moist air must be allowed to escape upward or outward, which calls for an open ridge and tempered incoming air, or forced ventilation.

The minimum square feet of surface area available per animal must be observed in design of structures and lots, as well as linear feeding space and adequate waterers, in order to minimize aerosol and direct contact exposure between animals. Square footage per 70-kg ewe should be 18 to 20 minimum, with 25 ft^2 per ewe-lamb pair and 30 ft^2 for a ewe with twins. As lambs grow, progressively more space is required.

Abrupt thermal change, whether from warm to cold or the reverse, is one of the most important stressors in temperate climates, especially in spring and autumn. The greater and more abrupt the thermal change, the more stressful to the sheep. To minimize thermal change, provide optional comfort zones for the sheep by allowing indoor-outdoor access, as well as by providing windbreaks.

Dust within buildings and lots and from adjacent fields should be minimized. Curtains on open-front structures, primarily used to limit intrusion of cold air in winter, have some efficacy in limiting dust aerosols. Curtains also darken the area, discouraging fly activity. Water sprinklers, thought to be cost-effective for diminishing dust in lamb feedlots in the semiarid high plains of Colorado, are contraindicated indoors for sheep because water spray elevates humidity and has adverse effects on wool quality. Bedding is of benefit within buildings, but it also contributes dust particulates to the environment. Windbreaks (trees, solid or fenestrated fences) are helpful in limiting the effects of dust on sheep, but solid windbreaks also reduce evaporative cooling in hot weather.

Transport should be limited to 10 to 12 hours nonstop or be interspersed with stops for offloading, rest, feed, and water. The unavoidable stress associated with transport and crowding is increased in hot, cold, or humid conditions.

Commingling should be limited even within the production unit. Subsets ("pens," breeding bands) should be kept intact as much as possible to reduce aerosol or nose-to-nose transmission of infectious agents.

Feed changes are more stressful to a sheep than formerly thought. At least 21 days and preferably longer should elapse during change from an all-forage ration to a high-energy (>50 per cent concentrate) ration. Further increases in percentage of concentrate should also be done incrementally. Sheep that have been deprived of food for any reason should be initially fed dry forage and fresh water (bland diet) and then given an increasing amount of concentrate over several feedings until full feed intake is attained.

Weaning is stressful for lambs. The social deprivation resulting from the withdrawal of the dam is evidenced by excitement, vocalizing, and agitated movement and behavior by lambs and ewes. They should be in "mixing" groups of more than 10 pairs prior to weaning, so that lambs identify and bond with agemates prior to weaning. It is important that ewes be moved out of sight and earshot at weaning and that lambs remain in the familiar environment to lessen the impact of this stressful experience. It is important that lambs have access to creep feed early on, and it is preferable that they be ingesting a substantial proportion of their daily caloric requirement as dry feed prior to weaning. Movement of weaned lambs to a new environment should be delayed for 10 to 14 days or longer after weaning. In spite of these stress-reducing strategies, lambs are at additional risk for respiratory disease after weaning, especially if commingled as they enter the feedlot. Adjustment to high-energy rations and to dust, chilling rain, or snow are stressors additive to those associated with weaning. Replacement ewe lambs, if spared the spartan conditions of the conventional lamb feedlot, may be at less risk by being in environments with more comfort zones from which to choose.

Forced exercise is stressful to penned, sedentary sheep and should be avoided. However, forced exercise as a diagnostic test may call attention to animals with OPP or other chronic lower respiratory disorder.

CLINICAL ASPECTS OF RESPIRATORY DISEASE

Respiratory disease in sheep is evidenced by reduced feed intake, reduced activity, visual evidence of depression, and separation from the flock. Serous nasal discharge, common in sheep, takes on diagnostic importance when the nares are left ungroomed or when the discharge becomes mucoid or purulent. Coughing or sneezing may be the first sign detected if more subtle early signs (reduced feed intake, depression, decreased activity) go undetected. Conjunctivitis with exudation may be evidence of a viral cause. When approaching a flock or pen of sheep, the veterinarian should pause briefly to listen for cough, sneeze, or other abnormal respiratory sound. When sheep are moved, coughing or sneezing may be elicited, although the presence of dust is a variable, which confounds the clinical interpretation. Stertorous sounds or wheezes may be audible if air movement in upper airways is constricted by mucus or exudate. Labored respiration is detected by the audible sounds produced, by exaggerated excursions of rib cage and abdomen, and by open-mouth breathing. Auscultation of larynx, trachea, and thorax will help localize the respiratory disorder within the tract.

The diagnostic technique of bronchoalveolar lavage, an alternative to necropsy for animals of genetic value, yields at least two types of diagnostic evidence: (1) the cellular response at the gas exchange region and (2) if bacteria are recovered in culture, antimicrobial sensitivity to drugs. Necropsy and culture of dead sheep and of those in extremis with severe respiratory disease are part of the disease prevention strategy.

The chronic respiratory disorders of adult sheep are often subclinical, becoming clinically apparent when superinfection occurs (usually *P. haemolytica* or *Actinomyces pyogenes*) or when the encroachment of cellular infiltrate on lung tissue becomes so extensive as to limit gas exchange. Some cases become evident only when affected sheep fail to keep up with the flock when driven or when respiratory effort becomes so labored as to interfere with eating and resting. Weight loss may ensue in either instance. OPP is the archetypal chronic respiratory disease of sheep. The lentivirus of OPP reduces macrophage function, which serves as a mechanism by which the organism evades immune surveillance, and in turn delays the immune response detectable in serum. Superinfection by *P. haemolytica* or other bacterium may precipitate the final exacerbation of respiratory signs, which may be misinterpreted as an acute episode if necropsy is not done.

FLOCK THERAPY

Therapy for respiratory disease in sheep is facilitated by transfer of sick sheep from the flock or pen of origin to a warm, dry, draft-free place. Individual treatment is by injection, in most instances, and includes antibiotic, nonsteroidal anti-inflammatory drugs, vitamins, and electrolyte solutions by gavage. Addition of antimicrobials to the feed or water for several days during processing into the feedlot is a cost-effective way to deliver the drug to feedlot lambs, but it is ineffective in treating the sick lamb that eats little or not at all. Because the prevalence of respiratory disease in transported lambs is high, because surface conditions are dusty in lamb feedlots during dry seasons of the year, and because some lambs have pre-existent lung lesions or are in the incubation stages of infectious respiratory disease when they arrive at the feedlot, the use of oxytetracycline at 300 mg/head/day on day 1 and decreasing to 50 mg/head/day by day 4, then discontinuing it, appears justified on medical and economic grounds.

Since the greatest risk factor in many production units is likely to be recently purchased sheep, therapy should be used in a prospective manner on that subset while in quarantine. Recognizing the sentinel case of respiratory disease, or the first few cases, may be the signal to treat all sheep in that subset or pen. Decisions are made primarily on the basis of clinical and gross necropsy evidence. If feed intake is sustained, oxytetracycline in the feed (300 mg/head/day) may be the most cost-effective and has a measure of efficacy against several common respiratory disease agents. Conversely, if feed intake is reduced, injection of long-acting oxytetracycline (20 mg/kg every 72 hours) may be elected because it has been shown to be effective against both *P. haemolytica* and *M. ovipneumoniae*, and sheep need to be handled only at 3-day intervals. Two or three treatments (i.e., 6 to 9 days total) are recommended. Procaine penicillin (44,000 IU/kg) subcutaneously s.i.d. for 4 to 6 days or ceftiofur sodium (i.e., 1.1 mg/kg for 5 days) reduces lesion scores and morbidity and mortality, granted that this dosage regimen requires agreement that it represents extralabel use. Both drugs require daily handling of the affected sheep. Lack of clinical response or bacterial culture and sensitivity testing that yields new data may require a change of therapy. The "one injection and stop" approach to treating sheep may yield bacterial resistance. Decisions to treat with antibiotic should be made with the realization that a full course of antibiotic therapy, once begun, should be continued for 2 days beyond the end of fever.

COST-EFFECTIVE MANAGEMENT STRATEGIES

Management strategies for minimizing losses due to respiratory disease in sheep must be developed as a joint decision-making process. The short- and midterm production goals and the current health status of the flock form the starting point for decision making. Structures, prevailing winds, drainage, population density, and other factors should be critically assessed for characteristics that contribute to flock health and profitability and for deficiencies that increase the risk of respiratory disease and production losses.

It is implicit that the management strategies that minimize risk of respiratory disease at the lowest cost should be put in place first. Because management strategies to prevent or minimize respiratory disease are part of the overall production strategy, it is recommended that the veterinarian utilize a software program to facilitate consultation with the producer. The power of the computer to account quickly for changes in a number of variables as they affect net return rapidly provides estimates of the potential financial impact of implementing agreed-upon strategies. By considering two or three scenarios and reviewing the print-outs, the veterinarian and producer can jointly agree on one or more strategies that can yield profound benefit to the production unit at an affordable price that fits the prevailing economic realities of the sheep industry.

BIBLIOGRAPHY

Alley MR, Clarke JK: The effect of chemotherapeutic agents on the transmission of ovine chronic non-progressive pneumonia. N Z Vet J 28:77–80, 1980.
Davies DH, Davis GB, McSporron KD, et al: Vaccination against ovine pneumonia: a progress report. N Z Vet J 31:87–90, 1983.
Gilmour NJL, Martin WB, Sharp JM, et al: The development of vaccines against pneumonic pasteurellosis in sheep. Vet Rec 3:15, 1979.
Gilmour NJL, Sharp JM, Gilmour JS: Effect of oxytetracycline therapy on experimentally induced pneumonic pasteurellosis in lambs. Vet Rec 111:97–99, 1982.
Gilmour NJL, Qurie M, Jones GE: Metaphylactic use of long acting oxytetracycline in pasteurellosis in lambs. Vet Rec 123:443–444, 1988.
Malone FE: Causes of mortality and loss of production in housed lambs. The Veterinary Annual 30:64–71, 1990.
Rodger JL: Parainfluenza 3 vaccination of sheep. Vet Rec 125:453–456, 1989.
Salsbury DL: Control of respiratory disease and border disease in sheep. Vet Med 79:401–404, 1984.
Thurley DC, Boyes BW, Davies DH, et al: Subclinical pneumonia in lambs. N Z Vet J 25:173–176, 1977.
Wells PW, Robinson GT, Gilmour NJL, et al: Vet Rec 114:266–269, 1984.

Parasites of the Respiratory System

ROBERT K. RIDLEY, DVM, PhD

LUNGWORMS

Although lungworms are found in cattle, sheep, pigs, and goats, the most important parasite of the respiratory system in food animals worldwide is *Dictyocaulus viviparus*, the only lungworm found in cattle. In the United States, dictyocauliasis has been reported sporadically from different parts of the country but is most often associated with cool, moist climates. *D. viviparus* larvae have been reported to survive winters on heavily contaminated pastures as far north as Canada, so extensive movement of cattle may result in clinical dictyocauliasis in areas where formerly it was not considered a problem. *D. filaria*, *Muellerius capillaris*, and *Protostrongylus rufescens* are found in sheep and goats. *D. filaria* has about the same distribution as *D. viviparus; Muellerius* occurs infrequently; and *Protostrongylus* is uncommon in domesticated animals in the United States and Canada. *Metastrongylus apri* is the most common lungworm found in pigs.

Life Cycle

Female *D. viviparus* in the trachea and bronchi produce embryonated eggs, which are coughed up, swallowed, and usually hatch while still in the digestive tract, so L_1 larvae are found in fresh bovine feces. Under favorable conditions, first-stage larvae develop to the infective third stage in less than a week. A coprophilous fungus (*Pilobolus* spp.) greatly facilitates the spread of larvae on pasture. The infective larvae ascend the fungus as it grows on the dung pat and invade the sporangia. When the sporangia rupture, the infective larvae are dispersed with the fungal spores. Cattle are infected when they ingest infective third-stage larvae from contaminated pastures. The third-stage larvae penetrate the intestine and migrate via the lymphatics to the mesenteric lymph nodes, where they molt to the fourth stage and gain access to the blood vascular system. From here they are carried to the lungs and penetrate the alveoli. Adult worms are found in the trachea and bronchi. It takes 3 or 4 weeks for worms to reach maturity and start producing larvae. Mature females are up to 80 mm long; males are smaller, with long, heavy spicules. The life cycle of *D. filaria* is essentially the same as that of *D. viviparus*.

The metastrongylid nematodes, unlike *Dictyocaulus*, have indirect life cycles and require intermediate hosts. *Muellerius* and *Protostrongylus* use mollusks (land snails or slugs), and *Metastrongylus* requires an earthworm. Transplacental transmission of *P. rufescens* apparently occurs in sheep, because larvae have been found in ovine fetuses and newborn lambs.

Pathogenesis

Larvae migrating through the alveoli and bronchioles produce an inflammatory response, which may block small bronchi and bronchioles with inflammatory exudate. The bronchi contain fluid and immature worms; later adult worms and the exudate they produce also block the bronchi. Secondary bacterial pneumonia and concurrent viral infection are often complications of dictyocauliasis. It has recently been found that prior infection with *Ostertagia* sp. and *Cooperia* sp. exacerbate subsequent lungworm infections in cattle, whether or not the worms were in the gut at the time. *D. viviparus* recovered from animals previously infected with these two gastrointestinal worms were more numerous and larger than lungworms recovered from cattle that did not have the *Ostertagia* and *Cooperia* infection. Although the mechanism of this is not fully known, it is tempting to speculate that other trichostrongylid nematodes can also influence the course of lungworm infection in cattle.

Clinical Signs

Clinical signs of dictyocauliasis range from none to a mild cough with no loss of condition through a more severe cough, rapid weight loss, and death. Clinical disease is most frequently seen in young animals, 4 to 6 months of age, running at pasture. Because the larvae migrate through the lymphatics, a good immunologic response is usually seen. The disease lasts only 3 or 4 weeks if few larvae are ingested and acute disease does not occur. Subacute forms of this verminous pneumonia do not result in heavy death losses, but the lungs may be badly affected. Treatment will rid the host of the parasites but does not necessarily result in resolving the lesions. *D. filaria* causes a severe parasitic bronchitis in sheep (husk, verminous pneumonia). *M. apri* produces similar signs in pigs.

Diagnosis

Although clinical signs in endemic areas may be suggestive of dictyocauliasis, definitive antemortem diagnosis depends on finding the first-stage larvae in fresh feces. (*Dictyocaulus* larvae are the only nematode larvae found in rectal samples of bovine feces.) Larval recovery is usually done with a Baermann exam, although some investigators feel that zinc sulfate flotation is equally or more effective. Practitioners should be aware that it is necessary to set up Baermann exams shortly after feces are passed because first-stage *Dictyocaulus* larvae become lethargic quickly and are not recovered in Baermann funnels after being subjected to refrigerator temperatures. In our laboratory, just holding fecal samples in obstetric sleeves at room temperture overnight significantly reduced the recovery of L_1 larvae by the Baermann technique. Obtaining rectal samples will obviate the need to distinguish L_1 *Dictyocaulus* larvae from free-living larvae found as normal inhabitants of soil. It should also be noted that larvae will not be found when the disease is due to immature worms.

Adults are easily found in the trachea and bronchi at necropsy, but finding immature stages usually necessitates dissecting the pulmonary tissue and either allowing it to set in physiologic saline or using the Baermann technique with physiologic saline.

Antemortem diagnosis of *Muellerius* and *Protostrongylus* also depends on finding larvae in the feces. In sheep it is necessary to differentiate between *D. filaria*, *Muellerius*, and *Protostrongylus*. *D. filaria* first-stage larvae are 0.5 mm in length and have a distinct "knob" on the anterior end. *Muellerius* and *Protostrongylus* L_1 larvae are shorter, about 0.3 mm in length.

Epidemiology

Arrested development (hypobiosis) is a phenomenon usually associated with *Ostertagia ostertagi*. It has also been found that *D. viviparus* can arrest in the lungs of animals early in the fifth stage (adult). Animals that harbor arrested stages do not show clinical signs and are "silent carriers." Arrested immature worms are thought to constitute a part of naturally acquired lungworm infections and result in pasture contamination when conditions become favorable for their survival. Because hypobiosis has been demonstrated in *D. viviparus*, one cannot assume that pastures are safe in spring after a severe winter. Silent carriers may carry the infection through other times when larvae would be unlikely to survive on pasture, for example, a hot, dry summer.

Because most animals at pasture carry both *Ostertagia* and *Cooperia* infestations, bringing cattle from areas where lungworms are endemic to areas where lungworms were formally not a problem may result in economic losses because of the synergistic effects of lungworm infection.

Comparatively few larvae, when ingested by susceptible animals, will result in unsafe pastures over the course of a grazing season. This is because the pasture will become so heavily contaminated with larvae that the infection will be potentially fatal if susceptible calves are introduced and allowed to graze.

Neither of the metastrongylid nematodes (*Muellerius* or *Protostrongylus*) is a major pathogen. Both require land snails or slugs as intermediate hosts, and these are not ingested in large enough numbers to cause serious disease.

Treatment

D. viviparus is one of the few parasites for which an effective vaccine is available, although not in the United States. The vaccine is composed of irradiated larvae that are not killed but that survive long enough to reach the mesenteric lymph nodes and elicit an immune response. Most irradiated larvae die before reaching the lungs; however, some do reach the lungs and produce eggs, so the use of the vaccine in areas not known to be contaminated with *Dictyocaulus* is contraindicated.

Approved anthelmintics for treating *D. viviparus* in nonlactating and beef cattle include albendazole,[1] fenbendazole[2] ivermectin,[3] levamisole,[4-6] and oxfendazole.[7] There are no approved anthelmintics for controlling lungworms in lactating dairy cattle. Ivermectin[8] is now approved as an oral drench for controlling *D. filaria* in sheep and as an injectable against adult *Metastrongylus* spp.[9] in swine. Fenbendazole[10] and levamisole[11] are also approved for use in swine. Albendazole and ivermectin are labeled for use against L_4 and adults of *D. viviparus*, but fenbendazole and levamisole also show efficacy against immature forms. There are no approved anthelmintics for controlling lungworms in goats, but *Muellerius* and *Protostrongylus* infections, because there are few worms involved, usually do not warrant anthelmintic intervention. Choice of anthelmintic will be dictated by whether gastrointestinal nematodes, especially inhibited *Ostertagia*, are present. Ivermectin for sheep is effective against all larval stages of nasal bots (*Oestrus ovis*).

OTHER PARASITES

Oestrus ovis

"Nose bots" are larvae of dipteran flies. These flies are active from late spring until autumn during the hot part of the day and larviposit around the nostrils of sheep. The larvae develop through second and third instars in the frontal and maxillary sinuses of the host. Third-instar larvae crawl out of the sinuses and pupate for 10 to 70 days in the ground. The complete life cycle takes from 2 to 10 months, so there is usually only one cycle per year. When the flies are active, sheep will seek shade, keep their noses to the ground, or try to protect their nostrils in the wool of other sheep. The first instar maggot causes a mucoid to mucopurulent nasal discharge. Because the second- and third-instar larvae have small keratinized oral hooks and ventral spines, these stages can traumatize the nasal mucosa and produce hemorrhages, causing blood in the nasal discharge. If the larvae die in situ they may become calcified or cause abscesses. Occasionally *Oestrus* larvae penetrate through the sinuses to the brain and cause death. Clinically, sheep infested with nose bots will sneeze and shake their heads in futile attempts to dislodge the larvae. Except for nasal secretions noted above, sheep infected with nose bots appear in good health.

Ascaris suum

Although ascarids do not occur as adults in the respiratory system of food animals, migrating larvae can cause verminous pneumonia ("thumps") when they reach the lungs. Ascarid infection is common in swine throughout the United States. *A. suum* females can produce up to 1 million eggs/day, which become infective in 10 to 14 days. Ingested eggs hatch in the small intestine, penetrate the intestinal wall, and are carried by the portal circulation to the liver and then to the lungs. In ascarid-naive pigs 4 to 5 months of age, L_3 larvae migrate to the lungs and cause focal hemorrhages 4 to 6 days postinfection. Clinical signs of verminous pneumonia due to ascarid migration include a soft, moist cough and a tendency toward

---

[1]Valbazen, Valbazen Paste, SmithKline Animal Health, West Chester, PA 19350.
[2]Panacur, Safe-Guard, Hoechst Roussel Agri-Vet Co., Somerville, NJ 08876.
[3]Ivomec, Merck Sharp and Dohme Research Laboratories, Rahway, NJ 07065.
[4]Tramisole, American Cyanamid Co., Wayne, NJ 07470.
[5]Levasole, Totalon, Pitman Moore Co., Kansas City, KS 66103.
[6]Ripercol, Cyanamid Agric. de Puerto Rico, Manati, PR 00701.
[7]Synanthic, Syntex Animal Health, Inc., Palo Alto, CA 94304.
[8]Ivomec for Sheep, Merck Sharp and Dohme Research Laboratories, Rahway, NJ 07065.
[9]Ivomec for Swine, Merck Sharp and Dohme Research Laboratories, Rahway, NJ 07065.
[10]Safe-Guard Premix, Hoechst Roussel Agri-Vet Co., Somerville, NJ 08876.
[11]Ripercol-L, Cyanamid Agric. de Puerto Rico, Manati, PR 00701.

abdominal breathing. Older pigs that are reinfected show fewer lung lesions and fewer clinical signs, indicating an immune response to the migrating larvae. Controversy exists as to whether larvae migrating through the lungs increase susceptibility to pneumonic pathogens. Recent evidence suggests that respiratory diseases contribute more significantly to average daily gain (ADG) and favorable feed conversion ratios than ascariasis does.

Cattle grazing areas previously occupied by pigs may become infected with *A. suum* and develop an acute, atypical pneumonia that may be fatal.

Continuous feeding of pyrantel tartrate[12] in the feed (96 g/ton) is effective in preventing migrating larvae from reaching the lungs. Ivermectin (300 µg/kg) for swine will also control migrating L_4 larvae.

---

[12]Banminth-48 Premix, Pfizer, Inc., Lee's Summit, MO 64063.

BIBLIOGRAPHY

Courtney CH, Sundlof SF: Veterinary Antiparasitic Drugs—1990. American Association of Veterinary Parasitologists; Institute of Food and Agricultural Sciences, University of Florida, Gainesville, FL.
Eddi CS, Williams JC, Swalley RA: Epidemiology of *Dictyocaulus viviparus* in Louisiana (U.S.A.). Vet Parasitol 31:37–38, 1989.
Gupta RP, Gibbs HC: Epidemiological investigations on *Dictyocaulus viviparus* (Bloch, 1782) infection in cattle. Can Vet J 11:149–156, 1970.
Kloosterman A, Ploeger HW, Frankena K: Increased establishment of lungworms after exposure to a combined infection of *Ostertagia ostertagi* and *Cooperia oncophora*. Vet Parasitol 36:117–122, 1990.

Respiratory Tract Diagnostic Methods

JEROME G. VESTWEBER, DVM, PhD

Respiratory signs can be associated with either respiratory or cardiovascular diseases. In addition, clinical respiratory signs may also be associated with systemic infectious diseases, toxemia, central nervous system disturbances, neoplasms of the thoracic cavity, poisoning, acid-base imbalance, diaphragmatic hernias, and pleuritis. Thus it is important to do a thorough physical examination and supportive laboratory tests to determine if respiratory signs are due only to primary respiratory tract disease.

The next decision in the diagnostic plan is determination of the involved respiratory tract segment. This may be established by observing the character of respiratory effort. The time ratio for inspiration and expiration is approximately 1:1, with a very short pause at the end of expiration. An increased inspiratory phase is commonly associated with upper respiratory tract disease and some forms of bronchopneumonia. An increased expiratory phase is commonly associated with pulmonary emphysema, pleuritis, hydrothorax, or diaphragmatic hernia. When both the inspiratory and the expiratory phases of respiration are increased, bronchopneumonia is the likely cause. Audible sounds are also helpful in establishing what segment is involved with disease. Normal breathing usually produces no audible sounds, whereas stenotic sounds are produced by constriction of the upper respiratory tract and are sometimes called stridor. Snorting can occur when there is nasal mucosal swelling, a collection of exudates, a foreign body, or a neoplasm. The sound produced by pharyngeal stenosis is called snoring and can be produced by pharyngeal constriction from diseases such as retropharyngeal lymph node enlargement, abscesses of the pharyngeal wall, or generalized pharyngeal cellulitis. Laryngeal stenosis produces roaring and is usually caused by inflammatory, edematous, purulent, or necrotic lesions of the laryngeal mucosa. Stenosis of the trachea can produce a loud purring sound, which can be localized by compression or auscultation along the trachea. This sound can be caused by extreme swelling of the tracheal mucosa or collapse of tracheal rings. Groaning may accompany expiration when there is extensive emphysema or another painful lesion within the thoracic or abdominal cavity.

AUSCULTATION AND PERCUSSION OF LUNGS

Auscultation and percussion are useful diagnostic procedures, provided pathologic interpretations can be made from the sounds. A good quality stethoscope should be used in quiet surroundings. A routine should be established for auscultating the lung field, keeping in mind that a major area of the lung beneath the front legs cannot be readily evaluated. At each site one should listen for at least one or two breath sounds. To amplify any abnormal breathing sounds, deep respiratory efforts can be produced by placing a plastic bag loosely over the muzzle of the animal. Progress cranial to caudal over the lung field in a horizontal plane, repeating the steps in a more dorsal plane, while making mental notes of audible differences in lung sounds between dorsal and ventral regions of the lung. The anatomic location of major bronchi should be kept in mind when interpreting lung sounds. The left lung field should be compared with the right because often one lung field is more severely involved.

Lung sounds can be divided into breath sounds and adventitious sounds, with the term breath sound applying to any sound that accompanies air movement through the tracheobronchial tree. Breath sounds vary randomly in intensity over a broad range depending on whether the sounds are produced over the larger airways or over the remaining lung parenchyma.

Adventitious sounds are extrinsic to the normal sound-production mechanism of the respiratory tract and are abnormal sounds superimposed upon the breath sounds. It has also been proposed that adventitious sounds be further classified as crackles and wheezes.

Crackles are discontinuous sounds, which have been thought to be produced by equalization of pressure or opening of an airway subserving an atelectatic region of the lung. The reopening of a collapsed airway appears to occur regularly, producing a characteristic shower of short, high-frequency sound. Late inspiratory crackles are often associated with pulmonary edema, interstitial diseases, and fibrosing alveolaritis, whereas early inspiratory or early expiratory crackles are associated with bronchopneumonia and tracheobronchial fluid accumulation.

Wheezes are continuous, musical adventitious sounds that are produced by narrowing and vibration of airway walls or by tissue masses/foreign bodies in close contact with airway walls. Inspiratory wheezes are associated with extrathoracic airway problems such as laryngeal paralysis, collapsing or stenosis of cervical trachea, or other extrathoracic airway obstructions. Expiratory wheezes are associated with intrathoracic airway problems such as pulmonary emphysema, collapsing or stenosis of intrathoracic trachea, and other intrathoracic airway obstructions.

A pleural friction rub is produced by roughened pleural

surfaces and heard during both inspiration and expiration. This sound is associated with a primary pleuritis, pneumonia, or secondary pleuritis. Emphysematous sounds are heard most frequently as a squeak or a whistle following the expiratory effort and are heard most commonly over a bullous area of emphysema.

The absence of respiratory sounds is as important to the diagnostician as the presence of abnormal sounds. No normal lung sounds imply that nonfunctional lung tissue is beneath the stethoscope, provided that the animal is not breathing very shallowly. Pleural effusion, pneumothorax, diaphragmatic hernia, or other space-occupying lesions of the thorax may be responsible for a silent lung.

Percussion is a useful diagnostic procedure when a systematic approach is established and proficiency is obtained. The procedure is useful for making a diagnosis of excessive pleural fluid, pulmonary consolidation, or pulmonary emphysema. Normal resonance will be replaced by dull solid sounds in cases of pleural fluid or pulmonary consolidation. Emphysema produces a tympani-like resonance during percussion.

VIRAL ISOLATION AND IMMUNOFLUORESCENT SPECIMENS FROM THE NASAL CAVITY

Mucous membranes of the nasal cavity are frequently the first tissues to be involved in a viral infection. In response to early infection, viral-infected, live, and dead mucociliary cells are sloughed into the lumen of the nasal cavity and are good specimens for viral isolation or immunofluorescent studies. Samples for virus isolation can be made from nasal secretions by brushing sterile cotton swabs against the wall of the nasal cavity and placing the swab in a viral transport medium[1] to be sent to a diagnostic laboratory. A specimen for immunofluorescence studies can be collected by introducing a chemical spatula approximately 8 to 10 cm into the nasal cavity and lightly rubbing the nasal septum to obtain virus-infected cells. The cells are then transferred gently to clean microscopic slides and submitted for immunofluorescent studies of the common respiratory viral agents.

TRANSTRACHEAL ASPIRATION

Transtracheal aspiration is a valuable method for retrieving cells for cytology, isolating pathogenic bacteria, and identifying the spectrum of antibiotic sensitivity. One technique for this procedure involves restraining the animal, preferably standing, with the head and neck extended dorsally. The ventral midcervical skin area is clipped, surgically prepared, and infiltrated with local anesthetic. One hand is used to grasp the trachea while a small 1-cm incision is made in the skin, an Edwards 5-1/2-inch (14-cm) 9-gauge bleeding trocar in a larger animal is introduced between the tracheal rings, and, depending on the size of the animal, a 90-cm polyethylene tube[2] (PE 260) is passed through the trocar into the trachea. Once the polyethylene tubing is within the trachea, the trocar is removed to prevent incising the tube and then passed distally to a horizontal segment of the trachea. Then 30 ml of sterilized physiologic saline solution is injected via a 15-gauge needle that is placed in the end of the polyethylene tubing. Retrieval of 5 to 10 ml of saline wash is sufficient for cytologic and bacterial identification. Numerous other sterile needle-catheter combinations for transtracheal aspiration are available for sample collection.

BRONCHOPULMONARY LAVAGE

Another method available for study of the cellular constituency or the microbiology of the lung involves bronchopulmonary lavage. The method involves elevating the head with a nose lead, grasping the tongue, and bringing it to the exterior of the mouth, and, with the aid of a laryngoscope, placing a guarded culture instrument[3] into the laryngeal lumen. The cap of the guarded culture instrument and the internal swab stylet are removed, and the external shell remains extending from the laryngeal lumen through the oral cavity to the exterior of the mouth. Depending on the size of the animal, sterile polyethylene tubing with a 2-cm latex rubber tip attached is passed through the guarded culture instrument into the trachea. Passage of the catheter is continued into the smallest airway attainable, which is usually in the right caudal lung lobe. Sterile saline (approximately 25 to 50 cc) can be injected and retrieved for cellular and microbiology studies. Bronchial lavage can also be done during bronchoscopy. This method offers an advantage, in that visual examination of the tracheobronchial tree can be carried out during bronchoscopy in addition to obtaining a bronchial lavage.

THORACOCENTESIS

Significant accumulations of fluid within the thoracic cavity are rare, but fluid can accumulate with fibrinous bronchopneumonia or pleuritis. Following surgical skin preparation, aspiration with an 8-cm 16-gauge needle is best accomplished on the right side of the chest in the fifth or sixth intercostal space, just dorsal or ventral to the humeroradial joint. Any excessive fluid can be removed if necessary, and fluid obtained can be cultured or examined for cell type. Caution needs to be taken to not allow entrance of air into the pleural cavity. If necessary, a thoracic drain tube can be inserted for the continued drainage of fluid and administration of medication.

LUNG TISSUE BIOPSY

It is possible to obtain lung tissue biopsy specimens for histopathologic examination. The necessary equipment consists of a trephine with stylet (13 cm in length and 5 to 6 mm in diameter) and electric hand drill capable of a minimum speed of 2400 rpm. An area of skin in the eighth or ninth intercostal space on either side is shaved, disinfected, and anesthetized. The trephine is inserted as far as the pleura, the stylet is removed, the drill is attached, and a 5-cm incision is made into the lung tissue. A core of lung tissue is aspirated with the aid of a large syringe, containing 5 ml of sodium citrate, and then immediately placed in fixative.

RADIOLOGY

Radiographs can be taken with the animal either standing or lying on its side with forelegs drawn forward. The entire thorax of calves can be done, but only part of the chest can

---

[1]Hank's Balanced Salt Solution, Gibco Laboratories, Grand Island, NY 14072.
[2]Intramedic Polyethylene Tubing, Clay Adams, Division of Becton, Dickinson and Co., Parsippany, NJ 07054.
[3]Kalayjian Industries, Inc., Long Beach, CA 90803.

be examined in adults; also, part of the chest may be covered by the forelimb.

Angiocardiography can be performed to determine the vascular filling of the lungs. This procedure is accomplished by passing a 9 French angiocatheter down the external jugular vein into the pulmonary artery, injecting diatrizoate meglumine[4] rapidly, and taking lateral radiographs at 0.5-second intervals starting at the time of injection.

Scintigraphy of the respiratory system, a nuclear technique used extensively in human medicine, can provide a measure of both total and regional ventilation plus perfusion of each lung. Intravenous injection of technetium-99m–labeled albumin will distribute to the lung capillary bed in direct proportion to the regional blood flow, whereas inhaled 81m krypton gas will allow visualization of pulmonary airways.

OTHER LABORATORY PROCEDURES AND TESTS

Seventy-two hours following the induction of experimental *Pasteurella haemolytica* pneumonia, the total white blood cell count, absolute immature band neutrophil counts, and blood fibrinogen were significantly increased and the neutrophil count was elevated. This supports the thesis that neutrophils are being mobilized to the lung and immature neutrophils are being called upon to contain the infection. Leukopenia or lymphopenia may be seen with an acute uncomplicated case of viral infection. Most of the changes in serum chemistry values associated with respiratory disease are minor and usually do not reflect definite diagnostic significance. With the availability of venous and arterial blood gas analysis, the status of pulmonary function can be determined. Arterial blood gas determinations of pO_2 levels are helpful in monitoring the progress of treatment. Other, more sophisticated lung function tests are confined mostly to research.

Following transtracheal aspiration or bronchopulmonary lavage, specimens for bacterial isolation can be cultured on blood agar or MacConkey agar. Aspirates can also be submitted for a Gram's stain. When available, minimal inhibitory concentrations of the effective antibiotics can be determined to indicate the dose and frequency required to obtain an adequate tissue level. Smears for cytologic evaluation of the aspirate can be made in several ways, but specimens may need to be centrifuged and smears made from the resulting sediment. Air-dried smears can be stained using the common blood stains such as new methylene blue, Wright's stain, Wright-Leishman stain, or Harleco's Diff-Quik.[5] Material obtained from the bronchial aspiration will include cellular elements that normally line the tracheobronchial tree; cells derived from inflammatory, hemorrhagic, congestive, neoplastic, or other pathologic processes; and background material composed of mucus, proteinaceous exudate, or degenerated cells. In many cases the cause of the disease process can be recognized and identified.

SEROLOGIC TESTS FOR VIRUSES AND BACTERIA

A serologic diagnosis can be made most accurately by paired serum samples taken at 2- to 4-week intervals and then demonstrating at best a fourfold rise in titer. A less accurate diagnosis could be made by finding a high titer with only one serum sample taken from 5 or more recovered animals.

Cattle

Infectious Bovine Rhinotracheitis (IBR)–Serum Neutralization

Maternal antibody titers will last from 2 to 6 months. Following aerosol exposure to IBR, cattle will develop serum antibodies to the virus by 21 days and maximum levels of serum antibodies (titers of 1:16 to 1:256) by 28 days after exposure. Re-exposure will result in a two- to fourfold increase in titer. Infective titers will last for 6 months to 1 year. Serum titers resulting from intranasal vaccination are commonly less than 1:4, whereas intramuscular vaccination results in serum titers of 1:4 to 1:16.

Bovine Virus Diarrhea–Serum Neutralization

Immunologic tolerance can exist and can result in a very low serum antibody titer or no titer, even though severe infection exists with the virus. Infective titers often range from 1:64 to greater than 1:256 and last for 1 year or longer. Vaccination titers for the commercial C24V and NADL vaccines range from 1:8 to 1:64 at 21 days following administration.

Parainfluenza-3 Virus

Circulating serum antibody titers after viral exposure most commonly range from 1:32 to 1:512, with maximal concentrations at 14 to 20 days following exposure.

Bovine Respiratory Syncytial Virus

Infective titers commonly range from 1:64 to 1:640. Vaccination titers will range from 1:64 to 1:512 at 21 days following vaccination.

DN599 (Herpes 4) Virus

Infective titers range from 1:10 to greater than 1:2400 by the indirect fluorescent antibody test.

Pasteurella haemolytica

Serum antibody titers to *P. haemolytica* measured with the indirect hemagglutination procedures are usually not significantly different among calves that develop respiratory tract disease as compared with those that remain healthy.

Mycoplasma spp.

Indirect hemagglutination titers of 1:20 or more are assumed to reflect recent or current exposure to *M. bovis* or *M. dispar*.

Haemophilus somnus

Titers of 1:256 to 1:512 (in nonvaccinated herds) may be a result of early active or chronic infection. Titers of 1:1040 to 1:4096 are indicative of recent active infection. Vaccination can result in titers of 1:64 to 1:128 and in increases to 1:256 after booster injection. Paired serum samples with fourfold changes of titer indicate active infection.

---

[4] Renografin-60, E. R. Squibb and Sons, Inc., Princeton, NJ 08540.
[5] Diff-Quik, American Scientific Products, Kansas City, MO 64116.

Swine

Pseudorabies and Swine Influenza

A titer of 1:4 for pseudorabies is considered positive in many states, whereas hemagluttination inhibition (HAI) titers of 1:360 to 1:20,000 are considered positive for swine influenza. An HAI titer of 1:1000 to 1:20,000 is considered positive for parvovirus, whereas vaccination will produce a titer of 1:1000 at 1 month (but this will drop to less than 1:400 by 60 days following vaccination).

Sheep

Parainfluenza-3, Ovine Progressive Interstitial Pneumonia, Bovine Viral Diarrhea, and Respiratory Syncytial Viruses

These viruses are currently considered to be important in respiratory disease and are being diagnosed by serology. In addition, the adenovirus, infectious bovine rhinotracheitis, and bluetongue viruses, which appear to have minor importance, can also be diagnosed.

BIBLIOGRAPHY

Dungworth DL, Hoare MN: Trephine lung biopsy in cattle and horses. Res Vet Sci 11:244, 1970.
Frank GH, Smith PC: Prevalence of *Pasteurella haemolytica* in transported calves. Am J Vet Res 44:981–985, 1983.
Goyal SM, Khan MA, McPherson SW, et al: Prevalence of antibodies to seven viruses in a flock of ewes in Minnesota. Am J Vet Res 49:464–467, 1988.
Kotikoff MI, Gillespie JR: Lung sounds in veterinary medicine. Part I. Terminology and mechanisms of sound production. Compend Contin Educ Pract Vet 5:634–639, 1983.
Kotikoff MI, Gillespie JR: Lung sounds in veterinary medicine. Part II. Deriving clinical information from lung sounds. Compend Contin Educ Pract Vet 6:462–467, 1984.
Martin SW, Lumsden JH: The relationship of hematology and serum chemistry parameters to treatment of respiratory disease and weight gain in Ontario feedlot calves. Can J Vet Res 51:499–505, 1987.
McGuirk SM: Internal medicine diagnostics—thoracic cavity. Bovine Proc 15:69, 1983.
Phillips RM: Interpretation of serological results received from the diagnostic laboratory. Proc Ann Conf Vet, Kansas State University, 1983, p H-1.
Rosendal S, Martin SW: The association between serological evidence of mycoplasma infection and respiratory disease in feedlot calves. Can J Vet Res 50:179–183, 1986.
Roudebush P, Ryan J: Breath sound terminology in the veterinary literature. J Am Vet Med Assoc 194:1415–1417, 1989.
Sanfacon D, Higgins R: Epidemiology of *Haemophilus somnus* infection in dairy cattle in Quebec. Can J Comp Med 47:456–459, 1983.
Vestweber JG, Klemm RD, Leipold HW, et al: Experimental *Pasteurella haemolytica* pneumonia: clinical and pathological studies. Am J Vet Res 50:1792–1798, 1990.

Respiratory Therapeutics
CHARLES A. HJERPE, DVM

The general objectives of respiratory system therapy are as follows:

1. Control of bacterial infections (discussed in the section on bacterial diseases).
2. Removal of causes of respiratory tract irritation.
3. Maintenance of normal intrapleural pressures.
4. Maintenance of airway patency.
5. Maintenance of tracheobronchial clearance.
6. Maintenance of adequate arterial oxygenation and carbon dioxide removal.

Table 1 presents drugs used for respiratory problems.

REMOVAL OF CAUSES OF RESPIRATORY TRACT IRRITATION

Animals affected with respiratory tract disease should not be exposed to irritants such as dust, smoke, or ammonia gas. If barns are used to house such animals, these structures must be adequately and uniformly ventilated so as to achieve a minimum of four air changes per hour. It is also important to avoid draftiness, extreme temperatures, and marked temperature fluctuations. Cattle affected with extrinsic allergic alveolitis (bovine farmer's lung) should not be fed moldy hay, especially within a closed air space, and dusty feeds should be avoided regardless of the etiology of the condition.

Medicinal cough suppression is rarely, if ever, necessary in the food animal species. It is usually contraindicated, as tracheobronchial clearance is assisted by the cough reflex. Administration of corticosteroids for control of respiratory tract irritation and coughing may lead to respiratory secretion retention. Administration of analgesics may have a similarly deleterious effect.

MAINTENANCE OF NORMAL INTRAPLEURAL PRESSURES

When pleural effusion is diagnosed, thoracentesis and drainage are indicated, although rapid refilling is to be expected. Indwelling chest tubes can be utilized when refilling is a problem. When thick exudates are present that cannot be removed with a chest tube, and when the condition is unilateral, thoracotomy can be performed in cattle by removing the lower portion of the fifth rib. The pleural space is flushed twice daily (for several weeks), until the wound closes by granulation.

Intrapleural instillation of antimicrobial drugs is unnecessary for treatment of infectious pleural disease, since all but polymyxin B cross the pleural membrane readily from the blood stream. Intrapleural administration of aminoglycoside antibiotics (dihydrostreptomycin, neomycin, kanamycin, gentamicin) is contraindicated because of the risk of respiratory arrest from neuromuscular blockade.

MAINTENANCE OF AIRWAY PATENCY

Glucocorticoids are used in the management of acute, severe necrotic laryngitis in cattle to help maintain airway patency while antimicrobial therapy is used to control the bacterial infection. Flumethasone is administered by intravenous or intramuscular injection in a dose of 1 mg/45 kg body weight. A single treatment with a glucocorticoid is usually sufficient.

Parasitic bronchitis in cattle can be treated with levamisole phosphate, administered by subcutaneous injection, or levamisole hydrochloride, administered orally as a drench, bolus, gel, or in feed in a dose of 8 mg/kg body weight. A levamisole cutaneous pour-on formulation requires a dose of 10 mg/kg body weight. Fenbendazole is effective as a drench, paste, or in feed in a dose of 5 mg/kg body weight. Albendazole is effective as a drench or paste in a dose of 10 mg/kg body weight. Ivermectin is effective in a dose of 200 µg/kg body weight when injected subcutaneously, or in a dose of 500 µg/kg body weight when administered as a pour-on foundation.

Table 1. DRUG LIST OF RESPIRATORY MEDICATIONS

Generic Name	Proprietary Name	Manufacturer/Distributor	Species	Classification	Dose	Route	Withdrawal Period Slaughter (days)	Milk (hr)
Acetylcysteine	Mucomyst	Meade Johnson Pharmaceutical Division 2404 W. Pennsylvania St. Evansville, IN 47721	Any	UA[a]	140 mg/kg (loading); 70 mg/kg (maintenance)	I[b]	—	—
Albendazole	Valbazen	SmithKline Beecham Animal Health Products 501 5th St. Bristol, TN 37620	Bovine	OTC[c]	10 mg/kg	O[d]	27	NA[e]
Doxapram hydrochloride	Dopram-V Injectable	A.H. Robins Co. 1407 Cumings Dr. Richmond, VA 23220	Any	UA	Variable[f] (0.2 mg/kg)	IV, SC	—	—
Epinephrine Injection, USP 1:1000	—	—	Any	UA	5 ml/454 kg	IV[g]	Zero	Zero
Fenbendazole	Safe-Guard	Hoechst-Roussel Agri-Vet Co. Sommerville, NJ 08876	Bovine, Porcine	OTC	5 mg/kg (bovine); 9 mg/kg fed over 3–12 days (swine)	O	8 (cattle) zero (swine)	NA
Flumethasone	Flucort Solution	Syntex Animal Health, Inc. 4800 Westown Pkwy., Suite 200 West Des Moines, IA 50265	Bovine	UA	5 mg/45 kg	IV, IM[h]	Zero	Zero
Furosemide diethanolamine	Lasix Injectable Solution	Hoechst-Roussel Agri-Vet Co. Sommerville, NJ 08876	Bovine	Rx[i]	500 mg/454 kg	IV, IM	2	48
Ivermectin	Ivomec	MSD AgVet P.O. Box 2000 Rahway, NJ 07065	Bovine, ovine, porcine	OTC	200 mcg/kg (bovine and ovine); 300 mcg/kg (porcine)	SC (bovine and porcine); O (ovine)	35 (bovine) 11 (ovine) 18 (porcine)	NA
Levamisole	Tramisole	American Cyanamid Co. One Cyanamid Plaza Wayne, NJ 07470	Bovine, ovine, porcine	OTC	8 mg/kg (O,SC) 10 mg/kg (PO[j])	O (bovine, ovine, porcine) SC, PO[j] (bovine)	2 (bovine-O); 3 (ovine and porcine-O); 6 (bovine-O-gel); 7 (bovine-SC); 9 (bovine-PO); 11 (porcine-O-gel)	NA

[a] UA = Unapproved drug.
[b] I = Inhalation administration.
[c] OTC = Over-the-counter food animal drug.
[d] O = Oral administration.
[e] NA = Not approved for use in lactating dairy cattle.
[f] Dosage is variable, depending on depth of anesthesia, respiratory volume, and respiratory rate.
[g] IV = Intravenous administration.
[h] IM = Intramuscular administration.
[i] Rx = Prescription legend food animal drug.
[j] PO = Pour-on cutaneous administration.

Parasitic bronchitis in sheep and swine is treated by oral administration of levamisole hydrochloride or fenbendazole or by subcutaneous injection (swine) or drenching (sheep) with ivermectin.

Tracheotomy may be indicated in cases of impending upper respiratory tract obstruction from necrotic laryngitis, actinobacillosis, pharyngeal abscessation, facial snakebite, nasal bone fractures, and so on. Laryngospasm and bronchospasm are not recognized as clinical entities in the food animal species.

MAINTENANCE OF TRACHEOBRONCHIAL CLEARANCE

A "clean," patent tracheobronchial tree is essential for normal gas exchange. Tracheobronchial exudates are cleared by the mucociliary apparatus, assisted by the cough reflex. Drying, thickening, and subsequent retention of tracheobronchial secretions may result from systemic dehydration, administration of nonhumidified oxygen, insertion of a tracheotomy tube, or prolonged treatment with anticholinergics. Use of corticosteroids may cause decreased tracheobronchial clearance and immunosuppression.

Clearance of thick exudates may be facilitated by inhalation therapy using ultrasonic nebulization of physiologic saline solution. The objective is to loosen and liquify the exudates by increasing the volume and reducing the viscosity of tracheobronchial fluids. Ultrasonic nebulizers produce tiny droplets that reach the lower respiratory tract. Mucolytic agents (such as acetylcysteine [Mucomyst]) and antibiotics can be administered, along with moisture, but are no longer considered efficacious and may be irritating. For nebulization to be effective, patients should be nebulized for 30 to 45 minutes on three to six occasions per day. Inhalation therapy is usually palliative rather than curative and is generally impractical in food animals because of the problems of restraint and the close supervision required. Newborn animals can be treated in nebulization cages designed for dogs and cats.

Steam humidification therapy is most effective in clearing nasal and laryngeal exudates, as little moisture actually reaches the tracheobronchial membrane. Bubble humidifiers are ineffective for therapeutic purposes. Expectorants are now considered to be ineffective for improving tracheobronchial clearance.

Maintenance of a normal state of systemic hydration and normal blood pressures are the most effective and practical strategies for assisting tracheobronchial clearance in food animal patients. Caution should be exercised, however, since overhydration by overzealous intravenous fluid therapy may result in pulmonary edema.

MAINTENANCE OF ADEQUATE ARTERIAL OXYGENATION AND CARBON DIOXIDE REMOVAL

Clinical signs that indicate possible need for oxygen (O_2) therapy include tachypnea, dyspnea, cyanosis, and tachycardia. However, an arterial partial pressure of O_2 value of less than 70 to 80 mm Hg is the definitive indicator of a possible need for O_2 therapy. O_2 therapy is indicated in anoxic anoxia from inadequate ventilation or severe lung disease. It is not likely to be beneficial in anemic anoxia, stagnant anoxia, or histotoxic anoxia. When stagnant anoxia results from hypovolemia or from peripheral vasodilation (shock), restoration of normal blood pressures by vigorous intravenous fluid therapy is indicated in addition to O_2 therapy.

O_2 therapy is usually impractical in food animals because of cost, problems of restraint, and the close supervision required. O_2 has been administered to valuable cattle by means of an O_2 therapy mask or nasal tube using flow rates of 12 L/minute and 4 to 8 L/minute/90 kg body weight, respectively. The nasal tube should be inserted to a point one third of the way from the lateral canthus of the eye to the base of the ear. The newborn can be treated in nebulization or oxygen cages designed for dogs and cats.

Hypoxia from inadequate ventilation is usually the result of anesthetic overdose and depression of the medullary respiratory center. Intubation and mechanical ventilation with O_2 or with a mixture of O_2 and 5 to 10 per cent carbon dioxide (CO_2) and/or intravenous administration of an analeptic, such as doxapram, is indicated. Use of combined O_2:CO_2 therapy can increase the depth of respirations, improve intake of O_2, improve pulmonary circulation, and reduce pulmonary congestion. In treating severe lung disease, ultrasonic nebulization therapy and O_2 therapy may be combined. O_2, together with artificial respiration, may be of value in helping to revive unconscious neonatal animals following dystocia.

MISCELLANEOUS OBJECTIVES IN RESPIRATORY SYSTEM MEDICATION

Epinephrine is specific for treatment of acute pulmonary edema from anaphylaxis in cattle. Epinephrine is administered in 1:1000 concentration by intravenous injection in a dose 5 ml/450 kg body weight.

Glucocorticoids appear to be of value in the treatment of atypical interstitial pneumonia and acute bovine pulmonary emphysema (3-methylindole toxicosis). Flumethasone is administered once daily by subcutaneous or intramuscular injection in a dose of 5 mg/45 kg body weight until expiratory dyspnea is controlled, or for 3 days. If dyspnea is present on day 4, flumethasone therapy is continued in a reduced daily dosage of 1 mg/45 kg body weight until dyspnea is controlled, or for 4 additional days. Virtually all animals that respond will do so within 7 days.

Diuretics such as furosemide may be of value, together with glucocorticoids, in the management of early cases of acute bovine pulmonary emphysema (3-methylindole toxicosis). Furosemide is administered twice daily by intravenous or intramuscular injection or oral boluses in a dose of 2.2 to 4.4 mg/kg body weight.

BIBLIOGRAPHY

Blood DC, Radostits OM: Veterinary Medicine, 7th ed. London, Bailliere Tindall, 1989, pp 361–363.
McKiernan BC: Principles of respiratory therapy. In Kirk RW (ed): Current Veterinary Therapy VIII: Small Animal Practice. Philadelphia, WB Saunders, 1983, pp 216–221.

SECTION 11
Diseases of the Circulatory System

DONALD R. CLARK, DVM, PhD, Diplomate, ACVIM, Consulting Editor

Cardiovascular Pathophysiology

DONALD R. CLARK, DVM, PhD, Diplomate, ACVIM

EVENTS OF THE CARDIAC CYCLE

Each heartbeat with its associated bioelectric and mechanical events is termed a cardiac cycle. The cardiac cycle is divisible into phases of ventricular systole (contraction or emptying) and ventricular diastole (relaxation and filling). The interrelated events of venous, atrial, ventricular, and arterial pressure along with ventricular volume, heart sounds, and the electrocardiogram are depicted in Figure 1.

HEART SOUNDS DURING THE CARDIAC CYCLE

Vibrations produced during a cardiac cycle give rise to heart sounds (Table 1). The first heart sound ("lubb") is associated with atrioventricular valve (mitral and tricuspid) closure as systole begins. The second sound ("dupp") is due to closure of the semilunar valves (aortic and pulmonic) as ventricular diastole begins. The third and fourth sounds, related to rapid ventricular filling and to atrial systole, respectively, are not ordinarily audible but may be heard in circumstances such as A-V block or congestive heart failure.

In heart failure, exaggeration of the normally inaudible sounds produces a triplicate sound or cadence described as a gallop rhythm. A gallop rhythm is convincing evidence of congestive right or left heart failure and thus is a significant clinical finding.

Table 1. ABNORMAL HEART SOUNDS AND THEIR LIKELY CAUSES

Sound	Likely Causes
Splitting of second	Systemic or pulmonic hypertension
Accentuation of third or fourth ("gallop rhythm")	Congestive heart failure
Systolic murmur	Anemia, atrial septal defect, ventricular septal defect, aortic or pulmonic stenosis, mitral or tricuspid regurgitation
Diastolic murmur	Aortic or pulmonic insufficiency
Continuous murmur	Patent ductus arteriosus

CARDIAC MURMURS

Additional sounds generated in the heart and great vessels are murmurs and result from turbulent flow of blood. The turbulent or disturbed blood flow most frequently occurs as a result of change in the structure of the heart and vessels. Murmurs are systolic if they occur between the first and second heart sounds and diastolic if they occur between the second and the following first sound. Continuous murmurs may span the entire cardiac cycle.

NORMAL AND ABNORMAL CARDIAC OUTPUT

At rest the heart pumps a basal volume of flow proportionate to the animal's body size. The cardiac index, a general estimate of basal output, is approximately 3 to 3.5 L/M²/minute. Increases from this index are promoted by exercise, as neural and humoral influences increase heart rate or stroke volume or both. The combination of increased cardiac output and greater extraction of oxygen allows oxygen delivery to tissues to increase during exercise by as much as 15-fold in healthy animals. Acute failure to deliver basal cardiac output produces

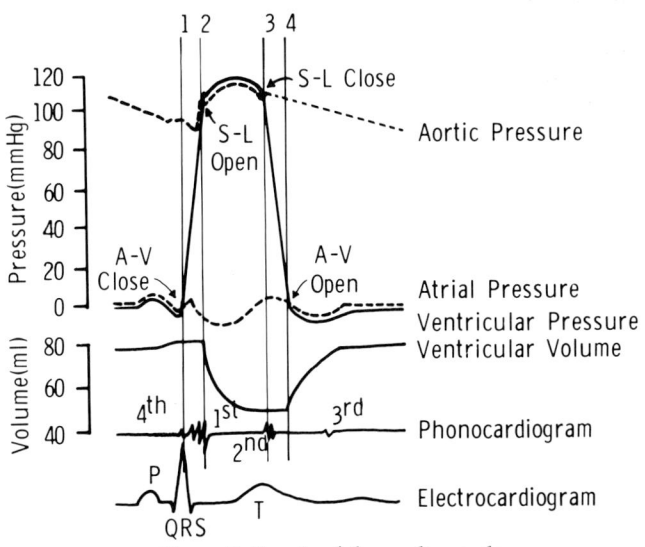

Figure 1. Events of the cardiac cycle.

circulatory shock; a more progressive and chronic inability to sustain adequate flow is the basis for congestive heart failure.

MICROCIRCULATION AND EDEMA

Fluid is forced from capillary walls into the interstitial spaces in the initial portion of the capillaries and reenters the capillary largely in the distal or venous end. The balance of hydrostatic and osmotic pressures assures that accumulation of interstitial fluids will not be excessive. Tissue edema results from abnormal increases in interstitial fluid protein concentration or from hypoproteinemia, either of which reduces the effective plasma colloid osmotic pressure. Edema may also result from an increased venous pressure as seen in congestive heart failure, or whenever lymph drainage is impaired.

BIBLIOGRAPHY

Ettinger SJ: Textbook of Veterinary Internal Medicine, 2nd ed. Philadelphia, WB Saunders, 1983.
Jubb KVF, Kenney PC: Pathology of Domestic Animals, 2nd ed. New York, Academic Press, 1970.

Diseases of the General Circulation

DONALD R. CLARK, DVM, PhD, Diplomate, ACVIM

CIRCULATORY SHOCK

Pathophysiology and Etiology

Circulatory shock is defined as a severe insufficiency in capillary perfusion. Usual causes of circulatory shock are marked depletion of extracellular fluid volume (hypovolemic), loss of effective cardiac pumping action (cardiogenic), or excessive alteration in the caliber of vessels (vasculogenic). The effective circulatory blood volume may be diminished by actual loss of blood or plasma or by sequestration of blood in widely dilated vessels. Table 1 provides an etiologic classification of shock.

Thus shock may result from such diverse causes as loss of blood (20 ml/kg or greater), acute emesis or diarrhea, myocardial depression, and vascular effects of circulating endotoxins from *Escherichia coli* and other organisms.

Clinical Signs of Circulatory Shock

Certain signs of circulatory shock relate to etiologic factors such as hypovolemia or endotoxin, while others result from physiologic responses, principally autonomic nervous system activity (Table 2).

Therapy of Circulatory Shock

Early and effective correction of circulatory volume deficit is mandatory in shock therapy. Repletion of circulating fluid volume is most urgent in hypovolemic shock. The need for large volumes of fluids in shock involves the following considerations: (1) fluid losses may be hidden or inapparent, (2) capillary permeability may be increased, (3) loss of vascular tone may necessitate a greater than normal filling volume, (4) limited vascular overfilling (hypervolemia) ensures optimal stroke volume and cardiac output and, (5) crystalloid or electrolyte solutions given intravenously are distributed largely to the interstitial compartment and are retained in vessels only to a limited extent, perhaps 25 per cent of the total. Fluids may be given according to some predetermined dosage or, better, in amounts and at rates shown to be appropriate by central venous pressure (CVP) monitoring. If plasma protein concentrations are not severely reduced, fluids may be safely given until CVP reaches 5 to 10 cm H_2O.

Blood, Plasma, and Plasma Expanders

Homologous blood may be of value if significant hemorrhage has occurred and before severe shock with capillary sludging and microthrombi formation related to disseminated intravascular coagulation (DIC) has ensued. If blood transfusions are elected, the blood administration should be accompanied by infusion of balanced electrolytes. Most effective is 20 to 40 ml/kg of whole blood accompanied by two to six times this volume of balanced electrolytes.

Plasma is quite satisfactory for expansion of the blood volume. Plasma expanders such as dextrans are also effective, particularly dextran 70 solutions. Dextran 70 offers advantages of enhancing fluid shifts into vascular spaces and of preventing capillary sludging and DIC during severe shock states. Its chief disadvantage is high cost of treatment in large animals. An effective dosage is 4 to 10 ml/kg along with electrolyte solutions.

Electrolyte Solutions

Treatment of shock should be based on volume expansion in order to achieve optimal cardiac filling, cardiac output, capillary perfusion, and urine output. Ideally this is accomplished by monitoring the CVP as fluids are administered. In this way fluids can be given vigorously until CVP reaches 5 to 10 cm H_2O. It is unlikely that pulmonary edema or other complications will occur if fluids are given under CVP guidance. Ringer's lactate is preferred to normal saline whenever large quantities of fluids are required, except if hyperkalemia exists. The lactacidemia in shock does not preclude administration of lactated Ringer's. The solution may be buffered by addition of 0.75 g $NaHCO_3$/L to raise the pH to 7.4.

If CVP is not monitored and fluid is given on an empirical

Table 1. ETIOLOGIC CLASSIFICATION OF SHOCK

A. Shock due to reduction in blood volume (hypovolemic)
 1. Loss of whole blood by external or internal hemorrhage.
 2. Loss of plasma by exudation at body surface or into body cavities.
 3. Loss of water and electrolytes by excessive sweating, diarrhea, diuresis, emesis, and transudation (e.g., acute intestinal obstruction).
B. Shock due to changes in venous capacitance or peripheral resistance (vasculogenic shock)
 1. Endotoxins and vasoactive agents of anaphylaxis.
 2. Vasomotor paralysis from central nervous system trauma or paralysis.
 3. Severe prolonged vasoconstriction from catecholamines.
C. Shock due to acute changes in cardiac pumping effectiveness (cardiogenic shock)
 1. Interference with effective cardiac filling. Cardiac tamponade, constrictive pericarditis, hydropericardium, positive pressure ventilation.
 2. Restricted ventricular emptying. Acute cor pulmonale, increased vascular resistance, ruptured chordae tendineae, toxic myocardial depression, cardiac dysrhythmias.

Table 2. PRINCIPAL SIGNS OF HYPOVOLEMIC CIRCULATORY SHOCK

1. Rapid, weak pulse
2. Diminution of heart sounds
3. Mucous membranes pale or ashen, cold and dry
4. Prolonged capillary refill time (≥3 sec)
5. Muscle weakness and depressed sensorium
6. Coldness of skin, particularly in extremities
7. Oliguria or anuria

dosage, 20 to 40 ml/kg is very conservative, and amounts as great as 1 to 3 blood volumes (100 to 300 ml/kg) are sometimes required. Dosage should be modified according to the severity of shock and patient response.

Hypertonic Solutions

A significant advance in hypovolemic shock therapy involving the use of intravenously administered solutions whose tonicity is eight times (2400 mOsm/L) that of plasma (approximately 300 mOsm/L). Most commonly a 7.5 per cent sodium chloride solution is chosen. Various studies have shown that hypertonic saline (HSL) (4 ml/kg), given over an approximate 8- to 10-min interval, is effective in restoring cardiac output, tissue perfusion, mesenteric blood flow, and urine output in hypovolemic shock patients. In many situations, especially field conditions, these solutions may be more convenient to store, transport, and use than the much larger volumes of isotonic electrolytes usually chosen. Indications for use of HSL include shock resulting from trauma, hemorrhage, sepsis, or severe gastrointestinal (GI) fluid loss. HSL may be especially useful whenever head trauma is a feature and the likelihood for cerebral edema is high. Contraindications would include dehydration, especially if the sodium concentration is high, and uncontrolled hemorrhage that may worsen with the HSL-induced volume shift to the extracellular compartment.

Although research and clinical experience in use of HSL in large animals is still limited, its usefulness and therapeutic value seem obvious at this point. Thus present information suggests that significant therapeutic benefits, in large as well as small animals, may be expected by the use of HSL in treatment of hypovolemic shock from a wide variety of causes.

The combination of 4 to 5 ml/kg HSL and 4 to 5 ml/kg of dextran 70 as the initial therapeutic step in severe shock, followed by infusions of balanced electrolytes in 30 minutes, may be a more optimal approach.

Cardiostimulatory and Vasoactive Drugs

Adrenergic drugs have limited usefulness in treatment of circulatory shock. Because they may be vasoconstrictive, arrhythmogenic, and likely to increase tissue oxygen demands, catecholamines are generally contraindicated in shock. The only important exceptions to the total avoidance of catecholamines is their usefulness in shock of anaphylaxis and in other shock states when they may appear critical for cardiac stimulation. Dopamine (Intropin[1]) and even more particularly dobutamine (Dobutrex[2]) have only modest vasoactive properties and can be used in an intravenous drip with greater safety than can other catecholamines.

[1]Available from Eli Lilly & Co., Indianapolis, IN 46206.
[2]Available from Arnar-Stone Laboratories, McGaw Park, IL 60085.

Steroids

Steroids in large or "pharmacologic" doses are indicated in shock, but only after repletion of fluid volume. If given earlier their vasodilatory action may produce a fall in arterial pressure and worsen venous pooling. An optimal dose of glucocorticoids is 4 to 6 mg/kg dexamethasone or 25 to 30 mg/kg prednisolone, or equivalent. Evidence exists that soluble steroid salts act more rapidly, but the cost differential makes their use questionable. Following volume repletion in shock, these agents represent an effective means of promoting tissue perfusion by arterial vasodilation.

Other Therapeutic Measures

Broad-spectrum antibiotics should be utilized whenever shock is the result of sepsis or trauma. It is advisable, however, to consider the potential cardiodepressant effect of the aminoglycoside antibiotics.

Heparin is sometimes employed at a dosage of 100 units/kg to treat or prevent DIC in shock. Cardiotonics other than catecholamines include glucagon (Glucagon USP-Lilly[1]) at a dosage of 50 μg/kg repeated at 30-minute intervals, and calcium gluconate at 10 to 20 mg/kg given slowly intravenously. Mannitol, given IV, at 1 to 3 g/kg may enhance urine flow in the hypotensive shock patient and minimize cerebral edema in head trauma. Metabolic acidosis in shock may be minimized by administration of sodium bicarbonate. Amount required may be estimated from blood gas analysis or alternatively by determining total carbon dioxide.

CONGESTIVE HEART FAILURE

Pathophysiology

Congestive heart failure is the chronic failure of the cardiac pump to meet circulatory requirements and is characterized particularly by expansion of the extracellular fluid (ECF) volume and by edema. With the failing myocardium the contractile vigor of the ventricles declines, resulting in a diminishing of cardiac output and setting in motion a series of compensatory mechanisms. The principal physiologic compensations are increases in heart rate and ECF volume. Heart rate changes are autonomically controlled; expansion of the ECF volume is principally due to increased sodium and water reabsorption by the underperfused kidneys. Increased activity of the renin-angiotensin-aldosterone mechanism provides one important means for enhancement of salt retention by renal tubules.

Heart failure may be principally either left-sided or right-sided, depending on which ventricle is most affected. In right-sided failure the systemic veins and capillaries distend as a consequence of the right heart being unable to move the venous return forward. Increased systemic capillary turgor and pressure result in tissue edema with a likelihood of ascites, hydrothorax, and migration of fluids to dependent, ventral areas. Cattle with brisket disease are classic examples of right heart failure. Left heart failure is marked by high pulmonary capillary pressure and pulmonary edema. Common causes of left heart failure include aortic or mitral valvular disease and myocardiopathies. Right heart failure is more generally attributable to increased pulmonary vascular resistance (cor pulmonale), pericarditis, and myocardiopathies. Cattle with moderately severe cor pulmonale induced by high altitude generally respond favorably to being moved to lower altitudes.

Treatment of Congestive Failure

The prognosis for successful recovery and expense of treatment may discourage intense therapy except in selected cases. In general, therapeutic regimens should include restriction of exercise and salt, diuretics, and digitalis glycosides. Aminophylline may be beneficial. Digitalis must be used with care and careful patient monitoring. Provisionally the dose for digitalization of the ox could be estimated as follows:

Intramuscularly   Digitoxin, USP   0.031 mg/kg.
Intravenously   Digoxin, USP   0.0088 mg/kg.

The digitalization procedure sometimes employed is to administer one third of the calculated dose daily until proper results are identified or until initial signs of toxicity are noted. Daily maintenance doses can be estimated at one eighth to one fifth of the digitalizing dose given in two divided doses and with careful and frequent examinations for evidence of toxicity.

Excessively high venous and capillary pressures and the accompanying edema and cardiac distension can commonly be relieved by saluretic diuretics. The use of angiotensin-converting enzyme inhibitors such as captopril (Capoten[1]) may also prove to be an effective means of reducing the degrees of hypervolemia.

ANAPHYLAXIS

Anaphylaxis is an acute, severe reaction to administration of an antigen to which an animal has been sensitized. Reactions involve the release of cellular histamine, kinins, and other vasoactive substances. The effects of these released substances, particularly histamine, is smooth muscle constriction, increased capillary permeability, and exocrine gland secretion. Results include urticaria, pruritus, hypotension, and bronchospasm. Respiratory distress and hypotensive shock may result.

Epinephrine is the drug of choice in treatment of anaphylaxis. Administration reverses the effects of histamine and limits the release of autacoids. Antihistamines act as competitive inhibitors of histamine at H1 receptors but do not alter the effects of histamine already released and acting. Corticosteroids potentiate the beneficial effects of epinephrine and, additionally, exert other nonspecific anti-inflammatory actions. While recognizably beneficial, neither antihistamines nor glucocorticoids are the first or primary drugs to use in acute hypersensitivity reactions.

In general, a regimen for therapy of anaphylaxis is as follows:

1. Epinephrine (1:1000) subcutaneously or intramuscularly: 0.5 to 1.0 ml/100 lb. Dilute to 1:10,000 if used intravenously; may be repeated at 15-minute intervals.
2. Corticosteroids intravenously or intramuscularly equivalent to dexamethasone at 0.25 to 1 mg/kg. Larger doses are tolerated, and the dose given may be doubled in severe cases.
3. Diphenhydramine (Benadryl[2]). Intramuscularly or intravenously at 0.5 to 1 mg/kg.

Adjunctive therapy may require intravenous electrolytes and bronchodilators such as aminophylline. Patients with severe and persistent collapse may require therapy as described above for circulatory shock.

---
[1]Available from E.R. Squibb, Princeton, NJ 08540.
[2]Available from Park, Davis and Co., Detroit, MI 48233.

SPONTANEOUS ATHEROSCLEROSIS IN SWINE

The pig is susceptible to spontaneous atherosclerosis, a process that can be accelerated by feeding a high-fat diet. The incidence of identifiable lesions has been reported to increase with age, ranging to 35 per cent in pigs over 3 years old. Although therapy for affected animals is not ordinarily feasible, brood animals to be maintained over a long period are known to be largely protected from atherosclerosis by receiving a high-protein, low-saturated-fat diet.

BIBLIOGRAPHY

Ettinger E: Textbook of Veterinary Internal Medicine, 2nd ed. Philadelphia, WB Saunders, 1983.
Gibbons A: Hypertonic Solutions in the Treatment of Shock. Proceedings of the 8th Annual Veterinary Forum, ACVIM, Washington, DC, 1990, pp 69–72.
Skold BH, Getty R: Spontaneous atherosclerosis of swine. J Am Vet Med Assoc 139:655, 1961.
Symposium on Drugs Affecting the Heart. J Am Vet Med Assoc 171:77–105, 1977.

Diagnostic Methods in Food Animal Cardiology

BIMBO WELKER, DVM, MS

The definitive diagnosis of cardiac disease in food animals can be hampered by the relative infrequency of occurrence and the lack of equipment usable in a field setting. Most affected animals, however, can be identified as having a diseased cardiovascular system, and a tentative diagnosis can usually be made by available field techniques. Specialized techniques are typically available at referral hospitals or universities for confirmation or differentiation of the disease process.

The first step in diagnosing diseases of the cardiac system involves recognition of the signs, clinical findings, and historical information that is suggestive of dysfunction.

SIGNS OF CARDIOVASCULAR DISEASE

Most signs are not specific for heart disease but rather can result from other disease processes. These should serve as a signal for further investigation of the cardiac system. Signs include edema, ascites, lethargy, wasting, diarrhea, coughing, syncope, and sudden death. A thorough physical examination and basic blood work will help determine if these signs are cardiogenic or noncardiogenic in nature.

CLINICAL FINDINGS

Murmurs, muffled heart sounds, arrhythmias, and abnormal jugular pulses are all findings that are highly suggestive of cardiac disease. Murmurs and arrhythmias are first detected by auscultation and, if necessary, can be more clearly defined by specialized tests.

AUSCULTATION

Proper auscultation requires a quality stethoscope, quiet environment, and adequate restraint of the patient to allow uninterrupted listening. Knowledge of auscultation sites is also important. The points of maximal intensity (PMI) for the various valves are as follows: *pulmonic valve*—left, third intercostal space, approximately 5 cm below the level of the shoulder; *aortic valve*—left, fourth intercostal space, above the level of the pulmonic valve; and *mitral valve*—left, fifth intercostal space, at or just dorsal to the level of the elbow. The tricuspid valve can best be heard on the right, at the third or fourth intercostal space, between the shoulder and elbow. The most common mistake in auscultation of large animals is listening at improper locations. The locations for auscultation of the pulmonic, aortic, and tricuspid valves will require that the stethoscope be pushed cranially into the axillary area.

Abnormalities noted with auscultation can be in the form of disturbances in blood flow (murmurs), changes in audibility of sounds, or alterations in rhythm.

Disturbances in Blood Flow or Murmurs

Normal heart sounds are produced by vibration of the cardiogenic structures as a result of energy imparted to them in the processes of the normal cardiac cycle. Anything that disturbs the usual flow of blood in the heart creates turbulence and can result in an audible murmur. Murmurs are characterized as either physiologic or pathologic in nature. Physiologic or functional murmurs are not associated with cardiac dysfunction but must be differentiated from those that are. Physiologic murmurs are typically of low to medium intensity, peak in early or midsystole, end before the second heart sound, do not radiate, and are variable in intensity from one auscultation to the next. They are usually found over the semilunar valves. The most common causes of physiologic murmurs include fever, excitement, and anemia.

Pathologic murmurs generally are those associated with a cardiac dysfunction. When a murmur is detected it should be characterized to better define it. The characteristics to be evaluated include location in the cycle; the PMI (side, intercostal space, and level); loudness or intensity (scale of 1 to 6); location in the cycle (systolic [from S_1 to S_2], diastolic [from S_2 to S_1], or continuous); and timing in the cycle (early, mid, late, or throughout). This information will allow the auscultator to approximate the structure(s) involved and speculate on the type of lesion present. If valves are involved in the pathology, the murmur can be classified as an ejection or regurgitant type. Ejection murmurs occur when blood is forced through a narrowed opening during systole. The PMI is usually over the semilunar valves and can occur during any stage of systole. Differentials include physiologic murmur, stenosis of semilunar valves, or congenital defects allowing blood to move across the septum. Regurgitant murmurs can occur during systole or diastole. Systolic regurgitant murmurs are evident with AV valve incompetence, while diastolic regurgitant murmurs are suggestive of semilunar valve incompetence.

Changes in Audibility of Sounds

The cardiac sounds can be heard in any large animal using proper auscultation techniques. Conditions such as obesity, thick chest walls, and poor technique should be ruled out when muffled sounds are encountered. If the sounds are decreased in amplitude, conditions considered should include fluid around the heart (hydropericardium) or in the chest (pleural effusion), masses positioned between the body wall and heart (abscesses or neoplasms), fluid within the lungs (congestive heart failure or pneumonia), and emphysema. In addition, electrolyte imbalances, such as hypocalcemia, can cause a decrease in amplitude and therefore an apparent muffling of sound.

Confirmation or clarification of the conditions that result in murmurs or muffled sound may require additional tests. Thoracocentesis/pericardiocentesis, echocardiography, and/or thoracic radiographs will be helpful.

Alterations in Rhythm

Rhythm disturbances occur as a result of abnormalities in impulse generation and/or conduction. The most common types of dysrhythmias in food animals include bradycardia associated with high vagal tone and decreased feed intake; ventricular premature contractions (VPCs) associated with conditions resulting in myocardial irritation (myocarditis, pericarditis, etc.); atrial premature contractions (APCs) associated with abnormalities in electrolyte or acid-base status, high vagal tone, or possibly irritation or disruption of the atrial musculature; and atrial fibrillation. Atrial fibrillation is classically associated with gastrointestinal disease and thought to result from acid-base, electrolyte or autonomic nervous system abnormalities. Differentiation of the type of dysrhythmia present is best accomplished by performing an electrocardiogram.

ELECTROCARDIOGRAPHY (ECG)

Because of the type of conduction system present in the heart of large animal species, the ECG is useful for evaluation of conduction disturbances and little else. A basic lead configuration that demonstrates all the components of the electrical cycle is adequate. A simple base-apex lead in the following configuration will suffice: the left area lead is attached to the left axillary area adjacent to the point of the elbow; the right arm lead is attached in the right jugular furrow in the midcervical region; and the chest lead is attached anywhere on the animal as a ground lead. This set-up run on lead I will result in a P-QRS-T configuration that is adequate for interpretation of dysrhythmias.

Common dysrhythmias will appear as follows: APCs—random P-QRS-T complexes will occur throughout the strip. Note that a P is associated with each configuration. VPCs—random QRS-T complexes occur throughout the strip. Note that a P *is not* associated with each configuration, and the configurations are shaped differently. Atrial fibrillation is characterized by having no P waves, a variation in the R-R interval, a variation in the amplitude of the QRS complexes, and the presence of F waves. Any of a number of other types of dysrhythmias are possible in food animals as in other species. At least with a rhythm strip in hand it can be studied and compared or sent for a second opinion.

ABNORMAL JUGULAR PULSES OR DISTENTION

Pulsation of the jugular vein can be demonstrated in the normal animal. The pulsations generally extend no higher than the midcervical region when the head is held level. These pulsations are a reflection of events occurring in the right atrium and ventricle. Abnormal pulsation, evidenced by extension farther up the neck and/or erratic configuration, occurs due to resistance to right heart filling. Resistance to filling may be due to abnormal electrical activity (dysrhythmias), obstruction to flow (heart base tumors or abscesses, pericardial effusion), or myocardial failure. Distention of the jugular veins may be another indication of filling problems. The normal jugular vein is thin walled and easily compressed. It should fill rapidly when held off at the thoracic inlet and empty rapidly when released. Persistence of jugular distension should be differentiated from an inflamed jugular vein (phlebitis) secondary to previously administered intravenous drugs. The most common causes of jugular distension or pulsation in ruminants include restrictive pericarditis or cardiac tamponade secondary to hardware, lymphosarcoma of the right atrium, tricuspid insufficiency resulting from endocarditis, jugular phlebitis, and dysrhythmias, in particular APCs, VPCs, and atrial fibrillation. Differentiation of these conditions may require an ECG, ultrasound, and/or a pericardiocentesis.

SPECIALIZED TESTS

The ECG may or may not be considered a specialized test depending on availability of equipment. It can still be considered a "cow-side" test, however, and used anytime dysrhythmias are suspected. Another specialized test that should be included in a list of field diagnostic methods is thoracocentesis/periocardiocentesis. This diagnostic test is indicated any time abnormal fluid is suspected in the chest or pericardium. The most common cause of pericardial effusion is traumatic pericarditis.

Pericardiocentesis

The technique for pericardiocentesis is as follows: in the standing cow, the skin just behind the elbow is clipped and surgically prepped. A 6- to 8-inch 18-gauge needle is inserted aseptically through the skin at the fifth or sixth intercostal space approximately level with the elbow. The needle is advanced *slowly* until pericardial fluid is obtained.

Complications can occur with pericardiocentesis, but the incidence is low. Complications include laceration of a coronary artery or the myocardium, ventricular premature beats, or ventricular fibrillation. Death due to cardiac tamponade may also occur. Once again, the incidence is low and pericardiocentesis is suggested in any case where effusion is suspected.

Echocardiography

The greatest advance in diagnostics of large animal cardiology has occurred with ultrasound. Ultrasound allows visualization of the cardiac structures for evaluation of individual components and their function. It should be prescribed for evaluation of patients with murmurs, suspected congenital defects, valvular dysfunction, muffled sounds, or unexplained dysrhythmias. It is an excellent, noninvasive method of evaluation. The disadvantages include the cost of the equipment and the specialized training required to perform the examination and interpret the data.

Radiography

Radiographic evaluation of the heart is limited to small ruminants and neonates of large animals. The information derived from radiographs even in these cases is at best supplemental to the ultrasound data. Radiographs are more likely to provide information regarding the status of the pulmonary tree relative to cardiac function or reveal evidence of thoracic effusion and possibly gross cardiac enlargement. Detailed information is rarely derived. Contrast studies in the smaller species or young may provide useful information where defective circulation is suspected (congenital defects).

Proper use of field methods should allow the practitioner to identify cardiac dysfunctions and generate a tentative differential list. Because of food animal economics, this may be all that is necessary to instigate treatment and arrive at a prognosis.

BIBLIOGRAPHY

Bonagura JD, Herring DS, Welker F: Echocardiography. Vet Clin North Am: Equine Pract 1:311–334, 1985.
Ducharme NG, Dill SG, Rendano VT: Reticulography of the cow in dorsal recumbency: an aid in the diagnosis and treatment of traumatic reticuloperitonitis. J Am Vet Med Assoc 182:585–588, 1983.
Fregin GF: Electrocardiology. Vet Clin North Am: Equine Pract 1:419–432, 1985.
Levine SA, Harvey WP: Clinical Auscultation of the Heart, 2nd ed. Philadelphia, WB Saunders, 1959.
Raphel CF, Fregin GF: Clinical examination of the cardiovascular system in cattle. Compendium of Continuing Education 2:S259–S264, 1980.

Acquired Diseases of the Heart
BIMBO WELKER, DVM, MS

The most common acquired cardiac conditions in food animals include traumatic pericarditis, bacterial endocarditis, lymphosarcoma, atrial fibrillation, and nutritional dystrophies. The food animal practitioner should be familiar with diagnosis, treatment, and prognosis of these five conditions, realizing that other, less common conditions may also occur.

TRAUMATIC RETICULOPERICARDITIS

Signs, Clinical Findings, and Diagnosis

Nonspecific signs suggestive of cardiac dysfunction and consistent with traumatic reticulopericarditis include lethargy, inappetence, rapid drop in production, and mild hyperthermia. The physical examination findings suggesting pericardial involvement include bilateral jugular distension or abnormal pulsation, a muffling of cardiac sounds, or a characteristic "washing machine" murmur. The signs and examination findings will vary depending on the volume of fluid accumulation within the pericardium and the rate of its development. The differentials for jugular distension or pulsation include any cause of decreased right heart filling, valvular dysfunction, arrhythmias, or cardiomyopathies. The muffled heart sounds must be differentiated from masses or fluid in the thorax that decrease the audibility of the sounds. Pleuritis is an important differential for pericarditis. Pericarditis can tentatively be differentiated from pleuritis by the auscultation characteristics. Pericarditis typically results in a muffling of heart sounds, an absence of lung sounds ventrally, and an increase in the audibility of lung sounds dorsally. In contrast, pleuritis results in a muffling of lung sounds ventrally, but not of heart sounds. In fact the heart sounds will radiate in a wider than normal area. The characteristic "washing machine" or splashing murmur is heard in cases of pericarditis where there is gas and fluid accumulation in the pericardium. Gas production will result if the organism involved is a gas producer. While this murmur is pathognomonic for pericardial disease, its absence does not rule it out.

The definitive diagnosis of pericardial disease must be made using pericardiocentesis and, if available, echocardiography. Pericardiocentesis will allow evaluation of the effusion. Fluid collected can be used for culture and sensitivity to determine appropriate antibiotic therapy. A false positive centesis can occur if the fluid obtained is actually from the thoracic cavity rather than the pericardial sac. Auscultation characteristics and performing the centesis at alternate locations might help alleviate this problem. Ultrasonography of the thorax provides the best method of establishing the location of the fluid.

A definitive diagnosis of traumatic reticulopericarditis can be made only by identifying penetration of a foreign body from the reticulum into the pericardial sac. This will require evidence of reticulitis at the time of a laparotomy and/or rumenotomy, identifying a foreign body on ultrasound within the pericardial sac, or visualizing a foreign body on thoracic radiographs. In a field setting and depending on economics, the most definitive method would be a laparotomy/rumenotomy exploratory. Both ultrasound and radiography can be costly and difficult to interpret even for specialists.

Nontraumatic or primary pericardial effusion may occur and should be considered as a differential when a foreign body or reticulitis cannot be identified. Hematogenous pericarditis has been reported in cattle. The characteristics of the fluid obtained from pericardiocentesis may be similar. A single isolate is likely to be found in cases of hematogenous pericarditis as compared to a mixed population found in traumatic reticulopericarditis. Transudation of fluid into the pericardial sac as a result of congestion or hypoproteinemia may also occur. The fluid characteristics should be confirmatory.

Etiology

Traumatic reticulopericarditis is the result of penetration of the reticular wall, diaphragm, and pericardial sac by a sharp metal object and of an ensuing septic inflammation. The condition occurs most commonly in older cattle. Dairy cows and beef cattle in feedlot conditions are at higher risk. Confinement and management practices increase their exposure and probability of ingesting foreign objects, such as wire and nails.

Ingested metal objects tend to settle into the first compartment or reticulum. During reticular contraction or episodes of increased abdominal pressure, such as parturition, the sharp object may be pushed through the wall. Because of the close anatomic relationship between the pericardium and the reticulum, an object penetrating the cranial wall may be directed into the pericardial sac. Penetration into the pericardial sac may inoculate the area with organisms. If the offending structure persists long enough to allow significant inoculation and the body defenses cannot overcome the insult, proliferation of the bacteria will occur. The result may be an acute, subacute, or chronic fibrinopurulent pericarditis. Absorption of bacterial toxins results in systemic signs of fever and malaise. Accumulation of fluid within the pericardial sac or thickening of the pericardium and epicardium will restrict myocardial function and result in the signs of heart failure.

Treatment and Prognosis

A diagnosis of traumatic reticulopericarditis should never be given anything better than a guarded (30 per cent) prognosis. The chronicity of the condition is a major factor in the possible outcome. Chronicity, however, may be difficult to ascertain. Acute cases may respond to prolonged antibiotic therapy and removal of the foreign object, if it is still present, via left laparotomy and rumenotomy. Repeated pericardiocenteses or pericardectomy for drainage and lavage have been useful in a few cases for short-term salvage. The best treatment is prevention. Environmental and management control to prevent exposure to metal objects combined with prophylactic magnet administration can help significantly reduce the incidence of traumatic reticulopericarditis.

Nontraumatic cases of pericarditis should be prognosed and treated similarly, except for the rumenotomy. A laparotomy may still be utilized as a diagnostic tool. The prognosis for any type of pericarditis is poor because of the involvement of and subsequent heart failure resulting from myocardial and epicardial impairment.

BACTERIAL ENDOCARDITIS

Signs, Clinical Findings, and Diagnosis

The clinical signs of bacterial endocarditis will vary depending on the stage of the disease. The most common complaints on admission are recurrent fever, anorexia, weight loss, and poor production. Lameness or stiffness may even be the predominant factor. In the early stages of the disease these signs can be present without evidence of cardiac malfunction. Of these nonspecific signs the identification of a recurrent fever should at least suggest the possibility of early bacterial endocarditis. As the disease progresses, some sign of cardiac abnormality usually develops. Early evidence includes tachycardia (80 to 120 beats/minute), murmurs, loud pounding heart sounds, arrhythmias, and/or pulse deficits. These signs, while more specific for cardiac disease, are not specific for endocarditis. Finding nonspecific signs, especially recurrent fever, in combination with a murmur is highly suggestive of bacterial endocarditis and warrants specific diagnostic investigation. As the disease process advances, signs of congestive heart failure will begin to appear. At this stage peripheral edema, jugular and mammary vein distension, dyspnea, pulmonary edema, and cachexia may appear. Eventually the cow may become recumbent and die.

Diagnosis of bacterial endocarditis in the early stages is difficult. Since clinical signs can occur without evidence of cardiac abnormalities, the practitioner must be sensitized to the very nonspecific signs, especially recurrent fever, and be alerted to conditions that may predispose to the disease, such as chronic infectious processes elsewhere in the body. Identifying a bacterial endocarditis at this stage or even at later stages requires a positive blood culture and/or echocardiographic detection of the lesion(s).

Proper blood culturing technique is critical for a correct diagnosis. Sampling should be done from multiple (minimum three) aseptically prepared sites. Arterial and venous sites are acceptable. Sampling from indwelling catheters is not recommended. Blood should generally be drawn during fever spikes to improve efficacy. It is important that two or more of the samples be positive to rule down the possibility of contamination from one site. Additionally, multiple negative cultures do not definitively rule out the disease.

Echocardiographic evaluation (if available) is a noninvasive and quick method of diagnosing endocarditis. False positives and negatives can occur. In the early stages the lesions may be very small and missed on ultrasound. Failure to identify the lesion is therefore not conclusive.

Etiology

Bacterial endocarditis in cattle is typically a sequela to a chronic infectious process at some distant site and to persistent bacteremia. Common sources of chronic or recurrent bacteremia in cattle include traumatic reticulopericarditis, liver abscesses, metritis, mastitis, omphalophlebitis, and musculoskeletal diseases. Circulating bacteria may colonize the valve leaflets either by direct adherence or by embolism of the valve capillaries. Typically the tricuspid valve is the most commonly involved. Any valve or combination of valves can be affected. *Actinomyces (Corynebacterium) pyogenes* and α-hemolytic *Streptococcus* spp. are the organisms most commonly isolated from these lesions.

The lesion produced on the valve leaflets will vary depending on chronicity. In acute cases the lesion may develop into a large, cauliflower-like (vegetative) growth on the free edge of the leaflet. As the disease becomes chronic the lesion becomes smaller and wart-like (verrucose) and the valves are shrunken and distorted.

The consequences of such valvular lesions result from either the interference with normal valve function or the showering of septic emboli. Large vegetative lesions can interfere with normal blood flow and cause cardiac dysfunction. Dysfunction is produced either by producing inefficient valves or by causing the myocardium to work harder to expel blood through the obstructed orifice. In addition, the vegetative lesions tend to fragment easily, sending emboli throughout the systemic circulation. These emboli can lodge and create abscesses at distant sites. Typical sites include the lungs, kidney, and joints. As the lesions become more chronic they are less fragile and the pathology produced is related primarily to the distortion of the valves. Inefficiency of the valves produces the clinical signs primarily related to cardiac failure.

Treatment and Prognosis

Any possibility of successful treatment of bacterial endocarditis requires early detection and long-term (minimum 4 weeks) antibiotic therapy. Treatment in the early stages before evidence of cardiac dysfunction, when it is most difficult to diagnose, will result in a fair (50 per cent) to good (70 per cent) prognosis for recovery. As the signs of right-sided heart failure develop (edema, jugular distension or pulsation), the prognosis progressively drops to poor. Even with successful treatment of the infection, any valvular disfiguration and subsequent murmurs or insufficiencies are likely to persist.

The selection of the antibiotic should optimally be based on culture and sensitivity results. During the interim period, considering the most common organisms involved, penicillin is a reasonable selection. Procaine penicillin G (minimum 20,000 units/kg b.i.d.) is safe and inexpensive for the long-term therapy required. If evidence of congestive heart failure is present, diuretics and a low-salt diet may be beneficial. Recovery is likely to be slow and gradual. Evidence of recovery will be an improvement in appetite, weight gain, and cessation of febrile episodes. Signs related to valve distortion, however, are likely to persist.

Prevention of bacterial endocarditis should be aimed at preventing or treating the chronic disease processes that produce the chronic bacteremic episodes.

ADULT LYMPHOSARCOMA

Signs, Clinical Findings, and Diagnosis

The clinical signs associated with infiltration of the heart by lymphosarcoma will vary depending on the structures involved and the degree of involvement. Characteristically the tumor begins in the right atrium but by no means is limited to this structure. As the tumor infiltrates the musculature of the heart and/or enlarges in size, function of the myocardium becomes impaired. Clinical signs of cardiomyopathy may ensue (brisket edema and jugular distension or pulsation). Disruption of the sinoatrial node in the right atrium may result in cardiac arrhythmias. These signs are not specific for lymphosarcoma and must be differentiated from other causes of cardiac malfunction. Traumatic reticulopericarditis and bacterial endocarditis are the most common.

A diagnosis of lymphosarcoma as the cause of cardiomyopathy or arrhythmia can be very challenging. If lymphosarcoma can be identified elsewhere in the body, a tentative diagnosis can be assumed. Echocardiographic examination can be useful in identifying masses associated with the cardiac structures. This may allow differentiation of lymphosarcoma from other common causes of cardiac dysfunction such as pericarditis and bacterial endocarditis. A pericardiocentesis may provide information if hydropericardium is suspected from auscultation of muffled heart sounds or from ultrasound. Occasionally, abnormal cell types may be identified in the fluid. Leukemia is a characteristic of only one third of clinical cases, but if identified is very significant. The primary differential to consider is persistent lymphocytosis (PL), a benign lymphoproliferative response to bovine leukemia virus (BLV). The definitive diagnosis of lymphosarcoma can be made only by histologic examination of tissues obtained by biopsy or at necropy. Serologic tests for BLV infection are available. Titers to the virus, however, cannot be interpreted as a diagnosis of bovine lymphosarcoma. Titers indicate exposure to or infection by the virus. Estimates suggest anywhere from 20 per cent to 60 per cent of cattle will have titers to BLV. A negative titer in an animal suspected of having a lymphosarcoma tumor is more valuable in ruling it out than a positive titer that only confirms exposure and seroconversion. Only 5 per cent of cattle infected with BLV develop lymphosarcoma.

Etiology

Adult bovine lymphosarcoma, also known as enzootic bovine lymphosarcoma (EBL), is a fatal systemic neoplasia of the lymphoreticular tissue. The heart is only one of many tissues that can be affected. The diverse types of tissues and organ systems that can be affected result in a potential myriad of presenting clinical signs. Seroepidemiologic studies indicate that BLV is the causative agent of EBL. BLV is a retrovirus.

The spread of BLV is mainly by contact. Transmission is most likely by infected lymphocytes through hematophagous arthropods (bloodsucking) and contaminated instruments (needles, syringes, etc.). While BLV and/or BLV-infected lymphocytes are present in the milk of most infected dams, transmission to the calf is infrequent. Maternal antibodies in the colostrum are believed to protect the calf during the nursing period. Prenatal transmission is also uncommon. Less than 20 per cent of infected calves born to BLV-infected dams are BLV positive at birth. Recent studies raise the possibility of transmission of BLV in semen. BLV-infected lymphocytes could conceivably be present in semen from bulls with inflammatory conditions of the urogenital tract.

Bovine lymphosarcoma affects both sexes and all breeds but is most common in adult dairy cattle. The majority of cases show up in the 5- to 8-year-old age group, with most being 3 years of age. There also appears to be a tendency to aggregate along familial lines.

Treatment, Prevention, and Prognosis

There are no effective treatments for lymphosarcoma to date, and therefore the prognosis is grave. The economic losses due to death, loss of productivity, and import regulations make this disease financially very significant.

Eradication of BLV infection and therefore EBL is feasible. Eradication programs should be based on accurate identification and removal of BLV-positive animals from the herd. A vaccine may be present in the future but at present is still experimental.

ATRIAL FIBRILLATION

Signs, Clinical Findings, and Diagnosis

Generally cows with atrial fibrillation (AF) do not present with signs specifically related to the cardiovascular system. The most common complaints associated with cows having AF are anorexia and poor production. Obviously these signs are very nonspecific and, in fact, probably more related to the underlying cause of the arrhythmia.

Atrial fibrillation will be detected during cardiac auscultation. Two characteristic features can be auscultated to diagnose tentatively the presence of this arrhythmia. This conduction disturbance creates an *irregularly irregular* rhythm. During auscultation absolutely no pattern can be detected in the intervals between beats. The heart rate will vary from normal to tachycardia with this disturbance. When the rate is very rapid the irregularity in intervals may not be easily appreciated. The other auscultatory finding is variation in intensity from beat to beat. This sound is referred to as "jungle drum" beats. Either or both of these auscultation findings are highly suggestive of atrial fibrillation in the cow.

The definitive diagnosis of atrial fibrillation requires electrocardiography. A rhythm strip or base-apex lead will suffice. The base-apex lead is performed by placing the left arm (LA) lead on the point of the left elbow, the right arm (RA) lead in the right jugular furrow, and the chest (C) lead as a ground lead anywhere on the animal. This arrangement recorded on lead I will describe a positive P wave, a positive QRS deflection, and a positive T wave in the normal animal. Criteria used to diagnose atrial fibrillation will include absence of P waves, the presence of F waves (baseline flutter), an irregular R-R interval, and variation in the amplitude of the QRS complex.

Etiology

Atrial fibrillation is one of the most common arrhythmias detected in cattle. It can and usually does occur without apparent underlying primary heart disease. It is therefore often referred to as a functional arrhythmia. The clinical significance of this is that if the underlying cause of the disturbance can be corrected, the arrhythmia may convert back to normal sinus rhythm. The most common underlying causes that tend to predispose to atrial fibrillation are gastrointestinal disorders. It should be noted, however, that atrial fibrillation has been associated with diseases of other systems. As a general rule, acid-base and electrolyte abnormalities frequently seen with these disturbances have been incriminated but not yet proven. Therapy is usually directed at these imbalances and correction of the primary disease process.

Primary heart disease must be considered a differential, especially in those that fail to respond to correction of the primary problem and its associated imbalances. Ultrasound may be useful in identifying gross abnormalities in the right atrium such as lymphosarcoma.

Treatment and Prognosis

Treatment of atrial fibrillation is warranted in any cow economically valuable enough to keep in the herd. Persistence of atrial fibrillation may lead to poor performance and progressive cardiac disease.

Treatment should first be directed at the suspected underlying disease, usually gastrointestinal, and the concomitant acid-base and electrolyte disorders. Once these are corrected, 40 to 50 per cent of cattle will self-convert to normal sinus rhythm within *5 to 7* days. Persistence of AF after this time is a criteria for therapeutic intervention. The treatment of choice is *quinidine sulfate* (44 mg/kg dissolved in 4 L distilled water) administered slowly intravenously (approximately 1 L/hour). Oral administration studies have not proven as effective. In most cases conversion will occur in *2 to 4 hours*. At whatever time conversion does occur the drug is stopped immediately. Cows converted using this technique generally remain in normal sinus rhythm. Quinidine can be toxic to the heart, and therefore the treatment should be monitored with an ongoing electrocardiogram. The ECG change suggestive of toxicity is a widening of the QRS. Side effects that are noted in all cases include ataxia, blepharospasm, diarrhea, increased frequency of defecation, and increase in rumen contractions. These effects are transient, lasting less than 12 hours.

In cases with very high heart rates the conversion may be facilitated by administering digoxin (1 mg/100 kg intravenously) prior to quinidine treatment.

A failure to respond to treatment suggests either inappropriate treatment or underlying heart disease. These cases typically have a poor prognosis for performance and may lead to progressive cardiac disease.

NUTRITIONAL MYODEGENERATION (WHITE MUSCLE DISEASE)

Signs, Clinical Findings, and Diagnosis

Nutritional myodegeneration or white muscle disease (WMD) presents as two distinct syndromes: a cardiac form and a skeletal muscle form. Both forms tend to affect the young but have been suspected in yearlings and adults. The cardiac form typically affects neonates in the first week of life. Signs are peracute to acute and usually result in severe debilitation or sudden death. Because the cardiac, diaphragm, and intercostal muscles are affected, animals may present with signs predominantly referable to the respiratory system. Cardiac murmurs and irregular heartbeats may be detected. Murmurs at this age require consideration of congenital anomalies as differentials. If the case presents without significant signs of cardiac dysfunction but with severe debilitation or sudden death, the differential list must include septicemia, pneumonia, diarrhea and dehydration, or toxicity.

WMD should be considered as a differential anytime these signs present in a neonate from a geographic area where the problem is endemic. The antemortem diagnosis of WMD should be based on *whole-blood levels of selenium* and *plasma levels of vitamin E*. Whole-blood selenium concentrations range from 0.07 to 0.1 ppm in normal naimals. The critical levels of vitamin E in *plasma* are 1.1 to 2.0 ppm. Vitamin E in plasma deteriorates rapidly and therefore needs to be put on ice immediately and stored at $-21°$ F ($\sim -11.6°$ C) if the analysis is not going to be performed immediately. The blood and plasma levels of selenium and vitamin E, respectively, do not assess body stores. Tissue samples taken by antemortem biopsy or at postmortem can be useful in evaluating body stores. Liver concentrations can be useful in establishing deficiencies. Liver levels of 0.9 to 1.75 µg/g DM (dry matter) for cattle and 0.9 to 3.5 µg/g DM for sheep are considered normal. A diagnosis of selenium and/or vitamin E deficiency can also be established or supported by ration analysis.

The postmortem findings are typical and include white streaks in the muscle bundles that represent bands of coagulation necrosis or, in chronic cases, may represent fibrosis and calcification. In calves the left ventricular wall and septum are most frequently affected.

Etiology

Deficiencies of selenium and/or vitamin E apparently result in destruction of cell membranes and proteins, leading to a loss of cellular integrity. Cell damage results from the presence of free radicals and peroxides. Normal cellular metabolism produces high levels of reactive forms of oxygen (free radicals) such as hydrogen peroxide, hydroperoxides, superoxides, and various other radicals. Vitamin E in the cell membrane scavenges these free radicals before they can combine with unsaturated fatty acids to form lipid hydroperoxides. Selenium as a component of the enzyme glutathione peroxidase (GSH-Px) destroys the peroxides that have already formed.

Certain regions of the United States and other countries are inherently low in selenium. The northeastern and eastern seaboard and the northwestern regions are particularly deficient. Acid soils, soils originating from volcanic rock, and high-sulfur soils or those treated with sulfur-containing fertilizers are likely to be low. In addition, forages may vary in selenium content. Legumes take up less than grasses, and all forages take up less selenium during rapid growth and in times of high rainfall.

Vitamin E deficiencies become a problem when animals are fed poor quality hay, straw, or root crops. Stored grains lose their vitamin E content with time. Cereal grains, green growing pastures, and properly prepared hays usually have adequate concentrations of vitamin E.

Selenium and vitamin E tend to have a sparing effect on one another. Adequate levels of vitamin E can decrease the level of selenium required in the diet. In contrast, low levels of vitamin E will increase the requirements of selenium.

Treatment and Prognosis

The calf that presents with signs of cardiac dysfunction as a result of vitamin E and/or selenium deficiency must be given a poor prognosis. Most animals die within 24 hours. If therapy is to be instituted it must be immediate and before signs advance. Injectable vitamin E/selenium (at 2.5 to 3.0 mg/45 kg), either intramuscularly or subcutaneously, is recommended.

Prevention of myocardial degeneration from WMD must be aimed at proper supplementation of the dam either by salt mix or by total ration supplementation and, if late in gestation, prepartum injectable vitamin E/selenium.

BIBLIOGRAPHY

Blood DC, Radostitis OM: Veterinary Medicine, 7th ed. Baltimore, Williams & Wilkins, 1989.
Ferrer JF: Bovine Lymphosarcoma. Compendium of Continuing Education S235–S241, 1980.
Ferrer JF, Marshak RR, Abt DA, Kenyon SJ: Relationship between lymphosarcoma and persistent lymphocytosis in cattle: a review. J Am Vet Med Assoc 175:705–708, 1979.
Krishnamurthy D, Nigam JM, Peshin PK, Kharole MV: Thoracopericardiotomy and pericardiectomy in cattle. J Am Vet Med Assoc 175:714–718, 1979.
Maas JP: Diagnosis and management of selenium-responsible diseases in cattle. Compendium on Continuing Education 5:S393–S400, 1983.
McGuirk SM, Muir WW, Sams RA: Pharmacokinetic analysis of intravenously and orally administered quinidine in horses. Am J Vet Res 42:938–942, 1981.
McGuirk SM, Muir WW, Sams RA, Rings DM: Atrial fibrillation in cows: clinical findings and therapeutic considerations. J Am Vet Med Assoc 182:1380–1386, 1983.
Miller JM: Bovine Lymphosarcoma. The Bovine Proceedings 20:34–36, 1988.
Power HT, Rebhun WC: Bacterial endocarditis in adult dairy cattle. J Am Vet Med Assoc 182:806–808, 1983.
Smith JA: Bacterial endocarditis in cattle. Bovine Clinics 3:8, 1983.
Stöber M: The clinical picture of the enzootic and sporadic forms of bovine leukosis. The Bovine Practitioner 16:119–129, 1981.

Hematology of Food Animals
MARLYN S. WHITNEY, DVM, PhD, DIPLOMATE, ACVP

Hematologic evaluation is useful for the assessment of many disease states. Primary alterations in hematologic parameters result from disorders within the hemic system itself. Perhaps more important, secondary hematologic alterations commonly occur as the result of abnormalities in other body systems, so hematologic evaluation can provide important diagnostic clues to many diverse conditions. Because similar hematologic abnormalities may occur in response to widely different processes, determination of hematologic parameters alone rarely provides a definitive diagnosis. However, when hematologic alterations are interpreted in conjunction with other patient information, such as the clinical history, physical examination findings, and other relevant laboratory data, appropriate diagnostic decisions can often be made. This article will emphasize general principles regarding the use and interpretation of hematologic tests. For in-depth discussions of the clinical signs, range of possible clinicopathologic alterations, and treatment of specific disorders, the reader may refer to appropriate sections of other articles in this volume. Hematology laboratory methodology is described elsewhere.[1,2,5]

LABORATORY EVALUATION OF THE HEMIC SYSTEM

Parameters Evaluated

The complete blood count (CBC), the most common hematologic procedure performed, serves as a broad screening test for hematologic abnormalities. If the CBC provides incomplete information regarding hematologic abnormalities, additional diagnostic procedures may be warranted.

A CBC aids assessment of any animal that has clinical indications of anemia, infection, inflammation, or bleeding disorders. Additionally, a CBC may provide useful diagnostic clues in animals with vague or nonspecific clinical signs. The CBC usually consists of the following: hematocrit, hemoglobin, red blood cell (RBC) count, total white blood cell (WBC) count, platelet count or estimate, and examination of a stained blood film to determine the WBC differential distribution and to evaluate individual blood cell staining characteristics and morphology. In addition, an estimate of the total plasma protein level is often done by refractometer, using plasma from the hematocrit tube. In many veterinary laboratories an estimate of the plasma fibrinogen level is included in the CBC for food animals since the fibrinogen level is a useful adjunct to the WBC count for identification of inflammatory responses in these species.

A bone marrow examination may assist in explaining CBC findings that cannot be explained by the patient's clinical history, physical examination findings, or other diagnostic test results. A bone marrow examination is indicated when the CBC identifies any unexplained peripheral blood cytopenia. Bone marrow examination is also used for evaluation of animals with suspected hematopoietic neoplasia, for the clinical staging of disseminated neoplasia of any type, and for monitoring the bone marrow status of animals undergoing chemotherapy with agents known to affect hematopoiesis.

In addition to a platelet count, the most common laboratory procedures for assessment of the hemostatic mechanism are the activated clotting time (ACT) and the activated partial thromboplastin time (PTT) for assessment of the intrinsic and common coagulation cascades, and the prothrombin time (PT) for assessment of the extrinsic and common coagulation cascades. If a thrombotic disorder, such as diffuse intravascular coagulation, is suspected, the PTT and PT may be supplemented with determinations of antithrombin III (ATIII) and plasma fibrinogen levels and a test to detect the presence in serum of excessive fibrin degradation products (FDP). Other tests used to evaluate hemostasis, such as determinations of specific coagulation factor levels, von Willebrand factor assays, and platelet function tests, are rarely requested for food animal patients, and the availability of these tests for these species is essentially restricted to a few hemostasis research laboratories.

For animals suspected of having iron deficiency or disordered iron metabolism, determination of serum iron and transferrin levels is helpful. The serum transferrin level is usually determined as the serum total iron binding capacity (TIBC). Body iron stores can be estimated by microscopic examination of Prussian blue–stained bone marrow specimens.

Although crossmatching is often not done for the first transfusion in food animals, animals receiving multiple transfusions should be crossmatched with the donor animals to lessen the risk of a transfusion reaction.

The Office Hematology Laboratory

The types of laboratory procedures performed in-house in an individual practice will be determined by the caseload of the practice, economic considerations, and the accessibility of reliable outside laboratories. It is well within the capability of most veterinary practices to perform in-house CBCs. Some practitioners may elect to perform additional hematologic procedures in their practice laboratories.

The methodology of hematologic procedures is described in detail elsewhere.[1, 2, 5] A centrifuge that can accommodate microhematocrit tubes is required for determination of the hematocrit. Cell counts can be performed either manually with a hemacytometer or with automated cell counters in those practices with a large enough caseload to make them cost-effective. Sample preparation for manual cell counting is most easily done using Unopette* blood dilution chambers. Dilution chambers are available for performing reasonably accurate WBC and platelet counts. Manual RBC counts are less accurate. For estimating the total plasma protein level, a high-quality, hand-held, temperature-compensated clinical refractometer is a worthwhile investment. If a heated water bath is available, the plasma fibrinogen level can be estimated refractometrically by the heat precipitation method. This method is suitable for detecting the elevated fibrinogen levels characteristic of inflammatory processes but is not sensitive or accurate enough to be reliable for detecting the decreased fibrinogen levels characteristic of consumptive coagulopathies. Various hemoglobinometers intended for office or field use are available. Romanowsky-type polychrome stains, such as Wright's and Wright-Giemsa's, are routinely used for staining blood smears and bone marrow aspirate smears. Commercially available quick stains such as Diff-Quik* are easy to use and give excellent results. New methylene blue stain is used to do reticulocyte counts on anemic animals. The ACT is a useful office screening test for detecting disorders in the intrinsic and common coagulation pathways.

Sample Collection and Handling

Samples for routine CBCs should be collected into tubes containing ethylenediaminetetraacetate (EDTA). Blood collection tubes should be filled to capacity. If tubes are filled to less than one half of their capacity, there will be excessive EDTA present in relation to the blood volume, and artifactual spiculation of erythrocytes may occur. Underfilling of EDTA tubes may cause a falsely high refractometric total protein estimation. Liquid EDTA has a high refractive index, and as the volume ratio of EDTA to plasma is increased, there is an increasing likelihood that a significant error in the protein reading will occur. Excessive EDTA may also cause a falsely decreased hematocrit owing to erythrocyte shrinkage.

If the CBC specimen is to be shipped to an outside laboratory, or if the CBC cannot be performed immediately in the office laboratory, a few blood smears should be made and allowed to air dry and the remainder of the specimen should be kept at refrigerator temperature until the cell counts are done. Platelet counts must be done within 2 hours of sample collection. If this cannot be done, platelet numbers can be estimated using the stained blood smear. While reasonably accurate WBC and RBC counts can be obtained on properly cooled specimens held for several days, accurate determination of the WBC differential distribution, estimation of platelet numbers, and assessment of blood cell morphology require that blood smears be made as soon as possible after sample collection. Staining can be delayed for several days if necessary. Once made, smears that are not stained immediately should be protected from water, dust, and flies (flies delight in eating the blood off of slides). Bone marrow aspirate smears should be handled in the same manner as blood smears. Bone marrow core biopsies are routinely fixed in formalin in the same manner as other tissue biopsies. (Caution: Blood and bone marrow aspirate smears should not be exposed to formalin vapors since this may impair staining of the specimens. Blood and bone marrow smears should be shipped separately from formalin-fixed tissues.)

Samples for coagulation tests should be collected by careful venipuncture and handled per the instructions of the laboratory performing the analysis. Plastic syringes and plastic or silicon-coated collection and storage tubes should be used. Sodium citrate is the most commonly used anticoagulant for PTT, PT, ATIII, and fibrinogen determinations. The volume ratio of blood to anticoagulant must be correct: nine parts blood to one part 3.8 per cent sodium citrate solution. Samples for FDP analysis are collected into special tubes intended specifically for that purpose. Specimens for most coagulation tests must be analyzed as quickly as possible after sample collection, or the plasma must be harvested as soon as possible and frozen at $-20°C$ until the analyses can be performed.

Samples for additional laboratory tests that may be required should be collected and handled per the instructions of the laboratory performing the analysis.

---

*Available from Becton, Dickinson and Co., Rutherford, NJ 07070.

*Available from Scientific Products Division, Baxter Healthcare Corporation, McGaw Park, IL 60085.

Hematologic Reference Ranges

Reference ranges for selected hematologic parameters of cattle, sheep, goats, and swine are presented in Table 1. These are ranges for adult animals. Animals less than 6 months of age tend to have somewhat lower hematocrits, RBC counts, hemoglobin levels, and plasma protein levels and somewhat higher total WBC counts. Neonates generally have a high hematocrit that decreases rapidly owing to colostrum ingestion. The hematocrit continues to decrease during phases of rapid growth, when body size is increasing faster than blood volume. Although fewer than 1 per cent of the circulating erythrocytes are reticulocytes in healthy adult swine, suckling pigs have moderate to marked reticulocytosis and metarubricytosis owing to intense erythrogenesis related to rapid body growth and attendant increase in blood volume. In all species lymphocyte counts tend to decrease with advancing age. Lactating animals, especially high-yield dairy cows, may have decreased hematocrits, RBC counts, and hemoglobin levels. Animals grazing at high altitude tend to have increased hematocrits, RBC counts, and hemoglobin levels. Whenever possible, reference ranges derived by the laboratory performing the hematologic tests should be used.

GENERAL PRINCIPLES OF HEMATOPOIESIS

General Information

With the exception of lymphocytes, blood cell formation in the normal healthy adult animal occurs only in the bone marrow. In normal adults much of the marrow space is hematopoietically inactive and filled with fat. Active bone marrow remains in the flat bones and in the ends of the long bones. If the marrow hematopoietic tissue itself is healthy and has a proper nutrient supply, it can expand again into the fat-filled areas in response to increased peripheral use, loss, or destruction of blood cells. The capacity to respond to increased need for blood cells varies with the species and is generally less in food animal species than in companion animals. If the marrow is unable to respond adequately, extramedullary hematopoiesis may occur in the spleen and/or liver.

Like all tissues, for proper function the hematopoietic tissue must have a blood supply adequate to bring in sufficient amounts of oxygen and nutrients and to carry away wastes. Humoral mediators arising in the peripheral tissues also must be carried by the blood to the marrow to signal the marrow to produce numbers of cells sufficient to meet changing peripheral demands. Developing blood cells are nurtured by other cells in the marrow, such as reticulum cells and macrophages. These cells perform such functions as physically supporting the hematopoietic cells and converting nutrients to the proper form for uptake by the developing blood cells.

The Effects of Disease on Hematopoiesis

The hematopoietic tissue is liable to the same basic pathologic processes as other tissues—namely hyperplasia, hypoplasia/aplasia, neoplasia (primary or metastatic), fibrosis, inflammation, and infarction. Hyperplasia, hypoplasia/aplasia, and hemtopoietic neoplasms may affect single or multiple components of the bone marrow. For example, following an episode of hemorrhage, an animal may develop hyperplasia of the erythroid compartment of the bone marrow, with the myeloid and megakaryocytic compartments remaining relatively normal. In this case there is an increased stimulus for erythrocyte production but less for leukocytes and platelets. In the case of toxins that damage the marrow stem cells that have not yet differentiated into specific cell lines, all three marrow compartments may become hypoplastic or aplastic simultaneously.

Lesions in the bone marrow may have either a diffuse or a focal distribution. Diffuse lesions will almost surely affect hematopoiesis and cause alterations in CBC findings, whereas focal lesions may have little or no effect on overall hematopoiesis. Hyperplastic and hypoplastic responses, primary hematopoietic neoplasms, and myelofibrosis usually have a diffuse distribution throughout the bone marrow. Osteomyelitis and bone marrow infarction may occur as focal lesions, but osteomyelitis may become multifocal and widespread in the case of bacterial infections that have spread hematogenously.

Table 1. HEMATOLOGIC REFERENCE RANGES

Parameter (Units)	Cattle	Sheep	Goats	Swine
Hematocrit (%)	24–46	27–45	22–38	32–50
Hemoglobin (g/dl)	8–15	9–15	8–12	9–16
RBC count ($\times 10^6/\mu l$)	5.0–10.0	9.0–15.0	8.0–18.0	5.0–8.0
Reticulocytes (% of RBC)	0	0	0	0–1
MCV (fl)	40–60	28–40	16–25	50–68
MCHC (g/dl)	30–36	31–34	30–36	29–34
Platelet count ($\times 10^5/\mu l$)	1.0–8.0	2.5–7.5	3.0–6.0	2.0–7.2
WBC count ($/\mu l$)	4000–12,000	4000–12,000	4000–13,000	11,000–22,000
Band neutrophils ($/\mu l$)	0–120	Rare	Rare	0–800
Segmented neutrophils ($/\mu l$)	600–4000	700–6000	1200–7200	2000–15,000
Lymphocytes ($/\mu l$)	2500–7500	2000–9000	2000–9000	3800–16,500
Monocytes ($/\mu l$)	25–850	0–750	0–550	0–1000
Eosinophils ($/\mu l$)	0–2400	0–1000	50–650	0–1500
Basophils ($/\mu l$)	0–200	0–300	0–120	0–500
Total plasma protein (g/dl)	6.0–8.5	6.0–7.5	6.0–7.5	6.0–8.0
Fibrinogen (g/dl)	1–7	1–5	1–4	1–5
Serum iron ($\mu g/dl$)	57–162	162–222		91–199
TIBC ($\mu g/dl$)	120–348	293–373		191–461
ATIII (% of normal canine pool)	130–153			
PT (sec)	22–55			11–12
PTT (sec)	44–64			34–39
FDP ($\mu g/ml$)	<10	<10	<10	<10
ACT	90–120			

Source: Derived from Duncan JR, Prasse KW: Veterinary Laboratory Medicine—Clinical Pathology, 2nd ed. Ames, IA, Iowa State University Press, 1986; Jain NC: Schalm's Veterinary Hematology, 4th ed. Philadelphia, Lea & Febiger, 1986; and the Clinical Pathology Laboratory of the Veterinary Teaching Hospital, Texas A&M University, College Station, TX. See text for expected variations due to age, elevation, etc.

- Obtain clinical history and perform physical examination
- Identify or confirm anemia with Hct or hemoglobin determination

If the cause of anemia is not evident from the above:
- Do a complete CBC
- Do a reticulocyte count and adjust it for the severity of the anemia to determine if the anemia is regenerative or nonregenerative
- Determine the MCV and MCHC
- Further narrow the list of etiologic possibilities using the diagnostic clues indicated below each type of anemia (1a–2b)

1 Regenerative Anemia*		2 Nonregenerative Anemia*	
• Adjusted reticulocyte count >2.0 • Normal to slightly increased MCV • Normal to slightly decreased MCHC • Basophilic stippling common in ruminants		• Adjusted reticulocyte count <0.5 • MCV and MCHC variable (see below) • Bone marrow evaluation may be necessary to differentiate between 2a and 2b	
1a Blood Loss	1b Hemolysis	2a Ineffective Erythropoiesis	2b Erythroid Hypoplasia
• Total protein decreased • ± Hypovolemia (severe acute hemorrhage) • ± Trauma • ± Hemorrhagic effusion • ± Hematuria • ± Melena or fecal occult blood • ± Evidence of endo- or ectoparasites • ± Evidence of hemostatic disorder • See Table 3 for causes	• Total protein normal or increased • ± Hyperbilirubinemia† • ± Bilirubinuria† • ± Hemoglobinemia† • ± Hemoglobinuria† • ± Abnormal RBC morphology (e.g., schistocytes,† spherocytes,‡ RBC ghosts,† agglutination) • ± RBC parasites • ± Spleno/hepatomegaly‡ • See Table 3 for causes	• Nuclear maturation arrest often causes increased MCV • Cytoplasmic maturation arrest often causes decreased MCV and/or decreased MCHC • MCV and MCHC may be normal • Erythroid compartment of marrow hyperplastic, but maturation sequence not complete • See Table 4 for causes§	• MCV and MCHC usually normal • Erythroid compartment of marrow hypoplastic or aplastic • See Table 4 for causes§

*If the corrected reticulocyte count is >0.5 but <2.0, the anemia may be a hemolytic or blood loss anemia that has not yet had sufficient time (4 to 6 days) to become regenerative.
†These findings suggest intravascular hemolysis.
‡These findings suggest extravascular hemolysis.
§Diagnosis of the anemia may be facilitated by a search for physical or laboratory evidence of the conditions listed in Table 4.

Hct = hematocrit; CBC = complete blood count; MCV = mean corpuscular volume; MCHC = mean corpuscular hemoglobin concentration; RBC = red blood cell.

Figure 1. Procedures for the assessment of anemia.

Neoplasms that metastasize to the bone marrow from other tissues may appear as focal, localized lesions that do not cause any widespread effects on blood cell production, or they may become so widespread in later stages as to have a diffuse distribution that essentially replaces the bone marrow. The latter situation may occur in the case of bovine lymphosarcoma, which may arise in the lymph nodes or other extramedullary tissue and subsequently metastasize to the bone marrow.

Lesions in virtually any tissue may have secondary effects on the hematopoietic tissues, and these in turn will affect the results of a CBC. It is common to have multiple processes simultaneously operant on the hematopoietic tissue.

DISORDERS OF THE ERYTHRON

Evaluation of the erythroid portion of the CBC is directed toward the detection and classification of anemia or polycythemia and toward the detection of any abnormalities in erythrocyte size, staining affinity, or morphology.

Anemia

Anemia is a common condition with diverse etiologies; it is a component of many diseases. The erythroid portion of the CBC is used to confirm the presence of anemia and, together with the remainder of the CBC data and the information obtained from the patient's history and physical examination findings, often provides the necessary clues for determining the cause of the anemia. A flow chart for the assessment of anemia is presented in Figure 1. The anemia is first classified as regenerative or nonregenerative. Especially in the case of nonregenerative anemias it is helpful to further classify the anemia with respect to RBC size (normocytic versus macrocytic or microcytic) and color (normochromic versus hypochromic). Classification of the anemia in this manner greatly shortens the list of etiologic possibilities.

Regenerative anemias are those in which marrow production and release of reticulocytes have increased to compensate for increased loss of erythrocytes via hemorrhage or hemolysis. In contrast, nonregenerative anemias result from a decreased ability of the bone marrow to produce and release erythrocytes in response to peripheral needs. They can result from an intrinsic problem in the hematopoietic tissue, such as the lack of an essential nutrient or the presence of a toxin, or from an abnormality in the humoral-signaling mechanisms that normally elicit an adequate level of erythropoiesis.

The reticulocyte count is used to determine if an anemia is regenerative or nonregenerative. With Wright's stain, reticulocytes appear as polychromatophils—erythrocytes that take up some blue stain as well as pink. Therefore Wright's–stained blood smears from animals with highly regenerative anemias show marked polychromasia. Accurate identification and enumeration of reticulocytes is best accomplished via the use of new methylene blue–stained smears. The reticulocyte count is expressed as the percentage of erythrocytes that display the blue reticulum characteristic of reticulocytes stained with new methylene blue. For accurate assessment of the adequacy of a regenerative response, the reticulocyte count must be adjusted according to the severity of the anemia. To adjust the reticulocyte count, divide the patient's hematocrit by the mean normal hematocrit for the species and multiply the result by the patient's reticulocyte count expressed as a percentage. For example, a cow with a hematocrit of 18 and a reticulocyte count of 10 per cent would have an adjusted reticulocyte count of $(18 \div 35) \times 10 = 5.1$. An adjusted reticulocyte count of greater than 2.0 indicates a regenerative response, while a value less than 0.5 indicates a nonregenerative response. Values between 0.5 and 2.0 may occur early in a regenerative response (before the marrow has had time to respond maximally) or as the result of secondary factors that impair a regenerative response. In cattle, and to a somewhat lesser degree in sheep and goats, regenerative responses are often characterized by prominent basophilic stippling of erythrocytes, as well as by reticulocytosis. Basophilic stippling is readily observable with Wright's stain. Nucleated red blood cells (nRBC) may be present in the circulation of animals with regenerative anemias, but they will be outnumbered by reticulocytes. Since nRBC may be present in the circulating blood in some nonregenerative anemias, their presence cannot be used to differentiate regenerative from nonregenerative anemias.

Calculated parameters that are used to further classify anemia are the mean corpuscular volume (MCV) and the mean corpuscular hemoglobin concentration (MCHC), calculated as follows: $MCV = (Hct/RBC\ ct) \times 10$, and $MCHC = (Hgb/Hct) \times 100$. In these formulas Hct is the hematocrit (per cent), RBC ct is the erythrocyte count in millions of cells/μl, and Hgb is the hemoglobin level in g/dl. The unit of the MCV is the femtoliter (fl), and the MCHC is expressed as g/dl.

An increased MCV (macrocytosis) may be a feature of a regenerative anemia since reticulocytes are somewhat larger than mature erythrocytes. The MCV and MCHC may or may not be affected in nonregenerative anemias. If a nonregenerative anemia is due to ineffective erythropoiesis, the MCV and/or the MCHC will often (but not always) be abnormal. An increased MCV in the absence of a regenerative response is indicative of ineffective erythropoiesis due to interference with mitosis of the developing erythrocytes. A decreased MCV (microcytosis) suggests interference with hemoglobin production, as does a decreased MCHC (hypochromasia). If a nonregenerative anemia is due to erythroid hypoplasia, the MCV and MCHC are almost always normal. See Table 4 for causes of ineffective erythropoiesis and erythroid hypoplasia.

True increases in MCHC do not occur. If the calculated MCHC is above the normal range, an error in determination of one of the parameters used in the calculation should be suspected. Hemolysis in the CBC specimen will cause a falsely elevated MCHC since only intact erythrocytes are included in the hematocrit reading and all the hemoglobin in the specimen is included in the hemoglobin measurement.

Abnormalities in erythrocyte size, morphology, and staining affinity should be noted when the blood smear is evaluated, as these often provide important diagnostic clues. The calculated MCV and MCHC should always be checked for accuracy by examination of the stained blood smear. For example, if the calculated MCV is decreased, the erythrocytes should appear microcytic on the blood smear. If there is a discrepancy between calculated values and what is seen on a blood smear, interpretation should be based on what is seen on the smear. See Table 2 for a list of selected morphologic abnormalities of erythrocytes and their diagnostic significance.

Table 2. POSSIBLE SIGNIFICANCE OF ALTERATIONS IN ERYTHROCYTE SIZE, STAINING, AND MORPHOLOGY

Size Changes	
Increased MCV	May be a feature of regenerative anemias; often present in ineffective erythropoiesis due to nuclear maturation defects
Decreased MCV	Often a feature of ineffective erythropoiesis due to disorders of hemoglobin synthesis (iron deficiency is most common cause)
Altered Staining Affinity*	
Polychromasia	Signifies increased release of immature RBCs (reticulocytes) into the circulation; therefore a feature of regenerative anemias
Hypochromasia	Often a feature of ineffective erythropoiesis due to disorders of hemoglobin synthesis (iron deficiency is most common cause)
Basophilic stippling	Commonly seen in regenerative anemias in ruminant species; in absence of regenerative anemia, may signify lead toxicity
Morphologic Abnormalities	
Nucleated RBCs	May be present in highly regenerative anemias (reticulocytes should outnumber nRBCs in this situation); in absence of regenerative anemia, consider bone marrow stromal damage (endotoxemia; heavy metal toxicity such as lead poisoning; neoplastic infiltration), extramedullary hematopoiesis
Acanthocytes	Liver disease; disordered lipid metabolism; sometimes seen in calves with pneumonia
Spherocytes	Immune-mediated hemolytic anemias; Heinz body hemolytic anemias
Schistocytes	Thrombotic disorders (including localized and diffuse intravascular coagulation); vasculitis, chronic renal disease, vascular tumors (hemangiosarcoma)
Ovalocytes	Characteristic of the family Camellidae; sometimes associated with myelophthisic syndromes
Heinz bodies	Hemolysis due to oxidant toxins (cruciferous plants, castor beans, rye grass, onions, copper); sometimes seen in cattle with postparturient hemoglobinuria (possibly associated with increased susceptibility to oxidants)

*Wright's-type stains.

Regenerative Anemias

As previously stated, these anemias are due to excessive loss of erythrocytes via hemorrhage or hemolysis. Table 3 lists causes of hemorrhage and hemolysis. If the bone marrow is healthy, erythroid hyperplasia occurs to compensate for peripheral erythrocyte losses. Because it takes 4 to 6 days for the bone marrow to increase circulating reticulocyte numbers significantly, a CBC performed early in the course of a hemorrhagic or a hemolytic anemia may give the false impression of a poorly regenerative or nonregenerative anemia. Regenerative anemias are often characterized by the presence of diagnostic clues that help to shorten the list of potential etiologies.

Blood loss anemias are usually characterized by a decrease in the plasma protein level since all components of blood, not just the cells, are lost via hemorrhage. A site of hemorrhage may be evident, or other clinical or laboratory evidence may suggest occult loss of blood. Severe acute bleeding episodes result in hypovolemia as well as hypoxia owing to a decreased erythrocyte mass. Affected animals may present with hypovolemic shock to compound the hypoxia owing to the anemia. The hematocrit of animals with acute hemorrhage will not fully reflect the severity of the erythrocyte loss until approximately 48 hours after bleeding has ceased. Intravascular fluid

Table 3. CAUSES OF REGENERATIVE ANEMIA IN FOOD ANIMALS

Hemorrhage*
Trauma
Surgery
Hemostatic disorders
Gastrointestinal ulcers
Parasitism: infestation with endoparasites or ectoparasites that feed on the blood supply
Hematuria
Vascular neoplasia (e.g., hemangiosarcoma)

Hemolysis
Intravascular
    Bacteria (e.g., *Leptospira* spp., *Clostridium perfringens* type A, *Clostridium hemolyticum*)
    RBC parasites (*Babesia*)
    Toxins (e.g., onions, rye grass, cruciferous plants, castor bean plants, copper)
    Immune-mediated hemolysis (e.g., neonatal isoerythrolysis occurring in calves of dams given bovine-origin vaccines against anaplasmosis, drug-induced immune-mediated hemolysis, autoimmune hemolytic anemia)
    Postparturient hemoglobinuria of cattle
    Intrinsic erythrocyte defects (e.g., bovine congenital erythropoietic porphyria)
Extravascular
    RBC parasites (e.g., *Anaplasma*, *Eperythrozoon*)
    Toxins (e.g., onions, rye grass, cruciferous plants, castor bean plants, copper)
    Immune mediated (e.g., drug-induced immune-mediated hemolysis, autoimmune hemolytic anemia)
    Intrinsic erythrocyte defects

*Chronic blood loss may lead to iron deficiency, causing the anemia to change from regenerative to nonregenerative.

is lost during hemorrhage, and compensatory shifts of body water from extravascular compartments to restore blood volume (and thereby dilute the remaining erythrocyte mass) take time.

Chronic blood loss anemia, as from chronic infestation with bloodsucking parasites or a chronically bleeding ulcer, progresses slowly. If chronic blood loss gradually depletes the body iron stores, the anemia may change from a regenerative anemia to a nonregenerative iron deficiency anemia (see below).

Hemolysis generally results in a stronger and somewhat quicker regenerative response than does hemorrhage because the components of the erythrocytes (iron and proteins) are not lost from the body and can be readily recycled. The plasma protein level is usually normal or increased.

Hemolysis can be either an intravascular or an extravascular phenomenon. The clinical and laboratory findings vary according to which type of hemolysis predominates in a particular case. In extravascular hemolysis, erythrocytes are phagocytized at an increased rate by macrophages in the spleen, liver, and perhaps other tissues. In intravascular hemolysis, the erythrocytes rupture in the circulating blood stream, releasing their hemoglobin into the plasma. Therefore splenomegaly and hepatosplenomegaly are most consistent with extravascular hemolysis, while hemoglobinemia and hemoglobinuria indicate intravascular hemolysis. Hyperbilirubinemia may occur with any hemolytic process but is more frequent in intravascular than extravascular hemolysis. Early in the course of hemolysis, hyperbilirubinemia is due to increased unconjugated (indirect reacting) bilirubin. As the process progresses, conjugated bilirubin may also increase. The blood smears of patients with intravascular hemolysis may contain fragmented erythrocytes (schistocytes) or the membranes of ruptured cells (erythrocyte "ghosts"). Heinz bodies may be seen on the erythrocytes of animals with intravascular or extravascular hemolysis owing to oxidant toxins. Blood smears of patients with extravascular hemolysis may contain spherocytes, but these are difficult to identify in food animals since their erythrocytes are normally small and lack a distinct central pallor.

Intravascular hemolytic episodes tend to cause a sudden rapid decrease in the hematocrit (aptly termed a hemolytic crisis), allowing the animal no time to compensate for the resultant anemia. Therefore these anemias tend to present with clearly evident clinical signs of anemia and its attendant hypoxia, and signs of a regenerative response may not yet be present in the peripheral blood. In contrast, anemias due primarily to extravascular hemolysis often progress slowly. As increased destruction of erythrocytes decreases the hematocrit, the bone marrow undergoes erythroid hyperplasia to compensate for the lost erythrocytes. However, high rates of erythrocyte destruction often prevent the marrow from fully compensating, so that the net effect is a slowly worsening anemia. The animal has time to compensate for the anemia with cardiac hypertrophy and adaptive alterations of erythrocyte metabolism. By the time medical attention is sought, the hematocrit may be quite low and a regenerative response should be evident.

Nonregenerative Anemias

These anemias are due to decreased production of erythrocytes either because of defects in the maturation of erythrocyte precursors (referred to as maturation arrest anemias, or ineffective erythropoiesis) or because of hypoplasia or aplasia of the erythroid compartment of the bone marrow. Since nonregenerative anemias are primarily the result of decreased erythrocyte production, and since erythrocytes have long life spans, nonregenerative anemias generally develop slowly. Slow development of anemia allows time for compensatory cardiovascular changes and alterations of erythrocyte metabolism, which help counteract the anemia by increasing the efficiency of oxygen delivery to the tissues. For this reason, nonregenerative anemias can become quite severe before clinical signs, such as exercise intolerance, become evident.

Causes of nonregenerative anemias are listed in Table 4. Sometimes etiologic clues can be identified by the CBC (the clues that may be provided by the MCV and MCHC have been discussed), but a bone marrow examination is often necessary for the complete evaluation of nonregenerative anemias. In those nonregenerative anemias due to ineffective erythropoiesis, the erythroid compartment of the marrow will be hyperplastic. However, the maturation sequence will be interrupted at some point, resulting in an increase of early precursors with few of the more mature cells of the maturation sequence present. In those nonregenerative anemias due to erythroid hypoplasia or aplasia, marrow erythroid cells of all stages of development will be decreased. The most common hypoplastic anemia is the anemia of chronic inflammation. This type of anemia can occur secondarily to chronic neoplastic as well as chronic inflammatory disorders. The anemia is usually mild, and bone marrow findings typically include myeloid hyperplasia, increased iron stores, and plasmacytosis, in addition to mild erythroid hypoplasia.

Polycythemia

Polycythemia is an increased erythrocyte mass per volume of blood. There are two kinds of polycythemia; relative and absolute. In relative polycythemia the hematocrit is increased because the aqueous portion of the blood is decreased. This situation is the result of dehydration and is by far the most common type of polycythemia seen. Rehydration resolves the problem. Absolute polycythemia is due to an actual increase

Table 4. CAUSES OF NONREGENERATIVE ANEMIA IN FOOD ANIMALS

Ineffective Erythropoiesis (Maturation Arrest Anemias)
Nuclear maturation arrests (disorders of nucleic acid synthesis)
  Vitamin B_{12} deficiency
  Cobalt deficiency*
  Folic acid deficiency
Cytoplasmic maturation arrests (disorders of hemoglobin synthesis)
  Iron deficiency
  Pyridoxine deficiency
  Copper deficiency
  Molybdenum toxicity
  Lead toxicity

Erythroid Hypoplasia/Aplasia
Anemia of chronic disease
  Chronic inflammation
  Chronic neoplasia
Inadequate erythropoietin production
  Chronic renal disease
  Hypothyroidism†
Cytotoxic bone marrow damage‡
  Radiation
  Bracken fern
Immune mediated
  Pure red cell aplasia
Myelophthisic syndromes
  Leukemia
  Metastatic neoplasia
  Myelofibrosis
Infections
  Trichostrongyles (nonbloodsucking)

*Because rumen microflora can synthesize vitamin B_{12}, vitamin B_{12} deficiency does not occur in ruminants unless they are grazing on cobalt-deficient soils (cobalt is required for vitamin B_{12} synthesis).
†Has been seen in cattle with hypothyroidism secondary to fluorosis.
‡Usually accompanied by leukopenia and thrombocytopenia.

in the total erythrocyte mass in the body. This can be the result of an appropriate response of the bone marrow to increased erythropoietin levels secondary to increased peripheral need for erythrocytes. Examples of this type of polycythemia include that associated with tissue hypoxia secondary to high altitude and that associated with pulmonary disease that interferes with oxygenation of hemoglobin. Polycythemia can also be the result of a response to a tumor, usually of renal origin, that is producing erythropoietin or an erythropoietin-like substance. Some cases of absolute polycythemia are the result of inappropriate production of erythrocytes not in response to increased erythropoietin levels. This situation is usually idiopathic and is sometimes a prelude to the development of a hematopoietic malignancy. Hereditary polycythemia has been seen in inbred Jersey cattle. Affected animals have hematocrits of 60 to 80, with no reticulocytosis and no lesions to explain a secondary polycythemia. They are weak, lethargic, and dyspneic and often die by 6 months of age. Survivors usually have a remission of clinical signs by the time they reach maturity.

DISORDERS OF THE LEUKON

The leukocytic portion of the CBC is used to detect leukocytosis or leukopenias and to determine which specific types of leukocytes are altered in number. Table 5 lists the causes of shifts in the absolute numbers of leukocytes. The morphology of the leukocytes should also be assessed. As is the case with the erythroid portion of the CBC, detection of abnormalities in the leukocytic compartment may not provide a specific etiologic diagnosis but usually provides diagnostically and prognostically useful information, especially when used in conjunction with other patient data.

Although differential leukocyte counts are often reported as the percentages of each type of cell present (relative numbers), interpretations should always be based on the absolute numbers of each type of cell in the circulating blood (derived by multiplying the percentages by the total WBC count). A relative neutrophilia can be due to either an absolute neutrophilia or an absolute lymphocytopenia, or a combination of the two. If the total number of leukocytes is sufficiently decreased, it is possible to have a relative neutrophilia even though there is an absolute neutropenia. In health, the food animal species have a higher proportion of lymphocytes than of neutrophils in circulation, so when a relative neutrophilia occurs it is sometimes called a "lymph-seg reversal." "Lymph-seg reversal," like "relative neutrophilia," is an ambiguous term that has no diagnostic usefulness until translated into terms of what the absolute numbers of neutrophils and lymphocytes are. Throughout this article, terms such as neutrophilia, neutropenia, lymphocytosis, etc., refer to absolute numbers of the leukocytes.

Morphologic abnormalities of leukocytes include the presence of increased numbers of immature neutrophils (a "left shift"), toxic changes in neutrophils, and reactive changes in lymphocytes. In addition, cells with morphology consistent with neoplastic transformation are sometimes seen in the circulating blood of animals with leukemia.

Table 5. CAUSES OF SHIFTS IN LEUKOCYTE NUMBERS

Neutrophilia
Epinephrine release (physiologic leukocytosis)*
Corticosteroid effects (stress leukogram)†
Inflammation
Infection (especially bacterial; also fungal, viral, parasitic)
Myelogenous leukemia

Neutropenia
Acute inflammation
Severe, overwhelming infection/inflammation (common with coliform infections, endotoxemia)
Bone marrow cytotoxicity (irradiation, bracken fern)
Myelophthisic syndromes

Lymphocytosis
Chronic viral infections
Epinephrine release (physiologic leukocytosis)*
Lymphoid leukemia
Persistent lymphocytosis of cattle (see text)

Lymphocytopenia
Acute viral infections
Mycoplasma infections
Septicemia
Corticosteroid effects†
Loss of lymph (ruptured thoracic duct, alimentary lymphosarcoma, enteric neoplasia, granulomatous enteritis, Johne's disease, protein-losing enteropathy)
Lymphosarcoma
Hereditary thymic aplasia (T cell deficiency) of Black-Pied Danish cattle

Monocytosis
Resolving inflammation
Chronic persistent inflammation
Acute inflammation
Tissue necrosis
Corticosteroid effects†

Eosinophilia/Basophilia
Endogenous or exogenous parasites that cause tissue reactions
Allergic reactions

*Associated with fear, excitement, strenuous exercise. Lymphocytosis may be a feature of physiologic leukocytosis in pigs. This response has been seen 3 to 5 hours after feeding in healthy pigs.
†Can be due to increased endogenous corticosteroid release or to administration of exogenous corticosteroids. Associated with pain and temperature extremes. In cattle also seen with displaced abomasum, milk fever, ketosis, dystocia, feed overload, and indigestion. In pigs also seen with parturition, strenuous exercise, and immediately after transport.

Disorders of the leukocytic portion of the hemic system may occur alone or in conjunction with abnormalities in the erythron and/or thrombon. Various combinations of increases and decreases in the circulating numbers of the different types of leukocytes occur, with some general patterns being associated inflammation, epinephrine effects, and corticosteroid effects. Two or more factors may simultaneously affect the leukogram.

Inflammation

Inflammation can cause neutrophilia or neutropenia, depending on the type, stage, and severity of the inflammatory process. During the acute phase of inflammation, neutrophil numbers may be normal or even decreased and there will often be a left shift. As the suppurative process progresses, an adequate bone marrow response results in neutrophilia followed by a disappearance of the left shift as the bone marrow reaches a higher steady state of neutrophil production. As inflammation subsides, neutrophil production slowly decreases to normal again. In general, localized suppurative inflammatory processes, such as abscesses and metritis, cause higher neutrophil counts than more diffuse inflammatory processes.

The magnitude of the left shift and the likelihood of the development of neutropenia in the acute phase of inflammation depends on the size of the bone marrow storage pool of mature neutrophils at the onset of inflammation, the severity of the inflammation, and the ability of the bone marrow to increase its production of neutrophils in the face of increased peripheral demands. In ruminants acute inflammation frequently causes a period of neutropenia, and a pronounced left shift may develop and persist for several days. Ruminants do not have a large bone marrow storage pool of mature neutrophils to draw upon, and they do not have as strong a neutrophilic response to suppurative inflammatory processes as many other animals do. However, by 3 to 5 days after the onset of inflammation, neutrophil numbers should start to increase and the left shift should lessen. A left shift that persists for more than 4 to 5 days without the development of a neutrophilia indicates that the bone marrow response to the inflammatory process is inadequate, and this warrants a guarded prognosis.

In severe inflammatory processes the bone marrow may be unable to respond adequately to the tissue demand for neutrophils, and the neutropenia will persist or worsen as the inflammatory process progresses. This is especially likely to happen during infections by bacteria that produce systemic toxins, such as endotoxin. Such toxins may damage the developing neutrophils in the bone marrow and prevent an adequate increase in neutrophil production. The morphologic alterations of neutrophils associated with toxicity include Doehle body formation, foamy cytoplasmic basophilia, and enlargement of neutrophils. Persistent or worsening neutropenias accompanied by neutrophil toxicity warrant a very poor prognosis.

Since ruminants may not develop a pronounced neutrophilic response during inflammation, fibrinogen determination is a useful adjunct to the leukogram for the detection of inflammation in ruminants. Hyperfibrinogenemia occurs during inflammation. Hyperfibrinogenemia also occurs with dehydration. The plasma protein:fibrinogen ratio can be used to help differentiate the hyperfibrinogenemia of inflammation from that of dehydration since all the plasma proteins will be proportionately elevated in dehydration and fibrinogen will be disproportionately elevated in inflammation. A protein:fibrinogen ratio of less than 10 is indicative of inflammation, while a value of greater than 15 is consistent with normalcy or dehydration.

Monocytosis and lymphocytosis are frequent features of chronic inflammatory leukograms. Monocytosis can also occur during the acute and subacute phases of inflammation, especially if tissue necrosis is present. Reactive lymphocytes are often seen during inflammation; the reactive changes signify antigenic stimulation and are seen in many infectious processes. Inflammatory responses involving hypersensitivity reactions often result in eosinophilia, sometimes in conjunction with basophilia. Parasitic diseases in which some stage of the parasite invades or migrates through tissues are likely to incite eosinophilia.

Corticosteroid Effects (The Stress Leukogram)

The classic findings associated with corticosteroid release or administration are mild to moderate neutrophilia, lymphocytopenia, monocytosis, and eosinopenia. These findings are commonly referred to as a "stress leukogram" since endogenous steroid release occurs in response to stress. The lymphocytopenia is probably the most consistent characteristic. The neutrophilia is due to decreased margination of neutrophils on the vascular walls, decreased migration of neutrophils into tissue, and increased release into the peripheral circulation of neutrophils from the bone marrow storage pool. The neutrophilia is usually mature (no left shift), but there may be a left shift if the corticosteroid response occurs in conjunction with inflammation. In fact it is common to see a corticosteroid response superimposed on an acute inflammatory response since increased endogenous steroid release commonly occurs during the acute phases of inflammation. The total WBC count of cattle typically reaches 8000 to 18,000/μl in response to steroids. Alterations in the leukogram are usually most pronounced 4 to 8 hours after steroid administration, and they are usually gone by approximately 24 hours after a single therapeutic dose or within 72 hours after a longer treatment regime.

Epinephrine Effects (Physiologic Leukocytosis)

Epinephrine release, which is usually the result of an animal being excited or fearful at the time of sample collection, causes a mature neutrophilia. In pigs lymphocytosis may occur as well. The effect is primarily the result of increased blood pressure and muscular activity, which cause the portion of the neutrophils that are normally marginated on the vascular walls to be dislodged into the flowing blood, and which may cause increased ejection of lymphocytes from the thoracic duct into the blood stream. Epinephrine has no effect on the bone marrow. Epinephrine effects are usually short-lived, disappearing soon after the animal becomes quiet.

Hematopoietic Neoplasia

The leukogram findings of animals with hematopoietic neoplasia are extremely variable. The proliferation of neoplastic cell lines in the bone marrow may crowd out the normal hematopoietic cells and cause anemia or other cytopenias. Neoplastic cells are often released from the bone marrow into the blood; their numbers in the blood can range from very low to extremely high. The most common hematopoietic neoplasms in food animals are those of lymphoid origin, and these are most common in cattle. Myeloproliferative diseases are rare in food animals.

Lymphoid leukemias in cattle are most often the result of the adult form of multicentric lymphosarcoma caused by bovine leukemia virus (BLV). The neoplasm often arises in the peripheral lymphoid tissue (lymph nodes, etc.) but may metastasize to the bone marrow. Neoplastic cells are found in the circulation in approximately 30 per cent of cases. Because the clinical course of the disease is usually rapid and the erythrocytes of cattle have long life spans (up to 160 days), severe anemia is usually not a sequela of lymphoid leukemia in cattle.

Bovine Persistent Lymphocytosis

BLV infection is also associated with another condition, called persistent lymphocytosis. Persistent lymphocytosis is defined as an increase in the absolute lymphocyte count beyond the normal level for the patient's age for at least 3 months. Only a small percentage of cattle with persistent lymphocytosis develop lymphosarcoma, but about 65 per cent of cattle with BLV-associated lymphosarcoma previously had persistent lymphocytosis.

Functional Disorders of Leukocytes

Functional disorders of leukocytes may be either hereditary or acquired. Few hereditary disorders have been seen in food animals. Some experimental work has been done in food animals (mostly cattle) to determine the effects of various infectious agents on the functions of leukocytes.

Chédiak-Higashi syndrome is a hereditary abnormality found in cattle of the Hereford and Angus breeds. It is a generalized cellular disorder characterized by abnormal fusion of cytoplasmic granules of leukocytes. The basic abnormality underlying the syndrome is unknown. Because the granules of melanocytes are also abnormally fused, affected animals have coat color dilution. Giant granules can usually be seen in the neutrophils and eosinophils on Wright's-stained blood smears from affected cattle. Leukocyte function is abnormal, so affected animals have increased susceptibility to infection. Platelet function is also abnormal, causing mild bleeding abnormalities. Affected animals may be neutropenic and thrombocytopenic. There is a propensity for lymphohistiocytic proliferation in the bone marrow, liver, and spleen of animals with Chédiak-Higashi syndrome, which contributes to pancytopenia and increased susceptibility to infection.

DISORDERS OF THE THROMBON AND HEMOSTATIC MECHANISMS

Disorders of the thrombon and hemostatic mechanisms may be either hereditary or acquired. A few hereditary disorders have been identified in food animals. Acquired disorders may be the result of bone marrow dysfunction in the case of thrombocytopenia or thrombocytosis, of increased platelet destruction or consumption in the case of thrombocytopenia, or of decreased synthesis, increased utilization, or increased loss in the case of deficiencies of coagulation factors and other proteins involved in the coagulation cascades. Platelet function defects may occur secondarily to various disease states, such as renal uremia.

Thrombocytopenia

Thrombocytopenia may result from decreased platelet production, increased platelet consumption, increased platelet destruction, or sequestration of platelets in the spleen. Decreased platelet production may result from bone marrow toxicity that affects the megakaryocytes or their progenitors. Increased platelet consumption is most commonly associated with thrombotic disorders, including diffuse intravascular coagulation (DIC). DIC is a potential sequela of many diseases. Increased platelet destruction due to an immune response directed against platelets is seen in some species of animals. Endotoxemia may cause splenic sequestration of platelets.

Thrombocytosis

Thrombocytosis is sometimes a feature of iron deficiency anemia. In iron deficiency anemia, circulating levels of erythropoietin are increased and erythropoietin has some thrombopoietic effect. Thrombocytosis may also be a feature of some forms of hematopoietic malignancy.

Thrombocytopathies

The platelets of cattle with Chédiak-Higashi syndrome have a dense granule storage pool deficiency, which affects platelet function and may lead to prolonged bleeding times. A familial thrombocytopathy has been seen in Simmental cattle. Affected animals have prolonged bleeding times, and mild to severe hemorrhage may occur, especially following trauma or surgery. A hereditary platelet function defect due to abnormalities in the platelet granules has been seen in pigs. Acquired platelet function defects may occur secondarily to various disease states, but these have not been extensively studied in food animals. Platelet function defects secondary to renal uremia may occur in food animals.

Disorders of Hemostasis

Both congenital and acquired deficiencies of the proteins involved in the hemostatic mechanism occur and may cause a bleeding diathesis. Acquired deficiencies may result from hepatic failure, rodenticide or moldy sweet clover poisoning, or the development of DIC.

The coagulation factor deficiency of hepatic failure is due to decreased protein synthesis by the liver and may result in prolongation of the PTT and PT. Poisoning with coumarins (found in many rodenticides and in moldy sweet clover hay) or with other rodenticides that are vitamin K antagonists may result in deficiencies of the vitamin K–dependent coagulation factors and prolong the PTT and PT. Diffuse intravascular coagulation is typically characterized by prolongation of the PT and PTT, thrombocytopenia, hypofibrinogenemia, decreased ATIII level, and increased fibrin degradation products.

Congenital disorders of hemostasis are seen in food animals. Hereditary deficiency of coagulation factor VIII has been seen in Hereford cattle, and factor XI deficiency has been seen in Holstein cattle. These disorders are characterized by an increased PTT; specific coagulation factor assays are used to identify and confirm the specific factor deficiency present. Some Poland-China cross and Yorkshire-Hampshire cross pigs have a hereditary deficiency of von Willebrand factor, resulting in a disease that is analogous to autosomal recessive type III von Willebrand disease of humans. Homozygotes have a moderate to severe bleeding tendency. Routine coagulation test results are often normal, but occasional animals have a slightly increased PTT. Von Willebrand factor assays are used to confirm the diagnosis. Heterozygotes are detectable by laboratory tests (von Willebrand factor assays) but are asymptomatic. A hereditary afibrinogenemia has been reported in Saanen goats. Affected newborn and young kids have a severe hemorrhagic diathesis characterized by hemarthroses and by bleeding from the umbilicus into the subcutaneous tissues and from the mucous membranes. The disorder is inherited as an incompletely dominant trait, with homozygous goats having no detectable fibrinogen and heterozygotes having decreased levels.

REFERENCES

1. Benjamin MM: Outline of Veterinary Clinical Pathology, 3rd ed. Ames, IA, Iowa State University Press, 1978.
2. Coles EH: Veterinary Clinical Pathology, 3rd ed. Philadelphia, WB Saunders, 1980.
3. Dodds WJ: Hemostasis. In Kaneko JJ (ed): Clinical Biochemistry of Domestic Animals, 4th ed. New York, Academic Press, 1989, pp 274–315.
4. Duncan JR, Prasse KW: Veterinary Laboratory Medicine—Clinical Pathology, 2nd ed. Ames, IA, Iowa State University Press, 1986.
5. Jain NC: Schalm's Veterinary Hematology, 4th ed. Philadelphia, Lea & Febiger, 1986.
6. Kaneko JJ: Porphyrins and the porphyrias. In Kaneko JJ (ed): Clinical Biochemistry of Domestic Animals, 4th ed. New York, Academic Press, 1989, pp 235–255.

Therapeutic Management of Cardiovascular and Hemolymphatic Diseases

PETER D. CONSTABLE, BVSc, MS, Diplomate, ACVIM, MRCVS

The aim of this article is to provide an overview of current therapeutic agents and techniques used in treating diseases of the cardiovascular and hemolymphatic systems. The emphasis will be placed on the treatment of specific conditions in cattle since therapy is more frequently attempted and documented in this species. However, many of the principles outlined below can be directly extrapolated for use in other ruminant species.

ANEMIA

The numerous causes of anemia are discussed in greater depth elsewhere in this volume. Central to the successful treatment of anemic conditions is characterization of the cause. The etiology is often readily apparent after consideration of the history and physical examination findings. Laboratory assessment of the regenerative response, through examination of various red blood cell indices, red blood cell fragility, total iron binding capacity, serum iron and ferritin concentrations, bone marrow response, body hemosiderin stores, and the normalcy of coagulation, may add useful information in selected cases. The clinician needs to be cognizant that characterization of the anemia should be attempted before blood transfusions are administered since the immunologic response to the infused blood will alter many of these tests.

From a therapeutic perspective anemia can be conveniently attributed to (1) acute blood loss, (2) chronic blood loss, or (3) chronic inflammation.

Acute Blood Loss

Acute hemorrhage is often life threatening. Immediate treatment is required to minimize further blood loss and rapidly increase venous return. It is important to realize that the cause of death after acute hemorrhage is usually hypovolemia rather than inadequate oxygen carrying capability. The immediate focus of treatment after severe hemorrhage should therefore be rapid restoration of perfusion pressure and plasma volume. This is best achieved by the rapid administration of balanced electrolyte solutions and hypertonic saline (HS) solutions once hemorrhage is controlled.

HS (2400 mOsm/L sodium chloride, equivalent to 7.2 per cent sodium chloride, 4 to 5 ml/kg intravenously over 2 to 10 minutes) has been used successfully to resuscitate sheep,[1] pigs,[2] horses,[3] and dogs[4] from hemorrhagic/hypovolemic shock. HS is believed to exert its beneficial effects primarily through rapid plasma volume expansion and associated increases in systemic arterial pressure, cardiac output, and urine production. HS also constricts venous capacitance beds and redistributes the cardiac output away from muscular and cutaneous vascular beds, facilitating perfusion of vital organ systems.[5] HS is therefore the treatment of choice for the initial resuscitation of animals in acute hemorrhagic shock. The advantages of HS in this setting are as follows:

1. It resuscitates animals rapidly and economically.
2. The hypertonicity of the solution ensures that it remains sterile and in solution over a wide range of environmental temperatures, providing a long shelf life.
3. The solution is not viscous and is easy to infuse intravenously.
4. It reverses some of the cellular abnormalities induced by hemorrhagic shock.
5. It rapidly restores cardiac output.
6. It minimizes the increase in pulmonary vascular resistance and edema observed with rapid isotonic crystalloid fluid administration.
7. It minimizes net water administered.

Contraindications to HS administration include hypernatremia, hyperosmolality, hypokalemia, severe acidosis, and inability to control hemorrhage. HS solutions should be infused at the dose and rate outlined above. Profound hypotension can result from extremely rapid intravenous injections of HS. It should be emphasized that this treatment is applicable only to the *initial* management of hemorrhagic shock, allowing sufficient time for the clinician to control hemorrhage definitively or obtain blood for transfusion. The dose rate of HS can usually be repeated once after 30 minutes if necessary, but additional treatments should not be contemplated because of the risk of hypernatremia.

Volume expansion with isotonic crystalloid fluids (such as normal saline) can improve oxygen delivery in animals with mild hemorrhagic shock. To ensure adequate resuscitation, the volume of isotonic saline administered should be approximately three times the volume of blood lost. Infusion of an adequate volume of isotonic fluid cannot usually be performed rapidly enough in large animals, and HS administration or blood transfusion should be considered as a more practical alternative.

Indications for blood transfusion following acute hemorrhage include (1) inability to control hemorrhage (such as bleeding from an abomasal ulcer), (2) lethargy, (3) weakness, (4) inappetence, (5) exercise intolerance, (6) elevated heart rate, (7) pale mucous membranes, and (8) late pregnancy, when hypoxia may result in fetal death. A good clinical examination is usually the best method of evaluating the severity of a bleeding episode and the necessity for blood transfusion. Laboratory determination of the hematocrit and plasma protein is not an accurate guide to the extent of hemorrhage since these do not change for some hours after the bleeding episode. The most accurate laboratory indicator of the need for blood transfusion is the oxygen tension in mixed venous blood, which is well approximated by determining the oxygen tension in jugular venous blood. Venous oxygen tensions less than 30 mm Hg indicate inadequate oxygen delivery to the tissues, regardless of tissue oxygen demand. Volume expansion with HS or isotonic fluid can improve oxygen delivery through increasing cardiac output; however, blood transfusions may be more beneficial in selected cases since they increase venous return *and* the oxygen carrying capacity of blood. Fresh blood is preferred in this case since stored blood has a decreased erythrocyte 2,3-diphosphoglycerate (DPG) concentration. This shifts the oxyhemoglobin dissociation curve to the left, potentially decreasing tissue oxygenation.

Iron supplementation is not required after one episode of acute blood loss since body iron stores are usually adequate and grazing ruminants ingest sufficient quantities of iron on a daily basis. Additional iron may be required by the animal when bleeding episodes have been frequent, as outlined below, or when anorexia is present.

Chronic Blood Loss

Chronic blood loss is a common occurrence in food animals and frequently results from severe internal or external parasitism. The anemia is usually microcytic and hypochromic. Because blood loss occurs over a prolonged period, the animal can successfully adapt to very low hematocrit values. Ruminants can frequently stand and graze with a hematocrit as low as 5 per cent, provided that the rate of blood loss is slow enough to allow compensatory mechanisms to be evoked.

Therapy should be directed primarily at removal of the cause of the chronic blood loss. Blood transfusions are generally not indicated in animals with chronic anemia because transfused red blood cells are short-lived (2 to 4 days). Additionally, transfused red blood cells interfere with the animal's normal bone marrow response to anemia. A possible benefit of transfusion is the provision of rapidly utilizable hemoglobin because these animals may have total depletion of their iron stores. Administration of iron may also be of additional benefit in rapidly replenishing body iron stores. This can take the form of oral administration or deep intramuscular injection of iron compounds.

Chronic Inflammation

Anemia of inflammatory disease is usually normocytic, normochromic, and mild in nature. It is characterized by low serum iron concentration, normal or decreased total iron binding capacity, and increased bone marrow iron stores.[6] The anemia results from sequestration of iron by the mononuclear phagocytic cell system as a defensive measure.[20] Blood transfusions and iron supplementation are contraindicated in the treatment of this disorder since excess iron may enhance the pathogenicity of the invading bacteria. Additionally, there is no depletion of total body iron stores, making iron supplementation superfluous.

Blood Transfusions

The objective of blood transfusion is to supply the animal with one of four factors: (1) red blood cells and therefore hemoglobin, (2) clotting factors, (3) immunoglobulin, or (4) protein. The techniques for collection are similar for all conditions, the exception being that clotting factors can be deactivated when blood is collected in glass. Blood should therefore be collected in plastic containers if it is being used in the treatment of coagulation disorders.

Blood is readily obtained from the jugular vein of a cow through a 10- or 12-gauge bleeding trocar. Placement of a choke rope will facilitate venous distension and hasten blood flow. Up to 15 per cent of the blood volume, corresponding to approximately 1.2 L blood/100 kg, can be removed safely over 15 to 20 minutes from the donor. Blood is most easily collected in an open-mouth glass jar containing 4 g sodium citrate/L blood to be collected. The blood is gently swirled during collection to ensure adequate mixing of the anticoagulant. Excess sodium citrate should not be added since hypocalcemia can be induced if the blood is administered rapidly to the recipient. The blood should be administered immediately or refrigerated at 4°C for up to 24 hours prior to use. Filters are not required for transfusion if fresh blood is used and anticoagulation has been adequate. To prevent transmission of infective agents to the recipient, the blood donor should be free of anaplasmosis and bovine leukemia virus (BLV).

Blood is usually administered intravenously, although in exceptional circumstances the intraperitoneal route may be used. Crossmatching of blood is unnecessary for the first blood transfusion but may be required for subsequent transfusions, particularly if the period between transfusions exceeds a week. The most practical way of ensuring compatibility of blood types is to monitor the recipient's response during the first 10 minutes of blood administration. Transfusion should be stopped if trembling, tachypnea, weakness, and salivation are observed. These responses are more common in neonates, in which they may result from a rapid rate of administration rather than an anaphylactic reaction. Treatment of transfusion reactions primarily involves discontinuing blood administration. Epinephrine and antihistamine given intramuscularly are of benefit in severe cases. Recommencement of blood transfusion, preferably from another donor, should be done only under close supervision and using slow infusion rates.

Iron Administration

Iron is most economically and safely administered orally, with ferrous salts being absorbed the most efficiently. Suggested daily oral dose rates of ferrous sulfate are as follows: cattle 8 to 15 g; sheep, goats, and swine 0.5 to 2 g. Treatment can be continued for up to 2 weeks.[7] Dark feces, reflecting the presence of unabsorbed iron, may be observed after oral dosing. Heavy oral dosing is not recommended since iron toxicity has been induced in piglets administered large doses (0.6 g/kg) of ferrous iron.[8]

Parenteral iron injections can be prohibitively expensive when administered to adult cattle, and anaphylactic reactions and cellulitis have occasionally been observed following iron injection. Caution should be exercised if multiple treatments are administered since iron cannot be rapidly excreted from the body and iron toxicity may result. Iron must be injected as a slow-release compound, usually iron dextran complex (100 mg/ml). Injection of quick-release salts containing iron, or intravenous injection of iron dextran, will result in rapid death, as the excess iron causes the rapid precipitation of blood protein.

Parenteral iron administration should be considered in animals with documented iron deficiency (microcytic, hypochromic anemia; low serum iron; and low ferritin concentrations with normal iron-binding capacity) and abnormal gastrointestinal function. Dose rates for ruminants are empirical, and additional treatments with iron should be given when indicated by the mean corpuscular hemoglobin concentration and total hemoglobin concentration. Neonatal pigs routinely require iron injections within the first week of life, since they are born with minimal iron stores and the sow's milk is low in iron. This subject is discussed in greater detail elsewhere. Parenteral iron administration is not routinely required in other neonates.

Vitamin B_{12}

There are very few indications for the use of vitamin B_{12} in the treatment of anemia in food animals. Vitamin B_{12} is synthesized in adequate quantities by ruminant bacteria and is required by all cells in the body for DNA synthesis. The adult ruminant liver usually has adequate stores of vitamin B_{12} that can maintain normal blood levels for at least 6 months. Supplementation of anemic animals with vitamin B_{12} should be considered only in ruminants with cobalt deficiency (causing absorbed vitamin B_{12} to be inactive) or inadequate liver stores (suckling ruminants, extremely prolonged anorexia). Vitamin B_{12} deficiency should be considered in ruminants with a macrocytic anemia that is not attributable to a regenerative response. Suggested intramuscular doses of cyanocobalamin are as follows: cows 2500 μg; calves 1000 to 1500 μg; sheep, goats, and swine 1000 μg. The dosage can be repeated in 7 days if necessary.

The two major advantages of vitamin B_{12} in the treatment of anemia are its low cost and pretty red color. Many veterinarians administer vitamin B_{12} in the belief that it does not hurt, it might help, and it looks like they are doing something. When administering vitamin B_{12} to an anemic animal, the veterinarian needs to determine whether he or she is treating the patient or the owner. It is likely that the majority of food animals receiving vitamin B_{12} injections do not require treatment.

Anabolic Steroids

These agents are useful adjunct treatments for anemia. The mechanism of action of anabolic steroids is through erythropoietin-mediated stimulation of red cell production and nonspecific stimulation of bone marrow. Anabolic steroids are most efficacious when therapeutic endeavors have been instituted against the etiologic agent, and the erythron is showing a regenerative response. However, less than one half of the human patients with refractory anemia respond to treatment with androgenic and anabolic steroids, suggesting that a variable response may also occur in food animals. Appropriate dose rates have not been developed; however, the following intramuscular dosages are suggested: testosterone propionate in oil, cow 100 to 300 mg, sheep and goat 25 mg, three times per week; testosterone phenylpropionate, cow 25 to 50 mg, sheep, goat, and pig 10 mg, every 10 days; testosterone enanthate, cow 250 mg, sheep, goat, and pig 100 mg, every 3 to 4 weeks; nandrolone phenylpropionate, cow 100 to 200 mg, sheep, goat, and pig 50 to 100 mg, every 7 to 10 days; nandrolone laurate, cow 100 to 200 mg, sheep, goat, and pig 50 to 100 mg, every 3 to 4 weeks; stanozolol, cow 250 to 350 mg, sheep, goat, and pig 25 to 50 mg, repeated weekly up to 4 doses; boldenone undecylenate, cow 500 to 700 mg, sheep, goat, and pig 50 to 100 mg, may repeat treatment in 3 weeks. Nearly all of these anabolic steroids are not approved for use in animals intended for food, with the exception of an ear implant containing testosterone propionate and estradiol benzoate. Androgenic compounds containing nandrolone are most widely used for the treatment of anemia in human patients.

ENDOCARDITIS AND THROMBOPHLEBITIS

These two conditions are considered together since the principles of treatment are similar and many cases of endocarditis arise from septic thrombophlebitis. The goals of treatment are (1) to prevent growth of the lesion and (2) to sterilize the lesion.

Inhibition of platelet aggregation and therefore thrombus growth has traditionally involved the administration of aspirin (100 mg/kg orally every 12 hours) or heparin (various doses recommended). Serious questions as to the efficacy of these treatments in food animals must be raised. Aspirin (acetylsalicylic acid) has recently been shown *not* to inhibit bovine platelet aggregation despite marked inhibition being observed in numerous other species.[9] It appears that even though thromboxane formation occurs when bovine platelets are activated, thromboxane synthesis does not appear to be the major biochemical pathway for platelet aggregation in the cow. Aspirin is therefore unsuitable for the treatment of thromboembolic problems in cattle.

Heparin has been used in food animals to prevent growth of a thrombus. Heparin cannot diminish the size of an existing thrombus. Full-dose intravenous heparin therapy is required to prevent extension of the thrombus since adequate concentrations of heparin must be present to neutralize thrombin. Doses required to do this must necessarily alter the coagulation cascade, and monitoring of the activated partial thromboplastin time (APTT) is required to ensure the adequacy of treatment. The traditional goal is to increase the APTT by one and a half to two times. Since the appropriate dose rate for heparin required for this effect has not been determined in ruminant animals, monitoring of the APTT is required to ensure a therapeutic effect.

Heparin has also been used in the prevention of hypercoagulable states such as disseminated intravascular coagulation, although correction of the inciting cause and adequate supportive care are probably of much greater importance. Low-dose heparin administration, usually via subcutaneous injection every 12 hours, is used to *prevent* hypercoagulable disorders. Dose rates for ruminant animals are currently unavailable. Speculation as to the appropriate dose rate is dangerous since the widely recommended low dose rate used in horses (40 IU/kg subcutaneously every 12 hours) has recently been shown to be inadequate when compared with the actual effective dose rate of 125 IU/kg subcutaneously every 12 hours.[10] In addition, marked individual and interspecies variations in dose response have been identified.[10] Monitoring of plasma heparin concentration and APTT is therefore the only accurate way of determining the effectiveness of heparin therapy in ruminants. In human medicine the empirical therapeutic range of low-dose heparin prophylaxis is 0.05 to 0.20 IU heparin/ml plasma; such therapy does not prolong the APTT. Dosage rates need to be adjusted in animals with hepatic or renal disease since heparin is metabolized by the reticuloendothelial system and excreted by the kidney. Because of problems in determining correct dose rates and the requirement for continued monitoring of the APTT, heparin therapy is currently not practical in food animal medicine.

Antibiotics are indicated for the treatment of endocarditis and thrombophlebitis in an attempt to sterilize the lesion. The duration of treatment is controversial, although a minimal duration of 3 weeks is suggested. Optimal treatment of endocarditis requires culture and susceptibility testing since a variety of bacteria can be associated with these disorders in ruminants and swine. In endocarditis, three samples of venous blood from different sites should be obtained aseptically over 1 to 2 hours before instituting antibiotic therapy. The blood should be cultured in a broth medium, with a minimal blood volume of 10 ml and a blood:broth ratio of 1:10 in order to minimize serum bactericidal activity.[11] The requirement of three cultures is not absolute, although a greater number of cultures increases the chance of successful culture and minimizes the potential for skin microflora contamination from confounding the result. In septic thrombophlebitis, ultrasound examination can be useful in identifying appropriate areas for aspiration and culture. *Fusobacterium necrophorum* and *Actinomyces pyogenes* (formerly *Corynebacterium pyogenes*) are almost always isolated from venous thrombosis in cattle.[12] If blood cultures and susceptibility determinations are not performed, procaine penicillin (22,000 IU/kg every 12 hours) is the antibiotic of choice for endocarditis and thrombophlebitis since the majority of bacterial isolates are penicillin sensitive.

ANTIARRHYTHMIC AGENTS

Cardiac arrhythmias are relatively common in sick ruminants. Most arrhythmias are not associated with structural heart disease and do not constitute a significant threat to the animal's well-being. Whenever cardiac arrhythmias are identified, the clinician should closely evaluate the animal for evidence of heart failure or cardiac murmurs (suggestive of organic heart disease) or gastrointestinal and metabolic abnormalities (suggestive of functional arrhythmias resulting from dysautonomia or electrolyte and acid-base abnormalities). Recent reports have implicated the pivotal role of increased vagal tone and gastrointestinal disorders in the genesis of supraventricular arrhythmias in cattle.[13, 14] The vast majority of arrhythmias in cattle respond to resolution of dysautonomia and electrolyte or gastrointestinal abnormalities, and therapy should therefore be directed primarily toward these areas.

Only four pharmaceutical agents (quinidine, lidocaine, digoxin, and atropine) are routinely used to treat cardiac arrhythmias in food animals. These drugs should be administered only when the arrhythmia is producing serious hemodynamic effects. Therapy needs to be closely monitored because marked variations in plasma concentrations occur following dosage. Both quinidine and digoxin are excreted in the milk, and adequate withdrawal times should be used if treated animals are slaughtered or their milk is sold for consumption.

Quinidine

Quinidine is categorized as a class 1a antiarrhythmic agent, possessing membrane stabilizing ability. It slows cardiac conduction, prolongs the effective refractory period, and decreases the excitability of myocardial tissue. Quinidine is considered the treatment of choice for sustained atrial fibrillation in cattle with normal or only partially compromised ventricular function. Because of the potential toxic effects of quinidine, treatment should ideally be confined to cattle that have normal gastrointestinal motility, acid-base status, and serum electrolyte concentrations. Quinidine may also be administered to cattle when atrial fibrillation is thought to be responsible for the clinical signs (lethargy, anorexia, poor milk production).[15] Since the majority of cattle with atrial fibrillation spontaneously convert to normal sinus rhythm, and fatalities can occur with intravenous quinidine infusions, quinidine should not be administered for at least 3 weeks after resolution of any concurrent disorders.

The therapeutic range of quinidine in animals is thought to be 2 to 3 µg/ml plasma,[16] and appropriate dosage schedules are presented in Table 1. Extremely large doses of quinidine are required for oral administration, necessitating slow intravenous infusion for effective and economical treatment.[16] Quinidine should be administered only intravenously under continuous electrocardiographic monitoring with frequent recordings performed at a paper speed of 50 mm/second. Widening of the QRS and QTc is considered a normal therapeutic response to quinidine since a high correlation between plasma quinidine concentration and QRS deviation exists.[17] Another normal response to quinidine infusion is an increase in the frequency of the ventricular response rate, which can progress to a transient, supraventricular tachycardia. Infusion should be stopped or slowed in this eventuality.[13] Treatment should be discontinued if the QRS is prolonged more then 25 per cent during administration, indicating that toxic levels of quinidine may be present. Blepharospasm, diarrhea, increased rumen motility, weakness, ataxia, and depression have been observed during quinidine infusion in cattle.[15, 16] Sodium bicarbonate (1 mEq/kg intravenously) should be administered if toxic signs are severe since it increases quinidine binding to albumin and lowers the plasma potassium concentration, decreasing the effect of quinidine on cardiac tissue.

Lidocaine

Lidocaine is classed as a 1b antiarrhythmic agent, possessing membrane stabilizing activity. Lidocaine decreases automatic-

Table 1. PHARMACOKINETIC DATA AND DOSE RATES FOR SELECTED ANTIARRHYTHMIC AGENTS IN CATTLE AND SHEEP

Antiarrhythmic Agent	Dose	$T_{1/2}$ (hr)	V_d (L/kg)	Cl_T (ml/m/kg)	Reference
Cattle					
Quinidine sulfate	49 mg/kg IV in 4 L water over 4 hr 42 mg/kg IV q 6 hr maintenance	2.3	3.8	19	16
	209 mg/kg oral loading dose 180 mg/kg oral q 6 hr maintenance				
Digoxin	0.022 mg/kg IV loading dose, then 0.0034 mg/kg IV q 4 hr maintenance, or 0.0086 mg/kg/hr continuous IV infusion	7.8	6.4	9.5	25
Digitoxin	0.050 mg/kg IV q 5–6 hr	2–3	NA	NA	30
Sheep					
Digoxin					
Ewes	0.025 mg/kg IV q 8 hr × 3 loading dose 0.005–0.015 mg/kg q 12 hr maintenance	15.2	27.6	17	22, 38
Lambs	0.04 mg/kg IV q 8 hr × 3 loading dose 0.008–0.025 mg/kg q 12 hr maintenance	13.7	35.5	22	22, 38
Lidocaine	1–2 mg/kg IV over 60 sec	1.0	1.3	38	39
	0.3–0.4 mg/kg/min IV infusion for 15 min followed by 0.1–0.2 mg/kg/min IV for 45 min				19

$T_{1/2}$ = Half-life; V_d = volume of distribution; Cl_T = total clearance; NA = not applicable.

ity and conduction velocity of cardiac tissue with only minimal alterations of the refractory period. Its electrophysiologic effects are dependent on an adequate potassium concentration; therefore it is less effective in the presence of hypokalemia. Lidocaine is considered the drug of choice for the treatment of ventricular arrhythmias and is usually administered as a bolus intravenous dose (over 10 seconds) of 1 to 2 mg/kg followed by continuous intravenous infusion (0.025 to 0.060 mg/kg/minute). If continuous intravenous infusion is not done, a second bolus of lidocaine (0.05 mg/kg) can be given 30 to 120 minutes after the first dose. Higher doses should be administered with caution since muscular spasm and shivering have been observed in ewes after 4 mg/kg lidocaine was administered over a 60-second period.[18] Absorption from intramuscular injections is too erratic for therapeutic purposes. The therapeutic blood concentration of lidocaine is 1.5 to 5 µg/ml.[19]

Lidocaine toxicity is manifested initially by neurologic abnormalities. These can occur when the blood lidocaine concentration exceeds 10 µg/ml.[19] Higher doses of lidocaine are required to produce deleterious cardiopulmonary effects. Lidocaine toxicity has been accidently induced in sheep by administration of lidocaine hydrochloride, 20 mg/kg subcutaneously. Typical signs of lidocaine toxicity (muscle tremors, dullness, opisthotonos, blindness, extensor rigidity, and convulsions) were observed within 15 minutes of administration. The neurologic signs abated within 90 minutes of injection and were not induced when 10 mg/kg was administered subcutaneously at a later date.[20] At least 5 mg/kg lidocaine can be administered subcutaneously to cattle before toxic signs are observed.[21] Lidocaine is rapidly metabolized and excreted; therefore the duration of neurologic signs should be short, provided that hepatic and renal blood flow is adequate for metabolism and excretion.

Digoxin

Digoxin exerts its antiarrhythmic effect indirectly through alterations in autonomic tone and cardiac contractility. Digoxin slows the sinus rate, depresses atrioventricular conduction, and prolongs the atrial effective refractory period. It is the antiarrhythmic agent of choice in food animals when heart failure is present. The therapeutic plasma concentration of digoxin is thought to be 0.8 to 2.0 ng/ml, with toxicity usually occurring at concentrations exceeding 2.5 ng/ml. Sheep may require lower plasma concentrations for successful therapy since toxic signs (third-degree AV block and ventricular premature complexes) have been identified in 6 of 12 sheep with plasma digoxin concentrations of 0.9 to 2.7 ng/ml.[22] Neonates require higher doses of digoxin on a body-weight basis than do adults.

Digoxin must be administered intravenously in ruminants since ruminal bacteria degrade orally administered digoxin[23] and intramuscular injections of digoxin produce severe muscle necrosis.[24] The half-life of digoxin in ruminants is much shorter than that observed in other species, necessitating frequent dosing. Appropriate dosages are outlined in Table 1. The constant intravenous infusion dose is the preferred method of digoxin administration in cattle since it prevents the attainment of toxic doses.[25] The doses stated differ significantly from those previously proposed, which appear to be inaccurate.[26, 27]

The requirement for frequent intravenous administration of digoxin makes long-term treatment impractical and uneconomic. An alternative method of digoxin administration is oral administration immediately following induced closure of the esophageal groove. This allows digoxin to by-pass the rumen and escape degradation. Esophageal groove closure is best accomplished by pharyngeal administration of 100 to 250 ml 10 per cent sodium bicarbonate solution in cattle or 5 ml 10 per cent copper sulfate solution in sheep,[28] and intravenous injection of 0.5 IU/kg lysine-vasopressin injection in goats.[29] Esophageal groove closure remains for up to 2 minutes following these treatments. This technique has successfully been used in the treatment of heart failure in sheep in our clinic, as demonstrated by the presence of therapeutic blood levels of digoxin in conjunction with clinical improvement.

Digitoxin is another cardiac glycoside that has been used in cattle. The therapeutic plasma level for digitoxin is thought to be 9 to 30 ng/ml.[30] Digitoxin has been administered to cattle by deep intramuscular injection (0.006 mg/kg every 24 hours maintenance);[31] however, this route and dose rate are not recommended. Another study[30] suggested the dosage schedule outlined in Table 1. Until adequate pharmacokinetic studies of digitoxin are performed, digoxin appears to be the cardiac glycoside of choice in ruminants.

Atropine

Atropine is a muscarinic receptor antagonist that is used in ruminants to inhibit bradycardic states resulting from administration of agents with vagomimetic activity, such as xylazine and calcium borogluconate. In cattle, atropine usually reverses second-degree AV block produced by excessive administration of calcium ions, converting the rhythm to sinus tachycardia.[32] Atropine is not routinely used in ruminants because prolonged inhibition of gastrointestinal motility predisposes the animal to free gas bloat. Suggested dose rates of atropine (as atropine sulfate) are 0.04 mg/kg intramuscularly (preferably), or 0.02 mg/kg intravenously. It should be administered only when cardiac output is thought to be inadequate as a result of bradycardia or second-degree AV block.

HEART FAILURE

Inotropic agents may be indicated on a short-term basis in food animals undergoing surgical procedures or in animals with heart failure in late gestation, where the birth of a viable fetus is desired. In contrast, long-term treatment of heart failure is rarely attempted since heart failure usually indicates severe, irreversible cardiac pathology that is incompatible with an economic, productive life. Despite these reservations, the treatment of selected cases of heart failure has been undertaken, albeit unsuccessfully, in cattle.[31, 33]

The most cost-effective treatment of heart failure in food animals involves stall rest, restriction of sodium intake, and furosemide administration. Minimizing exertion decreases cardiac work. Unrestricted access to salt blocks or consumption of high-salt forages can exacerbate the clinical signs of heart failure in cattle; however, it is usually impractical to formulate a low-sodium diet for affected animals. Furosemide is cheap and is administered orally (2 to 5 mg/kg every 12 to 24 hours) or intravenously (1 to 2 mg/kg every 12 to 24 hours). Dramatic clinical improvements have been observed in ruminants with heart failure within 1 day of instituting furosemide therapy. Prolonged therapy can lead to hypokalemia, necessitating periodic monitoring of serum potassium concentrations. This is particularly important when cardiac glycosides are administered since hypokalemia potentiates digoxin toxicity.

Specific inotropic agents (Ca^{+2}, digoxin, dopamine, and dobutamine) should be administered in selected cases. The serum calcium concentration should be closely monitored in ruminants with heart failure since lactating, anorexic animals are often hypocalcemic. Calcium is most economically administered as calcium borogluconate. Digoxin can be administered intravenously but is prohibitively expensive if prolonged treatment is anticipated (see above). Dopamine and dobutamine infusions (1 to 4 µg/kg/minute intravenously) are widely used as inotropic agents during general anesthesia; however, they are impractical for long-term use. Cattle with heart failure arising from mountain sickness (high-altitude disease) should be treated initially by immediate movement to a lower altitude. Unresponsive animals may improve after parenteral administration of furosemide and dexamethasone.[34] Digoxin and intranasal oxygen may also be of benefit in extremely valuable animals.

Nonspecific agents that could be used in the treatment of heart failure are aminophylline, nitroprusside, and nitroglycerin. Aminophylline is principally used as a bronchodilator; however, it also possesses weak inotropic and diuretic activity. Therapeutic blood levels have been achieved following oral administration of theophylline 20 mg/kg every 12 hours, although blood levels need to be monitored.[35] Vasodilators (such as nitroglycerin and nitroprusside) have been used in selected cases of heart failure without obvious success. The impression gained from using these agents is often one of delaying the inevitable.

ENZOOTIC BOVINE LEUKOSIS

The most common hemolymphatic proliferative disorder in cattle is enzootic bovine leukosis (EBL). Chemotherapy and immunotherapy of cattle with EBL (BLV-associated) have rarely been attempted. Two reports,[36, 37] however, have suggested that chemotherapy may induce short-term remission and alleviate clinical signs associated with rapid tumor growth. Chemotherapy may therefore be considered a short-term measure in the treatment of valuable breeding cattle with lymphosarcoma where the defined goal is embryo transfer or semen collection. However, before chemotherapy is initiated, the possibility that affected cattle are genetically susceptible to development of lymphosarcoma should be considered. Propagation of this genotype may therefore be undesirable.

Treatment of EBL has been attempted with L-asparaginase (10,000 IU/m² body surface area intravenously every 2 weeks for three treatments) and prednisolone (0.5 mg/kg intramuscularly every 24 hours for four treatments).[36] Short-term regression of clinical signs was observed after treatment, although the cow later relapsed and was euthanized 2 months later. L-Asparaginase deprives tumor cells of asparagine and therefore inhibits protein synthesis, since neoplastic cells lack adequate L-asparaginase synthetase activity.

Immunotherapy has also been used in leukemic cattle through the administration of adriamycin entrapped in liposomes conjugated with monoclonal antibodies directed against tumor-associated antigens of bovine leukemic cells. Successful short-term regression of tumors and a decrease in circulating tumor-associated antigen have been reported.[37] Immunotherapy utilizing a cell-wall extract of *Nocardia rubra*, a known immunopotentiator, has induced complete regression of enlarged subcutaneous lymphatic nodules in Holstein cattle.[37] The hypothesized mechanism of action was intralesional activation of macrophages, natural killer cells, and the subsequent elaboration of cytokines. These encouraging results suggest that short-term remission can be obtained in cattle with EBL, although optimal treatment regimes have yet to be developed. A major drawback to the use of selected chemotherapeutic and immunotherapeutic agents for the treatment of EBL is cost, since an initial course of L-asparaginase treatment in cattle currently exceeds $1000.

REFERENCES

1. Nakayama S, Sibley L, Gunther RA, et al: Small volume resuscitation with hypertonic saline (2,400 mOsm/L) during hemorrhagic shock. Circ Shock 13:149–159, 1984.
2. Maningas PA, Bellamy RF: Hypertonic sodium chloride solutions for the prehospital management of traumatic hemorrhagic shock. A possible improvement in the standard of care? Ann Emerg Med 15:1411–1414, 1986.
3. Schmall LM, Muir WW, Robertson JT: Hemodynamic effects of small volume hypertonic saline in experimentally induced hemolytic shock. Equine Vet J 22:273–277, 1990.
4. Velasco IT, Pontieri V, Rocha-e-Silva M, et al: Hyperosmotic NaCl and severe hemorrhagic shock. Am J Physiol 239:H664–H673, 1980.
5. Constable PD, Schmall LM, Muir WW, et al: Small volume hypertonic saline (2400 mOsm/L) treatment of calves in endotoxic shock: hemodynamic changes. Am J Vet Res 52:981–989, 1991.
6. McGillivray SR, Searcy GP, Hirsch VM: Serum iron, total iron binding capacity, plasma copper, and hemoglobin types in anemic and poikilocytic calves. Can J Comp Med 49:286–290, 1985.
7. Szabuniewicz M, McGrady JD: Anemia and hematinic drugs. In LM Jones, NH Booth, LE McDonald (eds): Veterinary Pharmacology and Therapeutics, 4th ed. Ames, IA, Iowa State University Press, 1977, p 481.
8. Campbell EA: Iron poisoning in the young pig. Aust Vet J 37:78–83, 1961.
9. Gentry PA, Tremblay RRM, Ross ML: Failure of aspirin to impair bovine platelet function. Am J Vet Res 50:919–922, 1989.
10. Gerhards H, Eberhardt C: Plasma heparin values and hemostasis in equids after subcutaneous administration of low-dose calcium heparin. Am J Vet Res 49:13–18, 1988.
11. Kasari TR, Roussel AJ: Bacterial endocarditis. Part 1. Pathophysiologic, diagnostic, and therapeutic considerations. Compend Contin Educ Pract Vet 11:655–659, 1989.
12. Ikawa H, Narushima T, Kohno T: Bacteriology of caudal vena caval thrombosis in slaughter cattle. Vet Rec 120:184–186, 1987.
13. Constable PD, Muir WW, Freeman L, et al: Atrial fibrillation associated with neostigmine administration in three cows. J Am Vet Med Assoc 196:329–332, 1990.
14. Constable PD, Muir WW, Bonagura J, et al: Clinical and electrocardiographic characterization of cattle with atrial premature complexes. J Am Vet Med Assoc 197:1163–1169, 1990.
15. McGuirk SM, Muir WW, Sams RA, et al: Atrial fibrillation in cows: clinical findings and therapeutic considerations. Am J Vet Res 182:1380–1386, 1983.
16. McGuirk SM, Muir WW, Sams RA: Pharmacokinetic analysis of intravenously and orally administered quinidine in cows. Am J Vet Res 42:1482–1487, 1981.
17. Heissenbuttel RH, Bigger JT: The effect of oral quinidine on intraventricular conduction in man: correlation of plasma quinidine with changes in QRS duration. Am Heart J 80:453–462, 1970.
18. Morishima HO, Heymann MA, Rudolph AM, et al: Transfer of lidocaine across the sheep placenta to the fetus. Am J Obstet Gynecol 122:581–588, 1975.
19. Morishima HO, Gutsche BG, Stark RI, et al: Relationship of fetal bradycardia to maternal administration of lidocaine in sheep. Am J Obstet Gynecol 134:289–296, 1979.
20. Scarratt WK, Troutt HF: Iatrogenic lidocaine toxicosis in ewes. J Am Vet Med Assoc 188:184–185, 1986.
21. Clarke ML, Hattey DG, Humphreys DJ: Veterinary Toxicology, 2nd ed. London, Balliere Tindall, 1982, p 111.
22. Berman W, Musselman J, Shortencarrier R: The physiologic effects of digoxin under steady state drug conditions in newborn and adult sheep. Circulation 62:1165–1171, 1980.
23. Jenkins WL: Ruminant pharmacology. In Booth NH, McDonald LE (eds): Veterinary Pharmacology and Therapeutics, 5th ed. Ames IA, Iowa State University Press, 1982, pp 607–619.
24. Steiness E, Svendsen O, Rasmussen F: Plasma digoxin after parenteral administration: local reaction after intramuscular injection. Clinical Pharmacol Ther 16:430–434, 1974.
25. Koritz GD, Anderson KL, Neff-Davis CA, et al: Pharmacokinetics of digoxin in cattle. J Vet Pharmacol Ther 6:141–148, 1983.
26. Howard JL: Table of common drugs: approximate doses. In Current Veterinary Therapy: Food Animal Practice. Philadelphia, WB Saunders, 1986, p 1205.
27. Adams HR: Digitalis and other inotropic agents. In Booth NH, McDonald LE (eds): Veterinary Pharmacology and Therapeutics, 5th ed. Ames IA, Iowa State University Press, 1982, pp 435–457.
28. Constable PD, Hoffsis GF, Rings DM: The reticulorumen: normal and abnormal motor function. Part II. Secondary contraction cycles, rumination, and esophageal groove closure. Compend Contin Ed Pract Vet 12:1169–1174, 1990.
29. Mikhail M, Brugere H, Le Bars H, et al: Stimulated esophageal groove closure in adult goats. Am J Vet Res 49:1713–1715, 1988.
30. Benthe HF, Dirksen HCG, Weissmuller A: Investigation of the plasma digitoxin concentration in cattle at different dosages. Bovine Pract 18:169–173, 1983.

31. Davis LE, Garb S: Treatment of a cow with congestive heart failure. J Am Vet Med Assoc 142:255–257, 1963.
32. Littledike T, Glazier D, Cook HM: Electrocardiographic changes after induced hypercalcemia and hypocalcemia in cattle: reversal of the induced arrhythmia with atropine. Am J Vet Res 37:383–388, 1976.
33. Fellers G, Ardington P, Cimprich R: Clinicopathologic conference. J Am Vet Med Assoc 166:700–706, 1975.
34. Johnson TS, Rock PB: Acute mountain sickness. N Engl J Med 319:841–845, 1989.
35. Langston VC, Koritz GD, Davis LE, et al: Pharmacokinetic properties of theophylline given intravenously and orally to ruminating calves. Am J Vet Res 50:493–497, 1989.
36. Masterson MA, Hull BL, Vollmer LA: Treatment of bovine lymphosarcoma with L-asparaginase. J Am Vet Med Assoc 192:1301–1302, 1988.
37. Onuma M, Yasutomi Y, Yamamoto M: Chemotherapy and immunotherapy of bovine leukosis. Vet Immunol Immunopathol 22:245–254, 1989.
38. Berman W, Musselman J, Shortencarrier R: The pharmacokinetics of digoxin in newborn and adult sheep. J Pharmacokin Biopharm 10:173–186, 1982.
39. Bloedow DC, Ralston DH, Hargrove JC: Lidocaine pharmacokinetics in pregnant and nonpregnant sheep. J Pharm Sci 69:32–37, 1980.

SECTION 12
Diseases of the Digestive System

GLEN F. HOFFSIS, DVM, MS, Diplomate, ACVIM, Consulting Editor

Introduction to the Ruminant Forestomach

PETER D. CONSTABLE, BVSc, MS, MRCVS,
Diplomate, ACVIM

The forestomach is a specialized fermentation vat consisting of 2 primary structures, the reticulorumen and the omasum, which are functionally separated by a sphincter, the reticulo-omasal orifice. Fermentation is controlled by the ruminant through forage selection, buffer addition (saliva), and continual mixing through specialized contractions of the forestomach. Reticuloruminal motility ensures a consistent flow of partially digested material into the abomasum for further digestion. This constant flow of digesta differs markedly from the intermittent flow observed in monogastric animals.

Sympathetic and parasympathetic nerves control reticuloruminal motility. Sympathetic innervation consists of numerous fibers from the thoracolumbar segment that join at the celiac plexus to form the splanchnic nerve. The splanchnic nerve can inhibit forestomach motility, but normally there is little or no tonic sympathetic drive to the forestomach. Parasympathetic innervation is via the vagus nerve, which promotes forestomach motility.[1,2] Different branches of the vagus nerve innervate distinct areas of the forestomach and abomasum; therefore damage to the nerve arising from abscessation, peritonitis, or lymphosarcoma should result in predictable alterations in forestomach and abomasal motility. Correlation of the area of vagal innervation with lesion location and the nature of the motility disturbance can usually suggest whether nervous damage is present (Table 1).

Table 1. STRUCTURES INNERVATED BY THE DORSAL AND VENTRAL VAGUS NERVE IN SHEEP

Dorsal Vagus Nerve	Ventral Vagus Nerve
Cardia	
Esophageal groove (caudal lip)	Esophageal groove (cranial lip)
Reticulum Caudal	Reticulum Cranial Medial Lateral
Reticulo-osmasal orifice	Reticulo-osmasal orifice
Omasum (majority)	Omasum (only ventral parietal surface)
Abomasum Visceral surface Pylorus	Abomasum Parietal surface Pylorus

RETICULORUMINAL MOTILITY

Four different specialized contraction patterns can be clinically identified in the reticulorumen:[3] (1) primary or mixing cycle, (2) secondary or eructation cycle, (3) rumination (associated with cud chewing and essentially a modification of the primary cycle), and (4) esophageal groove closure (associated with suckling milk). The motility pattern and function of each cycle should be understood, because specific disorders such as vagal indigestion, rumen bloat, and lactic acidosis often have characteristic alterations in forestomach motility.

Primary Contractions

Primary cyclic activity results in the mixing and circulation of the digesta in an organized manner. The contraction cycle begins with a biphasic reticular contraction, followed by sequential contraction of the dorsal and ventral ruminal sacs. This contraction sequence is initiated, monitored, and controlled by the gastric center in the medulla oblongata and mediated by the vagus nerve.[1,4] Numerous excitatory and inhibitory inputs are summated in the gastric center to determine both the rate and strength of contraction (Fig. 1).

Forestomach atony is defined as the complete absence of reticuloruminal motility. Atony can result from the absence of excitatory inputs or increase in inhibitory inputs to the gastric center, direct depression of the gastric center (associated with generalized depression and severe illness), or failure of vagal motor pathways.[5] Forestomach hypomotility refers to a reduction in the frequency or strength of primary contractions and is caused by either a reduction in the excitatory drive to the gastric center or an increase in inhibitory inputs. The distinction between primary contraction frequency and strength is important clinically, particularly in reference to therapy of reticuloruminal hypomotility. The *frequency* of primary contractions gives a rough indication of the overall health of the ruminant animal. In the cow, the primary contraction frequency averages 1 cycle/minute. The rate increases transiently during feeding and decreases during rumination and recumbency.[3] Because of this variability, auscultation should proceed for at least 2 minutes for determining the frequency of contractions. The *strength* and *duration* of each contraction is determined primarily by the nature of the forestomach contents, although alterations in serum electrolyte concentrations (particularly hypocalcemia) can also influence primary cyclic activity. The strength of contraction is subjectively determined by observing the movement of the left paralumbar fossa and assessing the loudness of any sounds associated with rumen contraction.

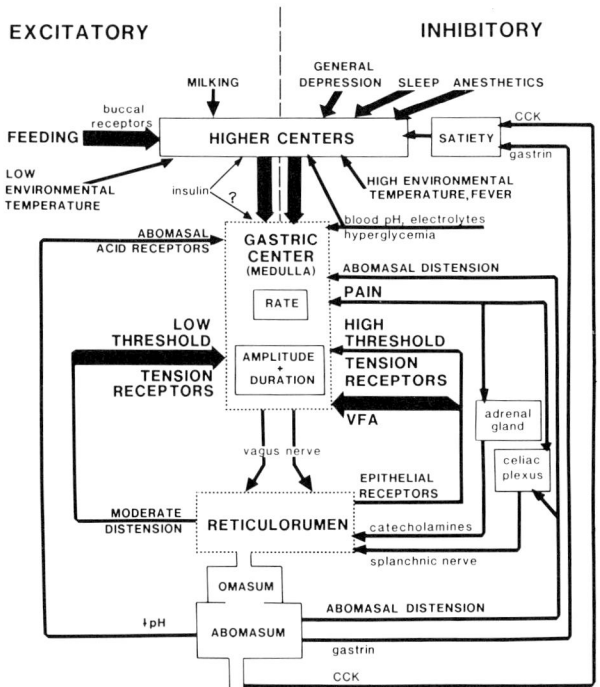

Figure 1. Control of reticuloruminal motility, indicating the major excitatory and inhibitory factors. (From Constable PD, Hoffsis GF, Rings DM: The reticulorumen: normal and abnormal motor function. Part 1. Primary contraction cycle. Compend Contin Educ Pract Vet 12:1008–1015, 1990.)

Excitatory Inputs to the Gastric Center

Mild reticuloruminal distention and chewing activity are major excitatory inputs to the gastric center, whereas milking, environmental cold, and a decrease in abomasal pH are weaker stimuli (Fig. 1). Feeding excites reticuloruminal motility via increased rumen volume and chewing activity. Prolonged anorexia decreases the reticulorumen volume, therefore decreasing this excitatory input. Agents such as epinephrine, serotonin, PGF2α, bradykinin, histamine, PGE2, and substance P can prevent the stimulatory response of mild forestomach distention.[6]

Inhibitory Inputs to the Gastric Center

The major inhibitory inputs to the gastric center are pyrexia, pain, moderate to severe rumen distention, and increased volatile fatty acid (VFA) concentration (Fig. 1). Pyrexia can result from high environmental temperatures or endogenous pyrogen release. Endogenous pyrogens directly affect the gastric center through a mechanism that is independent of the hypothalamic thermoregulatory center. Forestomach atony during endogenous pyrogen release results from a combination of 2 different pathways, a prostaglandin-associated mechanism (which can be prevented by administering nonsteroidal anti-inflammatory drugs) and a poorly understood temperature-independent mechanism.[7]

Pain is often associated with rumen hypomotility or atony. Painful stimuli act directly on the gastric center to inhibit motility, although modification of reticulorumen motility in response to painful stretching of viscera can be partially attributed to catecholamine release. The sympathetic nervous system response to pain can also stimulate splanchnic motor nerves, directly inhibiting reticulorumen motility.[1]

Moderate to severe forestomach distention exerts an inhibitory influence on reticuloruminal motility. Epithelial receptors located in the ruminal pillars and papillae of the reticulum and cranial rumen sac respond to mechanical stimulation (stretch) as well as changes in VFA concentration (see later).[4] These receptors are stimulated continuously during severe rumen distention.[1,5] The opposing actions of low-threshold (stimulatory) and high-threshold (inhibitory) tension receptors therefore help to control the fermentation process and maintain an optimal reticulorumen volume.

The ruminal VFA concentration also influences forestomach motility.[4,8] Volatile fatty acids in the reticulorumen exist in a dissociated and nondissociated form, the degree of ionization being governed by the rumen pH and the pKa of each particular acid.[5] Epithelial receptors detect the concentration of nondissociated VFA in rumen fluid, which is usually high enough to produce a mild tonic inhibitory input to the gastric center.[4] Rumen atony in lactic acidosis is thought to result initially from an elevated concentration of nondissociated VFA in rumen fluid, the decrease in rumen pH driving more of the VFA into a nondissociated form.

Reticuloruminal motility can also be inhibited by abomasal distention, sleep, central nervous system depression, hyperglycemia, water deprivation, and alterations in blood pH and electrolyte concentration.[1,3] The inhibitory effect of glucose should be remembered when anorectic ruminants are treated with intravenous dextrose solutions, because dextrose (1 g/kg, intravenously) decreases the frequency and strength of rumen contractions for up to 3 hours in sheep.[9]

Forestomach motility can also be influenced by the action of specific gastrointestinal hormones that do not appear to act directly on the gastric center. Plasma concentrations of cholecystokinin and gastrin are increased in sheep parasitized with *Ostertagia circumcincta* and *Trichostrongylus colubriformis*, and this increase is thought to contribute partially to the reduction in forestomach motility and feed intake observed in affected sheep. However, the role of these hormones in healthy ruminants is presently uncertain.[10]

Secondary Contractions

Secondary contraction cycles occur independently of primary contractions and at a lower frequency. They are concerned primarily with the eructation of gas, the rate being determined by the gas or fluid pressure in the dorsal ruminal sac.[2,3] Rumen contractions are essential for eructation.[3] Tension receptors in the medial wall of the dorsal ruminal sac initiate the reflex via the dorsal vagus nerve. Contractions start in the dorsal and caudodorsal ruminal sacs and then spread forward to move the gas cap anteriorly to the cardia region, which subsequently opens.[11] The cardia remains firmly shut if foam (frothy bloat) or fluid (laterally recumbent animals) contacts it. Free gas bloat is often observed in ruminants in lateral recumbency. Eructation occurs in these animals after they become sternally recumbent or stand, when fluid moves away from the cardia. Bloat can also result when peritonitis, abscesses, or masses distort the normal forestomach anatomy, preventing active removal of fluid from the cardia region. Esophageal obstructions, associated with intraluminal, intramural, or extraluminal masses, are also a common cause of free gas bloat. Passage of a stomach tube usually identifies these abnormalities, and forestomach motility is unimpaired unless the vagal nerve is damaged. Bloat is also observed in cattle with tetanus, the bloat probably arising from spasm of the esophageal musculature.

A persistent mild bloat is often observed in ruminants that have ruminal atony or hypomotility secondary to systemic disease. The bloat usually requires no treatment and disappears with the return of normal motility. Although the fermentation rate is lower than normal in these cases, rumen contractions are not strong enough to remove all of the gas produced.[5]

Auscultation of the left paralumbar fossa (which detects rumen motility) cannot differentiate secondary contraction cycles from primary contraction cycles, unless synchronous eructation is heard. However, when palpation of the left paralumbar fossa is coupled with reticular auscultation (by placing the bell of the stethoscope at the left costochondral junction between the seventh and eighth ribs), the 2 contraction cycles can be distinguished.[12] Reticular contractions (indicating a primary contraction) can usually be heard a few seconds before the dorsal ruminal sac contraction is seen or palpated. The reticular contraction is not easy to identify, and this technique requires practice. The absence of a reticular contraction before dorsal ruminal sac motility indicates a secondary contraction.

Rumination

Rumination is a complex process involving regurgitation, remastication, insalivation, and deglutition.[3] It is initiated by the "rumination area" located close to the gastric center in the medulla oblongata. Rumination allows further physical breakdown of food with the addition of large quantities of saliva (buffer) and is an integral part of ruminant activity. Rumination has been associated with a sleeplike state and appears to be an enjoyable experience.[5] The time spent ruminating each day appears to be determined by the coarseness of the rumen contents and the nature of the diet.[13] Rumination usually commences 30 to 90 minutes after feeding and proceeds for 10 to 60 minutes at a time, resulting in 8 to 9 hours per day (maximum of 10) spent in the activity.

Epithelial receptors located in the reticulum, esophageal groove area, reticuloruminal fold, and ruminal pillars detect coarse ingesta and initiate rumination.[2, 13] These epithelial receptors are unspecialized sensory nerve endings and therefore respond to a number of different stimuli.[4, 5] They can be activated by increases in ruminal VFA concentration or severe stretch (resulting in alterations in primary or secondary cycle activity) or mild mechanical "rubbing" (inciting rumination).[13] The epithelial receptors are ideally located to contact coarse ingesta, which usually float on top of the more fluid ventral ruminal contents. An intact dorsal or ventral vagus nerve is necessary for regurgitation to proceed.[3] The rumination reflex is not totally dependent on mechanical stimuli from the reticulorumen. Sheep fed a total liquid diet will occasionally exhibit a form of rumination, but with a much shorter chewing period.[13] Regurgitation follows an extra contraction of the reticulum before the normal biphasic contraction of the primary cycle.[2, 3] The glottis is closed, and an inspiratory movement lowers the intrathoracic pressure, which causes the distal esophagus to fill with rumen contents when the cardia relaxes. Reverse peristalsis carries the bolus up to the mouth, where it undergoes further mastication.[3] The extra reticular contraction is not essential for regurgitation because fixation or removal of the reticulum does not prevent cattle from ruminating.

It is often difficult to quantify the time spent ruminating; therefore only the absence or presence of rumination is normally noted. Rumination is often absent in sick ruminants. In these animals, the reappearance of rumination is considered a good prognostic sign because it often heralds an improvement in the clinical condition of the animal. Additional causes for a reduction or absence of rumination include reticuloruminal hypomotility or atony, central nervous system depression, excitement, pain, liquid rumen contents (no coarse fiber present to stimulate the epithelial receptors), mechanical damage to the reticulum (peritonitis), and a high rumen fluid osmotic pressure (>350 mOsm/L).[14] More unusual causes for the absence of rumination are chronic emphysema (difficulty in creating a negative thoracic pressure) and massive damage to the epithelial receptors that incite the reflex (seen in rumenitis). The effect of osmotic pressure on ruminal function is significant and should not be disregarded. In particular, electrolyte solutions administered orally to sick ruminants should be isotonic; hypertonic solutions will exacerbate dehydration unless adequate water is available for immediate consumption.

Esophageal Groove Closure

The esophageal groove reflex allows milk in the suckling preruminant to bypass the forestomach; milk is directed from the esophagus along the reticular groove and omasal canal into the abomasum. Milk initiates the reflex by chemical stimulation of receptors in the buccal cavity, pharynx, and cranial esophagus.[6] Once the reflex is established in neonates, sensory stimuli can cause esophageal groove closure without contact of milk with the chemoreceptors. Esophageal groove closure is therefore normal in calves given water in an identical manner to which the calf previously received milk or in calves abruptly changed from nipple to bucket feeding.[15] Reflex closure continues to operate during and after the development of a functional rumen, provided that the animal continues to receive milk. Esophageal groove closure has been observed in cattle up to 2 years of age and can probably be induced pharmacologically in older cattle.[16]

Esophageal groove closure can be induced by the oral administration of particular salt solutions. In adult sheep, 5 ml of a 10 per cent solution of copper sulfate consistently causes esophageal groove closure. This lasts for at least 15 seconds, during which time a second orally administered liquid will pass directly into the abomasum. Watery rumen contents favor the establishment of this reflex.[19] Repeated administration of copper sulfate should be avoided because of the high risk of copper toxicosis. Closure of the esophageal groove in cattle less than 2 years of age can be induced by oral drenching with solutions of sodium bicarbonate, sodium chloride, or sugar.[16] One hundred to 250 ml of a 10 per cent solution of sodium bicarbonate induces esophageal groove closure in 93 per cent of cattle.[16, 20] Closure is immediate and usually lasts for 1 to 2 minutes. Oral solutions administered during this time are directed into the abomasum, which avoids dilution in the rumen. In goats, closure is best induced by injection of vasopressin 1 IU/kg.[21] Reflex closure can be useful in the treatment of abomasal ulcers in younger animals, because magnesium hydroxide or Kaopectate can be given orally shortly after sodium bicarbonate solution.

The esophageal groove reflex is inhibited by abomasal distention, which causes milk to enter the rumen instead of the abomasum. Liquid administered to calves via an esophageal feeder will not induce groove closure; this should be remembered when colostrum is administered to newborn calves and oral fluids are given to diarrheic calves. In calves less than 3 weeks of age, overflow of fluid from the reticulorumen into the abomasum begins when 400 ml is administered. This means that the fluid volume administered by an esophageal feeder should exceed 400 ml if rapid absorption is required.[18]

Reticuloruminal contractions decrease or cease during suckling via a dopaminergic pathway.[17] Esophageal groove closure is also inhibited by dopamine administration. Because incomplete closure of the esophageal groove is thought to be involved with primary digestive disturbances in milk-fed calves, metoclopramide (an antidopaminergic agent) may therefore be of benefit in the treatment of digestive disturbances in suckling ruminants. The clinical effectiveness of this therapy is yet to be determined.

OMASAL MOTILITY

The omasum is a compact spherical organ comprising the omasal canal and omasal body. Motility of the omasal canal is coordinated with that of the reticulorumen, whereas omasal body contractions occur independently of and at a slower rate than reticuloruminal contractions. The function of the omasum is incompletely understood; however, it plays an important role in (1) transport of appropriately sized feed particles from the reticulorumen to the abomasum, (2) esophageal groove closure, (3) fermentation of ingesta, and (4) absorption of water, volatile fatty acids, and minerals.

The omasum is situated centrally in the anterior abdomen, which prevents direct examination through techniques such as palpation and percussion. Auscultation of omasal activity has been described.[23] The technique requires placement of the stethoscope on the right lateral thorax between the seventh and tenth ribs at the level of the shoulder joint. Flowing liquid sounds, indicating flow of ingesta along the omasal canal into the abomasal fundus, are heard approximately 12 seconds after the second reticular contraction. This is an extremely difficult technique that requires practice, because it is hard to be certain that omasal motility is directly responsible for the generated sound.

Definitive evidence of an omasal disorder therefore usually requires exploratory celiotomy or rumenotomy. Common diseases affecting the omasum include omasal impaction, omasal canal obstruction, and omasal erosions. Omasal canal obstructions usually result from ingestion of baling twine or plastic and are easily diagnosed during rumenotomy. Omasal erosions may be severe enough to lead to perforation of 1 or more omasal leaves. These erosions are commonly seen in healthy cattle and their etiopathogenesis is unknown, although inflammation resulting from *Fusobacterium necrophorum* infection is a likely cause.[24] Omasal lesions are also observed in cattle dying of diseases such as bovine virus diarrhea, infectious bovine rhinotracheitis, and rinderpest.

Omasal impaction is a clinical disease of controversial significance, primarily because the normal bovine omasum varies markedly in size and consistency. The disorder is characterized by anorexia, an extremely firm and enlarged omasum that may be painful on palpation, the absence of other pathologic abdominal conditions, and clinical improvement after softening of the omasum. Treatment consists of intraoperative kneading of the omasum until the contents become pliable. Four liters of mineral oil should be administered intraruminally for 3 to 5 days postoperatively to facilitate softening. Omasotomy is indicated in nonresponsive cases. The omasum is exteriorized through a midline abdominal incision, opened along the greater curvature, and flushed with water until it becomes soft and pliable. The omasum is closed with a 2-layer inverting pattern and the abdomen closed routinely.[25]

CLINICAL ASSESSMENT OF FORESTOMACH FUNCTION

Assessment of the primary contraction cycle should be part of the routine clinical examination of ruminant animals. Secondary contraction cycles, esophageal groove closure, and rumination need only be examined when problems associated with the gastrointestinal tract have been identified. Careful assessment of forestomach motility will help the clinician identify the nature of any dysfunction and provide a rational course for treatment. When assessing forestomach function, the clinician must determine (1) the rate and strength of rumen contractions, (2) the ruminal volume, (3) the nature of the rumen contents, and (4) the nature of the feces. This is best approached with use of the following sequential technique for the cow.

1. Visual Examination. The abdominal profile is critically examined to determine (1) if any distention is present and (2) the organ most likely to cause the distention. In addition, the left paralumbar fossa is inspected for periodic distention, and the frequency and strength of ruminal contractions are determined.

2. External Ruminal Palpation. The physical nature of the ruminal contents is assessed by ballottement and succussion of the left paralumbar fossa and flank region. Normal primary cyclic motility leads to a stratification of ruminal contents, with firmer fibrous material floating on top of a more fluid layer. The normal rumen therefore feels doughy in the dorsal sac and more fluid ventrally. Abnormal ruminal stratifaction, or an excessively firm or watery rumen, suggests that a forestomach disorder is present. Very watery rumen contents that splash and fluctuate on ballottement are suggestive of lactic acidosis, vagal indigestion, ileus, or prolonged anorexia. Firm rumen contents are observed with restricted water intake.

3. Auscultation. Identification of rumen contractions requires both auscultation and observation of the left paralumbar fossa. Sound is produced when fibrous material rubs against the rumen wall during contraction. Very little sound is produced when the rumen contains small quantities of fibrous material (i.e., watery rumen). In this case, observation of the left paralumbar fossa for periodic distention is needed to detect rumen motility. Rumen hypomotility or hypermotility is usually associated with a change in the type of sound heard during auscultation, with a distant bubbling replacing the normal close crescendo-decrescendo crackling sound. Auscultation should proceed for at least 2 minutes in 2 locations: (1) the left paralumbar fossa and (2) the seventh to eighth intercostal space at the costochondral junction. The former does not differentiate primary from secondary contraction cycles unless synchronous eructation is heard, whereas the latter does allow differentiation of the 2 basic cycles. Less than 2 contractions/2 minutes indicates hypomotility; greater than 5 contractions/2 minutes indicates hypermotility.

4. Internal (Rectal) Ruminal Palpation. The rumen (specifically dorsal and caudodorsal ruminal sacs) should be palpated during rectal examination and the volume and consistency determined. The results should then be compared with those obtained during external ruminal palpation. A portion of the ventral ruminal sac may be palpated on some cows by lifting the ventral abdomen dorsally with a horizontal bar placed at the level of the umbilicus.

5. Examination of Fecal Material. The size of digested plant fragments in ruminant feces provides an indirect measure of forestomach function, because solid matter normally stays in the rumen until the particle size is sufficiently small to pass through the reticulo-omasal orifice.[22] Excessively large fibers (>0.5 cm) or fine plant particles in the feces indicate rapid or prolonged rumen turnover time, respectively. The nature of the feces can also provide information on the diet; numerous corn kernels may provide evidence of excessive grain consumption.

6. Rumen Fluid Evaluation. Rumen fluid is easily obtained by passage of a stomach tube, although special collection instruments aid in sample collection and avoid saliva contamination. Samples should not be collected by percutaneous puncture of the rumen because of the associated risk of peritonitis. Fluid analysis is best performed on fresh samples.

Color. This is dependent on the diet; corn silage and straw diets produce yellow-brown rumen contents, concentrates produce an olive-brown color, and pasture produces a green color. A black-green color usually indicates ruminal stasis; a milky gray-brown color is often observed in lactic acidosis.

Odor. Rumen fluid normally has a slightly aromatic, unobjectionable odor. Acidic-sour smells are suggestive of lactic acidosis; rumen putrefaction produces a rotting odor.

Consistency. Rumen contents are normally slightly viscous. Excessive viscosity indicates significant saliva contamination, and the sample should be discarded because it is not a valid representation of rumen fluid. A watery sample with little particulate matter indicates anorexia and is usually associated with reduced protozoal and bacterial numbers. Rumen fluid that has numerous stable bubbles that do not coalesce is indicative of frothy bloat.

pH. Rumen pH is easily determined with the use of pH papers. The normal pH is 6 to 7. A pH value of 5.5 to 6 is seen in cattle on high-grain diets or early lactic acidosis. pH values less than 5.5 are virtually pathognomonic for lactic acidosis, although some cattle on high-grain diets can have rumen pH values down to 5.0. A reduced feed intake of 2 or more days' duration often increases rumen pH up to 7 or 8. Rumen pH values exceeding 8 are due to (1) saliva contamination (sample should be discarded), (2) severe putrefaction of ingested protein associated with prolonged rumen stasis, or (3) urea toxic effects.

Methylene Blue Reduction. This test measures the reducing ability of anaerobic ruminal bacteria. To a test tube containing 0.5 ml of a 0.03 per cent solution of methylene blue, 10 ml of fresh rumen fluid is added, and the time taken for the solution to clear is measured. In cattle, the clearance time is normally between 2 and 6 minutes, the faster rate being observed in cattle on high-grain diets. Clearance times greater than 10 minutes indicate inadequate anaerobic bacterial numbers, and rumen transfaunation is required. The clearance time is much faster in sheep (usually 1 to 4 minutes). This test is invalid at rumen pH less than 5.5.

Protozoa. One drop of fresh rumen contents is placed on a slide and examined under low power (40×). Normal rumen fluid contains greater than 40 protozoa per low-power field, with actively moving protozoa that can be broadly characterized into 3 sizes (small, medium, big). Low protozoal numbers (<8 per low-power field), nonmotile protozoa, or loss of population heterogeneity all indicate an abnormal intraruminal environment. Transfaunation is indicated if these abnormalities are identified, particularly if the methylene blue reduction time is prolonged. It is not usually necessary to identify the protozoal species present, but occasionally it is valuable to differentiate isotrichids (formerly holotrichs), which are usually the larger protozoa, from oligotrichs (entodiniomorphs), which are smaller and more resistant to pH values of less then 6. Protozoal energy stores can be assessed by adding 1 drop of Lugol's iodine to 1 drop of rumen fluid on a slide. Healthy protozoa are almost uniformly stained by iodine; protozoa that have been starved have diminished starch stores, evidenced by decreasing numbers of starch granules.

Chloride Concentration. The rumen fluid should be centrifuged and the supernatant submitted for determination of the chloride concentration, which is normally 10 to 25 mEq/L in cattle and <15 mEq/L in sheep. Elevated rumen chloride concentrations result from abomasal reflux (internal vomition), ileus, or high salt intake. Rumen chloride concentrations are extremely useful in localizing the site of gastrointestinal obstruction in ruminants with rumen distention, because high values indicate obstruction at or distal to the pylorus, whereas low values indicate obstruction at the level of the omasum or reticulo-omasal orifice. The physical examination will provide evidence as to whether this obstruction is functional or pathologic.

Rumen Osmolality. The rumen osmotic pressure is actively controlled by the ruminant and closely approximates serum osmotic pressure. A constant osmotic pressure ensures homeostatic conditions for ruminal microbes, which are susceptible to lysis or swelling if large and vapid variations in rumen osmolality occur.[14]

Gram Stain. Rumen fluid normally contains a large heterogeneous population of bacteria that are predominantly gram-negative. Lactic acidosis produces a more uniform bacterial population that is predominantly gram-positive.

Other Tests. A number of other laboratory tests, such as sedimentation time, cellulose digestion test, and total titratable acidity, have also been used in the examination of rumen fluid. These tests seldom add additional information other than that obtained from the preceding, and their routine use is not recommended.

SIMPLE INDIGESTION

Definition

Simple indigestion is a common disease primarily affecting nongrazing ruminants. The disorder is relatively easy to diagnose when a large number of ruminants become inappetent immediately after a change in feeding practices. It is much more difficult, however, to diagnose simple indigestion when only 1 animal is affected and the diet has been unchanged. In this case, simple indigestion is diagnosed by exclusion.

Pathogenesis

The cause of simple indigestion is presumed to be an altered ruminal microbial population, secondary to a rapid change in the intraruminal environment. The ruminal microbial population is normally in a continual state of flux, the population characteristics being determined by feeding frequency, nature of diet, and water intake. Diurnal variations in the rumen microbial population therefore occur. Because these variations are more pronounced in ruminants fed once or twice daily than in animals grazing pasture or fed a total mixed ration, indigestion is more likely to occur in intermittently fed ruminants.

Clinical Signs

The first indication of simple indigestion is a reduction in appetite, accompanied by a moderate decrease in milk production in lactating animals. The fecal consistency is usually altered, and typically a malodorous loose stool is voided within 12 to 24 hours of the onset of clinical signs. Reticuloruminal motility is depressed or absent, and rumination ceases. The rumen contents are more fluid on external palpation. Systemic signs of illness are not observed.

Diagnosis

Three criteria must be fulfilled before a diagnosis of simple indigestion can be made: (1) abnormal forestomach motility, (2) abnormal rumen contents, and (3) exclusion of all known diseases affecting the forestomach and gastrointestinal tract. Rumen fluid analysis aids in confirming the diagnosis of simple indigestion. Strong supportive evidence for a diagnosis is a recent change in feed substrate, feeding frequency, or quantity of feed available and more than 1 animal being affected.

Differential diagnoses that must be strongly considered when only 1 animal is affected are traumatic reticulitis, left displaced abomasum, and acetonemia. Traumatic reticulitis is usually accompanied by an abrupt and marked decrease in appetite and milk production, and abdominal pain and pyrexia are often present. Forestomach motility may appear decreased in cattle with left displaced abomasum, but the characteristic "ping" of the left displaced abomasum is usually identified during simultaneous auscultation and percussion. Acetonemia occurs most frequently in the first 6 weeks after parturition and is diagnosed by assessment of urine and milk acetoacetate concentration.

Treatment

The primary goal of treatment is rapid attainment of a normal intraruminal environment. This is most easily achieved through rumen transfaunation, which provides a balanced, buffered, nutrient-dense solution that also includes essential microorganisms. At least 3 L of freshly strained rumen juice are needed to transfaunate an adult dairy cow; 8 to 16 L is considered ideal. Rumen contents can be collected at the local abattoir or from cattle on the farm by passing a stomach tube and back-siphoning rumen juice. The latter process is time-consuming, and a number of cattle and special stomach tubes are required because the volume obtained varies from animal to animal. Stealing cuds from ruminating cattle has also been proposed as a means of obtaining rumen juice; however, this method is impractical for routine use and is incapable of producing adequate volumes. Probiotic agents may be of additional benefit to rumen transfaunation if imbalances in the small intestinal microbial population are suspected. Probiotic preparations contain certain bacterial species *(Lactobacillus, Streptococcus)* that "implant" in the small intestine, potentially preventing or reducing establishment of a pathogenic bacterial species in the intestinal tract. Further work is required to determine the optimal way of using probiotic agents. Good-quality grass hay and straw should be available to the anorexic animal, because sick ruminants often prefer these feeds to alfalfa or concentrates. Oral administration of specific alkalinizing or acidifying agents should not be routinely undertaken in cases of indigestion. Magnesium hydroxide or magnesium oxide (450 g per adult cow) should be administered only to cattle with a confirmed diagnosis of lactic acidosis. These compounds can cause a severe alkalemia and hypermagnesemia when they are administered to cattle with normal or high rumen pH; high rumen pH is frequently encountered in cattle with simple indigestion. Acetic acid (vinegar, 4 to 10 L) can be administered to cattle with putrefaction of the rumen associated with a high rumen pH.

Ruminatorics, such as nux vomica, ginger, tarter, and parasympathomimetics, have a very limited application in the present-day treatment of forestomach dysfunction. Parasympathomimetic agents, such as neostigmine or carbamylcholine, should not be used when rumen atony is present. Neostigmine requires vagal activity to be effective and therefore cannot incite normal primary contractions in atonic animals. Neostigmine may be of some benefit in hypomotile states because it increases the strength of the primary contraction without upsetting rhythm or coordination. Carbamylcholine causes uncoordinated, spastic, and functionless forestomach contractions, therefore having no place in the treatment of forestomach dysfunction

Simple indigestion can be prevented by increasing the feeding frequency, adding buffers to the feed (such as crude fiber or sodium bicarbonate), and avoiding rapid changes in feeding practices and substrate.

BIBLIOGRAPHY

Constable PD, Hoffsis GF, Rings DM: The reticulorumen: normal and abnormal motor function. Part I. Primary contraction cycle; and Part II. Secondary contraction cycles, rumination, and esophageal groove closure. Compend Contin Educ Pract Vet 12:1008–1015, 1169–1174, 1990.

Ruckebusch Y: Gastrointestinal motor functions in ruminants. *In*: Wood J (ed): Handbook of Physiology. The Gastrointestinal System. Bethesda, MD, American Physiological Society, 1990, pp 1225–1282.

REFERENCES

1. Leek BF: Reticulo-ruminal function and dysfunction. Vet Rec 84:238–243, 1969.
2. Kay R: Rumen function and physiology. Vet Rec 113:6–9, 1983.
3. Sellers AF, Stevens CE: Motor functions of the ruminant forestomach. Physiol Rev 46:634–659, 1966.
4. Leek BF, Harding RH: Sensory nervous receptors in the ruminant stomach and the reflex control of reticulo-ruminal motility. In McDonald IW, Warner ACI (eds): Digestion and Metabolism in the Ruminant. Armadale, NSW, Australia, New England Publishing Unit, 1975, pp 60–76.
5. Leek BF: Clinical diseases of the rumen: a physiologist's view. Vet Rec 113:10–14, 1983.
6. Ruckebusch Y: Pharmacology of reticulo-ruminal motor function. J Vet Pharmacol Ther 6:245–272, 1983.
7. van Miert ASJPAM: Fever and associated clinical haematologic and blood biochemical changes in the goat and other animal species. Vet Q 7:200–216, 1985.
8. Crichlow EC, Leek BF: Forestomach epithelial receptor activation by rumen fluids from sheep given intraruminal infusions of volatile fatty acids. Am J Vet Res 47:1015–1018, 1986.
9. Bowen JM: Effects of insulin hypoglycemia on gastrointestinal motility in the sheep. Am J Vet Res 23:948–954, 1962.
10. Grovum WL: Factors affecting the voluntary intake of food by sheep. 3. The effect of intravenous infusions of gastrin, cholecystokinin and secretin on motility of the reticulorumen and intake. Br J Nutr 45:183–201, 1981.
11. Dougherty RW, Habel RE, Bond HE: Esophageal innervation and the eructation reflex in sheep. Am J Vet Res 19:115–128, 1958.
12. Williams EI: A study of reticulo-ruminal motility in adult cattle in relation to bloat and traumatic reticulitis with and account of the latter condition as seen in general practice. Vet Rec 67:907–911, 1955.
13. Ash RW, Kay RNB: Stimulation and inhibition of reticulum contractions, rumination and parotid secretion from the forestomach of conscious sheep. J Physiol 149:43–57, 1959.
14. Welch JG: Rumination, particle size, and passage from the rumen. J Anim Sci 54:885–894, 1982.
15. Abe M, Iriki T, Kondoh K, Shibui H: Effects of nipple or bucket feeding of milk-substitute on rumen by-pass and on rate of passage in calves. Br J Nutr 41:175–180, 1979.
16. Riek RF: The influence of sodium salts on the closure of the esophageal groove in calves. Aust Vet J 30:29–37, 1954.
17. Beuno L, Sorraing JM, Fioramonti J: Influence of dopamine on rumino-reticular motility and rumination in sheep. J Vet Pharmacol Ther 6:93–98, 1983.
18. Chapman HW, Butler DG, Newell M: The route of liquids administered to calves by esophageal feeder. Can J Vet Res 50:84–87, 1986.
19. Monnig HO, Quin JI: Studies on the alimentary tract of the merino sheep in South Africa. II. Investigations on the physiology of deglutition, II. Onderstepoort J Vet Sci 5:485–499, 1935.
20. Wester J: The rumination reflex in the ox. Vet J 86:410–410, 1930.
21. Mikhail M, Brugere H, Le Bars H, et al: Stimulated esophageal groove closure in adult goats. Am J Vet Res 49:1713–1715, 1988.
22. Ulyatt MJ, Dellow DW, John CSW, et al: Contribution of chewing during eating and rumination and the clearance of digesta from the ruminoreticulum. *In* Milligan LP, Grovum WL, Dobson A (eds): Control and Digestion and Metabolism in Ruminants. Prentice-Hall, NJ, 1986, pp 498–517.
23. Asai T: Transfer of ingesta in the omasum of calves. Jpn J Vet Sci 37:609–613, 1975.
24. Brownlee A, Elliot J: Studies on the normal and abnormal structure and function of the omasum of domestic cattle. Br Vet J 116:467–473, 1960.
25. McDonald JS, Witzel DA: Three cases of chronic omasal impaction in the dairy cow. J Am Vet Med Assoc 152:638–640, 1968.

Choke

GERARD J. KOENIG, DVM, MS

DEFINITION

Esophageal obstruction in domestic farm animals is commonly referred to as choke. Cattle are most often affected because of their indiscriminant eating habits. Typical clinical signs include dysphagia, ptyalism, and anorexia; in cases of complete obstruction, bloat may be observed. Long-standing cases may result in dehydration and metabolic acidosis.

PATHOGENESIS

Choke can result from partial to complete obstruction of the esophagus. The most common cause is foreign bodies such as hedge apples, potatoes, sugar beets, ears of corn, apples or similar fruits, and turnips. Other less common etiologic agents include metal objects or pieces of cloth. These objects are often swallowed whole or in large chunks and are unable to pass the length of the esophagus because of their size. Obstruction usually occurs at the pharyngeal-esophageal junction, thoracic inlet, base of the heart, or just cranial to the cardia of the stomach. Sheep may suffer from choke if dry or pelleted grain is consumed rapidly which prevents lubrication by saliva. Boluses given to dehydrated cattle, especially calves, may result in choke.

CLINICAL SIGNS

Cattle with complete obstruction may exhibit sudden onset of severe distress, anxiety, frequent attempts to swallow, and ptyalism. Violent movements of the head with attempts to regurgitate, grunting, and protrusion of the tongue may be observed. Often ingested fluid and water will be coughed up or regurgitated through the nostrils. Bloat develops as a result of inability to eructate rumen gas.

Chronic obstructions cause depression and dehydration. Evidence of pain subsides with time. Continued loss of sodium bicarbonate and sodium phosphate in saliva leads to a metabolic acidosis and net loss of sodium from the body. Loss of salivary secretions and inability to drink water lead to dehydration.

DIAGNOSIS

The combination of foreign objects capable of obstruction located in an animal's ranging area with signs of dysphagia and ptyalism warrants a tentative diagnosis of choke. Sedation may be necessary for permitting proper examination. Precautionary measures (i.e., gloves or obstetric sleeves) should be taken if the possibility of rabies exists. An oral speculum may be used to allow examination of the oral and pharyngeal areas.

Inability to pass a tube into the rumen also suggests choke. If the obstruction is chronic in nature, care must be taken during passage of a stomach tube to prevent perforation of the esophagus. A mass may be visualized or palpable externally if it is present in the pharynx or along the left jugular furrow if it is present in the cervical esophagus. Evacuation of the accumulated liquid ingesta followed by esophagoscopy may reveal the nature of the obstruction. Survey and contrast radiography may be of value in ruling out other esophageal disorders.

Choke must be differentiated from causes of pharyngeal paralysis, other intraluminal disorders, and extraluminal structures that restrict dilation of the esophagus. Paralysis of the pharynx is seen in rabies and botulism.[1] Tetanus can result in bloat, dysphagia, and drooling.[1] Slaframine, larkspur, milkweed, and sneezeweed may induce ptyalism and bloat.[2] Trauma to the pharynx and esophagus may be seen with careless use of balling guns, dose syringes, stomach tubes, or deworming tubes.[1] Severe oral and esophageal erosions due to infectious causes (i.e., mycotic stomatitis, bovine virus diarrhea, malignant catarrhal fever, or other viral causes of stomatitis), chemical causes (i.e., T-2 toxin, stachybotryotoxin), or traumatic lesions from plants or foreign bodies may induce ptyalism.[1] Esophageal stricture from previous obstructions could resemble choke.[1] Megaesophagus may present with signs of expectoration, regurgitation, and intermittent bloat.[3] Animals with esophageal diverticulum may exhibit difficulty eating and reflux boluses of feed with saliva.[4] Primary neoplasms of the pharnyx and esophagus are rare.

Extraluminal compressive masses such as enlarged lymph nodes, abscesses, or primary neoplasms can cause difficulty in swallowing, excessive salivation, coughing, and bloat.[4] Developmental defects such as persistent right aortic arch are possible in young animals but rarely occur.[1] Cervical cellulitis may be associated with perivascular injections of irritating substances, or it may be a reaction to larval migration of *Hypoderma lineatum* particularly secondary to administration of larvicidal anthelmintics.[1]

TREATMENT

Emergency treatment may be necessary if bloat becomes life-threatening. Trocarization with a 14-gauge needle or installation of a temporary fistula will alleviate respiratory distress and allow treatment of the primary problem. If signs of metabolic acidosis or significant dehydration are detected, appropriate fluids should be administered. Removal of accumulated fluid with suction and keeping the muzzle pointed downward will reduce the risk of aspiration pneumonia. Sedation or downward traction on the head may be of benefit.

Obstructions due to grain often resolve spontaneously within several hours but can be dislodged with passage of a stomach tube or with fluid pumped against the blocked area. Some clinicians have made use of a 2-tube system that allows fluid to be pumped into the esophagus under pressure. A cuffed tube is passed into the esophagus and inflated. A smaller-bore stomach tube is passed into the cuffed tube, forming a tight seal. Mineral oil or water is then pumped into the esophagus. Food-type obstructions are usually broken apart in this manner. Dilation and lubrication of the esophagus often allows the passage of solid objects. Care must be taken to prevent aspiration pneumonia. Heavy sedation or general anesthesia and endotracheal intubation with a cuffed tube are recommended with this procedure.

The possibility of necrosis with devitalized tissues and resulting loss of strength must be considered with long-standing obstructions and therapy adjusted accordingly. Objects in the pharynx may be manually removed. Cervical esophageal obstructions may be externally manipulated toward the pharynx for manual removal.

More aggressive measures are necessary for intrathoracic obstructions and in cervical obstructions when manipulation fails. A large-bore stomach tube may be utilized in large cattle if a smooth, solid object is the suspected cause. Judicious use of a Hauptner probe, Thysgesen's probang, or a loop made by bending a 10- to 12-foot piece of #9 steel wire may dilate the esophagus ahead of the obstruction and allow passage of the object into the rumen. Alternatively, these instruments allow the object to be snared and pulled toward the pharynx. The inside loop of these instruments is sharpened (except the wire) and may cut the object into smaller pieces.

Rumenotomy is a viable option for intrathoracic obstructions near the cardia. A loop of stiff wire may be used to snare the object and bring it into the rumen. Utilizing a large-bore stomach tube, an assistant may be able to push the object toward the cardia, where it can be grasped.

Esophagotomy is indicated when sharp or irregular objects are lodged or other more conservative efforts have failed. Obstructions that have existed for 48 hours or more have a high likelihood of mucosal necrosis and ultimate breakdown or stricture formation as sequelae. Slaughter may be considered as an option in cases in which necrosis or severe damage is suspected. Administration of broad-spectrum antibiotics should be considered when slaughter is not an option.

The key to prevention is to make objects capable of causing esophageal obstruction inaccessible to livestock.

BIBLIOGRAPHY

Guard C: Choke and esophageal disorders. In Smith BP (ed): Large Animal Internal Medicine. St Louis, CV Mosby, 1990, pp 745–747.
Oehme FW: Textbook of Large Animal Surgery. Baltimore, Williams & Wilkins, 1988, pp 428–435.

REFERENCES

1. Blood DC, Radostits OM: Veterinary Medicine. London, Baillière Tindall, 1989, pp 167–176, 1309.
2. Evers RA, Link RP: Poisonous Plants of the Midwest and Their Effects on Livestock. Urbana, IL, University of Illinois Press, 1972.
3. Anderson NV, Vestweber JG: Hiatal hernia and segmental megaesophagus in a cow. J Am Vet Med Assoc 184:193–195, 1984.
4. Singh AP, Nigam JM: Radiography of bovine esophageal disorders. Mod Vet Pract 61:867–869, 1980.

Pharyngeal Lacerations and Retropharyngeal Abscesses in Cattle

D. MICHAEL RINGS, DVM, MS, Diplomate, ACVIM

DEFINITION

Injuries of the oropharynx are most often associated with trauma due to balling guns, Frick speculums, drench syringes, or boluses themselves. Often the operator has no idea that an injury has occurred until the cow becomes inappetent or the swelling in the throat area is seen. Although many lacerations are small and heal spontaneously with minimal clinical signs, identifiable pharyngeal lacerations cause much distress to affected cattle, resulting in significant weight loss or death.

CLINICAL SIGNS

Clinically affected animals are likely to develop swelling in the area immediately behind the mandibles and above the larynx. This swelling can cause difficult swallowing (dysphagia) or inspiratory dyspnea. Accompanying signs of bloat, excessive salivation, fetid breath, depression, and fever can be seen. Affected cattle frequently stand with the head and neck extended, and although many show a strong desire to eat and drink, they are unable to do so. The most severe lacerations may result in the dissection of phlegmon along muscle fascial planes down the neck and occasionally into the thoracic inlet.

DIAGNOSIS

Visual or digital examination of the posterior throat area would be necessary to confirm the presence of a pharyngeal laceration. Lacerations are most often found in the dorsal pharynx on either side of the larynx. Digital examination of the opening will sometimes reveal boluses in instances of balling gun trauma. Endoscopy of the pharyngeal area can be done as well. With retropharyngeal abscesses, no opening into the pharynx may be present; however, compression and displacement of the larynx may be seen via endoscopy. Radiographs of the retropharyngeal area are useful in identifying abscesses and can also be used to determine the presence and extent of dissecting lesions down the neck. Ultrasonography is useful in identifying abscesses located in soft tissue.

TREATMENT

Minor pharyngeal lacerations may not require treatment, whereas larger, deeper lacerations may require extensive and prolonged treatment. Removal of material embedded in the laceration will allow contraction of the wound and speed healing. This also prevents material from becoming walled-off, which might later become an abscess. It is not advisable to flush pharyngeal lacerations vigorously until the limits of the laceration have been established because of the risk of extending the infection farther down the neck. Systemic broad-spectrum antibiotics are indicated to control infection. Restricting oral intake is helpful in preventing reintroduction of material into the wound cavity. In animals exhibiting dysphagia, the passage of a nasogastric tube provides a useful means for maintaining the hydration of the patient. If the laceration is severe and the patient in poor physical condition, a rumen fistula should be considered so that additional nutritional supplementation can be easily given. Animals suffering from respiratory embarrassment may require a tracheotomy. Corticosteroids have been used to reduce inflammation.

Retropharyngeal abscesses require drainage. Percutaneous aspiration will provide immediate but temporary relief, but the abscess will likely re-fill with time. A ventral surgical approach is advisable for large, well-established abscesses for avoiding damage to vessels and nerves in the area as well as providing the best drainage into the oral cavity. It is advantageous to flush the area with disinfectants (dilute tamed iodine solutions) after drainage to prevent re-establishment of the abscess.

PROGNOSIS

It is difficult to assess an acute pharyngeal laceration accurately. The size of the laceration does not correlate well with the outcome of the case. Small lacerations tend to retain material and are more likely to result in retropharyngeal abscesses, whereas large lacerations empty more easily but are slower to heal. Most animals that return to eating and drinking on their own within a week have a good prognosis for survival but may incur significant weight loss. If phlegmon develops along the fascial planes of the cervical muscles, the prognosis decreases greatly. These tracts may localize at a point that can be drained or can continue into the mediastinum.

Cattle with retropharyngeal abscesses that have been drained from a ventral incision and experiencing no cranial nerve dysfunction are likely to return to normal function. Cattle that remain dysphagic after drainage are likely to have suffered cranial nerve damage, which may persist; salvage is advisable if antibiotic withdrawals can be met and the animal is neither debilitated nor febrile.

BIBLIOGRAPHY

Adams GP, Radostits OM: Balling gun–induced trauma of the pharynx in feedlot cattle. Can Vet J 29:389–390, 1988.
Davidson HP, Rebhun WC, Habel RE: Pharyngeal trauma in cattle. Cornell Vet 71:15–25, 1981.

Diseases of the Ruminant Forestomach
Lactic Acidosis (Rumen Overload, Rumen Acidosis, Grain Overload, Engorgement Toxemia, Rumenitis)

KARL W. KERSTING, DVM, MS
JAMES R. THOMPSON, DVM, MS
WALLACE M. WASS, DVM, PhD

DEFINITION

Several distinct syndromes are recognized. Ingestion of excessive quantities of highly fermentable carbohydrate feed leads to lactic acidosis with systemic dehydration and severe depression. It is by far the more common of the acute syndromes.

Ration ingredients characteristically involved include any of the common feed grains fed in quantities larger than those to which the animal has been accustomed. Finely ground grains are more likely to cause severe problems, but grinding is by no means a prerequisite. Other products known to have caused lactic acidosis in cattle include brewers' grains or distillery by-products such as corn gluten. Green corn, sweet corn, bakery bread, and apples and similar fruits have also been involved.

The propensity of a given feed to induce lactic acidosis is dependent on its content of precursors of lactic acid. Carbohydrates that can lead to accumulation of lactic acid are starch, maltose, sucrose, lactose, cellobiose, fructose, and glucose.[3]

Ingestion of large quantities of highly fermentable protein-aceous material causes excess ammonium ion production, leading to alkalosis with excitement and hyperesthesia. (Consumption of soybeans and soybean derivatives is the most common cause in the midwestern region of the United States.) Either or both syndromes are commonly observed wherever intensive livestock management is practiced.

A syndrome of chronic rumen acidosis has been described in which lactic acidosis may not be a prominent feature, the lactic acid generated having been metabolized by other microorganisms. The disorder occurs in beef or dairy cattle fed for high production and results from feeding high proportions of concentrate at the expense of appropriate quantities of fibrous roughage or from too rapid introduction to such high-energy rations. Associated findings in affected animals include low milk fat, reduced rate of gain, liver abscesses, chronic laminitis, ketosis, rumenitis or rumen parakeratosis, bloat, and obesity.

PATHOGENESIS

The normal ruminant forestomach can be correctly visualized as a continuous culture fermentation receptacle. The normal microflora constitutes the culture; the ration being fed constitutes the medium or substrate on which the culture grows. The fermentation end-products are normally acetic, propionic, and butyric acid, short-chain volatile fatty acids that are absorbed from the rumen as the animal's primary energy source. Bacterial cell protein is also produced and is digested further down the tract as an amino acid source. Water-soluble vitamins are additional by-products.

When the ration is abruptly changed to larger than normal quantities of highly fermentable carbohydrate, normal fermentation patterns change. Gram-positive streptococcus and lactobacillus organisms become predominant, and lactic acid (both D- and L-) becomes a principal fermentation end-product. Lactic acid production increases osmotic pressure within the rumen so that fluid is drawn into the rumen from the circulatory system and thus from other tissues as well (Fig. 1). The rumen pH drops, resulting in rumen stasis, and a large percentage of the normal rumen microflora is destroyed. Most of the gram-negative microorganisms and protozoa disappear. Symptoms become severe when the pH reaches 4 to 5.

The D- and L-lactic acids are converted to sodium lactate. In the rumen they contribute to hypertonicity. Some become absorbed into the circulation (mainly D-lactate because of its slower metabolism) and contribute to a depression of the blood pH. There is some absorption of lactate from the omasum and abomasum and some as a result of continuing fermentation in the intestinal tract. An osmotic gradient is also established within the intestine, drawing fluid into the lumen and contributing to the profuse diarrhea.

Chemical damage to the surface epithelium of the rumen mucosa occurs and later results in adherence of debris and penetration by particulate matter from the rumen ingesta, such as hair and sharp pieces of plant material. Bacterial and mycotic organisms begin to invade the rumen wall, and absorption patterns are changed.

The urine volume will usually be greatly decreased as a result of the dehydration, and secreted urine will be high in D-lactate and will be acidic.

The initial syndrome of acidosis is often followed by bacterial or mycotic rumenitis. Other possible sequelae are liver abscesses and peritonitis. Bloat may result from the decreased rumen motility and altered fermentation patterns. The development of acute, and later chronic, laminitis observed in some animals is thought to relate to the relative levels of histamine produced during the acute phases of the process.

Pregnant animals frequently abort some days or weeks after the acute phases of illness. Secondary rumenitis may cause an increased incidence of bloat, and this is thought to be a major cause of unexplained deaths in feedlots, commonly diagnosed as "sudden death syndrome."

The entire disease process is complex and variable, and a

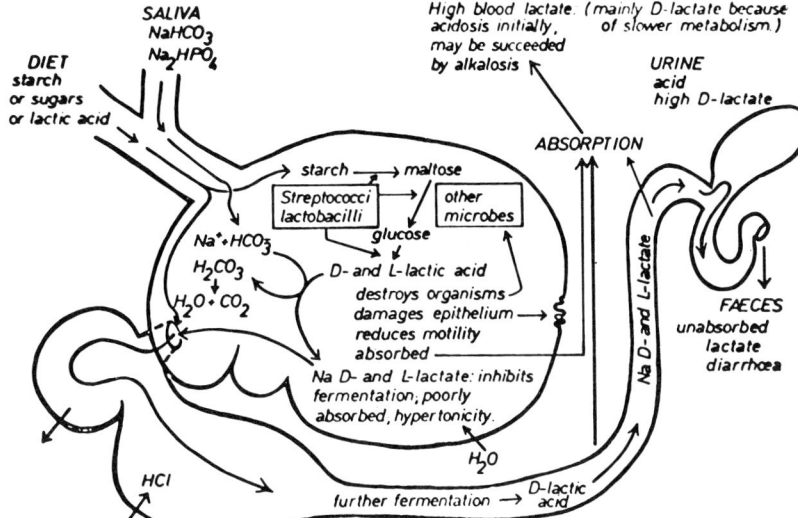

Figure 1. Schematic depiction of rumen lactic acidosis.

suggested additional component might be endotoxic shock from toxins released from the destruction of large numbers of gram-negative microorganisms from the rumen ingesta.[4,8]

CLINICAL SIGNS

The rapidity of onset of clinical signs varies and depends on the nature and quantity of the feed consumed and the adaptation of the animal to that feed. Unadapted animals may die from quantities of feed that are readily consumed by animals conditioned to the feed. On the other hand, even animals on "full feed" will overeat and develop acute lactic acidosis under some circumstances.

Usually, clinical signs will become apparent in 12 to 36 hours after engorgement on grain or similar material. Incoordination and ataxia are first noticed, followed by profound weakness and depression. Anorexia will be apparent, and affected animals appear blind. Rumen stasis is complete, with abdominal pain evidenced by occasional grunting and grinding of the teeth. Abdominal fullness and fluid distention of the rumen are observed.

Significant dehydration will become apparent within 24 to 48 hours. Fetid diarrhea develops but may not be observed in animals that die early. Profuse diarrhea may be considered a sign of improvement if the animals are not seriously depressed.

In severe cases, the animals may become recumbent in 24 to 48 hours because of weakness and toxemia. The respiratory rate will most likely be increased because of acidosis. Body temperature may be subnormal by the time other signs are observed. The pulse is usually weak and thready in character.

Recumbent animals will lie quietly, often with the head tucked to the side, as in parturient paresis. Crusty mucus will be present on the muzzle because the animal fails to clean its nostrils.

When a herd problem is observed, it is common to see several animals with profound depression and acute lactic acidosis. Animals with less severe cases will also be present and are likely to show only mild depression and diarrhea. Some animals may have acute laminitis with a characteristic lameness.

Acute deaths usually occur in 24 to 48 hours, but many animals have apparent recovery with later deterioration and death due to secondary complications. It is not unusual for losses to continue for 3 to 4 weeks in severely affected herds.

Some animals will partially recover but perform poorly in the feedlot because of chronic rumenitis, liver damage, or laminitis.

CLINICAL PATHOLOGY AND NECROPSY

Affected animals have hemoconcentration and acidic rumen content. The pH of ingesta aspirated from the rumen may be 4 or lower, and the urine pH may be as low as 5. Blood pH changes within a narrow range and requires more precise conditions and sophisticated equipment for measurement. Samples should be collected in heparinized tubes containing a layer of mineral oil, or the tubes should be completely filled, sealed, and then refrigerated (4° C) until measured. Accurate assessment of the blood pH requires that bicarbonate or total carbon dioxide be measured also. Values below 7.2 generally indicate severe acidosis and a poor prognosis.

If soybeans or other high-protein feeds have been consumed, rumen pH may be alkaline due to ammonia production. This will be reflected in the blood and urine pH as well.

Necropsy of acute cases demonstrates that the rumen is distended and filled with fluid content. The offending material is likely to be evident, but post-mortem measurements of pH levels are not likely to be valid because of rapid changes in the dead animal.

Rumen engorgement of slightly longer duration will be characterized by rumenitis. However, post-mortem autolysis occurs rapidly in the rumen, so observations on the rumen mucosa must be interpreted carefully.

DIAGNOSIS

Diagnosis will usually be based on history and clinical examination. The history alone is often sufficient, but often it may be misleading if the pattern of feed consumption is not known or not suspected. Laboratory evaluations, especially of the rumen ingesta, plasma, and urine pH, are particularly helpful.

The condition must be differentiated from polioencephalomalacia, urolithiasis, fulminating peritonitis, parturient hypocalcemia, and other diseases that cause profound depression.

TREATMENT

Animals with mild cases may recover without treatment; but in more severe forms, the damage to the animal may be so extensive that even with intensive therapy only limited success will be achieved.

Emptying of the rumen by oral lavage or rumenotomy is indicated if circumstances permit.

The oral administration of antacids such as magnesium carbonate or magnesium hydroxide is indicated, but they should be mixed in 2 to 3 gallons (8 to 12 L) of warm water and given by stomach tube to ensure dispersion throughout the rumen. Initial doses of up to 1 g/kg body weight (454 g for an adult bovine) should be followed by smaller doses repeated at 6- to 12-hour intervals. If the rumen has been evacuated, the initial dose should not exceed 0.5 lb (225 g).

It is important that dehydration and acidosis be corrected as well. Balanced electrolyte and 5 per cent sodium bicarbonate solutions should be given intravenously. A 450-kg animal with 10 per cent dehydration may require as much as 50 L of fluid over a 24-hour period. Sodium bicarbonate should be given at the rate of 0.5 mEq/kg body weight initially and repeated in 24 hours if necessary (1 g of sodium bicarbonate will supply 12 mEq of bicarbonate ion). Correction of blood pH to within the normal range is vital for survival of the animal even if the offending rumen ingesta are removed.

Oral administration of activated charcoal at the rate of 2 g/kg body weight is said to enhance clinical recovery from acute lactic acidosis. This effect may be achieved by inactivating endotoxin thought to be released by the destruction of gram-negative rumen microorganisms.[2]

Administration of antihistamines is considered to be of value by some. Recent field experience indicates that oral administration of thiabendazole in normal anthelmintic doses helps in controlling secondary mycotic rumenitis.

PREVENTION

Avoiding sudden and drastic changes in the ration is paramount in preventing rumen acidosis. Bunk-fed cattle need regular quantities of ration at regular intervals, and adequate bunk space must be available so that all animals have an opportunity to feed normally. The ration must include adequate roughage (generally not less than 10 per cent) regularly.

Animals on self-feeder programs are particularly vulnerable to excessive consumption, especially early in the feeding program. Every precaution must be taken to ensure that roughage is available (mixed in the feed if possible) and that animals are brought onto full feed slowly. Feeders must be checked regularly and not permitted to run low or stand empty so that excessive intake by hungry animals is avoided after the feeders have been refilled.

Progress has been made in the prevention of rumen lactic acidosis by pharmacologic means. The ionophore antibiotics including monensin, lasalocid, and salinomycin appear to be particularly useful in maintaining higher rumen pH and lower rumen lactate concentrations as well as in improving feed efficiency in treated as compared with control animals.[7]

Rumenitis (Ruminal Parakeratosis, Chronic Rumen Acidosis)

DEFINITION

The term *rumenitis* refers to a series of inflammatory changes that develop in the rumen mucosa and underlying tissues in cattle fed high-energy rations with inadequate roughage. Clinically, the syndrome includes the associated lesions of liver abscess and laminitis. The incidence may be as high as 100 per cent in cattle fed all-concentrate rations for prolonged periods or those that have not been carefully adapted to such rations. Rumenitis also occurs as a secondary stage of acute rumen engorgement with acidosis.

PATHOGENESIS

The association between liver abscess formation and ruminal lesions was first reported by Smith[9] and later by Jensen and colleagues.[10] A definite relationship between rumen adaptation to high-energy rations and the development of rumen lesions is now generally understood.

The exact pathogenesis of the rumen lesions has not been elucidated, but it is commonly accepted that the end-products of rumen fermentation accumulate and change in relative quantity, causing an increase in hydrogen ion concentration and leading to inflammation of the rumen mucosa.

Lactic acidosis is often not a prominent feature of this disorder, and affected animals may not go through an acute phase of illness. Some animals may perform very well, showing acceptable weight gains or producing high volumes of milk in the case of dairy cows. The rumen fluid may be moderately acidic, but in the absence of lactic acid that is probably metabolized by other microorganisms, the effects are mostly chronic and insidious.[6]

The sequence of events would appear to be (1) inflammation of the rumen mucosa, (2) adherence of debris to the mucosa, (3) ulceration and infection of deeper layers in the rumen wall, and (4) focal abscess formation in the rumen wall.

The appearance of abscesses in the liver follows sequentially. Chronic laminitis is a later sequela, but its relationship is uncertain and appears less well correlated with the preceding events. Other independent factors may be involved in the development of chronic laminitis. It is frequently observed in cattle fed high-energy rations for 60 to 90 days, but the incidence appears to be higher among females, and laminitis sometimes occurs in the absence of rumen and liver lesions. Likewise, there is nothing specific about the lesions in the rumen or the liver; the lesions in either could arise from other causes.

CLINICAL SIGNS

Cattle do not necessarily become clinically ill during the early stages of rumenitis and liver abscess formation. Feed consumption is usually good, and weight gains on all-concentrate rations for periods over 100 days are very acceptable. However, the addition of good-quality hay or silage for at least 10 to 20 per cent of the ration will often result in increased feed consumption and average daily gain.

Animals with advanced rumen and liver lesions may show reduced appetite and weight gains, usually late in the feeding period. Affected individuals show an apparent lack of fill, as evidenced by gauntness of the abdomen. Other clinical signs, possibly from developing peritonitis or septicemia, may be seen. There will be elongation and flatness of the hooves with a very apparent alteration in gait if there is a chronic laminitis.

An increase in the incidence of unrelated problems such as respiratory disease is likely in severely affected groups of cattle.

NECROPSY

Lesions are usually observed only at slaughter and result in the condemnations of livers and rumens. The rumen mucosa will have edema and clumping of papillae in mild cases. More advanced cases demonstrate matting and necrosis of papillae with diffuse ulcerations. Hair and debris will adhere to the mucosa. Extensive thickening of the rumen wall with abscessation is also observed.

There is increased thickness of the cornified portion of the rumen epithelium and increased numbers of vacuoles on histologic examination. The lesion is characteristic of an acid burn.

Abscesses will be observed on cut sections of the liver and are apparent as light-colored spots on the uncut surface in severe cases.

DIAGNOSIS

Chronic laminitis may be the first visible sign, but in many instances, its appearance accompanies or precedes a noticeable reduction in feed consumption and rate of gain.

The condition can be suspected in any group of cattle being fed for maximal gains on high-energy or all-concentrate rations, but confirmation often depends on examination of rumens and livers at slaughter.

TREATMENT

Treatment and prevention depend on the inclusion of adequate good-quality roughage in the ration. Stemmy hay is preferred as a roughage source and should equal at least 10 per cent of the dry matter in the ration. Chopped or finely ground hay is less effective in preventing rumenitis. Ensilage can be used, but greater quantities are necessary. Ground corncobs are commonly used as roughage but should be supplemented with some hay.

Antibiotics fed at disease prevention levels reduce the incidence of liver abscesses but have no effect on the development of rumen lesions.

Individual animals that survive acute rumen engorgement develop secondary rumenitis, often with severe mycotic involvement. Thiabendazole given daily (25 mg/kg body weight) is helpful in reducing the severity.

Ruminal Tympany (Bloat)

DEFINITION

Ruminal tympany, or bloat, refers to excessive accumulation of gas in the rumen. The gas may be in free form or may be mixed with ingesta in the form of froth. It occurs both on pasture and in feedlots and is a major cause of mortality in cattle wherever intensive farming is practiced. Additional losses include decreased milk production and reduced rate of gain. The reduced potential for using legume plants for pasture has a significant economic impact.

PATHOGENESIS

If the animal is able to eructate naturally, excessive production of gas in the rumen is of little consequence. This mechanism becomes ineffective under some circumstances, particularly when the cardia of the stomach becomes obstructed by froth.

Frothing of rumen ingesta occurs when the viscosity of the fluid is elevated. Under some conditions, several naturally occurring plant substances will have this effect. These include saponins, pectins, hemicelluloses, and certain proteins. The pH of the rumen contents is important in determining the stability of the foam. A pH of 6 is near optimum for maximal stability. Hypermotility of the rumen wall in the initial stages also contributes to the development of frothy bloat. Free-gas bloat is commonly associated with rumen atony.

The bloat occurring in animals on pasture is most typical of frothy bloat. However, feedlot bloat may also be frothy.

Succulent plants, particularly young growing legumes in the prebloom stage, are leading contributors to pasture bloat. Alfalfa pasture is commonly involved. Harvested crops are less likely to cause bloat. The presence or absence of moisture on the plants does not appear to be a significant factor.

Animal factors can be important as well; particular strains of cattle have been shown to be more susceptible. This is probably related to the ability to or capacity for producing saliva. Adaptation of animals to a particular feed is an important factor. There may be short-term increased susceptibility due to changes in rumen microflora, but as animals become adjusted to a particular pasture or ration, the long-term effect is toward decreased susceptibility.

Secondary bloat may be caused by an obstruction of the esophagus or the cardia of the stomach. Anything that causes rumen atony will also cause tympany of the rumen. This is frequently observed in parturient hypocalcemia and may be part of the rumen acidosis–rumenitis syndrome. Bloat may be a terminal event in animals that die after several days or weeks of severe chronic rumenitis subsequent to rumen acidosis.

Isolated cases of chronic bloat are commonly seen in feedlot animals, often with no apparent cause. Numerous cases of chronic bloat are sometimes observed in animals that have recently suffered a respiratory disease epidemic. This will follow the acute infection by a few days to several weeks. This secondary bloat has been attributed to the necessary heavy use of oral or parenteral antibiotics to treat the respiratory disease. Rumen microflora may be altered, and this may lead to excessive gas production.

Greatly enlarged mediastinal and bronchial lymph nodes are often observed at necropsy. Mechanical compression and partial obstruction of the esophagus by these abnormal structures are possible explanations for the bloat. It is also possible that the enlarged lymph nodes interfere with vagal innervation of the rumen, causing rumen atony and subsequent tympany.

CLINICAL SIGNS

Severe ruminal tympany is readily apparent to the trained observer. In mild cases, however, it is necessary to differentiate between the rumen simply filled with ingesta and one distended with gas. In the latter case, the skin over the left paralumbar fossa is very tight. The entire abdomen is distended, but the upper left quadrant will be distorted so that it protrudes above the level of the bone prominences in the lumbar region.

Animals in the early stages of bloat will exhibit signs of colic. Increased rumen motility will also be noted. Animals with advanced cases will show dyspnea with open-mouth breathing, and rumen movements will be absent.

It is usually necessary to pass a stomach tube to differentiate free-gas bloat from frothy bloat.

NECROPSY

Post-mortem bloat in ruminants that die from other conditions causes some confusion in diagnosis if other findings are negative.

When bloat is the primary cause of death, there will be congestion and hemorrhage in the anterior portions of the carcass and edema in the rear quarters, particularly in the scrotal and ventral perineal areas.

Also there will be congestion and possibly extravasated blood in the ventral sinuses of the spinal column and in the cranial cavity. The liver will be pale, and the lungs will show signs of compression. The rumen will be distended, but usually the contents will be less frothy than before death.

DIAGNOSIS

A preliminary diagnosis in the living animal is usually based on observation of the distended abdomen with extreme tightness of skin and distortion in the upper left quadrant. It may be necessary to pass a stomach tube to determine whether the bloat is frothy. Determination of the underlying cause will depend on complete clinical examination and careful evaluation of the history, particularly relative to recent consumption of feed or pasture plants.

Establishing a post-mortem diagnosis frequently a problem. It is necessary to rule out clostridial infections, lightning strike, and other causes of sudden death. The diagnosis will depend, in part, on the absence of local or systemic lesions of such conditions.

TREATMENT

Free-gas bloat can usually be treated by passing a stomach tube. If the bloat is frothy, the stability of the foam must be reduced before the gas can be removed. Any bland oil, such as mineral oil, is useful for this purpose. Oil mixed with detergent will disperse more rapidly in the rumen ingesta. Ordinary household detergents have been used for this purpose. Recommended dosages vary but are usually in the range of 0.5 to 1 lb (226 to 454 g) per animal. Chemicals such as poloxalene and dioctyl sodium succinate are also effective in lowering the viscosity of the fluid ingesta, thereby reducing the stability of the foam.

Silicones have been used for treatment and prevention of bloat but are probably less reliable than oils are. Orally administered turpentine is an old treatment that is reasonably effective but is highly irritating to the tissues and also imparts undesirable flavors to meat and milk.

It is important that the therapeutic agent be deposited in the region of the cardia or given in a sufficient quantity of fluid for ensuring that it is well dispersed in the rumen. In this way, a fluid line can be re-established and the obstruction relieved. Injection through the left flank into an atonic rumen is not likely to be adequate in severe cases.

In acute frothy bloat with the animal in severe distress, emergency rumenotomy may be necessary to save the animal's life.

Treatment of secondary bloat usually depends on removal of the primary cause. The bloat in parturient hypocalcemia will be rapidly relieved after the administration of intravenous calcium salts. Bloat in an animal that has become cast on its side or that is in dorsal recumbency will usually be relieved by shifting the animal to a more normal position.

Chronic bloat in feedlot animals can sometimes be treated by surgically establishing a small temporary rumen fistula, with or without the use of a prosthetic device. Rumen gas will escape through the fistula until it becomes closed by granulation tissue, usually in about 4 to 6 weeks. By then the primary condition will often have corrected itself, and an uneventful recovery is made.

PREVENTION

Gradual adaptation to high-performance rations is of primary importance for avoidance of bloat. Animals going into lush legume pasture should be given an ample prefeeding of dry hay. Access to the new pasture should be limited to short intervals until the animals are well adjusted to the new feed. In some instances, mowing the forage and leaving it down for 1 or 2 days before pasturing is the best practical approach for preventing bloat. The same conditions apply to animals in feedlots. The change from starter feed to full feed should be made very gradually over a 3- to 4-week period. Self-fed cattle are particularly vulnerable, and it is wise practice to feed animals from bunks until they are well adjusted to the ration that will be supplied in the self-feeder.

Materials used for the treatment of bloat have been used for prevention. These include detergents, mineral oil, and poloxalene in various formulations. To be effective, however, these materials must be consumed by the animal the same day that the bloat-causing ration is fed.

The ionophore antibiotic monensin, fed at 0.66 and 0.99 mg/kg body weight daily, reduced the severity of legume bloat. The effect was thought to be due to decreased protozoal numbers and resulting decreased gas production.[1, 5]

In feedlot bloat, feeding more coarse roughage will often correct the problem. In other instances, it may prove practical to include an inexpensive detergent at the rate of 10 to 20 lb per ton of concentrate ration.

It has been suggested that preventive and therapeutic levels of antibiotics included in the ration may cause bloat. However, many feeders routinely use tetracycline at rates of up to 5 mg/lb (11 mg/kg) body weight for 7 to 14 days to prevent respiratory disease outbreaks with no increased occurrence of bloat. Some digestive upset may result, however, if the animals are not gradually introduced to the drug over a period of 2 to 3 days. Withdrawal of the antibiotics from the ration should also be made gradually for avoidance of digestive disturbances such as bloat.

BIBLIOGRAPHY

Blood DC, Radostits OM, Henderson JR: Veterinary Medicine. London, Bailliere Tindall, 1983, pp 221–246.
Clark RTJ, Reid CSW: Foamy bloat of cattle: a review. J Dairy Sci 57:7, 1974.
Dougherty RW, Riley JL, Cook HM: Changes in motility and pH in the digestive tract of experimentally overfed sheep. Am J Vet Res 36:6, 1975.
Dunlop RH, Hammon PB: D-lactic acidosis of ruminants. Ann NY Acad Sci 119:1109, 1965.
Fell BF, Kay M, Whitelaw FG, Boyne R: Observations on the development of ruminal lesions in calves fed on barley. Res Vet Sci 9:458–466, 1968.
Garry FB: Managing bloat in cattle. Vet Med 85:643–650, 1990.
Harvey RW, Wise MB, Blumer TN, Barrick ER: Influence of added roughage and chlorotetracycline to all concentrate rations for fattening steers. J Anim Sci 27:5, 1968.
Hofirek B, Jagos P, Dvora R: Metabolic profile test of rumen fluid and its application in the diagnosis of rumen dysfunctions (abstract). Bovine Pract 11:90, 1976.
Jensen R: Diseases of Sheep. Philadelphia, Lea & Febiger, 1974, pp 209–262.
Jensen R, et al: Fatal abomasal ulcers in yearling feedlot cattle. J Am Vet Med Assoc 169:5, 1976.
Kay M, Fell BF, Boyne R: The relationship between the acidity of the rumen contents and rumenitis in calves fed on barley. Res Vet Sci 10:181, 1969.

Reid CSW: Causes and control of bloat. NZ J Agric 133:1, 1976.
Rowland AC, Wieser MF, Preston TR: The rumen pathology of intensively managed beef cattle. Anim Prod 11:499, 1969.
Wass WM, Thompson JR: Rumen acidosis in cattle on intensive feeding programs. Proceedings, XIVth World Congress on Diseases of Cattle. Dublin, Ireland, 1986, pp 1135–1139.

REFERENCES

1. Bartley EE, Nagaraja TG, et al: Effects of lasalocid or monensin on legume or grain (feedlot) bloat. J Anim Sci 56:1400–1406, 1983.
2. Buck WB: Proceedings, XVIII Conference, Rumen Function. Chicago, IL, 1985, p 1.
3. Cullen AJ, Harmon DL, Nagaraja TG: In vitro fermentation of sugars, grains and by-product feeds in relation to initiation of ruminal lactate production. J Dairy Sci 69:2616–2621, 1986.
4. Dougherty RW, Coburn KS, Cook HM, Allison MJ: Preliminary study of appearance of endotoxin in circulatory system of sheep and cattle after induced grain engorgement. Am J Vet Res 36:6, 1975.
5. Katz MP, Nagaraja TG, Fina LR: Ruminal changes in monensin- and lasalocid-fed cattle grazing bloat-provocative alfalfa pasture. J Anim Sci 63:1246–1257, 1986.
6. Garry FB: Diagnosing and treating indigestion caused by fermentative disorders. Vet Med 85:660–670, 1990.
7. Nagaraja TG, Avery TB, Galitzer SJ, Dayton AD: Prevention of lactic acidosis in cattle by lasalocid or monensin. J Anim Sci 53:206–216, 1981.
8. Mullenax CH, Keller RR, Allison MJ: Physiologic responses of ruminants to toxic factors extracted from rumen bacteria and rumen fluid. Am J Vet Res 5:16, 1944.
9. Smith H: Ulcerative lesions of bovine rumen and their possible relation to hepatic abscesses. Am J Vet Res 5:16, 1944.
10. Jensen R, Deane HM, Cooper LJ, et al: The rumenitis–liver abscess complex in beef cattle. Am J Vet Res 15:55, 1954.

Traumatic Reticuloperitonitis and Its Sequelae

ROBERT N. STREETER, DVM

Traumatic reticuloperitonitis (TRP) is a sporadic infectious disease of ruminants due to the penetration of the reticulum by ingested foreign material and the resultant contamination of various organs or body cavities. Cattle are principally affected because of their indiscriminant feeding behavior. The disorder occurs rarely in other ruminant species (sheep, goats, and llamas).[1,2] A variety of clinical syndromes can result, but they all have a common underlying pathogenesis. The following discussion focuses on the disease in cattle.

ETIOLOGY AND EPIDEMIOLOGY

Traumatic reticuloperitonitis is most often caused by linear metallic foreign bodies, with wires and nails being the most common inciting agents.[3,4] Nonferromagnetic objects are only occasionally responsible. Metallic debris is encountered more commonly in processed feeds and forages rather than on pastures; hence, the condition is seen more in confined cattle. Cattle can also acquire linear foreign material when they are exposed to construction sites or to deteriorating buildings and fences. Most cases occur in animals over 2 years of age.[4] The age predilection is likely due to differences in feeding practices between adult and young stock and to increased exposure occurring over time. Dairy cattle are more commonly affected than are beef cattle, which likewise reflects a difference in husbandry practices. Foreign material is frequently found in the reticulum of cattle, often without consequence. Scars within the reticulum or evidence of adhesions associated with TRP have been noted in up to 70 per cent of adult dairy cattle at post-mortem inspection.[5]

PATHOPHYSIOLOGY

Ingested particles enter the rumen after deglutition and, with ensuing ruminal contractions, come to rest within the reticulum. The "honeycombed" internal surface of the reticulum predisposes the objects to lodge within the cellulae reticullae, and with continued reticular contractions, they can be forced to penetrate the wall.

Perforation is usually in the cranioventral aspect of the reticulum and less commonly in a medial or lateral direction. Lesions due to intramural penetration without disruption of the serosal surface are frequently subclinical or result in a mild self-limiting disease. Once the foreign material penetrates the serosa, the accompanying enteric microflora initiates a local peritonitis, and clinical signs develop. Progression of the disease beyond this stage is variable. Among the possible outcomes are acute local peritonitis, chronic local peritonitis, diffuse peritonitis, perireticular abscess formation, hepatic involvement with liver abscessation, vagal neuritis and vagal indigestion, traumatic splenitis, and transdiaphragmatic migration with resultant pericarditis, mediastinitis, pleuritis, or pneumonia.

Characteristics of the foreign body may influence its migration. In an experimental model of TRP in which wires and nails were given simultaneously, the wires were far more frequently found both within the reticulum and to be perforating the wall.[6] Abdominal compression due to an enlarged rumen or advanced pregnancy has been postulated to be a predisposing factor to the development of transdiaphragmatic migration of foreign objects.[7]

CLINICAL SIGNS

Acute Localized Peritonitis

Acute localized peritonitis is common to all cases of TRP. The most consistent findings with this underlying lesion are an initial rise in body temperature and heart rate, evidence of abdominal pain, decreased or absent reticuloruminal motility, and rapid decline in appetite and milk production.

Pyrexia is usually moderate (39.5° to 40.5° C); in uncomplicated cases, the temperature returns toward normal within a few days. Likewise, the heart rate is moderately elevated in most cases of localized peritonitis (80 to 100 beats/minute) with a gradual decline over the following 4 to 7 days. Aberrations in respiratory parameters are variable and mild unless significant lung abscessation or pleuritis occurs. The only change in most cases is an increased rate and shallow depth of respiration due to pyrexia and pain. Manifestations of abdominal pain may be subtle or quite obvious. In severe cases, animals may resist movement, have a short stilted gait, stand with elbows abducted, have a markedly arched posture, audibly grunt with respiratory efforts or while walking, and prefer to remain standing or recumbent for long periods of time. Other signs include extended head and neck with tensed cervical and facial muscles, fasciculations of forelimb muscles, and odontoprisis. Maneuvers used to detect pain include pinching the withers, percussion over the area of the reticulum, and lifting of the cranioventral abdomen with the knee or a pole. Such manipulations may evoke an audible and visual response in severe cases, whereas in milder cases or those of some chronicity, the response can be detected only by simultaneous auscultation over the trachea. Typically, the outward signs of abdominal pain regress to the point at which they are difficult to detect after the third to fourth day of illness.

Evidence of abdominal pain is not specific for TRP and may be found in other disorders of the cranial abdomen such as abomasal ulcers, liver abscesses, rumenitis, abomasal lymphoma, and peritonitis from other causes. Discriminant palpation and percussion of the right and left abdomen may assist in ruling out potential causes by identification of a most painful locus over a particular organ. Also, thoracic pain can closely mimic that originating in the abdomen. Pain elicited on deep intercostal palpation and abnormal respiratory sounds on auscultation should alert the clinician to this possibility.

Reticuloruminal activity is invariably affected early in the course of the disease. Initially there is marked suppression or complete absence of ruminal contractions in the first few days. As motility returns, evidence of pain may coincide with contraction of the reticulum during the primary phase of the contraction cycle. Slight distention of the left paralumbar fossa due to an accumulation of gas in the rumen, resulting from less frequent eructation, may be noted. Occasionally, animals may be noted to vomit or drop their cud. Rumen contents may be firmer than normal as a result of dehydration and decreased motility. Feces are frequently scant and dry in the early stages of the disease. Defecation may be more frequent, small in volume, and accompanied by grunting or other evidence of abdominal pain. Diarrhea early in the course of the disease, especially when it is accompanied by symptoms of toxemia, should alert the clinician to the possibility of acute diffuse peritonitis or another diagnosis.

A precipitous drop in milk production and appetite are characteristic of TRP. These signs can be very helpful in distinguishing subacute TRP from a variety of diseases with similar vague signs of gastrointestinal atony such as left displaced abomasum, simple indigestion, and ketosis. The drop in milk yield is usually greater than 50 to 75 per cent during the first 24 hours in TRP, in contrast to the typically more gradual and less marked decline noted in these other maladies.[7]

The course of the disease with acute localized peritonitis is thus relatively short. Most uncomplicated cases will show progressive improvement over 3 to 5 days. If signs persist after this time, the development of chronic active peritonitis or other complications should be considered.

Chronic Localized Peritonitis

Chronic peritonitis may result from persistence of the foreign body or its tract leading to extension of the infection initiated by the original perforation. Clinical findings are similar to those seen with acute local peritonitis but are less extreme. There is less evidence of abdominal pain, and its detection can be difficult. Body temperature and heart rate may return to within normal range or be slightly elevated. Appetite and milk production usually remain subnormal. Feces continue to be scant, but the character may range from firm to loose depending on the animal's hydration status and degree of toxemia present.

Diffuse Peritonitis

Diffuse peritonitis is an uncommon result of TRP because of the inherent ability of the bovine to form adhesions in response to peritoneal injury. When it does occur, it is often a fulminating and highly fatal disease. Generalized peritonitis usually develops as a primary event directly after foreign body perforation, although cases may develop some time (weeks) after onset of typical TRP signs.[7] The course is usually short.

Animals may progress to prostration, recumbency, and death within 24 to 36 hours. Features distinguishing this from routine cases of TRP include very high heart rate (100 to 120+ beats/mintue), high fever (40° to 41° C) with rapid progression to hypothermia, rapid development of severe dehydration, diarrhea, profound depression, and recumbency. The prognosis for such cases is poor despite aggressive therapy.

Thoracic Sequelae: Pericarditis

Transdiaphragmatic migration of the foreign body occurs in a significant number of cases, and the result is often catastrophic. Diaphragmatic involvement is reported to occur in approximately 28 to 60 per cent of TRP cases, and pericarditis in 6 to 8 per cent.[4,8] The actual incidence may be significantly less because many mild cases of TRP may not be included in such surveys. Pulmonary or mediastinal abscessation and pleuritis may occur separately or in conjunction with pericarditis. Recognition of intrathoracic involvement in cases of TRP is important because it affects prognosis significantly and additional therapeutic measures should be considered in those animals undergoing treatment. The time span between reticular perforation and involvement of the pericardium is variable, ranging from a few days to weeks or months.

Clinical signs referable to traumatic pericarditis include most of those mentioned for acute localized peritonitis because some degree of peritoneal involvement invariably occurs. The signs displayed are due to a combination of pain, toxemia, and the development of congestive heart failure. The most consistent distinguishing clinical findings in animals with pericarditis are persistent tachycardia and abnormalities on cardiac auscultation. The heart rate of affected cattle is continually elevated, typically over 100 beats/minute. Pyrexia is present in cases suffering from toxemia but may be absent in subacute cases wherein congestive heart failure predominates. The auscultatory findings depend on the duration of the condition and the presence or absence of gas within the pericardial space. Gas may be present owing to its production by multiplying microorganisms. Initially, a pericardial friction rub is heard. This may be confused with a pleural friction rub if the inflamed portion of the pleura is in contact with the pericardium. With time, exudation into the pericardial sac occurs, with production of muffled heart sounds. Only if gas and fluid are present concurrently will characteristic "splashing" sounds be heard.

As exudate and gas accumulate within the pericardial space, cardiac tamponade develops. The clinical signs generated are due to right-sided failure because of the thinner wall and lower systolic pressure of the right side of the heart. Signs include venous distention, abnormal jugular pulses, and brisket edema. In severe cases, hepatic and portal congestion may lead to profuse diarrhea, ascites, and a palpable liver under the right costal arch. Peracute death due to laceration of a coronary vessel with resultant hemopericardium and cardiac tamponade can occur. Rarely, subcutaneous emphysema may be present over the lateral and dorsal thorax as gas produced within the mediastinum or pleura escapes to the subcutis.

Other Sequelae

A syndrome of omasal transport failure may occur in association with perireticular and liver abscesses subsequent to TRP.[9,10] The pathogenesis is thought to involve vagal nerve damage by resultant adhesions or from direct pressure applied by an abscess. Other forms of vagal indigestion are also potential sequelae to TRP; a variety of clinical manifestations have been described (see Vagus Indigestion).[11,12]

Involvement of the spleen in TRP is unusual. Less than 0.23 per cent of cases in a large survey involved the spleen.[4] This condition may be clinically silent, result in chronic low-grade sepsis and pyrexia, or lead to diffuse peritonitis if a large abscess is subsequently ruptured. Rarely, sepsis associated with TRP can serve as the precursor to the development of diseases such as endocarditis, septic arthritis, embolic pneumonia or nephritis, and amyloidosis.[13, 14] TRP is also reported to be a predisposing factor in the development of acquired diaphragmatic herniation in the bovine albeit an extremely rare occurrence.[15]

DIAGNOSTIC AIDS

Clinical pathologic techniques widely recognized as helpful in the evaluation of an animal suspected of having TRP include hematology and abdominocentesis. Serum biochemical profiles may be helpful in detecting other diseases present, but results are not routinely abnormal in TRP.

Changes in the leukogram in cases of TRP are affected by the duration of the disease and the sequelae present. The classic response is a leukocytosis, a neutrophilia, and a left shift (a regenerative response). However, many cases will have a normal total leukocyte count, and the differential count must be relied on to reflect the presence of the inflammatory process. The leukogram in uncomplicated cases returns toward normal within 3 to 5 days. In cases of diffuse peritonitis, the leukogram may reveal a leukopenia and degenerative left shift. Traumatic pericarditis tends to generate somewhat higher total counts (14,000 to 20,000 cells/μl) than do cases of acute or chronic localized peritonitis. Overall, leukograms are variable in TRP.

Elevation of plasma fibrinogen concentration is a fairly constant feature of inflammatory diseases in cattle.[16] Due to the influence of dehydration on this parameter, it is suggested that a ratio of plasma protein to fibrinogen less than 10:1 be used as a finding consistent with TRP.[17] Elevation of total plasma protein has been examined as a useful index for the suspicion of TRP.[18] High levels of total plasma protein (>10 g/dl) had a high positive predictive value (76 per cent) in determining the presence of TRP.

Examination of peritoneal fluid is a sensitive indicator of peritoneal inflammation. The total nucleated cell count and protein level in peritoneal fluid appear to be less reliable indicators of abdominal inflammation than is the differential cell count. The presence of greater than 40 per cent neutrophils and less than 10 per cent eosinophils in the sample is suggestive of peritonitis.[19] Cell counts greater than 6000/μl and protein levels greater than 3 g/dl have been used to predict the presence of peritonitis.[20] The presence of degenerate neutrophils and bacteria is also supportive. Culture of the sample also provides useful information regarding subsequent antimicrobial therapy.

Radiography of the cranioventral abdomen and caudal thorax is a useful diagnostic tool in the identification of TRP, pericarditis, and perireticular abscesses.[21, 22] Difficulties exist because of the size of the animal, which allows only a lateral view. Hence, the absolute location of the foreign body is difficult to determine. The procedure may be performed standing or with the patient in dorsal recumbency. Standing reticulography requires powerful equipment not available to most practitioners. Placement of the animal in dorsal recumbency provides the advantage of being able to use a portable unit on most cows. This also allows rumen gas to accumulate in the reticulum, which increases contrast and visualization of foreign material. Nonpenetrating foreign bodies may fall from the ventral reticulum during dorsal recumbency. Dorsal reticulography is not without risk, however, especially in acute cases (in which the procedure can lead to dissemination of the peritonitis) and in animals with compromised cardiovascular function (i.e., pericarditis).

Radiographically, foreign bodies that lie outside the reticulum, within but not on the floor of the viscus, are suggestive of TRP.[21] A gas shadow adjacent to the reticulum or a gas-fluid interface is indicative of an intra-abdominal abscess, but the sensitivity of detecting this with reticulography appears to be low. Gas within the abomasum may occasionally be confused with an abscess caudal to the reticulum.

Endoscopic examination of the cranial abdomen has been reported to be of benefit in the diagnosis of TRP; however, the specificity of this technique can be questioned.[23]

Diagnostic aids applicable to cases of pericarditis include electrocardiography, pericardiocentesis, and ultrasonography. Electrocardiographic changes seen with pericarditis in large animals include electrical alternans and diminished amplitude of the QRS complexes.[24, 25]

TREATMENT

The appropriate treatment for TRP will depend on the stage of the disease when treatment is requested, the sequelae that are present or are likely to develop, the value of the animal, and diagnostic and surgical facilities available to the clinician.

Medical management of TRP includes administration of parenteral antibiotics, provision of a reticular magnet, and strict confinement to a small area. The choice of antibiotics should be predicated on cultural examination of an abdominocentesis sample. If a sample is not available, the decision is based on the knowledge that this is a polymicrobial infection; agents commonly encountered include *Actinomyces pyogenes*, coliforms, and anaerobes (*Fusobacterium* and *Bacteroides* spp.). Consideration should be given to use of a drug with a short withholding time such that salvage may remain an option should therapy be unsuccessful. The utility of magnets used therapeutically is limited because they may remain within the rumen for extended periods after administration owing to the lack of rumen motility. Also, only foreign bodies in the ventral aspect of the reticulum are likely to be affected by a magnet. Strict confinement is used to allow adhesions to develop around the perforation, hence limiting the dissemination of sepsis. Elevation of the forequarters has been recommended for retarding forward migration of the foreign body.

Medical management gives favorable results in a high percentage of cases. The offending foreign body will often have returned to the lumen or have completely penetrated through the reticular wall and be inaccessible via rumenotomy by 2 to 4 days after the onset of signs. Hence, surgical intervention for removal of the foreign body may be unrewarding. It may, however, be indicated in valuable animals, especially if the offending foreign body is detected radiographically within the diaphragm or not in contact with a magnet. For the majority of cattle, surgical management is elected in cases not showing significant and continuing improvement after 3 to 4 days of conservative therapy.

Surgical removal of the foreign body is indicated in cases of chronic active peritonitis and for preventing further migration of a nonstabilized foreign body. Surgical management involves a left-sided laparotomy, exploratory, and rumenotomy.[26] Extreme care should be taken to palpate the cranioventral abdomen before the rumenotomy and only after exploration of the caudal and right abdomen so that the sepsis is not dispersed. Fibrinous adhesions should not be broken down, and retrieval of the foreign body should be performed only during the subsequent rumenotomy. If no adhesions are present around the reticulum and the contents can be accurately palpated with no associated lesions present, a rumenotomy may not be necessary. During the rumenotomy, the reticulum is examined for adhesions, and these areas are searched closely for a foreign body. If an abscess is located and is found to be firmly adherent to the wall of the reticulum, it is lanced through the wall of the reticulum at a point of firm attachment. This provides chronic active drainage of the area. Recurrence does not appear to be a significant problem.[9] If an abscess is not tightly adherent to a portion of the reticulum, a second surgery and drainage through a ventral approach may be indicated.

Cases of diffuse peritonitis require intensive therapy consisting of intravenous fluids, antibiotics, and anti-inflammatory agents, but the mortality is high despite aggressive therapy. If large quantities of exudate have accumulated within the peritoneum, its drainage via a catheter or teat tube placed in the ventral abdomen may be beneficial. Peritoneal lavage is difficult to accomplish in cattle owing to the size of the animal, the presence of the omentum, and large amounts of fibrin and subsequent adhesions.

Therapy for traumatic pericarditis is frequently unsuccessful and usually reserved for valuable individuals. Antibiotic considerations are similar to those for cases of TRP. Rumenotomy is indicated early in the disease to increase the probability of retrieving the foreign body. Drainage of the pericardial sac can be accomplished via pericardiocentesis, catheterization of the pericardium, or pericardiotomy. Pericardiocentesis will provide only short-term benefit. Placement of a pericardial catheter is more difficult but enables repeated drainage and lavage with antimicrobial solutions. Problems are frequently encountered when large fibrin clots present in the exudate cause occlusion of the catheter. Adhesions often develop within the pericardial sac, leading to compartmentalization and inability to achieve adequate drainage by this method. Use of proteolytic enzymes in the lavage solution may lessen these occurrences. The catheter is ideally left in place until the fluid retrieved is no longer septic.

Pericardiotomy via a fifth rib resection has the advantage of allowing more complete drainage of the pericardium. Occasionally, a foreign body that was inaccessible by rumenotomy may be removed by this approach. This technique must be employed before the exudate is resorbed and the pericardium adheres to the epicardium. A constrictive pericarditis may develop with time despite appropriate therapy. Surgical removal of the pericardium (pericardiectomy) is necessary to prevent this occurrence. This technique has been performed in the bovine, but its practicality is limited.[27]

Regardless of the techniques used, therapy for pericarditis is generally assumed to be a short-term salvage procedure capable of allowing the eventual slaughter of the animal or enabling short-term extension of the animal's reproductive life span.

PREVENTION AND CONTROL

With the widespread use of magnetic screening devices on feed-processing equipment, the incidence of TRP has been reduced. General farm cleanliness and discontinued use of baling wire may also decrease the incidence of TRP. The prophylactic use of rumen magnets has been demonstrated to be highly effective in preventing the occurrence of TRP due to ferromagnetic foreign bodies.[28, 29] Their use is probably indicated in individual valuable cattle and in herds known to have a significant problem with this disease. Animals are usually given the magnet between 1 and 2 years of age.

REFERENCES

1. Maddy KT: Traumatic gastritis in sheep and goats. J Am Vet Med Assoc 124:124–125, 1954.
2. Smith JA: Noninfectious diseases, metabolic diseases, toxicities, and neoplastic diseases of South American camelids. Vet Clin North Am [Food Anim Pract] 5:106, 1989.
3. Jagos P: The characteristics of foreign bodies in traumatic inflammations of cattle. Acta Vet (Brno) 38:545–552, 1969.
4. Editorial: Traumatic gastritis and "tramp iron." J Am Vet Med Assoc 125:331–332, 1954.
5. Maddy KT: Incidence of perforation of the bovine reticulum. J Am Vet Med Assoc 124:113–115, 1954.
6. Kingrey BW: Experimental bovine traumatic gastritis. J Am Vet Med Assoc 127:477–481, 1955.
7. Blood DC, Hutchins DR: Traumatic reticular perforation of cattle. Aust Vet J 31:113–123, 1955.
8. Blood DC, Hutchins DR: Traumatic pericarditis of cattle. Aust Vet J 31:229–232, 1955.
9. Fubini SL, et al: Failure of omasal transport attibutable to perireticular abscess formation in cattle: 29 cases (1980–1986). J Am Vet Med Assoc 194:811–814, 1989.
10. Fubini SL, et al: Vagus indigestion syndrome resulting from a liver abscess in dairy cows. J Am Vet Med Assoc 186:1297–1300, 1985.
11. Rebhun WC, Lesser FR: Vagus indigestion in cattle: clinical features, causes, treatments, and long-term follow-up of 112 cases. Compend Contin Educ Pract Vet 10:387–392, 1988.
12. Ferrante PL, Whitlock RH: Chronic (vagus) indigestion in cattle. Compend Contin Educ Pract Vet 3:S231–237, 1981.
13. Power HT, Rebhun WC: Bacterial endocarditis in adult dairy cattle. J Am Vet Med Assoc 182:806–808, 1983.
14. Johnson R, Jamison K: Amyloidosis in six dairy cows. J Am Vet Med Assoc 185:1538–1543, 1984.
15. Bristol DG: Diaphragmatic hernias in horses and cattle. Compend Contin Educ Pract Vet 8:S407–412, 1986.
16. McSherry BJ, et al: Plasma fibrinogen levels in normal and sick cows. Can J Comp Med 34:191–197, 1970.
17. Schalm OW, Jain NC, Carroll EJ: Plasma proteins, dysproteinemias, and immune deficiency disorders. In Jain NC (ed): Veterinary Hematology. Philadelphia, Lea & Febiger, 1986, p 960.
18. Dubensky RA, White ME: The sensitivity, specificity, and predictive value of total plasma protein in the diagnosis of traumatic reticuloperitonitis. Can J Comp Med 47:241–244, 1983.
19. Wilson AD, et al: Abdominocentesis in cattle: technique and criteria for diagnosis of peritonitis. Can Vet J 26:74–80, 1985.
20. Hirsch VM, Townsend HGG: Peritoneal fluid analysis in the diagnosis of abdominal disorders in cattle: a retrospective study. Can Vet J 23:348–354, 1982.
21. Fubini SL, et al: Accuracy of radiography of the reticulum for predicting surgical findings in adult dairy cattle with traumatic reticuloperitonitis: 123 cases (1981–1987). J Am Vet Med Assoc 197:1060–1064, 1990.
22. Ducharme NG, et al: Reticulography of the cow in dorsal recumbency: an aid in the diagnosis and treatment of traumatic reticuloperitonitis. J Am Vet Med Assoc 182:585–588, 1983.
23. Wilson AD, Ferguson JG: Use of a flexible fiberoptic laparoscope as a diagnostic aid in cattle. Can Vet J 25:229–234, 1984.
24. Hoffsis GF: Cardiovascular system. In Amstutz HE (ed): Bovine Medicine and Surgery. Santa Barbara, CA, American Veterinary Publications, 1980, pp 753–755.
25. Freestone JF, et al: Idiopathic effusive pericarditis with tamponade in the horse. Equine Vet J 19:38–42, 1987.
26. Ducharme NG: Surgery of the bovine forestomach compartments. Vet Clin North Am [Food Anim Pract] 6:371–397, 1990.
27. Nigam JM, Manohar M: Pericardectomy as treatment for constrictive pericarditis in a cow. Vet Rec 92:202–203, 1973.
28. Poulsen JSD: Prevention of traumatic indigestion in cattle. Vet Rec 98:149–151, 1976.
29. Carroll RE: The use of magnets in the control of traumatic gastritis of cattle. J Am Vet Med Assoc 129:376–377, 1956.

Diseases of the Abomasum and Small Intestine

GLEN F. HOFFSIS, DVM, MS, Diplomate, ACVIM
SHEILA M. McGUIRK, DVM, PhD, Diplomate, ACVIM
PETER D. CONSTABLE, BVSc, MS, MRCVS, Diplomate, ACVIM
D. MICHAEL RINGS, DVM, MS, Diplomate, ACVIM

Left Displaced Abomasum

GLEN F. HOFFSIS, DVM, MS, Diplomate, ACVIM
SHEILA M. McGUIRK, DVM, PhD, Diplomate, ACVIM

DEFINITION

The abomasum normally lies ventral to the rumen. Left displaced abomasum (LDA) occurs when the abomasum assumes an abnormal position on the left side of the abdomen between the rumen and the body wall (Fig. 1). First described in 1950,[1] it is one of the most frequently diagnosed diseases of dairy cows.

The disease is limited almost exclusively to dairy cattle, with the highest occurrence in cows of the middle-aged group (4 to 6 years of age) in early lactation. Approximately 80 per cent of all cases are diagnosed in the first month of lactation. The incidence has been estimated to be 0.35 to 1.94 per cent.[2,3] In some herds, the majority of cows in the herd have developed an LDA at some point during their life. The condition is rarely diagnosed in dairy bulls, young heifers, and beef cows. The incidence is also low in pregnant cows.

Although genetic factors have been investigated,[4] no significant differences were detected between the pedigrees of affected and unaffected cows.[5] The incidence is highest in confined cows that have minimal exercise.[6]

The precise etiologic origin of LDA is unknown, although it appears that primary factors that result in atony and gas distention of the abomasum can lead to displacement. The dietary factor associated with a high incidence of LDA is a low-roughage, high-concentrate diet.[6–9] Feeding high-concentrate diets increases production of volatile fatty acids in the rumen. High concentrations of volatile fatty acids directy affect forestomach smooth muscle by decreasing motility.[10] As motility decreases, carbon dioxide produced from the reaction between rumen bicarbonate and abomasal hydrochloric acid as well as methane and nitrogen accumulate in the abomasum gas.

Concurrent disease may also decrease abomasal motility. Hypocalcemia, metritis, mastitis, traumatic reticulitis, abomasal ulcers, fatty liver syndrome, and simple indigestion have been associated with LDA in over 25 per cent of affected cows.[6,11,12] Cows treated for these postpartum diseases will often develop an LDA during the course of the disease.

Mechanical etiologic factors may also be involved in LDA. During pregnancy, the gravid uterus may elevate the rumen and other viscera from the abdominal floor, allowing the abomasum to move slightly to the left of the midline. After parturition, with increased grain feeding, gas formation and atony may develop, and the displacement becomes complete. The shape of the cow's abdomen is suggested as another mechanical factor. The incidence in dairy cows may be higher than in beef cows because of their tendency to have proportionately larger and deeper bodies. Prolonged recumbency from lameness, hypocalcemia, or calving difficulty may cause malpositioning of the abomasum. Free-stall housing has also been incriminated because some cows have difficulty getting to their feet when the stalls are short. When the abomasum is dilated, struggling to rise may cause a malposition of the abomasum. Once gas is trapped within the abomasum, it will move and rise within the abdominal cavity. Displacement of the abomasum occurs only when the abomasum is dilated with gas.

CLINICAL SIGNS

Early signs of an LDA are usually subtle. Most cows are hypophagic, refusing grain but continuing to eat some hay. If the condition is not corrected, progressive weight loss will continue for several weeks, and the cow will usually be culled from the herd for poor body condition. Cows with LDA are rarely asymptomatic.[13] Clinical signs may be observed intermittently if the abomasum displaces and replaces repeatedly.

There is a progressive decline in milk production in cattle with LDA. Because of the digestive malfunction and the inability to consume or digest adequate nutrients to support milk production, most cows will be ketotic at some time during the course of the disease. Ketosis occurs when the energy deficit results in fat mobilization. The ketosis associated with LDA is a classic example of secondary (complicated) ketosis.

Feces may vary from more firm than normal (a sign typical of ketosis) to diarrhea. Cows with diarrhea have a much poorer prognosis than do those with normal or dry feces.[14] Many cows with LDA have normal feces.

Vital signs are usually normal in cattle with LDA unless there is concurrent disease such as metritis. Dehydration usually occurs only late in the course of the condition unless there are other disease problems. Atrial premature depolarizations or fibrillation occurs frequently in a wide variety of gastrointestinal diseases including LDA. The heart should always be carefully auscultated for determining whether an arrhythmia is present.

Auscultation of the left abdominal wall for several minutes may reveal spontaneous tinkling and gurgling sounds. Simul-

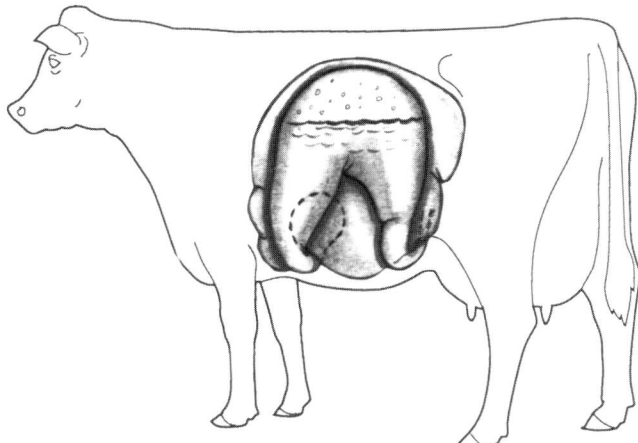

Figure 1. Left displaced abomasum (LDA). The presence of gas is indicated with circles to represent bubbles. The location of the gas cap is usually beneath the last rib and extends from the anterior aspect of the paralumbar fossa forward for a distance of 10 to 20 inches.

taneous auscultation and percussion of the paralumbar area will yield a high-pitched, tympanic resonance ("ping") similar to that produced by a pebble dropped into a well. The area of the resonant ping may be as small as 10 to 12 cm (4 to 5 inches) or as large as 45 cm (18 inches) in diameter. The location of the ping will vary depending on the position of the abomasum and the amount of gas trapped within the abomasum and rumen fill. The ping may extend forward to the ninth or tenth rib or as far ventrally as a line between the stifle and the shoulder joint. When LDA occurs in young heifers, the area of resonance is frequently low in the left flank just in front of the stifle. Therefore the clinician should always auscultate and percuss the entire left side of the abdomen. Rumen contractions, if present, are difficult to hear in the area occupied by the abomasum.

Occasionally an LDA will cause a visible distention of the left paralumbar fossa just caudal to the last rib. Palpation of this area will reveal a balloon-like structure that springs back when the hand is removed. In contrast, rumen gas usually causes a uniform bulge over the entire paralumbar fossa. A left displaced abomasum can rarely be palpated by rectal examination.

Many of the clinical signs exhibited by cows with LDA may be attributed to ketosis or concurrent diseases such as hypocalcemia, mastitis, metritis, peritonitis, abomasal ulcers, or hepatic lipidosis. Cows with persistent or unresponsive ketosis should be repeatedly and carefully examined for LDA.

CLINICAL PATHOLOGY

Most cows with LDA have a metabolic alkalosis. However, some have a normal acid-base balance or, occasionally, a metabolic acidosis. The proposed mechanisms for the acid-base imbalance are discussed hereafter (see Abomasal Volvulus). Serum electrolyte alterations are usually small. Whitlock reported values of 137 ± 0.6 mEq/L for sodium, 3.5 ± 0.1 mEq/L for potassium, 86 ± 4.0 mEq/L for chloride, and 27 ± 0.7 mEq/L for bicarbonate in 75 cows with left abomasal displacement.[15] Serum calcium concentration is usually slightly decreased. Serum phosphorus and magnesium levels may be normal or slightly increased. Electrolyte changes are discussed in more detail hereafter (see Abomasal Volvulus).

Serum glucose concentration may be decreased, increased, or normal. If serum glucose is elevated, glycosuria may be found. Ketonuria is often present, reflecting the ketonemia and elevation of serum nonesterified fatty acid concentration. Approximately 50 per cent of the cows with metabolic alkalosis have paradoxic aciduria,[16, 17] the mechanism of which is discussed hereafter (see Abomasal Volvulus).

DIAGNOSIS

Auscultation of the characteristic ping produced spontaneously or by simultaneous auscultation and percussion of the left paralumbar fossa is diagnostic for LDA.[18] Occasionally, it is difficult to distinguish the ping associated with rumen gas or pneumoperitoneum from that of the LDA when it is found in the characteristic location. In general, the rumen ping occurs over a wider area, and the pitch is lower. Rectal examination may determine that the rumen is filled with gas. The ping of a pneumoperitoneum can be produced on both sides of the abdomen along the transverse processes. The abdomen is usually not distended with pneumoperitoneum, a rare condition, except after abdominal surgery.

A Liptak test may distinguish a rumen from an abomasal ping. A needle (18-gauge × 5 cm) is inserted through an aseptically prepared site just ventral to the lowest extent of the ping. A few drops of fluid can be obtained and tested with pH paper. A pH less than 5 indicates that the abomasum has been entered, whereas a value greater than 5 suggests that the rumen has been entered.

Another way of differentiating a rumen from an abomasal ping is to pass a stomach tube into the rumen. An assistant can blow into the stomach tube while the clinician auscultates and percusses the left side of the abdomen. If the characteristics of the sound produced by air forced through the rumen fluid are similar to the sound obtained earlier by simultaneous auscultation and percussion, then the ping is most likely from the rumen. If these maneuvers elicit 2 distinctly different sounds, the abomasum is most likely the origin of 1 of the sounds. Rolling the cow provides another means of differentiating pings. If the ping disappears after rolling, the most likely cause was LDA (see Treatment).

TREATMENT

The goal in treatment of LDA is to return the abomasum to its normal position so that normal digestive function can resume. The sooner that this is accomplished, the quicker the cow will return to normal milk production and regain normal energy balance. Treatment should be accomplished as quickly, permanently, and inexpensively as possible.

Numerous conservative treatments have been tried. These are targeted at increasing gastrointestinal motility and abomasal tone. If treatment is successful, gas will be expelled, and the deflated abomasum will spontaneously return to its normal position. Calcium solutions, neostigmine, and saline cathartics have been used. These drugs have given mixed results, and even when the abomasum does return to its normal position, there is a high incidence of recurrence.

Nonsurgical replacement of the abomasum with or without concurrent drug treatment is another conservative approach. This has been done by forcing the cow to walk up a steep incline or transporting the cow in a truck. After transport, cows requiring treatment for LDA frequently have very little gas in the abomasum, and the ping may not be detectable. Invariably the ping will return. The LDA can be replaced more consistently by rolling the cow.[19] It is placed in right lateral recumbency by reefing, moved to dorsal recumbency, and rolled in a to-and-fro motion. Abdominal massage while rolling helps move the abomasum to the ventral midline. Finally, the cow is rolled to left lateral recumbency and allowed to rise from that position. Rolling is usually successful in replacing the abomasum except when adhesions prevent correction. However, the recurrence rate from rolling is high (approximately 75 per cent). Rolling cows for correcting LDA may be complicated by progression to an abomasal volvulus or severe intestinal volvulus.[20] Close monitoring during the procedure and auscultation of the right side of the abdomen after completion of the roll is recommended.

All surgical methods for the correction of the LDA involve fixation of either the omentum or the abomasum to the body wall.[20] The simplest procedure is the ventral closed-suturing technique, which is performed when the cow with LDA is rolled from right lateral recumbency to dorsal recumbency. When the characteristic ping can be auscultated in the right paramedian area, the abomasum is blindly sutured to the abdominal wall with a long needle.[21] A bar suture rather than a conventional suture has been recommended.[22]

The ventral paramedian abomasopexy is done with the cow in dorsal recumbency. After routine surgical preparation, a

20-cm (8-inch) paramedian incision to the right of midline beginning approximately 10 cm caudal to the xyphoid cartilage is made. The wall of the abomasum, which should be visible immediately under the incision, is incorporated in the closure of the abdominal wall.[23, 24]

The left flank abomasopexy is performed via a left paralumbar fossa laparotomy. A nonabsorbable suture, placed in the greater curvature of the abomasum, is carried along the parietal peritoneum to the right paramedian area and inserted through the abdominal wall. As the abomasum is gently pushed to its normal location, the sutures are grasped from the outside by an assistant, pulled until the abomasum is secured in its normal location, and tied.[25]

The right flank omentopexy is performed from a right paralumbar laparotomy.[26, 27] After deflation and replacement of the abomasum, the omentum near the pylorus is incorporated into the incision line to hold the abomasum in normal position.

Minimal treatment should be required after successful surgery. Most cows begin eating within hours of correction. Cows that are dehydrated may respond more rapidly with fluid therapy. Fluids can be easily administered orally. Solutions with a high chloride concentration or a balanced electrolyte solution can be used. A satisfactory fluid can be made by dissolving 150 g sodium chloride and 30 g potassium chloride in 10 L water. Approximately 40 L can be administered orally by stomach tube to most cows. Some cows will voluntarily drink the electrolyte solution, and in such cases it should be offered ad libitum. Oral fluids have an additional benefit in filling the rumen, thereby creating a barrier against redisplacement of the abomasum.

Special attempts to correct acid-base deficiencies are unnecessary in the uncomplicated LDA. Once the abomasum is surgically replaced, electrolyte and acid-base abnormalities will correct spontaneously within 12 hours with no treatment other than good feeding practices. Ringer's solution or an equivalent balanced electrolyte solution is preferred for intravenous treatment in the severely dehydrated cow.

PREVENTION

Because the precise etiologic factors for LDA are unknown, prevention is equally imprecise. Nutritional counseling is currently the most effective approach.[28] Dry cows should be separated from lactating cows so they can be fed according to their specific requirements. Dry cows should be maintained primarily on roughages for rehabilitating the digestive tract and reducing the level of volatile fatty acids. Roughages should provide 70 per cent or more of the total dry matter intake with no more than 30 per cent of the total ration on a dry matter basis as concentrates.[7, 28] Corn silage alone is not satisfactory for dry cows because it contains approximately 50 per cent concentrate on a dry matter basis. Corn silage provided ad libitum also leads to excessively fat cows (fat cow syndrome) that have a high incidence of LDA. Corn silage should not exceed 15 kg/cow/day during the dry period. Corn silage should be coarse-cut (>1/2 inch) to provide maximum coarseness in the diet. Good-quality grass hay, alone or with other feeds such as corn silage, is excellent for dry cows.[28]

In the late (2 weeks before parturition) dry period, cows should be gradually switched from the dry cow to lactating cow ration. Ration changes should be made gradually to allow the rumen flora to adapt. Dry cows should become accustomed to grain feeding before parturition to a level of approximately 5 kg of concentrates per head per day by parturition. Once cows are milking, concentrates should be gradually increased by about 1 kg/day to desired levels over several days.[28] Total mixed rations provide more constant rates of fermentation and gas production than do other feeding methods that allow cows to engorge periodically. Palatable feeds that provide adequate energy but promote ruminal activity are ideal for the peripartum period.

The prevention of postpartum diseases such as parturient hypocalcemia, retained placenta, and coliform mastitis will indirectly reduce the incidence of displaced abomasums. These and other diseases that decrease abomasal motility are responsible for the high incidence in many herds. Management practices that promote the general health of the herd and reduce stresses in the periparturient period often indirectly reduce the incidence of displaced abomasums.

Reducing mechanical obstacles may also aid in preventing displaced abomasums in some herds. Short free stalls may force cows to struggle in rising, causing a mechanical force that could be the final factor in causing a displaced abomasum. Steep or slippery entry and exit ramps for milking parlors may also have a similar effect. Any obvious obstacles should be corrected.

Right Displaced Abomasum and Abomasal Volvulus (Torsion)

GLEN F. HOFFSIS, DVM, MS, DIPLOMATE, ACVIM
SHEILA M. McGUIRK, DVM, PhD, DIPLOMATE, ACVIM

DEFINITION

The etiology and pathogenesis of right displaced abomasum (RDA) and right volvulus of the abomasum (RVA) are similar to those described for LDA. The 2 conditions differ only in mechanical aspects. The abomasum moves within the abdominal cavity once it is atonic and dilated with gas. Usually it moves to the left side of the rumen to become an LDA. The clinical signs of LDA are relatively mild and very predictable. If the abomasum travels to the right side of the abdominal cavity, the signs are very unpredictable and vary from mild to severe, depending on the amount of vascular compromise incurred by the abomasum.

RDA and RVA occur most frequently in dairy cows after parturition, as do LDAs.[29] However, RDA and RVA are found much more frequently than are LDAs in bulls, young animals, beef cows, and feedlot cattle. Occasionally the abomasum will initially displace to the left (LDA) and later move to the right, becoming an RDA or RVA or right omasal-abomasal volvulus (OAV).[20, 30] In North America, LDA occurs far more frequently than do RDA and RVA. Gabel reported 147 cases of LDA, compared with 18 cases of RVA during the same period.[29]

CLINICAL SIGNS

In RDA, the abomasum rises and rotates dorsally 90° to 180° from its normal position. This is not sufficient to occlude the vasculature or put undue pressure on nerves and organ attachments. Two slightly different types of rotation may result in RDA as illustrated in Figures 2 and 3. The clinical signs associated with RDA are identical to those of LDA.

With volvulus of the abomasum (RVA), the signs are more

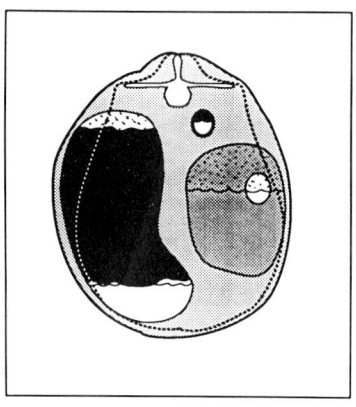 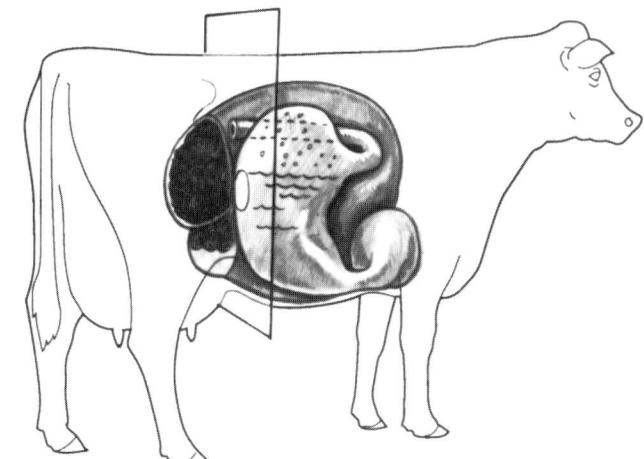

Figure 2. Right displaced abomasum (RDA). The abomasum may be rotated approximately 90° out of position as indicated. The presence of solid ingesta within the organ is represented as solid black. Fluid is represented as waves, and gas is represented as bubbles. The area of resonant "ping" corresponds to the size and location of the gas cap.

The cross-sectional view indicates abdominal contour in the condition, compared with normal as represented by the dotted line.

The square cross-sectional line on the lateral view is positioned at the midpoint of the paralumbar fossa. The point at which the line bisects organs is the portion of organs that can be palpated rectally.

pronounced and increase in severity as the degree of twist increases. These signs are attributed to pain, hypovolemia, and shock resulting from stretching of the organs and attachments, vascular impairment, and acid-base alterations.

The abomasum undergoes a complicated twist on the right side of the abdomen, but all of the specific conditions (RDA, RVA, OAV) involve varying degrees of the same general motion. The range of motion varies from the slight twist in RDA[31] (see Figs. 2 and 3) to the most extensive found in OVA[32] (see Fig. 5). In RVA (Fig. 4), the twist involves a 180° rotation counterclockwise as viewed from above and a second 180° counterclockwise twist as viewed from the rear. Because of the twisting in 2 planes, it is not purely either a volvulus or a torsion. Clockwise twists of the abomasum or omasum have never been observed by the authors and probably do not occur. If only the abomasum is involved, the twist is located in the abomasal wall just caudal to the omasum, and the duodenum will course posterior to the omasum. In OAV, the omasum is included with the abomasum in the volvulus. In this instance, the duodenum courses anterior to the omasum, and the twist is located at the reticulo-omasal junction (Fig. 5).

In RVA and OAV, the abomasum occupies a position lateral to the liver. The liver is compressed by the distended abomasum and may show surface pressure changes.

At the onset of volvulus, the cow usually has signs of discomfort and abdominal pain (see Abdominal Pain). Because the abomasum has partial or complete inflow and outflow obstruction, fluid and gas accumulate within a few hours, causing abomasal distention. The distention is most noticeable at the anterior ventral aspect of the right paralumbar fossa just behind the last rib.

If the abomasal vessels are sufficiently compromised, shock ensues, producing signs of rapid dehydration, cool extremities, and depression. The heart rate may be elevated to about 100 beats/minute or more. The cow does not eat or drink, and milk production ceases.

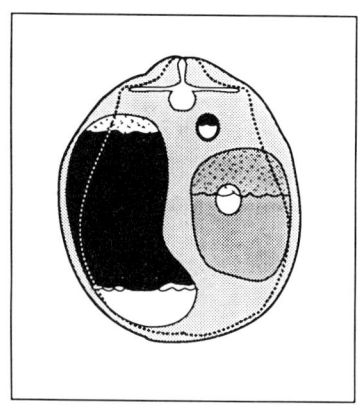 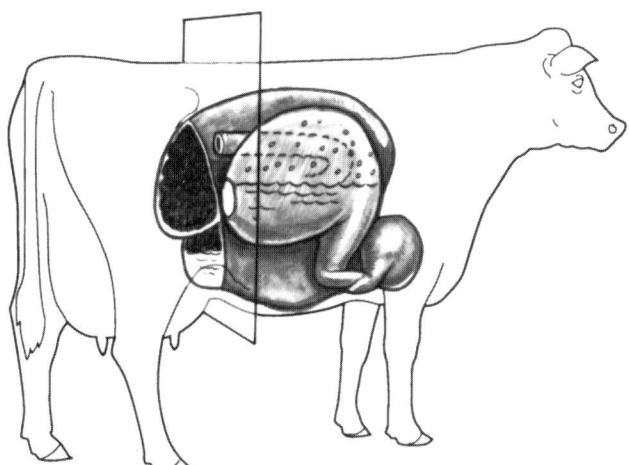

Figure 3. Right displaced abomasum (RDA). Rotation is approximately 180° counterclockwise as viewed from the rear. This entity and that represented in Figure 2 are different forms of right displaced abomasum, which are difficult to differentiate from each other clinically. Both are sometimes termed abomasal dilation.

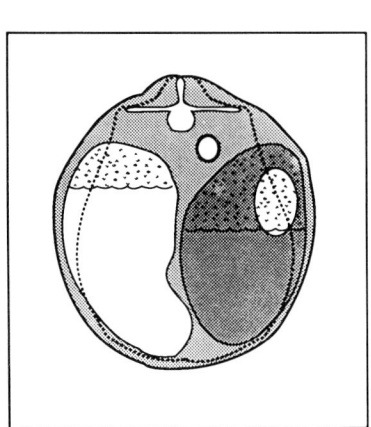 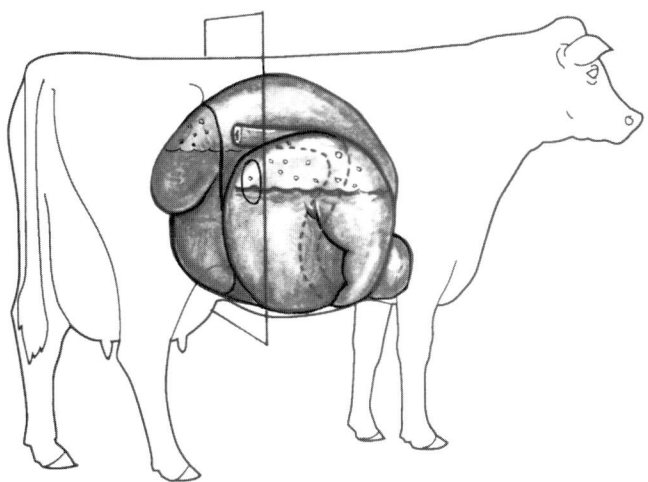

Figure 4. Abomasal volvulus (torsion) (AV). The abomasum is twisted 180° in a counterclockwise direction as viewed from the rear in addition to 180° in a counterclockwise direction as viewed from above. The abomasal contents are fluid, and, secondarily, rumen contents may become more fluid.

The fecal volume, consistency, and color may be normal for a short time after the volvulus occurs as the intestines empty. After several hours, the volume decreases and the character changes depending on abomasal outflow. The consistency of the feces is pasty, but diarrhea may be present in some cases. The feces are brown to black in color owing to extravasation of blood from the abomasal or duodenal wall, which is digested in the intestines. Fecal volume and consistency ultimately depend on the degree of abomasal outflow obstruction.

A large resonant ping will be located by simultaneous auscultation and percussion over the upper right rib cage.[33] The area begins behind the last rib and extends forward for 45 to 90 cm (18 to 36 inches). The area of resonance will become larger as the degree of volvulus and its duration increase (see Figs. 4 and 5). Ballottement with simultaneous auscultation of the right side of the abdomen posterior to the last rib often reveals high-pitched splashing sounds as the abomasal fluid is agitated. In pregnant cows, the resonant area may be further anterior and audible over a smaller area. As the abomasum is pushed farther forward, the diaphragm diverts it medially.

The abomasum can usually be palpated rectally with RVA or OAV and sometimes with RDA (see Figs. 3 to 5). With careful palpation, the posterior aspect of the dilated abomasum can be felt at the anterior aspect of the right paralumbar fossa. If the abomasum is palpable per rectum, volvulus should be suspected.

CLINICAL PATHOLOGY

The acid-base imbalance is more pronounced with RVA or OAV than with LDA or RDA. The majority of these cows will have a severe metabolic alkalosis. The venous blood gas values in one advanced case were pH, 7.53; P_{CO_2}, 50 mmHg; P_{O_2}, 33 mmHg; HCO_2, 40.5 mEq/L; base excess, +17.5 mEq/L. The metabolic alkalosis is generated by sequestration of abomasal hydrochloric acid (HCl) secretions in the abomasum or forestomachs.[34] Normally, hydrochloric acid is formed by the following reaction:

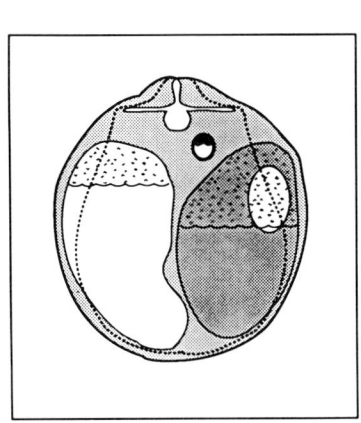 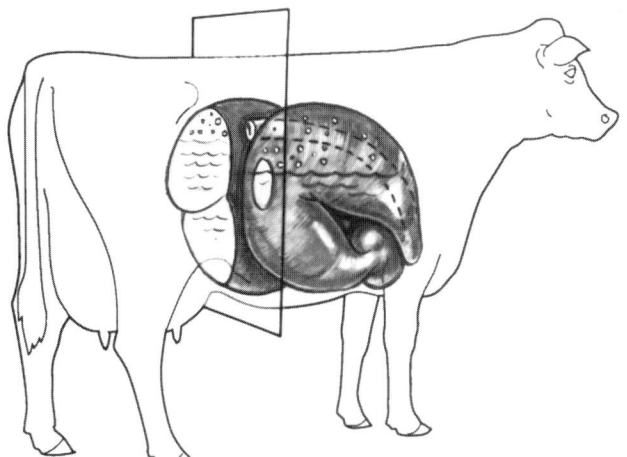

Figure 5. Omasal and abomasal volvulus (OAV). The abomasum is twisted 180° as viewed from the rear as well as 180° as viewed from above and is indentical to that illustrated in Figure 4. The only difference is that the twist includes the omasum, and the point of rotation is located at the reticulo-omasal junction rather than at the omasal-abomasal junction as in Figure 4. The duodenum crosses the reticulum in this condition.

NaCl + H$_2$O + CO$_2$ →
NaHCO$_3$ (plasma) + HCl (abomasum)

The hydrochloric acid must then move out of the abomasum to be absorbed in the intestine to buffer the sodium bicarbonate (NaHCO$_3$) in the plasma generated by this reaction. If the hydrochloric acid is not moved to the intestines for absorption, the sodium bicarbonate is not buffered, and a metabolic alkalosis ensues. Reflux of abomasal contents into the forestomachs may also aid in the genesis of the metabolic alkalosis in cattle with RDA.[35] This can be documented and quantitated by measuring the concentration of chloride in rumen fluid.

Some cows with RVA or OAV may have a metabolic acidosis. Acidosis may develop with hypovolemia and subsequent lactic acid production by ischemic peripheral tissues. Increased acid metabolite formation and absorption of endotoxins from the damaged gastrointestinal tract may contribute to the acidosis. Cows with RVA or OAV that have acidosis have a poor prognosis.

Electrolyte alterations are more pronounced in RVA and OAV than in simple abomasal displacements. In the case previously illustrated, serum electrolyte concentrations were sodium, 135 mEq/L; potassium, 2.8 mEq/L; chloride, 59 mEq/L; calcium, 8.3 mEq/L; phosphorus, 10.0 mEq/L; and magnesium, 2.5 mEq/L. The glucose concentration was 274 mg/dl.

Serum sodium concentration is usually within normal limits unless there is hypotonic water loss or renal sodium loss. Potassium concentrations are usually low from a combination of decreased dietary intake, abomasal sequestration, and metabolic alkalosis. There may be some urinary loss of potassium in spite of low serum levels. Serum chloride concentrations are often markedly low because chloride is sequestered in the abomasum and forestomachs. Serum calcium levels may be decreased from decreased dietary intake, decreased absorption, or increased formation of calcium soaps. Increased serum phosphorus concentration occurs frequently, but the precise mechanism is not known. Decreased elimination from the gastrointestinal tract and dehydration with decreased renal perfusion probably play a role.

Glucose levels are usually normal or elevated in cows with RVA and OAV. Many cows are hyperglycemic from massive glucocorticoid release secondary to the severe abdominal crisis. In most cases, the renal tubular threshold for glucose is exceeded and there is glycosuria.

Ketonemia and ketonuria are frequently found (see Left Displaced Abomasum). Paradoxic aciduria occurs frequently as the result of the dehydration, hypokalemia, or hypochloremia.[16, 17] With volume contraction, avid sodium retention results in formation of acid urine. The excretion of undetermined anions, most likely acid metabolites, may contribute to the paradoxic aciduria.[16, 17] There is no association between ketonuria and aciduria. The calculation of the anion gap [(Na$^+$ + K$^+$) − (Cl$^-$ + HCO$_3^-$)] provides an estimate of unmeasured anions and may help characterize the disease.

DIAGNOSIS

Diseases that cause resonant pings in the right paralumbar fossa must be differentiated from RVA and OAV.[33] Gas in the colon or duodenum will sometimes produce a ping. The resonant area is usually small (less than 15 cm in diameter) and located high in the paralumbar fossa. Pneumoperitoneum may result in resonance high in the right paralumbar fossa. These pings are incidental findings and are not responsible for clinical signs. A torsion of the cecum will produce a ping in the right paralumbar fossa. Cecal resonance is usually located in the dorsal and posterior aspect of the fossa (Fig. 6), compared with the anterior ventral aspect of the fossa with RVA and OAV. Intestinal obstructions may also cause pings in various locations on the right side of the abdomen (Fig. 7).

Diseases that cause acute abdominal pain and intestinal obstruction must also be differentiated from RVA or OAV. These are discussed in more detail hereafter (see Abdominal Pain). Diagnosis of RVA or OAV is based on the clinical signs of dehydration and shock, the presence of a large ping on the right side of the abdomen, compatible rectal palpation findings, and a scant tarry stool. Hypochloremia and metabolic alkalosis support the diagnosis. In some instances, it may help to aspirate fluid from the abomasum via the right flank. A small-gauge needle is inserted just below the area of the resonant ping. If the pH of the fluid is less than 4, the organ is most likely the abomasum. If the abomasum is very tightly distended, insertion of a needle may cause leakage of fluid or damage to the abomasal wall.

TREATMENT

Immediate surgery is indicated once RVA or OAV is diagnosed. Unlike LDA and RDA, a volvulus does not correct spontaneously and cannot be corrected by drug therapy, rolling, or the closed-suture technique. Time makes a great difference in the response of a cow to surgical correction. Delaying surgery increases the chances for irreversible damage to the wall of the abomasum or vagus nerve.

A laparotomy is done in the right paralumbar fossa in a standing animal[29] or the ventral paramedian site in a recumbent animal.[36] The paralumbar fossa approach offers the surgeon the best chance of maintaining his or her orientation and understanding the anatomy of the volvulus.

The abomasum is deflated, and then the left hand and forearm are used to push the dorsal aspect of the abomasum in an anterior and ventral direction as if being tucked under the reticulum. The omasum is gently cradled and pulled in a posterior and right lateral direction. After crossing the midline, the abomasum is essentially in an LDA position. The abomasum is then approached from the posterior and ventral part of the abdomen and pulled to the right of the midline. The omentum is used to retract the pylorus into view at the incision site, and an omentopexy is performed. Most RVA and OAV can be corrected without removing abomasal fluid. If fluid is not removed, there is less chance of abdominal contamination, correction is faster, and the abomasal hydrochloric acid is available for reabsorption. This is an advantage because the sequestered hydrochloric acid is available in precisely the correct dose.

Fluids should be administered intravenously during and after surgery, particularly if dehydration is apparent. The goal in fluid therapy is to replace the plasma and extracellular fluid deficit, provide chloride or potassium ions, and correct the metabolic alkalosis. Twenty or more liters of fluid will be necessary for correction of the fluid deficit in very dehydrated adult cows.[15] The first 8 L may be given as rapidly as possible in a severely dehydrated cow, whereas the remainder is given at the rate of about 5 L/hour until normal hydration is restored. A balanced electrolyte solution high in chloride concentration should be chosen. Ringer's solution or isotonic sodium chloride solution is preferred. Sodium bicarbonate and sodium lactate should not be used. Acidifiers, such as ammonium chloride, are not necessary whether abomasal contents are removed or not. After surgical correction, the acid-base and electrolyte status of most cows will return to normal within about 12 hours if abomasal contents are not removed and a balanced

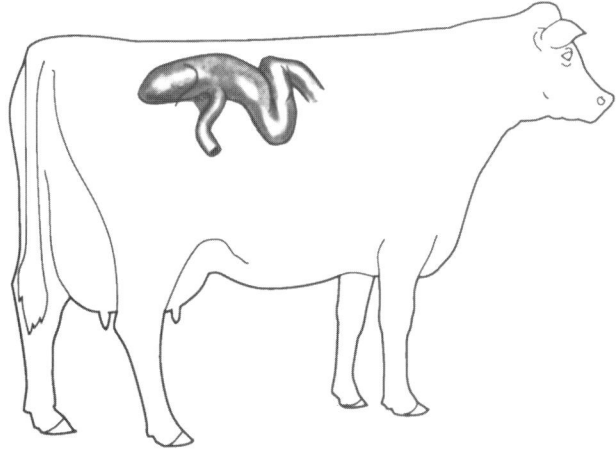

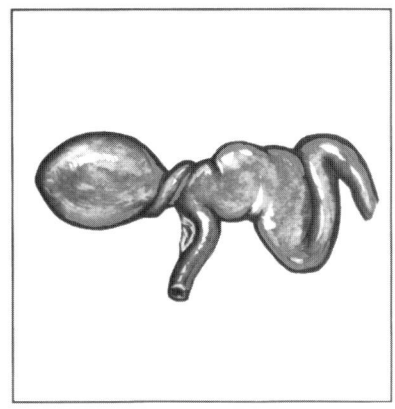 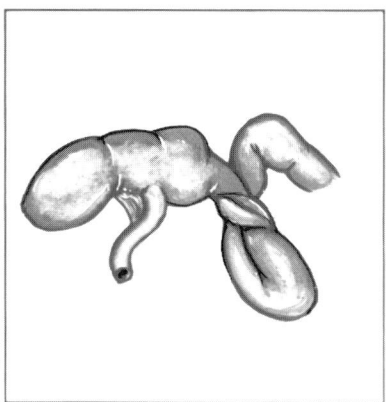

Figure 6. Cecal torsion and cecocolic volvulus. The normal position of the cecum, ileum, and colon is illustrated within the cow. The other drawings illustrate two different ways the cecum or colon twists. Sometimes the apex of the cecum extends in a forward direction to the level of the paralumbar fossa.

electrolyte solution is administered during and after surgery. In fact, in the authors' experience, some animals will have a mild acidosis 12 to 24 hours after surgery due to the absorption of sequestered hydrochloric acid. Antibiotics and glucose may be given to combat infection and ketosis in dairy cows.

PROGNOSTIC INDICATORS

Several investigators have attempted to establish parameters and values that may be used for accurately predicting survival of affected cattle. RVA and OAV are life-threatening diseases requiring intensive and skillful therapy for success. It is important to provide as accurate as possible estimates to the owner regarding the cost and prognosis of therapy.

The preoperative prognostic indicators evaluated by Constable et al.[37] indicated that hydration status, heart rate, duration of inappetence before surgery, and serum alkaline phosphatase activity were the best indicators of outcome (Table 1). The positive predictive value is the proportion of cattle with the test condition that have the predicted outcome (i.e., a positive predictive value of 0.96 indicates that 96 per cent of cattle with dehydration less than 4 per cent will be productive).

This study found that these indicators were superior to low serum chloride concentration and anion gap. The data also indicated that it is more difficult to predict a nonproductive animal than a productive animal.

The prognosis depends on the severity of the volvulus and the time lag between the onset and the correction. The abomasal fluid volume estimated at surgery can also be used to assess prognosis.[38] The fluid volume increases in direct proportion to the severity and duration of the twist. Constable

et al. reported a recovery rate of 74 per cent (normal and productive) in 80 cases of abomasal volvulus.[37] Diarrhea should be observed within 12 hours of surgery as the abomasal fluid enters the intestinal tract. Fecal consistency usually returns to normal in 1 or 2 days after surgery in successful cases. Some cows will have a decreasing volume of feces over the next week followed by abdominal distention. These signs are iden-

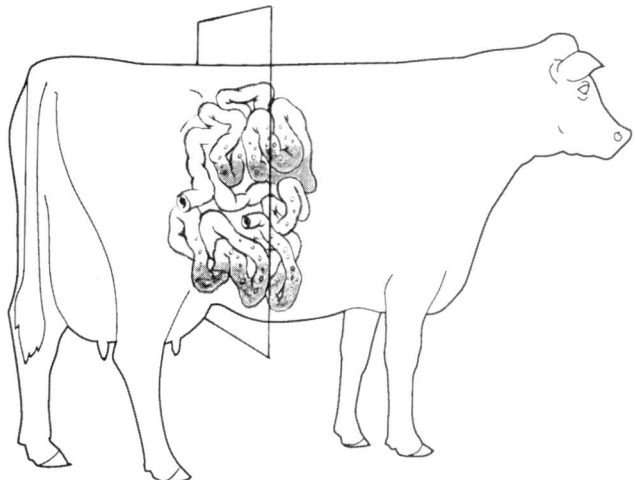

Figure 7. Intestinal obstruction. The small intestine is distended with gas and fluid proximal to the site of obstruction. The abdomen is distended on both sides, and small tympanic areas may be audible on the right side in various locations. Rectal examination reveals distended loops of intestine in a wide area extending into the pelvis.

Table 1. ABILITY OF PREOPERATIVE PROGNOSTIC INDICATORS TO SUCCESSFULLY PREDICT OUTCOME IN CATTLE WITH RIGHT VOLVULUS OF THE ABOMASUM

Test Condition	Positive Predictive Value
Ability to Predict Productive Animals	
Dehydration <4%	0.96
Heart rate ≤80 beats/minute	0.88
Duration of inappetence ≤24 hours	0.88
Serum creatinine ≤1.5 mg/dl	0.91
Serum alkaline phosphatase ≤100 IU/L	0.90
Serum chloride ≥95 mEq/L	0.90
Serum sodium ≥135 mEq/L	0.84
Ability to Predict Nonproductive Animals	
Heart rate >120 beats/minute	0.67
Dehydration ≥6%	0.52
Duration of inappetence >24 hours	0.39
Serum alkaline phosphatase >100 IU/L	0.55
Blood pH <7.35	0.50
Serum creatinine >1.5 mg/dl	0.48
Serum sodium <135 mEq/L	0.40
Serum chloride ≤79 mEq/L	0.38

tical to those described hereafter and indicate a poor prognosis (see Vagus Indigestion [Functional Pyloric Stenosis]).

PREVENTION

The prevention of abomasal volvulus is identical to that for LDA.

Vagus Indigestion

GLEN F. HOFFSIS, DVM, MS, Diplomate, ACVIM
SHEILA M. McGUIRK, DVM, PhD, Diplomate, ACVIM

DEFINITION

Vagus indigestion is a syndrome that is most common in adult cattle and only rarely occurs in cattle under 2 years of age. The history is characterized by bouts of indigestion and anorexia. In lactating cows, milk production does not reach the expected potential. The primary signs of weight loss, dehydration, abdominal distention, and decreasing volume of bowel movements gradually become worse over several weeks or months.

The cause of vagus indigestion is thought to be interference with vagus nerve function. The specific form of vagus indigestion may depend on the location of the involved segment of vagus nerve. Clinical vagus indigestion syndromes were reproduced experimentally by Hoflund through sectioning various parts of the vagus nerve.[39] The specific causes of vagus nerve malfunction are not entirely identified. Most cases are thought to be associated with adhesions, such as with traumatic reticuloperitonitis, distention, inflammation, or stretching of the vagus nerve. The vagus nerve courses through the diaphragm in the area of the reticulum, where adhesion, infection, and inflammation due to traumatic reticuloperitonitis or a perforated abomasal ulcer are most intense. The vagus nerve is easily damaged in this region. Other causes are actinobacillosis of the reticulum or rumen, inflammation of the mediastinal lymph nodes with diseases such as malignant lymphoma or tuberculosis, liver abscesses, diaphragmatic hernia, and pleuritis. Cattle that survive surgery for abomasal volvulus (RVA or OAV) but do not recover satisfactorily often develop signs of vagus indigestion.[40]

Because of vagus nerve malfunction, transport of ingesta through the ruminant forestomachs or abomasum is impaired. Fecal output gradually decreases, and the abdomen distends. The common features of the vagus indigestion syndromes are decreased fecal output, abdominal distention, dehydration, and weight loss.

CLINICAL SIGNS

The clinically recognized forms of vagus indigestion can be categorized as follows:

1. Ruminal distention with hypomotility or atony of the rumen (type I). There is an increase in the volume of rumen contents, which are more fluid than normal with a small gas cap at the top. This type of vagal indigestion resembles simple bloat except that the distention is caused by foamy rumen fluid rather than gas. No rumen sounds are audible, and the heart rate is normal or increased. There is a functional blockage between the omasum and the abomasum, which has been referred to as a failure of omasal transport.

2. Ruminal distention with hypermotility (type II). This is identical to type I except that the rumen has increased motility. The rumen wall can be seen to contract in waves, which are visible through the abdominal wall. Rumen contractions are poorly audible, so observation of the waves of contraction is important. The contractions are incoordinated primary or secondary rumen contractions, which often occur at the rate of 4 to 6/minute (normal 2/minute). In type I or type II, bradycardia may be present, with the heart rate as low as 40 beats/minute if there is anorexia.

3. Functional pyloric stenosis (type III). In this syndrome, abomasal emptying is impaired, causing accumulation of fluid or semisolid ingesta within the abomasum. Secondarily, the rumen distends with fluid. The fluid that accumulates in the forestomachs results from reflux of abomasal secretions into the rumen or failure of transport of ingested fluids and saliva through the abomasum. This category of vagus indigestion is sometimes further divided into a partial or complete pyloric stenosis.[39] This type of vagus indigestion frequently develops after surgery for abomasal volvulus.

In vagal indigestion type I and type II, the distended rumen will cause a symmetrically rounded left abdominal wall. If the rumen extends into the right side of the abdomen, the right abdominal wall will have a normal contour or may be slightly distended ventrally.

The abdomen assumes a characteristic shape with type III (functional pyloric stenosis). The right side of the abdomen is pear-shaped as viewed from the rear because the lower right quadrant of the abdomen is pushed outward by the distended abomasum and ventral sac of the rumen, whereas the paralumbar fossa remains normally contoured. The left side of the abdomen would appear symmetrically rounded like an apple because of rumen distention. The characteristic shape of an apple on the left side and a pear on the right side of the abdomen has been termed papple[35] (Fig. 8).

The clinical signs are similar in all 3 syndromes. The feces are decreased in volume and have a pasty consistency. There is dehydration, decreased milk production, and a gradual and progressive weight loss. In the later stages, the animal usually refuses feed. The temperature, pulse, and respirations are normal. Ingested water is not adequately absorbed from the rumen for maintenance of hydration.

On rectal examination, the rumen is greatly distended and

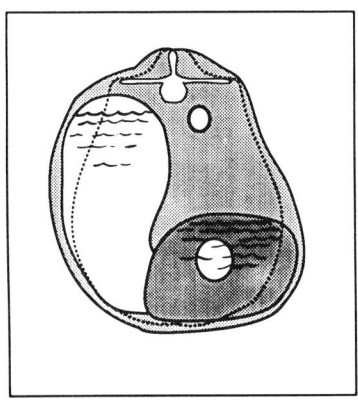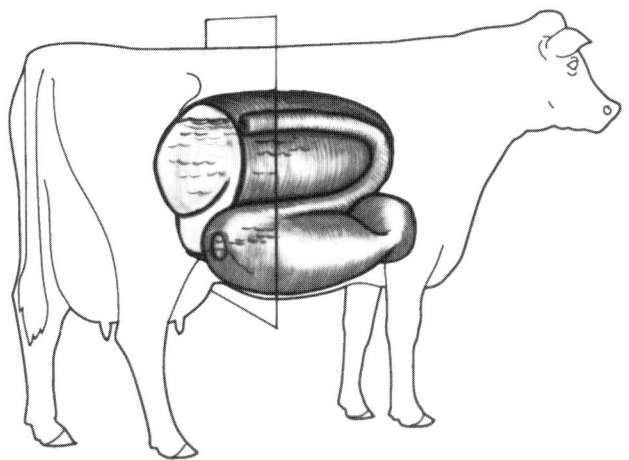

Figure 8. Vagus indigestion with functional pyloric stenosis. The abomasum is distended with contents that are fluid. The rumen and reticulum are secondarily filled with fluid. The left side of the abdomen is distended in a symmetric and round manner, whereas the right side is distended only in the lower right quadrant.

has a fluid consistency in all 3 syndromes. The posterior ventral blind sac of the rumen is so distended that it extends to the right side of the abdomen. The rumen has an L shape as viewed from the rear (Fig. 8). Although the abomasum is not usually palpable, rumen distention and the L shape can be determined on rectal palpation. The fluid consistency of the distended rumen and abomasum can be detected by ballottement of the abdomen.

CLINICAL PATHOLOGY

Dehydration often increases packed cell volume and total serum protein. Advanced cases may have prerenal uremia in response to dehydration and poor renal perfusion. In functional pyloric stenosis, hypochloremic metabolic alkalosis will be found. Serum chloride may be decreased to 40 to 50 mEq/L. An elevation in rumen chloride concentration (above 30 mEq/L) indicates abomasal fluid reflux into the rumen.[41] If the rumen chloride is normal, either abomasal emptying is not impaired or the abomasum has a functional obstruction but is retaining rather than refluxing secretion into the rumen. In type I and type II, the serum and rumen chloride levels are usually normal. Many affected cows will also be hypokalemic. When peritonitis is responsible for the vagal syndrome, the complete blood count may show a neutrophilic leukocytosis, hyperfibrinogenemia, and increased total protein and globulin concentrations.

DIAGNOSIS

The differential diagnosis of vagus indigestion should include the diseases that cause abdominal distention. Any disease that causes intestinal obstruction will eventually result in abdominal distention and must be differentiated by physical examination and laboratory findings. Accumulation of fluid within the abdominal cavity from ascites, peritonitis, or ruptured urinary bladder should be considered. These can be diagnosed by finding symmetric abdominal distention with characteristic abdominal paracentesis findings. The clinician must also consider hydrops allantois or amnion as a cause of the distention. These can be differentiated by rectal examination. Primary bloat can be differentiated from vagus indigestion because the onset is acute and the distention is due to ruminal gas rather than fluid. Frothy bloat is difficult to distinguish from vagus indigestion, although primary ruminal contractions are frequently not audible in vagus indigestion. In grain overload (D-lactic acidosis), there should be a history of exposure to a high-carbohydrate feed source. The onset of signs is acute, leading to toxemia and rapid dehydration with severe metabolic acidosis. Abomasal impaction should be differentiated from functional pyloric stenosis. Ballottement will indicate firm abomasal contents in primary abomasum impaction, whereas in vagus indigestion, the abomasal contents are usually fluid.

The diagnosis of vagus indigestion is based on the typical history and clinical signs. An atropine response test has been described as an aid in differentiating bradycardia related to vagus indigestion from primary heart disease or other causes of bradycardia. It is now believed that the bradycardia is not specific for this syndrome but is a consequence of anorexia and an associated increase in vagal tone.[42]

TREATMENT

Because most cattle are in poor physical condition when vagus indigestion is diagnosed, supportive therapy is important. A balanced electrolyte solution such as Ringer's solution should be administered intravenously for restoring any chloride deficit and correcting the dehydration. As much as 40 L over 1 or 2 days may be necessary. More specific fluid therapy and chloride replacement can be accomplished if blood-gas and electrolyte data are available. In vagus indigestion, fluid and electrolyte therapy must be given intravenously, because fluids administered orally are poorly absorbed and contribute to the rumen distention.

Once the animal is rehydrated, the clinician will be better able to assess the underlying causes of the disease. Hydration attempts are frequently unsuccessful because fluid sequesters in the forestomachs. An exploratory laparotomy and rumenotomy are usually indicated in valuable individuals. The abdomen can be explored for adhesions or abscesses in the area of the reticulum, tumors, or other possible causes. The rumen can be evacuated and the reticulum, esophageal groove, and omasal orifice explored for foreign material and masses. Occasionally, abscesses can be drained and adhesions removed for specific correction of the condition. In many cases, the underlying cause cannot be identified or corrected. If there is ruminal tympany, a rumen fistula can be created to allow continued escape of gas from the rumen on a semipermanent basis. It also provides easy access to the rumen for administration of cathartics or fluids.

Prognosis in vagus indigestion is guarded to poor regardless of the clinical syndrome. A few animals respond favorably to rehydration or exploratory rumenotomy; however, extensive treatment is usually given only to valuable cattle. Less valuable cattle should be slaughtered before any drugs are given and animals become weak or cachectic.

Abomasal Impaction

GLEN F. HOFFSIS, DVM, MS, Diplomate, ACVIM
SHEILA M. McGUIRK, DVM, PhD, Diplomate, ACVIM

DEFINITION

Abomasal impaction may be defined as the abnormal accumulation of solid ingesta in the abomasum. It is caused by a failure of the abomasal musculature to contract properly ("abomasal pump"), the ingestion of foreign material, or the ingestion of indigestible feeds. The history usually indicates a gradual onset of disease, and the disease frequently goes unnoticed until the terminal stages. Abomasal impaction is seen most commonly in commercial beef cattle fed marginal rations, but it also occurs in dairy cattle. Specific forms of abomasal impaction could be categorized as follows.

1. Primary abomasal impaction results from ingestion of excessive amounts of coarse, indigestible roughages. It occurs in beef cows in many parts of the country from attempts to reduce feed costs for maintenance through the winter months. Cows fed late-cut hay, straw, and corn stover during the winter months are particularly vulnerable. These poorly digested feeds accumulate in the abomasum and secondarily fill the reticulum and rumen. Because of the indigestibility, a negative energy balance develops. Because adequate nutrients are not absorbed, cows retain a good appetite and consume the offending feed until the physical capacity of the rumen limits further intake. Affected cows are usually unthrifty and in a state of starvation. Dairy calves may be similarly affected. Calves receiving inadequate nutrition from poor-quality milk replacers will sometimes eat bedding or other rough forages, which causes impaction of the abomasum.

2. Foreign material may become entrapped in the abomasum, causing primary impaction. Cows frequently eat the placenta after parturition. If a placenta becomes lodged in the pylorus, the abomasum may become impacted. Baling twine or similar foreign material may be ingested and entrapped in the abomasum. A concretion may form and lead to impaction. Unthrifty or louse-infected young cattle may ingest large quantities of hair by licking. The hair may form a trichobezoar in the abomasum, causing impaction.

3. Failure of the abomasal "pump" due to a lack of motility should be considered a secondary abomasal impaction. In vagus indigestion, the abomasum is sometimes filled with semisolid material resembling an impaction. After surgical correction of abomasal volvulus, the abomasal musculature or nervous innervation may be damaged sufficiently to impair emptying. Often the abomasal contents are fluid.

CLINICAL SIGNS

Abomasal impaction usually occurs in the winter in beef cows. Long hair tends to mask the poor body condition. The abdomen becomes progressively distended because of the abomasal ingesta, giving the cow a round, fat appearance. Cows that are casually observed by owners are often thought to be fat and healthy. Upon closer examination, they are found to be very thin. The disease may be advanced, and death may occur before owners realize that problems exist.

The major clinical signs are the characteristic shape of the distended abdomen (Fig. 9), poor body condition, and dehydration. The fecal output is reduced in volume, and the feces are hard and dry in most cases. The temperature, pulse, and respirations are normal.

CLINICAL PATHOLOGY

Hypochloremic metabolic alkalosis may occur but is not as predictable in abomasal impaction as in vagus indigestion. The catabolic state tends to produce metabolic acidosis, which

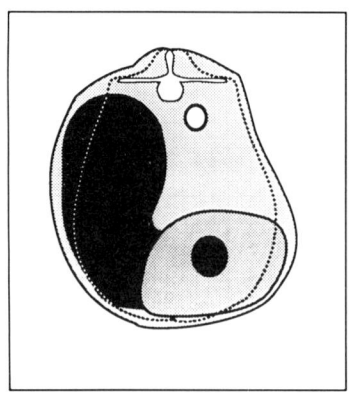
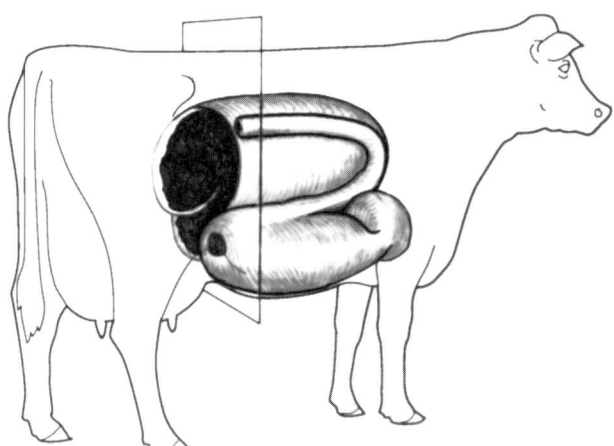

Figure 9. Abomasal impaction. The abomasum is engorged with firm feedstuffs, and the rumen and reticulum are secondarily filled with similar material. The shape of the abdomen is identical to that illustrated in Figure 8.

modifies the overall acid-base status in the animal. Dehydration increases the packed cell volume and total protein, but these changes may be masked by progressive anemia and hypoproteinemia resulting from starvation. As a result, total protein concentration and the packed cell volume may be in the normal range.

DIAGNOSIS

Abomasal impaction produces a characteristic "papple"-shaped distention of the abdomen and should be differentiated from vagus indigestion from other causes, which may have a similar type of distention. Ballottement or ultrasonography can distinguish the fluid contents of the abomasum and rumen with vagus indigestion, compared with the firm contents in abomasal impaction. The history of a gradual onset of clinical signs and feeding poor-quality roughages will help confirm the diagnosis. A rumen distended with firm ingesta and the L shape may be found on rectal examination. The abomasum is usually beyond reach.

Malignant lymphoma may cause thickening of the abomasal wall and accumulation of ingesta in the lumen. It can be differentiated in some cases by the presence of peripheral lymphadenopathy, abomasal ulceration, circulation of neoplastic lymphocytes, or serologic tests for bovine leukemia virus.

TREATMENT

Treatment of individual cattle is effective only in the early stages of the disease. In the earliest stages, saline cathartics, such as 0.5 kg of magnesium hydroxide or magnesium sulfate, may effectively evacuate the abomasum. Fecal softeners, such as mineral oil and dioctyl sodium sulfosuccinate (DSS), may also be effective in softening the mass of ingesta. The rumen may be physically evacuated by rumenotomy in advanced cases; the abomasum may be medicated by passing a stomach tube through the reticulo-omasal orifice and administering mineral oil or DSS directly into the abomasum. An indwelling nasogastric tube may be placed via rumenotomy for continued medication of the abomasal impaction.[43] Physical removal of the abomasal contents by abomasotomy may also be accomplished.[44]

As supportive treatment, intravenous or oral fluids containing glucose and amino acids can re-establish hydration and provide nutritional support for animals in advanced stages of the disease that are suffering from starvation. To be successful, therapy should begin early.

PREVENTION

The welfare of the remainder of the herd should receive major emphasis when abomasal impaction is diagnosed. Foreign material, such as twine, should be removed from the environment. Nutrition should be improved by limiting coarse roughages, increasing the amount of high-quality hay or silage, and, possibly, feeding concentrates. For calves, removing the bedding and improving the quality of milk replacer and starter rations are recommended.

Intussusception
GLEN F. HOFFSIS, DVM, MS, DIPLOMATE, ACVIM
SHEILA M. MCGUIRK, DVM, PHD, DIPLOMATE, ACVIM

DEFINITION

Intussusception occurs sporadically in cattle. There is no known breed, sex, or age group susceptibility. The pathophysiologic process in cattle is similar in most respects to that in other species. A major difference in cattle is that intussusception usually occurs in the jejunum and seldom occurs in the large intestine or ileocecal valve region.[45] The clinical course is more prolonged in cattle than in horses. In the authors' experience, cattle have survived complete obstruction from intussusception for as long as 12 days while exhibiting little more than depression. The precise etiologic agent has never been determined, and the history is not usually specific for the disease.

CLINICAL SIGNS

The animal will usually exhibit signs of acute abdominal pain and colic when intussusception first occurs. These signs gradually subside in 12 to 24 hours, and from then until death, progressive signs of depression, inactivity, and abdominal distention are observed. The animal does not eat or drink and becomes progressively more dehydrated.

The feces are normal in consistency, color, and volume at the onset of obstruction. After about 12 hours, a small amount of blood and mucus, originating at the site of obstruction, gradually traverses the intestinal tract and appears in the feces. Fecal volume gradually decreases for several days after obstruction but may not cease for 3 or 4 days. Because intussusception is usually in the jejunum, fecal output does not cease immediately. Feces are often fluid in the first 24 hours but gradually become firmer and by 3 or 4 days after obstruction will be dry or pasty. The feces are usually dark brown or black owing to the extravasation of blood at the site of intussusception.

Initially, the abdomen has a normal contour. Within about 12 hours, gas accumulation in the small intestine anterior to the area of obstruction (jejunum and duodenum) causes a progressive distention of the abdomen. The animal will have a symmetrically rounded shape on both the left and right sides of the abdomen. Auscultation and percussion of the right side of the abdomen may reveal small tympanic areas and areas with succussible fluid in various locations depending on where the gas-distended intestines contact the abdominal wall. Resonant areas are usually absent on the left side of the abdomen because of the rumen. Multiple loops of gas-distended small intestine located anterior to the pelvic inlet are found on rectal palpation (see Fig. 7). The intussusception itself is rarely palpable.

CLINICAL PATHOLOGY

There is hemoconcentration with an increase in the packed cell volume and total protein. The total leukocyte count may be increased in advanced cases with necrosis at the intussusception. Analysis of peritoneal fluid obtained by abdominal paracentesis may not indicate the nature of the disease because the necrotic segment is often shielded by the adjacent gut segment, the omentum, or adhesions.

The acid-base status is not predictable. If the intussusception is in the anterior small intestine, there is an ileus with sequestration of fluid in the abomasum, which leads to hypochloremic hypokalemic metabolic alkalosis (see Abomasal Volvulus). If the intussusception is in the caudal part of the intestinal tract, abomasal fluid can escape into the small intestine for a long time and be absorbed. In these cases, normal acid-base status may be found. As with all obstructive diseases, the animal may eventually become acidotic in the terminal stages.

DIAGNOSIS

The acute abdominal pain and abdominal distention associated with intussusception must be differentiated from abdominal pain caused by other diseases. Volvulus of the root of the mesentery and strangulated hernias are particularly similar and difficult to differentiate in the acute phase. Hernias can be differentiated by palpation. Volvulus of the root of the mesentery is usually distinguished by severe, generalized, small intestinal distention but occasionally cannot be diagnosed until surgery.

TREATMENT

The treatment for intussusception is surgical after initiation of appropriate fluid and electrolyte replacement. An approach from the right paralumbar fossa in the standing animal allows excellent exploration of the abdomen. The disadvantage of standing surgery is that the animal may attempt to lie down because of the intense pain that results from intestinal manipulation.

In the recumbent animal, the right paralumbar fossa or the ventral midline approach may be used. It is more difficult to explore the abdomen in recumbent cattle with abdominal distention; however, the exposure of the intussusception may be better. The animal is easier to control in the recumbent position while the intussusception is manipulated. Exteriorization may be difficult, and because tissues are friable, the site of intussusception may rupture. The intussusception must be reduced or resected and an intestinal anastomosis performed.

Supportive therapy is essential during and after surgery. Intensive fluid therapy is usually required to combat dehydration, electrolyte and acid-base imbalance, and shock.

Volvulus of the Root of the Mesentery
GLEN F. HOFFSIS, DVM, MS, Diplomate, ACVIM
SHEILA M. McGUIRK, DVM, PhD, Diplomate, ACVIM

DEFINITION

This occurs sporadically and is usually seen in diary cows; however, no specific age, sex, or breed predisposition has been found. The entire small intestine twists approximately 360° around the mesenteric root. The cause is unknown, although it has occurred after rolling of cows for correction of uterine torsion or LDA. It has also occurred after paramedian abomasopexy for correction of LDA.[45]

CLINICAL SIGNS

Acute abdominal pain and decreasing fecal output are seen. A progressive and symmetric distention of the abdomen will occur. Tympanic areas can sometimes be auscultated on the right side of the abdomen. On rectal examination, multiple gas-distended loops of small intestine will fill the abdominal cavity and extend into the pelvic cavity. The site of the twist in the mesentery is usually beyond reach. Acid-base balance and electrolyte concentrations may not be altered significantly because of the short course of the disease.

TREATMENT

Immediate surgery is indicated.[45] The abdomen should be explored from the right paralumbar fossa in the standing animal. Most cases cannot be definitively diagnosed without surgery because the twist cannot be palpated rectally. At surgery, the twist in the mesentery can be located in the dorsal abdomen anterior to the left kidney. The direction of the twist can be determined by palpation, and most cases can be corrected by manipulation within the abdomen. Portions of the intestine may have to be decompressed and exteriorized for correction of the twist to be facilitated. The prognosis is good when early diagnosis and surgery can be accomplished. Supportive therapy should include antibiotics and intravenous fluids.

Strangulated Inguinal Hernia
GLEN F. HOFFSIS, DVM, MS, Diplomate, ACVIM
SHEILA M. McGUIRK, DVM, PhD, Diplomate, ACVIM

DEFINITION

Strangulated inguinal hernia usually occurs in mature bulls. A loop of intestine may accidentally drop into the internal inguinal ring. A congenital enlargement of the internal ring probably predisposes to this condition. The side of involvement is almost always the left inguinal ring. Obstruction will not occur if the inguinal canal is large and the intestine can freely move within the ring and scrotum. In fact, some bulls may live for years with a large inguinal hernia without signs of intestinal malfunction. However, if the ring is small, the intestine will become entrapped, and ingesta will not pass. External enlargement of the scrotum may not be apparent if the ring is small and a small amount of intestine drops into the inguinal canal. Because the inguinal hernia is not always apparent externally, it is important to consider this when bulls with intestinal obstruction are examined.

CLINICAL SIGNS

The signs of acute abdominal pain, tympany, abdominal distention, and decreased fecal output seen in strangulated inguinal hernia are similar to those seen in volvulus of the root of the mesentery and intussusception. Sometimes an enlargement may be visible at the neck of the scrotum.

DIAGNOSIS

The diagnosis can be made in all cases by rectal palpation of the internal inguinal ring. In every case of intestinal obstruction in a bull, the inguinal rings should be thoroughly examined for a hernia.

TREATMENT

Immediate surgery is required with use of either a left paralumbar laparotomy on the standing bull or a ventral approach over the inguinal canal at the neck of the scrotum.

PREVENTION

The owner should be advised that inguinal hernias may be hereditary. The owner can then decide whether to continue using the bull for breeding.

Abdominal Pain

GLEN F. HOFFSIS, DVM, MS, DIPLOMATE, ACVIM
SHEILA M. McGUIRK, DVM, PhD, DIPLOMATE, ACVIM

DEFINITION

Abdominal pain is the result of afferent input from stretch receptors in the serosal surfaces of all intestinal, urinary, and reproductive organs and the peritoneum. They are also located in the mesenteric attachments of these organs. Anything that stretches these organs, such as visceral distention, torsion, or volvulus, will induce pain. Sometimes, manipulation of organs and mesentery during surgery causes pain. Direct trauma to the surface of the organ, as in traumatic reticuloperitonitis or ulceration of mucosal surfaces, produces pain. Ischemia of tissues involved with torsion, volvulus, intussusception, and strangulated hernias also causes pain. The manifestations of abdominal pain are similar in all cattle regardless of the specific cause. It is important to recognize these signs and to differentiate the probable origin. Signs of abdominal pain are often the primary reasons clients seek veterinary service for their affected animals.

CLINICAL SIGNS

Cattle with abdominal pain have the overall appearance of discomfort. Frequently, they may kick at their abdomen with their rear legs. Stretching, arching of the back, and frequent and alternate standing and lying down indicate discomfort. Cows may shift their weight from one hindleg to another in rapid fashion ("treading"). Cattle are sometimes reluctant to move and often have an anxious, wide-eyed expression. Affected cattle will usually isolate themselves from the remainder of the herd and refuse feed and water. Milk production will be decreased or negligible in lactating cows. Some assume a crouching position as though they are attempting to lie down. The heart rate is usually increased to approximately 100 beats/minute. Respirations are increased but shallow in character, giving the impression that deep respiratory movements are painful. Cattle may swish the tail or grind teeth.

DIFFERENTIAL DIAGNOSIS

Stretching and ischemia of the abomasal wall causes pain in abomasal volvulus. The diagnosis is based on a large area of resonant tympany (ping) audible on the right side of the abdomen. The abomasum is usually palpable by rectal examination. The abdominal pain in cecal volvulus results from stretching of the wall of the cecum. A ping is auscultated in the right paralumbar fossa, and the cecum can be identified by rectal examination.

Intussusception induces pain from stretching of the intestine and mesentery as well as distention of the intestine proximal to the obstruction. Tympany may be present at several sites on the right side of the abdomen. Finding bilateral abdominal distention and gas-distended loops of intestine on rectal examination help differentiate this condition.

Volvulus of the root of the mesentery results in abdominal pain because of stretching of the mesentery. Tympany, bilateral abdominal distention, and the rectal examination findings in torsion of the mesentery root are similar to those of intussusception. These 2 conditions are usually differentiated at surgery.

A strangulated inguinal or umbilical hernia causes pain from distention of the intestine with fluid proximal to the obstruction. In both conditions, gas-distended loops of intestine are found on rectal examination, and the abdomen has bilateral distention. Inguinal herniation can be definitively diagnosed by rectal examination of the internal inguinal rings. Umbilical hernias can be diagnosed by external palpation of the umbilical area.

Penetration of the foreign body causes pain in traumatic reticuloperitonitis. Localization of pain in the anterior abdomen, the presence of a low-grade fever, a sudden decrease in milk production, mild neutrophilia, and a history of exposure to foreign bodies help differentiate this condition.

Urolithiasis with urethral or bladder distention induces pain as a result of distention of the serosal surfaces of these structures. A history of lack of urination, the presence of a distended bladder on rectal palpation, and elevated blood urea nitrogen and creatinine concentrations help to diagnose urolithiasis. Blockage of the ureter with exudate results in pain in pyelonephritis. An abnormal urinalysis coupled with an enlarged ureter found on rectal palpation help with its differentiation.

Abomasal ulcers may induce pain from direct trauma to the abomasal wall or regional peritonitis from perforation. Ulcers usually bleed into the intestinal tract, resulting in dark, tarry stools (melena).

Abnormalities of the uterus frequently induce abdominal pain. Uterine torsion is the most notable uterine abnormality that consistently results in pain. This can be definitively diagnosed by rectal or vaginal examination. Diffuse peritonitis may also cause pain primarily owing to movement or disturbances of abdominal adhesions.

Differentiation of the various causes of abdominal pain is primarily accomplished by physical examination coupled with a skillfully obtained history. In some cases, clinical laboratory findings or exploratory surgery is necessary for a definitive diagnosis.

Acknowledgment

The authors greatly appreciate the helpful critique of Peter D. Constable.

Gastric Ulcers of Swine

PETER D. CONSTABLE, BVSc, MS, MRCVS, DIPLOMATE, ACVIM

DEFINITION

Gastric ulceration is a significant economic disease of intensive swine operations. Ulceration is usually restricted to the nonglandular region (pars esophagea), although in rare instances the glandular region (particularly the fundus) may become ulcerated.[46] The pathogenesis of ulceration in the 2 locations appears to be different.

PATHOGENESIS

Gastric ulceration in growing pigs of all breeds is often associated with the feeding of a finely ground ration (particle size <1.5 mm diameter). These diets increase the stomach water content, preventing establishment of the normal pH gradient within the stomach. The absence of gastric partitioning causes the pH at the pars esophagea to be relatively low and the pH at the fundus to be relatively high, which promotes additional acid secretion and therefore results in gastric hyperacidity. The stratified squamous epithelium that covers the pars esophagea is subsequently damaged by the abnormally low pH, with production of multiple superficial erosions, parakeratosis, and mucosal injury. The injury is confined to the pars esophagea because glandular secretions and buffering capacity protect the adjacent glandular regions. Deep ulceration with extensive hemorrhage or perforation may follow if feeding of a finely ground diet continues. Histamine, a powerful stimulant of gastric secretion in swine, can experimentally induce ulceration of the pars esophagea.[47] This finding supports the central role that gastric hyperacidity plays in ulcer development.

Ulceration of the fundic region, although much rarer than ulceration of the pars esophagea, can also occur in swine. Infection with swine fever and *Erysipelothrix rhusiopathiae* as well as *Hyostrongylus rubidus* infestation and glucocorticoid release have been associated with fundic ulceration.[46, 47]

CLINICAL SIGNS AND DIAGNOSIS

Gastric ulceration is usually asymptomatic and is a frequent incidental finding during necropsy or slaughter inspection. Studies have demonstrated that gastric ulceration has little or no effect on growth rate or feed efficiency in subclinically affected animals.[46]

The most common clinical sign of gastric ulceration is sudden death. The carcass of affected pigs appears extremely pale at necropsy, and the stomach and proximal small intestine contain a large volume of blood. Deep ulceration is usually confined to the pars esophagea in growing pigs, although lesions may also extend to the contiguous esophagus in a small proportion of cases. Anemia, weakness, inappetence, vomition, and melena may be present is more protracted cases, which potentially increases the difficulty of diagnosis. Debility associated with ulceration and fibrosis (cicatrization of the pars esophagea) has been infrequently observed. Pigs with this complication have a poor growth rate and regurgitate frequently.[48] Determination of plasma gastrin or pepsinogen concentrations is of no value in diagnosing the condition, because similar values are present in normal pigs and pigs with parakeratosis or ulceration of the pars esophagea.

TREATMENT

Specific antacid medication is impractical and uneconomical. Antacids have been widely recommended for the treatment of gastric ulceration in swine despite the absence of appropriate clinical studies. Their usefulness must be seriously questioned, because aluminum silicate (50 g, every 24 hours) does not protect swine against experimentally induced ulceration of the pars esophagea.[49] An additional drawback is the requirement for frequent treatments. Cimetidine (0.5 mg/kg, every 12 hours), an H_2-blocker, is a logical treatment for valuable breeding animals; however, pharmacokinetic studies have not been completed in swine. In addition, the wisdom in treating breeding stock for ulceration should be considered, because the heritability of the condition is moderately high (0.52).[50] This suggests that selection of breeding stock for resistance to ulceration should be effective; however, such selection is not widely undertaken.

Treatment of pars esophagea ulceration is more appropriately directed at ensuring normal partitioning of the gastric contents. This is best achieved by changing the diet to one of larger particle size (>3.5 mm in diameter) and higher fiber content. The addition of roughage through incorporation of at least 25 per cent ground oats in the ration is a practical method of increasing fiber content. The feeding of pelleted feed should be avoided if possible.[46]

Treatment of fundic ulceration is directed at minimizing concurrent stress and eliminating any existing parasite burden. Concurrent parasite infestations should be treated because they may induce ulceration. *Hyostrongylus rubidus* is best treated with dichlorvos, levamisole, or ivermectin.

PREVENTION

Gastric ulceration can be prevented by feeding a diet with an adequate particle size and fiber content, as outlined in the preceding. Major changes in diet formulation should be undertaken only when the economic losses from ulceration are serious, because diets high in particle size or fiber may be unattractive from an economic or manageability viewpoint. Other dietary modifications should include supplementation with vitamin E–selenium; diets deficient in these factors have been associated with an increased prevalence of ulceration.[46]

Sodium polyacrylate (5 to 20 g daily, per os) is effective in preventing experimentally induced ulcers.[49] Sodium polyacrylate is a polyionic, viscous compound that is thought to delay gastric emptying and reduce the free-acid content of gastric juice.[49] An early field study indicated that incorporation of sodium polyacrylate at 0.1 to 0.5 per cent in the diet effectively controlled esophagogastric ulceration, with resultant increased weight gain and feed conversion.[51] In contrast, a more recent study found that feeding 0.1 per cent sodium polyacrylate in conjunction with a finely ground diet did not prevent the development of parakeratotic lesions.[52] The reasons for the conflicting results are not presently clear.

Abomasal Emptying Defect of Sheep

D. MICHAEL RINGS, DVM, MS, DIPLOMATE, ACVIM

DEFINITION

Within the last 10 years, a syndrome of weight loss associated with distention of the abomasum has been recognized in sheep, especially Suffolks.[53] This problem occurs sporadically in sheep greater than 1 year of age, with the greatest incidence being 2 to 5 years. In addition to Suffolks, this problem has been diagnosed in the Hampshire, Columbia, and Corriedale breeds.

ETIOLOGY AND PATHOGENESIS

The mechanism responsible for abomasal emptying defect (AED) is, at present, undefined. Although the greatest number of affected animals occurs in the Suffolk breed, which suggests a breed predisposition, a previous study failed to show evidence of direct heritability.[54] A similar condition in Great Britain was associated with the scrapie agent[55]; however, no evidence of scrapie has been detected in affected sheep in the United States. The occurrence of this problem is not seasonal and has not been associated with any particular management or feeding program. Unlike abomasal impactions in cattle, which start at the pylorus, the distention in the abomasum of affected sheep is primarily confined to the body of the abomasum with the antral and pyloric areas uninvolved. Regardless of the inciting cause, failure of the abomasum to empty properly results in gradual distention of this organ. Distention probably results in neural feedback to the satiety center located in the hypothalamus, with resultant loss of appetite. The animal starves with a full stomach. Because the pylorus and antrum are unaffected, sufficient abomasal secretions are passed through to the duodenum to allow electrolyte absorption. Feedstuffs entering the abomasum contribute to the distention, which may exceed 18 L (normal <2 L).

CLINICAL SIGNS

Most animals with AED have a history of gradual weight loss from weeks to months. Weight losses are often inapparent with sheep in heavy fleece until the animal is emaciated. Although affected sheep lack a good appetite, the gregarious nature of this species causes owners to believe they are eating because affected sheep stay with the flock during feeding. Most AED sheep continue to pass feces of a normal, pelleted consistency. Body temperature and respiratory rates are normal, but tachycardia (>90/minute) is consistently seen.[56] Rumen motility varies from decreased (<2/2 minutes) to increased (>4/2 minutes). Ventral abdominal distention is visually apparent in more than 50 per cent of the animals, and careful ballottement of the right ventral abdominal quadrant usually suggests the presence of a distended viscus. AED has a chronic course but is ultimately fatal if untreated.

DIAGNOSIS

Suffolk sheep with a history of weight loss in which no apparent cause can be found should be examined for AED. Physical examination findings of weight loss, tachycardia, and a distended viscus in the right ventral abdominal quadrant would be strongly suggestive of AED. Laboratory determinations of serum chloride and potassium concentrations as well as analysis of blood gases will be normal; however, elevations in rumen chloride concentration (>15 mEq/L) are found in a majority of cases as a result of abomasal reflux. Sonograms of the right ventral quadrant immediately behind the liver will reveal an enlarged abomasum instead of the normal small bowel images. When sonography is unavailable, an exploratory celiotomy can be performed to confirm the diagnosis.

TREATMENT

AED has a poor prognosis with use of any of the previously reported treatment regimens; only approximately 30 per cent of treated sheep survive more than 6 months. Sheep diagnosed early in the course of the problem (before the abomasum becomes too distended) can be treated medically with a combination of metoclopramide hydrochloride* (0.1 mg/kg twice daily) subcutaneously and 2 to 4 ounces of mineral oil orally for 10 to 21 days. Improvement should be noted within 1 week of treatment. When the abomasum becomes distended beyond a 6 to 7 L volume, it is unreasonable to expect purely medical treatment to be effective. Abomasotomy and evacuation of the contents, accompanied by medical treatment, should be attempted in these sheep although the prognosis for recovery is even lower in these animals, compared with those requiring only medical treatment. Recent attempts to imbricate the abomasum at the time of evacuation have met with mixed results. The incidence of relapse among sheep that apparently respond to treatment (regain their appetites with distending) is high (≥75 per cent in 1 year).

REFERENCES

1. Begg H: Diseases of the stomach of the adult ruminant. Vet Rec 62:797, 1950.
2. Markusfeld O: The association of displaced abomasum with various periparturient factors in dairy cows: a retrospective study. Prev Vet Med A 4:172–183, 1986.
3. Trent A: Surgery of the bovine abomasum: surgery of the bovine digestive tract. Vet Clin North Am 6:399–447, 1990.
4. Stober M, Wegner W, Lunebrink J: Research on the familial occurrence of left-sided displacement of the abomasum in cattle. Bovine Pract 10:59, 1975.
5. Martin SW, Kirby KL, Curtis RA: A study of the role of genetic factors in the etiology of left abomasal displacement. Can J Comp Med 42:511, 1978.
6. Robertson JM: Left displacement of the bovine abomasum: epizoologic factors. Am J Vet Res 29:421, 1968.
7. Coppock CE, Noller CH, Wolfe SA, et al: Effect of forage-concentrate ratio in complete feeds fed ad libitum on feed intake prepartum and the occurrence of abomasal displacement in dairy cows. J Dairy Sci 55:783, 1972.
8. Coppock CE: Displaced abomasum in dairy cattle: etiological factors. J Dairy Sci 57:926, 1972.
9. Svendsen P: Etiology and pathogenesis of abomasal displacement in cattle. Vet Med 21(Suppl 1):1, 1969.
10. Ash RW: Inhibition of reticulo-rumen contractions by acid. Proceedings, Physiological Society, July 10 and 21, 1956, pp 75–76.
11. Wallace CE: Left abomasal displacement: a retrospective study of 315 cases. Bovine Pract 10:50, 1975.
12. Robb EJ, Johnstone C, et al: Epidemiological study of risk factors for abomasal displacement: a case control study (abstract). J Dairy Sci 69:105, 1986.
13. Ingling AL, Albert TF, Schueler RL: Left displacement of the abomasum in a clinically normal cow. J Am Vet Med Assoc 166:601, 1975.
14. Wallace CE: Prognostic significance of diarrhea in cows with left displacement of the abomasum. Bovine Pract 11:62, 1976.
15. Whitlock RH: Pathophysiology of lower gastrointestinal tract problems in the bovine. Proceedings, 9th Annual Convention, American Association of Bovine Practitioners, 1976, pp 43–48.
16. Gingerich DA: Paradoxical aciduria in bovine metabolic alkalosis. J Am Vet Med Assoc 166:227, 1975.
17. Gingerich DA, Murdick PW: Experimentally induced intestinal obstruction in sheep: paradoxical aciduria in metabolic alkalosis. Am J Vet Res 36:663, 1975.
18. Robertson JM: Diagnosis of left displacement of the bovine abomasum. J Am Vet Med Assoc 146:820, 1965.
19. Cote JF: Displaced abomasum: a method of correction. Can Vet J 1:58, 1960.
20. St. Jean GD, Hull BL, Hoffsis GF, et al: Comparison of the different surgical techniques for correction of abomasal problems. Compend Contin Educ 9:F377–383, 1987.
21. Hull BL: Closed suturing technique for correction of left abomasal displacement. Iowa State Univ Vet 3:142, 1972.
22. Grymer J, Sterner KE: Percutaneous fixation of left displaced abomasum, using a bar suture. J Am Vet Med Assoc 180:1458, 1982.
23. Lowe SE, Loomis WK, Kramer LL: Abomasopexy for repair of left displacement in dairy cattle. J Am Vet Med Assoc 147:389, 1965.

---

*Reglan, A. H. Robins Company, Richmond, VA 23220.

24. Robertson JM, Boucher WB: Treatment of left displacement of the bovine abomasum. J Am Vet Med Assoc 149:1423, 1966.
25. Ames SH: Repositioning displaced abomasum in the cow. J Am Vet Med Assoc 153:1470, 1968.
26. Hoffsis GF: Right paralumbar omentopexy for the correction of left displaced abomasum. Proceedings, 4th Annual Convention, American Association of Bovine Practitioners, 1971, p 1979.
27. Gabel AA, Heath RB: Correction and right-sided omentopexy in the treatment of left-sided displacement of the abomasum in dairy cattle. J Am Vet Med Assoc 155:632, 1969.
28. Staubus S: Management suggestions for preventing left displaced abomasums. Ohio State University, Dept of Dairy Science, personal communication.
29. Gabel AA, Heath RB: Treatment of right-sided torsion of the abomasum in cattle. J Am Vet Med Assoc 155:642, 1969.
30. Poulsen JSD: Clinical chemical examination of a case of left-sided abomasal displacement changing to right-sided abomasal displacement. Nord Vet Med 26:91, 1974.
31. Pearson H: The treatment of surgical disorders of the bovine abdomen. Vet Rec 92:245, 1973.
32. Habel RE, Smith DF: Volvulus of the bovine abomasum and omasum. J Am Vet Med Assoc 179:447, 1981.
33. Smith DR, et al: The identification of structure and conditions responsible for right side tympanitic resonance (ping) in adult cattle. Cornell Vet 72:180, 1982.
34. Hammong PB, Dzuik HE, Usenik EA, Stevens CE: Experimental intestinal obstruction in calves. J Comp Pathol Ther 74:210, 1964.
35. Whitlock RH: Bovine stomach diseases. In Anderson NV (ed): Veterinary Gastroenterology. Philadelphia, Lea & Febiger, 1980, pp 396–432.
36. Boucher WB, Abt D: Right-sided dilatation of the bovine abomasum with torsion. J Am Vet Med Assoc 153:76, 1968.
37. Constable PD, St. Jean G, et al: Preoperative prognostic indicators in cattle with abomasal volvulus: a prospective study in 80 animals. Am J Vet Res (in press).
38. Smith DA: Right-side torsion of the abomasum in dairy cows: classification of severity and evaluation of outcome. J Am Vet Med Assoc 173:108, 1978.
39. Neal PA, Edwards GB: Vagus indigestion in cattle. Vet Rec 82:296, 1968.
40. Rebhun WC: Vagus indigestion in cattle. J Am Vet Med Assoc 176:506, 1980.
41. Ferrante P, Whitlock R: Chronic (vagus) indigestion in cattle. Compend Contin Educ Pract Vet 3:S231, 1981.
42. McGuirk SM, Bednarski RM, Clayton MK: Bradycardia in cattle deprived of food. J Am Vet Med Assoc 196:894–896, 1990.
43. Baker JA: Abomasal impactions and related obstructions of the forestomachs in cattle. J Am Vet Med Assoc 175:1250, 1979.
44. Merritt AB, Boucher WB: Surgical treatment of the abomasal impaction in the cow. J Am Vet Med Assoc 150:1115, 1968.
45. Robertson JT: Differential diagnosis and surgical management of intestinal obstruction in cattle. Vet Clin North Am 1:377, 1979.
46. O'Brien JJ: Gastric ulceration (of the pars oesophagea) in the pig: a review. Vet Bull 39:75–82, 1969.
47. Zamora CS, Reddy VK, Johnson P, et al: Effect of histamine and prostaglandin E_2 on gastric blood flow in swine. Am J Vet Res 42:956–959, 1981.
48. Blackshaw JK: Effects of gastric ulceration on growth rate on intensively reared pigs. Vet Rec 106:52–54, 1980.
49. Kokue E, Kurebayashi Y, Shimoda M, et al: Evaluation of prophylactic activity of drugs on swine gastroesophageal ulcer induced by betazole-reserpine using the method of endoscopy. Jpn J Vet Sci 45:143–149, 1983.
50. Berruecos JM, Robison OW: Inheritance of gastric ulcers in swine. J Anim Sci 35:20–24, 1972.
51. Yamaguchi M, Takemoto K, Asano T, et al: Prevention of gastric ulcers in swine by feeding sodium polyacrylate. Am J Vet Res 42:960–962, 1981.
52. Roth FX, Kirchgessner M, Bollwahn W, et al: Fattening performance, nutrient digestibility, and gastric lesions in pigs in response to differing particle size of feed. 2. Effect of a supplement of sodium polyacrylate and coarse oat bran. Vet Med A 32:652–661, 1985.
53. Rings DM, Welker FH, Hull BF, et al: Abomasal emptying defect in Suffolk sheep. J Am Vet Med Assoc 185:1520–1522, 1984.
54. Ruegg PL, George LW, East NE: Abomasal dilatation and emptying defect in a flock of Suffolk ewes. J Am Vet Med Assoc 193:1534–1536, 1988.
55. Sharp MW, Collins DF: Ovine abomasal enlargement and scrapie (letter). Vet Rec 120:215, 1987.
56. Rings DM: Abomasal emptying defect in Suffolk sheep. In Proceedings, American College of Veterinary Internal Medicine, 1987, pp 759–762.

Diseases of the Large Intestine

PETER D. CONSTABLE, BVSc, MS, MRCVS,
Diplomate, ACVIM

The large intestine of the ruminant comprises the cecum, ascending colon (which contains the proximal loop, centripetal and centrifugal coils of the spiral loop, and distal loop), transverse colon, descending colon, and rectum. The ruminant large intestine allows additional microbial degradation of digesta to occur through fermentation in the cecum and proximal loop of the ascending colon.[1] The large intestine of the pig is similar to that of the ruminant, comprising cecum, ascending colon (centripetal and centrifugal coils), transverse colon, descending colon, and rectum. In ruminants and swine, the spiral loop is the major site for water reabsorption; the distal loop, transverse colon, descending colon, and rectum serve as a temporary store for excreta until defecation can proceed.

A number of surgical and medical diseases affect the large intestine of ruminants and swine. Large intestinal disorders that are considered in this article include cecal dilation, cecocolic volvulus, cecal torsion, colonic obstruction, atresia coli, rectal prolapse, rectal stricture, and atresia recti and ani. Large intestinal diseases caused by infectious agents, such as coccidiosis, winter dysentery, salmonellosis, and swine dysentery, are addressed elsewhere.

Cecal Dilation

DEFINITION

Cecal dilation is defined as an enlarged, gas-filled cecum without vascular compromise or obstruction to digesta flow. Cecal dilation is often accompanied by dilation of the proximal loop of the ascending colon. The condition is most commonly diagnosed in lactating dairy cows, although cecal dilation has also been reported in sheep and the goat.[2]

PATHOGENESIS

Normal cecocolic motility consists of regular coordinated peristaltic and antiperistaltic contractions of the cecum and proximal loop of the ascending colon (frequency approximately 1/minute in the cow) that result in a thorough mixing of the digesta. The pacemaker sites for these regular cecocolic contractions are the ileocecal junction and blind end of the cecum. Superimposed on this basic mixing pattern is the periodic discharge of ileal contents into the cecum as well as complete evacuation of cecocolic contents into the spiral loop. Cecal gas also passes on to the spiral loop in association with periodic cecocolic contractions.[1]

Cecal atony or hypomotility is a prerequisite for cecal dilation. Cecal motility is decreased in ileus and hypocalcemia.[3] The regular peristaltic and antiperistaltic contractions of the cecum and proximal colon are also markedly inhibited by a decrease in cecal digesta pH associated with an increase in cecal volatile fatty acid concentration.[4] The feeding of grain or lush alfalfa is therefore considered a causative factor in cecal dilation because it is accompanied by an increase in cecocolic fermentation.

CLINICAL SIGNS AND DIAGNOSIS

Cecal dilation often occurs secondarily to diseases such as mastitis, metritis, left displaced abomasum, and other gastrointestinal disorders, so the presence of a dilated and dislocated cecum does not necessarily indicate a pathologic condition of the large intestine. The clinical signs of cecal dilation are nonspecific and result from the concurrent disease process. A tympanic resonance is often detected in the right paralumbar fossa caudal to the tenth rib; however, the sound is usually not high-pitched and varies in quality over time. Rectal examination reveals a moderately distended large viscus in the posterior right abdominal quadrant or pelvic inlet and the presence of a normal quantity of fecal material in the rectum.

The major differential diagnoses are cecocolic volvulus or cecal torsion (see later). These conditions are differentiated from cecal dilation on the basis of heart rate, hydration status, resonant ping size, presence of abdominal pain, fecal characteristics, and extent of cecal distention determined during rectal palpation.

TREATMENT

Cecal dilation does not require surgical correction. Treatment should be directed toward resolution of concurrent disease and correction of any blood pH, or serum electrolyte abnormalities. The cow should be monitored periodically to ensure that cecocolic volvulus or cecal torsion does not develop. Dilation of the cecum can persist for months without any deleterious effect on milk production or appetite.[5]

Cecocolic Volvulus (Cecal Volvulus) and Cecal Torsion

DEFINITION

Dilation and displacement of the cecum and proximal loop of the ascending colon can result in severe distention, vascular compromise, and obstruction to digesta flow. This condition is defined as cecocolic volvulus. The term cecocolic volvulus is preferred to cecal volvulus, because the cecum and proximal loop twist about an axis through the mesenteric attachment of the colon.[3, 6-8] The term also conveys the integral role that dilation of the proximal loop plays in the etiopathogenesis.

Cecal torsion is defined as rotation of the cecum along its longitudinal axis. The colon is not involved in the twist.[3, 9] Because the ileum enters at the junction of the cecum and proximal loop of the ascending colon, cecal torsion can be readily differentiated from cecocolic volvulus at surgery by observing the site of the twist in relation to the ileocecal valve.

Cecocolic volvulus and cecal torsion occur most frequently in cattle,[10, 11] although cases have also been described in sheep.[2] Cecal torsion appears to occur much less frequently than does cecocolic volvulus.[3, 6, 11] Although the incidence of both conditions has increased markedly in cattle over the last 30 years, they do not occur as commonly as left displaced abomasum or abomasal volvulus.

PATHOGENESIS

Cecocolic volvulus is assumed to result from dilation and displacement of the cecum and proximal loop,[3, 6] although direct evidence is lacking. The same factors that produce cecal dilation are therefore thought to produce cecocolic volvulus and cecal torsion. The twist is located in the proximal loop of the ascending colon because this region is relatively fixed in position, being attached by the greater omentum and common intestinal mesentery dorsal to the descending duodenum.[8] The common mesentery will occasionally be so displaced by the cecocolic volvulus that volvulus of the entire intestinal tract ensues.[3] This is a rapidly fatal condition.

Cecal torsion results from dilation and rotation of the cecum at its apical end, because the distal third of the cecum is unattached and therefore free to move. Once a volvulus or torsion has been created, the pathophysiologic changes are identical to those observed with strangulating obstruction elsewhere in the intestinal tract.

CLINICAL SIGNS

The 2 conditions can be differentiated only during surgical correction. Cecocolic volvulus and cecal torsion occur most commonly in lactating dairy cows, particularly during winter and early spring. The majority of cases occur within 2 months of parturition. There does not appear to be any breed predilection among dairy cattle.[10, 11]

Most affected cattle exhibit signs of abdominal pain associated with a precipitous drop in milk production and appetite. Tachycardia and rumen hypomotility or atony are often present. A large gas-filled viscus is usually detected on simultaneous auscultation and percussion of the right paralumbar fossa. The ping normally fills the entire paralumbar fossa but does not extend as far proximal as the ninth rib. A tentative diagnosis is confirmed by rectal examination. Fecal material is usually absent, or much reduced in quantity. One or more large (>10 cm diameter) loops of distended large bowel are detected on careful palpation, with the distended colon or blind end of the cecum often filling the pelvic inlet. The small intestine may also be distended with fluid. The presence of more than 1 distended large viscus is suggestive of cecocolic volvulus.

The acid-base and electrolyte status is normal in acute cases. This is expected, because experimental occlusion of the ascending colon for 4 days has no effect on the acid-base or electrolyte status.[12] A mild hypochloremic hypokalemic metabolic alkalosis is present with more prolonged volvulus duration as a result of small intestinal distention and obstruction. Severe acid-base and electrolyte alterations are observed with advanced cases, associated with the onset of circulatory shock.

DIAGNOSIS

The diagnosis of cecocolic volvulus and cecal torsion is usually straightforward. The major differential diagnoses are cecal dilation and colonic obstruction. Cattle with cecal dilation usually have a concurrent disease, the distended cecum is not tense on palpation, feces are present in the rectum, signs of abdominal pain are not evident, and the heart rate is usually normal. Colonic obstruction can mimic cecocolic volvulus or cecal torsion, depending on the location of the obstruction, and exploratory celiotomy may be required for a definitive diagnosis to be made. Severe abomasal volvulus can be confused with these cecal disorders; however, the resonant right-sided ping is usually located in a more anterior location, and only 1 large distended viscus can be palpated rectally.

TREATMENT

The overall recovery rate with surgical intervention is 75 to 85 per cent.[10, 11] Surgical correction is best achieved through a standing right flank celiotomy, because this approach facilitates cecal emptying. Flunixin meglumine (1 mg/kg, intravenously) may be administered preoperatively to provide analgesia, because pain from surgical manipulation of distended and ischemic bowel can cause cattle to become recumbent during the procedure. Treatment with flunixin meglumine constitutes extra-label drug use, and appropriate withholding times should be observed. Severe distention of the large bowel is immediately observed after opening of the abdominal cavity, and the greater omentum is difficult to identify. Gas decompression of the large intestine is normally required before a thorough exploration of the abdomen can be performed. After decompression, the surgeon should determine whether the twist is primarily located in the proximal loop of the ascending colon (cecocolic volvulus) or cecum (cecal torsion). The direction of the twist is either clockwise or counterclockwise when it is viewed from the right-hand side.[10] The blind end of the cecum is gently exteriorized and a typhlotomy performed at the most ventral portion. Up to 20 L of a green-brown malodorous liquid can be removed. Proximal colonic contents are also evacuated by gently advancing the digesta to the typhlotomy site. The typhlotomy site is closed with a 2-layer inverting suture pattern and the cecum thoroughly rinsed with isotonic saline. The cecum is then returned to the abdominal cavity, and the twist is corrected. The cecum and ascending colon should then be carefully inspected for assessment of the nature and extent of damage. A partial typhlectomy should be performed if the cecum appears necrotic. The twist is usually located distal to the ileocecocolic junction, which makes direct visualization difficult in some cases. The ascending colon is usually the site of the most severe vascular damage, and resection of necrotic colon, although technically difficult, has been accomplished.[13] Severe damage to this area is more easily handled by infolding the necrotic portion if it is focal, bypassing the area with a side-to-side colocolic anastomosis, placing an omental patch over the necrotic area, or simply leaving the necrotic area in situ. Parenteral antibiotics and intravenous fluid therapy should be administered, as required. A profuse, watery diarrhea should be present within 12 hours of surgical correction. Failure to pass feces within 24 hours of surgery suggests that the volvulus has not been completely corrected, and a second surgery is indicated. A recurrence rate of at least 10 per cent has been reported,[10, 11] in which case partial typhlectomy should be performed at the second surgery. Recurrence may reflect a pre-existing anatomic abnormality, because marked abnormalities in the omental attachments to the large intestine have been observed in a bull with recurrent cecocolic volvulus.[14] Resection of the blind end of the cecum is not routinely performed at the initial surgery, because typhlectomy prolongs surgery time and increases the degree of contamination.[11] In addition, typhlectomy has not been proved to successfully prevent further episodes of cecal dilation and subsequent volvulus. Partial typhlectomy could potentially predispose the cow to further episodes of cecocolic dilation and displacement by altering normal cecocolic motility.

Colonic Obstruction

DEFINITION AND PATHOGENESIS

Obstruction of the colon can be either partial or complete, resulting from either intraluminal obstruction or extraluminal compression. Intraluminal obstruction is most frequently diagnosed in adult dairy cattle but is occasionally observed in suckling pigs and lambs.[15] Obstruction most commonly arises from enterolith impaction in the spiral colon, because this is the major site of water reabsorption and the colonic diameter is at its smallest. One report identified a colonic obstruction resulting from intussusception of the proximal loop of the ascending colon into the spiral loop.[16] Extraluminal compression can affect any portion of the colon. Fat necrosis (lipomatosis), lymphosarcoma, and adhesions resulting from localized peritonitis have all been associated with extraluminal colonic obstruction.[17]

CLINICAL SIGNS AND DIAGNOSIS

The clinical signs of complete colonic obstruction are identical to those observed in cecocolic volvulus or cecal torsion; in partial obstruction, the clinical signs reflect a gradual and progressive occlusion of the large intestine. Severe electrolyte or acid-base abnormalities are usually absent in partial obstruction, and dehydration is only mild. A tympanic resonance is heard over the right paralumbar fossa on simultaneous percussion and auscultation. Rectal palpation reveals the presence of scant, loose feces and distended loops of small and large intestine.

Definitive diagnosis of colonic obstruction is obtained at surgery. The major differential diagnoses are ileus, cecocolic volvulus, cecal torsion, and small intestinal intussusception. Ileus can be very difficult to differentiate from partial colonic obstruction without surgical exploration of the abdomen. The other 3 conditions are easily differentiated during surgery.

TREATMENT

The cause of the obstruction is identified during standing right flank exploratory celiotomy. An intraluminal obstruction is gently massaged until the enterolith is broken down, allowing colonic contents to move freely through the previously obstructed area. If the colonic contents are firm and impacted over a wider area, injection of dioctyl sodium sulfosuccinate directly into the impaction will aid softening. The colon can be incised for retrieval of a single object in the unlikely event that the obstruction cannot be broken down. Preplacement of retention sutures on either end of the proposed incision is helpful in preventing the colon from slipping back into the abdomen during colotomy.

In extraluminal compression, the location and extent of the lesion are determined at surgery, and attempts to free the colon should be made. If this cannot be safely accomplished, a side-to-side colocolic or ileocolic anastomosis should be performed at an accessible site after the cecocolonic contents have been removed through typhlotomy. Surgical anastomosis is most easily performed under general anesthesia, although successful outcomes have been obtained on standing cattle.[17] The voiding of a profuse watery diarrhea within 12 hours of surgery and a rapid improvement in appetite usually indicate a successful outcome.

Atresia Coli

DEFINITION

Atresia coli is defined as the absence of a colonic segment. The condition most commonly affects the spiral loop of the ascending colon in calves; however, atresia coli has also been identified in sheep and swine.[18]

PATHOGENESIS

Atresia coli occurs most often in Holstein calves; however, sporadic cases have been observed in Angus, Ayrshire, Hereford, Maine-Anjou, Shorthorn, Simmental, and crossbred calves.[19, 20] Atresia coli is believed to develop early in embryonic life as a result of vascular insufficiency to the developing spiral colon. An association between atresia coli and early pregnancy diagnosis (before day 42 of gestation) by amniotic palpation has been observed, which suggests that in utero trauma can damage the colonic blood supply.[21] The sporadic nature, the multiple breed involvement, the association with rectal palpation, the development in only 1 calf of a set of identical twins,[22] and the absence of atresia coli in 14 progeny of affected cattle[19, 23] all suggest a nonhereditary cause. A genetic predisposition to atresia coli cannot be presently ruled out, however, because the Holstein breed is overrepresented in reported case series.[19, 20]

CLINICAL SIGNS AND DIAGNOSIS

The absence of feces since birth coupled with progressive abdominal distention, inappetence, and depression over the first 2 to 4 days of life should alert the clinician to the possibility of atresia coli. Some calves exhibit a high stepping gait, which is suggestive of abdominal pain. Passage of a well-lubricated flexible tube per rectum is occasionally helpful in establishing the diagnosis; however, great caution must be taken because the distal colon is fragile and easily torn. Atresia is indicated by resistance at 10 to 20 cm of insertion associated with the absence of feces. Cytologic examination of rectal contents for the absence of squamous epithelial cells has been used as a presumptive test for atresia coli. This test requires lavage of the rectum with an isotonic solution, centrifugation, and staining of the sediment with new methylene blue.[24] This test is difficult to interpret in suspected cases of atresia coli and is therefore not recommended. Barium contrast enemas are also of limited value in aiding diagnosis; they are often nondiagnostic, can result in colonic rupture, and increase the cost of treatment.[19] Definitive diagnosis of atresia coli is made during right flank exploratory celiotomy. Surgical intervention is considered urgent because continued distention of the large intestine leads to ischemic necrosis, peritonitis, and perforation.

Differential diagnoses include acute intestinal accident, abomasal volvulus, neonatal septicemia, acute diffuse peritonitis, and atresia ani. Feces are present or have been voided some time previously in the first 4 conditions, whereas atresia ani is easily identified on close inspection of the perineum. Meconium impaction is not considered a differential diagnosis, because there do not appear to be any reports of this condition in calves.[19]

TREATMENT

Atresia coli is a fatal condition unless it is surgically corrected. Despite a poor initial success rate, recent advances in the surgical and medical management of affected calves have increased the long-term success rate to approximately 35 per cent.[19, 20] Calves that are able to stand, appear bright and alert, and have a normal temperature and immunoglobulin status are considered the best candidates for surgery. Failure of passive transfer is present in at least one third of affected calves, and plasma should be administered when needed.[19]

Surgical correction is best attempted under general anesthesia via a right flank celiotomy. The distended cecum is elevated out of the abdomen and the meconium removed through a stab incision. After closure of the typhlotomy site with a 2-layer inverting pattern, the colon is traced and the proximal atretic segment identified. The descending colon is identified by retrograde passage of a soft flexible tube through the anus. A portion of the proximal blind end of the colon is then resected and an end-to-side colocolic anastomosis performed. This technique minimizes postoperative motility disturbances and stenosis at the anastomotic site.[19, 20] An alternative surgical technique that may be useful in sick calves is colonic decompression followed by cecostomy.[25] This surgery can be performed quickly under local anesthesia. Colonic resection and anastomosis is performed at a later time when the calf is in better physical condition.

Postoperative treatment should consist of administration of broad-spectrum bactericidal antibiotics, frequent feedings of milk, and general supportive care. Calves can become severely dehydrated after infection by enteric pathogens because the spiral colon is often absent, which limits the capability of the large intestine to reabsorb water.

Rectal Prolapse

DEFINITION AND PATHOGENESIS

Rectal prolapse is a common condition affecting sheep, pigs, and cattle. Prolapse often results from an increase in intrapelvic pressure and therefore accompanies conditions such as tenesmus, diarrhea, frequent coughing, obesity, vaginal prolapse, and vaginal irritation. Housing in stalls with excessive slope from front to back may also predispose to rectal prolapse, although this has not been well substantiated. Excessively short tail docking predisposes sheep to rectal prolapse. Amputation of the tail at the sacrococcygeal junction results in marked atrophy of the tail musculature, which permits excessive movement of the rectum to occur.

DIAGNOSIS

The diagnosis of rectal prolapse is straightforward. Owners can occasionally confuse the condition with vaginal prolapse, particularly when the prolapse is self-reducing. Detailed questioning of the owner is sometimes required for differentiation of the 2 conditions.

TREATMENT

Rectal prolapses often recur despite treatment; therefore, salvage for slaughter (through prolapse replacement followed by pursestring suture) should be considered in animals of minimal genetic value. The techniques outlined in the following should be considered in animals that will be retained in the herd or flock.

Mild rectal prolapses that are often self-reducing are observed most commonly in sheep. These are best handled by administering a lumbosacral epidural (0.5 to 1 ml 2 per cent lidocaine per 50 kg body weight) and injecting an irritant solution (such as iodine-based solutions in mineral oil) perirectally at 9, 12, and 3 o'clock around the anus, at a depth up to 6 cm. Injections are not placed at the 6 o'clock position because of potential damage to the bladder and sex organs. A pursestring suture around the anus is placed and maintained for 5 days after injection, and the animal is fed a diet that results in soft feces in order to facilitate fecal voiding. The aim of the suture and injection is to promote perianal fibrosis, limiting movement of the rectum within the pelvis. The lumbosacral epidural will produce rear limb paralysis for up to 2 hours. A lumbosacral epidural is easier to perform in small ruminants than is a caudal epidural at the first intercoccygeal space.

Small, recent rectal prolapses in cattle and swine should be replaced and a pursestring suture placed approximately 1 cm outside the circumference of the anus. Caudal epidural injection of lidocaine (0.5 to 1 ml 2 per cent lidocaine per 100 kg at the first intercoccygeal space) may relieve straining for a few hours. After this time, the presence of the pursestring suture may incite further straining. If this occurs, the suture should be removed or long-term caudal epidural analgesia produced by injecting a mixture of equal volumes of 70 to 95 per cent ethyl or isopropyl alcohol and 2 per cent lidocaine. The volume of the alcohol–local anesthetic mixture should be determined by monitoring the response to a previous injection of lidocaine only. The duration and degree of response to the alcohol epidural is variable. Potential sequelae to administration of an alcohol epidural include paraphimosis in males, incontinence, and permanent paralysis of the tail. Overdosage can damage the sciatic nerves, producing prolonged rear limb paresis or paralysis.[26] Alternative techniques for control of tenesmus after rectal prolapse include continuous caudal epidural analgesia, insufflation of air into the peritoneal cavity, or tracheotomy.

Large rectal prolapses in cattle and pigs and recurrent rectal prolapses in sheep usually require amputation of the prolapsed segment. Amputation is best done immediately adjacent to the anus, because this will minimize the chance for postoperative stricture formation. Numerous methods have been developed for amputation of the prolapsed segment. These techniques require epidural analgesia, as outlined in the preceding, which is often accompanied by circumferential placement of strangulating sutures around the proposed site of amputation. The prolapsed portion is then amputated immediately or allowed to slough naturally. Another technique for amputation involves the use of prolapse rings.

Rectal Stricture

DEFINITION AND PATHOGENESIS

Rectal stricture can be congenital or acquired. Rectal and vaginal constriction is a congenital disorder of Jersey cattle that is inherited in an autosomal recessive manner. The condition is characterized by a nonelastic fibrous band at the junction of the rectum and anus in both sexes, in association with vestibular stenosis in females.[27]

Acquired rectal strictures are rare in ruminants, being caused by perirectal adhesion formation, lymphosarcoma, fat necrosis, full-thickness rectal tear, or previous amputation of a rectal prolapse. Acquired rectal strictures occur more commonly in swine, in which they result from damage to the arterial blood supply of the rectum (as a result of proctitis due to pathogens such as *Salmonella typhimurium*)[28] or bruising and laceration of the prolapsed rectum.[29]

CLINICAL SIGNS AND DIAGNOSIS

The stricture may be severe enough to prevent passage of feces, with resultant marked abdominal distention and progressive depression and inappetence. The rectal stricture may be palpated approximately 5 cm anterior to the anus.

TREATMENT

Surgical correction has been attempted with use of a modified pull-through technique. An incision is made dorsal to the anus, and the dorsal connective tissue of the rectum is dissected free until normal rectal tissue proximal to the stricture is reached. This section of rectum is pulled caudally to the perineal region, where it is sutured to the skin for creation of a new rectal opening. The rectal segment containing the stricture is then resected.[30]

Atresia Recti and Ani

DEFINITION AND PATHOGENESIS

Atresia ani occurs most frequently in swine, although it has also been observed in cattle, sheep, and goats.[31-33] It results when the membrane separating endodermal hindgut from perineal ectodermal tissue fails to perforate. Atresia ani is a hereditary condition in pigs and is probably an inherited defect in calves and sheep.[31-33] The mode of inheritance in pigs is thought to be polygenic.[33]

CLINICAL SIGNS

The clinical signs of atresia ani are similar to those observed with atresia coli but are slower in onset. Affected males usually die by 2 to 3 weeks of age unless surgical correction is performed. Females with atresia ani may reach breeding age without surgical correction, because a significant proportion of affected females have a common cloaca, with feces being voided through the vagina.

DIAGNOSIS

The diagnosis of atresia ani with or without rectovaginal fistula is easily made by examining the perineal region. Affected animals often have a number of other abnormalities such as horseshoe or polycystic kidney, cryptorchidism, spinal dysraphia, and coccygeal or sacral vertebral agenesis, which may be manifest as a corkscrew tail.[31] Because of the possibility that this is an inherited defect, surgical correction should be performed only on animals not intended for breeding.

TREATMENT

Epidural anesthesia or local infiltration is used to supply analgesia for surgical correction. The perineum is forced to bulge out by the application of gentle pressure in the flank region, and a circular skin incision (approximately 3 cm diameter in calves) is made in the appropriate location for the anus. A cruciate incision in the same location is not advised because of the greater potential for stricture formation.[31] The blind end of the rectum is identified and mobilized after blunt dissection. The rectum is pulled through the circular opening, sutured directly to the skin, and opened, and the contents are removed. Postoperative care consists of frequent milk feedings. The surgical site heals rapidly and without evidence of infection. The owner should be warned about stricture formation, which can be easily relieved by repeating the same pull-through technique.

Atresia recti is not as common as is atresia ani, although it may accompany the latter condition. Treatment of atresia recti by a colonic pull-through technique or colostomy is unlikely to be economic. There do not appear to be any successful reports of animals reaching adulthood after surgical correction of this condition.

REFERENCES

1. Ruckebusch Y: Gastrointestinal motor functions in ruminants. In Wood JL (ed): Handbook of Physiology. Gastrointestinal Tract II. Bethesda, MD, American Physiological Society, 1990, pp 1225–1281.
2. Waldeland H: Caecal dilatation and displacement in sheep. Vet Rec 111:455–456, 1982.
3. Pearson H: Dilatation and torsion of the bovine cecum and colon. Vet Rec 75:961–964, 1963.
4. Svendsen P, Kristensen B: Cecal dilatation in cattle. Nord Vet Med 22:578–583, 1970.
5. Duelke BE, Whitlock RH: Persistent cecal dilatation in a lactating dairy cow. Cornell Vet 66:301–308, 1976.
6. Dirksen G: Dilatatio et torsio caeci et ansae proximalis coli in cattle. DTW 15:409–416, 1962.
7. Espersen G: Dilatation and displacement of the abomasum to the right flank, and dilatation and dislocation of the cecum. Vet Rec 76:1423–1432, 1964.
8. Smith DF, Kolb D, Wilsman N, et al: Clinical and anatomic description of dilatation and dilatation with volvulus of the cecum and proximal loop of the ascending colon in adult cattle. Int Cong Dis Cattle II:1571, 1988.
9. Oehme FW: Torsion of the cecum in a cow. J Am Vet Med Assoc 150:171, 1967.
10. Whitlock RH: Cecal volvulus in dairy cattle. Int Cong Dis Cattle, I:60–63, 1976.
11. Fubini SL, Erb HN, Rebhun WC, et al: Cecal dilatation and volvulus in dairy cows: 84 cases (1977–1983). J Am Vet Med Assoc 189:96–99, 1986.
12. Hammond PB, Dziuk HE, Usenik EA, et al: Experimental intestinal obstruction in calves. J Comp Pathol 74:210–221, 1964.
13. Pankowski RL, Fubini SL, Stehman S: Cecal volvulus in a dairy cow: partial resection of the proximal portion of the ascending colon. J Am Vet Med Assoc 191:435–436, 1987.
14. Wynn Jones E, Johnson L, Moore CC: Torsion of the bovine cecum. J Am Vet Med Assoc 130:167–170, 1957.
15. Roneus O: Coprostasis in the spiral colon of piglets. Nord Vet Med 9:362–368, 1957.
16. Hamilton GF, Tulleners EP: Intussusception involving the spiral colon in a calf. Can Vet J 21:32, 1980.
17. Smith DF, Donawick WJ: Obstruction of the ascending colon in cattle: 1. Clinical presentation and surgical management. Vet Surg 8:93–97, 1979.
18. van der Gaag I, Tibboel D: Intestinal atresia and stenosis in animals: a report of 34 cases. Vet Pathol 17:565–574, 1980.
19. Constable PD, Rings DM, Hull BL, et al: Atresia coli in calves: 26 cases (1977–1987). J Am Vet Med Assoc 195:118–123, 1989.
20. Ducharme NG, Arighi M, Horney D, et al: Colonic atresia in cattle: a prospective study of 43 cases. Can Vet J 29:818–824, 1988.
21. Hess M, Leipold G, Muller W: Zur Genese des angeborenen Darmverschlusses des Kalbes. Monatsschr Vet Med 37:89–92, 1982.
22. Ducharme NG, Horney DF, Smith DF, et al: An investigation of the heritability of colonic atresia in calves. Int Cong Dis Cattle I:750–754, 1988.
23. Hoffsis GF, Brunner RR: Atresia coli in a twin calf. J Am Vet Med Assoc 171:433–434, 1975.
24. Johnson R, Ames NK, Coy C: Congenital intestinal atresia of calves. J Am Vet Med Assoc 182:1387–1389, 1983.
25. Berchtold VM, Mittelholzer A, Camponovo L: Atresia coli beim Kalb. DTW 92:395–398, 1985.
26. Skarda RT: Techniques of local analgesia in ruminants and swine. Vet Clin North Am 2:621–663, 1986.
27. McGhee CC, Leipold HW: Morphologic studies of rectovaginal constriction in Jersey cattle. Cornell Vet 72:427–436, 1982.
28. Wilcock BP, Olander HJ: The pathogenesis of porcine rectal stricture. II. Experimental salmonellosis and ischemic proctitis. Vet Pathol 14:43–55, 1977.
29. Saunders CN: Rectal stricture syndrome in pigs: a case history. Vet Rec 94:61, 1974.
30. Boyd JS, Taylor DJ: Surgery in rectal stricture in pigs. Vet Rec 114:386, 1984.
31. Dreyfuss DJ, Tulleners EP: Intestinal atresia in calves: 22 cases (1978–1988). J Am Vet Med Assoc 195:508–513, 1989.
32. Dennis SM, Leipold HW: Atresia ani in sheep. Vet Rec 91:219–222, 1972.
33. Norrish JG, Rennie JC: Observations on the inheritance of atresia ani in swine. J Hered 59:186–187, 1968.

Nematode Infections in Cattle, Sheep, Goats, and Swine

R. P. HERD, MVSc, PhD

CATTLE

Major Parasites

Although gastrointestinal parasitism in cattle may involve several species, the abomasal nematode *Ostertagia ostertagi* is the most pathogenic and economically important in temperate regions of the world, including most areas of the United States. It is consequently important to understand the life cycle, epidemiology, and pathogenesis of this parasite and to plan control strategies with *Ostertagia* as a major target. Control strategies effective against *Ostertagia* will also be effective against most other trichostrongylid worms. Although *O. ostertagi* has been incriminated in most outbreaks of ostertagiasis, *O. leptospicularis* and *O. bisonis* may also cause disease.

Life Cycle

Ostertagia species have a direct life cycle. Eggs passed in the feces hatch first-stage larvae (L_1), which develop and molt to become second-stage larvae (L_2), which in turn develop and molt to the third-stage infective larvae (L_3). This development may occur within a week under optimal conditions, and L_3 may then migrate from the dung pat to herbage if there is adequate moisture. After ingestion of infective L_3 by cattle, the parasitic cycle involves development through L_3–L_4–L_5 stages within the gastric glands. This usually takes 18 to 21 days, by which time the young adult emerges from the glands into the lumen of the abomasum. Under certain conditions to be discussed later, the parasite undergoes hypobiosis (arrested development, inhibited development) and does not develop to the adult stage for several months.

Epidemiology

Seasonal Development of Infective Larvae

In Britain, Western Europe, and northern United States, contamination of pastures with worm eggs starts early in the grazing season, but it is not until summer that conditions are ideal for rapid development of eggs to L_3. Hence, there is an explosive increase of potentially dangerous L_3 in summer resulting from eggs passed over a period of several months.

New populations of L_3 accumulate in the fecal pats through July, August, and September in northern temperate regions and become available to grazing cattle provided there is sufficient rainfall to assist the migration of L_3 from feces to herbage. This pattern may be modified in a dry summer when L_3 become trapped within the fecal mass and do not escape to herbage until autumn rains occur, which results in a big increase in pasture infectivity in the fall when L_3 are likely to become conditioned for arrest. Young, nonimmune cattle are often exposed to light infection in the first half of the grazing season and heavy infection in the second half.

Marked seasonal patterns of pasture infectivity also occur in the Southern Hemisphere and southern United States. In many regions, the hot dry summer or the alternating wet and dry weather in summer is adverse to larval survival. Even with irrigation systems, the alternating wet and dry conditions each day are lethal to larvae. In most regions with a mild winter, there is a progressive increase in pasture contamination and infectivity from autumn through spring because of the combination of high worm egg output and favorable environmental conditions. In summer, there is likely to be high mortality of pasture larvae and little transmission of infection.

Dairy cattle in confinement or beef cattle in feedlots are not exposed to significant numbers of infective larvae, although type II ostertagiasis can occur if cattle are harboring massive numbers of hypobiotic larvae when they are moved from pasture to confinement or feedlot. Although eggs may be passed in the feces of animals removed from pasture, it seems that conditions in confinement are inimical to development of eggs to infective larvae. It is possible that the high concentration of urine has an inhibitory effect in these situations. Infection with coccidia is often a bigger problem in confinement housing and feedlots.

Longevity of Infective Larvae

Although contamination of pastures with worm eggs may be continuous throughout the year, development to infective L_3, migration of L_3 from dung pats, and the subsequent survival of L_3 on herbage differ markedly throughout the year in response to prevailing weather conditions. The fecal pat with its high moisture content acts as an important reservoir of infection and provides a safe haven for L_3 during dry periods. The migration of L_3 from dung pats to herbage is intermittent and dependent on sufficient moisture to provide a continuous film of water. Once a dung pat has dried out, rainfall of 50 to 100 mm over 2 or more days is needed to induce migration. When rainfall is intermittent, migration tends to occur in waves. The L_3 rarely migrate more than a meter from the dung pat, but larvae may be spread over a wider area by temporary localized flooding after heavy rainfall, or by hooves, farm equipment, and insects. Preferred locations for L_3 are close to the ground on the undersides of legume leaves and in leaf axils of grasses that spread laterally.

In northern temperate regions, numbers of L_3 on pasture tend to be highest in summer and autumn after development from eggs passed in spring and summer. The L_3 survive until the following spring when rising temperatures trigger enhanced activity and death after exhaustion of food reserve. Infective L_3 of many trichostrongylid species survive well under winter snow and are then available to infect cattle turned out to pasture in early spring. The decrease in numbers in L_3 as they die in the spring is accentuated by the diluting effect of accelerated herbage growth. In southern temperate regions, numbers of L_3 on pasture escalate in autumn, winter, and spring if there is adequate warmth and precipitation but die off rapidly under hot conditions in summer.

Hypobiosis (Arrested Development, Inhibited Development)

Hypobiosis is a temporary cessation of development of a parasite at a precise point in its early life; in the case of *O. ostertagi*, this occurs at the early L_4 stage. It has been reported in a large range of nematode parasites (at least 30 species). It has important practical implications because it enables the parasite to survive in a dormant state during adverse periods, when it would otherwise be eliminated by host immunity or when its progeny would be destroyed by adverse seasonal conditions. This hypobiosis mainly occurs during the adverse winter in northern states and the adverse summer in southern states. Many arrested larvae later resume normal development when the internal or external environment has become more favorable. They then seed pastures with eggs, often at a time when pasture infectivity may be quite low (e.g., spring in the North, autumn in the South). A massive synchronous maturation of arrested larvae will cause clinical disease, such as type II ostertagiasis. This has been hard to control in the past because most available anthelmintics have been ineffective against hypobiotic larvae.

The patterns of worm transmission tend to be reversed in the northern and southern temperate zones. Major accumulations of pasture L_3 occur in summer in the North, whereas major mortality of L_3 occurs at that time in the South. Major accumulations of pasture L_3 occur in spring in the South, whereas major mortality occurs at that time in the North. Type I ostertagiasis mainly occurs in the first half of the year in the South and in the second half of the year in the North. Pre–type II ostertagiasis, the phase of arrested development, occurs in winter in the North and in summer in the South. Type II ostertagiasis, the clinical syndrome associated with the maturation of arrested larvae, occurs mainly in early spring in the North and early autumn in the South.

Host Immunity

Calves are most susceptible to worms during their first season at pasture but generally acquire a strong immunity during their second grazing season. Cattle exposed to *Ostertagia* infections normally have a strong immunity by the end of their second grazing season. Hence, the disease is mainly a problem of dairy replacement heifers at pasture or beef calves grazing contaminated pasture during the postweaning period. Adult cattle are little affected because of their acquired immunity. Nevertheless, problems can develop in cattle that have received minimal exposure to parasites as calves or in cattle suffering immunosuppression from a variety of causes, such as malnutrition, concurrent disease, or chemotherapy. Cattle raised indoors or on drylots will have little exposure to nematodes and may not develop strong immunity. In general, dairy calves develop immunity faster than do beef calves because of their greater exposure to parasites. Consequently, clinical parasitism is even less common in adult dairy cattle than in adult beef cattle.

Pathogenesis

The major lesions, biochemical changes, and clinical signs associated with ostertagiasis usually occur immediately after emergence of young adults from the gastric glands. Cellular changes are initially confined to the parasitized glands, but when young adults begin to emerge, the hyperplasia and loss of cellular differentiation become more generalized, giving the abomasal wall a Moroccan leather appearance. Destruction of parietal hydrochloric acid–producing cells often elevates the abomasal fluid pH from 2 to 7. This results in a failure to denature protein, failure to activate pepsinogen to pepsin, and loss of a bacteriostatic effect, which leads to the onset of diarrhea.

The hyperplastic and undifferentiated mucosa also becomes more permeable to macromolecules, which leads to elevated plasma pepsinogen levels (>3000 IU tyrosine) as nonactivated pepsinogen diffuses into the circulation. Plasma proteins also leak in the opposite direction from the circulation to the abomasal lumen. Necrosis and sloughing of surface epithelial cells may follow emergence of large numbers of worms, and congestion or edema of the abomasal folds may be encountered. The clinical consequences of all these changes are loss of appetite, ill-thrift, and diarrhea.

Clinical Disease

There are 2 main clinical forms of ostertagiasis, type I and type II.

TYPE I. This clinical entity results from the rapid acquisition of large numbers of L_3 that complete their development to the adult stage in 3 to 4 weeks. It occurs mainly in young cattle up to 18 months of age during their first season at pasture. It is most common from July to October in northern temperate regions and from January to April in southern temperate zones. Clinical signs coincide with the emergence of young adults from the gastric glands 3 weeks or more after cattle are exposed to heavily infected pastures. The main signs are anorexia, weight loss, diarrhea, and mortality. It is common for a large percentage of the group to be affected, in contrast to type II disease, in which only a small percentage show signs.

PRE-TYPE II. In this form, clinical signs are absent or mild in character, and the vast majority of Ostertagia worms (often >80 per cent) are arrested in their development at the early L_4 stage, slightly over 1 mm in length. Pre–type II ostertagiasis occurs in winter after acquisition of arrested-prone L_3 in late autumn in northern regions. In southern regions, pre–type II ostertagiasis occurs in late spring and summer after acquisition of arrested-prone L_3 in spring. It appears that hypobiosis of Ostertagia is largely a seasonal phenomenon triggered by falling temperatures in northern regions and other unknown stimuli in southern regions. Host immunity is thought to play a relatively minor role in this instance.

TYPE II. This clinical phase results from the emergence and maturation of large numbers of arrested larvae in the early spring in northern regions and early fall in southern regions. Clinical cases have been observed in grazing cattle, housed cattle, and feedlot cattle, most commonly 2 to 4 years of age. Diarrhea may be intermittent, coinciding with the emergence of successive waves of developing larvae. Anorexia, weight loss, hypoalbuminemia, moderate anemia, and submandibular edema (bottle jaw) may also occur. Clinical signs are usually seen in only a small percentage (<10 per cent) of animals coincident with massive emergence of larvae or loss of immunity.

Type II ostertagiasis can be differentiated from type I by the different seasonal occurrence, grazing history, older age of animals, small number affected, more protracted course, poorer prognosis, and insusceptibility to most anthelmintics. Although beef and dairy cattle both exhibit type II ostertagiasis, a higher proportion of hypobiosis has been reported in beef cattle production systems. On many dairy farms, the year-round pasture contamination by calves ensures continual transmission of worms, and there is probably less selection pressure for the parasite to undergo hypobiosis for ensuring survival.

Diagnosis

A detailed history is helpful in arriving at a correct diagnosis, because there is a lack of specificity in clinical signs and a poor correlation between fecal egg counts and worm burdens. Knowledge of seasonal conditions, grazing history, likely levels of pasture infectivity, nutritional and reproductive status, managerial practices, anthelmintic treatments, and the expected degree of immunity to worms is helpful in making a decision. For example, type I disease is most likely to be a herd problem in calves during their first grazing season, whereas type II disease affects only a small percentage of animals at the time when there is emergence and maturation of hypobiotic worms, that is, early spring (northern regions) and early fall (southern regions).

Clinical signs of anorexia, weight loss, diarrhea, rough coat, and submandibular edema are suggestive of but not specific for ostertagiasis. Fecal egg counts may remain low in some animals in clinical outbreaks of disease and give no indication of the number of immature worms, inhibited worms, or adult worms in which egg laying has been suppressed by anthelmintic treatment or host immunity. Furthermore, it is difficult to differentiate eggs of Ostertagia from those of most other trichostrongylid species *(Haemonchus, Cooperia, Trichostrongylus)* or hookworms *(Bunostomum)*. Plasma pepsinogen concentrations are sometimes better correlated with Ostertagia burdens than are fecal egg counts, but false-positives and false-negatives may occur.

The most positive way to make a diagnosis is by necropsy examination and total worm counts. The distinctive abomasal lesions can be observed and aliquots of abomasal contents and abomasal wall digests counted for worms. Adult Ostertagia are fine, hairlike worms of only 1 cm length and are easily missed on macroscopic examination, even when many thousands are present. A moribund animal or one that is profusely scouring sometimes expels many of its worms in the feces, so that the worm count is artificially low at necropsy. Whereas moderate worm burdens are pathogenic in young cattle, heavy worm burdens may be required to cause clinical disease in adult cattle.

Control Strategies

The question arises as to which herds or animals should be dewormed and which should not. This question must be answered on an individual herd basis and can be answered correctly only by the veterinary practitioner who is familiar with the farm and its livestock. There is no cut-and-dried recommendation that applies to every farm, and each one must be considered separately on its merits or lack of merits. The practitioner must make the decisions, drawing on his or her considerable knowledge of the farm, to provide a custom-made worm control program for each farm, instead of a blanket recommendation for all herds. There is also need to consider each class of cattle separately and to provide different control programs for bulls, dairy cows, replacement heifers, cow and calf herds, beef stockers or replacements, and feedlot cattle.

Treatment priorities for dairy cattle and beef cattle are summarized in Tables 1 and 2 respectively. When decisions are being made about treatment, 2 key questions should be asked:

1. What is the likely immune status of each group of cattle?
2. What is the likely degree of pasture infectivity and exposure to worms?

The answer to these 2 questions can be derived from the

Table 1. TREATMENT PRIORITIES FOR DAIRY CATTLE

Class of Cattle	Immune Status	Worm Exposure	Action
Bulls	Sex-related susceptibility	Variable	Treat
Cows at pasture	High	Low	No treatment
Problem herds	Low	High	Treat
Cows on concrete or drylot	Variable	Low	No treatment
Replacement heifers			
1st year at pasture	Low	High	Treat
2nd year at pasture	Variable	Variable	±Treat

practitioner's general knowledge of the farm, its grazing history, and seasonal conditions, aided by the use of quantitative fecal egg counts. Laboratory tests may be misleading if they are considered in isolation but can be of much value if the most appropriate technique is selected, and if the results are interpreted in relation to the history and management of the herd. Fecal egg counts are useful as a guide to the degree of immunity to worms and the severity of pasture contamination, but they do not measure the severity of infection. This subject is discussed later in this section.

Immune Status

The following basic facts will be helpful in decision-making.

- Well-fed beef or dairy cows usually have a high degree of acquired immunity to worms, which results in few worms (<3000) and low fecal egg counts (<10 eggs per gram [epg]).
- There is no evidence that low worm burdens in immune cows cause reduced milk production, in spite of advertising claims.
- If adult cattle have fecal egg counts in the hundreds, it generally means that they have lost, or never achieved, immunity. Thus, fecal egg counts are sometimes useful in assessing the immune status.
- Unlike lambing ewes, beef or dairy cows exhibit only a slight periparturient relaxation of immunity to worms. Hence, fecal egg counts may rise only slightly, from a mean of about 5 epg to about 20 epg after calving. This is epidemiologically insignificant.
- Young cattle under 2 years may have little immunity to worms, large worm burdens (>100,000), and high egg counts (>100 epg) and suffer severe production losses and mortality.
- There is a sex-related susceptibility to worms so that young bulls are more susceptible than are steers, which in turn are more susceptible than are heifers. Thus, production losses and mortality are likely to be greatest in young bulls.

Pasture Infectivity

The following facts are relevant to any decision taken.

- Pastures perpetuate parasites, so the greatest risk occurs in nonimmune cattle grazing pasture.

Table 2. TREATMENT PRIORITIES FOR BEEF CATTLE

Class of Cattle	Immune Status	Worm Exposure	Action
Bulls	Sex-related susceptibility	Variable	Treat
Cows at pasture	High	Low	No treatment
Suckling calves	Low	Low	No treatment
Problem herds	Low	High	Treat
Weanlings	Low	High	Treat
Feedlot	Variable	Low	Treat on arrival

- Cattle housed continually in confinement, stalls, loafing pens, drylots, or feedlots are rarely exposed to parasitic larvae, except for *Nematodirus* spp. and *Strongyloides*.
- The degree of pasture infectivity is strongly influenced by the previous grazing of a pasture. Young, untreated, nonimmune animals (especially young bulls) will cause the greatest pasture contamination with worm eggs.
- The degree of pasture infectivity is also strongly influenced by seasonal conditions. Warm, wet conditions favor hatching, development, and migration of infective larvae from feces to pasture. Drought conditions enhance larval mortality.
- Once a pasture becomes highly infective, the larvae survive long periods and pose a threat to all grazing animals. In the northern United States, larvae from one year commonly survive until late spring of the next year. In the southern United States, larvae survive well through autumn, winter, and spring but succumb to high summer temperatures.

Each Farm Is Different

Some examples of different farm scenarios are given in the following. Each farm needs to be considered as an individual entity, and fecal egg counts need to be done for fully evaluating the degree of immunity and pasture contamination.

- If a farm is well managed and the cattle are well fed, most adult cattle will have developed a strong protective immunity to worms and not require deworming. In the case of beef cows, they will not be a serious source of pasture contamination for their suckling calves. This can be checked by fecal egg counts. Low counts will indicate strong immunity and low pasture contamination; high counts will indicate that something is wrong.
- In some herds, problems may occur in only a few individuals that have failed to develop a strong immunity because of genetic or other factors. These few animals with high egg counts can be treated or culled.
- Occasionally, a whole group may fail to develop adequate immunity to worms through lack of exposure because they were raised in confinement, or in arid regions, or in drought conditions in which infective larvae failed to survive on pastures. They would later be susceptible to worms if they are moved to a contaminated pasture, exhibit high egg counts, and respond to treatment.
- Animals that were once strongly immune may lose immunity to worms through malnutrition, disease, or lack of exposure. Winter-starved adult cattle may lose immunity to worms and exhibit high fecal egg counts. In this situation, the adult cattle could be a serious source of pasture contamination for their nonimmune calves, and treatment of both cows and calves would be justified. Check fecal egg counts if in doubt.
- In a well-managed cow and calf operation, the suckling calves are nonimmune, but initially they will be exposed to little pasture infection because of low egg counts in their immune dams and limited reliance on pasture. Suckling calves also gain some protection from the milk diet, which alters ecologic conditions in the gastrointestinal tract to cause reduced establishment of worms and stunting of worm growth. In this situation, both cows and calves are likely to show low fecal egg counts.
- By weaning time, treatment of beef calves is usually warranted. A fecal egg count check, together with herd history, will immediately reveal valuable information about their immune status and the degree of pasture contamination. A control program is usually of vital importance in the immediate postweaning period. This is generally a period of high susceptibility combined with high pasture contamination and infectivity.

- Dairy replacement heifers in their first year of grazing are usually very susceptible to worms and likely to be exposed to serious pasture contamination if they are grazing pastures previously grazed by similar batches of calves. A preventive control program is usually essential, and its success can be monitored by fecal egg counts to check pasture contamination.

It is desirable that the veterinarian take control of the situation, consider each group of cattle separately, monitor fecal egg counts, and give the owner a comprehensive worm control program. Decisions should be based on what he or she sees on each farm, rather than on what is seen in advertisements, magazine articles, or nonrefereed journals. Such information can be inaccurate or misleading, often failing to give the whole story.

It is now widely accepted that young beef or dairy cattle are the most susceptible to nematode infections. Dairy replacement heifers are especially at risk during their first season at pasture, and beef calves are often exposed to high pasture infectivity in the immediate postweaning period. Control options for these 2 groups are summarized in Tables 3 and 4 respectively. These control strategies have been tested worldwide and resulted in substantial economic gains, sometimes in excess of $100 per animal. With regard to mature female cattle, there is no scientific justification for a blanket recommendation to deworm all beef and dairy cows. There is no guarantee of an economic benefit to the producer or any certainty of increased milk production, conception rates, or calf weaning weights. Each farm should be considered individually, and there is no blanket recommendation that applies to all farms.

Fecal Egg Counts

Fecal egg counts may be of great value in assessing both the immune status and the degree of pasture contamination if they are used and interpreted correctly. Samples should be monitored at key periods by quantitative egg counts of fresh fecal samples from a representative number of animals from each age group. Samples from 5 to 6 animals per group are often adequate, but a wide variation in counts of the sampled animals would indicate the need to sample a larger group. Samples should be kept refrigerated at 4° C to prevent hatching of eggs before the egg counts are done. Fecal egg counts considered in relation to the history and management of the farm provide an ongoing evaluation of the success of the program, the efficacy of the drugs used, and the need for any changes to ensure low pasture contamination. If pasture contamination is kept low, susceptible cattle will never be exposed to infection levels that cause clinical or subclinical disease.

It is useful to take fecal samples at key times. These may include the day of treatment, to check if the previous treatment was successful in suppressing fecal egg counts for the full interval between treatments. If cattle have high counts in the hundreds or thousands, it is not much use suppressing egg counts for a brief period, and then allowing egg counts and

Table 3. CONTROL OPTIONS FOR DAIRY REPLACEMENT HEIFERS

Single RRD* at turnout to pasture
Non-ivermectin dewormers at 3 and 6 weeks after turnout
Ivermectin† 3 and 8 weeks after turnout
Single "treat-and-move" to safe pasture
Alternate grazing with other species

*Rumen retention device.
†Not approved for heifers of breeding age.

Table 4. CONTROL OPTIONS FOR BEEF WEANLINGS

Single RRD* at weaning time
Treatment at weaning time; repeat at 3-week intervals with non-ivermectin dewormers if needed
Treatment at weaning time; repeat at 5-week intervals with ivermectin if needed
Single "treat-and-move" to safe pasture
Alternate grazing with other species

*Rumen retention device.

pasture contamination to return to pretreatment levels. Another key time is when cattle are moved to a new pasture. If it is found that they have high counts, they should be treated to ensure that little contamination is carried into the new pasture. In this way, clean cattle going into a safe pasture may be protected for months, instead of a few days only. Adult cattle need fewer egg count checks than do young cattle because of their immunity to worms, but a suspected loss of immunity may be detected by a rise in egg counts. Fecal egg counts of young cattle are especially valuable in the postweaning period, when it is usually vital to give strategic treatments for keeping pasture contamination low.

Quantitative Techniques

A quantitative fecal flotation technique, such as the readily available modified McMaster (Paracount-EPG) technique, or the homemade Cornell-McMaster technique, is needed in large animal practice. These techniques are simple, fast, and easy to use. They should be a part of every large animal practice and are not for "research only"! The modified McMaster slide is commonly used to measure fecal egg counts as low as 25 eggs per gram, which is all that is needed for private practice, because any counts below this are epidemiologically insignificant. It should be remembered that only a small percentage of the eggs passed in feces successfully complete development to the infective stage. A modified McMaster slide with a sensitivity of 8 eggs per gram is also available. If a higher sensitivity is needed to detect low egg counts for adult cattle or for research projects, the more laborious Wisconsin double centrifugal-flotation technique can be used.

Fecal egg counts are of major value in measuring pasture contamination and the risk of serious infection but of limited value in estimating the number of worms in the animal. Fecal egg counts are of little diagnostic value in cattle except when they deviate from the expected pattern. Thus, adult cattle usually have very low fecal egg counts (<10 epg) and contribute little to pasture contamination because of a strong acquired immunity to worms. However, high counts in the hundreds could indicate an absence of immunity and the need for treatment and changes in management. The lack of correlation between worm numbers and fecal egg counts occurs for a variety of reasons including host immunity, worm fecundity, ratio of male to female worms, age of worms, diurnal and seasonal variations in egg laying, and the presence of hypobiotic or migrating larval stages, which have yet to reach the egg-laying stage.

In one study with 59 calves infected with *Ostertagia, Trichostrongylus*, and *Cooperia* spp. in Colorado, the ratio of worms to eggs per gram of feces ranged from 4 worms per egg to 2796 worms per egg. Striking differences may also occur in worm fecundity between species. Thus, a female *Haemonchus* may lay about 10,000 eggs per day, compared with only 100 to 200 per day for low producers like *Ostertagia* or *Trichostrongylus*, or 50 per day for *Nematodirus*. As many as 1 million hypobiotic *Ostertagia* larvae have been recovered from the

Table 5. ANTHELMINTICS APPROVED FOR CATTLE

Anthelmintic	Trade Name	Spectrum	Dosage (mg/kg)	Safety Index
Albendazole	Valbazen	Nematodes, cestodes, trematodes	10	10
Coumaphos*	Baymix	Trichostrongylid spp.	2 (6×)	4
Fenbendazole	Panacur, Safe-Guard	Nematodes, cestodes	5, 10	20
Ivermectin	Ivomec	Nematodes, arthropods	0.2	30
Ivermectin-clorsulon	Ivomec-F	Nematodes, arthropods, trematodes	0.2/7	5
Levamisole	Levasole, Tramisol	Nematodes	8	3
Morantel tartrate*	Nematel, Rumatel	Nematodes	10	30
Morantel tartrate*	Paratect bolus	Nematodes	RRD†	30
Oxfendazole	Synanthic	Nematodes, cestodes	4.5	50
Phenothiazine	Various	Nematodes	220	1
Thiabendazole*	TBZ, Omnizole	Nematodes	44	10

*Approved for lactating dairy cattle.
†Rumen retention device releases about 200 mg/day for 60 days.

abomasum of cattle with pre–type II ostertagiasis. These larvae have the potential to cause severe damage and death when they emerge from the gastric glands but do not betray their presence by worm eggs.

Anthelmintics

Anthelmintics approved for cattle are shown in Table 5. Most modern drugs have high efficacy against the important gastrointestinal nematodes of cattle, and several of them (levamisole, ivermectin, albendazole, fenbendazole, oxfendazole) are also effective against lungworms. Ivermectin is the most efficient drug against hypobiotic (arrested) larvae. The newer benzimidazole drugs (albendazole, fenbendazole, oxfendazole) also have some activity against hypobiotic larvae, but this is variable. The efficacy appears to depend on the degree of hypobiosis. It has been shown that oxfendazole (4.5 mg/kg) has high efficacy against hypobiotic larvae in the South during periods of hypobiotic induction (February–April) and emergence (August–September), but efficacy is low during periods of peak arrest (May–July). The variable efficacy of oxfendazole was correlated with expected changes in larval metabolic activity. The newer benzimidazole drugs are also effective against tapeworms, and one of them, albendazole, is effective against mature flukes. For full details on antiparasitic drugs, the reader is referred to Courtney and Sundlof (1990) listed in the bibliography.

A variety of new delivery systems have been developed in recent years to simplify bovine parasite control. These devices are summarized in Table 6. The individual animal devices have the advantage that every animal gets the correct dosage. This is important for ensuring maximum worm kill and reduction in pasture contamination. It also avoids selection for drug resistance due to suboptimal anthelmintic dosage. The group dosing systems have considerable appeal because labor is minimal and they sometimes allow a worm control program to be initiated where it was previously impossible. There is, however, a variable intake of drug, especially in heavily parasitized animals with reduced appetite or thirst. One cannot be certain that every animal gets the correct dosage, and there is a risk that suboptimal dosages will speed up selection for drug resistance. A review on this subject by the author is listed in the bibliography.

Serious concerns have been raised in recent years about the ecotoxicity of ivermectin. The drug is almost totally excreted in the feces, in which it has a prolonged half-life and high potency against both arthropods and nematodes, at extremely low concentrations. It has adverse effects on a vast number of beneficial and nonpestiferous arthropod species that are essential to the ecosystem. Most of the 250 invertebrate species found in cattle feces are useful and nonpestiferous and aid in dung degradation, soil aeration, humus content, water percolation, recycling of soil nutrients, and pasture productivity. Several workers have observed significant changes in the dung-degrading fauna and delayed dung degradation of feces from ivermectin-treated animals, with resultant reduction in grazing area. More research is required to determine if strategic treatments can be given at safe periods to reduce these adverse ecologic effects. Ivermectin contamination of water may also pose a wildlife threat, because it is toxic at extremely low concentrations; the LC_{50} for rainbow trout is only 0.003 ppm.

SHEEP

Sheep in temperate nonarid regions frequently suffer severe clinical disease and production losses from worm infection. Generally, ewes and lambs are most susceptible to helminth infection, whereas dry ewes and wethers are more resistant. Consequently, ewes and lambs (pre- and postweaning) should be given the highest priority in parasite control programs and safe grazing strategies. High concentrations of sheep at pasture and high fecal egg counts often lead to dangerous levels of pasture infectivity. The periparturient rise in fecal egg counts is particularly important in lambing ewes, reaching much higher levels than in cattle. Sheep are less able than are cattle to withstand the pathogenic effects of many thousands of worms, and serious outbreaks of helminthiasis are common in sheep. A disastrous situation may occur if parasitized sheep are kept on a low plane of nutrition.

Parasite control is most satisfactorily achieved by reducing the exposure of sheep to infection by the integration of strategic anthelmintic treatments and judicious pasture management. This is dependent on a knowledge of the epidemiology for each region. This is lacking in many areas of the United States, and there is an urgent need for more research of this type.

Table 6. NEW DELIVERY SYSTEMS

System	Anthelmintic
Individual Animal Administration—Correct dosage	
Rumen retention device	Morantel (Paratect, Paratect Flex)
Pour-ons	Levamisole (Totalon), Ivermectin (Ivomec)
Rumen injector	Oxfendazole (Synanthic)
Group Administration—Variable dosage	
Medicated feed block	Fenbendazole (En-pro-al, Safe-Guard)
Medicated drinking water	Various drugs (Dosetroff)

Major Parasites

The trichostrongylid worms constitute the most important group of sheep worms in the temperate regions of the world. Three genera, *Haemonchus*, *Ostertagia*, and *Trichostrongylus*, are the most abundant and most harmful in the Northern and Southern Hemispheres. They are responsible for severe production loss, clinical disease, and mortality. *Haemonchus contortus*, a voracious bloodsucker, is the most damaging species in warm and wet regions, becoming less important in the colder zones where *Ostertagia* and *Trichostrongylus* spp. predominate. Nevertheless, *H. contortus* is a major problem for sheep in the nonarid regions of both northern and southern United States.

Life Cycle and Turnover

The trichostrongylid worms of sheep have a simple and direct life cycle. Eggs passed in feces hatch and develop through free-living L_1–L_2–L_3 stages within a week under optimal conditions. *Nematodirus* is an exception in that free-living development takes place entirely within the egg shell, and hatching may be delayed until the following year. The trichostrongylid L_3 is the infective stage, and parasitic development from L_3 to egg-laying adult normally takes 2 to 4 weeks. Under certain conditions, development of *Haemonchus*, *Ostertagia*, and *Nematodirus* spp. in the gastrointestinal tract may be arrested at the early L_4 stage for several months and then resume development later when conditions are more favorable. As with the cattle nematodes, hypobiosis has important implications for epidemiology and control.

It appears that *Ostertagia* and *Haemonchus* spp. have a short adult life span of only about 1 month and a rapid population turnover. Because of this short life span, the number of worms present in the animal depends on the current intake of infective larvae from pasture. If the intake of L_3 is decreased, as when sheep are moved indoors or to drylot, their worm burdens will rapidly drop. However, anthelmintic treatment of animals that continue to be exposed to new infection at pasture will be of little value. It merely removes an adult population soon to be lost, and the lost worms are quickly replaced by new infection. Anthelmintic treatment gives better protection against long-lived species such as *Trichostrongylus*. Thus, a single anthelmintic treatment may remove a large adult population of *Trichostrongylus* spp. that has accumulated over a long period, and it would be only partly replaced when treated animals were returned to contaminated pasture.

Epidemiology

Seasonal Development of Infective Larvae

The sheep nematodes, like those of cattle, exhibit marked seasonal patterns of infectivity with only 1 or 2 disease-producing generations of worms per year. In Britain, Western Europe, and northern United States, most eggs passed in spring and early summer complete their development to infective L_3 in midsummer, which results in an explosive increase of pasture infectivity at that time. In a dry summer, this may be delayed until autumn rains occur. Pasture infectivity then persists at high levels until the following spring, when L_3 start to die because of rising temperatures. Although L_3 on pasture successfully persist through the winter, any contamination of pasture after September rarely results in significant new infections. In the Southern Hemisphere and southern United States, major accumulations of L_3 on pasture occur from autumn through spring but decline rapidly in summer.

The Periparturient Rise

The periparturient rise (PPR) appears to be of considerable importance in sheep and swine but is absent or moderate in horses and cattle. It has serious practical implications for sheep nematode control. It occurs any time from 2 weeks before lambing until 12 weeks after lambing, irrespective of the season of lambing. At this time, there is a general reduction in the immune response to worms, so that resistance to incoming larvae, controls on worm fecundity, and the capacity to expel worms are all diminished. It is suspected that lactogenic hormones are indirectly involved in bringing about these changes. The epidemiologic significance of the PPR is that it ensures heavy pasture contamination with worm eggs at the time of birth of the new host generation and transmission of worms from one host generation to the next. Although conditions may not be immediately suitable for the development of eggs to L_3, there may be a dangerous accumulation of L_3 later when lambs are relying less on milk and more on pasture.

Hypobiosis (Arrested Development)

Hypobiosis has important practical implications because it enables the parasite to survive in a dormant state in the host during adverse periods when there is a hostile immunologic environment or when its progeny would not survive in the outside environment. In contrast to the turnover of normally developing worms, arrested larvae tend to accumulate and may reach very large numbers, apparently unaffected by host immune responses. If a sudden resumption of development to adult worms occurs, it may produce a dramatic increase in pasture contamination and large worm burdens in the host at a time when pasture infectivity may be quite low. Hypobiotic larvae are also of practical importance because they are unaffected by some anthelmintics.

A marked degree of winter hypobiosis has been observed in sheep in northern United States, with almost the entire worm burden of *H. contortus* (98 to 100 per cent), *O. circumcincta* (89 to 98 per cent), and *N. filicollis* (77 to 90 per cent) affected. At this time, the adult worm population was limited almost exclusively to *Trichostrongylus* spp. It appears that *Trichostrongylus* spp. have a long adult life span, which allows transmission from year to year, whereas *O. circumcincta* and *H. contortus* have short life spans and a greater reliance on survival from year to year in the hypobiotic state. Hypobiosis is especially important to *H. contortus*, whose free-living stages survive poorly on pasture during winter. There is little information available on the occurrence of hypobiosis in sheep in southern states.

Host Immunity

Immune competence against gastrointestinal helminth infection is slow to develop in sheep and may not be fully expressed until about 9 months of age. Thus, young sheep on infected pastures generally acquire heavy infections and exacerbate the situation by shedding large numbers of eggs in the feces. Although sheep eventually develop a strong resistance to *Nematodirus* spp. and moderate resistance to *Trichostrongylus* spp., resistance to *Haemonchus* and *Ostertagia* spp. is more labile, and outbreaks can occur in sheep of all ages. Immunologic unresponsiveness has been observed in the neonate, the periparturient ewe, and the nutritionally deprived. A genetic approach based on selection for responsiveness in young animals may offer the best approach to improvement of immunologic responsiveness of young animals to parasite antigens.

Pathogenesis

Infection with *H. contortus* results in anemia and hypoproteinemia owing to the voracious blood-sucking activities of adults and fourth-stage larvae (L_4). Sudden death may occur as a result of severe blood loss. In addition, the migration of larvae into the pits of the gastric glands and the attachment of adult worms to the mucosa cause abomasitis. There is a significant rise in abomasal pH and plasma pepsinogen levels soon after infection, but not to the same levels as those seen in ostertagiasis. The activities of the parasite are believed to interfere with the digestibility and absorption of protein, calcium, and phosphorus. In chronic cases, death may result from exhaustion of protein and iron stores.

The other trichostrongylid worms have a variety of effects. The pathogenesis of ostertagiasis type I and type II is similar to that described for cattle. *T. axei* causes abomasitis, whereas *Trichostrongylus* and *Nematodirus* spp. in the small intestine cause villous atrophy and plasma leakage into the intestine. Anorexia is an important feature and exacerbates the hypoproteinemia resulting from the protein-losing enteropathy. Deficiencies in digestion and absorption may be partly due to the loss of enzymes normally found on the microvilli, which results when villous atrophy occurs. Most sheep acquire multiple infections, and there is evidence of a synergistic effect between *O. circumcincta* and *T. colubriformis*, so that the combined effects are more pathogenic than one would expect from the sum of the effects of the 2 parasites given alone.

Clinical Disease

Sheep infected with *H. contortus* may die suddenly without showing clinical signs, especially if they have been driven. The main signs are marked anemia with pale skin and mucous membranes, anorexia, submandibular edema, and weakness. When driven, affected sheep may lag behind, stagger, go down, then rise and walk a little farther after rest. In most cases, there is no diarrhea; feces are drier and harder than normal and greatly reduced in quantity. In chronic cases, there is extreme weight loss, and the fleece may be lost. Sheep infected with other trichostrongylid worms show anorexia, ill-thrift, weight loss, diarrhea, dehydration, staggering, weakness, recumbency, and death. In some cases, there is a black scour. Lamb and yearling flocks are most seriously affected, and once mortality starts, a few animals may die each day.

Diagnosis

Gastrointestinal parasites are the most likely cause of ill-thrift and diarrhea in sheep and should always be considered, especially in sheep suffering malnutrition. Diarrhea without ill-thrift or loss of condition is not often due to worms. A detailed history including age, sex, reproductive status, likely immune status, managerial practices, and anthelmintic treatments is helpful in arriving at an accurate diagnosis.

Fecal egg counts are a useful aid to diagnosis in sheep under 12 months of age, but it is dangerous to make a diagnosis on the basis of a fecal egg count alone. A total worm count at necropsy should be done wherever possible. The trichostrongylid worms are fine, hairlike worms that can be easily missed by a cursory inspection, even when many thousands are present. In addition to examining aliquots of abomasal and intestinal contents under the microscope, it is desirable to examine digests of the abomasal wall for larval stages. The interpretation of the total worm count must take into consideration the fact that different species are pathogenic at different levels. Thus 1000 *H. contortus* may be just as pathogenic as 10,000 *O. circumcincta*.

Control Strategies

Many control programs are guided by guesswork, convenience, or desperation after mortality occurs, and they ignore reinfection, the PPR, hypobiosis, and selection for drug resistance. Many control programs give sheep a few days without worms before the process of reinfection returns their worm burdens to pretreatment levels. At that stage, over 95 per cent of the total worm population is likely to be in the environment, so that treatment removes less than 5 per cent of all worms, and sheep are subject to immediate reinfection. These haphazard treatments may stop some deaths, but they do not stop production losses. For reducing worm burdens on a more permanent basis, it is necessary either to give repeated anthelmintic treatments at short intervals (e.g., every 2 weeks) or to reduce the rate of infection by some form of integrated control combining the prophylactic use of anthelmintics with appropriate grazing management. The latter approach is preferable because it involves less drug cost, less labor cost, and less selection pressure for the evolution of drug resistance.

The modern epidemiologic strategies are summarized hereafter.

Prelambing Treatments

This is a key strategy for lambing ewes for the prevention of the potentially damaging PPR and clinical or subclinical disease in both ewes and lambs. When treatment is given to ewes in winter in northern regions, it is essential to use an anthelmintic (e.g., levamisole, ivermectin) that is effective against hypobiotic larvae, thus preventing maturation to adults and participation in the PPR. This treatment can be given at the time of winter housing or at any convenient period before the ewes go out to spring pasture. The object is to prevent them from contaminating spring pasture with worm eggs. Late-lambing ewes will require a second treatment just before or at lambing if they have already grazed spring pasture contaminated with overwintered larvae. In the case of both early- and late-lambing ewes, good results will be obtained only if ewes are kept indoors or in drylots or are moved to safe pastures after treatment for avoidance of immediate reinfection. These strategies do not work well if ewes are maintained on contaminated pastures. The "safe pasture" concept is discussed next.

Turnout of Lambs to Safe Pasture with No Treatment

Lambs raised indoors in a relatively parasite-free environment can be turned out to a safe pasture without the need for any anthelmintic treatment. A safe pasture is not necessarily "clean" or free of infective larvae, but is one in which infectivity is sufficiently low that the worm burdens of susceptible stock moved to it increase slowly. Regrowth after mechanical harvesting of hay, silage, or small grain crops can generally be considered safe. The use of electric fencing may facilitate maximal exploitation of safe pastures on many farms. Pastures previously grazed by cattle or other species are generally safe because of the small amount of cross-infection between species. Nevertheless, calves less than 6 months of age are susceptible to *H. contortus*. Rotational grazing is usually not effective for parasite control because of the prolonged survival of infective larvae on contaminated pastures.

Prophylactic Treatment in Spring in Northern Regions

The advantage of prophylactic treatment in the spring is that it prevents the occurrence of the summer build-up of pasture infectivity and resulting clinical and subclinical disease. When market lambs or ewe lamb replacements are turned out to spring pasture, they are immediately exposed to L_3 that have survived over winter on pasture. Suckling lambs acquire infection from progeny of hypobiotic worms carried by ewes in winter as well as from overwintered L_3. By midsummer, they may be exposed to a massive build-up of second-generation worms and clinical helminthiasis.

Studies in Ohio showed that 4 treatments at 3-week intervals, starting 3 weeks after spring turnout, were just as effective as 8 treatments at 3-week intervals for the entire grazing season. It was obvious that the early-season treatments were highly beneficial, whereas the late-season treatments were a waste of time and money. Studies in Ohio also demonstrated the value of prophylactic treatments in the spring for horses and dairy replacement heifers. In all 3 host-parasite systems, this strategy prevents the escalation of second-generation (disease-producing) worms.

Treat-and-Move Strategies

The rationale of this strategy is to extend the effectiveness of a single treatment by moving animals to a safe pasture to limit reinfection. Thus, if sheep are treated by July 1 and moved to a safe pasture in northern regions, they are unlikely to be exposed to the summer explosion in pasture infectivity. If they are treated and left on the same pasture, they will be exposed to heavy reinfection and derive little benefit from treatment. Thus, the move to a safe pasture is the key factor in this strategy. If a flock is moved to a safe pasture after treatment, it will enjoy several months of low worm burdens rather than only 2 or 3 worm-free days as the result of treatment alone. Infected sheep should not be allowed to graze a safe pasture; they must be treated before being allowed to graze. The treatment serves 2 purposes: it removes a potentially harmful worm burden from the sheep, and it protects a safe pasture from new contamination.

In the Ohio studies, this strategy initially worked well, but a marked rise in pasture infectivity was observed in early October. It appeared that there had been a build-up of *H. contortus* larvae aided by the high fecundity of this parasite and late-season rains favorable for development and survival of the free-living stages. It was concluded that a single treat-and-move strategy would provide safe pasture for a sufficiently long period for lambs to be marketed early, but a double treat-and-move system would be needed for lambs at pasture for longer periods of time. The latter would involve 2 anthelmintic treatments administered about 6 to 8 weeks apart and the use of 2 pastures ungrazed by sheep that year. There is a need to study the selection pressure for drug resistance with this system because it can be argued that the safe pasture may eventually become populated with the progeny of resistant survivors.

Anthelmintics

There are only 4 anthelmintics approved for use in sheep in the United States (ivermectin, levamisole, phenothiazine, thiabendazole) and 2 for goats (phenothiazine, thiabendazole). Sheep or goat nematodes have now developed resistance to all of these drugs in the United States. Widespread benzimidazole and phenothiazine resistance over many years led to excessive reliance on ivermectin and levamisole, with eventual selection for resistance to these drugs as well. The situation is likely to get worse in the future, although a new drug, moxidectin,* has shown high efficacy against *H. contortus*

---
*Available from American Cyanamid.

resistant to ivermectin in Texas. The use of anthelmintics approved for horses or cattle, but not sheep, is no solution to the problem. This is because of cross-resistance between levamisole and morantel (i.e., worms resistant to levamisole are resistant to morantel) and side-resistance between all benzimidazole and pro-benzimidazole drugs (albendazole, cambendazole, febantel, fenbendazole, mebendazole, netobimin, oxfendazole, thiabendazole). A cross-resistance between phenothiazine and benzimidazole drugs may explain why benzimidazole resistance occurred so quickly after thiabendazole superseded the use of phenothiazine in the early 1960s.

The future outlook for worm control of sheep and goats is bleak, unless action is taken to abandon traditional approaches and to develop new chemical and nonchemical strategies with less selection for drug resistance. The first need on any farm is to determine whether anthelmintic resistance has already occurred. The simplest way for the practitioner to do this is to do the fecal egg reduction test, which can be simply done with use of the McMaster slide kit described in the cattle section. Basically, fresh fecal samples from a representative sample of each test group (at least 5 animals per group) are counted for worm eggs at the time of treatment and 10 to 14 days later. If the interval is less than 10 days, the suppressive effects of drugs on worm egg production (without killing worms) may result in an overestimation of drug efficacy. If the interval is greater than 14 days, there is time for sheep to become reinfected and shed eggs from new worms. Modern broad-spectrum anthelmintics should cause a fecal egg reduction of at least 90 per cent if they are working effectively. This test gives the practitioner a good indication of resistance, but larval cultures, in vitro tests, and total worm counts at necropsy are needed for a complete evaluation.

The following strategies will help conserve anthelmintic efficacy and limit the drug resistance problem.

1. *Avoiding anthelmintic overkill at all times.* Suppressive treatment programs dosing sheep every 2 to 4 weeks will eliminate susceptible worms but leave only resistant worms to contaminate pastures.

2. *Developing strategic treatment programs as outlined in the preceding.* Fewer treatments, epidemiologically based, will be just as effective for worm control, be more economic than continuous treatments, and have reduced selection for drug resistance.

3. *Taking care in selecting the anthelmintic.* It is a waste of time and money to use a drug if worms have already developed resistance to it. This is where the fecal egg reduction test is useful. Remember, there may also be side-resistance to a string of related drugs, or cross-resistance to unrelated drugs that share a common mode of action.

4. *Using full anthelmintic dosage.* It is better to set the dosage for the heaviest animal rather than for the average animal of the group, in order to avoid underdosing of some animals. Reduced dosages are likely to allow survival of worms with partial resistance (heterozygotes). They may then mate with similar worms, producing offspring that are highly resistant (homozygotes).

5. *Treating all introductions.* Sheep from an outside farm with a resistance problem may introduce resistant worms to a clean farm. Double dosages or a combination of 2 anthelmintics may be a useful safeguard.

6. *Avoiding prolonged drug encounter.* This can occur with licks, blocks, or small-dose sustained-release rumen retention devices that have a gradual "tailing off" of drug concentration. It may also occur with ivermectin because of its persistence at low concentrations for several weeks after treatment.

7. *Rotation of anthelmintics.* An annual rotation of drugs of different chemical families (e.g., ivermectin, levamisole,

benzimidazoles) is recommended because frequent rotation of anthelmintic types has led to the selection of multiple drug resistance in the past. Do not include any drugs in the rotation to which worms have already developed resistance, or any drugs that are side- or cross-resistant.

8. *Synergism of anthelmintics.* Combinations of drugs sometimes result in synergistic increases in efficacy. For example, the experimental administration of both levamisole and mebendazole in sheep resulted in improved efficacy against benzimidazole-resistant worms in Australia. Chemical modification of existing drugs and novel delivery systems may also be used to enhance drug efficacy in the future.

9. *Breeding genetically resistant hosts.* New techniques of embryo splitting and transfer introduce the possibility of accelerating the selection of flocks genetically resistant to parasites. Heritability of resistance to worms appears to be high, and associations have been found between acquired resistance and certain lymphocyte antigen markers.

10. *Worming vaccines for sheep.* Several antigens of *H. contortus* and *T. colubriformis* have been identified as host protective and are being genetically engineered before their assessment in vaccination trials.

11. *Biologic controls of nematodes.* Studies with both dung beetles and nematode-killing fungi have given promising results and warrant further examination.

12. *Management strategies.* Lambing ewes, suckling lambs, and weanlings are the most susceptible to worms, whereas dry ewes and wethers are more resistant. It is therefore desirable to design management systems that save the safest pastures for the most susceptible groups. Movement of sheep to safe pastures, drylot, or indoors after pastures become highly infective is of more value than are anthelmintic treatments. Alternate grazing with cattle induces the same parasitologic benefits as leaving pastures ungrazed for long periods, but without the economic or agronomic disadvantages. Dry ewes and wethers, more resistant to worms, might be used in place of cattle. Alternate grazing with different animal species can provide excellent parasite control, whereas rotational grazing with a single species is of little or no value.

GOATS

The major nematode pathogens of sheep are also the major pathogens of goats, and recommendations for parasite control in goats are frequently based on data obtained in sheep. This approach is not always the most effective, because it ignores differences in management, grazing habits, epidemiology, and the pharmacokinetics of anthelmintics. Parasites are a minor problem where goats browse bushy herbage and avoid grazing close to the ground. Haemonchosis is a major problem where goats graze pasture in warm, humid areas, particularly in the South. *Ostertagia* is more important in northern and central states; *Trichostrongylus* spp. contribute to helminthiasis in both northern and southern regions. Signs of helminthiasis include anorexia, ill-thrift, weight loss, anemia, diarrhea, rough coat, and mortality. Angora goats appear to be especially susceptible to gastrointestinal nematodes under intense grazing conditions.

Suppressive anthelmintic treatment with a variety of dewormers is often relied upon during the peak transmission season but may lead to multiple drug resistance. It would be more logical to initiate some of the prophylactic strategies described for sheep so that better parasite control and production gains are obtained with less selection for drug resistance. These strategies include preparturient treatments for preventing the PPR, prophylactic treatments in spring in northern regions, and treat-and-move strategies with movement to safe pastures. This ensures protection for several months instead of several days. Safe pastures, such as regrowth after harvesting, provide safe grazing. This is not the case with rotational grazing, in which parasite populations may even be increased. However, improved nutritional status due to rotational grazing may help offset the deleterious effects of increased parasite numbers. Exposure to most nematodes is minimal with goats in confinement, but coccidiosis and *Strongyloides* infection are likely to be problems in nonimmune kids.

Anthelmintics

Goat owners face a special dilemma in the selection of effective anthelmintics for worm control for the following reasons.

1. Only 2 anthelmintics are approved for goats in the United States. These 2 drugs (thiabendazole, phenothiazine) both have a serious drug resistance problem, and they have been superseded by modern drugs.

2. The problems of drug resistance discussed for sheep are also applicable to goats and may be even more serious for goats.

3. It appears that goats metabolize some anthelmintics more rapidly than sheep do, so that higher dosages are needed than for sheep.

4. Poor results from underdosing goats with sheep dosages may sometimes have been mistakenly attributed to drug resistance.

5. On the other hand, the repeated use of low (sheep) dosages for goats is likely to have enhanced the selection for drug resistance.

6. The first report of ivermectin resistance in the United States appears to have been in Angora goats in east Texas after intensive ivermectin treatment at a dosage of 0.2 mg/kg for 5 years.

There is clearly a need for more research into the pharmacokinetics of anthelmintics in goats as well as for the development of alternative parasite control strategies based on nonchemical methods.

SWINE

Nematode parasites remain a serious limiting factor to successful swine production, although the prevalence and intensity of infection vary with the region, type of housing, and management system. An increasing trend for total confinement of pigs has been associated with a decline in the incidence of the stomach worms *(Hyostrongylus, Ascarops, Physocephalus)* as well as the thorny-headed worm *(Macracanthorhynchus hirudinaceus)* and lungworm *(Metastrongylus* spp.). However, the prevalence of some parasites in confined swine is as high as that in pastured swine. Problems often persist because of the incorrect choice of anthelmintics, inappropriate timing of treatment, and lack of fecal monitoring. In some regions, an increased incidence of *Strongyloides* has been associated with a change to permanent farrowing houses and liberal use of bedding.

Three intestinal species, *Ascaris suum, Oesophagostomum* spp., and *Trichuris suis*, remain as serious pathogens in swine both in confinement and at pasture. Newborn pigs in some areas suffer high mortality from *Strongyloides ransomi* transmitted via the colostrum. Liver condemnations due to *Ascaris suum* and *Stephanurus dentatus* have increased in some regions, and the stigma of trichinosis still persists over the swine industry in the United States.

Life Cycle and Epidemiology

Pigs become infected with ascarids *(Ascaris suum)* by ingestion of infective eggs. After hatching, L_3 penetrate the gut wall and commence the typical ascarid hepatic-tracheal migration. They reach the liver via the portal vein within 24 hours of infection, then pass via the blood stream to the heart and lungs. Larvae reach the lungs about a week after infection, break out of the capillaries into the alveoli, molt to L_4, and migrate up the bronchioles, bronchi, and trachea. They are coughed up and swallowed, molt to L_5 in the small intestine, develop to maturity, and pass eggs in the feces 6 to 8 weeks after infection. Female *Ascaris suum* produce enormous numbers of eggs, up to half a million eggs/worm/day. The eggs become infective in 10 to 30 days under optimal conditions and are very resistant to external conditions, remaining viable for up to 5 years if protected from desiccation.

Pigs become infected with the nodular worm *(Oesophagostomum* spp.) by ingestion of an infective larva (L_3). These invade the intestinal wall and are found in the mucosa and submucosa of the large intestine as early as 20 hours after infection. The third molt occurs in the gut wall, L_4 return to the gut lumen, molt to L_5, develop to maturity, and pass strongyle-type eggs in the feces 7 to 8 weeks after infection. There is little host reaction to primary infection, but nodule formation may be marked in subsequent infections of sensitized animals. Sows commonly exhibit a periparturient rise in fecal egg counts, reaching a peak 6 to 7 weeks after farrowing. Newborn pigs may be exposed to serious infection, because eggs can develop to infective L_3 within a week under optimal conditions.

The whipworm *(Trichuris suis)* life cycle is unusual in that eggs carry an infective L_1 (not L_3) when ingested by swine, and all larval molts occur within the host. Larvae spend 2 to 3 weeks migrating within the cecal and colonic mucosa before reaching the surface epithelium and maturing to egg-laying adults 6 to 7 weeks after infection. The long filamentous anterior end of the adult worm remains imbedded in the mucosa, forming subepithelial tunnels. The characteristic barrel-shaped, double operculated eggs become infective 3 weeks after being passed and can survive for up to 6 years in protected environments.

The threadworm *(Strongyloides ransomi)* can alternate between a free-living and a parasitic existence. Pigs may be infected prenatally, via colostrum, by ingestion of L_3, or by skin penetration of L_3. Transcolostral infection appears to be of considerable importance, with the greatest number of L_3 passed on the first day of lactation. Counts up to 50 L_3/ml of colostrum have been recorded. Sows apparently harbor arrested L_3 in their fat depots until farrowing time, when they migrate to the milk cisterns of the mammae. Sufficient larvae may be stored in the fat deposits of the sow to infect 4 consecutive litters. The prepatent period is only 4 days after prenatal or transcolostral infection and 7 to 10 days after other routes of infection. Embryonated eggs or L_1 are passed in the feces, and the parasite persists indefinitely in muddy areas.

Pathogenesis

Penetration of the intestinal mucosa by nematode larvae *(Ascaris, Oesophagostomum, Trichuris, Strongyloides)* or tunnelling by adults *(Trichuris)* provides a portal of entry for bacteria, spirochetes, and viruses. Further migration within the gut wall may cause extensive destruction of tissue *(Trichuris, Strongyloides)* or a host nodular reaction, caseation, and calcification *(Oesophagostomum)* leading to interference with digestion and motility. Local peritonitis and adhesions sometimes result in intussusception or necrosis. Emergence of whipworm *(Trichuris)* larvae may produce dysentery 3 weeks after infection, well before eggs are passed in the feces, and be misdiagnosed as swine dysentery or proliferative enteritis. These parasitic cases do not respond to antibiotic therapy. Outbreaks of necrotic enteritis may be activated in pigs carrying *Salmonella* infections.

Migration of larvae through the liver *(Ascaris)* may result in interstitial hepatitis or "milk spots" and cause large-scale condemnation of livers at abattoirs. Larvae of gastrointestinal nematodes migrating through the lungs *(Ascaris, Strongyloides)* cause alveolar injury with edema and consolidation. Pigs become more susceptible to other diseases such as enzootic pneumonia and swine influenza. Severe gastric ulcers with fatal bleeding have been associated with both experimental and natural infection of *A. suum*, although the underlying mechanisms are not clear. Anemia sometimes occurs in pigs heavily infected with *Trichuris* as a result of blood-sucking and tissue destruction. Hypoproteinemia may be associated with any parasite where there is marked anorexia or a protein-losing enteropathy. Death of young pigs sometimes results from invasion of the myocardium by skin-penetrating *Strongyloides*.

Clinical Disease

Ascariasis may be manifest in young pigs by ill-thrift, stunted growth, pot belly, and diarrhea. Adult worms may be vomited. Occasional cases of obstructive jaundice or intestinal obstruction and rupture occur. Larvae migrating through the lungs may cause "thumps" and elicit a soft cough. Nodular worms may cause weight loss and diarrhea in pigs of all ages but rarely death. The diarrhea is often khaki in color and contains undigested food. There may be a blood-stained mucoid diarrhea if massive numbers of larvae penetrate the gut wall. The bloody diarrhea of whipworm infection, starting 3 weeks after infection, may be confused with swine dysentery or proliferative enteritis. Affected pigs may also show anorexia, weight loss, straining, rectal prolapse, and a high mortality rate. Newborn pigs with a heavy threadworm infection may show stunted growth, pot belly, bloody diarrhea, and a high mortality rate.

Diagnosis

The history, clinical signs, fecal examinations, and response to treatment are likely to be of value in making a correct diagnosis. The age of the affected pigs and their likely exposure to infective eggs or larvae are important considerations. Ascariasis is a disease of young pigs, and older animals rarely show clinical signs although they may be an important source of contamination. Strongyloidiasis is mainly confined to baby pigs and may result from prenatal or transcolostral infection as well as from L_3 in the environment. The major nematode species *(Ascaris, Oesophagostomum, Trichuris)* have a prepatent period of 6 to 8 weeks, and it is possible for clinical signs to develop before the characteristic thick-shelled eggs *(Ascaris)*, strongyle-type eggs *(Oesophagostomum)*, or double operculated eggs *(Trichuris)* are passed in feces. By contrast, the smaller embryonated eggs of *Strongyloides* may be passed as early as 4 days after infection.

Fecal examinations are of value in determining which parasites are a major problem, but there is a poor correlation between fecal egg counts and worm burden. A small number of *Ascaris* females may produce millions of eggs, whereas *Trichuris* females are not prolific egg layers, and a low or modest egg count may be associated with severe disease. The most positive way to make a diagnosis is by necropsy examination so that the intensity of the worm infection and the degree of tissue destruction can be accurately assessed.

Control Strategies

The North Carolina Swine Parasite Control Program or its modifications can be used effectively in many regions. In this program, sows and gilts are given a broad-spectrum anthelmintic 5 to 10 days before breeding and again 5 to 10 days before farrowing for removing parasites from their digestive system, which serve as a source of the PPR and infection in the farrowing house. Boars are treated twice a year. Young pigs are treated at 5 to 6 weeks of age, and treatment is repeated 30 days later. Anthelmintics to consider include dichlorvos, levamisole, or ivermectin as single treatments, fenbendazole for 3 to 12 days, and pyrantel tartrate or hygromycin B as continuous additives to the feed during the period of greatest risk. Swine should be kept on well-drained open lots, on temporary pastures, or on clean concrete or slats. Treatment is normally not needed for pigs in a clean operation on raised decks, but treatment of breeders once yearly offers a safeguard against accidental infection.

A major control problem is the great survival capacity of ascarid and whipworm eggs. Sometimes the only solution is to move range pigs to fresh ground and cultivate the old ground for at least 3 years before reintroducing swine. In housing, thorough cleansing with hot detergents or high-pressure water can be used to prepare surfaces for disinfection with agents such as hot lye (95 per cent sodium hydroxide). The disinfectant should be applied to walls and left for 2 to 3 days and then hosed away before pigs are returned. It is advisable to scrub sows thoroughly with hot detergent and water to remove eggs before moving them into a farrowing pen that has been cleaned and disinfected. Sows should also be treated a few days before they enter the farrowing pen so that feces containing viable eggs and expelled worms will not be introduced. Likewise, if young pigs are to be returned to pasture after treatment, it is preferable to confine them on concrete for 1 to 2 days, and to destroy all feces and expelled worms before they are returned to pasture.

Feeder pigs can be given single treatments or continuous feed medication with pyrantel tartrate or hygromycin B. Where pigs are run on dirt and subject to continuous reinfection, it is more effective to provide a continuous feed additive. Baby pigs should be treated with thiabendazole, levamisole, or ivermectin at 5 and 10 days of age if threadworm (*Strongyloides*) is a problem. It is imperative to keep breeding stock on dry, well-drained surfaces, because *Strongyloides* is capable of reproducing in a free-living cycle and will persist indefinitely in muddy areas. If swine kidney worm (*Stephanurus dentatus*) is a problem, both adult and larval stages can be killed by fenbendazole and adults by levamisole. The "gilt only" farrowing system may also be considered, but it has the disadvantage of producing smaller litters.

Anthelmintics

Modern swine anthelmintics have high efficacy, high safety, and easy administration. Swine anthelmintics have high efficacy against the major parasites (Table 7). Most are adminis-

Table 7. MODERN ANTHELMINTICS APPROVED FOR SWINE

Parasite	Anthelmintic	Efficacy
Large roundworm (*Ascaris*)	Dichlorvos	95–100
	Fenbendazole*	95–100
	Hygromycin B	95–100
	Ivermectin	95–100
	Levamisole	95–100
	Pyrantel	95–100
Nodular worm (*Oesophagostomum*)	Dichlorvos	95–100
	Fenbendazole	95–100
	Hygromycin B	95–100
	Ivermectin	95–100
	Pyrantel	95–100
	Levamisole	80–100
Whipworm (*Trichuris*)	Dichlorvos	90–100
	Fenbendazole*	90–100
	Hygromycin B	85–100
Lungworm (*Metastrongylus*)	Fenbendazole	95–100
	Ivermectin	95–100
	Levamisole	90–100
Threadworm (*Strongyloides*)	Ivermectin†	95–100
	Thiabendazole	95–100
	Levamisole	80–95
Kidney worm (*Stephanurus*)	Fenbendazole	100 (adult and larvae)
	Levamisole	80–100 (adult only)

*Fenbendazole is effective against migrating ascarid larvae in the liver and lungs, and migrating whipworm larvae in the cecal and colonic mucosa.
†Ivermectin is effective against somatic *Strongyloides* L_3 so that treatment of sows 3 to 16 days before parturition prevents transfer of larvae from dam to piglets via the colostrum.

tered in the feed, but levamisole can also be given in the drinking water. Ivermectin is approved only for subcutaneous injection. A high safety index is essential when swine are treated on a herd basis and there is variation in individual drug consumption rates. The safety of dichlorvos, the only organophosphate approved for swine, has been enhanced by incorporation of the drug into slow-release resin pellets. Cataracts and deafness may occur in swine fed hygromycin B for prolonged periods. At 3 times the recommended dosage, transient salivation and vomiting may occur in pigs given levamisole. Coughing and vomiting may also occur as pigs infected with lungworms expel the parasites. Fenbendazole and ivermectin are both safe in swine, and there are no contraindications except for an 18-day withdrawal period for ivermectin.

BIBLIOGRAPHY

Armour J, Ogbourne CP: Bovine Ostertagiasis: A Review and Annotated Bibliography. Miscellaneous Publication No. 7 of the Commonwealth Institute of Parasitology, Commonwealth Agricultural Bureaux, Farnham Royal, Bucks, England, 1982, pp 1–93.
Blood DC, Radostits OM: Veterinary Medicine, 7th ed. London, Baillière Tindall, 1989, pp 1016–1070.
Courtney CH, Sundlof SF: AAVP Antiparasitic Drugs: A Comprehensive Compendium of FDA-Approved Antiparasitic Drugs. Gainesville, University of Florida, 1990.
Gibbs HC, Herd RP, Murrell KD (eds): Parasites: epidemiology and control. Vet Clin North Am [Food Anim Pract] 2:205–505, 1986.
Herd RP: New delivery systems simplify bovine worm control. Mod Vet Pract 69:85–91, 1988.
Herd RP: Cattle practitioner: vital role in worm control. Compend Contin Educ Pract Vet 13:879–888, 1991.

Tematode Infections in Cattle, Sheep, and Goats

R. P. HERD, MVSc, PhD

Fasciola hepatica is the most important trematode of livestock throughout the world. It is an increasing problem as new dams, irrigation projects, and improved water facilities provide new habitats for the lymnaeid snail intermediate hosts. Acute fluke disease causes high mortality in sheep, whereas chronic fluke disease causes substantial production losses in both cattle and sheep. Several studies suggest that effective control can result in increased mature cow body weights, conception rates, milk production, and calf weaning weights. Feedlot studies have demonstrated increased weight gains and feed conversion rates, with reduced liver rejection rates at abattoirs.

In the United States, *F. hepatica* occurs primarily in the Gulf Coast states and western states, whereas *F. gigantica* occurs in Hawaii. *Fascioloides magna* is an additional problem in the Gulf Coast states, Great Lakes region, and northwestern states where cattle, sheep, or goats share pastures with deer, elk, and moose natural hosts. *Dicrocoelium dendriticum*, the small black lanceolate fluke, is restricted to foci in New York State. The paramphistomes, or rumen flukes, appear to be of minor economic significance in the United States, although heavy infections can cause severe enteritis and mortality in cattle and occasionally in sheep and goats elsewhere. *Paramphistomum microbothrioides* (syn. *Cotylophoron cotylophorum*) is the most common species in the United States.

LIFE CYCLE

Trematodes have an indirect life cycle with a snail intermediate host. *F. hepatica*, *F. gigantica*, *F. magna*, and *P. microbothrioides* all have aquatic snail intermediate hosts. *D. dendriticum* has a land snail as its first intermediate host and a brown ant as its second intermediate host. One fluke egg passed by the cattle, sheep, or goat final host can give rise to thousands of infective cercariae or metacercariae. This has great epidemiologic importance and is in marked contrast to the situation with nematodes, in which 1 egg produces only 1 infective larva. Eggs of *Fasciola*, *Fascioloides*, and *Paramphistomum* spp. hatch in water to miracidia, which develop through sporocyst, redia, and cercaria stages after miracidia actively penetrate the appropriate snail intermediate host. Cercariae later emerge from the snail and encyst as metacercariae on herbage to be eaten by the final host. Eggs of *Dicrocoelium* are ingested by land snails, which later expel slime balls containing up to 400 cercariae. Whole colonies of brown ants may become infected by eating slime balls. The final host is infected by ingesting ants attached to herbage.

Most livestock are infected by ingestion of metacercariae from pasture, although prenatal infection with *F. hepatica* has been reported in a small percentage of calves. Metacercariae encyst in the small intestine, and young flukes migrate through the gut wall and peritoneal cavity to reach the liver in 4 to 6 days. They migrate in the hepatic parenchyma for 6 to 8 weeks, then enter the bile ducts and mature to egg-laying adults 10 to 12 weeks after infection. The life cycle of *F. gigantica* is similar to that of *F. hepatica*. *F. magna* completes the full life cycle only in deer, elk, or moose natural hosts. Adults are enclosed in thin-walled cysts in the hepatic parenchyma, and eggs escape via fistulae to the bile ducts. In cattle, young flukes become completely encapsulated by a host reaction in the liver, and there is no channel for release of eggs to the exterior. Thus diagnosis is not possible by fecal examination. In sheep and goats, young flukes tunnel extensively, causing severe damage to the parenchyma and ultimately host death. Immature paramphistomes develop in the duodenal mucosa but migrate through the abomasum to the rumen and reticulum as they mature. *Dicrocoelium* migrates up the bile ducts from the duodenum and matures in the bile ducts and gallbladder without invading the liver parenchyma.

EPIDEMIOLOGY

The initiation of effective trematode control programs and the proper timing of treatment are dependent on an understanding of the epidemiology of the disease. Livestock most likely to be affected with *F. hepatica* are those grazing in low-lying swampy areas, flood irrigation areas, or anywhere that surface water or small, slowly moving streams favor the propagation of lymnaeid snails. *F. hepatica* can survive for many years in sheep and shed up to 50,000 eggs per day, but cattle develop resistance and expel most flukes within a year. Cattle appear to have a degree of natural resistance to liver fluke as well as an ability to develop acquired immunity, whereas sheep and goats seem to be lacking in both. Pastures become infective with metacercariae as early as 2 months after being grazed by infected livestock. Metacercariae may survive on pastures for up to 1 year but die within 2 weeks under hot dry conditions. Housed animals will be protected against the disease unless they are fed hay with sufficient moisture to enable metacercariae to survive. Metacercariae are killed by ensilage.

In the Gulf Coast, warm and wet conditions in mild winters, spring, and early summer are highly favorable for massive proliferation of snails, hatching of fluke eggs, and development of cercariae within snails. Most fluke transmission occurs between the months of February and July. Transmission ceases with death of eggs, snails, and metacercariae in the first sustained drought of summer. By autumn, flukes transmitted in the spring are egg-laying adults and fully susceptible to approved flukicides. The extent of production losses is influenced by the level of nutrition and concurrent nematode infections. In the Gulf Coast states, peak fluke burdens, adult *Ostertagia* burdens, and nutritional stress may all coincide in the winter. Whereas warm, wet conditions favor snail and fluke proliferation, cold winter conditions (below 10° C) inhibit their reproduction. In some regions of the Pacific Northwest, peak fluke transmission is delayed because of death of metacercariae and infected snails during the freezing winter. Although the summers are of a semiarid nature, flood irrigation of pastures provides ample moisture for summer-autumn transmission. Considerable success has been achieved in predicting high- or low-risk years for fascioliasis from meteorologic data in both Britain and the Gulf Coast regions of the United States.

PATHOGENESIS

Acute fluke disease due to *F. hepatica* is caused by the sudden invasion of the liver by masses of young flukes. Severe destruction of parenchyma results in acute hepatic insufficiency as well as massive hemorrhage into the peritoneal cavity. Chronic fluke disease develops slowly and is caused by the activities of adult flukes in the bile ducts. In addition to cholangitis, biliary obstruction, and fibrosis, they cause anemia by their blood-sucking activities. Hypoproteinemia may result from seepage of plasma proteins from the damaged bile duct epithelium. The pathogenesis of *F. gigantica* is similar to that of *F. hepatica*. Migration of immature flukes through hepatic tissue and production of anaerobic necrotic tracts may trigger germination of latent spores of *Clostridium novyi* and exotoxin production that causes black disease. This occurs much more commonly in sheep than in cattle. Bacillary hemoglobinuria due to exotoxins of *Clostridium haemolyticum* may also be triggered by migrating liver flukes in cattle.

F. magna infection in cattle is usually clinically inapparent because of massive encapsulation of flukes, but their unrestricted tunnelling in sheep and goats can be rapidly fatal. It is reported that a single fluke can cause death. In the wildlife natural hosts, there is only minor liver damage because the adults are enclosed in thin-walled cysts. *D. dendriticum* is relatively nonpathogenic because of its small size, smooth cuticle, and failure to invade the liver parenchyma. It may, however, cause cirrhosis of bile ducts and condemnation of livers. Clinical paramphistomiasis is caused by massive numbers of immature flukes in the duodenal mucosa, whereas adult flukes in the rumen and reticulum cause little harm in most circumstances.

CLINICAL DISEASE

Acute liver fluke disease due to *F. hepatica* is seen in sheep and goats but rarely in cattle because of both natural and acquired immunity. It is caused by massive hemorrhage and tissue destruction after ingestion of large numbers of metacercariae. Acute fluke outbreaks are likely to occur in seasons of very high rainfall. Death is usually sudden or occurs within 48 hours of the onset of symptoms. Clinical signs include anorexia, dullness, weakness, pale membranes, dyspnea, ascites, abdominal pain, and alternating standing up and lying down. It may be possible to palpate an enlarged liver. The feces are dry and are not diarrheic. Outbreaks may last only 2 to 3 weeks but involve high mortality, especially if the fluke migration triggers further deaths from black disease. A subacute syndrome may also occur, with affected animals surviving for 2 weeks after the onset of clinical signs.

The chronic disease is a wasting condition caused by the blood-sucking activities of adult *F. hepatica* in the bile ducts. Sheep progressively lose weight over months and develop pale membranes, submandibular edema (bottle jaw), ascites, or rarely jaundice. Shedding of the wool may also occur. Cattle usually suffer the chronic disease only and experience weight loss, anemia, and a reduction of up to 10 per cent in milk yield. In Britain and the Pacific Northwest of the United States, most fluke infections are acquired by cattle in the autumn and early winter, and the effects on lactation and body condition become apparent in midwinter. The poor body condition can contribute to lowered reproductive performance and a higher percentage of barren cows. Subacute disease sometimes occurs in calves exposed to large numbers of metacercariae. Infection with *F. gigantica* causes clinical signs similar to those caused by *F. hepatica*. *F. magna* infection may cause a syndrome similar to chronic *F. hepatica* disease in cattle and acute *F. hepatica* disease in sheep. In tropical regions, paramphistomes may induce a severe enteritis with weight loss and diarrhea and may be clinically indistinguishable from ostertagiasis or Johne's disease. *D. dendriticum* infection is usually asymptomatic.

DIAGNOSIS

Clinical diagnosis of liver fluke disease is often complicated by the concurrent presence of gastrointestinal nematodes, which produce some of the same clinical signs. A common experience in the Gulf Coast is that of giving 1 or more treatments for nematodes with little effect. When a flukicide is given, a dramatic clinical improvement occurs. A history of access to snail habitats, seasonal conditions favorable for snail reproduction, and an unexpected drop in milk yield are all important indicators in endemic areas. In outbreaks of acute *F. hepatica* disease in sheep and goats, there will be no fluke eggs in the feces; and in cases of *F. magna* infection, patency is unlikely to be reached in domestic animals. In subacute disease due to *F. hepatica*, a few flukes may reach adult stage and pass small numbers of eggs in the feces. In chronic *F. hepatica* infection in cattle, sheep, and goats, variable numbers of eggs occur in the feces. The immature paramphistomes that cause clinical signs do not betray their presence by eggs.

It is desirable to use a sedimentation technique for the detection of fluke eggs, because they do not float well in most flotation solutions. *F. hepatica* eggs are large (up to 150 μm), operculated, thin-walled, and yellow-brown. Eggs of *F. gigantica*, *F. magna*, and *P. microbothrioides* all resemble *F. hepatica* eggs but are a little larger, and those of *P. microbothrioides* have a transparent gray-green appearance. Immature rumen flukes are sometimes passed in the feces. They are 3 to 4 mm in size and can be detected by sedimentation and decanting techniques. The eggs of *D. dendriticum* are quite distinctive, being small (up to 45 μm), dark brown, and operculated, and contain a miracidium when passed in the feces.

Researchers in the southern United States have identified several problems in the diagnosis of *F. hepatica* infection in cattle with use of the fecal sedimentation method: (1) it is time-consuming, requiring at least 10 samples per cattle group and 15 to 30 minutes per sample; (2) egg counts are low, usually less than 5 eggs per gram, even in heavily infected herds; (3) egg counts vary widely among animals in a herd, because most flukes and egg shedding occur in a few highly susceptible animals; (4) herd egg counts peak and wane according to seasonal transmission; (5) immature fluke infections cannot be detected; and (6) lack of standardization of techniques between laboratories prevents meaningful comparisons of data. The researchers reported a new method based on the use of 2 sieves.* It is twice as fast, less prone to technical variance, and suitable for use by veterinary practitioners. Currently, no serologic tests are accurate enough to improve on diagnosis by fecal examination in individual animals. Enzyme-linked immunosorbent assay (ELISA) tests are limited by low sensitivity and specificity and by the difficulty of differentiating current infection from previous infection.

In acute *F. hepatica* outbreaks, the main necropsy findings are an enlarged hemorrhagic liver covered with fibrinous strands, a large amount of blood-stained peritoneal fluid, and over 1000 immature flukes in the liver parenchyma. In the subacute disease, the liver is also enlarged and hemorrhagic, but some of the flukes will have reached the adult stage. The chronic disease is characterized by an emaciated carcass; a small, shrunken, fibrotic liver; and 200 or more adult flukes in the bile ducts. In cattle infected with *F. magna*, flukes are found within a thick capsule with heavy black pigmentation of the liver; whereas in sheep or goats, tunnels are seen in the parenchyma. In paramphistomiasis, immature flukes may cause thickening and hemorrhage of the duodenal wall but are sometimes overlooked because of their small size.

CONTROL STRATEGIES

Control is best achieved by strategic use of flukicides for removal of flukes before productivity is affected and for

---

*Flukefinder. Visual Difference, Inc., 5051 Old Pullman Road, Moscow, ID 83843–8835; (208) 882-6040.

Table 1. FLUKICIDES FOR *Fasciola* spp. IN CATTLE

Flukicide	Trade Name	Dosage (mg/kg)	Safety Index	Minimum Age of Fluke (Efficacy >90%)
Albendazole	Valbazen	10	10	Adults only
Clorsulon	Curatrem	7	5	8 weeks
Clorsulon-ivermectin	Ivomec-F	2/0.2		Adults only
Triclabendazole*	Fasinex	12	20	1 week

*Not approved in the United States.

prevention of egg shedding before large numbers of susceptible snails are present. In some situations, the use of molluscicides, grazing management strategies, and fencing or drainage of snail habitats may be successfully integrated with strategic treatments. The timing, frequency, and choice of flukicides are best determined after consideration of the epidemiology of fluke disease in each area. The most appropriate timing may not always coincide with the times when livestock owners normally handle their stock for other purposes. However, the returns from improved weight gains, feed conversion, conception rates, milk production, or calf weaning weights may justify a change in management procedure to allow more effective fluke control. There may also be a need to offset winter nutritional stress, because poorly nourished animals are more susceptible to the effects of liver fluke disease.

Studies in Louisiana suggest that an annual fall treatment with a flukicide is adequate for the sustained reduction of fluke burdens in low-risk and moderate years, as determined by climatic forecasts, but that a late spring or summer treatment may be needed in high-risk years or on farms with a history of severe liver fluke disease. The fall treatment is especially important in removing adult fluke burdens before the winter nutritional stress period, as well as in reducing environmental contamination with fluke eggs before the massive late winter–spring–early summer build-up of the snail population.

A summer treatment in the Gulf Coast may be superior in preventive value for both fluke and gastrointestinal nematodes, compared with spring treatments. Summer treatment with a broad-spectrum flukicide (e.g., albendazole) or combination of a narrow-spectrum flukicide (e.g., clorsulon) and an anthelmintic would remove a high proportion of flukes in the drug-susceptible mature or late-immature stages. This treatment would also remove peak numbers of hypobiotic larvae in southern states and prevent problems when they normally emerge in the subsequent fall. Removal of both worms and flukes from cattle would give prolonged protection because environmental transmission is at its lowest level in summer. The Gulf Coast researchers point out that although summer treatment does not coincide with the most convenient times for handling cattle, recent progress in new drug delivery systems (e.g., pulse-release rumen devices, medicated feed blocks) suggests that it may soon be feasible to treat cattle at critical times dictated by local epidemiologic factors. In the Pacific Northwest, a spring treatment at the start of the pasture season would eliminate many adult flukes before they contaminated pasture with eggs and thus reduce the summer-fall transmission potential.

Effective management systems include grazing systems that avoid high-risk areas during periods of high transmission potential and the fencing off or drainage of snail habitats if practical. Molluscicides, such as copper sulfate, may be of value when they are applied to relatively small snail habitats and integrated with strategic flukicide treatments. Toxic effects in nontarget species and phytotoxicity are important constraints to molluscicide use. Copper sulfate has been widely used in the past but has sometimes resulted in copper poisoning of livestock or killing of fish after drainage into nearby streams. Biologic approaches to snail control have also been attempted, including the release of sciomyzid marsh flies, but the results were disappointing.

FLUKICIDES

Flukicides for cattle are shown in Table 1. Albendazole is the only approved broad-spectrum drug in the United States with efficacy against gastrointestinal nematodes, lungworms, tapeworms, and adult liver fluke. However, it has little efficacy against immature *Fasciola* less than 12 weeks of age. It is consequently most effective in the fall when flukes are adult, but it is considerably less effective in the spring or early summer when a mixed, immature-mature population is present.

Clorsulon is effective against *Fasciola* spp. only but has activity against late-immature flukes (8 to 12 weeks). It can also be combined with modern anthelmintics such as benzimidazole drugs, levamisole, and ivermectin to provide a broad spectrum of activity. Unfortunately, the dosage of clorsulon in combination with ivermectin (Ivomec-F) is only 2 mg/kg (Table 1), which limits its usefulness to adult flukes only. Greater efficacy against late-immature flukes could be obtained by treating cattle with a combination of clorsulon (7 mg/kg) and anthelmintics at recommended dosages.

A new benzimidazole drug, triclabendazole, is so efficient against all stages of *Fasciola* spp., it introduces the possibility of complete elimination of fascioliasis by treatment at intervals of 8 to 10 weeks (within the prepatent period). It has high efficacy against *F. hepatica* from 1 day after infection and 100 per cent efficacy against flukes aged 6 weeks or older. It is also a very safe drug with a high safety index (Table 1). Most other flukicides are effective only against *F. hepatica* 8 weeks and older, by which time severe pathologic damage has already occurred.

Most drugs effective against *F. hepatica* are also effective against *F. gigantica*. Higher dosage rates are required for efficacy against *F. magna*, and 100 per cent efficacy is needed in sheep and goats because even a single migrating fluke can kill the host. Most benzimidazole drugs have activity against *D. dendriticum* at high dosage rates. Drugs recommended for paramphistome therapy (bithionol, brotionide, niclosamide, resorantel) are not approved for food animals in the United States.

BIBLIOGRAPHY

Blood DC, Radostits OM: Veterinary Medicine, 7th ed. London, Baillière Tindall, 1989, pp 1016–1070.
Courtney CH, Sundlof SF: AAVP Antiparasitic Drugs: A Compendium of FDA-Approved Antiparasitic Drugs. University of Florida, Gainesville, 1990.
Gibbs HC, Herd RP, Murrell KD (eds): Parasites: epidemiology and control. Vet Clin North Am [Food Anim Pract] 2:205–505, 1986.
Malone JB, Loyacano MS, Armstrong DA, Archibald LF: Bovine fascioliasis: economic impact and control in Gulf Coast cattle based on seasonal transmission. Bovine Pract 17:126–133, 1982.
Malone JB, Craig TM: Cattle liver flukes: risk assessment and control. Compend Contin Educ Pract Vet 12:747–754, 1990.

Cestode Infections in Cattle, Sheep, Goats, and Swine

R. P. HERD, MVSc, PhD

Gastrointestinal cestodes of food animals are of minor importance, but cystic larval stages of human and canid taeniids that occur in food animal intermediate hosts are of both economic and public health significance.

In the United States, *Moniezia* spp. of cattle, sheep, and goats are widely distributed owing to the ready availability of the oribatid pasture mite intermediate hosts. Livestock become infected by accidental ingestion of the mites, which are especially numerous on permanent pasture. The "fringed tapeworm" *(Thysanosoma actinioides)* is limited to western states because the appropriate intermediate host (psocid louse) is not so widely disseminated.

A discussion of cysticercosis and hydatidosis is outside the scope of a discussion of digestive system diseases, but it should be noted that *Taenia saginata* has become more common in the United States over the last decade as a result of the influx of migrant workers from enzootic areas, as a consequence of the use of raw sewage for the fertilization of pasture, and because of sewage contamination of irrigation water. There is a similar risk of the introduction of *T. solium* with migrant workers from Mexico and other enzootic areas. Cystic hydatidosis persists as a problem in sheep-raising areas in Utah, California, Arizona, and New Mexico, whereas alveolar hydatidosis is becoming more important in North Central states. Cysticercosis of sheep due to larval *T. ovis* and *T. hydatigena* causes carcass and organ rejection at abattoirs and adversely affects export markets.

LIFE CYCLE AND EPIDEMIOLOGY

Most cestodes of veterinary importance have an indirect life cycle with 1 intermediate host. There are no free-living larval stages. In the case of *Moniezia* and *Thysanosoma* spp., eggs disseminated from gravid proglottids passed in cattle, sheep, or goat feces are consumed by an arthropod intermediate host. The oncosphere or hexacanth embryo is released and burrows into the body cavity of the arthropod, where it develops to a cysticercoid (a small cyst with a single depressed scolex) within 100 to 200 days depending on the temperature. Each cysticercoid develops into a single tapeworm if the infected intermediate host is eaten by the appropriate final host.

Moniezia tapeworms are relatively short-lived. They start shedding eggs about 6 weeks after infection, then disappear from the host after about 3 months. The eggs have a poor survival capacity and are infective for mites for only about 3 months after being passed. Development of cysticercoids in mites takes several months depending on the temperature, and it appears that cysticercoids can overwinter in mites. The prevalence of *Moniezia* infection in livestock shows a seasonal fluctuation coinciding with the active period of the vectors. At present, it is not clear how much the transmission of tapeworm eggs is affected by wind, water, temperature, vectors, and fomites. Coprophagous flies probably play an important role in egg dissemination. Unlike *Moniezia*, *Thysanosoma* is a long-lived worm surviving for several years.

PATHOGENESIS

The intestinal tapeworms of cattle, sheep, and goats are not serious pathogens, although *Moniezia* infection is sometimes associated with poor growth and diarrhea. Adult tapeworms compete with the host for nutrients, interfere with gut motility, and excrete toxic substances. *M. expansa* has been associated with enterotoxemia outbreaks in lambs. It has been suggested that it causes sluggish bowel movements and conditions suitable for the production of *Clostridium perfringens* exotoxins. There is evidence that tapeworm-infected sheep may be more subject to fly-strike. Young animals are most susceptible to tapeworm infection, and it is possible that older animals develop an acquired immunity. *T. actinioides* infection is not of clinical importance, but its presence in the bile ducts can result in the condemnation of livers.

CLINICAL DISEASE

There is some controversy over the importance of tapeworm infection of food animals, with a tendency for farmers to overemphasize their importance and be more concerned about tapeworms than the more pathogenic nematodes and trematodes. At the same time, it is probably a mistake to ignore tapeworms totally and regard them as completely nonpathogenic. Most infections do not cause clinical disease, but heavy infections are sometimes associated with poor growth, diarrhea, or clostridial infections. Clinical signs are usually not seen in cysticercosis or hydatidosis of food animals unless large cysts disrupt vital organs.

DIAGNOSIS

Diagnosis is usually made by finding proglottids or the characteristic thick-walled eggs in feces. *Moniezia* eggs contain a distinctive hexacanth embryo in a piriform apparatus. The much smaller *Thysanosoma* eggs have no piriform apparatus. *Moniezia* is a large cestode (200 cm), and it is common to recover masses of them at routine necropsy of lambs in the spring. In spite of their spectacular volume, tapeworms are much less pathogenic than are the tiny hairlike trichostrongylid nematodes. The smaller *Thysanosoma* tapeworms (20 cm) are usually found in the duodenum or bile ducts at necropsy.

TREATMENT

Because control of the arthropod vectors is impractical, periodic treatment with cestocides is the main method of control. In the past, lead arsenate (0.5 g for lambs, 1 g for adult sheep, 0.5 to 1.5 g for calves) was the main drug employed. It has now been superseded by more efficient and safer pro-benzimidazole or benzimidazole drugs, including albendazole, cambendazole, febantel, fenbendazole, mebendazole, and oxfendazole. Preliminary studies suggest that albendazole and fenbendazole at dosages of 10 mg/kg and oxfendazole at 4.5 mg/kg have excellent activity against gastrointestinal cestodes. There are no highly effective chemotherapeutic agents for the control of larval cestodes in ruminants, but several drugs (e.g., praziquantel, mebendazole) have shown promising results under experimental conditions. At present, the best approach is to use drugs such as niclosamide and praziquantel to eliminate adult cestodes in the human and canid definitive hosts, with the object of reducing the environmental contamination with cestode eggs.

Drugs Affecting the Digestive System

LLOYD E. DAVIS, DVM, PhD

Digestive disturbances are among the problems most commonly encountered in food animal practice. Precise diagnoses often are difficult, and, hence, an understanding of the underlying pathophysiologic features of a particular case may be lacking. This has led, in the past, to the marketing and use of various nostrums that had questionable efficacy in correcting the underlying medical problems. Drugs in modern use act to increase or decrease motility or secretion or to exert effects locally within the lumen of the gastrointestinal tract.

DRUGS AFFECTING MOTILITY

Drugs modify motility and tone of the gastrointestinal tract by their direct action on autonomic receptors in smooth muscle or reflexly by causing distention of the bowel. These drugs and their dosage are listed in Table 1.

The cholinergic drugs increase gastric emptying and propulsive activity of the intestines and colon while at the same time inhibiting the smooth muscle of sphincters. Pilocarpine and arecoline act primarily at muscarinic sites and exert marked pharmacologic effects on the heart, glands, eyes, bronchioles, and urinary tract as well as stimulating motility of the gut. The effects of these drugs are readily antagonized by atropine. Carbachol has much less effect on the heart and bronchioles but stimulates nicotinic sites. This enhances its effects on the bowel, but fasciculation of skeletal muscle and stimulation of epinephrine release from the adrenal medulla may occur. The release of epinephrine may inhibit motility of the reticulorumen and intestine. These effects are dose-related, and the effects of carbachol are poorly antagonized by atropine.

Bethanechol is another synthetic choline ester that is more specific in its actions. It will stimulate the smooth muscle of the gastrointestinal tract and the urinary bladder with minimal effects on cardiovascular system or bronchioles. It has no nicotinic effects and is readily antagonized by atropine.

The anticholinesterases act at both muscarinic and nicotinic sites. All cholinergic receptors in visceral organs, ganglia, and skeletal muscle are stimulated. In addition to its ability to inhibit acetylcholinesterase, neostigmine also directly stimulates the cholinergic receptor. Because of their nicotinic actions, the effects of these drugs are only partially antagonized by atropine.

Cholinergic and anticholinesterase drugs should not be administered in the presence of mechanical obstruction of the gut, peritonitis, or doubtful viability of the intestinal wall. Whenever these drugs are employed, the therapist must have injectable atropine available to counteract excessive stimulation of the gut or untoward side effects.

The cathartics increase motility of the bowel by directly stimulating the smooth muscle, by activating receptors in the mucosa that reflexly release acetylcholine, or by modifying secretion and absorption of electrolytes and water. The drugs employed in food animals are listed in Table 1.

The irritant cathartics increase motility of the intestinal tract by directly stimulating smooth muscle in the wall of the bowel and by increasing secretion. The most commonly used drugs of this group are the anthraquinone derivatives. The pharmacologically inactive glycosides in aloin and senna are transported to the colon, where emodin, which stimulates motility, is released. This accounts for the delay of about 12 hours between ingestion and stimulation of defecation. The action of this group most nearly mimics the physiologic act of defecation. The compounds are absorbed to some extent and are excreted into the urine and milk. They will color alkaline urine red and acidic urine a dark yellow.

Castor oil is a nonirritating triglyceride of ricinoleic acid. After ingestion, castor oil is hydrolyzed in the small intestine to release ricinoleic acid, which increases secretion of electrolytes and water. The increased intraluminal volume stimulates motility of the small intestine, causing the elimination of liquid feces.

The irritant cathartics should not be administered to patients with possible obstruction, enteritis, or colitis. They should not be given to animals late in pregnancy because they may initiate parturition. Care should attend their use in lactating animals

Table 1. DOSAGE OF DRUGS THAT MODIFY GASTROINTESTINAL MOTILITY

Category and Drug	Cattle	Sheep and Goats	Swine	Comments
Cholinergics				
Pilocarpine	65–300 mg, SC	10–30 mg, SC	10–30 mg, SC	Stimulate motility
Arecoline	4–8 mg, SC	2–4 mg, SC	1–4 mg, SC	throughout
Carbachol	4 mg, SC	0.1–0.2 mg, SC	50 µg/kg, SC	gastrointestinal tract
Bethanechol	50 µg/kg, SC	50 µg/kg, SC		
Anticholinesterase				
Physostigmine	30–50 mg, SC	5–20 mg, SC	5–20 mg, SC	Stimulate motility
Neostigmine	1 mg/CWT	0.01–0.02 mg/kg	0.03 mg/kg	throughout
				gastrointestinal tract
Cathartics				
Senna	120–150 g	30–60 g	30–60 g	Stimulate colon only
Aloin	10–20g	2–4 g	1–2.5 g	Stimulate small intestine
Castor oil	—	—	20–150 ml	motility
Magnesium sulfate	250–1000 g	25–125 g	25–125 g	
Sodium sulfate	500–750 g	60 g	30–60 g	
Magnesium oxide	500 g	5–10 g	5–10 g	
Magnesium hydroxide susp.	1–4 L	20–150 ml	10–50 ml	
Liquid petrolatum	250–500 ml	100–200 ml	100–200 ml	Lubricant
Docusate	5–15 g	2–5 g	2–10 g	Surfactant
Anticholinergics				
Atropine	0.08 mg/kg	0.08 mg/kg	0.04 mg/kg	Inhibit motility
Methscopolamine	5 mg/CWT	5 mg/CWT	5 mg/CWT	
Opioids				
Morphine	—	—	0.25 mg/kg	Decrease propulsive
Paregoric	15–30 ml (calves)	—	—	movement but increase
Diphenoxylate	0.05 mg/kg	0.5 mg/kg	0.5 mg/kg	segmental resistance

SC = subcutaneously; CWT, hundredweight.

because active fractions are secreted into milk, and these may cause purgation in the nursing offspring.

The saline cathartics stimulate motility reflexly by distending the bowel. The magnesium and sulfate ions are poorly absorbed from the gut, thereby exerting an osmotic effect that causes movement of water from plasma into the lumen of the intestine. The increased volume stretches the mucosa and stimulates mechanoreceptors, which reflexly increases peristaltic activity.

Sodium sulfate is the most effective of the saline cathartics on a molar basis. It is inexpensive, safe, and best administered by stomach tube in a 6 per cent solution. Magnesium salts are effective and relatively inexpensive. Magnesium sulfate is generally employed in adults, whereas magnesium oxide or magnesium hydroxide may be used in calves, lambs, and piglets.

Drugs employed to lubricate the fecal mass in obstipation or impactions include liquid petrolatum ("mineral oil") and the surfactants. These substances are pharmacologically inert in usual doses, but docusate may stimulate motor activity of the intestine when it is administered at high dosage. They are administered orally or may be incorporated in enemata to soften fecal masses in the colon. The principal untoward effects of liquid petrolatum are interference with absorption of fat-soluble vitamins, inhibition of healing of wounds in the anorectal area, interference with normal defecatory reflexes, and foreign body reactions at the gut wall, liver, and mesenteric lymph nodes after absorption. Liquid petrolatum and surfactants should not be used simultaneously because emulsification of the oil might facilitate its absorption from the gut.

Appropriate uses of cathartics include (1) cleansing the bowel before elective surgery, (2) as an aid to eliminate parasites after administration of a vermifuge, (3) in poisoning to hasten elimination of unabsorbed toxin, (4) to facilitate reduction of impactions, and (5) to facilitate defecation in patients with prolapses or hernias where straining would be undesirable (use lubricants or surfactants). *Cathartics must not be given to patients showing signs of abdominal pain.*

Several drugs have been advocated for use as rumenatorics. Increases in frequency and amplitude of ruminal contractions have been observed after administration of physostigmine, carbachol, and arecoline. Marked inhibition of ruminal motility follows administration of epinephrine, histamine, atropine, and large doses of carbachol or arecoline. The larger doses of carbachol and arecoline stimulate the release of epinephrine from the adrenal medulla, which, in turn, inhibits the ruminal musculature. Veratrine is an alkaloid derived from *Veratrum album* that stimulates reticuloruminal activity at small doses and vomiting at larger doses. The status of the drug in the treatment of ruminal atony has not been established, but subcutaneous doses of 40 mg in cattle and 20 mg in sheep have been suggested.

Frequently, ruminal stasis is secondary to other conditions such as ketosis, acid-base disturbances, or infectious diseases. It is generally more rewarding to correct the underlying disturbances than to try to stimulate ruminal motility with drugs.

Drugs may be administered to decrease peristaltic activity or spasm within the gastrointestinal tract. The anticholinergic drugs occupy the cholinergic receptor at muscarinic sites and prevent the action of acetylcholine on smooth muscle and glands. Atropine blocks the effects of parasympathetic stimulation on smooth muscle, glands, and heart. At large doses, it readily crosses into the brain, where it produces excitement. Methscopolamine is a more polar compound that does not cross the blood-brain barrier and that blocks ganglia in the gut as well as exerting antimuscarinic effects. Inhibition of excessive motility or spasm of the gut is frequently incomplete because other mediators or autacoids such as serotonin, histamine, and prostaglandins may be involved in the abnormal activity of the gut.

The opioids—paregoric (camphorated tincture of opium), morphine, loperamide, and diphenoxylate—decrease propulsive activity, delay gastric emptying, and increase tone of the intestine and sphincters. The decrease in peristalsis occurs because of the spasmogenic effect of the opioids, which prevents the sequential contraction and relaxation characteristic of peristaltic movements. Tone of the colon is increased to the point of spasm, allowing time for desiccation of feces. Effective suppression of motility of the gut can be attained at doses that exert few systemic effects. It is questionable whether opioids should be administered for treatment of diarrhea. The fundamental problem in most cases of diarrhea is hypomotility and excessive secretion of fluid and electrolytes into the lumen of the bowel.

DRUGS AFFECTING SECRETION

The glands associated with the digestive system are regulated by the autonomic nervous system and by various hormones. Cholinergic drugs increase secretion of most glands, and anticholinergic drugs decrease their secretion (Table 2).

Acid secretion by the abomasum of ruminants and the stomach of swine is controlled by the vagus nerves and gastrin secreted by the argentaffin cells. The anticholinergic drugs will block gastric secretion mediated by vagal mechanisms but have no effect on gastrin- or histamine-induced secretion. The histamine H_2-receptor antagonists cimetidine and ranitidine decrease secretion induced by either histamine or gastrin. Their dosage and clinical use in food-producing animals remain to be established.

Of greater significance, as a practical matter, is the increased secretion of intestinal glands produced by enterotoxin-produc-

Table 2. DRUGS THAT MODIFY GLANDULAR SECRETION IN THE GASTROINTESTINAL TRACT

Organs	Drug	Action
Salivary	Pilocarpine	Increase
	Physostigmine	Increase
	Arecoline	Increase
	Atropine	Decrease
Gastric	Histamine	Increase acid secretion
	Pentagastrin	Increase acid secretion
	Betazole	Increase acid secretion
	Atropine	Partially decrease acid secretion
	Cimetidine	Decrease acid secretion
	Glucocorticoids	Decrease secretion of mucus
	Aspirin	Decrease secretion of mucus
	Phenylbutazone	Decrease secretion of mucus
Biliary	Bile salts	Increase bile formation
	Ouabain	Increase bile formation
	Theophylline	Increase bile formation
	Phenobarbital	Increase bile formation
	Magnesium sulfate	Increase bile formation
Pancreatic exocrine	Atropine	Decrease secretion
	Glucagon	Decrease secretion
	Bethanechol	Increase secretion
Intestinal	Bethanechol	Increase secretion
	Pilocarpine	Increase secretion
	Castor oil	Increase secretion
	Prostaglandins	Increase secretion
	Atropine	Decrease secretion
	Chlorpromazine	Decrease secretion
	Aspirin	Decrease secretion
	Flunixin meglumine	Decrease secretion
	Lidamidine	Decrease secretion

ing pathogens. The enterotoxins elaborated by *Vibrio* and *Escherichia coli* increase secretion by altering cyclic nucleotide and calcium concentrations within intestinal glands. The excess secretion over absorption of water and electrolytes results in diarrhea. These mechanisms have been the target for drug therapy of severe infectious diarrheas. Large doses of nicotinic acid affect cyclic nucleotide levels and have been shown to reduce scours in piglets. The search for new drugs that specifically antagonize the secretory effects of enterotoxins is being actively pursued. However, there are several new approaches to therapy that have been shown to be effective in diminishing secretion and mortality associated with infectious diarrhea.

Chlorpromazine (1 mg/kg, intramuscularly) decreases secretion and duration of diarrhea caused by *E. coli*. The mode of action is inhibition of the calcium-dependent regulator that stimulates secretion by the intestinal cells. Another effect of enterotoxins is to stimulate the production of prostaglandins, which in turn raise the intracellular concentration of cAMP, thereby causing secretion. Drugs such as aspirin and flunixin meglumine inhibit the production of prostaglandins and reduce mortality from coliform-induced diarrhea. For this purpose, aspirin was added to the feed or drinking water of piglets for providing a daily dose of 0.5 to 1.0 g during the period of 9 to 20 days postpartum.

Lidamidine is a newer drug with antiperistaltic and antisecretory activity that is effective against both prostaglandin- and enterotoxin-induced diarrheas. Experimentally, at a dose of 8 mg/kg, this drug completely protected animals against the cathartic effects of castor oil.

These newer approaches to the inhibition of secretion, together with appropriate fluid, electrolyte, and antibacterial therapy, should enable us to markedly reduce neonatal losses associated with infectious diarrhea.

DRUGS ACTING WITHIN THE LUMEN OF THE GASTROINTESTINAL TRACT

Many drugs that have been administered orally to ruminants and swine for local effects have been shown to have little therapeutic value. These include compounds such as nux vomica, gentian, cassia, tartar emetic, and capsicum. Mixtures containing such substances should be regarded as being obsolete unless they are being offered with placebo intent.

Surfactants, such as polyoxalene, are useful to reduce foaming of gastrointestinal contents as seen in frothy bloat of ruminant animals. They are best administered into the rumen via a stomach tube.

Adsorbents have been advocated for the treatment of gastroenteritis and diarrhea. They coat the surface of the inflamed mucosa and were thought to adsorb irritants and enterotoxins on their surface. Recently, it was found that adsorbents such as kaolin, attapulgite, and bentonite do not bind enterotoxin. The ion exchange resin cholestyramine avidly binds *E. coli* enterotoxin, but its efficacy is greatly reduced in the presence of milk. Bismuth subsalicylate possesses unique properties that are used in the treatment of enteritis. The bismuth is insoluble and exerts a demulcent effect by coating inflamed surfaces, and the salicylate exerts a local anti-inflammatory effect in the bowel.

Antacids such as calcium carbonate, magnesium hydroxide, aluminum trisilicate, sodium bicarbonate, and aluminum hydroxide have been employed in the treatment of gastric and ruminal hyperacidity. Care should be taken when these drugs are used in the treatment of ruminal acidosis because alkalization of the ruminal contents will enhance the absorption of histamine, ammonia, and other basic substances.

Antibiotics acting within the bowel are discussed elsewhere in the book.

SUMMARY

Although many drugs have been advocated for the treatment of various disorders of the digestive system, numerous agents have proved to be ineffective for their intended use. It is possible to modify motility and secretion, alter surface tension, and change pH with drugs. Many of the drugs employed exert widespread pharmacologic effects in the body, which must be understood for their safe use in management of disorders of the gastrointestinal tract.

BIBLIOGRAPHY

Constable PD, Hoffsis GF, Rings DM: The reticulorumen: normal and abnormal motor function. Part I. Primary contraction cycle. Compend Contin Educ Pract Vet 12:1008–1014, 1990.

Davis LE, Baggot JD: Gastrointestinal pharmacology. *In* Anderson NV (ed): Veterinary Gastroenterology. Philadelphia, Lea & Febiger, 1980, pp 277–310.

Jenkins WL: Drugs acting on the digestive system. *In* Booth NH, McDonald LE (eds): Veterinary Pharmacology and Therapeutics, 6th ed. Ames, IA, Iowa State University Press, 1988, pp 657–671.

Jenkins WL: Ruminant pharmacology. *In* Booth NH, McDonald LE (eds): Veterinary Pharmacology and Therapeutics, 6th ed. Ames, IA, Iowa State University Press, 1988, pp 672–684.

Yeoman GH: Recent advances in the chemotherapy of neonatal diarrhea in farm animals. *In* Recent Advances in Neonatal Diarrhea in Farm Animals. Bristol, TN, Beecham Laboratories, 1980, pp 43–52.

SECTION 13
Diseases of the Reproductive Tract

LOUIS F. ARCHBALD, DVM, PhD, MS, Consulting Editor

Bovine Mastitis

SEBASTIAN E. HEATH, Vet MB, MVSc, MRCVS,
Diplomate, ACVIM

The bovine udder may become compromised by bacterial contamination and occasionally by trauma, both of which cause mastitis. On a herd basis, the only significant cause of mastitis is bacteria. Bacterial mastitis becomes clinical when milk has a cell count greater than 500,000 cells/ml and an etiologic agent can be isolated. Mastitis is considered subclinical when milk merely has an elevated cell count, with or without isolation of a bacteriologic agent. Mastitis causes reduced productivity, over 70 per cent of which is the result of reduced milk production. Most mastitis (approximately 90 per cent) in a herd is subclinical; hence subclinical mastitis is the greatest source of economic losses. Since subclinical mastitis cannot be detected by physical examination, a primary concern of dairy herd management is the prevention of mastitis through a scientifically formulated milk quality/mastitis control program. Instituting a mastitis control program on a farm will provide a benefit-cost ratio of 3 to 5:1.

The level of infection in a herd depends on the rate and duration of infections. On average about 40 per cent of all cows in the United States are infected in one or more quarters of the udder at any one time. The estimated cost in lost production is $200/cow/year. Mastitis is caused by inadequate milking hygiene (75 per cent), equipment malfunction (20 per cent), and cow factors (5 per cent). The dollar cost of treating mastitis occupies only a minimal sum compared with the sum lost due to lost milk production. With increasing modernization of farming the individual cow can be considered as a production unit in the herd, with disease prevention being the most important aspect of health.

The susceptibility of the mammary gland to new intramammary infections varies throughout the lactational cycle. The highest incidence of new intramammary infections occurs during the first week after dry-off, although the highest level of exposure occurs during milking. It has been estimated that 42 per cent of all new intramammary infections become established during the dry period. However, many of these infections only become patent in the first 9 weeks of lactation.

The major immunologic defenses of the udder during the dry period involve the teat canal, neutrophils, macrophages, lactoferrin, and the lactoperoxidase-thiocyanate systems. To some extent all of these defenses become compromised during the dry period, making the udder more susceptible to new intramammary infections. The levels of antibacterial defenses that are most effective against different types of bacteria vary with the time of the dry period. Thus infections with different bacteria occur at different stages of the dry period.

At dry-off, the volume of milk produced per day continues at about the same rate as before for about 3 more days. During this time, the udder becomes distended with milk, leading to dilatation and shortening of the teat canal. This predisposes the teat canal to penetration by bacteria.

In addition, since milk is still being produced in the early dry period, the amount of citrate in the secretions is also high. Citrate binds iron but still allows the iron to be utilized by bacteria for growth. This binding of iron to citrate competes with chelation of iron by lactoferrin, which otherwise permanently binds iron, an essential growth factor for many bacteria. A high molar ratio of citrate to lactoferrin, therefore, is associated with low bactericidal activity. As involution progresses, the volume of milk produced declines, and so does the citrate-lactoferrin ratio. Also, the concentration of bicarbonate ions in the secretions increases, and this enhances the action of lactoferrin. As a result, the involuted mammary gland is quite resistant to new intramammary infection. In fact, spontaneous cure from infection may occur. Coliform infections from the early dry period are usually eliminated at this stage.

To reduce the potential for bacteria entering through the teat canal, it is advisable when drying a cow off to seal the teat with an antibacterial teat sealant. To reduce the potential for bacteria to multiply in the involuting gland, it is common practice to infuse a long-acting antibiotic preparation (dry cow therapy).

Once lactogenesis recommences at the end of the dry period, similar alterations to the involution phase of drying off occur, making the udder again more susceptible to new intramammary infection. A large volume of colostrum is produced in the last 3 days of pregnancy that dilutes lactoferrin and preoccupies macrophages with the removal of fat rather than bacteria. This is reflected in the relatively high incidence of environmental mastitides (coliforms, *Streptococcus uberis*).

The lactating cow possesses several additional protective mechanisms over the cow whose udder is in a transitional state of drying off or preparing for lactation. These include frequent removal of milk and potential pathogens and frequent cleansing and sanitizing of the udder.

In the lactating cow, the teat canal is the first and most important line of defense. The length and diameter of the teat canal are inversely proportional to the susceptibility of the gland to new infections by major pathogens. The teat canal is lined by keratin and may adsorb approximately 10^6 bacteria. Since it is periodically shed at milking, it removes adsorbed bacteria. Between milking it dries out, forming a seal to the teat entrance. Fatty acids dissolved in the keratin make it bactericidal.

If the keratin lining of the streak canal is damaged, bacteria encounter less resistance at colonizing the canal and infecting the gland. This may occur, for example, with high milking vacuums or if liners are used that are not specified for the machine. These factors can cause physical damage to the teat end by everting the teat canal and by causing vascular damage to the teat sphincter. This is seen clinically as an everted teat canal and as petechiae at the teat end after milking. Full insertion of intramammary tubes also damages the teat canal, leading to new infections and reduced cure rates. Nothing should be inserted into the teat canal that is longer than 1/4 inch.

It is normal for the teat canal to be dilated for approximately 2 hours after milking, making the udder very susceptible to infection at this time. Cows should be fed immediately after milking so that they remain standing for as long as possible and therefore avoid udder contact with the ground (the source of pathogens). Lame cows are more prone to mastitis probably because they lie down soon after milking while the teat canal is still dilated.

The second line of defense of the lactating gland is cell mediated. Cells in milk are collectively referred to as somatic cells. Normally, there are 0.5 to 2.0×10^5 cells/ml milk. These cells are primarily macrophages, epithelial cells, and some lymphocytes. The number of these cells does not usually change. When a mammary gland becomes inflamed, neutrophils permeate into the gland cistern in large numbers and increase the cell count in milk. Neutrophils then become the main cell in milk and are involved in bacterial killing. A low somatic cell count predisposes the udder to infection by opportunistic organisms, such as bacteria from the environment. In herds with low average somatic cell counts for all cows, the risk of mastitis caused by environmental bacteria appears to be higher than in herds with higher average somatic cell counts.

PATHOGENESIS

Of cows that suffer from clinical mastitis, about 80 per cent either remain infected for or become reinfected during the rest of lactation. Most infections that occur in the early stages of lactation are most significant economically, since milk production is highest at this time and more of the subsequent lactation will be affected.

Pathogens of the bovine udder are usually categorized as major or minor. The common major pathogens are *Streptococcus* spp., *Staphylococcus aureus*, coliforms, and *Mycoplasma* spp., which can be further subdivided into contagious (*Streptococcus agalactiae, Staphylococcus aureus, Mycoplasma*) and environmental (*Streptococcus uberis, Streptococcus dysgalactiae*, coliforms) organisms. The pathogenesis of mastitis is easiest to understand when divided into infections caused by gram-positive (invasive), gram-negative (noninvasive), and other organisms.

Gram-Positive Mastitis

After penetration of the teat canal there is an incubation lag of 3 to 5 days before clinical signs become evident. During this time there is a randomly distributed invasion of ductal and alveolar cells by bacteria. The bacteria are believed to release cytotoxic exotoxins. Invasion and death of ductal and alveolar cells causes intense edema, increased permeability of the blood–mammary gland barrier, and death of mammary secretory tissue. As inflammation progresses there is leakage of plasma proteins, which later organize into fibrin, so that the milk contains large clots and may become purulent. Ductal cell hyperplasia also develops. This, together with blocking of ducts by fibrin, leads to alveolar involution. Thus reduced milk secretion is the result of secretory cell death and involution caused by pressure buildup.

The ductal cells remain hypertrophied for several weeks after recovery, and the shedding of ductal epithelial cells is partly responsible for the prolonged elevation in somatic cell counts noted after subsidence of the infection. Other reasons for persistently elevated somatic cell counts in chronic cases of mastitis include the establishment of infected foci of infection and encapsulated abscesses. As secretory tissue is destroyed, complete recovery from gram-positive mastitis is rare, since such mastitis usually results in some degree of permanent glandular damage.

Gram-Negative Mastitis

Gram-negative pathogens are often referred to as coliforms. Their common mode of causing disease is by release of endotoxin. Endotoxin is part of the cell wall of all gram-negative bacteria. Since there are no known strains that are particularly virulent, milking management is the basis for control of these organisms.

With the exception of *Pseudomonas* spp., gram-negative organisms are not invasive. A suggested pathogenesis involves an initial incubation phase of about 10 hours, then phagocytosis by ductal epithelial cells and neutrophils, followed by release of endotoxin from the cell walls of dying bacteria. Cows are very susceptible to the effects of endotoxin, and systemic effects of small amounts of endotoxin will cause the cow to go into shock.

CLINICAL SIGNS

Gram-Positive Mastitis

Acute mastitis caused by gram-positive organisms results in pronounced elevations in somatic cell count. Acute streptococcal infections (*Streptococcus uberis, S. dysgalactiae*, and *S. agalactiae*) generally cause greater elevations in somatic cell count and greater reduction in milk production than infections caused by staphylococci. Chronic staphylococcal infections are associated with a greater degree of stromal fibrosis and atrophy than streptococcal infections, often resulting in nonfunctional quarters. Chronic infections may be difficult to detect clinically but may have a profound effect on the bulk tank milk cell count.

The acute disease associated with *Staphylococcus aureus* is the result of the effect of a variety of exotoxins, which, depending on their type and quantity, are associated with mild to severe inflammation, microabscesses, necrosis, and fistulous tracts (beta and delta toxins); avascular necrosis, local vascular thrombosis, gangrene (blue bag); and sloughing of the skin and teat (alpha toxin). All of the toxins can be absorbed systemically and result in life-threatening toxemia. Gangrenous mastitis is most commonly seen in early lactation and in younger cows. Chronic staphylococcal infections are more common in older cows and are associated with induration and fibrosis of the udder.

Gram-Negative Mastitis

The clinical signs of coliform mastitis are caused by endotoxin on the affected quarter and from systemic disease.

Uniform swelling of the affected quarter and watery milk are typical, with little fibrosis or induration. Coliform infections do not progress in severity but have a distinct clinical pattern from the outset to resolution; that is, they do not change from acute to chronic or vice versa. Because infection with coliforms is opportunistic, clinical signs are related to the size of the infective dose, and the bacteria are readily cleared from the udder once polymorphonuclear leukocytes infiltrate. The frequent association of peracute coliform mastitis in early lactation is related to a relatively poor ability of the polymorphonuclear leukocytes to become mobilized. This allows for uncontrolled proliferation of the organisms in the ducts and alveoli before they are killed by the late-arriving leukocytes.

Systemic endotoxemia can be peracute in onset (6 to 8 hours). Endotoxemic cows rapidly become critical patients. Treatments are primarily concerned with combating the life-threatening consequences of endotoxemia (diarrhea, electrolyte imbalances, hypovolemia, including hypocalcemia, coagulopathy, pulmonary edema) and preventing further exposure to endotoxins (frequent stripping of the affected quarter).

Clinically, coliform ("toxic") mastitis usually causes greater changes in milk than in the udder and may often go unnoticed. Damage is rarely permanent, that is, beyond the current lactation, since secretory tissue is not damaged directly.

Mastitis from Other Causes

Infection with minor pathogens (*Corynebacterium bovis, Staphylococcus epidermidis*) causes only mild inflammation of the udder, and elevations in somatic cell counts in milk may be noted. Some researchers speculate that these organisms have a predominant protective effect on the udder that outweighs any deleterious effect ascribed to them.

The pathogenesis of *Mycoplasma* mastitis is believed to involve hematogenous spread at some stage in the disease. There is an initial incubation phase of 2 to 3 days, followed by changes in the milk 1 to 2 days later. It commonly affects all four quarters simultaneously, or if it starts in one quarter it will often spread to other quarters. The milk becomes tannish brown with sandy flakes that float. Clinical onset is sudden and may be associated with arthritis and lameness. Chronic carriers are common and shed *Mycoplasma* into the environment in large numbers, resulting in progressive fibrosis of the udder and atrophy of the alveolar cells.

Leptospiral mastitis develops after hematogenous dissemination. Leptospiral infection causes a vasculitis. If this involves the udder, milk secretion is abruptly terminated ("milk drop syndrome"), and leakage of blood into the udder secretion is prominent. Thus the milk is brownish orange and its volume is small; the udder is typically flaccid ("flabby bag"), since milk production has dropped off dramatically.

Summer mastitis ("August bag") is usually a disease of the dry cow and periparturient heifers. It is usually a mixed infection with *Actinomyces pyogenes, Peptococcus indolicus*, and a microaerophilic or anaerobic bacterium. Invasion of the udder may be through the teat canal or after penetration of the skin by biting flies. Biting flies can injure the udder; horn flies (*Haematobia irritans*) then deposit the infectious bacteria into the injured tissue sites, from where the infection spreads. The pathogenesis is one of invasive necrosis, with extensive destruction of all mammary tissue. The infection does not follow anatomic tissue boundaries and often results in abscess formation and fistulous tracts. The affected quarters of the udder are invariably destroyed, so that salvage of the animal is the most important aspect of treatment in these cases. If the infection is acute, an overwhelming toxemia will result in shock, disseminated intravascular coagulopathy, abortion, and death in a very short time.

DIAGNOSIS

Individual Cows

The clinical diagnosis of mastitis in the individual cow is usually made by the milker. In the early stages of the disease, the most important clinical signs of mastitis are changes in the appearance and consistency of the milk (detected by foremilking) and swelling, heat, and edema of the affected quarter(s), often referred to as a "hot udder" (noticed while the udder is being prepared for milking). The importance of a clinical diagnosis of mastitis is to be able to separate the cow from the herd, to begin treatment as soon as possible, and to collect a pretreatment sample for microbiologic evaluation.

Once a diagnosis of mastitis is made, it is necessary to grade it clinically, since this has direct bearing on the choice of therapy. Different authors use different systems, but they all mean similar things. Clinical grades of mastitis are subacute (grade I), with only mild changes in either the milk or the udder, or acute (grade II), with gross changes in the milk and/or udder. In grade II mastitis the udder will be grossly enlarged and may be hot and painful; the milk will have large clots or be purulent. The cow is likely to have a body temperature of more than 2°F (>1°C) above normal. Peracute (grade III) mastitis is similar to grade II mastitis but with additional systemic disease. Subclinical mastitis is diagnosed by examining herd records. *Chronic mastitis* is the term applied to cases that remain infected for more than 100 days and/or have three or more quarter infections per lactation.

The ability of milkers to diagnose mastitis is an important part of a mastitis control program since it represents the first level of diagnosis. The efficiency with which milkers are doing this can be screened by several methods. These include examining the milk filter at the end of milking and examining the Dairy Herd Improvement Association monthly report for counting the number of cows with high somatic cell counts and the bulk tank somatic cell count.

The Herd

Adequate and pertinent records of udder health must be available to be able to diagnose a herd problem. Although the principles of control are similar, the diagnosis of a mastitis problem should be distinguished from a milk quality control program. The former deals with resolving an existing problem, whereas the latter is concerned with improving milk production and quality in a well-managed herd. The most commonly used parameters to make a diagnosis of mastitis in a herd are somatic cell counts and microbiologic evaluation of bulk tank milk.

Somatic Cell Counts

Somatic cell counts are reported as actual values or as their logarithmic derivations. Actual values are representative of the milk from which they are taken, such as a cow, a group of cows, or the bulk tank. They are used primarily to monitor milk quality, and occasionally to identify infected cows in a herd. Linear somatic cell counts are logarithmic derivations of the actual values. They are more suitable for identifying, quantifying, and localizing problems in herds.

Bulk Tank Somatic Cell Count

The bulk tank somatic cell count depends on the prevalence of infected quarters and on the severity of their condition. Since there can be considerable spurious variations between each sample, rolling averages (average of the previous three readings) are more meaningful. The bulk tank somatic cell count is measured directly on a sample from the bulk tank, hence it is an average of cows milked into the tank.

Often only a small percentage of the cows in a herd make up most of the bulk tank somatic cell count for the herd. Thus to evaluate this test it must be known which cows are included and which are excluded from the sample. If a farmer is good at detecting mastitic cows and does not let any of their milk into the tank, a low bulk tank somatic cell count may be evident, but there exist a high number of clinical cases. Likewise, if mastitis detection is poor, the bulk tank somatic cell count may be high but the apparent number of cows with mastitis in the herd may be low.

Linear Somatic Cell Count

The linear somatic cell count is a logarithmic derivation of the actual somatic cell count. A midpoint (geometric mean) of a range of actual somatic cell count is the linear somatic cell count score (Table 1). This converts the actual somatic cell count to a single-digit number and makes it easier to use. When one calculates averages for the herd or part of the herd, a logarithmic score minimizes the relative contribution of the individual cow, making the values more representative of the herd as a whole. Other advantages of the linear somatic cell count are a high linear correlation with milk production losses and the availability to veterinary practitioners through most Dairy Herd Improvement Association centers. Linear somatic cell counts can be reported for every cow in Dairy Herd Improvement Association–registered herds.

The somatic cell count for individual cows can be compiled into meaningful groups so that frequency distributions of problems in time and space can be identified. This is done in an attempt to characterize the patterns of disease and to determine the number of animals at risk. Most Dairy Herd Improvement Association reports provide the option of grouping cows by stage of lactation and age and also provide a herd average. Some test centers also allow veterinarians to access the data by modem and to compile their own lists. Examples of these lists include strings of cows within a herd, purchased cows, or cows at a certain level of production.

Bulk Tank Milk

The accurate interpretation of tests on the bulk tank milk must be considered in the context of the clinical and historical data of the farm. Most commonly, it is a tool to monitor milk quality. Other uses include assessment of the level of subclinical mastitis in a herd, identification of the pathogens in the herd, and as an indicator of the effectiveness of sanitation. Goals and targets for the various bulk tank parameters are listed in Table 2.

Microbial Identification

Identification of the organisms in bulk tank milk helps to identify which pathogens are on a particular farm and whether these have the potential to cause herd problems. For example, when *Streptococcus agalactiae*, *Staphylococcus aureus*, or *Mycoplasma* is found in bulk tank milk, there is a potential for outbreaks caused by these agents, as well as early initiation of a mastitis control program.

Mastitis pathogens are often grouped into contagious and environmental bacteria. This is based on their epidemiologic behavior, that is, on their ability to colonize the udder (Table 3). Contagious organisms are obligate parasites of the cow's udder, which serve as reservoirs of these organisms. Infections by these organisms are spread most commonly during milking and by infection from one cow to the next by contaminated fomites. Fomites include milking equipment, milkers' hands, rags, and sponges. Infections are invasive and persistent and readily become chronic if they are not treated early. Methods of reducing the spread of contagious organisms are aimed at preventing the contamination of healthy cows by infected ones at milking time.

Environmental organisms are opportunistic invaders of the mammary gland. Their reservoir is the environment, hence they will never be completely eradicated. It is not known exactly when these organisms are introduced to the gland, but it is likely to occur if cows are milked with wet and dirty udders or if they are moved to a heavily contaminated area soon after milking when the teat canal is still dilated.

Quantifying a Herd Problem

The most commonly used indices to quantify a mastitis problem in a herd are the number of clinical cases at any one

Table 1. COMPARISON OF THE VARIOUS MEASUREMENTS OF SOMATIC CELL COUNTS (SCCs)

Linear SCC (Score)	Midpoint SCC for Linear SCC ($\times 10^3$ cells/ml)	SCC range for Linear SCC ($\times 10^3$ cells/ml)	CMT (Score)
0	12.5	0–17	Negative
1	25	18–34	Negative
2	50	35–70	Negative
3	100	71–140	Negative
4	200	141–282	Trace
5	400	283–565	Trace
6	800	566–1130	1(–2)
7	1600	1131–2262	(1–)2(–3)
8	3200	2263–4525	3
9	6400	>4526	3

Table 2. TESTS AVAILABLE ON BULK TANK MILK, THEIR IDEAL VALUES, AND LEVELS AT WHICH HERD INTERVENTION IS LIKELY TO RESULT IN IMPROVED MILK QUALITY

Parameter	Ideal Level (Organisms/ml)	Intervention Level (Organisms/ml)
Parameters of Milk Quality and Handling		
Standard plate count (plain agar)	<5000	>10,000
Laboratory pasteurized count	≤10	>150
Somatic cell count (cells/ml)	≤200,000	>400,000
Parameters of Milking Technique and Hygiene		
Coliform count	≤10	>150
Contagious Bacteria (Major Pathogens)		
Staphylococcus aureus (coagulase-positive)	0	>300
Streptococcus agalactiae (cAMP-positive)	0	Positive
Mycoplasma spp.	0	Positive
Environmental Pathogens		
Streptococcus dysgalactia	<500	>1500
Streptococcus uberis	<500	>1500

Table 3. TYPICAL PATTERNS FOUND IN HERDS INFECTED WITH COMMON MAJOR PATHOGENS

Parameter	Organisms			
	Streptococcus agalactiae	Staphylococcus aureus	Mycoplasma spp.	Environmental Bacteria
Regular bulk tank somatic cell count	Fluctuates between moderate to high	≥400,000	≥400,000	≤200,000
Bulk tank milk microbiology	Positive	>300 organisms/ml; may find elevated Corynebacterium bovis count	Positive	Positive for Streptococcus uberis, Streptococcus dysgalactia, and coliforms; may find elevated Staphylococcus epidermidis count
Clinical cases	Few to moderate in number; most cases will be grade I, many subclinical cases	Moderate in number; may find high percentage of three-teated cows and cases of gangrenous mastitis	Moderate in number; most cases will be grade II and respond poorly to therapy	Low to moderate in number; most cases will be grade II or III; may find cases of toxic mastitis
Culling rate	Low	High	High	Low, but case-fatality rate may be high
Likely sources within the herd	Carrier cows in herd	Carrier cows; affected cows are not segregated; poor teat dipping; ineffective dry cow therapy	Introduction of positive cows to the herd; carrier cows; lack of segregation; ineffective mastitis detection	Dirty, wet udders are being milked; housing and calving areas may be filthy; poor teat dipping may also increase S. uberis
Control program	Eradicate	Segregate and/or cull affected cows; eradicate	Cull or segregate cows depending on circumstances; eradicate	Improve cleanliness of environment; improve udder preparation

time (prevalence), new cases over a defined time period (incidence), individual cow California Mastitis Test (CMT), herd CMT, bulk tank somatic cell count, herd linear somatic cell count, and frequency distributed linear somatic cell count of individual cows. The quantification of a problem will only be approximate; however, as long as the estimate of loss is realistic, to the manager, it serves the purpose of simple illustration.

The number of clinical cases at any one time is calculated from annual averages. The goal for dairy herds should be to have less than 1.0 per cent of cows clinically affected with mastitis (milk is withheld) at any one time (prevalence). Also, if recognition of cows with mastitis is early and treatment is prompt, appropriate, and successful, cows with mastitis should be out of the milking herd for about 1 week. This means that the incidence of mastitis should be less than 1.0 per cent of the milking herd per week or less than 4.0 per cent of the milking herd per month. Intervention is indicated when the incidence of clinical cases is more than 1.5 per cent per week. Since these values are annual averages, it is acceptable to see the incidence of mastitis in the dry season to be half the yearly average, whereas in the wet or housed season this value may double.

Individual clinical cases are also an important indicator of the level of disease within the herd. It has been estimated that for every clinical case there are another 15 to 40 subclinical cases in the herd. Subclinical cases, that is, cows with high somatic cell count but without grossly detectable changes in the udder or milk, are more prone to developing clinical mastitis than are other cows. Therefore, an increase in the number of clinical cases may be an indicator of worse to come, rather than being the problem itself.

The culling rate for mastitis, including mastitis-related low production (e.g., chronic cases and "3 titters") should be less than 6 per cent; intervention is indicated at greater than 8 per cent. The case-fatality rate should be less than 0.5 per cent.

The CMT score should be negative or trace for greater than or equal to 90 per cent of the herd. The bulk tank CMT should always be negative. The goal for the bulk tank somatic cell count is less than or equal to 300,000 cells/ml. Losses associated with elevations in the bulk tank somatic cell count are compiled in Table 4.

To quantify losses one has to compare production with obtainable goals for that farm. This is achieved by setting targets. Targets are set for each individual farm and are levels of production or disease that can be expected to be achieved within a given time period (e.g., 1 year). In milk quality control programs, targets can be set as a degree of improvement over the existing year or of improvement over state average or by comparison with similar herds. Practically, target levels lie somewhere between ideal and current standards and should be set so that they can be expected to be met within the given time frame.

CONTROL MEASURES

Control of mastitis in a herd is directed at preventing subclinical mastitis, since this is responsible for the greatest economic losses. Prevention of subclinical mastitis will also reduce the number of clinical cases. About 75 per cent of contagious mastitides occur during milking, as do a significant number of environmental infections. Nevertheless, this is not the only time at which mastitis can be prevented. The control of mastitis is a 24-hour-a-day occupation and must be implemented inside and outside of the milking parlor and at all stages of the cow's life. Prevention of mastitis includes strict and immaculate milking technique and hygiene, proper post-milking care, and control of the environment for both lactating and dry cows.

Implementation of a mastitis control program and the drive to meet targets involves the veterinarian in many ways. These include education of the farm managers and workers. The managers need to be made aware of how mastitis is initiated and maintained, how much mastitis in a herd is costing, and how it can be dealt with on a herd basis. Incentives for farm managers can be made by comparison of their performance

Table 4. ESTIMATED PRODUCTION LOSSES AND INFECTION RATES ASSOCIATED WITH DIFFERENT BULK TANK SOMATIC CELL COUNTS

Bulk Tank Somatic Cell Count ($\times 10^3$/cells/ml)	% Cows Affected	% Production Loss in Herd
<300	<20	0–2.5
300–500	20–40	2.5–7.5
500–800	40–70	7.5–15.0
>800	>70	15.0–25.0

Table 5. COMPOUNDS AND THEIR CONCENTRATIONS COMMONLY USED AS POST-MILKING SANITIZERS (POST-TEAT DIP)

Compound*	Concentration (% Solution)
Chlorhexidine	0.5
Sodium hypochlorite	4.0
Iodophors	1.0
Quaternary ammonium	0.5–1.0
Linear dodecyl benzene sulfonic acid	2.0
Bromine	0.2

*FDA-approved products are sold to be used unadulterated. Sodium hypochlorite is not an FDA-approved teat dip.

with targets. Milkers need to be educated and periodically reminded on how to milk cows hygienically and to able to detect mastitic cows early. They can also be inspired by incentives (e.g., based on bulk tank somatic cell count, bulk tank milk microbiology, and/or number of clinical cases) or threatened with sanctions (e.g., for dirty milk filters).

Milking Technique

Correct milking procedures follow three stages: premilking preparation, milking technique, and postmilking sanitation. Immaculate attention must be given to each of these to ensure hygienic collection of the milk, minimal spread of mastitis, and prevention of new intramammary infections. The goal of premilking preparation is for the cow to have a dry and clean udder that is ready for milking. Current recommendations include washing and drying the udder, predipping the teats and drying them off again, and using individual towels for each cow. Where climate permits, the cows' udders should be cleaned before the cows enter the milking parlor. Sprinkler systems are popular in warm climates and can reduce the workload in the parlor.

Good milking also relies on good liner fit and machine vacuum stability (i.e., on well-functioning equipment), since these reduce the introduction of bacteria into the udder. Design faults are rare in modern dairies and, contrary to common belief, are not a major cause of mastitis. On the other hand, defective replaceable and serviceable components may contribute to up to 20 per cent of cases of mastitis. The most common problem lies with the milk liners when they "slip" or "squawk." "Liner slip" is the entering of air between the liner and the teat into the inflation chamber and allows the liner to crawl up the teat (teat cup crawl). "Slipping" air flows at tremendous speeds. This produces droplets that fly around, impact, and rebound off the inside of the entire cluster. These high-speed droplets also impact with the teat ends of all quarters at high speed, resulting in penetration of the teat canal ("impacts"). The importance of dry udders becomes paramount in this context; if a wet udder allows contaminated fluid, "magic water," to accumulate around the rim of the liner and liner slip occurs, this water will be sucked into and dispersed around the entire inflation chamber, including its introduction to all four quarters. Injection of these droplets has been shown to occur in 40 to 80 per cent of quarters not affected by slip, if one quarter of a cluster is squawking. Therefore, if introduced material contains pathogens, mastitis commonly results.

Common causes of liner slip are avoided by proper positioning of the cluster and providing mechanical support for the cluster, replacing the liners at the end of their recommended life span, and cutting off the vacuum before removing the claws.

Post-milking Sanitation

After milking, the teats should again be sterilized using a product approved by the Food and Drug Administration. Common teat sanitizers are listed in Table 5. Dipping of teats after milking is the single most effective preventative measure against contagious forms of mastitis. It reduces the infection rate by contagious organisms (approximately 75 per cent), the infection rate of environmental streptococci, and the incidence of subclinical mastitis in a herd; that is, it is preventative not curative.

TREATMENT

Having to treat excessive numbers of cows with mastitis is admitting to a failure of a mastitis prevention program. Excessive numbers of cases requiring treatment can seriously impair the effective operation of a farm by consuming valuable time that could otherwise be spent on disease prevention. In addition, it must be remembered that treating individual cows has little bearing on the incidence of mastitis in a herd.

Treatment strategies vary with the clinical severity of the disease. The subacute case (grade I) requires only intramammary therapy for 3 days after each milking. An acutely affected cow (grade II) should be treated with systemic and intramammary antibiotics for a minimum of 3 days. The peracute cow (grade III) needs to be treated with systemic and intramammary antibiotics, oral or intravenous fluids, and anti-inflammatory drugs.

The selection of antibiotics should be based on the sensitivities of identified (gram-positive) pathogens on the farm. The choice of drugs should then be determined and prioritized by likely therapeutic benefit. Only compatible combinations of intramammary and systemic drugs should be used (Table 6).

Severe cases of mastitis respond well to anti-inflammatory

Table 6. COMMONLY AVAILABLE DRUGS TO TREAT MASTITIS WITH SYSTEMICALLY ADMINISTERED ANTIBIOTICS AND THEIR COMPATIBILITIES AND SUGGESTED DOSAGES

Intramammary Preparation	Compatible Systemic Drug	Dosage	Drug Withdrawal Time*
Ampicillin (Hetacillin)	Procaine penicillin G	20,000 IU/kg q24h IM	Milk: 96 hr Meat: 14 days
	Ampicillin	10 mg/kg q24h IM	Milk: 96 hr Meat: 6 days
	Amoxicillin	10 mg/kg q24h IM	Milk: 96 hr Meat: 6 days
Cloxacillin	Penicillins		
Penicillin and novobiocin	Penicillins		
Penicillin and dihydrostreptomycin	Penicillins		
Cephapirin	Penicillins		
Erythromycin	Erythromycin	12.5 mg/kg q24h IM	Milk: 96 hr Meat: 28 days
	Tylosin	12.5 mg/kg q24h IV	Milk: 96 hr Meat: 28 days
	Penicillins		
Oxytetracycline	Oxytetracycline	10 mg/kg q24h IV	Milk: 96 hr Meat: 14–28 days, depending on manufacturer
	Sulfonamides	200 mg/kg q24h PO	Milk: 72 hr Meat: 10 days
	Potentiated sulfonamides	48 mg/kg q48h IM	Milk: 72 hr Meat: 12 days

*Drug withdrawal times are guidelines only, since the dosages given are for extra-label use.

drugs (aspirin, 960 gr p.o. q12h; flunixin meglumine, 1 mg/kg IM/IV q24h) and hydrotherapy. Hydrotherapy is applied by standing a cow in a stall and spraying the affected quarter for 15 to 30 minutes twice a day with a firm and broad, but not painful, stream of water from a hose. All cases of mastitis respond favorably to frequent stripping of the affected quarters. This can be enhanced by repeated injections of oxytocin (5 to 10 units IM q4h). Fresh cows, especially first-lactation heifers, may have additional complications with udder edema. This can be treated with diuretics (e.g., furosemide 1 mg/kg IM q24h). Cows with hemorrhagic mastitis are often treated with vitamin K_1 (1 mg/kg IM q24h). Gangrenous mastitis (usually the result of a peracute infection with *Staphylococcus aureus*) may require amputation of the teat. This is done by clamping emasculators halfway down the cold and avascular teat and then cutting off the distal portion.

Cows that have not responded to 7 to 10 days of treatment are not likely to respond to any form of therapy and may be forming abscesses in the udder. Once these cases are clinically stable, recovery is usually adequate even when therapy is withdrawn. After milking a mastitic cow, the cluster should be sterilized before being used on the next cow.

BIBLIOGRAPHY

Jarrett JA: Symposium on bovine mastitis. Vet Clin North Am 6(2):231–431, 1984.
National Mastitis Council: Laboratory Handbook on Bovine Mastitis. Research Committee of the National Mastitis Council. Fort Atkinson, WI WD Hoard & Sons, 1987.
Sundlof SF, Riviere JE, Craigmill AL: Food Animal Residue Avoidance Databook: a Comprehensive Compendium of Food Animal Drugs. Gainesville, FL University of Florida, 1992.

Lactation Failure
S. K. LYLE, DVM

LACTATION FAILURE IN SWINE

Lactation failure is recognized in all food animal species and has profound economic significance owing to production losses that go beyond those incurred by the symptomatic dam. Classically in swine, lactation failure has been referred to as mastitis, metritis, and agalactia. This is probably a misnomer in that lactation failure most likely represents a multidisease complex, with mastitis, metritis, and agalactia being one aspect of this complex. Of greater frequency and economic impact is suboptimum milk production in sows (which is largely asymptomatic), resulting in increased neonatal losses and poor weight gains in piglets.

Diagnosis and Clinical Signs

Parameters in a herd that lead toward a diagnosis of lactation failure are increased death in piglets from starvation, crushing, or diarrhea; higher variation in weaned piglet weights compared with newly farrowed weights; and average weaning weights below the herd's target.[1] Identification and enumeration of these symptoms underscore the importance of records within the herd. Calculation of sow productive indices can be used to compare individual sows within the herd.[2] Examination of the herd for the presence of systemic disease, locomotor disturbances, and general condition of sows during gestation and lactation and examination of individual sows for function and number of teats, presence of mastitis, udder injuries, vulvar discharges, appetite, litter nursing behavior, and vigor may help to determine whether lactation failure is a herd or individual sow problem.

Symptomatic sows are usually anorectic, lethargic, hyperthermic (39.5° to 41°C), and constipated and have elevated respiratory and heart rates. Signs usually begin 1 to 3 days post partum. These sows spend most of their time lying down, frequently without the udder exposed for piglet nursing. When mastitis is present, affected glands are edematous and painful and skin discoloration is evident in white breeds. A malodorous, brown vulvar discharge is evidence of metritis.

Etiology

A multitude of factors are believed to increase the risk of agalactia. Sow genetics, selection criteria for replacement gilts, breeding age or weight, udder injuries facilitating entry of infectious agents to the gland, and overall health status of the herd can be important factors affecting lactation performance.[1] Endotoxemia plays a role in some cases of lactation failure, specifically in those sows that are anorectic and/or febrile. The source of endotoxin (usually from *Escherichia coli*) has been theorized to come from the alimentary tract (secondary to anorexia and gut stasis), the uterus (secondary to metritis, retained fetuses or placentae), or the mammary gland. Attempts to reproduce the disease experimentally by endotoxin infusion have given mixed results, but the intramammary or intrauterine route will produce agalactia.[3] However, postmortem examination of sows exhibiting symptoms of endotoxemia usually fails to demonstrate lesions in either the uterus or the gastrointestinal tract.[4]

In sows experiencing lactation failure, elevated levels of plasma 17β estradiol and cortisol and decreased serum prolactin and thyroxine values have been documented.[5] It is not known if these altered endocrine profiles represent a primary dysfunction or whether hormonal disturbances occur secondary to stress or endotoxemia.

Management factors that can predispose sows to the syndrome include elevated farrowing house temperature, inadequate ventilation, poor sanitation of farrowing crates, flooring systems, and nutrition. In the United States, the increased use of woven wire or welded metal floors (plastic-coated) has improved sanitation of the crate floor. In Europe, bedded stalls are still used in some operations, and their use has been shown to increase the incidence of coliform mastitis when compared with the incidence of disease in sows allowed access to outdoor runs for defecation/urination.[6] The complex effects of nutrition on lactation performance are more difficult to sort out. Overfeeding or underfeeding during gestation, inadequate calcium-phosphorus ratios, and vitamin E–selenium deficiency have been incriminated in increasing the incidence of lactation failure in a herd. Contamination of grain with ergot alkaloids (*Claviceps* spp.) or aflatoxins will cause agalactia or hypogalactia.

Treatment

Efforts to manage lactation failure depend somewhat on whether the problem exists as an individual sow problem or a herd problem. Agalactic sows can be treated with 5 to 20 IU of oxytocin every 2 hours to allow milk letdown and assist in preventing piglet starvation. Additional therapy directed against endotoxemia is frequently indicated. Such therapy consists of broad-spectrum antibiotics and nonsteroidal anti-inflammatory agents (flunixin meglumine, 100 to 250 mg IM twice daily, extra-label use) or corticosteroids (prednisolone, 50 to 100 mg). Furosemide (extra-label use) can be used for udder edema, and tranquilization (acepromazine, 10 to 20 mg, or azaperone (Stresnil), 5 to 7 ml, both extra-label use) is helpful in sows or gilts too agitated to allow nursing. Cross-fostering is probably the most practical method of decreasing losses in the piglets. When cross-fostering is not a viable option, oral supplementation with a mixture of 1 qt cow's milk, 1 oz syrup, and 1 oz corn oil should be fed at 10 per cent of the piglet's weight each day.

Prevention

Genetic improvement (by selection of replacement gilts from sows with top sow productive indices and culling of sows with lactation failure), limited feeding (2.3 kg/day) of a balanced corn-soy ration during gestation, laxative diets, vitamin E–selenium supplementation, adequate calcium-phosphorus ratios (e.g., large white breeds have increased dietary requirements), avoidance of fat sows or thin sows, vaccination to minimize the herd incidence of disease, diminishing stress in periparturient sows and gilts, induced farrowing, and forced exercise (if practical for the type of operation) have all been shown to be beneficial to decreasing the incidence of lactation failure in a herd.

LACTATION FAILURE IN OTHER SPECIES

Lactation failure in other food animal species can occur secondary to many systemic diseases, especially those producing fever, toxemia, or metabolic disturbances. *Mycoplasma mycoides* ss. *mycoides* can cause agalactia, abortion, depression, and diarrhea in does and polyarthritis and pneumonia in nursing kids. Although tylosin or tetracyclines may relieve symptoms in affected does, they probably do not eliminate the carrier state; therefore, culling of does infected with *Mycoplasma* spp. is recommended. Endophyte *(Acermonium coenophialum)*-infected fescue pastures have been associated with the production of agalactia or dysgalactia. Removal of the animals from infected pastures is the only known therapy.

REFERENCES

1. Bradford JR: Investigating and correcting suboptimum lactation performance in sows. Compend Cont Ed Pract Vet 12:269–273, 1990.
2. National Swine Improvement Federation: Guidelines for Uniform Swine Improvement Programs. St. Paul, MN, Institute of Agriculture, 1987.
3. Elmore RG, Martin CE, Berg JN: Absorption of *Escherichia coli* endotoxin from the mammary glands and uteri of early postpartum sows and gilts. Theriogenology 10:439–446, 1978.
4. Ross RF, Ornig AP, Woods RD, et al: Bacteriologic study of sow agalactia. Am J Vet Res 42:949–955, 1981.
5. Elmore RG, Martin CE: Mammary glands. *In* Leman AD (ed): Diseases in Swine, pp 175–181. Ames, IA, Iowa State Press, 1986.
6. Wegmann P, Bertschinger HU, Eng V: Relationship between contamination of the teat end with coliform bacteria and incidence of coliform mastitis (MMA). *In* 10th Congress of International Pig Veterinary Society, Brazil, 1988, p 302.

Retained Fetal Membranes
M. L. FAHNING, DVM, PhD

Most veterinarians agree that fetal membranes should be considered retained if they are not passed by 12 hours after calving. Few topics elicit as much discussion among practitioners and academicians as the subject of retained fetal membranes (RFM). Veterinarians have diverse opinions on how this condition is best handled and treated, and controversy exists between whether or not manual removal is indicated.

Economically, RFM represent one of the most significant abnormalities occurring during the postpartum period in cattle. The consequences of RFM result in an increased incidence of postpartum metritis, pyometra, and delayed conception. Schukken and associates[1] also reported that cows with RFM had a three times higher chance of developing subsequent mastitis than cows not experiencing this condition.

The incidence of RFM commonly falls in the 3 to 12 per cent range in the dairy cattle population. It is found less frequently in beef cattle. An increased incidence occurs in cattle following abnormal calving, as in twins, forced extraction, abortions, induced parturition, and premature births. The condition has also been associated with nutritional factors such as vitamin deficiencies (carotene, vitamins A and E), mineral deficiencies or imbalances (calcium and phosphorus), trace mineral deficiencies (selenium and iodine), and toxins in feeds (nitrate).

The exact cause of RFM has not been fully elucidated. In general, it is proposed that the condition of RFM is caused by a disturbance of the loosening mechanism in the placentomes. The normal loosening process actually begins days, weeks, and even months prior to parturition. The mechanism of collagen development in the placental epithelium and the maternal crypts begins months before parturition. The contractions of the uterus during the dilation and expulsion phases cause constant changing pressure, resulting in alternating ischemic and hyperemic conditions. It also results in changes in surface area of fetal chorionic villi. The attachment of the chorionic epithelium in the maternal crypts becomes impaired. Thus during the expulsion phase the first signs of mechanical detachment become evident.

Major pathologic conditions affecting placentome separation include immature placentomes associated with shortened gestation, edema associated with cesarean sections or uterine torsion, and placentitis associated with infections. Uterine atony associated with milk fever and hydropic conditions also contributes to the incidence of RFM, but uterine atony without any other disturbances in the loosening process is not a major factor in causing RFM.

A review by Paisley and co-workers[2] demonstrated the wide variety of treatment alternatives that exist for treating RFM. One of the earliest and most widely practiced forms of treatment for RFM has been manual removal. However, most of the scientific literature concludes that manual removal with or without chemotherapy results in reduced, rather than enhanced, fertility. Considerable trauma to the endometrium occurs even during conservative attempts at manual removal and is also associated with inhibition of the uterine defense mechanism. The use of intrauterine antiseptics and other therapeutic agents further inhibits uterine phagocytosis. This further delays uterine involution. Bolinder and colleagues[3] reported a higher incidence and more severe uterine infections after manual removal of RFM compared with untreated cows with RFM. Manual removal also prolonged the occurrence of the first functional corpus luteum by 20 days.

Drugs that increase uterine motility are frequently used in the treatment of this condition. These drugs include oxytocin, estrogen, ergot derivatives, calcium solutions, and prostaglandins. However, they have limited value in terms of results. The lack of response should not be surprising owing to the low incidence of uterine atony as a primary cause of RFM.

Administration of intrauterine antibiotics and antibacterials has been routine therapy for RFM for many years. However, their widespread use is not supported by most reports evaluating their use in relation to conception rates or days open.

The use of intrauterine therapy does decrease putrefaction and the associated fetid odor of RFM. Although this may be an important consideration aesthetically from the client's viewpoint, it still makes its use questionable economically because of the cost of treatment. In addition, the economics of withholding milk for human consumption are also a factor.

Prostaglandins administered during the immediate postpartum period (within 1 hour) have been advocated by some practitioners as a means of preventing or at least lowering the incidence of RFM; however, no good evidence exists to support this use of prostaglandins. Burton and co-workers[4] reported that neither prostaglandin $F_{2\alpha}$ nor an analogue of prostaglandin (fenprostalene) were uterotonic during the early postpartum period.

In summary, the results of most studies support the conclusion that no treatment is the best way to handle retained placenta in the cow. The cow should, however, be closely monitored for signs of systemic involvement so that if this occurs appropriate supportive therapy can be administered. Routine postpartum examination starting at about 2 weeks post partum as part of the routine fertility program should be practiced. Certainly some clients will demand manual removal of RFM, and these situations present veterinarians with an opportunity and challenge to educate the client.

Other species of food animals that experience RFM include sheep, goats and swine, but these species have a much lower incidence of RFM. Mortality resulting from RFM is relatively low. However, in swine the membranes are often retained in the apical portion of the uterine horns and are not usually visible externally. These animals often develop septic metritis, and mortality could be relatively high. In swine, if RFM are suspected, these animals should be given repeated doses of oxytocin (20 to 30 units every 2 to 3 hours) and broad-spectrum antibiotics.

REFERENCES

1. Schukken YH, Erb HW, Scarlet JM: A hospital-based study of the relationship between retained placenta and mastitis in dairy cows. Cornell Vet 79:319–326, 1989.
2. Paisley LG, Mickelsen WD, Anderson PB: Mechanisms and therapy for retained fetal membranes and uterine factors of cows: a review. Theriogenology 25:353–381, 1986.
3. Bolinder A, Seguin B, Kindahl H, et al: Retained fetal membranes in cows: manual removal versus nonremoval and its effect on reproductive performance. Theriogenology 30:45–56, 1988.
4. Burton MJ, Herschler RC, Dziuk HE, et al: Effect of fenprostalene on postpartum myometrial activity in dairy cows with normal or delayed placental expulsion. Br Vet J 143:549–554, 1987.

Metritis and Endometritis
GAVIN F. RICHARDSON, DVM, MVSc, BA

Pathologic uterine infections of cows can result in considerable economic loss to producers. These losses result from reduced reproductive efficiency, loss of production, cost of therapy, increased replacement costs, forced culling, and sometimes the adverse effects of systemic illness. Under the appropriate circumstances, veterinarians can reduce these economic losses by promoting good nutrition and encouraging proper sanitary practices at calving and during the early postpartum period.

Puerperal metritis occurs in the early postpartum period. In dairy cows, this period has been defined as the period following parturition when the pituitary gland is insensitive to gonadotropin-releasing hormone (GnRH) (the first 7 to 14 days). Retained fetal membranes, dystocia, trauma to the reproductive tract, emphysematous fetus, hydrallantois, and unsanitary conditions at parturition can all predispose to puerperal metritis. Affected cows can be anorectic, depressed, and toxic and can become dehydrated and/or go into shock. There is often a foul-smelling suppurative to reddish-brown vulvar discharge.

Pathologic uterine infections that persist into the intermediate postpartum period are referred to as metritis or endometritis. The intermediate period in dairy cows begins when the pituitary gland becomes sensitive to GnRH and lasts until the first ovulation (generally 10 to 30 days post partum). Metritis and endometritis can still be present in the postovulatory period (which lasts until uterine involution is complete at 40 to 45 days in normal cows). Endometritis can also result from pyometra or the introduction of pathogens during insemination (e.g., by breeding during the luteal phase).

Cows with metritis may have slightly elevated temperatures and may be somewhat anorectic or have reduced milk production. There will be subinvolution of the uterus and possibly a malodorous or purulent vaginal discharge.

Endometritis can be characterized by infertility and a purulent vulvar discharge, which is most often observed during estrus. Affected cows can exhibit shortened or prolonged estrous cycles because of excessive prostaglandin release or embryonic death, respectively. The uterus can be slightly enlarged and may contain a small amount of fluid; however, there may be no palpable abnormalities on transrectal examination.

Perimetritis occurs when uterine infections extend through the uterine wall. A localized or generalized peritonitis can result, and the uterus will often form adhesions to adjacent structures. Because of these adhesions the reproductive tract can be difficult to palpate or retract. Infertility can result, especially if the ovaries, oviducts, or ovarian bursae are involved or if an abscess drains into the uterine lumen. If the adhesions are extensive, they can compromise the ability of the uterus to expand, resulting in affected cows becoming chronic aborters. Attempts to break down the adhesions only result in the formation of more extensive adhesions.

ETIOLOGY

Actinomyces pyogenes is probably the most important aerobic organism involved in pathologic postpartum uterine infections. Gram-negative anaerobes that act synergistically with *A. pyogenes* to produce these infections include *Fusobacterium necrophorum* and *Bacteroides* spp. Infections with streptococci, staphylococci, *Pasteurella* spp., *Bacillus* spp., *Pseudomonas* spp., and so on rarely persist, cause permanent endometrial damage, or lead to impaired fertility. However, they may be responsible for acute septic metritis in some cows.

Escherichia coli may produce endotoxins. Less commonly, clostridial infections can produce severe or fatal disease. Other organisms that can cause endometritis include mycoplasmas, ureaplasmas, *Haemophilus somnus*, *Campylobacter fetus* ss. *venerealis*, *Brucella abortus*, *Tritrichomonas fetus*, and certain viruses; these will not be discussed in this section.

DIAGNOSIS

The diagnosis of postpartum endometritis can be difficult in a clinical setting. Examination of the vagina with a speculum may be the most effective method of selecting cows for the treatment of endometritis. This should be combined with an accurate history, visual inspection of the perineum, examination of the tail for evidence of vaginal discharge, and transrectal examination of the reproductive tract. Endometrial culture and biopsy can be used, but there are difficulties with interpretation. Furthermore, there have been reports of reduced fertility in cows during the breeding period immediately following postpartum endometrial biopsy. In most instances a decision must be made regarding therapy prior to the availability of culture or biopsy results. Nonetheless, culture and biopsy results can be useful in providing retrospective information.

The characteristics of vaginal discharge from a postpartum cow must be interpreted carefully to avoid misdiagnosis, incorrect therapy, or unnecessary therapy. Manual or speculum examination of the vagina in a sanitary manner may be necessary in order to insepct this discharge. The discharge of reddish-brown, nonodorous fluid that may contain flecks of debris or exudate during the first 10 to 18 days post partum may be normal lochia and not due to puerperal metritis. As long as the discharge does not become foul smelling, uterine involution usually proceeds normally. Purulent vulvar discharge in a postpartum cow may not be a sign of metritis or endometritis but may be a sign of an active uterine defense mechanism. A cloudy, mucous discharge at estrus is no more likely to be infected with pathogenic organisms than is clear mucus. Cows with slightly enlarged reproductive tracts and/or slightly abnormal discharges at 30 days post partum probably will not benefit from antimicrobial treatment.

A wide variation in the rate of uterine involution can make the results of a single clinical examination of the uterus prior to 21 days post partum difficult to interpret.

TREATMENT

Cows with severe metritis that are toxic, dehydrated, or in shock will require appropriate supportive therapy.

When administering antimicrobial therapy one must keep in mind that intrauterine infusions are often effective only in the lumen and endometrium. In the early postpartum uterus, the infusion of relatively large volumes (e.g., 250 to 500 ml) may be required to enhance the distribution of antibiotic throughout the uterus. In an involuted uterus, infusion volumes of 20 ml for heifers and 40 ml for cows are probably adequate.

Systemic therapy is required if septicemia is present or if the oviducts, ovaries, or deeper layers of the uterus are involved. In general, the duration and concentration of systemically administered antibiotics are less in the endometrium and uterine lumen than for antibiotics administered into the uterus. To ensure adequate concentrations of antibiotics in all parts of the reproductive tract, both local and systemic therapy may be required. Once instituted, intrauterine or systemic antibiotic therapy should be continued for a *minimum* of 3 days.

Penicillin-resistant organisms release penicillinase into the environment, which in turn can protect other sensitive organisms in the uterus. Sodium penicillin G is useful for intrauterine infusion at a dosage of 10 million IU only in the postovulatory period when bacterial populations are less diverse. This will result in therapeutic levels in the uterine lumen and endometrium for up to 24 hours. Procaine penicillin G can be used for systemic therapy (at a dosage of 22,000 IU/kg q12h) during the early postpartum period, because it is usually effective against bacteria likely to invade the endometrium from the uterine lumen.

When given intravenously at 11 mg/kg q12h, concentrations of oxytetracycline in the uterus are believed to be insufficient to affect *A. pyogenes*, especially in the early postpartum cow. However, systemic therapy with tetracyclines could empirically be effective against systemic infections.

Despite the lack of controlled studies, the intrauterine administration of tetracyclines has been described as an effective preventative measure for metritis in cows with retained fetal membranes as well as an effective treatment for postpartum metritis. Intrauterine dosages of 2 to 6 g of tetracycline daily or every second day appear to be adequate. The use of tetracycline preparations that are irritating to the uterus should be avoided. For example, powdered tetracyclines in solution and preparations containing propylene glycol can cause considerable endometrial irritation.

Intrauterine infusions of irritating solutions such as iodine probably should not be used to treat pathologic uterine infections. Producing additional inflammation in an already inflamed uterus is probably of no advantage and may even be detrimental.

The practitioner should always remember that intrauterine antiseptics and many antibiotics are capable of inhibiting phagocytosis for several days after application. This depressed leukocyte activity could be disastrous, especially if the organism involved is resistant to the antibiotic or antiseptic used. Furthermore, the pasteurized uterine secretions collected from a cow with retained fetal membranes severely inhibited the antibacterial activity of many antibiotics under both aerobic and anaerobic conditions. Another disadvantage of antibiotic therapy is that milk must be withheld from human consumption to avoid drug residues.

Infusing warm water or saline into the early postpartum uterus and then siphoning it off has been suggested as a means to remove infected materials and improve the condition of the cow. Although controlled studies to evaluate this form of therapy are lacking, the removal of most or all of the material from an infected uterus should logically be of benefit. Nonetheless, there can be several hazards or difficulties associated with this type of therapy. The uterus can be punctured or damaged during the procedure, irrigation fluid might flow into the oviducts and cause salpingitis, placental tissue and debris can block the hose during siphoning, and a large, dependent uterus may be difficult to empty satisfactorily. Initial infusion volumes of 1 L are recommended until it can be determined whether the fluid can be retrieved. After this, infusion volumes vary from 1 to 4 L and are continued until the effluent is relatively clear.

Cows with chronic endometritis are reported to benefit by flushing the uterus with saline during diestrus using techniques for the nonsurgical collection of embryos. This can be followed by the administration of prostaglandins and breeding at the induced estrus. For severe endometritis, flushing can be repeated every 48 hours, as indicated.

The positive effects of GnRH would logically result from its ability to stimulate the release of pituitary luteinizing hormone (LH), resulting in ovulation and the resumption of regular estrous cycles. This should increase the number of estrous periods prior to breeding and thus increase the fertility of postpartum dairy cows. However, GnRH therapy will only be effective if the pituitary is sensitive to GnRH (i.e., the cow should be approximately 10 or more days post partum) and if there is sufficient follicular development on the ovaries (follicles $\geq$ 10–15 mm). Cows treated with GnRH in the first 20 or so days post partum should be monitored closely for the development of pyometra.

Cows with retained fetal membranes and/or metritis may benefit from therapy with prostaglandin $F_{2\alpha}$ or its analogues (PGF). Cows with delayed uterine involution may have higher average progesterone levels than normal cows prior to the formation of the first corpus luteum. If this progesterone is from luteinized follicles, PGF therapy would be beneficial. PGF may also stimulate phagocytosis.

The PGF preparations currently used do not increase myometrial activity in the early postpartum cow, even when the uterus is primed with estrogen. There is also evidence that PGF is not essential for uterine involution. However, there are indications that PGF does stimulate ovarian activity in the postpartum period.

PGF is indicated in the treatment of postpartum endometritis. The optimal time for PGF therapy would be *after* day 7 of the estrous cycle when the corpus luteum is most responsive. This is because the successful resolution of endometritis has been associated with the occurrence of estrus. Nonetheless, there may also be a benefit to noncyclic cows. PGF may have a beneficial effect on the postpartum uterus that is independent of its luteolytic effect.

METRITIS AND ENDOMETRITIS IN OTHER FOOD-PRODUCING ANIMALS

Metritis and endometritis in sheep and goats can resemble these conditions in cows. In sows, urogenital infections can occur as endemic infections or as epidemics. Abnormal vulvar discharges can originate from infections of the urinary tract, vagina, uterus, or a combination of these tissues. Many different bacteria have been isolated from these infections, often in mixed cultures. Viruses, or even ureaplasmas, could also be involved. The boar may transmit some of the causative organisms venereally. History, clinical signs, and slaughterhouse inspections are commonly used methods of determining the site and nature of these infections. Record analysis will help identify key epidemiologic features of the problem. Uterine infections are commonly associated with reduced conception and farrowing rates and regular returns to estrus.

The principles of therapy for uterine infections in cows can be applied to small ruminants and swine. However, intrauterine infusions are more difficult in these smaller animals, GnRH therapy is unlikely to be of benefit, and PGF therapy may not be beneficial in sows. Proper sanitation and hygiene (including at breeding), culling affected animals, and good management practices will reduce the incidence of these infections much more effectively and economically than will therapy, especially in sows. Tetanus prophylaxis should be considered when treating uterine infections in small ruminants.

BIBLIOGRAPHY

Bretzlaff K: Rationale for treatment of endometritis in the dairy cow. Vet Clin North Am [Food Anim Pract] 3:593–607, 1987.
Dial GD, MacLachlan NJ: Urogenital infections of swine: I. Clinical manifestations and pathogenesis. Compend Cont Ed Pract Vet 10:63–70, 1988.
Dial GD, MacLachlan NJ: Urogenital infections of swine: II. Pathology and medical management. Compend Cont Ed Pract Vet 10:529–538, 1988.
Paisley LG, Mickelson WD, Anderson PB: Mechanisms and therapy for retained fetal membranes and uterine infections of cows: a review. Theriogenology 25:353–381, 1986.

Pyometra in Cattle
LOUIS F. ARCHBALD, DVM, PhD, MS

Pyometra is the accumulation of purulent exudate in the uterus. It is an infectious uterine disorder characterized clinically by retention of the corpus luteum and anestrus. Since there are no systemic manifestations of the disease, affected cows do not appear ill. However, these cows are economic liabilities since they often experience infertility and, in some instances, sterility. Spontaneous recovery from the disease is uncommon.

Pyometra should not be confused with chronic endometritis, in which there may be thickening or enlargement of the uterine wall and the presence of a purulent vulvar discharge. In most instances, these cows are cyclic, although there may be irregularities in the length of the estrous cycles.

OCCURRENCE

Pyometra occurs most often during the early postpartum period (15 to 60 days post partum). It may be a sequel to dystocia, retained fetal membranes, or acute septic metritis. It can also occur at various intervals after breeding. Such cases are associated with early embryonic death, which may result from an infection introduced at the time of breeding or one already present in the uterus at breeding. Insemination of cows during the luteal phase or of pregnant cows will often result in pyometra. The use of bulls infected with the protozoan *Trichomonas fetus* will often result in cases of pyometra.

ETIOLOGY

Postpartum pyometra is caused by infection of the uterus by a variety of microorganisms. These include hemolytic streptococci, hemolytic staphylococci, coliforms, *Actinomyces pyogenes*, and *Pseudomonas aeruginosa*. Occasionally, animals may be infected with clostridia or different types of fungi. *Actinomyces pyogenes* is probably the most common cause of bovine pyometra and can be the cause of pyometra in several cows within a herd.

Postbreeding pyometra, although relatively uncommon, is usually caused by the same microorganisms as those causing postpartum pyometra. However, a more common cause of postbreeding pyometra is the protozoan *Trichomonas fetus*.

CLINICAL SIGNS

Affected cows show no general signs of illness, even though the uterus contains a considerable amount of purulent material. Due to failure of the uterine luteolytic mechanism, the corpus luteum is retained and true anestrus is common. In some cases of postpartum pyometra a purulent vulvar discharge may be observed, particularly when the cow lies down. The consistency of the discharge is usually thick and mucoid. Its color may be yellow, creamy white, grayish white, greenish gray, or reddish brown. In other cows, the cervix is closed and there is no evidence of such a discharge.

On rectal examination the uterus is distended with fluid and there is a corpus luteum on one of the ovaries. The size of the uterus can correspond to that characteristic of any stage of pregnancy. Distribution of the fluid in the uterus may be bilaterally symmetric, or it may predominantly occupy one uterine horn. In cases of unilateral enlargement of the uterus, the corpus luteum may be observed on the contralateral ovary. It should be noted that a pyometra may occasionally exist even if no corpus luteum can be palpated. In addition, it is not uncommon to find that the corpus luteum is smaller than that observed during midcycle.

In most cases, vaginal examination will reveal varying degrees of enlargement of the cervical os and the presence of purulent material in the anterior vagina.

DIAGNOSIS

Mucometra, hydrometra, and pregnancy are the three most important conditions that must be differentiated from pyometra. Mucometra or hydrometra occurs most frequently in cases of chronic cystic follicles of the ovaries. However, cases of segmental aplasia of the tubular tract derived from the müllerian duct system should also be considered when mucometra or hydrometra is observed. The most diagnostic feature of pyometra is the absence of any positive signs of pregnancy—amnionic vesicle, fetal membranes, placentomes, and the fetus—in a fluid-filled uterus.

TREATMENT AND PROGNOSIS

Treatment of pyometra is directed toward reestablishment of the estrous cycle through destruction of the corpus luteum (luteolysis). This can be achieved by several different methods.

The most effective and safest method is by the use of exogenously administered prostaglandin and its analogues. The intramuscular administration of 25 mg of dinoprost tromethamine (Lutalyse)* has been shown to be effective in causing luteolysis and evacuation of uterine contents of cows with pyometra. Estrus is usually observed within 3 to 4 days following treatment, and complete uterine evacuation is observed in most cows at this time. Cloprostenol, a prostaglandin analogue, has also been shown to be effective when administered intramuscularly at the dosage of 0.5 mg.

Various estrogens can also be used as luteolytic agents in the treatment of pyometra. However, results are inconsistent, and cystic follicles, ovaritis, ovarian adhesions, and relaxation of the pelvic ligaments are disadvantages of this approach to treatment.

In some cases there may be lysis of the corpus luteum but rectal palpation of the uterus indicates continued presence of intrauterine fluid. Partial or complete cervical stenosis, possibly as a result of trauma at calving, should be considered in the etiology of this apparent lack of response to treatment.

Manual enucleation of the corpus luteum through the rectal wall is an effective but unacceptable method of destroying the corpus luteum. The major disadvantages of this method include excessive hemorrhage and subsequent ovarian adhesions. In addition, in some cases it may be difficult to identify the corpus luteum on the ovary using rectal palpation.

Manual draining of the uterus and intrauterine infusion with antibiotics following evacuation of uterine contents result in low clinical recovery rates and poor conception rates.

---

*Available from the Upjohn Company, Kalamazoo, MI 49001.

Bovine Vaginitis
GAVIN F. RICHARDSON, DVM, MVSc, BA

NECROTIC VAGINITIS

Necrotic vaginitis can occasionally occur as a result of trauma to the birth canal following dystocia or concurrent to metritis. The condition can be painful, and affected cows may arch their backs, strain, and become anorectic. A necrotic, diphtheritic inflammation of the vestibule and vagina occurs accompanied by a fetid, watery, reddish discharge. Some degree of vaginal stenosis may result.

Treatment consists of the local application of bland, oily antibiotic preparations two to three times daily. The infection must not be carried forward into the uterus. Antibiotics should also be administered systemically.

Cows with chronic tenesmus can be treated with a conventional epidural anesthetic. Epidural anesthesia can be prolonged by installing a catheter in the epidural space and capping it between infusions of local anesthetic. Prolonged epidural anesthesia using alcohol preparations in small increments, to effect (usually 3 to 8 ml is required), has been described; however, this procedure can lead to prolonged paralysis of the tail and its associated problems. Analgesics and sedatives may also be of benefit in these cows.

If severe pneumovagina is a problem, the dorsal portions of the vulvar lips can be sutured closed (Caslick's operation).

VESTIBULOVAGINITIS

Vestibulovaginitis most often occurs when a uterine and/or cervical infection is also present. It can also result from poor vulvar tone and poor perineal conformation. Vaginoscopy is essential to confirm the diagnosis of this condition.

Besides the organisms usually involved in uterine infections, mycoplasmas, ureaplasmas, *Haemophilus somnus*, and an enterovirus have also been associated with this disease. The "Epivag" virus causes infection of the entire tubular genital tract of cows in Africa.

If a uterine infection is also present, the therapy would be as described for metritis and endometritis. If poor perineal conformation is the cause, the dorsal portion of the vulva can be sutured closed (Caslick's operation). If indicated, bland, oily antibiotic preparations can be applied. Rest from sexual activity will aid healing and help prevent the possible spread of the disease. Good sanitation and the isolation of affected animals may also help prevent the spread of infection.

GRANULAR VULVITIS

Granular vulvitis is a transient, disseminated, lymphoid hyperplasia in the vulvar mucosa that disappears without treatment in 10 to 14 days. This represents a characteristic reaction of this area to various infectious organisms and irritants; it should not result in infertility unless pathogenic organisms such as ureaplasmas are involved.

Treatment is usually not required. However, in a natural breeding situation, rest from sexual activity for 2 to 4 weeks might be advisable in case a pathogenic organism is involved. If artificial insemination is used, the double-rod insemination technique should be used to prevent the possible transfer of pathogens into the uterus.

INFECTIOUS PUSTULAR VULVOVAGINITIS

Infectious pustular vulvovaginitis is caused by a herpesvirus very similar or identical to the one that causes infectious bovine rhinotracheitis. Vesicles are formed in the vagina that become pustules and eventually ulcers. The lesions may become secondarily infected with bacteria and/or coalesce. The condition in bulls is known as infectious pustular balanoposthitis. Pain is exhibited, and infertility can result from a reluctance to breed. If breeding should occur, there is an unproven potential for reduced conception and/or pregnancy rates.

The diagnosis is often based on clinical signs alone but can be confirmed by isolation of the virus.

Rest from sexual activity is recommended for 3 to 4 weeks or more to allow for healing and to prevent the spread of the disease. Oily antibiotic preparations can be applied to combat secondary bacterial infections and reduce the possibility of preputial adhesions in bulls. The use of infectious bovine rhinotracheitis vaccines to prevent the disease is questionable.

BIBLIOGRAPHY

Elmore RG: Food-animal regional anesthesia: Bovine blocks: continuous epidural anesthesia. Vet Med/Small Anim Clin 75:1174–1176, 1980.
Roberts SJ: Veterinary Obstetrics and Genital Diseases, Theriogenology, 3rd ed. Ann Arbor, MI, Edward Bros., 1986.

Bovine Ovarian Cysts

HOWARD L. WHITMORE, DVM, PhD, MS

Ovarian cysts (cystic follicles) are one of the most common abnormalities encountered by veterinarians. It has been reported that 5 to 15 per cent of dairy cows develop cystic follicles during the postpartum and breeding periods. Individual problem herds may have a much higher incidence (30 to 40 per cent) for short periods of time. Cystic follicles are traditionally defined as persistent fluid-filled structures on the ovary equal to or greater than 2.5 cm in diameter in the absence of a corpus luteum.

ETIOLOGY

The cause of cystic follicles is not completely known. A hormone imbalance occurs consisting of insufficient release of luteinizing hormone (LH) at the time of ovulation. The fact that LH works so well as a treatment for this condition lends credence to this hypothesis. Many factors are associated with cystic follicles, although their exact mechanism of action is not known. Cystic follicles are common in older high-producing cows. They are more common in the early postpartum period (15 to 45 days) and in cows having complications at calving time (metritis, milk fever). Some studies show that feeding high levels of concentrate high in protein is associated with cystic ovaries. Many managers of dairy herds believe that cysts are caused by something in the feed. Although some legume forages such as alfalfa and clover contain estrogen activity, analysis of these forages from problem herds often provides evidence that they are not the source of the problem.

TYPES OF OVARIAN CYSTS

Two types of pathologic ovarian cysts are generally described: follicular cysts and luteal cysts. Follicular cysts are thin-walled structures that may occur as single or multiple structures on one or both ovaries. Cows with follicular cysts may show signs ranging from constant estrus activity to nearly complete anestrus. The majority of cows show a modified low-grade estrus and tend to associate closely with other cows in normal estrus.

Luteal cysts are thick-walled structures because the walls have undergone partial luteinization. They tend to be single structures occurring in one ovary. Both types of cysts result from failure of ovulation. It is often difficult and not necessary to diagnose what type of cyst is present because both types of cysts are treated the same.

Cystic corpora lutea may develop following ovulation. They are similar to normal corpora lutea except they are larger and more fluctuant because they contain fluid in their central cavity. Cystic corpora lutea generally produce enough progesterone to support a pregnancy and so are considered nonpathologic structures.

DIAGNOSIS

Diagnosis of cystic follicles is based on the history and rectal palpation of the ovaries. The history often reveals signs of anestrus, low-grade estrus, or constant estrus (nymphomania). Cows that have been cystic for several months often show relaxation of the pelvic ligaments and the tail head, which results in a slight forward and ventral tilt of the pelvis.

Rectal examination of ovaries is important and is the primary method used to make the diagnosis. Studies show that experience is positively correlated with accurate diagnosis of cystic follicles. This is based on serum and milk progesterone assay and assumes that cows with fluid-filled structures equal to or greater than 25 mm with less than 1 ng/ml level of serum progesterone have follicular cysts. Cows with follicular cysts may have one or more thin-walled soft fluctuant cysts on one or both ovaries. Very little luteal tissue is present in the cyst walls, and they are usually easy to diagnose. Cows with luteal cysts tend to have one fluid-filled, thick-walled structure on one ovary. Veterinarians must palpate these structures very carefully to try to differentiate them from cystic corpus luteum or normal large corpora lutea. Luteal cysts do not have an obvious line of demarcation between luteal tissue and the ovary, do not have an ovulatory papilla, and generally have a few thinner-walled areas that are soft and fluctuant. Cystic corpora lutea have a line of demarcation between the ovary and the corpus luteum, have an ovulatory papilla in most cases, and have a more uniform firm liver-like consistency to their walls. Normal corpora lutea palpate the same as cystic corpora lutea except that normal corpora lutea have a smaller diameter and absence of fluid in their central cavity.

Veterinarians generally make an accurate diagnosis in most cases; however, there are times when it is difficult to differentiate a luteal cyst from a cystic corpus luteum or normal corpus luteum that does not have ovulatory papilla. This is the "borderline" gray area of diagnosis of cystic follicles. In these cases it may be helpful to perform a cow side milk progesterone test or to treat the cow with prostaglandin. Some veterinarians prefer to inject prostaglandin and observe for estrus for 5 to 7 days. If estrus is not observed in 5 to 7 days, then gonadotropin-releasing hormone (GnRH) is administered. Other veterinarians prefer to inject GnRH and prostaglandin at the same time in these questionable cases.

Sometimes cows in true estrus will have a normal preovulation follicle that is nearly 25 mm in diameter. In these cases it is helpful to closely palpate the horns of the uterus. The uterine horns of the cows with cystic follicles shorten by nearly 50 per cent and become very flaccid. The uterine horns of cows in estrus have increased tone and do not shorten.

TREATMENT

The two most common hormones used to treat cystic follicles are gonadotropin-releasing hormone (GnRH) and luteinizing hormone (LH). GnRH causes treated animals to release their own endogenous LH from their anterior pituitary. LH products consist of human chorionic gonadotropin (HCG) and anterior pituitary extracts. LH products have high levels of LH activity and provide the animal with an exogenous source of LH. Several studies have compared the response rate of GnRH and HCG for treating cystic follicles and report a 70 to 80 per cent cure rate for both GnRH and HCG, showing that they appear to work equally well.

Gonadotropin-Releasing Hormone

GnRH is a decapeptide hormone that is produced in the hypothalamus. GnRH is also produced synthetically, and several analogues are available. The standard dose of GnRH in the United States is 100 µg given intramuscularly. GnRH causes endogenous LH release for 2 to 4 hours after treatment. The LH release stimulates luteal tissue formation. The newly formed luteal tissue functions similar to a corpus luteum and results in a significant increase in blood progesterone concentration in 80 to 90 per cent of treated cows. Cows that respond to GnRH come into estrus in 5 to 30 days, with a peak between 19 and 23 days. Owners are advised to breed the animals on the first normal estrus 5 or more days after treatment. GnRH is probably the most common treatment for ovarian cysts used in the United States today.

GnRH may have advantages over HCG and anterior pituitary extracts because it is produced synthetically, has a lower molecular weight (~1500) so is less antigenic, and has a faster clearance rate. It is probably the treatment of choice if repeat treatments are necessary. A few cows may be misdiagnosed for ovarian cysts when they actually have a large functional cystic corpus luteum. In this situation, GnRH would not prolong the functional life span of the corpus luteum; however, HCG could prolong function of the corpus luteum and delay the next estrus for 5 to 10 days.

Exogenous Luteinizing Hormone

Human chorionic gonadotropin is a high-molecular-weight (~30,000) hormone rich in LH activity. It is obtained from the urine of pregnant women. The recommended dose of HCG is 5000 units intravenously and 10,000 units intramuscularly. These doses appear equivalent based on clinical response. HCG stimulates luteal tissue formation and increases blood progesterone concentration in 80 to 90 per cent of treated cows. Cows that respond positively to HCG treatment show normal estrus in 19 to 23 days, which is very similar to the response to GnRH.

Anterior pituitary extracts high in LH activity are usually obtained from sheep and swine. They are rich in LH but also contain follicle-stimulating hormone (FSH) and other pituitary protein hormones. These pituitary extracts have considerable antigenic properties, although the clinical significance has not been established. Anterior pituitary extracts are becoming more difficult to purchase commercially, and so their use for treating cystic follicles may be decreasing.

Simultaneous Administration of GnRH and Prostaglandins

One study evaluated the effect of simultaneous administration of GnRH and prostaglandins compared with GnRH alone in 75 cows with cystic follicles. The results revealed that intervals to first estrus and to conception, proportion in estrus by day 21 after treatment, and pregnancy rate by 90 days did not differ significantly between the groups. Based on these results, simultaneous administration of GnRH and prostaglandins to all cows with cystic follicles is not recommended and has no advantage over use of GnRH alone. Some veterinarians still prefer simultaneous administration of GnRH and prostaglandin in those borderline, difficult-to-diagnosis cases of either luteinized cysts or cystic corpora lutea.

Administration of GnRH Followed in 10 to 14 Days by Prostaglandin Therapy

The administration of GnRH causes significant luteinization in the ovary by 10 to 14 days following treatment. Prostaglandin could be given at 10 to 14 days to cause regression of the induced luteal tissue and induction of estrus within 2 to 5 days. The interval from initial treatment to estrus could then be shortened from an average of 23 days to an average of 16 days. However, maximum estrus detection efficiency must be achieved to obtain the benefit of this treatment scheme. If estrus is not observed after prostaglandin administration, the beneficial effect of such an approach cannot be realized.

Cows Requiring Repeat Treatments for Cystic Follicles

Most researchers report 70 to 80 per cent of cows with ovarian cysts respond to the initial treatment. Most cows that respond favorably come into estrus 19 to 23 days following initial treatment. Therefore, ovaries are not usually reexamined until 28 or more days after treatment. Some veterinarians prefer to reexamine ovaries 14 days after treatment to see if cysts have decreased in size and show increased luteinization. Cows with cysts that have not decreased in size are re-treated at day 14.

Cows that need repeat treatments are generally given a second or third dose of GnRH. One study reported that 225 cows treated with GnRH resulted in clinical recovery with onset of estrous cycles in 76, 78, and 66 per cent of cows, following first, second, and third treatment, respectively. Thus, there were only 12 of the 225 cows that failed to recover following three treatments. Cows not responding to two or three treatments of GnRH should be given exogenous LH such as HCG or anterior pituitary extracts.

Some difficult repeat cases may be treated with administration of a second dose of GnRH 4 or 5 days after the first dose. The theory here is that the first treatment of GnRH induces both LH and follicle-stimulating hormone (FSH) release. FSH stimulates some new follicles and granulosa cells. The second treatment of GnRH then results in additional luteinization of new granulosa cells. This theory has not been tested under controlled conditions.

BIBLIOGRAPHY

Archbald LF, Norman SN, Tran T, et al: Does GnRH work as well as GnRH and $PGF_{2\alpha}$ in the treatment of ovarian follicular cysts? Vet Med 86:1037–1040, 1991.

Dinsmore RP, White ME, English PB: An evaluation of simultaneous GnRH and cloprostenol treatment of dairy cows with cystic ovaries. Can Vet J 31:280–284, 1990.

Roberts SJ: Veterinary Obstetrics and Genital Diseases, 3rd ed, pp 478–491. North Pomfret, VT, David and Charles, 1986.

Whitmore HL, Hurtgen JP, Mather EC, Seguin BE: Clinical response of dairy cattle with ovarian cysts to single or repeat treatments of GnRH. J Am Vet Med Assoc 174:1113–1115, 1979.

Synchronization of Estrus

ROBERT A. GODKE, PhD
DANIEL P. RYAN, PhD

SWINE

Most swine in North America are maintained under controlled management conditions. Often the size of farrowing facilities and/or number of farrowing crates dictates to what extent producers are interested in estrus synchronization and artificial insemination in swine breeding herds.

Sows do not usually cycle during lactation. Producers have been synchronizing sows for years by weaning small groups of females and mating them at the synchronized postweaning estrus. For lactating sows in good body condition, this postweaning estrus is usually exhibited in 4 to 7 days. Injections of pregnant mare serum gonadotropin (PMSG) and human chorionic gonadotropin (HCG) have been used to increase synchrony of this postweaning estrus. When piglets are weaned between the fourth and sixth week of lactation, 750 to 1000 IU of PMSG can be administered intramuscularly or subcutaneously 8 to 12 hours after pig removal and 500 to 750 IU of HCG given intramuscularly to each female 56 hours following PMSG. With this treatment schedule, weaned sows are mated by appointment starting 24 hours after HCG treatment and 12 hours later, regardless of the signs of estrus.

PMSG (400 to 1000 IU) and HCG (200 to 750 IU) have been used clinically to induce estrus in anestrous sows. Although on occasion this approach has been successful, the problem(s) causing this situation needs to be corrected or sow breeding problems often continue. PMSG and HCG have also been used in attempts to induce estrus for early mating of prepubertal gilts. This approach is not recommended for ovulation induction in lightweight gilts ($\leq$165 days of age), since pregnancies in these sows usually fail owing to luteal insufficiency during the first 25 days of gestation.

Attempts have been made to synchronize gilts with daily intramuscular injections of progesterone for 18 to 22 days. Although the appropriate dose of progesterone inhibits the animals from exhibiting estrus during treatment and the sows usually exhibit estrus 2 to 5 days after treatment, this approach often results in polycystic ovaries and lowered post-treatment fertility. The second post-treatment estrus (21 days later), however, is generally considered to be fertile.

Daily feeding of 15 mg allyltrenbolone (Regumate)* for 14 to 18 days will synchronize estrus in cyclic gilts and sows within 4 to 8 days post treatment. Although this progestin is effective orally and fertility levels are good (60 to 70 per cent pregnancy rates), polycystic ovaries often occur in cyclic gilts. When this agent is individually fed, compared with group feeding, the interval from progestin withdrawal to the onset of estrus is more precisely synchronized among treated sows. At synchronized estrus, each sow can be hand mated once daily while in estrus or mated by appointment twice on the sixth and again on the seventh day after progestin withdrawal. This compound has yet to be approved for use in swine in the United States.

Unlike other farm animals, prostaglandins used alone are not effective for estrus synchronization in sows. The corpora lutea of cyclic sows are not responsive to prostaglandin $F_{2\alpha}$ ($PGF_{2\alpha}$) during the first 10 to 12 days of the estrous cycle. In contrast, $PGF_{2\alpha}$ will induce luteal regression in pregnant sows during the first trimester and near the end of the third trimester of pregnancy.

In the gilt the life span of corpora lutea can be prolonged by exogenous estrogen or by giving HCG on day 12 of the estrous cycle (estrus = day 0). In contrast, the prolonged luteal tissue is susceptible to exogenous $PGF_{2\alpha}$. One approach to synchronizing gilts is to administer 500 to 1000 IU of HCG intramuscularly on day 12 of the estrous cycle and then 10 to 15 mg $PGF_{2\alpha}$ or 1000 and 500 μg of cloprostenol (Estrumate†) intramuscularly 24 hours apart at least 12 days later to induce synchronized luteal regression.

Estrogen priming of endogenous corpora lutea and subsequent administration of $PGF_{2\alpha}$ can be used to synchronize estrus and ovulation in gilts. One approach is to administer 10 mg estradiol benzoate intramuscularly on days 10 through 14 of the estrous cycle to induce luteal maintenance. Then 10 days or later after the last estradiol injection, 10 mg of $PGF_{2\alpha}$ is given intramuscularly in a split dose 4 hours apart to induce luteal regression. A second scheme using estradiol benzoate and $PGF_{2\alpha}$ involves the intramuscular use of 5 mg of estradiol benzoate for 20 days, starting at any stage of the estrous cycle, and 10 mg of $PGF_{2\alpha}$ in a split dose 5 days following the last estradiol injection. With this method, sows are expected to exhibit estrus 4 to 7 days after the $PGF_{2\alpha}$ treatment.

Another approach to estrus synchronization and ovulation control in swine involves the artificial induction of accessory corpora lutea followed by prostaglandin treatment. Using this method, gilts at various stages of the estrous cycle are administered 1000 or 1500 IU of PMSG subcutaneously and 750 IU of HCG intramuscularly at 72 or 96 hours post PMSG. Twelve days after administration of HCG, 1000 and 500 μg of cloprostenol is administered intramuscularly 24 hours apart. With this procedure, a supplemental injection of 1000 IU of PMSG may be given at the time of the prostaglandin treatment to enhance follicular development and to increase the number of gilts in estrus. More than 85 per cent of the sows are expected to exhibit estrus following prostaglandin treatment, with pregnancy rates following hand mating of these animals expected to be greater than 80 per cent.

Another method of estrus synchronization of sows and gilts involves mating the animals (as a field group) to fertile boars in pasture lots for 22 to 25 days and then 12 days after the last day of boar exposure administering 15 mg of $PGF_{2\alpha}$ intramuscularly followed 12 hours later by 10 mg of $PGF_{2\alpha}$ intramuscularly or 1000 and 500 μg of cloprostenol intramuscularly 24 hours apart to induce luteolysis. Using this approach, all pregnant sows and gilts should be between days 12 and 37 of gestation at the time of $PGF_{2\alpha}$ treatment. Since exogenous $PGF_{2\alpha}$ is luteolytic in swine during early gestation, these animals will abort and return to estrus 4 to 7 days post treatment. Mating at this estrus results in no detrimental effects on pregnancy rates or litter size. This method would also allow the producer to test herd boars for fertility prior to the actual breeding season. Although this method is effective, swine producers often fail to see the logic in using this procedure, especially when they are paying to feed the animals during this lengthy estrus synchronization program.

One should not overlook that estrus can be enhanced and often group-synchronized to some degree in swine by management practices. When a mature boar is allowed daily exposure to maturing prepubertal gilts in adjacent pens, the onset of puberty often occurs 10 to 18 days earlier in the boar-exposed gilts over those without boar exposure. Apparently, sight, olfaction, and auditory interactions of the boar with the prepubertal gilts can produce an altered pattern in gonadotropin secretion, resulting in stimulated follicular development.

---

*Available from Hoechst-Roussel Pharmaceuticals, Somerville, NJ 08876.

†Available from Haver-Loekert, Shawnee, KS 66201.

When mature gilts have reached their genetic age of maturity but have not begun to cycle because of confinement rearing, they can be stimulated to start cycling as a group by separating and transporting them to an outside pasture. This method is most effective when gilts weigh greater than 230 pounds at the time of the change in environment. The pasture allows for free exercise, and the animals can be checked for estrus twice daily with a mature teaser boar. This procedure, often referred to as "transport heat," is not effective once these confined gilts have begun to cycle and corpora lutea are present. The practitioner may wish to collect blood samples (marginal ear vein) from a random group of these gilts on the feed floor to verify low circulating progesterone levels in these animals before recommending this procedure to the producer. A low dose of estradiol (≤ 1 mg IM) to these gilts at the time of moving has been shown to enhance the expression of estrus and more precisely synchronizes a group response.

Estrus may be induced in prepubertal gilts nearing ovarian transition by mixing or changing animals among groups or markedly changing the daily routine. An example of this might be the "county fair" syndrome, in which a disproportionate number of the young gilts come into estrus, expressing a strong immobility response the day of the show.

SHEEP AND GOATS

Early studies reported that estrus can be synchronized in sheep and goats during the breeding season by daily injections of progesterone. This approach is time consuming, labor intensive, and not practical for the producer.

However, ewes and does can be treated with vaginal pessaries impregnated with progestins. These pessaries can be pretreated with either crystalline progesterone or various potent progestins, including norgestomet, fluorogestone, and medroxyprogesterone. These pessaries are placed in the anterior vagina, adjacent to the cervix, with a vaginal speculum and plunger. The string attached to the pessary extends beyond the surface of the vulva for easy removal. The pessaries are left in place for 12 to 14 days in the ewe and 18 to 21 days in the doe. Fluorogestone can also be administered to ewes orally at 9 mg/day to synchronize estrus. However, social dominance behavior and a wider window of synchrony are often drawbacks with this approach.

During the breeding season, both ewes and does in good body condition treated with progestin pessaries for estrus synchronization have had pregnancy rates comparable to nontreated animals in the same flock using hand mating. These pregnancy rates, however, are variable and range from 30 to 70 per cent in various field trials using artificial insemination. It is evident that ewe and doe nutrition and management are of critical importance in conducting a successful flock estrus synchronization program.

To increase the number of animals exhibiting a synchronized estrus following progestin treatment, 400 to 800 IU of PMSG can be administered at the time of pessary removal. Using this approach, treated ewes and does are expected to exhibit estrus during a 48-hour interval. Following treatment, the animals are exposed to a group of fertile rams and bucks for natural mating or, with the aid of a teaser ram or buck, artificially inseminated twice at 12 and 24 hours for ewes and 18 and 24 hours for does after the onset of estrus. For fixed-time matings using fresh or frozen semen, ewes are inseminated twice at 48 and 60 hours and does are inseminated twice at 30 and 48 hours after progestin withdrawal.

More recently, norgestomet (SYNCROMATE B)* has been used successfully as an ear implant to synchronize estrus and ovulation in sheep and goats during the breeding season. Favorable results have been reported using one half of the standard 6-mg bovine implant to synchronize estrus in the ewe. A modified approach is to implant the cyclic ewe for 5 or 6 days and then administer 15 mg of $PGF_{2\alpha}$ or 125 µg of cloprostenol intramuscularly at the time of implant removal. This treatment allows for a reduction of the standard 12- to 14-day progestin-exposure interval and a more precise synchrony of estrus. One problem with the use of the ear implant is that marked changes in ambient temperature during the interval implants are in place may decrease progestin absorption from the implant. This may result in breakthroughs, with the ewes and does exhibiting estrus during treatment.

A newer progesterone-impregnated Silastic, T-shaped vaginal device has been developed for sheep in New Zealand. This vaginal implant, known as the controlled internal drug release (CIDR) device, functions similarly to the vaginal pessary. Pregnancy rates reported from field tests with the CIDR device in New Zealand and Australia compare favorably with those of nontreated control ewes. An application has been filed with the Food and Drug Administration for this device to become available to the livestock industry in the United States.

Prostaglandins can be used effectively for estrus synchronization of both cyclic sheep and goats. Since these agents induce luteal regression to synchronize estrus, they are only effective for this purpose during the luteal phase, between days 5 and 14 of the estrous cycle in ewes and between days 4 and 16 of the estrous cycle in does. The intramuscular use of 10 to 15 mg of $PGF_{2\alpha}$ IM or 125 µg of cloprostenol given 8 to 9 days apart in the ewe and 11 to 12 days apart in the doe will effectively synchronize estrus in these animals during the breeding season. In cyclic ewes or does, estrus is usually exhibited 2 to 3 days after the last prostaglandin injection. With this approach, natural mating with fertile rams or bucks or double insemination is recommended when fresh or frozen semen is used with this synchronization program. Pregnancy rates following prostaglandin treatment usually range between 55 and 85 per cent and are similar to those of nontreated female animals in the same flock.

Prostaglandins can also be used with flock management practices to group-synchronize ewes. One approach is to place a mature, vasectomized, teaser ram (wearing a marking harness) with the ewe flock during the transitional stage before the onset of the breeding season. The presence of the mature ram will often stimulate ewes in transition to exhibit estrus 6 to 12 days after the teaser ram has been introduced in the flock. A 15-mg dose of $PGF_{2\alpha}$ or 125 µg of cloprostenol and 400 to 500 IU of PMSG to these ewes (grouped 6 to 9 days after estrus) is administered intramuscularly. The ewes are mated naturally at estrus or subjected to double artificial insemination 12 hours apart. Serum progesterone levels can be evaluated from each animal prior to prostaglandin treatment to verify endogenous luteal function. This approach has become popular for those producing show lambs using frozen-thawed semen from a valuable stud ram.

Another method is to use a 14-day progestin treatment on ewes going through seasonal transition, allowing them to exhibit estrus, and then to administer prostaglandin 6 to 9 days after progestin-induced estrus. Placing the ewes on a good plan of nutrition for 30 to 40 days prior to transition and closely shearing the ewes are often of benefit when using these group-synchronization procedures.

One must keep in mind that prostaglandins do not synchronize acyclic or out-of-season ewes or does. Occasionally, however, the use of a 12- to 14-day progestin treatment plus PMSG treatment during the nonbreeding season has induced estrus and resulted in live offspring born out of season. This

---
*Available from Sanofi Animal Health, Inc., Overland Park, KS 66212.

procedure is often requested by an enthusiastic owner in hopes of producing out-of-season sale lambs. The procedure is somewhat more effective in the Mediterranean breeds of sheep and least effective in the larger meat breeds (Hampshire and Suffolk). In most cases, the treated ewe that produces out-of-season lambs rarely produces offspring from male exposure during the next natural breeding season. This procedure is not recommended for the commercial sheep producer at this time.

In general, animals that have supplemental nourishment (increase in dietary energy) for more than 30 days prior to treatment and are healthy at the time of treatment respond to synchronization agents better than those in poor condition. If plans are made to use estrus synchronization, artificial insemination at estrus is recommended over that of fixed-time mating for both ewes and does.

CATTLE

It has been demonstrated that daily injections of progesterone inhibit cyclic cows from exhibiting estrus. When such treatment is discontinued, estrus is usually exhibited within 2 to 5 days after the last daily injection of progesterone.

The results of testing progestational agents in field trials showed that the first-service pregnancy rates from the progesterone-treated cows were depressed 5 to 50 per cent below those of the control animals inseminated during a corresponding estrous cycle. Chronic, daily exposure to progesterone or progestin agents (>14 days) was blamed, in retrospect, for the inconsistent results in early estrus synchronization trials.

In the early 1970s the synthetic progestin norgestomet was revived by researchers for estrus synchronization of cattle. The synchronization scheme developed for cyclic heifers and nonlactating beef cows reduced the number of days that females were exposed to progesterone treatment. This approach involves the use of a small (6 mg) norgestomet implant placed subcutaneously on the caudal side of the ear. Concurrently, intramuscular injections of 3 mg of norgestomet and 5 mg of estradiol valerate are given to each animal. The ear implants are removed after 9 days, and the cows are mated approximately 12 hours after the onset of estrus or mated once or twice at a predetermined time after implant removal. Inseminating cows by appointment with this method is most often done between 48 and 72 hours after implant removal.

The norgestomet estrus synchronization scheme for nursing beef cows was initially called the "Shang" treatment. It consists of the same hormonal treatment described above for heifers and nonlactating cows but with the addition of short-term calf removal prior to insemination. Calves are removed and isolated from the cows for 48 to 72 hours, starting at the time of implant removal or 12 hours post implant removal. With this approach, cows are either mated at 12 hours after the onset of estrus or mated by appointment 48 to 60 hours after implant removal, without estrus detection. Calves are returned to their dams immediately after insemination. Removing the calves at 12 hours after implant removal and inseminating the cows 48 to 54 hours after implant removal has become one of the more popular methods used in field estrus synchronization programs.

Various calf removal schedules have been successful in inducing a fertile synchronized estrus as early as 30 days following calving in beef cows maintained under proper nutritional management. However, it is recommended that mature beef cows be at least 40 days post partum at the time of progestin treatment. Norgestomet has now been approved for synchronization of estrus and ovulation in nonlactating dairy heifers.

Major field trials using the short-term norgestomet scheme to synchronize estrus in cattle have resulted in pregnancy rates from first-service insemination that are similar to pregnancy rates from herdmate females inseminated during a corresponding estrous cycle.

$PGF_{2\alpha}$ is a naturally occurring 20-carbon fatty acid. Exogenous $PGF_{2\alpha}$ is often used for estrus synchronization in cows because it induces regression of the corpus luteum. It is always recommended that animals be examined for pregnancy before the administration of $PGF_{2\alpha}$, since this compound is an effective abortifacient during the first 120 days of pregnancy.

Early experiments revealed that $PGF_{2\alpha}$ administration during days 0 to 5 of the bovine estrous cycle (estrus = day 0) did not elicit signs of estrus. It was shown that $PGF_{2\alpha}$ would induce luteal regression followed by estrus and ovulation in cows when administered during the luteal phase of the estrous cycle (days 6 through 17). $PGF_{2\alpha}$ treatment between days 17 and 21 does not alter the length of the estrous cycle. Synchronization of estrus with $PGF_{2\alpha}$ has been successfully accomplished by several methods.

The first method involves palpation of all cyclic cows and heifers in the herd and administering a luteolytic dose (25 mg) of $PGF_{2\alpha}$ intramuscularly to those cows with a palpable corpus luteum. These cows are artificially inseminated at an appointed time or 8 to 12 hours after the onset of estrus. Cows without a corpus luteum at the first injection are then administered the same dose of $PGF_{2\alpha}$ 7 to 8 days after the first group was treated. These cows are inseminated at an appointed time or at estrus. This method, although quite effective, usually requires dividing the herd into two separate groups to manage animals more effectively during estrus detection and artificial insemination. This approach may not fit into the usual ranch management system because of the need for separate pasture lots and multiple insemination schedules. In addition, it is important that the practitioner be proficient in ovary palpation and in the identification of a corpus luteum on the ovary. The use of a single serum progesterone determination for each cow prior to treatment would be beneficial for allotting cows to each of the two treatment groups.

The second method involves treating all cycling cows with two separate intramuscular injections of $PGF_{2\alpha}$ 10 to 12 days apart. The animals are either artificially inseminated 8 to 12 hours after the onset of estrus or are mated by appointment (once or twice) 72 to 96 hours after the second dose of $PGF_{2\alpha}$. This approach is designed to eliminate the pretreatment palpation for a corpus luteum as needed with the first method. By treating with a second injection of $PGF_{2\alpha}$ 10 to 12 days later, those cows in which luteal regression occurred following the first treatment would be treated on days 7 to 9 of the subsequent cycle and those cows in which $PGF_{2\alpha}$ was not effective following the first injection would be in the middle of their estrous cycle (days 7 to 17 of the cycle) at the time of the second injection. It should not be overlooked that this method would double the cost of $PGF_{2\alpha}$ per animal over that of the first method. An option to reduce the cost of $PGF_{2\alpha}$ per cow in the herd with this method would be to inject all cyclic cows in the herd (without palpating) as in the second method and inseminate all those exhibiting estrus as in the first method. Then, all the remaining animals not exhibiting estrus during the 10 to 12 days after the first injection are reinjected with $PGF_{2\alpha}$ and inseminated at induced estrus or at an appointed time after the second $PGF_{2\alpha}$ injection.

The third approach calls for estrus detection during the first 5 days of the breeding season. Those animals detected in estrus are inseminated 8 to 12 hours after the onset of estrus. On the sixth day of the breeding season, all females in estrus are inseminated mid morning and the remaining cyclic animals are administered a luteolytic dose of $PGF_{2\alpha}$. The treated females are then inseminated at estrus by the standard A.M.–

P.M. method. Artificial insemination at a predetermined time after the PGF$_{2\alpha}$ injection is not recommended with this procedure because of the variability in the onset of estrus that usually occurs with this approach. One drawback with the third method is that an estrus detection period of 10 to 12 days is required to complete the synchronization procedure. However, the addition of the breeding bulls on days 1 to 6 of this procedure has become very popular in beef herds in the midwestern and western states.

The fourth synchronization method includes the use of a progestin agent along with a single prostaglandin treatment. With this method a norgestomet implant is placed subcutaneously in the ear of all cycling animals for 7 or 8 days, followed by an intramuscular injection of 25 to 30 mg of PGF$_{2\alpha}$ when the implant is removed. The progestin agent is given to prevent the onset of estrus for 7 to 8 days in those cows with regressing or a regressed corpus luteum, and the prostaglandin is administered to induce luteolysis in cows with remaining functional corpora lutea at the time of implant removal. The use of prostaglandin with this approach allows more flexibility for choosing the day of implant removal. This method, theoretically, allows the complete herd to be synchronized and inseminated during a 96-hour interval following implant removal. This means that all cows could be inseminated within 12 days after the first day of progestin treatment. With this method, cows can be inseminated at estrus using the standard A.M.-P.M. method or time mated (once or twice) at desired intervals.

A potent PGF$_{2\alpha}$ analogue, cloprostenol, is now available for cattle estrus synchronization procedures in the United States. An intramuscular dose of 500 µg will synchronize estrus and ovulation in cows and heifers similar to a dose of 25 mg of PGF$_{2\alpha}$. Another analogue, fenprostalene (Bovilene),* is available for use in cattle, with a recommended dose of 1 mg administered subcutaneously to induce luteolysis during the luteal phase of the estrous cycle.

First-service pregnancy rates from cows and heifers synchronized with prostaglandin and its potent analogues are usually comparable with pregnancy rates of herdmates inseminated during a corresponding estrous cycle.

BIBLIOGRAPHY

Bosu WTK, Serna J, Barker CAV: Peripheral plasma levels of progesterone in goats treated with fluorogestone acetate and prostaglandin F$_{2\alpha}$ during the estrous cycle. Theriogenology 9:371–390, 1978.
Carter PD, Parsonson IM: Control of reproductive function in cattle using cloprostenol. Aust Vet J 52:514–516, 1976.
Corteel JM, Gonzalez C, Nunes JF: Research and development in the control of reproduction. Proceedings of the Third International Conference on Goat Production and Disease, Tucson, Arizona, pp 584–601, 1982.
Dziuk PJ, Bellows RA: Management of reproduction of beef cattle, sheep and pigs. J Anim Sci 52(suppl 2):355, 1983.
Guthrie HD, Polge C: Treatment of pregnant gilts with prostaglandin analogue, cloprostenol, to control oestrus and fertility. J Reprod Fertil 52:271–273, 1978.
Haresign W: Ovulation control in sheep. In Crighton DB, Foxcroft GF, Haynes NB, Lamming GE (eds): Control of Ovulation. London, Butterworths, 1978.
Inskeep EK: Potential uses of prostaglandins in control of reproductive cycles of domestic animals. J Anim Sci 36:1149–1157, 1973.
Kraeling RR, Rampacek GB: Synchronization of estrus and ovulation in gilts with estradiol and prostaglandin. Theriogenology 8:103–112, 1977.
Momont H, Sequin B: Temporal factors affecting the response to prostaglandin F$_{2\alpha}$ products in dairy cattle. Proc Soc Theriogenol, pp 166–167, 1982.
Moody EL, Lauderdale JW: Fertility of cattle following PGF$_{2\alpha}$ controlled ovulation. J Anim Sci 45(suppl 1):189, 1977.
Richardson GF, Braun WF, Godke RA: Clinical uses of gonadotropin-releasing hormone and prostaglandin in cattle. Mod Vet Pract 15:533–538, 1982.
Schultz RH, Beerwinkle DR, Bierschwal CJ, et al: Synchronizing beef cows with cloprostenol (multi-location trial). J Anim Sci 45(suppl 1):206, 1977.

---

*Available from Syntex Animal Health, West Des Moines, IA 50315.

Stevenson JS, Davis DL: Estrous synchronization and fertility in gilts after 14- and 18-day feeding of Altrenogest beginning at estrus or diestrus. J Anim Sci 55:119, 1982.
Thatcher WW, Chenault JR: Reproductive physiological responses of cattle to exogenous prostaglandin F$_{2\alpha}$. J Dairy Sci 59:1366–1375, 1976.
Webel SK, Day BN: The control of ovulation. In Cole DJA, Foxcroft GR (eds): Control of Pig Reproduction. London, Butterworths, 1982.
Wiltbank JN, Mores S: Breeding at a predetermined time following Syncro-Mate-B treatment. National Association of Animal Breeders Beef Artificial Insemination Conference, Denver, pp 47–51, 1977.
Wiltbank JN, Sturges JC, Wideman D, et al: Control of estrus and ovulation using subcutaneous implants and estrogens in beef cattle. J Anim Sci 33:600–606, 1971.

Potential Problems with the Use of Artificial Insemination in Cattle

DALE PACCAMONTI, DVM, MS, Diplomate, ACT

A large part of the progress in the dairy industry in the past half century can be attributed to the success of artificial insemination. With the advent of techniques for the extension and freezing of semen, the number of potential offspring from a bull is much greater. While although artificial insemination bypasses the obvious problems of maintaining potentially dangerous bulls with unproven genetic qualities, it does have its own unique problems.

ESTRUS DETECTION

Inefficiency of estrus detection remains one of the major problems confronting the user of artificial insemination. The effort needed for estrus detection is one of the major reasons for the low acceptance of artificial insemination in the beef industry. In many cases, poor estrus detection is also the most difficult problem for a veterinarian to solve or correct for the herd owner. True anestrus is uncommon in the properly fed, healthy dairy cow after 45 days post partum. In most suspected cases the cows are actually pregnant or have pathologic conditions such as ovarian cysts or pyometra. In beef herds, anestrus is a significant problem, especially in herds with *Bos indicus* breeding. Rectal palpation, ultrasonography, and progesterone levels of anestrous animals will help to correctly diagnose the condition.

Failure of adequate estrus detection in a dairy herd can be verified by examination of the herd records.[1] The ratio of normal interestrus intervals to multiples of normal intervals is unaffected by early embryonic death and therefore reflects missed estrus periods. A parameter easily calculated during a herd visit is the percentage of cows presented for pregnancy check that are pregnant. Nonpregnant cows represent missed estrus, since they will have had at least one estrus between the time they were bred and when they were presented for pregnancy examination.

An estrus detection trial can be used with any beef or dairy herd to check detection efficiency. Nonpregnant cows are observed for a period of 24 days, and all estrus periods and services are recorded. The number of cows detected in estrus divided by the total number of cows is an estimate of the estrus detection efficiency, since normal cyclic cows should exhibit one or more estrus periods in this 24-day period. If a low percentage of cows are detected in estrus, rectal palpation of the internal genitalia should be performed to verify that the cows are cycling and not pregnant. The presence of a corpus luteum on one or both ovaries indicates that the cow is experiencing normal estrous cycles.

Concentrations of milk or serum progesterone can be helpful in verifying luteal function and the capabilities of the producer to detect estrus in the herd. The evaluation of progesterone concentrations in a group of cows to be mated can be used to ascertain the percentage of cows being serviced with high progesterone (i.e., cows not in estrus).

There are many aids that can be used to increase the efficiency of estrus detection. However, there is no substitute for visual observation of cows in estrus. The practitioner should be certain that observers are able to accurately recognize the signs of estrus. Observation periods of 30 to 45 minutes during the morning and the evening remain the optimum method for detecting estrus. In warm humid climates it is recommended that a third check be made during the night. Sole reliance on detection aids as the means of identifying animals in estrus results in a decrease in estrus detection efficiency. Aids often employed include estrus detector patches, tail paint or chalk, androgenized steers or heifers, and surgically altered bulls. Estrus expectancy charts and breeding wheels can be used to identify animals that are anticipated to return to estrus.

Detailed records are usually lacking in beef herds, and management practices in many of these herds make estrus detection difficult. Breeding at a predetermined time following the administration of prostaglandins or progestins has been proposed to circumvent the problem of estrus detection. However, results are often disappointing if cows are not palpated to verify ovarian activity before treatment. Progesterone determination can be incorporated into the protocol to select those cows to be included in an estrus induction program. Estrus synchronization often results in increased estrus activity among grouped animals.

TIMING OF INSEMINATION

Contrary to producer's beliefs, good results can be achieved from once-a-day artificial insemination service.[2] Animals detected in estrus by the morning should be inseminated that morning, and any others observed in estrus later on in the day should be mated the next morning. This recommendation is justified because animals exhibiting estrus early in the morning have likely been in estrus during the previous night and those not exhibiting estrus until later in the day are likely just coming into estrus.

HYGIENE

Equipment used for artificial insemination should be free from debris and contamination. When the equipment is prepared for insemination and thawing of semen, cleanliness should be of primary concern. The vulva of the cow should be properly cleaned before placement of the artificial insemination pipette. Double sheathing the artificial insemination gun will reduce contamination of the uterus from vaginal flora.

SEMEN QUALITY

Frozen semen prepared and stored according to Certified Semen Services (CSS) standards and purchased from a reputable dealer can usually be assumed to be of good quality. If questions arise as to the quality of frozen semen, a sample unit from the same batch should be evaluated following recommended procedures.[3]

Although there is the potential for disease transmission in artificial insemination since organisms can survive freezing, semen processed according to CSS standards should be relatively free of disease-producing organisms. Widespread use of a bull could increase the prevalence of a genetic defect. With current testing procedures most common genetic defects are noted before the bull is used widely by the industry.

SEMEN STORAGE AND HANDLING

Frozen semen should be maintained in liquid nitrogen until ready to use. When removing a straw of semen, the canes containing the semen should be raised no higher than necessary, since exposure to the warmer temperatures in the neck of the canister results in damage to the sperm. Semen should be transferred immediately from the tank to the thawing vessel and should be thawed according to the particular bull stud's directions. Lacking specific guidelines, a warm water thaw (95°F) for at least 40 seconds is recommended by the National Association of Animal Breeders for 0.5-ml straws. Thawing the straw in the pocket, in the cow, or in cold water will adversely affect the sperm. Semen should be used within 15 minutes of thawing. Thawed sperm cells are susceptible to cold shock so care should be taken to protect the semen until it is placed in the cow, including warming the artificial insemination gun prior to loading.

SEMEN PLACEMENT

It has long been recommended that semen be placed in the uterine body just inside the internal cervical os. Although this is a sound recommendation in theory, in practice it has probably been responsible for the failure of some inseminators to achieve good results. Placement of semen in the cervix is associated with a decrease in pregnancy rates compared with placement of the semen in the uterus. Studies have found that a large number of inseminators have difficulty fully penetrating the cervix. Inseminators who underwent retraining to place semen in either the uterine body or horn were initially equally capable of accurate placement. However, after 6 months those attempting placement in the body showed a significant reduction in accuracy, while those placing it in the horn retained their proficiency.[4] This would seem to indicate that the horn provides a more easily identifiable landmark than the cervix with a higher degree of repeatability.

Unintentional withdrawal of the insemination gun during semen deposition may occur in a significant number of inseminations. If the gun is placed in the uterine body initially, semen will be deposited in the cervix if it is withdrawn during insemination. However, if the gun is initially placed in the horn, even if the pipette is withdrawn during insemination, the semen will be deposited in the uterus. Semen placement can be evaluated on slaughterhouse specimens with the use of dye or radiographs to determine an inseminator's proficiency.

Spermatozoa can migrate from one horn to the other in the cow.[5] In heifers inseminated in one horn of the uterus, sperm was present in all parts of the uterus and oviducts, even in the contralateral oviduct distal to a surgical resection within 2 hours.[5] Therefore, assessment of the left-to-right pregnancy ratio is not a valuable parameter to determine inseminator proficiency. Placement of semen into the horn contralateral or ipsilateral to the ovulatory follicle does not influence pregnancy rates.[6] Reports that placement of semen in the horn was associated with an increase in pregnancy rates when compared with placement in the uterine body have not been substantiated. It is possible that when semen was placed in the horn it was definitely in the uterus, while when placed in the uterine body it may have been in the cervix. Depositing the semen in the uterus is the key factor; and if this can be achieved more consistently by horn placement than by body placement, then that target is preferable.

REFERENCES

1. Braun RK: Analysis of reproductive records using DHIA summaries and other monitors in large dairy herds. In Morrow DA (ed): Current Therapy in Theriogenology, 2nd ed. Philadelphia, WB Saunders, 1986, pp 414–418.
2. Gonzalez LV, Fuquay JW, Bearden HJ: Insemination management for a one-injection prostaglandin $F_{2\alpha}$ synchronization regimen: I. One daily insemination period versus use of the A.M./P.M. rule. Theriogenology 24:495–500, 1985.
3. Barth AD: Evaluation of frozen bovine semen. Proceedings of the annual meeting of the Society for Theriogenology, Coeur d'Alene, ID, 1989, pp 92–99.
4. Senger PL, Becker WC, Davidge ST, et al: Influence of cornual insemination on conception in dairy cattle. J Anim Sci 66:3010–3016, 1988.
5. Larsson B: Transperitoneal migration of spermatozoa in heifers. J Vet Med 33:714–718, 1986. Berlin and Hamburg, Germany, Paul Parey Scientific Publishers.
6. Momont HW, Seguin BE, Singh G, Stasiukynas E: Does intrauterine site of insemination in cattle really matter? Theriogenology 32:19–26, 1989.

Management of the Repeat Breeder Female

DWIGHT F. WOLFE, DVM, MS

Most veterinarians define a repeat breeder as a female animal that fails to conceive after three or more regularly spaced services in the absence of detectable abnormalities of the internal genitalia. The incidence of the problem in dairy herds ranges from 5.0 to 15.1 per cent, with an apparent average of 10.5 per cent of dairy cattle affected. The problem appears to be less frequent in beef cattle and small ruminants. Swine are also affected, and approximately 20 per cent of sows culled for reproductive failure are culled because of return to estrus following breeding.

A discussion of repeat breeders or conception failure must address normal reproductive expectancy. With normal healthy cycling cows a 63 per cent conception rate is expected on first service. Similar results are expected on each successive service such that 5 per cent of a normal healthy cycling cattle population can be expected to be repeat breeders based on the previous classification of failure of conception after three services (per cent nonpregnant = 37 per cent first service × 37 per cent second service × 37 per cent third service = 5 per cent nonpregnant).

ECONOMICS

Repeat breeding accounts for significant economic loss to the livestock producer. Each affected cow experiences an extended calving interval of at least three estrous cycles, or approximately 2 months. Although failure of conception may be less costly than abortion or the production of inferior offspring, in Holstein cattle in the United States this extension of the calving interval causes an 8.8 per cent reduction in the annual income above feed cost and an average loss of 0.15 calf and 144 kg of milk per cow. A similar reduction in production potential occurs in all livestock species owing to the extra maintenance expense and the reduced production.

FERTILIZATION FAILURE

Fertilization requires that viable, competent spermatozoa and ova arrive in the uterine tube at the appropriate time. Studies using planned slaughter after breeding indicate that in first-service heifers, the fertilization rate approached 100 per cent compared with 83 to 85 per cent in pluriparous, normal cows and only 60 per cent in repeat breeders.

CONGENITAL ANATOMIC DEFECTS CAUSING FERTILIZATION FAILURE

Segmental aplasia of Müller's ducts is one of the more common abnormalities causing fertilization failure. The developmental defects may involve the vagina, cervix, uterus, and uterine tubes. Imperforate hymen, imperforate cervix, aplasia of all or part of one or both uterine horns or uterine tubes, and double external or internal cervical ora are manifestations of this condition. Additional forms of the abnormality are didelphia, in which each uterine horn connects by a separate cervical canal, and uterus unicornis, in which only one uterine horn is present. Any manifestation of these conditions may cause fertilization failure by preventing the union of sperm and ova.

Diagnosis and Treatment

Most of these conditions can be confirmed by physical examination. Varying degrees of vaginal constriction, imperforate hymen, and anomalies of the external cervical os are detectable by speculum, endoscopy, ultrasound, or digital vaginal examination. Accumulation of normal cyclic secretions may occur anterior to an obstruction producing dilation of a portion of this tubular tract. Careful rectal palpation or ultrasound examination will distinguish this condition from pregnancy. The incidence of congenital anomalies is reported to be less than 1.0 per cent and because of the suspected heritable nature of these conditions, surgical repair is not recommended.

DEFECTS OF SPERM, OVA, OR ZYGOTE CAUSING CONCEPTION FAILURE

Chromosomal abnormalities of sperm or ova may prevent fertilization or cause conception failure through the creation of lethal gene products. Male and female animals heterozygous for a genetically balanced autosomal abnormality are usually phenotypically normal, but they can produce unbalanced products of meiosis that will create unbalanced embryos that may die in utero. Chromosomal abnormalities are reported in all the domestic animal species.

Polyploidy (more than the 2N number of chromosomes) can be caused by two or more sperm penetrating (polyspermy) and fertilizing (polyandry) one ova or by the suppression of the second polar body and fertilization of a diploid ova by one sperm (polygyny). The resultant polyploidy is usually lethal. The incidence of these conditions is more frequent in aged gametes. Fertilization of aged gametes seldom occurs under natural mating conditions. However, the improper timing of artificial insemination may allow aging of either sperm or ova prior to fertilization.

Diagnosis of Chromosomal Abnormalities

Chromosomal analysis of blood leukocytes from a heparinized venous blood sample by a cytogenetics laboratory will detect the presence of numerical or gross structural autosomal abnormalities. Balanced autosomal abnormalities that do not result in numerical or gross structural alterations require leukocyte culture to harvest cells during mitosis or meiosis. Diagnosis of lethal chromosomal aberrations is difficult and depends on cytogenetic studies of the embryo or parents of the embryo. Embryos should be submitted in tissue culture medium with 10 per cent serum and 100 IU penicillin and 100 mg streptomycin per milliliter.

ACQUIRED ABNORMALITIES CAUSING FERTILIZATION FAILURE

Ovarobursal Disease

Acquired lesions of the genital tract are usually due to infections or parturient trauma. Adhesions, mild to severe, between the ovary and fimbria may prevent entrance of ova into the uterine tube. The right ovary appears to be more frequently involved, but the condition may be bilateral. Mild lesions may not affect fertility.

The incidence of the disease is uncommon in heifers but increases with age. The adhesions may occur in all species but appear to be most common in cattle. Mycoplasmas have been isolated from a high proportion of ovarobursal lesions, and it has been suggested that there is a relationship between semen-borne mycoplasmas and this disease.

Diagnosis and Treatment

Diagnosis of ovarian adhesions is difficult. Careful rectal palpation of the ovaries may detect a small percentage of the fertility-limiting adhesions, and ultrasonography may enhance the accuracy of the diagnosis. Exploratory laparotomy or laparoscopy may be indicated in valuable females. Therapy is disappointing in the bilaterally affected cow. If the condition is unilateral, rectal palpation with breeding only when the ovulation occurs on the unaffected ovary may be rewarding. An alternative is surgical removal of the affected ovary, so that all subsequent ovulations are from the normal ovary. If this option is chosen, the contralateral ovary should be carefully examined during surgery to ensure that there is no pathologic condition that is undetectable by rectal palpation. As veterinary skill improves with laser surgery, these procedures should be amenable to dissolution of ovarobursal adhesions.

Occlusion or Inflammation of the Uterine Tube

Occlusion or inflammation of the uterine tube (oviduct) may prevent fertilization. These conditions may prevent sperm or ova transport to the ampulla or create an environment unsuitable for fertilization. Salpingitis, hydrosalpinx, pyosalpinx, or pachysalpinx may be sequelae to puerperal metritis. These conditions are not consistently palpable per rectum.

Diagnosis and Treatment

Two tests utilizing either phenolsulfonphthalein (PSP) or gamma-radiated starch powder have been advocated for assessment of uterine tube patency. The reader is referred to the second edition of this text for discussion of these techniques. Rectal palpation or ultrasonographic examination may detect occlusive disease of the uterine tube. Although these tests may detect patency of the uterine tube, none assess uterine tube function. Embryo transfer techniques may be used to assess patency and function of the uterine tubes with considerable accuracy by experienced veterinarians. Collection of fertilized ova in the uterine horn is definitive for uterine tube patency and function. If unfertilized ova are collected, uterine tube patency is assured, but other causes of fertilization failure should be considered.

IMPROPER TIMING OF INSEMINATION

Improper timing of insemination is one of the primary causes of fertilization failure. This situation rarely occurs with natural mating and is usually management induced by artificial insemination. As determined by progesterone levels, in some herds up to 20 per cent of inseminated cows are in the luteal phase of the cycle. If the problem is anticipated, the veterinarian should review the estrus detection program and then client education, palpation of cows by a veterinarian, serum or milk progesterone samples collected at the time of insemination, and the use of estrus detection aids such as heat detection patches, surgically altered teaser males, or androgenized heifers or steers should be considered. Additionally, improper semen handling or placement during artificial insemination may cause fertilization failure.

OVULATORY DISORDERS

Ovulation occurs 10 to 12 hours after the end of behavioral estrus in the cow, 12 to 36 hours after the onset of estrus in the doe, 24 hours after the onset of estrus in the ewe, and 24 to 42 hours after the onset of estrus in the sow. In superovulated female animals ovulation may occur over a 12- to 60-hour period.

It is generally believed that ovulatory defects are due to endocrine disturbances. The quantity and timing of luteinizing hormone (LH) release from the anterior pituitary gland determine when ovulation occurs. Inappropriate LH release, in relation to estrus, may lead to anovulation. The preovulatory follicle then becomes cystic. Cows with cystic ovarian disease experience irregularities of the estrous cycle and will not qualify in the classic description of the repeat breeder. Insemination or mating at this anovulatory estrus will result in fertilization failure.

Diagnosis of delayed ovulation is based on sequential rectal palpation or ultrasonography of the same follicle on the same ovary at more than 24 hours after estrus. Since ovulation in cows occurs 18 to 36 hours after the ovulatory LH peak, sequentially monitoring the temporal relationship of the LH peak to the time of ovulation over several estrous periods may establish normal ovulatory behavior for an individual cow. Treatment may involve repeated insemination every 12 to 24 hours until ovulation occurs. The veterinarian should use caution to avoid manual rupture of the follicle by palpation. Alternatively, gonadotropin-releasing hormone (GnRH: 100 µg intramuscularly) or human chorionic gonadotrophin (HCG: 3000 to 4500 units intravenously), given 6 hours before or at the time of insemination in the next ensuing estrus, may hasten ovulation.

SEMEN AND FERTILITY

Bulls with high and low conception rates have been identified through artificial insemination records. The reason for the variation in conception rates among bulls with apparently good semen quality is unknown. Fertilization failure or early embryonic death may result with a higher frequency from matings of bulls of low fertility. This condition presumably occurs in species other than cattle.

Careless handling of frozen semen can drastically lower fertilization rates. Proper care of the liquid nitrogen tank, proper handling of the semen from the tank to the cow, and proper insemination technique must be observed for optimum results. Infertility associated with faulty artificial insemination techniques is discussed elsewhere.

CONCEPTION FAILURE

Conception failure is the result of early embryonic death. In cows, early embryonic death must occur before day 16 to maintain regular estrous cycle lengths, and numerous studies indicate that the majority of embryonic losses are before day 15. In ewes and sows, embryonic death must occur by day 12 to maintain regular cycle length.

PHYSIOLOGIC CAUSES OF EARLY EMBRYONIC DEATH

Aging of the ovum may occur in delayed ovulating female animals or in those that are inseminated too late after ovulation. Generally, the aged ovum is still fertilizable but a defective zygote develops that undergoes early embryonic death.

HORMONE INFLUENCE

Improper balance of estrogen and progesterone during the early postovulatory period can affect ovum transport through the uterine tube. Excessive estrogen slows uterine tubal transport so that the ovum does not enter the uterus at the proper time. Excessive progesterone hastens ova transport. Either of these conditions may allow ova to leave the uterine tube at a time when the uterine environment is not synchronous with the physiologic needs of the ovum so that early embryonic death occurs.

Progesterone deficiency has been suggested as a cause of conception failure in many species. The primary source of progesterone during early pregnancy is the corpus luteum. Blood progesterone levels greater than or equal to 2 ng/dl are considered minimum for maintenance of pregnancy. Milk or blood progesterone studies indicate that 2 to 50 per cent of cows that ovulate and fail to conceive have low progesterone levels. Some cows with low progesterone levels do conceive, however. Diagnosis of luteal insufficiency is difficult. Palpation or ultrasonography of the corpus luteum for size and consistency is unreliable owing to the wide variation in corpus luteum size. Multiple, frequent blood or milk samples taken at varying times during the estrous cycle must be assayed to assess progesterone profiles for an individual cow.

Numerous empiric treatments have been used for progesterone insufficiency. Injections of HCG or GnRH from 1 to 10 days after breeding have been recommended to stimulate LH in the cow. Various regimens of exogenous progesterone have been administered to females of several species for pregnancy maintenance. One of the popular treatments in cows is 500 mg of repositol progesterone at 10 days after breeding and every 10 days thereafter. Administration of progesterone before the third day after breeding impairs fertility by probably increasing uterine tubal transit time for the embryo.

ENVIRONMENTAL INFLUENCES ON FERTILITY

Reduced conception rates in cows is well documented in the warm months of the year. Excessive solar radiation the day of insemination and high environmental temperature the day following insemination have a negative effect on conception rate. A rise of 0.5°C in body temperature causes a decline in conception rate. Ewes and sows subjected to high ambient temperature also suffer greater embryonic deaths. The elevated uterine temperature may cause fertilization failure by sperm or ova damage, or early embryonic deaths may occur. Provision of shade and free access to feed and water are suggested to improve hot weather fertility. Water mists and forced ventilation to increase evaporative cooling may be helpful in reducing thermal heat stress in swine and dairy cattle, but some studies using large numbers of animals have failed to demonstrate reduction of summer infertility through the use of these cooling methods.

NUTRITION

The effects of nutritional deficiencies and excesses on fertility are well documented. Little is known, however, of the pathogenesis. Energy restriction is probably the most common nutritional malady, and in heifers on inadequate energy diets a reduction of plasma progesterone levels and a reduction of normal fertilized ova have been documented. There is uncertainty as to whether the low energy intake may also alter sperm transport, fertilization, or growth and development of the early embryo. Low energy intake may also alter the endocrine function of the hypothalamus, anterior pituitary gland, or ovaries. There is some evidence that feeding excessive amounts of protein or nonprotein nitrogen to dairy cows is deleterious to conception.

NUTRITIONAL DEFICIENCIES

Several mineral deficiencies may be associated with failure of conception. Fertilization failure and early embryonic death have been associated with inadequate dietary copper, manganese, phosphorus, cobalt, and iodine. Vitamin A and β-carotene deficiencies may be significant causes of infertility. Diets may have adequate vitamin A yet be low in β-carotene. In cattle, delayed ovulation, silent estrus, and anovulation with follicular cyst formation have been associated with these deficiencies. Moreover, bovine luteal tissue has the highest β-carotene content of any tissue. Defective corpus luteum formation and ovarian steroidogenesis may be associated with β-carotene deficiency thus causing ovulatory abnormalities or early embryonic deaths owing to progesterone insufficiency.

Diagnosis of nutrient deficiencies requires thorough ration analysis and possibly serum profiles for affected cows. Vitamin A content of liver biopsy samples is most indicative of vitamin A stores in the body. Therapy consists of balancing the ration and supplying the appropriate nutrients in a form of high bioavailability. It appears that the reproductive efficiency of dairy cows may be improved with the addition of 300 mg of β-carotene per day, although the efficacy of this treatment is questioned by some researchers. The reader is referred to the Dietary Management section of this text for more detailed discussion of nutritional diseases.

AGE

It is generally agreed that fertility declines with age of the female. In cattle, heifers have higher fertilization rates than mature cows but also experience a higher incidence of early embryonic deaths. The number of repeat breeders is lowest in first-calf heifers and increases with age. It is reported that 13.3 per cent of cows older than 9 years of age are repeat breeders. This may be due to degenerative ovarian disease, endocrine deficits, or the accumulation of scar tissue with subsequent loss of function of the uterine tubes, uterus, cervix, or vagina.

UTERINE DISEASES

Postparturient metritis and endometritis have been incriminated as causes of conception failure in cattle. Many female animals, especially cows, suffer metritis in the early postpartum period. Even though many pathogenic or nonspecific organisms have been isolated from these cows, most of these cases heal spontaneously by the second- or third-postpartum estrus. Metritis and endometritis cause fertilization failure owing to sperm death in the hostile environment. Should fertilization occur, early embryonic death ensues because the uterine environment is detrimental to the embryo.

Diagnosis

Diagnosis of metritis is made by rectal palpation of an enlarged and/or fluid-filled uterus. Transrectal or transabdominal ultrasonography may be useful in sows, ewes, and does. Endometritis is more difficult to diagnose because by 30 days post partum only gross abnormalities are detectable by rectal palpation. Estrual mucus may have a cloudy appearance or contain flecks of purulent material. Examination of the vagina and cervix by speculum or endoscopy may reveal evidence of urovagina, pneumovagina, or other conditions that may incite endometritis. Material of the uterine lumen may be cultured to determine the presence of pathogenic organisms.

With the cow adequately restrained, the veterinarian should scrub and disinfect the vulva and perineal area. By rectal palpation, the cervix is grasped and stabilized. As an assistant parts the vulvar lips, a guarded culture swab is introduced through the cervix and into the body of the uterus. The sterile swab is advanced out of its protective sheath, the tip is gently manipulated within the uterus, and the swab is retracted back into the sheath. The swab is retracted from the cervix, and with the vulvar lips parted the guarded swab is withdrawn. In heifers, sows, ewes, and does, the guarded swab is positioned against the external os of the cervix and the swab is advanced into the uterus. The sample is refrigerated or packed on ice for immediate transport to the laboratory.

The degree of damage caused by endometritis cannot be determined by culture. Uterine biopsy, however, may be beneficial in assessing endometrial damage. By rectal palpation, the cervix is grasped and manipulated while the biopsy instrument is passed through the cervix and into the body of the uterus. The tip of the forceps is opened, and by rectal manipulation the uterine wall is pressed into the jaws of the forceps. The jaws of the forceps are closed, excising a small piece of endometrium. The forceps is withdrawn and the specimen is immediately placed into Bouin's solution, which produces fewer shrinkage artifacts than formalin, and sent to a laboratory with a staff experienced in interpreting endometrial biopsy specimens. A minimum of three samples should be collected, one sample from 3 to 6 cm anterior to the bifurcation on the medial surface of each uterine horn and a sample from the uterine body taken as near the cervix as possible. The samples collected 5 to 10 days after estrus are best, since samples collected during estrus are difficult to evaluate for endometritis. Abnormal samples may contain bacteria, inflammatory cell infiltrates, cystic endometrial glands, or lymph nodules. The degree of endometrial damage is determined by the extent of periglandular fibrosis. There is no therapy for endometrial fibrosis or atrophy.

Treatment

Therapy for metritis and endometritis may involve intrauterine or systemic therapy. Many practitioners opt for repeatedly shortening the estrous cycle with systemic prostaglandins. This technique uses the natural immunologic response of the uterus during the estrogen-dominated portion of the cycle. Additionally, advantages of this method are that it avoids trauma and possible contamination of the uterus by intrauterine infusion techniques; it is easily accomplished in heifers, ewes, and does in which intrauterine infusion may be difficult; and there is no milk withdrawal necessary in lactating dairy cows as may be required with some antimicrobial agents used for intrauterine infusion.

If intrauterine therapy is chosen, antibiotic selection should be based on results of culture and sensitivity testing. Mild antiseptics such as 3 to 5 per cent povidone-iodine in sterile saline or chlorhexidine suspension are often effective. Infusion of 2 to 5 ml of Lugol's solution in 30 ml of sterile saline is a popular treatment for chronic endometritis. This antiseptic solution is mildly irritating and causes a mild chemical curettage of the endometrium. Numerous substances have been used for intrauterine infusion for treatment of endometritis and, provided the substances are not exceptionally irritating to the uterus, improved fertility often occurs because of, or in spite of, the treatment. Appropriate withdrawal times should be observed for milk and meat when using antimicrobial compounds.

INFECTIOUS CAUSES OF INFERTILITY

Campylobacteriosis

Campylobacter fetus subsp. *venerealis* is a significant pathogen of cattle that may cause mild endometritis and salpingitis. Campylobacteriosis (formerly called vibriosis) primarily affects cows, although bulls can be carriers, and the disease generally manifests as a herd infertility problem.

From 10 to 14 days after infection, mild endometritis develops and in 25 per cent of the cases the infection enters the uterine tube. Infertility is due to early embryonic death, and salpingitis may cause fertilization failure at subsequent estrous cycles.

Diagnosis

Most infected cows return to estrus 30 to 35 days following insemination. There are no palpable abnormalities in infected cows, and the appearance of the estrual mucus is not diagnostic. Definitive diagnosis is by isolation of the organism from an actively infected cow. With the cow adequately restrained and the vulva and perineal area cleaned and disinfected, the cervix is immobilized by rectal palpation. The tip of a sterile, guarded infusion pipette is placed into the external os of the cervix, and cervicovaginal mucus is aspirated into the pipette through a sterile 10-ml syringe attached to the pipette. Cervical mucus, especially during diestrus, is quite viscous and may be difficult to aspirate into the pipette. Infusion of 2 to 5 ml of sterile saline into the cervix followed by aspiration may facilitate collection of the mucus sample, but undiluted mucus is preferred. One to 2 ml of mucus is adequate. The pipette is retracted into the speculum, and both are withdrawn from the vagina, avoiding vulvar contamination. The sample is immediately inoculated into a transport vial containing Clark's medium with an increased CO_2 concentration. If Clark's medium is unavailable, the mucus is placed in a sterile tube that can be sealed to avoid oxygen contamination. The sample is refrigerated and delivered to a laboratory as quickly as possible.

Treatment

Most infected cows spontaneously recover from the disease after 3 to 6 estrous cycles, if they are not reinfected. Therapeutic administration of a bacterin may be useful. A single subcutaneous injection of streptomycin, 22 mg/kg, has been beneficial in bulls. The reader is referred to the bacterial disease section of this text for further discussion.

Trichomoniasis

The protozoan *Trichomonas fetus* causes venereal disease characterized by vaginitis, metritis, or both in cattle. Infected cows remain infertile for 2 to 6 months, probably due to early embryonic death caused by endometritis.

Diagnosis

Occasionally, infected cows may exhibit postcoital pyometra. These animals are usually acyclic and are not discussed here. Definitive diagnosis of trichomoniasis is dependent on isolation of the organism. Examination of bull smegma is the preferred technique, but cervicovaginal mucus may be acceptable. The mucus is collected as previously described for campylobacteriosis, and culture is done in Diamond's medium. The trichomonads may be identified by direct microscopic examination of the mucus at $100\times$ magnification by an irregular jerky movement associated with continuous rolling. At $400\times$ magnification, the characteristic morphology of the protozoan can be easily identified. These are the presence of three anterior flagella and an undulating membrane.

Treatment

Treatment of infected cows is usually not necessary because in most cases spontaneous recovery occurs after several estrous cycles. Dimetridazole, 50 mg/kg orally for 5 days, is effective for treating infected bulls. Metronidazole, 10 mg/kg up to 75 mg/kg intravenously given once daily for 2 days, is also effective. Neither of these drugs is approved for use in cattle in the United States. The reader is referred to the protozoal disease section of this text for additional discussion.

SUMMARY

The repeat breeder problem is complex. Frequently several abnormal conditions are involved, and the veterinarian is challenged to diagnose the condition. Extensive diagnostic tests are available that should be used on selected valuable individual female animals or on herds with repeat breeder problems. Successful therapy is satisfying. Reliable prognoses on individual female animals accompanied by judicious culling should be economically rewarding to the producer.

Potential of Embryo Transfer for Infectious Disease Control

DAVID A. STRINGFELLOW, DVM, MS

Technologic advances and obvious economic and humane advantages have resulted in an increased demand for the use of embryo transfer to move genetic material between populations of livestock, including cattle, small ruminants, and swine. Research involving particular bovine pathogens has shown that embryo transfer can be an effective means for introducing germplasm into herds while preventing the introduction of infectious disease–producing agents. Specific evidence in other livestock species is less convincing, but based on an assessment of epidemiologic factors involved in embryo transfer, it is clear that the movement of embryos is innately safer than the movement of postnatal animals whenever the transmission of specific pathogens is a concern. Insurance that embryos are free of pathogens can be provided by screening the health status of donors, by special handling of embryos, or by a combination of these two methods. Reassurance of the disease control potential of embryo transfer is provided in an assessment of the epidemiologic factors involved in embryo transfer, a summary of results of studies concerning the transmission of specific pathogens through embryo transfer, and an outline of effective methods for ensuring that embryos are pathogen free.

EPIDEMIOLOGIC ASPECTS OF EMBRYO TRANSFER

For an infectious disease to be transmitted through embryo transfer, a series of essential events must occur. Initially, embryos must be exposed to a pathogenic agent, resulting in adherence of the agent to the embryo, infection of the embyro, or contamination of recovery fluids. Then sufficient quantities of the pathogen must survive the processes of embryo collection and transfer, resulting in introduction of an infective dose into the recipient. Each of these events can be thought of as links in a chain of infection. If a single link is broken, transmission of disease will not occur.

There are a variety of factors intrinsic to the process of embryo transfer that deter the spread of infectious diseases. There is a temporal limit to the potential for exposure of transfer stage embryos to pathogens because embryos are collected shortly after conception (7 days). Exposure to agents not regularly found in the reproductive tract within a week after estrus is especially unlikely to occur. The immune status of the donor's reproductive tract during the period of conception and early embryonic development also serve to limit exposure potential. If exposure does occur, infection of embryos or adherence of pathogens is prevented for many agents by the zona pellucida that surrounds transfer-stage embryos. Additionally, there are a variety of obstacles that must be overcome by the agent for transmission to occur. These include the dilution factors of recovery medium and the effects of antibiotic therapy, freezing and thawing, mechanical washing, and special treatments (i.e., enzymes). That each of these obstacles can be overcome with the result that an infectious agent can be transmitted through embryo transfer has not been documented in a naturally occurring circumstance in any livestock species.

EMBRYO–PATHOGEN INTERACTION: SPECIFIC RESEARCH

Early concerns about the potential for transmission of infectious agents through embryo transfer procedures resulted from work in laboratory animals, but there is little evidence for naturally occurring, vertical transmission of pathogens through the embryos of livestock. Numerous studies using zona pellucida–intact (ZP-I) bovine embryos have resulted in the declaration that these embryos can be transferred with a relative degree of safety. Bovine embryos have been exposed in vitro to akabane virus, bovine leukemia virus, bluetongue virus (BTV), bovine diarrheal virus, foot-and-mouth disease virus (FMDV), infectious bovine rhinotracheitis virus (IBRV), vesicular stomatitis virus (VSV), bovine cytomegalovirus (BHV-4), and *Brucella abortus* and subsequently washed and assayed for infectious agent. Only IBRV, VSV, and BHV-4 adhered to the zona pellucida of these embryos, and it has been shown that trypsin treatment is effective for removal of IBRV and BHV-4. In vitro studies with *Haemophilus somnus, Ureaplasma diversum, Mycoplasma bovis,* and *Mycoplasma bovigenitalium* have shown adherence of these organisms after recommended washing procedures were used. Of these, *H. somnus* was inactivated by the use of standard levels of antibiotics in embryo wash medium. Treatments to ensure freedom of ZP-I bovine embryos from the other agents have yet to be documented, but neither a significant exposure potential for transfer-stage embryos to these agents nor natural transmission of the agents through embryo transfer has been demonstrated, so the use of such treatments might be unnecessary.

Embryo–pathogen interactions have been less extensively studied in other livestock. There is experimental evidence that BTV, *Brucella ovis,* and *B. abortus* adhere to ZP-I ovine embryos after in vitro exposure to these agents, but the infectious agent did not remain when embryos were washed subsequent to exposures to *Campylobacter fetus* and border disease virus. It is noteworthy that transmission of disease was not demonstrated when ovine embryos were collected and transferred from donor ewes that were known to be infected with BTV, maedi/visna virus, and the agent of scrapie. Similarly, transmission of disease could not be demonstrated after transfer of caprine embryos collected from donors that were serologically positive for BTV or caprine arthritis-encephalitis virus.

Zona pellucida–intact porcine embryos have been exposed in vitro to African swine fever virus, FMDV, hog cholera virus (HCV), porcine parvovirus, pseudorabies virus (PRV), swine vesicular disease virus (SVDV), and VSV. Washing was not 100 per cent effective in removing any of these viruses, although there appeared to be a substantial beneficial effect for removal of FMDV and PRV. Additional treatment of ZP-I porcine embryos with trypsin after in vitro exposure to HCV, PRV, and VSV was reported to be effective for ensuring that the embryos were free from these viruses. In further attempts to determine the potential for transmission of viral pathogens, embryos were collected from donor swine that were infected with HCV, PRV, or SVDV and transferred to negative recipients. Seroconversion occurred in recipients receiving embryos from PRV-infected donors, but only in those situations in which the virus was artificially introduced directly into the uterus. Again, it is noteworthy that none of the diseases have been shown to be transmitted with embryos under "natural" circumstances.

PATHOGEN-FREE EMBRYOS

A conservative approach to certifying the pathogen-free status of embryos for transfer is to ensure that the donor is free of the specific infectious agents of concern. In cattle, for example, it is possible to collect serum samples from the donor on the day of embryo collection or earlier and at some time after collection while the embryos are stored in the frozen state. The measure of safety using this method is absolute if a reliable test for specific antibody to the pathogen of concern is available and sufficient time is allowed between collection of paired sera for the normal incubation period of the disease. This method is also effective for screening the health status of the sire of the embryos since the donor serves as a sentinel animal for agents that might be introduced with the semen at the time of insemination. Using this conservative approach, the former in vivo environment of the embryo is certified to be pathogen-free before the frozen embryo is actually thawed and transferred.

Substantial evidence has accrued that the testing of donors is not necessary if standard materials and methods that are described in the *Manual of the International Embryo Transfer Society* are used in handling embryos. The following methods that conform to the standards are suggested:

- *Washing of Embryos.* Only ZP-I embryos can be effectively washed. To ensure the efficacy of washing, embryos are examined over all surfaces, using a stereomicroscope set at a minimum of 50× magnification to ensure that the zonae pellucidae are intact (Fig. 1) and free of adherent material. This visualization is done before and after washing. Ten 35-mm sterile plastic Petri dishes containing 2 ml of Dulbecco phosphate-buffered saline (PBS) plus 2 per cent fetal bovine serum (FBS)* with antibiotics (PSF: 100 U penicillin [base], 100 μg streptomycin [base], and 0.25 μg amphotericin B per

---

*Filter sterilized, *Mycoplasma* tested, and virus screened.

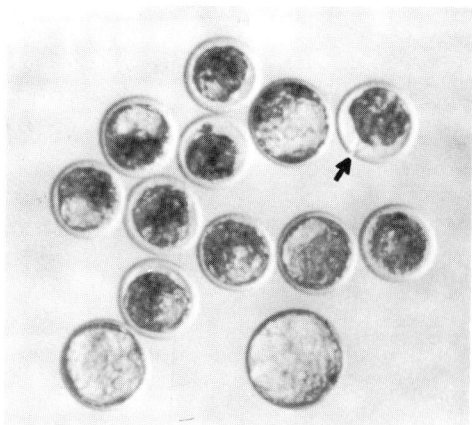

Figure 1. Day 7 bovine embryos enclosed by the zona pellucida (× 50). One embryo had a defective zona (*arrow*) and could not be certified to be pathogen-free after washing.

milliliter of medium) are used for washing of embryos. A separate, sterile 20-λ micropipette is used to carry groups of embryos between wash dishes. A hand-held micropipetter* that provides for easy exchange of pipettes and does not have a plunger that enters the pipette is essential to avoid contamination. The ratio of volume of medium containing embryos in the micropipette to volume of medium in each wash dish should be at least 1:100. While embryos are in each wash dish, the dishes are gently rotated with a circular motion, alternating between clockwise and counterclockwise motions to ensure adequate dilution and washing action. Embryos from a single donor animal are washed in groups of 10 or fewer.

Trypsin-treatment. Treatment of ZP-I embryos with the enzyme trypsin has been shown to be effective for removal/inactivation of certain viral pathogens that adhere to the zona pellucida. This treatment is required for embryos to be imported into certain countries. As in the standard washing technique, embryos are examined over all surfaces before and after treatment, using a stereomicroscope set at a minimum of 50× magnification to ensure that the zonae pellucidae are intact. Embryos from only one donor animal at a time are treated in groups of 10 or fewer. Equipment and techniques for pipetting as well as dilution factors are the same as presented under washing of embryos. The trypsin treatment involves the use of 2 ml of medium in twelve 35-mm Petri dishes. Dishes 1 to 5 contain PBS† plus 0.4 per cent bovine serum albumin plus PSF, dishes 6 and 7 contain 0.25 per cent trypsin in Hanks' balanced salt solution (pH, 7.6 to 7.8), and dishes 8 to 12 contain PBS plus 2 per cent FBS plus PSF. Generally, embryos are exposed to trypsin for about 2 minutes and all treatments are conducted at ambient temperature (approximately 25°C). It is known that exposure to trypsin for up to 5 minutes does not have a detrimental effect on the developmental capabilities of transfer-stage bovine embryos.

The development of additional treatments for embryos of livestock is underway. Future methods may include the use of various antibiotics, chemical disinfectants, enzymes, and specific antibodies. Although these new techniques will create a variety of options for ensuring the pathogen-free status of embryos, it should not be forgotten that current procedures already provide an extremely high degree of safety.

Embryo transfer has become widely available at reasonable cost to livestock producers in many parts of the world. When it is practical, transfer of embryos should be the preferred method for introducing germplasm into herds and flocks because of its potential for preventing the spread of infectious diseases.

EQUIPMENT AND SUPPLY LIST

Equipment

1. Micro-pipettor (No. 19803/0558) Minitub of America, Rt. 1 Box 3, Cambridge, IA 50046
2. 20-lambda Micropipettes (No. 21–175c) Fisher Scientific, 585 Alpha Drive, Pittsburgh, PA 15238

Supplies

1. Dulbecco phosphate-buffered saline (No. 310–4040AJ) Grand Island Biological (GIBCO), Grand Island, NY 14072

2. Bovine albumin fraction V solution (No. 670–5260AG) GIBCO, Grand Island, NY 14072
3. Fetal bovine serum (No. A1111L) HyClone Laboratories, Inc., 1725 South State Hwy 89–91 Logan, UT 84321
4. Penicillin-streptomycin-amphotericin B combination (No. 600–5240AG) GIBCO, Grand Island, NY 14072
5. Trypsin (10× liquid) (No. 610–5090AE) GIBCO, Grand Island, NY 14072
6. Hanks' balanced salt solution (No. 310–4020AG) GIBCO, Grand Island, NY 14072

BIBLIOGRAPHY

Conclusions of the research subcommittee of the International Embryo Transfer Society, Import/Export committee. Rev Sci Tech Off Int Epiz 8:567–568, 1989.

Echternkamp SE, Kappes SM, Maurer RR: Exposure of bovine embryos to trypsin during washing does not decrease embryonic survival. Theriogenology 32:131–137, 1989.

Hare WCD, Seidel SM (eds): Proceedings of the International Embryo Movement Symposium. Ottawa, International Embryo Transfer Society, 1988.

Stringfellow DA, Seidel SM (eds): Manual of the International Embryo Transfer Society, 2nd ed. Champaign, IL, International Embryo Transfer Society, 1990.

Abortion—An Approach to Diagnosis

DAN E. GOODWIN, DVM, PhD

Abortions in animals represent genetic and economic losses and frequently cause a serious disposal problem, especially if the abortion resulted from disease that is transmissible to other animals and humans. Although figures are not available to reveal losses caused by abortion in the United States, the U.S. Department of Agriculture collects and publishes information showing livestock production estimates (Table 1). This table should permit veterinarians in various states to estimate losses due to reproductive failure, a portion of which is a result of abortion. Comparison can be made among states as well as with the United States average shown at the bottom of the table. In Nebraska, for example, the table suggests that 8 per cent of cows eligible to calve in 1989 failed to produce a live calf; thus the reproduction failure rate was 8 per cent, a portion of which was due to abortion. The table also shows that Nebraska equaled the United States average of 8 per cent.

There is an indication that reproductive rates in cattle, sheep, and swine in the United States improved between 1982 and 1989. In Table 2 statistics show that inventory numbers have declined but reproductive rates per animal unit have increased.

The livestock owner who has never had an animal abortion problem has not been in business very long or owns only a few animals. Occasional abortions are to be expected and can sometimes be beneficial, for example, when the loss is caused by faulty genes that will not be perpetuated. Depending on economic and genetic considerations, single abortions may not be worthy of diagnostic investigation. Abortion losses of 2 to 3 per cent can be tolerated without undue concern in well-managed livestock operations. A practical solution to low-level abortion problems is to segregate and dispose of the aborting animals by slaughter; the loss of potentially valuable

---

*Micro-pipettor, Cat. No. 19803/0558, Minitub of America, Cambridge, IA 50046.

†Note: Calcium and magnesium are present in the prewashes when this treatment is used in our laboratory.

Table 1. UNITED STATES LIVESTOCK PRODUCTION BY STATE—1989

State	All Cows That Have Calved Jan. 1, 1989–1990 1000 Head		1989 Calf Crop		Breeding Ewes 1 yr and Older Jan. 1, 1989	Lamb Crop/100 Ewes 1 yr and Older Jan. 1, 1989	Dec. 1988–Nov. 1989†		
							Sows Farrowing	Pigs/Litter	Pig Crop
	1989	1990	1000 Head	%*	1000 Head	Number	1000 Head	Number	1000 Head
Alabama	940	930	800	86			15	7.7	117
Alaska	4.4	4.0	3.4	81	1.4	50	.05	8.5	.45
Arizona	355	350	290	82	185	70	6	8.2	49
Arkansas	1000	991	850	85			39	8.9	344
California	2022	2070	1850	90	632	87	7.8	7.5	58
Colorado	880	850	825	95	355	113	12	8.1	99
Connecticut	42	41	38	92	5.8	148	.23	7.1	1.6
Delaware	12	11	9	78			2.5	7.4	18
Florida	1300	1265	1000	78			9.8	7.7	74
Georgia	804	780	670	85			64	7.8	497
Hawaii	93	86	70	78			2.2	6.7	14.5
Idaho	700	700	660	94	220	123	3.7	7.7	28.5
Illinois	720	750	640	87	98	163	309	7.6	2356
Indiana	530	540	460	86	68	132	228	7.9	1788
Iowa	1520	1510	1440	95	293	131	715	7.8	5564
Kansas	1483	1488	1400	94	130	112	79	7.8	617
Kentucky	1275	1250	1160	92	25	124	59	7.6	446
Louisiana	670	710	580	84	12	92	3.8	6.7	25.3
Maine	56	59	57	99	11	145	.55	7.9	4.4
Maryland	169	162	155	94	23	100	10	7.2	72.3
Massachusetts	41	42	33	80	9.7	134	1.48	7.0	10.3
Michigan	470	475	440	93	72	132	67	7.8	522
Minnesota	1135	1075	1075	97	170	132	251	8.0	2005
Mississippi	780	780	690	88			11.5	7.4	84.8
Missouri	2230	2205	2050	92	87	126	163	7.5	1214
Montana	1405	1392	1350	97	434	115	13.5	7.6	102
Nebraska	1860	1860	1710	92	97	129	224	7.8	1748
Nevada	264	310	255	89	70	120	.83	7.8	6.4
New Hampshire	27	23	22	88	7.6	158	.33	7.2	2.3
New Jersey	41	36	32	83	9	111	.8	7.5	6
New Mexico	641	677	560	86	384	76	1.38	7.7	10.5
New York	859	865	830	96	57	118	6.5	7.7	49.8
North Carolina	450	470	440	96	9.5	116	153	8.1	1239
North Dakota	920	1000	1000	104	111	141	14.3	7.7	109.3
Ohio	738	734	645	88	165	121	116	7.9	923
Oklahoma	1950	2000	1930	98	94	96	11.8	7.4	87
Oregon	667	690	650	96	280	111	5.3	8.1	42.8
Pennsylvania	915	890	820	91	91	108	43	8.2	350
Rhode Island	3.5	3.5	3.5	100			.23	7.1	1.6
South Carolina	327	315	265	83			24.5	7.3	177.5
South Dakota	1650	1645	1670	101	430	120	98	7.7	762
Tennessee	1240	1215	1100	90	8.1	120	47	7.7	357
Texas	5700	5700	5000	88	1250	92	28	7.2	201.5
Utah	418	413	360	87	405	106	1.3	7.6	9.6
Vermont	184	181	169	93	17	147	.38	7.0	2.6
Virginia	805	840	780	95	95	137	23.8	7.9	187
Washington	575	600	520	89	51	147	3.4	8.0	26.8
West Virginia	271	270	245	91	62	111	1.7	7.2	12.3
Wisconsin	1890	1940	1900	99	66	152	70	7.7	540
Wyoming	695	660	640	94	555	103	1.1	8.0	8.5
US	43,727	43,854	40,142	92	7187.1	108	2948	7.79	22,971

Sources: Crop Reporting Board, Statistical Reporting Service, USDA, Washington, DC: cattle—released Feb. 2, 1990; sheep and goats—released Feb. 2, 1990; hogs and pigs—released Jan. 3, 1990.

*Percentage estimates for calf crop are based on the assumption that the 1989 calf crop was produced by the average of the Jan. 1, 1989, and the Jan. 1, 1990, inventory of all cows that calved.

†The figures for Sows Farrowing, Pigs/Litter, and Pig Crop are averages calculated from the following quarterly reports: December, 1988–February, 1989; March–May, 1989; June–August, 1989; and September–November, 1989.

Table 2. COMPARISON OF U.S. LIVESTOCK PRODUCTION FOR THE YEARS 1982 AND 1989

	1982	1989
Cattle		
All cows that have calved ($\times 1000$)	50,331	43,727
Calf crop (%)	89	92
Sheep		
Breeding ewes 1 year and older ($\times 1000$)	8,788	7,187
Lamb crop/100 ewes 1 year and older ($\times 1000$)	97	108
Swine		
Sows farrowing ($\times 1000$)	5,702	2,948
Pigs/litter ($\times 1000$)	7.38	7.79

Sources: Crop Reporting Board, Statistical Reporting Service, USDA, Washington, DC: cattle—released January 28, 1983, and February 2, 1990; sheep and goats—released January 26, 1983, and February 2, 1990; hogs and pigs—released December 22, 1982, and January 3, 1990.

breeding animals is usually offset by the removal of defective genes and destructive pathogens.

Whenever losses continue or abortion storms occur there is no question about the need for a thorough investigation of the problems by the owner and the practicing veterinarian and, if indicated, by the diagnostic laboratory staff. Although diagnoses are sometimes hard to establish, a thoughtful and accurate history, thorough clinical examination, and persistent laboratory investigation of numerous materials will usually yield facts that can be assembled to arrive at a diagnosis. The obstacles that sometimes stand in the way of successful investigations of abortions have been outlined by Kirkbride[1] as follows:

1. Abortion is frequently the result of an event that occurred weeks or months earlier; and the cause, if it was ever present in the conceptus, is often undetectable by the time of abortion.

2. The fetus is often retained in utero for hours and days after death, resulting in autolysis that hides lesions.

3. Fetal membranes, which are commonly affected first and most consistently, are frequently unavailable for examination.

4. Toxic and genetic factors that may cause fetal death or abortion are not always discernible in the specimens available for examination.

5. Many causes of bovine abortion are unknown, or there are no routine diagnostic procedures for identifying them.

HISTORY

The value of a thorough history cannot be overstated. Veterinarians should gather essential information in a systematic way so that the livestock owner, the veterinarian, and, if necessary, the diagnostic laboratory staff will have a map to follow as they consider diagnostic approaches. Questions should be asked objectively. Asking leading questions should be avoided since the animal owner may be influenced to give misleading answers. After information is obtained about the owner's name and address, animal species, breed, and number of animals at risk, written answers need to be obtained for the questions listed in the abortion questionnaire (Fig. 1).

The history may yield answers that will give a strong indication of the cause of abortion. If such is the case, then the veterinarian should direct the investigation at confirming this. It may require the collection of selected specimens for submission to a diagnostic laboratory. When accompanied by the written history and a request for specific tests, the specimens may generate the facts that will permit a diagnosis to be rendered.

CLINICAL SIGNS

If the history does not yield strong indications about the cause of abortion, the veterinarian should plan a broader investigation that would include an inspection of the animal's environment, clinical examination of aborting animals, and perhaps clinical examination of male and female herdmates. At the conclusion of the broader investigation, veterinarians may have obtained additional facts that will direct attention toward specific causes of abortion. At the least, they should have sufficient information at this point to suggest that the cause will fit into one of the following categories:

- Venereal infections
- Nonvenereal ascending infection
- Septicemia
- Anemia
- Nutritional problem

1. Are breeding records available to show length of estrous cycles and the numbers of services required for conception? (If practical, photocopies of the records should be obtained.)
2. How many abortions have occurred?
3. Is this a new problem or a continuing one?
4. When did the abortions begin?
5. At what stages of gestation have abortions occurred?
6. Does the problem occur chiefly in young animals in their first pregnancy or in animals of all ages?
7. Do aborting animals appear to be sick before or after aborting?
8. Is dystocia a problem?
9. Are fetuses dead (fresh or autolyzed?) or alive at time of abortion?
10. Are aborted fetuses of normal size for their gestational age?
11. Do they show developmental abnormalities?
12. Do they show signs of skin disease?
13. Are term newborn animals weak?
14. Have mummies been aborted?
15. How long does it take for placentas to be expelled?
16. Do placentas show any abnormalities?
17. Have new breeding animals (male or female) been introduced in the past year?
18. Have aborting animals been hauled, worked, or otherwise stressed recently?
19. Were aborting animals treated with steroid drugs recently?
20. Is artificial insemination/embryo transfer practiced?
21. If so, what is the source of semen/embryos? (Sire health programs and semen/embryo processing techniques may need to be ascertained.)
22. Are clean-up sires used as a follow-up to artificial insemination? (Their breeding history and soundness may need to be ascertained.)
23. What type of vaccines/bacterins are used; at what ages and frequency are they used; and who manufactured them? (Dose level, expiration date, and methods of administration may need to be determined if history indicates abortions have resulted from vaccine breaks/vaccine infections/vaccine misuse.)
24. What is the type and source of (1) pasture, (2) hay, (3) protein supplement, (4) grain, (5) mineral supplement, (6) water?
25. What fertilizer applications were made to pastures/fields in the past year?
26. What heating/cooling methods are used in animal housing? (Carbon monoxide levels may need to be determined.)
27. What have previous abortion investigations disclosed?
28. What do you believe has caused the current abortion problem?

Figure 1. Answers from the livestock owner will assist the veterinarian and, if necessary, the diagnostic laboratory in investigating abortion problems.

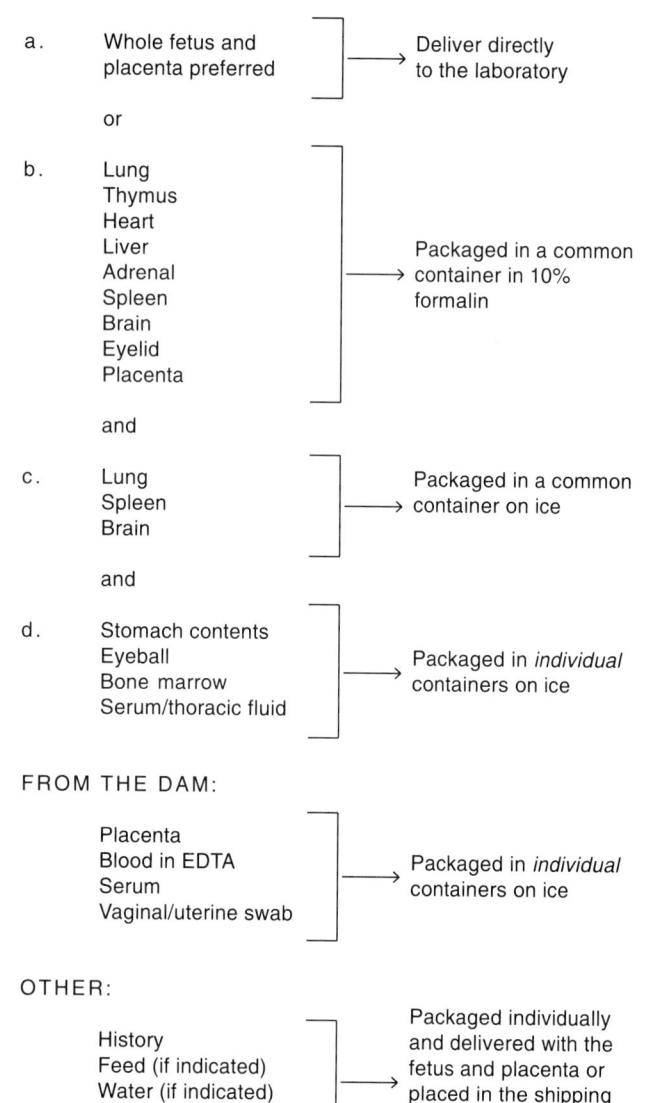

Figure 2. Materials to be submitted to the diagnostic laboratory for abortion investigation.

- Trauma
- Genetic defect
- Toxic problem
- Endocrine abnormality
- Other

Depending on the category, the veterinarian may render a clinical diagnosis that will stand without the need for any additional investigation. Trichomoniasis, anaplasmosis, modified live-virus vaccine administration, trauma, and carbon monoxide poisoning are examples of abortion causes that can frequently be recognized without diagnostic laboratory assistance. Laboratory investigations should never be used as a substitute for a poor history or for a poor clinical investigation.

MATERIALS FOR LABORATORY EXAMINATION

If it appears that laboratory assistance is needed and can be medically and economically justified, then specimens should be obtained for laboratory investigation. Laboratory staffs that are presented with good materials and good histories generally try harder to find productive answers. Rotten tissues and sorry histories frequently yield rotten and sorry results. The best specimens are freshly aborted fetuses and placentas. Dam serum samples delivered to the laboratory without delay along with a thorough written history or with a person who can provide the laboratory with a thorough history are also helpful. Because the average success rate for abortion diagnosis is around 25 per cent, it stands to reason that the laboratory staff is more likely to identify causative agents if it is able to examine several fetuses. Accordingly, if they are available, three to four fetuses and placentas and appropriate serum samples should be submitted. The failure of a laboratory staff to isolate pathogens from several fetuses is probably significant: it suggests that the diagnostic search should lead to other considerations (e.g., genetic, endocrine, or toxic).

If it is impractical to submit whole fetuses, then the veterinarian should conduct necropsy examinations, collect clean or sterile fresh and fixed specimens, record the necropsy observations, and send the history, necropsy report, and specimens to the laboratory without delay. Gloves should always be worn during necropsy examinations to protect against infections from *Brucella, Salmonella, Chlamydia,* and other pathogens. The veterinarian must assume the responsibility for protecting assistants who help with necropsy examination and specimen collection and shipment. The concern for protecting others must also extend to unwary postal and express service employees and laboratory employees who ultimately receive the package of abortion materials. Leaking packages traveling through public transport systems may sometimes constitute a serious public health hazard.

Any organ or tissue that appears to be abnormal should be collected, along with generous portions of placenta, lung, thymus, heart, liver, adrenal gland, spleen, tied-off stomach and its contents, brain, bone marrow, eyelid, eyeball, and fetal blood or thoracic fluid (aqueous humor from the eyeball is useful for diphenylamine testing for nitrate; eyelids are useful for histopathologic demonstration of fungal spores; fetal blood and thoracic fluid may be of value for serologic testing). Fresh specimens of placenta and gastrointestinal tract should never be placed in the same containers with other tissues.

A serum sample collected from the dam should be submitted with the knowledge that single samples may have limited value. Another sample collected 2 to 3 weeks later will extend the usefulness of serologic tests. When this is impractical or impossible, the veterinarian might consider submitting samples from several animals that have aborted recently along with samples from several animals that appear to be normal. A comparison of titers for various abortion diseases may allow inferences to be drawn that will point toward a specific disease as the abortion cause. The value of negative serologic results should not be overlooked since it is sometimes important to know that specific diseases are probably not present. The value of serologic investigations in individual herds can sometimes be enhanced by comparing test results from current serum samples with results obtained from reference serum samples that may have been collected several months or even years earlier. Some diagnostic laboratories routinely hold aliquots of serum samples for 1 to 2 years. Veterinarians should inquire if they are available. They may also want to advise livestock owners to consider having blood collected from selected valuable animals while they are healthy, so that serum can be held in the owner's freezers as reference standards for investigation of subsequent diseases that may develop. Serum samples should be stored in sterile tubes free of residues that may be toxic for cell cultures used in some serologic tests. Brucellosis tubes and some commercial tubes are not satisfactory.

If the veterinarian believes that it is indicated, he or she may wish to submit a blood sample in ethylenediaminetetraacetic acid (EDTA) from the dam or fetus for hematologic studies. Other samples that may be of value include vaginal and uterine swabs and feed, water, or other materials from the animal's environment that might be related to the abortion problem. A summary of diagnostic materials that may be needed for the investigation is presented in Figure 2.

CONCLUSIONS

It is apparent that abortion investigations can require remarkable amounts of time, tedious work, and careful thought on the part of the animal owner, the veterinarian, and diagnostic laboratory personnel. The animal owner who expects a blood sample collected from a recently aborted animal to yield information that will explain the abortion is usually going to be disappointed. The animal owner who is willing to spend the time and money for a thorough investigation is usually going to be rewarded with a presumptive or positive diagnosis that will permit effective treatment and preventive measures to be applied. Because of the limitations discussed previously, laboratory diagnostic success rates will probably never rise out of the minority range; however, the facts elucidated by the laboratory investigation combined with the facts contributed by the owner's history and the veterinarian's clinical examination will usually allow the veterinarian to render a useful diagnosis in the majority of the cases that are investigated.

REFERENCE

1. Kirkbride CA: Diagnostic approach to abortion in cattle. Compend Cont Ed Pract Vet 4(8):S341–S346, 1982.

Elective Termination of Pregnancy

PHILIP G. A. THOMAS, BVSc, MACVSc,
DIPLOMATE, ACT

Maintenance of pregnancy in domestic animals relies on a constant source of the hormone progesterone, which is secreted by the corpus luteum and placental tissues. Interrupting pregnancy can be achieved by eliminating progesterone support for the pregnancy, by manually disrupting the conceptus, or by evacuating uterine contents.

COW

Induction of abortion is indicated following accidental breeding ("mismate"), in feedlot heifers, and in pathologic conditions of pregnancy, such as fetal maceration, fetal mummification, hydramnios, hydroallantois, and prolonged gestation.

Intrauterine infusion will cause embryonic death and manual evacuation of uterine contents. Suitable solutions include 50 ml of 0.5 per cent aqueous iodine or 2 g of tetracycline in saline. Infusion will not be effective until 5 days following estrus when the developing embryo descends from the oviduct into the uterus. At this time, irritating solutions may cause luteolysis, in addition to their manual effect, resulting in early return to estrus. Infusion after the 11th day after estrus may lengthen the estrous cycle.

Manual rupture of the amniotic vesicle by rectal manipulation is possible once the vesicle can be palpated at 30 to 35 days of gestation. After 60 days of gestation and until 3 or 4 months of gestation, when the vesicle can no longer be isolated within the fluid-filled chorioallantois, it may be possible to terminate pregnancy by manually decapitating the fetus. The mean time to abortion is 25 days, and fetal membranes may be palpable for 2 to 4 weeks following such an approach.

During the first 5 months of pregnancy in the cow, progesterone secreted from the corpus luteum maintains pregnancy. Between 150 and 250 days of gestation, the placenta acts as an additional source of progesterone. In the last month of gestation, placental progesterone declines and pregnancy is again maintained by luteal progesterone.

Interrupting Normal Pregnancy

Removal of progesterone support for pregnancy can be achieved in the first 5 months of gestation by manual enucleation of the corpus luteum. However, this practice can induce adhesions of the ovary and ovarian bursa and occasionally cause severe hemorrhage and even death. Most manual techniques have become unnecessary since the availability of exogenous prostaglandins.

Luteolysis may be accomplished by the administration of estrogens. Within the first 4 days following breeding, 40 to 80 mg of diethylstilbestrol (DES) or 4 to 8 mg of estradiol cypionate (ECP) will terminate pregnancy by altering the oviductal environment and changing the transport time through the oviduct for the developing embryo. One hundred to 150 mg of DES or 10 to 20 mg of ECP is 60 to 80 per cent effective in terminating pregnancy during the first 5 months of gestation. Abortion occurs within 3 to 7 days of treatment. Estrogen treatment results in estrous behavior, vulvar swelling, a mucopurulent discharge, relaxation of parts of the posterior reproductive tract, and opening of the uterotubal junction. Ascending infection and salpingitis are possible sequelae, and return to fertile estrus may be longer than following prostaglandin treatment.

Daily intramuscular administration of 100 to 200 IU of oxytocin between days 2 and 7 following estrus will block luteal development, prevent pregnancy, and cause early return to estrus.

Pregnancy may be interrupted by intramuscular administration of 25 mg of prostaglandin $F_{2\alpha}$ ($PGF_{2\alpha}$) or 375 µg of the prostaglandin analogue cloprostenol (Table 1). Cloprostenol is 90 per cent effective in inducing abortion up to 150 days of gestation. The bovine corpus luteum will not reliably respond to a single luteolytic dose of prostaglandin or its analogues until 6 days following estrus. Prostaglandins alone will cause abortion until 5 months of gestation.

Exogenous glucocorticoids reduce placental progesterone after 150 days of pregnancy. However, they will not reliably induce abortion as a single therapeutic agent until the last month of pregnancy.

Between 5 and 8 months of pregnancy, a combination of $PGF_{2\alpha}$ or an analogue with 25 mg of dexamethasone is necessary to terminate both luteal and extraovarian sources of progesterone. Abortion follows within 5 days. This combination is about 95 per cent effective, although repeated injections are occasionally necessary. Behavioral estrus of 8 to 12 hours' duration is common before or during abortion.

There are several side effects associated with therapeutic abortion. Induced abortion after the fourth month of gestation results in an 80 per cent incidence of retained fetal membranes. Research has demonstrated that prostaglandin administration at the time of induced parturition does not reduce the incidence of retained fetal membranes. Two to 4 per cent of feedlot heifers aborted with a combination of prostaglandin and dexamethasone will develop fetal mummification. These mummies are usually expelled following re-treatment with prostaglandin. Acute toxic metritis is an unusual sequel to induced abortion.

In the last month of pregnancy, either dexamethasone or prostaglandin alone will induce premature parturition within 2 to 3 days. Retained fetal membranes may occur if parturition is induced more than 2 weeks before term.

Interrupting Abnormal Pregnancy

Fetal mummification may be treated with either prostaglandin or estrogens. Expulsion of the mummy usually occurs in 24 to 72 hours. Occasionally, mummies can become lodged in the vagina and require manual removal. Twenty per cent of mummies do not respond and require re-treatment or hysterotomy. Treatment of fetal maceration is less rewarding. Estrogen requires an intact endometrium to be effective, and maceration may be accompanied by endometrial damage. Cervical dilation is often poor and manual removal not possible. Cows experiencing fetal maceration have a poor prognosis for fertility.

Hydroallantois is characterized by a rapid accumulation of large volumes (up to 150 liters) of watery fluid in late gestation owing to abnormal placentome function. In hydramnios, a smaller amount of fluid (20 to 80 liters) accumulates slowly from midgestation, usually as a result of a fetal anomaly. Pregnancy may be terminated in cows with hydramnios or hydroallantois with simultaneous administration of prostaglandin and dexamethasone. Following treatment, prognosis for fertility is good in cases of hydramnios but postabortion complications are common following treatment for hydroallantois. In such cases, prognosis for fertility and life are poor. Slaughter is usually the best alternative for cows with hydroallantois.

EWE

Pregnancy in the ewe is supported by luteal progesterone for only the first 50 days of gestation. The corpus luteum of the ewe is sensitive to prostaglandins 5 days after estrus. Until 50 days of gestation, luteolysis and abortion may be accomplished by the intramuscular administration of 10 to 20 mg of $PGF_{2\alpha}$. Abortion follows in 2 to 3 days, and during the breeding season the ewe may be bred again. Dexamethasone (10 mg) will cause fetal death and abortion after 85 days of gestation. Esters of estradiol (5 to 10 mg ECP) may be effective throughout gestation.

DOE

In the doe, pregnancy is maintained entirely by luteal progesterone. Luteolysis is, therefore, reliably induced throughout gestation by the intramuscular administration of 2.5 to 10 mg of $PGF_{2\alpha}$ or an equivalent amount of a synthetic analogue. Abortion will follow within 5 days of injection. Repeated injections are occasionally necessary.

Therapeutic abortion may be followed by repeated short duration estrous cycles. Reduced fertility is often observed during such estrous cycles. However, if therapeutic abortion is accomplished early in the breeding season, it is possible to rebreed the doe in the same season.

Table 1. COMMON DRUG DOSES

Drug	Supplier	Species	Dose
Dexamethasone (Azium)	Scherring Corp. Kenilworth, NJ 07033	Bovine Ovine Caprine	25 mg IM 15 mg IM 15 mg IM
Prostaglandin $F_{2\alpha}$ (Lutalyse)	The Upjohn Co. Kalamazoo, MI 49001	Bovine Ovine Caprine	25 mg IM 15 mg IM 8 mg IM
Cloprostenol (Estrumate)	BayVet Division of Cutter Laboratories, Inc. Shawnee Mission, KS 66201	Bovine	500 µg IM
Fenprostalene (Bovilene)	Diamond Laboratories, Inc. Des Moines, IA 50304	Bovine	1 mg SC

SOW

Therapeutic abortion is infrequently used in the sow. Pathologic pregnancies, usually mummification of part of a litter, do not routinely require treatment, and the short duration of gestation in the pig precludes the need for therapeutic abortion for other reasons. Elective abortion is used for estrus synchronization, both as a management tool and in artificial breeding programs. Pregnancy in the sow is dependent on luteal progesterone. Therefore, prostaglandins will terminate pregnancy from day 12 of the estrous cycle. For estrus synchronization, sows are bred and then aborted between day 16 to 40 of pregnancy with 5 to 10 mg of $PGF_{2\alpha}$ or 500 µg of cloprostenol. A more effective synchrony may be achieved by repeating the injection 12 hours later. Typically, sows abort 30 to 45 hours after treatment and return to fertile estrus within 4 to 10 days. Conception rate at first estrus is up to 90 per cent.

Glucocorticoids will not readily induce abortion in sows. The use of estrogenic compounds should be avoided since they are luteotrophic and their administration on days 11 and 12 of the cycle will cause pseudopregnancy.

New products are constantly being evaluated for their efficacy as abortifacients. Currently, prostaglandins seem the ideal therapeutic agent for species with luteal-dependent pregnancy. Two new experimental drugs might aid elective pregnancy termination in the future. Epostane inhibits the action of 3β-hydroxysteroid dehydrogenase, the enzyme that converts pregnenolone to progesterone. Thus there is reduction of progesterone production by the corpus luteum or the placenta. RU 38.486 is a competitive blocker of progesterone receptors. Its use results in reduced progesterone activity at target cells in the uterus.

BIBLIOGRAPHY

Morrow DA (ed): Current Therapy in Theriogenology 2. Philadelphia, WB Saunders, 1985.

Diseases of the Male Internal Genitalia

R. L. CARSON, DVM, MS, Diplomate, ACT
R. S. HUDSON, DVM, MS, Diplomate, ACT

Disease of any of the internal genitalia of male food animals is rare. The one exception is disease of the vesicular glands of the bull. The incidence of vesiculitis varies from a sporadic 2 to 5 per cent in adult bulls to 5 to 50 per cent in groups of young bulls, suggesting contagion. Most acute cases occur in bulls either younger than 2 years old or older than 9 years old; however, evidence of inactive infection can be found in many middle-aged bulls. In addition to the direct effect of vesiculitis on reproduction, it is frequently the most obvious manifestation of a serious and complex disease syndrome, including elusive infections in other pelvic genitalia and concomitant or sequential epididymitis, orchitis, and periorchitis.

In bulls, the relative ease of examination of the vesicular glands and the more obvious response to insult may account for vesiculitis being reported more often than infections of other accessory genitalia. Although ampullitis, prostatitis, and bulbourethral adenitis appear frequently with vesiculitis at necropsy, ampullitis is less readily diagnosed clinically and prostatitis is almost never diagnosed. Greater size and firmness of the ampullae may escape detection, and the dense capsule of the bull prostate precludes enlargement. The bulbourethral glands are not palpable.

ETIOLOGY AND PATHOGENESIS

Numerous microorganisms have been associated with vesiculitis, including *Brucella abortus, Actinomyces pyogenes, Escherichia coli, Pseudomonas, Proteus mirabilis, Actinobacillus seminis, Actinomyces bovis, Nocardia farcina, Haemophilus, Salmonella, Chlamydia*, and certain viruses. The infectious agent often eludes identification. In some cases, especially in outbreaks among young bulls, infectious bovine rhinotracheitis or enteroviruses appear to initiate the insult and predispose the animal to opportunistic bacterial infections. *Chlamydia psittaci* has been reported to cause seminal vesiculitis in the buck. The predilection of *Brucella* for genital tissue includes the seminal vesicles of all the food animal species. The presence of *Brucella suis* in the seminal vesicles of boars without microscopic lesions causes concern in seminal transmission.

The pathogenesis of vesiculitis is not clear. The outbreaks in groups of young bulls may be related to normal homosexual activity with ascending infection or oral and nasal entry of organisms and hematogenous spread. Likewise, extragenital foci of infection, especially in the lungs, appear to be a source of blood-borne infection. Ascending infection in the rare cases of generalized urinary tract disease must be considered. Often there is a concurrent vesiculitis and epididymitis and occasional orchitis, but it is difficult to determine which comes first. In practice, the veterinarian may not be able to determine the origin or route of infection.

Studies point to increased susceptibility of the seminal vesicles associated with discrete unpalpable congenital abnormalities, but bulls with satisfactory service records and no evidence of vesiculitis may have palpable unilateral hypoplastic or aplastic seminal vesicles or ampullae.

DIAGNOSIS

Overt clinical signs rarely arise. Acute vesiculitis may cause signs of localized peritonitis, tenesmus, and obscure rear limb lameness. The condition is usually discovered on routine rectal palpation or after purulent exudate is found in the semen. Acutely affected vesicular glands are initially swollen, possible painful, and often devoid of the normal lobulation. Advanced disease may cause abscess formation and fibrosis. In cases of inactive vesiculitis the glands will be fibrotic and lack normal lobulation. Caution is required in that there is normal variation in the size of the vesicles within and among bulls. Also, some diseased organs elude even careful palpation. Old bulls typically have firmer vesicular glands than young bulls.

Culture of fluid massaged from the vesicular glands and collected through a hygienically inserted sterile urethral catheter is preferable to culture of semen, which always contains contaminants. Even so, the vesicular fluid may be adulterated with the products of other organs.

PATHOGENESIS

Acute vesiculitis may regress spontaneously or may progress to a chronic state of bacterial infection. Abscess formation and fibrosis may form adhesions extending to other organs or form tracts extending to the inguinal rings. Cases of long duration usually involve other foci of genital infection.

The effect of solitary vesiculitis on reproduction is difficult to assess. Greater viscosity of vesicular fluid may reduce gross motility of sperm. Reports of more sperm abnormalities probably reflect concurrent disease in the testes or epididymides. Survival of frozen-thawed semen is reduced.

Concern for transmission of disease through coitus or artificial insemination is logical, but the extent of risk is unknown. Many bulls with vesiculitis have been used without detectable suppression of herd fertility. In short, bulls with vesiculitis are classified as unsound but may not be infertile. The threat of infection to other genitalia, especially to the testes and epididymides, outweighs the threat of vesiculitis alone.

TREATMENT AND CONTROL

Spontaneous recovery in many young bulls does not permit a good evaluation of treatment. Most young bulls with acute vesiculitis respond favorably to broad-spectrum antibiotic therapy if adequate dosage and duration of treatment are used. However, many bulls with well-established bacterial infections resist antibiotic therapy. Confirmed and suspected chlamydial infections seem to respond to daily intravenous oxytetracycline, 5 mg/lb for 10 days. Regression of swelling is often dramatic. Surgical removal of the vesicles through the ischiorectal fossa is often disappointing. Easily replaceable bulls of marginal quality should be culled.

It may be that the recommendation to cull all bulls with the disease based on possible predisposition by congenital abnormalities merits consideration. The idea, however, is unlikely to gain popularity among producers working in free enterprise systems.

Vaccination against infectious bovine rhinotracheitis prior to close group housing of young bulls and other management practices that help control infectious diseases of other bodily systems are believed to help reduce the prevalence of vesiculitis.

BIBLIOGRAPHY

Arthur GH, Noakes DE, Pearson H: Veterinary Reproduction and Obstetrics. London, Baillière Tindall, 1982.
McCaulay AD: Seminal vesiculitis in bulls. In Morrow, DA (ed): Current Therapy in Theriogenology. Philadelphia, WB Saunders, 1980.

Diseases of the Testis and Epididymis
DWIGHT F. WOLFE, DVM, MS

The scrotum is a protuberance of the abdominal wall and encloses the testes and epididymides. The external surface of the scrotum is composed of irregularly undulating epidermis that is relatively free of hair, although some breeds of sheep do have wool covering this skin. The corium contains elastic fibers, collagen bundles, and bundles of smooth muscle cells running in parallel, oblique, and perpendicular orientation. The corium also contains a rich plexus of blood vessels and lymphatic vessels and large sebaceous and apocrine sweat glands.

The subcutis consists of a multidirectional network of smooth muscles and connective tissue. The tunica dartos comprises the smooth muscle layers of the corium and the subcutis. It is connected by loose connective tissue, the scrotal fascia, to the tunica vaginalis parietalis.

The testis must be maintained 2°C to 7°C cooler than core body temperature, and the scrotum functions as a protector and thermoregulator for the testes. In the bull and ram there is a temperature gradient of 4°C to 6°C from the base to the apex of the scrotum. Contraction or relaxation of the tunica dartos and cremaster muscles assists with maintenance of this temperature gradient.

EXAMINATION OF THE SCROTAL CONTENTS

The scrotum should be examined and palpated for evidence of dermatitis, fibrosis, or varicosities that may interfere with thermoregulation. The testis and adnexa should be freely movable within the vaginal cavity, and the tunica albuginea of the testis should be smooth and entire. Each testis should be palpated for the presence of cystic, fibrous, or calcified lesions within the parenchyma. The head, body, and tail of the epididymis and the ductus deferens should be entire and free from granulomatous lesions. The pampiniform plexus should be palpated for varicosities. Any dysymmetry between the right and left testis and epididymis should be noted. There should be no fluid accumulation within the vaginal cavity. Scrotal circumference, or, in boars, testicular length and width, should be determined and compared with normal for the species, age, and breed.

DEVELOPMENTAL ANOMALIES

Among fertile male animals of various breeds and species there is wide variation in testicular size correlated with scrotal circumference, sperm output, age, and body weight. Scrotal circumference measurement affords practical evaluation of testicular size and has been standardized for bulls and rams by the Society for Theriogenology.

Developmental anomalies of the testis usually manifest as hypoplasia when one or both testes are small (<30 cm scrotal circumference in postpubertal bulls) and more obscure defects if a variable portion of one testis is involved. Moderate hypoplasia causes subfertility but not sterility. Small, nonstimulated testes at puberty are associated with a primary deficiency of gonadotropins. The site of developmental failure may be the testis, hypothalamus, or pituitary. Testicular hypoplasia therefore has an insidious effect on breeding performance with the affected male being unable to settle adequate numbers of females in a limited breeding season. The condition is probably heritable in food animal species and must be differentiated from testicular atrophy. Testicular atrophy is an acquired condition that develops over time, and history and repeated examinations are key to the diagnosis. Testicular atrophy may result from postpubertal gonadotropin failure, which results in testes with shrunken tubules from loss of germinal epithelium. There is no treatment for testicular hypoplasia.

Blind or aberrant efferent ductules cause sperm stasis and extravasation with resultant sperm granulomas. With time, granulomas in the epididymal head produce occlusion of the epididymal duct, with resultant increased retrograde pressure on the seminiferous epithelium and testicular degeneration.

Aplasia of any portion of the epididymis blocks sperm

transit. However, blockage in the body or tail of the epididymis does not increase retrograde pressure on the seminiferous epithelium and therefore testicular function is not affected. Thus the testicle may appear normal. Bilateral granulomatous occlusion or epididymal aplasia may constitute irreversible sterility.

TESTICULAR DEGENERATION

Alteration of thermoregulation causes the most commonly diagnosed disease of the testes. Cryptorchid or ectopic testes are degenerate for this reason. Any local thermal interference causing insulation of the scrotum, such as dermatitis, hydrocele, periorchitis, or prolonged recumbency from lameness or systemic disease, rapidly induces testicular degeneration. The condition may appear after a short febrile episode and is common during prolonged hot and humid weather. Scrotal frostbite affects many males, and boars may acquire testicular degeneration from prolonged exposure to cold floors or, infrequently, torsion of a testis. Local inflammatory conditions such as orchitis or epididymitis cause testicular degeneration.

At least a portion of the progressive degeneration that attends aging is likely caused by multiple insults over time. A large proportion of old bulls, rams, and bucks with testicular degeneration have distal fibrosis of the testis, indicating probable vascular lesions.

If not reversed, testicular degeneration may progress to spermiostasis, inspissation of sperm, granuloma formation, fibrosis, and calcification. These degenerative changes are permanent.

Diagnosis

Degeneration often appears as a loss of normal turgidity and elasticity as the testis is palpated superficially and gently. Deep, firm palpation of fibrosis or calcification indicates advanced testicular degeneration with a guarded prognosis for return to fertility. Many of the previously discussed local causes of testicular degeneration are readily evident, but often the cause of the condition escapes detection.

Serial semen evaluations through the course of unchecked degeneration show a nonspecific progression from a minor increase in sperm abnormalities to oligospermia, to an increase in major head and midpiece abnormalities, and to the appearance of primordial germ cells. In degeneration without obvious cause and with incomplete history, evaluation of but a few ejaculates often fails to assist in differentiating the condition from moderate hypoplasia.

Radiography provides a valuable aid to palpation findings of fibrotic areas or masses, indicating especially the degree and pattern (isolated or diffuse) of calcification. Diagnostic radiography is not deleterious to spermatogenesis.

Real-time ultrasonography may be helpful in characterizing local or diffuse lesions in the testis. Anechoic areas within the testicular parenchyma indicate solid masses while hyperechoic areas indicate cystic lesions. The veterinarian should not confuse the anechoic mediastinum testis as a pathologic lesion.

In the stallion testicular biopsy is used for diagnosis of testicular disease. This procedure is more risky in boars and ruminants owing to the potential for development of sperm granulomas following the biopsy. Violation of the blood-testis barrier or escape of the haploid germ cells from the tubular tract initiates an inflammatory reaction with resultant granuloma formation.

Treatment

There is no specific treatment for testicular degeneration. Known factors inciting the degenerative process should be remedied, and hormone therapy should be avoided. Young sires with moderate degeneration frequently recover 60 to 90 days after the insult.

ORCHITIS AND PERIORCHITIS

Orchitis occurs in a small percentage of breeding males and usually is a unilateral condition. Systemic infections are the most common cause of orchitis, but trauma or neoplasia occasionally initiate the disease. The primary route of infection is by hematogenous spread, but extension of infection from the urogenital tract may occur. Infection and inflammation of the testis and surrounding tunica vaginalis is caused by a myriad of agents, including *Brucella abortus, Actinomyces pyogenes, Escherichia coli, Pseudomonas, Proteus mirabilis, Actinobacillus seminis, Actinomyces bovis, Nocardia farcinca, Haemophilus, Salmonella, Chlamydia, Mycoplasma*, and several cocci. Orchitis due to bovine herpesvirus and cytopathogenic enterovirus has been reported in bulls. Periorchitis due to mesothelioma has been diagnosed in bulls. Careful examination of the peritoneum by rectal palpation or abdominocentesis with cytologic assessment may assist with diagnosis of this neoplasm.

Acute inflammation of the testis or tunica causes swelling and pain, and frequently an alteration of gait is noted. The tunica vaginalis prevents excessive swelling of the testis, and severe enlargement is usually caused by fluid and fibrin accumulation in the vaginal cavity. Suppurative organisms may cause abscess formation. Chronic inflammation results in testicular degeneration, and unilateral inflammation may reduce or destroy spermatogenesis in the contralateral testis owing to interference with normal thermoregulation of that testis.

Diagnosis

Orchitis may be evident by testicular palpation as an alteration from normal turgidity. Gross distention of the vaginal cavity that prevents testicular palpation indicates periorchitis. Mild inflammatory changes may be detected by thermography, which detects variations from normal thermal patterns of the scrotum. Radiography may be useful, but ultrasonography of the scrotum and its contents is more useful for detection of these soft tissue diseases.

Treatment

Gentle cold water sprays for 30 minutes twice daily help reduce the damaging inflammatory heat. The use of systemic antimicrobial agents is questionable. Although systemic antibiotics may traverse the normally impervious blood-testis barrier, reduced tissue perfusion makes antibiotic penetration unlikely and probably ineffective.

Early in the course of unilateral inflammation of a testis concern should be directed to the contralateral testis. Although surgical removal of a mildly inflamed testis and adnexa might be overtreatment, careful aseptic hemicastration is indicated when the prognosis for the affected side is poor. Minimal additional inflammatory insult is caused by the surgery. A healthy or completely restorable remaining testis can be expected to compensate for 60 to 80 per cent of the original sperm output of two testes. The decision for hemicastration should be made early in the course of therapy to shorten recuperation time prior to return to fertility.

EPIDIDYMITIS

The tail of the epididymis is vulnerable to infection, especially in rams but also in bulls and bucks. This problem is less common in boars. Unilateral caudal epididymitis without testicular involvement is common in bulls. The opportunistic microorganisms of orchitis may be involved, although one author indicates that *Brucella abortus*, *Mycobacterium tuberculosis*, and *Actinomyces pyogenes* are the major causative agents in bulls. Concomitant infections of the testis and/or pelvic genitalia are common.

In adult rams *Brucella ovis* causes a specific severe epididymitis that is responsible for significant loss of flock reproductive efficiency. The organism may exist in the epididymis without palpable enlargement, or there may be extreme swelling and fibrosis even with draining sinus tracts through the scrotum. The testes may be involved. Transmission is by genital, oral, and respiratory routes and is enhanced by the animal's sampling of urine of other rams. The condition is often bilateral and causes sterility.

A separate epididymitis affecting ram lambs is attributed to a group of lamb epididymitis organisms, which mostly are *Brucella* species but do not include *B. ovis*. The epididymitis appears to acquire particular vulnerability in the peripubertal hormonal environment. Both ascending infections from sodomy and oral infections from filthy environments are suspected as inciting causes. Infertility is the result.

Diagnosis

Palpation of swollen, painful, indurated epididymal tails is the best method of diagnosis. In endemic flocks, palpation several times a year helps identify new cases. Acute inflammation in bulls causes resistance to even gentle palpation.

Brucella ovis epididymitis of rams usually produces numerous leukocytes in the ejaculate and is relatively easily cultured from semen. Large numbers of leukocytes accompany detached sperm heads and low motility. Leukocytes in semen are not uniformly characteristic of epididymitis.

Control

There is no good widely documented treatment for infectious epididymitis. Many bulls appear to recover spontaneously; unilateral castration is considered in severe cases.

Ram epididymitis requires palpation of epididymides, separation of clinically affected rams, and culling. Vaccination is of marginal value: it may reduce palpable lesions but usually not the inflammation and leukocyte content of semen. Lamb epididymitis appears to be controlled at times by feeding of tetracycline. There is no vaccine.

BIBLIOGRAPHY

McEntee K: Pathology of the testis and epididymis of the bull and stallion. Proc Annu Conf Soc Theriogenol 80–91, 103–109, 1979.

Roberts SJ: Veterinary Obstetrics and Genital Diseases, 3rd ed. Ann Arbor, MI, Edwards Bros., 1986.

Wolfe DF, Hudson RS, Carson RL, Purohit RC: Effect of unilateral orchiectomy on semen quality in bulls. J Am Vet Med Assoc 186:1291–1293, 1985.

Diseases of the Penis and Prepuce

R. L. CARSON, DVM, MS, Diplomate, ACT
R. S. HUDSON, DVM, MS, Diplomate, ACT

The frequency and wide variety of significant lesions of the penis and prepuce of food animals dictate careful examination by the veterinarian. This may be done by close observation of the animal during coitus, during service with an artificial vagina, or during stimulation with an electroejaculator. Alternatively, the penis may be extended manually, which may be the preferred method when a lesion is suspected since the aforementioned methods often worsen a preexisting condition. Manual extension is easily done in the standing restrained ram or buck; bulls may require that an assistant place a hand in the rectum to help relax the retractor penis muscles. Once the technique of manual extension is mastered, there is little or no need for tranquilizers, which carry the risk of postexamination penile injury. Some boars resist manual manipulation and require sedation or anesthesia.

BULL

Balanoposthitis primarily affects young bulls and may be due to infectious bovine rhinotracheitis or to nonspecific abrasions sustained during excessive service. The associated pain may cause bulls to refuse to serve. Healing is usually spontaneous, and service may be resumed in 2 weeks. Infectious bovine rhinotracheitis is venereally transmitted, and affected bulls may shed virus in semen. Intranasal vaccination may offer some degree of protection from this disorder.

Viral papillomas (warts) are found frequently on the penis but not on the prepuce of young bulls in groups. Abrasions admit the virus, and the wart grows rapidly and may surround the tip of the penis. Surgical removal is simple, the primary concern being preservation of the urethra and the glans penis. Ligating and suturing, if needed, are preferable to thermocautery, which may cause deep and serious necrosis. Vaccine, even if available, is of marginal value.

Young bulls commonly display a matted ring of hair surrounding the free portion of the penis. The hair comes from body coat hair of other bulls that have been mounted. The ring should be removed to avoid a deep annular laceration that might create a urethral fistula, a cavernosal fistula, or penile amputation.

Persistent frenulum, a congenital band-like attachment of the prepuce to the tip of the penis along the median raphe, is usually found in virgin bulls. The frenulum, not to be confused with a persistent prepubertal preputial adhesion, may cause ventral deviation of the erect penis. The impotence thus induced in *Bos taurus* breeds may not affect *Bos indices* breeds that have excessive prepuce. Strong evidence for heritability dictates culling affected bulls from purebred herds. Otherwise, the frenulum is easily ligated at each end and excised.

Deep lacerations of the dorsum of the penis may interrupt the sensory nerve supply, which is essential for intromission and ejaculation. Scars from lacerations should alert the examiner to possible impotence. Sensation may be tested by stimulation of the glans and dorsum with an electric prod while holding the retractor penis muscles. A positive response is a surprisingly mild contraction of the muscles. A better test is actual mating.

Deep lacerations of the glans and free portion may result in fistulae into the corpus cavernosum, which could result in erection failure or bleeding during erection, the blood being toxic to sperm. Immediate suturing after injury is indicated. Careful longitudinal wedge resection of the fistulae, separate closure of the tunica albuginea and skin, and 3 weeks of rest from sexual activity are usually successful. Fistulae of the glans are especially resistant to closure and require longitudinal resection, curettage of the cavity of the fistula, and deep suturing.

Lacerations or fistulae of the urethra, if more than 5 cm from the terminus, may reduce effective deposition of the ejaculate. Healing of sutured defects is categorically difficult because of the naturally vigorous wave-like movement of urination. A drastic but effective solution is concomitant ischial urethrotomy with indwelling catheter. After healing of the distal urethra, the ischial urethra is allowed to heal spontaneously.

Spiral and ventral deviations of the penis prevent intromission and are observed during mating. Deviations usually appear in 3- to 4-year-old bulls, after a period of satisfactory service. Both types occur as defects of the penile apical ligament. Spiral deviations may be repaired by surgically implanting a 2×12 to 2×15 cm homologous graft of fascia lata between the tunica albuginea and apical ligament through a midline incision on the dorsum of the penis. Repair of ventral deviations may be attempted with the same procedure, with reduced success.

Rupture of the corpus cavernosum penis (hematoma) is a common and serious breeding accident. It is often caused by innately vigorous sexual behavior and is characterized by circumscribed symmetric swelling surrounding the penis just cranial to the neck of the scrotum. The prepuce is usually dark purple from extravasated blood and will often be prolapsed. The injury will heal spontaneously in many cases, when accompanied by systemic antibiotics and 60 days of rest from sexual activity. However, surgical closure of the rent in the tunica albuginea provides less risk of recurrence and of some serious sequelae.

Surgery performed 1 to 2 days after injury allows easier repair. Under general anesthesia or deep sedation in right lateral recumbency with aseptic conditions, an incision of the cranioventral skin is made over the lateral aspect of the bulge of the hematoma. Subcutaneous tissue incision exposes the blood clot, which is removed. The affected portion of the penis is exposed and pulled through the incision in the skin. Multiple layers of peripenile elastic tissue are incised longitudinally and laterally to the penis to expose the tunica albuginea. The usually transverse rent will be found predictably at the dorsal aspect of the distal bend of the sigmoid flexure. Distraction of the torn edges may be 2 cm. The frayed edges are excised and sutured with a boot lace pattern using No. 1 polyglycolic acid suture. The multiple elastic layers are closed with a single simple continuous suture of 3–0 gut. Loose clots in the cavity are rinsed free with sterile saline at 37°C. The wall of the hematoma is sutured with 1–0 gut without closing space, and then the skin incision is closed. Maximal healing requires 60 days of rest from sexual activity.

Because of the violence of the injury and frequent sequelae, the prognosis for rupture of the tunica albuginea is guarded, whether conservatively or surgically managed. Sequelae are peripenile adhesion, hematogenous abscess, disruption of the sensory nerve supply, and vascular shunts at the rupture site. These shunts that cause erection failure may be repaired by the technique for fresh rupture.

Failure of erection may arise from post-hematomal shunts or congenital and uncorrectable multiple shunts in the free portion of the penis. Both types of shunts may be confirmed by serial contrast radiography of the corpus cavernosum. Obstructive cavernositis, intracorporeal thrombosis, and dystrophic calcification are conditions that also cause erection failure. All are difficult to diagnose during life and are irreparable.

Preputial injuries, usually sustained in service, appear most frequently in *Bos indices* breeds and their crossbreeds, particularly in those bulls with excessively pendulous sheaths, long prepuces, and wide preputial orifices. Initial injury is one of contusion and/or laceration. Mild injuries may require little more than 2 weeks of rest but may become major wounds if the animals are left in service, thus extending breeding time loss as much as 2 months or more with possible complete loss of breeding use. The typical progression of the condition is traumatic edema, preputial prolapse, increased edema, attempted coitus, and laceration (splitting), usually on the ventrum of the prepuce.

Care of prolapse with or without laceration involves cleansing, applying of a lanolin-based protectant ointment, and bandaging with stockinette and adhesive elastic tape. Latex rubber tubing inserted into the preputial lumen and incorporated into the bandage provides urine drainage. The bandage protects the injury, reduces edema, and should be changed every 3 days or as needed. When reduction of edema allows reversion of the prepuce, bandaging without stockinette continues until the prepuce remains in place spontaneously.

If the prepuce is too long for containment or if a granulating deep laceration prevents the return to normal function, circumcision is indicated. One technique involves (1) full extension of the penis and prepuce, which may require cutting across stenotic areas of prepuce, (2) applying a latex rubber tourniquet at the preputial orifice, (3) resecting sufficient prepuce between proximal and distal annular incisions to reduce excessive length, (4) removing fibrotic tissue but still allowing full penile extension, (5) ligating all severed vessels, (6) removing the tourniquet and completing hemostasis, and (7) suturing superficial elastic tissue and skin with simple, interrupted stitches using 1–0 gut. A bandage similar to that described for simple prolapse is applied. The bandage should be removed in 3 days and the stitches removed in 10 days. Bulls usually can return to service in 60 days.

Retropreputial abscesses result from deep preputial laceration and immediate, complete retraction of the prepuce. The condition is common in *Bos taurus* breeds. Without prolapse, the injury may not be discovered until function is severely compromised by formation of peripenile adhesions. Abscesses should be drained through the original laceration in the prepuce and never through the skin of the sheath. The prognosis is poor, but spontaneous recoveries occur in 60 to 90 days in a small proportion of affected bulls. Surgical excision of peripenile adhesions has been unrewarding.

Bulls regularly serving the artificial vagina occasionally sustain an avulsion of the prepuce from its attachment to the free portion of the penis. The prepuce is severely distracted and, contrary to the usual contraindication for suturing fresh but contaminated preputial wounds in range bulls, these avulsions should be repaired immediately.

BOAR

Penile congenital defects in the boar include persistent frenulum, which may be managed surgically as in the bull. Erection failure may be caused by heritable micropenis and cavernosal venous shunts that are irreparable.

Failure of penile extension may also be caused by infrequent or habitual "balling" in which the penis is inserted in the preputial diverticulum. Young boars may be corrected by forcing dismounting when the action is noted. Repeated mounting often results in correct extension. If the practice persists, culling should be considered in that there is some evidence of heritability. Surgical extirpation of the diverticulum is discouraged.

Lacerations of the distal portion of the penis are common in boars and usually result from biting females or other boars during breeding activity. Lacerations heal with 2 weeks of rest from sexual activity and no treatment. Severe wounds may require daily application of topical antibiotic ointments or, rarely, surgical closure. Occasionally cavernosal or urethral fistula may follow severe lacerations. Preputial injuries are rare in boars.

RAM AND BUCK

Penile and preputial injuries are quite rare in rams and bucks and usually can be managed similarly to those in bulls. Occasionally the urethral process may be grossly traumatized or blocked with urinary calculi. Amputation of the process is simple and appears to have no suppressant effect on fertility.

Posthitis (pizzle rot) is a chronic necrotizing disease of the preputial orifice. Considered to be caused by the interaction of *Corynebacterium renale* infection and the high (4 per cent) urinary urea content of a high protein diet and reduced water intake, the condition is a serious cause of impotence. Early in the course of the disease, the orifice is ulcerated and exudes thick purulent debris. The condition may progress to fill the entire preputial cavity with exudate and necrotic tissue and occlude the prepuce. Early-stage disease may respond to thorough cleansing and regular application of penicillin ointment. Systemic treatment is ineffective.

BIBLIOGRAPHY

Hudson RS: Diagnosis of disturbances of mating ability in bulls. Auburn Vet 37:81–84, 1981.
Hudson RS: Diseases of the penis and prepuce: *In* Howard JL (ed): Current Veterinary Therapy 2: Food Animal Practice. Philadelphia, WB Saunders, 1986.

Dairy Herd Reproductive Efficiency

LOUIS F. ARCHBALD, DVM, PhD, MS, Diplomate, ACT

Dairy herd reproductive efficiency is usually defined in terms of a calving interval of less than 13 months for 90 per cent of the herd, with an annual herd culling rate of less than 6 per cent. Infertility is defined as failure to conceive following a reasonable number of services (e.g., three to four artificial insemination services) or failure to conceive within a reasonable period of time after calving (e.g., 130 to 140 days post partum) or both.

The author sincerely appreciates permission to use some of the information on this topic previously presented in the second edition of this book by Edward T. Henry, DVM, in the preparation of the current article.

FACTORS AFFECTING REPRODUCTIVE EFFICIENCY

Two most important factors that affect reproductive efficiency of a dairy herd are estrus detection rate and breeding or conception efficiency. This statement presupposes that artificial insemination is the major means of conception and calving is mainly year round.

Estrus Detection Efficiency

Estrus detection efficiency is defined as the percentage of eligible cows that are actually seen or detected in estrus. A detection rate of 70 to 80 per cent should be the goal of every manager of a dairy herd if reproductive efficiency is to be achieved. The time of day and quality of the time spent in heat detection are of critical importance. Early morning and late evening (when combined) are the two periods in a 24-hour day that yield a high percentage of detected estrus.

A major factor that contributes to the efficiency with which cows are detected in estrus is the human. Under the conditions of artificial insemination, a human assumes the responsibility of the bull for detecting cows in estrus. Research has shown that the human is a poor substitute for the bull in this regard.

Previous research has shown that the interval from calving to first ovulation averages about 3 weeks (usually unaccompanied by detectable estrus), while the first detected estrus is usually about 5 weeks post partum. It is generally assumed that complaints by dairy managers that cows are not cyclic most likely represent inadequate estrus detection rather than true anestrus. However, care should be taken with this assumption, especially during the hot summer months when cows may not readily exhibit signs of estrus and when they do the length of the estrus period may be shortened. Rectal palpation of the ovaries for the presence of a corpus luteum, determination of milk or plasma progesterone, or both can be used to determine whether cows are actually cyclic and are being missed in estrus.

Some of the factors that can be used to evaluate estrus detection efficiency are listed in Table 1.

The 24-day estrus detection rate is an excellent method to use. It can easily be implemented by the dairy manager to determine how efficiently estrus periods are being detected. Cows must achieve several criteria before they can be evaluated using this method. First, they should be at least 30 days post partum; second, they should be free of any pathologic conditions (e.g., cystic follicles, pyometra); and third, they should not be pregnant. It should be remembered that pregnancy is a genuine reason for cows to experience anestrus.

Using this method, a 24-day period is considered. A list of cows most likely to exhibit estrus within the next 24 days is obtained. At the end of this period, the number of cows observed in estrus is divided by the total number of cows eligible to cycle. For example, if there were 50 eligible cows and only 15 were observed in estrus during the 24-day period,

Table 1. PARAMETERS USED TO EVALUATE HEAT DETECTION EFFICIENCY

Parameter	Value
Days (d) in milk at first breeding	60–65 days
24-Day detection rate	80–85%
% Cows pregnant at examination	80–85%
% Cows detected in estrus by 60 d post partum	>85%
% Cows artificially inseminated by 90 days post partum	>90%

Value listed is the desired goal for that parameter.

then estrus detection efficiency is 30 per cent. A positive characteristic of this method is that it takes only 24 days to determine the degree of estrus detection efficiency by the dairy manager.

The per cent cows pregnant at pregnancy examination is also a very good parameter for evaluating estrus detection efficiency. It can be easily calculated at the end of the routine reproductive visit. In addition, it provides some information about conception rates in the herd. However, its primary value lies in its ability to determine estrus detection efficiency.

Conception Rate

Conception rate can be directly affected by the following factors: accuracy of estrus detection, competency of the inseminator, fertility of the herd (female), and fertility of the semen sample (bull).

Accuracy of Estrus Detection

The accuracy of estrus detection is defined as the percentage of cows exhibiting true physiologic estrus. Using natural service, the bull readily detects estrus. However, with artificial insemination the accuracy of estrus detection is vitally important, since insemination of cows not in estrus, or at the wrong time during estrus, usually results in failure of conception. Recent research using milk progesterone concentrations to accurately time insemination has shown that many cows are inseminated when not in estrus. In fact, determination of milk progesterone concentrations in cows suspected of being in estrus may be a valuable adjunct to improving accuracy of estrus detection.

Competency of the Inseminator

The competency of the inseminator can be considered to be the most significant factor contributing to conception efficiency. It has been demonstrated that conception rates can vary as much as 22 per cent among artificial insemination technicians. The technician's major responsibilities are related to the proper handling of the semen from the time of removal from the tank to correct placement in the uterus of the cow. Other considerations include temperature fluctuations and proper handling of the straw, ampule, and inseminating gun. Of the factors listed in Table 2, competency of the inseminator is considered to be the most important.

Fertility of the Herd (Female)

A major factor in fertility of the herd is to have as many cows as possible cycling and free of reproductive disease when they enter the breeding program. Of extreme value is the existence of a routine reproductive program in the herd to identify and correct any potential and actual reproductive problems. In addition to being free of pathologic conditions (e.g., cystic follicles, pyometra etc.), early resumption of cyclic activity within the first 30 days post partum has been shown to have a significant effect on fertility. Recent research has shown that the use of exogenous GnRH is beneficial in establishing cyclicity in cows experiencing abnormal postpartum ovarian function within the first 30 days post partum.

Fertility of the Semen Sample (Bull)

Fertility of the semen sample has been shown to have a significant effect on conception rates. It should not be considered dogma that each straw or ampule of semen from different bulls has the same fertility. Previous research has demonstrated that the first service conception rate can vary as much as 36 per cent among bulls used in artificial insemination (range 34 to 70 per cent).

Some of the factors commonly used to evaluate conception rates are listed in Table 3.

MONITORING INFERTILITY IN THE HERD

There are a number of parameters that can be used to determine if the herd is experiencing an undue amount of infertility. These parameters are listed in Table 4.

Of the parameters listed in Table 4, days open, days in milk, calving interval, and herd reproductive status index are the more common and traditional ones used to assess reproductive performance. Calving interval is a good one, but in addition to being a historical parameter, its derivation requires two parturitions. Similar to days open, calving interval only considers cows that conceived.

Herd reproductive status index is a good measure of the influence open cows impose on meeting the goals of reproductive efficiency. It accounts for all cows that go beyond a specified period of time (e.g., 100 or 120 days post partum) and have not conceived. As long as this number stays high (>65 days), then probably there are only a few cows that are outside the reproductive goals relative to days open.

Since in many dairies calving is done on a year-round basis, calculating the percentage of herd diagnosed pregnant per

Table 2. FACTORS AFFECTING CONCEPTION PERFORMANCE

Factors	Value
Inseminators	22%
Bulls	15%
Cystic follicles	8%
Retained placenta	12%
Age of cow	0
Uterine infections	8%

Source: Darlington RL: Research summary of factors affecting conception to first service in dairy cows: III. Clinical factors—cystic ovaries, retained placenta, uterine infections and milk fever. Proceedings of the annual meeting of the Society for Theriogenology, Spokane, WA, 1981.

Table 3. PARAMETERS USED TO EVALUATE CONCEPTION RATE

Parameters	Value
First-service conception rate	50–55%
Services per conception	1.5–1.8
% Cows pregnant by three or less services	85–88%
% Cows returning for four or more services	<15%

Value listed is the desired goal for that parameter.

Table 4. PARAMETERS USED TO DETERMINE INFERTILITY IN THE HERD

Parameter	Value
Calving interval	12–12.7 months
Days open	95–105 days
Days in milk (for herd)	160–175 days
Herd reproductive status index	>65
% of herd diagnosed pregnant per month	8–9%
% Cows open more than 150 days	<10%
% Annual culling for infertility	<6%

Value listed is the desired goal for that parameter.

Table 5. PARAMETERS USED TO EVALUATE REPRODUCTIVE FAILURES

Parameter	Value
% Cows open more than 150 days	<10%
% Cows returning for fourth or more artificial insemination	<15%
% Annual culling for infertility	<6%
Herd reproductive status index	>65

Value listed is the desired goal for that parameter.

month is a useful tool. To maintain an equal number of lactating cows, the rate of calving should equal the rate of drying off and should include a small percentage for culling. This means that there should be equal numbers of new pregnancies per month. In other words, 8 to 9 per cent of the cows in the herd should become pregnant every month.

Many of the parameters listed earlier can be used to evaluate the performance of cows that conceived and eventually calved. However, other parameters should be used to evaluate reproductive failures in the herd (Table 5). It should be mentioned that all dairy herds will experience some degree of infertility. However, when the actual figures exceed the ones listed in Table 5, investigation into the possible causes should be performed.

BIBLIOGRAPHY

Archbald LF, Norman SN, Bliss EL, et al: Incidence and treatment of abnormal postpartum ovarian function in dairy cows. Theriogenology 34:283, 1990.

Barr HL: Influence of estrus detection on days open in dairy herds. J Dairy Sci 58:246, 1975.

Beerwinkle LG: Heat detection programs and techniques. Proceedings of the National Association of Animal Breeders, Eighth Conference on Artificial Insemination of Beef Cattle, Denver, CO, 1974.

Darlington RL: Research summary of factors affecting conception to first service in dairy cows: III. Clinical factors—cystic ovaries, retained placenta, uterine infections and milk fever. Proceedings of the annual meeting of the Society for Theriogenology, Spokane, WA, 1981.

Davidson JN, Farver TB: Conception rates of Holstein bulls for artificial insemination on a California dairy. J Dairy Sci 63:621, 1980.

Henry ET: Dairy herd reproductive efficiency. In Howard JL (ed): Current Veterinary Therapy 2: Food Animal Practice, p 803. Philadelphia, WB Saunders, 1986.

King GJ, Hurnik JF, Robertson HA: Ovarian function and estrus in dairy cows during early lactation. J Anim Sci 42:688, 1976.

Senger PL, Hillers JK, Mitchell JR, et al: Research summary of factors affecting conception to first service in dairy cows: I. Bulls, inseminators and semen quality. Proceedings of the annual meeting of the Society for Theriogenology, Spokane, WA, 1981.

Stevenson JS, Call EP: Influence of early estrus, ovulation and insemination on fertility in postpartum Holstein cows. Theriogenology 19:367, 1983.

Thatcher WW, Wilcox CJ: Postpartum estrus as an indicator of reproductive status in the dairy cow. J Dairy Sci 56:608, 1973.

Evaluation of Reproductive Efficiency in Beef Cattle Herds

W. DUANE MICKELSEN, DVM, MS, Diplomate, ACT

STEVEN E. WIKSE, DVM, Diplomate, ACVP

ECONOMICS AND GOALS

Unlike the managers of dairy herds, the beef cattle producers derive most of their income from calves born into the herd, making fertility the most important trait of beef cattle. Fertility has been shown to be five times more important than the next important disease condition in cattle, and in fact fertility was five times more important than growth rate and ten times more important than carcass quality.

Although there were 37 million beef cows of reproductive age in the United States in 1983, only 27.4 million calves (74 per cent) were weaned. Data from Montana research station beef herds indicate that net calf crops are approximately 71 per cent. Cows not pregnant at the end of the breeding season accounted for 17.4 per cent of the losses, which together with prenatal deaths (6.4 per cent), death from birth to weaning (2.9 per cent), and fetal deaths (2.3 per cent) reduced the potential net calf crop by 29 per cent. In a Washington study, using 8,184 beef cows and heifers that had been on a routine reproductive herd health program for at least 10 years, 10 per cent were not pregnant.

If calves from 75 per cent of cows exposed to bulls are weaned at 500 lbs, the average weaning weight is 375 lbs. However, if 95 per cent of the cows wean a calf, the average weaning weight is 475 lbs. For 100 cows, this amounts to about $8,500 at present market prices.

The necessary selling price per 100-lb calf weight to break even with various calf crops (at weaning) and the average weaning weights, assuming an annual cow cost of $300, are shown in Table 1. Ideally, cows should wean calves that weigh 50 to 60 per cent of the dams' weight. To do this calves must be born early in the calving season.

The reproductive goals of a well-managed beef ranch should be a 63-day breeding season, more than 95 per cent of cows exposed to bulls pregnant at pregnancy examinations, less than 2 per cent abortion losses in cows diagnosed pregnant, and delivery of a live, vigorous calf by at least 93 per cent of cows exposed to bulls. Impaired fertility is present when these goals are not met. In the United States, beef cattle producers achieved 10 to 30 per cent less than the above objectives.

Veterinary practitioners can influence the reproductive efficiency of beef herds by expanding their activities beyond the traditional services of pregnancy diagnosis and evaluation of bull semen. This can be done by a more total herd production management involvement that encompasses identification and correction of management and nutritional deficiencies. Practitioners must be familiar with the causes of, and methods to increase, reproductive efficiency.

Most herd disease and production problems are caused by many factors, and many are primarily determined by management practices and reproductive efficiency.

HERD FERTILITY EVALUATION

Basic information recorded at the fertility examination should be the cow's identification number, age, breed, body condition score, and estimated days pregnant or, if nonpregnant, its ovarian and uterine findings. Additional data are breeding pasture and bull or bull battery identification. At this

Table 1. NECESSARY SELLING PRICE PER HUNDREDWEIGHT TO BREAK EVEN WITH VARIOUS PER CENT CALF CROPS AND AVERAGE WEANING WEIGHTS ASSUMING AN ANNUAL COW COST OF $300

Calf Crop (weaned)	Average Weaning Weights (lb)				
	350	*400*	*450*	*500*	*550*
100	85.72	75.00	66.67	60.00	54.55
90	95.24	83.32	74.08	66.67	60.60
85	101.00	88.24	78.45	70.59	62.24
80	107.15	93.76	83.32	75.00	68.19
70	122.44	107.15	95.24	85.76	77.92

time, records of calving dates, breeding season length, culling programs, age groups, incidence of dystocia, vaccination history, and breed records should be obtained and recorded (Fig. 1).

The length of the breeding season greatly influences herd reproductive performance. Sixty-three days is recommended for cow herds. Longer breeding seasons (up to 5 months) are management deficiencies that result in a lack of selection for reproductive efficiency. Thirteen- to 15-month-old heifers should be mated for 42 days and rebreeding should begin 2 to 3 weeks prior to the cow herds. These practices will ensure earlier rebreeding in future seasons. Although shortening the breeding season may result in cash flow problems the first year, the overall results of shortening the breeding season indicate that net calf crop, actual weaning weight, and total weight of calf weaned per cow all increase.

A culling program that removes from the herd cows that are nonpregnant or that will calve late has proven to increase herd fertility through selection pressure for reproductive efficiency.

The age of the animals is important, since the 4- to 9-year-old group has a higher pregnancy rate than do heifers, first-lactation cows, and cows older than 9 years of age (Table 2). This is probably related to energy deficiencies in these age groups, since body condition scores average 3.5 (on a scale of 1–9, with 9 being very fat) in nonpregnant cows and heifers and 4.5 in pregnant cows at the pregnancy examination. Body condition scores are directly related to the nutritional status of the herd and should be obtained on all cows examined for infertility. Cows in poor body condition have a delayed return to estrus compared with cows in good body condition. As body condition scores decrease, there is a delay in days to rebreeding.

The type of pasture, or feed, the cattle are on from calving to breeding is important. Cows should eat quality forage that is high in energy and protein. Inadequate energy intake affects primarily heifers and first-calf cows because they are still growing. Their growth, coupled with the energy requirements of gestation and lactation, increase their need for energy sources. Inadequate nutrition can cause a negative energy

Herd owner _____ Date _____

1. ID system used _____
2. Birth dates and weights recorded? (Y,N)
3. Herd vaccination history: *Campylobacter, Leptospira, Trichomonas,* infections bovine rhinotracheitis, BVD, pinkeye
4. Was crossbreeding used? (Y,N)
5. Breeding season length _____ Date bull in _____; Out _____
6. Bulls semen tested? (Y,N); Only new bulls (Y,N)
7. Total number bulls used in herd _____
8. Total cows exposed to bulls _____ Cow/bull ratio: _____
   _____ <18 mo _____ 3 yr _____ 4—9 yr _____ >9 yr
9. Cows added/sold between breeding and calving: _____
   a. Were these animals serologically screened? (Y,N)
   b. For which diseases?
10. Yearling heifers bred prior to cows? (Y,N)
11. Calves born alive _____
12. Calves born first 3 weeks _____; second 3 weeks _____; third 3 weeks _____; fourth 3 weeks _____
13. Calves died first 5 days post calving _____
14. Percentage dystocia: heifers _____ cows _____
15. Calves lost birth to weaning _____
16. Calves weaned _____; weighed? (Y,N)
17. Cows died in past year _____
18. Calving % = $\dfrac{\text{calves born alive}}{\text{cows pregnant}}$
19. Net calf crop = $\dfrac{\text{number of calves weaned}}{\text{number cows exposed}}$
20. Have internal and external parasite control procedures been used? (Y,N) Date _____
21. Pregnancy status: Number tested _____ Number pregnant _____ Number open _____
    Number open _____ <18 mo _____ 3 yr _____ 4—9 yr _____ >9 yr _____
    % open _____ <18 mo _____ 3 yr _____ 4—9 yr _____ >9 yr _____
    Body condition score of herd: Thin (1–3) _____ Moderate (4–6) _____ Fleshy (7–9) _____
22. Number with body condition score <4 _____
23. Number culled for the following reasons:
    open _____ teeth _____ feet _____ eyes _____ udder _____
24. Results of female reproductive examinations:
    a. Number of pregnant cows and heifers at various stages of gestation
       1) 30–60 days _____
       2) 60–90 days _____
       3) 90–120 days _____
       4) 120–150 days _____
       5) >150 days _____
    b. Nonpregnant cows status
       1) LSRSUN (noncycling): left and right ovaries static; uterus normal
       2) LCL3RSUN (cycling nonpregnant): left ovary has corpus luteum greater than 20 mm; right ovary static; uterus normal
       3) LSRCL3 U pyometra (trichomoniasis): left ovary static; right ovary has corpus luteum greater than 20 mm; pyometra present

Figure 1. Form for obtaining a herd fertility evaluation. (From Mickelson WD: Vet Med 85:418–427, 1990.)

Table 2. BREAKDOWN OF NONPREGNANT HEIFERS AND COWS BY AGE GROUP

	Group 1 (18–24 mo)	Group 2 (30–36 mo)	Group 3 (4–9 yr)	Group 4 (>9 yr)
Noncycling, nonpregnant	189 (18.2%)	169 (14.8%)	27 (0.4%)	70 (15.0%)
Cycling, nonpregnant	28 (2.7%)	134 (11.7%)	124 (2.2%)	29 (6.2%)
Total in group	1035	1137	5548	464

Source: Mickelsen WD, et al: Survey of the prevalence and types of infertility in beef cows and heifers. J Am Vet Med Assoc 189:51–54, 1986.

balance after calving, inhibiting estrus and lowering conception rates.

A live calf, born unassisted, should be of paramount importance to the cow-calf producer. The incidence of dystocia should be determined since conception rates for all cows experiencing calving problems is reduced by 15.9 per cent. Since the two main causes of dystocia are calf birth weight and dam pelvic area, calving ease bulls should be used and heifers should be selected for large pelvic areas. Prolonged stage 2 of parturition and poor sanitation increase time to rebreeding and reduce conception rates, but early assistance in calf delivery and proper sanitation procedures have been shown to enhance subsequent conception.

It is important to find out if bulls used are of different ages and breeds in the same breeding pasture. Studies have shown that the dominant bull, or bulls, in a group, sire 60 to 100 per cent of the calves. Pregnancy rates in a herd could be severely reduced if an older, dominant bull became infertile from illness or injury. The bulls should be tested for fertility prior to the breeding season since approximately 20 per cent of all bulls of the beef breeds are not suitable for breeding programs.

The ratio of bulls to cows has an influence on herd fertility. Optimal ratios vary with the size and geography of the breeding area. In the western United States and Canada, one bull per 20 cows is often used in rough terrains, but in open range stocking rates of one bull per 30 to 50 cows are effective if semen quality, libido, and mating ability are not impaired.

The effect of crossbreeding on reproductive efficiency has been well documented. Weaning weight per cow exposed to breeding increased from the combined efforts of heterosis on survival and growth of calves and by increased reproduction and milk production on first-generation cross (F_1) cows. In the western United States the Hereford × Angus cow consistently produces more pounds of calf and becomes pregnant earlier the next breeding season than purebred cattle of either breed.

EXAMINATION OF THE COW

Fifty to 100 per cent of nonpregnant cows and 5 to 10 per cent of pregnant cows should be routinely examined on a fertility investigation if the herd is not on a routine herd health program. Examination per rectum of the internal genitalia of nonpregnant animals may reveal answers to the etiology of infertility. The ovaries of noncycling females measure less than $2 \times 0.5 \times 0.5$ cm in length, height, and width, respectively, and contain no functional structures. The uterus is small, with uniform thinning of the walls. The primary cause of anestrus is energy deficiency. In cyclic animals, one ovary will usually contain a corpus luteum, which causes a doubling or tripling of the size of the ovary compared with the opposite ovary. Other palpable characteristics of the uterus include tone and edema, depending on the number of days examined post estrus.

If the uterus feels normal on palpation and there is a corpus luteum on the ovary, the cows are experiencing normal estrous cycles and bull problems, dystocia, or infectious diseases such as trichomoniasis and campylobacteriosis should be suspected.

Trichomoniasis can be substantiated by isolation of the organism. When introduced into a susceptible herd, trichomoniasis and campylobacteriosis can result in pregnancy rates as low as 50 to 60 per cent. Chronically infected herds are likely to exhibit suboptimal fertility.

Projected calving dates from pregnancy examinations obtained 35 days or more after the breeding season have the potential to offer a systematic herd evaluation if breeding records are not available. By estimating the stages of pregnancy by rectal palpation, an estimate can be made on cyclic activity and conception during the previous breeding season. Projected calving dates also allow time for nutritional or other management decisions to be made before the next breeding season.

Palpation for pregnancy with projected calving dates is most accurate the first 120 days of gestation. After that time period, there will be individual palpation variances. The use of both placentomes and fetal size may improve accuracy of estimation in later stages of gestation.

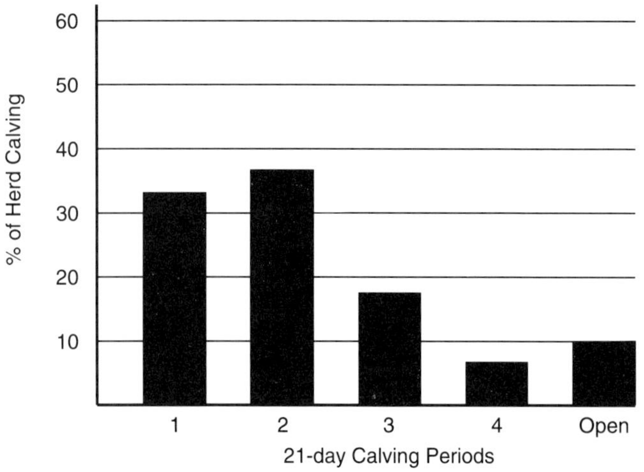

Figure 2. Calving percentage for cows in a 200-herd before the causes of infertility were diagnosed. (From Mickelsen WD: A beef herd infertility investigation: case report. Proceedings of the Annual Meeting of the Society for Theriogenology, Hastings, NB, 1989, pp 115–120.)

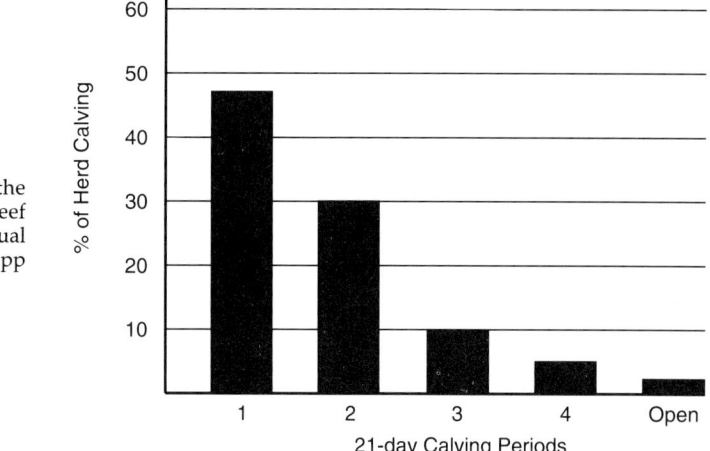

Figure 3. Calving percentage for the herd in Figure 2 after the causes of infertility were corrected. (From Mickelsen WD: A beef herd infertility investigation: case report. Proceedings of the Annual Meeting of the Society for Theriogenology, Hastings, NB, 1989, pp 115–120.)

EVALUATING REPRODUCTIVE MANAGEMENT

The goal is that 70 per cent of cows should calve in the first 21-day period. Herds under excellent management calve up to 75 per cent of the cows during the first 21-day period and have a 95 per cent pregnancy rate in a 63-day breeding season. Failure to reach these goals results in decreased weaning weights per cows exposed for breeding. Too few cows in estrus during the first 21 days of the breeding season and low first-service conception rates directly affect weaning weights and pregnancy rates. Assuming the calf will gain 1.5 to 2 lbs/day from birth to weaning results in a weaned calf that will weigh 30 to 40 pounds less for every 21-day cycle delay in becoming pregnant.

The total breeding percentage reflects the reproductive performance of the herd. Further grouping of information to analyze breeding efficiency by cow age groups, by body condition scores, and by pasture or bull battery is necessary. The second criterion is the period breeding percentage, which is based on pregnancy rates, or calving dates, by 21-day intervals throughout the breeding season. The primary emphasis should be placed on factors that influence the first 21-day breeding interval, primarily the percentage of cows with normal cycles at the start of the breeding season. Cow age, postpartum interval, and cow body condition affect this percentage.

The calving percentage can be analyzed by dividing the number of calves born alive by the number of cows pregnant. Ideally this figure should be 98 per cent or greater in herds that have been examined for pregnancy at least 35 days after the breeding program ends. The net calf crop is calculated by dividing the number of calves weaned by the number of cows exposed to bulls. The net calf crop should be greater than 90 per cent.

From these reproductive indices plus calculating the calving patterns into 21-day periods for the whole herd, heifers, first-lactation heifers, 4- to 9-year old cows, and older cows, reproductive patterns and indices (Figs. 2 and 3) can then aid in diagnosing the causes of impaired fertility. In addition, female genital examinations may further confirm whether animals are cyclic and nonpregnant, in which case bull problems, dystocia, trichomoniasis, or campylobacteriosis may be suspected. If the animals are not cyclic, nutritional deficiencies (primarily low energy) are usually at fault.

The mean length of the interval between parturition and conception and the percentage of calves weaned relative to the number of cows or heifers exposed for breeding are general measures of reproductive performance.

In most herds there may be multifactoral causes contributing to the herd problem, which should then be listed, followed by recommendations for their alteration or elimination by managerial changes. Many recommendations are possible, such as increasing energy intake during the last trimester of gestation, placement of heifers and first-lactation heifers into separate feeding groups, inclusion of new vaccines in the immunization schedule, routine pregnancy determination, and breeding soundness evaluation of bulls. The degree of expected improvement in production and cost-effectiveness should also be discussed. Improved production record-keeping may be advised to document the actual success and economic outcome of management changes.

These herd management changes can be conveyed to the producer either verbally or in writing. Written reports can be accumulated from year to year and will aid in the evaluation of the overall performance of the reproductive program. Computerized programs offer the veterinarian even better evaluation of the herd's management programs.

BIBLIOGRAPHY

Bellows RA, Patterson DJ, Burfening PJ, et al: Occurrence of neonatal and postnatal mortality in range beef cattle: II. Factors contributing to calf death. Theriogenology 28:573–586, 1987.

Patterson DJ, Bellows RA, Burfening PJ, et al: Occurrence of neonatal and postnatal mortality in beef cattle: I. Calf loss incidence from birth to weaning, backward and breech presentations and effects of calf loss on subsequent pregnancy rate of dams. Theriogenology 28:557–571, 1987.

Spire MF: Breeding season evaluation of beef herds. In Howard JL (ed): Current Veterinary Therapy 2: Food Animal Practice, pp 808–811. Philadelphia, WB Saunders, 1986.

Management of Reproduction of Sheep and Goats

RANDALL S. OTT, DVM, MS, DIPLOMATE, ACT

Effective management of reproduction of sheep and goats is essential to the profitability of livestock enterprises using these species. Cost-effective production of sheep and goats is accomplished with a population viewpoint. Initial and contin-

---

Use of some treatment regimens described in this article lack official regulatory approval. Refer to label instructions for proper usage.

ual selection of proper genetics, combined with judicious culling, is the backbone of successful flock management.

Selection of a breed, or crossbreed, that is the best match for available environmental, nutritional, and managerial resources is the important first step. Selective preference should be given to offspring of those animals that perform well without requiring therapy or costly management practices. Synchronization of estrus, artificial insemination, and embryo transfer have the potential for greatly accelerating genetic change. Intensive mating practices, feeding regimens, and vaccination programs must be continually reviewed to ensure that the benefits derived are greater than the costs incurred.

The most important tool for increasing the reproductive capacity of the flock is the selection of highly fertile male animals. Recognition of the correlation between male and female fertility, combined with the magnification of the male animal's contribution to the flock's gene pool (which is substantial even in natural mating systems), underscores the necessity of selective preference for highly fertile rams and bucks. The most important trait of breeding rams and bucks is large scrotal circumference for age. This provides an indirect measurement of early puberty and testicular size that is positively related to sperm production. Other important traits include serving capacity (the male animal's ability to inseminate the female animal) and testicular health.

As a service for clients, the fitness of individual rams and bucks may be assessed for breeding purposes. Highly fertile animals increase production by causing conception in more ewes and does and by fertilizing more ova per female animal. Breeding soundness examinations can be valuable to help diagnose breeding problems in the flock. Finding that the rams or bucks are satisfactory breeders may "rule out" this parameter and cause one to look for other causes, such as infections, subfertility of ewes or does, or nutritional deficiencies. A breeding soundness examination may confirm a suspected case of male infertility and allow the owner to receive compensation or a replacement animal from the seller if the sire is under warranty. Guidelines for breeding soundness examinations of rams and bucks are available from the Society for Theriogenology.

SHEEP

Most ewes are bred by natural service, although selective or hand mating and artificial insemination are used in certain situations. A suggested mating system for maximum ewe fertility is the use of three rams in each breeding unit. More ewes are detected in estrus when three rams are working together. Breeding pastures should be large enough so that dominant rams do not prevent subordinate rams from mating. A limit of 50 ewes per ram has been recommended. Rams are frequently harnessed with tupping crayons so that ewes that have been served by the ram can be identified. The crayon color should be changed every 14 to 15 days. Introduction of the ram to the breeding flock at the beginning of the breeding season can result in partial synchrony of ovulation in the ewes several days later. Ewes tend to ovulate without showing signs of estrus, whereas does have been reported to exhibit signs of estrus without ovulation at the beginning of the breeding season.

Ewes are serviced two to six times per estrus. When more than one ram is present, multiple sire matings occur. Rams with good libido may mate 20 to 30 times a day. The duration of estrus in the ewe ranges from 10 to 40 hours with an average of about 24 hours. The length of the estrous cycle in sheep is 16 to 17 days. Ewes in estrus actively seek the ram. The need to learn how to find and successfully compete for the ram is believed to account for the poor performance of maiden ewes in pasture mating.

A common practice in sheep breeding is to flush the ewes just before and during the breeding season. Flushing ewes is believed to stimulate more ovulations during the early and late breeding season but is probably of little benefit during the middle of the season. Failure to meet energy requirements during gestation may result in pregnancy toxemia (ketosis) in late gestation in ewes carrying more than one offspring.

Early born ewe lambs can cycle and conceive in their first breeding season. Bringing ewe lambs into production as early as possible decreases maintenance costs before the start of production and increases lifetime production. To accomplish early breeding, lambs must be large enough (65% of mature weight is suggested) and in good condition. Age at puberty varies greatly among breeds. Female offspring from rams selected for large scrotal circumference for age reach puberty at a younger age.

Care should be taken that animals added to the flock come from herds in which owners practice disease control. A program of reproductive disease prevention includes sanitation, early diagnosis of disease, and proper vaccination programs.

Determination of pregnancy in ewe lambs enables the nonpregnant ones to be culled and marketed while they can still command slaughter lamb prices. Real-time ultrasonography has been reported as an accurate and cost-effective method of pregnancy determination in large flocks.

DAIRY GOATS

A common condition that causes infertility in dairy goats is intersex or hermaphroditism. Female hermaphrodites may have a vulva of normal size, but the clitoris is enlarged and the vagina is short or atretic. A penile clitoris, or even an ovotestis, may occur in does that otherwise appear phenotypically female. Hermaphroditism and congenital hypoplasia of the reproductive tract are commonly observed in naturally hornless (polled) goats and are more likely to occur when both parents are polled. Despite phenotypic variation, intersex goats are usually genetic females with a normal female chromosome (60,XX) complement.

Selective or hand mating is the usual practice in dairy goat herds. It is not desirable to allow odorous bucks to run free with milking does. The duration of estrus in does is 32 to 40 hours. Does are usually mated at the onset of estrus and at 12-hour intervals until estrus subsides. In artificial insemination programs, does are inseminated when they first accept mounting by a teaser buck and also 12 hours later.

Whether hand-mating or artificial insemination is practiced, proper detection of estrus is the most important aspect of goat breeding. Does actively seek the presence of the buck when in estrus. Bucks are sometimes descented at the time of dehorning by burning and destroying the odor glands located posteriorly and medially to the horn buds. This is probably a bad practice as does, when given a choice, will usually prefer a scented buck to a deodorized one. As in sheep, the presence of bucks can initiate and even synchronize cyclic activity of does at the beginning of the breeding season. Detection of estrus in does is best accomplished with the use of a buck. An intact buck should be penned in an area where does in estrus can be observed congregating near the pen.

Signs of estrus in does are tail wagging, bleating, and urinating near the buck. There may be swelling of the vulva and a mucous discharge from the vulva. The reaction of the buck to the doe being teased is an indication of estrus in does.

Some does show few signs of estrus other than limited tail wagging and standing for mounting by the buck, and these signs may be present only after teasing. Does will occasionally stand for mounting by other does; however, the level of homosexual activity in goats is low in reproductively normal does.

The length of the estrous cycle of dairy goats is 20 days. Abnormally short (5 to 8 days) estrous cycles may occur in does early in the breeding season. False pregnancy may occur in the doe with a large volume of clear fluid being passed at "parturition."

CONTROL OF REPRODUCTION IN SHEEP AND GOATS

Sheep and goats are considered "short-day breeders" since they initiate reproductive activity in response to decreasing length of daylight. Both are classified as seasonally polyestrous and become anestrus as a result of either pregnancy or the end of the breeding season.

Control of the time of breeding allows control of the time of lambing and kidding and control of milk production in does. Progestagens have been the most widely used agents for ovulation control. Fluorogestrone acetate has been administered by the intravaginal route using an impregnated polyurethane sponge. Vaginal pessaries are left in place for 14 days in ewes and for 21 days in does, and an injection of pregnant mare serum gonadotropin (PMSG) is given at the time of removal. In goats, an 11-day regimen has proved successful when preceded by prostaglandin $F_{2\alpha}$ ($PGF_{2\alpha}$) and PMSG administration on day 9.

$PGF_{2\alpha}$, or its analogues, will induce luteolysis in the cycling ewe or doe during the breeding season. A dose of 2.5 mg has been shown to be adequate for induction of estrus in the doe. In ewes, dosages ranging from 6 to 15 mg have been used for estrus induction. Fertility at the induced estrus has been reported to be normal in goats; however, some workers have reported reduced fertility in sheep.

Control of the time of parturition in sheep and goats enables closer supervision of lambing and kidding during planned periods when labor could be used more efficiently. In one study, dexamethasone (16 mg) administered to ewes on day 143 of gestation resulted in lambs on days 144 to 146, with the largest litters being delivered earliest. The use of exogenous $PGF_{2\alpha}$ has been demonstrated to be the drug of choice to induce parturition in goats. Does receiving either 2.5 mg or 5.0 mg $PGF_{2\alpha}$ on day 144 gave birth to kids within 28 to 57 hours. Retained fetal membranes have not been reported to be associated with induced parturition in ewes or in does.

A number of factors, including light, temperature, and the presence of the male, influence the onset of the breeding season. However, photoperiod is believed to be the most important factor. Control of photoperiod using artificial lighting has received much attention in research with sheep. However, this method does not have much application in either sheep or goats. In the United States, the breeding season for sheep and goats generally extends from August to February. Breed differences and geographic area account for wide variations. Some goat dairies have practiced exposure of breeding animals to total darkness for 17 hours daily after the beginning of June to induce early onset of cyclic activity. There is interest in developing breeds and strains of both species that under proper management might reproduce without seasonal restrictions, thus allowing accelerated lambing in ewes and year-round milk production in does.

BIBLIOGRAPHY

Ott RS: Dairy goat reproduction. Compend Cont Ed Pract Vet 4:S164–S172, 1982.
Ott RS: Management of noninfectious problems in reproduction of the ewe and female goat. *In* Laing JA, Morgan JB, Wagner WC (eds): Fertility and Infertility in Veterinary Practice, 4th ed., pp 113–119. London, Ballière Tindall, 1988.
Ott RS, Memon MA: Sheep and Goat Manual. Society for Theriogenology, Hastings, NB, 1980.

Reproductive Management Problems in Swine

MARTIN L. VAN DER LEEK, BVSc, MS, MRCVS
H. NEIL BECKER, DVM, MS

Profitability in swine production is largely determined by herd feed conversion because feed costs comprise 60 to 75 per cent of total production costs. In farrow-to-finish operations, a large portion of this feed bill goes toward maintenance of the breeding herd. Optimizing breeding herd reproductive efficiency is therefore crucial to maintain or improve herd profitability.

Reproductive problems are rarely caused by a single factor. The investigation of a primary complaint often identifies the need for a more extensive or herd reproductive analysis. Infectious diseases are commonly blamed for reproductive inefficiency but rarely are the primary cause. Veterinarians need to look beyond infectious disease etiologies, examining all aspects of reproductive management. Noninfectious causes have become increasingly important as a result of intensification.

Producers may request veterinary assistance when confronted with a specific reproductive problem, or they may seek regular veterinary input into reproductive management. This article, although concentrating on a problem-oriented approach, provides an outline for the veterinarian interested in assessing herd reproductive performance. The herd approach is also valuable for appreciating the relationship between a specific problem and herd reproductive efficiency.

PROBLEM-ORIENTED APPROACH TO REPRODUCTIVE FAILURE

Primary complaints commonly encountered are outlined in Table 1.

When investigating infertility it is important to ascertain at what time during the reproductive cycle the loss is occurring (prior to or after conception). The distinction between conception rate and farrowing rate is important and will allow the veterinarian to focus the investigation. The result of postconception loss is determined by the time of death of embryos/fetuses and number of viable embryos/fetuses remaining. Implantation occurs 12 days after conception, and four viable embryos are required at this time for maintenance of pregnancy. Two live fetuses are required for a pregnancy to be carried to term. Embryonic death prior to day 12 with fewer than four viable embryos remaining will result in a regular return to estrus. Embryonic death prior to day 12 with at least four embryos surviving will manifest as reduced litter size. Embryonic death between day 12 and day 30 will result in

Table 1. PROBLEM-ORIENTED REPRODUCTIVE PROBLEM SOLVING

Primary Complaint	Factors	Comments and Recommendations
Anestrus (gilts)	Boar exposure	Expose to mature boar daily from 135 to 160 days-of-age, 15 minutes of daily exposure sufficient; fence-line contact often most practical
	Estrus detection	Enhanced by use of a mature boar, 15 minutes of exposure sufficient, continuous exposure not recommended
	Nutrition	Gilts should be fed to achieve goal (see Table 3) without overconditioning
	Housing	Recommended stocking rate = 8 sq ft/pig, keeping group size < 50; adequate ventilation
	Ambient temperature	Extremes adversely affect feed intake; supplemental heat recommended in the winter, cooling in the summer (shade, water cooling system—drip cooling, water back-up; air conditioning—zone cooling)
	Season and photoperiod	16–18 hr of daylight required to induce cycling; expose gilts to normal daylength patterns throughout the year
	Endocrine status	Perform serum progesterone analysis for evidence of luteal activity
	Developmental defects	Hermaphrodites, immature and malformed tracts, cystic ovaries; perform slaughtercheck
	Mycotoxins	Precocious puberty (swollen vulvas common); test feed, perform slaughtercheck
	Breed	Landrace mature earlier
	Induction of estrus	Natural methods: 1. transportation stress (limited to gilts 190 days and older), 2. regrouping, 3. vasectomized boar
		Hormonal treatments: 1. synthetic progesterone, allyl trenbolone (Regumate, Hoescht-Roussel Pharmaceuticals) fed for 14 days, then withdrawn will induce estrus in up to 90% of gilts within 4 to 7 days (not currently available in the US); 2. injectable PMSG/HCG combination (P.G. 600, Intervet America Inc.) will induce estrus in up to 70% of gilts 4 to 7 days after a single injection (available in the US).
Postweaning anestrus	Nutrition	High energy ration (>17 Mcal/sow/day) and sufficient protein (>689 g/sow/day) required throughout lactation (NRC recommendations, 1988)
	Lactation length	Optimum = 18 to 24 days for intensive operations; for each 10-day reduction in lactation there is a potential 1-day increase in the wean-to-estrus interval; may not be flexible due to facility limitations (often shortened because of a lack of farrowing crates and increased because of poor nursery facilities)
	Parity	First litter gilts often delayed
	Season	Common during late summer and early fall (especially in primiparous sows)
	Ambient temperature	See anestrus (gilts)
	Estrus detection	Consider boar exposure, housing (individually housed sows show estrus sooner) and detection procedures
	Metritis	Postmortem, slaughtercheck
Regular returns	Timing of mating	Breed 12 to 24 hr after onset of estrus; "in heat in the morning, breed in the afternoon; in heat in the afternoon, breed the following morning"
	Number of matings/estrus	Two or more matings at 12 to 24-hr intervals
	Type of mating	Homospermic (single boar) vs. heterospermic (multiple boars): use of multiple boars during estrus period improves the chance that the effect of a subfertile boar will be canceled by the subsequent use of a fertile boar; natural vs. artificial insemination comparable results can be achieved with artificial insemination, provided personnel are competent and the technique is correct; hand vs. pen mating: pen mating may yield better results if heat detection is a problem
	Boar usage	≤6 times/week (hand mating), 5 to 7 sows/boar (pen mating: continuous farrowing), 2 to 3 sows/boar (pen mating: batch farrowing)
	Quality of mating	Personnel should manage two or less matings/man at one time (hand mating); observe quality of floor surface
	Infectious disease	Porcine parvovirus, pseudorabies virus
	Endometritis	Postmortem, slaughtercheck
	Ambient temperature	Temperatures in excess of 90°F adversely affect embryonal survival (embryo is most susceptible during first 30 days) and sperm production (delayed effect); provide shade, water cooling system (drip cooling, water back-up), air conditioning (zone cooling)
	Breed	White breeds generally have higher conception rates
Delayed returns	Season	Late summer; usually no change in litter size
	Ambient temperature	Delayed effect of temperature extremes
	Infectious disease	Parvovirus, pseudorabies virus, Lelystad virus (mystery swine disease), leptospirosis (including *L. bratislava*) and eperythrozoonosis; isolation (60–90 days) and serologic testing of new introductions (use of antibiotics during this period not recommended)
	Housing	Provide least stressful environment
	Nutrition	Excess energy intake during early gestation may cause embryonal death
	Mycotoxins	See anestrus (gilts)
Failure-to-farrow (following positive pregnancy check)	Pregnancy diagnosis	Observe for return to estrus at 18 to 24 days; use accurate amplitude depth, or both amplitude depth and Doppler ultrasound devices at 30-day intervals
	Abortion	Failure of personnel to observe abortions
	Mycotoxins	See anestrus (gilts)
	Infectious disease	Reproductive (especially pseudorabies virus) and systemic disease
	Season	Summer to early fall
	Developmental defects	Cervical hypoplasia in gilts
Small litters	Parity	Maximum litter size from parity 3 to 6; breed gilts on second cycle
	Lactation length	For each 1 day decrease in lactation length below 28 days there is a potential 0.1 pig loss
	Infectious disease	Reproductive diseases (particularly PPV and enteroviruses)
	Timing of mating	See regular returns
	Number of matings/estrus	See regular returns
	Type of mating	See regular returns
	Boar usage	See regular returns
	Boar fertility	Semen evaluation or review of records (difficult if heterospermic matings are used)
	Ambient temperature	See anestrus (gilts)

Table 1. PROBLEM-ORIENTED REPRODUCTIVE PROBLEM SOLVING *Continued*

Primary Complaint	Factors	Comments and Recommendations
Abortions	Infectious diseases	Reproductive (particularly leptospirosis, pseudorabies, mystery swine disease [PEARS] and brucellosis) and systemic disease; laboratory submission of fetal and placental tissue, serology of dam
	Mycotoxins	See anestrus (gilts)
	Season	Summer to early fall and winter; likely associated with feed intake
	Nutrition	Underfeeding
	Parity	Common in sows beyond parity 6
Stillbirths	Parity	More common in gilts and sows beyond parity 6
	Calcium deficiency	Feed analysis for both calcium and phosphorus
	Infectious disease	Reproductive disease (leptospirosis, mystery swine disease (PEARS) and pseudorabies virus)
	Prolonged labor	Confirm that personnel know when and how to intervene; overconditioned sow/gilts
	Mycotoxins	See anestrus (gilts)
Mummies	Parity	See stillbirths
	Infectious disease	Parvovirus, pseudorabies virus, Lelystad virus, encephalomyocarditis virus, enteroviruses, influenza
	Mycotoxins	See anestrus (gilts)
Vaginal discharges	Urogenital infection	Sanitation, facility design; vaginal or preputial diverticulum culture may be helpful; medicate breeding herd ration, use an antibiotic preputial wash

Source: Adapted from Thacker BJ: Detection and diagnosis of swine reproductive failure. *In* Morrow DA (ed): Current Therapy in Theriogenology, 2nd ed. Philadelphia, WB Saunders, 1986.

delayed returns to estrus. However, embryonic death after day 30, when skeletal calcification begins, will result in fetal maceration/mummification.

Fetal tissues submitted to a diagnostic laboratory are generally used to demonstrate the presence of infectious agents by isolation in culture, by fluorescent antibody techniques, or by serology. Since fetal immunocompetence occurs at about 70 days, it is preferable to submit younger fetuses to avoid the potential interference of fetal antibodies with isolation or fluorescent antibody tests. Fetal age can readily be determined using the crown–rump length. A fetus having a crown–rump length of more than 17 cm is considered to be older than 70 days.

HERD APPROACH TO EVALUATION OF REPRODUCTIVE PERFORMANCE

When assessing herd reproductive efficiency a number of components need to be evaluated (Table 2). A farm walk may identify obvious problems, but an analysis of the breeding herd records is often required to pinpoint problems. The importance of adequate, accurate records cannot be overstated. The advent of the computer age and the availability of software packages for monitoring herd production has facilitated record-keeping and simplified record analysis. A portable computer, used to illustrate herd trends graphically and to demonstrate the financial impact of an intervention, can be a powerful and persuasive tool. Table 3 lists target values and the interference level (the level that warrants remedial action) for parameters used to monitor reproductive performance.

Although a number of parameters are used to measure overall reproductive performance, *pigs weaned/sow/year* is commonly used. This parameter is the product of the *litters/sow/year* and the *number of pigs weaned/litter*. The factors

Table 2. COMPONENTS OF A HERD REPRODUCTIVE EVALUATION

Herd inspection	Facilities, ventilation, temperature, sanitation, body condition, gilt pen stocking density, vaginal discharges, litter sizes, newborn piglet weights
Record analysis	See Table 3 for parameters of interest and Figure 1 for possible approach
Breeding management	Estrus detection, timing of mating, number of services/mating, boar usage, lactation length, boar exposure, type of mating, quality of mating, vaccination program, pregnancy detection
Herd serology	Pseudorabies virus, brucellosis, leptospirosis, Lelystad virus, encephalomyocarditis virus, porcine parvovirus, eperythrozoonosis; repeat annually*
Postmortem	Sow/boar deaths, fetal and placental tissues, slaughtercheck*
Ration analysis	See Section 4, Dietary Management

*Monitoring pathology in slaughtered stock: guidelines for selecting sample size and interpreting results. Booklet available from U.S. Department of Agriculture, Animal Plant Health Inspection Service, Veterinary Services, NAHMS, 555 South Howes, Fort Collins, CO 80521. Also useful for determining sample sizes for herd serology.

Table 3. TARGETS OF REPRODUCTIVE PERFORMANCE

Parameter	Target	Interference Level	US Values*
Litters/sow/year	2.4	2.0	2.2
Live pigs/litter	10.5	10.0	10.2
Pigs weaned/litter	9.5	9.0	8.7
Farrowing rate	90.0%	80.0	81.2
Wean-to-service	7.0 days	9.0	9.7
Regular returns	4.0%	12.0	9.2†
Delayed returns	1.0%	2.5	
Litters < 8 pigs	10.0%		
Abortions	1.0%	2.5	
Stillbirths	5.0%	8.0	
Mummies	0.5%	1.0	
Sexual maturity	First estrus at 5 to 8 months (aver. = 7), 220 lbs		
Sow inventory	Weekly farrowings × 26		
Gilt inventory	Matings/week × 1.2 to 1.5 × weeks in gilt pool (factor depends on % of selected gilts eventually mated)		
Boar inventory	Female inventory ÷ 20		
	or		
	desired No. matings/service × crates-to-fill		
	farrowing rate × desired No. matings/boar/time		
Number bred/week	Expected farrowings ÷ farrowing rate		
Sows	80–85% of total breedings		
Gilts	15–20% of total breedings		

*Data from Stein TE: Interpreting production data from swine breeding herds. Agri-Practice 11:30–34, 1990.
†Per cent of repeat services.

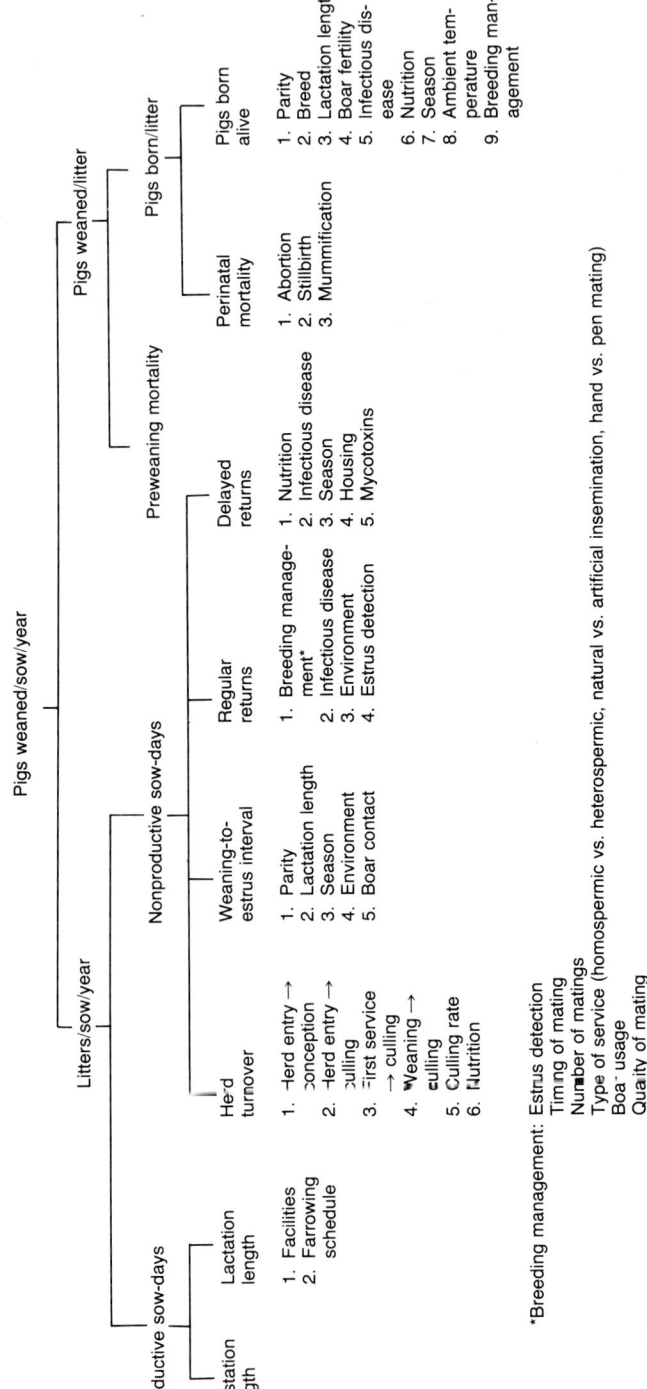

Figure 1. Algorithm for factors affecting pigs weaned/sow/year. (Adapted from Stein TE: Problem-oriented population medicine in swine breeding herds. Compend Cont Ed Pract Vet 10:871–878, 1988.)

that influence pigs weaned/sow/year are best represented in the form of an algorithm as in Figure 1. Other parameters used to assess herd reproductive performance include pigs/crate/year, pounds of pork/sow/year, and number of sow days/pig produced.

Most consultants, and software packages, distinguish between productive and nonproductive sow-days, as outlined in Figure 1. A nonproductive sow day is defined as any day a sow or gilt of breeding age is present in the breeding herd and is not either gestating or lactating. Since the gestation length is fixed and the lactation length is often inflexible, owing to facility or management constraints, nonproductive sow-days have the greatest impact on the litters/sow/year. The cost of a nonproductive sow-day has been estimated at $1.43 for intensively managed, confinement operations. Of the factors affecting nonproductive sow-days, those determining herd turnover have the most significant impact on litters/sow/year. These need to be addressed if herd reproductive performance is to be improved.

The practitioner interested in herd evaluation is urged to consult the many references available. Some are listed in the bibliography. Other reference sources include the American Association of Swine Practitioners and various regional meetings and workshops offered by veterinary schools.

BIBLIOGRAPHY

Clark LK, Leman AD: Factors that influence litter size in swine: parity 3 through 7 females. J Am Vet Med Assoc 191:49–58, 1987.
Clark LK, Leman AD: Factors that influence litter size in swine: parity one females. J Am Vet Med Assoc 192:187–194, 1987.
Clark LK, Leman AD: Diagnosing reproductive problems in swine. In Proceedings of the annual meeting of the American Association of Swine Practitioners, pp 191–196. St Louis, MO, 1988.
Dial GD: Optimizing reproductive performance and establishing new horizons for sow productivity. In Proceedings of the annual meeting of the American Association of Swine Practitioners, pp 151–174. Indianapolis, IN, 1987.
Dial GD: Differential diagnosis of reproductive failure in commercial swine herds. In Proceedings of the George A. Young Swine Conference, Lincoln, NB, 1988.
Dial GD: Diagnostic techniques for troubleshooting reproductive failure in commercial swine herds. In Proceedings of the George A. Young Swine Conference, Lincoln, NB, 1988.
Leman AD, Fraser D, Greenley W: Factors affecting nonproductive sow-days. In Proceedings of the 11th Congress of the International Pig Veterinary Society, Luzanne, Switzerland, 1990.
Leman AD, Straw B, Glock RP, et al: Diseases of Swine, 6th ed, Ames, IA, Iowa State University Press, 1986.
Polson P, Dial G, Marsh W: A biological and financial characterization of nonproductive days. In Proceedings of the 11th Congress of the International Pig Veterinary Society, Luzanne, Switzerland, 1990.
Radostits OM, Blood DC: Herd Health. Philadelphia, WB Saunders, 1985.
Rueff LR: Diagnosing and improving suboptimal reproductive performance. In Proceedings of the annual meeting of the American Association of Swine Practitioners, pp 197–214. St Louis, MO, 1988.
Stein TE: Swine reproductive performance: data collection, analysis and interpretation. In Morrow DA (ed): Current Therapy in Theriogenology, 2nd ed, pp 996–1001. Philadelphia, WB Saunders, 1986.
Stein TE: Problems-oriented population medicine in swine breeding herds. Compend Cont Ed Pract Vet 10:871–878, 1988.
Stein TE: Interpreting production data from swine breeding herds. Agri-Practice 11:30–34, 1990.
Terpstra C, Wensvoort G, Pol JMA: Experimental reproduction of porcine epidemic abortion and respiratory syndrome (mystery swine disease) by infection with Lelystad virus. Koch's postulates fulfilled. Vet Q 13:131–136, 1991.
Thacker BJ: Swine breeding herd records, In Morrow DA (ed): Current Therapy in Theriogenology, 2nd ed, pp 1068–1078. Philadelphia, WB Saunders, 1986.
Thacker BJ: Detection and diagnosis of swine reproductive failure. In Morrow DA (ed): Current Therapy in Theriogenology, 2nd ed. Philadelphia, WB Saunders, 1986.
Tubbs RC: Factors that influence the weaning-to-service interval in sows. Compend Cont Ed Pract Vet 12:105–115, 1990.
Wensvoort G, Terpstra C, Pol JMA, et al: Mystery swine disease in the Netherlands: the isolation of Lelystad virus. Vet Q 13:121–130, 1991.

Therapeutic Management of Reproduction

R. S. YOUNGQUIST, DVM

CATTLE

Estrus Synchronization

Estrus synchronization is used in beef and dairy herds to facilitate artificial insemination and to shorten the breeding season when using natural service by bulls with excellent semen quality and libido. Luteolysis can be induced by treatment with prostaglandin $F_{2\alpha}$ ($PGF_{2\alpha}$; dinoprost tromethamine [Lutalyse]*) or one of its several synthetic analogues (cloprostenol [Estrumate]†; fenprostalene [Bovilene]‡), or the luteal phase of the estrous cycle can be artificially prolonged by administration of a progestin (Tables 1 and 2).[1,2]

Prostaglandin $F_{2\alpha}$

Treatment with $PGF_{2\alpha}$ between days 5 and 17 of the estrous cycle is followed by luteolysis, follicular development, estrus, and ovulation between 2 and 5 days after administration. Estrus occurs sooner after $PGF_{2\alpha}$ treatment in heifers compared with cows. Response to $PGF_{2\alpha}$ and degree of synchrony after treatment vary with the stage of the estrous cycle; cows treated after day 10 of the estrous cycle are more likely to respond, but cows treated on days 5 through 10 are in estrus sooner after treatment and are more closely synchronized than those treated between days 11 and 17. In most trials, fertility at the synchronized estrus is similar to that of nonsynchronized (nontreated) controls. Cows and heifers not in the luteal phase of the estrous cycle cannot respond to $PGF_{2\alpha}$ administration. Thus, the most common reason for apparent failure of $PGF_{2\alpha}$ synchronization is acyclicity at the time of treatment.[3] Cows that are selected for synchronization must be free of any genital abnormality, must not be pregnant, and must be experiencing normal ovarian cycles. After treatment with $PGF_{2\alpha}$, cows should be observed for estrus and inseminated according to the "A.M.–P.M. rule" (cows first detected in estrus in the morning are inseminated that evening, while cows first detected in estrus in the evening are inseminated the next morning). Several schemes have been advocated for the use of $PGF_{2\alpha}$ in synchronization programs.[4]

Double-Injection Programs

PROGRAM A. Two injections of $PGF_{2\alpha}$ are given at an 11-day interval. Estrus is expected 2 to 5 days after the second injection, and cows are inseminated at the usual time relative to the onset of estrus. If one of the goals is to avoid estrus detection, cows can be inseminated once at 72 to 80 hours after the second injection or twice at 72 and 96 hours after the second injection. However, some reduction in pregnancy rates must be expected.

PROGRAM B. Cows detected in estrus after the first injection of $PGF_{2\alpha}$ can be inseminated in the usual manner. Only those that are not detected in estrus are given a second injection 11 days after the first injection and are then inseminated as in program A.

---

*Available from the Upjohn Company, Kalamazoo, MI 49001.
†Available from Mobay Corporation, Animal Health Division, Shawnee, KS 66201.
‡Available from Syntex Animal Health, Inc., West Des Moines, IA 50265.

Table 1. SELECTED INDICATIONS FOR ENDOCRINE THERAPY FOR MANAGEMENT OF REPRODUCTION IN FOOD-PRODUCING ANIMALS

Drug	Cattle	Sheep	Goats	Swine
Prostaglandin	Estrus synchronization; induced parturition; induced abortion; unobserved estrus; pyometra; mummified fetus; luteal ovarian cysts	Estrus synchronization (during the breeding season); induced abortion	Estrus synchronization (during the breeding season); induced abortion; induced parturition	Estrus synchronization (after abortion only); induced parturition
Gonadotropin-releasing hormone	Ovarian follicular cysts; repeat breeders; fertility enhancement; postpartum therapy			
Progestins	Estrus synchronization	Estrus synchronization; nonseasonal breeding	Estrus synchronization; nonseasonal breeding	Estrus synchronization
Gonadotropins	Superovulation	Nonseasonal breeding; superovulation	Nonseasonal breeding; superovulation	Induce puberty; postfarrowing anestrus
Corticosteroids	Induced parturition	Induced parturition	Induced parturition	

Single-Injection Programs

PROGRAM C. Cows are examined per rectum and only those with a mature corpus luteum are treated with $PGF_{2\alpha}$. Estrus is detected from days 2 through 5 after injection, and cows are inseminated. Since rectal palpation of the ovaries may not be a reliable method for detecting a functional corpus luteum, enzyme immunoassay for progesterone determination (Ovusure)* may be a useful adjunct for identifying cows that are likely to respond to $PGF_{2\alpha}$.

PROGRAM D. Estrus is detected and cows are inseminated for the first 6 days of the breeding season. Cows not inseminated by the sixth day are injected with $PGF_{2\alpha}$ and inseminated at the usual time relative to estrus. In herds that do not appear to have normal estrous cyclicity (5 per cent in estrus per day or 25 to 30 per cent inseminated by the sixth day) the $PGF_{2\alpha}$ treatment can be delayed or abandoned.

Progestins

The luteal phase of the estrous cycle can be artificially prolonged by administration of exogenous progestins and then abruptly terminated to mimic natural regression of the corpus luteum. Since all treated cows undergo termination of the artificial luteal phase simultaneously, estrus and ovulation are synchronized.

Norgestomet–Estradiol Valerate

An implant containing 6 mg of norgestomet (Syncro-Mate B)† is placed subcutaneously in the ear of cows to be synchronized and left for 9 days. Simultaneously, an intramuscular injection of 5 mg of estradiol valerate and 3 mg of norgestomet is given. Removal of the implant mimics corpus luteum regression and is followed by estrus within 36 to 60 hours. Cows are inseminated relative to detected estrus or by appointment at 48 to 56 hours after implant removal. Pregnancy rates following insemination at detected estrus or insemination by appointment are reported to be similar.

This scheme appears to induce cyclicity in some anestrous cows and prepubertal heifers. However, subsequent pregnancy rate in these animals is variable and likely to be low. Treatment with norgestomet–estradiol valerate induces estrus in ovariectomized females. Thus, signs of estrus are independent of ovarian function in treated animals.[5] Calf removal for 48 hours at the time of implant removal has also been suggested as a method for improving synchrony and increasing induction of estrus in anestrous cows.

Melengestrol Acetate–Prostaglandin $F_{2\alpha}$

Estrus can also be synchronized by the combined use of melengestrol acetate (MGA, an orally active progestin approved in the United States only as a growth stimulant for heifers) and $PGF_{2\alpha}$. Feeding MGA (0.5 to 0.6 mg/head/day) for 9 days and intramuscular injection of $PGF_{2\alpha}$ on the last day of MGA feeding will synchronize estrus in cyclic cows and induce estrus in anestrous cows. However, pregnancy rates tend to be higher when cows are cycling before synchronization.[6] Fertility at the synchronized estrus may be reduced after cows are treated with short-term feeding of MGA and $PGF_{2\alpha}$ on the last day of MGA feeding. Reduced pregnancy rates are avoided when MGA is fed for 14 days and $PGF_{2\alpha}$ is injected 17 days after the last MGA treatment. The length of this treatment period, however, may render the method impractical.[7]

Anestrus/Subestrus

Failure of cows to display, or managers to observe, signs of estrus contributes significantly to reproductive inefficiency in herds using artificial insemination. Approximately 90 per cent of dairy cows examined because of a history of anestrus have evidence of progressive ovarian changes. By 60 days after calving, nearly 90 per cent of dairy cows have initiated normal estrous cycles, but only about 60 per cent are detected in estrus.[8] Estrus in dairy cows averages 12 to 16 hours (range, 6 to 24 hours). Sixty-five per cent of cows are in estrus for less than 16 hours, and 25 per cent are in estrus for less than 8 hours.

$PGF_{2\alpha}$ is widely used in the treatment of unobserved estrus.[9] (See Tables 1 and 2.) Between approximately days 5 and 17 of the estrous cycle, the corpus luteum is responsive to a luteolytic dose of $PGF_{2\alpha}$. Following treatment, plasma progesterone concentrations decline rapidly and reach less than 1 ng/ml within 24 hours. Estrus occurs an average of 3 days (range, 2 to 5 days) after treatment. Treatment with $PGF_{2\alpha}$ has no direct effect on fertility. The benefits of $PGF_{2\alpha}$ treatment are limited by inaccurate identification of ovarian structures by palpation, failure of the cow to respond to the drug, and failure of the manager to observe estrus in treated cows. Treatment with $PGF_{2\alpha}$ results in earlier conception and reduced days open but cannot overcome poor estrus detection.[10] Timed insemination (80 hours after treatment) may be considered in herds with low rates of estrus detection, but pregnancy

---

*Available from Elanco Products Co., Indianapolis, IN 46206.
†Available from Sanofi Animal Health, Inc., Overland Park, KS 66210.

Table 2. SELECTED DRUGS USED FOR REPRODUCTIVE MANAGEMENT OF FOOD-PRODUCING ANIMALS

Drug	Manufacturer	Species	Dose and Route of Administration
Dinoprost tromethamine (Lutalyse)	Upjohn Company, Kalamazoo, MI	Bovine Ovine Caprine Porcine	25 mg/animal IM 5–16 mg/animal IM 8–20 mg/animal IM 10–15 mg/animal IM
Cloprostenol (Estrumate)	Mobay Corporation, Animal Health Division, Shawnee, KS	Bovine Caprine Porcine	500 µg/animal IM 125 µg/animal IM 175 µg/animal IM
Fenprostalene (Bovilene)	Syntex Animal Health, Inc., West Des Moines, IA	Bovine Porcine	1 mg/animal SQ 500 µg/animal SQ
Norgestomet/ estradiol valerate (Syncro-Mate B)	Sanofi Animal Health, Inc., Overland Park, KS	Bovine Ovine Caprine	6 mg norgestomet implant; 3 mg norgestomet and 5 mg estradiol valerate injection IM 3–6 mg norgestomet implant; 1.5–3 mg norgestomet and 2.5–5 mg estradiol valerate injection IM 6 mg norgestomet implant
Gonadotropin-releasing hormone (Cystorelin)	Sanofi Animal Health Inc., Overland Park, KS	Bovine	100 µg/animal IM
Gonadotropin-releasing hormone (Factrel)	Ft. Dodge Laboratories, Ft. Dodge, IA	Bovine	100 µg/animal IM
Dexamethasone	Tech America Group, Inc., Elwood, KS	Bovine Ovine Caprine	20–25 mg/animal IM 16 mg/animal IM 16 mg/animal IM
Triamcinolone	Solvay Veterinary, Inc., Princeton, NJ	Bovine	30 mg/animal IM
Betamethasone	Schering Corporation, Kenilworth, NJ	Bovine	20 mg/animal IM
Pregnant mare serum gonadotropin/ human chorionic gonadotropin (PG-600)	Intervet America, Inc., Millsboro, DE	Porcine	400 IU PMSG and 200 IU HCG/gilt IM

rates in cows inseminated by appointment are lower than those in cows bred at observed estrus.[11, 12]

Repeat Breeders

Repeat breeders are those cows that have been unsuccessfully inseminated three or more times, exhibit normal estrous cycles and have no detectable reproductive abnormalities on rectal palpation. Causes that have been suggested for repeat breeding include fertilization failure, early embryonic death, anatomic defects, infections of the reproductive tract, delayed ovulation, luteal phase deficiency, improper estrus detection and timing of insemination, and inadequate semen quality.[13] The pregnancy rate of dairy cows has been improved under some conditions by intramuscular administration of 100 µg of gonadotropin-releasing hormone (GnRH; Cystorelin,* Factrel†) at the time of the third or subsequent insemination in both normal and repeat breeder cows.[14–16] (See Tables 1 and

---
*Available from Sanofi Animal Health, Inc., Overland Park, KS 66210.
†Available from Ft. Dodge Laboratories, Ft. Dodge, IA 50501.

2.) Treatment with GnRH at earlier inseminations, however, does not appear to enhance pregnancy rates.[17, 18] Dairy herds with efficient reproductive management are less likely to benefit from GnRH administration at insemination, but the practice may be profitable under some conditions.[19] Fertility of repeat breeder cows has also been improved by saline lavage of the uterine cavity using a procedure similar to that used for nonsurgical recovery of embryos.[20]

Induced Abortion

Induced abortion is indicated in cases of unwanted or abnormal pregnancy. In cattle, the corpus luteum is maintained throughout gestation but the placenta is capable of secreting sufficient progesterone to maintain pregnancy in some animals after the fourth to fifth month. (See Tables 1 and 2.) Lysis of the corpus luteum with $PGF_{2\alpha}$ is an effective means of inducing abortion during the first 4 months of pregnancy. Expulsion of the fetuses occurs an average of 5 days (range, 2 to 10 days) after treatment. When abortion is induced between the fourth and eighth month of gestation, placental secretion of progesterone can be terminated by concurrent intramuscular administration of a 16α-substituted synthetic corticosteroid such as dexamethasone (20 to 25 mg) or flumethasone (10 mg). Abortion during the second or third trimester may be complicated by dystocia, retained fetal membranes, and metritis.[21, 22]

Induced Parturition

Induced parturition may be indicated in cases in which an oversized fetus is anticipated, in cases in which it is desirable to allow late-calving cows a longer postpartum rest period, and in cases of excessive udder edema. Calves delivered up to 2 weeks before term can be expected to survive and have normal passive transfer of antibodies from maternal colostrum.[23–26]

Short-acting corticosteroids were among the first drugs used to induce parturition in cattle.[27] Administration of synthetic corticosteroids mimics the fetal release of cortisol, which is believed to initiate parturition at term by reducing placental progesterone secretion and triggering release of prostaglandin, which subsequently results in luteolysis. (See Tables 1 and 2.)

Treatment of cows with intramuscular administration of dexamethasone (20 to 30 mg), flumethasone (5 to 10 mg), betamethasone (20 mg), or triamcinolone (30 mg) within the last 2 weeks of gestation results in delivery in an average of 48 hours (range, 24 to 72 hours). Cows that have not calved by 72 hours after the initial treatment should be re-treated. Retained fetal membranes is a common sequel to induced parturition, and the prevalence is inversely related to the degree of fetal maturity (i.e., the more mature the fetus, the less likely will parturition be followed by retained fetal membranes). Cows with retained fetal membranes generally do not require treatment unless they develop metritis, and their future reproductive performance is usually unimpaired.

Intramuscular administration of $PGF_{2\alpha}$ to cows during the last 2 weeks of pregnancy results in luteolysis and fetal delivery 24 to 72 hours after injection. (See Tables 1 and 2.) Calf viability and the prevalence of retained fetal membranes are similar to those following corticosteroid-induced parturition.[28, 29]

Postpartum Hormonal Therapy

Abnormalities such as genital tract infections, anestrus, and ovarian follicular cysts are common during the postpartum period of dairy cows. A number of investigators have attempted to reduce the prevalence of postpartum diseases and enhance reproductive function by routine treatment of all cows in the herd during the early postpartum period. Recently, most interest has centered on the use of GnRH and $PGF_{2\alpha}$.

Gonadotropin-releasing Hormone

Gonadotropin-releasing hormone is a small peptide hormone secreted by the hypothalamus and passes through the hypophyseal portal system to the anterior pituitary to stimulate release of gonadotropins: follicle-stimulating hormone (FSH) and luteinizing hormone (LH). Pituitary responsiveness to GnRH is low at parturition but increases after calving. Administration of GnRH at 2 weeks post partum can result in release of sufficient LH to induce ovulation in milked dairy cows.[30, 31] (See Tables 1 and 2.)

Cows treated with GnRH to induce ovulation 2 weeks post partum had fewer ovarian cysts and enhanced fertility when compared with untreated herdmates.[32] Other trials have demonstrated that cows treated with GnRH had increased first-service pregnancy rates and fewer days open when early (approximately 40 days) postpartum rebreeding was practiced. Treatment with GnRH at 2 weeks post partum has also been shown in some trials to improve reproductive performance of cows affected by puerperal abnormalities such as dystocia, retained fetal membranes, uterine infections, hypocalcemia, and ketosis.[33] The mechanism by which GnRH might improve reproductive performance is unclear. Administration of GnRH at 15 days after calving did not affect the rate of uterine involution or reduce uterine bacterial infections.[34] Cows with inactive ovaries at 6 weeks post partum that were treated with GnRH had fewer days open and required fewer services per conception than did similar cows not treated with GnRH.[35]

Induction of ovulation during the early postpartum period with GnRH was found to have some negative effects on reproduction.[36] Longer intervals to first estrus and pregnancy followed treatment with GnRH because of an increased prevalence of pyometra and prebreeding anestrus in a dairy herd experiencing an above average number of postpartum uterine infections.

Prostaglandin $F_{2\alpha}$

During the immediate postpartum period, serum concentrations of $PGF_{2\alpha}$ and its metabolites are elevated. The uterus is apparently the major source of $PGF_{2\alpha}$, and cows affected with puerperal uterine infections produce more $PGF_{2\alpha}$ than do normal cows. It has been suggested that this massive production of $PGF_{2\alpha}$ is related to the process of uterine involution.[37] However, treatment with exogenous $PGF_{2\alpha}$ during the postpartum period does not appear to alter the rate of uterine involution. There may not be an absolute requirement for $PGF_{2\alpha}$ because uterine involution was not delayed in cows in which prostaglandin synthesis was suppressed by the use of a prostaglandin synthetase inhibitor.

Several clinical trials have shown that administration of $PGF_{2\alpha}$ during the postpartum period may enhance the reproductive performance of dairy cows that are otherwise unaffected by periparturient diseases.[38, 39] (See Tables 1 and 2.) The mechanism by which reproductive performance is improved is unclear but appeared to be unrelated to the luteolytic effect of $PGF_{2\alpha}$. There appears to be some other beneficial effect(s) because the reproductive performance of cows with low serum progesterone concentrations (and thus no corpus luteum on their ovaries) is more markedly improved than that of cows with high serum progesterone concentrations at the time of treatment. Administration of $PGF_{2\alpha}$ to cows affected by periparturient diseases such as dystocia, retained fetal membranes, uterine infections, and metabolic diseases appeared to improve their reproductive performance.[40–42] However, recent research has shown that prostaglandin treatment of postpartum cows that had experienced dystocia and/or retained fetal membranes had no beneficial effect on fertility during the succeeding postpartum period.[43]

SHEEP

Nonseasonal Breeding

Most breeds of sheep are seasonally polyestrous during short photoperiods. In the northern hemisphere the breeding season is between late summer and early autumn. Typically, ewes mated at this time lamb during late winter and spring. The gestation period of sheep is approximately 5 months. Thus, in theory, ewes are capable of producing two lamb crops per year. Lambing can be accelerated by a system of exposing nonpregnant ewes to rams for 5 equally spaced 30-day periods. Ewes can then lamb at intervals as short as 7.2 months.[44]

Photoperiod

Photoperiod can be altered to initiate estrous cycles during the anestrous season. Using this scheme ewes are exposed during late winter to 16 hours of light per day (to simulate the long days of summer). The extra light is removed 60 days prior to the intended breeding season to mimic the onset of shorter days typical of autumn.

Another year-round lighting scheme allows a breeding season every 8 months. Ewes are exposed to 4 months of long days (16 hours of light and 8 hours of dark) followed by 4 months of short days (9 hours of light and 15 hours of dark).

Ram Effect

Introduction of either an intact or a vasectomized ram into a flock of ewes during the transitional breeding season advances the onset of the breeding season. Most ewes ovulate by 3 to 6 days after introduction of rams. The induced ovulation is seldom accompanied by estrus, but the subsequent estrus period 17 to 24 days later is ovulatory and fertile. The ram effect is lost when rams are kept with ewes throughout the year.

Melatonin

Melatonin implants are available in some sheep-producing countries (but not in the United States) and are used to stimulate early onset of the breeding season in ewes and rams. Treatment is initiated 4 to 6 weeks prior to the intended breeding season.

Progestins

A combination of norgestomet and estradiol valerate, as used to synchronize estrus in cattle, has been administered to ewes during the anestrous season and during the breeding season.[45] (See Tables 1 and 2.) An intramuscular injection containing estradiol valerate and norgestomet and a subcutaneous implant containing norgestomet is administered on the first day of treatment. Doses of norgestomet–estradiol valerate combination for injection ranging from one-eighth to the full dose intended for cattle are reported. Similarly, success is reported to follow use of one-half the cattle dose on entire norgestomet implants. Implants are removed after 9 to 14 days, and estrus is expected within 3 days. Gonadotropins administered at the time of implant removal include a single intramuscular dose of 375 to 750 IU of pregnant mare serum gonadotropin (PMSG; also known as equine chorionic gonadotropin) or 9 mg IM of FSH in six divided doses, two times a day for 3 days.

Other progestins that have been used by oral administration, intramuscular injection, subcutaneous implant, and intravaginal sponges include progesterone (5 to 25 mg/day IM, 10 to 400 mg/vaginal sponge, 100 to 600 mg/implant), chlorgesterone acetate (1 to 3 mg/day per os), fluorogesterone acetate (10 to 60 mg/vaginal sponge), melengestrol acetate (0.1 to 2 mg/day per os), and medroxyprogesterone acetate (10 to 60 mg/vaginal sponge, 10 to 60 mg/day per os, 10 to 60 mg/implant). Ewes are treated for 12 to 15 days after which the progestin is acutely withdrawn. PMSG (375 to 750 IU) is administered at the end of progestin treatment. None of these products is approved for use in sheep in the United States.

Immunization

Ovulation and lambing rates have been improved by immunizing ewes against androstenedione. In countries where these products are approved for use in sheep (they are not available in the United States), two injections are given initially, 8 and 4 weeks before introduction of rams. In subsequent years, a single booster is given 3 to 4 weeks before rams are joined with the ewes. Fecundity is not improved when ewes are in poor body condition.

Estrus Synchronization

The estrous cycles of ewes can be synchronized to facilitate artificial insemination or to shorten the breeding season in flocks using natural mating. (See Tables 1 and 2.) When rams are used to mate synchronized ewes, a 1:10 ram-to-ewe ratio is recommended.

Prostaglandin $F_{2\alpha}$

$PGF_{2\alpha}$ will not induce luteolysis until 4 to 6 days after ovulation. Schemes similar to those used in cows could be used to synchronize ewes during the breeding season. However, the interval between doses in two-injection schemes is 9 days because the length of the estrous cycle of ewes is shorter than that of cows. Reported doses of dinoprost tromethamine range from 5 to 16 mg per ewe. Ewes generally exhibit estrus 2 to 4 days after the second injection of $PGF_{2\alpha}$. Fertility following estrous synchronization using $PGF_{2\alpha}$ has been shown to be comparable to untreated controls in most trials. Since there are no corpora lutea in the ovaries during the nonbreeding season, $PGF_{2\alpha}$ cannot be used to synchronize estrus at this time.

Progestins

Progestins administered for approximately the length of a normal estrous cycle suppress gonadotropin release and ovarian function. When the progestin is withdrawn, follicular development, estrus, and ovulation follow. Potent synthetic analogues of progesterone such as fluorogestrone acetate (30 mg for 14 days) and medroxyprogesterone acetate have been administered by subcutaneous implants, but intravaginal sponges are more commonly used. Estrus synchronization using progestins can be used during either the breeding or the nonbreeding season. If progestins are used during the nonbreeding season, PMSG (375 to 750 IU) is given on the day of sponge removal to stimulate follicle growth.[46]

Induced Parturition

Lambing can be induced in ewes during the last week of pregnancy using either 16 mg of dexamethasone[47] or 15 mg of estradiol benzoate.[48] (See Tables 1 and 2.) Because ewes rely on placental and not luteal progesterone to maintain pregnancy after the 50th day of gestation, $PGF_{2\alpha}$ is not effective for inducing parturition after that time. Retained fetal membranes following corticosteroid-induced parturition is not as common in ewes as it is in cows.

GOATS

Nonseasonal Breeding

Since the breeding season of goats is comparable to that of sheep, it can be similarly modified using management techniques and exogenous hormones (in countries where they are approved). (See Tables 1 and 2.)

Nonhormonal Methods

The breeding season can be advanced by 2 to 3 months if does are exposed to 19 hours of light per day for 70 days beginning in mid to late winter. After such exposure to artificial light, does are exposed to ambient lighting for 42 days, at the end of which bucks are placed in the herd. Estrous cycles follow approximately 20 days later. Introduction of bucks into the herd during the transitional breeding season results in synchronization of estrus and ovulation within 5 to 7 days.[49]

Hormonal Methods

Stimulation of estrus and ovulation during the nonbreeding season requires progesterone priming prior to treatment with gonadotropins.[50] Progestins can be administered either by intramuscular injection, intravaginal sponges, or by subcutaneous implants. Vaginal sponges containing medroxyprogesterone acetate (60 mg for 14 days) and fluorogestrone acetate (30 to 40 mg for 12 days) and subcutaneous implants containing norgestomet (6 mg for 16 to 17 days) have been used to deliver progestins. Gonadotropin treatments include 700 to 1000 IU PMSG 48 hours before sponge removal alone or in combination with human menopausal gonadotropin (75 to 150 IU) at sponge removal. Melatonin (2 mg daily for 3 months) maintains sexual activity in goats during the nonbreeding season.

Estrus Synchronization

During the breeding season, estrous cycles of does can be synchronized by suppressing follicular development and ovulation with progestins or by luteolysis with $PGF_{2\alpha}$. (See Tables 1 and 2.)

Progestins

Progestins used to stimulate estrous cycles during the nonbreeding season can also be used during the breeding season. Most successful procedures for estrus synchronization with progestins include administration of PMSG (400 to 1000 IU) concurrent with, or 24 hours before, implant or sponge removal.[52]

Prostaglandin $F_{2\alpha}$

The estrous cycle of does with functional corpora lutea can be synchronized by administration of two doses of $PGF_{2\alpha}$ (8 mg dinoprost tromethamine; 125 µg cloprostenol) at an interval of 10 days.[52]

Induced Abortion

Although therapeutic abortions are only occasionally indicated in does, $PGF_{2\alpha}$ is an effective abortifacient should mismating occur. (See Tables 1 and 2.) Since does require luteal progesterone throughout gestation, $PGF_{2\alpha}$ is an effective abortifacient any time after the first week of pregnancy. Treatment with 15 to 20 mg dinoprost tromethamine is followed by fetal expulsion in 2 to 3 days. Short, anovulatory estrous cycles can follow abortion. Thus, rebreeding should be delayed following such treatment.

Induced Parturition

Induced parturition may result in improved survival of both does and kids as well as be an important facet in control of certain diseases such as caprine arthritis-encephalitis. Accurate breeding records are an absolute requirement for successful induction. Since the doe requires luteal progesterone throughout gestation, $PGF_{2\alpha}$ is an effective agent for inducing parturition.[53] Does treated on day 144 of gestation deliver between 27 and 55 hours (average, 30 to 35 hours) after $PGF_{2\alpha}$. Dexamethasone (16 mg) has been used to induce parturition, but $PGF_{2\alpha}$ is more effective. (See Tables 1 and 2.)

SWINE

Estrus Synchronization

Synchronization of estrus in sows and gilts facilitates the use of artificial insemination, allows more efficient use of facilities and labor, and may permit more precise scheduling of activities during the work week. In addition, breeding at a synchronized estrus simplifies application of other management techniques such as electronic or chemical pregnancy diagnosis and induced farrowing. Management techniques and pharmacologic agents can be used to control and synchronize estrous cycles of sows and gilts.[54, 55] (See Tables 1 and 2.)

Management Techniques

Boar Exposure and Relocation

Exposure of gilts that are approaching puberty to a mature boar stimulates follicular growth and hastens the onset of estrus. Most gilts raised in confinement without exposure to boars remain prepubertal until 6 months of age. Relocation of gilts to a breeding pen and mixing of animals from different groups stimulate follicular growth and a synchronous estrus 3 to 5 days later. The estrous cycle of gilts that have reached puberty is not affected by relocation and boar exposure. Relocation may also be useful in treating prolonged postweaning anestrus in sows.[56]

Group Weaning

Ovarian function is suppressed in lactating sows. Follicular growth is initiated at weaning, and a relatively synchronous estrus occurs 4 to 9 days after weaning. The time from weaning to estrus in sows weaned more than 10 days after farrowing is inversely proportional to the length of lactation (i.e., longer lactations are followed by shorter intervals from weaning to estrus). Weaning after very short lactations (<10 days) is followed by a long interval to estrus (>14 days) and reduced reproductive performance.

Pharmacologic Agents

Prostaglandin $F_{2\alpha}$

In swine, corpora lutea are sensitive to $PGF_{2\alpha}$-induced luteolysis only after days 12 to 14 of the estrous cycle. Thus $PGF_{2\alpha}$ can only be used successfully to synchronize sows when the stage of the estrous cycle is known. Pregnancy prevents natural regression of corpora lutea. Consequently, corpora lutea in the ovaries of sows more than 2 weeks pregnant can be regressed with exogenous $PGF_{2\alpha}$.[57] One scheme that can be used to synchronize estrus with $PGF_{2\alpha}$ involves breeding of postpubertal gilts and treatment with $PGF_{2\alpha}$ to induce abortion after two weeks of pregnancy. This is followed by a fertile estrus in 4 to 10 days. Pregnancy rates at the first post-abortion estrus are similar to those at spontaneous estrus. Doses of $PGF_{2\alpha}$ used to induce abortion are 15 mg of dinoprost tromethamine followed in 12 hours by a second 10-mg dose; 1.0 mg of cloprostenol followed in 24 hours by a second 0.5-mg dose; and a single cloprostenol dose of 0.5 mg.[58]

Progestins

Follicular growth and ovulation can be suppressed in postpubertal gilts by treatment with altrenogest*, an orally active synthetic progestin. Gilts are fed 15 to 20 mg altrenogest per day for 14 to 18 days. Withdrawal of altrenogest is followed by follicular growth and a synchronous estrus in 2 to 8 days. Sixty-five to 80 per cent of treated gilts exhibit estrus within a period of 2 days. Fertility of gilts synchronized with altrenogest is similar to that of untreated controls. Altrenogest is approved for use in swine in some countries but has not been approved for treatment of swine in the United States.

Gonadotropins

Pregnant mare serum gonadotropin stimulates follicular growth, estrus, and ovulation when corpora lutea are not present in the ovaries. HCG is used in some treatment strategies to induce ovulation. Gilts as young as 160 days of age respond to intramuscular administration of 500 to 1000 IU of PMSG, followed in 48 to 96 hours by intramuscular injection of 500 to 750 IU of HCG. In these young animals, however, ovulation is followed by premature luteal failure and less than 60 per cent are able to maintain pregnancy. Synchronous estrus can be induced in peripubertal gilts that are 5½ to 6 months of age by administration of a single intramuscular injection of 400 IU of PMSG and 200 IU of HCG (PG-600).† Since the ovaries of lactating sows rarely contain corpora lutea, a single intramuscular injection of PMSG (1500 IU) on the day of weaning, or PMSG followed in 80 to 96 hours by an intramuscular injection of HCG (1000 IU) has been used to synchronize estrus and reduce the prevalence of postweaning anestrus in sows. Partial weaning for one to three 12-hour periods prior to gonadotropin treatment may improve response.

---

*Available from Hoechst-Roussel, Somerville, NJ 08876.
†Available from Intervet America, Millsboro, DE 19966.

Induced Farrowing

Induced farrowing in swine has the potential to avoid or reduce the number of unattended farrowings, thus resulting in more live pigs per litter. In addition, continuous farrowing can be avoided and the farrowing house manager has more opportunities to cross-foster neonatal pigs. $PGF_{2\alpha}$ will induce luteal regression and abortion any time after day 12 to 14 of pregnancy, but normal pig survival can be anticipated if sows are treated no more than 72 hours prior to their expected farrowing date.[59-61] Since the average gestation length varies from herd to herd, it should be computed from contemporary herd records prior to undertaking induced farrowing. In herds with an average gestation length of 114 days, $PGF_{2\alpha}$ is administered intramuscularly on day 111 or 112 of pregnancy. Sows should be selected for induction only if they are accurately identified and their breeding date is known.

Most sows farrow between 20 and 30 hours after treatment (range, 12 to 36 hours). Doses of $PGF_{2\alpha}$ used to induce farrowing are 10 mg of dinoprost tromethamine, 175 µg of cloprostenol, and 500 µg of fenprostalene. Oxytocin given 20 hours after $PGF_{2\alpha}$ will shorten the time to farrowing (1 to 3 hours after oxytocin injection). Large doses of oxytocin (>30 IU) may cause dystocia and uterine inertia, but smaller doses (<10 IU) cause fewer undesirable side effects.

More precise control of farrowing has been reported to follow induction of parturition with a combination of cloprostenol and xylazine (Rompun).*[62] Sows were injected intramuscularly with 250 µg cloprostenol 3 days prior to their expected date of parturition. Cloprostenol treatment was followed in 20 hours by intramuscular injection of 2 mg/kg xylazine. The interval from xylazine treatment to delivery of the first pig was 1.5 ± 0.3 hours. Xylazine treatment of sows caused emesis and sedation in some treated animals (70% and 40%, respectively) but did not affect other parameters associated with farrowing, such as stillbirths or piglet survival.

Gonadotropin-Releasing Hormone

Under some circumstances, pregnancy rates in cattle have been improved by treatment with GnRH at the time of insemination. Treatment of gilts and sows with 50 µg of GnRH at the time of first detection of estrus did not, however, improve their reproductive peformance.[63]

REFERENCES

1. Kiracofe G: Estrus synchronization in beef cattle. Compend Contin Educ Pract Vet 10:57–61, 1988.
2. Rice LE: Reproductive management of beef herds using estrus synchronization. In Bovine Reproduction, Proceedings of a Symposium, pp 21–28. Princeton Junction, NJ, Veterinary Learning Systems, 1987.
3. Seguin BE, Momont HW, Fahmi H, et al: Single appointment insemination for heifers after prostaglandin or progestin synchronization of estrus. Theriogenology 31:1233–1238, 1989.
4. Schultz RH: Synchronization of estrus: A. Prostaglandin/prostaglandin analogues and GnRH. In Abbitt B (ed): Cow Manual, pp 104–113. Hastings, NB, Society for Theriogenology, 1987.
5. McGuire WJ, Larson RL, Kiracofe GH: Syncro-mate B induces estrus in ovariectomized cows and heifers. Theriogenology 34:33–37, 1990.
6. Beal WA, Good GA: Synchronization of estrus in postpartum beef cows with melengestrol acetate and prostaglandin $F_{2\alpha}$. J Anim Sci 63:343–347, 1986.
7. Patterson DJ, Kiracofe GH, Stevenson JS, Corah LR: Control of the bovine estrous cycle with melengestrol acetate (MGA): a review. J Anim Sci 67:1895–1906, 1989.
8. Ball PJH: Milk progesterone profiles in relation to dairy herd fertility. Br Vet J 138:546–551, 1982.
9. Young IM: Selection of specific categories of dairy cows for oestrus induction with dinoprost. Vet Rec 113:319–320, 1983.
10. Fetrow J, Blanchard T: Economic impact of the use of prostaglandin to induce estrus in dairy cows. J Am Vet Med Assoc 190:384–386, 1987.
11. Stevenson JS, Lucy MC, Call EP: Failure of timed inseminations and associated luteal function in dairy cattle after two injections of prostaglandin $F_{2\alpha}$. Theriogenology 28:937–946, 1987.
12. Whittier WD, Gwazdauskas FC, McGilliard ML: Prostaglandin $F_{2\alpha}$ usage in a dairy reproduction program for treatment of unobserved estrus, pyometra and ovarian luteal cysts. Theriogenology 32:693–704, 1989.
13. Lafi SQ, Kanenne JB: Risk factors and associated economic effects of the repeat breeder syndrome in dairy cattle. Vet Bull 58:891–903, 1988.
14. Lucy MC, Stevenson JS: Gonadotropin-releasing hormone at estrus: luteinizing hormone, estradiol, and progesterone during the periestrual and postinsemination periods in dairy cattle. Biol Reprod 35:300–311, 1986.
15. Roussel JD, Beatty JF, Koonce K: Gonadotropin releasing hormone therapy in functional infertility of dairy cattle. Theriogenology 30:1115–1119, 1988.
16. Stevenson JS, Frantz KD, Call EP: Conception rates in repeat-breeders and dairy cattle with unobserved estrus after prostaglandin $F_{2\alpha}$ and gonadotropin-releasing hormone. Theriogenology 29:451–461, 1988.
17. Lewis GS, Caldwell DW, Rexroad CE, et al: Effect of gonadotropin-releasing hormone and human chorionic gonadotropin on pregnancy rate in dairy cows. J Dairy Sci 73:66–72, 1990.
18. Mee MO, Stevenson JS, Scoby RK: Influence of gonadotropin-releasing hormone and timing of insemination relative to estrus on pregnancy rates of dairy cattle at first service. J Dairy Sci 73:1500–1507, 1990.
19. Weaver LD, Daley CA, Goodger WJ: Economic modeling and the use of gonadotropin-releasing hormone at insemination to improve fertility in dairy cows. J Am Vet Med Assoc 192:1714–1719, 1988.
20. Coe PH: Uterine flush as therapy for repeat breeder cows. Agri-Practice 5:29–32, 1984.
21. Barth AD: Induced abortion in cattle. In Morrow DA (ed): Current Therapy in Theriogenology 2, pp 205–209. Philadelphia, WB Saunders, 1986.
22. Oetzel GR, Ball L, Mortimer RG, Olson JD: Pregnancy palpation and therapeutic abortion. In Abbitt B (ed): Cow Manual, pp 27–35. Hastings, NB, Society for Theriogenology, 1987.
23. Drost M: Induction and synchronization of parturition. In Abbitt B (ed): Cow Manual, pp 132–134. Hastings, NB, Society for Theriogenology, 1987.
24. Barth AD: Induced parturition in cattle. In Morrow DA (ed): Current Therapy in Theriogenology 2, pp 209–214. Philadelphia, WB Saunders, 1986.
25. Welch RAS, Day AM, Duganzich DM, Feathersome P: Induced calving: a comparison of treatment regimes. N Z Vet J 27:190–194, 1979.
26. Barragry TB: The pharmacological induction of parturition. Irish Vet J 29:71–75, 1975.
27. Adams WM: The elective induction of labor and parturition in cattle. J Am Vet Med Assoc 154:261–265, 1969.
28. Floyd JG, Ott RS, Zinn GM: Induction of parturition in beef cows with alfaprostol. Agri-Practice 9(4):10–12, 1988.
29. Day AM: Cloprostenol for termination of pregnancy in cattle: the induction of parturition. N Z Vet J 25:136–139, 1977.
30. Kesler DJ, Garverick HA, Youngquist RS, et al: Effect of days postpartum and endogenous reproductive hormones on GnRH-induced LH release in dairy cows. J Anim Sci 45:797–803, 1977.
31. Zaied AA, Garverick HA, Bierschwal CJ, et al: Effect of ovarian activity and endogenous reproductive hormones on GnRH-induced ovarian cycles in postpartum dairy cows. J Anim Sci 50:508–513, 1980.
32. Britt JH, Harrison DS, Morrow DA: Frequency of ovarian follicular cysts, reasons for culling, and fertility in Holstein-Friesian cows given gonadotropin-releasing hormone at two weeks after parturition. Am J Vet Res 38:749–751, 1977.
33. Brown MD: Postpartum use of GnRH in dairy cows. Mod Vet Pract 66:27–29, 1985.
34. Holt LC, Whittier WD, Gwazdauskas FC, et al: Involution, pathology and histology of the uterus in dairy cattle with retained placenta and uterine discharge following GnRH. Anim Reprod Sci 21:11–23, 1989.
35. Archbald LF, Norman SN, Bliss EL, et al: Incidence and treatment of abnormal postpartum ovarian function in dairy cows. Theriogenology 34:283–290, 1990.
36. Etherington WG, Bosu WTK, Martin SW, et al: Reproductive performance in dairy cows following postpartum treatment with gonadotropin-releasing hormone and/or prostaglandin: a field trial. Can J Comp Med 48:245–250, 1984.
37. Thatcher WW: Role of prostaglandins during the periparturient period in the cow. In Proceedings of the Society for Theriogenology, pp 55–68. September 16–17 1988.
38. Young IM, Anderson DB: Improved reproductive performance from dairy cows treated with dinoprost tromethamine soon after calving. Theriogenology 26:199–208, 1986.
39. McClary DG, Putnam MR, Wright JC, Sartin JL Jr: Effect of early postpartum treatment with prostaglandin $F_{2\alpha}$ on subsequent fertility in the dairy cow. Theriogenology 31:565–570, 1989.
40. Steffan J, Adriamanga S, Thibier M: Treatment of metritis with antibiotics or prostaglandin $F_{2\alpha}$ and influence on ovarian cyclicity in dairy cows. Am J Vet Res 45:1090–1094, 1984.

---
*Available from Mobay Corp., Animal Health Division, Shawnee, KS 66201.

41. Benmrad M, Stevenson JS: Gonadotropin-releasing hormone and prostaglandin $F_{2\alpha}$ for postpartum dairy cows: estrus, ovulation, and fertility traits. J Dairy Sci 69:800–811, 1986.
42. Studer E, Holtan A: Treatment of retained placentas in dairy cattle with prostaglandin. Bovine Practitioner 21:159–160, 1986.
43. Archbald LF, Tran T, Thomas PGA, Lyle SK: Apparent failure of prostaglandin $F_{2\alpha}$ to improve the reproductive efficiency of postpartum cows that had experienced dystocia and/or retained fetal membranes. Theriogenology 34:1025–1034, 1990.
44. Magee B: Star accelerated lambing. *In* Symposium on Diseases of Small Ruminants, pp 47–56. Corvallis, OR, American Association of Small Ruminant Practitioners, 1990.
45. Bretzlaff K, Kimberling C, Simons J: Accelerated lambing. Soc Theriogenol Newsletter 11(4):8–9, 1988.
46. Ott RS, Memon MA: Control of reproduction. *In* Ott RS, Menon MA (eds): Sheep and Goat Manual, pp 19–23. Hastings, NB, Society for Theriogenology, 1980.
47. Wagner WC, Thompson FN, Evans LE, Molokwu ECI: Hormonal mechanisms controlling parturition. J Anim Sci 38(Suppl 1):39–57, 1974.
48. Restall BJ, Herdegen J, Carberry P: Induction of parturition in sheep using oestradiol benzoate. Aust J Exp Agr Anim Husb 16:462, 1976.
49. BonDurant RH: Induction of estrus in does by introduction of buck or photoperiod manipulation. *In* Morrow DA (ed): Current Therapy in Theriogenology 2, pp 579–581. Philadelphia, WB Saunders, 1986.
50. Amoah EA, Gelaye S: Superovulation, synchronization and breeding of does. Small Ruminant Res 3:63–72, 1990.
51. Smith MC: Synchronization of estrus and the use of implants and vaginal sponges. *In* Morrow DA (ed): Current Therapy in Theriogenology 2, pp 582–583. Philadelphia, WB Saunders, 1986.
52. Ott RS: Prostaglandins for induction of estrus, estrus synchronization, abortion and induction of parturition. *In* Morrow DA (ed): Current Therapy in Theriogenology 2, pp 583–585. Philadelphia, WB Saunders, 1986.
53. Williams CSF: Practical management of induced parturition. *In* Morrow DA (ed): Current Therapy in Theriogenology 2, pp 588–589. Philadelphia, WB Saunders, 1986.
54. Day BN: Control of estrus and ovulation in swine. Agri-Practice 10(3):11–15, 1989.
55. Clark LK, D'Allaire S, Leman AD: Reproductive system. *In* Leman AD, Straw B, et al (eds): Diseases of Swine, 6th ed, pp 101–143. Ames, Iowa State University Press, 1986.
56. Almond GW, Dial GD, Dixon D: Stress induced estrus in previously anestrous sows. *In* Proceedings of the 10th Congress of the International Pig Veterinary Society, Rio de Janeiro, Brazil, August 14–17. Am Assoc Swine Pract, Des Moines, IA, 1988.
57. Guthrie HD, Polge C: Treatment of pregnant gilts with a prostaglandin analogue, cloprostenol, to control oestrus and fertility. J Reprod Fertil 52:271–273, 1978.
58. Dial GD, BeVier GW: Pharmacological control of estrus and ovulation in the pig. *In* Morrow DA (ed): Current Therapy in Theriogenology 2, pp 912–914. Philadelphia, WB Saunders, 1986.
59. Hurtgen JP: Induction of parturition in swine. *In* Morrow DA (ed): Current Therapy in Theriogenology 2, p 927. Philadelphia, WB Saunders, 1986.
60. Simons J: An overview of parturition induction in swine. Soc Theriogenol Newsletter 8(5):6–7, 1985.
61. Wevar VCA, Bosch RA, Perettil H, Vivas A: Induction of parturition in sows with a synthetic prostaglandin (prosoluin) under intensive field conditions: comparison of three different treatments. *In* Proceedings of the 10th Congress of the International Pig Veterinary Society, Rio de Janeiro, Brazil, August 14–17. Am Assoc Swine Pract, Des Moines, IA, 1988.
62. Ko JCH, Evans LE, Hsu WH, Hopkins SM: Farrowing induction with cloprostenol-xylazine combination. Theriogenology 31:795–799, 1989.
63. Kirkwood RN, Thacker PA: The influence of a premating injection of gonadotropin-releasing hormone on sow and gilt fertility. Can Vet J 30:959–960, 1989.

SECTION 14
Diseases of the Urinary System

JIMMY L. HOWARD and THOMAS C. RANDOLPH,* DVM, Consulting Editors

Therapeutic Management of Urinary Diseases

VERNON C. LANGSTON, DVM, PHD*

As with all diseases, the treatment of a urinary disorder is dependent on the pathophysiologic mechanisms involved. Because these mechanisms often overlap, so do the treatments. It is thus necessary to realize what objectives are attainable. Table 1 lists the common urinary diseases and the therapies employed.

CONTROL OF INFECTION

Although the general principles of rational antimicrobial therapy apply equally to urinary tract infections, there are special considerations that must be taken into account. First, in choosing an antimicrobial, it should be remembered that different drugs concentrate in urine to varying degrees. Thus, organisms that might normally be resistant to a drug at systemic concentrations can be successfully treated in cystitis or pyelonephritis. For example, ampicillin trihydrate does not normally produce plasma concentrations therapeutic against most *Escherichia coli* infections; however, *E. coli* cystitis can usually be treated by relatively small doses of this formulation. Indeed, cystitis caused by certain *E. coli* can even be treated with large doses of penicillin G, a drug to which similar systemic bacteria would almost certainly be resistant. Care should be taken to ensure that laboratory categorizations of sensitivity are based on urine and not serum concentrations.

Urinary pH also affects the activity of the antimicrobial.

*Deceased.

Because herbivores normally maintain an alkaline urine, antibiotics such as gentamicin perform well without the assistance of a urinary alkalizer. However, agents such as the penicillins are more active in an acidic environment, and in selected cases such as *Corynebacterium renale* infections, urinary acidification may be of value. Acidification of the urine of food animals is absolutely essential if methenamine is to be used as a urinary antiseptic.

Urinary tract infections can be notoriously resistant to treatment. It is generally recommended that first-time treatments last at least 10 days. If significant bacteriuria persists after 3 days of therapy, resistance is probable, and a change in the antimicrobial might be indicated. For recurrent infections, treatment for 3 to 6 weeks is usually required, and even then the prognosis for cure may be guarded. In dealing with extremely resistant organisms, irrigation of the bladder with drugs that would otherwise be too costly or toxic for systemic administration may be an option. It is important not to overlook contributing factors such as urinary calculi that may restrict urinary flow from the renal pelvis, thereby aggravating a pyelonephritis (calculi lodged in ureter) or serving as a nidus of infection in cystitis. Water and salt should always be provided, and animals that refuse to drink should receive isotonic fluids orally or parenterally for maintaining hydration and fluid diuresis. A repeat urinalysis 1 to 2 weeks after ending therapy is prudent for the detection of relapses. Care to avoid catheterization-induced reinfection is essential.

In selecting an antimicrobial for long-term use, preference should be given to those drugs with minimal toxicity and residue potential. If culture and sensitivity results are lacking, penicillin G is commonly used in combatting gram-positive organisms (e.g., *Corynebacterium renale*), whereas a cephalosporin such as ceftiofur or a potentiated sulfonamide might be more appropriate when a gram-negative or *Staphylococcus* sp. is suspect. An aminoglycoside could also be used in the latter instance; however, its toxicity and residue potential may limit the duration of therapy.

Table 1. COMMON URINARY DISEASES AND THEIR TREATMENTS

Disease	Control Infection	Alter pH*	Diuresis	Induce Micturition	Relax Urethral Tone
Cystitis	+	+	Fluid‡		
Pyelonephritis	+	+	Fluid		
Urolithiasis					+
Urolithiasis prevention		+	Increase water intake		
Bladder paralysis				+	
Renal failure			+		

*Dependent on specific disease entity.
‡"Fluid" refers to forced fluid diuresis.
+May be employed in treatment.

ALTERATION OF URINARY pH

The need to alter pH of the urine in urinary tract infections has already been addressed. Another indication is urolithiasis, in which acidification may help prevent formation of struvite calculi. Ammonium chloride is given orally at 50 to 100 mg/kg twice daily (or 0.5 per cent of the ration) for prevention of urolithiasis in steers and sheep. It should not be used in patients with hepatic failure, renal failure, or metabolic acidosis. In the rare instance in which urinary alkalization is needed, sodium bicarbonate is usually administered.

INDUCTION OF DIURESIS

Fluid diuresis is commonly employed in the treatment of urinary tract infections and in the prevention of urolithiasis. The promotion of high urine output will in essence "wash out" bacteria, cellular debris, crystals, and small calculi. Because forced fluid diuresis is not practical for the long-term prevention of urolithiasis, increased water intake (and subsequent urine production) is accomplished by the addition of salt to the diet at 4 per cent (single-source diet) to 12 per cent (creep-fed calves). It has also been suggested that the increase in chloride ions may decrease the incidence of some forms of urolithiasis. Ammonium chloride has a transient (1- to 3-day) diuretic effect but should be thought of primarily as a urinary acidifier.

In those instances in which rehydration has failed to reestablish urinary flow (e.g., renal shutdown from shock or nephrotoxicity), aggressive diuresis with use of large doses (e.g., 5 to 10 mg/kg) of intravenous furosemide may be required. Alternatives to furosemide include the osmotic diuretics such as mannitol (0.25 to 1 g/kg intravenously over 5 minutes) or dextrose. If administration of an osmotic diuretic fails to induce adequate urine flow, the dose should not be repeated because overhydration and hyperosmolality may result in pulmonary edema. Congestive heart failure also represents a contraindication to the use of the osmotic diuretics. Dimethyl sulfoxide (DMSO) given intravenously as a 20 per cent solution at 0.5 to 1 g/kg also acts as a potent diuretic although appreciable hemolysis may occur. Dopamine infusion at 2 to 5 µg/kg/minute may also be helpful in oliguria although it requires continuous intravenous infusion and monitoring. Although the thiazide diuretics are quite effective in nonrenal diseases such as udder edema or early congestive heart failure, they usually are not capable of inducing urine production in refractory renal cases.

It deserves mention that the commonly used sedative xylazine has a significant diuretic action. In those instances in which bladder rupture is imminent, sedation with an alternative to xylazine may be preferable.

INDUCTION OF MICTURITION

It is often difficult to diagnose urinary tract disease ante mortem without a sample of urine. Although perineal stimulation ("feathering") and catheterization are effective means of accomplishing this in the female, obtaining a urine sample from a male is more difficult. Diuretic induction of urine flow with subsequent urination is commonly used, although this prohibits determination of urine specific gravity and will dilute many constituents. If a more representative urinalysis is desired, bethanechol may be administered subcutaneously at 0.075 mg/kg for directly inducing contraction of the detrusor muscle. Usually the animal will urinate within 20 minutes of injection. Bethanechol has been used in other species for the management of bladder paralysis postobstruction or after spinal lesions. Urinary or gastrointestinal obstruction represents a strict contraindication to the use of bethanechol. Intravenous injection can cause pronounced bradycardia and collapse.

RELAXATION OF URETHRAL TONE

Occasionally, relaxation of urethral tone has been advocated as an aid in the treatment of urolithiasis. Aminopropazine is most commonly used for this purpose. It should be noted that this drug acts only on smooth muscle. If the obstruction is in the proximal urethra, there may be benefit; if, however, the blockage occurs at the sigmoid flexure, an area lined by skeletal instead of smooth muscle, aminopropazine is of doubtful utility. Some blockages may be cleared by backflushing the urethra. If this is attempted, use of a local anesthetic as the flushing solution (e.g., 0.5 per cent lidocaine) will relieve urethral spasm.

AVOIDANCE OF DRUG-INDUCED NEPHROTOXICITY

A variety of therapeutic agents are potentially nephrotoxic. Chief among these are the aminoglycoside, sulfonamide, and tetracycline antimicrobials and the nonsteroidal anti-inflammatory drugs (NSAIDs).

Nephrotoxicity from the aminoglycoside antibiotics is well known by most practitioners. Although they are largely restricted to extracellular fluid spaces, the unique ability of the renal tubular cells to concentrate aminoglycosides leads to the tubular nephrosis and long withdrawal times associated with these antibiotics. The nephrotoxic potential is variable among members of this class: from highest to lowest, neomycin, gentamicin, amikacin and kanamycin, tobramycin, and streptomycin. The following are suggested guidelines for minimizing aminoglycoside-induced nephrotoxicity.

1. Do not use neomycin parenterally because it is the most nephrotoxic of the aminoglycosides.
2. Ensure that the animal is adequately hydrated at all times. Dehydration significantly increases the risk of toxic effect.
3. Avoid prolonged use (>3 to 5 days) of the aminoglycosides whenever possible because toxicity is proportional to total dose administered.
4. Increases in blood urea nitrogen or creatinine occur only after substantial kidney damage has occurred. Sequential urinalyses (when feasible) for detecting proteinuria and casts may be a better indicator of early problems.
5. In valuable animals, therapeutic drug monitoring is a useful aid in decreasing the incidence of nephrotoxicity.

Nephrotoxicity associated with the sulfonamides is due to crystalluria. This is primarily a problem with the older sulfonamides, such as sulfathiazole, when they are used in species that produce an acidic urine. As long as hydration is well maintained and the newer agents (or triple sulfonamide preparations) are used, crystalluria is rarely a concern. One extralabel practice that may cause concern is that of administering oral triple sulfonamide solutions intravenously. These solutions often contain large amounts of sulfathiazole. With oral administration, the plasma concentrations rise slowly and cause few problems; however, if they are given intravenously, the kidney is presented with unusually large concentrations of a relatively insoluble sulfonamide that may precipitate.

The tetracyclines have long been known to be capable of causing azotemia by their antianabolic properties. Also, a Fanconi-like syndrome is associated with the use of outdated tetracyclines. Most of the tetracycline-induced nephrotoxic effects have, however, been seen when large-dose (i.e., 20 mg/kg twice daily) oxytetracycline was administered to animals suffering from *Pasteurella* pneumonia or coliform mastitis. It now appears that the endotoxemia associated with either disease acts synergistically to induce proximal tubular damage.

The NSAIDs are not generally considered to be potent nephrotoxins, however, they can induce severe tubular damage, especially if other nephrotoxins are given concomitantly (e.g., an aminoglycoside) or if hypotension or dehydration is present. Pathologically this is manifested as a renal papillary necrosis or interstitial nephritis.

Other potentially nephrotoxic therapeutic agents include monensin, vitamin D, and vitamin K_3.

Urolithiasis in Food Animals
(Urinary Calculi, Waterbelly, Calculosis)

JAMES G. FLOYD, JR., DVM, MS, DIPLOMATE, ACT

Urolithiasis is a disease of significant economic importance in domestic food animals resulting from urinary tract obstruction by mineral-protein calculi. Urolithiasis in cattle produces losses from death and from condemnation of carcasses contaminated by urine. One estimate places the loss to the United States cattle industry at approximately 0.6 per cent of annual production.[1]

Castrated male ruminants between 5 and 18 months old are primarily affected by urinary calculi and fall into 2 main classes: (1) feedlot animals with grain as a high percentage of their diets and (2) pastured animals grazing grasses high in silicates.[1,2] Swine are rarely afflicted with urolithiasis, although the condition is sporadically found in all ages and types of hogs. Older swine occasionally are found with calculi located in the renal pelvis.[3]

Treatment of urolithiasis involves restoration of urinary flow, repair of damaged and contaminated tissues with time, and, in most cases, salvage of the animal. Total recovery of normal urinary excretory and reproductive functions after treatment for urolithiasis is possible but not the rule; therefore slaughter is often the most cost-effective course of action.

PATHOGENESIS

Urolithiasis develops in ruminants as a result of mineral precipitation and binding onto an organic matrix, concretion of the crystallized matrix into uroliths, and partial or total occlusion of the ureter or urethra by the urolith.[4] The proteinaceous matrix that serves as a nidus for mineral crystallization can be desquamated epithelial cells or other urinary tract cellular and organic debris. This debris may collect as a result of inflammation, infection, and parenteral administration or ingestion of exogenous estrogenic substances that promote hypertrophy and keratinization of secondary sex glands, such as diethyl stilbestrol. Higher levels of mucoproteins in the urine associated with rations high in concentrates and low in roughages may act as a cementing factor that enhances calculus formation.[4]

Male ruminants are predisposed to calculosis because their urethral diameter is smaller than that of females. Although urolithiasis occurs in intact bulls and rams,[2,5,6] males castrated as young animals are more at risk because their urethral diameter does not develop as fully owing to their lack of exposure to androgens. Urolithiasis rarely occurs in females, although there are reported cases of female calves with ruptured bladders resulting from calculi.[7] Ureterolithiasis has been reported in a mature cow as a sequel of nephrolithiasis.[8]

Interactions of several dietary and physiologic factors determine the type of urinary calculi that are formed by ruminants. Urine pH is a major determining factor of calculus composition. Acid urine promotes the formation of silicate, oxalate, and xanthine calculi. Alkaline urine favors the formation of calcium and magnesium phosphates and carbonates, triple phosphates (calcium, ammonium, and magnesium phosphate calculi), and iron carbonate.[3] Normal urine pH of ruminants is 7.0 to 9.5.[3,9] When urine pH increases to the 8.5 to 9.5 range, calcium carbonate and phosphate crystals begin to precipitate.[3,9] As pH rises, urine colloids lose their ability to behave as a protective gel, and mineral precipitation, particularly phosphates and carbonates, is facilitated.[4]

Diet is another main determinant of the type of urinary calculi that may develop. Feedlot cattle and sheep on grain-based feedlot rations that are high in phosphorus tend to develop phosphate (calcium, ammonium, and magnesium) calculi. Cattle on western United States range pastures with grasses high in silica tend to form silicious calculi.[1] Carbonates (calcium, ammonium, and magnesium) tend to be the predominant calculi formed in the urine of grazing animals when grass silica concentrations are not high, such as on clover pastures and with plants high in oxalates.[3,4] Oxalate calculi in steers on feed have been associated with fescue (*Festuca* spp.) seed screenings in the diet.[10] Xanthine calculi have been reported in sheep in New Zealand but are not common in the United States.[4] Elevated dietary magnesium has been experimentally shown to cause urolithiasis in growing male calves.[11]

Management factors can contribute to the incidence of urolithiasis. Water deprivation from frozen pumps or tanks can cause relative concentration of urinary mineral solutes and increase the likelihood of their precipitation. Dehydration in times of drought can also promote urolithiasis by urinary concentration. Estrogenic implants and vitamin A deficiency have also been implicated.[4] The estrogenic substance implicated was diethyl stilbestrol (DES) in at least one report of a high incidence of fatal urolithiasis.[4] The risk of calculosis is not reported to be high from estrogenic implants in approved usage after the banning of DES. The considerable economic advantage in feed conversion and weight gain these implants offer to stocker and feeder steers offsets any slight increase in risk that might be associated with them.

The gross appearance of calculi differs depending on their predominant chemical composition. Phosphatic calculi tend to be numerous and very small, forming a gritty urinary "sludge."[3] These calculi are often noticed as "grit" or "sand" on the preputial hairs of male cattle, sheep, or goats. These calculi are smooth and have a softer consistency than do silicate calculi.[12] Silicious calculi tend to be single and form rough, hard, white stones of 4 to 7 mm.[3,12]

The course of urolithiasis depends on the location and degree of urinary tract occlusion. Uroliths can be present in the kidney, urine, bladder, or urethral mucosa without necessarily causing obstruction of urinary outflow. Nephroliths do not usually cause clinical problems unless portions of the stone are passed, resulting in ureteral obstruction and hydronephrosis.[4, 8, 12] Clinical disease occurs when urinary outflow is significantly obstructed, which usually occurs when a calculus lodges in the urethra.[12] Predilective sites of entrapment in the urethra are the ischial arch, the proximal flexure of the penis, and the urethral orifice. In small ruminant males, the urethral process is often the site of obstruction.

CLINICAL SIGNS

Clinical signs accompanying partial occlusion of urinary outflow are uneasiness, signs of abdominal pain, stranguria, dribbling urine, and hematuria. The urethra at the point of calculus obstruction often becomes inflamed and swollen, further decreasing the size of the lumen and exacerbating the occlusion. With total occlusion, the animal displays signs of colic, teeth grinding, rear leg stamping, circling motion of the tail, and decreased feed consumption.[1, 13] Rectal palpation may reveal a pulsating urethra and distention of the bladder.[1] Cystourethrography has been utilized as a diagnostic tool for differentiation of urolithiasis from cystitis in small ruminants;[14] however, this technique is probably only applicable in referral institutions.

DIAGNOSIS

Within 48 hours after a total obstruction of the lower urinary tract, a rupture of the bladder or urethra will likely occur. These animals will have a distended abdomen ("waterbelly") with a transmitted fluid wave apparent on ballottement. The differential diagnosis includes bloat, ascites, pneumonia, peritonitis, and pneumonia. Azotemia will develop over a period of days, with coma and death as the sequelae.[4] If the urethra ruptures, the subcutaneous tissues of the ventral abdomen become infiltrated with urine, especially in the preputial region. The differential diagnosis includes penile hematoma and preputial abscessation.[13] Necrosis and sloughing of the skin over these areas will occur if the animal does not die sooner, with drainage of urine from the deeper tissues resulting in a more prolonged course of disease.[4] Serum urea nitrogen concentrations in cases of bladder or urethral rupture have been reported up to 200 mg/dl.[12]

TREATMENT

Treatment of urolithiasis depends on the type of animal affected, the type of calculi, and the stage of the disease. Clients will often desire more aggressive treatment of intact males they value as sires, despite a relatively poor prognosis in more advanced cases. A reasonable course of action in feedlot steers or wethers in early stages of clinical urolithiasis is immediate slaughter before bladder or urethral rupture. This salvages the animal and reduces costs of surgery and treatment, which is prudent in light of likely recurrence of multiple phosphatic calculi in animals on feedlot diets.[12] After bladder or urethral rupture with urine infiltration of the ventral abdominal region, relief of the obstruction is necessary to relieve azotemia and acidosis. Tissue repair allowing the tissues to become edible may then occur, and the animal may be salvaged, which may take several weeks.[12]

If the urethral process of wethers, rams, or bucks is the site of obstruction, it may easily be amputated with scissors or a blade. This will sometimes relieve the obstruction, although in feedlot animals the calculi are often multiple and may also be lodged in other sites. Removal of calculi through retrograde passage of a catheter from the glans penis is not usually successful in male goats and sheep because the urethral diverticulum present at the level of the ischial arch precludes passage of normal catheters past that point.[6] The urethral diverticulum has been successfully avoided by the use of a pre-curved catheter utilized for retrograde cystourethrography.[14] Repair of a ruptured bladder was accomplished in a ram through celiotomy with intraoperative normograde urethral flushing with a catheter through the bladder rupture before it was repaired.[6] In this fashion, the ram was preserved as a breeding animal. Economic considerations preclude this treatment in most small ruminants, however.

If urethral obstruction can be relieved, a ruptured bladder will often heal without surgical repair. Ischial urethrotomy and catheterization has been an effective method of obstruction removal. Catheters inserted through ischial urethrotomy incisions have been installed to drain near the urethrotomy site[15] or passed into the bladder with the other end inserted distad along the urethra to emerge and drain at the prepuce.[12] The latter method is preferred in bulls whose continued breeding ability is desired. In that case, the catheter can be removed after several days when normal urinary function is restored. The former method is suitable for salvage of animals for slaughter. In a similar fashion for salvage, an ischial approach can be utilized for penile amputation and suturing of the penile stump to the skin.[12] After ischial urethrostomy in animals desired to be kept as pets, such as some small ruminants, long-term success has not been favorable.[16] The lack of long-term success in most small ruminant cases has prompted the recommendation they not be kept longer than 3 to 4 months.[17]

Stone removal at the proximal sigmoid flexure of the penis can be accomplished through a prescrotal approach in a laterally recumbent animal. In some cases, use of a Bachus towel clamp to crack the stone will allow the pieces to pass. If this fails after 1 or 2 attempts, then a urethrotomy over the site of obstruction should be done.[12] This method may also allow a breeding bull to be preserved as a sire.

PREVENTION

Successful prevention of urolithiasis may be accomplished through dietary management. In feedlot steers on high-phosphorus diets, increased feeding of calcium can prevent calculosis.[18, 19] Calcium to phosphorus ratios of 1.2:1 are normally recommended by the National Research Council, but increasing the ratio up to 2:1 in cattle and up to 2.5:1 in sheep has been advocated as anti-calculogenic.[4, 20] Mineral supplementation in sheep is more successful mixed in the feed than if offered free choice.[20]

Adding up to 4 per cent salt (NaCl) to the feedlot ration has been effective in steers and lambs as a method of increasing urine volume in the presence of adequate drinking water.[4, 20] The urine diluting effect of salt may also be used as a preventive in cattle grazing high-silica grasses. It has been recommended that calves be creep-fed with a high-salt supplement during the last 60 days before weaning by starting out with a salt-free supplement and gradually increasing to one with 12 per cent salt.[4]

Lowering the urine pH by feeding urine acidifiers such as ammonium chloride has been effective. Recommendations for daily amounts range from 7.1 to 10 g to sheep and 45 g to steers.[4, 20]

Managers should always be aware of the role of a reliable source of palatable water at all times in the prevention of calculosis. This is particularly critical in cold weather because of the danger of a freeze.

REFERENCES

1. Jensen R, Mackey DR: Diseases of Feedlot Cattle, 3rd ed. Philadelphia, Lea & Febiger, 1979, pp 262–267.
2. Ogaa JS, Agumbah GJO, Patel JH, et al: Massive obstructive urolithiasis in a bull used for artificial insemination. Vet Rec 117:664–666, 1985.
3. Jubb KFV, Kennedy PC: Pathology of Domestic Animals, 2nd ed. New York, Academic Press, 1970, pp 322–326.
4. Blood DC, Radostits OM, Henderson JA: Veterinary Medicine, 6th ed. London, Baillière Tindall, 1983, pp 360–366.
5. Murray MJ: Urolithiasis in a ram. Compend Contin Educ 7:S269–S273, 1985.
6. Tulleners EP, Hamilton GF, Farrow CS: Surgical repair of ruptured urinary bladder in a ram. J Am Vet Med Assoc 177:708–709, 1980.
7. Gera KL, Nigam JM: Urolithiasis in bovines. Indian Vet J 56:417–423, 1979.
8. Divers TJ, Reef VB, Roby KA: Nephrolithiasis resulting in intermittent ureteral obstruction in a cow. Cornell Vet 79:143–149, 1988.
9. Sorensen DK: Urinary system. In Amstutz HE (ed): Bovine Medicine and Surgery, 2nd ed. Santa Barbara, CA, American Veterinary Publications, 1980, pp 841–846.
10. Waltner-Toews D, Meadows DH: Urolithiasis in a herd of beef cattle associated with oxalate ingestion. Can Vet J 21:61–62, 1980.
11. Kallfelz FA, Ahmed AS, Wallace RJ, et al: Dietary magnesium and urolithiasis in growing calves. Cornell Vet 77:33–45, 1986.
12. Walker DF: Surgery of the urinary tract. In Walker DF, Vaugahn JT (eds): Bovine and Equine Urogenital Surgery. Philadelphia, Lea & Febiger, 1980, pp 59–66.
13. Powe TA: Diseases of the urinary system. In Howard J (ed): Current Veterinary Therapy—Food Animal Practice 2. Philadelphia, WB Saunders, 1986, pp 816–818.
14. van Weeren PR, Klein WR, Voorhout G: Urolithiasis in small ruminants II. Cysto-urethrography as a new aid in diagnosis. Vet Q 9:79–83, 1987.
15. Winter RB, Hawkins LL, Holterman DE, et al: Catheterization: an effective method of treating bovine urethral calculi. Vet Med December 1987, pp 1261–1268.
16. van Weeren PR, Klein WR, Voorhout G: Urolithiasis in small ruminants I. A retrospective evaluation of urethrostomy. Vet Q 9:76–79, 1987.
17. Oehme FW, Tillmann H: Diagnosis and treatment of ruminant urolithiasis. J Am Vet Med Assoc 147:1331–1339, 1965.
18. National Research Council: Nutrient Requirements of Beef Cattle, 6th ed. Washington, DC, National Academy Press, 1984.
19. Huntington GB, Emerick RJ: Oxalate urinary calculi in beef steers. Am J Vet Res 45:180–182, 1984.
20. Pierson RE, Kimberling C: Commercial lamb feedlot management. In Howard J (ed): Current Veterinary Therapy—Food Animal Practice 2. Philadelphia, WB Saunders, 1986, p 179.

Urinary Disorders Associated with the Neonate

RICHARD F. RANDLE, DVM, MS

CONGENITAL DEFECTS

The occurrence of congenital anomalies associated with the urinary system in ruminant species is rare. Often congenital defects are multiple and are associated with more than one body system. A variety of urinary system defects have been recorded and include hydronephrosis, polycystic kidneys, renal dysgenesis, renal agenesis, hypospadias, ectopic ureter, and patent urachus.

Patent Urachus

At birth, the urachus should close rapidly in association with rupture of the umbilical cord. Situations that cause delayed or incomplete closure of the urachus can result in this condition. Congenital patent urachus in ruminants is rare; however, infections of other umbilical structures or the urachus itself may result in incomplete closure and lead to an acquired patent urachus after birth. Aggressive manipulation of the umbilical cord at parturition may predispose to an acquired patent urachus.

Patent urachus is most often diagnosed by direct visualization of urine dripping from the urachus or a persistently wet umbilical stump. Retrograde or intravenous contrast radiography may also be used as an aid in diagnosing a patent urachus.

The usual therapy is surgical removal of the entire urachus. The associated arteries and veins are typically ligated and removed as well. A common sequela of a patent urachus is cystitis secondary to ascending infections; therefore systemic antimicrobials are indicated. Conservative therapy may be considered and consists of medical management of infection and cauterization of the urachus with such agents as silver nitrate, iodine, or phenol. A potential problem exists with this therapy in that cauterization of the urachus at the umbilical stump may trap organisms higher up in the urachus and lead to infection and urachal abscessation necessitating surgery later.

Polycystic Kidneys

The most commonly reported congenital defect seen in most species is polycystic kidneys. Typically, the condition is unilateral, and no clinical signs appear because of compensation by the other kidney. If the defect is extensive and bilateral, the animal is usually stillborn or dies in the perinatal period. Often other congenital anomalies are found in these animals.

Most often this condition is reported as a finding at necropsy. The affected kidney is enlarged and composed of either a few large cysts or numerous small cysts. A grossly enlarged kidney may be encountered on rectal examination in adult large ruminants. Ultrasonography may aid in the diagnosis of polycystic kidneys.

Renal Oxalosis

Renal oxalosis results from excessive deposition of calcium oxalate crystals in the glomeruli, tubules, and collecting ducts. This condition has been described in aborted fetuses and neonatal calves that have not been exposed to a known oxalate source. Calves with renal oxalosis have a frequent occurrence of cardiac and musculoskeletal defects such as arthrogryposis, osteopetrosis, and chondrodysplasia, which suggests a metabolic disorder involving glycine.

Hypospadias

Hypospadias has been recorded most commonly in small ruminants. The condition is found to be associated with hermaphroditism in goats. It has also been reported as a finding along with other congenital defects in newborn lambs.

OMPHALITIS

Inflammation of the umbilical arteries, umbilical vein, urachus, or surrounding tissues is termed omphalitis. These structures combine to form the umbilicus, which represents the vestige of the fetal maternal connection. The umbilical vein, which carries oxygenated blood from the placenta to the fetus via the liver and ductus venosus, becomes the round ligament of the liver. The two umbilical arteries, which carry waste materials from the fetus to the placenta, become the round ligaments of the bladder. The remnant of the urachus becomes incorporated into the apex of the bladder.

Pathogenesis

At parturition, the umbilical arteries retract into the abdomen and close by smooth muscle contraction in response to increased partial pressure of oxygen in the blood while the umbilical vein and urachus remain outside of the abdomen. The vein closes rapidly by smooth muscle contraction, and the urachus shrinks and dries within a few days.

Of the umbilical structures, the urachus is the most commonly infected in calves, with *Actinomyces pyogenes* being the most commonly identified organism involved. *Escherichia coli*, *Proteus*, *Enterococcus*, *Streptococcus*, and *Staphylococcus* species have also been identified as causative agents; therefore antimicrobial therapy should be based on culture results.

Clinical Signs

Clinical signs associated with omphalitis may be varied. Usually the animal is presented with a history of purulent drainage from the umbilicus at 1 to 2 weeks of age. The umbilicus may be enlarged, firm, hot, and painful on palpation. In approximately 25 per cent of the cases, there is an associated umbilical hernia. The animals may have concurrent systemic infections such as bacteremia, septic arthritis, pneumonia, diarrhea, uveitis, or peritonitis. Some animals show no evidence of drainage or inflammation at the umbilicus but are febrile, appear depressed, and are tender in the abdomen on palpation. Other clinical signs include dysuria, pollakiuria, and cystitis as a result of direct communication between the urachus and the bladder or interference with filling and emptying of the bladder.

Diagnosis

Infections of the umbilicus are easily identified in the presence of a draining tract or enlarged umbilicus. For determining the extent of urachal involvement, a metal probe or radiopaque contrast material can be placed in the draining tract and radiographs taken. Radiographic findings include a cranioventrally positioned bladder and a radiopaque structure ventral to the bladder. Deep palpation above the umbilicus with the animal either standing or in lateral recumbency may reveal an abdominal mass or painful areas. Ultrasonography may also be used as an aid in determining the involvement of the various umbilical structures. Omphalitis should be considered in neonates with a normal appearing umbilicus but that are unthrifty or have a fever of unknown origin.

Treatment

The treatment of choice is exploratory laparotomy and surgical excision of the abscesses. Urachal infections extending into the bladder require excision of the apex of the bladder and ligation of the umbilical arteries. In the absence of systemic involvement, prognosis is good, and recovery is usually uneventful.

Prevention

The control of umbilical infections centers on good sanitation and hygiene at parturition. The use of astringents and disinfectants on the umbilicus at birth is widely practiced, but there is limited evidence that this is of significant benefit.

BIBLIOGRAPHY

Baxter GM: Umbilical masses in calves: diagnosis, treatment, and complications. Compend Contin Educ 11:505–513, 1989.

Dennis SM: Urogenital defects in sheep. Vet Rec 105:344–347, 1979.
Fetcher A: Renal disease in cattle. Part I. Causative agents. Compend Contin Educ 7:S701–S708, 1985.
Smith BP: Large Animal Internal Medicine. St. Louis, CV Mosby, 1990, pp 370–372.
Trent AM, Smith DE: Surgical management of umbilical masses with associated umbilical cord remnant infections in calves. J Am Vet Med Assoc 185:1531–1534, 1984.

Renal Toxicants
DENNIS J. BLODGETT, DVM, PhD

Primary renal toxicoses in food animal veterinary medicine occur relatively infrequently. Oak toxicosis is by far the most common renal toxicosis diagnosed and is discussed in some detail. Other primary renal toxicants are listed in tabular form according to the species that are most likely affected (Tables 1 to 3). Toxicants capable of producing secondary renal lesions are also listed in these tables. Therapeutic drugs associated with renal problems in food animals are discussed in another section.

OAK POISONING

Occurrence

More than 60 species of oak *(Quercus)* are found in North America. Oak species range from shrubs to large trees and are classified as either white or black oaks. The acorns of white oaks mature in 1 year, whereas the black oaks require 2 years for acorn development. The species of oak does not vary the clinical syndrome. All species of oak should be considered toxic.

Oak toxicoses occur as seasonal problems. In the southwestern United States, shin oak *(Q. harvardi)* and Gamble's oak *(Q. gambelli)* cause problems in the spring of the year when new buds and leaves are heavily ingested. Much of the rest of the United States has problems in the fall when animals ingest acorns. More cases occur after summer droughts when forage is scarce or heavy rains dislodge acorns. Cases in the fall usually cease several weeks after the first hard frost. Young buds and acorns have a higher tannin concentration than do mature leaves and are more palatable.

Oak poisoning affects cattle primarily, although sheep and goats are also susceptible. Calves seem more susceptible than are adult cattle. Swine are fairly resistant to oak poisoning. Oak poisoning has a low-moderate morbidity with a moderate-high case mortality of approximately 35 to 80 per cent.

Toxic Principle

Tannin or its metabolites are believed to be the toxic components of oak buds and acorns. Most of the tannin content of acorns resides in the shell. Tannin is a gallotannin that is hydrolyzed in the rumen to gallic acid and pyrogallol. Gallic acid is a polyhydroxyphenol compound capable of precipitating proteins. Pyrogallol is a glucose ester to which several gallic acid moieties are bound. Pyrogallol, unlike gallic acid, is incapable of precipitating proteins, although it has a higher oral toxicity in rabbits than does either gallotannin or gallic acid. Rabbits dosed with tannic acid (gallotannin), gallic acid, or pyrogallol developed lesions similar to those of cattle poisoned by oak. Lesions were not evaluated histologically,

Table 1. BOVINE NEPHROTOXICANTS

Source	Epidemiology	Clinical Signs	Pathology	Comments
Oak (*Quercus* spp.)	See text	See text	See text	See text
Soluble oxalates	See Table 2	See Table 2	See Table 2	See Table 2; much fewer reports in cattle than in sheep owing to management differences
Redroot pigweed (*Amaranthus retroflexus*)	Found throughout US; onset 3–7 days; drylot or pasture exposure to large quantities of the plant in summer to early fall	See Table 3	See Table 3	Unknown toxicant; gross and histologic lesions inseparable from those of oak toxicosis
Cantharidin (blister beetles, *Epicauta* spp.)	Toxic blister beetles throughout US; primary problems in crimped alfalfa hay from the southwest (i.e., OK, TX, AK, KS); onset time few hours; morbidity and mortality very dependent on dose of blister beetles	Salivation, lacrimation, urination, defecation, anorexia, rumen atony, pollakiuria, colic, shock, hematuria	Increased packed cell volume, leukocytosis, hypocalcemia, increased serum urea nitrogen and creatinine, hematuria, decreased urine specific gravity; esophageal and gastrointestinal hyperemia and ulceraton, pale swollen kidneys, congested and hemorrhagic ureters and bladder; tubular degeneration/necrosis	Rare toxicant in cattle
Ochratoxin	Rare mycotoxin of grain or grain silage (e.g., wheat, barley, sorghum, corn, rye and oats); see Table 3 for onset, morbidity, and mortality	Depression, anorexia, diarrhea, dehydration	Hyperphosphatemia, hypocalcemia, increased serum urea nitrogen; perirenal edema, enteritis; see Table 3 for histopathologic findings	3 cases reported in IA and WY; silages containing 1–6 ppm ochratoxin A
Bovine Toxicants Producing Secondary Renal Lesions				
Lead	Variety of sources involved (e.g., grease, used motor oil, batteries, caulking, linoleum, paint chips, silage contaminated with soil of high lead concentration); onset times of 2 days to several weeks depending on availability and dose; morbidity low-moderate, mortality moderate-high	Depression, blindness, anorexia, rumen atony, colic, constipation or diarrhea, bruxism, ataxia, hyperirritability, muscle tremors, convulsions possible	Blood lead >0.35 ppm; lead source sometimes still visible in digestive tract; brain edema, cerebral congestion, laminar cortical necrosis; gastroenteritis, hepatocyte degeneration and necrosis, proximal tubule degeneration and necrosis, thickening and hyalinization of glomerular capsules; possible acidophilic intranuclear inclusions in hepatocytes and tubular epithelium	Common toxicosis in cattle; primary systems affected are central nervous system and gastrointestinal; blindness is reversible, convulsions are more likely with very bioavailable lead sources (e.g., grease); see CNS toxicant section for treatment
Arsenic (inorganic)	Variety of sources (as found in some herbicides, rodenticides, and insecticides and in ashes of treated wood); onset <24 hours; morbidity low-high, mortality high	Weakness, trembling, ataxia, depression, colic, rumen atony, diarrhea, prostration; course of disease: hours to several days	Hyperemia of abomasum and sometimes duodenum, petechiae of GI serosa, congestion of liver, kidneys and lungs; edema and necrosis in mucosa and submucosa of abomasum and duodenum, hepatic and proximal tubular degeneration and necrosis	Fairly common bovine toxicosis, primarily a gastrointestinal syndrome; cattle attracted to salty taste of arsenic salts; many cases die before diarrhea is evident; herbicide-treated foliage retains its toxicity
Zinc	Environmental contamination or misformulation of diet; milk replacer implicated previously; chronic toxicosis has onset time >2 weeks; high morbidity, low-moderate mortality	Pica, anorexia, diarrhea, bloat, polydipsia possible	Possible anemia and hemolysis, ulcers in abomasum, enteritis and congestion of small intestine, possible pale and shrunken kidneys; degeneration and necrosis of pancreatic acinar cells, degeneration and necrosis of proximal tubular epithelium, cast formation possible; hepatocyte necrosis	Infrequent bovine toxicosis, primarily a gastrointestinal syndrome; dietary concentrations >700 ppm toxic especially for young animals
Bracken fern (*Pteridium aquilinum*)	Found in forested areas throughout US; onset time 1–3 months; onset several weeks after removal of source possible; morbidity usually low, mortality high	Depression, rough coat, anorexia, hemorrhagic diarrhea, elevated temperature (104–109° F), hematuria, epistaxis; course of disease: 1–4 days	Leukopenia, thrombocytopenia, anemia (late); petechiae, ecchymoses, and frank hemorrhage throughout body organs and within body cavities; hypoplasia of bone marrow, possible hyperplasia/carcinoma of urinary bladder epithelium	Infrequent bovine toxicosis, primarily a bleeding syndrome in cattle; plant is toxic green or dry; unknown radiomimetic toxin

Table 2. OVINE AND CAPRINE NEPHROTOXICANTS

Source	Epidemiology	Clinical Signs	Pathology	Comments

Soluble oxalates
  Halogeton (*Halogeton glomeratus*)
  Greasewood (*Sarcobatus vermiculatus*)
  Curly dock (*Rumex crispus*)
  Rhubarb (*Rheum rhaponticum*)
	Most problems due to sodium oxalate in halogeton found in arid regions of western US (i.e., NV, UT, ID, WY and CO); halogeton is found along roadsides and other disturbed areas, produces acute toxicosis within a few hours of ingestion; high morbidity and mortality possible	Tachypnea, dyspnea, depression, frothing, incoordination, prostration, rumen atony with bloat, coma, tetany, and convulsions possible; course of disease: 1–48 hrs	Hypocalcemia; increase in serum urea nitrogen and aspartate aminotransferase; pale and swollen kidneys, hemorrhagic and edematous rumen wall, hyperemia of abomasal and intestinal mucosa, ascites; numerous calcium oxalate crystals in kidney tubules and rumen wall	Parenteral calcium administration will not prevent death; oxalates inhibit carbohydrate metabolism enzymes (i.e., lactic and succinic dehydrogenase); preventive measures include not driving hungry or thirsty animals past dense stands of halogeton and supplementing dicalcium phosphate

Oak (*Quercus* spp.)	See text	See text	See text	See text
Cantharidin	See Table 1	See Table 1	See Table 1	See Table 1; rare reports in sheep
Ovine Toxicants Producing Secondary Renal Lesions				
Copper	Chronic copper accumulation over weeks to months; sporadic occurrences in flock often associated with stress (i.e., vaccination, shipping, etc.); morbidity <10%, mortality >80%	Depression, anorexia, jaundice, prostration, hemoglobinuria, coma	Hemolysis, decreased packed cell volume, hemoglobinuria; mottled yellow-brown liver, icterus, enlarged spleen, coffee-colored urine, gun-metal–colored kidney; hepatic necrosis, hemoglobin casts in kidney tubules	One of most common ovine toxicoses, seen when dietary copper-molybdenum ratios >10:1; poor prognosis for treatment chelation with penicillamine

however. Lesions produced by tannic acid in rabbits were most like the lesions produced when rabbits were fed oak.

Because the exact toxic principle is unknown, the mechanism of action in oak toxicosis can only be hypothesized. One theory is that phenolic groups of gallotannin or gallic acid will bind to proteins in saliva, dietary components, digestive enzymes, or gastrointestinal epithelium. Binding of the phenolic compounds to epithelium has an astringent action. Bound phenolic groups that reach the abomasum may be released by the change in pH. The free phenolic compounds may be absorbed, causing further destruction of plasma proteins, endothelial cells, and renal tubular epithelium. Endothelial cell damage would promote fluid extravasation and edema. Damage to renal tubular epithelium would cause interstitial edema and increased back pressure of glomerular filtrate, yielding perirenal edema.

Deer are believed to be resistant to acorn poisoning because of a high concentration of proline in their saliva. Browsing animals in general have relatively larger salivary glands and higher concentrations of proline in the saliva than do grazers such as cattle and sheep. Tannin bound to proline is hypothesized to pass through the gastrointestinal tract unhydrolyzed. Goats, a partial browsing species, are more resistant than are cattle and sheep to oak poisoning.

Clinical Signs

Animals usually have ingested oak buds or acorns for 3 to 14 days (average 1 week) before clinical signs are apparent. The renal and gastrointestinal systems are predominantly affected. Initially the animal presents with anorexia, depression, and weakness. A mucous nasal discharge may be present. The rumen is atonic, and initially the animal is constipated with dark brown mucus-covered feces. Later in the course of the disease, black tarry diarrhea may develop. Animals are often gaunt and emaciated with an elevated lumbar spine. Ventral edema may be apparent anywhere from the jaw to the perineum. Polydipsia, polyuria, and dehydration may occur. Terminally, the animal is recumbent. Epistaxis has also been noted. The course of the disease usually ranges from 2 to 12 days, with 3 to 7 days being average.

Pathology

Anorexia, rumen atony, and renal damage produce many clinical pathologic abnormalities. Azotemia and increased serum creatinine are consistent findings with the ratio usually being 10:1 or greater. Hypochloremia is also a consistent finding as a result of trapping of chloride in an atonic gastrointestinal tract. Hyponatremia is also common owing to renal loss from decreased reabsorptive capability. Hypocalcemia results from decreased ingestion and an inverse relationship with phosphorus. The reason for hyperphosphatemia is poorly understood, because the kidney plays only a minor role in phosphorus excretion in ruminants. Hypermagnesemia may be present from decreased elimination associated with decreased glomerular filtration. Magnesium serum concentrations greater than 3.5 mEq/L are usually prognosticators of death. A general trend toward hypokalemia is present in most animals because of decreased intake and increased salivary potassium excretion with concurrent hyponatremia under the influence of aldosterone. However, hyperkalemia has been noted in some of the more acute oak toxicoses. Alkalosis is more common than is acidosis, although acidosis is sometimes found in animals with severe diarrhea. The alkalosis is the result of a functional abomasal atony, which produces a sequestration of hydrochloric acid in the abomasum and forestomachs. Bicarbonate ions are substituted for chloride ions in circulation, causing an alkalosis. Sometimes plasma fibrinogen concentrations are elevated, especially in chronic cases. Prolonged plasma thromboplastin times are also noted. The urine specific gravity is less than 1.020 and is often in the isosthenuric range of 1.008 to 1.014. Proteinuria may also be present.

Necropsy findings also relate primarily to the gastrointestinal tract and the kidneys. The gastrointestinal tract may have congestion, hemorrhage, and ulceration. Ulceration is especially likely in the abomasum and small intestine. The subserosal area of the gastrointestinal tract may have petechial to

Table 3. PORCINE NEPHROTOXICANTS

Source	Epidemiology	Clinical Signs	Pathology	Comments
Redroot pigweed (*Amaranthus retroflexus*)	Found throughout US; onset 3–7 days after ingestion, primarily in confinement-raised swine turned into unused drylot in summer to early fall; morbidity 5–90%, mortality ≥75%	Initial incoordination, weakness, trembling, and knuckling of hindlegs; sternal recumbency, paresis, and flaccid paralysis; alert, good appetite, and normal temperature early; terminally coma, ventral edema, and distended abdomen; course of disease: approximately 48 hr	Hyperkalemia, increased serum urea nitrogen, increased creatinine; perirenal edema; pale, normal to small kidneys with subcapsular petechiae; thoracic and abdominal fluid accumulation; proximal tubular nephrosis, necrosis and dilation of distal and convoluted tubules, proteinaceous casts, oxalate crystals in tubules sometimes observed	Unknown toxicant; plant also contains soluble oxalates and nitrate; less common toxicosis than in years past with less access of swine to drylot; chronic cases possible
Vitamin D Cholecalciferol (vitamin D_3) Ergocalciferol (vitamin D_2)	Dose-dependent onset time of 2 days to several weeks; feed formulated >1000× too high; morbidity 75–100%, mortality ≤25%	Lethargy, emesis, anorexia; rough hair coat and lameness with more chronic problems; course of disease: 1 day to weeks	Hypercalcemia, hyperphosphatemia, hypermagnesemia, possible increase in serum urea nitrogen; hyperemic gastric mucosa; edematous, firm, and congested lungs; multifocal pinpoint pale spots in renal cortex; chronic cases with fractures of bones (esp. femurs and ribs); necrosis and mineralization in kidneys, gastric mucosa, lungs, heart, and small blood vessels of lungs and heart	Cumulative toxicant, vitamin D_3 more toxic than vitamin D_2; unclear whether mineralization is primarily dystrophic (secondary to necrosis) or metastatic; fairly uncommon toxicosis
Ochratoxins (esp. ochratoxin A)	Rare mycotoxin of grain (e.g., wheat, barley, sorghum, corn, rye, and oats); onset time 2 days to several weeks; morbidity may approach 100%, mortality usually <35%	Polydipsia, polyuria, decreased weight gain, enteritis, and anorexia (large doses)	Isosthenuria, proteinuria, increased serum urea nitrogen, possible increase in aspartate aminotransferase; pale and swollen kidneys, gastric and intestinal hyperemia; proximal tubular necrosis and dilation; chronically, renal interstitial fibrosis and glomerular sclerosis; possible intestinal mucosal, lymphoid, and hepatic necrosis	Feed concentrations >0.2 ppm toxic; toxin binds strongly to proximal tubules; $T_{1/2}$ in porcine approximately 3–5 days; few reported cases
Porcine Toxicants Producing Secondary Renal Lesions				
Cocklebur (*Xanthium strumarium*)	Found throughout US; onset 1–2 days after ingestion; primarily due to cotyledon ingestion in field in spring, sometimes due to seed contamination of feed	Depression, sternal recumbency, jaundice, enteritis, coma	Increased serum liver enzymes and bilirubin; mottling and possible enlargement of liver; hepatic necrosis and possible secondary kidney tubular necrosis with proteinaceous casts	Carboxyatractyloside is toxicant; few confirmed cases

ecchymotic hemorrhages. Acorns or oak foliage may or may not be present owing to the delay in onset time. Ventral subcutaneous edema may be severe. Often ascites and hydrothorax are present. The perirenal area is edematous and often tinged with blood. The kidneys are pale and normal to swollen in size with petechial subcapsular hemorrhages. At times, the liver may appear pale and mottled.

Histopathologic findings include coagulative necrosis of the proximal tubules forming acidophilic granular casts of epithelial and protein debris. Many tubules may be dilated in the cortical and medullary regions. Bowman's capsules may be normal or fluid-filled. Sometimes there is a swelling or thickening of capsular and glomerular epithelium. Chronic cases have mononuclear cell infiltrates and fibrous connective tissue production in the cortex.

Diagnosis

A tentative diagnosis of oak toxicosis is based on the presence of renal failure, compatible clinical signs, and evidence of oak bud or acorn consumption. Renal failure is diagnosed by the presence of azotemia or dehydration in conjunction with low urine specific gravity. Prognosis in individual cases correlates with return of appetite and decreases in creatinine and serum urea nitrogen. The prognosis is guarded at best, considering 2/3 to 3/4 of the kidney tubules are affected before increases in serum urea nitrogen and creatinine and a decreased urine specific gravity are seen.

Treatment

Therapy is aimed at restoration of renal perfusion, extracellular fluid volume, and rumen motility. Renal perfusion and severe dehydration should ideally be corrected by intravenous fluid administration. Deficits of sodium, chloride, and calcium electrolytes are expected. The trend in most cases is toward hypokalemia, although some individual animals have hyperkalemia. In lieu of laboratory electrolyte results, normal saline with added calcium and potassium should be used. Oral fluid therapy, although less efficacious, may be more practical in certain situations than is intravenous administration. Oral fluids should be balanced in electrolytes and preferably low in magnesium.

Rumen motility is often difficult to re-establish. Loss of rumen fermentation necessitates parenteral vitamin B supplementation and transfaunation. A high-quality legume forage should be made available for the herd with just a little grain supplement on the side. Animals that remain anorexic may benefit from oral propylene glycol to supplement their energy needs. Even with better-quality feed available, many animals will continue to seek out acorns.

Prevention

Preventive methods are more rewarding than are therapeutic attempts. A pelleted ration with 10 per cent calcium hydroxide (slaked lime) will partially prevent oak toxicosis when it is fed at the rate of 0.9 kg/head/day in calves and 1.8 kg/head/day in adult cattle during problem seasons. The mechanism of action is unknown. An untested method would be to supplement diets with feedstuffs high in proline (e.g., corn gluten meal, meat and bone meal, dehulled soybean meal) during these times. Certainly, pastures or ranges with less oak species should be utilized in the spring in southwestern United States and in the fall elsewhere in the country.

OTHER TOXICANTS

See Tables 1 to 3.

BIBLIOGRAPHY

Divers TJ, Crowell WA, Duncan JR, Whitlock RH: Acute renal disorders in cattle: a retrospective study of 22 cases. J Am Vet Med Assoc 181:694–699, 1982.
Dollahite JW, Pigeon RF, Camp BJ: The toxicity of gallic acid, pyrogallol, tannic acid, and *Quercus harvardi* in the rabbit. Am J Vet Res 23:1264–1266, 1962.
Fetcher A: Renal disease in cattle. Part II. Clinical signs, diagnosis, and treatment. Compend Contin Educ 8:S338–S345, 1986.
Kasari TR, Pearson EG, Hultgren DD: Oak (*Quercus garryana*) poisoning of range cattle in southern Oregon. Compend Contin Educ 8:F17–F29, 1986.
Kingsbury JM: Poisonous Plants of the United States and Canada. Englewood Cliffs, NJ, Prentice-Hall, 1964, pp 444–446.
Osweiler GD, Carson TL, Buck WB, Van Gelder GA: Clinical and Diagnostic Veterinary Toxicology, 3rd ed. Dubuque, IA, Kendall/Hunt Publishing Co, 1985.
Panciera RJ: Oak poisoning in cattle. *In* Keeler RF, Van Kampen KR, James LF (eds): Effects of Poisonous Plants on Livestock. New York, Academic Press, 1978, pp 499–506.
Robbins CT, Mole S, Hagerman AE, Hanley TA: Role of tannins in defending plants against ruminants: reduction in dry matter digestion? Ecology 68:1606–1615, 1987.
Spier SJ, Smith BP, Seawright AA, et al: Oak toxicosis in cattle in northern California: clinical and pathologic findings. J Am Vet Med Assoc 191:958–964, 1987.

Infectious Pyelonephritis and Pyelonephritis in Cattle
RICHARD F. RANDLE, DVM, MS

Pyelonephritis may occur in a number of ways including secondary to an ascending infection from the lower urinary tract, by spread from embolic nephritis of hematogenous origin, or as a result of specific infectious processes such as that caused by *Corynebacterium renale* in cattle. The most common route is secondary to ascending infections.

PATHOGENESIS

The primary factors involved in the development of pyelonephritis are the presence of infection in the urinary tract and the stagnation of urine allowing progression of the infection up the tract. Ureteral reflux from the bladder may be involved in the process. The infection ascends from the bladder via the ureters and invades the renal pelvis. Infection of the renal pelvis results in erosion of the papilla, necrotic debris in the renal pelvis, and a suppurative nephritis involving the tubular and interstitial structures of the affected lobes. The infection may be either unilateral or bilateral.

Corynebacterium renale and *Escherichia coli* are the organisms most commonly responsible. Other organisms involved include *Corynebacterium pilosum*, *Corynebacterium cystitidis*, and a number of gram-negative organisms. The *Corynebacterium* spp. are normal inhabitants of the skin and have shown the ability to adhere to bovine urinary bladder, vagina, and vulval epithelium. These organisms are also capable of survival in the environment for long periods of time. Transmission most likely results from direct manipulation of the urogenital tract. Venereal transfer is possible in light of the fact that these organisms have been isolated from the prepuce of healthy bulls.

CLINICAL SIGNS

Cattle affected with pyelonephritis typically exhibit hematuria, pyuria, dysuria, fever, and occasionally colic signs. The presence and severity of these signs can vary considerably early in the course of the disease. As the condition becomes chronic, gross urine abnormalities abate somewhat, and the animal exhibits more generalized signs of chronic disease including inappetence, loss of condition, and loss of production over a period of weeks.

Rectal examination may reveal thickening of the bladder wall and ureters. Affected kidneys may show enlargement, loss of lobulation, and pain on palpation. These changes are most easily detected in the left kidney. Ultrasonography may be used to detect involvement of the various structures. The right kidney is best imaged from the right paralumbar fossa, whereas the left kidney, ureters, and bladder are best imaged via rectal probe.

DIAGNOSTIC FINDINGS

Urinalysis findings include hematuria, pyuria, and bacteriuria. Culture of urine is necessary for confirming the causative agent. Blood evaluation usually indicates an inflammatory leukogram and an elevated fibrinogen. Evidence of azotemia or uremia is usually not present unless there is bilateral involvement or the animal is in the terminal stages of the disease.

NECROPSY FINDINGS

Major necropsy findings are confined to the urinary tract. The affected kidney appears grossly enlarged, and lobulations may appear less evident than normal. Necrotic areas on the surface of the kidney may be present. Abscesses and necrotic debris are evident in the renal pelvis. Affected ureters are thick-walled and contain blood, pus, and mucus. The bladder wall is thickened, and the mucosa is hemorrhagic, edematous, and possibly ulcerated.

TREATMENT AND PROGNOSIS

The treatment of choice in cases of *Corynebacterium* infection is penicillin. Prognosis, in most instances, is good provided therapy is instituted early and extensive structural damage to the urinary tract has not occurred. Infections caused by other organisms are best treated with antimicrobials on the basis of results of culture and sensitivity of urine.

Animals infected with *C. renale* require more aggressive therapy, and the prognosis in these animals is guarded. Treatment with procaine penicillin for an extended period of time (2 to 4 weeks) is recommended. Initial response to therapy may be good, but relapse is common, and clearing of the infection is difficult. In unilateral infections in valuable animals, a nephrectomy may be warranted provided the functional ability of the other kidney is established.

Adjunct therapy should include intravenous fluid therapy in severely affected patients. Animals should be encouraged to drink plenty of fresh water for maintaining or increasing urine output to clear the urinary tract of debris and organisms. Availability of salt will aid in increasing thirst and ensuring adequate water intake. Urinary acidifiers have been used and may be of value in the treatment of pyelonephritis. The adhesive abilities of *Corynebacterium* have been shown to be pH-dependent, with less adhesion occurring in an acid pH. Ammonium chloride at 50 to 100 mg/kg twice daily has been recommended.

PREVENTION AND CONTROL

No specific control measures are advocated, but isolation of affected animals, removal of contaminated bedding, and careful hygiene associated with examination of the urogenital tract may reduce environmental contamination and transmission of the disease. Artificial insemination may be considered but, in most instances, is not economically justifiable.

BIBLIOGRAPHY

Blood DC, Radostits OM: Veterinary Medicine, 7th ed. London, Baillière Tindall, 1989, pp 399–400, 574–575.
Johnson R, Grymer J, Gerloff B, Dunstan R: Nephrectomy as treatment for pyelonephritis in a cow. Compend Contin Educ 6:S356–S359, 1984.
Smith BP: Large Animal Internal Medicine. St. Louis, CV Mosby, 1990, pp 888–889.
Takai S, Yanagawa R, Kitamura Y: pH-Dependent adhesion of piliated *Corynebacterium renale* to bovine bladder epithelial cells. Infect Immun 28:669–674, 1980.
Tulleners EP, Deem DA, Donawick WJ: Indications for unilateral nephrectomy: a report on four cases. J Am Vet Med Assoc 179:696–700, 1981.
Yanagawa R: Causative agents of bovine pyelonephritis: *Corynebacterium renale, C. pilosum, C. cystitidis. In* Pandy R (ed): Progress in Veterinary Microbiology and Immunology, vol 2. Basel, Kagar, 1986, pp 158–174.

Cystitis, Pyelonephritis, and Miscellaneous Diseases of Swine

RODERICK C. TUBBS, DVM, MS, Diplomate, ACT

CYSTITIS

Cystitis is an inflammatory condition of the urinary bladder. It appears to occur more frequently in the female, apparently because of the shorter urethra, compared with the male's, which predisposes the female to ascending urinary tract infections. Females are also predisposed to trauma of the urethra and anterior vagina at coitus and parturition, with many cases of cystitis in sows occurring after breeding and after farrowing. Solid-floored or solid-backed gestation crates have also been suggested as predisposing factors to cystitis in sows, because sows will often sit on the floor or come in contact with the back of the crate, allowing direct access to the lower urinary tract by fecal contaminants and other microorganisms. Other possible predisposing factors include decreased water intake, infrequent micturition, and incomplete emptying of the bladder at micturition. Feet and leg injuries, poor body conformation, poorly designed facilities, and systemic illness all may contribute to an unwillingness by the sow to stand, drink, and urinate frequently. Sows that urinate from the sitting or recumbent positions may fail to empty the bladder completely.

Clinically, cystitis is characterized by pollakiuria, dysuria, oliguria, and, depending on the severity of the individual case, variable amounts of hematuria, pyuria, and bacteriuria. Urethritis usually accompanies cystitis and may account for some of the pain, grunting, and straining seen in association with urination. The most consistent diagnostic sign associated with cystitis is the frequent passage of blood-stained, turbid urine.

Most of the organisms associated with cystitis in sows are normal inhabitants or contaminants of the vagina and vestibule. These include *Escherichia coli, Proteus mirabilis, Staphylococcus* spp., *Streptococcus* spp., *Klebsiella*, and enterococcus. A specific primary pathogenic organism that causes cystitis and pyelonephritis in swine (*Eubacterium suis*, formerly *Corynebacterium suis*) is discussed separately.

Laboratory tests for confirmation of a clinical diagnosis of cystitis include urinalysis for the presence of protein (a high level in the urine indicates inflammatory reaction in the urinary tract, if collection methods have precluded contamination from the lower genital tract) and inflammatory cells as well as culture of properly collected urine for the presence of microorganisms. One author has suggested that urine pH may be used as a diagnostic and prognostic indicator for urinary tract disease in the sow.[1] A slightly acid urine pH is considered normal. The pH is reported to be higher than 7.5 in problem herds, and in one survey, sows with urine pH of 8.5 or above frequently lost pregnancies, were culled, or died.

Necropsy lesions of cystitis include the expected components of the inflammatory response in acute cases: swelling, edema, hyperemia, and possibly hemorrhage of the mucosal surface of the bladder. The lesions progress in subacute and chronic cases, until the entire bladder wall becomes grossly thickened, and the mucosal surface is rough and coarsely granular.

Treatment of cystitis consists of systemic administration of appropriate antibiotics based on culture and sensitivity testing. Treatment should be continued for 7 to 14 days. In swine, treatment is often initiated with procaine penicillin at 22,000 to 33,000 IU/kg intramuscularly once or twice per day until the results of culture and sensitivity testing are available. It should be noted that this dosage is higher than the label indicates for penicillin in swine; therefore appropriate veterinary-client-patient relationships should exist, and extended withdrawal times for slaughter should be observed. More specific antibiotic therapy may be selected on the basis of laboratory findings. Ampicillin is preferred by some clinicians as initial treatment and should be administered at label dosages twice per day. Prognosis is fair to good if treatment is initiated early in the course of the disease, and guarded to poor if the disease has progressed to a more chronic condition before therapy is initiated.

PYELONEPHRITIS

Pyelonephritis is inflammation of the renal pelvis and kidney. It usually occurs secondary to cystitis as a continuation of an ascending urinary tract infection. It may also result from hematogenous origin.

Predisposing factors, early clinical signs, and organisms involved are similar to those described for cystitis, with the exception that by the time the infection has ascended to the kidneys, clinical signs may be more severe; and in addition to the hematuria and pyuria observed with cystitis, systemic signs such as depression, fever, inappetence, and weight loss may be a more profound part of the clinical presentation. As with cystitis, the frequent passage of blood-stained, turbid urine is the most reliable clinical evidence of pyelonephritis. renal function tests such as blood urea nitrogen may be beneficial in determining the extent of kidney damage due to pyelonephritis but will be elevated only when more than 75 per cent of the nephrons are nonfunctional.[2] At necropsy, mucosal lesions in the ureters and kidneys are similar to those described as occurring in the bladder with cystitis. Treatment for pyelonephritis is very similar to that for cystitis. The prognosis for pyelonephritis is much more guarded than that for cystitis.

Eubacterium suis

Eubacterium suis is a gram-positive anaerobic bacillus and is a specific pathogen affecting the urinary tract[3] and possibly the reproductive tract in female swine. Clinical signs are very similar to those caused by other organisms associated with cystitis and pyelonephritis, except that *E. suis* may cause severe illness with sudden onset and death within hours or days after the clinical signs are first noticed. Other cases may have a more protracted course such as that seen with cystitis and pyelonephritis caused by commensal or contaminant microorganisms.[3] *E. suis* has also been associated with a chronic course of disease known as the "thin-sow" syndrome. This syndrome must be differentiated from weight loss and emaciation associated with underfeeding, parasites, and other chronic diseases.

A major feature of *E. suis* in pigs is its association with the male.[4] The organism apparently is a common inhabitant of the lower urinary tract, particularly the preputial diverticulum, in male swine. Most boars are asymptomatic, but occasional hematuric episodes may be observed. The high rate of recovery of the organism from asymptomatic males and its association with clinical signs in females have been the basis of the suggestion that the organism is venereally transmitted. Proper handling of specimens (urine, preputial swabs), proper environmental conditions for culture, and the use of selective media are necessary to achieve good culture results.[3–5]

Treatment of *E. suis* can be effective if it is applied early in the course of the disease and for an appropriate length of time. Procaine penicillin at 22,000 to 33,000 IU/kg once or twice per day for 7 to 14 days is a commonly used antibiotic regimen. Extended slaughter withdrawal times should be used for the extra-label dosage. Ampicillin has also been used with good results and is the preferred treatment of some clinicians but needs to be administered twice per day. Response may be evident as early as 3 to 4 days after initiation of therapy if treatment is begun early in the course of the disease. As with other causes of cystitis and pyelonephritis, sanitation in the breeding and gestation areas is critical to control of *E. suis*. Penicillin and ampicillin injections have been used at the time of parturition and at the time of breeding as prophylactic measures in problem herds, with equivocal results. Chlortetracycline at 400 g/ton of feed for 2 weeks followed by 200 g/ton for another 4 to 6 weeks has been used as adjunctive therapy for both treatment and prevention. Because of the potential for venereal transmission of *E. suis*, flushing the boar's preputial cavity with chlorhexidine, tetracycline, or other antibiotics has been attempted in an effort to prevent cystitis and pyelonephritis in sows. Positive treatment results have been reported in some cases but may in fact be associated with a general increase in attention to sanitation, breeding, and management practices. Selective culling of suspected problem boars may be justified, particularly if individual boars cause excessive trauma with bleeding from the lower urogenital tract of the sow at mating.

MISCELLANEOUS DISEASE OF THE URINARY SYSTEM OF SWINE

Diseases of the urinary system other than cystitis and pyelonephritis are rarely diagnosed in swine, either because they are masked by the clinical signs of a primary disease or because they do not cause clinical signs unless extensive lesions are present, and even then it is often difficult or impossible to differentiate them from the more common conditions of cystitis and pyelonephritis. Other diseases or conditions that have been reported or could potentially occur in swine include renal ischemia, glomerulonephritis, nephrosis, hydronephrosis, interstitial nephritis, embolic nephritis, urolithiasis, and cystic kidneys. A more detailed discussion of these conditions can be found in the second edition of this text and in other standard reference textbooks.

BIBLIOGRAPHY

Blood DC, Radostits OM: Veterinary Medicine, 7th ed. London, Bailliére Tindall, 1989, pp 396–402, 575.
Jones JET: Urinary system. In Leman AD, et al (eds): Diseases of Swine, 6th ed. Ames, IA, Iowa State University Press, 1986, pp 162–167.
Jones JET: Corynebacterial infections. In Leman AD, et al (eds): Diseases of Swine, 6th ed. Ames, IA, Iowa State University Press, 1986, pp 619–621.
Powe TA: Diseases of the urinary system. In Howard JL (ed): Current Veterinary Therapy: Food Animal Practice 2, 2nd ed. Philadelphia, WB Saunders, 1986, pp 816–817.

REFERENCES

1. Muirhead M: Sow urine pH mortality key. Int Pigletter 9:43, 1990.
2. Duncan JR, Prasse KW: Veterinary Laboratory Medicine Clinical Pathology. Ames, IA, Iowa State University Press, 1977, p 115.
3. Walker RL, MacLachlan NJ: Isolation of *Eubacterium suis* from sows with cystitis. J Am Vet Med Assoc 195:1104–1107, 1989.
4. Pijoan C, Lastra A, Leman A: Isolation of *Corynebacterium suis* from the prepuce of boars. J Am Vet Med Assoc 183:428–429, 1983.
5. Dagnall GJR, Jones JET: A selective medium for the isolation of *Corynebacterium suis*. Res Vet Sci 32:389–390, 1982.

SECTION 15 ☐ ☐ ☐ ☐ ☐ ☐
Diseases of the Eye

CECIL P. MOORE, DVM, MS, Diplomate, ACVO, Consulting Editor

Ophthalmic Examination Techniques for Food and Fiber Animals

DANIEL M. BETTS, DVM, MS, Diplomate, ACVO

PRELIMINARY CONSIDERATIONS

An ophthalmic examination is indicated whenever a complete physical examination is warranted. In addition to those instances in which overt ocular or orbital disease symptoms occur, a thorough evaluation of the eyes, orbits, and periorbital areas should be done whenever systemic or generalized disease, regardless of its etiologic origin, is suspected. Because many systemic diseases have ocular manifestations, a thorough inspection of the eyes can be helpful in differentiating infectious, metabolic, toxic, neoplastic, and nutritional conditions. Prepurchase or soundness evaluation should include a thorough ophthalmic examination. Some special instrumentation and careful restraint are necessary, but neither should be an excuse for neglecting an ophthalmic examination. Correctly done, an ophthalmic examination should provide significant information leading to a more precise diagnosis and effective treatment. Taking time to examine the eyes routinely is not excessively time-consuming. It permits the veterinarian to practice the technique so it becomes easy and productive; it affords the opportunity to learn variations of normal appearances of eyes; and it leads to an appreciation of the variety of lesions that occur in the eyes of different species and breeds.

The reader is encouraged to consult recent veterinary ophthalmology texts for descriptions and interpretation of the abnormal findings that may be encountered in performing an ophthalmic examination. It is beyond the scope of this article to describe the spectrum of lesions that may be observed. Without a sound appreciation of the range of normal variations and the nature of pathologic changes in the eye, there is a great chance that disease, especially early signs of disease, will be overlooked or misinterpreted.

It is tempting to work without records in dealing with food animals, but keeping good records, including histories, can be invaluable for working with complicated problems or unresponsive or progressive disease conditions. Unfortunately, these are not always anticipated, so every case should be documented from the start. When multiple-person practices may be providing services by different doctors at different times, it may be imperative to keep complete records of history, findings, conclusions, treatment, and progress. Special forms may be helpful in organizing the examination, reminding the doctor of all the observations to be made and providing an easy method of rapidly recording the findings. Drawing and labeling a diagram of the lesions will facilitate record-keeping and later evaluation of progress.

GETTING THE HISTORY

When questioning animal owners or caretakers regarding the anamnesis, the clinician should make no assumptions. Details should be noted no matter how insignificant they may seem at the start. Begin with age, breed, sex, stage of gestation, and use of the animal if these are not obvious. Because the caretaker is usually eager to talk about the immediate problem, inquire about the initial symptoms and the changes that followed. Questions should be asked about the presence of pain, vision loss, and behavior changes. Ask caretakers for their ideas about the cause of the problem. Find out what has been done to treat the problem, if treatment changed the appearance of the eye, or if pain or vision status changed with treatment.

Because ocular problems can be caused by hereditary disorders, especially in purebred animals, ask about related animals having similar problems. Inquire about the ration of the animal and look at the feed if the appearance of the animal is not consistent with the described ration. Check the vaccination history, including products and dates; also ask about recent diseases of any kind in any of the animals of the herd or flock. Include questions about the environment (i.e., housing, bedding, air quality, stresses of temperature extremes and crowding), physical hazards including electricity, and exposure to potential toxins. Other questions may arise as the clinician proceeds with his or her examination. Questions should be asked in terms that can be readily understood by the caretaker, and questions should be avoided that imply a correct or preferred answer.

Historical information, even more than results of the examination, may indicate that other animals in the herd or flock have been involved or affected. Check other related or similarly managed animals even if the caretaker does not think others are affected.

INSTRUMENTS AND SUPPLIES FOR THE EXAMINATION

It is most convenient to carry ophthalmic instruments and supplies in a special box or grip for farm calls and have a specially designated place for them in the examination area of the hospital. If they are readily available, they are more likely to be used. In addition to the usual supplies of syringes, needles, cotton balls and gauze pads, and other personal choices for examination room supplies, the items listed in Table 1 are recommended.

INITIAL ASSESSMENT OF APPEARANCE AND VISION

With the animal free in its natural environment, look for evidence of either unilateral or bilateral blindness. An obstacle course with hay bales is useful. If monocular blindness is suspected, confirm it by patching the sighted eye. Note the carriage of the head and ears and the use of the nose for tactile as well as olfactory sensation. In addition to observing visual behavior, note the gross appearance of the head, face, and eyes. Look for evidence of abnormalities in the position and movement of the eyelids, periorbital swellings or depressions, and the amount and nature of any ocular discharges or periocular exudates. Check carefully the position, size, and prominence of the eyes relative to the lids and orbits. Note the position and movement of each nictitans. Compare the right and left sides for symmetry.

RESTRAINT FOR EYE EXAMINATION

Physical and chemical restraint for a close-up and detailed examination of the eyes is influenced by the needs of the veterinarian and the specific patient being examined. The least restraint that will allow safe and expedient completion of the task is preferred. A chute, stanchion or crate, and halter, nose lead, or snare, depending on the species, size, and temperament of the patient, may be required. Chemical restraint for all of the large mammals can be accomplished with xylazine* given intravenously. Because large ruminants tend to go recumbent with xylazine, physical restraint must allow for this possibility. Dosages are 0.025 to 0.22 mg/kg—only 10 per cent of the recommended equine dose! Therefore, the clinician must be careful not to overdose ruminants. It is prudent to have tolazoline or yohimbine available for reversing the effect of xylazine if necessary. A palpebral nerve block for preventing blepharospasm during the examination is usually not necessary when xylazine is used. Sedation may interfere with the animal's response to provocation of the palpebral, corneal, or menace reflexes, but the pupillary and oculocephalic reflexes are not hindered.

ASSESSMENT OF NEUROPHTHALMIC REFLEXES

The palpebral reflex is elicited by tapping the medial canthus with a fingertip. The ophthalmic branch of the trigeminal nerve (V) is the sensory nerve. The normal response is closure of the lids mediated by the facial nerve (VII) and retraction of the globe mediated by the abducens nerve (VI).

The corneal reflex is induced by touching the cornea. A safe technique is to touch the cornea with a strand of moistened cotton. The sensory and motor nerves as well as the anticipated response are the same as for the palpebral reflex.

A crude estimation of vision can be made by moving the hand vertically in front of the eye and observing a blink, retraction of the globe, or head movement. Absence of response to a menacing gesture may be related to retina or optic nerve dysfunction on the afferent side and lesions affecting the motor nerves discussed previously for palpebral and corneal reflexes. In addition, the examiner must be aware that air currents or contact with facial hair may lead to a false-positive response. Apathy, central nervous system depression, or sedation may lead to a false-negative response.

In moving the animal's head from side to side and up and down, the examiner may stimulate nystagmus with rapid eye movement in the direction of the head movement. Sensory input for the oculocephalic reflex begins in the semicircular canals of the inner ear and is conducted to the brain stem by the vestibular branch of the auditory nerve (VIII). The dorsal, ventral, and medial rectus muscles are innervated by the oculomotor nerve (III), and the lateral rectus muscle is innervated by the abducens nerve (VI).

The pupillary light reflex (PLR) is best evaluated in a darkened room or stall and requires a bright focal light source (dim penlights are unsatisfactory) directed through the pupil to the central fundus for at least a few seconds. Ruminants' pupils respond more slowly to light stimulation than do the pupils of dogs or cats. In comparison to ruminants, pigs' pupils respond relatively quickly. Closing the lids for several seconds and then releasing them to observe for pupillary dilation from the absence of light and then constriction with stimulation from room light is a poor test. A uniformly bright light pointed along the visual axis, from the same distance and for the same length of time in each eye, will allow a reasonable assessment of the magnitude of the response. The retina and optic nerve are the afferent origins of the reflex. Most PLR fibers decussate at the optic chiasm, continue in the contralateral optic tract, and exit into the midbrain.

The motor nerve to the iris sphincter is the parasympathetic

Table 1. INSTRUMENTS AND SUPPLIES RECOMMENDED FOR LARGE ANIMAL OPHTHALMIC EXAMINATION

Instruments
Magnifying head loupe with 2–2.25× power (Donnegan Optical Co, Kansas City, MO)
Ophthalmic diagnostic set with fiberoptic transilluminator and direct ophthalmoscope interchangeable heads on rechargeable battery handle (Welch-Allyn or Propper)
20 diopter aspheric lens (Welch-Allyn)
Dressing forceps, serrated tips, 6-inch
Nasolacrimal cannula, 20-gauge
I-slit (No. 2043, Concept)
Kimura spatula (Storz, V. Mueller, or Scanlon); a scalpel blade (back edge) may be substituted

Supplies
Eyewash: Dacriose (IO Lab, Division of Johnson & Johnson) or alternative formulation:
  Boric acid ½ oz
  Sodium bicarbonate ½ oz
  Sodium chloride ½ g
  Glycerin 2 oz
  Roccal conc. 10 drops
  Water qs to 1 gallon
Fluorescein-impregnated paper strips (Fluor-I-Strips, Ayerst)
Schirmer tear test strips (SMP Division, Cooper Laboratories)
  Alternative: #42 Whatman filter paper, cut strips 7.5 × 60 mm
Tropicamide (Mydriacyl, Alcon)
Proparacaine (Maurry Biological)
Culturette and Mini-tip Culturette (Becton Dickinson)
#3 Fr, #5 Fr, and #8 Fr open-end male urinary catheter
Lidocaine (Xylocaine, 2%, Astra)
Xylazine (Rompun, 100 mg/ml, Haver/Diamond)

All items, except the Kimura spatula, are available through most veterinary supply distributors.

---

*Xylazine is not approved for use in food animals. When it is used, milk must be discarded for several days and animals must not be slaughtered for several days after xylazine administration. Clearance times have not been determined.

nerve originating in the Edinger-Westphal nucleus adjacent to the oculomotor nerve nucleus. This parasympathetic nerve remains in close proximity to the oculomotor nerve until it enters the ciliary ganglion in the orbit. The postganglionic fibers diverge and enter the globe at multiple locations and pass into the iris. Because decussation occurs in as many as 3 locations on the afferent side, there is relatively equal distribution of the efferent impulse in the motor nerves to the iris of both eyes after stimulation of 1 fundus. This accounts for the indirect pupillary light response in the opposite eye. Owing to the closeness of the oculomotor nucleus to the Edinger-Westphal nucleus and the oculomotor nerve to the preganglionic parasympathetic nerve, it is quite unlikely that PLR abnormalities would originate in this portion of the reflex arc without concurrent abnormalities of ocular motility. Because the PLR is mediated at subcortical levels, a normal PLR does not imply that vision is present. The absence of a PLR does not imply blindness either, because the efferent side of the reflex, including the iris itself, may be defective but not interfere with vision.

Interpretation of deficits in the neurophthalmic reflexes must be made in conjunction with a complete ophthalmic examination in order to localize the lesion in the sensory tissue, the afferent or efferent nerves, the brain, or the end organ (e.g., the iris) in which the response should occur.

DETAILED EXAMINATION OF THE EYE

Once the animal is restrained, the veterinarian should review the gross appearance of the head, face, and eyes and the position and movement of the eyelids. Then with a general idea of the presence or absence of ocular, orbital, or periorbital lesions, a detailed examination should be initiated. The examiner should look before manipulations or palpation. In addition to closely observing the detailed appearance of problem areas already noticed, the examiner should also look for abnormalities in tissues that did not appear abnormal on initial assessment. Because small or subtle changes may be hard to see, the room lights should be dimmed to improve the contrast and to avoid glare. A magnifying head loupe and a bright uniform light such as a transilluminator should be used. The light is directed onto the eye from all angles to enhance shadows and contrasts.

As the examiner moves closer, he or she proceeds with a systematic examination beginning with the eyelids and continuing with the conjunctiva, nictitans, sclera, cornea, anterior chamber, iris, pupil, lens, and anterior vitreous. Each tissue of the eye is examined thoroughly. When the eye and orbit are examined, abnormalities of structure or function are noted, that is, changes in size, shape or contour, position and movement, color, clarity or transparency, texture, and reflectivity. Findings are described precisely and recorded.

It may be helpful to cut long tactile hairs from the eyelids before starting the examination. Touching them with a light source or fingers may provoke blepharospasm and resistance. As much as possible, the examiner should avoid touching the eyelids during the anterior segment examination. It is very difficult to hold open the eyelids of large ruminants especially if the eye is painful. Larger swine may be a challenge because the eyelids fold up beneath the bony orbital margin and are not accessible for manipulation. Small ruminants are fairly easily manipulated. The upper lid may be elevated most easily by placing the side of the thumb firmly near the margin of the lid and rolling the thumb upward as you press against the orbital rim. The lids should not be forced open or everted until the examiner is certain that there is not a deep corneal wound that might rupture if inadvertent pressure is applied to the globe. A topical anesthetic for relief of surface pain may be helpful in getting an animal to relax and open the lids. A palpebral nerve block may be necessary in order to proceed with the examination. Two to 5 ml of 2 per cent lidocaine injected subcutaneously along the dorsal margin of the zygomatic arch, beginning at the supraorbital process, will block the palpebral nerve and paralyze the orbicularis oculi muscle.

When exudates or the pathologic changes on the conjunctiva, cornea, or lids suggest that bacterial or fungal culturing may be productive, samples should be taken before any solutions to clean, dilate, or anesthetize are placed onto the conjunctiva. Gross debris should be wiped away from the lids with a clean, dry gauze pad or cotton ball. A commercial culturing system, such as the Culturette,* comes with an ampule of sterile transport medium. This ampule can be broken within the plastic tube to moisten the sampling swab, which improves efficiency in recovering microorganisms. The swab should be manipulated into the conjunctival sac without contacting the lids or lashes. The author believes that cultures from the dorsal conjunctival sac should yield significant pathogens, whereas the ventral cul-de-sac may contain other incidental bacteria.

Corneal ulcers should be cultured carefully with the moistened cotton tip rotated on the edge of the lesion. A Miniculturette* is easier to direct precisely with minimal risk to deep ulcers or descemetoceles. Laboratory personnel who inoculate the agar plates should be advised that the sample may be limited to the tip of the swab. In a hospital environment, culture media may be inoculated directly with tissue or debris scraped from a lesion, usually a corneal ulcer, with the edge of a Kimura spatula. Sterilization of the spatula may be accomplished in the flame of a disposable lighter. A Gram stain of a slide preparation may provide early information on the nature or the mix of the bacterial population so that appropriate antibacterials may be started before the culture and sensitivity results are available.

The lens, vitreous, and fundus are more easily viewed if the pupil is dilated. At the appropriate time, as early in the examination as possible, several drops of 1 per cent tropicamide are instilled into each eye. It will take 15 to 20 minutes to dilate the pupil for a view of the perimeter of the lens. Atropine is a poor drug to use to dilate a pupil for posterior segment examination. It may take an hour or more to dilate the pupil, and it will persist for 1 to several days. Although the size and shape of lens opacities may be determined with the transilluminator, a slit-beam light is optimal for this purpose. The biomicroscope is ideal, but a disposable I-slit light† is an excellent alternative. Slit-beam illumination is also useful in examining corneal thickness and locating opacities within the cornea and viewing exudates or flare in the anterior chamber. The depth of the anterior chamber is easily seen with the slit beam. The anterior vitreous is the deepest portion of the globe that can be examined clearly with the transilluminator and head loupe.

The direct ophthalmoscope is still the most commonly used instrument for examining the fundus. Ophthalmoscopes with nickel-cadmium rechargeable batteries and a halogen light bulb give a more consistent white light for true color viewing than do the older flashlight batteries and bulbs that yield a yellowish-white light. This instrument provides great magnification but a small field of view. Keeping both eyes open and working in a darkened room help the examiner avoid the distortion from involuntary accommodation. A viewing dis-

---

*Becton Dickinson, Franklin Lakes, NJ 07417–1883.
†Concept, 12707 U.S. Rte. 19 South, Clearwater, FL 33516.

tance of 1 to 2 inches with a lens setting of 0 to −2 D (diopters) is appropriate. The direct ophthalmoscope may also be used for a highly magnified view of surfaces in the anterior segment by use of different lens settings, that is, a +10 D for the iris and anterior lens capsule, and a +15 D or +20 D for the cornea or conjunctiva. The viewing distance is kept at 1 to 2 inches.

A preferable ophthalmoscopic technique, and a safer one for the examiner, is to perform monocular indirect ophthalmoscopy by holding the transilluminator at your cheek and directing the light into the patient's eye. With the other hand at arm's length, a 20 D aspheric lens is held 1 to 2 inches in front of the cornea. Focus is achieved by moving the lens slightly forward or back until the image of the fundus appears in the frame of this lens. The image is inverted, but with a little practice one will quickly adapt. The greater field of view allows a better perspective of the entire fundus. This technique of monocular indirect ophthalmoscopy is far superior to attempts to evaluate the fundus with the transilluminator alone, even if the head loupe is used.

A binocular indirect ophthalmoscope provides the best 3-dimensional view of the fundus but is expensive, and most are hampered by electric cords and attached transformer.

Ancillary diagnostic procedures are often indicated after the initial observations. The examiner should be careful not to do something that would interfere with another procedure. For example, bacteriostatic preservatives in anesthetic or mydriatic solutions will inhibit microbial growth in cultures. Therefore, culture samples should be taken before any solutions are applied to the eye. Because pupillary light reflexes are diminished or abolished after application of mydriatics, PLRs are checked before mydriatic instillation. Tearing may increase significantly after manipulation of the lids or conjunctiva; topical anesthetics will decrease reflex tearing and potentially decrease a Schirmer tear test value. Any fluids added to the eyes may enhance a Schirmer reading. Therefore, the Schirmer test should be performed first, if it is indicated. Ointments may cause a problem with the examination because they may obscure the view of intraocular structures.

Palpation of the lids and periorbital structures is important if there are swellings, filling defects, or exophthalmos. Retropulsion for determination of the presence of orbital masses or abscesses is accomplished by pushing the globe posteriorly with digital pressure on the upper eyelid. Intraocular pressure can be crudely estimated by placing the tips of the index fingers on the upper eyelid and depressing alternately with one, then the other finger, noting the indentability of the globe. Schiøtz tonometry does not work in large animals, but accurate intraocular pressures can be measured with more sophisticated instruments, such as the MacKay-Marg tonometer, Glaucotest, or Tonopen instruments. Because of their cost, these are generally used only by specialty practitioners.

The nictitans may be elevated for inspection of its margin and most of its anterior surface by depressing the globe from the dorsolateral aspect. For examination of the base and posterior surface, a topical anesthetic is applied, and after 2 to 3 minutes, a thumb forceps with serrated tips is used to grasp well onto the center of the free margin. It can be everted for examination for foreign material embedded in the third eyelid or in the conjunctival cul-de-sac. While the nictitans is everted, the cornea, anterior chamber, and iris should be inspected.

Most of the conjunctiva and cornea may be observed by flexing and extending the animal's neck and turning the head to one side or the other. Animals tend to gaze in the direction of the long axis of the body, so they will turn the eyes opposite to the rotation of the head, thereby revealing much of the anterior surface of the globe. This also facilitates the examination of the intraocular structures, including the fundus.

Samples for cytologic examination of conjunctival or corneal lesions may be taken with a saline-moistened swab or by gently scraping the edge of a Kimura spatula across the suspect tissue and distributing the sample on a clean glass slide. The back edge of a scalpel blade is a suitable substitute for the spatula. A topical anesthetic is required for scrapings. Dif-Quik stain is simple to perform and an effective stain for routine cytologic use.

Fluorescein dye is helpful in delineating breaks in the corneal epithelium. The dye may not be essential for observing deep lesions with obvious boundaries, but its use is never contraindicated. If in doubt about the presence of an ulcer or the re-epithelization of an ulcer crater, fluorescein should be used to determine the extent of the wound. Solutions of fluorescein should be avoided, especially in farm animals, because ocular secretions with *Pseudomonas* bacteria may contaminate the bottle and survive in the fluorescein to be subsequently inoculated in other animals.

The individually wrapped dye-impregnated paper strips (Fluor-I-Strips) are the only safe way of delivering dye to the cornea. The strip is folded longitudinally before it is removed from the paper envelope. The folded strip is held by the undyed end, and several drops of an eyewash solution are placed in the fold. The dye solution is dispensed from the end of the strip onto the cornea in the vicinity of the suspected ulcer, then the eye is irrigated thoroughly for removal of all excess dye and stained mucus. The dye is water-soluble, so it will not adhere to any intact epithelial surface, but where the epithelium is damaged, the underlying corneal stroma will retain the dye. Where there is undermined epithelium, the dye will disclose the extent of the lesion. With a magnifier head loupe and transilluminator, the cornea is examined for retained dye. A cobalt blue filter on the tip of the light will intensify the appearance of the dye where there is only faint retention.

A deficiency of tears leading to keratoconjunctivitis sicca is rare in ruminants or swine. Occasionally, conjunctivitis may be so severe that tear ducts are swollen shut or scarred, and the flow of the secretion onto the surface of the eye is reduced. The Schirmer tear test is done to estimate the production or flow of the aqueous portion of the tear film. There are different methods suggested for large animals because of the large amount of tears they normally produce. First, exudates or excess tears are carefully wiped away from the medial canthus. A standard 5×40 mm strip is folded at the notch cut on the side of the strip and hooked over the central portion of the lower lid. The degree of wetting is measured from the fold in the strip. The accepted normal for cattle is 24 mm in 30 seconds. Alternatively, a 7.5×60 mm strip of #42 Whatman filter paper folded 10 mm from the end may be used. This method yields at least 20 mm in 60 seconds in normal cattle and at least 15 mm in sheep and goats. Tear tests should be done before a topical anesthetic solution is applied to the eye.

Obstruction of the nasolacrimal drainage apparatus is indicated by persistence of a tear streak from the medial canthus. The puncta can be cannulated on the medial canthi of the upper and lower lids of small ruminants and pigs. With a 6-ml syringe filled with an eyewash solution and attached to a lacrimal cannula, the upper punctum can be located with a careful ventrally directed sweeping motion along the inner surface of the lid margin. Usually the punctum can be visualized. A topical anesthetic is required. With the cannula inserted 5 to 10 mm, a few milliliters of solution can be forced through the upper canaliculus and into the lacrimal sac. Most of it will then flow through the lower canaliculus and out the punctum on the lower lid. While irrigating the nasolacrimal duct, the examiner should look for exudates, foreign matter, or *Thelazia*. When patency of the upper loop is established, the lower lid is compressed against the orbital margin with the thumb while more solution is forced down the nasolacrimal apparatus. If it is patent, the solution will appear in the nostril immediately. Obstructions may occasionally be dislodged with gentle pressure. Sedation and retrograde flushing may be required.

In larger ruminants, it is much easier to insert a #5 Fr or #8 Fr open-end male urinary catheter into the nasal opening of the nasolacrimal duct and flush retrograde. The opening is found in the lateral wall near the floor of the nostril. The alar fold is lifted, and the catheter is inserted several centimeters and flushed with 8 to 10 ml of eyewash solution up through the duct and into the conjunctival sac. A noselead or halter is adequate restraint for this procedure.

Llamas, guanacos, and alpacas may spit when the nostril is manipulated. It is prudent to sedate them and work from the side. Cannulating the puncta at the lid margins seems to be less provocative.

Aspiration of material from the retrobulbar space is performed for cytologic examination or culture for differentiating causes of exophthalmos. This may be done quickly and easily with use of a sterile 3- or 4-inch 18-gauge needle by bending it in a slight arc and inserting it into the orbital space at the dorsal edge of the zygomatic arch posterior to the supraorbital process. It is directed medially with the concavity of the arc facing posteriorly. If the coronoid process of the mandible is encountered, the needle is redirected anteriorly into the retrobulbar space. When the suspected mass is probed, a 12-ml syringe is attached to the needle hub and suction applied slowly until material appears in the syringe. The plunger is then released slowly. The needle may be repositioned and suction reapplied until a suitable sample is collected. Thorough head restraint and sedation with xylazine is necessary.

For obtaining samples for culture or cytologic examination in cases of severe iritis or panophthalmitis, aqueous paracentesis may be useful but requires general anesthesia. Because of the risk of intraocular damage, this procedure should not be attempted by the inexperienced. A 22-gauge, 1-inch hypodermic needle attached to a 3-ml syringe is inserted into the lateral cornea immediately inside the limbal zone. The needle is passed into the anterior chamber parallel to the plane of the iris. This may require considerable effort, especially in mature animals. In soft, inflamed eyes, it is easy to misdirect the needle. A sample of 0.1 to 0.2 ml of exudate or aqueous is sufficient. The needle should not be manipulated excessively so that the needle track is distorted or torn. When the needle is withdrawn, the track may leak a few drops, but it will seal quickly with fibrin.

Attempts to clear the anterior chamber of blood or exudates or to lower intraocular pressure by anterior chamber paracentesis are all contraindicated. Hemorrhage and displacement of intraocular structures are likely to complicate these efforts. Neoplasms should be approached very cautiously because needle puncture will often lead to uncontrolled hemorrhage. Tumors should be evaluated and managed in consultation with an experienced veterinary ophthalmologist. Traumatizing a neoplasm could lead to metastasis that might not otherwise have occurred.

Several instruments and techniques are available for more complete or detailed examination of the eyes of animals, but their availability is usually limited to veterinary ophthalmologists. When preliminary findings indicate more extensive work-up or interpretation is needed, consultation should be pursued. Where the value of the animal or the concern of the owner warrants, examination with a slit-lamp biomicroscope or binocular indirect ophthalmoscope and tonometry, gonioscopy, electroretinography, fluorescein angiography, aqueous or vitreous centesis, or diagnostic ultrasonography may be merited.

TREATMENT TECHNIQUES

Cleaning the eyes is often overlooked or done inadequately, usually owing to a lack of a suitable eyewash bottle. A 6- or 8-ounce plastic goosenecked wash bottle that will direct a sizable stream of a buffered saline solution is inexpensive but effective. Avoid a fine needle-like stream from a pump spray bottle because the excessive pressure may be painful even to normal cornea or conjunctiva. Additionally, it may damage the cornea or severely startle the animal. Commercial preparations in suitable squirt bottles are available (Dacriose). Do not hold the bottle so close that the animal can jump or swing its head and injure the eye on the tip. Likewise, do not touch any tissue, tears, or exudate and risk aspirating contaminated fluids back into the bottle. Exudates and mucus can be wiped from the conjunctiva or lid margins with a gauze pad or cotton ball. Cotton torn from a roll is too loose and will leave too much fiber behind unless it is thoroughly moistened. Dry or very lightly moistened cotton balls or gauze pads are more efficient for picking up mucus or exudates. Be careful not to abrade the cornea. Wetting the cotton or gauze does not significantly reduce the risk.

TOPICAL MEDICATIONS

Ointments and solutions can be applied from the tube or bottle, but often the squinting or head movement of the patient makes it difficult or risky for both the animal and the person administering the treatment. Ointments may be applied to the clean gloved fingertip and then wiped off with a quick swipe across the medial canthus or one of the lid margins. Solutions may be squirted onto the ocular surfaces from a tuberculin syringe. Break the needle shaft from the hub of a 23- or 25-gauge needle and attach it to the syringe. Usually 0.1 ml of the solution is adequate. Because of the size of the area being treated and the dilution in the larger tear volume, large animals require several drops of medication or the equivalent of a 1- to 1½-inch strip of ointment. When using ointments, be certain that the vehicle melts at a low enough temperature (quickly enough) that it does not get squeezed out and off the eye when the animal blinks. Powders and aerosol sprays are easy to use but are very irritating and, therefore, should not be used in animal eyes.

For safe and reliable delivery of liquid medications to the eye of larger animals, a subpalpebral lavage or nasolacrimal lavage can be very handy. Because of the difficulty in placing lavage tubing through the thick upper lid of the bovine and the risk of the tubing's abrading the cornea, a nasolacrimal unit is preferred by the author.

The opening of the nasolacrimal duct is located on the ventrolateral aspect of the nostril. A polyethylene tube (0.060 inch outside diameter, i.e., Intramedic PE 100 (0.600 inch outside diameter) is inserted 5 to 7 inches or until it encounters resistance to further passage. A small flag of adhesive tape is fixed to the tubing and sutured with 4–0 nylon or silk to the mucous membrane as near to the opening of the duct as possible. The patency of the tube is confirmed before suturing is initiated. If a saline or eyewash solution cannot be flushed readily into the conjunctival sac, withdraw the tubing slightly and try again. Occasionally, exudates in the duct will plug the tubing and require initial thorough flushing. The tubing is positioned snugly under the alar fold where it leaves the nostril and is secured with tape flags and sutures to the animal's face and poll. It may be terminated as far away as the withers, but the shortest reasonable length of tubing is preferred. Taping the end to a halter works well. Thread a blunted 20-gauge needle carefully into the tubing. An injection cap will fit on the needle hub. Medication can be injected into the tubing and flushed through with an eyewash "chaser." For medications that remain stable within the tubing, a quantity sufficient to fill the tubing and to irrigate the eye is used. This may require an additional 0.1 to 1.5 ml of irrigating solution. Acetylcysteine may be a problem in this regard because it is unstable at room temperature.

Some interesting slow-release reservoirs and pumps have been used to facilitate continuous slow medicine application through lavage systems, but their limited availability and expense often make them impractical.

Drug delivery systems utilizing slow release of medication from sustained-release devices such as contact lenses have been investigated and developed over the past 15 years. Materials development has been fruitful, but placement and retention of the devices has not been as successful. Collagen shields* that protect traumatized corneas for 2 to 3 days until they dissolve are known to absorb drugs and release them as the shield dissolves. Although they are currently available only in sizes for dogs and cats, in the future they are expected to be available for large animals. Retention is not a problem because the lens will conform and adhere to the cornea regardless of its curvature or contour. Collagen shields should not be placed over infected wounds.

SUBCONJUNCTIVAL INJECTIONS

Subconjunctival injections are used to deposit a reservoir of medication that can lead to higher drug concentrations in the anterior segment of the eye for a prolonged period of time depending on the drug formulation. There are many variables that affect the fate of drugs given in this manner. Absorption directly into the eye from the injection site is minimal. Much of the drug is taken up through the vasculature and lymphatics and escapes into the general circulation. This is of little value to the eye. A small but significant portion will leak from the injection site through the needle track and mix in the tear film. The persistent presence of a small amount of drug over several hours to a few days may be more effective than are the pulsating higher concentrations of topical applications given only a few times a day. A more significant volume will leak back onto the surface when the drug is given subconjunctivally than when injected deep beneath Tenon's capsule at the surface of the sclera.

Subconjunctival injections are frequently administered by everting a lid and injecting beneath the palpebral conjunctiva. Because the eyelid vasculature removes the drug quickly, intrapalpebral "subconjunctival" injections have little value for treating intraocular disease except for the small portion of the drug that may leak back onto the surface of the eye. Deep injections into the base of the membrana nictitans are similarly lost, especially in swine, in which there is a large venous plexus deep to the medial canthus. It is preferable to place the drug as near to the lesion as possible. Although more effort and care is required, injections under the bulbar conjunctiva are potentially more effective. A 25-gauge needle is used to inject up to 1 ml in cattle and up to 0.5 ml in small ruminants on the dorsal or lateral aspect of the globe. A lid retractor is helpful but not necessary.

---

*Opticor. Pitman-Moore, Inc., Washington Crossing, NJ 08560.

TARSORRHAPHY AND NICTITANS FLAP

When long-term protection of the cornea is indicated, a nictitans flap can be placed. Because it is difficult to manipulate lids and nictitans in cattle, a tarsorrhaphy with the nictitans incorporated is an easy and effective procedure. Catgut sized 0 to 2–0 with a swaged-on needle is used in a vertical mattress pattern, with incorporation of a partial-thickness bite into the anterior of the nictitans where the suture crosses the palpebral space. This will elevate the nictitans to cover the cornea within the space between the lid edges. In sheep, goats, and small pigs, a conventional nictitans flap to the upper eyelid or dorsal bulbar conjunctiva is easier and preferred. In camelids, the globe is large and prominent and the nictitans is very difficult to stretch across the globe unless the animal is deeply sedated or anesthetized.

NERVE BLOCKS

The palpebral nerve block is a useful procedure for facilitating examination and treatment. In the ruminants, a 1- to 1½-inch 20- or 22-gauge needle is inserted subcutaneously along the dorsal margin of the zygomatic arch beginning at the junction of the supraorbital process with the zygomatic arch. Cattle will need 5 to 10 ml and smaller ruminants 3 to 5 ml. Local anesthesia of the eyelids may be accomplished with up to 5 to 7 ml of lidocaine infiltrated into each eyelid quadrant.

A Peterson eye block will anesthetize and paralyze all portions of the globe, orbit, and adnexa innervated by the oculomotor, trochlear, abducens nerves, and maxillary and ophthalmic branches of the trigeminal nerve. A curved 3- to 4-inch 18-gauge needle is inserted through the skin in the posterior angle of the junction of the supraorbital process and the zygomatic arch. Three milliliters of anesthetic is injected as the needle is advanced medially. The concavity of the arc in the needle is turned posteriorly, and the needle is directed slightly ventrally. When the coronoid process of the mandible is contacted, the needle tip is "walked" off the anterior border until it can be advanced deep into the orbit. When the needle strikes the bone of the medial floor of the orbit (at a depth of 3 to 4 inches in large ruminants and 2 to 3 inches in smaller ruminants), 8 ml of lidocaine is injected in sheep, goats, llamas, guanacos, and alpacas, and 15 to 20 ml in mature cattle. The Peterson eye block is sufficient for enucleation when it is combined with xylazine and butorphanol. It is not normally needed for examination or to facilitate treatment.

Infectious and Parasitic Eye Diseases of Cattle

CECIL P. MOORE, DVM, MS, Diplomate, ACVO
ROBERT B. MILLER, DVM, PhD

INFECTIOUS EYE DISEASES

Infectious Bovine Keratoconjunctivitis

Infectious bovine keratoconjunctivitis (IBK or "pinkeye") affects cattle worldwide and results in substantial economic loss to cattle producers (an estimated $150 to $300 million per year in the United States). Economic losses associated with

IBK result from (1) reduced growth rate, (2) decreased milk production, (3) costs of treatment including labor costs, (4) reduced value of affected cattle, and (5) death losses.

Etiology

Moraxella bovis, a gram-negative coccobacillus, is recognized universally as the primary cause of IBK. However, this is a complex disease with multiple factors affecting the pathogenicity of *M. bovis* strains, the transmission, and the clinical course of the disease. Contributing factors in spontaneous cases include exposure to ultraviolet light, high numbers of face flies, environmental irritants (dust, wind, tall grass, weeds, pollens), concurrent infections (IBR, *Mycoplasma* spp.), exposure of susceptible calves to infected or carrier animals, close confinement, and breeds or strains of cattle with increased susceptibility (e.g., nonpigmented eyes). In some instances, marginal nutritional status (e.g., vitamin A deficiency) may also be a contributing factor.

Transmission and Pathogenesis

M. bovis organisms are harbored in nasal and ocular secretions and may be transmitted by direct contact, aerosols, and fomites. Although a number of fly species may transmit *M. bovis*, the face fly *(Musca autumnalis)* is the primary mechanical vector for IBK. Asymptomatic cattle may act as carriers, shedding the bacteria primarily in nasal secretions. Pathogenic forms of the *M. bovis* organism that cause clinical disease (i.e., conjunctivitis and keratitis) are piliated strains that generally produce hemolysins. Ultraviolet light may stimulate conversion of nonhemolytic, nonpiliated organisms to pathogenic forms. A rapid logarithmic growth phase of the organism accompanies this transformation. Whereas hemolytic strains are usually isolated from summer epidemics, nonhemolytic strains may be identified in winter outbreaks.

Pathogenesis of spontaneous disease often involves ultraviolet light damage to the central, superficial corneal epithelium. Adherence of organisms occurs as pili bind to surface receptors of corneal epithelial cells. Production of destructive substances by the virulent *Moraxella* organisms (dermonecrolysins, hemolysins) and release of degradative enzymes by inflammatory cells (hydrolases, proteases, and collagenases) result in progressive necrosis of the corneal epithelium and subsequently the corneal stroma. Enzymatic disruption and breakdown of stromal collagen may result in descemetocele formation and corneal perforation. The most severe disease typically occurs in young susceptible cattle. The clinical course reflects the rate and extent of corneal necrosis and the rapidity with which reparative processes, primarily fibrovascular infiltration and corneal remodeling, occur.

Clinical Findings

Lesions and clinical signs include (generally in order of occurrence) epiphora, photophobia, conjunctivitis, blepharospasm, focal axial corneal opacity (edema), central corneal ulcer, miosis, aqueous flare, mucopurulent ocular discharge, extensive corneal necrosis (with or without staphyloma formation), circumlimbal corneal neovascularization, dense granulation tissue, and corneal fibrosis. The clinical course of IBK is usually about 3 weeks, although resolution may be delayed up to 1 month or longer in more extensive cases. In most cases, healing results in corneal scarring and opacities that clear considerably over several weeks or months. In severe cases, blinding sequelae may include keratoconus, panophthalmitis, buphthalmos (glaucoma), or phthisis bulbi.

Differential Diagnosis

Differential diagnoses for IBK include other causes of infectious conjunctivitis (e.g., infectious bovine rhinotracheitis [IBR], mycoplasmal infection), causes of uveitis (e.g., malignant catarrhal fever, immune-mediated), thelaziasis, ocular foreign bodies, corneal granulation tissue, photosensitization, and neoplasia (squamous cell tumor).

Infectious bovine keratoconjunctivitis typically manifests as a central corneal ulceration and differs clinically from the conjunctivitis (without ulceration) caused by IBR. It is recognized that IBK is more severe in cattle concurrently infected with IBR. Furthermore, IBK may be more severe in cattle that have been vaccinated with a modified live virus IBR intranasal vaccine before *Moraxella* infection.

Other infectious agents, including adenovirus, *Mycoplasma*, *Branhamella (Neisseria)*, and *Listeria*, have been recovered from eyes showing clinical signs closely resembling *Moraxella*-induced IBK. However, these organisms have not demonstrated fulfillment of Koch's postulates in causing lesions characteristic of IBK. It is probable that the presence of 1 or more of these ocular infectious agents will predispose an animal to subsequent *M. bovis* infection.

Diagnosis

Clinical diagnosis of IBK is often based on the seasonal occurrence of disease, the characteristic clinical signs, and a high incidence of ocular lesions in young animals. Definitive diagnosis is based on positive bacterial culture and identification of *M. bovis*, a nonmotile, aerobic, diplobacillus that grows optimally at 37° C. Samples are optimally collected from a corneal ulcer with use of a sterile swab moistened with Amies or Stuart's transport medium. Swabs should be plated directly or placed in additional transport media, which should then be packed in ice. Brain-heart infusion agar with 5 per cent ovine or bovine red blood cells is the appropriate medium for supporting growth of *M. bovis*. Because overgrowth by other bacteria may readily occur, cloxacillin (1 to 2.5 µg/ml) is frequently added to the media as an inhibitor. Pathogenic forms of *M. bovis* usually demonstrate a rough colony morphology and are hemolytic. Crystal violet dye may be used to differentiate questionable colonies, because pathogenic organisms will stain with this dye whereas nonpathogenic organisms will not stain. Such staining apparently does not interfere with subsequent subculturing. A fluorescent antibody test can be used to identify *M. bovis* in tears or from cultures.

Treatment

A number of different treatments have been recommended for IBK. Fortunately, the bovine cornea has a remarkable ability to regenerate and heal extensive lesions. This healing capacity plus a generally wide range of antibiotic susceptibilities for *M. bovis* allows most treatments to be effective when they are administered promptly and with appropriate frequency. IBK may be effectively treated by administering antibiotics topically, subconjunctivally, or systemically.

Commercially available topical ophthalmic antibiotics that may be used in food animals and are effective in treating IBK are gentamicin, triple antibiotic (neomycin, bacitracin, and polymyxin B), and oxytetracycline ointments. Topical nitrofurazone is also effective. Reports from Great Britain indicate that a single dose (125 mg) of topical benzathine cloxacillin in oil* achieves therapeutic levels for 2 to 3 days and accelerates

---
*Orbenin. Beecham Labs, Bristol, TN.

resolution of ocular lesions. This might seem to be paradoxic in view of the fact that addition of cloxacillin to selective culture medium for *M. bovis* isolation has also been advocated. Whereas therapeutic levels of benzathine cloxacillin are greater than 2.5 µg/ml for most *Moraxella* organisms, inhibitory levels for other commonly encountered ocular surface aerobes are between 1 and 2.5 µg/ml.

Topical antibiotic should be applied 3 times daily for several days. Both eyes should be treated; however, care must be taken to avoid mechanical transmission of *M. bovis* between eyes. Although topical antibiotics are effective, the need for frequent application may, in most instances, render this method impractical. Drugs that may be subconjunctivally administered and to which *M. bovis* is generally susceptible in vitro are ampicillin or amoxicillin (50 mg), kanamycin (100 mg), penicillin (500,000 units), and gentamicin (20 mg). Studies of subconjunctivally injected antibiotics in tears of normal calves indicate that peak levels occur within 1 hour and reduce over 8 hours to below therapeutic levels. This occurred with oil-based and aqueous suspensions of amoxicillin, oil-based benzathine cloxacillin, and kanamycin.

These findings suggest the need for subconjunctival injection of a drug 2 or 3 times daily if continual therapeutic levels in the tears are to be achieved. A long-acting oxytetracycline (OTC) in the same study produced therapeutic tear concentrations for more than 72 hours after subconjunctival injection. However, because this product produced severe chemosis and conjunctival necrosis in calves injected subconjunctivally, this method of administering long-acting OTC is *not* recommended for field use.

A single intramuscular injection of long-acting OTC (20 mg/kg) in calves with acute IBK shortened the duration of clinical signs and reduced the rate of shedding of *M. bovis*. Oxytetracycline binds to ocular surface cells, and its effectiveness against *M. bovis* infection appears to be dependent more on its distribution to surface tissues than on its diffusion into the tears. Therapeutically, 2 intramuscular injections 48 to 72 hours apart are recommended when long-acting OTC is administered. In addition to its efficacy in treating diseased eyes, intramuscular long-acting OTC will also eliminate the carrier state of *M. bovis*.

Most sulfonamides at dosages high enough to produce therapeutically effective serum concentrations (i.e., 100 mg/kg) produce tear concentrations bacteriostatic for *M. bovis*. In calves with artificially induced IBK, a single dose of sulfamethazine (sulfadimidine) at 100 mg/kg eliminated ocular and nasal *M. bovis* infections. Intravenously administered sulfamethazine (100 mg/kg) remains in the precorneal film at effective therapeutic levels for 24 hours. A single injection may be effective in eliminating *M. bovis* from infected eyes. Sulfamethazine given orally or intravenously at a dose of 100 mg/kg for 1 to 3 days may be an effective alternative to topical IBK treatment.

Although antibiotics constitute the primary therapy for IBK, topical or subconjunctival atropine is indicated in cases in which reflex miosis or anterior uveitis is present. Topical 1 per cent atropine ointment is recommended 2 times daily for several days for stimulating mydriasis and reducing pain from ciliary spasm. As an alternative to topical instillation of atropine ointment, 0.25 ml (0.1 mg) of small animal injectable atropine (0.4 mg/ml) may be injected subconjunctivally. Corticosteroids are not recommended until late in the healing stages, that is, when corneal neovascularization has replaced necrotic stroma and filled in stromal defects. Other supportive therapy includes a third eyelid flap, temporary tarsorrhaphy, or an eye patch. These measures are aimed at protecting the eye from ultraviolet light and environmental irritants. A third eyelid flap or temporary tarsorrhaphy is indicated when deep stromal ulceration is noted or in cases in which descemetocele or staphyloma formation is present.

Locally administered corticosteroid therapy has been widely used in the treatment of IBK. Because corticosteroids potentiate collagenase activity, topical or subconjunctival use of these drugs in the active ulcerative phase of IBK can stimulate loss of stromal collagen and result in corneal perforation. In addition, local immunosuppression may increase the rate of shedding of *M. bovis* organisms in lacrimal fluids. Corticosteroids may be used to reduce vascularization and granulation tissue after an ulcer has healed. However, no studies have been reported showing that regression of corneal vascularization and granulation after IBK is substantially improved by steroid treatment.

With treatment early in the course of the disease, the prognosis for vision in most cases of IBK is good. Because the severity of the disease tends to be greater in young animals, the sequelae are consequently often more severe.

Prevention

Prevention of IBK involves improved management practices, vaccination, and elimination of carrier animals. *M. bovis* spreads rapidly through a herd, infecting virtually all susceptible animals. Therefore, when possible, it is important to segregate and treat affected animals at the earliest signs of an outbreak. Newborn calves and new animals introduced into the herd may be treated with a single topical instillation of 1.5 per cent silver nitrate solution or topical antibiotic ophthalmic ointment (gentamicin, triple antibiotic, or tetracycline–polymyxin B).

Before and during fly season, face fly populations may be reduced by using insecticides. Pyrethrin-impregnated ear tags applied to both ears of all cattle before the fly season begins will reduce the transmission and incidence of IBK. Insecticide-containing face rubbers or dust bags with 5 per cent coumaphos can be used during fly season. Fly control needs to be done on an areawide basis to be most effective. Manure removal to curtail breeding of *Musca autumnalis* is also recommended.

Adequate shade should be provided to reduce exposure to ultraviolet light. Optimally, self-applicating fly control devices should be installed near shady areas. Avoid overcrowding by providing ample space for animals when they are housed and fed together. Clipping pastures will reduce ocular irritation to grazing animals. For minimizing direct transmission of infective organisms, disinfect equipment and hands after treatment or care of infected animals.

The role of IBR vaccination in the management of herd outbreaks of IBK has been a topic of some debate. Because IBR may cause conjunctivitis and predispose cattle to IBK, prevention of IBR may reduce the incidence and severity of *M. bovis* infections. However, IBR vaccine should not be administered in the face of an IBK outbreak.

A number of adjuvanted bacterins containing pili antigens and multiple strains of *M. bovis* are commercially available. Pili and associated attachment antigens play an important role in adhesion of the bacterium to epithelial cells. With the most recently developed oil-adjuvanted bacterins, only a single injection is recommended 3 to 6 weeks before the onset of vector (fly) season. Calves may be vaccinated between 21 and 30 days of age. Vaccination alone does not eliminate the disease. Conflicting results have been reported from vaccine efficacy studies. Whereas most have demonstrated decreased incidence and reduced severity of IBK in vaccinated calves, others have shown no difference between vaccinates and nonvaccinates. Improvements in vaccines have evolved around incorporation of additional antigens that stimulate antibodies against the corneal damaging activity (relative enzyme activity) of *M. bovis*.

Reduction in the number of carrier animals may be achieved by the administration of systemic antimicrobial agents. Oxytetracycline and sulfamethazine appear to be 2 antibacterials that are effective and practical for use on a herd basis. Similar to the therapeutic doses discussed earlier, sulfamethazine may be given orally or intravenously at a dose of 100 mg/kg. Alternatively, intramuscular long-acting oxytetracycline at a dose of 20 mg/kg may also be administered. For elimination of carriers, all adult cattle in the herd should be treated with 1 of these drugs during the nonvector season and before calving.

Infectious Bovine Rhinotracheitis (Conjunctival Form)

Endemic conjunctivitis from infectious bovine rhinotracheitis (IBR), caused by bovine herpesvirus, may occur either as the primary manifestation of the infection or in association with respiratory or reproductive forms of the disease. Affected animals are febrile (39° to 41° C) and anoretic. Lactating cows experience a substantial decrease in milk production. Abortions have been reported several weeks after signs of conjunctivitis have abated.

IBR conjunctivitis may be unilateral or bilateral. Ocular discharge is initially serous but becomes mucopurulent in 2 to 4 days. Multifocal areas of epithelial necrosis and lymphocytic infiltration (white plaques) may be noted on the palpebral conjunctiva during the first week of the disease. During the second week of infection, the multifocal lesions may coalesce into larger areas of necrosis. The conjunctivitis is most severe during this phase of the disease as characterized by extreme conjunctival hyperemia, large conjunctival ulcers, diphtheritic membrane formation, and copious mucopurulent discharge.

In severe cases, a secondary keratitis occurs characterized by peripheral corneal edema and mild perilimbal corneal neovascularization. Corneal ulceration generally does *not* occur secondary to IBR conjunctivitis. This is an important differentiating feature from IBK, which typically produces a central corneal ulceration. In some animals, anterior uveitis may be manifest as mild ocular hypotony, slight iris congestion, and moderate miosis. Affected animals with severe bilateral disease may become transiently nonvisual. Healing of ocular lesions usually begins during the third week after acute infection, and lesions spontaneously resolve by the end of week 4 or 5.

IBR conjunctivitis is diagnosed by (1) its association with systemic illness, (2) characteristic ocular lesions, (3) virus isolation, (4) fluorescent antibody testing of conjunctival scrapings, and (5) serologic examination. The most reliable means for definite diagnosis is culture of affected eyes during the first week of infection and inoculation of bovine cell cultures. Fluorescent antibody techniques may be used on conjunctival scrapings, and serologic testing may be helpful if blood samples are collected during the acute and convalescent stages of the disease.

Because several animals are usually affected simultaneously, individual treatment is generally not possible or practical. If individual treatment of ocular lesions is possible, empiric therapy consists of a broad-spectrum topical antibiotic (without corticosteroid) 3 to 4 times daily for control of secondary bacterial invaders. Although specific antiviral ophthalmic drugs are commercially available, they have not been routinely used in bovine patients because of the costs and the need for frequent topical administration (i.e., 5 times daily).

Antibiotics may be administered subconjunctivally; however, this would not appear to offer any advantage over topical antibiotics because therapeutic levels of most antibiotics are not present in the tears for more than 8 hours after subconjunctival administration. If anterior uveitis is present, topical atropine 1 per cent should be administered to effect (mydriasis). Therapy is continued until clinical improvement or spontaneous healing has been observed.

Because of substantial economic losses resulting from the occurrence of various forms of IBR in a herd, the disease should be prevented by annual vaccination. Bovine vaccination programs are discussed elsewhere in the text.

Other Causes of Infectious Conjunctivitis or Keratitis

Pasteurella and *Mycoplasma* infections also cause bovine conjunctivitis. *Pasteurella* sp. infections in calves cause conjunctivitis in addition to rhinitis, pharyngitis, and pneumonia. In calves with lower respiratory disease from *Pasteurella* infection, mucopurulent ocular discharge and conjunctivitis are frequent clinical findings. Treatment is aimed primarily at the pneumonia and, therefore, involves administration of systemic antibiotics, that is, oxytetracycline, sulfonamides, penicillin, ampicillin, amoxicillin, erythromycin, or a quinoline (e.g., ceftiofur). Although topical ophthalmic antibiotics are effective in treating the conjunctivitis, they are not routinely administered because of labor costs involved.

Mycoplasma bovoculi and *Ureaplasma* sp. have been isolated from herds with epizootic conjunctivitis. *M. bovis*, *M. laidlawii*, and *M. bovirhinus* are less commonly reported. Mycoplasmal ocular disease is relatively mild and is characterized by serous discharge and conjunctival hyperemia. Although keratitis is uncommonly associated with pure mycoplasmal infections, *M. bovoculi* will enhance the pathogenicity of *M. bovis*, resulting in extensive corneal lesions. In suspected cases of mycoplasmal ocular disease, eyes should be cultured with use of swabs moistened with sterile modified Hayflick broth.

Outbreaks of mycoplasmal conjunctivitis tend to occur seasonally, with the highest incidence in the warm months presumably due to the combination of a young susceptible population and the high prevalence of face flies. Although the disease is usually self-limiting over a course of 3 to 5 weeks, topical oxytetracycline ointment applied 3 times daily or intramuscular injection of long-acting oxytetracycline is effective in shortening the course of the disease. There is no effective vaccine for mycoplasmal disease.

Other causes of infectious bovine ocular surface disease are *Branhamella catarrhalis*, *Corynebacterium pyogenes*, *Leptospira* spp., *Acinetobacter* sp., *Moraxella ovis*, *Aspergillus fumigatus*, bovine adenovirus, and bluetongue virus.

Infectious Uveitis

Systemic infections caused by a number of different bacterial organisms may result in uveitis in cattle. Neonatal septicemias caused by *Escherichia coli*, *Corynebacterium* sp., *Klebsiella* sp., *Listeria* sp., *Salmonella* sp., and *Streptococcus* sp. may result in septic uveitis in calves. Ocular findings typical of uveitis are corneal edema, episcleral vascular injection, cloudy ocular media (inflammatory cells and fibrin), constricted pupil, and iris congestion. Calves typically develop ocular lesions during the first 2 weeks postnatally. Neonatal septicemias are characterized by pyrexia, weakness, depression, multiple organ involvement (e.g., swollen joints), umbilical abscesses, pneumonia, enteritis, meningitis, or endotoxemia. In neonatal septicemia cases, lack of colostral antibody is an important predisposing factor.

The most prevalent form of bacterial uveitis in adult cattle is associated with primary suppurative disease of other organs with resultant septicemia, that is, mastitis, metritis, and endocarditis. Ocular involvement in these diseases is usually manifest as a fibrinous anterior uveitis. In contrast, ocular lesions of thromboembolic meningoencephalitis (TEME), caused by *Haemophilus somnus*, are typically found in the posterior uvea. Acute septic TEME most commonly occurs in feedlot cattle and may cause a thromboembolic chorioretinitis that results in funduscopically visible exudates and hemorrhages. In cases in which an infected animal survives the acute septicemia, foci of chorioretinal exudates may subsequently be noted as areas of necrosis and chorioretinal scarring. Retinal detachments may result from retinal edema and subretinal exudates. Blindness may occur from ocular lesions or septic thrombosis of brain tissues.

Systemic antibiotics and supportive care are the mainstays of treating animals with bacterial septicemias. Ocular therapy for septic uveitis consists of topical antibiotics or antibiotic-corticosteroid combinations (if no ulceration is present) and 1 per cent atropine ophthalmic ointment 4 times daily. Systemic nonsteroidal anti-inflammatory agents may also be useful in treating the uveitis, although these agents have not been widely used in ruminants for this purpose. Even after successful treatment, sequelae of uveitis include synechiae and chorioretinal scars.

Granulomatous uveitis in cattle is presently uncommon because of the low incidence of bovine tuberculosis. It has been reported that 5 per cent of cattle with generalized tuberculosis have granulomatous uveitis. Although the anterior uvea is primarily involved initially, the disease may progress to a generalized ophthalmitis and solid retinal detachment. Systemic mycoses are other possible causes of granulomatous uveitis in cattle.

Malignant catarrhal fever (MCF) virus causes disseminated vasculitis and thrombosis in domestic and wild ruminants. Ophthalmitis is common and is a characteristic feature of the "head and eye" form of the disease. In addition to a high fever (40° to 42° C), mucopurulent rhinitis, conjunctivitis, uveitis, and mucosal erosions are typical clinical findings of acute MCF. Ophthalmic lesions include conjunctival and ciliary injection, miosis, iris congestion and hyperemia, corneal edema, and exudates in the anterior chamber. Although not usually visible clinically, retinal vasculitis is also often present. Ophthalmic and systemic treatment is empiric, and because the disease is almost always fatal, therapy is usually impractical.

No specific diagnostic test is available for MCF. The absence of central corneal ulceration helps to distinguish MCF from IBK, and the severity of ocular lesions is worse than would be expected with IBR and mycoplasmal or bluetongue infections. In areas where MCF and rinderpest are endemic, these diseases may appear to be similar, and differentiation based on clinical lesions can be difficult.

Prognosis for recovery from MCF is poor. Affected animals should be isolated and especially should be kept away from sheep. There is no vaccine for MCF.

Miscellaneous Infectious Eye Diseases

Bovine Viral Diarrhea

Ocular discharges have been reported in acute or chronic cases of bovine virus diarrhea (BVD), a togavirus infection. Animals congenitally affected with BVD during the second trimester may suffer cerebellar hypoplasia or ocular lesions. With in utero infections, retinal inflammation and necrosis may result in retinal folds (dysplasia), rosettes, or separation. Other ocular abnormalities may include microphthalmia, leukocoria (cataracts), and optic neuritis. Calves may be born blind with nystagmus and abnormal pupillary light responses.

Diagnosis of BVD-associated congenital ocular disease is based on clinical findings and positive BVD titers. Precolostral serum samples from affected calves are submitted for serum virus neutralization titer or virus isolation, which can be performed from buffy coat cells of a whole blood sample.

Listeriosis

Listeria monocytogenes causes encephalitis in cattle and may also cause ocular signs including facial paralysis and ptosis that is often unilateral on the side of the central lesion. Conjunctivitis, medial strabismus (from involvement of the abducens nucleus), and central blindness are also manifestations of listeriosis. In chronic cases, uveitis with hypopyon may occur. In neonatal calves, an acute, rapidly fatal encephalitis characterized by opisthotonos, nystagmus, and corneal opacity may occur. Diagnosis of listeriosis is based on clinical signs and isolation of *L. monocytogenes* from tissues at necropsy. Early treatment with broad-spectrum systemic antibiotics may be effective in some cases.

Bovine Leukosis

A progressive unilateral or bilateral exophthalmos may occur in cattle with lymphosarcoma. Chemosis and exposure keratitis may occur. Generalized lymphadenopathy may accompany the orbital infiltrates. Differential diagnoses include frontal or maxillary sinusitis, nasal neoplasia, postorbital abscess, and actinomycosis. Diagnosis is based on clinical findings, a complete blood count, cytologic examination of orbital aspirates, and bovine leukosis virus agar-gel immunodiffusion test. A temporary tarsorrhaphy may be inserted as a palliative measure for protecting the cornea. Enucleation or exenteration is rarely indicated owing to the poor prognosis for an affected animal, although tissues may be obtained for confirmatory histopathologic examination.

PARASITIC EYE DISEASE

Ocular Thelaziasis

Ocular thelaziasis occurs in approximately one third of the cattle in North America and the British Isles. The 3 species occurring in cattle are *T. rhodesi*, *T. gulosa*, and *T. skrjabini*. *T. californiensis* occurs in sheep and wild ruminants. Adult *Thelazia* worms, which are 1 to 2 cm long, inhabit the conjunctival sac, including the recesses around the third eyelid, and ducts of the lacrimal system. *Musca autumnalis* serves as the biologic vector for bovine *Thelazia* spp. Most *Thelazia* infestations are subclinical; however, lacrimation and mild conjunctivitis are sometimes present. On close examination of affected eyes, a mild superficial keratitis may also be noted. In addition to producing mildly irritating metabolites, the parasite has serrated cuticles that may physically injure the ocular surface. Diagnosis is based on direct visualization of the *Thelazia* in the conjunctival sac or nasolacrimal flushes. *Thelazia* worms are motile unless topical anesthetic is used.

Because *Thelazia* spp. are highly commensal parasites, treatment is usually not necessary. Worms may be removed manually after instillation of topical anesthetic solution. Parasiticides, administered either topically or systemically, appear to be effective in killing the adult worms. Treatment with a topical ophthalmic organophosphate (e.g., echothiophate iodide*) has been recommended. Oral levamisole (15 mg/kg), oral fenbendazole (10 mg/kg), or topical ivermectin formulated into eye drops (2 μg/ml) is lethal to *Thelazia* worms. Systemic ivermectin at the recommended dose is not consistently effective against conjunctival *Thelazia*. Reinfestation is probable unless vector control is achieved. The use of insect repellents and general fly control measures should reduce the prevalence of face flies and, therefore, the incidence and recurrence of thelaziasis.

BIBLIOGRAPHY

Coleman RE, Gerhardt RR: Isolation of *Moraxella bovis* from the crops of field-collected face flies. J Agric Ent 4:92–94, 1987.

English RV, Nasisse MP: Ocular parasites. *In* Smith B (ed): Large Animal Internal Medicine. St. Louis, Mosby Year Book, 1990, pp 1244–1247.

George LW, Smith JA, Kaswan R: Distribution of oxytetracycline into ocular tissues and tears of calves. J Vet Pharmacol Ther 8:47–54, 1985.

George LW, Ardans A, Mihalyi J, et al: Enhancement of infectious bovine keratoconjunctivitis by modified-live infectious bovine rhinotracheitis virus vaccine. Am J Vet Res 49:1800–1806, 1988.

Gerber JD, Selzer NL, Sharpee RL, Beckenhauer WH: Immunogenicity of a *Moraxella bovis* bacterin containing attachment and cornea-degrading enzyme antigens. Vet Immunol Immunopathol 18:41–52, 1988.

Miller RB, Fales WH: Infectious bovine keratoconjunctivitis: an update. Vet Clin North Am [Large Anim Pract] 6:597–608, 1984.

Moore LJ, Rutter JM: Attachment of *Moraxella bovis* to calf corneal cells and inhibition by antiserum. Aust Vet J 66:39–42, 1989.

Rebhun WC: Orbital lymphosarcoma in cattle. J Am Vet Med Assoc 180:149–152, 1982.

Rebhun WC: Ocular manifestations of systemic diseases in cattle. Vet Clin North Am [Large Anim Pract] 6:623–639, 1984.

Rebhun WC, Smith JS, Post JE, et al: An outbreak of the conjunctival form of infectious bovine rhinotracheitis. Cornell Vet 68:297–307, 1978.

Rosenbusch RF, Knudtson WU: Bovine mycoplasmal conjunctivitis: experimental reproduction and characterization of the disease. Cornell Vet 70:307–320, 1980.

Smith PG, Blankenship T, Hoover TR, et al: Effectiveness of two commercial infectious bovine keratoconjunctivitis vaccines. Am J Vet Res 51:1147–1150, 1990.

*Phospholine Iodide. Ayerst Laboratories, New York, NY 10017.

Selected Eye Diseases of Sheep and Goats

CECIL P. MOORE, DVM, MS, DIPLOMATE, ACVO
LAURIE MILLS WALLACE, DVM, MVSc

Those ocular disorders of sheep and goats that may be most often encountered by the clinician or generally are of greatest economic importance are considered here. Disease categories presented include (1) congenital and neonatal, (2) infectious, and (3) parasitic diseases. Ocular neoplastic diseases are discussed elsewhere in this text.

CONGENITAL AND NEONATAL DISEASES

Craniofacial Anomalies

Ingestion of the plant *Veratrum californicum* by pregnant ewes on the fourteenth day of gestation may result in cyclopia in lambs. Other severe craniofacial malformations, including anencephaly, hydrocephalus, and cerebral hypoplasia, may occur in one or more of the fetuses carried by the ewe. Prolonged gestation is common in ewes carrying affected lambs. Fetal death is also a result of ingestion of *V. californicum* and is indicated by a return to estrus. During the first trimester of gestation, ewes should be restricted from grazing alpine pastures where this plant is known to grow.

Microphthalmia and Multiple Ocular Defects

Trexel sheep, which are common in Great Britain and Europe, have produced lambs with microphthalmia and multiple congenital ocular anomalies. Defects associated with the microphthalmic globes include microcornea, aphakia, aniridia, and optic nerve hypoplasia. An autosomal recessive inheritance pattern is reported. Because of increasing interest in this breed in the United States, these anomalies may possibly become more common in North America.

Prolonged consumption of plants containing more than 3 ppm selenium may cause chronic selenium toxicosis in sheep. Toxic effects may also result from overzealous treatment of selenium deficiency. Fetal malformations are a common result, because the fetus shares in the deposition of selenium. Ocular manifestations include anophthalmos and microphthalmia with multiple ocular cysts. Similar ocular defects have been reported with apholate toxicity in sheep.

Bluetongue-Associated Anomalies in Sheep

Bluetongue, an arbovirus transmitted by *Culicoides* gnats, affects adult sheep and causes extensive vasculitis that results in lameness, swelling of the face, pulmonary edema, and death.

Controlled studies and field observations have established the pathogenicity of the bluetongue virus for the ovine fetus. Developmental ocular anomalies were noted in the fetuses of ewes vaccinated with modified live bluetongue virus on day 40 (controlled experiment) and during the fifth and sixth weeks of gestation (field observation). Typical central nervous system abnormalities noted in these fetuses included hydrocephalus and cerebellar hypoplasia. Retinal necrosis and retinal rosette-like lesions were postinflammatory changes noted within affected retinas. It is interesting to note that fetuses from ewes experimentally vaccinated with modified live virus vaccine between days 50 and 75 of gestation also developed lesions of retinitis and choroiditis.

The practical significance of these observations is 2-fold: (1) ocular and cranial fetal anomalies are components of spontaneous cases of bluetongue, and (2) administration of modified live bluetongue virus vaccine to pregnant ewes is not advised, particularly during the second trimester of gestation.

Entropion

Eyelid inversion, or entropion, is the most common neonatal ocular disease of sheep. Although the mode of inheritance is unclear, entropion is considered to be a significant genetic problem in some flocks and may affect a high percentage of lambs 1 to 3 weeks of age. However, in neonatal lambs or kids with normal eyelid conformation, entropion may develop secondary to systemic illness, for example, septicemia or dehydration from bacterial or viral enteritis.

Entropion is painful and can cause corneal opacification from rubbing by eyelashes, periocular hair, and wool. Initial clinical signs are lacrimation and photophobia that progresses to conjunctivitis, keratitis, enophthalmos, and blepharospasm. Bilateral involvement can result in blindness, inefficiency in nursing and foraging, difficulty moving with the flock or herd, and increased vulnerability to predators. Because vigor and feed intake are reduced, growth and weight gain are suboptimal in affected lambs.

Treatment for entropion consists of 1 or more of the following techniques for everting the eyelid: (1) injection of a repositol liquid (such as a penicillin suspension) into the eyelid to produce a subcutaneous bleb; (2) crimping the skin just external to the eyelid margin with mosquito hemostats or wound clips; (3) eversion of affected eyelids with 2 to 3 vertical mattress sutures placed into the eyelid skin; or (4) surgical resection of a skin crescent followed by wound closure (Hotz-Celsus procedure). Injection and crimping techniques are less time-consuming than are suture methods. When an eyelid is injected or crimped, natural growth and facial development combined with fibrosis at the treated site usually prevent recurrence of the entropion.

In addition to alleviating the frictional irritation by everting the eyelid, if management conditions permit, topical antibiotic ointment (triple antibiotic, gentamicin, erythromycin, or tetracycline) should be applied 2 to 3 times daily for control of secondary infections and for lubrication of the ocular surface. Medical treatment is particularly important in cases of severe ulcerative keratitis in which both antibiotic and 1 per cent atropine are indicated. Atropine should be administered once daily (or repeated until mydriasis results) for a duration of 5 days.

In severe or nonresponsive cases of entropion, suturing the eyelids to prevent recurrence of the inversion may be necessary. Placement of nonabsorbable everting sutures without skin resection is effective in providing immediate relief from entropion. Sutures are left in place for 2 to 3 weeks to allow the cornea to heal and to allow growth that favors normal eyelid position and function. Surgical removal of an elliptic skin strip and suturing the resultant wound is infrequently necessary but may be used for refractory cases.

Ectropion

Mild drooping or eversion of the eyelid is occasionally seen in sheep as a conformational variation. Although this may predispose some animals to recurrent conjunctivitis, most do not exhibit discernible ocular disease. A congenital upper eyelid eversion has been described in exotic piebald sheep.

Eyelid trauma and overzealous correction of entropion are the most common causes of severe ectropion, which may result in exposure and drying of the ocular surface and chronic keratoconjunctivitis. Surgical correction is necessary for correction and involves either an eyelid shortening procedure or a V-Y blepharoplasty. The reader is referred to an ophthalmic surgery text for further information of these procedures.

Neonatal Uveitis

Neonatal sheep and goats may become septicemic with an associated uveitis. Hematogenous spread of organisms, such as *Mycoplasma* spp., coliforms, *Staphylococcus* spp., *Pasteurella multocida*, or *Corynebacterium* spp., may result in fibrin and inflammatory cell accumulation in the anterior chamber with miosis and iris edema. When lesions are bilateral, opacification may be sufficient to result in blindness. Treatment includes systemic antibiotics, oral or parenteral fluid therapy, and topical treatments with 1 per cent atropine and an antibiotic-corticosteroid combination. In these cases, administration of atropine may need to be repeated 2 to 3 times daily for the desired mydriasis to be achieved.

INFECTIOUS DISEASES

Infectious Ovine Keratoconjunctivitis

Microorganisms incriminated as causing infectious keratoconjunctivitis of sheep are chlamydia, mycoplasmas, and aerobic bacteria.

Chlamydia psittaci is the etiologic agent of ovine chlamydial conjunctivitis. Two strains of *C. psittaci* occur naturally. One causes conjunctivitis and polyarthritis, and a second causes enzootic abortion. When infected with the strain that causes conjunctivitis, lambs have a higher prevalence of ocular disease than do adult animals, and 80 per cent of lambs will have bilateral involvement. Although some lambs develop arthritis, they may have conjunctivitis without joint involvement.

Chlamydial conjunctivitis is highly contagious and spreads rapidly by direct contact, insect transfer, and contact with contaminated discharges. Organisms are shed in tear and nasal secretions and may persist in ocular tissues for several months after remission of ocular signs.

Early clinical findings of chlamydial ocular infection are petechial hemorrhages, conjunctival lymphoid follicles, and corneal edema. Severe conjunctival hyperemia, neutrophilic infiltrates of the cornea, and corneal ulcerations may occur after the fifth day. In more severe cases, corneal neovascularization occurs as a later sequel to infection.

Diagnosis is based on cytologic evaluation of stained conjunctival scrapings from acutely infected animals. Gram-negative, basophilic (Wright's or Giemsa's stains) intracytoplasmic inclusions within conjunctival epithelial cells are diagnostic of chlamydia. However, because inclusions may be seen in less than 50 per cent of affected animals, positive cultures or immunofluorescence testing of conjunctival scrapings may be used as alternative methods for diagnosis. Chlamydial organisms can be cultured from conjunctival scrapings as well as from blood taken from sheep with polyarthritis and conjunctivitis.

Although the disease is usually self-limiting in 2 to 3 weeks, topical and systemic tetracycline therapy may be initiated to speed resolution of keratoconjunctivitis. Injection of long-acting oxytetracycline (10 to 20 mg/kg) or addition of oxytetracycline to feed (80 mg/head/day) may be beneficial in reducing the severity of the disease and decreasing numbers of organisms shed from ocular tissue.

Mycoplasma and several different genera of aerobic bacteria have been isolated from sheep with infectious ovine keratoconjunctivitis. *Mycoplasma conjunctivae* and *Branhamella (Neisseria) ovis* are the most important causes of nonchlamydial conjunctivitis in sheep. *M. conjunctivae* is considered to be the most important etiologic agent in outbreaks of infectious ovine keratoconjunctivitis in the United Kingdom. *B. ovis* is a gram-negative diplococcus that is similar to *Moraxella* species. This agent has been cultured from normal sheep and goats and animals with keratoconjunctivitis. *B. ovis* may occur secondarily to either *C. psittaci* or *M. conjunctivae* and may complicate the ocular disease, causing more serious lesions such as corneal ulceration.

Outbreaks of nonchlamydial keratoconjunctivitis may occur in the spring and carry into the summer months. Lambs 6 to 8 weeks of age appear to be most susceptible. Clinical signs include lacrimation, injected conjunctival vessels, and keratitis. However, only a small percentage of infected animals develop a noticeable keratitis.

Although a rickettsial keratoconjunctivitis, presumably caused by an agent identified as *Colesiota* (or *Rickettsia*) *conjunctivae*, has been reported in sheep, the existence of such an infectious agent has recently been challenged. Because the organism was identified only by conjunctival scraping and not by culture, it is probable that in earlier reports various forms of epithelial inclusions of *Chlamydia psittaci* were misinterpreted as being rickettsial organisms.

Mycoplasmal Keratoconjunctivitis and Keratouveitis of Goats

Mycoplasma agalactiae causes systemic disease affecting the eyes, joints, mammary glands, or gravid uteri of goats. Transmission occurs by direct contact with infected animals or their secretions or by contact with contaminated fomites. Clinical findings include fever, lameness, mastitis, keratoconjunctivitis, and uveitis. Blindness may be noted if the ocular media are totally opaque bilaterally. Diagnosis is based on clinical signs and the isolation of *M. agalactiae* from blood, milk, joint fluid, or tears. Treatment involves the use of systemic antibiotics (tetracycline, tylosin, or erythromycin) and the isolation of infected animals.

In young goats, *M. mycoides* subsp. *mycoides* infection causes fever, keratoconjunctivitis, arthritis, mycoplasmaemia, and death. *M. mycoides* subsp. *mycoides* has been isolated from an epidemic of mastitis, arthritis, and keratoconjunctivitis in goats. *M. conjunctivae* causes conjunctivitis, photophobia, circumlimbal infiltrates, and corneal opacities in goats without systemic signs or with only mild respiratory disease. *Acholeplasma oculi* (or *oculusi*) has been isolated from goats in epidemics of keratoconjunctivitis. *A. oculi* and *M. arghinini* have produced mild keratoconjunctivitis experimentally. The ocular disease is characterized by lacrimation, conjunctival vascular injection, and, in some cases, lymphoid follicular development. Keratitis with neovascularization and anterior uveitis may also occur, and choroiditis and hyalitis have been described. Differential diagnoses include other agents known to cause keratoconjunctivitis (such as *Branhamella* sp.) and infectious bovine rhinotracheitis (IBR) as well as noninfectious causes such as trauma.

Depending on the stage of disease, conjunctival scrapings may reveal neutrophils, lymphocytes, plasma cells, or necrotic epithelial cells. Organisms, when observed, appear in epithelial cell cytoplasm as basophilic coccobacillary structures that must be differentiated from pigment granules. Mycoplasmal organisms can be cultured and identified from conjunctival swabs.

Mycoplasmal keratoconjunctivitis of goats is generally self-limiting. Even in complicated cases, a full resolution of lesions may be observed in 3 to 4 weeks. Recurrence is sometimes noted. Topical or systemic tetracycline therapy may be used to reduce the severity and hasten progression of the clinical course. Injectable and topical therapy may be combined. In outbreaks in which a number of animals must be treated, administration of injectable long-acting oxytetracycline (10 to 20 mg/kg) or addition of oxytetracycline to the feed (80 mg/head/day) may be the most practical method of treatment. In cases of severe ulcerative keratitis, applying topical 1 per cent atropine to effect and protecting the eye from the environment with a temporary tarsorrhaphy or third eyelid flap are recommended.

Introduction of new animals into a herd often precedes a herd outbreak. For this reason, isolation and, in some instances, treatment of new animals is important before contact with the herd.

Scrapie-Associated Retinopathy in Sheep

The scrapie agent, which causes central nervous system degeneration in sheep, has been associated with multifocal retinitis in 2 animals. Retinal lesions were characterized funduscopically as multifocal hyper-reflective areas in the tapetal fundus. The histologic correlates were focal subretinal eosinophilic deposits of complex lipid material. The precise relationship to the scrapie agent was not established.

Infectious Bovine Rhinotracheitis Keratoconjunctivitis in Goats

The herpesvirus causing infectious bovine rhinotracheitis (IBR) can infect goats and cause eye disease. In a case in which IBR was isolated from ocular and nasal discharges, ocular findings included conjunctivitis and keratitis. Keratoconus was also observed several days after onset of severe respiratory disease.

PARASITES

Elaeophoriasis

"Sorehead" is a parasitic disease of domestic and wild ruminants caused by the filarid parasite *Elaeophora schneideri*. In deer, the most common host, the adult parasites are found in the common carotid and internal maxillary arteries. In these sites, microfilaria are produced and migrate into the capillaries of the face and head. *Hybomitra* and *Tabanus* flies transmit the microfilaria to new hosts.

Although *Elaeophora* infections are generally asymptomatic in deer, in small domestic ruminants and elk, the microfilaria in the facial and ocular capillaries cause an immunologic reaction. Adult sheep are most commonly affected and develop alopecia, ulcerations, and encrusted lesions of the face. In North America, elaeophoriasis is most prevalent in the fall and winter in the western ranges where sheep are grazed at high altitudes.

Affected sheep may develop anterior uveitis and chronic keratoconjunctivitis with epiphora, blepharospasm, conjunctival hyperemia, chemosis, and corneal opacities. Clinical signs of anterior uveitis are nonspecific and include miosis, exudates in the anterior chamber, and synechia formation. Cataracts can also occur in affected animals. Funduscopic lesions are consistent with chorioretinitis and optic neuritis, including retinal edema, retinal vascular attenuation, pigmentary changes in the tapetal and nontapetal fundus, papilledema, and optic disk atrophy. Diagnosis is based on clinical signs and demonstration of microfilaria in skin or conjunctival biopsy specimens.

Drugs that may be used to treat elaeophoriasis are oral piperazine (50 mg/kg) or diethylcarbamazine (100 mg/kg) or intravenous stibophen (35 ml). The efficacy of ivermectin against *E. schneideri* is not known. Treatment of heavily parasitized animals can be fatal because of occlusion of the carotid arteries with adult worms. Keratitis and uveitis are treated symptomatically.

Toxoplasmosis

The intracellular protozoan parasite *Toxoplasma gondii* can cause intraocular disease in small ruminants, that is, anterior uveitis and chorioretinitis (primarily retinitis). However, the acquired form of toxoplasmosis in ruminants is often asymptomatic, and ocular lesions are relatively uncommon. Funduscopic changes are nonspecific, and in the early stages of disease, fundic lesions are typical of acute neuroretinitis (i.e., retinal edema and papillitis). Chronic changes include retinal degeneration, clumping of the retinal pigment layer, and choroidal scarring and optic disk avascularity. Orbital pain and swelling may result from parasitic invasion of extraocular muscles and orbital fat. Diagnosis and treatment of toxoplasmosis are discussed elsewhere.

Nasal Bots

Larva of the arthropod *Oestrus ovis*, the sheep botfly, can aberrantly migrate up the nasolacrimal duct and enter the conjunctival sac, causing local inflammation. Conjunctival migration is accompanied by epiphora, conjunctival erythema, and chemosis. Finding of the larva within the conjunctival sac is diagnostic. Treatment consists of mechanical removal and topical or systemic organophosphates.

BIBLIOGRAPHY

Egwu BO, Faull WB, Bradbury JM, Clarkson MJ: Ovine infectious keratoconjunctivitis: a microbiological study of clinically unaffected and affected sheep's eye with special reference to Mycoplasma conjunctivae. Vet Rec 125:253–256, 1989.

Greig A: Ovine keratoconjunctivitis. In Practice 11:110, 113, 1989.

Jensen R: Diseases of the eye. *In* Kimberling CV (ed): Jensen and Swift's Diseases of Sheep, 3rd ed. Philadelphia, Lea & Febiger, 1988, pp 183–185.

Hopkins JB, Stephenson RH, Storz J, et al: Conjunctivitis associated with chlamydial polyarthritis in lambs. J Am Vet Med Assoc 163:1157–1160, 1973.

Hosie BO: Infectious keratoconjunctivitis in sheep and goats. Vet Annu 29:93–97, 1989.

Mohanty SB, Lillie MG, Corselius NP, Bech JD: Natural infection with infectious bovine rhinotracheitis virus in goats. J Am Vet Med Assoc 160:879–880, 1972.

Moore CP, Whitley RD: Ophthalmic diseases of small domestic ruminants. Vet Clin North Am [Large Anim Pract] 6:641–665, 1984.

Wyman M: Eye diseases of sheep and goats. Vet Clin North Am [Large Anim Pract] 5:657–675, 1983.

Ophthalmology of South American Camelids: Llamas, Alpacas, Guanacos, and Vicuñas

JULIET RATHBONE GIONFRIDDO, DVM, MS
DEBORAH S. FRIEDMAN, DVM, Diplomate, ACVO

The growing popularity of South American camelids (llamas, guanacos, vicuñas, and alpacas) as companion animals has established them as species important to veterinary practice. In spite of the significant economic value of llamas in the United States (where they currently number about 20,000) and their importance in South America for food, wool, transportation, and fuel, llamas' eyes have not received much attention. The veterinarian is at a disadvantage when called upon to treat ocular diseases in the llama because there are few anatomic descriptions of camelid eyes, and their ocular anatomy differs significantly from that of other domestic species.

Most veterinary work has centered on llamas and guanacos, but because the eyes of vicuñas and alpacas are probably very similar, the information given in this article can be extrapolated to include these other closely related species.

ANATOMY

Llama eyes are large and prominent. They are only slightly smaller than equine and bovine eyes despite the considerably smaller body size of the llama (Table 1) and are framed with long lashes and 3 sets of long vibrissae. The lacrimal caruncle is pigmented dark brown or nonpigmented and is covered with sparse, fine, white or black hair.

The eyelids are tightly adherent to the globe, which makes examination of the conjunctival fornices difficult. Unlike all other domestic animals, no meibomian gland duct openings are present on the eyelid margin. Meibomian glands are also apparently absent in the camel but are replaced by sebaceous glands on the lacrimal caruncle.[5,9] This is probably the case in the llama as well.

Magnification is helpful in observation of the lacrimal punctae. They are located several millimeters inside the eyelid edge at the medial canthus. The inside of the punctum is usually nonpigmented, but it is surrounded by pigmented palpebral conjunctiva. Application of fluorescein dye to the tear film of the llama, as in most domestic animals, usually results in passage of the dye through the nasolacrimal ducts to the external nares. The dye will not appear at the nares if the ducts are plugged: if blocked, the lacrimal punctae may be cannulated with a Teflon intravenous catheter and flushed with sterile saline.

The prominence of the llama eye is enhanced by the lack of visibility of any sclera. The margins of the cornea (limbus) match the shape of the palpebral fissure, so that although the eyelids cover almost none of the cornea, they cover the bulbar conjunctiva and sclera almost entirely. This differs significantly from the bovine, in which large amounts of sclera are exposed. Usually the conjunctiva overlying any exposed areas of sclera is pigmented so that no white is evident. The limbus is almost always marked with a dark brown pigment band that ends sharply on its corneal side and less abruptly on its scleral side. This band is approximately 2 to 3 mm wide and usually surrounds the entire cornea.

About 3 to 4 mm of the leading edge of the nictitating membrane (which is either pigmented or unpigmented) is visible at the medial canthus. The outer surface of the nictitating membrane can be examined by gentle retropulsion of the globe while the eyelids are simultaneously held open. The T cartilage of the nictitating membrane is readily visible. The membrane on either side of the cartilage is thin and almost transparent.

The elaborate structure of the iris is one of the most striking features of the llama eye (Fig. 1). On the dorsal and ventral margins of the pupil, the posterior pigment epithelium of the iris is proliferated and folded vertically. This structure (which may be termed the pupillary ruff) is analogous to the corpora nigra of other large animal species but is significantly larger and consists of a folded sheet of tissue rather than globular masses. The dorsal folds are taller than the ventral ones, and the central folds are taller and wider than the medial and lateral ones. When the pupil is dilated, the folds of the ruff

Table 1. COMPARISON OF AVERAGE LLAMA EYE SIZE WITH THAT OF THE EQUINE AND BOVINE (in millimeters)

	Equine[1]	Bovine[1]	Llama[2]
Anterior-posterior axis	43.68	34	38
Horizontal axis	48.50	41.90	39
Vertical axis	47.50	40.82	38

[1]Data from Martin et al, 1980.[17]
[2]Data from Friedman, 1989.[9]

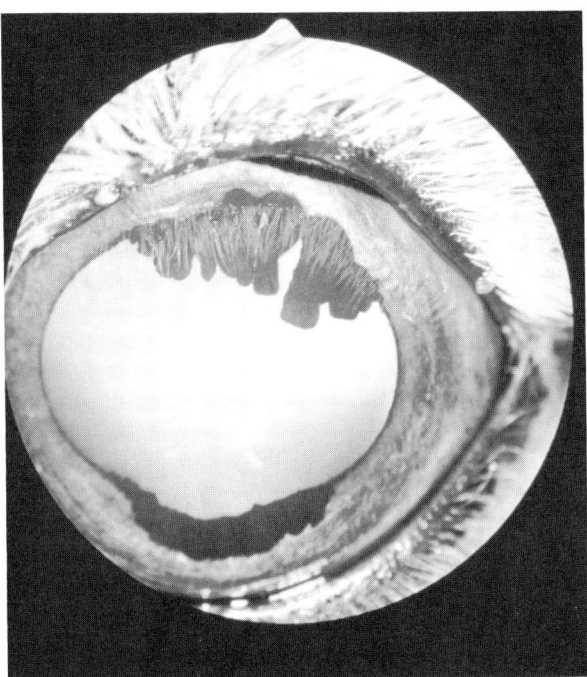

Figure 1. Frontal view of llama eye showing prominent pupillary ruff.

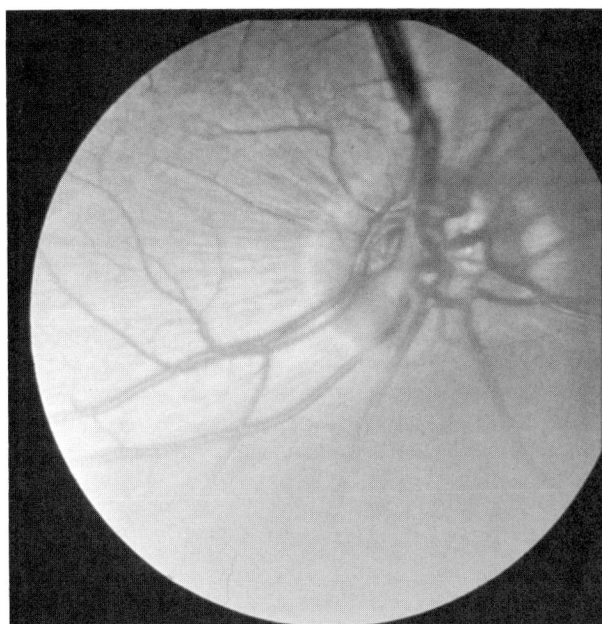

Figure 2. Llama fundus showing the lack of a tapetum and the myelination around optic nerve axons as they extend into the eye.

bunch together and slide up slightly, under the peripheral iris. In bright sunlight, the dorsal and ventral pupillary ruff meet and almost intermesh, but they do not meet in normal room light. Iris pigmentation is usually various shades of brown and occasionally blue. Streaks of blue often show through the brown pigment, representing areas of sparser pigmentation. White or black freckles are sometimes observed on the iris. The pupil is roughly oval with the long axis oriented horizontally. The medial and lateral portions of the pupil are smooth, round, and darkly pigmented. The medial hemicircle of the pupil has a greater diameter than the lateral one does, but the pupil is nearly round when maximally dilated. Persistent pupillary membranes are common, especially near the pupillary margin. Neonatal llamas occasionally have thin, gray, fibrinous strands spanning 1 or 2 folds of the pupillary ruff.

Unlike all other ungulates except the Suidae, the Bactrian camel and the dromedary, the fundus of the domestic South American camelid lacks a tapetum.[5, 9] This results in a red fundic reflex rather than yellow or green as in other animals. The fundus color is usually either red and brown or blue and brown. The red represents the choroid, visible through the retinal pigment epithelium.

The optic disk and retinal vasculature are similar to those of the bovine (Fig. 2). A large Bergmeister's papilla (hyaloid remnant) commonly protrudes from the disk. About 5 pairs of large retinal vessels emerge from the disk. The largest vessels emerge dorsally and wind around each other and are sometimes elevated from the surface of the retina. Two pairs of horizontal vessels are usually accompanied by myelin, which extends several disk diameters peripherally into the fundus. The myelin has a white feathered appearance. Ventrally, either a single vessel exits and divides into 2 branches, or 2 vessels leave the disk separately. The vessels are often dotted with pigment as they exit from the optic disk, and in some llamas a vascular pulse may be observed on the surface of the disk.

The bony orbit of the llama, like that of the horse and ox, is complete and made up of the frontal, lacrimal, zygomatic, maxillary, palatine, temporal, and sphenoid bones. Only the first 3 make up the orbital rim itself. There is a large notch dorsally in the frontal bone that is palpable in the living animal. About 2 cm rostral to the medial orbit is a 2-cm diameter opening into the nasal cavity bounded by the nasal, frontal, lacrimal, and maxillary bones. This opening is not present in other domestic animals and is probably associated with a scent gland.

EXAMINATION

Ocular examination is optimally undertaken with the llama restrained in stocks and the head held gently over a padded bar (Fig. 3). Because most llamas object violently to facial contact, it is useful to control head movement by wrapping a towel behind the ears and under the chin. Some llamas will tolerate an ophthalmic examination in sternal recumbency. A quiet environment greatly facilitates the examination. Liquids

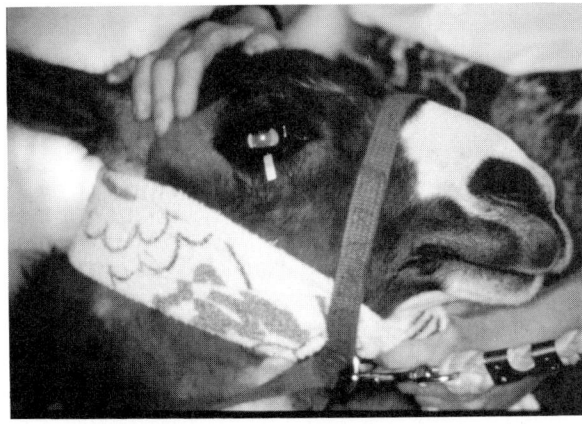

Figure 3. Schirmer tear test strip in place under the lower eyelid of the llama eye. Note restraint of the head with a folded towel.

such as 1 per cent tropicamide, topical anesthetic, and fluorescein dye may be easily applied to the eye during examination with a "squirt gun" made from a 3-ml syringe and a 22-gauge needle broken at the hub.

A complete ocular examination should include an external eye and anterior segment examination under magnification, reflex responses, a Schirmer tear test for tear production, measurements of intraocular pressure, and funduscopy. The menace reflex for testing vision may be elicited by a sudden hand movement across the visual axis (while avoiding the long vibrissae). The llama should blink, jerk the head, or jump back. Direct and indirect pupillary light reflexes in the llama are slow, and movement of the iris is minimal.

The Schirmer tear test may be done by placing the filter paper strip in the lower conjunctival fornix for 60 seconds. Tear production is measured in millimeters per minute, and the mean value is 19. Most llamas tolerate this test without struggling.

The intraocular pressure is most easily measured with a Tonopen applanation tonometer and averages 14 mm Hg with this instrument. Topical anesthetic should be used to facilitate tonometry. However, its detergent action on the tear film may result in a temporary dimpled appearance of the cornea, which can prevent clear observation of the fundus. For dilating the pupil for examination of the fundus, 1 application (about 0.25 ml) of 1 per cent tropicamide will cause mydriasis within 20 to 45 minutes.

MICROBIOLOGY OF THE NORMAL CAMELID EYE

Numerous species of bacteria (Table 2) and fungi (Table 3) have been isolated from the conjunctiva of the normal camelid eye. These organisms are similar to those reported from the normal eyes of other species,[15, 25, 28–31] and many of the organisms isolated from camelids have been implicated as opportunistic pathogens in other animals.[10, 16, 18]

In 1 study, a large percentage of camelids had *Pseudomonas* organisms in their conjunctival sacs during the winter.[11] This differs from the flora of other species. Although none of these isolates was *Pseudomonas aeruginosa* (a common cause of rapidly progressing corneal ulcers in many species[13, 18]) any *Pseudomonas* organism may have the potential to become pathogenic secondary to other ocular disease or trauma.[2]

Table 2. PERCENTAGE OF CAMELIDS POSITIVE FOR BACTERIA

	Llama (n = 147)	Alpaca (n = 17)	Guanaco (n = 37)
Gram-Positive Organisms			
Coagulase-negative			
Staphylococcus spp.	50	60	51
Coagulase-positive			
Staphylococcus spp.	7	6	8
Bacillus spp.	35	35	32
Streptococcus spp.	22	47	11
Corynebacterium spp.	15	—	8
Streptomyces spp.	11	41	7
Gram-Negative Organisms			
Pseudomonas spp.	14	35	52
Pasteurella spp.	0.6	6	22
Branhamella spp.	0.6	29	—
Moraxella spp.	0.6	—	—

This table represents a combination of data from 2 studies (Friedman, 1989;[9] Gionfriddo et al, 1991[11]). Only the major bacteria found in the largest numbers are reported.

Table 3. PERCENTAGE OF CAMELIDS POSITIVE FOR FUNGUS

Fungus	Llama (n = 109)	Alpaca (n = 17)	Guanaco (n = 20)
Aspergillus spp.	33	30	35
Fusarium spp.	29	4	5
Rhinocladiella spp.	9	2	—
Alternaria spp.	7	—	—
Mucor spp.	7	1	—
Penicillium spp.	3	1	—
Curvularia spp.	3	—	—

This table represents a combination of data from 2 studies.[9, 11] Only the fungi found in the largest numbers are reported.

Because numerous potential pathogenic bacterial organisms are harbored in the camelid conjunctival sac, topical antibiotic administration should be instituted before ocular surgery or after corneal or conjunctival injury.

Other types of microorganisms have not been found in camelid conjunctival sacs. In 2 independent studies,[9, 11] no *Mycoplasma* organisms were isolated. This is surprising because mycoplasma are ubiquitous in the environment[27] and are isolated from normal eyes of many other species.[27, 32] Neither viral nor chlamydial isolation has been attempted.

CAMELID OCULAR DISEASE

Conjunctiva and Cornea

Despite the large size and prominent position of their eyes, camelids seem to have relatively few external ocular injuries or disease. However, corneal contusions, abrasions, ulcerations, and foreign body penetrations have been observed.[7, 12] Corneal or conjunctival lacerations and ulcers should be treated in the same manner as in other species. Lacerations may be sutured directly with small-gauge suture material. The successful use of conjunctival flaps or grafts or nictitating membrane flaps for repair of corneal injuries has not been reported in camelids. Ingram and Sigler[14] used a conjunctival pedicle flap to try to prevent the rupture of a descemetocele in a cria (neonatal llama). The sutures quickly pulled loose from the cornea, and the cornea ruptured. This failure was probably due to the necrotic condition of the cornea and does not necessarily predict the usefulness of this technique in captive camelids.

Bacteria have been isolated from several cases of conjunctivitis and keratoconjunctivitis in llamas. In many cases, it is unknown whether these bacteria were the primary cause of the disease or secondary invaders. *Moraxella liquefaciens* was isolated from an ulcerated cornea of a llama and was thought to be a primary pathogen.[3] *Staphylococcus aureus* was isolated from the inflamed conjunctiva of the same animal. *Staphylococcus epidermidis* was found in the ulcerated cornea of a cria that had undergone cataract surgery.[14] This infected ulcer perforated, leading to phthisis bulbi. *Klebsiella pneumoniae*, *Moraxella* sp., *Bacteroides* sp., *Bacillus* sp., and *Streptococcus* sp. organisms have been isolated from llamas with conjunctivitis.[12] Clinical signs of bacterial conjunctivitis include hyperemic conjunctiva, serous or mucopurulent ocular discharge, and blepharospasm.

Ulcerative keratitis in llamas is caused primarily by injury and secondary bacterial invasion of the wound. Primary bacterial invasion of the cornea (as with *Moraxella bovis* in cattle) has not been documented. The llama with a corneal ulcer usually presents with blepharospasm, epiphora, and corneal edema. Because small corneal scratches may be missed on cursory examination, fluorescein dye staining should be performed on all cases of corneal injury and suspected ulcerative keratitis.

Microbiologic culture and sensitivity are recommended in cases of conjunctivitis, keratitis, and ulcerative keratitis. The value of culturing both corneal lesions and the conjunctiva was demonstrated by Brightman et al.[3] when these 2 inflamed areas yielded different bacteria. Most cases of external ocular bacterial infections respond well to appropriate topical antibacterial therapy. Antibiotic ointments may be placed in the inferior conjunctival fornix. If the camelid is uncooperative or if the condition requires frequent medication, an indwelling catheter (such as small-gauge polyethylene tubing) may be placed into the nasal orifice of the nasolacrimal duct. It is then threaded gently up the nasolacrimal duct until resistance is met, or the llama blinks, which indicates that the tubing has reached the eye.[7] The tubing is then affixed to the skin of the face near the nostril by placing a butterfly of tape around the tubing and suturing the tape to the skin. The tubing can be brought back along the face and sutured to the skin of the forehead and neck. A blunt needle inserted into the distal end of the tubing serves as an injection port for solutions through the tubing and into the eye. The needle hub is capped to prevent contamination between medications.

Parasitic conjunctivitis has been attributed to both flies and nematodes. *Thelazia californiensis*, a spirurid nematode, has been found in the conjunctival sac of deer, dogs, cattle, sheep, elk, foxes, rabbits, llamas, and humans.[7] *T. californiensis* has traditionally been reported to cause only mild conjunctivitis in llamas.[7] However, 2 llamas in Wisconsin had severe keratoconjunctivitis and corneal ulceration that was associated with *T. californiensis* infection.[9] The nematode completes its life cycle in muscoid flies and is transmitted between animals by these flies. The primary sign of infection is epiphora. The nematode may be seen in the eye on the surface of the conjunctiva or cornea, or it may be beneath the nictitating membrane or in the nasolacrimal duct.[7] Treatment involves mechanical removal of the nematode under topical anesthetic. Alternatively, diethylcarbamazine or ivermectin drops may be instilled into the conjunctival sac.[7] In llamas, as in cattle and horses, flies may feed on lacrimal secretions and cause conjunctival irritation. Therefore fly control is important for minimizing this form of conjunctivitis.

Fungal keratitis or conjunctivitis is rare in camelids although small numbers of colonies of *Rhondotorula, Acremonium, Scopulariopsis*, and *Aspergillus* have been cultured from llamas with conjunctivitis. The animals also had large numbers of bacteria in their eyes, and bacterial infection was probably the primary cause of the conjunctivitis.[12]

Reports of noninfectious corneal abnormalities are rare in camelids. Bilateral corneal edema has been reported in a female guanaco and its female offspring. This was thought to be a congenital, hereditary defect. It was associated with other ocular abnormalities and was probably a corneal endothelial dystrophy.[1]

Lens

Abnormalities of the camelid lens are observed frequently. Mature, hypermature, and immature cataracts as well as luxated lenses and lens colobomas have been seen. A large proportion of llamas have small focal cataracts. One way to diagnose these cataracts is to stand at arm's length and shine a penlight at the dilated pupil. The cataract will appear black against the red reflection from the fundus. Whether these cataracts progress to maturity or if they are hereditary is unknown. A lens coloboma associated with a cataract and corneal edema was reported in a guanaco.[1]

Cataract removal has been performed in llamas with limited success. In the 1 published report of a cataract surgery, lens extraction was followed by severe corneal edema, secondary bacterial ulcerative keratitis, and phthisis bulbi.[14] Another lens removal surgery in a young llama, done by the discission and aspiration technique, had complications of severe corneal edema, uveitis, and keratoconus.[19, 26] With frequent applications of topical corticosteroids, these symptoms resolved slowly.

The corneal edema that is seen as a complication of cataract surgery in llamas is probably due to a highly sensitive corneal endothelium in these animals and to a high degree of postoperative inflammation. The inflammation may be minimized by pre- and postoperative topical and systemic corticosteroids and nonsteroidal anti-inflammatory drugs. However, the limited success rate of cataract surgery in llamas and the potential severity of the postsurgical complications preclude its use in general veterinary practice.

Uvea and Posterior Segment

Congenital defects of the uvea and posterior segment have been seen in the llama. These include iris hypoplasia and coloboma, and optic disk and peripapillary colobomas. On histopathologic examination of the eyes of 3 neonatal llamas, a proliferative fibrotic uveitis was seen and was associated with a peripapillary coloboma. This condition was also accompanied by vitreous fibrosis and ossification, cataracts, retinal dysplasia, and retinal detachment.[4] Large optic disk colobomas were observed in one 10-month-old llama.[9] These colobomas caused no apparent visual deficit.

Equine herpesvirus I (EHV-I) causes severe ocular disease in camelids. Only 1 outbreak has been reported in the literature,[24] although others have been confirmed. Camelids acquire EHV-I virus by contact with members of the Equidae family, including horses, donkeys, and zebras. Vaccination of llamas for EHV-I with the equine vaccine has been attempted, but its efficacy is unknown.

Acute ocular signs were common in the published case of 21 alpacas and 1 llama with EHV-I.[24] The animals became blind and had severe uveitis, vitritis, chorioretinitis, and optic neuritis. Four animals also exhibited neurologic signs including nystagmus, head tilt, and paralysis. Two animals died. Treatment with a variety of antibiotics, steroids, nonsteroidal anti-inflammatory drugs, diuretics, vitamin A, and thiamine failed to restore vision. Diagnosis was made histologically after identification of eosinophilic inclusions in the brain and by virus isolation from brain tissue. Chronic ocular lesions in the recovered animals included vitreal fibrous traction bands, retinal detachment, retinal degeneration, and optic nerve atrophy with myelin loss. Animals that survived did not recover vision.

In 1989, a similar outbreak was observed in Illinois in a herd of llamas.[9] Twenty-eight llamas were exposed to 4 zebras with rhinitis. Within 10 to 17 days, 17 of the 28 llamas developed neurologic signs, including blindness, deafness, head tilt, and circling. In 3 animals, these signs progressed rapidly to recumbency and death. Ophthalmic examination showed severe anterior uveitis and chorioretinitis characterized by fluffy subretinal exudates, severe retinal hemorrhage, and retinal detachments. Histologic examination revealed numerous cells with intranuclear inclusions throughout the brain and inner retina. EHV-I was isolated from culture of brain tissue of 2 llamas and buffy coats of 1 zebra. The neurologic signs resolved in all but 1 llama. Ocular inflammation improved without treatment but left severe retinal detachments. Six animals remained blind.

A case of 1 blind llama without neurologic signs was reported by Paulsen et al.[21] Fundic examination revealed retinal degeneration with attenuated vessels, pale optic disks, optic nerve atrophy, and white foci (scars). Differential diagnosis included elaeophoriasis, primary retinal degeneration, toxicosis, hypovitaminosis A, toxoplasmosis, polioencephalomalacia, equine herpesvirus, and parelaphostrongylosis. Histologic examination of the brain showed a perivascular mononuclear cell infiltrate composed primarily of lymphocytes, but no herpesvirus inclusion bodies were seen. Tissue virus isolation was not attempted. Herpesvirus could not be identified as the cause owing to the negative serum titer and lack of inclusion bodies in the brain. However, these tests may have been negative because of the chronic nature of the condition, and EHV-I may have been the etiologic agent of the blindness in this animal.

Twelve cases of a "uveitis syndrome" in camelids have been seen.[8] These animals had histories of either respiratory or gastrointestinal symptoms (colic) and severe panuveitis. Most of the animals died. At necropsy, *Klebsiella* pneumonia was diagnosed in 1 animal, and *Pseudomonas* pneumonia was diagnosed in another. However, neither of these bacteria was thought to be the primary cause of uveitis in the llamas, and the etiologic agent of the panuveitis in the 12 animals remains obscure. Viral immunosuppression (such as by a lentivirus) that led to secondary bacterial invasion has been suggested but not confirmed.

Disseminated aspergillosis has also been implicated as a cause of neurologic disease and chorioretinitis in a zoo-housed, wild-caught alpaca.[22] The alpaca exhibited blindness with hemorrhage, mottling and elevation of the retina, retinal vasculitis, and optic neuritis. On post-mortem examination, *Aspergillus* was identified in the lung and eye.

It is clear that much remains to be discovered about llama eyes. Research into the etiology of various ocular diseases, especially the mode of inheritance of suspected hereditary problems (such as cataracts and colobomas), will be important to the veterinary practitioner advising llama owners on breeding programs. Documentation of diseases that camelids share with other species and that may cause ocular disease (especially uveitis) in camelids is an important future endeavor. In the meantime, practitioners must include most of the causes of ocular diseases of both domestic ruminants and horses in their differential diagnoses of eye problems in camelids.

REFERENCES

1. Barrie KP, Jacobson E, Peiffer RL: Unilateral cataract with lens coloboma and bilateral corneal edema in a guanaco. J Am Vet Med Assoc 173:1251–1252, 1978.
2. Bistner SI, Roberts SR, Anderson RP: Conjunctival bacteria: clinical appearances can be deceiving. Mod Vet Pract December:45–47, 1969.
3. Brightman AH, McLaughlin SA, Brumley B: Keratoconjunctivitis in a llama. VMSAC 76:1776–1777, 1981.
4. Dubielzig RR: Personal communication, 1990.
5. Duke Elder S: System of Ophthalmology, vol I. The Eye in Evolution. St. Louis, CV Mosby, 1958, pp 458, 470.
6. El-bab MRF, Misk NA, Hifny A, Kaasem AM: Surgical anatomy of the lens in different domestic animals. Anatomia Histol Embryol 11:27–31, 1982.
7. Fowler ME: Medicine and Surgery of South American Camelids. Ames, IA, Iowa State University Press, 1989.
8. Fowler ME: Personal communication, 1990.
9. Friedman DS: Unpublished data, 1989.
10. Gerding PA, McLaughlin SA, Troop MW: Pathogenic bacteria and fungi associated with external ocular disease in dogs: 131 cases (1981–1986). J Am Vet Med Assoc 93:242–244, 1988.
11. Gionfriddo JR, Rosenbusch R, Kinyon JM, et al: The bacterial and mycoplasmal flora of the normal camelid conjunctival sac. Am J Vet Res 52:1061–1064, 1991.
12. Gionfriddo JR: Unpublished data, 1990.
13. Hugh R, Gilardi GL: Pseudomonas. *In* Lenette EH (ed): Manual of Clinical Microbiology, 3rd ed. Washington DC, American Society for Microbiology, 1980.
14. Ingram KA, Sigler RL: Cataract removal in a young llama. Proceedings, 1983 Annual Meeting, American Association of Zoo Veterinarians, Tampa, FL, 1983.
15. Lundvall RL: The bacterial and mycotic flora of the normal conjunctival sac in the horse. Proceedings American Association of Equine Practitioners, 1967, pp 101–107.
16. Mitchell JS, Attleberger MH: Fusarium keratomycosis in the horse. Vet Med Small Anim Clin November:1257–1273, 1973.
17. Martin CL, Anderson BG: Ocular anatomy. *In* Gellat KN (ed): Textbook of Veterinary Ophthalmology. Philadelphia, Lea & Febiger, 1980, pp 12–121.
18. Moore CP, Fales WH, Whittington P, Bauer L: Bacterial and fungal isolates from equidae with ulcerative keratitis. J Am Vet Med Assoc 182:600–603, 1983.
19. Murphy C: Personal communication, 1990.
20. Jenkins D: Alpacas and llamas are susceptible to an equine disease. Llamas 30:15–16, 1985.
21. Paulsen ME, Young S, Smith JA, Severin GH: Bilateral chorioretinitis, centripetal optic neuritis, and encephalitis in a llama. J Am Vet Med Assoc 194:1305–1308, 1989.
22. Pickett JP, Moore CP, Beehler BA, et al: Bilateral chorioretinitis secondary to disseminated aspergillosis in an alpaca. J Am Vet Med Assoc 187:1241–1243, 1985.
23. Rahi AHS, Sheikh H, Morgan G: Histology of the camel eye. Acta Anat 106:345–350, 1980.
24. Rebhun WC, Jenkins DH, Riis RC, et al: An epizootic of blindness and encephalitis associated with a herpes virus indistinguishable from equine herpesvirus I in a herd of alpacas and llamas. J Am Vet Med Assoc 192:953–956, 1988.
25. Samuelson DA, Andresen TL, Gwin RM: Conjunctival fungal flora in horses, cattle, dogs and cats. J Am Vet Med Assoc 184:1240–1242, 1984.
26. Scherlie P: Personal communication, 1990.
27. Smith PF: The Biology of Mycoplasmas. New York, Academic Press, 1971.
28. Spadbrow P: The bacterial flora of the ovine conjunctival sac. Aust Vet J 44:117–119, 1968.
29. Urban M, Wyman M, Rheins M, Marraro RV: Conjunctival flora of clinically normal dogs. J Am Vet Med Assoc 161:201–206, 1972.
30. Whitley RD, Burgess EC, Moore CP: Microbial isolates of the normal equine eye. Equine Vet J Suppl 2:138–140, 1983.
31. Wilcox GE: Bacterial flora of the bovine eye with special reference to the *Moraxella* and *Neisseria*. Aust Vet J 46:253–257, 1970.
32. Wolf ED, Amass K, Olsen J: Survey of conjunctival flora in the eye of clinically normal, captive exotic birds. J Am Vet Med Assoc 183:1232–1233, 1983.

Food Animal Ocular Neoplasia

STEVEN M. ROBERTS, DVM, MS, Diplomate, ACVO

ROBERT KAINER, DVM, MS

Food animal ocular neoplasia has received little attention in comparison to companion animal ocular neoplasia. Available information deals with the most common neoplasms of large animals, squamous cell carcinoma and lymphosarcoma. Uncommon tumors have little literature documentation other than occasional case reports, inclusion in epidemiologic surveys, or mention in textbooks. This is not to suggest there is little interest in all food animal neoplasms. However, one must often extrapolate tumor behavior and treatment information from common food animal and companion animal tumor data. Frequently, economic considerations, intended use, and life expectancy of food-producing animals dictate the management approaches. Significant economic losses associated with bovine ocular squamous cell carcinoma and lymphosarcoma have prompted investigative studies into etiologic agents, pathophysiologic mechanisms, treatment modalities, and overall prognosis of these diseases.

Table 1. CLINICAL SIGNS AND DIFFERENTIAL DIAGNOSIS OF OCULAR NEOPLASIA IN FOOD ANIMALS

Clinical Signs	Bovine	Caprine	Ovine
Buphthalmia	IBK OSCC Ocular melanoma Ocular trauma	Ocular trauma	Ocular melanoma Ocular trauma
Corneal mass	Enzootic adult lymphosarcoma IBK Interstitial keratitis Ocular dermoid OSCC	Keratomycosis Ocular dermoid OSCC	Keratomycosis Ocular dermoid OSCC
Exophthalmos	Enzootic adult lymphosarcoma Nasal and paranasal sinus neoplasia Nonprogressive bilateral exophthalmos OSCC Oral, maxillary, and mandibular neoplasia Retrobulbar neoplasia Sporadic bovine leukosis	Nasal and paranasal sinus neoplasia OSCC Oral, maxillary, and mandibular neoplasia	Nasal adenocarcinoma Nasal and paranasal sinus neoplasia OSCC
Facial masses	Enzootic adult lymphosarcoma Dermal melanoma Fibroma Fibrosarcoma Nasal and paranasal sinus neoplasia Ocular dermoid Ocular melanoma OSCC Papillomatosis Retrobulbar neoplasia Sebaceous cyst Sporadic bovine leukosis	Dermal melanoma Fibroma Fibrosarcoma Histiocytoma Lymphosarcoma Nasal and paranasal sinus neoplasia OSCC Papillomatosis	Fibroma Fibrosarcoma Lymphosarcoma Nasal and paranasal sinus neoplasia Ocular melanoma OSCC Papillomatosis
Intraocular mass	Ectopic lacrimal gland Ocular melanoma OSCC	OSCC Ocular trauma	OSCC Ocular trauma
Nasolacrimal duct obstruction	Nasolacrimal duct occlusion Nasal and paranasal sinus neoplasia	Nasolacrimal duct occlusion Nasal and paranasal sinus neoplasia	Nasolacrimal duct occlusion Nasal and paranasal sinus neoplasia
Nictitans protrusion	Horner's syndrome Lymphosarcoma Ocular trauma Nasal and paranasal sinus neoplasia	Horner's syndrome Ocular trauma Nasal and paranasal sinus neoplasia	Horner's syndrome Ocular trauma Nasal and paranasal sinus neoplasia
Ocular discharge	Conjunctivitis Ocular trauma Lymphosarcoma Nasal and paranasal sinus neoplasia Retrobulbar neoplasia	Conjunctivitis Lymphosarcoma Nasal and paranasal sinus neoplasia	Conjunctivitis Lymphosarcoma Nasal and paranasal sinus neoplasia
Ocular pain	Brain stem neoplasia Ocular dermoid OSCC Orbital lymphosarcoma Sporadic bovine leukosis	Brain stem neoplasia Ocular dermoid OSCC	Brain stem neoplasia Ocular dermoid OSCC
Periorbital or eyeball mass	Ectopic lacrimal gland Fibroma Fibrosarcoma Ocular dermoid Ocular melanoma OSCC Retrobulbar neoplasia	Fibroma Fibrosarcoma Dermal melanoma Nasal and paranasal sinus neoplasia Ocular dermoid OSCC Papillomatosis	Fibroma Fibrosarcoma Dermal melanoma Nasal and paranasal sinus neoplasia Ocular dermoid OSCC Papillomatosis

IBK = infectious bovine keratoconjunctivitis; OSCC = ocular squamous cell carcinoma.

A wide variety of neoplastic conditions, either primary or secondary, can involve the eye and periocular tissues. Anatomic location of the tumor frequently determines the spectrum of clinical signs that develop. The basic tissue changes will consist of tissue distortion, desiccation of ocular tissues, and loss of function. Anatomic location of the tumor becomes influential in selection of treatment modalities. In some situations, tumor treatment is to provide palliative relief for the animal or remove the problem from the herd by culling affected individuals. In other situations, treatment has the goal of curing the animal. In many instances, emphasis is not on histologic diagnosis, as important as this may be, but rather on elimination of economic loss. However, a histologic diagnosis may influence specific treatment recommendations, as with benign versus malignant lesions or squamous cell carcinoma versus lymphosarcoma. Table 1 lists clinical signs and differential diagnoses frequently associated with adnexal and ocular neoplasia.

BOVINE OCULAR SQUAMOUS CELL CARCINOMA

Bovine ocular squamous cell tumors (OSCT) represent the most important neoplasm of food animals. The designation

OSCT, by common usage, includes both benign and malignant epithelial neoplasms of the eye or adnexa. The proper terminology for benign lesions is premalignant, keratoacanthomatous, or papillomatous. The terms "epithelioma of the eye" and "ocular squamous cell carcinoma" (OSCC) imply a malignant lesion. An estimated 12.5 per cent of the bovine carcass condemnations in federally inspected slaughter houses in the United States result from this neoplasm. The tumor develops at the epithelial surfaces of the conjunctiva, cornea, and eyelid margins. Thus disease typically affects the corneoscleral junction, nictitating membrane, and palpebral conjunctiva at the eyelid margin.

Clinical Signs

Gross appearance of OSCT depends on the anatomic location and stage of malignancy. Benign tumors are small, white, elevated, hyperplastic plaques or papillomatous structures with verrucous or exophytic surfaces. The lateral and medial limbus are the most frequently involved sites. Tumors located at the corneoscleral junction grow slowly owing to the natural barrier presented by the dense and poorly vascularized tissue in this region. Metastasis is slow with corneoscleral lesions. Malignant tumors are more irregular, nodular, pink, erosive, and necrotic. With tumor necrosis, a characteristic foul odor is often detectable. Benign keratoacanthomas or "wickers" are light brown, hornlike crusts along the lid margins that may become coated with lacrimal secretions. Frequent confusion of benign lesions with OSCC occurs, especially on the part of lay persons.

OSCT may develop through a series of benign stages, hyperplastic plaques, and papillomas to carcinoma in situ. Also, de novo carcinoma may develop as a small lesion. Over a course of months to years, the lesions become invasive OSCC. Malignant lesions involve, in decreasing order of prevalence, the lateral limbus, eyelid margins (especially the lower), nictitating membrane, and medial canthal regions. This neoplasm is locally invasive, with extensive orbital involvement possible if lesions remain untreated. Clinical signs associated with metastatic disease are not common, although parotid or lateral retropharyngeal lymph nodes may become infiltrated with neoplastic cells. In most cases, metastasis to vital organs will eventually occur; therefore, either lesions must be treated early or severely affected animals should be culled.

Diagnosis

It is often possible to make a presumptive diagnosis on the basis of the gross appearance of the lesions. Definitive diagnoses based on tissue samples allow grading of tumor malignancy. Collection of tissue samples for cytologic or histopathologic examination requires only simple instrumentation and techniques. After topical anesthesia, cytologic samples are collected with a spatula. Samples are spread carefully on a slide and fixed with polyethylene glycol spray or 95 per cent ethanol immersion. Fixation of biopsy specimens is by immersion in 10 per cent neutral buffered formalin. Biopsy specimens usually provide a more consistent diagnosis than do cytologic preparations. Collection of fine-needle aspirates from regional lymph nodes may be useful in some cases for detection of metastatic spread.

Benign lesions typically consist of superficial, anucleated, keratinized squamous cells. The few deeper epithelial cells present will contain enlarged nuclei and coarsely clumped chromatin. In histologic evaluation of benign lesions, no neoplastic invasion across the epithelial basement membrane occurs. Malignant lesions consist of pleomorphic epithelial cells of bizarre shapes, large hyperchromatic nuclei containing coarse clumps of chromatin, and prominent nucleoli. In histologic evaluation of malignant lesions, neoplastic invasion occurring across the epithelial basement membrane, keratin-pearl formation, and marked anaplasia are seen.

Treatment

When possible, lesions should be treated early. However, not all early lesions require treatment because precancerous lesions may undergo spontaneous regression in 30 to 50 per cent of cases. Malignant tumors rarely undergo spontaneous regression. Studies about the response of OSCT to particular forms of treatment must consider the type of lesions undergoing treatment for correct interpretation of treatment response data. Treatment options can consist of one or more of the following modalities: radiation therapy, biologic response modifiers or immunotherapy, surgical excision, cryosurgery, and hyperthermia. Small lesions are more successfully treated than are large lesions. Whereas small lesions respond to any of these modalities, large lesions involving multiple tissues require aggressive intervention and thus an increased cost for treatment. As with any form of neoplasia, retreatment is essential at the first sign of tumor recurrence. Except with radiation therapy, it is possible and frequently necessary to treat tumors repeatedly for achieving remission or cure. Some tumors will fail to respond to treatment regardless of the modality or combination of modalities used.

Radiation Therapy

Radiation therapy typically consists of brachytherapy with use of radioactive implants such as cesium-137, cobalt-60, gold-198, or iridium. Such therapy is effective and expensive; it requires qualified personnel and compliance with radiation safety regulations. Lesions at the corneoscleral junction respond to treatment with a beta irradiation source such as a strontium-90 probe. A superficial keratectomy for debulking lesions raised above the normal corneal surface increases the therapeutic effect of the beta irradiation. This is because absorption of 50 per cent of the electrons occurs for each millimeter of tissue penetration by emissions of the strontium-90 probe. Thus effective radiation treatment is possible for lesions only a few millimeters thick. Strontium-90 irradiation is useful for partial-thickness corneal lesions and superficial eyelid lesions.

Biologic Response Modifiers

Biologic response modifiers exert an antitumor effect by mobilizing nonspecific immune mechanisms against the neoplasm. This is possible because malignant transformation also causes loss of normal cell-surface antigens, production of new cell-surface antigens, and cell membrane changes. These antigenic changes help evoke an immune response involving principally the cell-mediated arm of the immune system, although many complex effector cell populations also interact. The response relies heavily on response amplification by interleukins and lymphokines or cytokines.

Bacterial products or chemical immunomodulators can cause nonspecific immunostimulation. Such bacterial products include *Propionibacterium acnes* (formally *Corynebacterium parvum*) (ImmunoRegulin*) and mycobacterium cell-wall fraction (Normagen†; Regressin-V‡). Chemical immunomodulators in-

---
*Immuno Vet, Tampa, FL 33630.
†Fort Dodge Laboratories, Fort Dodge, IA 50501.
‡Vetrepharm Research Inc., Athens, GA 30601.

clude levamisole and H_2-receptor blockers such as cimetidine. Specific active immunotherapy includes tumor cell vaccination with allogenic OSCC extracts and the potential future use of interferon and cytokines such as tumor necrosis factor.

Drawbacks to biologic response modification, as a cancer treatment, relate to heterogeneity of tumor cell populations, changing antigenic properties of tumors, and fluctuation in host immune system capacity. Despite the problems with biologic response modification in cancer treatment, bovine OSCC does respond to mycobacterium cell-wall preparations and allogenic OSCC extracts. Tumor regression in 25 per cent and 33 per cent of the cases treated occurs with mycobacterium cell-wall preparations and allogenic OSCC extracts, respectively.

Surgical Excision

Surgical excision of OSCT is perhaps the most common treatment. Small or well-circumscribed lesions are removable by local excision with or without adjunctive hyperthermia or cryosurgery procedures. Involvement of the nictitating membrane may warrant amputation of this eyelid, a procedure that rarely results in large animal ocular complications. Focal involvement of the cornea is amenable to local excision, by superficial keratectomy, followed by radiation, hyperthermia, or cryosurgical treatment. Tumors involving multiple regions of the eye and adnexa or those extending into the orbit require extensive surgical excision. Recommended treatment for involvement of only the globe and eyelids is an enucleation. For orbital involvement, recommended treatment is exenteration, performed with or without resection of the involved salivary glands and lymph nodes.

Cryosurgery

Cryosurgery is an excellent treatment choice for small or superficial neoplasms. Perform cryosurgery after topical, regional, or general anesthesia. Induce topical anesthesia of the globe and conjunctiva by instilling several drops of 0.5 per cent proparacaine hydrochloride solution into the conjunctival sac every 20 to 30 seconds for several minutes. Regional anesthesia by injection of 2 per cent lidocaine into the subconjunctival, retrobulbar, or adnexal tissues allows more aggressive tissue manipulations. For all forms of cryosurgery, animal restraint is with a squeeze chute and halter. A slotted ocular retractor is useful to proptose the globe, thus simplifying treatment. In preparation for cryosurgery, protect the surrounding normal tissues by using Styrofoam strips, plastic spoons or spatulas, and opthalmic or nitrofurazone ointment. When spray freezing, protect adjacent normal tissues from run-off of liquid cryogen.

The preferred cryosurgical procedure uses a double freeze-thaw technique: rapid freeze to $-25°$ C, unaided thaw to $5°$ C, and rapid refreeze to $-25°$ C, with either spray tips or probes delivering the cryogen to tissues. Liquid nitrogen ($-196°$ C) is the most potent, available, and economic cryogen for food animal use. Less potent cryogens, such as freon ($-50°$ C) or carbon dioxide ($-80°$ C), are useful on small tumors. Use of freon is questionable because of detrimental environmental effects. Cryosurgery is successful in treating OSCT lesions less than 2 to 3 cm in diameter and 1 to 2 mm in thickness. After cryosurgery, the treated tissues become swollen, depigmented, and necrotic and will exude a serous to mucopurulent discharge. Tumor tissue and some normal tissue will slough in 1 to 2 weeks. Healing is by second intention and is usually uneventful. Secondary leukoderma, leukotrichia, and cicatrix are common. If the tumor regrows, then retreatment is indicated.

Radiofrequency Current Hyperthermia

Radiofrequency current (RFC) hyperthermia is also an effective, simple, and economic modality especially for early treatment of benign lesions. In particular, lesions less than 2.5 cm in diameter respond well. Treatment can be performed with use of surface probes, piercing probes, or a combination of the two. RFC will penetrate tissue to a depth of 2 to 3 mm. Tumors thicker than 5 cm are debulked before treatment with surface or piercing probes. Tumors that regrow may be subsequently retreated with RFC.

RFC instruments pass a 6.78 MHz current through the tissues, causing heat generation. A thermistor or thermocouple in one of the probes feeds back to the RFC generator to maintain a tissue temperature of $50°$ C. Hyperthermia treatment for 30 seconds at $50°$ C is lethal to tumor cells but not normal cells. This results from tumor cells becoming hypoxic and having a decreased ability to repair damage. Normal cells are less susceptible to hyperthermia damage because of good oxygen tension and, if damaged, are capable of more effective repair. Depending on the device used, an audible tone emitted at 1-second or 2-second intervals will allow timing of the treatment delivery. Anesthesia and restraint techniques are used as outlined for cryosurgical treatment of OSCT lesions. If the tumor surface is dry, it should be moistened with several drops of physiologic saline solution to improve RFC conduction. For ensuring good tissue contact, surface probes are applied with use of firm pressure. The probe application pattern is a series of multiple overlapping sites. The entire lesion and several millimeters of surrounding normal tissue are treated. For large lesions, hyperthermia treatment sites should form a grid pattern. After treatment in an overlapping fashion, the probe is applied in a pattern perpendicular to the direction of the initial orientation. One must realize that the tissue between the probes is the region heated to $50°$ C. As with cryosurgery, a slotted ocular retractor is helpful in stabilizing the globe for treating corneal and scleral lesions.

During the treatment, tissues become pale or gray and the superficial layers slough, leaving an ulcerative surface. Treatment of the cornea results in leukoma and superficial ulceration. After treatment, tissues will become swollen, the treated tumor tissue will slough, and some adjacent epithelium will slough. Second intention healing is usually rapid and uneventful. Early treatment warrants a favorable prognosis because 90 per cent of the lesions resolve. The willingness of the animal owner to present the animal for follow-up treatment if the tumor recurs influences the overall cure rate.

Epidemiology

The etiology is multifactorial, with genetic, environmental, and viral factors documented or suspected. Sunlight is particularly important as a causing factor. Papillomas can transform to dysplastic tissue and then become OSCC. Thus, suspicion exists that papillomavirus can cause OSCC. Malignant lesions also develop de novo. Overall, a wide variety of cattle breeds develop OSCT. The breed most frequently diagnosed with the disease is the Hereford, both purebred and crossbred. The disease also occurs in cattle with similar patterns of periocular pigmentation such as the Simmentals. Selective breeding for partially or fully pigmented periocular skin or culling affected animals reduces the prevalence of this neoplasm. The prevalence of OSCT, including nonmalignant, precancerous tumors involving Hereford herds, can approach 20 to 40 per cent in regions with abundant sunlight. As many as 10 per cent of these tumors can be malignant. Cattle owners and prospective buyers should be aware of the guidelines for OSCT carcass condemnation followed by federally inspected slaughter plants (see Table 2).

LYMPHOSARCOMA

Bovine lymphosarcoma is a fatal systemic disease of the lymphoreticular tissue with associated ocular manifestations related to orbital tumor involvement. Adult or enzootic lymphosarcoma is the most common and devastating neoplasm of dairy cattle. Bovine leukemia virus is the cause. De novo lymphosarcoma in cattle, unrelated to the bovine leukemia virus–induced disease, also occurs. Goats also develop de novo lymphosarcoma. The etiologic agent of de novo lymphosarcoma is unknown.

Clinical Signs

The adult form of bovine lymphosarcoma causes formation of lymphoid masses at the following sites of predilection: abomasum, right side of the heart (especially the right atrium), kidney, uterus, peripheral and visceral lymph nodes, and retrobulbar portion of the orbit. Less frequently involved is the spleen, bone marrow, gallbladder, liver, and extradural spinal cord. In one case report, a Holstein cow with generalized lymphosarcoma developed intraocular changes as the presenting sign of disease. Typically, clinical signs in cattle or goats are variable and depend on the organs and body systems involved.

Ocular signs are the result of neoplastic lymphoid cell infiltration behind the globe resulting in exophthalmos, exposure keratitis, and finally proptosis. Commonly, the natural exophthalmos of dairy breeds may allow subtle exophthalmos to go undetected. It is also a mistake to assume the plethora of clinical signs associated with exposure keratitis represents primary ocular disease. Corneal signs include edema, vascularization, ulceration, and epidermalization. Conjunctival changes include hemorrhage, chemosis, and ocular discharge. Frequently, ocular changes develop quickly once the degree of exophthalmos has reached a critical point, thus drawing acute attention to the problem. A thorough physical examination will typically reveal lymph node enlargement, weight loss, anemia, and reduced milk production as well as the preceding ocular signs. Differential considerations for exophthalmos include orbital cellulitis, trauma, retrobulbar hemorrhage, retrobulbar soft tissue masses, chronic sinusitis, and sinus neoplasia.

Diagnosis

The finding of enlarged lymph nodes or other areas of lymphocytic infiltration on physical examination is suggestive of lymphosarcoma. Definitive diagnosis hinges on histologic identification of neoplastic lymphocytes in tissues from biopsy, fine-needle aspiration, or necropsy. Abnormal hematology and serum chemistry values parallel the systemic nature of this disease. About 33 per cent of bovine cases will have a leukemic hemogram. If lymphosarcoma is a differential diagnosis, perform serologic testing for bovine leukemia virus. The most common serologic screening method is an agar-gel immunodiffusion test, although a more sensitive and specific radioimmunodiffusion test is also available.

Treatment

In light of the systemic involvement with lymphosarcoma, treatment must be systemic if it is to be more than palliative. Before implementation of chemotherapy, the overall goals and logistics of treatment, bioavailability of oral drugs, and economic issues need consideration. If the goal is to improve the animal's overall condition long enough to deliver a calf, collect superovulated ova, or collect semen for long-term storage, chemotherapy is potentially possible. Palliative enucleation or orbital exenteration represents a less costly treatment approach. In certain situations, valuable animals may warrant chemotherapy and palliative surgery. Most cattle die, either in terminal stages of disease or through euthanasia, from multicentric lymphosarcoma within 6 months of the original diagnosis.

A published report of chemotherapy in a cow used L-asparaginase (10,000 IU/m^2) intravenously and prednisolone (0.5 mg/kg) intramuscularly. To reduce the chance of anaphylaxis, L-asparaginase was given intramuscularly. Another effective means of inducing bovine remissions uses a protocol shown to be effective in canine lymphosarcoma. The protocol drugs and dosages are cyclophosphamide (250 mg/m^2) per os or intravenously, vincristine (0.75 mg/m^2) intravenously, and prednisone (1 mg/kg) per os or intramuscularly. The frequency of chemotherapy is vincristine and cyclophosphamide given on weeks 1, 4, and 7 and then every 3 weeks, and prednisone daily for 21 days, then every other day. Alternatively, some veterinarians give prednisone only during the initial induction period.

Assuming the average bovid has a body surface of 5 m^2, the approximate costs per treatment would be $200 for L-asparaginase, $58 for parenteral cyclophosphamide, $56 for oral cyclophosphamide, $140 for nongeneric vincristine, $46 for generic vincristine, and $7 for parenteral prednisone acetate. Factors that must be considered before selection of a course of treatment include the overall goals of treatment, possible drug effects on germ cells, expected and unexpected systemic side effects in treated animals, possible teratogenic effects on a fetus, and potential effects on neonates before weaning.

Table 2. GUIDELINES FOR INSPECTION, ANTE-MORTEM AND CARCASS, AND DISPOSAL OF ANIMALS, CARCASSES, AND PARTS AFFECTED WITH NEOPLASIA

Epithelioma of the Eye
1. Any animal found on ante-mortem inspection to be affected and the eye has been destroyed or obscured by neoplastic tissue and which shows extensive infection, suppuration, and necrosis, usually accompanied with foul odor, or any affected animal with cachexia, regardless of extent, shall be condemned.
2. Carcasses of animals with the eye or orbital region affected will be condemned if the affection has
   a. involved the osseous structures of the head with extensive infection, suppuration, and necrosis;
   b. metastasized from the eye or orbital region to any lymph node (including the parotid lymph node), internal organs, muscles, skeleton, or other structure, regardless of the extent of the primary tumor; or
   c. regardless of extent is associated with cachexia or evidence of absorption or secondary changes.
3. Carcasses of animals affected to a lesser degree than above may be passed for human food after removal and condemnation of the head, including the tongue, provided the carcass is otherwise normal.

Neoplasms
1. An individual organ or other part of a carcass affected with a neoplasm shall be condemned. If there is evidence of metastasis or that the general condition of the animal has been adversely affected by the size, position, or nature of the neoplasm, the entire carcass shall be condemned.
2. Carcasses affected with malignant lymphoma shall be condemned.

From Code of Federal Regulations, Title 9, Chapter 3, Parts 309.6, 311.11, and 311.12 (1–1–90 edition).

Epidemiology

Adult or enzootic bovine lymphosarcoma occurs in herds and geographic clusters. It is most prevalent in adult cattle over 3 years of age. Prevalence peaks in the 5- to 8-year-old group. Sporadic bovine lymphosarcoma is rare and occurs at random in cattle less than 3 years of age. Orbital involvement infrequently occurs with sporadic bovine lymphosarcoma. The true prevalence of adult bovine lymphosarcoma is difficult to define. Federally inspected abattoirs condemn 20 cattle per 100,000 slaughtered for lymphosarcoma. Such data are misleading, because slaughter cattle populations inaccurately represented dairy cattle. Cattle in America and European countries may have herd infection rates with bovine leukemia virus of 80 per cent or greater. Thus, the disease may be more widespread than is suggested by national and international data. Table 2 lists the United States Federal Regulations for disposition of animals affected with lymphosarcoma.

Bovine leukemia virus spreads by direct contact, most likely by transmission of infected lymphocytes. To decrease the spread of bovine leukemia virus requires control of blood-sucking insects and use of proper aseptic technique. Animal health professionals must handle needles, syringes, and blood-contaminated instruments correctly. Prompt removal of infected animals from the herd is necessary for an effective eradication program. Because the etiologic agent of lymphosarcoma in other food animal species is unknown, there are no specific preventive or control recommendations.

MISCELLANEOUS TUMORS

Many other neoplastic conditions can involve the eye and surrounding tissues. Primary as well as secondary tumors, either from metastasis or local extension, may occur. Examples are local adnexal papillomas reported in cattle and mastocytomas reported in cattle, sheep, and goats. However, any tumor of the nasal and paranasal cavities has the potential to cause ocular involvement as the result of orbital spread (e.g., enzootic adenocarcinoma in sheep). Although not common, exophthalmos secondary to such orbital invasion is possible. Central blindness could result from neoplasia involving the occipital cortex or optic radiation. Midbrain and brain stem involvement could also cause cranial nerve deficits attributable to the eye. Examples include pupillary light response abnormalities, impaired ocular autonomic innervation, and impaired extraocular muscle function. One report documents facial paralysis and secondary ulcerative keratitis in a cow with an intracranial schwannoma.

The literature has not documented well ocular neoplasia other than squamous cell tumors and lymphosarcoma. Information about treatment and prevention is conspicuously missing from food animal practice literature. Frequently, euthanasia or enucleation is the treatment given. However, in select cases, treatment modalities extrapolated from companion animal practice and human medicine may warrant consideration. Regardless of the course of treatment selected, histologic confirmation of neoplasia and follow-up are necessary to generate accurate epidemiologic and prognostic data.

BIBLIOGRAPHY

Bailey CM, Hanks DR, Hanks BS: Circumocular pigmentation and incidence of ocular squamous cell tumors in Bos tarsus and Bos indicus × Bos tarsus cattle. J Am Vet Med Assoc 196:1605, 1990.
Craig DR, Roth L, Smith MC: Lymphosarcoma in goats. Compend Contin Educ 8:S190, 1986.
Evermann JF, DiGiacoma RF, Ferrer JF, Parish SM: Transmission of bovine leukosis virus by blood inoculation. Am J Vet Res 47:1885, 1986.
Ferrer JF: Bovine lymphosarcoma. Compend Contin Educ 2:S235, 1980.
Ford LN, Jennings PA, Spradbrow PB, Francis J: Evidence for papillomaviruses in ocular lesion in cattle. Res Vet Sci 32:257, 1982.
Grier RL, Brewer WG, Paul SR, Theilen GH: Treatment of bovine and equine ocular squamous cell carcinoma by radiofrequency hyperthermia. J Am Vet Med Assoc 177:55, 1980.
Guard CL, Rebhun WC, Perdrizet JA: Cranial tumors in aged cattle causing Horner's syndrome and exophthalmos. Cornell Vet 74:361, 1984.
Heeney JL, Valli VEO: Bovine ocular squamous cell carcinoma: an epidemiological perspective. Can J Comp Med 49:21, 1985.
Johnson R, Coy CH, Perry RL, et al: Nasal squamous-cell carcinoma in a sheep. Mod Vet Pract 63:897, 1982.
Kainer RA, Stringer JM, Lueker DC: Hyperthermia for treatment of ocular squamous cell tumors in cattle. J Am Vet Med Assoc 176:356, 1980.
Kainer RA: Current concepts in the treatment of bovine ocular squamous cell tumors. Vet Clin North Am [Large Anim Pract] 6:609–622, 1984.
Kainer RA: Bovine ocular squamous cell tumors. In Howard JL (ed): Current Veterinary Therapy, Food Animal Practice 2. Philadelphia, WB Saunders, 1986, p 833.
Klein WR, Bier J, Van Dieten JS, et al: Radical surgery of bovine ocular squamous cell carcinoma (cancer eye): complication and results. Vet Surg 13:236, 1984.
Masterson MA, Hull BL, Vollmer LA: Treatment of bovine lymphosarcoma with L-asparaginase. J Am Vet Med Assoc 192:1301, 1988.
Meek LA, Cooley AJ, Whitley RD: Intraocular lymphosarcoma as the presenting sign of generalized lymphosarcoma in a Holstein cow. Compend Contin Educ 9:F239, 1987.
Mitcham SA, Kasari TR, Parent JM, et al: Intracranial schwannoma in a cow. Can Vet J 25:138, 1984.
Rebhun WC: Orbital lymphosarcoma in cattle. J Am Vet Med Assoc 180:149, 1982.
Rings MD, Rojko J: Naturally occurring nasal obstructions in 11 sheep. Cornell Vet 75:269, 1985.
Rosenthal RC, Mac Ewen EG: Treatment of lymphoma in dogs. J Am Vet Med Assoc 196:774, 1990.
Russell WC, Brinks JS, Kainer RA: Incidence and heritability of ocular squamous cell tumors in Hereford cattle. J Anim Sci 43:1156, 1976.
Wilcock BP: The eye and ear. In Jubb KVF, Kennedy PC, Palmer N (eds): Pathology of Domestic Animals. New York, Academic Press, 1985, p 386.

Neuro-ophthalmology in Food Animals

B. KEITH COLLINS, DVM, MS, Diplomate, ACVO

The neuro-ophthalmic examination should be performed as a routine part of the general physical examination. It can be done quickly and provides clues to the diagnosis of diseases that affect both the ocular and nervous systems. Numerous diseases of food animals may feature neuro-ophthalmic abnormalities (see Table 1). A proper assessment of these abnormalities is important for diagnosis and prognosis and may be a determining factor in whether the animal is treated or shipped for slaughter. Seldom is a neuro-ophthalmic abnormality specific for a given disease condition, but its presence or absence may narrow the differential diagnosis. This article presents neuro-ophthalmic anatomy, examination techniques, and a brief discussion of diseases that may feature neuro-ophthalmic abnormalities in food animals.

OPHTHALMIC NEUROANATOMY

A basic knowledge of neuro-ophthalmic anatomy is required for proper interpretation of clinical signs. This section presents the cranial nerves (CN) that innervate the eye and ocular adnexa; explains how they function to integrate eye movements; and also describes anatomy of the pupillary light reflex, which is mediated, in part, by the parasympathetic nervous system. Sympathetic innervation to the eye is also discussed (see also Horner's Syndrome). The reader is referred to other sources for a more detailed discussion of neuro-ophthalmic anatomy.[1-3]

OPTIC NERVE (CN II). The optic nerve is an accumulation of nerve axons arising from the retina. It projects neurologic impulses originating in the ganglion cells of the retina to higher visual centers where they are perceived as vision. The optic nerve is a tract of the central nervous system and is covered by meninges. It is, therefore, susceptible to disease conditions that might cause meningitis. A complete lesion of the optic nerve causes blindness of the affected eye.

OCULOMOTOR NERVE (CN III). The oculomotor nerve has both motor and parasympathetic components. The parasympathetic nerve fibers are intimately associated with, but distinct from, the motor fibers. The parasympathetic nerve fibers innervate the intraocular muscles, including the iris sphincter and ciliary body muscles (see Pupillary Light Reflex Pathway). The motor fibers of CN III innervate most of the striated extraocular muscles including the *dorsal, medial,* and *ventral rectus* muscles, the *ventral oblique* muscle, and the *levator palpebrae superioris* muscle. The dorsal, medial, and ventral rectus muscles move the globe in each of these directions, respectively. Contraction of the ventral oblique muscle causes *extorsion* of the globe, that is, rotation of the dorsum of the globe laterally from the 12 o'clock position. The levator palpebrae superioris muscle elevates the upper eyelid in conjunction with sympathetically innervated smooth muscle (see also Horner's Syndrome).

A lesion of the parasympathetic component of CN III causes a widely dilated and unresponsive pupil; this paralysis of the intraocular muscles is called *internal ophthalmoplegia*. A lesion of the motor component of CN III causes impaired ocular motility and deviation of the globe (i.e., a ventral or ventrolateral strabismus); this paralysis of the extraocular muscles is called *external ophthalmoplegia*. The term external ophthalmoplegia most commonly refers to deficits of CN III but may also include deficits of CN IV and CN VI. Drooping of the upper eyelid (i.e., ptosis) also occurs with CN III deficits. Internal or external ophthalmoplegia may occur alone or in combination as *complete ophthalmoplegia*.

TROCHLEAR NERVE (CN IV). The trochlear nerve provides motor innervation to the *dorsal oblique* muscle only. Contraction of this muscle causes *intorsion* of the globe, that is, rotation of the dorsum of the globe medially from the 12 o'clock position. A lesion of the trochlear nerve causes a persistent extorsion of the globe, because the action of the ventral oblique muscle is then unopposed. In species that have a horizontally elongated pupil, such as ruminants, this is easily visualized as a deviation of the medial pupil in a dorsal direction (also called a dorsomedial strabismus).[4] In animals with a round pupil, such as the pig, extorsion is not as readily apparent. Funduscopic examination may be helpful, whereby the superior retinal vasculature appears deviated laterally.

TRIGEMINAL NERVE (CN V). The trigeminal nerve has 3 branches, namely, the ophthalmic, maxillary, and mandibular. The ophthalmic and maxillary branches are exclusively sensory nerves. Smaller branches of the *ophthalmic* nerve innervate the globe, nictitans, most of the upper eyelid, medial canthus, and lacrimal gland. The *maxillary* branch innervates the dorsolateral upper and lower eyelids and the lateral canthal area. Lesions of the ophthalmic branch are of greatest significance because they cause a decreased responsiveness to irritating ocular stimuli, possibly resulting in reduced lacrimation and dry eye, and reduced sensation to blink with exposure keratitis. The *mandibular* branch has sensory functions, but it also provides motor innervation to the muscles of mastication. It does not affect the eye directly. However, because the temporalis muscle lines the medial orbit, atrophy of this muscle secondary to a mandibular branch lesion may cause some degree of enophthalmos.

ABDUCENT NERVE (CN VI). The abducent nerve provides motor innervation to the *lateral rectus* and *retractor bulbi* muscles. A lesion of CN VI will cause a medial strabismus and eliminates the animal's ability to retract the globe into the orbit.

FACIAL NERVE (CN VII). The facial nerve is a mixed nerve having motor and parasympathetic components. It provides motor innervation to the *orbicularis oculi* and *retractor anguli oculi* muscles and parasympathetic innervation to the lacrimal gland. A lesion of CN VII causes paralysis of the eyelids and may cause reduced tear secretion.

VESTIBULOCOCHLEAR NERVE (CN VIII). The vestibular portion of the vestibulocochlear nerve relays sensory input from receptors in the inner ear to the vestibular nuclei, which together with the cerebellum help maintain proper balance. The medial longitudinal fasciculus is the pathway of the brain stem that relays this information regarding balance (or head position) to nerve nuclei innervating the extraocular muscles (i.e., CN III, IV, and VI). This causes a normal, rhythmic, yet involuntary movement of the eyes (i.e., a nystagmus) when the head is moved from side to side, or up and down. The reader is referred to the sections on conjugate eye movements and nystagmus.

SYMPATHETIC INNERVATION. Normal sympathetic innervation to the eye is a 3-neuron pathway beginning in the hypothalamus.[1,3] Upper motor neuron (or central) axons descend from the hypothalamus, through the midbrain, and within the spinal cord to synapse on the lower motor neurons in the cranial thoracic spinal cord segments T1 to T3. Preganglionic axons arising from these segments course rostrally to synapse in the ipsilateral cranial cervical ganglion. In ruminants, the cranial cervical ganglion is located close to the base of the cranium, medial to the tympanic bulla.[5] Postganglionic axons arising from the cranial cervical ganglion course rostrally to innervate the iris dilator muscle, smooth muscle of the orbit, nictitans, and upper eyelid, and the ocular and ipsilateral facial vasculature.

PUPILLARY LIGHT REFLEX PATHWAY. The pupillary light reflex (PLR) is an integral part of the neuro-ophthalmic examination, and it is used to assess the functional integrity of the retina, CN II, and the parasympathetic component of CN III. It is presented here because of the complex neuroanatomic pathways involved in this reflex.

The pathways for the PLR and vision are the same to the level of the midbrain. Briefly, the PLR begins when light falls on the retina, causing a photochemical reaction in the photoreceptor cells (rods and cones), which is in turn converted into a nervous impulse in the retinal bipolar cells. This signal continues through axons of the retinal ganglion cells, which collectively turn posteriorly at the *optic disk* to form the *optic nerve* (CN II). The optic nerve traverses the orbit, enters the optic foramen, and joins the contralateral optic nerve at the *optic chiasm* where a large percentage of nerve fibers cross over, or *decussate,* to the opposite *optic tract* (Fig. 1).

The percentage of nerve fiber decussation at the optic chiasm is related to the degree of frontal (or lateral) placement of the globes. In domestic food animals, the globes are more laterally placed than in small domestic animals, and the percentage of fiber decussation is proportionately greater. The mean percentages of decussation in domestic food animals have been reported as follows: cattle, 82.9 per cent; sheep, 88.9 per cent; and pigs, 87.8 per cent.[6] The clinical significance of this decussation is that a greater percentage of the retinal axons

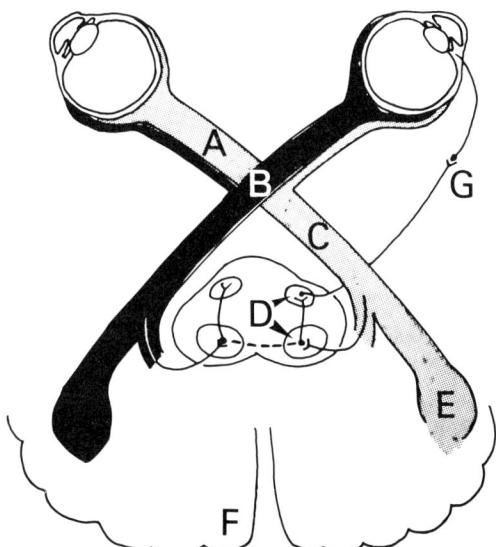

Figure 1. Neuroanatomy of the pupillary light reflex. *A,* optic nerve; *B,* optic chiasm; *C,* optic tract; *D,* midbrain with pretectal nucleus *(large arrow)* and parasympathetic oculomotor nucleus *(small arrow)*; *E,* lateral geniculate body of the thalamus; *F,* visual cortex; *G,* efferent parasympathetic pathway.

from one side project to the opposite visual cortex (e.g., left visual field is perceived in the right cortex).

Nerve fibers that contribute to the PLR (i.e., pupillomotor fibers) leave the optic tract to synapse in the pretectal nuclei of the midbrain. Most of the nerve axons that arise from the pretectal nuclei will decussate again and synapse in the contralateral parasympathetic oculomotor nucleus (called Edinger-Westphal nucleus in humans). This completes the afferent arc of the PLR (Fig. 1).

The efferent PLR pathway is mediated by the parasympathetic component of CN III. Preganglionic axons that arise from the parasympathetic oculomotor nucleus proceed rostrally to synapse in the ipsilateral ciliary ganglion adjacent to the optic nerve. Postganglionic axons arising from the ciliary ganglion innervate the ipsilateral ciliary body and iris musculature.

Nerve fibers that remain in the optic tract are responsible for vision. They proceed toward the *lateral geniculate body* (LGB) of the thalamus and are projected via the *optic radiations* to the *occipital* (or visual) cortex of the brain (Fig. 1). Because the nerve fibers that mediate the PLR are subcortical, animals with cortical blindness typically have normal PLRs.

HIGHER VISUAL CENTERS. Light stimuli projected via the lower afferent visual pathways are perceived in the occipital (or visual) cortex as vision. A lesion of the optic tracts, LGBs, optic radiations, or visual cortices may, therefore, cause blindness. Because of decussating nerve fibers, blindness occurs predominantly in the eye opposite the site of the lesion. A blind eye that is ophthalmoscopically normal and has normal PLRs is characteristic of a central (or cortical) blindness.

NEURO-OPHTHALMIC EXAMINATION

An accurate and thorough history should precede the clinical examination. The history may provide immediate clues as to whether the general physical and neuro-ophthalmic signs are the result of nutritional deficiency (e.g., vitamin A deficiency), toxicity (e.g., lead poisoning), or another disease condition.

Next, the animal should be examined in an unrestrained state and in its natural environment, if possible, for assessment of its general physical, mental, and visual status. A decreased visual status may be evidenced by separation from the flock or herd, or a hesitancy to pass through gates or a chute. However, animals with marked visual deficits may appear visual in a herd or flock situation, because they may cue on other animals. General physical examination findings are correlated with results of the ocular and neuro-ophthalmic examinations in order to arrive at the diagnosis.

The neuro-ophthalmic examination should include an assessment of the menace and palpebral reflexes, the conjugate eye movements, and the PLRs as described next. Evaluation of the corneal reflex may also be required in instances in which trigeminal sensory deficits are suspected. Abnormal eye movements (see Nystagmus) or deviations of the globe (see Strabismus) should be noted. Neuro-ophthalmic findings must be interpreted with respect to other ocular findings (e.g., uveitis, retinal disease), because concurrent primary ocular or orbital disease may be responsible for the perceived or real neuro-ophthalmic abnormality.

MENACE REFLEX. The menace reflex is used to assess the integrity of the retina, CN II, and CN VII as well as the animal's ability to perceive a menacing gesture (i.e., the visual cortex). A vertical hand movement in front of the animal's eye should normally elicit a rapid blink response and will often cause the animal to move its head away from the examiner. An absent menace reflex indicates either an inability to see the gesture (lesion of the retina, CN II, optic chiasm, optic tract, LGB, optic radiation, or cortex) or an inability to blink (lesion of CN VII). An absent menace reflex may also occur with cerebellar disease, although vision remains normal in this instance.[2,3] The menace reflex is a learned reflex, and neonatal animals may have a slow or absent reflex for the first few weeks of life.

PALPEBRAL REFLEX. The palpebral reflex is used to assess the integrity of CN V and CN VII. It is performed by alternately tapping the medial and lateral canthi, and the normal response is rapid closure of the eyelids. An absent palpebral reflex indicates either a sensory (lesion of CN V) or motor (lesion of CN VII) deficit. Animals may have a substantial sensory deficit and yet maintain a normal or near-normal palpebral reflex. This occurs if the animal's vision is normal, whereby a menace reflex is simultaneously elicited.

CORNEAL REFLEX. The corneal reflex is used to assess the integrity of CN V and CN VII in a manner similar to the palpebral reflex, but the stimulus is different. In this instance, a cotton-tipped applicator is gently tapped on the unanesthetized cornea. The normal response is rapid eyelid closure. Some retraction of the globe by the retractor bulbi muscle may also be noted, and this is mediated by CN VI.

CONJUGATE EYE MOVEMENTS. The normal ocular movements that occur with movement of the head are called *conjugate eye movements.* This has also been called vestibular or physiologic nystagmus, or a doll's head reflex.[2] Conjugate eye movements (mediated via CN III, IV, VI, and VIII) are elicited only when the head is moving. The rapid phase of ocular movement is always in the direction of head movement. Lesions of the vestibular apparatus, the medial longitudinal fasciculus, the cranial nerves that innervate the extraocular muscles, or the extraocular muscles themselves will disrupt the normal conjugate eye movements.

ASSESSMENT OF THE PUPILLARY LIGHT REFLEXES. The PLRs should be evaluated using a strong penlight and, preferably, a rechargeable 3.5-volt halogen light source equipped with a Finoff transilluminator.* A darkened or semidarkened

---

*Welch-Allyn, Skaneateles, NY 13153.

Table 1. NEURO-OPHTHALMIC MANIFESTATIONS OF SELECTED DISEASES IN FOOD ANIMALS

Condition	Species	Neuro-Ophthalmic Signs
Arsanilic acid	Pigs	Blindness from optic nerve and tract disease, and possibly central blindness as well
Blindgrass (*Stypandra imbricata*)	Sheep, goats	Central retinal degeneration, optic disk atrophy, optic tract lesion
Bluetongue	Sheep	Necrotizing retinopathy occurs in fetal lambs if the ewe is vaccinated in the first half of pregnancy
Bovine viral diarrhea	Cattle	Posterior segment changes are limited to the fetus or neonate and include retinitis and/or degeneration, optic neuritis and/or atrophy
Bright blindness (*Pteridium aquilinum*)	Sheep	Progressive retinal degeneration
Hog cholera	Pigs	Retinitis with perivascular cuffing, optic neuritis
Horner's syndrome	Any species	Miosis, ptosis, nictitans prolapse, and enophthalmos; ptosis is most consistent in food animals; vision is present with no intraocular inflammation
Ketosis (severe)	Cattle, sheep	Cortical blindness with normal PLRs
Lead poisoning	Cattle, sheep	"Snapping" of the eyelids, cortical blindness with usually normal PLRs, and less commonly nystagmus or mydriasis
Listeriosis	Cattle, sheep	Absent blink reflex, ptosis and exposure keratitis from CN VII palsy, decreased ocular sensation from CN V palsy, nystagmus or strabismus from CN VIII palsy, or medial strabismus from CN VI palsy
Locoweed (*Astragalus* sp.)	Cattle, sheep	Visual impairment believed related to cytoplasmic vacuolation of nerve tissue in the brain and retina
Male fern	Cattle	Papilledema progressing to optic neuritis with peripapillary hemorrhages and, later, optic atrophy
Organophosphate or carbamate toxicity	Any species	Miosis
Otitis media	Calves	Absent blink reflex, ptosis and exposure keratitis secondary to CN VII palsy
Polioencephalomalacia	Cattle, sheep	Cortical blindness, bilateral extorsion of the pupils (i.e., dorsomedial strabismus), PLRs usually intact; papilledema may occur
Pseudorabies	Pigs	Retinitis, optic neuritis, nystagmus
Rabies	Any species	The signs are variable; affected cattle are usually visual and may appear "wild-eyed," and focal retinitis is reported
Scrapie	Sheep	Central blindness due primarily to optic tract and geniculate body lesions, but retinitis may also be present
Stanchion trauma	Cattle	Bilateral CN VII palsy with absent blink reflexes and secondary exposure keratitis
Tetanus	Cattle, sheep	"Flashing" or protrusion of the nictitans due to spasm of the retractor bulbi muscle
Thromboembolic meningoencephalitis (TEME)	Cattle	Exudative chorioretinitis, retinal vasculitis, hemorrhage, and detachment; cranial nerve signs may occur with brain stem infarction
Toxoplasmosis	Any species	Chorioretinitis, optic neuritis
Vitamin A deficiency	Cattle, sheep, goats	Signs vary with age but may include night blindness progressing to day blindness, papilledema, retinal degeneration, detachment, and/or hemorrhages; PLRs usually absent

environment is optimal for assessing the PLRs. Light directed into the ipsilateral eye should elicit rapid constriction of the pupil, and this is called the *direct* PLR. Simultaneously, the contralateral pupil should also constrict, and this is called the *indirect* PLR. Simultaneous observation of the indirect PLR is more difficult in food animals because of the laterally placed eyes. It may be helpful to have an assistant observe the contralateral eye, with use of a weaker light source (so as not to elicit a direct PLR), and note the response.

Abnormalities of the PLRs may be neurologic or non-neurologic in origin.[3] Neurologic causes of a slow or absent PLR may occur with a lesion of the afferent pathway (e.g., the retina, optic nerve, or optic chiasm) or the efferent parasympathetic pathway (e.g., CN III paralysis). With a unilateral *afferent* lesion, both the direct PLR and the indirect PLR to the opposite eye are slow or absent, and the ipsilateral eye is blind. With a unilateral *efferent* parasympathetic lesion, the direct PLR is absent, but the indirect PLR to the opposite eye is present, and the ipsilateral eye is visual. Non-neurologic causes of a slow or absent PLR include intraocular disease (e.g., uveitis), functional abnormalities of the iris (e.g., posterior synechiae, iris atrophy), pharmacologic blockade (e.g., mydriasis from atropine therapy or plant toxicity), or pharmacologic stimulation (e.g., miosis from organophosphate toxicity). The reader is referred to other sources for a more comprehensive review of the PLR.[2, 3]

SPECIFIC NEURO-OPHTHALMIC ABNORMALITIES

This section presents common differential considerations based on a single presenting neuro-ophthalmic finding, but the reader must be aware that multiple neuro-ophthalmic abnormalities often occur. Table 1 lists diseases that may feature neuro-ophthalmic abnormalities. The reader is referred to appropriate chapters within the text for complete discussion of specific disease conditions.

Strabismus

Strabismus is an abnormal deviation of the globe. Normal doll's head movement of the eyes may simulate a positional strabismus, particularly in cattle that are restrained in a chute with the head tied up; the eye rotates ventrally in this instance. The examiner must be cognizant of this because it may complicate neuro-ophthalmologic assessment of the animal. Strabismus may occur as a congenital defect, or it may be acquired from extraocular muscle palsy, neurologic deficit, or secondary to a space-occupying orbital mass (e.g., orbital lymphosarcoma).

A bilateral inherited convergent (i.e., esotropia) or divergent (i.e., exotropia) strabismus has been reported in several breeds of cattle in the absence of other ocular dysfunction.[7] Esotropia occurs commonly in Jerseys and Shorthorns and may occur in other breeds. Exotropia occurs in certain lines of Jersey, Ayrshire, Brown Swiss, and Holstein cattle.

The most common infectious disease causes of strabismus include *listeriosis* and *thromboembolic meningoencephalitis* (TEME) by virtue of involvement of the cranial nerve nuclei (see cranial nerve abnormalities). Medial strabismus is common with listeriosis owing to involvement of the abducens nucleus and subsequent loss of lateral rectus muscle function. *Polioencephalomalacia* may cause a bilateral dorsomedial strabismus (or persistent extorsion) because of disease affinity for the trochlear nerve nuclei (refer also to section on cortical blindness). Strabismus from polioencephalomalacia occurs more commonly in calves.[7] *Vestibular disease* may cause a ventral or ventrolateral strabismus with CN VIII dysfunction.[8]

Nystagmus

Nystagmus is an involuntary and rhythmic movement of the eyes and, as already described, occurs normally with movement of the head (i.e., conjugate eye movements). If nystagmus occurs in the absence of head movement, it is considered abnormal. It is characterized by a slow and a rapid phase of contraction (or movement) and is named according to direction of the rapid phase (e.g., right or left). It is further described as horizontal, vertical, or rotatory in direction. Abnormal nystagmus may be congenital or acquired.

Vestibular disease may cause a spontaneous or positional (e.g., when the head is extended or flexed) nystagmus. Horizontal or rotatory nystagmus may occur with either peripheral or central vestibular disease, but vertical nystagmus occurs only with central vestibular disease. In peripheral disease, the fast phase of contraction is directed away from the side of the lesion and does not change with head posture, whereas in central disease the direction may vary. A positional strabismus (usually ventral) may also be noted with vestibular disease.[8]

Conditions resulting in *congenital blindness* may cause a unique type of nystagmus, whereby the ocular movements are randomly directed and usually lack a distinct slow or fast phase. This is referred to as a *searching, wandering,* or *pendular* nystagmus. Pendular nystagmus has also been reported in otherwise normal cattle.[9]

Cranial Nerve Signs

Localizing cranial nerve signs may occur with a variety of diseases, notably listeriosis, TEME, space-occupying lesions, polioencephalomalacia (see Strabismus), and secondary to trauma. With any of these conditions, the neuro-ophthalmic findings are determined by the brain stem nuclei or cranial nerves involved.

Listeriosis, caused by *Listeria monocytogenes,* is probably the most common cause of single or multiple cranial nerve deficits in cattle, sheep, and goats. Unilateral facial nerve paralysis is common, causing an absent blink reflex and exposure keratitis, in addition to ipsilateral facial drooping. Deficits of the trigeminal, abducent, and vestibulocochlear nerves may also occur. This may result in diminished or absent corneal or palpebral reflexes with deficits of CN V, medial strabismus with deficits of CN VI, and nystagmus or strabismus with deficits of CN VIII.

TEME, caused by *Haemophilus somnus,* may result in cranial nerve lesions in cattle due to infarcts of the brain stem. However, primary ocular disease, particularly posterior segment inflammation, is more common with TEME than with listeriosis and serves as a useful differentiating feature. Concurrent visual deficits are common with TEME.[7, 10]

Stanchion trauma is the most common cause of bilateral eyelid paralysis in cattle.[7] This occurs when the animal pulls backward within the stanchion and traps its head, with resultant trauma to the facial nerves. Relevant ocular signs include loss of the blink reflex with secondary exposure keratitis. The prognosis for recovery is good and generally occurs in 1 to 2 weeks.

Horner's Syndrome

Horner's syndrome is a condition of sympathetic denervation to the eye. The clinical manifestations of Horner's syndrome are not as florid in ruminants as in small domestic animals. In cattle, sheep, and goats, the most consistent and obvious sign is ptosis (i.e., drooping) of the upper eyelid.[5] Increased temperature of the face and ear on the affected side may also be noted, and this is most readily detected by palpating the base of the ear. Additional but more subtle signs may include miosis and nictitans prolapse. An absence of ipsilateral sweating is also reported in cattle with central or preganglionic Horner's lesions but not in sheep or goats. This is manifest as a dry nose on the affected side; it is most easily detected by first cleaning and drying the nose to facilitate observation of new sweat formation. Alterations of facial temperature and sweating do not occur with postganglionic Horner's lesions, such as might occur with orbital disease.[5]

Clearly, disruption of the sympathetic pathways at any location en route to the eye, either central, pre-, or postganglionic, may cause Horner's syndrome. Causes may include trauma, neoplasia, and focal infection or abscesses. Concurrent clinical signs, such as muscle atrophy of the forelimb (e.g., with a preganglionic lesion), or exophthalmia (e.g., with a postganglionic lesion), should aid in localizing the lesion. In cattle, direct trauma or perivascular irritation to the vagosympathetic trunk after venipuncture have been suggested as the most common causes of Horner's syndrome.[7]

Abnormalities of the Pupil (Miosis or Mydriasis)

Different degrees of pupillary responsiveness occur with visual *afferent* lesions depending on the extent of retinal or optic nerve involvement. Dysfunction of the visual *efferent* system may also occur, and this is manifest by intense and often persistent pupillary constriction (i.e., miosis) with dysfunction of the sympathetic system, or dilation (i.e., mydriasis) with dysfunction of the parasympathetic system. Contrary to blindness typical of afferent lesions, vision is usually normal with efferent lesions.[3]

Horner's syndrome is one cause of persistent miosis. Additional causes include *organophosphate* and *carbamate* toxicity, for which additional systemic signs should be apparent.

Pharmacologic blockade is a non-neurologic cause of mydriasis that mimics neurologic dysfunction and must, therefore, be considered in the differential diagnosis. Pharmacologic blockade from prior topical ophthalmic therapy with *atropine* will cause mydriasis for variable periods of time, often for days or weeks. Atropine is a parasympatholytic drug that inhibits contraction of the iris sphincter muscle. The history is important in making the diagnosis. Exposure to certain *plants* containing belladonna alkaloid derivatives (e.g., jimsonweed, deadly nightshade) can cause mydriasis through a similar pharmacologic action.[3]

Internal ophthalmoplegia is a neurologic cause of mydriasis. This occurs with lesions affecting the parasympathetic component of CN III (see anatomy of the PLR). Pharmacologic testing is beneficial in confirming the diagnosis in small animals and may similarly be useful in food animals.[3]

Retina–Optic Nerve Disease

Extensive retina or optic nerve disease will manifest clinically as blindness, with absent menace reflexes, and slow or absent direct PLRs of the affected eye. Retina and optic nerve disease often occur simultaneously. Ophthalmoscopic examination usually confirms the diagnosis, because the diseased retina or optic nerve can be viewed directly. Infectious, nutritional, metabolic, or toxic disorders and, rarely, inherited retinopathy should be considered.

Thromboembolic meningoencephalitis (TEME) of cattle, caused by *Haemophilus somnus*, is a common infectious cause of blindness from retinal involvement. Findings may include exudative chorioretinitis, multifocal retinal vasculitis with thrombosis and infarction, retinal hemorrhage, and retinal detachment.[10] Some consider the retinal vasculitis and infarction pathognomonic of TEME.

Vitamin A deficiency may cause blindness in cattle, sheep, and goats, although most reports have been in feedlot cattle.[11-13] The degree of visual impairment varies with the age of the animal and the severity of deficiency. Young, rapidly growing animals are most susceptible to deficiency. Blindness may be the predominant or only clinical symptom,[12] and the exact cause of blindness may vary with age of the animal.[11]

Swelling of the optic disk (i.e., papilledema) precedes blindness. Papilledema occurs secondary to increased cerebrospinal fluid (CSF) pressure. The CSF pressure increases because absorption by the arachnoid villi cells is reduced in vitamin A deficiency.[11-13] Papilledema alone is not sufficient to cause blindness unless it is chronic. Animals supplemented with vitamin A in the acute stage of deficiency have a favorable visual prognosis.

Night blindness (i.e., nyctalopia) may be observed in the early stages and is a prelude to retinal degeneration. Nyctalopia occurs because vitamin A is required for regeneration of rhodopsin, the primary visual pigment required for night vision. Nyctalopia is reported in experimental animals, but day blindness is more likely to be noticed first in a clinical situation.[11] Continued deficiency can cause retinal degeneration, hemorrhage, and detachment that are visible ophthalmoscopically.[11,12] Nyctalopia may be reversible with vitamin A therapy, but day blindness associated with advanced retinal degeneration will not reverse.

In young animals, optic disk atrophy may occur secondary to bony constriction of the optic nerves.[11-13] Bone remodeling and resorption is a normal growth process in the optic canals. Vitamin A deficiency causes a narrowing of the optic canals from a combination of abnormally increased bone growth dorsally and a cessation of normal resorption ventrally. This results in a narrowing of the canals with compression and necrosis of the optic nerves.

Bright blindness is a progressive retinal degeneration (PRD) that occurs in ewes grazing on bracken fern *(Pteridium aquilinum)*.[10,14,15] This type of PRD is endemic to regions of the United Kingdom and occurs most commonly in the fall and in sheep 2 to 4 years of age. Ophthalmoscopic examination reveals signs of PRD including retinal vascular attenuation, tapetal hyper-reflectivity, and optic disk atrophy. The bright tapetal reflectivity visible through a widely dilated and unresponsive pupil accounts for the name of this condition. Thiaminase is believed to be the toxic principle of bracken fern–induced PRD.[15]

Blindgrass (Stypandra imbricata) is a perennial herb that grows in western Australia. Permanent blindness occurs in sheep and goats having grazed on pastures with blindgrass and survived the acute illness. The toxic principle of the plant is unknown. The pathogenesis is poorly understood, but lesions primarily include a central retinal degeneration and degeneration of axons in the optic nerves and optic tracts.[16]

Arsanilic acid has been used as a food additive for pigs to stimulate growth and control swine dysentery. Chronic overdosage or administration during times of restricted water intake may cause blindness.[10,17] A parenchymatous neuropathy occurs with demyelination and axonal destruction of the optic nerves and tracts. Optic disk atrophy may be visible ophthalmoscopically. The electroretinogram is normal, but the visual evoked responses are absent. Blindness may also be central in origin with possible damage to the LGB, optic radiations, or visual cortex.[18]

Central (Cortical) Blindness

The hallmark signs of cortical blindness include absent menace reflexes, usually normal PLRs, and ophthalmoscopically normal eyes. Numerous disease conditions may result in cortical blindness either alone or together with other neuro-ophthalmic signs. These include lead poisoning or other chemical toxicoses, parasitic migrations, polioencephalomalacia, ketosis, infectious diseases, plant toxicities (e.g., locoweed), abscesses, and trauma. Concurrent clinical signs are important for differential diagnosis, and the reader is referred to appropriate chapters.

Lead poisoning occurs most commonly in cattle. Visual dysfunction can exist in the acute or subacute forms of the disease; chronic forms of the disease are uncommon. Blindness occurs owing to cerebrocortical swelling and necrosis, and this is most severe in the occipital lobes.[19] Although normal PLRs are typical of cortical blindness, mydriasis is reported with lead poisoning.[10,19]

Polioencephalomalacia (or cerebrocortical necrosis) is a thiamine-responsive disorder that occurs most commonly in feedlot cattle and lambs.[10] Although the pathogenesis is poorly understood, blindness occurs as a result of cortical swelling and necrosis. Blindness is often the first clinical sign observed and the last to resolve with therapy.[7] Ophthalmoscopic examination is typically normal, although papilledema is reported. PLRs are also usually normal, but severe cerebrocortical swelling may cause compression of the brain stem or cranial nerves with subsequent alterations of the PLRs.[10] The prognosis for return of vision is favorable with early thiamine treatment. The reader is referred to the section on strabismus.

Ketosis (pregnancy toxemia) may cause cortical blindness in cattle and small ruminants.[7,15] The prognosis for return of vision is usually excellent with appropriate therapy, but permanent blindness is reported.[7]

REFERENCES

1. deLahunta A: Veterinary Neuroanatomy and Clinical Neurology, 2nd ed. Philadelphia, WB Saunders, 1983.
2. Slatter D, deLahunta A: Neuro-ophthalmology. *In* Slatter D (ed): Fundamentals of Veterinary Ophthalmology, 2nd ed. Philadelphia, WB Saunders, 1990.
3. Collins BK, O'Brien D: Autonomic dysfunction of the eye. Semin Vet Med Surg [Small Anim] 5:24–36, 1990.
4. Shell LG: The cranial nerves of the brain stem. Prog Vet Neurol 1:233–245, 1990.
5. Smith JS, Mayhew IG: Horner's syndrome in large animals. Cornell Vet 67:529–542, 1977.
6. Herron MA, Martin JE, Joyce JR: Quantitative study of the decussating optic axons in the pony, cow, sheep, and pig. Am J Vet Res 39:1137–1139, 1978.
7. Rebhun WC: Ocular manifestations of systemic diseases in cattle. Vet Clin North Am [Large Anim Pract] 6:623–639, 1984.
8. Schunk KL: Diseases of the vestibular system. Prog Vet Neurol 1:247–254, 1990.
9. McConnon JM, White ME, Smith MC, et al: Pendular nystagmus in dairy cattle. J Am Vet Med Assoc 182:812–813, 1983.
10. Williams LW, Gelatt KN: Ocular manifestations of systemic disease. Part III. Food animals. *In* Gelatt KN (ed): Veterinary Ophthalmology. Philadelphia, Lea & Febiger, 1981.
11. Divers TJ, Blackmon DM, Martin CL, et al: Blindness and convulsions associated with vitamin A deficiency in feedlot steers. J Am Vet Med Assoc 189:1579–1582, 1986.
12. Paulsen ME, Johnson L, Young S, et al: Blindness and sexual dimorphism associated with vitamin A deficiency in feedlot cattle. J Am Vet Med Assoc 194:933–937, 1989.
13. Booth A, Reid M, Clark T: Hypovitaminosis A in feedlot cattle. J Am Vet Med Assoc 190:1305–1308, 1987.

14. Watson WA, Barnett KC, Terlecki S: Progressive retinal degeneration (Bright Blindness) in sheep: a review. Vet Rec 91:665–670, 1972.
15. Moore CP, Whitley RD: Ophthalmic diseases of small domestic ruminants. Vet Clin North Am [Large Anim Pract] 6:641–665, 1984.
16. Main DC, Slatter DH, Huxtable CR, et al: *Stypandra imbricata* ("Blindgrass") toxicosis in goats and sheep: clinical and pathologic findings in 4 field cases. Aust Vet J 57:132–135, 1981.
17. Vestre WA: Porcine ophthalmology. Vet Clin North Am [Large Anim Pract] 6:667–676, 1984.
18. Witzel DA, Smith EL, Beerwinkle KR, et al: Arsanilic acid–induced blindness in swine: electroretinographic and visually evoked responses. Am J Vet Res 37:521–524, 1976.
19. Baker JC: Lead poisoning in cattle. Vet Clin North Am [Food Anim Pract] 3:137–147, 1987.

SECTION 16
Neurologic Diseases of Food Animals

JIMMY L. HOWARD, DVM, MS, Consulting Editor

Cerebellar Disease in Cattle
MAURICE E. WHITE, DVM

The cerebellum coordinates and regulates movement. The cerebellar nuclei facilitate brain stem neurons but are themselves regulated by inhibitory signals from Purkinje's cells in the cerebellar cortex, which receive information from several neuronal systems. Since the cerebellum does not initiate movement, loss of voluntary movement is not a clinical sign of uncomplicated cerebellar disease; instead there is a general lack of coordination of muscle groups. Ataxia with preservation of strength, spasticity, a dysmetric usually hypermetric gait, and often a loss of balance are present. Newborn calves with congenital cerebellar disease may be unable to stand, and adults with progressive disease may reach the point where they cannot stand without assistance. A head tremor that worsens when the animal reaches for food or water (intention tremor) is commonly present. Because ocular muscles are coordinated by cerebellar nuclei, there is sometimes nystagmus. With severe disease opisthotonos can occur. Affected animals often appear to be anxious, wide-eyed, and hyperexcitable. A unique finding in some animals with cerebellar disease is a reduction or absence of the menace (blink) response despite normal vision and facial muscle strength. Before careful examination this might give the observer the impression that the animal is blind. Almost all cerebellar disease in cattle is bilateral, but in the occasional animal with unilateral disease, signs are commonly ipsilateral to the lesion. To summarize, the presence of ataxia, spasticity, and dysmetria in a strong, bright, and alert animal, often in association with tremor, nystagmus, and a decreased menace response in a sighted animal, suggests cerebellar disease.

This article will cover diseases that cause cerebellar signs; they are divided into three categories: (1) diseases in which signs are present at or near birth; (2) late onset disease; and (3) generalized neurologic disease with a major cerebellar component.

CONGENITAL CEREBELLAR DISEASE

Bovine Virus Diarrhea–Induced Cerebellar Degeneration with Hypoplasia

The most common cerebellar disease in North American cattle is probably congenital cerebellar degeneration due to infection with bovine viral diarrhea (BVD) virus between days 120 and 160 of gestation. Affected calves show signs of cerebellar disease from birth, occasionally in association with ocular lesions such as cataracts, retinal inflammations, and retinal hemorrhages. At necropsy there are uniform reductions in cerebellar size and multiple histologic lesions, including cavitation of white matter, disorganization of cortical structure, dysmyelination, and other changes. Several affected calves are sometimes born in a herd over a short time span, reflecting exposure to BVD during the spread of the agent; the owner often does not recall any signs of BVD in adult cattle during the time the fetuses were exposed. Diagnosis is usually made on the gross and histologic changes found at necropsy of affected calves. Evidence of a titer to BVD in the calf's precolostral serum would help confirm the diagnosis but is difficult to obtain under routine management conditions. Although there is no treatment, mildly affected calves often learn to compensate for the disorder.

Sporadic Congenital Cerebellar Ataxia with Hypomyelinogenesis

Cerebellar disease associated with hypomyelinogenesis of the cerebellum, brain stem, and spinal cord and with degeneration of Purkinje's cells and other neurons has been reported in several breeds, including Ayrshire, Jersey, Shorthorn, Hereford, Angus, Angus-Shorthorn, and Sofia Brown. Severe whole-body tremor and dysmetric ataxia might be present at birth or begin at 2 to 3 weeks of age. Most cases are suspected to be due to autosomal recessive inheritance. Diagnosis is by histologic examination and by exclusion of BVD-induced disease.

Absence of the Cerebellar Vermis

Sporadic cases involving the absence of the caudal portion of or the entire cerebellar vermis have been seen in cattle, sometimes associated with hydrocephalus. The cause is unknown.

Multiple Central Nervous System Malformation

Cerebellar degeneration is occasionally seen in association with other central nervous system malformations, such as hydranencephaly, in which cerebellar disease is part of a syndrome of multiple neurologic defects. Akabane virus and bluetongue virus can cause this syndrome, and idiopathic outbreaks have also been reported. Diagnosis is by evidence of viral infection if possible, and confirmation may require necropsy.

Neurofilamentous Degeneration of Horned Hereford Calves

A syndrome developed in a herd of Horned Hereford cattle that was characterized by the inability of calves to rise at birth and the presence of fine tremors, most prominent in the hind limbs and neck. Calves seemed otherwise normal and alert. Stimulation of calves led to worsening of signs, and progressive muscle weakness developed after stimulation and movement. In some there was loss of voice. At necropsy there was histologic evidence of neurofilamentous neuronal degeneration of multiple cell groups in the central nervous system and of ganglion cells in the peripheral and autonomic nervous systems. The affected herd was inbred, and this syndrome may be hereditary in origin.

Inherited Congenital Myoclonus of Polled Hereford Calves

Polled Herefords and their crossbreeds are occasionally affected at birth by a neurologic disease characterized by extensor spasm and inability to stand. There are no pathologic or biochemical lesions in the nervous system. Some calves react to noise or touch with vigorous extension of the neck and legs; contractions last a minute or two. The disease is inherited as an autosomal recessive. There is no treatment.

Maple Syrup Urine Disease of Calves

Polled Hereford, Hereford, and possibly other breeds can have "maple syrup urine disease." This syndrome is due to branched-chain keto acid decarboxalase deficiency, and there is a "burnt sugar" aroma of the urine. Signs start 1 to 3 days after birth and include dullness and opisthotonus. The disease is probably inherited as an autosomal recessive. There is widespread spongy vacuolation of brain tissue. There is no treatment.

LATE ONSET CEREBELLAR DISEASE

Cerebellar Abiotrophy

Late onset cerebellar degeneration or abiotrophy was seen in Holstein calves. Signs were first noted at 3 to 8 months of age and were progressive, with eventual loss of the ability to stand unassisted despite normal strength. There were no gross lesions at necropsy, but histologic examination showed degeneration of Purkinje's cells and neurons of the cerebellar nuclei. Affected calves with complete pedigrees traced to a single sire on both sides of the pedigree within three generations, and the condition was believed to be inherited as a recessive characteristic. The popularity of this genetic line in Holsteins has declined in recent years, and the disease now appears to be rare. There is a report of a similar syndrome in a Charolais calf. There is no treatment.

Solanum Poisoning

Some plants of the Solanaceae family, including *Solanum dimidiatum* in the United States, *S. fastigiatum* and *S. bonariensis* in South America, and *S. kwabense* in Africa, cause cerebellar degeneration when they are ingested in large quantities by cattle. Such affected animals show signs of severe cerebellar disease, which are precipitated by excitement. Animals seem normal when left to graze quietly, but signs develop rapidly when they are disturbed; the sudden development of ataxia, opisthotonos, tremor, and nystagmus can cause the animal to fall into what appears to be a seizure. At necropsy there is vacuolation and degeneration and loss of Purkinje's cells, with axonal spheroids in the cerebellar granular layer and white matter in some cases. The disease has been reproduced by prolonged feeding of toxic plants. Morbidity and mortality can be high, with cattle dying because of loss of body condition, accidents secondary to severe ataxia, and falling. Recovery seems to be rare, even when animals are removed from pastures containing these plants, but some compensation occurs.

Familial Convulsions and Ataxia

Familial convulsion and ataxia syndrome is a disorder of Angus cattle, in which it might be a dominant inherited trait, and has also been described in Charolais and Polled Hereford cattle. Newborn or young calves up to 8 months of age develop intermittent seizures that might be precipitated by excitement; in some cases multiple seizures over a period of 3 to 12 hours are followed by residual ataxia and dysmetria. If the animal survives to 15 months of age seizures decrease, and most survivors are normal at 2 years of age. At necropsy there is generally histologic evidence of degeneration of the cell bodies and axons of Purkinje's cells.

Cerebellar Neoplasia

Neoplasms of the cerebellum are rare in cattle. The most frequently described cerebellar tumor in cattle is medulloblastoma, which has been diagnosed in calves between 1 and 9 months of age and was reported in a pair of twins. With signs of progressive asymmetric cerebellar disease developing at such a young age, it is probable that the tumor starts in utero. Confirmation of the diagnosis is made at necropsy.

Parasitic Infections

Coenurosis

Invasion of the cerebellum by the intermediate stage of *Taenia multiceps* might produce signs of progressive cerebellar disease.

Hypoderma bovis

Injury due to larvae of parasites such as *Hypoderma bovis* is rare.

Cerebellar Trauma

Cerebellar trauma without accompanying signs of involvement of other parts of the brain is rare. The onset of signs in trauma is sudden, and there might be external signs of injury and/or blood in the cerebrospinal fluid. Animals can learn to compensate following cerebellar injury.

GENERALIZED NEUROLOGIC DISEASE WITH A PROMINENT CEREBELLAR COMPONENT

Polioencephalomalacia

Thiamine-responsive polioencephalomalacia is one of the most common ruminant neurologic diseases. The lesions are widespread, and the cerebellum is affected along with cerebral tissue. Signs of cerebellar involvement, such as ataxia, dysmetria, and tremor, may be present along with the signs of cerebral involvement (especially cerebrocortical blindness) that usually predominate. Response to thiamine treatment is diagnostic.

Dallis, Bahia, Tabosa, or Galleta Grass Poisoning

Some grasses can become infected by the fungus *Claviceps* and when ingested can cause neurologic disease, including cerebellar disease, in cattle. *C. paspali* in dallis grass *(Paspalum dilatatum)* or bahai grass *(P. motatum)*, and *C. cinera* in tabosa grass *(Hilaria mutica)* or galleta grass *(H. jamesii)*, have been associated with this syndrome. Morbidity can be 30 to 50 per cent within 2 to 3 days of a herd of cattle being placed in an infected pasture. Signs are often worse when the animal is excited. There is no specific treatment, but recovery usually occurs from 3 days to 3 weeks after removal of animals from affected pasture.

Phalaris Staggers, Tryptamine Alkaloid Poisoning

Chronic grazing of pasture containing *Phalaris* herbage can cause a neurologic syndrome. On histology there are yellow-brown pigment granules in nervous and other tissue. There is no specific treatment; supportive therapy and a change of diet are indicated.

Ryegrass Poisoning

In New Zealand, Australia, and South Africa, consumption of ryegrass *(Lolium rigidum)* or of ryegrass seed infested with nematode galls containing toxins produced by *Corynebacterium rathayi* can cause neurologic and hepatotoxic disease. This can be fatal, although signs often resolve 2 to 3 days after ryegrass is removed from the diet. *L. perenne* has been associated with neurologic disease in the United States. There is no specific treatment.

Swainsona Poisoning

The toxic alkaloid swainsonine, found in the leguminous plant *Swainsona* in Australia, is a potent inhibitor of mannosidase and causes neurologic abnormalities in animals that eat 50 per cent of their food ration as *Swainsona* for 6 to 8 weeks. Vacuolation of tissue due to accumulation of mannoside is seen on histology.

Storage Diseases

GM1 gangliosidosis in Friesians; α-mannosidosis in Angus, Murray Grey, and Galloway; β-mannosidosis in Salers; and glycogenosis in Brahman and Shorthorn cattle are storage diseases in which intraneuronal lesions develop because of enzyme deficiencies. Signs such as ataxia and tremor might be seen early in these conditions, but most progress to include more diffuse signs of central nervous system involvement, such as seizures or blindness. Diagnosis is made by enzymatic studies, and confirmation is at necropsy.

Peripheral Vestibular Disease

Middle and inner ear infections cause some of the most common neurologic disorders seen by practitioners. In one study, one of every five weaned calves in a feedlot had evidence of otitis media. Peripheral vestibular trauma can also occur. Damage to the peripheral vestibular receptors in the ear leads to signs of ataxia with preservation of strength. Facial weakness due to facial nerve impairment and head tilt are also present in most cases. When both ears are affected, the clinical signs resemble those of cerebellar disease. There are wide head excursions that look like a tremor, but there is no spasticity and no dysmetria. The inability to blink, which develops owing to facial weakness, can be mistaken for the loss of menace response occurring with cerebellar disease. *Pasteurella multocida* and *Actinomyces pyogenes* are commonly isolated from patients with otitis media, and treatment with antibiotics is usually effective.

Bovine Spongiform Encephalopathy

A very important, widespread, new clinical syndrome of progressive neurologic disease, including signs of cerebellar disease, has been described in adult cattle in Great Britain. There is an insidious onset of signs that ultimately leads to slaughter 1 week to 14 months later. Histology shows bilaterally symmetrical degenerative changes in the brain stem and gray matter that resemble those seen in diseases such as scrapie in sheep. There is no treatment.

BIBLIOGRAPHY

Abbit B, Jones MZ, Kasari TR, et al: Beta-mannosidosis in twelve Salers calves. J Am Vet Med Assoc 198:109–113, 1991.
Alroy J, Orgad U, Ucci AA, Gavris VE: Swainsonine toxicosis mimics lectin histochemistry of mannosidosis. Vet Pathol 22:311–316, 1985.
Baird JD, Wojcinski ZW, Wise AP, Godkin MA: Maple syrup urine disease in five Hereford calves in Ontario. Can Vet J 28:505–511, 1987.
Donnelly WJC, Sheahan BJ: GM1 gangliosidosis of Friesian calves: a review. Irish Vet J 35:45–55, 1981.
Healy PJ, Harper PAW, Dennis JA: Phenotypic variation in bovine alpha-mannosidosis. Res Vet Sci 49:82–84, 1990.
Jensen R, Maki LR, Laverman LH, et al: Cause and pathogenesis of middle ear infections in young feedlot cattle. J Am Vet Med Assoc 182:967–972, 1983.
Jones TJ: Cerebellar abiotrophy in a Charolais calf. Bovine Practitioner 23:163–164, 1988.
Leipold HW: Congenital defects of current concern and interest in cattle: a review. Bovine Practitioner 17:101–114, 1982.
McClintock AE, O'Neil AE: A possible case of inherited abnormalities of the central nervous system of cavles by an AI sire. Vet Rec 94:382–383, 1974.
Nicholson SS: Tremorgenic syndromes in livestock. Vet Clin North Am: Food Anim Pract 5:291–300, 1989.
O'Sullivan BM, McPhee CP: Cerebellar hypoplasia of genetic origin in calves. Aust Vet J 51:469–471, 1975.
Proceedings of an international roundtable on bovine spongiform encephalopathy. J Am Vet Med Assoc 196:1673–1690, 1990.
Riet-Correa F, Mendez MDC, Schid AL, et al: Intoxication by *Colanum fastigiatum* var. *fastigiatum* as a cause of cerebellar degeneration in cattle. Cornell Vet 73:240–256, 1983.
Riond J-L, Cullen JM, Godfrey VL, et al: Bovine viral diarrhea virus–induced cerebellar disease in a calf. J Am Vet Med Assoc 197:1631–1637, 1990.
Rousseaux CG, Klavano GG, Johnson ES, et al: "Shaker" calf syndrome: a newly recognized inherited neurodegenerative disorder of Horned Hereford calves. Vet Pathol 22:104–111, 1985.
Scarrett KW, Gamble DA: Cerebellar medulloblastoma in a calf. Compend Contin Educ Pract Vet 5:S627–S630, 1983.
White ME: A cerebellar abiotrophy of calves. Cornell Vet 65:476–491, 1975.
White ME, Lewkowicz J, Mohammed HO: CONSULTANT diagnostic database. Ithaca, NY, Cornell University, 1991, On-line.
Whittington RJ, Morton AG, Kennedy DJ: Cerebellar abiotrophy in crossbred cattle. Aust Vet J 66:12–15, 1989.

Inflammatory Neurologic Diseases of Small Ruminants

MARY C. SMITH, DVM

Neurologic diseases are among the most frustrating problems of sheep and goats. When a weak, disoriented, or convulsing animal is first examined, it is often difficult to differentiate between metabolic or toxic conditions and primary neurologic disease. Pregnancy toxemia, hypoglycemia, enterotoxemia, acidosis, hypocalcemia, and transport tetany are among the disease processes that have an apparent neurologic component. Polioencephalomalacia (described elsewhere in this volume) is so common in sheep and goats that the experienced veterinarian routinely administers thiamine (100 to 300 mg) to any animal showing vague or perplexing signs. Alert animals with posterior paresis are no easier to evaluate. While the trained neurologist is pinpointing which segment of the spinal cord is involved, the average practitioner, although very serious about performing a complete neurologic examination, is still struggling to separate the weakness of starvation or white muscle disease or the pain and dysfunction of polyarthritis from true spinal cord disease.

There is no easy way out of this dilemma. A veterinarian cannot afford to treat the patient with one drug at a time until a response to therapy confirms a diagnosis. If his or her best guess happens to be wrong, the patient may well die because of irreversible damage to nervous tissue. This is especially true of polioencephalomalacia and listeriosis. If a "shotgun" approach to therapy is adopted and the patient recovers, the veterinarian has gained experience with neurologic disease in general, not with any specific condition. If the patient dies, a complete necropsy, including histologic examination of brain and spinal cord, must be performed to arrive at even a tentative diagnosis. Unfortunately the laboratory is far away, sheep rot quickly, and the metabolic or nutritional problems that mimic neurologic disease often leave no lesions. So another hole is dug or another coyote fed, and the frustration increases.

The many neurologic diseases to which sheep and goats are susceptible have been reviewed in a 1983 symposium on sheep and goat medicine. This article will be limited to consideration of common conditions that, because of their inflammatory nature, can be diagnosed, if not cured.

HISTORY AND EXAMINATION

The diagnosis of neurologic diseases of small ruminants is often based on history and signalment as much as on physical examination. The age, diet, and stage of production strongly influence the prior probability (likelihood before further testing) of neurologic diseases. After a physical examination and neurologic evaluation have been completed, the clinical signs (as compared with textbook descriptions of various diseases) are used to modify the prior probability and create a ranked list of possible diagnoses.

Cerebrospinal fluid (CSF) analysis can be used to narrow the list of differential diagnoses. A lumbosacral tap is not always easily performed but is of minimal danger to the patient. No sedation is required for the animal with marked paraparesis, while struggling animals can be briefly quieted with 2 to 4 mg xylazine HCl/50 kg intravenously. Note that this drug is unapproved for small ruminants, and larger doses may be fatal to animals with central neurologic disease. The animal may be restrained with the pelvic limbs hanging over the edge of a table or bale or in lateral recumbency with the spinal column flexed. The lumbosacral area is clipped and prepared with alternating povidone-iodine and alcohol swabs. A 20-gauge 1 1/2-inch or 18-gauge 3 1/2-inch spinal needle is inserted into the depression just caudal to the level of the tubera coxarum. It is advanced through the supraspinous ligament toward the center of the lumbosacral space. Alternatively, CSF may be removed from the atlanto-occipital site if the head is flexed ventrally; the animal may be standing or in lateral recumbency. The needle enters the skin exactly on the midline at the level of the cranial border of the wings of the atlas and is directed slightly forward while being slowly advanced. At least 1.5 ml fluid should be collected and placed in an EDTA vacutainer for determination of protein concentration and total white blood cell (WBC) count and differential. If the sample is very bloody, a new tap should be performed 2 days later. In most instances of inflammatory central nervous system (CNS) disease, the protein and/or WBC concentrations will be increased. Minimal or no changes in these values (protein <40 mg/100 ml and 0 to 4 WBC/mm^3) are expected with toxic, metabolic, or non-neurologic diseases.

POST-DEHORNING ENCEPHALOMALACIA

This is a problem of the young goat kid. There is a history of recent disbudding using heat or paste cautery or cryosurgery. Sometimes the previously normal animal is obtunded and has to be taught to drink milk again. In other instances it is found dead a few days or weeks after disbudding, and the owner may suspect enterotoxemia. Owing to the thinness of the calvarium and the absence of a cornual sinus at the appropriate age for disbudding (about 1 week), the cerebrum is easily damaged by excessive heat or cold. Treatment consists of corticosteroids to reduce swelling of the cerebrum and antibiotics to protect against bacterial penetration of the brain through damaged bone. Tube feeding is performed several times a day until the ability to suckle returns. Meningitis or cerebral abscess formation and tetanus are possible sequelae. Tetanus antitoxin (250 IU subcutaneously) is indicated prophylactically if the kid did not receive colostrum from a doe vaccinated with tetanus toxoid during late pregnancy.

MENINGITIS

There are several situations in which meningitis may occur independent of disbudding. Septicemia in the neonatal lamb or kid, perhaps originating from an omphalophlebitis, may lead to meningitis. A septic arthritis or anterior uveitis may also be present. Fever, nystagmus, convulsions or depression, and pain on manipulation of the neck may occur. Older animals may develop a pituitary abscess after a septicemic episode.

In adult animals a migrating nose bot (*Oestrus ovis*) may penetrate the calvarium and cause inflammation or abscessation in the brain. Clinical evidence of the parasite in this or other members of the flock (nasal discharge, sneezing) is expected. This neurologic condition has always been infrequently recognized but should become even rarer with increased use of ivermectin for parasite control in small ruminants.

Yet another situation involves acute onset of meningitis without an obvious pre-existing focus of infection. The animals are growing or mature, frequently die in less than 24 hours from the onset of signs, and may represent a herd or flock problem. The literature is scanty, but the most commonly isolated organism appears to be a *Streptococcus*. It has been postulated that one or more members of the herd are asymptomatic carriers. In one herd of goats, seen by the author, the outbreak ceased after all animals were injected with benzathine penicillin to which the isolated *Streptococcus* was sensitive.

Aggressive antibiotic therapy should be instituted at once. Penicillin, tetracycline, or trimethoprim-sulfamethoxazole are possible choices. Anticonvulsants should be used if indicated; cooling with ice water is advised if the body temperature is above 42°C (108°F). If facilities permit, CSF should be obtained to document the presence of a purulent meningitis and to attempt culture of the causative organism. Because animals in convulsions due to polioencephalomalacia may develop an elevated temperature, thiamine must be part of the therapy for suspected meningitis.

LISTERIOSIS

Listeria monocytogenes is the most common bacterial cause of brain stem inflammation in small ruminants. The organism has traditionally been associated with silage feeding because it has the capability of multiplying in spoiled (high pH) silage at cold temperatures. In areas where silage feeding is not practiced, listeriosis still occurs, and thus other sources of the organism, such as hay, wet pasture, or intestinal carriers, should be considered.

If the *Listeria* organism is instilled into the conjunctival sac or inoculated into oral mucous membranes, it travels along cranial nerves such as the trigeminal nerve to the medulla. Several fever spikes may occur before the onset of neurologic signs, 2½ to 4 weeks after inoculation. Those signs observed will depend on the cranial nerves and brain stem nuclei affected by the inflammatory process. Rolling or circling; torticollis; paralysis of the ear, eyelid, or lip muscles; and salivation are possible signs. While some animals do indeed show a "classic" unilateral facial paralysis with circling, others may have a dropped jaw and dysphagia. Blindness, the hallmark of advanced polioencephalomalacia, is not often present in listeriosis, but facial nerve paralysis may result in a decreased menace response. Depression is common and helps to distinguish central brain stem disease from the facial nerve paralysis and vestibular signs resulting from otitis media. The body temperature is often normal in later stages. Some animals die so rapidly that they are not observed ill; in these, the diagnosis rests upon brain culture and histologic demonstration of microabscesses and glial nodules in the brain stem. Perivascular cuffing and meningeal infiltration with mononuclear cells and a few neutrophils and eosinophils also occur.

Although young lambs and kids can be experimentally or naturally infected, most animals with listeriosis are over 6 months of age. In sheep, breaks in the oral mucous membranes associated with loss and replacement of incisor teeth may be an important avenue for infection to reach cranial nerves. Stress or nutritional inadequacies may lower an animal's resistance to this organism; thus listeriosis sometimes occurs as a sequela to the dehorning of an adult goat. Most authors believe that the disease is more common during the winter than in other seasons. As the winter is also the time for advanced pregnancy, differentiation from pregnancy toxemia is important. Facial nerve paralysis does not occur with pregnancy toxemia, but ketonuria can be expected once the late pregnant animal is off feed due to listeriosis. It should be noted that glucosuria, a sign that clinicians associate with enterotoxemia, is common in any animal with central neurologic disease, especially if convulsing.

Examination of CSF will document the inflammatory nature of a suspected case of listeriosis but cannot be used to rule out caprine arthritis-encephalitis (CAE) virus infection or cerebrospinal nematodiasis. Typically there is an elevation in both cells and protein, with the increase in cell numbers being relatively greater (cells:protein ratio >1). However, completely normal CSF is sometimes obtained from an animal with listeriosis.

The prognosis is guarded at best if signs have advanced to the point where walking or swallowing is not possible. Treatment with antibiotics must be aggressive. Initial intravenous sodium penicillin can be followed by 44,000 IU/kg procaine penicillin G subcutaneously s.i.d. or b.i.d. Tetracycline (10 g/kg daily) is an alternative treatment. Antibiotics should be continued for at least 7 to 10 days. If no improvement occurs in 2 weeks, the down or dysphagic animal should be euthanized. Corticosteroids should be avoided, as they predispose to relapses. In a small herd or flock of valuable animals, prophylactic penicillin for 3 days might help other animals that are incubating the disease, but this has not been confirmed by controlled testing.

The stall should be well bedded; some animals benefit from a canvas sling. If facial nerve paralysis prevents closure of the eyelids, ophthalmic ointments and protective bandages or suturing of the lids will limit exposure keratitis. (This keratitis often obscures a primary uveitis.) Force feeding with a slurry or gruel of cooked cereal, alfalfa pellets, or blended vegetables using a spoon, turkey baster, or stomach tube is necessary if the animal cannot eat unassisted. Fluids (including rumen fluid, if available) are supplied by stomach tube to maintain hydration. Baking soda (1 to 2 tablespoons/day) is added if loss of saliva has led to acidosis. When monetary concerns and facilities permit, intravenous fluid therapy, including sodium bicarbonate, to correct deficiencies identified by laboratory testing would be ideal. The animal should be handled with gloves because of the possibility that the encephalitis is due to rabies.

CAPRINE ARTHRITIS-ENCEPHALITIS VIRUS

The neurologic disease caused by the CAE virus was first described (in 1974) under the name of viral leukoencephalomyelitis, but the original term has fallen out of favor. This retrovirus infection can involve exactly the same brain stem nuclei that are affected by listeriosis. Differentiation by clinical signs is not possible when only the brain stem is involved. Animals with CAE may be febrile. However, CAE commonly involves the spinal cord, whereas listeriosis almost never does. Also, CAE most commonly affects young kids 2 to 4 months old, an age when listeriosis is rare. On the other hand, CAE does occur in adult goats, and a similar disease can be seen in sheep infected with the chronic progressive pneumonia virus. Consideration of age merely helps the clinician to estimate the probability of one disease or the other.

The CAE virus is usually acquired through consumption of unpasteurized goat colostrum or milk containing infected macrophages. Infection by other routes in closely confined animals also occurs. Most (but not all) animals with clinical signs of CAE have a positive agar gel immunodiffusion test to the virus. Many infected, blood test–positive goats never develop clinical neurologic disease due to CAE. Also, young kids that received heat-treated (1 hour at 56°C) colostrum from infected does may have antibody but no CAE infection. Thus the blood test is useful to diagnose and monitor infection in the herd but cannot be used to confirm or deny presence of the clinical disease in an individual animal in an infected herd. CSF changes are similar to those seen with listeriosis, except that there is typically a relatively smaller increase in cells; the cells:protein ratio is generally less than 1.0.

There is no effective treatment for CAE. Signs may wax and wane, but usually they progress until euthanasia is indicated. Gross lesions are often visible in the brain and/or spinal cord by this time. These are single to multifocal areas of discoloration. Histologically, primary demyelination and perivascular mononuclear cell infiltrations are present. The skills of a trained pathologist, seriously considering both diseases, are necessary to distinguish CAE from listeriosis; before 1974 most cases were labeled listeriosis.

Because CAE is untreatable and the diagnosis is uncertain before necropsy, treatment for other possible neurologic diseases is indicated. In addition, if dysphagia is the predominant sign in a kid or lamb, vitamin E and selenium should be administered because of the possibility of white muscle disease.

CEREBROSPINAL NEMATODIASIS

In the United States the nematode generally implicated when parasite remnants or tracts are found in the CNS of sheep or goats is *Parelaphostrongylus tenuis*. The natural host of the adult worm is the white-tailed deer; numerous snails and slugs on pasture grazed by deer carry the infective larval stage. The larvae of *P. tenuis* migrate to the spinal cord of small ruminants that ingest the snails or slugs. A brief sojourn in the dorsal gray columns is normal and apparently asymptomatic in the deer, but inflammation and malacia may attend aberrant migration through the spinal cord or brain of sheep and goats, as well as llamas, alpacas, elk, and moose.

The clinical signs of *P. tenuis* migration vary with the number of larvae and the portion of the CNS invaded. If the parasite is migrating through the medulla, signs mimic those of listeriosis or CAE. Most affected animals are over 6 months of age, but this does not narrow the list of differential diagnoses. Exposure to pasture several months earlier is a prerequisite, although presence of the deer may have escaped notice.

Examination of CSF is quite helpful, as approximately 70 per cent of samples from goats clinically affected with *P. tenuis* contain eosinophils. However, the other 30 per cent are indistinguishable from CSF samples obtained from either listeriosis or CAE. In regions where coenurosis is a common cause of neurologic disease (often accompanied by papilledema and unilateral blindness), eosinophils in the CSF should prompt careful palpation or radiographic evaluation to detect the presence of parasitic cysts in the cerebrum.

Treatment of cerebrospinal nematodiasis is empirical; controlled clinical trials have not been performed. Various anthelmintics have been used, and some animals have appeared to respond to fenbendazole (15 mg/kg/day for 3 days), levamisole (8 mg/kg; subcutaneous administration achieves higher plasma levels than does the oral route), and diethylcarbamazine. More recently ivermectin has become popular with practitioners attempting to treat this disease in small ruminants. Although the drug normally does not reach the CNS of mammals, it might cross the blood-brain barrier where the parasite has evoked a localized inflammatory response. Ivermectin is now commonly given along with another drug such as fenbendazole. Ivermectin apparently does not reach the *P. tenuis* larvae during most of the early migration period. Nonpregnant animals are treated with dexamethasone for the first few days to limit the inflammation associated with destruction of the parasite.

SPINAL CORD DISEASE

If clinical signs can be localized to the spinal cord and CSF evaluation supports a diagnosis of inflammatory disease, CAE and *P. tenuis* migration are the most common etiologies. If CSF is unremarkable or cannot be analyzed, traumatic injury to the spinal cord and enzootic ataxia (copper deficiency) are important differentials.

The young kid with paraparesis or hemiparesis (often initially mistaken for lameness) that progresses to tetraparesis is apt to be afflicted with CAE. However, radiographs will help to rule out a vertebral body abscess. These abscesses are most common in animals with previous omphalophlebitis and may be located in a vertebra above the heart or above the kidneys. Lambs with an ascending paralysis beginning at the perineum may have a postdocking infection of the cauda equina. Treatment of these conditions is rarely successful.

The older lamb or kid or the adult with spinal cord disease again may have CAE or *P. tenuis*. As with brain stem disease, the presence of eosinophils in the CSF is highly suggestive of parasitic migration. Another clinical sign that has been associated with *P. tenuis* is the self-excoriation by the animal of a narrow, vertically oriented strip of skin, presumably due to irritation to a dorsal nerve root by the parasite. Some animals that have been treated for cerebrospinal nematodiasis stabilize or improve but retain a gait deficit for the rest of their lives. The goat with CAE of the spinal cord is not expected to recover. With either disease, signs referable to the brain may occur later in the clinical course, and histology will establish the diagnosis.

BIBLIOGRAPHY

Alden C, Woodson F, Mohan R, et al: Cerebrospinal nematodiasis in sheep. J Am Vet Med Assoc 166:784–786, 1975.

Barlow RM, McGorum B: Ovine listerial encephalitis: analysis, hypothesis and synthesis. Vet Rec 116:233–236, 1985.

Brewer BD: Neurologic disease in sheep and goats. Vet Clin North Am: Large Anim Pract 5:677–700, 1983.

Mayhew IG, deLahunta A, Georgi JR, et al: Naturally occurring cerebrospinal parelaphostrongylosis. Cornell Vet 66:56–72, 1976.

Norman S, Smith MC: Caprine arthritis-encephalitis: review of the neurologic form in 30 cases. J Am Vet Med Assoc 182:1342–1345, 1983.

Robinson WF, Ellis TM: Caprine arthritis-encephalitis virus infection: from recognition to eradication. Aust Vet J 63:237–241, 1986.

Scarratt WK: Ovine listeric encephalitis. Compend Contin Educ Pract Vet 9:F28–F32, 1987.

Smith MC: Diagnostic value of caprine cerebrospinal fluid analysis (abstract). *In* Proceedings of the 3rd International Conference on Goat Production and Diseases, 1982, p 294.

Sundquist B, Jönsson L, Jacobsson S, et al: Visna virus meningoencephalomyelitis in goats. Acta Vet Scand 22:315–330, 1981.

Tirgari M, Howard BR, Boargob A: Clinical and radiographical diagnosis of coenurosis cerebralis in sheep and its surgical treatment. Vet Rec 120:173–178, 1987.

Wright HJ, Adams DS, Trigo FJ: Meningoencephalitis after hot-iron disbudding of goat kids. Vet Med/Small Anim Clin 78:599–601, 1983.

Note: See *Current Veterinary Therapy 2* for additional articles on the subject.

SECTION 17
Diseases of the Musculoskeletal System

BRUCE L. HULL, DVM, MS, Diplomate, ACVS, Consulting Editor

Introduction to the Musculoskeletal System
BRUCE L. HULL, DVM, MS, Diplomate, ACVS

Examination of the musculoskeletal system should begin with observation of the animal in motion. If this is not possible, the animal should be observed while quietly standing. At rest the animal will shift its weight away from affected limbs. Lowering the head with extension of the neck forward will shift weight away from the rear legs, while elevating the head with flexion of the neck will shift weight away from the forelegs. In rear-leg lameness the weight is shifted forward, giving the shoulders a very prominent appearance. Front-leg lameness causes the animal to support most of its weight on the rear legs, giving a sickle-hocked appearance.

If a single digit is involved, the animal will stand base wide or base narrow to protect the affected claw. The classic example is bilateral medial claw sole abscesses, which lead to a cross-legged stance.

When in doubt one should always start the examination for lameness with the cow's foot, as 90 per cent of all bovine lameness is located distal to the fetlock. Of these foot lameness cases, approximately 90 per cent are located in the rear feet.[1] Rear-foot lameness problems are most often seen in the lateral toes, while front-foot lameness is most likely in the medial toes.

REFERENCES

1. Pinsent PJN: The management and husbandry aspects of foot lameness in dairy cattle. Bovine Pract 16:61–64, 1981.

Sole Abscesses
BRUCE L. HULL, DVM, MS, Diplomate, ACVS

A sole abscess is located between the sensitive laminae and the horny sole of the foot. The purulent exudate in these abscesses varies in color from pinkish-yellow to gray-brown and is usually under considerable pressure. Depending on duration, a variable amount of the sole is undermined.

ETIOLOGY

Abscesses result from damage to the integrity of the sole. This damage may be caused by foreign bodies, puncture wounds, laminitis, white-line separation, and cracks due to overgrown claws. As these breaks in the integrity of the sole are contaminated, they lead to bacterial growth beneath the sole.

CLINICAL SIGNS

The prime sign of a sole abscess is severe pain. This pain is often severe enough to cause the animal to be "three-legged lame." Owing to this lameness and its sudden onset, sole abscesses have often been confused with fractures. With sole abscesses the animal is reluctant to bear weight on the affected toe. This will lead to a base-wide or base-narrow stance to relieve pressure on the involved toe. Because sole abscesses are most frequent in the lateral toe of the rear foot, the base-wide stance and gait of the animal can easily be confused with that of a stifle injury.

A simple sole abscess is usually not associated with any swelling or inflammation above the coronary band. However, later in the course of the disease a sole abscess may break out and drain at the coronary band. Anytime a draining lesion is found at the coronary band, one should evaluate the PII-PIII joint for osteomyelitis.

Hoof testers may be employed to evaluate pain over a given digit or even an area of a digit. Radiographic evaluation is not indicated and is often unrewarding in the diagnosis of a sole abscess.

Although the signs and symptoms as described may make one suspicious of a sole abscess, the diagnosis is dependent on a foot trim. The foot trim should include following out any black lines or puncture wounds that may be encountered. Although these may appear small and insignificant, they often lead to a large sole abscess.

TREATMENT

While following out black lines or puncture wounds, dry lines will often become moist shortly before the abscess is opened. Opening the abscess will drain the pus, which is often under considerable pressure and may be accompanied by gas. Often there is a thin layer of new sole deep to the abscess.

Because this new sole is thin and soft, care must be taken in removing the undermined sole so that the sensitive laminae are not exposed. All undermined sole should be removed. If undermined sole is left, inadequate drainage may occur owing to occlusion by a pack of manure or mud, and the abscess may reform. The undermined sole is usually removed with a hoof knife or a hoof groover.

Although all undermined sole should be removed, the wall of the claw should be left intact to serve as a weight-bearing surface. This wall should be trimmed so that it extends only about 1 cm below the reforming sole. A long wall promotes the accumulation of manure and mud over the pared-out abscess. After paring off the undermined sole, the foot may be wrapped with an antiseptic ointment. If the wrap becomes soaked with manure and urine, wrapping is undesirable. Consequently it is probably preferable to leave the abscess open and treat it with a drying agent. It is usually best to clean this abscess area every day or two and apply a drying agent such as Kopertox[1] for 7 to 10 days.

Following this treatment there is usually dramatic relief from the lameness within 12 to 24 hours. The animal is usually back to normal and needs no further treatment after 7 to 10 days. If the lameness persists the diagnosis should be reevaluated or the lameness should be reexamined.

BIBLIOGRAPHY

Greenough PR, MacCallum FJ, Weaver AD: Lameness in Cattle, 2nd ed. Philadelphia, JB Lippincott, 1981.
White ME, Glickman TL, Embree IC, et al: A randomized trial for evaluation of bandaging sole abscesses in cattle. J Am Vet Med Assoc 178:375–377, 1981.

---

[1]Available from Fort Dodge Laboratories, Fort Dodge, IA 50501.

Vertical Wall Cracks
BRUCE L. HULL, DVM, MS, DIPLOMATE, ACVS

Vertical wall cracks, also called quarter cracks, are usually seen on the cranial aspect of the claws of the front feet. These cracks are a loss of the continuity of the hoof wall. The cracks start at the coronary band and extend for a variable distance toward the wear surface.

ETIOLOGY

Vertical wall cracks are most common in the front feet of beef bulls. Dry weather and hoof brittleness are definitely involved in the pathogenesis. Laminitis has been suggested as a cause but is certainly not a consistent finding. Occasionally damage to the coronary band due to external trauma may initiate a vertical wall crack. Since overly dry or brittle hooves are the prime cause of vertical wall cracks, a higher incidence of the condition can be expected in the late summer or early fall.

CLINICAL SIGNS

Vertical wall cracks range in severity from partial thickness cracks that are incidental findings to deep cracks that become infected and lead to septic laminitis. The range in lesion severity is accompanied by a wide range of clinical signs, from a normally moving animal to an abnormally moving or even severely lame animal. In any animal having vertical wall cracks, hoof testers should be used to ascertain if the lameness is indeed caused by the cracks.

TREATMENT

If an animal with vertical wall cracks is not lame, one should not be too vigorous in treatment. Excessive grooving out of the cracks will expose the sensitive laminae and lead to lameness. A good foot trim with special emphasis on shortening the toes is indicated to help relieve abnormal stress on the hoof wall. Also, the hoof wall should be sealed (grease, tar, Kopertox,[1] or varnish) to help it retain moisture and become more pliable. Resealing is indicated periodically until the crack grows out.

In addition to these procedures, any lame animal should have the crack cleaned out and widened with a hoof groover. Often this treatment will reveal an abscess (septic laminitis). Abscesses are most prevalent distally and in some cases may extend into sole abscesses. If the abscess can be pared out nicely and leave a dry defect in the hoof wall, this defect can be filled with hoof acrylic. However, if the defect has draining tracts it should be kept open.

When fissures extend from the coronary band to the wear surface, a wooden block should be applied to the normal digit with hoof acrylic. This block prevents excessive pull on the hoof wall as the cracks start to heal.

BIBLIOGRAPHY

Amstutz HE: Hoof wall fissures. Mod Vet Pract 59:906–908, 1978.
Greenough PR, MacCallum FJ, Weaver AD: Lameness in Cattle, 2nd ed. Philadelphia, JB Lippincott, 1981.
Petersen GC, Nelson DR: Foot diseases in cattle. Part II. Diagnosis and treatment. Comp Cont Ed 6:565–573, 1984.

---

[1]Available from Fort Dodge Laboratories, Fort Dodge, IA 50501.

Horizontal Wall Cracks
BRUCE L. HULL, DVM, MS, DIPLOMATE, ACVS

Horizontal wall cracks have also been called "thimble toe." The loss of continuity of the hoof wall is parallel to the coronary band and extends around the circumference of the toe. The heel area is usually not involved, or perhaps grows out before being recognized as a clinical problem. The lesion usually affects all eight toes of an animal.

ETIOLOGY

Horizontal wall cracks usually follow a severe systemic infection that has been accompanied by an acute febrile response. This febrile episode causes imperfect horn growth at the coronary band that later splits or separates. This imperfect hoof does not usually separate until it nears the wear surface (2 to 3 cm from the coronary band) and begins to have stresses applied to it as the animal walks. Nutritional deficiencies and metabolic diseases are also considered to be a cause by some investigators. Once the split occurs, the distal shell of the hoof is attached only by the sensitive laminae. As the animal walks, this shell moves back and forth, causing pain. In addition to the pulling on the sensitive laminae, dirt and manure may work into the cracks and cause a septic laminitis.

CLINICAL SIGNS

Before the split occurs, clinical signs are minimal. A small horizontal groove may be noted on the hoof, but the animal shows no pain. Once the split occurs, the animal becomes very sore and is often reluctant to move because walking causes the shell of the hoof to move and pull against the sensitive laminae. This stage may be accompanied by weight loss and sudden drop in milk production.

TREATMENT

The treatment of choice is a foot trim. The trim should be accompanied by removal of any undermined wall to prevent dirt and debris from accumulating. In doing this, care should be taken to avoid injury to the sensitive laminae. Also the toe should be "dubbed" as short as possible. This helps prevent the shell of the toe from rocking back and forth on the sensitive laminae as the animal walks. Although this treatment will alleviate pain, it usually takes 4 to 6 weeks for the new hoof wall to reach the wear surface and for the outer shell to fall off. Occasionally another foot trim, as described, will be needed during this time.

BIBLIOGRAPHY

Amstutz HE: Hoof wall fissures. Mod Vet Pract 59:906–908, 1978.
Greenough PR, MacCallum FJ, Weaver AD: Lameness in Cattle, 2nd ed. Philadelphia, JB Lippincott, 1981.

Rusterholz Ulcer

BRUCE L. HULL, DVM, MS, Diplomate, ACVS

A Rusterholz ulcer is a lesion at the junction of the sole and bulb that starts as a bruise, develops into a devitalized area, and later produces granulation tissue and even osteoarthritis. This lesion is usually located near the axial border of the involved toe and overlies the attachment of the flexor tendons. The ulcerated area is characterized by the presence of a mass of granulation tissue protruding through the sole. This granulation tissue is the result of the piston-like effect of PIII, forcing the sensitive laminae out through the defect in the sole. Rusterholz ulcers are most common in the lateral toes of the rear feet of mature animals.

ETIOLOGY

Although Rusterholz ulcers may occur in pastured animals, they are more frequent in animals confined on concrete. Wet concrete appears to be associated with a higher incidence of Rusterholz ulcer cases. Chronic bruising is definitely associated with their pathogenesis. Some workers have incriminated nutritional problems, especially calcium-phosphorus imbalance, genetics, and conformation as possible causes. The role of these various etiologic factors is not completely understood at present.

CLINICAL SIGNS

The lameness associated with Rusterholz ulcers is usually severe and sudden in onset. As this condition often involves the lateral toe of the rear foot, the animal usually walks and stands base wide to relieve pressure on the lateral digit. Stanchioned animals will often stand back so that only the toe bears weight on the curb of the manure gutter.

Hoof testers will elicit pain when applied over the bulb-to-sole junction of the affected digit. As with sole abscesses, the final diagnosis must be made in conjunction with a foot trim. The foot trim may reveal granulation tissue, a crack in the sole, or merely a discolored area of the sole. As with a sole abscess, the crack or discolored area must be pared out to reveal the lesion. Although a true sole abscess is possible in this area (axial sole and wall junction), a Rusterholz ulcer characterized by its granulation tissue is usually found.

Untreated Rusterholz ulcers often lead to weakness and necrosis of the flexor tendon near its attachment to PIII. This weakening eventually (3 to 4 weeks) causes a rupture of the tendon attachment. When the tendon ruptures, the toe of the hoof suddenly tips upward owing to the absence of flexion of PIII.

TREATMENT

Treatment of a Rusterholz ulcer is time-consuming and frustrating. After paring out all of the undermined sole, one must gently probe the granulation tissue for fistulous tracts. These tracts, if found, must be explored for evidence of deep abscesses or osteomyelitis. The presence of deep tracts, especially in suspected cases of osteomyelitis, is reason for radiographic evaluation of the foot. If PII-PIII joint involvement is found, digit amputation is the most economical treatment, although drainage and ankylosis should be considered in valuable animals.

The granulation tissue that protrudes through the sole must be debrided to the level of the sole and cauterized to prevent excessive hemorrhage. The sole around the ulcer must be "feathered" so that it is thinner and more pliable near the ulcer and thicker away from the ulcer. This thinned sole near the ulcer allows it to give with the piston-like effect of PIII while healing is taking place.

Although bandaging the foot, or drying it as is done with a sole abscess, may lead to a successful outcome, this is very tedious and time-consuming. It is certainly preferable to apply a wooden block to the normal digit with hoof acrylic.[1] Alternatively, a plaster block and cast may be applied to the normal digit. In either case this relieves pressure on the affected digit. Relief of pressure allows the animal a more pain-free recovery period but, more important, prevents the piston-like effect of PIII, which would lead to new granulation tissue. A block or cast also alleviates stretch on the flexor tendon, which may be weak.

Antiseptic dressings or drying agents such as Koppertox[2] should be used in conjunction with a wooden or plaster block.

---

[1] Available as Technovit from Jorgensen Laboratories, Loveland, CO 80537.
[2] Available from Fort Dodge Laboratories, Fort Dodge, IA 50501.

Even with the help of a block, a Rusterholz ulcer will take 3 to 6 weeks to heal.

BIBLIOGRAPHY

Greenough PR, MacCallum FJ, Weaver AD: Lameness in Cattle, 2nd ed. Philadelphia, JB Lippincott, 1981.
Petersen GC, Nelson DR: Foot diseases in cattle. Part II. Diagnosis and treatment. Comp Cont Ed 6:565–573, 1984.
Rebhun WC, Pearson EG: Clinical management of bovine foot problems. J Am Vet Med Assoc 181:572–577, 1982.

Verrucose Dermatitis

BRUCE L. HULL, DVM, MS, Diplomate, ACVS

Verrucose dermatitis is a proliferative lesion that appears "wart-like" and usually originates above the bulbs of the heel. Rarely this lesion can be seen on the dorsal surface of the foot above the interdigital area. Verrucose dermatitis is a distinct clinical entity and should not be confused with heel warts (recently described) or stable foot rot, which actually originates in the interdigital area and is often an erosive lesion.

ETIOLOGY

Although *Fusobacterium necrophorum* can be cultured from verrucose dermatitis, it is a mixed bacterial and fungal problem that is precipitated by filth and moisture. It is often associated with long toes and shallow heels, which causes the bulbs of the heels to be constantly exposed to water and manure.

CLINICAL SIGNS

Verrucose dermatitis is almost exclusively found on the rear feet. The wart-like growths characteristic of this lesion are often matted together by an exudation of dried serum. Although the lesion may extend as high as the dewclaws, it rarely causes lameness.

TREATMENT

A foot trim should always be performed as part of the treatment for verrucose dermatitis. This trim should be aimed at shortening the toes while preserving as much heel as possible. One should also consider either cleaning the environment or removing the affected animal from the environment until the lesion heals.

The wart-like lesion and the affected skin should be radically excised and heat cautery used to control hemorrhage. A dry antiseptic dressing should then be applied until healing is complete. The foot and bandage should be kept dry during the healing process.

Aseptic Laminitis of Cattle

A. DAVID WEAVER, PhD, FRCVS

Laminitis (pododermatitis aseptica diffusa), commonly termed "founder," occurs in acute, subacute, subclinical, and chronic forms. Laminitis is believed to be an important component of many manifestations of digital lameness. Occasionally acute laminitis is primary; however, more commonly, acute laminitis is secondary to rumen acidosis, which in itself may cause a clinically obvious digestive disturbance. Rarely in cattle is acute laminitis secondary to severe septic metritis or acute mastitis.

Affected cattle tend to be either dairy heifers or cows receiving high levels of concentrate feeding or intensively reared steers on a carbohydrate-rich fattening ration.

CLINICAL SIGNS AND DIAGNOSIS

The signs of severe acute laminitis are a generalized stiffness, arched back, mild pyrexia, tachycardia and tachypnea associated with the painful stance, reduced feed intake, and sweating. The hind legs may be extended forward, the forelegs may be close together or crossed, and a constant paddling movement may be evident. Some severe cases may be unwilling to rise. Others are reluctant to move and have a shortened stride. Edematous swelling may be seen around the coronary band. The feet are warm to the touch and painful on percussion. Histologic changes at this stage reveal severe changes in the dermal laminae, including edema, congestion, thrombosis, and a loss of onychogenic substance in the stratum germinativum and stratum spinosum. Increased pulsation in the digital arteries suggests a vascular hypertension, although within the claw a stagnant hypoxia is associated with venous hypotension. Differential diagnosis of acute aseptic laminitis includes septic laminitis, bilateral solar ulceration, and generalized systemic conditions such as pleuritis, pericarditis, and reticulo-peritonitis.

Subacute laminitis is a less dramatic form of acute laminitis, and diagnosis depends on a thorough clinical examination. Subclinical laminitis, which is being increasingly recognized, can be diagnosed only by observation of claw changes. The solar horn texture becomes soft and yellowish. Hemorrhages may be seen in the sole and wall, the latter in the form of pink lines parallel to the coronet. The white line may show hemorrhage or a yellow serous exudate, particularly in the dorsal half of the claw. Solar hemorrhage is seen as fine streaks or "paintmarks" within the horn itself, while bruising is located between the corium and sole horn. The multiple paintmark streaks are not painful to hoof testers.

Certain specific digital disease of the horn, including solar ulceration, heel erosions, under-run sole, and excessive horn wear, are believed to be a secondary effect of an attack of subclinical or acute laminitis some months previously (Fig. 1).

Chronic laminitis produces well-recognized changes in shape and texture of the digital horn. The dorsal angle is reduced from about 55° (normal) to 35° to 45°, and the dorsal wall may be concave. The coronary band may be flakey, and the periople may have lost its sheen. Horizontal lines (growth arrest lines) extend around the circumference of the claw, parallel to the coronet. The sole tends to be flat, resulting in a greater tendency to solar bruising. The areas of hemorrhage are dark gray or black when weeks or months old and more red if relatively fresh. The abaxial and, to a lesser extent, the axial white line are widened. More chronic cases have marked

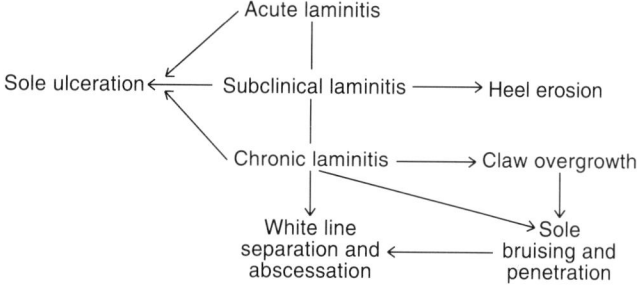

Figure 1. Possible effects of acute laminitis on the bovine claw.

overgrowth of the toe, and the abaxial wall tends to overgrow the sole.

TREATMENT AND PREVENTION

Treatment of acute laminitis should be considered an emergency. The primary aim is to get the animal moving in order to promote improved circulation within the claw. If the animal is recumbent, a digital nerve block may be given to abolish pain temporarily. If feasible, standing the animal in cold water will stimulate the circulation. Medical treatment is debatable in the absence of controlled studies. Corticosteroids (dexamethasone 10 to 20 mg intravenously or intramuscularly s.i.d.), antihistamines, and, more recently, antiprostaglandins have been recommended in the early stages of an acute attack. Antiprostaglandins may control the endotoxic pododermatitis. Flunixin meglumine (1 mg/lb intravenously s.i.d.), phenylbutazone (2 to 4 mg/lb orally every second day), and aspirin (50 mg/lb orally b.i.d.) have been given. With or without treatment, many cases fail to recover and are culled owing to poor production or to the development of secondary complications.

Chronic laminitis can be alleviated only by repeated and careful claw trimming. Attempts must be made to restore normal weight-bearing onto the walls and off the heels. This requires removal of the excessive growth at the toe and on the dorsal part of the sole to increase the dorsal angle. The overgrowth of the abaxial wall must be trimmed away, and any pathology (abscessation, white-line impaction) underlying the double sole must be corrected.

The lack of success in treating laminitis makes it important to educate farmers to adopt prophylactic measures. Prevention depends on good husbandry, and in particular on making all feed changes slowly. It is also helpful if heifers are given plenty of space for exercise on concrete rather than confining them to a small area.

The likely development of laminitis as a herd problem is reduced by encouraging movement, such as by positioning feed bunks at several well-separated points. In a herd at risk for laminitis, the minimum daily amount of long-stemmed hay that should be fed is 8 to 10 lb/head.

Claw trimming should be carried out twice a year on the entire milking herd, paying attention not only to cows with obvious claw deformities such as corkscrew claw and double sole, but also to those where the dorsal wall angle is less than 45°.

BIBLIOGRAPHY

Andersson L: Synovial fluid in laminitic dairy cows. Report of 2nd Symposium on Bovine Digital Disease. Skara, Sweden, September 1978.
Greenough PR: An illustrated compendium of bovine lameness. Mod Vet Pract 68:6–10, 1987.

Interdigital and Digital Dermatitis

A. DAVID WEAVER, PhD, FRCVS

INTERDIGITAL DERMATITIS

Interdigital dermatitis and digital dermatitis affect the skin in and around the interdigital space but are distinct entities.

Interdigital dermatitis (bovine contagious interdigital dermatitis) is a moist, superficial, relatively mild condition in which *Fusobacterium necrophorum*, although present, is not the primary etiologic agent. The transmissible causal agent is *Bacteroides nodosus*, which is seen microscopically as uniformly large barbell- or club-shaped gram-negative organisms. Direct smears must be examined, as culture of *B. nodosus* is difficult. *F. necrophorum* is subsequently responsible for the necrosis. The lesion can affect any age of animal and is usually associated with moist conditions in continuously housed animals.

The initial lesion, seen as a superficial break in the integument, does not cause lameness. Lameness develops as undermining of the axial wall and heel horn proceed. Later, interdigital skin necrosis and sloughing take place. It is believed that this lesion can spread onto the heel horn to cause "pockmarks" and transverse fissures as a result of necrosis of the horn. Such heel lesions are common, yet the frequent absence of interdigital changes at this time may indicate that these changes have resolved spontaneously.

The major differential diagnosis is interdigital phlegmon, which invariably starts in the deeper tissues and involves the skin only after producing a marked interdigital swelling (see Interdigital Phlegmon [Interdigital Necrobacillosis]).

Interdigital dermatitis is best controlled by footbathing affected cattle twice daily, 2 days a week, using 3 to 5 per cent formalin or 2 to 5 per cent copper sulfate. Severe cases of lameness may be successfully treated with antimicrobials as advised for interdigital phlegmon.

DIGITAL DERMATITIS

Digital dermatitis (also termed digital papillomatosis, "hairy warts") was originally reported from the Po Valley in Italy nearly 20 years ago but is now recognized in several other European countries and the United States. It causes sporadic or epidemic lameness problems in dairy herds and is occasionally seen in beef cattle. Often the disease appears to be introduced into a herd through purchased animals. The etiology is not known.

Clinical Signs and Diagnosis

The typical lesion is seen in the plantar skin, just proximal to the heels of one or both hind legs, predominantly in calved heifers and infrequently in older dairy stock. In the first stage, there is a moist, circumscribed, exudative lesion about 1 to 2 cm in diameter. It has a foul odor and is very sensitive to touch. Some hair is lost, and the peripheral hairs tend to be erect. After the skin is cleaned, a moist, red, granulating area is evident. Lesions expand in all directions and distally cause damage to the perioplic heel horn with underrunning of the heel and extensive heel horn necrosis. Some lesions also involve the skin proximal to the dorsal end of the interdigital space. The interdigital space is usually not involved (compare interdigital dermatitis).

The granulating lesion grows to become strawberry-like, then dries up to develop nonsensitive papillomatous fronds 1 to 2 cm long (dermatitis verrucosa) before slowly regressing spontaneously, often in the dry period. Affected cattle are typically confined, tending to be overcrowded, and mud with slurry on the concrete floor is probably a predisposing factor. The condition does not appear in grazing cattle.

The degree of lameness varies from slight to severe. A unilaterally affected heifer or cow often is more obviously lame than one with lesions in several legs.

Etiology

Despite the possible viral nature of this apparently infectious agent, no virus particles have been reported and immunoperoxidase staining has proved negative.

Bacteroides nodosus has been isolated from the surface of lesions in the United States, but its significance is doubtful.

Treatment and Prevention

Surgical removal by scalpel or cryotherapy is effective, and recurrence is unlikely; however, such treatment is impractical in herd outbreaks.

Curettage and one or more applications of a topical aerosol containing oxytetracycline and gentian violet have been successful in some herds in the United Kingdom. Other forms of successful treatment have included topical application of 37% formalin via aerosol, and parenteral antibiotic medication (procaine penicillin, 18,000 IU/kg intramuscularly once a day [s.i.d.] for 3 days, ceftiofur, 2 mg/kg intramuscularly s.i.d. for 3 days) in the United States.

Herd outbreaks have been treated with variable success using footbaths. Formalin footbaths alone are generally unsuccessful. Baths containing 2 to 4 g/L tetracycline, 0.5 to 1 g/L dimetridazole (Emtryl-Salsbury), or 20% zinc sulfate have been advocated for treatment, with the herd being walked through twice daily for 2 days every week.

Preventive footbathing should be a similar regimen. Use of an autogenous vaccine prepared from resected lesions on affected cattle has been unsuccessful in both treatment and prevention.

BIBLIOGRAPHY

INTERDIGITAL DERMATITIS

Rebhun WC, Pearson EG: Clinical management of bovine foot problems. J Amer Vet Med Assoc 181:572–577, 1982.

DIGITAL DERMATITIS

Rebhun WC, Payne RM, King JM, et al: Interdigital papillomatosis in dairy cattle. J Am Vet Med Assoc 177:437–440, 1980.
Blowey RW, Sharp MW: Digital dermatitis in dairy cattle. Vet Rec 122:505–508, 1988.
Blowey RW, Weaver AD: A color atlas of diseases and disorders of cattle. London, Wolff, 1991.

Interdigital Phlegmon (Interdigital Necrobacillosis)
A. DAVID WEAVER, PhD, FRCVS

Synonyms for interdigital phlegmon include acute footrot and foul and interdigital pododermatitis. This infectious condition is associated with *Fusobacterium necrophorum*. The role of other organisms, including *Bacteroides melaninogenicus* and *B. nodosus*, is unclear. The discrepancy may be due to problems in culture of these two bacteria and the absence, in some cases, of a satisfactory experimental model.

ETIOLOGY

Interdigital phlegmon is generally a sporadic condition encountered more commonly in adult cattle of dairy breeds. Major predisposing factors include sharp, irregular contact surfaces such as stony tracks and stubble fields, which, by causing microtrauma to many susceptible animals, may lead to incidents involving lameness in several animals within a few days. Interdigital dermatitis (*B. nodosus*) infection predisposes some cows to the development of interdigital phlegmon following the infection of superficial erosive lesions. The prevalence is increased by high rainfall periods and wet seasons of the year. Most studies have found that a greater number of hind- than forelimb digits are affected.

The prevalence in feedlot cattle can be occasionally high owing to the adverse conditions pertaining equally to dairy cattle—namely the regular movement of many close-packed cattle through narrow gateways, in yards, and around troughs in conditions that favor interdigital microtrauma and maintenance of high populations of infective organisms in the environment.

CLINICAL SIGNS

In contrast to interdigital dermatitis, the initial lesion affects much of the depth of the interdigital skin, which swells within 24 hours of the onset of infection to cause a slight separation of the toes and a symmetric hyperemic swelling above the heel bulbs. A longitudinal fissure then develops in the swollen interdigital skin, extending along part or the entire length of the space and, depending on severity, involving the deeper layers of skin or confined to the more superficial tissues. Cases are occasionally encountered ("blind foul") where no fissure develops. The amount of caseonecrotic tissue between the lips of the fissure increases for 48 to 72 hours, and it eventually sloughs. A pronounced and characteristic odor of necrobacillosis is perceived. Cellulitis and edema spread proximally from the coronary band to the pastern and fetlock region to cause a diffuse swelling, which also involves the skin above the heel bulbs. The degree of lameness varies from mild to severe, the severity being related to the extent of involvement of the deeper structures. Cattle show mild pyrexia with reduced feed intake, milk yield, and loss of flesh. The condition also affects fertility by making estrus more difficult to detect, as cows prefer recumbency and do not stand to be mounted.

Many milder, untreated cases of interdigital phlegmon will resolve spontaneously. More severe cases result in continuing lameness for several weeks as, following slough of a wedge of interdigital skin, infection is limited, granulation tissue develops, and the wound slowly undergoes epithelialization. Complications arise if the necrobacillary infection spreads more deeply to involve the adjacent axial aspect of the pedal joint, the navicular bursa, and the deep flexor tendon sheath, leading to septic arthritis, septic navicular bursitis, abscessation of the heel, and septic tenosynovitis. These complications cause severe lameness, pain on separation and flexion of the claws, and considerable swelling proximal to the coronary band.

Another late complication of interdigital phlegmon during the healing process is the occasional development of a thickened interdigital skin fold leading to interdigital skin hyperplasia. This fold is subject to trauma by the ground surface;

and, as it grows, it may develop areas of pressure necrosis between the axial surfaces and the axial horn.

DIAGNOSIS

Diagnosis depends on recognition of the characteristic interdigital lesion extending through the skin and accompanied by a foul odor. The foot must be cleansed, brushed, and carefully inspected to rule out the major differential diagnoses of perforating interdigital foreign body and interdigital dermatitis. The foreign body may have produced a small wound or may still be lodged in the subcutis. Interdigital dermatitis, unlike interdigital phlegmon, usually involves a superficial lesion with little surrounding swelling and tends to affect two or more feet to a varying degree.

Differential diagnosis of interdigital phlegmon also includes sole abscess, severe sole bruising and hemorrhage, interdigital hyperplasia ("corn"), and fracture of PIII.

TREATMENT

In early cases (<48 hours lameness), local treatment is particularly helpful in controlling the spread of necrobacillosis and encouraging rapid resolution. After cleaning the foot, all necrotic tissue in the interdigital space should be removed, preferably with a dry sponge, and a local astringent (5 per cent copper sulfate) or antibacterial dressing is applied to the area. Systemic therapy is recommended for all but the most minor lesions and may include sulfa drugs (sodium sulfadimidine, 150 to 200 mg/kg intravenously s.i.d. for 1 to 3 days), procaine penicillin G (22,000 IU/kg intramuscularly b.i.d. for 3 days), or oxytetracycline (10 mg/kg intravenously once only). If possible, affected cattle should be kept in dry conditions until the lesion is healing well.

In multiple case outbreaks in beef cattle, sulfonamides may be given in drinking water (sulfathiazole, 454 g/379 L for 3 days; or sulfamethazine, 454 g/758 L for 3 days) or feed (chlortetracycline, 2.2 mg/kg body weight for 7 days, followed by 1.1 mg/kg for 7 days). Appropriate withdrawal periods should be observed before slaughter.

When deeper structures have become involved in a septic process, drainage or claw amputation procedures are usually indicated. Radiology is useful in defining the extent of osteomyelitis. Most such cases involve a secondary infection with *Actinomyces* (formerly *Corynebacterium*) *pyogenes*.

CONTROL AND PREVENTION

Control is primarily a policy of sound management. Injuries to the interdigital space should be minimized by well-maintained and smooth-surfaced tracks and gateways and the provision of concrete aprons around water troughs and feed bunks. Muddy and poorly drained areas where cattle tend to stand should be fenced off or appropriately modified.

Prophylactic use of a footbath will drastically reduce the incidence of interdigital disease. Footbaths should contain 2 to 5 per cent formalin, and cattle should be walked through such a bath four times weekly. The bath should be emptied after every 800 cow passages. A prewash bath containing water is advantageous. Alternative footbaths contain 5 per cent copper sulfate solution, and mixtures of 2 per cent formalin with 5 per cent copper sulfate have also been advocated. Other footbaths have used zinc sulfate or 10 per cent copper sulfate in slaked lime. Caution is needed, from both animal health and environmental standpoints, in the disposal of footbath wastes.

Oral ethylenediamine dihydroiodide (EDDI) at a dose of 10 mg/head/day has been recommended for feedlot cattle, but its efficacy in preventing interdigital phlegmon is uncertain. EDDI is not approved in the United States as an additive in dairy rations.

The efficacy and economic value of commercial vaccines against interdigital phlegmon that contain whole cells or fractions of *F. necrophorum* with a mineral oil adjuvant are not yet clear. About 60 per cent protection was provided by a product containing concentrated, cell-free supernatant used in calf trials in Australia. The reduction of the incidence of interdigital dermatitis by footbathing or the use of an autogenous vaccine against *B. nodosus* may help the control of both interdigital dermatitis and interdigital phlegmon.

BIBLIOGRAPHY

Clark BL: Foot abscess of cattle. *In* Egerton JR, Yong WK, Riffkin GG (eds): Foot and Foot Abscess of Ruminants. Boca Raton, FL, CRC Press, 1989, pp 69–79.
Greenough PR, MacCallum FJ, Weaver AD: Lameness in Cattle, 2nd ed. Bristol, England, Wright Scientechnica, 1981, pp 151–158.
Weaver AD, Andersson L, Banting A, et al: Review of disorders of the ruminant digit with proposals for anatomical and pathological terminology and recording. Vet Rec 108:117–120, 1980.

Fescue Foot

GERARD J. KOENIG, DVM, MS

Fescue foot is one of several syndromes observed in cattle grazing tall fescue (*Festuca arundinacea*) pastures. It is a noninfectious, cool-season disease characterized by soreness and lameness in one or more feet, poor hair coat, and dry gangrene of the extremities (tail, feet, and ears). The disease is strikingly similar to ergotism but occurs in the absence of the ergot fungus *Claviceps*.

Tall fescue is a cool-season perennial grass grown in a large area of North America, especially in the eastern United States. It is considered a high quality forage except in instances when a form of toxicosis develops. Toxic syndromes have been associated with an endophytic infection of the grass by the clavicipitaceous fungus *Epichloe typhina* (or *Acremonium coenophialum*).

The full role of the endophytic fungus in tall fescue toxicosis has yet to be worked out, but investigators believe that the endophyte produces a toxin or toxins either alone or in combination with the grass. Evidence is mounting that fungus-infected tall fescue contains ergopeptine alkaloids, which are believed to cause vasoconstriction and the fescue foot syndrome.

Not all tall fescue pastures are infected with the endophyte fungus, and individual plants in infected pastures may be free of the disease. There are also varieties of tall fescue that are endophyte resistant. Transmission of the fungus through the seed appears to be the major source of pasture infection. Storage of seed at environmental temperature for 1 to 2 years appears to reduce the percentage of infected seed.

CLINICAL SIGNS

Early clinical signs usually appear 3 to 15 days after turning cattle onto toxic forage. Pastures with low toxicity may require longer periods of exposure. There is a wide range of clinical signs seen in cattle with fescue foot, varying from loss of weight and a rough hair coat to sloughing of feet, tail, and ears. The early signs are nonspecific, resembling any of a number of diseases, and include weight loss, reduced rate of gain, and an arched back. Other signs may include scouring and lameness. As the disease progresses, the animal may appear tranquilized, may tremble, and may show elevated body temperature, increased respiratory rate, increased heart rate, and occasional absence of rumen motility.

Changes occur primarily in the hindfeet and hindlegs and include soreness and swelling at and distal to the fetlock, knuckling, reddening between the dewclaws and hooves, altered hoof growth, and loss of hair from the coronary band. A red line forming at the coronary band of the hindfoot is considered a characteristic sign. A line of demarcation forms in severe cases between healthy tissue and the gangrenous hoof, with ultimate sloughing of the necrotic area. Forelimbs are occasionally involved also. Affected animals are reluctant to move and often only nibble feed. As a result of decreased feed intake, moderate to severely affected animals are often emaciated.

The tail may show changes, including discoloration, hair loss, necrosis, and sloughing of the tip. Lameness may or may not be associated with tail lesions. Under extreme conditions the ear tips may slough.

Abortions are rare in affected cattle, and pregnant cows are often nursed through parturition to salvage the calf.

Severity of lesions determines the outcome of the disease. Recovery in animals with no gross lesions is often slow when they are removed from toxic forage. Animals with more severe lesions will rarely recover completely and should be slaughtered or euthanized.

DIAGNOSIS

There are no consistent hematologic or serum chemistry changes in affected animals. Diagnosis is usually based on grazing history, season (usually cool or cold), and clinical signs. Fungus detection in tall fescue pastures is achieved by demonstration of mycelium through staining of either the seed or the sheath tissue or use of an enzyme-linked immunosorbent assay (ELISA) to determine the presence of the fungus and the quantity of endophyte mycelium in seeds. The ELISA test does not differentiate between other nontoxic but closely related fungi.

Conditions characterized by lameness and/or gangrene of the extremities must be ruled out. These include ergotism, chronic selenium poisoning, frostbite, infectious pododermatitis, and trauma.

PREVENTION

All animals grazing tall fescue pastures where the endophyte status is unknown should be monitored daily for early signs compatible with fescue foot, especially in cooler seasons. Animals with clinical signs should be removed from contaminated pastures and placed on different feed. Providing shelter during extremely cold temperatures minimizes additional stress and prevents secondary frostbite.

Pastures composed of fescue mixed with legumes are less likely to produce the disease than are pure stands of tall fescue. Intensive grazing or removal of mature vegetable growth reduces the potential for toxicity. Heavy nitrate fertilization and drought conditions can exacerbate the problem by increasing toxin levels. Replacement with resistant varieties is an alternative in problem pastures.

Dilution of the toxin by feeding nontoxic hay, grain, or protein supplement while animals are consuming toxic grass appears to be a rational approach to the problem. Toxic tall fescue cut for hay appears to remain toxic and should not be fed.

BIBLIOGRAPHY

Bush L, Boling J, Yates S: Animal Disorders. *In* Buckner RC, Bush LP (eds): Tall Fescue. Madison, WI, American Society of Agronomy, 1979, pp 248–264.

Hemken RW, Bush LP: Toxic Alkaloids Associated with Tall Fescue Toxicosis. *In* Cheeke PR (ed): Toxicants of Plant Origin, Vol. 1. Boca Raton, FL, CRC Press, 1989, pp 281–289.

Interdigital Fibroma
BIMBO WELKER, DVM, MS

DIFFERENTIALS AND DIAGNOSIS

Differentials for interdigital skin lesions include corns, foot rot, trauma, and interdigital papillomas. Corns are easily identified by their characteristic appearance. They appear as a relatively smooth surfaced protrusion of the interdigital skin. Gross evaluation of resected masses reveals a preponderance of dense fibrous tissue. Histologically the lesions are found to contain evidence of subacute or chronic inflammation with hyperkeratosis and parakeratosis. The gross and histologic appearances are subject to variation depending on the presence or absence of trauma or infection. While foot rot and trauma may cause inflammation and swelling of the interdigital skin, the characteristic hyperplasia will be absent. Papillomas of the interdigital skin differ in gross appearance, usually having a rough surface with wart-like projections.

ETIOLOGY

Hyperplasia of the interdigital skin occurs in response to chronic irritation. Irritation may be in the form of chronic infection (i.e., foot rot), trauma, or secondary to moist environmental conditions. Stretching of the interdigital skin as a result of abnormal foot conformation (i.e., splay toes), poor foot care, or bad trimming can cause proliferation. Excess fat in the interdigital space may result in protrusion into the space and subsequent proliferation. While heredity may play a role, hyperplasia of the interdigital skin is more likely an acquired problem.

The literature suggests a higher incidence in beef breeds. The most common breeds reported are Holstein and Hereford. No sex predilection has been verified, but it is generally accepted that it is more common in males. The lesion in males tend to occur more in the forelimbs, with weight distribution being the key predisposing factor. The dairy cow tends to develop lesions more commonly in the rear foot. Housing practices, that is, free stall stanchions, may cause the rear feet to be exposed to more moisture, urine, and manure than the front feet.

CLINICAL SIGNS

Hyperplastic tissue in the interdigital space does not necessarily cause lameness. In the author's experience a significant number of corns are not associated with lameness. The importance of this is that the practitioner should not incriminate hyperplastic tissue as a cause of lameness without evidence of sensitivity or obvious inflammatory changes. As a general rule, once the mass extends halfway down the hoof wall, lameness is seen. Other factors play a more important role in determining if pain is associated with a corn. Corns located in the palmar/plantar aspect of the interdigital space are more likely to be painful because of the "pinching" action of the claws. Corns that are infected, ulcerated, or traumatized should be viewed as probable cause of lameness. The degree of lameness associated with a corn can vary from minimal to severe. Severe lameness is usually associated with infected or traumatized corns or where deep tissue sepsis has occurred. Deep tissue sepsis will be evidenced by swelling, heat, and pain above the coronary band.

TREATMENT

All corns are not associated with lameness. The significance of a corn in any given case should be established. If there appears to be a correlation because of size, location, evidence of infection, or trauma, and there is sensitivity to manipulation, the lesion should be treated. If there is evidence of deep tissue involvement, the therapeutics and prognosis will change and should be adjusted accordingly.

Small corns may spontaneously regress if the inciting irritating factors are removed. These cattle should be put in a clean, dry environment. The lesions should be cleaned and bandaged if ulcerated, traumatized, or superficially infected. Abnormal hoof growth or conformation should be corrected. If the conservative therapy is ineffective, culling or surgical resection is advised. Large lesions that are sensitive to palpation or are infected, traumatized, or ulcerated are best treated by surgical resection. The animal is appropriately restrained and local anesthesia is provided. A regional intravenous block or a three-point local infiltration technique will suffice. The interdigital space should be thoroughly cleaned. An elliptic incision is made through the interdigital skin at the base of the mass. The incision should incorporate all diseased or involved tissue. The full-thickness elliptic incision should allow the proliferative mass to be elevated and easily dissected free of the underlying fat pad. There is no need to remove the fat pad unless it is redundant. If it protrudes past the cut skin edges it should be gently elevated and trimmed. After removal of the mass the interdigital space should be bandaged for protection and hemostasis. A gauze pad impregnated with an antibacterial ointment is packed into the interdigital space and secured using a figure-eight bandage. The animal should be kept in a clean, dry environment for 2 weeks, at which time the bandage can be removed. By 2 weeks the wound should have a healthy bed of granulation tissue and minimal risk of infection. Further bandaging is usually unnecessary. Systemic antibiotics are not routinely used. Use of systemic antibiotics may be indicated if there is evidence of deep tissue involvement.

PREVENTION

There may be familial or hereditary predispositions to the formation of corns. In these cases culling and restocking may be the most practical solution. Prevention is directed at minimizing the factors that irritate the interdigital skin. Routine foot trimming and a clean, dry environment will reduce the factors that cause direct irritation as well as decrease the risk of secondary irritation due to infectious causes.

BIBLIOGRAPHY

Greenough PR, MacCullum FJ, Weaver AD: Lameness in Cattle, 2nd ed. Philadelphia, JB Lippincott, 1981, pp 162–168.
Howard JL: Current Veterinary Therapy, 2nd ed. Philadelphia, WB Saunders, 1986, pp 899–900.
Peterson GC, Nelson DR: Foot diseases in cattle. Part II. Diagnosis and treatment. Comp Cont Ed 6:5565–5573, 1984.
Rebhun WC, Pearson EG: Clinical management of bovine foot problems. J Am Vet Med Assoc 181:572–577, 1982.

Contagious Foot Rot of Sheep

D. MICHAEL RINGS, DVM, MS

Ovine contagious foot rot (CFR) is a leading cause of lameness in sheep throughout the world. The infection, which may be either acute or chronic, is the result of the synergistic relationship between *Fusobacterium necrophorum* and *Bacteroides nodosus*. Infected animals may be asymptomatic to severely lame. Variation in the clinical signs and course of the disease can be attributed to the differences in the pathogenicity of the *B. nodosus* strain present, differences in breed susceptibility, or both. Among the common sheep breeds, Merinos show a high susceptibility.

ETIOLOGY AND PATHOGENESIS

Although a number of different bacteria have been cultured from CFR lesions, only *F. necrophorum* and *B. nodosus* consistently produce disease. *F. necrophorum* is an anaerobic, gram-negative bacteria commonly found in the environment of sheep. This organism propagates well under warm, moist conditions. Exposure of the feet, especially the interdigital area, to prolonged periods of moisture softens the skin and predisposes to superficial infections with *Fusobacterium*. *B. nodosus*, also an anaerobic, gram-negative bacteria, enters as a secondary invader at the skin-horn junction, where it proteases cause separation of the corium from the skin and basal epithelium. *F. necrophorum* accompanies *B. nodosus* and causes both severe inflammation and necrosis. Axial and abaxial hoof walls, as well as the sole, may become undermined by the infection.

CLINICAL SIGNS

Sheep infected with CFR vary in clinical signs from totally asymptomatic to severe lameness causing recumbency. Adult sheep have a higher incidence of CFR than do lambs, and morbidity in susceptible flocks may approach 70 per cent. The mildest form of CFR, a superficial skin infection in the interdigital space, is termed foot scald or scald. Affected sheep are not always lame but will show increased sensitivity to palpation of the interdigital area. When lameness is encountered, one or more feet may be infected concurrently. Slight limping, carriage of the foot, walking on the knees, or recumbency can all be seen in affected sheep. Minimal soft tissue inflammation may be visible externally, but pressure applied to the hoof walls or the sole will invoke a pain response. Chronically infected sheep often have malformed hooves, with cracks and crevices present in the hoof wall. Black fetid exudate, found upon opening of infected areas, is characteristic of this infection. In severely affected sheep the infection may extend to the PII-PIII joint, resulting in osteoarthritis. Draining tracts are frequently encountered at the coronary band as a sequela to the osteoarthritic form.

DIAGNOSIS

The clinical examination of infected sheep with characteristic lesions of CFR in a flock with multiple animals affected is usually sufficient to establish the diagnosis. Laboratory confirmation is difficult owing to the specialized cultural requirements of *B. nodosus*. Grams's stain of exudate from a *B. nodosus* lesion should show large, barbell-shaped, gram-negative bacteria.

TREATMENT AND CONTROL

F. necrophorum is free living in the environment of sheep and thus difficult to avoid; however, *B. nodosus* cannot survive for more than a few weeks in the environment, so a continuing problem with CFR can occur only if sheep carrying *B. nodosus* exist in the flock. Identification and separation of diseased from healthy animals is the first step in limiting the spread of the disease. Thorough to radical foot trimming may be necessary to expose the infection sufficiently to allow disinfection of the foot via footbaths. A number of chemicals have been used in footbaths, including 10 per cent formalin in water, 10 to 20 per cent copper sulfate in water, and 10 per cent (W/V) zinc sulfate in water. The zinc sulfate solution appears to be the most efficacious of this group and also the least toxic. Infected sheep should be made to stand in the footbath for 5 or more minutes two to three times per week until clinical signs are eliminated. Weekly trips through the baths will help prevent return of CFR. Sheep should be placed in clean surroundings for 2 to 3 weeks following an outbreak to prevent reinfection.

A number of antimicrobials have been used to treat infected sheep. These include penicillin, tetracycline and oxytetracycline, tylosin, and erythromycin. Dosages in excess of labeled dose may be required to reach therapeutic levels. Although interdigital injection of antibiotics has been practiced for years, it has no advantage over parenteral injection.

Recently a pilus vaccine[1] against *B. nodosa* was introduced into the United States after years of use in Australia. The currently available vaccine contains 10 strains that cross-react with 14 of the 20 *B. nodosa* strains found in the United States. Vaccination has been shown to reduce the incidence of CFR in flocks by 45 to 61 per cent, with the most significant reduction in previously infected ewes (92 per cent). The pilus antigen vaccine has also shown therapeutic effects in some infected sheep by reducing the clinical recovery period. The currently available vaccine contains an oil adjuvant that frequently causes swelling and sterile abscess formation at the site of injection. A two-dose course 6 weeks to 6 months apart is given initially, followed by either a semiannual booster or a single injection given prior to foot rot season.

---

[1]Footvax, available from Coopers Animal Health Inc., Kansas City, KS 66103.

BIBLIOGRAPHY

Egerton JR, Cox PT, Anderson BJ, et al: Protection of sheep against footrot with a recombinant DNA-based fimbrial vaccine. Vet Microbiol 14:393–409, 1987.
Hindmarsh F, Faser J, Scott K: Efficacy of a multivalent *Bacteroides nodosus* vaccine against foot rot in sheep in Britain. Vet Rec 125:128–130, 1989.
Kimberling CV: Jensen and Swift's Diseases of Sheep, 3rd ed. Philadelphia, Lea & Febiger, 1988, pp 317–321.
Lewis RD, Meyer HH, Gradin JL, Smith AW: Effectiveness of vaccination in controlling ovine footrot. J Anim Sci 67:1160–1166, 1989.
Outteridge PM, Stewart DJ, Skerman TM, et al: A positive association between resistance to ovine footrot and particular lymphocyte antigen types Aust Vet J 66:175–179, 1989.
Skerman TM: Footrot in Ruminants. *In* Stewart DJ, et al (eds): Proceedings of a Workshop. Melbourne, Australia, CSIRO, 1985.

Septic Arthritis
GUY ST. JEAN, DVM, MS, Diplomate, ACVS

Septic arthritis in food animals is observed secondary to (1) hematogenous infection, (2) traumatic injury or a septic hoof lesion with local introduction of infectious organisms and (3) iatrogenic inoculation associated with joint aspiration or injection.

Hematogenous origin infectious arthritis is commonly observed in young animals. Umbilical infection is a common site of a septic foci, but septic arthritis may be associated with any systemic infection. Organisms circulating in the blood gain access to the joint either via the vessels to the metaphysis or epiphysis or via the blood supply to the synovial membrane. Hematogenous origin septic arthritis is often polyarticular, with larger joints (hock, stifle, carpus, and fetlock) involved. Traumatic septic arthritis from direct penetration of a foreign body into the joint is commonly associated with mature animals and affects only the damaged joint(s). Organisms associated with septic arthritis are many and varied. Viruses, such as caprine arthritis-encephalitis, mycoplasma, and chlamydia, as well as bacteria, have been implicated as agents causing septic arthritis.

DIAGNOSIS

A prompt diagnosis of septic arthritis is important because of the progressive destructive nature of the disease. The signs associated with septic arthritis include severe lameness, distension of the joint capsule, and heat of the involved joint. Pain on palpation of the joint and a diminished range of motion are often observed. A low-grade fever, depression, and anorexia may be present. In young animals, umbilical stump lesions, pneumonia, and diarrhea may be noted.

Radiographic lesions will seldom be present in acute cases of septic arthritis. Radiographs should be performed to rule out the possibility of traumatic damage to the subchondral bone or osteomyelitis and to establish a baseline for future evaluation. As septic arthritis progresses, radiographic evidence of degenerative joint disease with bone lysis and periosteal proliferation may be noted. Radiographs of advanced cases of septic arthritis may reveal spontaneous ankylosis of a joint.

Synovial fluid evaluation is the most definitive way to diagnose infectious arthritis. Aseptic techniques must be used in performing arthrocentesis to avoid contamination of the sample or introduction of infectious organisms into the joint.

Results of synovial fluid analysis in cases of infectious arthritis include an increased volume of fluid, a yellow to brown flocculent fluid with a lack of viscosity, protein greater than 2 g/100 ml, white blood cell count greater than 30,000 cells/ml with 90 per cent or greater being neutrophils. A positive bacterial culture confirms the diagnosis, but a negative culture may indicate chronic infection or prior treatment with antibiotics. To improve culture results, synovial fluid should be placed on an aerobic culturette and in blood culture medium and the samples cultured immediately upon arrival at the laboratory.

TREATMENT

Treatment of septic arthritis involves eliminating the causative organism and removing the lysosomal enzymes and proteinaceous material that can damage the articular cartilage. Delay in treatment reduces the prognosis by allowing further periarticular fibrosis and articular damage. Broad-spectrum antibiotics administered systemically will produce adequate intra-articular levels. Treatment should be started before results of bacteriologic culture are available. Sodium ampicillin is often used by the author as the first treatment and is administered for 2 to 3 weeks. In cases where the primary source of infection is the umbilicus, surgical resection is indicated.

If systemic antibiotics and synovial aspiration do not bring improvement in 36 hours, joint lavage is indicated. Intermittent joint lavage using two 14-gauge needles introduced into the joint space using aseptic technique with the animal under heavy sedation or light anesthesia may be used in early cases before intra-articular fibrin deposition has occurred. Distention of the joint with the lavage solution infused under pressure is performed to distend the synovial membrane and disrupt adhesions. Large quantities of balanced polyionic fluid are used and allowed to circulate freely through the joint. Periodically blocking the outflow needle helps distend and lavage the entire joint. One to two liters of balanced polyionic solution should be used to lavage a septic joint. An alternative method of joint lavage is arthroscopy. Arthroscopy offers large ingress/egress portals, allowing administration of large volumes of fluid, ability to identify and remove fibrin clots, and evaluation of articular cartilage. When the inflammatory process becomes chronic, fibrin clots become too large to be removed by anything other than an arthrotomy. The joint is opened and lavaged, fibrin clots are removed, and the abnormal synovial membrane is removed. The open joint must be protected from environmental contamination by a sterile bandage until the joint closes by second intention.

Arthrotomy may be performed for joint debridement, curettage of infected cartilage, and removal of necrotic bone. If indicated, a bone graft and immobilization of the joint for 6 to 8 weeks may be incorporated in the treatment to produce arthrodesis and a pain-free limb. This procedure may be used successfully in many advanced cases of septic arthritis.

Administration of nonsteroidal anti-inflammatory drugs is indicated to reduce the pain associated with septic arthritis and to encourage early return to normal function. If possible, the joint affected should be supported with bandages and splints to make the animal more comfortable and avoid flexural deformity. Immobilization should be done only 8 hours/day to avoid reduction in the range of motion of the joint.

BIBLIOGRAPHY

Bertone AL, McIlwraith CW, Jones RL, et al: Comparison of various treatments for experimentally induced equine infectious arthritis. Am J Vet Res 48:519–529, 1987.
Montgomery RD, Long IR, Milton JL, et al: Comparison of aerobic culturette, synovial membrane biopsy and blood culture medium and detection of canine bacterial arthritis. Vet Surg 18:300–303, 1989.
Van Huffel X, Steenhaut M, Imschoot J, et al: Carpal joint arthrodesis as a treatment for chronic septic carpitis in calves and cattle. Vet Surg 18:304–311, 1989.
Verschooten F, DeMoor A, Steenhaut M, et al: Surgical and conservative treatment of infectious arthritis in cattle. J Am Vet Med Assoc 165:271–275, 1974.

Stifle Injuries and Patellar Luxations

WILLIAM H. CRAWFORD, DVM, MVSc,
Diplomate, ACVS

Animals with injury to the stifle may vary in their degree of lameness. Reluctance to flex the joint owing to pain results in a shortened stride, with the toe of the affected limb being dragged at the caudal phase of the stride. Various degrees of joint distension may be present. Acute injuries tend to have fluid (synovia and/or blood) swellings. Fibrous periarticular swellings may be associated with chronic injuries to the stifle.

Visual evidence of joint instability is present when the tibia subluxates cranial to the femur as the animal bears weight. Crepitation may be noted within the joint as the leg is manipulated or as the joint is palpated while the animal walks. Varus or valgus deviation of the limb originating from the stifle may be present if collateral ligament injury has occurred. An increase in the range of axial tibial rotation is present when collateral or cruciate ligament injuries are present.

A thorough examination of the injured stifle and comparison with the normal joint will help to identify which structures may be abnormal. Identification of the patella; medial, middle, and lateral patellar ligaments; tibial crest; medial collateral ligament; lateral and medial trochlea; and origin of the long digital extensor tendon and peroneus tertius should be made by palpation. Distended joint spaces should be identified as being on the medial or lateral side of the joint and subjectively evaluated for increased heat.

PATELLAR LUXATIONS

Proximal patellar luxation (upward fixation) is seen sporadically in lactating dairy cattle and more frequently in cattle of Zebu breeding and in Asian Buffalo. Usually an incomplete upward fixation occurs where the patella does not remain within the supratrochlear fovea. The toe of the affected limb drags, as the caudal phase of the stride is slightly prolonged. Stifle flexion occurs as a sudden, jerky motion that results in hyperflexion of the joint.

The etiology of the proximal patellar luxation is unknown. However, trochlea malformation, muscle tone, conformation, and nutrition are factors that should be considered.

Medial patellar desmotomy is indicated for proximal patellar luxation. The medial patellar ligament is transected near its point of insertion on the tibial crest.

Lateral patellar luxation may be unilateral or bilateral. This condition occurs in calves and adult cattle. The displaced patella may be palpated on the lateral surface of the joint. When calves with the bilateral form stand, the hindend is in a crouched position due to the inability of the stifles to extend.

Traumatic injury to the medial patellar ligament and/or the

medial femoropatellar ligament allows the patella to luxate laterally. In the congenital form, malformation of the patella and trochlea may be present. In neonatal calves it is important to determine whether the luxation is a primary condition or if it is secondary to femoral nerve injury.

Correction of traumatically induced lateral patellar luxation may be achieved by imbricating the torn medial femoropatellar ligament and joint capsule. The patella is reduced by placing the joint in extension. It may be necessary to relieve lateral tension on the patella by incising the retinaculum and fascia on the dorsolateral surface of the joint.

Congenital lateral patellar luxation in calves may be corrected if the condition is the result of laxity of the medial femoropatellar ligament. Plication of the medial joint capsule and retinaculum with release of the lateral femoropatellar ligament are indicated. If the condition is the result of congenital deformity of the trochlea, trochleoplasty may be considered. The prognosis for successful treatment is guarded.

Medial patellar luxation occurs rarely. The large medial trochlea and substantial lateral femoropatellar ligament prevent medial displacement of the patella unless a fracture or severe deformity is present.

FEMORAL NERVE PARALYSIS

Injury to the femoral nerve may occur during dystocia. One study reports on beef calves of the exotic breeds that became "hip-locked" in an anterior presentation, suffering femoral nerve injuries. Affected calves cannot extend the stifle of the injured leg, and if the condition is bilateral they are usually unable to stand. The quadriceps muscles are flaccid in the first few days following injury, and in 7 to 10 days marked atrophy of these muscles is noted. The diagnosis can be confirmed by doing electromyography 7 to 10 days following the injury.

The prognosis for calves with femoral nerve paralysis is guarded and dependent on the degree of nerve injury. If complete disruption of the nerve has not occurred, and if fibrosis does not inhibit reinnervation, quadriceps muscle tone may return within a 4-week to 6-month period.

CRUCIATE LIGAMENT INJURY

Cranial cruciate ligament (CCL) injuries are a serious and relatively common occurrence in dairy and beef cattle. Acute injuries occur from falls associated with slippery footing, estrous behavior, or ataxia from metabolic disease. In bulls and cows with chronic injuries, the CCL may be stretched or partially torn. In bulls the chronic form of the injury is thought to be related to the forces generated when the stifle is extended during mounting and copulation. It has been suggested that degenerative joint disease may precede CCL injury in cattle. Caudal cruciate ligament injuries are rare in cattle and are usually seen in conjunction with rupture of the CCL.

Examination of cattle with suspected CCL injury should begin by watching the animal walk. Most cattle with ruptured cranial cruciate ligaments are only partially weight bearing during the acute phase of the injury, but as the injury becomes chronic the degree of weight bearing increases. The affected limb has a shortened stride, and if there is weight bearing, instability of the stifle may be visualized as the tibia is displaced cranially relative to the femur.

If the patient is weight bearing and if the tibia is subluxated cranially, a drawer sign may be elicited. The examiner's shoulder is placed against the caudal midthigh to stabilize the femur, and the tibia is pulled caudally by exerting pressure at the level of the tibial crest. In cattle with a ruptured CCL, movement of the tibia relative to the femur can be detected.

Moderate joint effusion may be detected when the joint is palpated. If there is excessive effusion in acutely affected animals, or if there is marked fibrosis in chronic cases, instability of the joint and a positive drawer sign may be difficult to appreciate.

Radiographic examination of the stifle may provide further diagnostic information. In a lateral to medial view of a normal bovine stifle, the image of the tibial intercondylar eminence is completely overlapped by the image of the femoral condyles. However, if the tibia is displaced, the image of the intercondylar tibial eminence will be displaced cranial to the image of the femoral condyles. The cranial to caudal radiographic view is important to evaluate meniscal spaces. Radiographs should be examined for evidence of fractures of the intercondylar eminence, avulsion fractures at the insertion of the CCL and the collateral ligaments, ligamentous ossification within the CCL, and evidence of degenerative joint disease.

Conservative management of CCL ruptures is usually unsatisfactory. Instability of the femorotibial joint results in maceration of the menisci, with subsequent loss of hyaline cartilage and erosion of the subchondral bone of the femoral condyles.

Surgical procedures have been developed to manage this injury. Providing stability to the joint will reduce the rate of progression of degenerative joint disease. The simplest procedure is to do an extra-articular plication of the dorsal retinaculum. A greater degree of stability may be achieved by replacing the torn CCL with an intra-articular autograft constructed from tissues of the lateral patellar ligament and the medial fascia of the gluteobiceps muscle. The prognosis for surgically treated patients will vary from poor to fair depending on concurrent damage and the weight of the animal.

COLLATERAL LIGAMENT INJURY AND LAXITY

Traumatic injury to the medial collateral ligament is usually associated with trauma. Synovial effusion, reduced weight bearing, and a shortened cranial phase of the stride are seen in cattle with collateral ligament injuries. Swelling and pain are noted when the site of the medial collateral ligament is palpated. In addition, the medial side of the femorotibial joint can be felt to open as the distal limb is passively abducted. Injury to the lateral collateral ligament is rare and difficult to assess owing to the greater musculature and collateral support on the lateral side of the stifle. Radiographs may reveal an avulsion fracture at the origin or insertion of the affected collateral ligament.

Uncomplicated traumatically ruptured collateral ligaments of the stifle may heal if the patient is confined to a box stall for 6 to 8 weeks. If the injury is more severe, imbrication of the periarticular tissues may prove beneficial.

OSTEOCHONDROSIS

Osteochondrosis is a syndrome in which focal areas of thickened retained cartilage with minimal surrounding ossification are formed owing to failure of endochondral ossification. Rapidly growing individuals of all domestic species appear to be susceptible to this condition. Of the food animal species, swine are the most commonly affected. In animals with clinical lameness due to osteochondrosis, cartilage defects are seen in the articular cartilage.

In most cases the disease is not of significant consequence. In dairy cows the lameness may become significant enough to affect production. Bulls may suffer lameness severe enough to limit their ability to breed.

The patient may have a history of mild lameness or slight gait abnormality with a sudden exacerbation of serious lameness and marked synovial effusion. The sudden onset of severe lameness and increased synovial effusion usually follow an incidence of increased activity in yearling and 2-year-old animals. Secondary degenerative joint disease will also result in increased lameness. If there is severe deformity of the trochlea and patella, this may lead to luxation of the patella.

In cattle, the stifle appears to be the joint most frequently affected with clinical lameness related to osteochondrosis. Subchondral cystic lesions may be located within either the femoral condyle or the tibial plateau. These lesions may be considered incidental findings when not associated with lameness.

Diagnosis of stifle osteochondrosis is based on lameness, increased synovial effusion, and radiographic evidence of subchondral cystic lesions or osteochondral fragments associated with irregular contours of the femoral trochlea. Synovial fluid analysis will help distinguish subchondral cystic lesions from focal osteomyelitis.

Treatment of trochlear osteochondrosis has been done by arthroscopic debridement and removal of the poorly attached fragments. Postoperative box-stall confinement for 3 months is recommended to allow fibrocartilage to replace the diseased hyaline cartilage. Subchondral cystic lesions found on the tibial plateau are difficult to treat, as they are usually covered by the meniscal cartilage.

The prognosis for soundness in bulls with lameness resulting from osteochondrosis is guarded.

DEGENERATIVE JOINT DISEASE

Degenerative joint disease (DJD) causes varying degrees of lameness in all food animals. The condition is most important from a production standpoint in aged cows and bulls. The response of articular cartilage, bone, and periarticular soft tissues to injury and infection is the same in all species. The end result of the DJD cascade is articular cartilage loss, eburnation of subchondral bone, periarticular osteophytes, and chronic synovitis. Mineralization of the joint capsule may be observed in advanced cases of DJD.

Management of DJD should be directed toward prevention, as treatment is often unrewarding. It also appears that DJD may precede acute rupture of the cranial cruciate ligament. Phenylbutazone and aspirin may help alleviate the pain and lameness, but the disease is progressive.

SYNOVITIS

Heifers between 1 and 2 years of age may be presented with a unilateral synovitis of the stifle. It has been proposed that this may be associated with antigens to brucella or is secondary to a quiescent subchondral osteomyelitis. In evaluating these joints, osteochondrosis must be ruled out by radiology. Joint taps routinely reveal extremely high cell counts (50,000+) but are negative on culture.

Some have advocated the use of broad-spectrum antibiotics and anti-inflammatories; however, superior results seem to be obtained by arthrotomy accompanied by a radical synovectomy. Once the hyperplastic synovium has been removed, the prognosis is generally good for return to function.

BIBLIOGRAPHY

Bartels JE: Femoral-tibial osteoarthrosis in the bull: I. Clinical survey and radiological interpretation. J Am Radiol Soc 16:151–158, 1975.
Bartels JE: Femoral-tibial osteoarthrosis in the bull: II. A correlation of the radiographic and pathologic findings of the torn meniscus and ruptured cruciate ligament. J Am Radiol Soc 16:159–172, 1975.
Crawford WH: A surgical technique for the intra-articular repair of cranial cruciate ligament injuries in cattle. Vet Surg 19:380–388, 1990.
Ducharme NG, Stanton ME, Ducharme GR: Stifle lameness in cattle at two veterinary teaching hospitals: a retrospective study. Can Vet J 26:212–217, 1985.
Hanson RR, Peyton LC: Surgical correction of intermittent upward fixation of the patella in a Brahman cow. Can Vet J 28:675–677, 1987.
Krishnamurthy D, Bhargava AK, Tyagi RPS: Roentgenographic observations on bovine stifles with impaired (subluxation) patellar functions. Ind Vet J 52:64–68, 1975.
Leitch M, Kotlikoff M: Surgical repair of congenital luxation of the patella in the foal and calf. Vet Surg 9:1–4, 1980.
Meagher DM: Bilateral patellar luxation in calves. Can Vet J 15:201–202, 1974.
Moss EW, McCurnin DM, Ferguson TH: Experimental cranial cruciate replacement in cattle using a patellar ligament graft. Can Vet J 29:157–162, 1988.
Nelson DR, Kosch DB: Surgical stabilization of the stifle in cranial cruciate ligament injury in cattle. Vet Rec 111:259–262, 1982.
Tryphonas L, Hamilton GF, Rhodes CS: Perinatal femoral nerve degeneration and neurogenic atrophy of quadriceps femoris muscle in calves. J Am Vet Med Assoc 164:801–806, 1974.

Coxofemoral Luxations

ERIC TULLENERS, DVM, Diplomate, ACVS

HISTORY

Coxofemoral luxation is the most common luxation observed in dairy cattle.[1-3] The injury is usually caused by trauma and is almost always unilateral. In newborn calves coxofemoral luxation may occur as a result of forced extraction. Adult cattle are most commonly affected and often incur the injury in falls; after calving, possibly because of weakness, pelvic ligamentous laxity, and metabolic disturbances such as acetonemia and hypocalcemia; or while being ridden during estrus.[1-3]

LAMENESS EVALUATION

In neonatal calves and immature cattle, cranial dorsal coxofemoral luxations are most common. In adult cattle the direction of luxation is fairly evenly distributed between cranial dorsal and ventral, with most of the ventral luxations being in a caudal ventral direction.[1-3]

Animals suffering from cranial dorsal luxations are usually ambulatory but are most often non–weight bearing or are severely lame on the affected limb. The limb is externally rotated (stifle and foot turned outward) and, if weight bearing, the animal's toe touches. When viewed from the rear of the animal, the cranial dorsal aspect of the affected side of the pelvis is asymmetric and prominent because of the abnormal position of the greater trochanter. There is a visible and palpable increase in the distance between the greater trochanter and the tuber ischii as compared with the normal side. There is usually minimal soft tissue swelling, and in most instances the limb can be easily flexed. Manipulating the limb does not normally elicit the severe pain, crepitus, and grating characteristic of a fracture; however, the head of the femur has a noticeably abnormal position and range of motion. It is often helpful to examine the animal while it is recumbent, with the affected limb uppermost. An assistant grasps the metatarsus, flexes the limb, and holds it in a moderately abducted position. The assistant then rotates the limb in a circular motion around its longitudinal axis while the examiner presses firmly with the palm of the hand over the greater trochanter to feel the abnormal position and movement of the femoral head and greater trochanter.

Cattle with ventral luxations prefer to remain recumbent and usually rest with the limb in an abnormally abducted position. Cattle with ventral luxations may have serious complicating musculoskeletal injuries such as extensive muscle and ligamentous tearing or, less commonly, fracture of the greater trochanter, and they may be unable to stand. A diagnosis of ventral luxation can be supported by palpating the greater trochanter in an abnormal caudal or cranial and ventral position and by executing the same manipulative tests previously described. The limb can also be abducted to an abnormal extent. The femoral head may be palpable per rectum or per vaginum located cranial to the ilium or pubis in cattle with cranioventral luxation, or in the obturator foramen in cattle with caudal ventral luxation.[2,3]

A definitive diagnosis of coxofemoral luxation can be made by obtaining pelvic radiographs, but this is impractical and unnecessary in most instances. The differential diagnosis for an acute, severe injury localized to the hip region should include fracture of the pelvis or, more commonly, fracture of the capital femoral physis, femoral neck, greater trochanter, or proximal femur. Coxofemoral subluxation, septic arthritis, degenerative joint disease (coxitis), and osteochondrosis should also be considered.

TREATMENT

Most cattle do not thrive with a chronic coxofemoral luxation, so immediate treatment or slaughter is usually indicated. Excisional femoral head and neck arthroplasty is not a viable option for long-term productivity in most cattle.

Nonsurgical closed reduction is most likely to be successful if performed within 12 hours or, at most, 24 hours after injury, making client education and early detection critical. Success with closed reduction has been reported from 43 to 75 per cent[2,3] To attempt closed reduction, the animal should be restrained in lateral recumbency, with the affected limb uppermost, and heavily sedated with 0.22 mg/kg xylazine given intravenously. Larcombe and Malmo[2] describe their technique as follows:

The position of the cow's pelvis is fixed by a rope passed under the cow's thigh in the inguinal region and tied to a solid object. A second rope is tied to the lower part of the affected limb above the fetlock. Traction is applied using a block and tackle. Initially the direction of pull is in a line which passes through the displaced femoral head and the acetabulum. During traction, the femur is rotated by pushing down on the stifle and lifting the hock. If the femur moves and a sudden "clunk" is felt, the traction is immediately relaxed and the leg examined to see if the dislocation has been reduced. If the greater trochanter of the femur is in its normal anatomic position relative to the pelvic landmarks and the leg can be easily flexed without crepitus, then the replacement has been successful. If not, the process is repeated. If the dislocation is not reduced by this method, the femur is rotated in the opposite direction and if this does not work, prolonged traction is applied so that the head of the femur is pulled away from the pelvis, the leg is rotated as described above and the traction rapidly released. In many cases the dislocation is reduced as the leg is relaxed. In approximately 30% of cases it is necessary to try different directions of traction before the dislocation is reduced.

In a small number of cases (less than 5%) it is necessary to place a lever under the most proximal part of the femur. This allows the proximal femur to be lifted while the leg is rotated under traction. This assists in reducing the dislocation by lifting the head of the femur over the lip of the acetabulum.

Jubb and associates[3] delineate the following prognostic factors concerning closed reduction:

Factors demonstrating a statistically significant ($P<0.05$) influence on outcome were: ability to stand with the dislocation (85% vs. 11%), age less than 3 years vs. age 3 years or more (81% vs. 23%), dislocation in a cranial direction vs. dislocation in a caudal direction (82% vs. 31%), duration of dislocation less than 12 hours vs. duration of dislocation at least 12 hours (56% vs. 8%), occurrence during estrus vs. occurrence when not in estrus (77% vs. 30%), body weight less than 400 kg vs. body weight at least 400 kg (63% vs. 30%).

Open reduction can be successfully accomplished through a cranial lateral approach[5] but requires general anesthesia, assisted traction, and facilities where aseptic surgery can be performed. Open reduction may be successful when closed reduction fails because it allows for hematoma evacuation, it allows for removal of fibrin, tissue fragments, and joint capsule, and the surgeon can be completely confident that the femoral head has been replaced into the acetabulum. In one study involving 22 cattle, 95 per cent of the luxations could be reduced via a surgical approach.[1] In this study most cattle with cranial dorsal luxations were ambulatory before surgery, none had concomitant musculoskeletal injuries, and 75 per cent survived long term. Eight-three per cent of cattle with ventral luxations were unable to stand before surgery, and only 33 per cent survived long-term. Calves had a better long-term survival rate (75 per cent versus 50 per cent) and a lower reluxation rate (17 per cent versus 40 per cent) compared with adults. As with closed reduction, the most common cause of failure was reluxation.

In summary, coxofemoral luxation is a very serious, usually incapacitating orthopedic injury. Treated as an emergency, within 24 hours of the injury, closed reduction should be attempted initially. While still associated with a guarded prognosis, open surgical reduction is the treatment of choice for animals with luxations of greater than 24-hour duration. The prognosis is extremely poor for animals that are weak, recumbent, and unable to rise even momentarily. Most of these animals remain recumbent even with the luxation reduced, or they usually reluxate while struggling to rise.

REFERENCES

1. Tulleners EP, Nunamaker DM, Richardson DW: Coxofemoral luxations in cattle: 22 cases (1980–1985). J Am Vet Med Assoc 191:569–574, 1987.
2. Larcombe MT, Malmo J: Dislocation of the coxo-femoral joint in dairy cows. Aust Vet J 66:351–354, 1989.
3. Jubb TF, Malmo J, Brightling P, et al: Prognostic factors for recovery from coxo-femoral dislocation in cattle. Aust Vet J 66:354–358, 1989.
4. Greenough PR, MacCallum FJ, Weaver DA: Lameness in Cattle. Philadelphia, JB Lippincott, 1972, pp 255–260.
5. Piermattei DL, Greeley RG: An Atlas of Surgical Approaches to the Bones of the Dog and Cat. Philadelphia, WB Saunders, 1979, pp 132–133.

Spondylitis
BRUCE L. HULL, DVM, MS

Spondylitis means inflammation of the vertebrae. When applied to the disorder in cattle, it is generally synonymous with ankylosing spondylitis, as ankylosis and its sequelae are the causes of the clinical syndrome.

ETIOLOGY

Spondylitis is seen mostly in mature bulls housed in confinement situations. The lesion has also been observed in older cows. Degeneration of the intervertebral disc, allowing excessive intervertebral motion, is probably the initiating cause. This excessive motion in turn stimulates new bone formation around the vertebral bodies. New bone formation is most extensive ventrally but also occurs laterally. The exostosis typically affects the last two or three thoracic and first two or three lumbar vertebrae. However, the entire lumbar spine back to and including the lumbosacral joint may be involved.

CLINICAL SIGNS

Although bridging exostosis may be palpated rectally along the ventral surface of the vertebral bodies, this is not what causes the clinical signs. In fact, palpation of exostosis on the ventral surface of the vertebral bodies could almost be considered a normal finding in an older bull. In one study, 21 of 25 middle-aged dairy bulls showed evidence of vertebral osteophytosis.[1] In some animals exostosis becomes extensive enough to actually bridge the vertebral bodies and to form a splint along these bodies.

Fracture of this splint of exostosis leads to the clinical signs. Some reports indicate that the splint fractures after a clumsy mount or after a slip. In some cases the splint may fracture with no apparent predisposing trauma. The clinical signs generally appear suddenly and vary in severity, depending on the extent of the injury. Mild signs include difficulty in rising, reluctance to mount, and a stiff gait. The stiffness of gait may be quite severe, to the point that the animal drags its rear feet. In its most severe form, spondylitis causes a complete posterior paralysis and even absence of spinal reflexes.

Rectal palpation of the exostosis is a helpful diagnostic sign; however, not all cases of spondylitis extend into the posterior lumbar region.

TREATMENT

Treatment, especially in more severely affected animals, is probably hopeless, and the destruction of the animal should be considered. Mildly affected animals may respond to stall rest and analgesics; however, the symptoms are very likely to recur, often more severely. As the signs are the result of spinal cord trauma, high doses of prednisolone for an extended period may give some relief to early cases. If used, the dose is usually 0.5 mg/lb for 5 to 10 days followed by half this dose for another 5 to 10 days.

REFERENCE

1. Weisbrode SE, Monke DR, Dodaro ST, et al: Osteochondrosis, degenerative joint disease and vertebral osteophytosis in middle-aged bulls. J Am Vet Med Assoc 181:700–705, 1982.

Fractures

N. KENT AMES, DVM, MS

Fractures are a common problem facing the food animal veterinarian. With a thorough knowledge of the skeletal anatomy, the principles of fracture repair, and the nonathletic nature of most food animals, treatment is often rewarding. The type of therapy will be determined by the value, function, size, temperament, and concurrent diseases of the animal, plus the location and type of the fracture. The ability of the veterinarian and the facilities available to the veterinarian must also be considered.

FIRST AID TO THE FRACTURE PATIENT

When a fracture case is encountered, a thorough physical examination should be completed to determine concurrent disease and potential complications. Nerve damage and muscle damage are common concurrent diseases that may complicate the case and decrease the prognosis. Appropriate therapy must be initiated early for optimal results. Radiographs in two planes are essential to determine the location and character of the fracture and to aid in determining the method of fixation. All open fractures should be cleansed and debrided within the first few hours to prevent contaminated wounds from becoming infected. Debridement should be performed in a sterile manner using surgical gloves and sterile instruments and materials. Splints made from a polyvinyl chloride (PVC) pipe that is split sagitally, or a similar rigid material, are very effective as a temporary immobilization device. The splint should be well padded, and the joint should be *immobilized above and below the fracture*. A modified Robert Jones bandage or Thomas splint may also be used for temporary immobilization. If an animal is to be transported before fracture repair is attempted, adequate immobilization of the fracture is necessary to prevent the creation of an open fracture, to prevent further soft tissue damage, and to minimize discomfort to the patient.

PRINCIPLES OF FRACTURE REPAIR

The principles of fracture repair in food animals are similar to those in other species. The fracture must have anatomic reduction and rigid fixation, and the animal must continue to have normal body functions.

Reduction should be accomplished without delay to prevent muscle contracture and overriding of the fracture fragments. Holes drilled into the hoof with wire passed through them will allow traction to be placed on the affected limb, which facilitates reduction of the fracture. General anesthesia, open reduction, plus the use of a fracture distractor may be necessary to reduce some fractures in large animals successfully. The healing time will be decreased as a result of the correct anatomic reduction of a fracture.

It is documented that internal fixation with bone plates, screws, intramedullary pins, and wire gives excellent fixation of fractures. Internal fixation can be used in fractures that cannot be effectively immobilized with external fixation, allowing early return of function to the affected limb. The major disadvantages of internal fixation are insufficient strength, difficult surgical procedure, cost, and the potential of sepsis. The use of bone plates and screws in very young animals is often unrewarding owing to the soft nature of their bones and thin cortices, which allow screws to loosen and migrate. Intramedullary pins are effective and are available in sizes up to a ½ inch in diameter. The use of stack-pinning techniques may be more effective than use of a large solitary pin, which will allow rotational instability.

Kirschner devices and cross-pinning have met with some success. The major problems associated with these devices are infection and loosening of the devices owing to soft bones and thin cortices.

Many fractures in food animals can be successfully treated

with external fixation. Casts are very effective on fractures below the carpus and hock.

When placing a cast on the leg, the animal must be adequately restrained. General anesthesia is the method of choice; however, tranquilization and sedation plus physical restraint may be adequate. The leg should be clean and dry before a cast is applied. Stockinette can be applied over the leg, and felt or cast padding placed at the coronary band, under the dewclaws, over the accessory carpal bone, and at the top of the cast. Resin casts have the advantage of being strong, lightweight, and waterproof. A walking-bar incorporated into the cast that passes under, but not in contact with, the foot and extends up both sides of the leg will transfer the weight to the top of the cast and reduce concussive forces on the fracture. It will also strengthen the cast. Care must be taken during the application of casts to assure that the leg is aligned in both the cranial-caudal and medial-lateral planes. Any animal that has a cast should be confined and observed daily for signs of complications. These signs include cast breakage, increased lameness, and drainage or foul smells from under the cast. If any of these signs are present, the cast should be removed immediately and the limb reevaluated. Casts on adult animals may last from 4 to 6 weeks. However, casts on rapidly growing animals may need to be changed on a 2 to 3-week schedule for calves and a 1 to 2-week schedule for lambs and goats.

The modified Thomas splint and other forms of splints have the advantages of availability, ease of application, and low cost. However, they may be heavy and cumbersome to the patient, and inability to use them on particular fractures is a factor that limits their usage. They must be well padded to avoid pressure wounds of the axillary and inguinal area.

Large animal patients must be able to stand comfortably after fracture repair. Animals that remain recumbent for more than a few days postoperatively have a poor prognosis for recovery. Analgesics may be indicated to control the pain associated with the fracture. Although food animals generally do not tolerate mechanical assistance with hip lifts and slings, the animal should be assisted to its feet early during the convalescence period.

If the prognosis for recovery is extremely poor, if the value of the animal does not justify the cost of treatment, or if the animal is suffering inhumanely, euthanasia or salvage for meat is an option. Ultraconservative treatment, which consists of stall rest with little or no direct therapy of the fracture, may be possible in *select cases*. Fractures surrounded by heavy muscle masses, that is, the femur or humerus, with minor displacement may be considered for ultraconservative treatment if the patient can stand and carry on normal body functions while protecting the fracture.

LOCATION AND TYPE OF FRACTURE

Fractures of the first and second phalanges are generally treated with casts, but fractures of the third phalanx may be treated by elevating the affected digit above the ground with a wooden block or shoe placed on the normal claw. Arthritis and infections are common complications in phalangeal fractures. Ankylosis of the proximal or distal interphalangeal joint may be the only alternative to alleviate the associated lameness.

Fractures of the metacarpal and metatarsal bones are very common in calves and generally can be immobilized with external fixation alone. However, in unstable fractures, internal fixation with or without external fixation may be necessary. The prognosis of healing metacarpal or metatarsal fractures is favorable when proper reduction and adequate stability are provided.

Because the radius and tibia are relatively easy to approach surgically, open reduction and internal fixation are possible with fractures of these bones. It is very difficult to immobilize the stifle and elbow joint adequately with casts; therefore it is difficult to repair fractures of the tibia and radius with casts and satisfy the basic principle to immobilize the joint above and below the fracture. Thomas splints may be effective in tibial fractures when applied with significant tension to reduce and immobilize the fracture.

Fractures of the femur present special problems. The majority of femoral fractures in cattle are seen in neonates as a result of dystocia or trauma from the dam. These fractures are commonly in the distal diaphysis and are severely displaced. Straight bone plates are effective if adequate fixation of the distal fragment can be maintained. Right-angle plates are a useful alternative if straight plates are ineffective. Adequate stability of the femur is difficult to accomplish with external fixation. Intramedullary pins are effective when placed in the femur if the fracture is simple and midshaft. Bone plates often provide the most rigid fixation; however, ultraconservative therapy has been effective in selected cases that meet the necessary requirements.

The humerus may be the most difficult long bone to repair in food animals. The radial nerve and the brachialis muscle make the approach difficult. Fortunately humeral fractures are relatively rare, and the fracture may heal spontaneously with stall rest and ultraconservative treatment. Bone plates and screws afford rigid fixation in the spiral oblique fractures commonly found in the humerus.

Rib fractures are often diagnosed in food animals, but treatment is seldom attempted. The prognosis is generally favorable unless the fracture is traumatizing the underlying structures.

The distraction forces that accompany fractures of the olecranon and calcaneus require special attention. Internal fixation with plates and screws is indicated, although it is often inadequate because the resulting repair may be unstable. These fractures generally have a guarded prognosis.

Fractures of the pelvis are relatively rare in food animals, and treatment is seldom attempted. Fracture of the calcanela tuber, or "knocked-down-hip," does occur and results in a severe conformation blemish with little functional damage. Although the prognosis is generally favorable, complications may develop, including sequestration, abscessation, and fistulation.

Mandibular fractures occur and heal satisfactorily with the use of internal fixation. Intramedullary pins lend themselves well to mandibular fracture repair in food animals. Plates and screws also are effective methods of repair. Fractures of the symphysis can be wired together easily and effectively. The major complications are associated with osteomyelitis and dysmasesis during convalescence.

Fractures of the carpal and tarsal bones create a number of complications. Arthritis is a common sequela, as are infection and sequestration. The prognosis remains guarded.

COMPLICATIONS OF FRACTURE TREATMENT

Inadequate stabilization and osteomyelitis are major complications in fractures of food animals and can result in nonunion, malunion, and delayed union. The inability to stand and walk and tendon, ligament, and joint problems of the sound limb are common secondary complications that result from the size and weight of the animal. Muscle atrophy, arthritis, nerve and vascular injuries, and pressure necrosis are less common yet severe complications of food animal fractures.

BIBLIOGRAPHY

Adams OR: Lameness in Horses, 2nd ed. Philadelphia, Lea & Febiger, 1972.
Ames NK: Comparison of methods for femoral fracture repair in young calves. J Am Vet Med Assoc, 179:456–459, 1980.
Catcott EJ, Smithcors JF (eds): Equine Medicine and Surgery, 2nd ed. Wheaton, IL, American Veterinary Publications, 1972.
Gibbons WJ, Catcott EJ, Smithcors JF, (eds): Bovine Medicine and Surgery. Wheaton, IL, American Veterinary Publications, 1970.
Greenough PR, MacCallum FJ, Weaver AD: Lameness in Cattle. Philadelphia, JB Lippincott, 1972.
Smith HA, Jones TC, Hunt RD: Veterinary Pathology, 4th ed. Philadelphia, Lea & Febiger, 1972.

Tendon Injuries
N. KENT AMES, DVM, MS

Tendons are a highly specialized tissue made of collagen strands aligned in a linear fashion, which accounts for their flexibility, high tensile strength, and elasticity. The blood supply is minimal compared with that of muscle; however, tendons have an abundant nerve supply.

The healing process of tendons is dependent on a good blood supply, absence of infection, and adequate immobilization. However, because of the specialized make-up of tendons, healing is often complicated by adhesions, weakness, and stretching of the healed wound.

Tendon injuries in food animal species may be congenital or acquired. Contracted tendons are a congenital condition commonly seen by the practitioner. Acquired tendon injuries are usually the result of external trauma or rupture. The flexor tendons are often lacerated or severed in the metatarsal region as a result of trauma. The most notable tendon ruptures involve the gastrocnemius and peroneus tertius tendons in cattle.

CONTRACTED TENDONS

The majority of contracted tendons seen in calves are noted within the first few days following birth. The clinical signs vary in severity from a slight "bucking" of the carpus to severe flexion of the carpus and fetlock joint with inability to straighten the limb. Contracted tendons occur most commonly in the forelimbs, but all limbs may be affected. They may occur with other congenital or heritable abnormalities such as cleft palate and arthrogryposis. Therefore a calf with contracted tendons should have a thorough examination to rule out other problems before therapy is initiated.

Therapy in mild cases may require stretching of the tendons by manually extending the joints and by forced exercise. More severe cases will require continuous pressure on the tendons in the form of splints. The splint should extend from just above the level of the ground to the elbow in the forelimb and the hock in the rear limb. Polyvinyl chloride (PVC) pipe that is split sagittally, or a similar firm material, makes an excellent splint.

The splint should be well padded and tight enough to place some tension on the tendons. The toes should be left unbandaged to support the weight of the calf and further stretch the tendons. Splints may be left in place for 1 to 3 days, then changed and tightened. Severe cases may require a tenotomy to initially extend the leg. Tenotomies must be performed under aseptic conditions. The prognosis of contracted tendons is generally favorable unless the condition requires tenotomy.

Older animals may acquire contracted tendons as a result of disuse of limbs. This disuse is often secondary to previous tendon injury, fracture, nutritional deficiencies, and very rapid growth. The treatment is similar to congenital contracted tendon except that the inciting cause must be corrected and the prognosis is generally poorer.

RUPTURED TENDONS

Spontaneous rupture of tendons rarely occurs in food animals owing to their enormous tensile strength and to the general lack of stress they receive. Occasionally circumstances are created when a tendon will rupture.

Cows with postpartum paralysis may exert sufficient force while attempting to stand to rupture the gastrocnemius muscle or tendon. Likewise, trauma to the peroneus tertius may occur when an animal slips or falls with a rear leg extended in a backward direction.

Rupture of the gastrocnemius may be unilateral or bilateral. It is diagnosed primarily by physical examination. There is an obvious lameness with increased flexion of the hock and a knuckling of the fetlock, which often leads to a misdiagnosis of a fetlock problem. The hock is dropped as viewed from behind, and the angle of the stifle joint is increased to nearly 180°. Palpation may reveal a soft fluctuant swelling in the area of the rupture. It is unclear if this is a true tendon rupture or perhaps tendon-muscle separation. The prognosis is generally poor except in very mild cases that may respond to stall rest.

Rupture of the peroneus tertius is also diagnosed by physical examination. The classical rupture of the peroneus tertius will allow flexion of the stifle joint while extending the hock joint. This allows wrinkling of the Achilles tendon. If the animal can stand and walk, the prognosis is favorable and treatment is seldom attempted.

LACERATED TENDONS

Tendon lacerations commonly occur in the posterior aspect of the metatarsal region as a result of the animal kicking or its being struck with a sharp object. Because these wounds are traumatic and grossly contaminated, they require extensive debridement using sterile technique to remove all contaminated and devitalized tissue. After proper debridement it may be advantageous to delay suturing the laceration until sepsis is under control. Occasionally a large gap occurs between the tendon ends that cannot be closed. It is then necessary to allow the wound to heal by second intention. If the flexor tendons are cut, the leg should be immobilized in flexion to decrease the size of the gap and allow healing, which may require up to 3 months. Casts, splints, and shoes have all been used to place the leg in flexion. The major complications seen in tendon lacerations are sepsis and weakness of the healed tendon. The tendon must continue to be supported after the casts or splints are removed to allow the healed tendon to stretch slowly.

A method theorized to strengthen the healing tendon is carbon fiber implantation, which acts as a scaffold for the fibroblasts to align themselves and extrude collagen in a linear fashion. The resulting scar would emulate normal tendon.

Carbon fiber tendon implants have been used successfully in food animals, although much more investigation is needed to substantiate any claims.

BIBLIOGRAPHY

Ames NK, Coy CH: Repair of Bovine Tendon Lacerations with Carbon Fiber Implants. Proceedings XII World Congress on Diseases of Cattle. The Netherlands, 1982, p 1263-1265.
Goodship AE, Brown PN, Yeats JJ, et al: An assessment of filamentous carbon fiber for the treatment of tendon injury in the horse. Vet Rec 106:217-221, 1980.
McCoullagh KG, Goodship AE, Silver IA: Tendon injuries and their treatment in the horse. Vet Rec 105:54-57, 1979.
Valdez H, Clark RG, Hanselka DV: Repair of digital flexor tendon lacerations in the horse, using carbon fiber implants. J Am Vet Med Assoc 177:427-435, 1980.
Williams IF, Heaton A, McCullagh KG: Cell morphology and collagen types in equine tendon scar. Res Vet Sci 28:302-310, 1980.

Osteomyelitis
BIMBO WELKER, DVM, MS

Osteomyelitis in food animals usually results from hematogenous spread of infection or contamination of bone from exogenous sources as a sequela to trauma. The clinical manifestations, treatment, and prognosis of osteomyelitis will depend on the route of infection, the age and immune status of the animal, the virulence and susceptibility of the organism, and the chronicity of the problem.

PATHOPHYSIOLOGY

Hematogenous infection of bone is more common in neonates but can occur in adults. In the neonate this is usually a sequela to failure or partial failure of passive transfer. The most typical site of infection is the joint, but involvement of the metaphyseal bone region may occur. The metaphyseal side of the growth plate is susceptible because of the arrangement of the blood supply to that area. Small *loops* of capillaries in this region result in sluggish blood flow conducive to bacterial invasion, proliferation, and cellular infiltration, which cause occlusion of the vessels and ischemic necrosis of the bone. With age and blood flow pattern changes the subchondral bone becomes more susceptible, potentially resulting in collapse of articular cartilage. Long bones are most commonly involved, but other bones are susceptible (i.e., vertebra).

Open fractures, deep wounds, foreign bodies, and soft tissue infection with secondary osteomyelitis are all common sources of infection in ruminants. The sequence of events leading to osteomyelitis is the same as with hematogenous spread, but the location of the infection is not dictated by blood flow patterns.

The organisms most commonly isolated from cases of osteomyelitis from exogenous contamination in ruminants include coliforms, *Staphylococcus* spp., *Streptococcus* spp., and *Actinomyces* spp. (formerly *Corynebacterium*). *Pasteurella* spp. and *Salmonella* spp. are reported to be more typical of infection from hematogenous spread.

The presence of bacteria in bone does not always result in osteomyelitis. Osteomyelitis is more likely to occur if the immune status is compromised or if there is devitalized tissue present at the site of inoculation. Organisms thrive on avascular bone and devitalized tissue. Once infection occurs, the body may mount a response and totally eliminate the problem or at least wall it off. If the problem is not controlled by the body, the disease process may progressively destroy surrounding bone.

CLINICAL SIGNS

Young animals with hematogenous osteomyelitis will show signs of lameness in the affected limb. The area may be painful to palpation, swollen, and warm to the touch. Because of the close proximity to joints, the primary differential diagnosis is septic arthritis. Radiographic evaluation is necessary to differentiate metaphyseal osteomyelitis and septic osteoarthritis. Hematogenous spread to vertebral bodies is more likely to produce signs suggestive of neurologic disease.

Osteomyelitis secondary to trauma should be suspected when there has been obvious exposure of bone, when wounds fail to respond to conservative wound management, or when the degree of pain and lameness is in excess of what might be expected.

Radiographic evaluation is the method of choice for identifying bone infection. The infected area will be characterized by bone lysis, possible sequestra, or walled-off abscesses.

TREATMENT

Early aggressive wound debridement and antibiotic therapy should be instituted in any case where bone infection is a possible sequela. Examples include wounds exposing or involving bone, and cases of hypo- or agammaglobulinemia. If a culture and sensitivity are available, the antibiotic should be selected accordingly. If not, the antibiotic regime should be broad in spectrum, have good bone-penetrating ability, and be generally effective against the most common organisms encountered. More established cases of osteomyelitis require aggressive surgical debridement, long-term antibiotics (2 to 5 weeks), and support of the limb. Analgesics may also be beneficial to overall patient care. Careful consideration of milk and meat withdrawals is required for all drugs administered.

The prognosis for osteomyelitis depends on severity, chronicity, and aggressiveness of therapy. As a rule, early cases treated appropriately have a favorable prognosis. Cases of isolated sequestra secondary to trauma tend to respond well to surgical removal, debridement, and antibiotic therapy. However, cases of well-established chronic bone infection are less rewarding and generally less economical to treat. Cases of hematogenous osteomyelitis involving multiple areas or hematogenous spread to other organs should be cautiously prognosed.

BIBLIOGRAPHY

Greenough PR, MacCullum FJ, Weaver AD: Lameness in Cattle, 2nd ed. Philadelphia, JB Lippincott, 1981, pp 328-322.
Martens RJ, Auer JA, Carter GK: Equine pediatrics: septic arthritis and osteomyelitis. J Am Vet Med Assoc 188:582-585, 1986.
Slatter DH: Textbook of Small Animal Surgery, Vol. 2. Philadelphia, WB Saunders, 1985, pp 2020-2030.

SECTION 18
Dermatologic Diseases

DANNY W. SCOTT, DVM, Diplomate, ACVD, Consulting Editor

Parasitic Dermatoses

EDMUND J. ROSSER JR., DVM, DIPLOMATE, ACVD

The focus of this chapter is to discuss parasitic skin diseases observed in food animals that are commonly observed in a practice situation in the United States. A more comprehensive review of the subject can be found elsewhere.[1]

Parasitic skin diseases are one of the most common forms of skin disease observed in veterinary dermatology but are a frequently overlooked problem in food animals. This is unfortunate since there are a myriad of problems associated with these disorders. Pruritus is one of the common problems, often resulting in restlessness, aggressiveness, excoriation of the hide and hide damage, loss of wool, secondary infections, and myiasis. Indirectly this can result in a decrease in daily feed consumption and a decrease in weight gain, milk production, or wool density. Other problems associated with parasitic skin diseases include anemia, abnormal estrous cycles, increased susceptibility to respiratory disease, and even death. Several of these ectoparasites also serve as important vectors of numerous infectious diseases. With all of these factors taken into consideration, one can appreciate that considerable financial loss will be associated with these various problems.

MANGE

Psoroptic Mange

Psoroptic mange (body mange, common scab, sheep scab) is a U. S. Department of Agriculture (USDA) reportable and quarantinable disease in both sheep and cattle owing to the often debilitating effects of this disease. It is believed that psoroptic mange in sheep has been eradicated in the United States.[2,3] Another form of psoroptic mange (ear mites, ear mange) commonly affects the ears of goats and less frequently of sheep and is not a reportable disease.

Etiology and Pathogenesis

Psoroptes ovis mites cause the body mange form of psoroptic mange in sheep and cattle. They are surface dwelling, nonburrowing mites believed to feed on tissue fluids with subsequent crust and scab formation. *Psoroptes* spp. have not been shown to be infectious to humans.

In cattle, mite activity seems to be related to the formation of ulcers.[4] This microscopic ulcer formation may be related to mite feeding activity possibly through a combination of physical and chemical damage and immunologic host response. This reaction is associated with a large influx of plasma cells, eosinophils, and mast cells into the superficial perivascular dermal region and upper dermis with mast cell degranulation. Thus psoroptic scabies may be partially mediated by an allergic dermatitis reaction.[4,5] The scab formed above the ulcers contains many neutrophils and may serve as the pathway for massive movement of neutrophils and development of concurrent neutropenia.

Psoroptes cuniculi mites are associated with the ear mange form of psoroptic mange that most commonly occurs in goats and rarely in sheep.

The life cycle of *Psoroptes* mites is completed entirely on the host and occurs within 10 to 12 days.[1,6] The mites are capable of survival away from their host for 10 to 21 days, depending on the environmental conditions. The optimum environmental conditions for growth and development are moisture and cool temperatures. When these environmental conditions are present, animals are often being housed indoors with closer confinement, leading to a greater incidence of this form of mange in fall and winter. During hot and dry weather periods, mite survival time decreases and mites survive by residing in body-fold regions such as the perineal, inguinal, and interdigital regions. Transmission of the disease is through direct contact or mite-contaminated fomites with an incubation period from 2 to 8 weeks.

Clinical Signs

In cattle, psoroptic mange is most commonly noticed in the western states and Great Plains region. The chief complaint is intense pruritus, usually first affecting the withers, neck, base of tail, and rump. The lesions that develop are papules, pustules, crusts, scabs, excoriations, alopecia, and lichenification. The condition may progress to a generalized dense crusting dermatosis with exudation and secondary infections. Severely affected animals may show weakness, weight loss, cachexia, and even death.

In sheep, psoroptic mange is believed to have been eradicated in the United States. The chief complaint is intense pruritus, usually first affecting the lateral trunk and rump. The lesions that develop are papules, pustules, and yellowish crusts. The wool often becomes matted with crusts, and large areas of wool may be shed. Severely affected animals may show weakness, weight loss, cachexia, and even death. *Psoroptes cuniculi* mites have been a rare cause of ear mange in sheep.

In goats, *P. cuniculi* mites are commonly found in the external ear canal and may not be associated with the development of any clinical signs. When disease does develop there can be varying degrees of head shaking, ear scratching, changes in behavior, accumulation of excess cerumen, and crusts, scabs, and alopecia affecting the pinnae. Severely affected animals may develop otitis media and/or otitis interna and yellowish brown crusts on the poll, face, pastern, and interdigital regions.

Diagnosis

Historical and physical findings are what first lead one to suspect the diagnosis of psoroptic mange. The differential diagnosis includes sarcoptic mange, chorioptic mange, psorergatic mange, keds, and pediculosis. Confirmation of the diagnosis is by demonstration of the mites through skin scrapings, ear swabs, otoscopic examination, or skin biopsy. Body mange–associated mites are usually readily found in skin scrapings and may be found on skin biopsy. Histopathologic examination of skin biopsy specimens reveals a superficial perivascular dermatitis reaction with eosinophils, mast cells, plasma cells, lymphocytes, and macrophages, which may include a mixed cellular diffuse superficial dermal infiltrate. In addition, ulceration, eosinophilic microabscesses, superficial dermal edema, and serosanguineous crusts with neutrophils, eosinophils, and bacteria can be seen. In cattle, severely affected animals may have a leukopenia, marked neutropenia, eosinophilia, mild anemia, decreased albumin, and increased fibrinogen and γ-globulin levels.[7]

Ear mange–associated mites are more difficult to demonstrate. Evaluation often requires sedation or anesthesia of the animal and thorough otoscopic examination and microscopic examination of skin scrapings and ear swab samples from deep within the external ear canal.

Treatment and Control

The USDA-recommended treatment of choice for psoroptic mange in cattle is ivermectin given as a single subcutaneous injection at 200 μg/kg.[8] All affected or exposed animals on the premises are required to be treated along with a 14-day isolation period from unaffected animals. Ivermectin has been a well-tolerated drug in cattle and has not been associated with any teratogenic effects or decreases in breeding performance.

It is believed that psoroptic mange has been eradicated in sheep in the United States. If it is reported it would then be treated based on state-approved insecticide usage and quarantine procedures. Treatment usually entails vat-dipping, which is most effective if done within 2 weeks after shearing and repeated in 10 to 14 days. At present, ivermectin has shown varying results in the treatment of psoroptic mange in sheep.

Psoroptic ear mange of goats can be successfully treated with many of the commercially available otic preparations used in the treatment of ear mites in dogs and cats. Two commonly used preparations are (1) 1 part rotonone (Canex) to 3 parts mineral oil and (2) Tresaderm otic. Initially the ears canals should be thoroughly cleaned (preferably while under sedation or anesthesia at the time of otoscopic examination) and then medicated every 3 days for a total for 3 weeks. Ivermectin may also prove to be a useful treatment alternative since it has been shown to be effective in the treatment of ear mites in horses, dogs, cats, and rabbits.

Sarcoptic Mange

Sarcoptic mange (barn itch, scabies, head mange) is a pruritic skin disease of major importance to the swine industry and is also known to occur in cattle and rarely in goats and sheep. The disease is a USDA reportable disease in cattle and sheep. It is believed that sarcoptic mange has not yet been reported in sheep in the United States.[1, 3]

Etiology and Pathogenesis

Sarcoptes scabiei mites are burrowing mites that form tunnels in the epidermis and feed on tissue fluids and possibly epidermal cells. Controversy exists as to the specific mite involved as the causative parasite in the development of sarcoptic mange in various species. Some researchers believe that there is a separate species of *Sarcoptes* mite for each species of animal affected. However, the most prevalent view is that the same species of mite has undergone certain biologic and physiologic adaptations for the various species of animals affected.[9, 10] Certainly some varieties are more host-specific than others, but one should always anticipate the possibility of transfer of mites from one animal species to the other or from animals to humans.

In the food animal population, the pathogenesis of sarcoptic mange has been most closely examined in swine.[11] It appears that a hypersensitivity reaction to the mite is involved. In young piglets that are newly infected, this sensitization process takes several weeks, at which point pruritus and crusting of the pinnae are noticed. This is followed by a more generalized pruritus with an erythematous and papular eruption. During this stage there is blood and tissue eosinophilia, an intradermal skin test positivity to mite antigen is noted, and mites become increasingly more difficult to find. The chronic form of sarcoptic mange occurs when animals are in poor condition at the time of infection (poor feeding, management, and hygiene) or there is an underlying immunodeficiency disorder.

The life cycle of *Sarcoptes* mites is completed entirely on the host and occurs within 10 to 21 days. Regarding the survival of this parasite off of its host, the conventional view has been that the mites are very sensitive to drying and usually only survive a few days. However, studies show that survival of mites off of the host may last longer and that the environment can be considered a potential source of reinfestation over several weeks.[12] This has led to the addition of treatment of the environment in many scabies treatment protocols. Therefore, transmission of the disease can be through direct contact or mite-contaminated fomites. The disease is most commonly noticed during times of low temperature and high moisture.

Clinical Signs

In swine, sarcoptic mange is a common problem throughout the United States. The chief symptom is pruritus that first affects the ears with the presence of crusts and excoriations. In some instances an aural hematoma may develop. This is usually followed by a generalized pruritus, with the appearance of an erythematous and papular eruption over the trunk (especially the rump, flanks, and abdomen). If left untreated, diffuse lichenification, excoriations, and crusting may develop. Chronic scabies (hyperkeratotic mange, Norwegian scabies), which is much less common, occurs primarily in adult animals with thick asbestos-like scabs most often on the ears, head, and neck and less often on the legs.

In cattle, sarcoptic mange occurs throughout the United States and is most common and severe under conditions of poor feeding, poor housing, poor hygiene, and overcrowding. The chief symptom is pruritus, usually first affecting the face, neck, brisket, shoulders, inner thighs, rump, and tail base region. The lesions that develop are papules, crusts, excoriations, alopecia, and lichenification. If left untreated, the condition can become generalized.

In goats, sarcoptic mange is relatively rare and again presents as pruritus. It affects the ears, face, and neck and occasionally the limbs, with alopecia, crusting, and lichenification being most commonly observed.

In sheep, it is believed that sarcoptic mange has not yet been reported in the United States. The main symptom is pruritus that affects the ears, face, and limbs and tends to spare the wooled areas. Lesions noticed are crusts, excoriations, alopecia, and lichenification.

Diagnosis

The history and physical examination should first lead one to suspect the diagnosis of sarcoptic mange. The differential diagnosis includes psoroptic mange, chorioptic mange, psorergatic mange, lice, keds, and fly bite dermatitis. Confirmation of the diagnosis is by demonstration of the mite through skin scrapings, ear swabs, vacuum cleaner and filter sampling technique,[13] or skin biopsy. Of these four methods the vacuum cleaner and filter sampling technique and examination of ear swabs have been most useful. Histopathologic examination of skin biopsy specimens reveals varying degrees of a superficial perivascular dermatitis reaction with numerous eosinophils, eosinophilic microabscesses, leukocytic exocytosis, and ulceration. Since this mite may not be found by any of the above techniques, the disease may need to be presumptively diagnosed by a response to empiric scabicidal treatment. In cases of chronic scabies (hyperkeratotic mange) the mites are usually easily demonstrated using any of the previously mentioned techniques.

Treatment and Control

The recommended treatment of choice for sarcoptic mange in swine is ivermectin given as a single subcutaneous injection at 300 µg/kg. In some eradication programs this injection is repeated in 2 weeks and every pig on the premises is treated.[14] Since the environment may serve as a source of reinfection, the premises should be sprayed 5 days after ivermectin treatment with a state-approved and effective scabicidal spray (e.g., amitraz). Afterward, any incoming stock should be treated on arrival to the premises and initially isolated from the rest of the herd. Ivermectin has also been shown to be effective against *S. scabiei* in swine when it is administered orally at a dosage of 100 to 200 µg/kg/day for 7 consecutive days.[15]

In cattle, sarcoptic scabies is a USDA reportable disease. Guidelines have been established for isolation, quarantine, and treatment. Spray-dipping and vat-dipping have been the conventional treatment modalities using coumaphos, phosmet, or hot lime sulfur. However, it has been shown that ivermectin has been proven effective when given as a single subcutaneous injection of 200 µg/kg or applied as a topical solution to healthy (i.e., unaffected) areas of bovine skin at a dosage of 500 µg/kg.[16] However, when the solution was applied over areas of crusting and thickening, the ivermectin treatment was less effective in rendering a cure.

In sheep, sarcoptic mange has not yet been recognized in the United States and is listed as a reportable disease.

In goats, sarcoptic mange has been treated with various topical scabicidal dips and sprays. Ivermectin has been shown to be effective when given as a single subcutaneous injection at 200 µg/kg.

Chorioptic Mange

Chorioptic mange (tail mange, leg mange, symbiotic scab, foot mange, scrotal mange) is the most common form of mange in cattle and also occurs in goats and sheep. Chorioptic mange in sheep has been eradicated in the United States.

Etiology and Pathogenesis

Chorioptes mites are surface-dwelling mites that feed on epidermal debris. Controversy exists as to the specific mite involved as the causative parasite in the development of chorioptic mange in various species. There is some indication that only one species of mite, *Chorioptes bovis,* is responsible for chorioptic mange in cattle, goats, and sheep. However, many still believe that there are separate species of mites for each host affected: *C. bovis* (cattle), *C. caprae* (goats), and *C. ovis* (sheep). *Chorioptes* spp. have not been shown to be infectious to humans.

The pathogenesis of chorioptic mange is believed to involve a hypersensitivity reaction by the host since the mite can be demonstrated in apparently normal cattle and sheep.

The life cycle of *Chorioptes* mites is completed entirely on the host and occurs within 14 to 21 days. Regarding the survival of this parasite off of its host, the conventional view has been that the mites usually survive only a few days. However, similar to what has been shown for *Sarcoptes* mites, it appears that *C. bovis* mites may be able to survive off of the host for longer periods of time and that the environment should be considered a potential source of reinfestation for 10 weeks.[1] Therefore, transmission of the disease can be through direct contact or mite-contaminated fomites. The disease is more active and mite populations are greater during colder weather. In the warmer months, when animals are turned out to pasture, the disease often undergoes spontaneous remission and mite numbers become smaller. However, this decrease in activity of the disease does not occur in summer if the cattle are confined indoors.

Clinical Signs

In cattle, chorioptic mange occurs most frequently in stabled dairy cattle in the northeastern United States. Pruritus may be present but is variable in intensity and is rarely as severe as in psoroptic or sarcoptic mange. During the winter the lesions are usually confined to the perineum, posterior udder, and thigh region with papules, small crusts and scabs, erythema, excoriations, and alopecia. In more chronic cases the skin becomes lichenified. During the summer the disease process is less active and crusted lesions and mites are localized to the coronary band region, interdigital region, and muzzle. In addition, a rapidly spreading syndrome characterized by coronitis, intense pruritus, foot rot–like lesions, muzzle lesions, weight loss, and a drop in milk production has been described.[2]

In goats, chorioptic mange occurs most frequently in stabled goats in the northeastern United States. Pruritus is usually marked and affects the feet, hind legs, udder, scrotum, tail, and perineal area and less commonly the neck and flank. Papules, crusts, scabs, alopecia, erythema, oozing, and ulceration may develop.

In sheep, chorioptic mange is believed to have been eradicated in the United States. The clinical signs can be very similar to those seen in chorioptic mange of cattle and goats. In rams, a scrotal dermatitis can occur with yellowish exudates and crusts. There is a concurrent increase in testicular temperature with resultant testicular atrophy, decreased spermatogenesis, and infertility.

Diagnosis

The history and physical examination should first lead one to suspect the diagnosis of chorioptic mange. The differential diagnosis includes sarcoptic mange, psoroptic mange, and diseases associated with anal or perineal pruritus (e.g., pin worms, food allergy, lice). Confirmation of the diagnosis is by demonstration of the mite through skin scrapings in which the mite is usually easily found.

Treatment and Control

Treatment of chorioptic mange in cattle has included whole body spraying with 0.25 per cent crotoxyphos applied once or 2 per cent lime sulfur applied weekly for 4 weeks. Recently, ivermectin has been applied as a topical solution at a dosage of 500 µg/kg and was effective.[16]

In goats, chorioptic mange has been treated with whole-body dips or sprays with 0.25 per cent crotoxyphos, 0.25 per cent coumaphos, or 0.2 per cent trichlorfon applied twice at 10- to 14-day intervals. Whole-body dips or spraying with 0.2 per cent lime sulfur applied weekly for 4 weeks is also effective. The most effective treatment for chorioptic mange in goats has been a single whole-body dip using a 0.3 per cent fenvalerate (a synthetic pyrethroid) solution.[17]

In sheep, chorioptic mange is a USDA-reportable disease. Guidelines have been established for isolation, quarantine, and treatment. Vat-dipping has been the conventional treatment modality using coumaphos, phosmet, or lime sulfur after shearing the sheep.

Psorergatic Mange

Psorergatic mange (itch mite, sheep itch mite, cattle itch mite) is an uncommon skin disease that can occur in sheep and cattle in the United States. Psorergatic mange in sheep is believed to have been eradicated in the United States.

Etiology and Pathogenesis

Psorergatic mites burrow at various levels within the stratum corneum but not to the level of the stratum spinosum.[18] Most of the mites are located within or near the superficial region of the hair follicle opening. It has been proposed that *Psorergates ovis* mites feed on epidermal lipids. The parasite is host specific with *P. ovis* affecting sheep and *P. bos* affecting cattle. *Psorergates* mites have not been shown to be infectious to humans.

The pathogenesis of psorergatic mange is poorly understood, but a hypersensitivity reaction to mite excreta has been suspected.

The life cycle of *Psorergates* mites is completed entirely on the host and occurs in 4 to 5 weeks. It is believed that the mites usually cannot survive for more than a few days off the host. Transmission of the disease is through direct contact (especially after sheep have been shorn and they are in close contact after shearing) or contaminated fomites (especially clippers). The disease is more active and mite populations are greater during the winter and spring.

Clinical Signs

Psorergatic mange in cattle is a relatively rare disease. The disease is usually nonpruritic with mild patchy alopecia and scaling. Occasionally *P. bos* mites can be isolated from clinically normal cattle.

The Merino is the most commonly affected breed of sheep. The chief complaint is intense pruritus, manifested by rubbing and biting of the wool and resultant raggedness, matting, and chewed and shed areas of wool. The skin in affected areas has excess scaling. The most severely affected areas are areas that can be reached by the sheep's mouth, especially the lateral chest, flanks, and thighs.

Diagnosis

Historical and physical findings are what first lead one to suspect the diagnosis of psorergatic mange. The differential diagnosis in sheep includes lice, keds, and psoroptic and sarcoptic mange, and in cattle it includes lice and shedding. Confirmation of the diagnosis is by demonstration of the mites through skin scrapings or the vacuum cleaner and filter sampling technique.[13] The mites can be difficult to find; therefore, whenever possible samples should be taken in winter or spring when mite populations are highest. In sheep the wool should be clipped close to the skin over areas of chewing and excess scaling before taking samples.

Treatment and Control

In sheep, psorergatic mange is a USDA-reportable disease. Guidelines have been established for isolation, quarantine, and treatment. The most commonly used treatments are whole-body dips or sprays, which are most effective when performed in the summer within 2 weeks of shearing and repeated in 14 days. Effective insecticides include 2 to 3 per cent lime sulfur, 0.2 per cent malathion, 0.3 per cent coumaphos, and 0.03 to 0.3 per cent diazinon. Ivermectin was shown to be effective in one study when it was given as two treatments, 1 month apart.[6]

In cattle, owing to minimal lesions and apparent lack of economic losses, the disease is usually left untreated. However, 2 to 3 per cent lime sulfur dips/sprays or ivermectin have been effective treatments.

Demodectic Mange

Demodectic mange (follicular mange, demodicosis) is a dermatitis affecting the hair follicles of cattle, goats, swine, and rarely sheep.

Etiology and Pathogenesis

Demodex mites are considered normal residents of mammalian skin that reside in the hair follicles and sebaceous glands. The mites are host specific with *D. caprae* in goats, *D. bovis* in cattle, *D. phylloides* in swine, and *D. ovis* in sheep. Since *Demodex* mites are considered normal residents of the skin, demodectic mange is not considered to be a contagious disease.

The pathogenesis of demodectic mange in food animals is poorly understood. In cattle, it has been shown that the normal population of *Demodex* mites is transferred from the dam to the offspring during the first 2 to 3 days of life through direct contact with the dam. Much controversy exists as to the reason for the development of demodicosis in food animals, but multiple factors have been considered, including hereditary predisposition, effects of stress, poor nutrition, concurrent diseases, and any factors that may result in suppression of the immune system of the host. In addition, demodectic mange may occur in an apparently normal animal.

The life cycle of *Demodex* mites is completed entirely on the host and is believed to be completed in 20 to 35 days. *Demodex* mites are not capable of survival off of their host for more than several days. In cattle, the disease is most commonly observed in late winter and early spring.

Clinical Signs

In cattle, demodectic mange occurs most frequently in dairy cattle in the United States, with the Holstein breed being most commonly affected. The disease is usually nonpruritic and is characterized by papules, pustules, and small nodules over the brisket, withers, neck, and shoulder region. Other areas that may be affected include the back, flanks, face, and intermandibular region, and the mange may become a generalized skin disease. The clinical disease is variable in appearance from small papules that are only evident on palpation of the skin to small nodules that are clearly visible. Occasionally there may be areas of alopecia, and in severe cases there is abscess formation, ulceration, fistula, crusting, and the development of secondary bacterial infection.

In goats, demodectic mange occurs throughout the United States. The disease is nonpruritic, with the most common lesions being papules and nodules affecting the face, neck, shoulders, and sides. Although rare, the disease can become an extensive and generalized disease with ensuing death.

In swine, demodectic mange is of minor significance and is often clinically unnoticed until the time of slaughter. The disease is nonpruritic, with small papules initially affecting the snout and eyelids. The lesions may spread along the ventral neck and trunk with pustules, nodules, and secondary bacterial infection developing. Occasionally there may be scaling and nodular lesions containing a white and caseous material localized to the mammary gland and flank region.

In sheep, demodectic mange is an extremely rare disease. The disease is nonpruritic with alopecia, erythema, and scaling of the face, neck, shoulders and back. The formation of pustules, crusts, and scabs may be present on the coronets, nose, tips of ears, and periorbital region.

Diagnosis

The differential diagnosis for demodectic mange includes bacterial folliculitis, dermatophytosis (ringworm), and dermatophilosis (rain scald). Confirmation of the diagnosis is by demonstration of the mites through skin scrapings or skin biopsy. In performing a skin scraping over papular lesions, the skin should be pinched and squeezed first, followed by a deep scraping to the point of showing a small amount of blood. Nodular lesions should be incised and drained, with examination of the exudate usually revealing numerous *Demodex* mites. Histopathologic examination of skin biopsy specimens reveals hair follicles with numerous *Demodex* mites, in many instances to the point of the formation of a follicular cyst. Additionally there may be perifolliculitis, folliculitis, furunculosis, and granulomatous inflammation.

Treatment and Control

In general, demodectic mange in food animals is asymptomatic with minimal lesions and no apparent economic losses and therefore is usually left untreated. Because of the possible heritability of the disease, severely affected animals should be culled from the herd. Treatment with whole-body dipping with a 2 per cent trichlorfon (Neguvon) solution every other day for 3 treatments has been reported to be effective in cattle, swine and sheep. In goats, individual nodules can be incised, drained, and infused with tincture of iodine or rotenone in alcohol. Generalized demodicosis in goats has been treated with ronnel in propylene glycol (180 ml of 33 per cent ronnel in 1000 ml of propylene glycol) applied to one third of the body daily until cured or amitraz (10.6 ml Mitaban in 2 gallons of water) as a whole-body dip repeated every 14 days for 2 to 3 treatments.

Trombiculidiasis

Trombiculidiasis (chiggers, harvest mite, leg itch) is a pruritic dermatitis of sheep and cattle in the United States.

Etiology and Pathogenesis

Trombiculid larvae normally parasitize small rodents and feed off of tissue fluids but are also capable of parasitizing various food animals (especially sheep and cattle). The larvae usually feed for 7 to 10 days and then drop off the host and undergo further development. The adult and nymphal stages are free-living parasites that feed on other arthropods, invertebrates, and plant life. The most common mite associated with trombiculidiasis in the United States is *Trombicula (Eutrombicula) alfreddugesi*. Trombiculid larvae are also capable of parasitizing humans.

The pathogenesis of trombiculidiasis is believed to involve a hypersensitivity reaction to larval salivary antigens. Trombiculid larvae are most active in the late summer and fall, and the disease is noticed most often in animals that have been grazing in pasture or wooded areas.

Clinical Signs

In cattle and sheep, trombiculidiasis is a pruritic dermatitis most often affecting the distal limbs, face, and muzzle and may also affect the neck, ventral chest, and abdomen. The lesions that develop include crusts, excoriations, edema, and exudation. In sheep, the first signs noticed are often stamping of their feet and biting of the legs. In heavy infestations of sheep there can be severe edema of distal extremities, decreased feed consumption, and weight loss.

Diagnosis

The history and physical examination should first lead one to suspect the diagnosis of trombiculidiasis. The differential diagnosis includes psoroptic mange, chorioptic mange, sarcoptic mange, contact dermatitis, photosensitization, forage mites, biting flies, and dermatophilosis. Confirmation of the diagnosis is by demonstration of larvae either grossly (since they are naturally pigmented and often orange) or through skin scrapings.

Treatment and Control

Trombiculidiasis requires repeated infestation to develop into a continuous entity. Therefore, owing to its short season in most regions of the United States, the disease usually undergoes spontaneous remission. In severe cases, dipping or spraying with 2 per cent lime sulfur, 0.25 to 0.5 per cent malathion, 0.06 to 0.3 per cent coumaphos, 0.03 to 0.1 per cent diazinon or 0.25 per cent chlorpyrifos has been used on a single application basis.

LICE INFESTATION

Louse infestation (pediculosis) is a common parasitism of the skin observed in cattle, sheep, goats, and swine in the United States.

Etiology and Pathogenesis

Lice are divided into two categories based on their anatomy and feeding behavior. Biting lice (suborder: Mallophaga) have mouth parts adapted for biting and chewing, which allows feeding on epithelial cells. Sucking lice (suborder: Anoplura) have pointed heads and mouth parts adapted for sucking tissue fluids and blood from the host. Lice are host specific, with the following list of species being most common.

Cattle:
- Sucking lice—*Haematopinus eurysternus, Linognathus vituli, Solenopotes capillatus*
- Biting louse—*Damalinia bovis*

Sheep:
- Sucking lice—*Linognathus ovillis, Linognathus pedalis*
- Biting louse—*Damalinia ovis*

Goats:
- Sucking louse—*Linognathus stenopsis*
- Biting louse—*Damalinia caprae*

Swine:
- Sucking louse—*Haematopinus suis*

The life cycle of lice is completed entirely on the host and occurs in 2 to 4 weeks under optimum conditions with the eggs (nits) being deposited and glued to the hair shafts. Usually lice do not survive for more than 1 week off of the host. Survival of lice and their reproducibility are greatly affected by ambient temperatures. The optimum temperature range is very narrow, and temperatures either too cold or too hot may kill lice or decrease reproduction. The lowest populations of lice are encountered during the summer. The disease is more active and louse populations are greater during the winter, probably owing to crowding of animals, poorer nutrition, and thicker hair coats or wool density. Transmission of the disease is through direct contact or contaminated fomites.

The pathogenesis of pediculosis relates to the direct ability of lice to be mechanically irritating to the skin. In the case of sucking lice there is the capability of causing anemia and the ability to serve as a vector for various infectious diseases.

Clinical Signs

In cattle, pediculosis may be an incidental finding on physical examination and not associated with any clinical disease. The most common clinical feature is pruritus demonstrated by excess rubbing, scratching, and grooming. This results in a dull, dry hair coat, patchy alopecia, and excoriations. Formation of hairballs may be a problem in infested calves owing to continuous licking. Biting lice most commonly affect the neck, withers, and tailhead region. Sucking lice are found on the poll, head, neck, shoulders, tail, and inguinal and axillary regions. Sucking lice may also cause anemia.

In sheep, pediculosis is usually pruritic, with signs of biting and chewing of affected areas, matting and loss of wool, and foot stamping. Biting lice most commonly affect the neck and back region, whereas sucking lice are found on the face or lower legs. Severe infestations with *Linognathus pedalis* (foot lice) may cause lameness.

In goats, pediculosis is usually pruritic, with clinical signs very similar to those described in sheep. Severe damage to the coat can occur especially in Angora goats. Both biting and sucking lice may be found on the neck, ventral and lateral trunk, and inguinal region. Additional problems may include weight loss, decreased milk production, and anemia.

In swine, pediculosis is usually pruritic and affects the ears, jowl, neck, flanks, and inguinal and axillary regions. Heavy infestations in young pigs may cause anemia and decreased weight gain. *Haematopinus suis* also serves as an important vector in the transmission of swinepox. The incidence of pediculosis in swine has been decreasing, possibly owing to the increased use of ivermectin in the treatment of sarcoptic mange.

Diagnosis

The diagnosis of pediculosis is initially based on historical findings and physical examination. The differential diagnosis includes sarcoptic mange, psoroptic mange, chorioptic mange, psorergatic mange, and keds. Confirmation of the diagnosis is by demonstration of the lice or nits on physical examination since they are often readily visible, or through microscopic examination of skin scrapings.

Treatment and Control

The effective treatments for lice in food animals are numerous. In general, sprays and dips are most useful during warmer weather and should be repeated in 14 days. During the less favorable winter months, pour-ons, powders, and dusts are most practical. Powders and dusts are usually applied once weekly for 3 to 4 weeks. Ivermectin has been shown to be effective against sucking lice in cattle and swine when given as a single subcutaneous injection at 200 to 300 µg/kg. To control the disease, treatment of animals should coincide with a thorough cleansing of the environment and insecticide spraying of the premises.

KED INFESTATION

Ked infestation (sheep ked, sheep tick) is a pruritic skin disease of sheep and is occasionally found in goats.

Etiology and Pathogenesis

The ked is a blood-sucking, wingless, hairy insect with a sac-like and leathery body referred to as *Melophagus ovinus*. The ked is somewhat host specific in that it only parasitizes sheep and goats. The life cycle of the ked is completed entirely on the host and occurs in 5 to 6 weeks under optimum conditions. The female ked does not lay eggs but produces a fully developed larvae that attaches to wool or hair. The life expectancy of the female ked is 4 to 5 months, in which time 10 to 15 larvae are produced. Although keds may survive up to 14 days off of their host under optimal conditions, most will die in 3 to 4 days.

The ked is found in highest numbers in the fall and winter, and the numbers decrease markedly in the summer (hot, dry climates can be free of keds). Transmission of the disease is primarily through direct contact, and rarely does the environment serve as a source of reinfestation. Sheep or goats in poor condition (poor feeding, debilitation) are more readily infested. In normal animals a natural resistance can be acquired over time. Keds can serve as a vector in the transmission of bluetongue virus.

Clinical Signs

In sheep and goats, ked infestation is most commonly noticed in the colder and wetter areas of the United States. The chief symptom is pruritus affecting the neck, sides, rump, and abdomen. Subsequent rubbing, biting, and chewing at the wool results in matting and loss of wool. Feces from the ked causes a staining of the wool and reduces its value. Heavy infestations may cause anemia and weight loss.

Diagnosis

The diagnosis of keds is usually confirmed by physical examination, since the insects are sufficiently large (4 to 7 mm) to be seen without a microscope. The differential diagnosis includes sarcoptic mange, psoroptic mange, chorioptic mange, psorergatic mange, lice, trombiculidiasis, and forage mites.

Treatment and Control

The treatment of keds is effective when using the agents and principles as described in the discussion of the treatment of lice infestation. In sheep, shearing removes 80 to 90 per cent of adults and almost all of the pupae, and dipping or spraying is most effective if performed within the next 2 to 4 weeks. Ivermectin has also been mentioned to be effective in eliminating keds.

MYIASIS

Hypodermiasis

Hypodermiasis (hypodermosis, warbles, cattle grubs) is a common disease in cattle causing damage to the hide, anaphylactic reactions, and damage to the nervous system and esophagus.

Etiology and Pathogenesis

Hypodermiasis in cattle is due to the larval development stages of *Hypoderma bovis* and *H. lineatum*. The adult stage is a fly that deposits eggs onto the hair shafts of cattle for further development. The flies of *H. lineatum* deposit eggs on the legs of cattle (especially around the heels of the forelegs) leaving up to 15 eggs on a single hair; *H. bovis* flies deposit eggs over the rump and upper hindleg region leaving 1 egg per hair shaft. The adult flies are most active during spring to late summer, with *H. lineatum* preferring a warmer climate and being most active in the southern United States; *H. bovis* prefers cooler climates and is most active in the northern United States. Hatching of eggs occurs in 4 to 6 days, and the larvae penetrate the skin into the subcutaneous tissue. This process requires enzymatic digestion by the larvae, which is facilitated by larval proteases and collagenase.[19] *H. lineatum* migrates through the connective tissue to the distal one third of the esophagus and rests (winter resting site) in the loose connective tissue of the submucosa. *H. bovis* migrates through the connective tissue to the thoracolumbar spinal canal and rests (winter resting site) in the epidural adipose tissue between the dura mater and periosteum. This migration is usually completed in 4 weeks, followed by further feeding and growth for 2 to 4 months at the winter resting site. After this time further migration begins toward the dorsum of the body, and the larvae reach the subcutaneous tissue over the back region in the spring (spring resting sites). The larvae then perforate the skin to form a breathing pore and the second and third larval instar stages are completed over 1 to 2 months. These larval stages of development are accompanied by a granulomatous inflammatory reaction by the host and are referred to as the "warble" stage. When development is complete the larvae enlarge the breathing pore, drop from the host to the soil, and pupate. A completed life cycle from one generation to the next occurs within 9 to 12 months.

Clinical Signs

In cattle, the adult *Hypoderma* flies are primarily a nuisance and may result in cattle running from swarms of flies. During the spring, subcutaneous nodules develop that form a central hole (breathing pore) and are located over the back. These nodules contain the larvae or "warble." Other clinical signs that may be associated with *Hypoderma* larvae include anaphylactic reaction due to rupture of a third larval instar within a subcutaneous nodule ("warble"); posterior paresis and ataxia from the death of *H. bovis* larvae in the spinal canal; dysphagia, failure of eructation, and bloat from the death of *H. lineatum* larvae in the esophagus; and anaphylactic reaction due to death of connective tissue migrating larvae in a sensitized animal. Posterior paresis and esophageal-related problems can be averted by avoiding the use of systemically active insecticides when the larvae are known to be in the spinal canal or esophagus. In general this stage of larval migration occurs for *H. bovis* from October to March in the northern United States and from as early as August until March in the southern United States. However, this may vary slightly from state to state and from one year to the next depending on changes in weather patterns.

Diagnosis

The diagnosis of hypodermiasis in cattle is based on history and physical examination and the appearance of the characteristic subcutaneous nodules containing larvae over the dorsum of the animal. The differential diagnosis includes infectious granulomas, neoplasms, and epidermoid and dermoid cysts. Early detection of the disease, during the first instar larval stage, is possible using intradermal skin testing to *Hypoderma* antigens and enzyme-linked immunosorbent assay testing to measure *Hypoderma* antigen-specific antibody production.[19–21]

Treatment

The treatment of hypodermiasis in cattle has most commonly involved the use of systemically acting organophosphate compounds shortly after the end of the adult fly season. These products need to be used in strict accordance with manufacturer's recommendations to avoid signs of organophosphate toxicity. Methods of use have included pour-ons, sprays, oral dosing, impregnated ear tags and leg bands, and a feed additive. Ivermectin has also been shown to be effective when applied as a topical solution[22] at a dosage of 500 µg/kg or as a single subcutaneous injection at a dosage of 200 µg/kg. However, further investigations have shown that the LD_{50} for *Hypoderma* larvae is only 0.04 µg/kg and the LD_{90} is 0.105 µg/kg. Therefore conventionally used dosages of ivermectin are thousands of times higher than that necessary for the control of *Hypoderma* larvae and a dosage as low as 0.2 µg/kg is effective.[23] An acquired immunity to *Hypoderma* infection can occur. Based on this observation, vaccines containing various *Hypoderma* antigens have been tried and result in a decreased survival rate of migrating *Hypoderma* larvae in vaccinated versus nonvaccinated cattle.[19]

Cutaneous Myiasis

Cutaneous myiasis (calliphorine myiasis, blowfly strike) is most commonly a disorder of sheep and can result in serious losses in productivity and wool.

Etiology and Pathogenesis

Cutaneous myiasis in sheep in the United States is caused by the blowflies *Phormia regina* and *P. terrae-novae*. The adult blowfly lays its eggs in wounds, soiled or wetted wool, and carcasses, and the larvae hatch over the next several days. The larvae continue to grow over the next several days to weeks (depending on environmental conditions) and then fall to the ground and pupate. Cutaneous myiasis is most severe during times of large fly populations and the presence of susceptible sheep. Large fly populations occur during prolonged periods of warm, humid weather. The initial event is evoked by flies classified as primary flies that deposit eggs on live animals. The flies may be attracted to an already present wound or intact skin that is wet or soiled and has a favorable environment for bacterial growth. Proliferation of *Pseudomonas* spp. in the wool and on the skin attracts blowflies and stimulates oviposition. The larvae of these flies can subsequently pierce the skin and then create favorable conditions for invasion by secondary flies.

Clinical Signs

In sheep, cutaneous myiasis can be a disease of great economic importance and most severely affects Merino sheep because of their heavy skin folds. In general, sheep affected with blowfly strike are restless and anorectic and move around with their head held close to the ground. The lesions are usually pruritic and/or painful, and sheep will bite, kick, rub, and shake the affected areas. The lesions formed are malodorous and become ulcerated, and the wool may be lifted above the surrounding normal wool. Severely affected sheep may die of toxemia and septicemia. Blowfly strike is often classified according to the anatomic site affected:

- Wound strike—occurs on any preexisting wound
- Breech, crutch, or tail strike—often follows scalding of the area from diarrhea or urine
- Pizzle strike—soiling of the sheath of rams and wethers with urine
- Poll strike—following fighting wounds or in sheep with excess folding of skin around the poll
- Body strike—affects the dorsum of the body after prolonged wetting and development of fleece rot

Diagnosis

Diagnosis is based on history and physical examination and demonstration of the larvae (maggots) in the affected areas. Larvae should be specifically identified as to genus and species and differentiated from screwworm larval myiasis, which is a reportable disease in the United States.

Treatment and Control

The primary efforts in the treatment of cutaneous myiasis should be directed toward control methods and prevention of the disease. This includes breeding of sheep for less wrinkling and a flatter breech; surgical removal of breech folds (Mule's operation) at the time of castration or tailing; crutching in midseason (clipping the wool from around the tail and breech); ringing (clipping wool from around the bell and sheath of rams); and use of an effective intestinal parasite control program to decrease diarrhea.

When weather conditions are optimal (prolonged warm, humid weather), routine spraying or dipping with organophosphates or pyrethroids is helpful in controlling adult flies and larvae. For individually affected sheep the lesions should be cleaned and debrided, followed by the application of a topical ointment containing an effective insecticide (malathion, coumaphos).

Screwworm Myiasis

Screwworm myiasis can be a severe and devastating disease of cattle, sheep, and swine and is a reportable disease in the United States.

Etiology and Pathogenesis

Screwworm myiasis is caused by the blowfly *Cochliomyia hominivorax*, which is an obligatory parasite of warm-blooded animals and birds that lays its eggs only on wounds of live animals and not carcasses. Adult flies lay large clusters of eggs at the edges of a fresh wound and are most active during periods of hot, humid weather. The larvae hatch in 10 to 12 hours and penetrate the tissue surrounding the wound. Larvae develop and mature over the next 3 to 7 days and then fall off of the host onto the ground and pupate. Under optimum conditions the life cycle is completed in 3 weeks. The invading larvae produce a liquefaction necrosis of the tissues, and anemia, hypoproteinemia, toxemia, and death can occur.

Clinical Signs

When compared with cutaneous myiasis, many of the initial signs of screwworm myiasis are similar; however, this form of myiasis is even more devastating. The larval invasion of screwworm larvae is more extensive than for other maggots, and the larvae burrow deep into healthy tissue rather than feeding on more superficial and necrotic tissue.

Diagnosis

Diagnosis is based on history and physical examination and on the demonstration of the larvae (maggots) in wounds. Larvae should be specifically identified as to genus and species (usually by submitting larvae preserved in 70 per cent alcohol to a qualified laboratory).

Treatment and Control

The primary efforts in the treatment of this disease have been directed toward control of the screwworm blowflies. In the United States, eradication of *C. hominivorax* was accomplished by the release of male flies that were sterilized by irradiation. Occasional screwworm myiasis occurs in the southern United States (primarily in Texas) since the disease still occurs in Mexico and Central America. The basic treatment recommendations for individually affected animals is as described for cutaneous myiasis.

HELMINTH INFESTATION

Onchocerciasis

Onchocerciasis (worm nodule disease) occurs in cattle in the United States and can cause ocular and skin lesions.

Etiology and Pathogenesis

Cutaneous onchocerciasis in cattle is caused by the adult worms of *Onchocerca gutturosa* and *O. lienalis*.[24, 25] The adult worms of *O. gutturosa* normally live in the ligamentum nuchae, and the adults of *O. lienalis* reside in the gastrosplenic ligament. However, these adult worms may also develop in the subcutaneous connective tissue where they may cause nodules. The microfilaria migrate into the dermis and are most numerous on the ventral midline (especially umbilical region), dorsal cervical midline, and facial area. These microfilaria are ingested by *Simulium* spp. and *Culicoides* spp., which serve as intermediate hosts in which the larvae develop into an infective stage. Subsequent feeding of these *Simulium* spp. and *Culicoides* spp. on other cattle results in the deposition of these infective larvae. These larvae then migrate to either the ligamentum nuchae or gastrosplenic ligament where they develop into adults, thus completing the life cycle.

Clinical Signs

Cutaneous onchocerciasis in cattle is characterized by the presence of asymptomatic subcutaneous nodules affecting the shoulder, stifle, and hip regions.

Diagnosis

The diagnosis of cutaneous onchocerciasis is based on history and physical findings and on the demonstration of the adult worm within an excised subcutaneous nodule. Histologic examination reveals a granulomatous to pyogranulomatous response, usually with evidence of the outer cuticle of the adult worm within the granuloma. The differential diagnosis includes bacterial or fungal granulomas, demodicosis, and neoplasia.

Treatment and Control

Surgical excision of individual nodules is the only treatment available since the adult worms of *Onchocerca* have not yet been effectively treated by any systemic parasitic agent.

Stephanofilariasis

Stephanofilariasis is a common skin disease in cattle of minor aesthetic and economic importance in the United States.

Etiology and Pathogenesis

Stephanofilariasis in cattle in the United States is caused by *Stephanofilaria stilesi*. Lesions often occur on the skin of the ventral abdomen. Adult worms form cyst-like structures at the base of hair follicles. Microfilaria are present in the surrounding dermis and lymphatics and are ingested by *Haematobia irritans* (horn fly) during feeding on the ventral abdomen, which serves as the intermediate host. The larvae develop within the fly into the infective stage and are then deposited in cutaneous wounds.

Clinical Signs

Stephanofilariasis in cattle is characterized by varying degrees of papules, crusts, small ulcers, alopecia, hyperkeratosis, and leukoderma. Lesions are most commonly located on the ventral abdomen or ventral chest. The disease is most often observed in the western and southwestern United States in beef cattle breeds.

Diagnosis

The diagnosis of stephanofilariasis in cattle is based on history and physical examination and on the demonstration of the adult worm within cystic structures at the base of hair follicles on skin biopsy.

Treatment and Control

Since stephanofilariasis is of such little economic importance, treatment is usually neither undertaken nor recommended. Infections due to *S. stilesi* have been noted to undergo spontaneous remission over a 2- to 3-year time period.

REFERENCES

1. Scott DW: Large Animal Dermatology, pp 207–283. Philadelphia, WB Saunders, 1988.
2. Mullowney PC: Dermatologic diseases. In Howard JL (ed): Current Veterinary Therapy 2: Food Animal Practice, pp 906–953. Philadelphia, WB Saunders, 1986.
3. Loomis EC: Epidemiology and control of ectoparasites of small ruminants. Vet Clin North Am [Food Anim Pract] 2(2):397–409, 1986.
4. Stromberg PC, Guillot FS: Pathogenesis of psoroptic scabies in Hereford heifer calves. Am J Vet Res 50:594–601, 1989.
5. Stromberg PC, Fisher WF: Dermatopathology and immunity in experimental *Psoroptes ovis* (Acari: Psoroptidae) infestation of naive and previously exposed Hereford cattle. Am J Vet Res 47:1551–1560, 1986.
6. Blood DC, Radostits OM (eds): Diseases caused by arthropod parasites. In Veterinary Medicine, 7th ed, pp 1071–1099. London, Baillière Tindall, 1989.
7. Stromberg PC, et al: Systemic pathologic responses in experimental *Psoroptes ovis* infestation of Hereford calves. Am J Vet Res 47:1326–1331, 1986.
8. Strickland RK, Gerrish RR: Infestivity of *Psoroptes ovis* on ivermectin-treated cattle. Am J Vet Res 48:342–344, 1987.
9. Arlian LG, Runyan RA, Estes SA: Cross infestivity of *Sarcoptes scabiei*. J Am Acad Dermatol 10:979–986, 1984.
10. Arlian LG, Vyszenski-Moher, DL, Cordova D: Host specificity of *S. scabiei* var. *canis* (Acari: Sarcoptidae) and the role of host odor. J Med Entomol 25:52–56, 1988.
11. Martineau GP, Van Neste D, Charette R: Pathophysiology of sarcoptic mange in swine: I. Compend Cont Ed Pract Vet 9:F51–F58, 1987.
12. Arlian LG, Estes SA, Vyszenski-Moher DL: Prevalence of *Sarcoptes scabiei* in the homes and nursing homes of scabietic patients. J Am Acad Dermatol 19:806–811, 1988.
13. Klayman E, Schillhorn van Veen TW: Vacuum cleaner method for the diagnosis of ectoparasitism. Mod Vet Pract October 1981, pp 767–771.
14. Hogg A: The control and eradication of sarcoptic mange in swine herds. Agri-Practice 10:8–10, 1989.
15. Alva-Valdes R, et al: Efficacy of an in-feed ivermectin formulation against gastrointestinal helminths, lungworms, and sarcoptic mites in swine. Am J Vet Res 50:1392–1395, 1989.
16. Barth D, Preston JM: Efficacy of topically administered ivermectin against chorioptic and sarcoptic mange of cattle. Vet Rec 123:101–104, 1988.
17. Wright FC, Guillot FS, George JE: Efficacy of acaricides against chorioptic mange of goats. Am J Vet Res 49:903–904, 1988.
18. Sinclair A: The epidermal location and possible feeding site of *Psorergates ovis*, the sheep itch mite. Aust Vet J 67:59–62, 1990.
19. Berkenkamp SD: Hypodermosis: I. Comp Food Anim 12:740–746, 1990.
20. Pruett JH, Barrett CC: Induction of intradermal skin reaction in the bovine by fractionated proteins of *Hypoderma lineatum*. Vet Parasitol 16:137–145, 1984.
21. Prieto M, et al: Effect of ivermectin treatment on anti–hypodermin C titers of Asturiana cattle naturally infected with *Hypoderma lineatum*. Vet Parasitol 35:211–218, 1990.
22. Alva-Valdes R, et al: Efficacy of ivermectin in a topical formulation against gastrointestinal and pulmonary nematode infections and naturally acquired grubs and lice in cattle. Am J Vet Res 47:2389–2392, 1986.
23. Berkenkamp SD: Hypodermosis: II. Compend Cont Ed Pract Vet 12:881–887, 1990.
24. Ferenc SA, et al: *Onchocerca gutturosa* and *Onchocerca lienalis* in cattle: effect of age, sex, and origin on prevalence of onchocerciasis in subtropical and temperate regions of Florida and Georgia. Am J Vet Res 47:2266–2268, 1986.
25. Harty TM: *Onchocerca gutturosa* and *Onchocerca lienalis* in cattle: variation in length of microfilaria by site of recovery. Am J Vet Res 50:169–172, 1989.

Fungal Dermatoses
LINDA MEDLEAU, DVM, MS, Diplomate, ACVD
ZORANA RISTIC, DVM
NORMA E. WHITE-WEITHERS, DVM

DERMATOPHYTOSIS

Dermatophytes are a group of taxonomically related fungi with affinity for cornified epidermis, hair, horn, nails, and feathers. The dermatophytes that most frequently cause skin disease in large animals are members of the genera *Microspo-*

rum and *Trichophyton*. More than 30 species of *Microsporum* and *Trichophyton* have been identified, but only a few of them commonly affect large animals (Table 1).

Depending on their natural habitat, species of dermatophytes may be categorized as geophilic, zoophilic, or anthropophilic. Geophilic dermatophytes such as *M. gypseum* inhabit soil where they probably decompose keratinous debris. Zoophilic dermatophytes *(M. canis, T. mentagrophytes, T. verrucosum, T. equinum)* are not known to live in soil but are specialized parasites that live on the skin of animals. *Microsporum nanum* is both geophilic and zoophilic because it parasitizes pig skin and grows in soil from pig yards. Anthropophilic dermatophytes are primarily parasitic on humans and do not readily cause infections in animals.

Animals become infected with geophilic dermatophytes when they are exposed to contaminated soil. Infections with geophilic fungi tend to occur sporadically and are not readily contagious between animals. Infections with zoophilic dermatophytes are more common, especially in young animals kept in close contact with each other. Although high humidity and temperature, trauma, and poor nutrition may be predisposing factors, close confinement seems to be more important in the spread of this disease. Dermatophytosis occurs more often when animals are housed in crowded conditions for long periods, and outbreaks often occur during the winter. Infection may spread directly by contact with clinically infected or asymptomatic carrier animals or indirectly by contact with contaminated fomites (e.g., posts, gates, troughs, stanchions). Because immunologic status determines animal susceptibility, young animals are predisposed to infection. An infection that becomes widespread in winter usually clears up spontaneously after the animals are turned out to pasture in the spring. This may be the result of better nutrition and/or from the direct influence of light.

Lesions usually appear 1 to 2 weeks after exposure. Extensive hyphal growth and spore formation in the stratum corneum results in hyperkeratosis. Fungal hyphae also invade the ostium of hair follicles, proliferate on the surface of hair, and migrate downward to the hair bulb. Infected hairs become brittle, dry, and lusterless and break off. Ring-shaped lesions develop when the fungal invasion spreads centrifugally from its point of initial invasion. In cattle, lesions are characteristically circular, scaly, and hairless and are usually distributed on the neck, head, and trunk. Pruritus and pain are usually absent. In goats, the ears, head, neck, and limbs are typically affected. Lesions resemble those seen in cattle. In sheep, circumscribed alopecic lesions with thick, grayish crusts are most often found on the head and ears, and occasionally on the legs and around the tail. Affected sheep may have intense pruritus, leading to the development of secondary excoriations. Involvement of fleeced skin is rare, but when it does occur it is usually characterized by the development of nonpruritic raised plaques to which wool is still attached. After the plaques break off, well-defined, circumscribed, erythematous, scabby lesions remain that may become confluent. Lesion appearance in swine depends on the species of infecting dermatophyte. In *M. nanum* infections the lesions appear mainly behind the ears and on the trunk and are characterized by annular areas of reddish brown discoloration covered with superficial, dry, brown crusts. In *T. mentagrophytes* and *T. verrucosum* infections, the back, flanks, and head are usually affected. Lesions are characterized early by small, gray papules covered with scales that form reddish pseudoscabs that coalesce into raised, circumscribed, and erythematous lesions.

Direct microscopic examination and culture of skin scrapings and hairs from the periphery of lesions are necessary to confirm a clinical diagnosis of dermatophytosis. Skin scrapings are placed in a drop of 20 per cent potassium hydroxide solution, gently warmed, and examined under the microscope with reduced lighting. Hyphae and conidia (spores) may be present in scales and on hairs.

For culture, hairs and scales within and adjacent to lesions should be selected. Culture specimens should be transported in an envelope or Petri dish. Sealed glass or plastic containers should not be used because moisture can accumulate that permits growth of contaminating fungi and bacteria. Dermatophyte Test Media (DTM) is the most commonly used culture media for isolating dermatophytes in veterinary practice. Dermatophyte Test Media is available commercially in glass screw-capped containers (Fungassay)* or in dual compartment plates with DTM on one side and plain Sabouraud's dextrose agar on the other (Sab-Duets).† Dermatophyte Test Media contains the pH indicator phenol red, chlortetracycline, and gentamicin to inhibit bacterial growth, and also cyclohexamide, which inhibits some saprophytic fungi. When cultured on DTM, dermatophytes prefer to utilize protein, which causes the media to turn red. The red color change occurs simultaneously with the appearance of colony growth. Color change and colony growth usually occur within 7 days of culture inoculation. Dermatophyte colonies are white, cream, or buff colored. Saprophytic fungi may also grow on DTM cultures. Saprophytes prefer to utilize carbohydrates so that as the colony appears the media remains yellow. After all carbohydrates are utilized, saprophytes may then utilize protein. However, colony growth will be well established before the color change occurs, indicating that the fungus is not a dermatophyte. Consequently, DTM cultures should be examined daily for 2 weeks to determine if any color change occurs with colony growth or afterward. Also, darkly colored colonies are saprophytes regardless of when color change occurs.

Most dermatophytes grow well at room temperature (28°C to 30°C), but *T. verrucosum* grows best at 37°C. Also, most strains of *T. equinum* require nicotinic acid (niacin) and all strains of *T. verrucosum* require thiamine to produce macroconidia. Therefore, it is recommended that 2 drops of sterile, injectable vitamin B complex solution be applied to the surface of culture media prior to inoculation. Some strains of *T. verrucosum* also require inositol in the medium to form macroconidia.

Positive identification of cultured fungi should be made by examining slide preparations of the fungal colony. The sticky surface of acetate tape is touched to the surface of the fungal colony just proximal to its advancing periphery. The tape is then pressed, sticky side down, on a microscope slide with a drop of lactophenol cotton blue stain and examined under the microscope. Characteristic appearances of macroconidia and microconidia for several dermatophyte species are listed in Table 2.

Spontaneous recovery in cattle and sheep usually occurs within 6 to 12 weeks, but treatment is indicated if lesions

Table 1. DERMATOPHYTES OF VETERINARY IMPORTANCE THAT CAUSE SKIN DISEASE IN LARGE ANIMALS

	Cattle	Sheep	Goats	Swine
Microsporum canis	Rare	Rare	Rare	Rare
M. Gypseum	Rare	Rare	Rare	Rare
M. nanum	Rare			Common
Trichophyton equinum	Rare			
T. mentagrophytes	Occasional	Occasional	Occasional	Occasional
T. verrucosum	Common	Occasional	Occasional	Rare

---
*Available from Pitman Moore, Mundelein, IL 60060.
†Available from Bacti-Labs, Mountain View, CA 94042.

Table 2. MICROSCOPIC MORPHOLOGY OF DERMATOPHYTE SPECIES

Species	Macroconidia	Microconidia
Microsporum canis	Long, spindle shaped Rough, thick wall Asymmetric knob More than six compartments	Club or pear shaped
M. gypseum	Cucumber shaped Rough, thin wall Up to six compartments	Club shaped
M. nanum	Egg-shaped Rough surface One to three compartments	Club shaped
Trichophyton mentagrophytes	Cigar shaped Smooth, thin wall	Globe shaped Singly or in grape-like clusters
T. verrucosum	String bean shaped	Tear shaped
T. equinum	Club shaped Smooth, thin wall	Pear to globe shaped Stalked along hyphae

worsen or if halting the spread of dermatophytosis is desired. In the early stages of an outbreak when affected animals are few in number, the lesions can be treated topically. Crusts from the lesions are scraped or brushed off with a soft brush. Removed crusts are burnt so that they do not contaminate the environment. A topical antifungal product is then applied to the lesions and rubbed in. Topical products that can be used for localized lesions include povidone-iodine ointment and thiabendazole paste. Lesions should be treated once a day until they resolve. When infection is widespread, antifungal solutions that are sprayed on the bodies of all animals every 1 to 2 weeks should be used. Sprays of 400 pounds pressure should be used to remove crusts and scales so that the antifungal solution can penetrate the lesions. If there is no reinfection, lesions should resolve in 8 to 16 weeks. Topical products that can be used for treating generalized dermatophytosis include 2 to 5 per cent lime sulfur solution, 3 per cent captan, iodophors, and 0.5 per cent sodium hypochlorite. Sprays containing 100 ppm of natamycin have also been reported to be effective. Lime sulfur solution and iodophors may stain or be irritating to the skin. Captan is not approved for use in food animals and is a potent contact sensitizer in humans.

Systemic therapy is occasionally used in conjunction with topical treatment. Sodium iodide (1 g/14 kg body weight) as a 10 per cent solution administered intravenously at weekly intervals has been reported to be effective in farm animals. Orally administered griseofulvin has also been reported to be beneficial. Good response to griseofulvin has been noted in calves treated with 5 to 7.5 mg/kg/day for 7 days and in pigs treated with 1 g/100kg/day for 30 to 40 days. Griseofulvin is not approved for use in food animals.

Fungal spores can remain viable for years, and contaminated objects are a potential source for reinfection. To control an outbreak of dermatophytosis, the premises should be cleaned and treated with 5 per cent sodium hypochlorite solution, 3 per cent captan, or 2.5 to 5 per cent phenolic disinfectant.

A live vaccine (LTF-130) prepared in the Russian Republic from the mycelium of *T. verrucosum* has been used to successfully treat cattle in Europe and Scandinavia. This vaccine works prophylactically, giving protection for 3 to 5 years, and therapeutically to produce remissions within a few weeks of administration. Best results are achieved when newly infected herds with few clinical cases are vaccinated. Results are poorer in herds with a long-standing problem.

MYCETOMA

A mycetoma is a chronic fungal or bacterial granulomatous infection of the skin and subcutaneous tissues characterized by tumefaction, draining sinuses, and granules. Discharges are usually mucopurulent and contain granules composed of fungal or bacterial colonies and filaments. Mycetomas are either eumycotic or actinomycotic.

Eumycotic mycetomas are caused by fungi that normally inhabit the soil and vegetation. These fungi can be dematiacious (black grained) or nonpigmented (white grained). Infections are usually associated with penetrating wounds. Eumycotic mycetomas are rare in food animals, although black-grained mycetomas caused by *Drechslera rostrata* and *Helminthosporium speciferum* have been reported in cattle. All affected cattle had nasal granulomas that were ulcerated, suppurative, and fibrotic. Some also had ulcerated nodules on the rump, thighs, ears, tail, and/or vulva.

The actinomycotic mycetomas are caused by bacteria belonging to the genera *Nocardia*, *Actinomyces*, and *Actinobacillus*. These bacteria are environmental saphrophytes and can also be normal inhabitants of respiratory and digestive tracts in animals. The mode of infection is through wound contamination.

Nocardiosis in cattle usually causes mastitis. Skin disease (bovine farcy) has also been reported. Bovine farcy is characterized by painless, firm, subcutaneous nodules that tend to occur on the limbs, head, and neck but can be anywhere. Lesions may ulcerate and discharge odorless thick cheesy gray or yellow exudate. Lymphadenitis and regional lymphadenopathy are usually present.

Bovine actinomycosis is a chronic disease that usually involves the mandible and maxilla (lumpy jaw). Affected cattle develop painless, bony swellings of the jaw with abscesses and fistulous tracts containing small amounts of viscid, yellow pus and yellow-white "sulfur granules." Actinomycosis in sows is characterized by chronic suppurative mastitis, granulating ulcers on the udder, and granulomatous nodules or abscesses on the abdomen.

Actinobacillosis is seen in cattle, sheep, and rarely swine. In cattle the disease usually involves the tongue, which becomes swollen and hard (wooden tongue), and, less frequently, other tissue such as skeletal muscle and liver. Cutaneous actinobacillosis without tongue involvement has also been reported in cattle. Affected animals had ulcers and nodules in the mouth and on the head, chest, flanks, and thighs. In sheep, actinobacillosis is a purulent disease of the skin, lymph nodes, lung, and soft tissues of the head and neck. Epididymitis is also common in rams. In swine, actinobacillosis may be associated with soft tissue infections of the mammary glands and head, endocarditis, osteomyelitis, pneumonia, and suppurative joint lesions.

The diagnosis of mycetoma is based on cytology, culture, and biopsy. Swabs from draining sinuses or smears of crushed granules may reveal fungal or bacterial elements on cytology. In eumycotic mycetomas, pigmented or hyaline fungi with hyphae ranging from 2 to 4 μm in diameter are seen. In actinomycotic mycetomas, the bacterial organisms are well visualized with Gram's stain. *Nocardia* species appear as beaded gram-positive, thin (0.5 to 1 μm) branching filaments and bacillary forms. The organisms are also partially acid fast. *Actinomyces* species appear as small (1 μm) filaments, rods, and cocci that are gram positive and non-acid fast. Actinobacilli are gram-negative bacilli. Skin biopsy specimens reveal nodular to diffuse suppurative, pyogranulomatous, or granulomatous dermatitis, in which granules containing masses of the fungal or bacterial organism are seen. Fungal culture on plain Sabouraud's dextrose agar and bacterial culture on brain heart infusion agar should be performed for definitive identification of the organism.

Surgical excision and amputation are recommended for eumycotic mycetomas in humans and small animals. No treatment has been reported in food animals. For actinomycotic mycetomas, iodides, sulfonamides, triple sulfas, tetracycline, streptomycin, penicillin, and isoniazid have been used in food animals with variable results.

PHAEOHYPHOMYCOSIS

Phaeohyphomycosis is a subcutaneous infection caused by dematiacious (dark pigmented) fungi. These fungi are soil and vegetation inhabitants that gain entrance to the body through wounds. Phaeohyphomycosis is extremely rare in food animals.

The fungi *Dreschslera rostrata* and *Phaeosclera dematiodes* have been isolated in cattle and *Peyronella glomerata* has been isolated from goats. Lesions consisted of raised nodules with draining tracts that grossly resembled mycetomas.

The diagnosis of phaeohyphomycosis is based on biopsy and culture. Histologically, a suppurative, granulomatous, or pyogranulomatous nodular dermatitis is present. The presence of dark-walled septate hyphae differentiates phaeohyphomycosis from mycetomas, which contain granules but not septate hyphae. For culture, tissue exudate or biopsy specimens should be placed on plain Sabouraud's dextrose agar. Cultures should be incubated at 25°C to 30°C. Depending on the organism, growth may be rapid or slow. Identification is based on the microscopic morphology of the fungus.

Surgical excision or amputation, amphotericin B, 5-fluorocytosine, ketoconazole, and local hyperthermia have all been tried in small animals and humans with variable results. No treatment has been reported in food animals.

PYTHIOSIS

Pythiosis or phycomycosis is a chronic subcutaneous fungal infection that usually affects the distal extremities and/or the ventrum. It is caused by a *Pythium* species, *Hyphomyces destruens,* and occurs most commonly in tropical and semitropical climates.

Pythiosis has been reported in horses, dogs, and cattle. It also occurs in plants, where it destroys their roots ("wet feet"). In horses it is also known as "swamp cancer," "Florida horse leech," or "Gulf Coast fungus," since it occurs most often in the states bordering the Gulf of Mexico. Pythiosis has also been reported in Australia, New Guinea, Indonesia, Japan, Brazil, and Colombia. Because *Pythium* species require high environmental temperature and humidity for their growth and reproduction, infections occur most often during the summer and fall in tropical and temperate areas.

Pythium species are aquatic fungi with aquatic motile zoospores, which seem to be chemotactically attracted to damaged plant and animal tissue. The strong association between *Pythium* infection and the exposure to standing fresh water explains why lesions are usually found on the animal's legs and ventral abdomen. Antecedent trauma may offer zoospores the chance to invade damaged tissue.

Pythiosis in food animals is rare, with only six cases in beef calves reported. In all six calves, lesions were confined to the distal extremities, especially the fetlocks and the ventral abdomen, and were characterized by focal ulceration with dermal thickening, draining tracts, and watery purulent exudation. When the skin above the fetlocks was affected, diffuse periarticular swelling was also noticed. Coral-like bodies containing large masses of hyphae ("kunkers," "leeches"), typically found in fistulae in equine pythiosis, were not present in the infected calves.

The diagnosis of pythiosis is based on biopsy and culture. In bovine pythiosis, skin biopsy specimens reveal multifocal pyogranulomas or granulomas surrounded by dense fibrous connective tissue. In the center of the granulomas smooth-walled, branching 4- to 8-μm hyphae are found. Hyphae are partially surrounded by refractile granular material (Splendore-Hoeppli phenomenon). The hyphae stain easily with hematoxylin and eosin, Giemsa methenamine silver, or Gridley's stain.

Pythium species can be cultured on Sabouraud's dextrose agar or on 0.5 per cent vegetable extract agar. Tissue specimens should be washed vigorously in water, minced into 1-mm cubes, implanted in agar, and incubated at 37°C; identification is based on morphology of the hyphae.

Treatment of cutaneous pythiosis is indicated as lesions are discovered. In horses, surgical extirpation with several "retrims" in combination with intravenous amphotericin B therapy has been reported. The expense of amphotericin B, however, is a major limiting factor in the treatment of pythiosis in food animals. Immunotherapy with a phenolized *Pythium* vaccine was successfully used in horses that had lesions for less than 2 months, if the lesions were surgically removed at the beginning of the treatment.

Of the calves with pythiosis, two were treated with systemic tetracyclines, penicillin, sodium iodide, levamisole, topical povidone-iodine scrubs, and a *Pythium* vaccine with minimal to no improvement.

ASPERGILLOSIS

Aspergillus species are ubiquitous and can be found in soil and decaying vegetation in most parts of the world. *Aspergillus* is a monomorphic mold that produces large numbers of microconidia (spores) that are released into the environment and disposed by air. Humans and animals are more or less constantly exposed to these spores, but infection is uncommon. Aspergillosis usually occurs secondary to some other predisposing factor such as stress, excessive exposure to fungal contamination, prolonged antibiotic or corticosteroid therapy, or underlying immunodeficiency disease.

In food animals, aspergillosis has been most often associated with pulmonary disease, gastroenteritis, mastitis, and abortions. Cutaneous infections are rare, but aspergilli have been isolated from a subcutaneous granuloma in a Holstein-Friesen cow, from multiple cutaneous plaques on aborted calves, from granulomatous skin lesions in a male goat, and from papular skin lesions in pigs.

Aspergilli are common fungal contaminants in the laboratory and can be routinely cultured from the skin of normal animals. A presumptive diagnosis of aspergillosis can be made only if an *Aspergillus* species is repeatedly isolated from clinical material collected on successive days. Cultures are performed on Sabouraud's dextrose agar.

The best method of diagnosing aspergillosis is to substantiate cultural results by finding histologic evidence that the organisms are in tissue specimens. Aspergilli stain with hematoxylin and eosin; are highlighted with periodic acid–Schiff, Giemsa's methenamine silver, acid orcein–Giemsa (AOG), or Gridley's stain; and are characterized by narrow, septate, hyaline, branching hyphae with terminal bullous dilatations.

No treatment has been reported in large animals.

YEAST DERMATITIS

There are few reports of yeast dermatitis in food animals. Cutaneous lesions associated with *Candida albicans* infection have been reported in pigs exposed to wet conditions. Affected pigs developed small, discrete, circumscribed skin lesions that coalesced to form large areas of moist, exudative dermatitis on the lower limbs, thighs, and ventral aspects of the abdomen. Lesions resolved a few weeks after the pigs were moved to dry housing.

Yeast dermatitis resembling candidiasis has also been described in goats. Affected goats had generalized exfoliative dermatitis characterized by alopecia, scaling, crusting, lichenification, and greasiness. Budding yeasts and pseudohyphae were demonstrated in skin biopsy specimens, but fungal cultures were negative. Affected animals were killed or lost to follow-up before treatment could be initiated.

BIBLIOGRAPHY

Blood DC, Radostits OM, Henderson JA: Veterinary Medicine, 6th ed. London, Baillière Tindall, 1983.

Fraser CM (ed): The Merck Veterinary Manual, 6th ed. Rahway, NJ, Merck and Co., 1986.

Penny RHC, Muirhead MR: Skin. *In* Lehman AD, Straw B, Glock RD, et al (eds): Diseases of Swine, 6th ed, pp 82–100. Ames, Iowa State University Press, 1986.

Timoney JF, Gillespie JH, Scott FW, Barlough JE: Hagan and Bruner's Microbiology and Infectious Diseases of Domestic Animals, pp 366–424. Ithaca, NY, Comstock Publishing Associates, 1988.

Scott DW: Large Animal Dermatology, pp 136–202. Philadelphia, WB Saunders, 1988.

Bacterial Skin Diseases

S. D. WHITE, DVM, Diplomate, ACVD

Bacterial skin diseases of food animals are among the more devastating diseases in terms of economic loss. Numerous bacteria have been noted to cause skin disease in cattle, sheep, goats, pigs, and llamas; only the more important and common diseases are covered here. For other diseases the reader is encouraged to consult the sources listed in the bibliography.

DERMATOPHILOSIS

Dermatophilosis is a common superficial, pustular, crusting, and/or ulcerative dermatitis of cattle, sheep, goats, swine, and llamas caused by *Dermatophilus congolensis*.

Etiology and Pathogenesis

D. congolensis is a gram-positive facultative anaerobic actinomycete whose natural habitat is unknown. Attempts to isolate the bacteria from soils have been unsuccessful. *D. congolensis* has been isolated only from the skin of infected animals. The three most common factors in the initiation and development of dermatophilosis are skin damage, moisture, and (theoretically) the presence of asymptomatic, chronically infected carrier animals. Moisture causes the release of the infective, motile, flagellated loose spore form of the organism. Important sources of skin damage include biting flies and arthropods, prickly vegetation, and maceration. The distribution of clinical lesions (e.g., dorsum, distal extremities) often mirrors these environmental insults or sources of moisture (e.g., rain, mud, moist or unclean stalls). Crusts from infected animals are important potential sources of infection and reinfection. Dermatophilosis is a contagious disease. The incubation period averages about 2 weeks but may vary from 1 day to 5 weeks.

Clinical Signs

No age, breed, or sex predilections to dermatophilosis have been noted. Infections may infect a single animal or a majority of the herd.

The primary lesions in dermatophilosis are follicular and nonfollicular papules and pustules. However, these lesions rapidly coalesce and become exudative, which results in groups of hairs becoming matted together, resembling a paintbrush. Close examination shows the proximal portions of these hairs to be embedded in dried exudate. When these paintbrush-like mats are plucked off, areas of purulent or ulcerated skin are revealed. Active lesions contain a thick, creamy, whitish, yellowish or greenish pus that adheres to the skin surface and to the undersurface of the crusts. Acute active lesions of dermatophilosis are often painful, but the disease is rarely pruritic, except in llamas. The healing/chronic stage of the disease is characterized by dried crusts, scaling, and alopecia that may resemble dermatophytosis (ringworm).

In goats, the lesions of dermatophilosis are commonly seen on the pinna and tail of kids and the muzzle, dorsal midline, and scrotum of adults. Lesions may be limited to the distal limbs, resembling the "strawberry foot rot" form of dermatophilosis found in sheep.

In sheep, the most common clinical forms of dermatophilosis are crusts occurring from the coronary bands to the tarsi and carpi with underlying bleeding, fleshy masses of tissue (strawberry foot rot); pyramidal crusts over the topline and flanks (so-called mycotic dermatitis); and crusts on the ears, nose, and face of lambs.

In cattle, dermatophilosis may affect the rump and topline; face and ears (especially in calves [milk scald] and bulls); brisket, axilla, and groin; udder and teats or scrotum and prepuce; distal limbs; and perineum and tail. Animals with over 50 per cent of their body affected often show rapid weight loss and dehydration and die.

Dermatophilosis has been noted in the llama, usually over the dorsum, sides, or distal extremities during warm, rainy weather. Lesions are generally not painful but may be pruritic.

Dermatophilosis is very rare in swine. Affected pigs have a generalized exudative crusting dermatitis. Dual infections with *D. congolensis* and *Staphylococcus hyicus* have been reported. It should be remembered that dermatophilosis is a zoonosis, although human infections are relatively rare.

Diagnosis

The differential diagnosis of dermatophilosis is extensive, including dermatophytosis, staphylococcal folliculitis and furunculosis, viral infections, zinc-responsive dermatosis, and pemphigus foliaceus. In general, cutaneous crusts in food animals should be considered dermatophilosis until proven otherwise. Definitive diagnosis is based on direct smear, skin biopsy, and culture. Direct smears of pus or saline-soaked and minced crust may be stained with new methylene blue, Diff-Quik, or Gram stains. *D. congolensis* appears as fine branching and multiseptate hyphae that divide transversely and longitudinally to form cuboidal packets of coccoid cells arranged in parallel rows within branching filaments (railroad track appearance). In the healing or chronic stages of the disease, direct smears are rarely positive. Skin biopsy usually reveals varying degrees of folliculitis, intradermal pustular dermatitis, and superficial perivascular dermatitis. Intracellular edema with keratinocytes may be striking. Surface crust is characterized by alternating layers of orthokeratosis or parakeratosis and leukocytic debris (palisading crusts). *D. congolensis* is usually seen in the keratinous debris on the surface of the skin and within hair follicles. The organism is best visualized with Giemsa's, Brown and Brenn's, or acid orcein-Giemsa stains. A nodular to diffuse dermatitis resulting from granulomatous inflammation may be noted occasionally. *D. congolensis* grows well in blood agar when incubated in a microaerophilic atmosphere with increased carbon dioxide. However, the culture can be unsatisfactory as a result of rapid overgrowth of secondary invaders and contaminating saprophytes and in the chronic nonexudative stage. In such instances, incubating the crusts for several hours in saline and subsequently culturing this "broth" may be helpful.

Treatment

Recommended topical therapy includes the iodophors, 2 to 5 per cent lime sulfur, 0.5 per cent zinc sulfate, 0.2 per cent copper sulfate, and 1 per cent potassium aluminum sulfate (alum). The first three substances may stain hair and wool. Topical solutions are applied as total body washes, sprays, or dips for 3 to 5 consecutive days and then weekly until healing has occurred. In flocks of sheep where elimination of dermatophilosis is impractical, routine summer and fall protective dips with a 0.5 per cent zinc sulfate or 1 per cent potassium aluminum sulfate are reported to be effective.

The most commonly used systemic antibiotics in the treatment of dermatophilosis are penicillin and streptomycin. Various regimens have been recommended; the most common of these for cattle, sheep, goats, and llamas is 5000 IU/kg procaine penicillin G and 5 mg/kg streptomycin daily for 4 to 5 days. In addition, every attempt should be made to remove and dispose of crusts, to keep the animals dry, to give good quality nutrition, and to control the biting arthropod population.

STAPHYLOCOCCAL INFECTIONS

Most investigators recognize three clinically important coagulase-positive species of staphylococci: *Staphylococcus aureus, S. intermedius,* and *S. hyicus.* The relative percentage of the first two staphylococcal species isolated from lesions may vary among animal species. However, differences in antimicrobial susceptibility patterns between *S. aureus* and *S. intermedius* are probably not significant. *S. hyicus* is usually clinically important only in swine. When possible, bacterial cultures should always be performed in cases of staphylococcal pyoderma. It is my impression that the number of penicillinase-resistant coagulase-positive staphylococci species in food animals is increasing.

Impetigo

Impetigo is defined as a superficial pustular dermatitis that does not involve hair follicles. It occurs in goats, sheep, and cattle. Predisposing factors may include the stress of parturition, moist and filthy environments, and trauma. No age or breed predilections are apparent, but female animals appear to be predisposed to infection. Lesions occur most commonly on the udder, with the base of the teats and the intramammary sulcus most often affected. Occasionally, lesions may spread to the teats, ventral abdomen, medial thighs, perineum, and ventral surface of the tail. Superficial vesicles readily become pustular, rupture and leave erosions, and yield a brown crust. Pruritus and pain are rare, and affected animals usually suffer no systemic disturbance unless staphylococcal mastitis ensues. The differential diagnosis includes dermatophilosis, dermatophytosis, and viral infections. The definitive diagnosis is based on direct smear, skin biopsy, and culture. Skin biopsy reveals subcorneal pustular dermatitis with cocci often visible within the pustules. Therapy with daily topical medicines (chlorhexidine, iodophors) usually results in rapid healing within a few days. Systemic antibiotics are rarely needed but when indicated should be based on results of culture and sensitivity testing. Impetigo may be spread by the milker to other cattle and goats. Affected animals should be milked last, single-service paper towels should be used, and the hands of the milker should be washed after contact with infected animals.

Exudative Epidermitis

Exudative epidermitis is an acute generalized exudative vesiculopustular disease of suckling pigs caused by *Staphylococcus hyicus.* Research suggests that this disease may be caused not by *S. hyicus* infection per se but by some toxins elaborated by the microorganism. This is quite similar to the staphylococcal scalded skin syndrome in humans. Because *S. hyicus* can be isolated from the skin, ears, and nostrils of most normal pigs, many authors believe that clinical disease requires some combination of the bacteria and predisposed piglets (skin trauma, inadequate nutrition, other diseases, or stress). The incidence of this disease is not high, but the disease can be a severe problem on individual farms. Exudative epidermitis is most commonly seen in suckling pigs of 1 to 7 weeks of age with no breed or sex predilection. Morbidity varies from 10 to 90 per cent and mortality from 5 to 90 (average 20) per cent. The disease is nonseasonal, and hygiene and management are often good in affected herds. The incubation period is 3 to 4 days.

Clinically, exudative epidermitis may be divided into peracute, acute, and subacute forms. In the peracute form, a dark brown, greasy exudate appears periocularly, followed by a vesicopustular eruption on the nose, lips, tongue, gums, and coronets. Red-brown macules then appear behind the ears and on the ventral abdomen and medial thighs. The entire body is then covered by erythema, a moist greasy exudate, and thick brown crusts, hence the older term *greasy pig disease*. The feet are frequently affected, with erosions of the coronary band and heel. Conjunctivitis is common, and excessive exudation may result in the adherence of eyelids and blindness. The piglets show progressive depression, anorexia, and polydipsia and usually die within 3 to 5 days. Pruritus, pain, and fever are usually absent.

The acute form follows the general pattern of the peracute form. The skin becomes thicker and wrinkled, and the total body exudate then becomes hardened and cracked, resulting in a furrowed appearance. Death often occurs within 4 to 8 days.

In the subacute form, skin lesions are often confined to the head and ears and are less exudative. The piglets are usually healthy otherwise and recover spontaneously.

The differential diagnosis of exudative epidermitis includes swine parakeratosis, streptococcal pyoderma, biotin deficiency, and viral infections. The definitive diagnosis is based on skin biopsy and culture. Skin biopsy reveals subcorneal vesicular pustular dermatitis. A mild to moderate degree of acantholysis may be seen. With special stains, gram-positive cocci may be seen within the vesicles and pustules. *S. hyicus* may be cultured from vesiculopustular and consistently from the conjunctiva. Necropsy findings in pigs with exudative epidermitis include dilatation of ureters and renal pelves as a result of ureteral obstruction caused by edema, cellular infiltration, hyperplasia, and mucoid degeneration of ureteral epithelium; serous lymphadenitis, and mild catarrhal gastroenteritis.

The efficacy of any treatment for exudative epidermitis decreases as the duration and severity of the infection increases. Clinical and experimental evidence suggests that vitamin B (especially biotin) supplementation is helpful in therapy and prevention. Antimicrobial susceptibility tests should be performed in cases of exudative epidermitis owing to regional differences in antibiotic resistance. In penicillin-susceptible strains, early treatment with penicillin (5000 IU/kg twice daily), given intramuscularly for 3 to 5 days, may be effective. Tylosin (8 mg/kg), given intramuscularly for 2 to 3 days, has also been reported to be beneficial. Topical treatment with a cleansing, degreasing, and antimicrobial agent is also helpful. If conjunctivitis is severe, an antibiotic eye ointment is helpful. Affected piglets should be kept isolated, and exposed piglets should also be treated. Reducing factors predisposing to skin injuries and scrupulous hygiene will often limit an outbreak of exudative epidermitis.

Folliculitis and Furunculosis

Staphylococcal folliculitis (inflammation of the hair follicle) and furunculosis (a folliculitis that has broken through the wall of the hair follicle and now involves the surrounding dermis) are common in goats, sheep, and llamas, and uncommon in cattle and swine. The primary skin lesion of folliculitis is a follicular papule. Pustules may arise from these papules. Erect hairs are frequently noticed over a papule that is more easily felt than seen. These lesions often progressively enlarge and then become encrusted. The chronic healing phase is characterized by progressive flattening of the lesion and a gradually expanding circular area of alopecia and scaling. Hairs at the periphery of these lesions are often easily epilated, thus mimicking dermatophytosis (ringworm). Some lesions progress to furunculosis. This stage is distinguished by varying combinations of nodules, draining tracts, ulcers, and crusts. Scarring and occasionally leukoderma and leukotrichia may follow.

In goats, staphylococcal folliculitis and furunculosis have no age, breed, or sex predilection. Skin lesions are most commonly seen on the face, pinna, udder, ventral abdomen, medial thigh, perineum, and distal limbs. Deeper lesions are often warm and painful. Severe infections, especially with secondary mastitis, may produce pyrexia, anorexia, depression, and septicemia.

Staphylococcal folliculitis and furunculosis are also common in sheep. They may occur as benign pustular dermatitis (plooks) in otherwise healthy 3- to 4-week-old lambs, especially on the lips and perineum, which spontaneously regresses within 3 weeks. The condition also occurs as a severe facial dermatitis (facial and periorbital eczema, eye scab) in sheep of all ages, but especially in adult ewes just prior to lambing. Pustules, nodules, ulcers, and black scabs develop on the face, pinna, and horn base. This facial form appears to be contagious, and spread through a flock has been attributed to infections of head abrasions while animals are feeding in troughs or fighting.

In llamas, staphylococcal folliculitis usually presents as focal, usually nonpruritic, asymmetric areas of alopecia causing an exudation. The head or distal extremities are most commonly involved. In a limited number of animals, *Staphylococcus intermedius* has been the most consistently recovered organism on culture.

Staphylococcal folliculitis and furunculosis are uncommon in cattle. Trauma and poor hygiene are believed to be initiating factors. Lesions are most commonly found on the tail and perineum and less commonly on the scrotum and face. Pruritus and pain are variable.

In swine, staphylococcal folliculitis and furunculosis are also uncommon. No breed or sex predilection is apparent. The condition is most frequently seen in pigs younger than 8 weeks of age, and asymptomatic erythematous pustular dermatitis covers much of the body, especially the hind quarters, abdomen, and chest. The dermatosis usually regresses spontaneously within 3 weeks.

The most important differential diagnosis of staphylococcal folliculitis/furunculosis on the general body surface includes dermatophilosis and dermatophytosis. Definitive diagnosis is based on direct smears, skin biopsy, and culture. Skin biopsy reveals varying degrees of perifolliculitis, folliculitis, and furunculosis, with extensive tissue eosinophilia often accompanying the furunculosis. Bacteria may be visible with special stains.

Therapy of staphylococcal folliculitis/furunculosis varies with severity and stage of the disease. Most cases require topical cleansing, drying, and systemic antibacterial therapy. The author recommends daily applications of chlorhexidine for 5 to 7 days and then twice weekly until the infection is resolved. The choice of systemic antibiotics is best made on the basis of culture and sensitivity testing.

CORYNEBACTERIUM PSEUDOTUBERCULOSIS INFECTIONS

Corynebacterium pseudotuberculosis is a gram-positive, pleomorphic short rod. This bacterium requires various predisposing factors to become established as an infection; good management practices may be the most important means of controlling infections. The most common manifestation of *C. pseudotuberculosis* involving the skin in food animals is caseous lymphadenitis of sheep and goats. This is a common disease in these species and is the most frequent cause of abscesses. As a general rule, any abscess associated with a lymph node of a sheep or goat should be assumed to be due to *C. pseudotuberculosis* until proven otherwise. Lesions of caseous lymphadenitis are characterized by abscesses of lymph nodes and nodules and draining tracts in the skin. The purulent discharge is usually thick, creamy or cheesy, and yellowish, greenish, or tan. Confirmation of a tentative diagnosis can readily be made by examination of a Gram-stained smear (gram-positive pleomorphic rods) and confirmed by submitting a sample of pus to a diagnostic laboratory. A closed abscess can be sampled with a syringe and a fine needle. Since the pus is usually very thick, the syringe and needle are sent to the laboratory for flushing and later cultivation of the organism. The skin biopsy specimen shows nodular to diffuse dermatitis associated with tuberculoid granulomatous inflammation. An outer fibrovascular capsule is usually present. It may be possible to identify the organisms with tissue Gram's or Brown and Brenn's stain.

Although *C. pseudotuberculosis* is sensitive to a wide variety of antibiotics in vitro, treatment of caseous lymphadenitis with antibiotics is not very successful in vivo. The most common method of treating superficial abscesses is to wait until they are sufficiently large and "ripe" and simply open them surgically and allow them to drain thoroughly. The skin should be clipped and cleaned at the site, a vertical, bold incision made, and the contents completely expressed. This is followed by careful flushing of the abscess cavity with hydrogen peroxide or chlorhexidine. The cavity may be flushed daily or packed with swabs to ensure complete drainage. Sheep and goats with opened abscesses should be isolated from the herd until the wound has healed completely. During the summer a suitable insect repellent should be applied to open abscesses. The pus from draining abscesses contains large numbers of bacteria that can survive for long periods (months) in the environment. It is desirable to open abscesses and house animals with open abscesses in places not frequented by other animals in the herd. Isolation stalls or a shed where animals are unlikely to become contaminated at a later date are recommended. All pus-contaminated swabs and other material should be removed and disposed of. The clinician should remember that human infection with *C. pseudotuberculosis*, although rare, can occur. Care should be taken to minimize the chances of any human contamination by infected pus.

An alternative to simple abscess drainage is complete removal of the abscess. This may be used in certain selected cases such as in show animals or animals that cannot be isolated. This procedure enables the return of the animal immediately to the flock. The abscesses seldom recur, at least not at that site.

When a large number of animals in the flock are affected, one must rely on general principles of hygiene and preventive medicine. Vaccination programs are controversial.

SPIROCHETOSIS

The spirochete *Borrelia suilla* is believed to be a secondary invader of dermatoses of swine, often associated with poor hygiene and skin trauma (abrasions, lacerations, fight wounds, surgical sites). Bilateral ulcerative spirochetosis of the ears is often associated with the trauma of sarcoptic mange or the vice of ear biting. Young pigs, especially 2 to 3 weeks post weaning, are most commonly affected. Although any region of the body may be involved, lesions are most frequently seen on the head, ears, gums, shoulders, side of the body, and scrotum (after castration). The lesions are characterized by initial erythema and edema, which are followed by necrosis and ulceration or swelling and fistulae. A grayish brown, glutinous pustular discharge is typical. The central area of large swelling often sloughs out. Ear lesions frequently begin bilaterally at the base of the pinnae and extend distally and slough off, leaving a ragged bleeding margin. The major differential diagnoses include other infectious granulomas and various forms of necrosis (pressure, septicemia). Definitive diagnosis is based on direct smears, biopsy, and culture. Direct smears or dark-field illumination of wet preparations from lesions reveal spirochetes. Skin biopsy reveals varying degrees of necrosis, ulceration and granulation tissue, granulomatous inflammation, and vasculitis. Spirochetes are best visualized histologically with silver stains.

Porcine spirochetosis has been reported to respond to several days of injectable penicillin, 3 to 5 days of oral or injectable sulfonamides, or several days of potassium iodide given orally at a dosage of 1 g/35 kg, up to 2 g total dose. Ulcerative lesions on the pinna are reported to respond rapidly to topical tetracycline. Control measures should include improved sanitation and management.

CLOSTRIDIAL INFECTIONS

Clostridial species are ubiquitous anaerobic spore-forming gram-positive rods. They produce a wide variety of toxins and diseases.

Malignant edema (gas gangrene) is an acute wound infection of cattle, sheep, horses, and swine caused by various *Clostridium* species, including *C. septicum, C. sordellii,* and *C. perfringens*. Clinical signs appear within 12 to 48 hours of infection. There is a local lesion at the site of infection consisting of a soft, doughy swelling (pitting edema) with marked local erythema. As the disease progresses, the swelling becomes tense and occasionally hot and painful and the skin becomes dark and taut and eventually sloughs. Emphysema (crepitus) may or may not be present. Lesions may occur anywhere, especially in the inguinal, abdominal, cervical, shoulder, and head areas. A high fever is usually present. Affected animals are weak and depressed, may show muscle tremors and lameness, and usually die within 1 to 2 days.

Blackleg is an acute infectious disease of cattle, sheep, and swine caused by *C. chauvoei*. Clinical signs appear within 12 to 48 hours of infection. The early lesion is a hot painful swelling that progresses to a cold, painless, edematous, and emphysematous swelling. The skin is discolored and becomes dry and cracked. Lesions occur most commonly on an upper limb, the rump, and the neck. Affected animals have a high fever, are depressed and anorectic, and often die within 2 days.

Clostridial swelled head (big head) is an acute wound infection of sheep and goats usually caused by *C. novyi* and less commonly by *C. sordellii*. It is usually seen in rams and bucks at 1 to 2 years of age, especially in the summer and early fall when fighting is common. Lesions begin around the eyes and head and may spread to the neck and consist of subcutaneous edema and fluid exudation. Emphysema is quite rare. Affected animals are pyrexic and toxemic and usually die within 2 to 3 days.

Dermatohistopathologic findings in clostridial infections include diffuse subcutaneous and dermal edema and cellulitis with large numbers of degenerative neutrophils and bacteria. The latter are best visualized with special stains. Septic thrombi may be seen in subcutaneous blood vessels. The clinical signs of these diseases (e.g., swelling followed by necrosis, subcutaneous emphysema) are fairly suggestive of clostridial infection. The organisms may be isolated from lesions; however, owing to the rapid onset of these diseases and rapid death of the animal, any treatment attempted must be administered on an emergency basis. Early surgical drainage and debridement with administration of high levels of penicillin (50,000 IU/kg) or tetracycline (10 to 20 mg/kg) can be tried, but these measures are often futile. In endemic areas, it is recommended that cattle and sheep be vaccinated and that they be excluded from pastures known to be heavily contaminated by these organisms.

ERYSIPELAS

Erysipelas is an infectious disease of swine caused by *Erysipelothrix insidiosa (rhusiopathiae)*. The organism is a gram-positive pleomorphic facultative anaerobe. Erysipelas is worldwide in distribution and a serious economic problem in swine operations. Erysipelas occurs in acute, subacute, and chronic clinical forms. In the acute form, fever, depression, anorexia, and lameness are accompanied by bluish-purplish discoloration of the skin, especially of the abdomen, ears, and extremities. Pinkish to red macules and papules may also be seen. In the subacute phase, erythematous papules and wheals (urticaria) enlarge and become square, rectangular, or rhomboid shaped (diamond skin disease). These lesions often develop a purplish center and either regress spontaneously or progress to the chronic phase. The chronic phase is characterized by necrosis and sloughing, resulting in dark dry firm areas of skin that peel away. Occasionally the ears, tail, and feet may slough as well. Dermatohistopathologic findings include marked dermal vascular dilatation and engorgement in the acute phase and a neutrophilic vasculitis (arteritis) and suppurative hidradenitis in the subacute and chronic phases. The organisms may occasionally be visualized in sections stained with Gram's stain. Penicillin (11,000 IU/kg/day) is the antibiotic of choice for treatment. Pigs at risk may also be protected by penicillin therapy. Vaccinations are recommended to prevent herd outbreaks. Humans are susceptible to infections with *E. insidiosa*. The disorder, termed *erysipeloid*, is an occupational disease in humans who come into contact with animals, such as veterinarians. Lesions are most commonly seen on the hands and fingers and consist of a slowly progressive discrete, violaceous to erythematous and usually painful cellulitis.

BIBLIOGRAPHY

Cameron RDA: Skin diseases of the pig. Sydney, University of Sydney Postgraduate Foundation in Veterinary Science, 1984.
Fubini SL, Campbell SG: External lumps on sheep and goats. Vet Clin North Am [Large Anim Pract] 5:457–476, 1983.
Lofstedt J: Dermatologic diseases of sheep. Vet Clin North Am [Large Anim Pract] 5:427–448, 1983.
Rosychuk RAW: Llama dermatology. Vet Clin North Am [Food Anim Pract] 5:203–215, 1989.
Scott DW: Large Animal Dermatology. Philadelphia, WB Saunders, 1988.

Viral Skin Diseases

DANNY W. SCOTT, DVM, Diplomate, ACVD

Cutaneous lesions may be the only feature associated with a viral infection, or they may be part of a more generalized disease. A clinical examination of the skin often provides valuable information that assists the veterinarian in the differential diagnosis of several viral disorders.

An in-depth discussion of all the viral diseases—especially their extracutaneous clinical signs and pathology and their elaborate diagnostic and control schemata—is beyond the scope of this section. The reader is referred to appropriate sections of this text for details.

POXVIRUS INFECTIONS

The Poxviridae are a large family of DNA viruses. The genera include orthopoxvirus (cowpox, vaccinia), capripoxvirus (sheeppox, goatpox, bovine lumpy skin disease), suipoxvirus (swinepox), parapoxvirus (pseudocowpox, bovine papular stomatitis, contagious viral pustular dermatitis), and other unclassified poxviruses (ovine viral ulcerative dermatosis).

Pox lesions in the skin have a typical clinical evolution, beginning as erythematous macules and becoming papular and then vesicular. The vesicular stage is well developed in some pox infections and transient to nonexistent in others. Vesicles evolve into umbilicated pustules with a depressed center and a raised, often erythematous border. This lesion is the so-called pock. The pustules rupture and form a crust. Healed lesions often leave a scar.

Many of the poxviruses of food animals can produce skin lesions in humans: vaccinia, cowpox, goatpox, pseudocowpox, bovine papular stomatitis, and contagious viral pustular dermatitis. The most commonly zoonotic of these are contagious viral pustular dermatitis (orf, contagious ecthyma), pseudocowpox, and bovine papular stomatitis (milker's nodule).

VACCINIA. The orthopoxvirus that causes vaccinia is known to infect cattle and swine, producing syndromes clinically identical to cowpox and swinepox, respectively.

COWPOX. Cowpox is a rare disease of cattle in Europe. Tenderness of the teats is followed by the typical cutaneous sequence of events leading to pocks. The classic thick, red crust, ranging in diameter from 1 to 2 cm, is reported to be pathognomonic. In typical cases of cowpox, lesions are confined to the teats and udder. In severe cases, lesions may be seen on the medial thighs, perineum, vulva, scrotum of bulls, and mouth of nursing calves.

SHEEPPOX. Sheeppox is the most serious of the pox diseases and occurs in Africa, Asia, and the Middle East. Skin lesions follow a typical pock evolutionary sequence and have a predilection for the eyelids, cheeks, nostrils, ears, neck, axillae, groin, prepuce, vulva, udder, scrotum, and ventral surface of the tail.

GOATPOX. Goatpox occurs in Africa, Asia, Europe, and the United States. Skin lesions may or may not follow a typical pock evolutionary sequence and have a predilection for the head, neck, ears, axillae, groin, perineum, and ventral surface of the tail. Some outbreaks are characterized by only muzzle and lip lesions, whereas others involve only the udder, teats, scrotum, prepuce, perineum, and ventral tail.

BOVINE LUMPY SKIN DISEASE. Lumpy skin disease is an acute to subacute infectious disease of cattle in Africa. There is a sudden appearance of multiple papules and nodules. The lesions are firm, well circumscribed, and flattened and may be generalized or fairly localized. The neck, chest, back, legs, perineum, udder, and scrotum are commonly affected. Although the lesions can persist for months, they usually proceed to necrosis and disappear within 4 to 12 weeks. A narrow moat forms around the lesions and separates them from normal skin. These so-called sitfasts then slough, leaving crateriform ulcers that heal by scarring.

SWINEPOX. Swinepox occurs worldwide and is endemic to areas of intensive swine production. Skin lesions follow the typical gross pock sequence and occur most commonly on the ventrolateral abdomen and thorax and the medial thighs and forelegs.

PSEUDOCOWPOX. Pseudocowpox is a common parapoxvirus infection of cattle throughout the world. Typically, the first clinical signs are focal edema, erythema, and pain of affected teats. A small orange papule develops, followed by the formation of a dark-red crust. The edges of the lesions extend peripherally, and the central crust may appear umbilicated. Peripheral extension of the lesion continues, and the central area of the crust begins to desquamate, leaving a slightly raised crust commonly called a ring or horseshoe scab. This type of crust is said to be pathognomonic. Lesions occur on the teats and udder and, occasionally, the medial thighs and perineum.

BOVINE PAPULAR STOMATITIS. In bovine papular stomatitis, which is found worldwide, initial lesions are erythematous macules, which evolve into papules. These papules then undergo central necrosis and become encrusted and often papillomatous. Lesions occur most commonly on the muzzle, nostrils, and lips and occasionally on the sides, abdomen, hind legs, scrotum, and prepuce. Bovine papular stomatitis has also been incriminated as a cause of the so-called rat-tail syndrome in cattle.

CONTAGIOUS VIRAL PUSTULAR DERMATITIS. Contagious viral pustular dermatitis is a cosmopolitan disease (contagious ecthyma, soremouth, orf) of sheep and goats. Lesions usually occur on the lips, muzzle, nostrils, and eyelids. In severe cases, they may be seen on the genitals, perineum, coronets, interdigital spaces, pasterns, fetlocks, and oral cavity. Skin lesions follow a typical pock progression but are quite proliferative.

OVINE VIRAL ULCERATIVE DERMATOSIS. Ovine viral ulcerative dermatosis occurs throughout the world and is also known as ovine venereal disease and lip and leg ulcer. Granulating ulcers, 1 to 5 cm in diameter, containing pus and adherent crusts are present in the skin between the upper lips and nostrils, on the craniolateral aspects of the feet above the coronets, and interdigitally.

HERPESVIRUS INFECTIONS

INFECTIOUS BOVINE RHINOTRACHEITIS. Infectious bovine rhinotracheitis occurs worldwide and is caused by bovine herpesvirus 1. Skin lesions include erythema, pustules, necrosis, and ulceration of the muzzle or the vulva or both. Rarely, pustules, crusts, oozing, alopecia, and lichenification may be seen in the perineal and scrotal areas.

BOVINE HERPES MAMMILLITIS. Bovine herpes mammillitis occurs worldwide and is caused by bovine herpesvirus 2. Skin lesions may be confined to one teat or involve several and may extend to the udder and perineum. Classically, the disease is sudden in onset, with swollen, tender teats. Vesicles may be seen, but in many cases, the epithelium simply sloughs. The severity of the dermatitis varies from lines of erythema, often in circles, which enclose dry skin or papules with occasional ulceration, to annular red to blue plaques, which evolve into shallow 0.5- to 2-cm ulcers, to large areas of bluish discoloration, necrosis, slough, ulceration, and serum exudation.

BOVINE PSEUDOLUMPY SKIN DISEASE. This skin disorder is also caused by bovine herpesvirus 2 and is found worldwide. Skin lesions are similar in distribution and appearance to those of true lumpy skin disease but are located much more superficially in the skin (slightly raised plaques with a central depression and superficial necrosis).

BOVINE HERPES MAMMARY PUSTULAR DERMATITIS. This type of dermatitis, associated with bovine herpesvirus 4, has been reported from the United States. Lesions consist of multiple 1- to 10-mm vesicles and pustules on the lateral and ventral aspects of the udder.

BOVINE MALIGNANT CATARRHAL FEVER. This sporadic, acute, highly fatal systemic disease affects cattle in most parts of the world. Skin lesions include erythema, scaling, necrosis, and ulceration of the muzzle, the face, and, occasionally, the udder, teats, vulva, and scrotum. In addition, purplish discolorations, papules, crusts, thickening, oozing, and necrosis may affect the skin of the perineal, axillary, inguinal, and back regions. Similar dermatologic lesions may occur at the coronet, horn–skin junction, and caudal pastern area and may result in sloughing of hooves or horns.

PSEUDORABIES. Pseudorabies (Aujeszky's disease, "mad itch") is an acute, rapidly fatal herpesvirus infection that is worldwide in distribution. In ruminants and occasionally in swine, pseudorabies causes an intense, localized, unilateral pruritus with frenzied, violent licking, chewing, rubbing, and kicking at the affected area. Any part of the body may be affected, especially the head, neck, thorax, flanks, and perineum. Severe excoriations are produced.

TOGAVIRUS INFECTIONS

HOG CHOLERA. Hog cholera is a highly infectious disease of swine caused by a pestivirus that remains a problem in South America, parts of Europe, Asia, and Africa. Early cutaneous lesions consist of erythema and then purplish discoloration of the abdomen, snout, ears, and medial thighs. Areas of necrosis may develop on the pinnae, tail, and vulva. Chronically diseased swine develop a characteristic purplish blotching of the pinnae and generalized hypotrichosis.

BOVINE VIRUS DIARRHEA. Bovine virus diarrhea (mucosal disease) occurs worldwide and is caused by a pestivirus. Skin lesions begin as discrete erosions, which may coalesce and lead to necrosis of the muzzle, lips, and nostrils. Similar lesions may be present on the vulva, prepuce, coronet, and interdigital space. Occasionally, crusts, scales, and alopecia occur on the perineum, medial thighs, and neck.

OVINE BORDER DISEASE. Ovine border disease is a congenital infectious disease reported in most parts of the world. It results in an abnormal fleece (hairy shakers, fuzzies) and frequently a darkly pigmented area of fleece on the back of the neck.

PICORNAVIRUS INFECTION

FOOT-AND-MOUTH DISEASE. Foot-and-mouth disease is a highly contagious infectious disease (aphthous fever) of cattle, sheep, goats, and swine. Clinical signs include vesicles and bullae, which rupture to leave painful erosions in the mouth and on the muzzle, nostrils, coronet, interdigital spaces, udder, and teats. Occasionally, hooves may be sloughed.

VESICULAR EXANTHEMA. Vesicular exanthema, a calicivirus infection of swine, has not been reported in the United States since 1959. Clinical signs include vesicles and painful erosions on the snout, legs, oral mucosa, coronet, interdigital spaces, and occasionally the udder and teats.

SWINE VESICULAR DISEASE. An acute infectious disease, swine vesicular disease occurs in Africa, Asia, and parts of Europe. Vesicles and erosions are seen on the snout, lips, coronet, and occasionally the belly and legs.

MISCELLANEOUS VIRAL INFECTIONS

VESICULAR STOMATITIS. Vesicular stomatitis is an infectious disease of swine and cattle that is enzootic in North, Central, and South America. Vesicles progress rapidly to painful erosions of the oral cavity, lips, muzzle, feet, and occasionally the prepuce, udder, and teats.

RINDERPEST. Rinderpest is an acute, highly contagious systemic disease of ruminants and swine in Africa and Asia. Skin lesions are characterized by erythema, papules, oozing, crusts, and alopecia over the perineum, flanks, medial thighs, neck, scrotum, udder, and teats. Occasionally, a generalized exfoliative dermatitis is seen.

BLUETONGUE. An insect-borne infectious disease of sheep, goats, and cattle, bluetongue occurs throughout the world. Sheep and goats develop erythema, edema, and occasionally ulceration of the muzzle, lips, and oral mucosa. In addition, some animals develop coronitis with a dark red to purple band in the skin above the coronet. Cattle develop edema, dryness, cracking, and peeling of the muzzle and lips. Ulceration and crusting may be seen on the udder and teats. The neck, chest, flanks, back, and perineum may become scaly, wrinkled, alopecic, and fissured and may develop areas of moist superficial dermatitis.

AFRICAN SWINE FEVER. African swine fever is a peracute, fatal, highly contagious infection of swine in Africa and also in Europe. Severely affected swine develop a red to reddish-blue to purplish discoloration of the skin of the snout, ears, belly, legs, sides, and rump.

BOVINE EPHEMERAL FEVER. Transmitted by insects, bovine ephemeral fever affects cattle in Africa, Asia, and Australia. Clinical signs may include widespread subcutaneous emphysema and periarticular edema.

CAPRINE VIRAL DERMATITIS. This virus infection is an acute highly fatal disease of goats in India. The entire cutaneous surface, including the lips, gums, and tongue, is covered with papules and nodules that become necrotic, then ulcerated.

SWINE PARVOVIRUS VESICULAR DISEASE. Outbreaks of parovirus-related vesicular disease have been reported in swine in the midwestern United States. Lesions consist of vesicles and erosions on the snout and coronet and in the interdigital space and the mouth.

SCRAPIE. Scrapie is a vertically and horizontally transmissible disease of sheep and goats in many parts of the world. Clinical signs include intermittent, bilaterally symmetric pruritus, which often begins over the tail head and progresses cranially to involve the flanks, thorax, and occasionally the head and ears. Chronic rubbing and biting lead to alopecia, excoriations, and even hematomas.

BIBLIOGRAPHY

Scott DW: Large Animal Dermatology. Philadelphia, WB Saunders, 1988.

Protozoal Skin Diseases
DANNY W. SCOTT, DVM, DIPLOMATE, ACVD

Parasitic protozoa are an important cause of food animal disease in many areas of the world. Some of these protozoal diseases have an associated dermatosis, but the cutaneous disorders are of minimal importance compared with disorders that involve other organ systems. For detailed information on other clinicopathologic, diagnostic, and therapeutic aspects of these diseases, see the appropriate sections of this textbook.

TRYPANOSOMIASIS

Trypanosoma brucei has been reported to cause urticarial plaques over the neck, chest, and flanks of cattle in Africa.

SARCOCYSTOSIS

Affected cattle may lose the tail switch (rat-tail) and develop alopecia of the pinnae and distal extremities. Sarcocystosis may cause a poor hair coat and patchy alopecia in goats.

BESNOITIOSIS

Besnoitiosis (globidiosis) is reported to affect cattle and goats in Africa, Asia, southern Europe, and South America. In cattle, warm, painful, edematous swellings are present predominantly over the head, ears, distal extremities, and genitalia. These same areas then become alopecic, thickened, and folded (elephantiasis).

In goats, besnoitiosis (dimple) is characterized by thickening, folding, alopecia, fissuring, and oozing of the skin on the legs, ventrum, and scrotum. In addition, subcutaneous papules may be present over the hindquarters.

THEILERIASIS

Theileria parva is the cause of East Coast fever in cattle in Africa. The disease may be associated with the development of papules and nodules over the neck and trunk. *T. annulata* is a cause of bovine theileriasis in Asia, southern Europe, and northern Africa. Cutaneous lesions may be seen and include wheals or papules that begin on the face, neck, and shoulders and then become generalized. The lesions are firm, and pruritus may be intense.

BIBLIOGRAPHY

Franc M, Gourreau JM, Ferrie J: La besnoitiose bovine. Point Vét 19:445–455, 1987.
Scott DW: Large Animal Dermatology. Philadelphia, WB Saunders, 1988.

Immunologic Skin Diseases
DANNY W. SCOTT, DVM, DIPLOMATE, ACVD

Immunologic skin disorders typically affect only one animal in a group and, thus, are of minimal concern from an economic or production standpoint. For detailed information on immunologic skin disorders, the reader is referred to the bibliography.

URTICARIA

Urticarial reactions are characterized by localized or generalized wheals, which may or may not be pruritic and which may or may not exhibit serum leakage. The lesions are cold swellings that pit with digital pressure. Characteristically, the wheals are evanescent lesions, with each individual lesion persisting only a few hours. Urticarial lesions may assume bizarre shapes (serpiginous, linear, arciform, papular).

In cattle, urticaria has been reported in association with insect and arthropod stings and bites, infections, systemic medicaments (penicillin, streptomycin, oxytetracycline, chloramphenicol, neomycin, sulfonamides, diethylstilbestrol, carboxymethylcellulose, hydroxypropyl methylcellulose), biologicals (various vaccines and toxoids, especially for leptospirosis, *Brucella abortus* strain 19, foot-and-mouth disease, shipping fever, salmonellosis, rinderpest, and contagious pleuropneumonia), physical trauma (dermatographism), hypodermiasis, feedstuffs (pasture plants, moldy hay or straw, or potato and walnut leaves), and plants (stinging nettle). Lesions are most commonly seen on the face, ears, and trunk. Milk allergy is a unique autoallergic disease of cattle, especially Jerseys and Guernseys, which become sensitized to the casein in their own milk. The disorder is believed to be familial and is triggered by circumstances that cause milk retention or unusual engorgement of the udder with milk.

In swine, urticaria has been reported in association with insect and arthropod stings and bites, infections (especially erysipelas), topical applications (especially parasiticides), feedstuffs, systemic medicaments, plants (stinging nettle), and biologicals. Lesions are most commonly seen over the trunk and proximal limbs.

Therapy for urticaria includes elimination and avoidance of known etiologic factors and symptomatic treatment with systemic glucocorticoids (0.1 mg/kg dexamethasone IV or IM, or 1 mg/kg prednisone or prednisolone IV or IM) or nonsteroidal anti-inflammatory agents (aspirin, 5 mg/kg; phenylbutazone, 2 mg/kg; flunixin meglumine, 1 to 2 mg/kg). Antihistamines are rarely beneficial.

ATOPY

Atopy is a genetically determined pruritic dermatitis in which the animal becomes sensitized to inhaled environmental allergens. Atopy has been presumptively diagnosed in Suffolk sheep. These animals had recurrent seasonal (spring, summer, fall) pruritic skin disease. The face, ears, ventrum, and distal limbs were chiefly affected. Secondary lesions, developing over time, included excoriations, alopecia, lichenification, and hyperpigmentation. Intradermal skin testing revealed numerous positive reactions to various plant pollens and molds. Treatment was not initiated in these sheep, although systemic glucocorticoids, systemic antihistamines, or hyposensitization would be therapeutic options.

FOOD HYPERSENSITIVITY

Food hypersensitivity is an extremely rarely reported cause of pruritic skin disease in food animals. Incriminated substances have included wheat, maize, soybeans, rice bran, and clover hay in cattle and pasture plants in swine. Affected animals manifested generalized pruritus with or without papules, plaques, or wheals. Diagnosis would be established by feeding a hypoallergenic diet for 4 weeks (until the symptoms have resolved), then readministering the original diet (whereupon the clinical syndrome is reproduced within 1 to 7 days). Treatment would require avoiding offending foodstuffs.

DRUG ERUPTIONS

Drug eruptions are rarely reported in food animals. Drugs responsible for skin eruptions may be administered orally, topically, or by injections. Any drug may cause an eruption, and there is no specific type of reaction for any one drug. Thus, drug eruption may mimic virtually any dermatosis (e.g., urticaria, vasculitis, vesicobullous dermatitis, erythema multiforme, generalized pruritus, exfoliative dermatitis). The only reliable test for the diagnosis of drug eruption is to withdraw the drug and observe for the disappearance of the eruption in 10 to 14 days.

PEMPHIGUS FOLIACEUS

Pemphigus foliaceus is a rare autoimmune dermatosis of goats. Pustules and/or vesicles are the primary skin lesions but are difficult to find among the secondary lesions of annular erosions with epidermal collarettes, annular crusts, oozing, scaling, and alopecia. Lesions are most prominent on the face, ears, and limbs but may be generalized. Affected goats may or may not have pruritus and may or may not exhibit signs of systemic illness (fever, anorexia, depression, weight loss). Diagnosis is confirmed by skin biopsy (subcorneal pustules or vesicopustules containing numerous acantholytic keratinocytes and neutrophils), bacterial and fungal cultures (negative), and, if available, direct immunofluorescence testing (immunoglobulin with or without complement deposited in the intercellular spaces of the epidermis in primary skin lesions). The disease is chronic and incurable, thus necessitating long-term control with systemic glucocorticoids or injectable gold salts (aurothioglucose).

BOVINE EXFOLIATIVE ERYTHRODERMA

A cow with severe exfoliative erythroderma was studied. Her calves and an unrelated calf that were fed her colostrum developed exfoliative erythroderma. From birth to 4 days of age, the calves developed erythema and vesicles on the muzzle. Between 4 and 50 days of age, the calves developed generalized erythema, scaling, easy epilation, and alopecia. By 4 months of age, the calves had recovered. Skin biopsy specimens revealed intraepidermal pustules containing neutrophils. An immune-mediated disorder associated with colostrum was postulated.

BIBLIOGRAPHY

Bassett H: Bovine exfoliative dermatitis: a new bovine skin disease transferred by colostrum. Irish Vet J 39:106–107, 1985.
Scott DW: Large Animal Dermatology. Philadelphia, WB Saunders, 1988.
Scott DW, Campbell SG: A seasonal pruritic dermatitis in sheep resembling atopy. Agri-Practice 8(6):46–49, 1987.
Scott DW, Smith MC, Smith CA, et al: Pemphigus foliaceus in a goat. Agri-Practice 5(4):38–45, 1984.

Environmental Skin Diseases
DANNY W. SCOTT, DVM, Diplomate, ACVD

Environmental disorders are common and often a cause of substantial economic loss in livestock production. In many instances (chemical toxicoses, mycotoxicoses, hepatotoxic plant toxicoses) the dermatologic abnormalities are clinically spectacular and of important diagnostic significance but are of rather trivial overall importance prognostically, therapeutically, and financially compared with abnormalities in other organ systems. For detailed clinicopathologic information on these disorders, the reader is referred to the appropriate sections of this book.

MECHANICAL INJURIES

Intertrigo

Intertrigo is a superficial inflammatory dermatosis that occurs in places where skin is in apposition and is thus subject to the friction of movement, increased local heat, maceration from retained moisture, and irritation from accumulation of debris. When these factors are present to a sufficient degree, dissolution of stratum corneum, exudation, and secondary bacterial injection are inevitable.

Intertrigo is most commonly seen in dairy cattle and dairy goats. Congestion of the udder at parturition is physiologic but may be sufficiently severe to cause edema of the belly, udder, and teats. In most cases, the edema disappears within 2 to 3 days after parturition, but, if extensive and persistent, it can lead to intertrigo where the skin of the udder contacts the skin of the medial thighs. Erythema is followed by oozing, erosion, crusting, secondary bacterial infection, and, in severe cases, necrosis and a foul odor.

Udder-thigh intertrigo is generally treated with gentle antiseptic soaps (chlorhexidine) and astringent rinses (aluminum acetate) two or three times daily. In severe cases, diuretics (chlorothiazide, 0.5 g IV q12h; furosemide, 0.5 g IV q12h) and frequent massage are beneficial for reducing udder edema. When the dermatosis is no longer moist and exudative, dusting with powders two or three times daily helps to reduce friction. Healing is usually complete within 4 to 12 weeks.

Hematoma

A hematoma is a circumscribed area of hemorrhage into the tissues. It arises from vascular damage associated with sudden, severe, blunt external trauma (e.g., a fall) or with more prolonged physical trauma (e.g., head shaking because of irritation from ear mites). The lesions are usually acute in onset, subcutaneous, and fluctuant and may or may not be painful.

Hematomas are commonly seen in swine, usually over the shoulders, flanks, and hindquarters, following severe nonpenetrating trauma. Aural hematomas, most frequently seen in lop-eared breeds of swine, are associated with head shaking (from sarcoptic mange, pediculosis, or meal in the ears from overhead feeders) or ear biting. Vulvar hematomas are seen in the postpartum gilt and sow, associated with trauma from faulty farrowing crate doors or large piglets at farrowing. In cattle, hematomas may be seen over the stifle, ischial tuberosity, lateral thorax, point of the shoulder, and middle of the back.

Diagnosis is based on history and physical examination. Needle aspiration and cytologic examination reveal blood. Most hematomas are simply allowed to organize and partially resolve. Occasional herd outbreaks of hematomas, in which 10 per cent of the sows died of massive hemorrhage, have been reported. Increasing the level of vitamin K in the feed corrected the problem.

Gangrene

Gangrene is a clinical term used to describe severe tissue necrosis and sloughing. The necrosis may be moist or dry. The pathologic mechanism of gangrene is an occlusion of either arterial or venous blood supply. Moist gangrene is produced by impairment of lymphatic and venous drainage plus infection (putrefaction) and is a complication of decubital ulcers associated with bony prominences and pressure points in recumbent animals. Moist gangrene presents as swollen, discolored areas with a foul odor and progressive tissue decomposition. Dry gangrene occurs when arterial blood supply is occluded, but venous and lymphatic drainage remain intact and infection is absent (mummification).

The causes of gangrene include external pressure (pressure sores, rope galls, constricting bands, and porcine skin necrosis), internal pressure (severe edema), burns (thermal, chemical, friction, radiation, or electrical), frostbite, envenomation (snake bite), vasculitis, ergotism, fescue toxicosis, and various infections (salmonellosis, streptococcosis, spirochetosis, necrobacillosis, erysipelas, malignant catarrhal fever, bovine herpes mammillitis, bovine lumpy skin disease, and staphylococcal and clostridial infections).

Subcutaneous Emphysema

Subcutaneous emphysema is characterized by free gas in the subcutis. Possible causes include air entering through a cutaneous wound (from an accident or surgery), lung punctured by the end of a fractured rib, internal penetrating wounds (traumatic reticuloperitonitis), rumen gases migrating from a rumenotomy or rumenal trocarization, extension from pulmonary emphysema, extension from tracheal rupture, gas gangrene infections, and bovine ephemeral fever.

Subcutaneous emphysema is characterized by soft, fluctuant, crepitant subcutaneous swellings. The lesions are usually non-painful, and the animals are not acutely ill, except in the case of gas gangrene (clostridial infections).

Diagnosis is based on history and physical examination. Treatment is directed at the underlying cause. Sterile subcutaneous emphysema requires no treatment unless it is extensive and incapacitating, when multiple skin incisions may be necessary.

Black Pox

Black pox is a sporadic condition seen in dairy cattle. It is believed to be a traumatically induced teat disorder caused by poor milking machine techniques. *Staphylococcus aureus* is consistently cultured from the lesions but is presumed to be a secondary invader.

Lesions occur most commonly on the tip of the teat and are characterized by crateriform ulcers with raised edges and a black spot in the pitted center. The affected area may spread to involve the teat sphincter, whereupon mastitis is a possible sequela.

Black pox is usually quite intractable to topical and systemic medicaments. The milking machinery should be carefully analyzed as to pressure and technique.

THERMAL INJURIES

Burns

Burns are occasionally seen in livestock and may be thermal (barn, forest, and brush fires or accidental spillage of hot solutions), electrical (electrocution or lightning strike), frictional (rope burns or abrasions from falling), chemical (improperly used topical medicaments or maliciously used caustic agents), and radiational. The reader is referred to the appropriate section of this book for discussion of the pathophysiology of burns and the management of severely burned animals with extracutaneous complications.

Burns are most commonly seen over the dorsum, face, or teats and udder. Animals with burns over more than 50 per cent of their body usually die. First-degree burns involve the superficial epidermis, are characterized by erythema, edema, and pain, and generally heal without complication. Second-degree burns affect the entire epidermis, are characterized by erythema, edema, pain, and vesicles, and usually re-epithelialize with proper wound care. Third-degree burns include the entire epidermis, dermis, and appendages and are characterized by necrosis, ulceration, anesthesia, and scarring. Fourth-degree burns involve the entire skin, subcutis, and underlying fascia, muscle, and tendon.

In a study of Australian dairy cattle with teat burns (from brush fires), mature cows were more likely to return to normal function than heifers (78 vs. 40 per cent). Major post-burn complications included occlusion of teat orifice, twisted and distorted teats, and mastitis.

Frostbite

Frostbite is more common in neonates; animals that are sick, debilitated, or dehydrated; animals with heavily pigmented skin; and animals having pre-existing vascular insufficiency. Also at risk are dairy cattle and goats turned out into cold weather after udders and teats have been washed but inadequately dried off.

Frostbite most commonly affects ears, tails, teats, scrotum, and feet. Mild cases present as erythema, scaling, and alopecia. Severe cases present as necrosis, dry gangrene, and sloughing. The affected skin is usually anesthetic.

Therapy varies with the severity of the frostbite. In mild cases, treatment is usually not needed. In more severe cases, rapid thawing in warm water (41°C to 44°C) is indicated as soon as possible after it is known that refreezing can be prevented. Rewarming may be followed by the application of bland, protective ointments or creams. In very severe cases with necrosis and sloughing, symptomatic therapy with topical wet soaks and systemic antibiotics is indicated, and surgical excision is postponed until an obvious boundary between viable and nonviable tissue is present. Once-frozen tissue may be increasingly susceptible to cold injury.

PRIMARY IRRITANT CONTACT DERMATITIS

Primary irritant contact dermatitis is common in livestock and has numerous causes. The dermatologic findings reflect the mode of encounter with the contactant. Primary irritants have one thing in common: they invariably produce dermatitis if they come into direct contact with skin in sufficient concentration for a long enough period. Moisture is an important predisposing factor, since it decreases the effectiveness of normal skin barriers and increases the intimacy of contact between the contactant and the skin surface.

Commonly incriminated causes of primary irritant contact dermatitis include body excretions (feces, urine), wound secretions, caustic substances (acids, alkalis), crude oil, diesel fuel, turpentine, improperly used topical parasiticides (sprays, dips, wipes), irritating plants, wood preservatives, bedding, and a filthy environment.

Because direct contact is required, the face, distal extremities, and ventrum are most commonly affected. The dermatitis varies in severity (depending on the nature of the contactant) from erythema, papules, edema, and scaling to vesicles, erosions, ulcers, necrosis, and crusts. Pruritus and pain are variable. Severe irritants or self-trauma can result in alopecia, lichenification, and scarring. Leukotrichia and leukoderma can be transient or permanent sequelae.

In most instances, the nature of the contactant can be inferred from the distribution of the dermatitis: muzzle and distal extremities (plants and environmental substances such as sprays, fertilizers, and filth); a single limb (topical medicament); face and dorsum (sprays, dips, wipes); perineum and rear legs (urine, feces); and ventrum (bedding, filth). Salt produces large, irregularly shaped erythematous plaques in contact areas of swine. Pentachlorophenol (a component of waste motor oil, fungicides, wood preservatives) produces severe contact dermatitis in swine. During breeding season, buck goats urinate on their own face, beard, and forelimbs producing urine scald. A dermatitis may be seen on the muzzle, lips, and ear tips of kids and calves fed milk or milk replacer from pans and buckets. "Transit erythema" is a contact dermatitis of swine associated with exposure to lime. A severe contact dermatitis was reported in swine receiving tiamulin orally for the prevention of dysentery. It was hypothesized that the contactant was tiamulin and/or a metabolite in feces and/or urine.

Diagnosis is based on history, physical examination, and recovery when the offending contactant is removed. The contact irritant must be identified and eliminated. Residual contactant and other surface debris can be removed with copious amounts of water and gentle cleansing soaps. Moist, oozing dermatoses will benefit from the application of astringent soaks (aluminum acetate, magnesium sulfate). Other measures for treatment of symptoms, depending on the presence and severity of secondary bacterial infection or pruritus, may include topical or systemic antibiotics or glucocorticoids. In most instances, when the irritant is removed, the dermatitis will improve markedly within 7 to 10 days.

PORCINE SKIN NECROSIS

Porcine skin necrosis is becoming increasingly common as more swine are kept under intensive husbandry systems with minimal bedding. Necrotic lesions usually occur bilaterally over bony prominences and other areas easily damaged by environmental contact or fighting. The occurrence of most forms of porcine skin necrosis has been associated with rough concrete flooring, alkaline pH (alkalis and lime-washed pens), and contact dermatitis (formalin and calcium hypochlorite disinfectants, other caustic agents). Porcine ear necrosis is believed to be precipitated by fighting and bite wounds, which may become secondarily infected with *Staphylococcus hyicus* and β-hemolytic streptococci. Severe bacterial infection leads to vasculitis, thrombosis, and necrosis.

Although most forms of porcine skin necrosis are epidemic, mortality is negligible with most forms. In most instances, the initial skin lesion seen in piglets is a reddish brown macule or patch over a joint or other prominent cutaneous site where contact is made with the ground. The lesions are always bilateral and may be seen within a few hours after birth. The lesions progress through necrosis, erosion, and ulceration, reaching maximum severity in about 7 days. A blackish brown crust forms over the lesions, which begin to heal after about 3 weeks and are usually healed within 5 weeks of their onset. Lameness and local infections may or may not be seen. The knees are most commonly affected, followed in decreasing order of frequency by the fetlocks, hocks, elbows, coronets, chin, sternum, vulva, stifles, and rump.

Teat necrosis is also a herd problem, often being bilateral and affecting the cranial pair of teats most frequently. Tail biting and tail necrosis are often noted. A small abraded area appears on the dorsal or ventral surface of the tail root soon after birth and proceeds to necrose, ulcerate, and encircle the tail root, resulting in sloughing of the entire tail.

Ear necrosis begins as ear biting at the margins of the pinnae. Early lesions may resolve completely or evolve through a vesicular, exudative, and crusted phase (*S. hyicus* infection) and terminate as a scalloping of the ear margins. Sporadically, severe cellulitis develops (β-hemolytic streptococci) and progresses through vasculitis, thrombosis, and severe necrosis and ulceration. This severe form may be accompanied by sloughing of the entire pinna, bacteremia, polyarteritis, and pneumonia.

Diagnosis is based on history and physical examination. In most instances, therapy is of no benefit. Severe cellulitis of the ear is reported to respond to tylosin (100 g/ton of food), ampicillin (10 to 20 mg/kg/day per os), or sodium selenite (0.3 ppm in feed). Prevention is the key. Ensuring proper bedding and freedom from exposure to irritating chemicals is paramount. Gauze pads covered with adhesive tape applied over susceptible anatomic sites as soon as possible after birth will significantly reduce the incidence of skin necrosis in piglets.

OVINE FLEECE ROT

Under natural and experimental conditions, continued wetting of sheep, such that saturation of the skin surface persists, will produce fleece rot. Approximately 1 week of continual skin wetting is sufficient to produce the disorder. The seasonal incidence of fleece rot hence coincides with months of maximum rainfall. Certain sheep show a predisposition to fleece rot, which may be attributed to variations in physical characteristics of the fleece and skin that exist among sheep of different breeds and strains and even among individual sheep. Predisposing factors include increased staple length, less compact fleeces, low wax (sebum) content of fleece, and high suint content of fleece. Subsequent to wetting of the skin, a marked proliferation of bacteria, especially *Pseudomonas* spp., produces a superficial exudative dermatitis and fleece discoloration. Considerable economic losses are accrued owing to depreciation of fleece value.

Lesions are most common over the withers and along the back. Initially, the skin in affected areas assumes a deep purple hue. This is followed by the exudation and accumulation of seropurulent material, which causes the characteristic band of matted fleece. The wool in affected areas is saturated and may be easily epilated. Discoloration of the wool by green, blue, brown, orange, or pink bands may occur at any level of the staple. The area of fleece rot emanates putrid odors, which attract gravid blow flies. Affected sheep are otherwise healthy.

Diagnosis is based on history and physical examination. Therapy is not usually undertaken and is usually of no benefit. Chemical drying of the fleece decreases wetness and the incidence of fleece rot. Immunization of sheep with a cell-free vaccine containing high concentrations of soluble antigens from *P. aeruginosa* was reported to reduce the severity of fleece rot. Prevention, through selecting sheep for inherent resistance to fleece rot, would appear to be the most logical approach to dealing with the problem.

CHEMICAL TOXICOSES

A number of chemical toxicoses are known to produce cutaneous abnormalities. In most instances, these skin changes are diagnostically valuable cutaneous markers of important systemic diseases. Details of pathophysiology, diagnosis, and management of these toxicoses are presented elsewhere in this book.

Selenosis

Chronic selenosis may be seen in cattle, sheep, and swine and is suspected to be the cause of alopecia in the flanks and beards of goats. Typically, animals develop sore feet and lameness, which begins in the hind feet and progresses to involve all four feet. The coronary band area becomes tender, and transverse cracks and separations appear in the hoof. In severe cases, hooves may become necrotic and slough. The hair coat is rough, and there is progressive loss of especially the long hairs of the tail and fetlock regions.

Molybdenosis

Molybdenosis produces copper deficiency in ruminants. A rough, brittle, faded hair coat and varying degrees of pruritus may be seen. Black hairs often turn red or gray, especially around the eyes, producing a "spectacled" appearance. In sheep, wool loses its crimp, becoming straight and steely. The tensile strength of wool is reduced.

Arsenic Toxicosis

Arsenic toxicosis may produce a dry, dull, rough, easily epilated hair coat, progressing to alopecia and severe seborrheic skin disease. Occasionally, focal areas of skin necrosis and slow-healing ulcers may be seen.

Mercurialism

In cattle, mercurialism may be associated with a generalized loss of body hair and then a loss of the long hairs of the tail and fetlocks.

Chlorinated Naphthalene Toxicosis

The cutaneous changes of chlorinated naphthalene toxicosis in cattle begin over the withers and the sides of the neck and extend cranially, caudally, and ventrally. The skin becomes progressively more hyperkeratotic, scaly, thickened, alopecic, and fissured. Pruritus is absent. Horns may become loose and develop asymmetric growth.

Thallotoxicosis

In swine, thallotoxicosis may produce generalized alopecia and erythema and necrosis and oozing of the skin around the eyes and mouth.

Polybrominated and Polychlorinated Biphenyl Toxicosis

In cattle, polybrominated biphenyl toxicosis produces hematomas and abscesses over the back, abdominal veins, and rear legs and matting of the coat and alopecia over the lateral thorax, neck, and shoulders. In swine, polychlorinated biphenyl toxicosis produces erythema of the snout and anus.

Iodism

Cutaneous manifestations of iodism include variable degrees of scaling (seborrhea sicca) with or without partial alopecia, which are most prominent over the dorsum, neck, head, and shoulders.

PHOTODERMATITIS

Photodermatitis is ultraviolet light–induced inflammation of the skin. Phototoxicity is a dose-related response of all animals to light exposure (e.g., sunburn). Photosensitivity implies that the skin has been rendered increasingly susceptible to the damaging effects of ultraviolet light. Photoallergy is a reaction to a chemical (systemic or contact) and ultraviolet light in which an immune mechanism can be demonstrated. Photocontact dermatitis occurs when contactants cause photosensitivity or photoallergy. Phytophotodermatitis is caused by contact with certain plants.

Sunburn is a phototoxic reaction caused by excessive exposure to ultraviolet light B in animals that have lightly pigmented, thinly haired skin. Dairy goats that are light skinned may develop sunburn, especially on the lateral aspects of the udder and teats, when turned outside in summer. The skin becomes erythematous and scaly and if severely burned may exude, necrose, and crust. White pigs may develop sunburn especially along the back and behind the ears. Severely affected swine may slough their pinnae and tails.

Photosensitization of livestock, particularly sheep, goats,

Table 1. PRIMARY PHOTOSENSITIZATION AND THAT DUE TO ABERRANT PIGMENT SYNTHESIS AND UNCERTAIN ETIOLOGY IN LIVESTOCK

Source	Photodynamic Agent
Primary	
Plants	
St. John's wort (*Hypericum perforatum*)	Hypericin
Buckwheat (*Fagopyrum esculentum, Polygonum fagopyrum*)	Fagopyrin, photofagopyrin
Bishop's weed (*Ammi majus*)	Furocoumarins (xanthotoxin, bergapten)
Dutchman's breeches (*Thamnosma texana*)	Furocoumarins
Wild carrot (*Daucus carota*) and spring parsley (*Cymopterus watsonii*)	Furocoumarins
Cooperia pedunculata	Furocoumarins
Parsnips (*Pastinaca sativa*) or celery (*Apium graveolens*)	Furocoumarins
Perennial rye grass (*Lolium perenne*)	Perloline
Burr trefoil (*Medicago denticulata*)	Aphids
Chemicals	
Phenothiazine	Phenothiazine sulfoxide
Thiazides	?
Acriflavines	?
Rose bengal	?
Methylene blue	?
Sulfonamides	?
Tetracyclines	?
Aberrant Pigment Synthesis	
Bovine protoporphyria	Protoporphyrin
Bovine erythropoietic porphyria	Uroporphyrin I, coproporphyrin I
Uncertain Etiology	
Clover, alfalfa, lucerne, vetch, oats, field pennycress	?

Table 2. HEPATOGENOUS PHOTOSENSITIZATION IN LIVESTOCK

Source	Hepatotoxin
Plants	
Burning bush, fireweed (*Kochia scoparia*)	?
Kleingrass, dikkor (*Panicum coloratum*)	?
Ngaio tree (*Myoporum* spp.)	Ngaione
Lechuguilla (*Agave lecheguilla*)	Saponins
Caltrops, goat head, geeldikkop (*Tribulus terrestris*)	Saponins
Rape, kale (*Brassica* spp.)	?
Coal-oil brush, spineless horsebrush (*Tetradymia* spp.)	?
Sacahuiste (*Nolina texacana*)	?
Salvation Jane (*Echium lycopsis*)	Pyrrolizidine alkaloids, (echiumidine, echimidine)
Lantana (*Lantana camara*)	Triterpene (lantadene A)
Heliotrope (*Heliotropium europaeum*)	Pyrrolizidine alkaloids (lasiocarpine, heliotrine)
Ragworts (*Senecio* spp.)	Pyrrolizidine alkaloids (retorsine, jacobine)
Tarweed, fiddle-neck (*Amsinckia* spp.)	Pyrrolizidine alkaloids
Crotalaria, rattleweed (*Crotalaria* spp.)	Pyrrolizidine alkaloids (monocrotaline, fulvine, crispatine)
Millet, panic grass (*Panicum* spp.)	?
Ganskweed (*Lasiospermum bipinnatum*)	?
Vervain (*Lippia rehmanni, L. pretoriensis*)	Triterpenes (icterogenin, rehmannic acid)
Bog asphodel (*Narthecium ossifragum*)	Saponins
Alecrim (*Holocalyx glaziovii*)	?
Vuursiektebossie (*Nidorella foetida*)	?
Anthanasia trifurcata	?
Asaemia axillaris	?
Mycotoxicoses	
Pithomyces chartarum (on pasture, esp. rye)	Sporodesmin
Anacystis (Microcystis) spp. (blue-green algae in water)	Alkaloid
Periconia spp. (on Bermuda grass)	?
Phomopsis leptostromiformis (on lupines)	Phomopsin A
Fusarium spp. (on moldy corn)	T-2 toxin (diacetoxyscirpenol)
Aspergillus spp. (on stored feeds)	Aflatoxin
Infection	
Leptospirosis	Leptospires
Liver abscess	Bacerial toxins
Parasitic liver cyst (flukes, hydatids)	Parasites
Rift Valley fever	Virus
Neoplasia	
Lymphosarcoma	Malignant lymphocytes
Hepatic carcinoma	Malignant hepatocytes
Chemicals	
Copper, phosphorous, carbon tetrachloride, phenanthridium	

and cattle under range conditions, can be a major obstacle to production. Although photosensitized animals seldom die, resultant weight loss, damaged udders, refusal to allow the young to nurse, and the occurrence of secondary infections and fly strike may lead to severe economic losses. There are three features basic to all types of photosensitization: (1) the presence of a photodynamic agent within the skin, (2) the concomitant exposure to a sufficient amount of ultraviolet light A, and (3) the lack of pigment in skin with a thin haircoat. Photosensitization is classified according to the source of the photodynamic agent: primary (a preformed or metabolically derived photodynamic agent reaches the skin by ingestion, injection, or contact), hepatogenous (elevated blood phylloerythrin levels in association with liver disease), aberrant pigment synthesis (porphyria), and uncertain etiology. The major causes of photosensitization in livestock are listed in Tables 1 and 2.

The dermatologic findings in photosensitization are essentially identical, regardless of the cause. Cutaneous lesions are often restricted to light-skinned, sparsely haired areas but, in severe cases, may extend into the surrounding dark-skinned areas as well. The eyelids, lips, face, pinnae, perineum, udder, teats, and coronary bands are commonly involved. There is usually an acute onset of erythema, edema, and variable degrees of pruritus and/or pain. Vesicles and bullae may be seen, which often progress to oozing, necrosis, and ulceration. In severe cases, the pinnae, eyelids, tail, teats, and feet may slough. In New Zealand, a vesicobullous disease resembling foot-and-mouth disease was seen in swine fed parsnips or celery infected with the fungus *Sclerotinia sclerotiorum*.

MYCOTOXICOSES

Ergotism

Ergotism typically produces lameness of the hind limbs followed by swelling at the coronary bands, which progresses to the fetlocks. The feet become necrotic, cold, and anesthetic, and a distinct line separates viable from dead tissue (usually just above the coronary band). The front feet, pinnae, tail, and teats may be similarly affected and, in severe cases, may slough. Occasionally, large areas of skin (shoulder, lateral thorax, neck, muzzle) may be affected.

Fescue Toxicosis

Fescue toxicosis in cattle produces cutaneous changes similar to those described for ergotism.

Stachybotryotoxicosis

Stachybotryotoxicosis produces focal areas of necrosis and ulceration, especially of mucocutaneous areas, in cattle, sheep, and swine.

MISCELLANEOUS PLANT TOXICOSES

Leucaenosis

Leucaenosis in livestock may produce a gradual loss of the long hairs of the tail and fetlock or a sudden, fairly generalized alopecia. Hoof dystrophies and laminitis may be seen.

Hairy Vetch Toxicosis

Hairy vetch toxicosis produces cutaneous lesions in cattle. Early lesions include papules and plaques that ooze a yellowish pus-like material that becomes encrusted. Lesions begin on the udder, tailhead, and neck and spread to the face, trunk, and limbs. Pruritus is often marked and associated with considerable alopecia.

ZOOTOXICOSES

Snake Bite

Snake bites occur most commonly on the nose, head, neck and legs. The exact site of envenomation is rarely visible. Shortly after the bite, pronounced swelling obliterates the fang marks. Erythema and edema may progress to necrosis and slough. The affected area is usually painful.

Hyalomma Toxicosis

The cutaneous manifestations of *Hyalomma* toxicosis in livestock are characterized by a moist dermatitis that may be confined to the pinnae, face, neck, axillae, or groin but is often generalized. The skin is erythematous, edematous, oozing, and foul smelling. The hair coat becomes matted and is easily epilated, leaving a raw surface. The skin is painful. Cattle with nonpigmented hooves show distinct erythema of the coronets. In animals that do not die, the skin becomes dry, scaly, thickened, and alopecic.

DERMATITIS, PYREXIA, AND HEMORRHAGE IN DAIRY COWS

This syndrome has often been associated with the ingestion of diureidoisobutane. Initial cutaneous manifestations include a pruritic papulocrustous dermatitis on the head and neck that spreads to the back, udder, tailhead, perineum, and distal extremities. Rubbing, kicking, and licking produce excoriations and alopecia.

BIBLIOGRAPHY

André-Fontaine G, Bouisset S, Ganiere JP, et al: Photosensibilisation leptospirosique: mythe ou réalité. Point Vét 20:247–249, 1988.
Bridges CH, Camp BJ, Livingston CW, et al: Kleingrass (*Panicum coloratum* L.) poisoning in sheep. Vet Pathol 24:525–531, 1987.
Coppock RW, Mostrum MS, Simon J, et al: Cutaneous ergotism in a herd of dairy calves. J Am Vet Med Assoc 194:549–551, 1989.
Gourreau JM, Ducroz G, Ducroz J, et al: Le syndrome dermatite prurigineuse de la vache laitière. Point Vét 18:135–140, 1986.
Hammond AC, Allison MJ, Williams MJ, et al: Prevention of leucaena toxicosis of cattle in Florida by ruminal inoculation with 3-hydroxy-4-(1 H)-pyridone–degrading bacteria. Am J Vet Res 50:2176–2180, 1989.
Harwood DG, Hogg RA: Haematomata in cattle. Vet Rec 21:400, 1987.
Kellerman TS, Coetzer JAW: Hepatogenous photosensitivity disease in South Africa. Onderstepoort J Vet Res 52:157–173, 1985.
Laperle A: Dermatite aiguë chez des porcs traités à la tiamuline. Méd Vét Québec 20:20–22, 1990.
Martin T, Morgan S: What caused the photosensitivity in these dairy heifers? Vet Med 82:848–851, 1987.
Montgomery JF, Oliver RE, Poole WSH, et al: A vesiculo-bullous disease in pigs resembling foot and mouth disease: I. Field cases. NZ Vet J 35:21–26, 1987.
Montgomery JF, Oliver RE, Poole WSH, et al: A vesiculo-bullous disease in pigs resembling foot and mouth disease: II. Experimental reproduction of the lesion. NZ Vet J 35:27–30, 1987.
Morton JM, Fitzpatrick DH, Morris DC, et al: Teat burns in dairy cattle: the prognosis and effect of treatment. Aust Vet J 64:69–72, 1987.
Rowe LD, Norman JO, Currier DE, et al: Photosensitization of cattle in southeast Texas: identification of phototoxic activity associated with *Cooperia pedunculata*. Am J Vet Res 48:1658–1661, 1987.
Schneider DJ, Green JR, Collett MG: Ovine hepatogenous photosensitivity caused by the plant *Nidorella foetida* (Thunb.) D.C. (Asteraceae). Onderstepoort J Vet Res 54:53–57, 1987.

Scott DW: Large Animal Dermatology. Philadelphia, WB Saunders, 1988.
VanAmstel SR, Reyers F, Oberem PT, et al: Further studies on the clinical pathology of sweating sickness in cattle. Onderstepoort J Vet Res 54:45–48, 1987.
Vestweber JGE, Al-Ani FK, Johnson DE: Udder edema in cattle: effects of diuretics (furosemide, hydrochlorothiazide, acetazolamide, and 50% dextrose) on serum and urine electrolytes. Am J Vet Res 50:1323–1328, 1989.

Congenital and Hereditary Skin Diseases

DONNA WALTON ANGARANO, DVM,
DIPLOMATE, ACVD

There are a variety of dermatoses of food animals that have been classified as congenital and hereditary in nature. (There are a multitude of references in the literature regarding congenital and hereditary skin diseases. The interested reader is referred to *Large Animal Dermatology* by Scott for an extensive reference list.) Since these diseases are inherited, their diagnosis is of great significance. Practitioners need to be aware of the clinical appearance and method of inheritance of these dermatoses so that appropriate modifications may be made in breeding programs to decrease the frequency of occurrence. There is no specific therapy available for the majority of these diseases.

HYPOTRICHOSIS

Hypotrichosis has been most often reported in cattle, although it has also been recognized in sheep, goats, and swine. The reports in cattle are numerous and confusing. Each report with slight variation has been given a separate name. Table 1 is a summary of the various reports of this condition in cattle. It must be remembered that congenital hypotrichosis and alopecia may be inherited but may also occur as a result of illness (especially bovine viral diarrhea), nutritional deficiencies (especially iodine), or other conditions occurring during pregnancy. Hypotrichosis in cattle has been reported to increase susceptibility to sunburn, cold weather, bacterial dermatitis, and dermatophytosis.

There are a few isolated reports of ovine congenital hypotrichosis. Viable hypotrichosis was observed in the Polled Dorset. Hair was missing from the face and limbs. Skin biopsy specimens revealed a decrease in follicle numbers along with the presence of a keratosebaceous material within the hair follicles. This was believed to be a simple autosomal recessive trait.

Two forms of hypotrichosis have been described in swine. One form of congenital hypotrichosis is believed to be a simple autosomal recessive characteristic. Newborn pigs have a complete or almost complete lack of hair. Skin biopsy specimens show hypoplastic follicles and glands. The second form of porcine hypotrichosis (goiter type) has been reported in Mexican Hairless and German swine. This is an autosomal dominant trait that is lethal in the homozygous form. In addition to hypotrichosis, affected swine have hoof abnormalities, persistent foramen ovale, and enlarged thyroids. Iodine supplementation is not an effective treatment.

There are only anecdotal reports of hypotrichosis in the goat.

HYPERTRICHOSIS

Hereditary, congenital hypertrichosis has been reported as an autosomal dominant trait in European Friesian cattle. This condition is correlated with polypnea and decreased production during hot weather.

Congenital hair whorls in pigs are believed to be the result of an interaction between two dominant factors. Affected pigs are born with tufts of hair occurring on the neck, rump, or along the spinal column.

"Hairy shaker" or border disease of sheep is congenital but not hereditary. The disease is caused by an in utero togavirus infection. Maternal hyperthermia may also result in congenital, nonhereditary, hypertrichosis in lambs.

An abnormally curly coat has been reported as a hereditary defect in cattle. It is a viable, autosomal dominant trait in Ayrshire calves and an autosomal recessive trait in Swedish cattle and Polled Hereford calves. The presence of a congenital, tight, curly hair coat in Polled Hereford calves in Australia has been associated with cardiomyopathy. Affected calves die before reaching 6 months of age.

ICHTHYOSIS

Ichthyosis fetalis (bovine harlequin fetus) is a severe form of ichthyosis that has been reported in Norwegian Red Poll, English Friesian, and Brown Swiss cattle. Affected calves are stillborn or die shortly after birth. They have no hair and are covered by large, thick, horny scales that are divided by deep fissures. This is inherited as a simple autosomal recessive characteristic.

A milder form of ichthyosis, ichthyosis congenita, has been seen in German Pinzgauer, Holstein, and Chianiana calves. These calves are viable; however, the condition may be associated with ocular (cataract) and aural (microtia) anomalies. Hyperkeratosis may be present at birth or develop over the course of several weeks. The condition is believed to be the result of a sublethal, autosomal recessive trait.

There have been single reports of ichthyosis in swine and a llama. The lesions described in the llama were similar to bovine ichthyosis congenita.

Topical medications and systemic retinoid therapy are used to treat human ichthyosis. Although these treatments may be effective, their use is not practical in food animals. Treatment was attempted in the llama. Topical agents were ineffective, and etretinate, a synthetic retinoid, appeared to have some clinical effect. Unfortunately, the llama developed bacterial septicemia before thorough clinical evaluation of etretinate could be attained.

CUTANEOUS ASTHENIA

Cutaneous asthenia is a group of congenital, hereditary diseases of collagen, characterized by the clinical appearance of hyperextensive and fragile skin. The severity of the clinical signs is variable. Many names have been used to describe the clinical syndrome, including collagen dysplasia, dermatosparaxis, cutis hyperelastica, and the Ehlers-Danlos syndrome. Several of these syndromes may be distinguished clinically and genetically. In most cases, skin fragility and hyperelasticity result in gaping wounds and numerous thin, cutaneous scars.

In cattle and sheep, the syndrome is most often associated with a lethal, autosomal recessive trait. The clinical symptoms are the result of a deficiency of aminopropeptidase (procollagen peptidase, procollagen N-protease). Deficiency of this

Table 1. BOVINE HYPOTRICHOSIS

Name	Breed(s)	Inheritance/Sex	Clinical Signs
Lethal hypotrichosis	Holstein-Friesian Japanese cattle	Autosomal recessive Either	Die within hours Hair only on muzzle, eyelids, ears, tail, pastern Biopsy: Normal number of follicles, normal sebaceous glands, arrector pili muscles; hypoplastic follicles without hair, abnormal apocrine glands
Semi-hairlessness	Hereford Polled Hereford	Autosomal recessive Either	Calves viable Fine, curly hair at birth and later sparse and wiry; skin wrinkled, scaly Biopsy: Dysplastic follicles without hair
Viable hypotrichosis	Guernsey Jersey Hereford (1 case)	Autosomal recessive Either	At birth, hair on eyelids, ears, legs, and tail, may develop truncal hair Biopsy: Dysplastic follicles with no or little hair; abnormal apocrine glands; large dermal arteriovenous anastomoses
Streaked hypotrichosis	Holstein-Friesian	Sex-linked dominant Female	Lethal in males Hair lacking in streaks over hips, sides, legs
Tardive hypotrichosis	Friesian	Sex-linked recessive Female	Normal at birth Symmetric, progressive hair loss at 6 weeks to 6 months; begins on face
Symmetric alopecia	Holstein-Friesian	Autosomal recessive Either	Normal at birth Symmetric, progressive hair loss at 6 weeks to 6 months; begins on face Biopsy: Normal follicles without hair
Baldy calf syndrome	Holstein	Autosomal recessive Female	Lethal in males Normal at birth Die by 6 to 8 months Signs start at 1 to 2 months of age with generalized alopecia, scaling, lameness, loss of condition; tips of ears curl medially Horns fail to develop Some calves have low serum zinc levels
Hypotrichosis	Hereford Polled hereford	Autosomal dominant Either	Hair loss variable at birth; hairs thin, soft, curly May have impaired hoof development Biopsy: Hypoplastic follicles, arrector pili muscles; biochemical defect in formation of trichoprotein
Hypotrichosis	Jersey Guernsey		Hypophyseal hypoplasia
Hairlessness	Friesian		Abnormal thyroid glands One herd (31 calves)
Hypotrichosis and partial anodontia	Normandy-Maine-Anjou-Charolais	Sex-linked recessive Male	At birth, hairless and toothless Several weeks later fine downy hair and molars develop Macroglossia, defective horns, hypoplastic testes Die by 6 months of age Biopsy: Abnormal dermal papillae, dermal vasculature, apocrine and sebaceous glands
Hypotrichosis and incisor oligodontia	Holstein-Friesian	Autosomal dominant Either	Partial hypotrichosis on face and neck Missing four to six incisors
Hypotrichosis and incisor anodontia	Friesian	X-Linked, incomplete dominant Male	Males are severely affected; fine silky hairs on face, neck, ears, thorax, spine, tail, inner thighs; normal hair on abdomen; normal eyelashes, vibrissae, and tail brush Missing incisors Dams mildly affected; short grey coats Biopsy: Abnormal number of guard hairs; hairs all in telogen; normal glands and arrector pili muscles

enzyme results in a packing defect and abnormal cross-linking of collagen fibrils.

Bovine cutaneous asthenia has been reported in Belgian blue and white cattle with a clinical description of skin fragility and in Hereford cattle with clinical signs of hyperelasticity, skin fragility, and delayed wound healing. There have been isolated reports of cutaneous asthenia in Charolais and Simmental calves. Both animals had skin fragility along with joint laxity. One report of a Japanese Holstein revealed skin fragility and delayed wound healing. Cutaneous edema is an additional feature occurring shortly after birth in many bovine cases.

Ovine cutaneous asthenia has also been described in several breeds. In Norwegian Dala sheep the skin was extremely fragile. White Dorper sheep also show extremely fragile skin without joint abnormalities; however, in this breed, clinical signs were not evident until 3 to 8 weeks of age. Border Leicester-Southdown crossbred lambs demonstrated extreme skin fragility and joint laxity. Romney sheep may have concurrent fragility of the gastrointestinal tract and arteries.

A milder form of cutaneous asthenia has been reported in Merino sheep. In these cases there is no evidence of hyperextensibility of the skin or joint laxity. The clinical signs are those of skin fragility observed at the time of shearing. Laboratory studies have shown this to be a biochemically distinct form of the disease, since aminopropeptidase activity is present. These sheep possess a hereditary skin anomaly; however, it is mild enough to not be readily apparent until the animal reaches adulthood (when handled at shearing).

Porcine cutaneous asthenia is most often referred to as cutis hyperelastica. Affected pigs are generally viable; however, they have hyperextendable skin and scattered circular or oval depressions over the trunk. The condition was reported in a litter of Large White and Essex crossbred pigs. Joint laxity was not a feature.

In most cattle and sheep, cutaneous asthenia is fatal because bacterial septicemia is a common sequela. In swine and Merino sheep, affected animals may be viable with milder clinical signs. No therapy is available, other than avoidance of trauma.

APLASIA CUTIS

Aplasia cutis, also known as epitheliogenesis imperfecta, is characterized by focal ulceration with the absence of epithelium. The prognosis is variable, depending on the size of the lesion. Severely affected animals generally develop septicemia and die. Mild cases may heal by scar formation or surgical intervention.

Bovine aplasia cutis has been reported as a simple autosomal recessive characteristic in Ayrshire, Dutch Black Pied, Swedish Red Pied, German Yellow Pied (Simmental), Shorthorn, Angus, Jersey, and Holstein-Friesian cattle. Lesions are usually present on the extremities, although the muzzle and oral cavity may be affected. Hoof abnormalities may be present, and brachygnathia and atresia ani have been associated with aplasia cutis in Jersey cattle. Affected calves are frequently born prematurely. Laboratory studies of epidermal and dermal tissues from an affected calf revealed not only epidermal abnormalities but also a metabolic defect of dermal fibroblasts, suggesting that aplasia cutis may be a connective tissue disease.

Aplasia cutis is relatively rare in sheep. The condition is probably inherited (as in other species); however, evidence to support this is lacking. Oral lesions are most frequently reported along with separation of the hooves.

Yorkshire, Berkshire, and Wessex pigs have been observed with aplasia cutis. Lesions may be solitary or multiple and are usually located on the back, oral cavity, or extremities. Hydroureter and hydronephrosis have been associated with porcine aplasia cutis.

FOCAL CUTANEOUS HYPOPLASIA

Essex, Large White and Essex–Large White crossbred pigs have been reported to have focal cutaneous hypoplasia. Multiple, hairless, shallow depressions were evident over the trunk. The lesions were bilaterally symmetric in two of three reported cases.

EPIDERMOLYSIS BULLOSA

Epidermolysis bullosa has been reported as an hereditary disease in cattle and sheep. Although the cause of the disease is unknown, affected animals are known to develop bullous eruptions and ulceration in response to cutaneous trauma.

Epidermolysis in Simmental cattle is believed to be an autosomal dominant trait. In Brangus, the condition may be autosomal recessive. Erythema or ulceration may be present in the oral cavity, on the face, on the extremities, or over joints.

Ovine epidermolysis bullosa (red foot disease) has been observed in Suffolk, South Dorset Down, and Scottish Blackface lambs. Affected lambs tend to shed their hooves in addition to having the clinical signs as described in cattle.

Skin biopsy specimens reveal dermoepidermal separation with a lack of inflammation. Mortality is high, primarily owing to secondary septicemia. Avoidance of trauma is the major therapeutic option.

FAMILIAL ACANTHOLYSIS

There is a single report from New Zealand of 10 Angus calves with familial acantholysis. The condition was believed to be inherited as an autosomal recessive trait. At birth, affected calves had bullous eruptions and ulceration of the oral cavity, lips, nasolabium, and distal extremities. There was partial sloughing of the hooves. Skin biopsy specimens revealed intraepidermal separation with acantholysis. Affected calves were euthanized.

HEREDITARY ZINC DEFICIENCY

Zinc deficiency and associated parakeratosis has been well recognized in swine, sheep, and cattle. Although young animals of any of these species may be affected, only in cattle is the disease inherited. Friesian, Danish Black Pied, and Shorthorn cattle have been observed to transmit this lethal, autosomal recessive trait. Clinical signs are not usually present at the time of birth but are evident by a few weeks of age. Cutaneous lesions consist of progressive alopecia and scaling beginning near the mouth and becoming generalized. Systemic signs, especially diarrhea and rhinitis, may also be present.

The mechanism of this disease is believed to be related to an inability to absorb zinc through the intestinal wall. The bovine disease (lethal trait A46, hereditary parakeratosis, Adema disease) is analogous with acrodermatitis enteropathica in humans.

Laboratory studies of affected calves have shown lymphocytes to be normal at birth. However, as plasma zinc levels decrease and clinical signs become apparent, both B and T lymphocytes decrease in number and activity. Thymic hypoplasia is a consistent necropsy finding of affected calves.

Many reports indicate complete and rapid response to zinc replacement therapy. Treatments vary from 0.5 g of oral zinc oxide given daily to 2 g of oral zinc sulfate given per week. Relapse follows cessation of treatment. It has been suggested that oral oxyquinolines may also improve absorption of zinc. Initial improvement, followed by clinical deterioration, was reported in a Friesian calf. Plasma zinc concentrations were unchanged even during clinical improvement.

DERMATOSIS VEGETANS

Dermatosis vegetans is an autosomal recessive characteristic that is unique to Landrace and Landrace crossbred pigs. Cutaneous lesions may be present at birth or develop during the first few days of life. Circumscribed, erythematous papules and crusting dermatitis are present on the ventrum. As lesions spread peripherally, they become papillomatous in appearance. The coronary band is affected and becomes edematous. Hoof deformities occur, especially on the forefeet.

The general body condition deteriorates and most affected pigs succumb to a giant cell pneumonia by 5 or 6 weeks of age. Occasional pigs survive, and the lesions regress spontaneously. Skin biopsy specimens reveal an intraepidermal pustular dermatitis with eosinophils and parakeratosis. No effective therapy is known.

PORCINE JUVENILE PUSTULAR PSORIASIFORM DERMATITIS

So-called pityriasis rosea has been well documented as a self-limiting disease of young pigs. Unfortunately, the disease is not comparable to the human disease of the same name. Porcine juvenile pustular psoriasiform dermatitis has been proposed as a more accurate and descriptive name. The disease is believed to be familial, although the mode of inheritance is unknown.

Clinical signs appear at 2 to 3 weeks of age. The major importance is the clinical similarity to dermatophytosis. Lesions begin as erythematous papules on the ventrum and thighs that gradually enlarge and coalesce to form plaques. There is central clearing and depression covered with a bran-like scale. Lesions spontaneously resolve in 6 to 8 weeks.

LYMPHEDEMA

Congenital lymphedema due to a genetic malformation of lymphatic vessels has been observed in Ayrshire cattle. The condition is believed to be an autosomal recessive trait in cattle and is associated with the presence of secondary ear lobes. An Ayrshire-Friesian crossbred calf with congenital lymphedema and a unilateral accessory ear lobe was recently reported. This may dispute the proposed mode of inheritance.

The extent of lymphedema is variable. In severe cases, dystocia is a concern and affected calves may be stillborn. In milder cases, there is swelling of the extremities with otherwise normal body condition and growth rate.

ALBINISM

Albinism, which has been observed in Icelandic sheep and several breeds of cattle, may be partial or complete. Albinism has been attributed to both dominant and recessive inheritance. Complete albinism may be the result of a homozygous state. The condition has been described in Guernsey, Austrian Murboden, Shorthorn, Brown Swiss, and Charolais cattle.

CHÉDIAK-HIGASHI SYNDROME

Chédiak-Higashi syndrome is a pigmentary disorder with a recessive mode of inheritance. It has been observed in Hereford, Japanese Black, and Brangus cattle. Clinically, affected animals demonstrate a dilution of their hair color, a tendency to hemorrhage, and an increased susceptibility to infection.

In general, Chédiak-Higashi syndrome is characterized by partial oculocutaneous albinism, photophobia, increased susceptibility to infection, platelet pool storage deficiency, lack of natural killer cell activity, impaired microtubular function, and the occurrence of large, pleomorphic granules that are present in the cytoplasm of leukocytes and most granule-producing cells. These large granules are probably lysosomes, and this syndrome may represent a lysosomal storage disease.

PORPHYRIA

Porphyria is a form of photosensitization in which there is a hereditary abnormality of porphyrin synthesis. Exposure to ultraviolet light A results in tissue damage. There are two types of recessively inherited porphyria reported in cattle.

Bovine protoporphyria occurs in crossbred Limousin cattle. Affected cattle develop photodermatitis as a result of a deficiency of heme synthetase activity. Bovine erythropoietic porphyria is seen in several breeds of cattle including Shorthorn, Holstein-Friesian, and Hereford. Affected cattle have a deficiency of uroporphyrinogen III cosynthestase activity. Clinical signs are photodermatitis, anemia, growth retardation, and discolored teeth and urine. Teeth and urine fluoresce a bright red or orange on Wood's lamp examination.

There are reports of Southdown and Corriedale lambs with inherited liver insufficiency that have developed photosensitization.

HEREDITARY GOITER AND HYPOTHYROIDISM

Hereditary goiter and hypothyroidism have been reported in Afrikander cattle, Merino sheep, and Saanen-Dwarf crossbred goats. Affected animals have abnormal hair coats (wool) along with other signs of hypothyroidism.

WATTLES

Wattles (tassels) are teat-like projections having a fibrocartilaginous core. These projections occur singularly or in pairs and extend from the ventral neck. They are believed to be inherited as an autosomal dominant trait in swine.

CYSTS AND NEOPLASMS

A variety of inherited cysts and neoplasms have been observed in food animals. Most of these are single reports of a congenital occurrence. The most recognized hereditary neoplasia of food animals is the observation of melanomas in swine. Both miniature Sinclair and Duroc pigs have been observed to have congenital, familial melanomas.

BIBLIOGRAPHY

Ayers JR, Leipold HW, Padgett GA: Lesions in Brangus cattle with Chédiak-Higashi syndrome. Vet Pathol 25:432–436, 1988.
Belknap EB, Dunstan RW: Congenital ichthyosis in a llama. J Am Vet Med Assoc 197:764–767, 1990.
Bryden DI: Skin diseases of cattle. Sydney, Australia, University of Sydney Postgraduate Foundation in Veterinary Science, 1989.
Frey J, Chamson A, Gourreau J, et al: Collagen and lipid biosynthesis in a case of epitheliogenesis imperfecta in cattle. J Invest Dermatol 93:83–86, 1989.
Jubb TF, Malmo J, Morton JM, et al: Inherited epidermal dysplasia in Holstein-Friesian calves. Aust Vet J 67:16–18, 1990.
Kawaguchi T, Fukazawa H, Naito Y, et al: Dermal dysplasia characterized by collagen disorder-related skin fragility in a cow. Am J Vet Res 49:965–971, 1988.
Morrow CJ, McOrist S: Cardiomyopathy associated with a curly hair coat in Poll Hereford calves in Australia. Vet Rec 117:312–313, 1985.
Mulei CM, Atwell RB: Congenital lymphoedema in an Ayrshire-Friesian crossbred female calf. Aust Vet J 66:227–228, 1989.
O'Brien JK: Inherited parakeratosis in two Friesian calves. Vet Rec 119:205–206, 1986.
Perryman LE, Leach DR, Davis WC, et al: Lymphocyte alterations in zinc-deficient calves with lethal trait A46. Vet Immunol Immunopathol 21:239–248, 1989.
Scott DW: Large animal dermatology, pp 334–357. Philadelphia, WB Saunders, 1988.
Van Halderen A, Green JR: Dermatosparaxis in White Dorper sheep. J South African Vet Assoc 59:45, 1989.
Vogt DW, Carlton CG, Miller RB: Hereditary parakeratosis in Shorthorn beef cattle. Am J Vet Res 49:120–121, 1988.
Webb RF, Bourke CA: Dermatosis vegetans in pigs. Aust Vet J 64:287–288, 1987.
Wijeratne WVS, O'Toole D, Wood L, et al: A genetic, pathological and virological study of congenital hypotrichosis and incisor anodontia in cattle. Vet Rec 122:149–152, 1988.

Nutritional, Endocrine, and Keratinization Abnormalities

WILLIAM H. MILLER, JR., VMD

Traditionally, textbooks have provided separate coverage for nutritional, endocrine, or idiopathic disorders that cause skin lesions. Since all of these disorders can cause seborrheic skin lesions, a group of striking but nonspecific changes, it is best to consider all of these conditions together.

The skin and hair coat of animals is formed by the orderly proliferation, differentiation, and keratinization of basilar epidermal cells and hair matrix cells, respectively. The quality and sheen of the coat is influenced by the structure of the hair or wool and the nature and amount of surface lipids. The pigmentation of the skin and hair is directly influenced by the number and activity of the melanocytes but also secondarily by the structure of the hair, which can alter the absorption and refraction of incident light.

Skin and hair or wool growth is influenced by a wide variety of factors, including genetic makeup, systemic and local hormones, and a wide variety of nutrients. Abnormalities in any of these factors or their influence on other nutrients or hormones can cause seborrheic changes in which the skin initially is flaky and the coat is dull and dry. With time, the skin will thicken and have a crusted appearance and hairs will be lost. Although the skin over the animal's entire body is influenced by the same factors, food animals tend to show their lesions first or most severely on the face, head, distal limbs, and feet. Although certain disorders such as copper deficiency in cattle have a textbook appearance, one should be cautious in hastily defining the cause of the animal's seborrheic changes. Many different underlying events all can produce the same changes so the entire case should be reviewed carefully.

NUTRITIONAL DERMATOSES

Worldwide, nutritional diseases are of moderate to high incidence. For good health, immunologic competence, and normal skin, the animal must have a sufficient intake of calories, proteins, vitamins, and minerals. Pigs also require essential fatty acids. Deficiency in any one nutrient or imbalances in the animal's ration, either intentional or unintentional, can cause cutaneous and noncutaneous signs of illness. Cutaneous signs usually appear first, but they may be so mild that they are overlooked until the animal is showing systemic signs of illness.

Caloric, Protein, and Fatty Acid Deficiency Dermatoses

Marasmus (total starvation) or kwashiorkor (near total protein deficiency) can be caused by inadequate food intake, debilitating internal disease, or some combination thereof. Animals with either of these conditions are cachectic, are more susceptible to infections, and have dull, dry, brittle hair coats that are lost easily and will not regrow. The skin is thin, inelastic, and heals poorly. In these animals, the diagnosis of profound malnutrition is straightforward.

A more common condition is inadequate protein intake. Since approximately 30 per cent of an animal's protein intake is used to maintain the skin and hair coat, marginal protein deficiency will first be manifested in the skin. Signs will be as described above but usually less severe. Interestingly, malnourished pigs grow a longer, thicker, and heavier hair coat in which the hairs are wispy and may curl. Protein-deprived sheep produce less wool and wool that is produced is weaker and finer.

As long as ruminants have a sufficient intake of protein and carbohydrate, fats are not required in their diets. The only reference to a fat-associated dermatosis in ruminants is in calves fed a high-fat (15 to 20 per cent) milk replacer. The calves develop an alopecic, scaling dermatosis of the muzzle, periocular region, base of the pinnae, and limbs after eating the milk replacer for 2 to 3 weeks. Many calves also have signs of muscular disease. Reduction of the fat content to 10 per cent or administration of vitamin E–selenium results in rapid recovery. In all probability, the dermatosis was a secondary vitamin E deficiency induced by the fat intake.

Pigs fed fat-deficient diets will lose weight and develop generalized hair loss and scaling with the accumulation of a brownish exudate on the ears, axillae, and flanks. As long as the intake of linoleic acid is between 0.5 and 1 per cent of the caloric intake, the seborrhea does not develop. Unless pigs are fed substandard or spoiled foods, the fat deficiency seborrhea should not be seen. Fatty acid deficiency may, however, play some part in swine parakeratosis.

Vitamin Imbalances

Water-soluble vitamin deficiencies are rare in normally maintained ruminants. A vitamin C–responsive dermatitis has been described in calves. The condition occurs in young (16 to 75 day old), barn-fed, apparently well-kept dairy calves during the fall and winter. Aside from their skin disease, the calves usually are healthy. They develop widespread moderate to severe scaling, crusting, and alopecia, and their legs are erythematous with purpuric lesions. If left untreated, the dermatitis will resolve spontaneously in 2 months but the calves fail to thrive. With one to two subcutaneous injections of 3 g of ascorbic acid, the calves recover quickly and completely.

Biotin, niacin, pantothenic acid, and riboflavin deficiencies have been recognized and/or experimentally induced in pigs, especially when a high corn diet is fed. In all of these deficiencies, the pigs are ill and have a generalized seborrheic skin disease. With a biotin deficiency, the pigs also develop a stomatitis and pododermatitis with cracking of soles and hoof walls. A dark brown exudate accumulates around the eyes in pantothenic acid deficiency.

Fat-soluble vitamin deficiencies are also uncommon in food animals. Vitamin A deficiency can occur when animals are fed poorly supplemented concentrates with little or no access to green foodstuffs. Vitamin A–deficient animals have ocular, neurologic, reproductive, and dermatologic changes. Their coats are rough, dry, faded, and shaggy, and they have widespread seborrhea. The hooves can overgrow, are dry and brittle, and can have multiple, vertical cracks.

It is difficult to separate signs of vitamin E deficiency from those of selenium deficiency. Unless the animal is receiving excess amounts of fat, as previously discussed, signs of deficiency probably are due to imbalances in both nutrients. Although decreased wool growth has been associated with vitamin E–selenium deficiency in sheep, the primary dermatologic condition associated with those nutrients has been reported in goats in selenium-deficient areas. Affected animals develop periorbital alopecia and have a dull, dry, brittle coat and a generalized, dry, flaky seborrhea. An injection of vitamin E and selenium resolves the condition in 2 to 4 weeks, and twice-yearly injections prevent relapses.

Mineral Imbalances

Mineral imbalances probably account for more dermatologic conditions in food animals than all other nutrients combined. This high frequency relates to the ease in which pastures can be depleted of vital minerals and to mineral interactions. To further complicate matters there is species variability in susceptibility to deficiencies or excesses of minerals and serum mineral levels can be influenced by nonnutritional disorders. Trace mineral deficiencies can be difficult to document by blood test, and clinical disease can occur in the presence of normal blood levels.

Although all trace minerals are important for health, cobalt, iodine, selenium, copper, and zinc appear to be most important for the skin. Since calcium, iron, and molybdenum, to name a few, can influence the absorption and utilization of the other trace minerals, the entire ration, including the water, of the animal should be evaluated carefully. Selenium deficiency was discussed previously, and iodine deficiency is dealt with in the section on endocrine disorders. Cobalt-deficient animals have rough, faded hair coats, and sheep produce less and a poorer quality wool.

Copper deficiency is most important in cattle and sheep and can be due to inadequate intake or excessive intake of other minerals, especially molybdenum. It has been estimated that approximately 0.9 per cent of cattle in the United Kingdom develop signs of copper deficiency. Copper-deficient cattle have rough, dry coats that lighten in color and an exfoliative pododermatitis with heel cracks. Black hairs turn red or gray, while brown hairs turn yellow. Since the periocular hairs lighten the most, the animal has a masked or spectacled appearance. When the copper deficiency is secondary to molybdenum excess, gastrointestinal signs predominate. Copper-deficient sheep produce abnormal wool. It is straight and stringy with decreased strength and elasticity and can be abnormally colored. Early on, the pigment change can be episodic, giving the hair a banded look (achromotrichia). Later, the pigment loss can be uniform. Treatment involves correction of mineral imbalances and copper supplementation.

Zinc deficiency appears to be very important in food animals and can be due to a primary insufficiency or, even more importantly, to the ingestion through food or water of other substances such as calcium, iron, and phytates that inhibit zinc absorption. In cattle, zinc deficiency has been recognized as an inherited trait in certain breeds and as a spontaneous disorder in others. In the hereditary form, signs occur at 4 to 8 weeks of age whereas they can occur at any time in other cattle. Affected animals are prone to infections, especially pododermatitis, do poorly, and have a dull, rough, faded coat with scaling, crusting, and alopecia, especially of the face, ears, neck, mucocutaneous junctions, and distal limbs. The coronary bands can be inflamed and crusted, and the hooves can be overgrown and deformed. When high-calcium diets are fed to dry cows or young heifers, the first sign of the secondary zinc deficiency can be tail twitching with licking and chewing at the tailhead. Zinc-deficient sheep produce abnormal wool, eat their wool, and, in advanced cases, have thick, wrinkled skin with parakeratotic hyperkeratosis of the face, feet, and scrotum. Deficient goats develop a pruritic, crusting dermatitis that is most severe on the face and feet. Zinc-deficient sheep and goals also are prone to develop infectious pododermatitis. In cattle, sheep, and goats, the deficiency state is corrected and prevented by feeding a well-balanced diet that may or may not include zinc supplements.

Parakeratosis in swine is a transient disorder of young (7 to 10 weeks of age), rapidly growing feeder pigs. Zinc deficiency, either primary or secondary, is most often implicated, but fatty acid deficiency also may play a role. Affected pigs first develop erythematous macules and papules on their ventrum, and then the lesions become widespread. As the lesions age, they become scaly and crusty such that in advanced cases the pigs have a crusty dermatitis of their face, ears, tail, ventrum, and distal limbs. When diseased, the pigs have a reduced appetite and grow more slowly. Mild to moderately affected animals will improve in 10 to 14 days, while more severe cases can take up to 45 days. Therapy and, more importantly, prevention revolves around dietary modification to ensure that zinc and essential fatty acid levels are adequate and that calcium and phytate levels are not excessive.

ENDOCRINE DISORDERS

Hypothyroidism is the only endocrine dermatosis that has been recognized or experimentally induced in all food animals. The hypothyroid state can have a genetic basis but usually is due to a primary or secondary iodine deficiency. Although adults in the herd can show signs of disease (poor coat, decreased reproductive efficiency), neonatal animals are most severely affected and mortality usually is high. The animals are born weak with a generalized hypotrichosis or alopecia, diffuse hyperkeratosis, and puffy, thick skin. Palpable enlargement of the thyroid glands usually is found.

Since a variety of nonthyroidal illnesses such as starvation are known to lower triiodothyronine and thyroxine levels in food animals, baseline thyroid elevations in these animals are worthless. If iodine deficiency is suspected, iodine levels can be measured. Because of the high mortality rate in neonatal hypothyroid animals, treatment is not undertaken. Prevention is of paramount importance, and this is done by correcting the iodine deficiency in the parents.

Naturally occurring or iatrogenic hyperadrenocorticism has not been reported in food animals. Husbandry and economic considerations preclude the chronic use of corticosteroids in most food animals. Goats with pemphigus foliaceus have been successfully treated with high doses of prednisolone (2.2 mg/kg) with no adverse effects. When corticosteroids are given to sheep, their wool production decreases and the wool fibers are shorter and thinner than normal. This suggests that food animals are susceptible to the protein catabolic and antimitotic effects of chronic corticosteroid administration as are other animals.

SEBORRHEIC DISORDERS

Seborrheic disorders are those in which there is an abnormality in epidermal and follicular keratinization. The disorders included here are either of a genetic or an uncertain etiology. When an adult animal develops a seborrheic condition, it is a cutaneous manifestation of some other disorder. As the dermatology of food animals advances, the number of idiopathic conditions should decrease.

Ichthyosis

Ichthyosis has been reported in cattle and swine. Since there is a genetic basis for the disorder, signs are present at birth or develop shortly thereafter. Severely affected animals, such as calves with ichthyosis fetalis, are born dead or die shortly thereafter and have a severe, widespread scaling and crusting dermatosis. Calves with ichthyosis congenita are healthy at birth and have or will shortly develop a generalized hypotrichosis and scaling that will be most severe on the muzzle, limbs, and ventrum. The primary differential diagnosis in these calves is hypothyroidism. Since calves with ichthyosis congenita are otherwise healthy and have no obvious goiter, the tentative diagnosis of ichthyosis should be straightforward and can be confirmed by skin biopsy. Treatment is inappropriate, and the parents should be culled.

Swine Hyperkeratosis

Intensely managed boars and sows of any age or breed can develop a dorsally distributed seborrheic disorder. Most affected animals have a brownish scaly dermatosis over the neck and shoulder region, but the entire dorsum and flank regions can be involved. Manual removal of the scale shows that the underlying skin appears normal. The condition is not pruritic, and the animals are healthy otherwise.

No cause for the condition has been identified, but fat supplementation with cod liver oil (1 gallon/50 sows/week) will reduce the incidence. The response to fat supplementation could indicate that this is a nutritional dermatosis, but swine hyperkeratosis may also be a seborrheic condition associated with stress. Stress is known to increase eicosanoid synthesis, which in turn can increase epidermal turnover. Cod liver oil, with its high content of marine lipids, can influence eicosanoid production and thus could decrease the stress-induced epidermal hyperproliferation.

FARROWING HOUSE DERMATOSIS OF SOWS

An idiopathic dermatosis of farrowing sows has been described. The sows are normal until they enter the farrowing house, when they develop a nonpruritic rash consisting of multiple, scaly, annular, erythematous macules and patches. The hairs in the involved areas discolor to brown. Lesions occur predominantly on the trunk and only in white areas. Piglets are never affected and boars rarely so. The dermatosis resolves spontaneously when the sows leave the farrowing house.

When fungal cultures were taken, *Microsporum nanum* was isolated from over 50 per cent of the tested sows, but the organism could not be seen in skin biopsy specimens. Histologically, the dermatosis is a hyperplastic condition with perivascular accumulation of lymphocytes and eosinophils, typical of a hypersensitivity condition. No irritants or allergens could be identified in the farrowing house to explain the dermatosis. Since the condition is nonpruritic, does not effect productivity, and resolves spontaneously, it is considered a cosmetic problem, whose only impact might be on the value of the sow at sale.

EXFOLIATIVE DERMATITIS OF PYGMY GOATS

An exfoliative dermatitis has been recognized in Pygmy goats in which the animal shows hair loss, scaling, and crusting around the eyes, lips, and chin. The ears, poll, ventrum, and other areas also may be involved. All animals in the herd can be affected and the lesions wax and wane in severity. Histologically, the condition is a psoriasiform dermatitis of unknown cause. The condition responds poorly to all treatments except corticosteroids.

BIBLIOGRAPHY

Abraham MJ, Valasala KV, Rajan A: Clinical features of experimental hypothyroidism in calves. Kerala J Vet Sci 17:52–70, 1986.
Blood DC, Radostits OM: Veterinary Medicine: A Textbook of the Diseases of Cattle, Sheep, Pigs, Goats and Horses, 7th ed, pp 475–500, 1150–1228. Philadelphia, Baillière Tindale, 1989.
Hanson LJ, Sorensen DK, Kernkamp HCH: Essential fatty acid deficiency: its role in parakeratosis. Am J Vet Res 19:921–930, 1958.
Hutcheson DP: Nutrient requirements of diseased, stressed cattle. Vet Clin North Am [Food Anim Pract] 4:523–530, 1988.
Jefferies AR: Alopecic exfoliative dermatosis in goats. Vet Rec 121:576, 1987.
Lofstedt J: Dermatologic diseases of sheep. Vet Clin North Am [Large Anim Pract] 5:427–448, 1983.
Manning TO: Noninfectious skin diseases of cattle. Vet Clin North Am [Large Anim Pract] 6:175–186, 1984.
Miller WH: Fatty acid supplements as anti-inflammatory agents. In Kirk RW (ed): Current Veterinary Therapy X, pp 563–565. Philadelphia, WB Saunders, 1989.
Mullowney PC, Hall RF: Skin diseases of swine. Vet Clin North Am [Large Anim Pract] 6:107–127, 1984.
Nockels CF: The role of vitamins in modulating disease resistance. Vet Clin North Am [Food Anim Pract] 4:531–542, 1988.
Osweiler GD, Carson TL, Buck WB, VanGelder GA: Clinical and Diagnostic Veterinary Toxicology, 3rd ed, pp 87–142. Dubuque, IA, Kendall/Hunt Publishing Co, 1985.
Penny RHC, Muirhead MR: Skin. In Leman AD, et al (eds): Diseases of Swine V, p 76. Ames, Iowa State University Press, 1981.
Reuter R, Bowden M, Besier B, et al: Zinc response alopecia and hyperkeratosis in angora goats. Aust Vet J 64:351–352, 1987.
Rijnberk A, DeVijlder JJM, VanDijk JE, et al: Congenital defect in iodothyronine synthesis: clinical aspects of iodine metabolism in goats with congenital goiter and hypothyroidism. Br Vet J 133:495–503, 1977.
Scott DW: Large Animal Dermatology. Philadelphia, WB Saunders, 1989.
Scott DW, Samuelson M, Smith CA: Clinicopathologic Studies on a Chronic, Recurrent Dermatosis of Sows. Agri-Practice 10:43–49, 1989.

Disorders of Pigmentation and Epidermal Appendages
DANNY W. SCOTT, DVM, Diplomate, ACVD

DISORDERS OF PIGMENTATION

Hyperpigmentation

Hyperpigmentation (melanosis) is frequently encountered as an acquired condition, usually associated with chronic inflammation and irritation. Hyperpigmentation may affect only the skin (melanoderma), only the hair (melanotrichia), or both.

Lentigo is an idiopathic macular melanosis of swine. Annular, well-circumscribed, deeply and evenly pigmented macules are present, especially over the trunk. These lesions may be seen in combination with cutaneous melanoma.

Hypopigmentation

Hypopigmentation (hypomelanosis), amelanosis (achromoderma, achromotrichia), and depigmentation are not synonymous. Hypopigmentation refers to a decrease in normal melanin pigmentation. Amelanosis indicates a total lack of melanin. Depigmentation means a loss of pre-existing melanin. *Leukoderma* and *leukotrichia* are clinical terms used to indicate acquired depigmentation of skin and hair, respectively.

ALBINISM. Albinism is an autosomal recessive disorder of melanin synthesis that affects the skin, hair, and eyes. Affected animals have white skin and hair, pink eyes, and photophobia.

Albinism is rarely diagnosed in food animals and has been most completely studied in Icelandic sheep. In albinism, electron microscopic examination of skin shows that melanocytes are present but melanin synthesis is defective.

CHÉDIAK-HIGASHI SYNDROME. The Chédiak-Higashi syndrome is an autosomal recessive partial oculocutaneous albinism of Hereford cattle. Affected cattle also have photophobia, increased susceptibility to infections, hemorrhagic tendencies, and an average life span of about 1 year.

Light and electron microscopic examinations of skin reveal abnormally large and clumped melanosomes, which are delivered with difficulty to keratinocytes.

LEUKODERMA. Leukoderma is an acquired depigmentation of the skin that follows various traumatic and inflammatory injuries to the skin, such as pressure sores, regressing viral papillomatosis, freezing, and burns (chemical, thermal, radiation). Leukoderma has also been reported to follow contact with phenols and rubber. Many rubbers contain monobenzyl ether of hydroquinone (antioxidant), which inhibits melanogenesis.

VITILIGO. Vitiligo is an idiopathic acquired depigmentation. There are no preceding or concurrent signs of cutaneous inflammation or injury. Vitiligo has been reported in cattle (some cases of which may have a hereditary basis) and in swine with cutaneous melanoma (in which the condition may be immune mediated).

In cattle, especially Holstein-Friesians, vitiligo begins as a more-or-less symmetric development of well-circumscribed, annular areas of depigmentation. The depigmented areas are usually less than 1 cm in diameter (macule) but may occasionally be much larger (patch). Hairs may become depigmented as well. The muzzle, lips, and periocular areas are most commonly affected, but lesions may be seen on many mucocutaneous junctions, the hooves, and even the general body surface. Pruritus and pain are absent, and affected animals are usually healthy otherwise.

The diagnosis of vitiligo is confirmed by a skin biopsy that demonstrates a complete absence of melanin and melanocytes. Prognostically, the depigmentation may wax and wane in intensity but is usually permanent. There is no effective therapy.

LEUKOTRICHIA. Leukotrichia is an acquired depigmentation of the hair that follows various traumatic and inflammatory injuries to the skin. Precocious hereditary graying has been reported in Holstein-Friesian cattle in the Netherlands and is called "blau."

Porcine Erythema and Cyanosis

Swine frequently develop noninflammatory erythema or cyanosis of the skin for a number of reasons. Erythema may be seen with dermatosis erythematosa (especially ventrum, flanks, ears), sunburn (especially dorsum), transit erythema (especially ventrum), carbon monoxide poisoning (generalized), viral infections (especially ears, tail, and extremities with hog cholera and African swine fever), and bacterial infections (especially ears, tail, and extremities with streptococcosis, erysipelas, and actinobacillosis). Cyanosis may be seen with benign periportal cyanosis (sows at farrowing time, generalized), porcine stress syndrome (blotchy, then coalesced on dependent side), bacterial infections (especially ears, tail, and extremities with *Haemophilus parasuis* or *H. pleuropneumoniae* infections, *Escherichia coli* enteritis, hemagglutinating encephalomyelitis, salmonellosis, pasteurellosis, erysipelas, actinobacillosis), thiamine deficiency, and organophosphate or carbamate poisoning (generalized).

DISORDERS OF EPIDERMAL APPENDAGES

Hypotrichosis

Hypotrichosis implies a less than normal amount of hair. The condition may be regional or multifocal but is usually generalized. It has been reported in all food animal species and is usually hereditary.

Curly Coat

Abnormal curliness of the hair coat has been reported as an inherited condition in cattle and swine.

Hypertrichosis

Hypertrichosis implies a greater than normal amount of hair. It has been reported as an inherited condition in cattle and swine and with in utero border disease infection in lambs. Hypertrichosis may also be seen focally as a result of local injury or irritation. The hair in these focal areas may become excessive, thicker, stiffer, and darker than normal.

Hair Follicle Dysplasia

Hair follicle dysplasias have been reported in black-and-white and tan-and-white ("buckskin") Holstein cattle. Although the etiopathogenesis has not been elucidated, it is probable that heredity plays an important role.

Affected animals are born with normal hair coats but begin to lose the hair in the black- or tan-haired areas very early in life. These areas are hypotrichotic, often containing dull, stubbled hairs and a mild degree of scaling on the surface of the skin. The white-haired areas are normal. Affected cattle are otherwise healthy.

Diagnosis is based on skin biopsy, which shows dysplastic hair follicles and hair shafts, and abnormal melanin clumping within hair follicle outer root sheaths, hair shafts, and piliary canals. There is no effective therapy.

Abnormal Shedding

Normal shedding in food animals is basically controlled by photoperiod and, to a lesser extent, environmental temperature. Thus, most animals in temperate regions shed, to one degree or another, in spring and fall. In some animals, especially individual cattle or goats, abnormal spring shedding may result in excessive hair loss. Areas of marked hypotrichosis or alopecia may develop on the face, shoulders, and rump or may be fairly generalized and symmetric. The skin in affected areas is normal, and the animals are otherwise healthy. The pathogenesis of abnormal shedding is not understood.

Abnormal shedding may be confused with anagen defluxion, telogen defluxion, alopecia areata, or endocrine skin disease. However, affected animals spontaneously and completely recover within 1 to 3 months.

Anagen Defluxion

In anagen defluxion, a circumstance (antimitotic drugs, infectious diseases, endocrine disorders, metabolic diseases) interferes with anagen (the growth phase of hair follicles), resulting in hair follicle and hair shaft abnormalities. Hair loss occurs within days, as the growth phase continues. This is typical of the sudden hair loss that occurs within days of a very high fever, systemic illness, and malnutrition in calves, lambs, and kids. Hair loss is usually symmetric and widespread.

Diagnosis is based on microscopic examination of affected hairs. Anagen defluxion hairs are characterized by irregularities and dysplastic changes. The diameter of the shaft may be irregularly narrowed and deformed, and breaking often occurs at such structurally weak sites, resulting in ragged points.

Anagen defluxion spontaneously resolves when the constitutional stress is relieved.

Telogen Defluxion

In telogen defluxion, a stressful circumstance (high fever, pregnancy, shock, severe illness, surgery, anesthesia) causes the abrupt, premature cessation of growth in anagen hair follicles and the sudden synchrony of many hair follicles in catagen, then telogen (the resting phase of hair follicles). Two to 3 months later, a large number of telogen hairs are shed as a new wave of hair follicle cyclic activity begins. Hair loss is usually symmetric and widespread.

Diagnosis is based on microscopic examination of affected hairs. Telogen defluxion hairs are characterized by a uniform shaft diameter and a slightly clubbed, nonpigmented root end that lacks root sheaths. Telogen defluxion spontaneously resolves within 1 to 2 months of its appearance.

Alopecia Areata

Alopecia is a recently recognized, apparently rare disorder of cattle. There are no apparent age, breed, or sex predilections. The cause and pathogenesis are unknown.

Clinically, alopecia areata is characterized by focal or multifocal, well-circumscribed, annular patches of noninflammatory alopecia. The skin in affected areas appears normal. The face, neck, and trunk are most commonly affected. Pruritus and pain are absent, and affected animals are otherwise healthy. When hair regrows, it may be a lighter color than normal (leukotrichia).

The differential diagnosis includes other causes of annular alopecia: dermatophytosis, dermatophilosis, demodicosis, stephanofilariasis, staphylococcal folliculitis, and sterile eosinophilic folliculitis. All of these are characterized by various gross inflammatory changes: erythema, oozing, crusts, scales, and so forth, which are not seen with alopecia areata. Definitive diagnosis is based on skin biopsy (peribulbar lymphocytic perifolliculitis).

The prognosis appears to vary according to the distribution of lesions. Animals having localized lesions may undergo spontaneous remission within months to 2 years. Animals with widespread lesions may fail to recover. There is no effective therapy.

BIBLIOGRAPHY

Miller WH, Jr, Scott DW: Black-hair follicular dysplasia in a Holstein cow. Cornell Vet 80:273–277, 1990.
Ostrowski S, Evans A: Coat-color-linked hair follicle dysplasia in "buckskin" Holstein cows in central California. Agri-Practice 10:12–13, 1989.
Paradis M, Fecteau G, Scott DW: Alopecia areata (pelade) in a cow. Can Vet J 29:727–729, 1988.
Scott DW: Large Animal Dermatology, pp 387–398. Philadelphia, WB Saunders, 1988.
Scott DW, Guard CL: Alopecia areata in a cow. Agri-Practice 9:16–19, 1988.

Miscellaneous Skin Diseases
DANNY W. SCOTT, DVM, DIPLOMATE, ACVD

BOVINE STERILE EOSINOPHILIC FOLLICULITIS

Sterile eosinophilic folliculitis is a recently reported, apparently rare disorder of cattle. There are no apparent age, breed, or sex predilections. The cause and pathogenesis are unknown.

The disorder is nonseasonal in occurrence and is characterized by a more-or-less symmetric papulocrustous eruption. Lesions progress to annular areas of alopecia, crusting, scaling, and plaques. The head, neck, and trunk are commonly affected. Pruritus is usually mild to absent. The lesions are usually not painful, and affected animals are otherwise healthy. Typically, only one animal in a herd is affected.

The differential diagnosis includes other causes of annular, alopecic, crusty lesions: dermatophytosis, dermatophilosis, demodicosis, stephanofilariasis, *Pelodera* dermatitis, and staphylococcal folliculitis. Definitive diagnosis is based on exfoliative cytology (predominantly eosinophils, no intracellular microorganisms), skin biopsy (eosinophilic folliculitis and/or furunculosis, special stains for microorganisms negative), and negative cultures for bacteria and fungi.

The natural course of the disease is unknown. Although the condition is known to clear with topical or systemic glucocorticoid administration, relapses occur when therapy is stopped.

PORCINE DERMATOSIS ERYTHEMATOSA

Porcine dermatosis erythematosa is a poorly characterized dermatosis. The etiology and pathogenesis are unknown, and meaningful clinicopathologic studies have apparently not been conducted.

The dermatosis is reported to be quite common in white pigs and can occur in swine grazing new pasture or in fattening pigs and breeding stock housed entirely indoors. There is striking acute erythema over large areas of the body, including the ears, sides, and abdomen. There is no pruritus or pain, and affected swine are usually otherwise healthy.

Therapy is unnecessary, since complete, spontaneous recovery occurs within a few days.

BIBLIOGRAPHY

Scott DW: Large Animal Dermatology, pp 404–408. Philadelphia, WB Saunders, 1988.
Scott DW, Walton DK, Guard CL: Sterile eosinophilic folliculitis in cattle. Agri-Practice 7:8–14, 1986.

Neoplastic Skin Diseases
DANNY W. SCOTT, DVM, DIPLOMATE, ACVD

Veterinary oncology has come into its own as a specialty. Detailed information on the various aspects of the pathogenesis, immunology, and pathology of neoplasia is available in other publications and is not presented here. This chapter serves as a clinical overview of the most common cutaneous neoplasms and nonneoplastic tumors in food animals.

In general, the risk of cutaneous neoplasia increases with age. Specific sex predilections for cutaneous neoplasia are evident in female goats (udder papillomatosis, squamous cell carcinoma), female sheep (squamous cell carcinoma), and male swine (scrotal hemangioma). Breed predilections for cutaneous tumors are presented in Table 1.

The skin is one of the most common sites of neoplasia in food animals. The most common cutaneous neoplasms, by animal affected and in approximate descending order of frequency, are papilloma, squamous cell carcinoma, melanoma, and mast cell tumor (cattle); squamous cell carcinoma, papilloma, and melanoma (goats); squamous cell carcinoma and

Table 1. BREED PREDILECTIONS FOR CUTANEOUS TUMORS

Breed	Tumor
Shorthorn cattle	Papillomatosis
Saanen goats	Udder papillomatosis
Hereford cattle	Squamous cell carcinoma
Ayrshire cattle	Squamous cell carcinoma
Angora goats	Squamous cell carcinoma, melanoma
Merino sheep	Squamous cell carcinoma, follicular cyst
Berkshire swine	Scrotal hemangioma
Yorkshire swine	Scrotal hemangioma
Angus cattle	Melanoma
Suffolk sheep	Melanoma
Duroc-Jersey swine	Melanoma
Sinclair miniature swine	Melanoma
Nubian goats	Wattle cyst

papilloma (sheep); and melanoma, hemangioma, and squamous cell carcinoma (swine).

The key to appropriate management and accurate prognosis of cutaneous neoplasms is *specific diagnosis*. This can be achieved only by biopsy and histologic evaluation. Exfoliative cytology (aspiration and impression smear) is easy and rapid and often gives valuable information on neoplastic cell type and differentiation. However, exfoliative cytology is inferior to, and no substitute for, biopsy and histopathology.

EPITHELIAL NEOPLASMS

Papillomatosis

Papillomatosis (warts, verrucae) is common in cattle, uncommon in goats and sheep, and rare in swine. In most instances, papillomatosis is known to be caused by DNA papovaviruses. In cattle, there are at least six types of papovaviruses that tend to have site specificity on the animal. In general, papovaviruses are host-specific infectious agents that are transmitted by direct and indirect (fomite) contact. The incubation period varies from 2 to 6 months.

In cattle, papillomatosis is common and is caused by at least six different types of DNA papovaviruses. Bovine papovavirus type 1 (BPV 1) causes typical fibropapillomas on the teats and penises of animals younger than 2 years of age. These lesions often spontaneously regress within 1 to 12 months. BPV 2 causes typical fibropapillomas on the head, neck, and dewlap of animals younger than 2 years of age. These lesions are usually multiple, gray, firm, hyperkeratotic, pedunculated, or broad-based, are 1 mm to several centimeters in diameter, and often spontaneously regress within 1 to 12 months. BPV 3 causes so-called atypical warts in cattle of all ages. These lesions are low, flat, circular, and nonpedunculated, have delicate frond-like projections on their surfaces, and may occur anywhere on the body, including the teats. BPV 3–induced papillomas do *not* regress spontaneously. BPV 4 causes papillomas in the gastrointestinal tract. BPV 5 causes so-called rice grain warts on the teats of cattle of all ages. These lesions are small, white, and elongated and do *not* regress spontaneously. Interdigital papillomatosis is a chronic problem in housed dairy cattle and has no age or breed predilections. Typical fibropapillomas occur on the dorsal and ventral aspects of the interdigital spaces, especially on the hind legs, and are often associated with pain, lameness, weight loss, decreased milk production, and decreased estrus detection. These lesions do *not* regress spontaneously. Viral etiology is suspected but not proved.

In sheep, papillomatosis is uncommon and has no apparent age, breed, or sex predilections. The disease is caused by a DNA papovavirus. Lesions are usually verrucous and multiple and occur most frequently on the hairy skin of the face and legs. Ovine papillomas have the potential of transforming into squamous cell carcinomas.

In goats, papillomatosis is uncommon and no age predilection is apparent. Viral etiology is suspected but not proved. Caprine papillomatosis occurs in two clinical forms, and the lesions are usually verrucous. In one form, lesions occur commonly on the face, neck, shoulders, and forelegs and have no apparent sex or breed predilections. These lesions usually regress spontaneously, and transformation into squamous cell carcinoma may occur.

In swine, papillomatosis is rare and no age, breed, or sex predilections are apparent. Viral etiology is suspected but not proved. Lesions may be solitary or multiple and occur on the face, genitalia, and limbs.

The literature on the therapeutic management of papillomatosis is confusing and contradictory. Most of the confusion centers around two major points: (1) the failure to consider the self-limiting nature of many forms of papillomatosis and (2) the relatively recent discovery that there are many types of papovaviruses that produce papillomatosis in food animals. In cattle, papillomatosis caused by BPV 1 and BPV 2 usually regresses spontaneously, as does papillomatosis of sheep and papillomatosis of the head, neck, and forelegs in goats. Spontaneous remission usually occurs within 1 to 12 months, and animals that have persistent lesions should be suspected of having inappropriate immune responses. On the other hand, cattle with papillomatosis caused by BPV 3 or BPV 5, cattle with interdigital papillomatosis, and goats with papillomatosis of the udder have persistent disease, with spontaneous regression occurring rarely.

For lesions that must be removed for aesthetic or health reasons, surgical excision or cryosurgery is effective. It has been anecdotally stated that surgical excision, cryosurgical removal, or crushing of larger lesions may cause other lesions to regress. There is no scientific support for such a statement.

Many topical agents have been tried on individual lesions when surgery was impractical. The most commonly recommended agents include podophyllin (50 per cent podophyllin; 20 per cent podophyllin in 95 per cent ethyl alcohol; 2 per cent podophyllin in 25 per cent salicylic acid) and dimethyl sulfoxide (undiluted medical grade DMSO). These agents are usually applied once daily until remission occurs.

The subject of vaccination (autogenous or commercial) in the treatment and prevention of papillomatosis is very confusing, mostly because experimental and clinical trials were conducted prior to the recognition of the numerous types of papovaviruses involved in papillomatosis. When one allows for the different types of papovaviruses, the following generalizations seem justified. Autogenous vaccines and commercial bovine wart vaccines are ineffective for the treatment of caprine udder papillomatosis and ineffective for the treatment or prevention of bovine papillomatosis caused by BPV 3 and BPV 5 and of bovine interdigital papillomatosis. Vaccines containing BPV 1 and BPV 2 are effective for the prevention but not the treatment of bovine papillomatosis caused by BPV 1 and BPV 2.

General therapeutic adjuvants in all cases of papillomatosis, when feasible, include isolation of affected animals from noninfected animals, reduction of cutaneous injuries associated with the environment, and disinfection of the environment (e.g., with formaldehyde or lye).

Uncomplicated papillomatosis is usually of little concern, except in valuable animals in competitive shows or overseas sales. Economic losses can occur through hide damage, secondary infection or myiasis, and carcass condemnation. In cattle, it has been stated that animals with papillomatosis affecting over 20 per cent of their bodies have a poor prognosis.

Squamous Cell Carcinoma

Squamous cell carcinomas are common malignant neoplasms of food animals. The etiology of squamous cell carcinoma is not clear in all cases, but in most instances it is related to the chronic exposure of poorly pigmented, poorly haired skin to ultraviolet light. In some instances, squamous cell carcinomas may arise from viral papillomas or follicular cysts.

In goats, squamous cell carcinomas occur in adult to aged animals, with does and Angoras being predisposed. The tumors are usually solitary and occur most commonly on the perineum, vulva, and udder of female animals and on the ears of both sexes. The lesions may be ulcerative and/or proliferative, and metastasis is not uncommon. Caprine squamous cell carcinomas are known to arise from papillomas of the udder, especially in Saanens.

In sheep, squamous cell carcinomas occur in adult to aged animals with ewes and Merinos being predisposed. The lesions may be solitary or multiple and commonly occur on the pinnae, eyelids, muzzle, lips, and perineal region. The lesions may be ulcerative and/or proliferative, and metastasis may occur. Ovine squamous cell carcinomas are believed to occasionally arise from viral papillomas and follicular cysts, and vulvar squamous cell carcinomas occur most frequently in ewes that have had a radical Mule's operation to reduce susceptibility to fly-strike.

In cattle, squamous cell carcinomas occur in adult to aged animals with no sex predilection. Breed predilections include poorly pigmented animals, especially Herefords and Ayrshires. The lesions most commonly occur at mucocutaneous junctions, especially periocular and vulvar. Lesions may be ulcerative and/or proliferative, and metastasis is not uncommon.

In swine, squamous cell carcinomas occur in adult to aged animals with no sex or breed predilections. Lesions may be single or multiple and ulcerative and/or proliferative and occur especially on the pinnae and trunk. Metastasis may occur.

The therapy of choice is wide surgical excision. Other treatment modalities that may be successful in selected cases include cryosurgery, radiofrequency hyperthermia, and radiation therapy.

MESENCHYMAL NEOPLASMS

Hemangioma

Hemangiomas are benign tumors arising from the endothelial cells of blood vessels. They are uncommon in swine and cattle and rare in sheep and goats. The cause of hemangiomas is unknown.

In swine, hemangiomas occur most commonly in the scrotum of mature Yorkshire and Berkshire boars. The condition may be genetically determined. Lesions are usually multiple, beginning as tiny purple papules and progressing to hyperkeratotic, hyperpigmented, verrucous papules and plaques. Profuse hemorrhage may occur when lesions are traumatized.

In cattle, hemangiomas usually occur in mature animals but may occur congenitally. Lesions may be single or multiple and may occur anywhere on the body. So-called angiomatosis has been described in mature dairy and beef cattle in the United States and Europe. One or several black to reddish gray to pink, soft, sessile to pedunculated masses, 0.5 to 2.5 cm in diameter, are most commonly found over the back. These lesions are often initially detected because of recurrent hemorrhage, which can be profuse.

The therapy of choice of hemangiomas is surgical excision.

Mast Cell Tumor

Mast cell tumors are uncommon in cattle and rare in swine. Mast cell tumors may be benign or malignant, and they arise from cutaneous mast cells. The cause of these tumors is unknown.

In cattle, mast cell tumors occur in animals 6 months to 7 years of age, with no breed or sex predilections. Lesions are usually multiple, 1 to 40 cm in diameter, firm to fluctuant, and dermal or subcutaneous in location; they may or may not be ulcerated or alopecic. They can occur anywhere, especially over the neck and trunk. The majority of bovine mast cell tumors are malignant and metastatic.

In swine, mast cell tumors have been reported in animals 6 to 18 months of age, with no breed or sex predilections. Lesions may be single or multiple, 2 to 20 mm in diameter, firm to fluctuant, dermal to subcutaneous in location, and may occur anywhere on the body. Porcine mast cell tumors may be limited to the skin or may involve internal organs.

The therapy of choice is wide surgical excision when practical. Cryosurgery and radiation therapy are treatment options.

LYMPHORETICULAR NEOPLASIA

Lymphosarcoma

Cutaneous lymphosarcoma is a rare malignancy of cattle and is extremely rare in sheep, goats, and swine. In cattle, enzootic lymphosarcoma is caused by the bovine leukemia virus, but most cases of bovine cutaneous lymphosarcoma are sporadic and not associated with this retrovirus.

In cattle, cutaneous lymphosarcoma usually occurs in young adult animals, 1 to 4 years of age, with no sex or breed predilections. The lesions are usually multiple, are 1 to 8 cm in diameter, and may occur anywhere on the body, especially the neck and trunk. The overlying skin may be normal (urticaria like) or alopecic, crusted, hyperkeratotic, and ulcerated (ringworm like). Initially, affected cattle are otherwise healthy. Frequently, the cutaneous lesions spontaneously regress. However, remission is usually followed by relapse and fatal internal involvement.

Effective therapy has not been reported.

MELANOCYTIC NEOPLASMS

Melanoma

Melanomas are benign or malignant neoplasms arising from melanocytes or melanoblasts. Melanomas are common in certain breeds of swine, uncommon in cattle and goats, and rare in sheep. The cause of melanomas is unknown. In Sinclair miniature and Duroc-Jersey swine, melanomas appear to have a genetic basis.

In cattle, melanomas occur in animals of any age, newborn to aged, with no sex predilection. Dark-haired breeds appear to be predisposed, especially Angus. Lesions may be solitary or multiple and black to gray, are frequently ulcerated, and may occur anywhere on the body, especially the head, neck, and distal limbs. Most bovine melanomas are benign, although metastasis can occur.

In goats, melanomas occur most commonly in adult to aged animals with does being predilected. Angoras appear to be predisposed to develop these tumors. Lesions may be solitary or multiple and black to gray to brown, are frequently ulcerated, and occur most commonly on the perineum, tail, udder, pinnae, and coronets. Caprine cutaneous melanomas often metastasize.

In sheep, melanomas usually occur in adult to aged animals with no sex predilection. Suffolks appear to be predisposed. Lesions are often multiple and subcutaneous, are black to gray, and tend to occur in pigmented skin. Metastases are frequent.

In swine, melanomas occur in animals of any age, newborn to adult, with no sex predilection. Duroc-Jersey and Sinclair miniature swine are genetically predisposed to develop these tumors. The incidence of melanomas in some swine herds can reach 20 per cent, and littermates may be affected. Lesions may be solitary or multiple and may occur anywhere on the body, especially the trunk. In general, the lesions may be flat, well circumscribed, and evenly pigmented (lentigo or melanocytic nevus stages) or raised, black, and frequently ulcerated (melanoma stage). The smaller, flatter lesions often spontaneously regress, and regression may be associated with the development of vitiligo. Larger, raised lesions are often metastatic.

Surgical excision, where feasible, is the only effective therapy.

CYSTS

Cysts are uncommon in goats and sheep and rare in cattle and swine. These cysts are benign, nonneoplastic lesions characterized by an epithelial wall, with keratinous to amorphous contents.

Follicular cysts develop by retention of follicular or glandular products resulting from congenital or acquired loss or obliteration of follicular orifices. The cysts may be solitary or multiple, firm to fluctuant, well circumscribed, smooth, and round, and the overlying skin is often normal in appearance. Cysts that have been traumatized or ruptured can develop foreign body granuloma or secondary infection. Follicular cysts are most commonly seen in adult sheep and may have an inherited basis in Merinos. Lesions occur without apparent sex or site predilection and can cause aesthetic damage, damage to hides and fleece, and increased difficulty in shearing. Secondary squamous cell carcinomas may develop in the cyst walls.

Wattle cysts occur in goats. These cysts are believed to be developmental abnormalities, possibly arising from the branchial cleft. Nubian goats and Nubian crossbreeds are most commonly affected, and the lesions may have a hereditary basis. The cysts are present at the base of the wattle at birth but may not be noticed until the animal is 2 to 3 months of age. They are usually rounded, smooth, soft, and fluctuant, and the overlying skin is normal in appearance.

The treatment of choice for all cysts, when necessary, is surgical excision.

BIBLIOGRAPHY

Gourreau JM, Leclercq H, Scott DW, Mialot M: Mélanocytome chez un taurillon normand. Bull Acad Vét Fr 63:213–235, 1990.
Moulton JE: Tumors in Domestic Animals II. Berkeley, University of California Press, 1990.
Ramadan RO, El Hassan AM, Taj El Deen MH: Malignant melanoma in goats: a clinicopathological study. J Comp Pathol 98:237–246, 1988.
Scott DW: Large Animal Dermatology, pp 419–467. Philadelphia, WB Saunders, 1988.
Theilen GH, Madewell BR: Veterinary Cancer Medicine II. Philadelphia, WB Saunders, 1987.

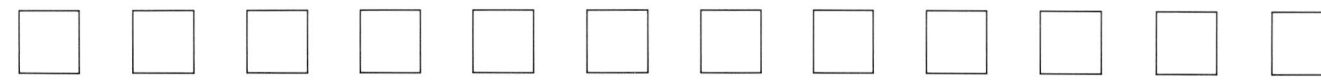

APPENDIX

- A Partial List of Reference Ranges
- Availability of Some Common Products
- Addresses of Some Companies Manufacturing Common Drugs
- Table of Common Drugs: Approximate Doses
- Conversion Tables

A Partial List of Reference Ranges

WALTER E. HOFFMANN, DVM, PhD

Reference ranges often depend on age, sex, breed, and other factors as well as emotional and physiologic stresses, such as transporting, pregnancy, and lactation at the time of sampling. Therefore, it is best for the reference ranges to be determined utilizing animals that most nearly fit the description of those from which samples will be taken for diagnostic purposes. Reference values are also dependent on the method of analysis, so it is most appropriate for reference values to be determined in the laboratory in which diagnostic samples will be analyzed. The values given here are from adult animals, unless otherwise indicated, and are derived from standard texts. These values should be used as only a very general point of reference, and more definitive reference ranges can be obtained from the laboratory conducting the analysis.

Table 1. REFERENCE VALUES FOR ADULT ANIMALS

	Cattle[1]	Sheep[1]	Goats[1]	Swine[1]	Llamas[2]
Erythrocytes					
Erythrocytes ($10^6/\mu L$)	5–10	9–15	8–18	5–8	11.3–17
Hemoglobin (g/dl)	8–15	9–15	8–12	10–16	12.6–17.8
PCV	24–46	27–45	22–38	32–50	28–39
MCV	40–60	28–40	16–25	50–68	20–27.5
MCH	11–17	8–12	5.2–8	17–21	—
MCHC	30–36	31–34	30–36	30–34	43.3–46.5
Reticulocytes (%)	0	0	0	0–1	—
RBC diameter	4–8	3.2–6	2.5–3.9	4–8	—
Fibrinogen (g/L)	3–7	1–5	1–4	1–5	1–4
Leukocytes					
Leukocytes (μL)	4000–12,000	4000–12,000	4000–13,000	11,000–22,000	7200–21,400
Neutrophil (bands)	0–120	rare	rare	—	0–360
Neutrophil (bands, %)	0–2	0–0.5	—	—	—
Neutrophils (seg)	600–4000	700–6000	1200–7200	—	4600–16,300
Neutrophils (seg, %)	15–45	10–50	30–48	28–47	—
Lymphocytes	2500–7500	2000–9000	2000–9000	—	1000–7800
Lymphocytes (%)	45–75	40–75	50–70	39–62	—
Monocytes	25–840	0–750	0–550	—	0–1000
Monocytes (%)	2–7	0–6	0–4	2–10	—
Eosinophils	0–2400	0–1000	50–650	—	0–3200
Eosinophils (%)	2–20	0–10	1–8	0.5–11	—
Basophils	0–200	0–300	0–120	—	0–400
Basophils (%)	0–2	0–3	0–1	0–2	—
Neutrophil/lymphocyte ratio	0.45/1	0.48/1	0.65/1	0.7/1	—
Platelets ($10^3/\mu L$)	100–800	250–750	300–600	130–950	200–600

PCV = packed cell volume; MCV = mean corpuscular volume; MCH = mean corpuscular hemoglobin; MCHC = mean corpuscular hemoglobin concentration; RBC = red blood cell.

Table 2. REFERENCE VALUES FOR YOUNG ANIMALS

	Calves (3–16 wk)	Kids	Piglets (3–4 mo)	Llama (Juv)
	Avg ± 1 SD	Avg ± 1 SD	Range	Range
Erythrocytes				
Erythrocytes ($10^6/\mu L$)	9.5 ± 1		6.4–8	—
Hemoglobin	11.2 ± 1.5		11.5–13.3	9–14
PCV	35.9 ± 3.8		38–44	26–34
Leukocytes				
Leukocytes (μL)	10,715 ± 3,047	13,530 ± 246	18.9–33.8	12,000–15,200
Neutrophils (bands)	24 ± 56	—	—	—
Neutrophils (bands, %)	0.23 ± 0.5	—	1–3	—
Neutrophils (segs)	2,872 ± 1,331	4,440 ± 160	—	6,500–8,500
Neutrophils (segs, %)	26.2 ± 8.8	—	17–42	—
Lymphocytes	6,861 ± 2,179	9,130 ± 210	—	3,200–5,000
Lymphocytes (%)	64.1 ± 8.6	—	46–77	—
Monocytes	794 ± 270	—	—	300–800
Monocytes (%)	8.2 ± 4.2	—	1–8	—
Eosinophils	106 ± 342	—	—	500–1,800
Eosinophils (%)	0.7 ± 2	—	.5–8.5	—
Basophils	54 ± 76	—	—	0–300
Basophils (%)	0.5 ± 0.6	—	0–1.5	—

Table 3. SERUM ENZYME ACTIVITY (U/L)

Enzyme	Cattle[3]	Sheep[3]	Goats[3]	Pigs[3]	Llamas[2]
Alkaline phosphatase	0–488	68–387	93–387	118–395	—
Transaminase (SGOT)	78–132	—	167–513	32–84	106–317
Gamma-glutamyltransferase	16–26	—	—	—	7–32
Sorbitol dehydrogenase	4.3–15.3	5.8–27.9	14–23.6	1–5.8	—
Lactic dehydrogenase	692–1,445	238–440	123–392	380–634	—

Table 4. SERUM CONSTITUENTS

	Cattle[3]	Sheep[3]	Goats[3]	Pigs[3]	Llamas[2]
Glucose (mg/dl)	45–75	50–80	50–75	85–150	90–156
BUN (mg/dl)	10–30	8–20	10–20	10–30	12–39
Creatinine (mg/dl)	1–2	1.2–1.9	0.8–1.8	1–2.7	1.5–3.3
Bilirubin (mg/dl)	0.01–0.47	0.1–0.42	0–0.1	0–0.6	0–0.1
Calcium (mg/dl)	9.7–12.4	11.5–12.8	8.9–11.7	7.1–11.6	7.5–11
Phosphorus (mg/dl)	5.6–6.5	5.0–7.3	—	5.3–9.6	3–9.5
Sodium (mEq/L)	132–152	139–152	142–155	135–150	147–158
Potassium (mEq/L)	3.5–5.8	3.9–5.4	3.5–6.5	4.4–6.7	4.1–6.6
Chloride (mEq/L)	97–111	95–103	99–110	94–106	105–122
Magnesium (mg/dl)	1.8–2.3	2.2–2.8	2.8–3.6	2.7–3.7	2–3.5
Total protein (g/dl)	6.74–7.46	6–7.9	6.4–7	7.9–8.9	5.4–7.5
Albumin (g/dl)	3.05–3.55	2.4–3.0	2.7–3.9	1.8–3.3	3.4–4.4
Globulin (g/dl)	3–3.48	3.5–5.7	2.7–4.1	5.3–6.4	1.7–3.5

BUN = blood urea nitrogen.

REFERENCES

1. Jain NC: Schalm's Veterinary Hematology, 4th ed. Philadelphia, Lea & Febiger, 1986.
2. Garry F: Clinical pathology of llamas. *In* Johnson LW (ed): Vet Clin North Am 1989.
3. Kaneko JJ: Clinical Biochemistry of Domestic Animals, 3rd ed. New York, Academic Press, 1980.

Availability of Some Common Products

Product	Company
Abate	American Cyanamid Co.
Acepromazine	Fort Dodge Laboratories
Acetest Tablets	Ames Company
Acetobols	Parnell Laboratories
Albacillin	The Upjohn Company
Albamast	The Upjohn Company
Albendazole	SmithKline Beecham Animal Health Products
Albon	Hoffmann-LaRoche Laboratories
Alcaine Ophthalmic Solution	Alcon Laboratories, Inc.
Altosid	Zoecon Industries, Inc.
Ambilhar	Ciba Pharmaceutical Co.
Ames Media	Reginal Media Labs.
Amphyl	National Laboratories Corp.
Amprolium	MSD AGVET
Anaplaz	Fort Dodge Laboratories
AnaSed	Lloyd Laboratories
Ancobon	Hoffmann-LaRoche Laboratories
Anthrax Spore Vaccine	Colorado Serum Company
Antivenin (Crotalidae)	Wyeth Laboratories
Antrycide	Imperial Chemical Ltd. (ICI)
Antrypol	Imperial Chemical Ltd. (ICI)
Anvax	Jensen-Salsbery Laboratories
Aquamephyton	MSD AGVET
Aqua-Pen and Four-Pen	G. C. Hanford Mfg. Co.
Arbo III	Armour Baldwin Laboratories
AS 700	American Cyanamid Co.
Atgard	Shell Chemical Co.
Atipamezole	Farmos Group Ltd
Atroban	Pitman-Moore, Inc.
Aureomycin	American Cyanamid Co.
Aureomycin Soluble Powder	American Cyanamid Co.
Aureomycin Sulmet Soluble Powder	American Cyanamid Co.
Aureo S 700	American Cyanamid Co.
Aurimite	Schering-Plough Animal Health
Azium	Schering-Plough Animal Health
Atroban Ear Tags	Cooper Animal Health
Bailey Ejaculators	Western Serum Co.
BAL	Hynson, Wescott & Dunning, Inc.
Banamine	Schering-Plough Animal Health
Banminth	Pfizer Laboratories
Baymix	Bayvet Division of Cutter Laboratories
Baytril	Haver/Diamond Scientific
Benadryl	Parke-Davis
Benzelmin	Syntex Animal Health, Inc.
Berenil	Hoechst-Roussel Agri-Vet
Betadine	Purdue Frederick Co.
Betamethasone	E. R. Squibb & Sons Inc.
Betasone	Schering-Plough Animal Health
Betavet Soluspan Aqueous Suspension	Schering-Plough Animal Health
Bicillin Fortified	Wyeth Laboratories
Biodry	The Upjohn Company
Biolyte	The Upjohn Company
Biosol	The Upjohn Company
Bloat Guard	SmithKline Beecham Animal Health Products
Bo-Se	Schering-Plough Animal Health
Bovaflavine	Farbwerke Hoechst, AG
Bovate	Hoffmann-LaRoche, Inc.
Bovatec	Hoffmann-La Roche, Inc.
Bovi-clox	E. R. Squibb
Bovilene	Syntex Animal Health, Inc.
Bovishield	SmithKline Beecham Animal Health
Braunamid	B. Braun Melsungen, AG
Bright-Line	American Optical Corporation
Butterfly Tubing	Abbott Laboratories
C-76	Frigitronics Incorporated
Cable Wire Suture	United Surgical Supplies Co.
Calcium Gluconate 23% Solution	Rx Veterinary Products
Calf-Guard	SmithKline Beecham
Calf-oid	The Upjohn Company
CalfSpan	SmithKline Beecham Animal Health
Cambendazole	MSD AGVET
Canex	Pitman Moore, Inc.
Cap-chur Rifle	Palmer Chemical & Equipment Co., Inc.
Caricide	American Cyanamid Co.
Carmilax	SmithKline Beecham Animal Health
Caseous D-T	Colorado Serum Company
CattleMaster	SmithKline Beecham Animal Health
Cefa-Dri	Bristol Laboratories
Cefa-Lak	Bristol Laboratories
Centrine	Fort Dodge Laboratories
Chap-Guard Plus	AgriLaboratories
Chapless Teat Dip	Anchor Laboratories
Chlorasan Uterine Boluses	Franklin Laboratories, Inc.
Chloromycetin Ophthalmic	Parke-Davis
Chlorpyrifos	Fort Dodge Laboratories
Chorionic Gonadotropin	Steris
Ciodrin	Shell Chemical Co.
Ciovan	Shell Chemical Co.
Ciovap	SDS Biotech Corporation
Combiotic	Pfizer, Inc.
Combot	Haver/Diamond Scientific
Compudose	Elanco Products Company
Concord-V	Haver/Diamond Scientific
Co-Ral	Cutter Animal Health
Co-Ral Pour-on	Haver/Diamond Scientific
Corid	MSD AGVET
Cortisate 20	Schering-Plough Animal Health
Cort-Sol	The Butler Company
Coumaphos	Bayvet-Cutter Laboratories
Cry-O-Dine Iodine Disinfectant	Crystal

Product	Company
Cryogun	Brymill Corporation
Crystiben	Solvay Animal Health, Inc.
Cuprate	Burns-Biotec Laboratories
Curatrem	MSD AGVET
Cystorelin	Sanofi Animal Health, Inc
Dacriose Solution	Smith, Miller & Patch Division
Dairiclox	SmithKline Beecham Laboratories
Dairy Bomb	AgriLaboratories
Dantrium	Norwich-Eaton Pharmaceuticals
Darco G-60	Atlas Chemical
Deccox	Rhodia, Inc.
Delnav	Anchor Laboratories
Del-Tox	Burroughs Wellcome Co.
Dental Wedge	Jorgenson Laboratories
Depo-Medrol	The Upjohn Company
Depo Pen	G. C. Hanford Mfg. Company
Dermethrin	Fort Dodge Laboratories
Dexamethasone	Sussex Drug Products Company
Dextrose 5%	Rx Veterinary Products
Diphenhydramine	
Di-Quat 10-S	The Butler Company
Diquel	Jensen-Salsbery Laboratories
Discovery	Franklin Laboratories
Diuril	MSD AGVET
D-L Batyl Alcohol	Sigma Chemical Company
Domoso Solution	Syntex Animal Health, Inc.
Dopram V	A. H. Robins Company
Dry Clox	Bristol Laboratories
Dry-Mast	Anchor Laboratories
Dursban	Fort Dodge Laboratories
Ear Force	Bio-Ceutic Division
ECOLI Guard	Haver/Diamond Scientific
ECOLI Guard Cow-Sow	Cutter Animal Health
ECP	The Upjohn Company
Ectiban	ICI Americas, Inc.
Ectiban EC	Rx Veterinary Products
Ectrin	Fermenta Animal Health Company
Electroid 7	Coopers Animal Health, Inc
Electrosulf-3	Affiliated Laboratories
Eltradd	Haver/Diamond Scientific
Emblax Powder	Haver/Diamond Scientific
Emtryl	Salsbury Laboratories
Eqvalan	MSD AGVET
Ery-Mune C	Anchor Laboratories
Erythro-200	Abbott Laboratories
Erythrocin Lactobionate	Abbott Laboratories
Estradiol	Sigma Chemical Company
Estrumate	ICI United States, Incorporated
Ethidium	Imperial Chemical Ltd. (ICI)
Etorphine	D-M Pharmaceuticals
EVA	SmithKline Beecham Animal Health
Expar	Coopers Animal Health, Inc.
FarrowSure	SmithKline Beecham Animal Health
Fenbendazole	Hoechst-Roussel Agri-Vet
Fenthion	Bayvet-Cutter Laboratories
Fenvalerate	SDS Biotech Corporation
Fermicillin	Fermenta Animal Health Company

Product	Company
Fermicon 7/MB	Bio-Ceutic Division
Finaplex	Hoechst-Roussel Agri-Vet Company
Fingajet	Hoechst-Roussel Agri-Vet
Flagyl	G. D. Searle and Company
Flo-Cillin	Bristol Laboratories
Flucort	Syntex Animal Health, Inc.
Formula #1200	G. C. Hanford Mfg. Co.
Formula A-34	Masticure Products Co., Inc.
Forte-Topical	The Upjohn Company
FSH-LH	Armour Baldwin
Fulvicin	Schering-Plough Animal Health
Fungicidin	Parlam
Fungizone	E. R. Squibb
Furacin Dressing	SmithKline Beecham Animal Health
Furacin Soluble Powder	SmithKline Beecham Animal Health
Furacin Solution	Norwich-Eaton Pharmaceuticals
Furosemide Injection	Phoenix Pharmaceuticals, Inc.
Gallimycin Dry Cow	AgriLaboratories
Gallimycin 36	Abbott Laboratories
Ganaseg	E. R. Squibb
Garamycin Ophthalmic	Schering Corp.
Gecolate	Summit Hill Laboratories
Genecol	Schering-Plough Animal Health
Gentocin	Schering Corporation
Glauber's Salt	Fisher Scientific
Glucagon	Eli Lilly Company
Glyceryl Guaiacolate	Summit Hill Laboratories
Gonadovet	Jensen-Salsbery Laboratories
Gonamone	Fort Dodge Laboratories
Granulex-V	SmithKline Beecham Animal Health
Guardian Ear Tags	American Cyanamid Co.
GX-118	Starbar
Halox	Burroughs Wellcome Company
Hava-Span	Haver/Diamond Scientific
Havidote	Haver/Diamond Scientific
Heifer-oid	Bio-Ceutic Division
Hetacin-K	Bristol Laboratories
Hetacin-K Intramammary Infusion	Fort Dodge Laboratories
Hetrazeen	Heterochemical Corporation
Hexasol 40	Whitney and Company
Hi-Amine	Pitman-Moore, Inc.
Histavet-P	Schering-Plough Animal Health
Horizon I + VAC 3	Cutter Animal Health
Horizon IX	Haver/Diamond Scientific
Huchar C	West Virginia Pulp & Paper Co.
Hydrozide Injection	MSD AGVET
Hygromix	Elanco Products
Hypnodil	Janssen Pharmaceuticals
Hypothermia (Radio-frequency Current) Equipment (Thermaprobe)	Hatch Co. or (Megatherm) Western Instrument Co.
Imidocarb	Burroughs Wellcome Company

Product	Company
Imizol	Burroughs Wellcome Company
Immobilon	Rickett and Colman Pharmaceutical Div.
Immunoregulin	Ribi Immunochem Research
Inhibitor	Zoecon Corporation
Injacom	Hoffmann-La Roche, Inc.
Injacom 100 + B	Hoffmann-La Roche, Inc.
Injectable Laxative	VEDCO, Inc.
Innovar-Vet	Pitman-Moore, Inc.
Iron Dextran	Med-Tech, Inc.
Isotox	Rhone-Poulenc
Ivomec	MSD AGVET
Ivomec F	MSD AGVET
Kantrim	Bristol Laboratories
Kenalog	E. R. Squibb
Keflin	Eli Lilly and Company
Ketaset	Bristol Laboratories
Ketostix	Ames Co.
Kopertox	Ayerst Laboratories
Korlan	Dow Chemical Company
K-Y Lubricating Jelly	Pitman-Moore, Inc.
Kymar	Burns-Biotec Laboratories
LA-200	Pfizer, Inc.
Labstix	Ames Co.
Lactated Ringer's Solution	Sanofi Animal Health, Inc.
Lasix	Hoechst-Roussel Agri-Vet
Levamisole	AgriLaboratories
Levasol	Pitman-Moore, Inc.
Lincomix	The Upjohn Company
Lindane Screwworm and Ear Tag Killer	Pitman-Moore, Inc.
Lindex	Tech America
Linspray	Norden Laboratories
Lintox	Zoecon Corporation
Lintox-D	Zoecon Corporation
Liquamast	Pfizer, Inc.
Liquamycin	Pfizer, Inc.
Lomadine	May & Baker Ltd.
Longicil	Fort Dodge Laboratories
Loridine	Elanco Products Company
Loxon	Burroughs Wellcome Co.
Lubrivet	The Butler Company
Lutalyse	The Upjohn Company
Lysoff	Cutter, Mobay, etc.
Marlate	E. I. DuPont de Nemours & Co., Inc.
Maxitrol Ophthalmic	Alcon Labs., Inc.
Maxidex Ophthalmic	Alcon Labs., Inc.
Mannitol	Abbott Laboratories
Mecadox Premix-10	Pfizer, Inc.
Menadione	Heterochemical Corporation
Methoxychlor and Malathion	Anchor Laboratories
Meticortin	Schering-Plough Animal Health
Metofane Anesthetic	Pitman-Moore, Inc.
Metrazol	Knoll Pharmaceutical
MGA	The Upjohn Company
MGA 200 Premix	The Upjohn Company
Mich Wound Clips	Propper Mfg.
Mikedimide	Parlam Corp.
Monoacetin	Fisher Scientific
Monoject	Sherwood Medical Industries
Moorman's Apralan	Moorman's Manufacturing Co.
Moorman's Dairy Dewormer	Moorman's Manufacturing Co.
Moorman's Fly Spray	Moorman's Manufacturing Co.
Morantel	Pfizer, Inc.
Moor Ma Fume	Moorman Manufacturing Co.
Morumide	SmithKline Beecham Animal Health
Moxidectin	American Cyanamid Co.
Multistix	Ames Co., Division of Miles Laboratories
Mycobiotic	Difco
Mycosel	Baltimore Biologics
Mycostatin	E. R. Squibb
Mydramide	BioProducts, Inc.
Mydriacyl	Alcon Laboratories
Naganol	Bayer
Naquasone Bolus	Schering-Plough Animal Health
Nasalgen	Jensen-Salsbery Laboratories
Naxcel	The Upjohn Company
Neguvon	Haver/Diamond Scientific, Cutter Animal Health, Mobay, or Bayvet
Nematel	Pfizer, Inc.
Neo-Aristovet	American Cyanamid Co.
Neomix 325 Soluble Powder	The Upjohn Company
Neomycin 325	AgriLaboratories
Neo-Synephrine HCl drops	Winthrop Laboratories
Neo-Terra	Pfizer, Inc.
NFZ Soluble 9.2	Hess and Clark, Inc.
Nicotinamide	Fisher Scientific
Nitrofurazone Dressing 0.2 %	AgriLaboratories
Nizoral	Janssen Pharmaceutical
Nolvalube	AVECO, Fort Dodge Laboratories, etc.
Nolvasan	Fort Dodge Laboratories
Nolvasan 5% Teat Dip	Fort Dodge Laboratories
Nolvasan Antiseptic Ointment	AVECO Co., Inc., Fort Dodge Laboratories, etc
Nolvasan Solution	AVECO Co., Inc.
Nolvasan Udder Wash Concentrate	Fort Dodge Laboratories
Nomagen	Fort Dodge Laboratories
Norit	American Norit
Novidium	May and Baker Ltd.
Nuchar	West Virginia Pulp & Paper
Ocusert	Ocusert-Alzo Pharmaceuticals
Omnizole	MSD AGVET
1-Stroke Environ	Vestal Laboratories
Ophthaine	E. R. Squibb
Ophthetic Ophthalmic Solution	Allergan Pharmaceuticals, Inc.
Optimizer D	Y-Tex Corp.
Optivisor	Donegan Optical
Orbenin-DC	SmithKline Beecham Animal Health
Organic Iodide	The Butler Company
Orthocide	Chevron Chemical Co.
Overtime	Bioceutic Laboratories
Ovine Ecthyma Vaccine	Colorado Serum Company
Oxfendazole	Suntex, Incorporated
Oxytetracycline HCl	Fermenta Animal Health Company

Product	Company
Oxyvet-100 Injection	Pfizer, Inc.
Panacur-American	Hoechst-Roussel Agri-Vet
Panolog	E. R. Squibb, Solvay Animal Health
Pentobarbital Sodium	Fort Dodge Laboratories
Pentothal	Abbott Laboratories
Permectrin II	Anchor Laboratories or Boehringer-Ingelheim
Permethrin	ICI Americas, Inc.; or Boehringer-Ingelheim, Anchor Laboratories, Bio-Ceutic, etc.
Permount	Fisher Scientific
Phosmet GX 118	Zoecon Corp.
PG-600	Intervet America, Inc.
Plastic Insemination Pipette	NASCO
Polyflex	Bristol Laboratories, Aveco, Fort Dodge Laboratories, etc.
Polyotic Soluble Powder and Oblets	American Cyanamid Co.
Pour-on Insecticide	Tech America; Kaw Valley
Povidone Scrub	The Butler Company
Predef 2X	The Upjohn Company
Prednefrin Forte Ophthalmic Solution	Allergan Pharmaceuticals, Inc.
Prevent	Pro-Vet
Probiocin	Microbial Genetics
Pro-Fixx	Scientific Products
Pro-Immune	Schering-Plough
Prolate	Zoecon Corporation
PromAce	AVECO, Fort Dodge Laboratories, etc.
Promazine	Fort Dodge Laboratories, Inc.
ProSystem 2,1,4,3	Ambico
Quartermaster	Hamilton Laboratories
Rabon	AgriLaboratories; Fermenta Animal Health
Ralgro	International Minerals and Chemical Corp.
Ravap	Fermenta Animal Health Company
Re-Covr	Solvay
Regu-Mate	Hoechst-Roussel Agri-Vet Company
Re-Sorb	SmithKline Beecham Animal Health
Revalor-S	Hoechst-Roussel Agri-Vet Company
Revive	Tech America
Revivon	Rickett and Colman Pharmaceuticals
Ribigen	Ribi Immunochem Research Inc.
Ridamite	Ormont Drug and Chemical Co. Inc.
Ringer's Solutions	Abbott Laboratories
Ripercol	American Cyanamid Co.
Robaxin	A. H. Robins Company
Roccal-D	The Upjohn Company
Rompun	Haver/Diamond Scientific
Rumalax	AgriLaboratories
Rumatel	Pfizer, Inc.
Rumensin	Elanco Products Company
Saber	Pitman-Moore, Inc.
Safe-Guard	Hoechst-Roussel Agri-Vet
Saffan	Schering-Plough Animal Health
Samorin	May and Baker Ltd.
Sandril (Reserpine)	Eli Lilly and Company
Scarlet Drench Powder	Haver/Diamond Scientific
ScourGuard 3	SmithKline Beecham Animal Health
Scourlyte	Schering-Plough Animal Health
Sebbafon	Winthrop Laboratories
Seletox	Schering-Plough Animal Health
SEZ	American Cyanamid Co.
Simax	Zoecon Corporation
Siteguard G	Coopers Animal Health, Inc.
Solu-Delta-Cortef	The Upjohn Company
Somato-Staph Bacterin	Anchor Laboratories
Spanbolet II	Norden Laboratories
Sparine	Wyeth Laboratories
Special Formula 17900-Forte	The Upjohn Company
Spotton	Haver/Diamond Scientific
Staphage Lysate (SPL)	Delmont Laboratories, Inc.
Starbar Insecticide Cattle Ear Tag	Starbar
Stewart's Media	Reginal Media Laboratories, Inc. (Remel)
Stiglyn	Pitman-Moore, Inc.
Stresnil	Pitman-Moore, Inc.
Strongid Paste	Pfizer, Inc.
Strongid-T	Pfizer, Inc.
Sulfabrom	MSD AGVET
Sulfa-Lite	Bio-Ceutic
Sulfa-Max 111	AgriLaboratories
Sulfa-Span	Cutter Animal Health
Sulmet Oblets	American Cyanamid Co.
Surge	Babson Brothers Company
Surital	Parke-Davis and Company
Synanthic	Syntex Animal Health, Inc.
SYNCRO-MATE B	Sanofi Animal Health, Inc.
Synovex C	Syntex Animal Health, Inc.
Synovex H	Syntex Animal Health, Inc.
Synovex S	Syntex Animal Health, Inc.
Tactik	F & B Chemicals Pty. Lyd. or Schering Corp.
Taractan	Hoffmann-La Roche Laboratories
TBZ	Merck & Co., Inc.
Technovit	Jorgensen Laboratories
Telazol	A. H. Robins Company
Telmin	Pitman-Moore, Inc.
Terminator	Fermenta Animal Health Company
Terramycin Injectable	Pfizer, Inc.
Tetacycline HCl Soluble Powder	The Butler Company
Thiabendazole Paste	MSD AGVET
Thorazine	Pitman-Moore, Inc.
Tiguvon	Bayvet Division of Cutter Laboratories, Inc.
TODAY	Bristol Laboratories
Tomahawk	Pitman-Moore, Inc.
Tomanol	Intervet Pty. Ltd.

Product	Company	Product	Company
Tonophosphan	Hoechst U.K. Ltd.	Valsyn GEL	Eaton Laboratories
Toxiban	Vet-A-Mix	Vanodyne-FAM	Vanodyne International Ltd.
Tramisol	American Cyanamid Co.	Vapona	Fermenta Animal Health
Traxel-2	Bayvet Division of Cutter Laboratories	Vebonol	Ciba-Geigy Ltd.
		Vetafil	Dr. S. Jackson
Tresaderm	MSD AGVET	Vetalar	Fort Dodge Laboratories
Tribrissen	Burroughs Wellcome Co.	Vetalog	Solvay Animal Health, Inc.
Trichlorfon	AgriLaboratories	Vetalog Parenteral	Solvay Animal Health, Inc.
Trypamidium	Specia	Vetibenzamine	Ciba-Geigy Ltd.
Tween 20	Fisher Scientific	Vetidrex	Ciba Pharmaceutical
Tygon	Norton, Plastics and Synthetics Div.	Vetisulid	E. R. Squibb
		Vetrophin	Abbott Laboratories
Tylan Injectable 200	Elanco Products Company	Vigilante	American Cyanamid Co.
Tylosin	Elanco Products Company	Vitamin K_1	MSD AGVET
Udder Balm	VEDCO	Voren	Boehringer Ingelheim
Uddermate	Anchor Laboratories	Warbex	American Cyanamid Co.
Valbazen	SmithKline Beecham, Norden	XLP-30	SDS Biotech Corporation
Valium	Hoffmann-La Roche Laboratories	Yobine Injection	Lloyd Laboratories
		Yomasan	Haver/Diamond Scientific

Addresses of Some Companies Manufacturing Common Drugs

Abbott Laboratories
Professional Veterinary Products
North Chicago, IL 60064

AgriLaboratories
6221 North K Highway
St. Joseph, MO 64505

Affiliated Laboratories
Myerstown, PA 17067

Alcon Laboratories, Inc.
Fort Worth, TX 76101

Allergan Pharmaceuticals
Irvine, CA 92713

Ambico, Inc.
P.O. Box 522
902 Sugar Grove Avenue
Dallas Center, IA 50063

American Animal Health, Inc.
2619 Skyway Drive
Grand Prairie, TX 75051

American Cyanamid Company
One Cyanamid Plaza
Wayne, NJ 07470

American Hoechst Corporation
Agricultural Division
Route 202–206
North Somerville, NJ 08876

American Optical Corporation
Buffalo, NY 15215

Ames Company
Div. of Miles Laboratories
Elkhart, IN 46514

Anchor Laboratories
2621 North Belt Highway
St. Joseph, MO 64502

Atlas Chemical
See ICI United States, Inc.

AVECO Co., Inc.
800 5th Street NW
Fort Dodge, IA 50501

Ayerst Laboratories
685 Third Avenue
New York, NY 10017

Babson Brothers Company
1880 Country Farm Drive
Naperville, IL 60566–7096

Baltimore Biologics
Cockeysville, MD 21030

Bayer
Bayerwerk, Federal Republic of Germany

Bayvet-Cutter Laboratories
P.O. Box 390
Shawnee Mission, KS 66201

Bio-Ceutic Division
Boehringer-Ingelheim Animal Health, Inc.
2621 North Belt Highway
St. Joseph, MO 64502

Bio Products, Inc.
369 Bayview Avenue
Amityville, NY 11701

Boehringer-Ingelheim
Sydney, Australia
or
2621 N. Belt Highway
St. Joseph, MO 64502

Bristol Laboratories
P.O. Box 657
Syracuse, NY 13201

Burns-Biotec
8530 K Street
Omaha, NB 68127

Burns Veterinary Supply
2019 McKenzie Drive
Suite 109
Carrollton, TX 75006

Burroughs Wellcome Company
50 Park Drive
Research Triangle Park, NC 27708

The Butler Company
5000 Bradenton Avenue
Dublin, OH 43017–0753

Chevron Chemical Co.
Ortho Division
San Francisco, CA 94119

Ciba Pharmaceutical
556 Morris Ave
Summit, NJ 07901

Ciba-Geigy Animal Health
P.O. Box 18300
Greensboro, NC 27419

Colorado Serum Company
4950 York Street
Denver, CO 80216

Coopers Animal Health, Inc.
A Pitman-Moore Company
421 East Hawley Street
Mundelein, IL 60060

Crystal Chemical Corp.
101-02 37th Avenue
Corona, NY 11368

Cutter Animal Health
Mobay Corporation, Animal Health Division
12707 West 63rd Street
P.O. Box 390
Shawnee, KS 66201

Delmont Laboratories, Inc.
P.O. Box 269
Swarthmore, PA 19081

D-M Pharmaceuticals
P.O. Box 1584
Rockville, MD 20850

Donegan Optical Co.
Kansas City, MO 64108

Dow Chemical Company
Indianapolis, IN 46268

E. I. DuPont de Nemours & Co., Inc.
Wilmington, DE 19698

Durvet, Inc.
P.O. Box 279
Highway 40 Eastbound
Blue Springs, MO 64015

Eaton Laboratories
17 Eaton Ave.
Norwich, NY 13815

Elanco Products Company
Division of Eli Lilly and Company
P.O. Box 1750
Indianapolis, IN 46206

EVSCO Pharmaceuticals
Affiliate of IGI, Inc.
P.O. Box 209 (Harding Hwy.)
Buena, NJ 08310

F & B Chemicals Pty. Ltd.
102/160 Rowe St.
Eastwood NSW 2122
Australia

Farbwerke Hoechst AG
Frankfurt, Germany

Fermenta Animal Health Company
10150 N. Executive Hills Blvd
Kansas City, MO 64190

Fisher Scientific
Pittsburgh, PA 15219

Fort Dodge Laboratories
Div. American Home Products
P.O. Box 518
800 Fifth Street NW
Fort Dodge, IA 50501

Franklin Laboratories, Inc.
Div. American Home Products
P.O. Box 669
Amarillo, TX 79105

Frigitonics, Inc.
Shelton, CT 06484

GLA Company
Agricultural Electronic Division
4743 Brooks Street
Montclair, CA 91763

Glaxo Laboratories
Greenford Middlesex, England

Grand Laboratories, Inc.
RR 3, Box 36
Freeman, SD 57029

Hamilton Laboratories
Spring Street Rd. #2
Hamilton, NY 13340

G. C. Hanford Mfg. Company
304 Oneida Street
Box 1017
Syracuse, NY 13201

Hatch Company
Loveland, CO 80537

Haver/Diamond Scientific
Mobay Corporation, Animal Health Division
12707 West 63rd Street
Shawnee, KS 66201

Hess and Clark, Inc.
Seventh and Orange Streets
Ashland, OH 44805

Heterochemical Corporation
Valley Stream, NY 11580

Hoechst U.K. Ltd.
Middlesex, United Kingdom

Hoechst-Roussel Agri-Vet Company
Animal Health Products
Route 202-206
Box 2500 BEDI
Somerville, NJ 08876–1258

Hoffmann-La Roche, Inc.
Roche Chemical Division
340 Kingsland Street
Nutley, NJ 07110

Hynson, Wescott, and Dunning, Inc.
Charles and Chase Sts.
Baltimore, MD 21201

ICI United States, Inc.
3411 Silverside Road
P.O. Box 751
Wilmington, DE 19897

Immunovet Incorporated
5910-G Breckenridge Parkway
Tampa, FL 33610

International Minerals and Chemical Corp. (IMC)
Terre Haute, IN 47808

Intervet America, Inc.
P.O. Box 318
Millsboro, DE 19966

Intervet Pty. Ltd.
34 Hotham Parade
Artarmon NSW 2064
Australia

Janssen Pharmaceutical
New Brunswick, NJ 08903

Jensen-Salsbery Laboratories
P.O. Box 167
Kansas City, MO 64141

Jorgenson Laboratories
1450 N. Van Buren Ave
Loveland, CO 80538

Kaw Valley
1801 S. 2nd Street
Leavenworth, KS 66248

Lextron, Inc.
630 "O" Street
P.O. Box 88
Greeley, CO 80632

Lloyd Laboratories
A Division of Vet-A-Mix
604 West Thomas Avenue
Shenandoah, IA 51601

Eli Lilly and Company
307 E. McCarty Street
Indianapolis, IN 46225

May and Baker Ltd.
Dageham, United Kingdom

B. Braun McIsungen AG
West Germany

MSD AGVET
Division of Merck & Co., Inc.
P.O. Box 2000, WBF 475
Rahway, NJ 07065-0912

Microbial Genetics
A Division of Pioneer Hi-Bred Int'l, Inc.
4601 Westown Parkway
Suite 120
West Des Moines, IA 50265

Moorman Manufacturing Co.
Quincy, IL 62301

Nasco
Fort Atkinson, WI 53538

National Laboratories
225 Summit Avenue
Montvale, NJ 07645

Norden Laboratories
601 W. Cornhusker Highway
Lincoln, NB 68521

Ocusert-Alzo Pharmaceuticals
Palo Alto, CA 94303

Norton, Plastics and Synthetics Division
Akron, OH 44309

Norwich-Eaton Pharmaceuticals
Norwich, NY 13815

Palmer Chemical and Equipment Co., Inc.
Douglasville, GA 30134

Parke-Davis and Company
Joseph Campau at the River
Detroit, MI 48232

Parlam Division
Ormont Drug and Chemical Co., Inc.
520 South Dean Street
Englewood, NJ 07631

Parnell Laboratories Pty. Ltd.
6 Norman Street
Peakhurst NSW 2210
Australia

Pfizer, Inc.
Animal Health Division
235 East 42nd Street
New York, NY 10017-5755

Phoenix Pharmaceuticals, Inc.
3336 Pear Street
P.O. Box 7, Fairleigh Station
St. Joseph, MO 64506-0007

Pitman-Moore, Inc.
421 East Hawley Street
Mundelein, IL 60060

Pro Vet Companies
P.O. Box 2286
Loves Park, IL 61131

Purdue Frederick
100 Connecticut Avenue
Norwalk, CT 06856

Reginal Media Laboratories, Inc. (REMEL)
12076 Santa Fe Drive
P.O. Box 14428
Lonexa, KS 66215

Rhodia, Inc.
Ashland, OH 44805

Rhone Merieux, Inc.
115 Transtech Drive
Athens, GA 30601

Rhone-Poulenc Animal Nutrition North America
500 Northridge Road
Suite 620
Atlanta, GA 30350

Rickett and Colman Pharmaceutical Division
Hull, England

A. H. Robins Company
1407 Cummings Drive
Richmond, VA 23770

Ribi Immunochem Research, Inc.
P.O. Box 1409
Hamilton, MT 59840

Rx Veterinary Products
15 W. Putman
Portersville, CA 93257

Salsbury Laboratory
2000 Rockford Rd.
Charles City, IA 50616

Sanofi Animal Health, Inc.
7101 College Blvd.
Overland Park, KS 66210

Schering-Plough Animal Health
P.O. Box 529
Kenilworth, NJ 07033

Scientific Products
McGraw Park, IL 60085

SDS Biotech Corporation
1100 Superior Avenue
Cleveland, OH 49114

G. D. Searle and Company
P.O. Box 5110
Chicago, IL 60680

Shell Animal Health
P.O. Box 3871
Houston, TX 77001

Shell Chemical Company
San Ramon, CA 94503

Sherwood Medical Industries
St. Louis, MO 63103

Sigma Chemical Company
St. Louis, MO 63178

SmithKline Beecham Animal Health
Whiteland Business Park
812 Springdale Drive
Exton, PA 19341

Smith, Miller & Patch
Division, Cooper Laboratories
Cedar Knolls, NJ 07927

Solvay Animal Health, Inc.
1201 Northland Drive
Mendota Heights, MN 55120-1139

Specia
Rhone Merieux, 69002
Lyon, France

E. R. Squibb & Sons, Inc.
P.O. Box 4000
Princeton, NJ 08540

Starbar
A Division of Zoecon Corporation
12200 Danton Drive
Dallas, TX 75234

Summit Hill Laboratories
P.O. Box 535
Navesink, NJ 07752

Sussex Drug Products Company
Edison, NJ 08817

Syntex Animal Health, Inc.
Subsidiary of Syntex Agribusiness, Inc.
4800 Westown Parkway
Suite 200
West Des Moines, IA 50265

TechAmerica
P.O. Box 338
Elwood, KS 66024

The Upjohn Company
Animal Health Division
7000 Portage Road
Kalamazoo, MI 49001

United Surgical Supplies Company
Mamaroneck, NY 10543

Vanodyne International Ltd. Eccles
Manchester M30 OWT, England

VEDCO, Inc.
Route 6, Box 35A
St. Joseph, MO 64504

Vestal Laboratories
St. Louis, MO 63166

Veta-A-Mix Animal Health
604 West Thomas Avenue
Shenandoah, IA 51601

Western Serum Co.
Denver, CO 80201

Western Instrument Co.
Denver, CO 80201

Winthrop Laboratories
90 Park Avenue
New York, NY 10016

Wyeth Laboratories
P.O. Box 8299
Philadelphia, PA 19101

Zoecon Corporation
12200 Denton Drive
Dallas, TX 75234

Table of Common Drugs: Approximate Doses

Name of Drug	Ruminants	Swine
Acepromazine	0.05 to 0.1 mg/kg IV, IM, or SC	0.1 to 0.2 mg/kg IV, IM, or SC
Acetazolamide	6 to 8 mg/kg orally in food or water	Same
Acetic acid (5% solution)	In 20% glucose give 1 to 4 L orally for urea toxicity	None
Acetylsalicylic acid (aspirin)	10 to 20 mg/kg	Same
Adrenal corticotropic hormone (ACTH) (Adrenomone)	200 units daily IM	Same
Albacillin	Intramammary infusion	None
Albamast (L)	Intramammary infusion (Novobiocin, 150 mg)	None
Albendazole	Cattle: 7.5 mg/kg oral paste	None
Ammonium chloride	200 mg/kg orally for urolithiasis prevention	None
Amphetamine (5% solution)	0.5 to 4 mg/kg IV, SC, or IP	Same
Ampicillin	4 to 10 mg/kg IM or IV	Same
Amprolium	10 mg/kg orally	100 mg/kg/day in food or water
Antivenin (Crotalidae) polyvalent	10 to 200 ml IV	Same
Aquamephyton	10 to 50 mg IV, IM, or SC	10 to 30 mg IV, IM, or SC
Atropine sulfate	0.1 to 1.0 mg/kg IV, IM, or SC	Same
Bacitracin plus polymyxin B	B.: 10,000 units and P.: 5 to 10 mg subconjunctival injection	None
BAL	4 mg/kg q 4 h IM until recovery	Same
D-L Batyl alcohol	0.5 to 1.0 g/adult animal daily IV as bone marrow stimulant	None
Baymix crumbles	60 g/100 kg orally on feed for 6 consecutive days	None
Bemegride (Mikedimide)	10 to 20 mg/kg IV	Same
Betavet soluspan	1 to 5 ml intra-articular	Same
Bicillin	1 ml/35 kg SC only	None
Biosol	5 to 10 mg/kg orally; 2 to 4 boluses, intrauterine	Same ½ to 1 bolus, intrauterine
Biosol-M (liquid)	1 ml/18 kg/day orally	Same
Butacaine sulfate (1% solution)	Topically in eye; duration 30 to 60 min	Same
Butazolidin	5 to 10 mg/kg orally, IV	None
Calcium EDTA (20% solution)	Max. safe dosage is 75 mg/kg/day IV drip	None
Calcium gluconate (23% solution)	1 ml/kg IV, SC, IM	Same
Calcium hydroxide (Slaked lime)	0.5 mg/kg daily as a 15% supplement in feed	None
Calcium hypophosphite	30 mg in 100 ml in 10% glucose IV	None
Cambendazole	20 mg/kg orally	None
Carbomycin	2.5 mg as a subconjunctival injection	None
Caricide	50 to 100 mg/kg	Same
Carmilax	1 to 4 bolets orally; 100 to 454 g powder in 4 L water	None
Cefa-Lak (sodium cephapirin)	Infuse one syringe into each infected quarter, 200 mg	None
Cephaloridine (Loridine)	10 mg/kg q 12 h IM or SC	Same
Cephapirin benzathine (Cefa-Dri)	300 mg/tube for mastitis	None
Charcoal, activated	2 to 9 g/kg in a concentration of 1 g charcoal in 3 to 5 ml water orally	None
Chloral hydrate	50 to 70 mg/kg IV	4 to 6 ml of 5% solution/kg IV
Chloramphenicol	20 to 50 mg/kg q 8 h orally; 10 mg/kg q 12 h IM or IV; 50 to 100 mg as a subconjunctival injection	Same
Chloropent injection	0.4 to 1.0 ml/kg IV	None
Chlorothiazide (Diuril)	4 to 8 mg/kg once or twice daily given orally for adult cattle	None
Chlorpromazine (Thorazine)	0.22 to 1.0 mg/kg IV; 1.0 to 4.4 mg/kg IM	0.55 to 3.3 mg/kg IV; 2.0 to 4.0 mg/kg IM
Chlortetracycline	6 to 10 mg/kg IV or IM; 10 to 20 mg/kg orally	Same
Choline chloride	Adult cow: 50 g daily orally; 25 g in 10% solution SC	None
Chorionic gonadotropin solution	Bov.: 5000 units IV; Cap.: 3000 units IV	2000 to 3000 units IV
Chorisol	2500 to 5000 USP units IV (cattle); 10,000 USP units IM	None
Cloprostenol	Adult cow: 0.5 mg IM	None
Cloxacillin (Dairi-Clox)	200 mg/tube for mastitis	None
Cloxacillin, benzathine (Dry-Clox; Bovi-Clox)	500 mg/tube for mastitis	None
Copper glycinate	60 mg for calves; 120 mg for mature cattle SC for Cu def.	None
Copper sulfate	0.4% solution; 2 to 4 L orally for phosphorous toxicity; 1 g/adult cow daily orally for the Cu def.	None
Co-Ral Pour-On	0.3 mg/kg—pour uniformly along back	None
Depo-Medrol	20 to 240 mg intrasynovial injection	Same
Dexamethasone	1 to 10 mg IV or IM	Same
Diazepam	0.5 to 1.5 mg/kg IV or IM	Same
Diethylstilbestrol	Abortifacient in cattle; 40 to 80 mg IM; 100 to 175 mg in late pregnancy	None
Digoxin	0.2 to 0.6 mg/kg IV	None
Dimercaprol (BAL)	10% solution in oil; 2.5 to 5.0 mg/kg IM every 4 hours for 2 days; t.i.d. on 3rd day; then b.i.d. for next 10 days or until recovery	None
Dipyrone (Novin)	5 ml/50 kg IM, IV, or SC	Same
Diquel	0.55 to 1.10 mg/kg IV or IM	1.25 to 4.4 mg/kg IV or IM
Doxapram (Dopram V)	5 to 10 mg/kg IV	Same
Dry-Clox	Infuse contents of one syringe into each infected quarter (Benzathine cloxacillin, 500 mg)	None

Name of Drug	Ruminants	Swine
Electrosulf-3	0.22 g/kg	Same
Eltradd IV-4000	Dissolve one packet in 4 liters of water—give 50 to 100 mg/kg/day IV or SC	Same
Emblax powder	Mix 454 g with 4 liters of water—administer intrarumenally	None
Epinephrine (1:1000 solution)	0.02 to 0.03 mg/kg SC, IM, or IV	Same
Ergonovine maleate	Cows: 1 to 3 mg; ewes and goats: 0.4 to 1.0 mg	Sows: 0.4 to 1.0 mg
Erythromycin (Erythro-100-200)	2 to 5 mg/kg IM, SC	Same
Erythromycin	300 mg/tube for mastitis	None
Erythromycin, novobiocin, plus polymyxin B	E.: 100 mg; N.: 15 mg; P.: 5 to 10 mg as a subconjunctival injection	None
Estradiol cyclopropionate	Adult cow: 4 to 8 mg IM abortifacient late pregnancy 20 mg IM. Repeat for 2 to 3 days	1 to 3 mg not for abortifacient
Fenbendazole	Cattle: 5 mg/kg oral suspension	None
Fenthion (Tiguvon) (Spotton)	30 ml/100 kg pour-on; 4 ml/150 kg one-spot	None
Finajet (Trenbolone acetate)	Cattle: 125–250 mg; sheep: 30 mg IV or IM	None
Flo-Cillin	2 ml/70 kg	None
Flucort solution	1.25 to 5.0 mg daily IV or IM	Same
FSH-P	Cattle: 10 to 50 mg; sheep and goats: 5 to 25 mg	5 to 25 mg
Fungicidin	Apply liquid liberally morning and night	Same
Furacin dressing	Apply directly on the lesion	Same
Furacin soluble powder	Dust on lesion directly	Same
Furaltadone (Valsyn Gel (L,O))	500 mg/tube for mastitis	None
Furosemide (Lasix)	2.2 to 4.4 mg/kg q 12 h IV	Same
Gallimycin 36 Sol. (L,D)	Intramammary infusion (erythromycin, 300 mg)	None
Glucagon	25 to 50 µg/kg IV	None
Glucose (40% solution)	Cattle: 500 ml; sheep: 50 ml IV	50 ml IV
Glycerol monoacetate (Monoacetin)	0.1 to 0.5 mg/kg IM hourly for several hours for fluoroacetate poisoning	None
Glyceryl guaiacolate (Gecolate) (5% solution)	110 mg/kg IV	None
Gonadotropin, pituitary (Vetrophin)	3 to 5 mg IV	None
Gonadotropin-releasing hormone (Gonadorelin)	100 µg IV	None
Gonadovet	Cows: 50 to 100 units; sheep and goats: 25 units	Sows: 50 units
Griseofulvin	20 mg/kg/day once daily orally for 6 weeks	Same
Halox drench	Add one packet to one liter of water; 1 ml/2.5 to 3.5 kg; do not use on goats	None
Hava-Span	1 bolus/50 to 100 kg	None
Hetacillin (Hetacin)	5 to 15 mg/kg IM or SC	Same
Hi-Amine	Cattle: 15 to 20 g/day for 2 to 3 weeks; sheep: 7.5 to 15 g/day for 2 to 3 weeks	None
Hydrochlorothiazide	0.25 to 5.0 mg/kg IV or IM	None
Hygromix	None	Mix in feed according to label
Hypnodil	None	Give to effect
Injacon	Cattle: 0.5 to 6 ml/head IM; sheep and goats: 0.25 to 2 ml/head IM	0.25 to 3 ml/head IM
Injacon 100 + B complex	Cattle: 2.5 to 10 ml/head IM; sheep and goats: 1 to 5 ml/head IM	1 to 5 ml/head IM
Innovar-Vet	None	1 ml/12 to 25 kg IM
Insulin	Adult cow: 150 to 200 units every 36 hr SC	None
Iron-dextran injection	None	100 to 200 mg IM for 1-to-3-day-old pigs
Isoflupredone acetate (Predef)	0.1 to 0.15 mg/kg	None
Jenotone	2 mg/kg q 12 h IM or SC	Same
Kanamycin (Kantrim)	6 mg/kg q 12 h IM; 10 to 20 mg subconjunctival	Same
Ketamine (Ketaset)	2.0 mg/kg IV	2.0 to 3.0 mg/kg IV
Kopertox	Apply to hoofs	Same
Kymar aqueous	Cattle: 25,000 USP units q 24 h IM; sheep: 5000 to 10,000 USP units	None
Levamisole (L-tetramisole) (Levasole)	3.3 to 8.0 mg/kg SC; 5.5 to 11.0 mg/kg drench or bolus	8 mg/kg in feed or water
Liquamast	Injection into udder immediately after milking (Oxytetracycline HCl, 426 mg)	None
Luteinizing hormone (PLH)	Sheep and goats: 2.5 mg IV; cows: 25 mg IV	5 mg IV
Magnesium gluconate	0.44 mg/kg of a 15% solution IV or SC	None
Magnesium lactate	2.2 ml/kg of a 3.3% solution IV or SC	None
Magnesium oxide	1 g/45 kg orally as a supplement to prevent grass tetany; 2 to 3 g/45 kg orally for acid antidote	None
Magnesium sulfate	0.44 ml/kg of a 20% solution IV or SC for grass tetany; 1 to 2 g/kg orally as cathartic	Same for cathartic
Mannitol (20% solution)	5 to 10 ml/kg IV	Same
Menadione (Vitamin K)	0.5 to 2.5 mg/kg q 12 h IM; 5 mg/kg orally	None
Methocarbamol (Robaxin)	110 mg/kg IV	None
Methoxyflurane	Induce 1%; maintain 0.5%	Same
Methylene blue	1 to 4% solution; 4.4 to 8.8 mg/kg IV drip for nitrate poisoning	None
Metrazol	10 mg/kg IV or 100 mg orally	Same
Milk of magnesia	3.0 to 30.0 ml/45 kg orally	Same
Mineral oil	Cattle: 1 to 4 liters orally; sheep and goats: 100 to 500 ml orally	50 to 100 ml orally
Molybdate (ammonium or sodium salt)	50 to 100 mg/head/day orally in copper toxicosis	None
Molybdenumized superphosphate	Apply 114 g per acre to molybdenum deficiency pastures	None

Name of Drug	Ruminants	Swine
Neguvon Pour-On	30 ml/100 kg—apply along the back	None
Neo-Aristovet	Apply to lesion once or twice daily	Same
Neomycin	7 to 12 mg/kg q 12 h orally	Same
Neostigmine methylsulfate	Solution 1:2000 to 1:5000; 1.1 to 2.2 mg/50 kg SC or IV	Same
Neo-Terramycin	1 to 3 boluses/50 to 100 kg orally	Same
Nicotinamide	2 to 3 mg/kg every 4 h	None
Nitrofurazone (0.2% ointment or solution)	Topically	Same
Norgestomet (SYNCRO-MATE B)	Cow: day one—6 mg ear implant plus daily injections of 5 to 6 mg IM 7 days	None
Novobiocin (Albamast [L]) (Biodry [D])	150 mg/tube for mastitis infusion; 400 mg/tube for mastitis infection	None
Oleandomycin	1.25 mg as a subconjunctival injection	None
Orbenin-DC (D)	Intramammary infusion (Benzathine Cloxacillin, 500 mg)	None
Oxfendazole	None	3 mg/kg orally
Oxytetracycline HCl	6 to 11 mg/kg IV or IM; 10 to 20 mg/kg q 6 h orally	Same
Oxytocin	20 to 100 USP units (1 to 5 ml) IM or IV	20 to 50 USP units IM or IV
D-Penicillamine (Cuprimine)	Antidote for copper and mercury; dose for humans: 15 to 50 mg/kg daily in divided doses orally	None
Penicillin		
Pen G, procaine	40,000 units/kg q 24 h IM	Same
Pen G and Pen benzathine	40,000 units/kg once	Same
Penicillin G + streptomycin	P.: 500,000 units; S.: 50 mg as a subconjunctival injection	None
Pentobarbital	30 mg/kg IV to effect	Same
Pentylenetetrazol (Metrazol)	6 to 10 mg/kg IV mild stimulant; 10 to 20 mg/kg IV barbiturate antidote	Same
Phenylbutazone	4 to 8 mg/kg orally; 2 to 5 mg/kg IV	Same
Piperazine	100 to 200 mg/kg orally	Same
Pituitary gonadotropin	5 mg/adult cow IV	None
Poloxalene (Therabloat)	100 mg/kg orally	None
Posterior pituitary extract	Cow: 10 to 20 USP units IV, IM	5 to 20 USP units IV, IM
Potassium chloride	50 g daily orally; 1.0 mEq/kg/hr IV drip	None
Potassium permanganate	Solution 1:5000 to 1:10,000 for lavage	None
Pralidoxime chloride	20 mg/kg IV for organic phosphate poisoning	None
Prednisolone sodium succinate (Solu-Delta-Cortef)	0.2 to 1.0 mg/kg IV or IM	Same
Progesterone suspension	Cows: 150 to 200 mg IM	None
Promazine (Sparine)	0.44 to 1.0 mg/kg IV or IM	Same
Proparacine HCl (Ophthaine)	0.5% solution; topically in the eye	Same
Propiopromazine (Tranvet)	0.22 to 1.0 mg/kg IV or IM	Same
Propylene glycol (50% solution)	Cattle: 500 ml; sheep 50 ml orally	None
Prostaglandin F_2 alpha	Cow: 25 to 30 mg IM; ewe and doe: 8 to 10 mg IM—often second injection in 11 to 12 days	None
Protamine sulfate (heparin antagonist)	100 mg/adult animal IV in a 1% solution for Bracken fern toxicosis	None
Saffan	None	2 to 3 mg/kg IV
Scarlet drench powder	200 to 400 ml as a drench	None
Selenium tocopherol (BO-SE)	5.0 to 7.0 ml/100 kg SC or IM	Same
Sodium acetate phosphate	Cattle: 60 gm in 300 ml water IV	None
Sodium bicarbonate (7.5% solution = 0.89 mEq/ml of bicarbonate)	2 to 5 mEq/kg IV for 4 to 8 h period	Same
Sodium formaldehyde sulfoxylate	5% solution as lavage as mercury poisoning antidote	None
Sodium nitrate (1% solution)	16 mg/kg IV, follow with 30 to 40 mg/kg IV sodium thiosulfate for cyanide poisoning	None
Sodium sulfate (Glauber's salt)	1 to 3 g/kg orally	None
Sodium thiosulfate	As arsenic antidote: 10 to 20% solution; 30 to 40 mg/kg IV or orally	None
Soframycin	250 to 500 mg as a subconjunctival injection	None
Spectinomycin	None	10 mg/kg orally q 12 h
Spiramycin	10 to 20 mg as a subconjunctival injection	None
Sulfabromomethazine (Sulfabrom)	130 to 200 mg/kg orally	None
Sulfachlorpyridazine (Vetisulid)	65 to 95 mg/kg orally	45 to 75 mg/kg orally
Sulfadimethoxine (Albon)	55 mg/kg orally (initial dose); 27.5 mg/kg orally (daily)	Same
Sulfaethoxypyridazine (SEZ)	200 to 400 mg/kg	Same
Sulfa-Lite	214 mg/kg initially followed by 107 mg/kg for the next 3 to 5 days	Same
Sulfamethazine	200 mg/kg orally (initial dose); 100 mg/kg orally (daily)	Same
Sulfisoxazole diolamine (Gantrisin)	Ophthalmic ointment	Same
Synovex-S	Steers: implant pellet in ear last 60 to 150 days of fattening period	None
Synovex-H	Heifers: implant pellet in ear last 60 to 150 days of fattening period	None
Tannic acid	5 to 25 g in 2.0 to 4.0 L of water orally	None
Taractan	None	0.3 to 1.0 mg/kg IV; 3.3 mg/kg IM
Tetracaine	0.5% solution; topically in eye; duration 20 to 30 min	Same
Tetracycline HCl (polyotic)	11 mg/kg orally	None
Thiabendazole	40 to 60 mg/kg	None
Thiabendazole paste	75 mg/kg	None
Thiamine	For polio: 0.25 to 0.5 g IM or IV for 3 to 5 days	None
Thiamylal sodium (Suritol)	3 to 5 mg/kg IV	Same
Triamcinolone (Vetalog)	0.02 to 0.04 mg/kg IM; 6.0 to 18.0 mg intra-articular	None

Name of Drug	Ruminants	Swine
Tribrissen	30 mg/kg daily orally	Same
Tripelennamine HCl (Re-Covr)	1 mg/kg IV or IM	Same
Tropicamide (Mydriacil)	0.5 to 1.0% solution; topically in eye; one drop in eye followed in 10 min with another drop	Same
Tylosin (Tylan)	2 to 4 mg/kg IM	Same
Valium	None	5.5 to 8.5 mg/kg IM
Valsyn Gel (L,D)	Intramammary infusion (Furaltadone, 500 mg)	None
Vebanol	200 to 300 mg IM	None
Vetame	Cattle: 0.1 to 0.2 mg/kg; Sheep: 1.0 mg/kg IM or IV	0.88 to 1.3 mg/kg IM or IV
Vitamin E—Selenium	0.1 mg/kg Se and 1.36 IU/kg vitamin E IM	Same
Vitamin K (Aquamephyton)	1 mg/kg IV or IM	Same
Xylazine (Rompun)	Cattle: 0.05 to 0.33 mg/kg IM; sheep: 0.01 to 0.22 mg/kg IM	None
Zeranol (Ralgro)	Cattle: 36 mg SC (ear); lambs: 12 mg SC (ear)	None

Conversion Tables

Table 1. HOUSEHOLD MEASURES

Measure	Approximate Equivalents	
	Metric	*Apothecaries*
1 drop	1/20 ml	1 minim
1 teaspoon	5 ml	1+ dram
1 dessertspoon	8 ml	2 drams
1 tablespoon	15 ml	½ ounce
1 wineglass	60 ml	2 ounces
1 glass	250 ml	8 ounces

From Kirk RW, Bistner SI: Handbook of Veterinary Procedures and Emergency Treatment, 3rd ed. Philadelphia, WB Saunders Co, 1981

Table 2. CONVERSION FACTORS

1 milligram	= 1/65	grain	(1/60)*
1 gram	= 15.43	grains	(15)
1 kilogram	= 2.20	pounds	[avoirdupois]
	= 2.68	pounds	[Troy]
1 milliliter	= 16.23	minims	(15)
1 liter	= 1.06	quarts	(1+)
	33.80	fluid ounces	(34)
1 grain	= 0.065	gm	(60 mg)
1 dram	= 3.9	gm	(4)
1 ounce	= 31.1	gm	(30+)
1 minim	= 0.062	ml	(0.06)
1 fluid dram	= 3.7	ml	(4)
1 fluid ounce	= 29.57	ml	(30)
1 pint	= 473.2	ml	(500−)
1 quart	= 946.4	ml	(1000−)

From Kirk RW, Bistner SI: Handbook of Veterinary Procedures and Emergency Treatment, 3rd ed. Philadelphia, WB Saunders Co, 1981
*Figures in parentheses are commonly employed approximate values.

Table 3. APPROXIMATE CONVERSIONS—POUNDS TO KILOGRAMS

Pounds	Kilograms
11	5
22	10
33	15
44	20
55	25
66	30
88	40
110	50
132	60
154	70
176	80
198	90
220	100
242	110

Table 4. CONVERSION FROM FAHRENHEIT TO CENTIGRADE THERMOMETRIC READINGS

Cent. Deg.	Fahr. Deg.	Cent. Deg.	Fahr. Deg.	Cent. Deg.	Fahr. Deg.	Cent. Deg.	Fahr. Deg.
−40	−40.0	−4	24.8	32	89.6	68	154.4
−39	−38.2	−3	26.6	33	91.4	69	156.2
−38	−36.4	−2	28.4	34	93.2	70	158.0
−37	−34.6	−1	30.2	35	95.0	71	159.8
−36	−32.8	0	32.0	36	96.8	72	161.6
−35	−31.0	+1	33.8	37	98.6	73	163.4
−34	−29.2	2	35.6	38	100.4	74	165.2
−33	−27.4	3	37.4	39	102.2	75	167.0
−32	−25.6	4	39.2	40	104.0	76	168.8
−31	−23.8	5	41.0	41	105.8	77	170.6
−30	−22.0	6	42.8	42	107.6	78	172.4
−29	−20.2	7	44.6	43	109.4	79	174.2
−28	−18.4	8	46.4	44	111.2	80	176.0
−27	−16.6	9	48.2	45	113.0	81	177.8
−26	−14.8	10	50.0	46	114.8	82	179.6
−25	−13.0	11	51.8	47	116.6	83	181.4
−24	−11.2	12	53.6	48	118.4	84	183.2
−23	−9.4	13	55.4	49	120.2	85	185.0
−22	−7.6	14	57.2	50	122.0	86	186.8
−21	−5.8	15	59.0	51	123.8	87	188.6
−20	−4.0	16	60.8	52	125.6	88	190.4
−19	−2.2	17	62.6	53	127.4	89	192.2
−18	−0.4	18	64.4	54	129.2	90	194.0
−17	+1.4	19	66.2	55	131.0	91	195.8
−16	3.2	20	68.0	56	132.8	92	197.6
−15	5.0	21	69.8	57	134.6	93	199.4
−14	6.8	22	71.6	58	136.4	94	201.2
−13	8.6	23	73.4	59	138.2	95	203.0
−12	10.4	24	75.2	60	140.0	96	204.8
−11	12.2	25	77.0	61	141.8	97	206.6
−10	14.0	26	78.8	62	143.6	98	208.4
−9	15.8	27	80.6	63	145.4	99	210.2
−8	17.6	28	82.4	64	147.2	100	212.0
−7	19.4	29	84.2	65	149.0	101	213.8
−6	21.2	30	86.0	66	150.8	102	215.6
−5	23.0	31	87.8	67	152.6	103	217.4
						104	219.2

From Catalogue 65, Hospital and Surgical Equipment. V. Mueller, Chicago.

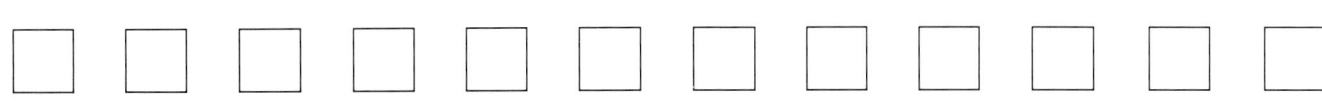

INDEX

Note: Page numbers in *italics* indicate illustrations. Page numbers followed by t refer to tables.

Abdomen, congenital defects of, 96
  distention of, in abomasal impaction, 732, *732*, 733
    in urolithiasis, 820
    in vagus indigestion, 730–731, *731*
  fluid in, in African swine fever, 486
  pain in, 735
  ultrasonography of, 27t, 28
Abducens nerve, anatomy of, 852
  in opthalmic examination, 830
Abomasum, displacement of, prevention of, dietary fiber in, 210
    to left, *723*, 723–725
    to right, 725–728, *726*
  drug administration to, esophageal groove closure in, 708
  emptying defect of, 736–737
  impaction of, *732*, 732–733
  protein in, 235t
  ulcer of, 708, 735
  volvulus of, 725–730, *727*, *729*, 730t, 735
Abortion, border disease and, 463
  borreliosis and, 516
  broomsnakeweed toxicity and, 347–348
  brucellosis and, 551–552, *552*, 554
  campylobacteriosis and, in cattle, 511
    in sheep, 155, 508, 509
  chlamydiosis and, 455
  diagnosis of, 787–791, 788t, *789*, 789t, *790*
  epizootic, 455
  fungal infection and, 525–526
  in goats, prevention of, vaccination in, 164
  in mystery pig disease, 485
  in pigs, 805–807, 807t
  induction of, in cattle, 791–792, 792t, 811, 811t
    in goats, 792, 792t, 811t, 814
    in pigs, 793, 814
  leptospirosis and, 543–545
  listeriosis and, 582, 583
  nocardiosis and, 521
  parvovirus and, in cattle, 432
    in pigs, 484–485
  ponderosa pine toxicity and, 347
  pseudorabies and, 480
  Q fever and, 622, 623
  rhinotracheitis virus and, 418
  viral infection and, diagnosis of, 416t
Abscess, in actinobacillosis, 535

Abscess *(Continued)*
  in lymphadenitis, in *Corynebacterium* infection, 537–538
  in vertical wall crack, 865
  myocardial, in *Haemophilus somnus* infection, 546, 547, *548*
  of jowl, streptococcal, 577–578
  of liver, in omphalitis, 103
    in rumenitis, 716, 717
  of sole, 864–865
  preputial, in bull, 797
  retropharyngeal, 713, 714
  umbilical, 102
Acanthocytes, 694t
Acantholysis, familial, 909
Acepromazine, dosage of, 930t
  for bovine bonkers syndrome, 327
  for lactation failure, in pigs, 769
  in capture of ruminants, 63
  preanesthetic, 61t, 66
Acetamides, in herbicides, toxicity of, 387, 388t
Acetazolamide, dosage of, 930t
Acetic acid, dosage of, 930t
  for indigestion, 711
Acetobols, for bovine ephemeral fever, 449
Acetonemia, in cattle, 309–312, *310*, 311t
  in sheep, 221
Acetyl promazine, for tetanus, 568
Acetylcysteine, for phenol toxicity, 411
  for tracheobronchial patency, 679t, 679–680
Acetylsalicylic acid (aspirin), 9t, 10
  and gastrointestinal secretion, 761
  dosage of, 930t
  for bovine ephemeral fever, 449
  for laminitis, aseptic, 868
  for mastitis, 767–768
  for thrombophlebitis, 701
  for urticaria, 901
Acholeplasma infection, 457–458
Achromoderma, 913
Acidosis, cerebrospinal fluid, sodium bicarbonate infusion and, 3
  in feedlot sheep, 161t, 162, *162*
  in listeriosis, 862
  lactic, 714–716, *715*
    in dairy cattle, 212
    magnesium for, 711, 716
  metabolism in, 18

Acidosis *(Continued)*
  ruminal, chronic, 716–717
  with dehydration, in calves, 2, 3
  in cattle, 6
Acorns, toxicity of, 348, 351t, 372–374, 373t, *374*
  to kidney, 822–826
Acremonium coenophialum, in fescue toxicity, 370, 870
Acridine derivatives, for babesiosis, 587t
Acroteriasis congenitale, 94
Actaea species, toxicity of, 350t
ACTH, dosage of, 931t
  in stress response, 17–19
Actinobacillosis, 534–535
  and mycetoma, 892–893
  and pneumonia, 549–551, 550t, 665, 667, 668t, 669
Actinomycosis, 536–537
  and mycetoma, 892–893
  in omphalitis, 101, 102, 102t
  in sinusitis, 639
  uterine, 770, 771
Adenitis, bulbourethral, 793
Adenomatosis, pulmonary, 477–478, 637
Adenovirus infection, in cattle, 429–430
  in goats, 461–462
  in pigs, 483–484
  in sheep, 461–462
Adrenal cortex, hyperfunction of, and skin lesions, 912
Adrenocorticotropic hormone, dosage of, 930t
  in stress response, 17–19
Adsorbents, for gastrointestinal disorders, 761
Aesculus species, toxicity of, 351t
Afibrinogenemia, in goats, 698–699
African swine fever, 486–488, *487*, *488*
  respiratory signs of, 668t
  skin lesions in, 899
Agalactia, 768–769
Agar gel immunodiffusion test, for bovine leukemia virus, 451
Agave lecheguilla toxicity, and photosensitization, 363
Agglutination testing, for brucellosis, 553, *553*
  for rotavirus infection, 104
Agkistrodon species, bites of, 411
Agrostemma species, toxicity of, 351t

935

Akabane disease, in cattle, 442–443
  in sheep and goats, 470
Alanine, in metabolism, in stress, 18
Albacillin, dosage of, 930t
Albamast, dosage of, 930t, 932t
Albendazole, dosage of, 930t
  for bronchitis, parasitic, 678, 679t
  for cestode infestation, 758
  for fluke infestation, 757, 757t
  for nematode infestation, 748, 748t
  in anthelmintic therapy, 49
  in llamas, 176, 176t
Albinism, 95, 910, 913
Albon. See *Sulfadimethoxine (Albon)*.
Alcelaphine herpesvirus, and catarrhal fever, malignant, 421, 421–422, 422
Alcohol, for rectal prolapse, 742
  in anesthesia, for tenesmus, in vaginitis, 773
Aldrin, in water supply, 376t
Alfadolone (Saffan), dosage of, 932t
  in anesthesia, 67
Alfalfa, energy concentration in, 191t, 191–192, 193t
  heat damage to, in storage, 342
  in dairy cattle feed, 212, 213, 213t, 214t
  in goat feed, 273, 275t
  protein in, metabolism of, 228t, 230, 235t, 239, 240
Alfaxolone (Saffan), dosage of, 932t
  in anesthesia, 67
Algae blooms, toxicity of, 292–293
Aliphatics, in herbicides, toxicity of, 387, 388t
Alkali disease, in selenium poisoning, 366, 367
Alkaline phosphatase, blood level of, 920t
Alkalosis, in oak poisoning, 824
  metabolic, in abomasal displacement, 724, 727–728
  with dehydration, in cattle, 6
Allergy, and pneumonia, in cattle, on feedlot, 138–140
  and rhinitis, drugs for, 638
  antihistamines for, 9, 9t
  to drugs, 25
Allerton virus, in lumpy skin disease, 427
Allium species, toxicity of, 350t
Allspice, toxicity of, 350t
Allyltrenbolone, for estrus synchronization, 776
Aloin, and gastrointestinal motility, 759, 759t
Alopecia, 915
  plant toxicity and, 364, 906
Alpacas. See *Camelids*.
Alpha-naphthyl thiourea, toxicity of, 385t, 386
Altrenogest, in estrus synchronization, 814
Aluminum, for fluoride toxicosis, 402
  in water supply, 376, 376t
Aluminum silicate, for gastric ulcers, 736
Aluminum sulfate, with potassium, for dermatophilosis, 895
Alveoli, epithelialization of, 634
  macrophages in, 634–635, 653
Amanita phalloides, toxicity of, 355, 356
Amaranthus species, toxicity of, 350t, 352
  to kidney, 823t, 825t
Amblyomma ticks, and immunosuppression, dermatophilosis with, 523, 524
  as vectors, of heartwater, 628, 629, 632

Amelanosis, 913
Amianthum muscaetoxicum, toxicity of, 350t
Amicarbalide, for babesiosis, 587t
Amikacin, for omphalitis, 102t
Amino acids. See also *Protein*.
  dietary requirement for, 196, 197
  metabolism of, in stress, 18
  structure of, 224, 232, 232
Aminoglycosides, nephrotoxicity of, 818
Aminophylline, for bronchospasm, with regurgitation, in anesthesia, 59
  for heart failure, 704
Amitraz, for mange, demodectic, 886
Amitrole, toxicity of, 390t, 392
Ammi majus, and photosensitization, 363
Ammonia, and pneumonia, in pigs, 666
  efflux of, in ruminants, 199
  in dairy cattle feed, 267–268
  in hypomagnesemic tetany, 319
  in protein synthesis, 197–198, 236–239
  toxicity of, 231, 327
Ammonium chloride, dosage of, 930t
  for pyelonephritis, infectious, 827
  in prevention of urolithiasis, 818, 820
Ammonium tetrathiomolybdate, for copper toxicosis, 398
Amoxicillin, for keratoconjunctivitis, infectious, 835–836
  for mastitis, 767t
  for omphalitis, 102t
  for pneumonia, 658t, 659t, 660
Amphetamine, dosage of, 930t
Amphotericin B, for fungal infection, 529
  in embryo transfer, 786–787
Ampicillin, dosage of, 930t
  for *Actinobacillus* pleuropneumonia, 550, 550t
  for cystitis, 828
  for ear necrosis, 903
  for *Eubacterium suis* infection, 520
  in pyelonephritis, 828
  for keratoconjunctivitis, infectious, 835–836
  for mastitis, 767t
  for omphalitis, 102t
  for pasteurellosis, in cattle, 557, 557t
    in pigs, 559, 560
  for pneumonia, 557, 557t, 658t, 659t, 660
  for streptococcosis, 577, 578
Amprolium, dosage of, 930t
  for coccidiosis, 602, 603t
  as feed additive, 186
    for stocker calves, 131
  in llamas, 176, 176t
Ampullitis, 793
Amsinckia species, toxicity of, 344, 347
Anabasine, as teratogen, 360
Anabolic steroids, as growth promotants, 180–183, 181t–184t, 294
  for acetonemia, 311, 311t
  for anemia, 701
  for toxemia of pregnancy, 313, 313t, 315
Anagen, defluxion in, 914–915
Analgesia. See also *Anesthesia*.
  regional, 77–88
    classification of, 77
    drugs for, 79, 79t
    of eyelids, 86–87, 87
    of eyes, 87–88, 88
    of horn, 84–85, 85
    of limbs, 85, 85–86, 86
    of penis, 84
    of udder, 86, 86

Analgesia (Continued)
  spinal, 79–83, 81–84
    spinal anatomy in, 77–79, 78, 78t
Anaphylaxis, 684
  after insect bites, 413
Anaplasmosis, diagnosis of, 589–591
  epidemiology of, 588–589
  management of, 591–595, 593t, 595t
    in outbreaks, 595–596
  pathogenesis of, 589
Anasarca, in besnoitiosis, 596–598, 597, 598
AnaSed, preanesthetic, 60–62, 61t
Ancobon, for fungal infection, 529
Anemia, 693–695, 694t–696t
  in anaplasmosis, 589–592
  in eperythrozoonosis, 614, 615
  in hemoglobinuria, postparturient, 323–325
  respiratory signs of, 668t
  treatment of, 699–701
Anencephaly, 92
Anesthesia, 58–76. See also *Analgesia*.
  and bloat, 59–60
  and eyeball rotation, 74, 75
  and hyperthermia, malignant, 74–75
  barbiturates in, 63–65, 64
  dissociative agents in, 66–67
  downer cow syndrome after, 322
  drug residues after, 58
  endotracheal intubation for, 70–72, 71, 71t, 73, 74
  fluid therapy in, 75–76
  guaifenesin in, 65–66
  in ophthalmic examination, 834
  inhalation, 67–72, 68–71, 71t, 73, 74
  ketamine in, 65–67
  pentobarbital in, 64
  premedication with, 60–63, 61t
  regurgitation in, 59
  respiration in, 58–59
  salivation in, 60
  stages of, 72–74
  xylazine in, 65–67
Anestrus, in cattle, 810–811
  in pigs, 806t
Aneurysms, of pulmonary artery, 647, 648, 649, 651, 652
Angiocardiography, in respiratory disease, 677
Angiomatosis, 917
Angora goats, herd management of, 163, 166
  nutrition for, 273–276, 274t, 275t
Anguina species, in ryegrass toxicity, 357
Ankylosing spondylitis, 877–878
Anophthalmia, 93
Anorexia, in cholera, in pigs, 495–496
Antacids, for gastric ulcers, 736
  for gastrointestinal disorders, 761
Anthelmintic therapy, 47–51
  for lungworm, 674
  for nematode infestation, in cattle, 748, 748t
    in goats, 752
    in pigs, 754, 754t
    in sheep, 751–752
  in llamas, 176, 176t
Anthrax, 565–567, 566t
Antibacterial drugs, and fungal mastitis, 527
Antibiotics. See *Antimicrobials* and specific drugs, e.g., *Penicillin*.

Antibodies, fluorescent testing for, in viral infection, 414, 416t
immune response to, 12–13
Anticholinergics, and gastrointestinal motility, 759t, 760
Anticholinesterase drugs, and gastrointestinal motility, 759, 759t
Anticoagulants, in rodenticides, toxicity of, 383, 384t, 385t
Antigens, immune response to, 12–13
Antihistamines, 8, 8–9, 9t
Anti-inflammatory drugs, nonsteroidal, 8, 9t, 9–10. See also *Acetylsalicylic acid (aspirin)*.
nephrotoxicity of, 819
Anti-lewisite, British, dosage of, 930t
for arsenic toxicosis, 395
Antimicrobials. See also specific drugs, e.g., *Chlortetracycline*.
and adverse reactions, 20–25, 22t–24t
as feed additives, 184–186, 185t–187t
for pigs, 282–283
dosages of, 931t–933t
for *Actinobacillus* pleuropneumonia, 550, 550t
for actinomycosis, 536, 537
for anaplasmosis, 592, 593, 593t, 595
for anthrax, 566
for babesiosis, 587, 587t
for bacillary hemoglobinuria, 571
for blackleg, 570
for campylobacteriosis, 508–510, 512–515, 785
for chlamydiosis, 456, 457
for coccidiosis, 602, 603t
for *Corynebacterium* infection, 538–540
for cystitis, 827–828
for dermatitis, digital, 869
for dermatophilosis, 523, 895
for dysentery, 561, 561t
for edema, malignant, 570
for ehrlichiosis, 617
for endocarditis, 688, 701–702
for entropion, 840
for eperythrozoonosis, in pigs, 616
for erysipelas, 580
for *Escherichia coli* infection, 518
for *Eubacterium suis* infection, 520
for foot rot, 873
for *Haemophilus parasuis* infection, 507
for *Haemophilus somnus* infection, 549
for heartwater, 631, 632t
for keratoconjunctivitis, infectious, in cattle, 835–837
mycoplasmal, in goats, 841
for leptospirosis, 545
for listeriosis, 583, 862
for mastitis, 767t, 767–768
for meningitis, 861–862
for mycoplasmosis, 458, 841
for nocardiosis, 522
for omphalitis, 102t, 102–103
for osteomyelitis, 881
for pasteurellosis, in cattle, 556–558, 557t
in pigs, 559, 560
for pasture fever, 621, 621t
for petechial fever, 619t, 620
for phlegmon, 870
for pneumonia, 642–643, 656–664, 657t–659t
for polyarthritis, 116
for pulmonary edema and emphysema, 646–647

Antimicrobials (*Continued*)
for pyelonephritis, 828
for salmonellosis, 109, 564–565
for septic arthritis, 874
for staphylococcosis, 579, 896
for streptococcosis, 577
for tetanus, 568
for tick-borne fever, 621, 621t
for toxoplasmosis, 625
for trichomoniasis, 785
for trypanosomiasis, 606–607, 607t
for tuberculosis, 532–533, 533t
for urinary tract infection, 817
for uterine infection, 771
in prevention of abortion, in borreliosis, 516
in respiratory therapy, 678–679, 679t
in sheep, 672
ionophore, toxicity of, 329–331
residues of, tests for, 31, 31t, 32t
Antithrombin III, measurement of, 691, 692t
Antitoxin, for botulism, 569
for tetanus, 568
Antitrypsin factor, in protein digestion, 225–226
Antivenin, dosage of, 930t
for snakebite, 412
Antrycide, for trypanosomiasis, 607, 607t
Antrypol, for trypanosomiasis, 607, 607t
Ants, stinging, 412t, 412–413
ANTU, in rodenticides, toxicity of, 385t, 386
Anus, atresia of, 742–743
Aplasia cutis, 909
Apocynum species, toxicity of, 350t, 352, 353
Aquamephyton. See *Vitamin K₁ (Aquamephyton)*.
Arachidonate, in stress response, 17
Arachnoidea, anatomy of, 77, 78
Arachnomelia, 94
Arecoline, and gastrointestinal motility, 759, 759t
Arginine, dietary, 280t
Arhinencephaly, 92
Arnold-Chiari malformation, 92
Aroclors (polychlorinated biphenyls), toxicity of, 405–407, 904
Arrhythmia, atrial fibrillation in, 689
auscultation of, 685
drugs for, 702t, 702–703
lymphosarcoma and, 688
Arrowgrass, cyanide in, 344, 347
Arsanilic acid, in prevention of eperythrozoonosis, 616
toxicity of, 395–396
to eyes, 854t, 856
Arsenate, for cestode infestation, 758
Arsenic, in water supply, 376, 376t
toxicity of, 394–396
in herbicides, 388t, 391
to kidney, 395, 823t
to skin, 904
Arteritis, umbilical, 101, 102, 821–822
Arthritis, chlamydial infection and, in cattle, 456
in erysipelas, 579, 580
in mycoplasmosis, in cattle, 458
in pigs, 505
of multiple joints, in piglet, 115–116
septic, 873–874
with encephalitis, viral, in goats, 167, 472, 472–474, 473, 862–863

Arthrogryposis, in cattle, 93
in sheep, Cache Valley virus and, 93, 474–475, 475
Artificial insemination. See *Insemination, artificial*.
Ascariasis, 752–754, 754t
drugs for, 49, 50
of respiratory tract, 666, 668t, 674–675
Ascarops strongylina infestation, dichlorvos for, 50
Ascites, in African swine fever, 486
ultrasonography of, 28
Asclepias species, toxicity of, 344–345, 348, 350t, 352, 353
Ascorbic acid (Vitamin C), deficiency of, skin lesions in, 911
in immunotherapy, 16
L-Asparaginase, for leukosis, enzootic, 704
for lymphosarcoma, 850
Aspartate aminotransferase, in downer cow syndrome, 322
in fat cow syndrome, 316
Aspergillus species, infection with, 524, 525, 527–528
ocular, in camelids, 846
of skin, 893
toxins of, 336, 337
Aspiration, and pneumonia, in anesthesia, 59
in petroleum toxicity, 407–409
from retrobulbar space, in ocular examination, 833
transtracheal, diagnostic, 676, 677
Aspirin. See *Acetylsalicylic acid*.
Asthenia, cutaneous, 907–909
Astragalus species, as teratogens, 360
toxicity of, 348
ocular signs of, 854t
selenium in, 366, 366, 367
to nervous system, 357
Astrovirus infection, in cattle, 452–453
in sheep, 474
Ataractics, preanesthetic, 60, 61t
Ataxia, cerebellar, with hypomyelinogenesis, 858
enzootic, in copper deficiency, 397
with convulsions, familial, 859
Atelectasis, pathology of, 636
Atgard (dichlorvos), for nematode infestations, in pigs, 754, 754t
for parasitosis, external, 53t
in anthelmintic therapy, 50
Atherosclerosis, spontaneous, 684
Atony, of forestomach, 706
ruminal, and bloat, 707–708
Atopy, 901
Atrazine, toxicity of, 389t, 392
Atresia ani, 742–743
Atresia coli, 96, 740–741
Atresia recti, 742–743
Atrial fibrillation, 689, 702
Atroban, for lice, in goats, 165
for parasitosis, external, 54t–57t
Atropine, and gastrointestinal motility, 759t, 760
dosage of, 930t
for arrhythmia, 703
for entropion, 840
for insecticide poisoning, 382
for keratoconjunctivitis, infectious, 836
for uveitis, infectious, 838
neonatal, 840
preanesthetic, 60, 66, 67
Aujeszky's disease. See *Pseudorabies*.

Aureomycin, for eperythrozoonosis, 176, 176t
Auscultation, of heart, 681, 681t, 684–685
  of lungs, 675–676
    in pneumonia, 642
    in pulmonary edema and emphysema, 643–646
  of ruminal contractions, 709
Autoimmune disorders, 15
Avatec. See *Lasalocid.*
Avermectins. See *Ivermectin (Ivomec).*
Avocado, toxicity of, 351t
Azaperone, preanesthetic, 61t
Azium. See *Dexamethasone.*

B lymphocytes. See *Lymphocytes.*
Babesan, for babesiosis, 587t
Babesiosis, 584–587, 587t
  vs. anaplasmosis, in cattle, 591
Baccharis, toxicity of, 350t
Bacillary hemoglobinuria, 571
Bacille Calmette-Guérin, in vaccination, against tuberculosis, 533
Bacillus anthracis infection, 565–567, 566t
Bacitracin, dosage of, 930t
  for dysentery, 561t
Back, fat of, ultrasonography of, 27, 29
Backgrounding, 130–134, 132t, *133*, *134*
Bacteroides nodosus infection, and dermatitis, of foot, 868, 869
  in foot rot, in sheep, 872, 873
Bahia grass, in *Claviceps* poisoning, in cerebellar disease, 860
Baking soda. See *Sodium bicarbonate* (baking soda).
BAL, dosage of, 930t
Balanoposthitis, 796
Bamboo, toxicity of, 351t
Banamine. See *Flunixin meglumine.*
Baneberry, toxicity of, 350t
Bang's disease, 551
Banminth (pyrantel), for ascariasis, in prevention of pneumonia, 675
  for nematode infestation, 754, 754t
  in anthelmintic therapy, 50–51
Barban, toxicity of, 387–391, 388t
Barbiturates, in anesthesia, 63–65, *64*
Barium, in water supply, 376, 376t
Barley, toxicity of, 350t
Basophils, in hypersensitivity, 15
  laboratory measurement of, 692t, 919t, 920t
  stippling of, in anemia, 694, 694t
Batyl alcohol, dosage of, 930t
Baycox, for coccidiosis, 602, 603t
Baymix. See *Coumaphos (Baymix).*
Bee stings, 412, 412t
Beetles, blister, toxicity of, 413
  to kidney, 823t
Beets, toxicity of, 350t
Bemegride, dosage of, 930t
Benadryl, for anaphylaxis, 684
  for inflammation, 9t
Benefin, toxicity of, 388t, 391
Benfluralin, toxicity of, 388t, 391
Bensulide, toxicity of, 390t, 392
Benzimidazoles, for nematode infestation, 748, 748t
  in anthelmintic therapy, 49–50
Benzoics, in herbicides, toxicity of, 387, 388t
Berenil, for babesiosis, 587, 587t

Berenil *(Continued)*
  for trypanosomiasis, 606, 607, 607t
Berne virus infection, 451–452
Besnoitiosis, 596–598, *597*, *598*, 900
Beta agonists, in growth promotion, 188
Beta carotene. See *Vitamin A.*
Beta species, toxicity of, 350t
Beta-hydroxybutyrate, in toxemia of pregnancy, 314
Betamethasone, for acetonemia, 311, 311t
  for inflammation, 11, 11t
Betavet soluspan, dosage of, 930t
Bethanechol, and gastrointestinal motility, 759, 759t
  in induction of micturition, 818
Bicarbonate sodium. See *Sodium bicarbonate.*
Bicillin, dosage of, 930t
Bile, secretion of, drugs affecting, 760t
Bilirubin, blood level of, elevated, in anemia, 695
  reference values for, 920t
Bio-Cox, toxicity of, 329–330
Biodry (novobiocin), dosage of, 931t, 932t
Biologic response modifiers, for ocular squamous cell carcinoma, 848–849
Biolyte oral rehydration solution, 5t
Biopsy, of liver, in fat cow syndrome, 317, 317t
  of lung, 676
Biosol, dosage of, 930t
Biotin, deficiency of, skin lesions in, 911
  nutritional requirement for, in pigs, 280t, 281–282
Biphenyls, polybrominated, toxicity of, 403t, 403–404, 404t, 904
  polychlorinated, toxicity of, 405–407, 904
Bipyridyliums, in herbicides, toxicity of, 387, 388t
Bird's-foot trefoil, toxicity of, 350t
Bishop's weed, and photosensitization, 363
Bismuth subsalicylate, as adsorbent, in gastrointestinal tract, 761
Bites, by insects, 412t, 412–413
  by snakes, 411t, 412–413, 906
Bittersweet, toxicity of, 350t
Black disease, 572–573
Black locust, toxicity of, 351t
Black patch disease, of red clover, in salivary syndrome, 338–339
Black pox, 902
Blackleg, 569–570, 897
Bladder, in *Corynebacterium renale* infection, 539
  in *Eubacterium suis* infection, 519–521
  inflammation of, in pigs, 817t, 827–828
  rupture of, lithiasis and, 820
  ultrasonography of, 28
Bladderpod, toxicity of, 350t
Blind staggers, in selenium poisoning, 366, 367
Blindgrass, toxicity of, 854t, 856
Blindness, causes of, 854t, 855, 856
Blister beetles, toxicity of, 413
  to kidney, 823t
Blisters, in foot-and-mouth disease, 438, *438*
Bloat, 717–718
  anesthesia and, 59–60
  in feedlot cattle, 138
  petroleum toxicity and, 407–409
  physiology of, 707–708

Bloat *(Continued)*
  xylazine and, preanesthetic, 62
Blood, arterial, oxygenation of, maintenance of, 680
  coagulation of. See *Coagulation.*
  laboratory evaluation of, 690–692, 692t
  normal values for, 919t–920t
  packed cell volume of, in dehydration, 2
  testing of, for viral infection, 415–417
  transfusion of, 6–7
    for hypogammaglobulinemia, 13
    for shock, 682
    in anemia, 699–700
Blood cells, production of, 692–693
  red, decreased level of, 693, 693–695, 694t–696t
    elevated level of, 695–696
    laboratory count of, 690–692, 692t, 919t, 920t
  white, disorders of, 696t, 696–698
    laboratory count of, 690–692, 692t, 919t, 920t
Blood pressure, arterial, in spinal analgesia, 80–81
  decreased, preanesthetic tranquilizers and, 60
Bloody scours, in pigs, 560–562, 561t
Blowflies, skin infestation by, 888–889
Blue eye disease, of pigs, 502–504
Bluetongue, and congenital defects, 436, 839
  in cattle, 435–437
  in sheep, 465–467
  skin lesions in, 899
Boar. See also *Pig(s).*
  nutrition in, 284
  penile disorders in, 797–798
Boldenone undecylenate, for anemia, 701
Bones, congenital defects of, 94
  fluorosis of, 399–402, *401*
  fracture of, 878–880
  infection of, hematogenous, 881
  marrow of, hematopoiesis in, 692–693
    in anemia, 695, 696t
Bonkers syndrome, 231, 327
Boophilus ticks, as vectors, of babesiosis, 584–587
Border disease, 462–464, 899
Boron, in water supply, 376, 376t
Borreliosis, in cattle, 515–516
  in pigs, 897
Bot infestation, nasal, 48–49
  and meningitis, 861
  ocular, 842
  of respiratory tract, 674
Botanical hydrocarbons, for external parasitosis, 51
Botulism, 568–569
Bovate. See *Lasalocid.*
Bovi-Clox, dosage of, 931t
Bovilene. See *Fenprostalene.*
Bovine. See also *Cattle* and specific disorders and pathogens, e.g., *Diarrhea, bovine viral* and *Herpesvirus.*
Bovine bonkers syndrome, 231, 327
Bovine somatotropin, 42–46, *43*, *44*
Bowenia species, toxicity of, 357
Box plant, toxicity of, 350t
Bracken fern, toxicity of, 350t
  to eyes, 854t, 856
  to kidney, 823t
Branhamella ovis infection, and conjunctivitis, 840

Brassica species, toxicity of, 350t
Braxy, 572
Breda virus, bovine, 451–452
Breeding, of cattle, dairy, 144–145, 145t, 150–152, 152t
    timing of, in large herd, 127, *127*
      in heifers, 129
      in small herd, 123–124
    of goats, 165–166
    of llamas, 173
    of pigs, 168–171
    of sheep, 154t, 154–159, 156t
Bright blindness, 854t, 856
British anti-lewisite, dosage of, 930t
    for arsenic toxicosis, 395
Brodifacoum, toxicity of, 383, 384t
Bromadiolone, toxicity of, 383, 384t
Bromocil, toxicity of, 390t, 392
Bronchi, inflammation of, 636
    parasitic, 678–679, 679t
    lavage of, in diagnosis, of respiratory disease, 676
    patency of, maintenance of, 679t, 679–680
    physiology of, 633–634
Bronchioles, inflammation of, 636
    physiology of, 634
Bronchopneumonia. See also *Pneumonia*.
    in cattle, 653–656
      control of, 660–664
      steroids contraindicated in, 419
      treatment of, 656–660, 657t–659t
    pathology of, 637
Bronchospasm, with regurgitation, in anesthesia, 59
Broomsnakeweed, toxicity of, and abortion, 347–348
Brown Swiss cattle, congenital neuromuscular disease in, 92
Brucellosis, 551–555, 552t, 552–554
    and epididymitis, 796
    and vesiculitis, 793
    vaccination against, and pneumonia, 663
Buck. See also *Goats*.
    fertility of, 804
    penile disorders in, 798
Buckeye, toxicity of, 351t
Buckwheat rash, 362
Buffers, as feed additives, 187
Bulbourethral glands, inflammation of, 793
Bull. See also *Cattle*.
    campylobacteriosis in, 510–512
    inguinal hernia in, strangulation of, 734–735
    nutrition for, 257, 258t
    penile disorders in, 796–797
    trichomoniasis in, 608–612, *609*
    vesiculitis in, 793–794
Bullous epidermolysis, 909
Bunchflower, toxicity of, 350t
Bunostomum infestation, 49, 50
Buparvaquone, for theileriosis, 628
Buphthalmia, 847t
Bupivacaine, in regional analgesia, 79t
Burning bush, toxicity of, 350t
Burns, of skin, 902
Bushbuck, petechial fever in, 618
Butacaine sulfate, dosage of, 930t
Butaphosphan, for downer cow syndrome, 323
Butazolidin. See *Phenylbutazone*.

Butorphanol, with xylazine, preanesthetic, 60–62
Buttercup, toxicity of, 351t
Buxus species, toxicity of, 350t
BZD virus, in lumpy skin disease, 427

Cache Valley virus infection, 93, 474–475, *475*
Cadmium, in water supply, 376, 376t
Calcaneus, fracture of, 879
Calcium, blood level of, decreased, in dairy cattle, in pregnancy, 212
    in downer cow syndrome, 323
    with milk fever, 304–309, 307t
    reference values for, 920t
    for fluoride toxicosis, 402
    for heart failure, 703–704
    in urolithiasis, 819, 820
    nutritional requirement for, 200–203, 202t
      in cattle, 251, 252t
        beef, 123t
          in pregnancy and lactation, 206t, 207, 208t, 209
        dairy, 268, 270t, 271t
          in pregnancy and lactation, 211–213, 213t, 214t
      in goats, 273, 274t, 275t, 277, 278
      in pigs, 170, 171, 279, 280t
        in pregnancy and lactation, 214–216
      in sheep, in pregnancy and lactation, 218
    supplemental, for grazing cattle, 295–296, 298, 299t
Calcium borogluconate, for milk fever, 306–307, 307t, 309
Calcium ethylenediaminetetraacetate, dosage of, 930t
Calcium gluconate, dosage of, 930t
    for shock, 683
Calcium hydroxide, dosage of, 930t
    in prevention of oak toxicity, 374, 826
Calcium hypophosphite, dosage of, 930t
    for hemoglobinuria, postparturient, 325, 325t
Calculi, urinary, 817t, 817–820
    and pain, 735
    in cattle, on feedlot, 141
    in lambs, 157
Calf (calves). See also *Cattle*.
    anthelmintic therapy in, 47
    blood tests in, reference values for, 920t
    Breda virus infection in, 451–452
    cold stress in, 116–118
    congenital defects in, 89–97
    delivery of. See *Calving*.
    diarrhea in, 103–109
      coronavirus infection and, 106, 440
    drug residues in, 34–35
    enterotoxemia in, clostridial, 573–575
    fluid replacement in, 2t, 2–5, 5t
    immunity in, colostrum and, 97–100, *99*
    nutrition in, in stress, 178–180, 179t
    omphalitis in, 101–103, 102t
    rhinotracheitis in, 418–419
    rotavirus infection in, 104–105, 439–440
    skeletal malformation in, lupine and, 346
    stocker, management of, 130–134, 132t, *133, 134*
    tetany in, hypomagnesemia and, 321

Calf Antibiotic and Sulfonamide Test, 31, 31t
Calf Span, for pneumonia, in cattle, 657t
Calici-like viruses, bovine, 453
Calicivirus infection, in pigs, 488–489
California Mastitis Test, 765t, 766
Calliphora species, skin infestation by, 888–889
Calmette-Guérin bacillus, in vaccination, against tuberculosis, 533
Calves. See *Calf (calves)*.
Calving, hemoglobinuria after, 323–326, 325t
    in dairy replacement program, 148
    nutrition after, 261
    on feedlot, 141
    timing of, in large herd management, 126, *126*, 126t, *127*, 129
Calycanthus, toxicity of, 350t
Cambendazole, dosage of, 930t
Camelids, eyes of, anatomy of, 842t, 842–843, *843*
    disorders of, 844–846
    examination of, 833, 834, *843*, 843–844
    normal microorganisms in, 844, 844t
    herd health management of, 172–177, 175t, 176t
Campylobacteriosis, and diarrhea, in neonatal ruminants, 109
    and enteropathy, proliferative, 513–515
    and infertility, 784–785
    in pregnant ewe, 155
    nonvenereal, 507–510
    venereal, 510–513
Campylognathia, 94
Candidiasis, 525–528
    of skin, 894
Cantharidin, toxicity of, 413
    to kidney, 823t
Caprine. See also *Goats* and specific disorders, e.g., *Rift Valley fever*.
Caprine arthritis-encephalitis virus, 167, 472, 472–474, 473, 862–863
Caprine viral dermatitis, 900
Captan, for dermatophytosis, 892
Carbachol, and gastrointestinal motility, 759, 759t
Carbadox, for dysentery, 561t
Carbamates, toxicity of, and miosis, 854t, 855
    in herbicides, 387–391, 388t
    in insecticides, 381–382, 382t
Carbamylcholine, for indigestion, 711
Carbocaine, in regional analgesia, 79t
Carbofuran, toxicity of, 382t
Carbomycin, dosage of, 930t
Carbon dioxide, removal of, in respiratory therapy, 680
Carcinoma, papillomatosis and, 462
    pulmonary, 477–478
    squamous cell, ocular, 847t, 847–850, 850t
    of skin, 917
Cardio-. See also *Heart*.
    of atrial fibrillation, 689
Cardiomyopathy, lymphosarcoma and, 688–689
Cardiotoxic plant(s), 352t, 352–354, 353t
    yew as, 371–372
Carelessweed, toxicity of, 350t
Caricide, dosage of, 930t
Carmilax, dosage of, 930t
β-Carotene. See *Vitamin A*.

Carpal bones, fracture of, 879
Carpal joints, swelling of, caprine arthritis-encephalitis virus and, 472, 472, 473, 473
Casein, digestion of, 226, 228t
Caseous lymphadenitis, in *Corynebacterium* infection, 537–538
Cashmere goats, herd management of, 163, 166
  nutrition for, 278
Cassia species, toxicity of, 350t
Castor bean, toxicity of, 351t
Castor oil, and gastrointestinal motility, 759, 759t
Castration, of calf, feeder, 180
  growth stimulant with, 122
  of lamb, 157
  pneumonia after, in pig, 667
Cataracts, congenital, 93
Catarrhal fever, malignant, 421, 421–422, 422
  and pneumonia, 653–654
  ophthalmitis in, 838
  skin lesions in, 899
  vs. bovine viral diarrhea, 433
Cathartics, and gastrointestinal motility, 759t, 759–760
Cats, toxoplasmosis in, 623, 625
Cattle, abortion in, induced, 791–792, 792t, 811
  blood tests in, reference values for, 919t–920t
  diet for. See *Diet*.
    protein in. See *Protein*.
  disorders in. See specific disorders, e.g., *Volvulus*, and affected structures, e.g., *Kidney(s)*.
  drug residues in, 34
  fluid replacement in, 5–6, 7
  neonatal. See *Calf (calves)*.
  range-fed, 285–293
    mineral supplementation for, 291–302
  reproduction in, in beef herd, 800t, 800–803, 801–803, 802t
    in dairy herd, 798t–800t, 798–800
    management of, 809–812, 810t, 811t
    estrus detection in, for artificial insemination, 779–780, 798, 798–799
    estrus synchronization in, 778–779, 809–810, 810t, 811t
    rate of, 787, 788t, 789t
  somatotropin in, 42–46, 43, 44
  wild, capture of, 62–63
CDAA, in herbicides, toxicity of, 387, 388t
Cecum, dilation of, 738–739
  torsion of, 739, 740
  volvulus of, 728, 729, 735, 739–740
Cefa-Dri, dosage of, 930t
Cefa-Lak, dosage of, 930t
Ceftiofur, for dermatitis, digital, 869
  for erysipelas, 580
  for omphalitis, 102t
  for pneumonia, in cattle, 658t, 659t, 659–660
    in pasteurellosis, 557t
    in pigs, in actinobacillosis, 550t
  for respiratory disease, in sheep, 672
Celastrus scandens, toxicity of, 350t
Cephaloridine, dosage of, 930t
Cephapirin, dosage of, 930t
Cerebellum, cortical atrophy of, congenital, 93
  diseases of, in cattle, 858–860

Cerebrospinal fluid, acidosis of, sodium bicarbonate infusion and, 3
  analysis of, in nematodiasis, 863
  in neurologic inflammation, 861
  sodium transport in, in toxicosis, 328
Cerebrum, cortical disorders of, ocular signs of, 854t, 856
Cervix uteri, congenital defects of, 97
  ultrasonography of, 27t, 28–29
Cestode infestations, 757–758
Cestrum species, toxicity of, 350t
Chabertia infestation, 48, 49
Charcoal, activated, dosage of, 930t
  for cardiotoxic plant poisoning, 354
  for herbicide poisoning, 393
  for insecticide poisoning, 381, 382
  for lactic acidosis, 716
  for photosensitization, hepatogenous, 363
  for rodenticide poisoning, 383
  for yew poisoning, 372
Chédiak-Higashi syndrome, 13, 698
  albinism in, 95
  skin lesions in, 910, 913–914
Chemical residues, in meat and milk, 29–42
Chemotherapy, for lymphosarcoma, 850
Cherry, toxicity of, 351t
Cherry laurel, toxicity of, 368
Chickens, monensin toxicity in, 330
  tuberculosis in, spread of, to pigs, 529, 530
Chiggers, skin infestation by, 886
Chinaberry, toxicity of, 351t
Chlamydiosis, in cattle, 455–457
  and pneumonia, 654
  in goats, vaccination against, 164
  in sheep, and keratoconjunctivitis, 840–841
Chloral hydrate, dosage of, 930t
  for acetonemia, 311
  preanesthetic, 63
Chloramben, toxicity of, 387, 388t
Chloramphenicol, dosage of, 930t
  residues of, 30, 32t
Chlordane, in water supply, 376t
Chlorfenac, toxicity of, 390t, 392
Chlorgesterone, in estrus stimulation, 813
Chlorhexidine, for staphylococcal folliculitis, 896
Chloridazon, toxicity of, 390t, 392
Chloride, blood level of, 920t
  nutritional requirement for, 200, 202
    in cattle, beef, in pregnancy and lactation, 207, 208t, 209, 210
      dairy, 270t
      in pregnancy and lactation, 212, 213, 213t, 214t
    in pigs, 279, 280t
      in pregnancy and lactation, 215
    in sheep, in pregnancy and lactation, 218
  ruminal, measurement of, 710
  supplemental, for grazing cattle, 295
Chlorinated hydrocarbons, for external parasitosis, 51, 52t, 53t, 56t, 57t
  toxicity of, 380–381
Chlorinated naphthalene, toxicity of, 904
Chloropent, dosage of, 930t
Chlorothiazide, dosage of, 930t
  for intertrigo, 902
Chloroxuron, toxicity of, 390t
Chlorpromazine, and gastrointestinal secretion, 761

Chlorpromazine *(Continued)*
  dosage of, 930t
  preanesthetic, 61t
Chlorpropham, toxicity of, 387–391, 388t
Chlorprothixene (Taractan), dosage of, 933t
  preanesthetic, 61t
Chlorpyrifos, for parasitosis, external, 52, 52t, 55t
  for trombiculidiasis, 886
  toxicity of, 381, 382t
Chlortetracycline, as feed additive, 186, 187t
  dosage of, 930t
  for anaplasmosis, 592, 593, 593t, 595
  for chlamydiosis, intestinal, in cattle, 456
  for *Eubacterium suis* infection, in pyelonephritis, in pigs, 828
  for mycoplasmosis, in cattle, 458
  for phlegmon, interdigital, 870
  for pleuritis, fibrinous, with pleuropneumonia, 664
  for pneumonia, 658, 661, 663
    in feedlot management, of lambs, 160, 161
  preventive use of, against abortion, in borreliosis, 516
    against pasteurellosis, 558
Chlorthal-dimethyl, toxicity of, 390t, 392
Chlorthiamid, toxicity of, 388t, 391
Choke, 712–713
Chokecherry, toxicity of, 347, 368
Cholecalciferol. See also *Vitamin D*.
  in milk fever, 268, 305, 307t, 308
  toxicity of, in rodenticides, 383–385, 384t, 385t
    to kidney, 825t
Cholera, in pigs, 495–496
  ocular signs of, 854t
  respiratory signs of, 668t
  skin lesions in, 899
Choline, dosage of, 930t
  for fat cow syndrome, 317
  nutritional requirement for, in pigs, 280t, 282
    in pregnancy and lactation, 215
Cholinergic drugs, and gastrointestinal motility, 759, 759t
Chorionic gonadotropin. See *Gonadotropin, human chorionic*.
Chorioptes mites, skin infestation by, 884–885
Chorisol, dosage of, 930t
Chromium, in water supply, 376, 376t
Chromosomal abnormalities, and conception failure, 781–782
  and congenital defects, 90
Cicuta species, toxicity of, 346, 350t
  to central nervous system, 358
Cimetidine, for gastric ulcers, 736
Circling disease, 580–583, 581, 583t
Citrate, in milk, in mastitis, 762
Citrinin, toxicity of, 337
Claviceps species, in ergotism, 334–336, 351t
  in cerebellar disease, 860
  in fescue toxicosis, 370, 906
  in skin disease, 906
Cloprostenol, dosage of, 930t
  for estrus synchronization, in cattle, 779
    in pigs, 776
    in sheep and goats, 777
  for pyometra, 773

Cloprostenol (Continued)
　in induction of abortion, 792, 792t, 793
　　in pigs, 811t, 814
　in induction of parturition, in pigs, 815
Clorsulon, for fluke infestation, 50, 757, 757t
　for nematode infestation, 748t
　in anthelmintic therapy, in llamas, 176, 176t
Clostridium infection, and bacillary hemoglobinuria, 571
　and blackleg, 569–570, 897
　and botulism, 568–569
　and braxy, 572
　and edema, malignant, 570, 897
　and necrotic hepatitis, 572–573
　and tetanus, 567–568
　of skin, 897
　vaccination against, in goats, 164
Clostridium perfringens infection, and diarrhea, in neonatal ruminants, 106–107
　in piglet, 112–114
　and enterotoxemia, 573–575
　in lamb, newborn, 156–158
　　prevention of, in feedlot management, 160, 161
　vaccination against, in llamas, 174
Clotrimazole, for fungal infection, 527, 529
Clotting. See Coagulation.
Clover, red, in salivary syndrome, 338–339
　sweet, toxicity of, 358–359
　toxicity of, 351t
Cloxacillin, dosage of, 930t
　for keratoconjunctivitis, 835–836
Coagulation, disorders of, 698–699
　in rodenticide toxicity, 383
　in sweet clover poisoning, 359
　intravascular disseminated, in shock, 683
　laboratory testing of, 691, 692t
Coal tar, toxicity of, 409–411
Coat, curly, 907, 911
Cobalt, deficiency of, skin lesions in, 912
　in water supply, 376, 376t
　nutritional requirement for, in cattle, 251, 252t, 260t, 270t
　　in pigs, 215
　　in sheep, 218
　supplemental, for grazing cattle, 296, 296t, 299t
Coban. See Monensin.
Coccidiosis, 525, 528, 599, 599–603, 600t, 601, 603t
　and diarrhea, in piglet, 112, 113
　feed additives for, 184, 186
　in cattle, on feedlot, 140
　in goats, 165
　in llamas, 176, 176t
　in sheep, 156
　in stocker calves, 131
Coccyx, articulation of, with femur, luxation of, 876–877
Cochliomyia hominivorax, skin infestation by, 889
Cocklebur, toxicity of, 350t, 351t, 352
　to kidney, 825t
Coenurosis, cerebellar, 859
Coffee tree, Kentucky, toxicity of, 351t
Coforta, for downer cow syndrome, 323
Cold, exposure to, and frostbite, 902–903
　in calves, 116–118

Cold (Continued)
　in goats, 166
　in lambs, 156
Cole's tube, in inhalation anesthesia, 70–71, 71
Colesiota conjunctivae infection, and keratoconjunctivitis, 840–841
Coliform bacteria, fecal, in water supply, 375
Colistin, in culture medium, for Eubacterium suis, 520
Collagen dysplasia, 95
Collagen shields, in ocular medication, 834
Collateral ligament, medial, trauma to, 875
Colon, ascending, volvulus of, 739–740
　atresia of, 96, 740–741
　obstruction of, 740
Colostrum, and passive immunity, 97–100, 99, 118
　in dairy replacement rearing, 148, 149t
Compartment syndrome, in downer cow, 322
Complement, in immune response, in respiratory tract, 635
Complement fixation test, for brucellosis, 553
Compudose, as growth stimulant, 181t–183t, 182
Conception, failure of, 781–785
　rate of, in cattle, dairy, 799, 799t
Congenital defects, 89–97
　bluetongue virus and, 436
　border disease virus and, 463
　Cache Valley virus and, 474–475, 475
　causes of, 89–90
　classification of, 91
　frequency of, 91
　of abdomen, 96
　of bone, 94
　of central nervous system, 92–93
　of eye, 93
　　in sheep and goats, 839–840
　of gastrointestinal tract, 96
　of hair, 95
　of heart, 95–96
　of joints, 94–95
　of muscle, 93–94
　of reproductive system, 96–97
　of skin, 95, 907–910, 908t
　of urinary tract, 96, 821
　toxic plants and, 346, 359–361
Conium maculatum, as teratogen, 360–361
　toxicity of, 346, 350t
Conium species, toxicity of, to central nervous system, 358
Conjunctiva, disorders of, in camelids, 844–845
　examination of, 832
　inflammation of, adenovirus infection and, 430
　　chlamydial infection and, 456
　　in bovine rhinotracheitis, 418
　　in goats, 164
　　in mycoplasmosis, 458, 479
　　infectious, in cattle, 834–837
　　in sheep, 840–841
　injection under, 834
　petechiae of, in heartwater, 629, 630
Constipation, dietary management of, 170
Contact dermatitis, 903
Convallaria majalis, toxicity of, 350t, 353
Conversion factors, 934t

Convulsions, familial, with ataxia, 859
　in heartwater, 629–630, 630
Cooling waters, industrial, toxicants in, 377–378
Cooperia nematode infestation, 47–50
Cooperia pedunculata lily, toxicity of, and photosensitization, 363
Copper, deficiency of, 397
　in hemoglobinuria, postparturient, 324–326, 325t
　skin lesions in, 912
　in water supply, 376, 376t
　mining of, water pollutants from, 378, 378t
　nutritional requirement for, in cattle, 251, 252t, 260t, 270t
　　in pigs, 280t, 281, 283
　　in sheep, 154, 218
　supplemental, for grazing cattle, 296t, 296–297, 299t
　toxicity of, 396–398, 616
　　to kidney, 824t
　　vs. enterotoxemia, clostridial, 575
Copper glycinate, dosage of, 930t
Copper sulfate, and esophageal groove closure, 708
　as growth stimulant, 283
　dosage of, 930t
　for dermatophilosis, 895
Copperhead bites, 411
Co-Ral Pour-On, dosage of, 930t
Corid. See Amprolium.
Corn, interdigital, 871, 872
　nutrients in, 196–197, 197t, 201t, 201–203, 202t
　　in dairy cattle feed, 211–213, 213t
　protein in, metabolism of, 226, 228t, 229t, 230, 235t–237t, 236, 239, 243t
　toxicity of, 352
Corn cockle, toxicity of, 351t
Cornea, anatomy of, in llamas, 842
　disorders of, in camelids, 844–845
　examination of, 831, 832
　inflammation of, with conjunctivitis. See Keratoconjunctivitis.
　masses in, differential diagnosis of, 847t
　opacification of, in catarrhal fever, malignant, 421, 422
　in paramyxovirus infection, 503
　protection of, nictitans flap for, 834
　reflex of, examination of, 830, 853
　ulceration of, in conjunctivitis, 835, 837
Cornell system, in feed protein estimation, 240–244, 241, 242, 243t
Cornual nerve, anesthetic block of, 84–85, 85
Coronavirus infection, and diarrhea, 106, 440
　respiratory, 498–500
Corpus cavernosum, rupture of, 797
Corpus luteum, cysts of, 774–775
　in pyometra, 772, 773
Corriedales, glycogen storage disease in, 93
Cortisol, secretion of, 10
Corydalis species, toxicity of, 350t
Corynebacterium infection, 536–541
Corynebacterium pseudotuberculosis infection, and ulcerative lymphangitis, 538–539
　of skin, 896–897
Corynebacterium pyogenes infection, in omphalitis, 101, 102, 102t
Corynebacterium renale infection, and posthitis, 540–541, 798

Corynebacterium renale infection (Continued)
  and pyelonephritis, 539–540, 826, 827
  of urinary tract, 817
Corynebacterium suis (*Eubacterium suis*) infection, 519–521
  and pyelonephritis, 828
Cottonmouth bites, 411
Cottonseed, gossypol in, toxicity of, 331–332
  nutrients in, 201, 201t, 202t
  protein in, metabolism of, 228t, 229t
Cough, in pigs, differential diagnosis of, 667, 668t
  physiology of, 634
  suppression of, 678
Coumaphos (Baymix), dosage of, 930t
  for mange, psorergatic, 885
  for nematode infestation, 748t
  for parasitosis, external, 52t–53t, 56t, 57t
  for psorergatic, 886
Coumarin, in sweet clover toxicity, 359
Counter, toxicity of, 382t
Cow. See *Cattle*.
Cow cockle, toxicity of, 351t
Cowdria ruminantium infection, and heartwater, 628–632, 629t, *629–631*, 632t
Cowpox infection, and mammillitis, 423–425, *424*, 424t
  of skin, 898
Coxiella burnetii infection, in Q fever, 622–623
Coxofemoral joint, luxation of, 876–877
Crackles, respiratory, auscultation of, 675
  in pneumonia, 642
Cranial cruciate ligament, trauma to, 875
Cranial nerves, disorders of, ocular signs of, 854t, 855
  in opthalmic examination, 830–831, 851–854
Creatine kinase, in downer cow syndrome, 322
Creatinine, blood level of, 920t
  clearance of, in estimation of drug excretion, 24
Creosote, toxicity of, 410
Cresols, toxicity of, 409–411
Creutzfeldt-Jakob disease, 454
Crooked calf syndrome, lupine and, 346, 360
Crotalaria species, toxicity of, 347, 350t, 351t
Crotalid bites, 411–412
  antivenin for, 412, 931t
Crotoxyphos, for mange, chorioptic, 885
Cruciate ligament, cranial, trauma to, 875
Crush syndrome, in downer cow, 322
Crutching, before lambing, 156
Cryosurgery, for papillomavirus, 431
  for squamous cell carcinoma, ocular, 849
Cryptococcosis, 525, 527
Cryptorchidism, 96, 795
Cryptosporidiosis, 612–613
  and diarrhea, in neonatal ruminants, 107–108
Crysticillin. See *Penicillin*.
Culicoides species, as bluetongue vectors, in cattle, 435–437
  in sheep, 465–467
Culling, of cattle herd, and dairy production, 146
  chuteside, 125

Culling (Continued)
  of sheep herd, 154–155
Cuprimine (D-penicillamine), dosage of, 932t
  for copper toxicosis, 398
Cuprate, for hemoglobinuria, postparturient, 325, 325t
Cuprax, for hemoglobinuria, postparturient, 325, 325t
Curatrem (clorsulon), for fluke infestation, 50, 757, 757t
  for nematode infestation, 748t
  in anthelmintic therapy, in llamas, 176, 176t
Curly coat, 907, 911
Curly dock, toxicity of, to kidney, 824t
Cutter Gold, for parasitosis, 55t
Cyanide, in arrowgrass, 344, 347
  in plants, 367–368
  in prepared feeds, toxicity of, 344
  in rodenticides, toxicity of, 385t, 386
  in sorghum, after herbicide application, 393
Cyanocobalamin (vitamin B_{12}), for anemia, 701
  nutritional requirement for, in pigs, 280t, 282
    in pregnancy and lactation, 215, 216
Cyanosis, with erythema, 914
Cycas species, toxicity of, 357
Cyclo-oxygenase inhibitors (NSAIDs), 8, 9t, 9–10. See also *Acetylsalicylic acid (aspirin)*.
  nephrotoxicity of, 819
Cyclophosphamide, for lymphosarcoma, 850
Cyfluthrin, for parasitosis, 55t
λ-Cyhalothrin, for parasitosis, 55t
Cymopterus species, skin reactions to, 362–363
Cypermethrin, for parasitosis, 55t
Cysticercosis, 758
Cystitis, *Corynebacterium renale* and, 539
  Eubacterium suis and, 519–521
  in pigs, 817t, 827–828
Cystorelin. See *Gonadotropin-releasing hormone*.
Cysts, cutaneous, 910, 918
  ovarian, in cattle, 774–775
Cytoecles species. See *Ehrlichiosis*.
Cytokines, in immunotherapy, 16
  metabolic effects of, 18–19
Cytomegalovirus infection, 481–482

Daft lamb disease, 93
Dairi-Clox (cloxacillin), dosage of, 931t
  for keratoconjunctivitis, 835–836
Daji, 628–632, 629t, *629–631*, 632t
Dalapon, toxicity of, 387, 388t
Dallis grass, in *Claviceps* toxicity, cerebellar, 860
Damalinia lice, skin infestation by, 887
Dandy-Walker syndrome, 92
Danofloxacin, for *Actinobacillus pleuropneumonia*, 550t
Dantrolene, in prevention of malignant hyperthermia, 74, 75
Daphne species, toxicity of, 350t
Datura species, toxicity of, 350t, 351t
DDT, in water supply, 376t
  toxicity of, 381

Death camas, toxicity of, 346, 351t
Death cap mushroom, toxicity of, 355, 356
Decoquinate (Deccox), for coccidiosis, 602, 603t
  as feed additive, 186
  in goats, 165
  in llamas, 176, 176t
  preventive use of, in sheep, 156
  in stocker calves, 131
Degenerative joint disease, of stifle, 876
Dehorning, encephalomalacia after, 861
  in feeder calves, 180
  sinusitis after, 639
Dehydration, in calves, 2t, 2–6, 5t
Delphinium species, toxicity of, 346, 350t
  after herbicide application, 393
Demodex mites, skin infestation by, 885–886
Deoxynivalenol, toxicity of, 332–334
Depigmentation, 913, 914
Depo-Medrol, dosage of, 930t
Dermatitis, caprine viral, 900
  contact, 903
  digital, 868–869
  exfoliative, in pygmy goats, 913
  in feedlot cattle, 140
  interdigital, 868
  plant toxicity and, 362–364
  pustular, psoriasiform, 909–910
  viral, 898–899
  ultraviolet light and, 904–906, 905t
  verrucose, 867
  with fever and hemorrhage, 906
Dermatophilosis, 522–524, 894–895
Dermatophytosis, 890–892, 891t, 892t
Dermatosis erythematosa, 915
Dermatosis vegetans, 909
Dermoids, ocular, 93
Dexamethasone, dosage of, 930t
  for acetonemia, 311, 311t
  for anaphylaxis, 684
  for *Haemophilus somnus* infection, 548
  for hemoglobinuria, postparturient, 325, 325t
  for inflammation, 9t, 10–11, 11t
  for insect bites, 413
  for laminitis, aseptic, 868
  for rhinitis, allergic, 638
  for shock, 7, 7t, 683
  for toxemia of pregnancy, 313, 313t
  for urticaria, 901
  in induction of abortion, 792, 792t
  in induction of parturition, in cattle, 811, 811t
    in goats, 805, 811t, 814
    in sheep, 805, 811t, 813
Dextran 70, for shock, 683
Dextrose, and ruminal motility, 707
  in rehydration, 4, 5t
Diacetoxyscirpenol, toxicity of, 332, 333
N,N-Diallyl-2-chloroacetamide, in herbicides, toxicity of, 387, 388t
Diamidine derivatives, for babesiosis, 587t
Diampron, for babesiosis, 587t
Diaphragm, hernia of, respiratory signs of, 668t
  in anesthesia, 58
Diarrhea, adenovirus infection and, 483–484
  astrovirus infection and, 474
  bacterial, antibiotics for, as feed additives, 186, 187t
  bovine Breda virus and, 452
  bovine viral, 432–434

Diarrhea *(Continued)*
   and cerebellar degeneration, 858
   and congenital defects, 90, 93
   and ocular disease, 838
   and pneumonia, 653–654, 660–663
   and skin lesions, 899
   serologic test for, 677
  coronavirus infection and, 106, 440
  epidemic, viral, 500–501
  Escherichia coli infection and, 517, 518
  in cryptosporidiosis, 612, 613
  in dairy replacement calves, 149t, 149–150
  in dysentery, 560–562, 561t
  in enterotoxemia, clostridial, 573, 574
  in feedlot cattle, 140
  in lamb, newborn, 157
  in neonatal ruminants, 103–109
  in paratuberculosis, 533, 534
  in piglet, 111–115
  in rotavirus infection, in cattle, 439
    in neonatal ruminants, 104–105
    in piglets, 112–114
    in pigs, 497–498
    in sheep, 467
  in salmonellosis, 563
  transmissible gastroenteritis virus and, 499
Diazepam, dosage of, 930t
  preanesthetic, 61t
Diazinon, for mange, psorergatic, 885
  for parasitosis, external, 55t
  for trombiculidiasis, 886
  toxicity of, 382t
Dicamba, toxicity of, 387, 388t
Dicentra species, toxicity of, 350t
Dichlobenil, toxicity of, 388t, 391
Dichlorodiphenyl trichloroethane (DDT), in water supply, 376t
  toxicity of, 381
Dichlorvos, for nematode infestations, 754, 754t
  for parasitosis, external, 53t
  in anthelmintic therapy, 50
Diclazuril, for coccidiosis, 602, 603t
Dicrocoelium dendriticum infestation, 755–757
Dictyocauliasis, 47–50, 673–674
Dicumarol, in sweet clover poisoning, 359
Dieldrin, in water supply, 376t
  toxicity of, 381
Diet. See also *Feed.*
  and urolithiasis, 819, 820
  as aid to management, of abomasal displacement, 725
  of *Eubacterium suis* infection, 521
  deficiencies of, and infertility, 783–784
  disorders of, and myodegeneration, 689–690
   and skin lesions, 911–912
  energy requirement in. See *Energy.*
  for calves, in stocker herd, 131, 132t
   in stress, 178–180, 179t
  for cattle, 250t, 250–252, 252t
   beef, 122, 122t, 123t, 127–128, 128t
    in breeding herd, 253t–256t, 253–260, 258t–260t
    in pregnancy and lactation, 204–210, 206t, 208t
   dairy, 260–272
    and milk production, 144, 144t
    in pregnancy and lactation, 210–214, 213t, 214t

Diet *(Continued)*
   in replacement rearing, 149, 149t–151t, *150, 151*
  for goats, 272–278, 274t, 275t
  for lambs, 156–157
  for llamas, 174–175, 175t
  for pigs, 170, 171, 278–285, 280t, 282t
   in pregnancy and lactation, 214–216
  for sheep, in pregnancy and lactation, 156, 216–221, 220
  grain in, and lactic acidosis, 714
  in prevention of acetonemia, 309, 311–312
  mineral requirements in, 200–203, 202t
  protein requirement in. See *Protein.*
  ration formulation in, 200–203, 201t, 202t
Diethylcarbamazine, for elaephoriasis, 841
Diethylstilbestrol, as growth stimulant, 181
  dosage of, 930t
  for abortion induction, 792
Diflubenzuron, for parasitosis, 56t
Digestive tract. See *Gastrointestinal tract.*
Digital dermatitis, 868–869
Digital nerves, anesthetic block of, 85, *85*
Digitalis, toxicity of, 350t, 353
Digitoxin, for arrhythmia, 702t, 703
  for heart failure, congestive, 684
Digoxin, dosage of, 930t
  for arrhythmia, 702t, 703
  for heart failure, congestive, 684
  with quinidine, for atrial fibrillation, 689
Dihydrostreptomycin, for campylobacteriosis, 512
  for dermatophilosis, 523
Dihydrotestosterone undecyclenate, for acetonemia, 311t
  for toxemia of pregnancy, 313, 313t, 315
Dimercaprol, dosage of, 930t
Dimethyl sulfoxide, as diuretic, 818
  for inflammation, 9t, 12
Dimethylarsinic acid, toxicity of, 388t, 391
Dimetridazole, for dermatitis, digital, 869
  for dysentery, in pigs, 561t
  for enteropathy, proliferative, in campylobacteriosis, 514
  for trichomoniasis, 785
Diminazene, for babesiosis, 587, 587t
  for trypanosomiasis, 606, 607, 607t
Dimple, 900
Dinitroanilines, in herbicides, toxicity of, 388t, 391
Dinitrocresol, toxicity of, 410
Dinitrophenol, toxicity of, 410
Dinoprost tromethamine, for pyometra, 773
  in induction of abortion, 811t, 814
  in induction of parturition, in pigs, 811t, 815
Dinoseb, toxicity of, 389t, 391
Diphenamid, toxicity of, 387, 388t
Diphenhydramine, for anaphylaxis, 684
  for inflammation, 9t
Diphenoxylate, and gastrointestinal motility, 759t, 760
Diphtheria, in feedlot cattle, 138
Diprenorphine, in capture of ruminants, 63
Dipyrone, 9t, 10
  dosage of, 930t
Diquat, toxicity of, 387, 388t
Diquel, dosage of, 930t
  preanesthetic, 61t

Disseminated intravascular coagulation, in shock, 683
Diureidoisobutane, toxicity of, 906
Diuretics, for urinary tract disorders, 818
  in respiratory therapy, 679t, 680
Diuril (chlorothiazide), dosage of, 930t
  for intertrigo, 902
Diuron, toxicity of, 390t
DN 599, serologic test for, 677
Dobutamine, for heart failure, 704
Dock plant (*Rumex* species), toxicity of, 351t, 364
  to kidney, 824t
Docking, of lambs, 157
Docusate, and gastrointestinal motility, 759t
Does. See *Goats.*
Dogbane, toxicity of, 350t, 352, 353
Domoso (dimethyl sulfoxide), as diuretic, 818
  for inflammation, 9t, 12
Dopamine, as diuretic, in urinary disorders, 818
  for heart failure, 704
Doppellender, 93
Dopram (doxapram), as antagonist to xylazine sedation, 62
  dosage of, 930t
  for hypoxia, 679t, 680
Dorset sheep, globoid cell leukodystrophy in, 93
Downer cow syndrome, 321–323
  milk fever in, 306
  on feedlot, 140
Doxapram, as antagonist to xylazine sedation, 62
  dosage of, 930t
  for hypoxia, 679t, 680
Doximplant, for heartwater, 632t
Doxycycline, for anaplasmosis, 592, 593
  for heartwater, 631
Doxymycin, for heartwater, *632*
Drechslera rostrata, skin infection by, 892, 893
Droncit, in anthelmintic therapy, in llamas, 176t
Droperidol, preanesthetic, 61t
Drugs. See also specific agents, e.g., *Phenylbutazone*, and classes, e.g., *Steroids.*
  adverse reactions to, 20–25, 22t–24t
  approximate dosages of, 930–933
  and skin eruptions, 901
  biologic half-life of, 41, *41*
  companies marketing, 921–925
   addresses of, 926–929
  residues of, after anesthesia, 58
   in meat and milk, 29–42
    agencies regulating, 30–32, 37
    extra-label use and, 33
    laboratory tests for, 31–33, 32t
    new drug development and, 40, *40–41, 41*
    pharmacokinetics in, 42
    prevention programs for, 36–37
    risk assessment in, 42
    therapies associated with, 39–40
    withdrawal times and, 33t, 33–34
Dry-Clox (cloxacillin), dosage of, 930t
  for keratoconjunctivitis, 835–836
Dry cow, management of, 146, 148, 261, 262t
Drylot, in stocker calf management, 130
Dura mater, anatomy of, 77, *78*

Dursban (chlorpyrifos), for parasitosis,
    external, 52, 52t
  for trombiculidiasis, 886
  toxicity of, 381, 382t
Dutchman's breeches, toxicity of, 350t
Dwarfism, 94
Dyfonate, toxicity of, 382t
Dysentery, 560–562, 561t
Dyspnea, differential diagnosis of, 667,
    668t

Ear, catheterization of, in rehydration, 6,
    7
  necrosis of, 903
Ear Force (permethrin), for lice, in goats,
    165
  for parasitosis, 54t–57t
Ear tags, for parasitosis, 55t
Eating disorders, in feedlot cattle, 140
Echocardiography, 27, 27t, 686
Ecthyma, contagious, 460–461, 461
  vaccination against, 164
Ectiban (permethrin), for lice, in goats,
    165
  for parasitosis, external, 54t–57t
Ectopia cordis, 96
Ectrin (fenvalerate), for lice, in goats, 165
  for mange, chorioptic, 885
  for parasitosis, 55t, 57t
Ectropion, 840
Edema, circulatory causes of, 682
  in mastitis, 768
  lymphatic, congenital, 910
  malignant, clostridial infection and, 570,
    897
  neuraxial, 92
    treatment of, 11, 12
  pulmonary, 643–647, 644, 645
    pathology of, 636–637
  with lactation failure, 769
Edinger-Westphal nucleus, in pupillary
    light reflex, 830–831
Ehrlichiosis, in cattle, 616–617, 617t
  and petechial fever, 618–620, 619,
    619t
  in pigs, 618
  in sheep, 617–618
  in tick-borne fever, 620, 620–621
Eimeria infestation. See Coccidiosis.
Elaephoriasis, ocular, in sheep, 841
Elderberry, toxicity of, 351t
Electrical power plants, cooling waters
    from, toxicants in, 377–378
Electrocardiography, 685
  of atrial fibrillation, 689
Electrolytes, balance of, 1
  for shock, 682–683
  in abomasal displacement, 724, 728–729
  replacement therapy with, in calves, 2–
    5, 5t
  with fluid therapy, in anesthesia, 75
  in diarrhea, in neonatal ruminant, 104
Electrosulf-3, dosage of, 931t
Elephant skin disease, 596–598, 597, 598,
    900
Eltradd IV-4000, dosage of, 931t
Emblax powder, dosage of, 931t
Embolism, pulmonary, with vena caval
    thrombosis, 648
  with meningoencephalitis, in Haemophilus somnus infection, 546–549, 547
  in pneumonia, 662, 664

Embolism (Continued)
  ocular signs of, 838, 854, 854t, 856
Embryo, transfer of, in infectious disease
    control, 785–787, 786
Emphysema, of lung, pathology of, 636,
    637
  with edema, 643–647, 644, 645
  subcutaneous, 902
  with gangrene, 569–570
Encephalitis, adenoviral, 484
  in Haemophilus somnus infection, 546–
    549, 547
  in listeriosis, 580–583, 581, 583t
  Japanese, 496–497
  viral, with arthritis, in goats, 167, 472–
    474, 862–863
  with meningitis, thromboembolic, in
    pneumonia, 662, 664
  ocular signs of, 838, 854, 854t, 856
  with myelitis, chlamydial infection and,
    456–457
  enteroviral, 490–491
  in paramyxovirus infection, 503
  with vomiting and wasting, 492–493
Encephalocele, 92
Encephalomalacia, after dehorning, 861
  with polio, cerebellar, 859–860
  in lamb, 157
Encephalomyocarditis, viral, 493–494
Encephalopathy, spongiform, 454–455,
    860
  with hepatic insufficiency, 356
Endocarditis, bacterial, 687–688
  treatment of, 701–702
Endometritis, 770–772
  and infertility, 784, 785
  in chlamydiosis, 456
Endophytic fungus, in fescue, 209
  toxicity of, to feet, 870–871
Endothal, toxicity of, 390t, 392
Endotoxemia, and shock, 7, 7t
  in lactation failure, 768–769
  in mastitis, 763–764
Endotracheal intubation, for anesthesia,
    70–72, 71, 71t, 73, 74
Endrin, in water supply, 376t
Energy, intake of, and milk production,
    43, 43–45
  metabolism of, in stress, 17–18
  nutritional requirement for, 189–191,
    190, 200–203, 201t, 202t
  in cattle, 191t, 191–194, 193t, 250,
    250t
    beef, 122, 123t
      for weight gain, 245
      in breeding herd, 253t–256t, 254,
        255, 258t, 258–259, 259t
      in pregnancy and lactation, 205–
        209, 206t
    dairy, 194, 261–264, 262t, 263, 264,
        264t, 265t, 270t, 271t
      in pregnancy and lactation, 210,
        212–213, 213t, 214t
  in goats, 273–278, 274t, 275t
  in pigs, 195–196
    in pregnancy and lactation, 214–216
  in sheep, 194–195
    in pregnancy and lactation, 217,
        219, 220t, 221
  supplementation with, for grazing cattle, 292
English ivy, toxicity of, 350t
Engorgement toxemia, 714–716, 715
Enguruti, 628–632, 629t, 629–631, 632t

Enrofloxacin, for Actinobacillus
    pleuropneumonia, 550t
Enteritis, in campylobacteriosis, 508–510
Enteropathy, proliferative, in
    campylobacteriosis, 513–515
Enterotoxemia, and diarrhea, in neonatal
    ruminants, 106–107
  clostridial, 573–575
  in feedlot cattle, 140
  in feedlot sheep, 161t, 162, 162
  in lambs, 158
  vaccination against, in goats, 164
  in llamas, 174
Enterovirus infection, and
    encephalomyelitis, 490–491
  and reproductive failure, 493
Entropion, 839–840
Envenomation, 411t, 411–413, 412t, 906
  antivenin for, 412, 931t
Environmental Protection Agency, in
    regulation of residues in food
    animals, 30, 37
Enzyme-linked immunosorbent assay, for
    Escherichia coli infection, 104
  for rotavirus infection, 104
Eosinophils, blood level of, elevated, with
    folliculitis, sterile, 915
  measurement of, 692t, 919t, 920t
Eperythrozoonosis, in llamas, 176, 176t
  in pigs, 614–616
  in sheep, 613–614
Ephemeral fever, 449–450
  skin lesions in, 900
Epicauta species, toxicity of, 413
  to kidney, 823t
Epichloe typhina, in fescue toxicity, 370, 870
Epidemic diarrhea virus, in pigs, 500–501
Epidermitis, exudative, staphylococcal,
    578–579, 895–896
Epidermolysis bullosa, 909
Epididymis, aplasia of, 794–795
  inflammation of, 796
  in brucellosis, 552, 552
Epidural space, anatomy of, 77, 78
  injection into, for analgesia, 80–83, 81,
    82
Epinephrine, dosage of, 931t
  effect of, on leukocytes, 697
  for anaphylaxis, 684
  for epistaxis, 639
  for rhinitis, allergic, 638
  for shock, after insect bites, 113
  in regional analgesia, 79
  in respiratory therapy, 679t, 680
  in stress response, 17
Epistaxis, 638–639
Epitheliogenesis imperfecta, 909
Epithelioma, ocular, 847t, 847–850, 850t
Epithelium, tumors of, 916t, 916–917
Epostane, in abortion induction, 793
Equine herpesvirus I, in ocular disease, in
    camelids, 845–846
Ergocalciferol. See Vitamin D.
Ergonovine maleate, dosage of, 931t
Ergotism, 334–336, 351t
  in cerebellar disease, 860
  in fescue toxicosis, 370, 906
  skin lesions in, 906
Eructation, physiology of, 707
Erysipelas, 579–580, 897–898
Erythema, with cyanosis, 914
  with dermatosis, 915
Erythrocytes, decreased level of, 693, 693–
    696, 694t–696t

Erythrocytes *(Continued)*
　elevated level of, 695–696
　laboratory count of, 690–692, 692t, 919t, 920t
　production of, 692–693
Erythroderma, exfoliative, 901
Erythromycin, dosage of, 931t
　for mastitis, 767t
　for omphalitis, 102t
Escherichia coli infection, 517t, 517–519
　and diarrhea, in neonatal ruminant, 103, 105–106, 109
　　in piglet, 111–115
　and polyarthritis, in piglet, 116
　and pyelonephritis, 826
　in lambs, newborn, 156, 157
　in omphalitis, 101, 102, 102t
　of urinary tract, 817
Esophageal groove, closure of, 708–709
Esophagus, inflammation of, in papular stomatitis, 426, *426*
　obstruction of, 712–713
Estradiocyclopropionate, dosage of, 931t
Estradiol, as growth stimulant, 181t–184t, 181–183
　for abortion induction, 792
Estradiol benzoate, for estrus synchronization, in pigs, 776
　in induction of parturition, in sheep, 813
Estradiol valerate, with norgestomet (Syncro-Mate B), in estrus management. See *Norgestomet*.
Estrogens, as growth stimulants, 181t–184t, 181–183
　excess of, and conception failure, 783
　in milk fever, 305
Estrumate. See *Cloprostenol*.
Estrus, in cattle, detection of, for artificial insemination, 779–780
　　in dairy cow, 798t, 798–799
　　management of, 778–779, 809–810, 810t, 811t
　　　melengestrol acetate for, as feed additive, 186–187
　in goats, 804–805
　　management of, 165, 166, 777–778, 811t, 813–814
　in pigs, management of, 776–777, 811t, 814
　in sheep, 804
　　management of, 158–159, 777–778, 812–813
Ethidium, for trypanosomiasis, 606, 607t
Ethoprop, toxicity of, 382t
Ethyl dipropylthiocarbamate, toxicity of, 389t, 391
Ethylenediamine dihydroiodide, for phlegmon, interdigital, 870
Ethylenediaminetetraacetate, dosage of, 931t
　in blood count, 691
Ethylisobutrazine (Diquel), dosage of, 931t
　preanesthetic, 61t
Etorphine, in capture of ruminants, 63
Eubacterium suis infection, 519–521
　and pyelonephritis, 828
Euflavine, for babesiosis, 587t
Eupatorium rugosum, toxicity of, 349, 350t
Euphorbia species, toxicity of, 350t
Ewe. See *Sheep*.
Exanthema, vesicular, 488–489, 899
Excenel. See *Ceftiofur*.

Exfoliative dermatitis, in pygmy goats, 913
Exfoliative erythroderma, 901
Exophthalmos, differential diagnosis of, 847t
　leukosis and, 838
Expar (permethrin), for lice, in goats, 165
　for parasitosis, external, 54t–57t
Eye(s), analgesia of, 87–88, *88*
　anatomy of, in camelids, 842t, 842–843, *843*
　　nerves in, 851–853, *853*
　cleaning of, 833
　congenital defects of, 93
　　in sheep and goats, 839–840
　disorders of, in camelids, 844–846
　　neurologic, 854t, 854–856
　examination of, 829–834, 830t, 853–854
　　in camelids, 833, 834, *843*, 843–844
　in catarrhal fever, malignant, 421, *422*, 838
　in paramyxovirus infection, 502–504
　infectious diseases of, in cattle, 834–838
　　in sheep and goats, 840–841
　neoplasia of, 846–851, 847t, 850t
　parasitic diseases of, in cattle, 838–839
　　in sheep and goats, 841–842
　rotation of, anesthesia and, 74, *75*
　subconjunctival injection of, 834
　topical medication for, 833–834
Eyelid(s), analgesia of, 86–87, *87*
　eversion of, 840
　examination of, 831, 832
　inversion of, 839–840

Face, masses in, differential diagnosis of, 847t
Facial nerve, anatomy of, 852
　in palpebral reflex, 830
Factrel. See *Gonadotropin-releasing hormone*.
Fagopyrism, 362
False hellebore (*Veratrum* species), as teratogen, 361, 839
　toxicity of, to heart, 353
　　to nervous system, 358
Famphur, for parasitosis, external, 53t
Farcy, 521
Farrowing, 170, 171
　dermatosis with, 913
　induction of, 815
　nutrition in, 216
Fascioliasis, 755–757, 757t
　black disease with, 572, 573
　clorsulon for, 50, 757, 757t
Fat, on back, ultrasonography of, 27t, 29
Fat cow syndrome, 315–317, 316t, 317t
　diet for, 261–262, 262t, *263*
　milk fever in, 306
Fatty acids, deficiency of, and skin lesions, 911
　dietary, for pigs, 280t, 282
　volatile, in reticuloruminal motility, 707
Feces, coliform bacteria of, in water supply, 375
　nematode egg count in, 747–748, 750
　nitrogen loss in, 225, 228
　testing of, for viral infection, 415, 416t
Feed. See also *Diet*.
　additive(s) to, antibiotics as, 184–186, 185t–187t
　　buffers as, 187
　　for estrus control, 186–187

Feed *(Continued)*
　for pigs, 282–283
　for stress, 187–188
　probiotics as, 176
　sarsaponin as, 187
　yeasts as, 187
　heat-damaged, 341–343
　hypersensitivity to, 901
　mold-damaged, 341–343
　protein in, measurement of, 224–225, 233–234
　　Cornell system for, 240–244, *241*, *242*, 243t
　　Iowa State system for, 234–236, *235*, 235t–237t
　　Wisconsin system for, 236–240, *238*, 240t, 241t
　toxicity of, ammonia in, 327
　　gossypol in, 331–332
　　ionophores in, 329–331
　　plants in, 343–345, 344t
　　sodium ions in, 328–329
Feedlot, calves on, nutrition in, 178–180, 179t
　cattle on, management of, 135–142, *136–139*, 140t, *141*
　　pneumonia in, control of, 660–662
　sheep on, management of, 159t–161t, 159–162, *161*, *162*
Feet. See *Foot*.
Femoral nerve, paralysis of, 875
Femoropatellar ligament, medial, trauma to, 874–875
Femur, articulation of, with coccyx, luxation of, 876–877
　with tibia, trauma to, 874–876
　fracture of, 879
Fenac, toxicity of, 390t, 392
Fenbendazole, dosage of, 931t
　for bronchitis, parasitic, 678, 679, 679t
　for cestode infestation, 758
　for nematode infestation, cerebrospinal, 863
　　in cattle, 748, 748t
　　in pigs, 754, 754t
　for thelaziasis, ocular, 839
　in anthelmintic therapy, 49
　in llamas, 176, 176t
Fenoprop, toxicity of, 391t
Fenprostalene, for estrus synchronization, in cattle, 779
　in induction of abortion, 792t
　in induction of parturition, 815
Fentanyl citrate (Innovar-Vet), dosage of, 931t
　preanesthetic, 61t
Fenthion, dosage of, 931t
　for lice, in llamas, 177
　for parasitosis, external, 52, 53t, 57t
Fenuron, toxicity of, 390t, 392
Fenvalerate, for lice, in goats, 165
　for mange, chorioptic, 885
　for parasitosis, 55t–57t
Fertility. See also *Infertility*.
　in cattle, beef, 800–803, *801–803*
　　dairy, 799t, 799–800, 800t
Fertilization, failure of, 781–785
Fescue, endophytic fungus in, 209
　toxicity of, 370–371
　　and skin lesions, 906
　　to foot, 870–871
Fetal membranes, retained, 769–772
Fetterbush, toxicity of, 350t

Fetus, examination of, after abortion, 789–791
  in pigs, 807
  harlequin, 907
Fiber, dietary, for dairy cattle, in pregnancy and lactation, 210, 213, 213t
  for pigs, and reduced intake, 196
Fibrillation, atrial, 689, 702
Fibrin degradation products, measurement of, 691, 692t
Fibrinogen, in inflammation, 697
  measurement of, 690, 691, 692t
Fibroma, interdigital, 871–872
Fibropapillomas, viral infection and, 431
Fiddleneck (*Amsinckia*), toxicity of, 344, 347
Finajet. See *Trenbolone*.
Finaplix. See *Trenbolone*.
Fire ants, stings of, 412t, 412–413
Fireweed (*Amsinckia*), toxicity of, 344, 347
Fistulas, penile, 796–797
Flavivirus infection, and encephalitis, 496–497
Fleece, hairy, in border disease, 463
Fleece rot, 904
Fleeceworms, external parasiticides for, 53t, 56t
Flies, as vectors, of anaplasmosis, 588, 593–595
  of keratoconjunctivitis, 835, 836
  bites of, and mastitis, 764
  external parasiticides for, 51–58, 52t–57t
Flo-Cillin. See *Penicillin*.
Flucort. See *Flumethasone (Flucort)*.
Flucytosine, for fungal infection, 529
Fluid. See *Water*.
Fluke infestations, 755–757, 757t
  drugs for, 47, 50
Flumethasone (Flucort), dosage of, 932t
  for acetonemia, 311t
  for inflammation, 11, 11t
  in induction of parturition, 811
  in respiratory therapy, 678, 679t, 680
Flunixin meglumine, 9t, 10
  before surgery, for cecocolic volvulus, 740
  for endotoxemia, with lactation failure, 768
  for laminitis, aseptic, 868
  for mastitis, 767–768
  for pulmonary edema, 646
  for shock, 7, 7t
  for urticaria, 901
Fluometuron, toxicity of, 390t, 392
Fluorescent antibody testing, for viral infection, 414, 416t
Fluoride, in water, 376, 376t
  geothermal, 379, *379*
  nutritional requirement for, 268
  toxicity of, 398–402, 399t, *400*, *401*
  in sheep, 219
Fluoroacetate, in rodenticides, toxicity of, 385t, 386
5-Fluorocytosine, for fungal infection, 529
Fluorogesterone, in estrus management, in goats, 777
  in sheep, 777, 813
Flushing, of ewes, 221
Focal cutaneous hypoplasia, 909
Fog fever, 643–647, *644*, *645*
Folacin, nutritional requirement for, 280t, 282

Follicle-stimulating hormone, dosage of, 932t
Follicles, cysts of, 918
  dysplasia of, 914
  inflammation of, eosinophilic, sterile, 915
  staphylococcal, 896
Follicular cysts, ovarian, 774–775
Fonofos, toxicity of, 382t
Food and Drug Administration, in regulation of residues in food animals, 30–31, 37
Food Safety and Inspection Service, in regulation of residues in food animals, 31, 31t, 37
Foot, abscess of, on sole, 864–865
  analgesia of, *85*, 85–86, *86*
  dermatitis of, 868–869
    infectious, in feedlot cattle, 140
  examination of, 864
  fescue toxicity in, 370, 371, 870–871
  fibroma of, interdigital, 871–872
  in selenium toxicity, 366, *367*
  phlegmon of, 869–870
  ulcer of, Rusterholz, 866–867
  wall cracks of, horizontal, 865–866
    vertical, 865
Foot rot, chlortetracycline for, as feed additive, 187t
  in sheep, 872–873
  strawberry, 522
Foot-and-mouth disease, 437–439, *438*
  in goats, 464
  in pigs, *494*, 494–495, *495*
  in sheep, 464, *464*
  skin lesions in, 899
Forage. See *Pasture* and *Rangeland*.
Foramen rotundum orbitale, in eyelid analgesia, 87, *87*
Foreign bodies, ingestion of, and reticuloperitonitis, 719–722, 735
Forestomach. See also *Omasum* and *Rumen*.
  function of, assessment of, 709–710
  indigestion in, 710–711
  innervation of, 706, 706t
  lactic acidosis in, 714–716, *715*
  motility of, 706–709, *707*
Formalin, for nocardiosis, 522
Foxglove, toxicity of, 350t, 353
Fractures, 878–880
Freemartinism, 97
Frenulum, persistent, 796
Friction rub, pleural, auscultation of, 675–676
Frostbite, 902–903
FSH-P, dosage of, 931t
Fundus, gastric, ulceration of, 735–736
  ocular, anatomy of, in llamas, 843, *843*
  examination of, 831–832
Fungicidin, dosage of, 931t
Fungizone (amphotericin B), for fungal infection, 529
  in embryo transfer, 786–787
Fungus (fungi), endophytic, in fescue, 209, 370, 371
  toxicity of, to feet, 870–871
  feed damage by, 341–343
  infection with, and abortion, 525–526
    and mastitis, 526–527
    drugs for, 529
    etiology of, 524–525
    nasal, 528–529
    ocular, in camelids, 845, 846

Fungus (fungi) (*Continued*)
  of skin, 890–894, 891t, 892t
  toxins of. See *Mycotoxin(s)*.
Furacin (nitrofurazone), dosage of, 931t, 933t
  for coccidiosis, 602, 603t
Furadan, toxicity of, 382t
Furaltadone, dosage of, 931t
Furosemide, dosage of, 931t
  for cholecalciferol toxicity, 385
  for edema, in mastitis, 768
    with lactation failure, 769
  for heart failure, 703
  for intertrigo, 902
  for urinary tract disorders, 818
  in respiratory therapy, 679t, 680
Furunculosis, staphylococcal, 896
Fusarium species, toxins of, 332, 333
Fusobacterium necrophorum infection, in dermatitis, of foot, 868, 869
  verrucose, 867
  in foot rot, in sheep, 872, 873

Gallbladder, in African swine fever, 487
  ultrasonography of, 27t, 28
Galleta grass, in *Claviceps* toxicity, cerebellar, 860
Gallimycin, dosage of, 931t
Gallop rhythm, 681
Gallotannins, in oak toxicity, 372–374, 822–824
Gamma globulin, deficiency of, 13
Gamma glutamyl transpeptidase, blood level of, 920t
Ganasag (diminazene), for babesiosis, 587, 587t
  for trypanosomiasis, 606, 607, 607t
Gangliosidosis, 92
  cerebellum in, 860
Gangrene, 902
  clostridial infection and, 897
  emphysematous, 569–570
  in ergotism, 334–336
Gantrisin, dosage of, 933t
Gard Star Plus (permethrin), for lice, in goats, 165
  for parasitosis, 54t–57t
Gasoline, toxicity of, 407–409
Gastrocnemius tendon, rupture of, 880
Gastroenteritis, transmissible, 498–500
  in piglet, 112–115
Gastrointestinal tract. See also specific structures, e.g., *Rumen*.
  congenital defects of, 96
  disorders of, in feedlot cattle, 140, 140t
  in arsenic toxicity, 394–395
  in oak toxicity, 824–825
  infection of, adenoviruses in, 430
    candidal, 528
    in African swine fever, 487
    transmissible gastroenteritis virus in, 498–500
      in piglet, 112–115
    viral, diagnosis of, 416t
    zygomycotic, 528
  innervation of, 706, 706t
  lumen of, drugs active in, 761
  motility of, 706–709, *707*
    drugs affecting, 759t, 759–760
  parasitosis of, cestode, 757–758
    nematode, in cattle, 743–748, 746t–748t

Gastrointestinal tract *(Continued)*
  in goats, 752
  in pigs, 752–754, 754t
  in sheep, 748–752
  trematode, 755–757, 757t
 pH in, and drug absorption, 21
 secretion in, drugs affecting, 760t, 760–761
 ultrasonography of, 28
Gazelle, Thomson's, petechial fever in, 619
Gecolate, dosage of, 931t
Gelsemium sempervirens, toxicity of, 350t
Genitalia. See also specific structures, e.g., *Uterus*.
 abnormalities of, and female infertility, 781–785
 campylobacteriosis of, 510–513
 congenital defects of, 96–97
 fungal infection of, and abortion, 525–526
 infection of, in bovine rhinotracheitis, 418
  viral, diagnosis of, 416t
 male, disorders of, internal, 793–794
  scrotal, 794–796
  posthitis of, in *Corynebacterium renale* infection, 540–541
 mycoplasmosis of, in cattle, 458
  in sheep and goats, 479
 trichomoniasis of, in cattle, 608–611, *609*
 tuberculosis of, 532
 ultrasonography of, 27t, 28–29
Gentamicin, for *Actinobacillus* pleuropneumonia, in pigs, 550t
 for dysentery, 561t
 for keratoconjunctivitis, 835–836
 for omphalitis, 102t
 residues of, 32t, 35–36
Geothermal water, toxicants in, 377–380, *378, 379*
Giant cell pneumonia, in dermatosis vegetans, 909
Giant rain lily, and photosensitization, 363
Giardiasis, and diarrhea, 109
Gilts. See also *Pig(s)*.
 development of, in herd management, 169–171
 estrus synchronization in, 776–777
 nutrition of, in pregnancy and lactation, 214–216, 284
Glasser's disease, 506–507
Glauber's salt (sodium sulfate), and gastrointestinal motility, 759t, 760
 dosage of, 933t
 for oak toxicity, 374
Globidiosis (besnoitiosis), 596–598, *597, 598*, 900
Globoid cell leukodystrophy, 93
Gloxazone, for anaplasmosis, 592, 593t
Glucagon, dosage of, 931t
 for shock, 683
Glucocorticoids. See *Steroids*.
Gluconeogenesis, 92
 in acetonemia, 310, *310*
 in piglet, 119
Glucose, and ruminal motility, 707
 blood levels of, in calves, 3
  reference values for, 920t
  reduced, in acetonemia, 310, *310*
   in piglet, 119–120
   in toxemia of pregnancy, 312, 313

Glucose *(Continued)*
 dosage of, 931t
 for acetonemia, 311, 311t
 for fat cow syndrome, 317
 for toxemia of pregnancy, 313t, 313–315
 in rehydration, 3–4
 metabolism of, immune response and, 19
Glutamate pyruvate transaminase, blood level of, 920t
Glutamic-oxaloacetic transaminase, blood level of, 920t
Glutamine, in metabolism, in stress, 18
Glutathione, blood level of, 154
Glycerol, for toxemia of pregnancy, 313, 313t
Glycerol monoacetate, dosage of, 931t
Glyceryl guaiacolate, dosage of, 931t
Glycogen storage diseases, 92–93
 cerebellum in, 860
Glycosides, cardioactive, in plants, 352–354, 353t
Glyphosate, toxicity of, 390t, 392
Goatpox, *459*, 459–460, 898
Goats, abortion in, induced, 792, 792t, 811t, 813–814
 blood tests in, normal values for, 919t–921t
 disorders in. See specific disorders, e.g., *Arthritis*, and affected structures, e.g., *Eye(s)*.
 estrus in, 804–805
  synchronization of, 777–778, 811t, 813–814
 herd health management in, 162–167
 horns of, analgesia of, 84–85, *85*
 neonatal. See *Kid*.
 nutrition of, 272–278, 274t, 275t
Goiter, hereditary, 910
 in pigs, 280
 in range-fed cattle, 297
Golden chain tree, toxicity of, 351t
Goldenrod, rayless, toxicity of, 348–349
Gonadorelin. See *Gonadotropin-releasing hormone*.
Gonadotropin, human chorionic, dosage of, 931t
 for ovarian cysts, in cattle, 775
 for ovulatory disorders, 782
 in estrus management, in goat, 165
 in pigs, 776, 811t, 814
 human menopausal, in estrus stimulation, in goats, 813
 pituitary, dosage of, 931t, 932t
 pregnant mare serum and, in estrus management, in goats, 165, 777–778, 805, 813
  in pigs, 776, 811t, 814
  in sheep, 158, 777–778, 805, 813
Gonadotropin-releasing hormone, dosage of, 931t
 for ovarian cysts, 774–775
 for ovulatory disorders, 782
 in reproductive management, in cattle, 811, 811t, 812
 in pigs, 815
 in uterine infection, 770, 771
Gonadovet, dosage of, 931t
Gossypol, toxicity of, 331–332
Grain overload, and lactic acidosis, 714–716, *715*
Granulocytopathy syndrome, 13
Granuloma, in nasal infection, fungal, 528–529

Granuloma *(Continued)*
 in uveitis, infectious, 838
Grass traps, in stocker calf management, 130–131
Grazing. See *Pasture* and *Rangeland*.
Greasewood, toxicity of, 347, 364
 in sheep, 221
 to kidney, 824t
Griseofulvin, dosage of, 931t
 for dermatophytosis, 892
Groundsel *(Senecio vulgaris)*, toxicity of, 343, 344, 347, 350t, 352
Growth, decreased, in eperythrozoonosis, 614, 615
 stimulation of, 294
  copper sulfate in, 283
  for stocker calves, 132–133
  in ruminants, 180–183, 181t–184t, 188, 188t
  with castration, of calf, 122
Growth hormone, 42–46, *43, 44*, 188
 in response to estrogen, 181
Grub infestation, 888
 external parasiticides for, 51–58, 52t–54t
 ivermectin for, 48
Guaifenesin, in anesthesia, 65–66
Guanacos. See *Camelids*.
Gutierrezia species, toxicity of, and abortion, 347–348
GX118 (phosmet), for parasitosis, external, 54t, 57t
Gymnocladus dioica, toxicity of, 351t

Haematopinus infestation, 48, 887
Haemonchus infestation, 47–50
 in goats, 165
 in sheep, 749–752
Haemophilus infection, in pneumonia, 635, 641–643, 664
 with meningoencephalitis, thromboembolic, 664
 vs. uveitis, 838
Haemophilus parasuis infection, 506–507
Haemophilus somnus, bacterin of, in prevention of thromboembolic meningoencephalitis, 662
 infection with, 546–549, *547, 548*
 serologic test for, 677
Hair, congenital defects of, 95
 depigmentation of, 914
 excess of, hereditary, 907, 914
 lack of, hereditary, 907, 908t, 914
 loss of, 915
 shedding of, abnormal, 914–915
Hair follicles, cysts of, 918
 dysplasia of, 914
 inflammation of, eosinophilic, sterile, 915
 staphylococcal, 896
Hairy vetch, toxicity of, 363–364, 906
Halofuginone, for theileriosis, 628
Halogeton, toxicity of, 345–347, 364
 in sheep, 221
 to kidney, 824t
Halothane, in anesthesia, 68
Halox drench, dosage of, 931t
Halquinol, for enteropathy, proliferative, in campylobacteriosis, 514–515
Haplopappus heterophyllus, toxicity of, 348–349
Harlequin fetus, 907
Harvest mites, skin infestation by, 886

948 □ INDEX

Harvester ants, stings of, 412, 412t
Hava-Span, dosage of, 931t
  for pneumonia, 657t
Head, swelling of, clostridial infection and, 897
Heart, auscultation of, 681, 681t, 684–685
  congenital defects of, 95–96
  diseases of, diagnosis of, 684–686
  electrocardiography of, 685, 689
  imaging of, in respiratory disease, 677
  insufficient function of, respiratory signs of, 668t
  lymphosarcomatous infiltration of, 688–689
  physiology of, 681, 681t, 681–682
  radiography of, 686
  toxins to, plant-derived, 352t, 352–354, 353t
    from yew, 371–372
  ultrasonography of, 27, 27t, 686
Heart failure, congestive, 683–684
  treatment of, 703–704
Heartwater, 628–632, 629t, 629–631, 632t
Heat. See *Temperature*.
Heavenly bamboo, toxicity of, 351t
Hedera helix, toxicity of, 350t
Heifer. See also *Cattle*.
  development of, in beef herd, nutrition in, 256t, 256–257, 258t
    in large herd management, 128t, 128–129, 129t
  estrus suppression in, 186
  pregnancy in, in dairy replacement program, 151–152, 152t
Heifer-oid, as growth stimulant, 181t
Heinz bodies, 694t, 695
  in postparturient hemoglobinuria, 324, 325
Helenium species, toxicity of, 349, 350t, 351t, 352
Hellebore, false (*Veratrum* species), as teratogen, 361, 869
  toxicity of, to heart, 353
    to nervous system, 358
Helminthiasis. See also specific parasitoses, e.g., *Ascariasis*.
  of skin, 889–890
  treatment of, 47–51
Helminthosporium species, in nasal infection, 638, 639
Hemagglutinating encephalomyelitis virus infection, 492–493
Hemangioma, 917
Hematocrit, measurement of, 690, 691, 692t
Hematoma, cutaneous, 902
  of corpus cavernosum, 797
Hematopinus suis louse, in swine pox, 482, 483
Hematopoiesis, 692–693
  in anemia, 695, 696t
  neoplasia in, 697–698
Hemlock, as teratogen, 360–361
  toxicity of, 346, 350t
  to central nervous system, 358
Hemoglobin, measurement of, 690, 691, 692t
  normal values for, 919t, 920t
Hemoglobinuria, bacillary, 571
  postparturient, 323–326, 325t
Hemolysis, in anemia, 694–695, 695t
  in copper toxicosis, 397–398
Hemoptysis, vena caval thrombosis and, 647, 648, 649, 651

Hemorrhage, and epistaxis, 638–639
  and shock, 682
  in African swine fever, 486, 487, 487, 488
  in anemia, 694–695, 695t
    management of, 699–700
  in *Haemophilus somnus* infection, 547–548
  in mastitis, 768
  in proliferative enteropathy, in campylobacteriosis, 513, 514
  in sarcocystosis, 626
  viremia in, diagnosis of, 416t
  with dermatitis and fever, in dairy cattle, 906
  with septicemia, in pasteurellosis, 555–556
Hemostasis, 698–699
Hemp, toxicity of, 353
Heparin, for thrombophlebitis, 701
  in prevention of disseminated intravascular coagulation, in shock, 683
Hepatitis, enzootic (Rift Valley fever), in cattle, 441t, 441–442
  in sheep and goats, 469–470
  necrotic, infectious, 572–573
Hepatotoxic plants, 354t, 354–356
  and photosensitization, 354t, 355, 363, 363t
Heptachlor, in water supply, 376t
  toxicity of, 381
Herbicides, organic, toxicity of, 386–393, 388t–390t
Herd, health management in, embryo transfer in, 785–787, 786
  of camelids, 172–177, 175t, 176t
  of cattle, beef, in large herds, 124–130, 125t, 126, 126t, 127, 128t, 129t
    in small herds, 121–124, 122t–124t
    on feedlot, 135–142, 136–139, 140t, 141
    stocker calves in, 130–134, 132t, 133, 134
    dairy, for production, 142t–146t, 142–147, 143, 145
    replacement rearing in, 147–153, 148t–152t, 150–152
  of goats, 162–167
  of pigs, 167–172
  of sheep, 153–159, 154t–156t
    on feedlot, 159t–161t, 159–162, 161, 162
  reproductive efficiency in, in cattle, beef, 800t, 800–803, 801–803, 802t
    dairy, 798t–800t, 798–800
  reproductive management in, in goats, 803–805
    in pigs, 805–809, 806t, 807t, 808
    in sheep, 803–805
Hereford cattle, cerebellar diseases in, 859
  horned, neurofilamentous degeneration in, 859
  shaker syndrome in, 92
Hermaphroditism, 97
  in goats, 804
Hernia, congenital, 96
  diaphragmatic, respiratory signs of, 668t
  inguinal, strangulation of, 734–735
  umbilical, vs. omphalitis, 102
Herpesvirus, and pseudorabies, in pigs, 480

Herpesvirus (Continued)
  bovine, and catarrhal fever, malignant, 421, 421–422, 422
    and mammillitis, 419–420, 420
    and pneumonia, 653–654, 660–663
    and rhinotracheitis, 417–419
  caprine, 459
  equine, in ocular disease, in camelids, 845–846
  in skin infection, 899
  ovine, 459
  type 4, serologic test for, 677
Hetacillin, dosage of, 931t
  for mastitis, 767t
Hi-Amine, dosage of, 931t
Hilaria grasses, in *Claviceps* toxicity, cerebellar, 860
Hippocastaneum species, toxicity of, 351t
Histamine, in inflammation, 8, 8
Histavet-P, for inflammation, 9t
Histidine, dietary, for pigs, 280t
Histoplasmosis, 525, 528
Hog cholera, 495–496
  ocular signs of, 854t
  respiratory signs of, 668t
  skin lesions in, 899
Hogs. See *Pig(s)*.
Holly, toxicity of, 350t
Holstein-Friesian cattle, syndactyly in, 94
Homidium, for trypanosomiasis, 606, 607t
Honker syndrome, in cattle, on feedlot, 138
Hoof. See *Foot*.
Hordeum vulgare, toxicity of, 350t
Horizontal wall cracks, 865–866
Horned Hereford cattle, neurofilamentous degeneration in, 859
Horner's syndrome, 854t, 855
Horns, analgesia of, 84–85, 85
  removal of, encephalomalacia after, 861
    in feeder calves, 180
    sinusitis after, 639
Horse chestnut, toxicity of, 351t
Horsebrush, toxicity of, 348, 355
Horses, Berne virus infection in, 451–452
  monensin toxicity in, 329–331
  pregnant mare serum gonadotropin of, in estrus management, in goats, 165, 777–778, 805, 813
    in pigs, 776, 811t, 814
    in sheep, 158, 777–778, 805, 813
  tying up syndrome of, vs. lathyrism, 345
Household measures, 934t
Human chorionic gonadotropin. See *Gonadotropin, human chorionic*.
Human menopausal gonadotropin, in estrus stimulation, in goats, 813
Humerus, fracture of, 879
Humidity, Weather Safety Index of, 124, 124t
Hyacinth, toxicity of, 350t
Hyalomma ticks, toxicity of, to skin, 906
Hyaluronidase, in regional analgesia, 79
Hydatidosis, 758
Hydranencephaly, 92
  Cache Valley virus infection and, 475
Hydrangea, toxicity of, 350t
Hydrocarbons, botanical, for external parasitosis, 51
  chlorinated, for external parasitosis, 51, 52t, 53t, 56t, 57t
  toxicity of, 380–381
  in petroleum, toxicity of, 407–409

Hydrocephalus, 92, 93
Hydrochlorothiazide, dosage of, 931t
Hydrocortisone, for inflammation, 11t
Hydrocyanic acid, toxicity of, 367–368
Hydrotherapy, for mastitis, 768
β-Hydroxybutyrate, in toxemia of pregnancy, 314
1,25-Hydroxycholecalciferol. See *Vitamin D.*
Hygromix, dosage of, 931t
Hygromycin B, for nematode infestations, 754, 754t
Hymenoxys richardsonii, toxicity of, 349
Hyostrongylus rubidus infestation, 49
Hyperadrenocorticism, and skin lesions, 912
Hyperbilirubinemia, in anemia, 695
Hypercapnia, in anesthesia, 59
Hyperfibrinogenemia, in inflammation, 697
Hyperglycemia, in milk fever, 304, 306
Hypericum species, and photosensitization, 362
  toxicity of, 350t
Hyperkeratosis, 913
Hyperparathyroidism, in oxalate poisoning, 364, 365
Hyperpigmentation, 913
Hypersensitivity, 14t, 14–15
  to food, 901
Hyperthermia, malignant, anesthesia and, 74–75
  radiofrequency current, for ocular squamous cell carcinoma, 849
Hypertonic saline, for hypovolemia, in anemia, 699
  for shock, 683
Hypertrichosis, 907
Hyphomyces destruens, skin infection by, 893
Hypnodil, dosage of, 931t
Hypobiosis, in nematodes, 744, 749
Hypocalcemia, in dairy cattle, in pregnancy, 212
  in downer cow syndrome, 323
  with milk fever, 304–309, 307t
Hypochromasia, in anemia, 694, 694t
Hypoderma infestation, 48
  cerebellar, 859
  of skin, 888
Hypogammaglobulinemia, 13
Hypoglycemia, in acetonemia, 310, *310*
  in piglet, 119–120
  in toxemia of pregnancy, 312, 313
Hypomagnesemia, and tetany, 318–321
  in cattle, range-fed, 296
  in milk fever, 305–308
Hypomelanosis, 913–914
Hypomyelinogenesis, cerebellar ataxia with, 858
Hypophosphatemia, in hemoglobinuria, postparturient, 324–326, 325t
  in milk fever, 304, 306, 307
Hypopigmentation, 913–914
  oculocutaneous, 93
Hypospadias, 96, 821
Hypotension, tranquilizers and, preanesthetic, 60
Hypothermia, in calf, 117–118
  in piglet, 119–120
Hypothyroidism, and skin lesions, 912
  hereditary, 910
  in border disease, 463
  iodine deficiency and, in pigs, 280

Hypotrichosis, 95, 907, 908t, 914
Hypovolemia, and shock, 682t, 682–683, 683t
  in anemia, 699–700
Hypoxemia, in anesthesia, 58–59
Hypoxia, treatment of, 680

Ichthyosis, 907, 912–913
Icterus, in eperythrozoonosis, 614, 615
Ilex species, toxicity of, 350t
Ill-thrift, eperythrozoonosis and, 613, 614
Imidazoles, for fungal infection, 529
  in bovine bonkers syndrome, 327
Imidocarb, for anaplasmosis, 592, 593, 593t
  for babesiosis, 587, 587t
Imidothiazoles, in anthelmintic therapy, 50
Imizol, for babesiosis, 587t
Immobilon, in capture of ruminants, 63
Immune response, and metabolic changes, 16–19
  in respiratory tract, 634–636
  suppression of, *Amblyomma* tick infestation and, in dermatophilosis, 523, 524
Immune system, colostrum in, 97–100, *99*
  disorders of, 13–16, 14t
  skin lesions in, 900–901
  function of, 12–13
Immunodeficiency, 13–14, 14t
Immunodiffusion test, agar gel, for bovine leukemia virus, 451
Immunofluorescent studies, of respiratory disease, nasal mucosal specimens in, 676
Immunoglobulins, 12–13
  in colostrum, 98–100
  in hypersensitivity, 14–15
  production of, lungs in, 635
Immunotherapy, 15–16
  for bovine leukosis, enzootic, 704
Impetigo, staphylococcal infection and, 895
Inclusion body rhinitis, 481–482
Indian hemp, toxicity of, 353
Indigestion, 710–711
  vagus nerve in, 730–732, *731*
Industrial cooling waters, toxicants in, 377–378
Infertility, 781–785
  in dairy cattle, 799t, 799–800, 800t
  in goats, 804
  in pigs, 805–807, 806t, 807t
    enteroviral infection and, 493
Inflammation, 8, 8–12, 9t, 11t. See also specific disorders, e.g., *Dermatitis.*
  leukocytes in, 696t, 697
Influenza, 501–502
  respiratory signs of, 668t
  serologic test for, 678
Infratrochlear nerve, anesthetic block of, 84–85, *85*
Inguinal hernia, strangulation of, 734–735
Inhibitor, for parasitosis, external, 56t
Injacon, dosage of, 931t
Innovar-Vet, dosage of, 931t
  preanesthetic, 61t
Insect bites, 412t, 412–413
Insecticides, toxic, carbamate, 381–382, 382t
  chlorinated hydrocarbon, 380–381

Insecticides *(Continued)*
  organophosphorus, 381–382, 382t
Insemination, artificial, in cattle, beef, in small herd, 121
  dairy, 799
    in replacement program, 150–151
  in control of campylobacteriosis, 512
  trichomoniasis in, 608, 611
  improper timing of, and conception failure, 782
Insulin, dosage of, 931t
Interferon, in immune response, 635
Interleukins, in metabolism, 17–19
Intersexuality, 97
  in goats, 804
Intertrigo, 901–902
Intestine(s), campylobacteriosis of, 508–510
  and proliferative disease, 513–515
  chlamydial infection of, in cattle, 456
  intussusception of, 733–735
  large, disorders of, 96, 738–743
  obstruction of, in volvulus, 728, *729*
  secretions of, drugs affecting, 760t, 760–761
Intravascular coagulation, disseminated, in shock, 683
Intussusception, 733–735
Iodine, for abortion induction, 791
  for rectal prolapse, 741–742
  nutritional requirement for, 200, 202
    in cattle, 251, 252t, 260t, 270t
      in pregnancy and lactation, 207, 208t, 212
    in pigs, 280t, 280–281
      in pregnancy and lactation, 215
    in sheep, in pregnancy and lactation, 218
  supplemental, for grazing cattle, 296t, 297, 299t
  topical, for actinobacillosis, 535
  toxicity of, to skin, 904
Ionophores, as feed additives, 184–185, 185t
  for coccidiosis, 602, 603t
  toxicity of, 329–331
Iowa State system, in feed protein estimation, 234–236, *235*, 235t–237t
Ipomoea species, toxicity of, 351t
Ipronidazole, for dysentery, 561t
Iris, anatomy of, in llamas, 842–843, *843*
  toxicity of, 350t
Iron, binding of, in mastitis, 762
  for anemia, 700–701
  for eperythrozoonosis, in pigs, 616
  in copper metabolism, 397, 398
  nutritional requirement for, in cattle, 251, 252t, 260t, 270t
    in pigs, 279–280, 280t
  serum measurement of, 691, 692t
  supplemental, for grazing cattle, 296t, 297, 299t
Iron-dextran, dosage of, 931t
Isocil, toxicity of, 390t, 392
Isoflupredone, dosage of, 931t
  for inflammation, 9t, 11, 11t
Isoflurane, in anesthesia, 68
Isoleucine, dietary, for pigs, 280t
Isometamidium, for trypanosomiasis, 606–607, 607t
Isoniazid, for tuberculosis, 532–533, 533t
Isopyrin, for bovine ephemeral fever, 449
Isospora infestation. See *Coccidiosis.*

Ivermectin (Ivomec), for ascariasis, in prevention of pneumonia, 675
for bronchitis, parasitic, 678, 679, 679t
for fluke infestation, 757, 757t
for hypodermiasis, 888
for louse infestation, of skin, 887
for mange, chorioptic, 885
psoregatic, 885
psoroptic, 883
sarcoptic, 884
for nematode infestation, cerebrospinal, 863
in cattle, 748, 748t
in goats, 752
in pigs, 754, 754t
in sheep, 751–752
for parasitosis, external, 51, 52, 53t, 56t, 57t
in llamas, 175–177, 176t
for thelaziasis, ocular, 839
in anthelmintic therapy, 48–49
Ivy, toxicity of, 350t, 351t
Ixodid ticks. See *Ticks*.

Jaagsiekte, 477–478
Japanese encephalitis, 496–497
Jaws, actinomycosis of, 536, 639
congenital defects of, 94
fracture of, 879
Jenotone, dosage of, 931t
Jessamine, toxicity of, 350t
Jimsonweed, toxicity of, 351t
Johne's disease, 533–534
Joints, congenital defects of, 94–95
coxofemoral, luxation of, 876–877
inflammation of. See *Arthritis*.
stifle, injuries of, 874–876
Jowl, abscess of, streptococcal, 537–538
Jugular vein, distention of, 686
pulsation of, abnormal, 685–686
Juvenile pustular psoriasiform dermatitis, 909–910

Kaboa, 628–632, 629t, *629–631*, 632t
Kale, and hemoglobinuria, postparturient, 324
toxicity of, 350t
Kallikrein, in babesiosis, 585
Kalmia species, toxicity of, 350t
Kanamycin, dosage of, 931t
for keratoconjunctivitis, 835–836
Kaopectate, for abomasal ulcer, esophageal groove closure with, 708
Karakul sheep, gray coat in, 95
Keds, external parasiticides for, 56t
skin infestation by, 887–888
Kentucky coffee tree, toxicity of, 351t
Keratinization, disorders of, 95, 909, 911–913
Keratitis, in camelids, 844–845
Keratoconjunctivitis, adenovirus infection and, 430
examination for, 832
in goats, 164
infectious, in cattle, 834–837
in goats, 841
in sheep, 840–841
mycoplasmosis and, in cattle, 458
in sheep and goats, 479
Keratogenesis imperfecta, 95

Keratouveitis, mycoplasmal, in goats, 841
Kerosene, toxicity of, 407–409
Ketamine, dosage of, 931t
in anesthesia, 66–67
for abscess extirpation, in caseous lymphadenitis, 538
for scar removal, in posthitis, 540
with guaifenesin and xylazine, 65–66
in capture of ruminants, 62–63
Keto acid decarboxylase, branched chain, deficiency of, 859
Ketoconazole, for fungal infection, 529
Ketoprofen, 10
Ketosis, glucocorticoids for, 9t, 11
in cattle, 309–312, *310*, 311t
in pregnancy, in cattle, 313t, 314–315
in sheep, 221, 312–314, 313t
ocular signs of, 854t, 856
vs. milk fever, 306
Khadar, 628–632, 629t, *629–631*, 632t
Kid. See also *Goats*.
arthritis-encephalitis virus in, 472–474, 862–863
blood tests in, reference values for, 920t
encephalomalacia in, after dehorning, 861
immunity in, colostrum and, 97–100, *99*
nutrition in, 277, 278
omphalitis in, 101–103, 102t
Kidney(s), disease of, and drug disposition, 24
Eubacterium suis infection of, 519
hemorrhage of, in African swine fever, 487, *487*, *488*
inflammation of, in cattle, in *Corynebacterium renale* infection, 539–540
in pigs, 817t, 828
infectious, 826–827
oxalosis of, in neonate, 821
polycystic, 821
toxicity to, 822–826, 823t–825t
citrinin in, 337
drug-induced, 818–819
ochratoxins in, 336, 823t, 825t
ultrasonography of, 27t, 28
Kidney worm infestation, anthelmintics for, 49, 50
in pigs, 752–754, 754t
Kochia scoparia, toxicity of, 350t
Kopertox, dosage of, 931t
for abscess, of sole, 865
Kuru, 454
Kwashiorkor, 911
Kymar aqueous, dosage of, 931t

Laburnum anagyroides, toxicity of, 351t
Lacrimal system, examination of, 832–833
obstruction of, 847t
Lactation, failure of, 768–769
in cattle, acetonemia in, 309–312, *310*, 311t
beef, nutrition in, 204–210, 206t, 208t, 253, 253t–255t, 255
dairy, herd management for, 142t–146t, 142–147, *143*, *145*
nutrition in, 210–214, 213t, 214t, 260–272
energy requirement in, 193t, 194
mammillitis in, 419–420, *420*
protein requirement in, 198–200
somatotropin and, 42–46, *43*, *44*
in pigs, energy requirement in, 196

Lactation (*Continued*)
in ergotism, 335
nutrition in, 216, 284
in sheep, acetonemia in, 221
energy requirement in, 195
nutrition in, 216–221, 220t
Lactic acid, as purgative, in botulism, 569
Lactic acidosis, 714–716, *715*
in dairy cattle, 212
magnesium for, 711, 716
Lactic dehydrogenase, blood level of, 920t
Lactobacilli, as feed additives, 187
Lactoferrin, in milk, in mastitis, 762
Lamb. See also *Sheep*.
arthrogryposis in, Cache Valley virus infection and, 475, *475*
congenital defects in, 89–97
diarrhea in, rotavirus infection and, 105
enterotoxemia in, clostridial, 573–575
immunity in, colostrum and, 97–100, *99*
neonatal management of, 156–157
omphalitis in, 101–103, 102t
weaning of, 157–158
in limited forage conditions, 221
in prevention of respiratory disease, 671–672
Lameness, coxofemoral luxation and, 876–877
in feedlot cattle, 140
physical examination in, 864
Rusterholz ulcer and, 866
Laminitis, aseptic, 867–868, *868*
in rumenitis, 716, 717
Lantana, toxicity of, 350t
Large intestine, disorders of, 96, 738–743
Larkspur, toxicity of, 346, 350t
after herbicide application, 393
Larvicides, external, 56t
Larynx, inflammation of, 636, 639–640
obstruction of, 640
physiology of, 633
Lasix. See *Furosemide*.
Lasalocid, as feed additive, 184, 185, 185t
for coccidiosis, 602, 603t
preventive use of, in sheep, 156
preventive use of, against pulmonary edema, 646–647
toxicity of, 329–330
Latex agglutination test, for rotavirus infection, 104
Lathyrus, toxicity of, 345, 350t
Laurel, toxicity of, 350t
Lavage, bronchopulmonary, in diagnosis, of respiratory disease, 676
for septic arthritis, 874
Lead, in water supply, 376, 376t
toxicity of, to eyes, 854t, 856
to kidney, 823t
vs. hypomagnesemic tetany, 320
Lechequilla, toxicity of, and photosensitization, 363
Lens, disorders of, in camelids, 845
examination of, 831
Lentigo, 913
Leptospirosis, 541t, 541–545
vaccination against, in goats, 164
Leucaena species, toxicity of, 364, 906
Leucine, dietary, for pigs, 280t
Leucothoe species, toxicity of, 350t
Leukemia, 696–698
Leukemia virus, bovine, 450–451
and lymphosarcoma, in cardiomyopathy, 688–689
treatment of, 704

INDEX □ 951

Leukocytes, disorders of, 696t, 696–698
 normal reference values for, 919t, 920t
Leukocytosis, in reticuloperitonitis, traumatic, 721
Leukoderma, 914
Leukodystrophy, globoid cell, 93
Leukoencephalomyelitis, viral, in goats, 862–863
Leukosis, bovine, and exophthalmos, 838
 enzootic, 704
Leukotrichia, 914
Leukotrienes, in inflammation, 8, 8
Levamisole, dosage of, 931t
 for bronchitis, parasitic, 678, 679, 679t
 for nematode infestation, cerebrospinal, 863
  in cattle, 748t
  in pigs, 754, 754t
  in sheep, 751–752
 for thelaziasis, ocular, in cattle, 839
 in anthelmintic therapy, 50
 in llamas, 176t
 in immunotherapy, 16
Lice, as vectors, of swine pox, 482, 483
 external parasiticides for, 51–58, 52t–54t, 56t, 57t
 in goats, 165
 in llamas, 176–177
 skin infestation by, 886–887
Lidamidine, and gastrointestinal secretion, 761
Lidocaine, for arrhythmia, 702t, 702–703
 for rectal prolapse, 741–742
 for urethral spasm, 818
 in regional anesthesia, 79, 79t
  of eye, 88
   in ophthalmic examination, 834
  of eyelid, 86, 87
  of horn, 84
  of limbs, 85, 86
  of udder, 86
  penile, 84
  spinal, 82, 83
Life Guard H. E. oral rehydration solution, 5t
Light, in management of estrus, in ewe, 158–159
 pupillary response to, anatomy of, 852–853, 853
  examination for, 830–831, 853–854
 sensitization to, toxic plants and, 354t, 355, 362–363, 363t
 ultraviolet, and dermatitis, 904–906, 905t
Ligustrum species, toxicity of, 350t
Lily, giant rain, and photosensitization, 363
Lily of the valley, toxicity of, 350t, 353
Limbs. See also Foot.
 analgesia of, 85, 85–86, 86
 injuries to, 874–876
Lime, dosage of, 930t
 in prevention of oak toxicity, 374, 826
Lime sulfur, for dermatophilosis, 895
 for dermatophytosis, 892
 for mange, chorioptic, 885
  psorergatic, 885
 for trombiculidiasis, 886
Lincomycin, for dysentery, 561, 561t
 for erysipelas, 580
 for polyarthritis, 116
Lindane, for parasitosis, external, 53t
 in water supply, 376t
Linognathus louse infestation, 48, 887

Linoleic acid, dietary, for pigs, 280t, 282
Lintox HD-Prolate, for parasitosis, 54t
Linuron, toxicity of, 390t, 392
Lipoproteins, metabolism of, in stress, 17–19
Liptak test, in abomasal displacement, 724
Liquamast, dosage of, 931t
Liquamycin. See Oxytetracycline (Terramycin).
Liquid Duster (permethrin), for lice, in goats, 165
 for parasitosis, external, 54t
Listeriosis, 580–583, 581, 583t
 neural inflammation in, 862
 ocular signs of, 838, 854, 854t
 vs. Haemophilus somnus infection, 548
Lithiasis, of urinary tract, 817t, 817–820
 and pain, 735
 in feedlot cattle, 141
 in lambs, 157
Liver, abscess of, in omphalitis, 103
 in rumenitis, 716, 717
 disease of, and drug disposition, 24–25
 failure of, coagulation factor deficiency in, 698
 fatty, 315–317, 316t, 317t
 in African swine fever, 486–487
 inflammation of, in Rift Valley fever, in cattle, 441t, 441–442
  in sheep and goats, 469–470
 necrotic, infectious, 572–573
 insufficiency syndrome of, 355–356
 necrosis of, in Rift Valley fever, 469–470
 plants toxic to, 354t, 354–356
  and photosensitization, 354t, 355, 363, 363t
 trematode infestation in, 755–757, 757t
 ultrasonography of, 27t, 28
Llamas, blood tests in, reference values for, 919t
 eyes of, anatomy of, 842t, 842–843, 843
  disorders of, 844–846
  examination of, 833, 834, 843, 843–844
  normal microorganisms in, 844, 844t
 herd health management of, 172–177, 175t, 176t
Lobelia, toxicity of, 350t
Locoweed (Astragalus), as teratogen, 360
 toxicity of, 348
  selenium in, 366, 366, 367
  to nervous system, 357
  ocular signs of, 854t
Locust, black, toxicity of, 351t
Lolium species, toxicity of, to nervous system, 357, 860
Lomadine, for babesiosis, 587t
Loridine, dosage of, 931t
Lorsban (chlorpyrifos), for parasitosis, external, 52, 52t, 55t
 for trombiculidiasis, 886
 toxicity of, 381, 382t
Lotrimin, for fungal infection, 527, 529
Lotus corniculatus, toxicity of, 350t
Louse. See Lice.
Lumbosacral puncture, for cerebrospinal fluid sampling, 861
Lumpy jaw, in actinomycosis, 536
Lumpy skin disease, 427–429, 428, 429, 898
Lung(s), adenomatosis of, 477–478
 adenovirus infection of, 484
 aspergillosis of, 528
 atelectasis of, pathology of, 636

Lung(s) (Continued)
 auscultation of, 675–676
 bacterial infection of, 654
 biopsy of, 676
 clearance mechanisms of, 653
 edema of, acute, 643–647, 644, 645
  pathology of, 636–637
 effusion of, drainage of, 678
 emphysema of, pathology of, 636, 637
 hemorrhage of, and epistaxis, 638–639
  in African swine fever, 487, 487
 inflammation of. See Pneumonia.
 physiology of, 634–635
 radiography of, 676–677
 tuberculosis of, 532
 ultrasonography of, 28, 28
 viral infection of, 653–654
Lungworm infestation, Dictyocaulus species in, 47–50, 673–674
 Metastrongylus species in, 49, 50, 752, 754t
 respiratory signs of, 668t
Lupine, as teratogen, 346, 360, 361
 toxicity of, 346
  in sheep, 221
  to central nervous system, 358
Lutalyse, for pyometra, 773
 in induction of abortion, 792t, 811t, 814
 in induction of parturition, 811t, 815
Luteal cysts, 774–775
Luteinizing hormone, dosage of, 931t
 imbalance of, and ovarian cysts, 774–775
 in ovulatory disorders, and conception failure, 782
Luxation injury, coxofemoral, 876–877
 patellar, 874–875
Lycopersicon esculentum, toxicity of, 350t
Lyme borreliosis, in cattle, 515–516
Lymph nodes, Corynebacterium pseudotuberculosis infection of, 896–897
 hemorrhage of, in African swine fever, 487
Lymphadenitis, cervical, streptococcal, 577–578
 in Corynebacterium infection, 537–538
Lymphangitis, ulcerative, Corynebacterium pseudotuberculosis infection and, 538–539
Lymphedema, congenital, 910
Lymphocytes, deficiency of, tests for, 14t
 in immune function, 12–13
 in lung, 635
 laboratory measurement of, 692t
 reference values for, 919t, 920t
Lymphocytopenia, 696, 696t
Lymphocytosis, 696t, 698
Lymphosarcoma, 917
 bovine leukemia virus and, 450–451, 704
 cardiac infiltration by, 688–689
 ocular involvement in, 838, 847t, 850t, 850–851
Lyonia species, toxicity of, 350t
Lysine, dietary, 171, 279, 280t, 283
Lysoff (fenthion), dosage of, 931t
 for lice, in llamas, 177
 for parasitosis, external, 53t
Lysozymes, in immune response, in respiratory tract, 635

Macrocytosis, in anemia, 694, 694t

952 □ INDEX

Macrophages, alveolar, 634–635, 653
Macrozamia species, toxicity of, 357
Mad cow disease (spongiform encephalopathy), 454–455, 860
Mad itch. See *Pseudorabies*.
Maedi-visna, 470–471
Magnesium, blood level of, normal values for, 920t
   deficiency of, and tetany, 318–321
   in milk fever, 305–308
   nutritional requirement for, in cattle, 251, 252t, 260t, 270t
      beef, 208t, 208–210
      dairy, 212, 213t, 214t
     in pigs, 215
     in sheep, 218
   supplemental, for grazing cattle, 296, 299t
Magnesium gluconate, dosage of, 931t
Magnesium hydroxide, for abomasal impaction, 733
   for abomasal ulcer, esophageal groove closure with, 708
   for lactic acidosis, 711, 716
Magnesium lactate, dosage of, 931t
Magnesium oxide, dosage of, 931t
Magnesium sulfate, and gastrointestinal motility, 759t, 760
   dosage of, 931t
   for cardiotoxic plant poisoning, 354
   for phenol toxicity, 411
Magnets, in prevention of reticuloperitonitis, traumatic, 721, 722
Malathion, for lice, in goats, 165
   for mange, psoregatic, 885
   for trombiculidiasis, 886
Male fern, toxicity of, ocular signs of, 854t
Maleberry, toxicity of, 350t
Malignant catarrhal fever. See *Catarrhal fever*.
Malta fever, 551
Mammillitis. See also *Mastitis*.
   herpetic, 419–420, 420, 899
   vs. vaccinial, 424, 424t
   vaccinial, 423–425, 424, 424t
Mandible, actinomycotic infection of, 536
   congenital defects of, 94
   fracture of, 879
Manganese, nutritional requirement for, in cattle, beef, 260t
      dairy, 270t
     in pigs, 280t, 281
      in pregnancy and lactation, 215
   supplemental, for grazing cattle, 294, 296t, 297, 299t, 300
Mange, chorioptic, 884–885
   demodectic, 885–886
   in llamas, 177
   ivermectin for, 48, 49
   parasiticides for, 51–58, 52t–54t, 56t, 57t
   psorergatic, 885
   psoroptic, 882–883
   sarcoptic, 883–884
Mannitol, dosage of, 931t
   for shock, 683
   for urinary tract disorders, 818
Mannosidosis, 92–93
   cerebellum in, 860
Maple syrup urine disease, 92, 859
Marasmus, 911
Marcaine, in regional analgesia, 79t
Mare serum gonadotropin, in estrus management, in goats, 165, 777–778, 805, 813

Mare serum gonadotropin *(Continued)*
   in pigs, 776, 811t, 814
   in sheep, 158, 777–778, 805, 813
Marrow, hematopoiesis in, 692–693
   in anemia, 695, 696t
Mast cell tumors, 917
Mastitis, and lactation failure, 768
   arthritis-encephalitis virus and, 473
   fungal infection and, 526–527
   herpetic, 419–420, 420, 899
   in cattle, 762–768, 765t–767t
   in *Corynebacterium bovis* infection, 541
   in goats, 167
   in maedi-visna, 471
   in mycoplasmosis, in cattle, 457–458
     in goats, 479
     in sheep, 479
   in nocardiosis, 521, 522
   in pseudocowpox, 425, 425–426
   in sheep, 156
   staphylococcal, 578, 579
   streptococcal, 575–576
   vaccinia and, 423–425, 424, 424t
Maxilla, actinomycosis of, 536, 639
Maxillary nerve, anesthetic block of, 86–87, 87
Mayapple, toxicity of, 351t
Meat, residues in, 29–42. See also *Drugs, residues of*.
Mebendazole, in anthelmintic therapy, in llamas, 176t
Mecoprop, toxicity of, 391t
Medial collateral ligament, trauma to, 875
Medial femoropatellar ligament, trauma to, 874–875
Medial patellar ligament, trauma to, 874–875
Medroxyprogesterone, in estrus stimulation, in goats, 813
   in sheep, 813
Melanoma, 917–918
Melanosis, 913
Melanthum virginicum, toxicity of, 350t
Melatonin, in estrus stimulation, in goats, 813
   in sheep, 812
Melengestrol, in estrus management, as feed additive, 184, 186–187
   in cattle, 810
   in sheep, 813
Melia azedarach, toxicity of, 351t
Melilotus species, toxicity of, 358–359
Melophagus ovinus, skin infestation by, 887–888
Menadione. See *Vitamin K*.
Meninges, anatomy of, 77, 78
Meningitis, in sheep and goats, 861–862
   streptococcal, in pigs, 577
Meningoencephalitis, in *Haemophilus somnus* infection, 546–549, 547
   thromboembolic, in pneumonia, 662, 664
     ocular signs of, 838, 854, 854t, 856
Meningoencephalocele, 92
Menispermum canadense, toxicity of, 350t
Mepivacaine, in regional analgesia, 79t
Mercury, in water supply, 376, 376t
   toxicity of, to skin, 904
Mesenchymal tumors, 917
Mesentery, volvulus of, 734, 735
Metabolic alkalosis, in abomasal displacement, 724, 727–728
Metabolism, disorders of, 304–326
   hormonal regulation of, in stress, 16–19

Metacarpal bones, fracture of, 879
Metastrongylus infestation, 49, 50, 752, 754t
   respiratory signs of, 668t
Metatarsal bones, fracture of, 879
Methionine, dietary, 280t
Methocarbamol, dosage of, 931t
Methoprene, for parasitosis, external, 56t
Methoxamine, for hypotension, tranquilizer-induced, 60
Methoxychlor, in water supply, 376t
Methoxychlormalathion, for parasitosis, external, 56t, 57t
Methoxyflurane, dosage of, 931t
Methscopolamine, and gastrointestinal motility, 759t, 760
Methylarsinate, toxicity of, 388t, 391
Methylene blue, dosage of, 931t
   for hemoglobinuria, postparturient, 325, 325t
   in assessment of ruminal bacteria, 710
3-Methylindol, in pulmonary edema, 643–647, 644
Metobromuron, toxicity of, 390t, 392
Metoclopramide, for abomasal emptying defect, 737
Metrazol, dosage of, 931t, 932t
Metritis, 770–772
   and infertility, 784, 785
Metronidazole, for trichomoniasis, 785
   in culture medium, for *Eubacterium suis*, 520
Miconazole, for fungal infection, 529
Micotil, for pneumonia, in pasteurellosis, 557, 557t
Microcytosis, in anemia, 694, 694t
Microphthalmia, 93
   in sheep, 839
Microsporum species, skin infection by, 890–892, 891t, 892t
Micturition, induction of, 818
Midges, as bluetongue vectors, in cattle, 435–437
   in sheep, 465–467
Mikedimide, dosage of, 931t
Milk, digestion of, esophageal groove closure in, 708–709
   production of. See also *Lactation*.
     herd health management for, 142t–146t, 142–147, 143, 145
     reduced, in leptospirosis, 542
     somatotropin and, 42–46, 43, 44
Milk fever, 304–309, 307t
   dietary management of, 268
   downer syndrome after, 322
Milk of magnesia, dosage of, 931t
Milking, technique of, and mastitis, 762, 766–767, 767t
Milkvetch, toxicity of, 348
Milkweed, toxicity of, 344–345, 348, 350t, 352, 353
Mine tailings, toxicants in, 377–380, 378, 378t
Mineral oil, dosage of, 931t
   for abomasal emptying defect, 737
   for bloat, 718
   for oak toxicity, 374
Minerals. See also specific elements, e.g., *Sodium*.
   imbalances of, skin lesions in, 911–912
   in water, consumption of, by range-fed cattle, 292, 295
   nutritional requirement for, 200–203, 202t

Minerals (Continued)
  in cattle, 251, 252t
    beef, 206t, 207–210, 208t
    dairy, 211–214, 213t, 214t
  in pigs, 279–281, 280t, 283
    in pregnancy and lactation, 214–216
  in sheep, 217–219, 220t
  supplementation with, for cattle, grazing, 291–302
    range-fed, 293–302
Mink, polychlorinated biphenyl toxicity in, 406
Mint, purple, toxicity of, 350t, 352, 368–369
Miosis, 854t, 855
Mistletoe, toxicity of, 351t
Mitaban, for mange, demodectic, 886
Mites, and mange, 882–886. See also Mange.
Mocap, toxicity of, 382t
Modikulogo, 628–632, 629t, 629–631, 632t
Modiola caroliniana, toxicity of, 351t
Mold, feed damage by, 341–343
Molinate, toxicity of, 389t, 391
Molybdenum, and copper deficiency, with postparturient hemoglobinuria, 324
  dosage of, 931t
  in copper metabolism, 396–398
  nutritional requirement for, in cattle, 251
    in sheep, 218
  supplemental, for grazing cattle, 296–297
  toxicity of, 397
    to skin, 904, 912
Monensin, as feed additive, 184–185, 185t
  for coccidiosis, 602, 603t
    in goats, 165
  for toxoplasmosis, 625
  preventive use of, against bloat, 718
    against pulmonary edema, 646–647
  toxicity of, 329–331
Moniezia species, infestation by, 47, 49, 757–758
Monistat, for fungal infection, 529
Monoacetin, dosage of, 931t
Monocytes, blood level of, 692t, 919t, 920t
  elevated, in inflammation, 696t, 697
Monteban, toxicity of, 329–330
Monuron, toxicity of, 390t, 392
Moonseed, toxicity of, 350t
Morantel, for nematode infestation, 748t
  in anthelmintic therapy, 50
Moraxella bovis infection, and keratoconjunctivitis, 835–837
Morning glory, toxicity of, 351t
Morphine, and gastrointestinal motility, 759t, 760
Mosquitoes, as vectors, of eperythrozoonosis, 614, 615
  of Rift Valley fever, 441, 469
Mouth, inflammation of. See Stomatitis.
Mucomyst (acetylcysteine), for phenol toxicity, 411
  for tracheobronchial patency, 679t, 679–680
Mucosa, infection of, bovine viral diarrhea in, 432–434
  rinderpest in, 445
  viral, diagnosis of, 416t
Mucous membranes, of respiratory tract, pathologic reactions in, 636

Mucus, in respiratory tract, functions of, 634
Müller's ducts, aplasia of, and conception failure, 781
Mummification, fetal, 807t
  enteroviral infection and, 493
Murmurs, cardiac, 681, 681t, 685
  in pericarditis, traumatic, 686–687
Muscle(s), congenital defects of, 93–94
  damage to, in downer cow syndrome, 322
  degeneration of, in selenium deficiency, 689–690
    in goats, 164
    in sheep, 154
  hypertrophy of, 93
Muscular dystrophy, 93–94
Musculoskeletal system, disorders of, 864–881
  in feedlot cattle, 140t, 140–141
  examination of, 864
Mushrooms, toxicity of, 355, 356
Mustard seeds, toxicity of, 351t
Mycetoma, 521, 522, 892–893
Mycobacterial infection, and paratuberculosis, 533–534
  and tuberculosis, in cattle, 531–533, 533t
  in pigs, 529–531
Mycoplasmosis, and lactation failure, 769
  in cattle, 457–458
    and mastitis, 763, 765, 765t, 766t
    and ocular inflammation, 837
    and pneumonia, 654
  in goats, 478–479
    and ocular inflammation, 841
  in pigs, 504–505
    and pneumonia, 665t, 665–667, 668t
    with pasteurellosis, 560
  in sheep, 478–479
    and ocular inflammation, 840
  serologic test for, 677
Mycosis. See Fungus (fungi).
Mycostatin (nystatin), for fungal infection, 529
  with mastitis, 527
Mycotoxin(s), and salivary syndrome, 338, 338–339, 339
  and skin lesions, 905t, 906
  citrinin as, 337
  ergot, 334–336, 351t, 370, 906
    in cerebellar disease, 860
  in prepared feeds, 344
  ochratoxin as, 336–337
  trichothecene, 332–334, 340–341
Mydriacil (tropicamide), dosage of, 933t
  in ocular examination, in llama, 843–844
Mydriasis, 855
Myelin, deficiency of, with cerebellar ataxia, 858
  in response to analgesics, 78, 79t
  of optic nerve, in llamas, 843, 843
Myeloencephalopathy, progressive degenerative, 92
Myiasis, 888–889
Myocardium, abscess of, in Haemophilus somnus infection, 546, 547, 548
  viral infection of, 493–494
Myoclonus, congenital, in polled Hereford cattle, 859
Myodegeneration, selenium deficiency and, 689–690
  in goats, 164
  in sheep, 154

Mystery pig disease, 485

Nagana (trypanosomiasis), 604t, 604–607, 607t
  of skin, 900
Naganol, for trypanosomiasis, 607, 607t
Nairobi sheep disease, 468–469
Nalidixic acid, in culture medium, for Eubacterium suis, 520
Nandina domestica (heavenly bamboo), toxicity of, 351t
Nandrolone, for anemia, 701
Naphtha, toxicity of, 407–409
Naphthalene, chlorinated, toxicity of, 904
Naptalam, toxicity of, 389t, 391
Narasin, toxicity of, 329–330
Nasal bot infestation, 48–49
  and meningitis, 861
  ocular, 842
  of respiratory tract, 674
Nasal cavity, bleeding from, 638–639
  fungal infection of, 528–529
  inflammation of, 636, 638
  obstruction of, 639
  physiology of, 633
  secretions from, testing of, for viral infection, 415–417
  viral isolation from, in diagnosis, 676
Nasolacrimal system, examination of, 832–833
  obstruction of, 847t
Natamycin, for dermatophytosis, 892
  for fungal infection, 529
  with mastitis, 527
Navel ill, 101–103, 102t
Naxcel. See Ceftiofur.
Necrobacillosis, interdigital, 869–870
Neethling virus, in lumpy skin disease, 427
Neguvon. See Trichlorfon (Neguvon).
Neisseria ovis infection, and conjunctivitis, 840
Nematel, for nematode infestation, 748t
  in anthelmintic therapy, 50
Nematode infestation, anthelmintics for, 47–50
  cerebrospinal, 863
  in cattle, 743–748, 746t–748t
  in goats, 165, 751, 752
  in pigs, 752–754, 754t
  in sheep, 748–752
  ocular, in camelids, 845
Neo-Aristovet, dosage of, 932t
Neomycin, dosage of, 932t
  residues of, test for, 32t
Neonate. See Calf, Kid, Lamb, and Piglet.
Neostigmine, and gastrointestinal motility, 759, 759t
  dosage of, 932t
  for indigestion, 711
Neo-Terramycin, dosage of, 932t
Nephritis, Eubacterium suis infection and, 519
  in cattle, 817t, 826–827
    Corynebacterium renale infection and, 539–540, 826, 827
  in pigs, 817t, 828
Nephrotoxicity, 822–826, 823t–825t
  drug-induced, 818–819
Nerium oleander, toxicity of, 344, 351t
  to heart, 353, 354

Nervous system, anatomy of, 77–79, 78, 78t
  blocking of. See *Analgesia* and *Anesthesia*.
  congenital defects of, 92
  damage to, in downer cow syndrome, 322
  degeneration of, in scrapie, 475–477
  disorders of, cerebellar, 858–860
    in feedlot cattle, 141
    in heartwater, 629–631, 630, 631
    in paramyxovirus infection, 503
  edema of, 92
    dimethyl sulfoxide for, 12
    glucocorticoids for, 11
    in Akabane disease, 443
    in bovine rhinotracheitis, 418
  inflammation of, in sheep and goats, 860–863
  malformations of, Cache Valley virus infection and, 474, 475
  plants toxic to, 356t, 356–358
    cardiac effects of, 352t, 352–353
  streptococcal infection of, 577
  viral infection of, diagnosis of, 416t
Neutrophils, blood levels of, decreased, 696, 696t, 697
  elevated, 696, 696t, 697
    in reticuloperitonitis, 721
  reference values for, 692t, 919t, 920t
  function of, in lung, 635
Niacin, nutritional requirement for, in cattle, 252
  in pregnancy and lactation, 212
  in pigs, 280t, 282
    in pregnancy and lactation, 215, 216
Nickel, in water supply, 376, 376t
Nicotiana species, as teratogen, 360, 361
  toxicity of, 351t, 358
Nicotinamide, dosage of, 932t
Nictalopia, 856
Nictitans, anatomy of, in llamas, 842
  examination of, 832
  flap of, for corneal protection, 834
  protrusion of, differential diagnosis of, 847t
Night blindness, 856
Nightshade (*Solanum* species), toxicity of, 351t
  and cerebellar degeneration, 351t
Nitarsone, toxicity of, 395–396
Nitralin, toxicity of, 388t, 391
Nitrate, in water supply, 376, 376t
  plants accumulating, 344
    after herbicide application, 393
  toxicity of, 231
Nitriles, in herbicides, toxicity of, 388t, 391
Nitrite, in water supply, 376, 376t
Nitro compounds, in plants, neurotoxicity of, 357
Nitrofen, toxicity of, 388t, 391
Nitrofurazone (Furacin), dosage of, 931t, 932t
  for coccidiosis, 602, 603t
Nitrogen. See also *Protein*.
  nonprotein, for dairy cattle, 27t, 266–268
    in ruminants, 230–231
  urea, blood level of, reference values for, 920t
3-Nitro-4-hydroxy phenylarsonic acid, for eperythrozoonosis, 616

3-Nitro-4-hydroxy phenylarsonic acid (*Continued*)
  toxicity of, 395–396
4-Nitrophenylarsonic acid, toxicity of, 395–396
Nizoral, for fungal infection, 529
Nocardiosis, 521–522, 892–893
Nodules, in lumpy skin disease, 428, 428
  in poxvirus infection, in sheep and goats, 459–460
Nofel, 616, 617
Nonsteroidal anti-inflammatory drugs, 8, 9t, 9–10. See also *Acetylsalicylic acid*.
  nephrotoxicity of, 819
Norea, toxicity of, 390t
Norgestomet, dosage of, 932t
  in estrus management, in cattle, 778, 779, 810, 811t
    in goats, 165, 777, 811t, 813
    in sheep, 158, 777, 811t, 812–813
Novidium, for trypanosomiasis, 606, 607t
Novin, 9t, 10
  dosage of, 930t
Novobiocin, dosage of, 931t, 932t
Novocain (procaine), in regional analgesia, 79, 79t, 82
Nutrition. See *Diet*.
Nystagmus, 855
Nystatin, for fungal infection, 529
  with mastitis, 527

Oak, toxicity of, 348, 351t, 372–374, 373t, 374
  to kidney, 822–826
Ochratoxin, toxicity of, 336–337
  to kidney, 336, 823t, 825t
Oculomotor nerve, anatomy of, 852
  in ophthalmic reflexes, examination of, 830–831
Oesophagostomum infestation, 47–51
  in pigs, 752–754, 754t
Oestrus ovis larval infestation, 48–49
  and meningitis, 861
  ocular, 842
  of respiratory tract, 674
Oil, toxicity of, 407–409
Oleander, toxicity of, 344, 351t, 353, 354
Oleandomycin, dosage of, 932t
Olecranon, fracture of, 879
Olifantsvelsiekte (elephant skin disease), 596–598, 597, 598, 900
Oliquindox, for enteropathy, proliferative, in campylobacteriosis, 514–515
Omasum, motility of, 709
  volvulus of, with abomasal volvulus, 725–730, 727
Omnizole. See *Thiabendazole*.
Omphalitis, 101–103, 102t, 821–822
Onchocerciasis, of skin, 889–890
Onderstepoort, for heartwater, 632t
Ondiri disease, 618–620, 619, 619t
Onions, toxicity of, 350t
Ophthaine, dosage of, 932t
Ophthalmia, in catarrhal fever, malignant, 421, 422, 838
Ophthalmic nerve, anesthetic block of, 86–87, 87
Ophthalmitis, in camelids, 844–846
  in cattle, 834–839
  in sheep and goats, 840–842
Ophthalmoplegia, oculomotor nerve lesions and, 852
Ophthalmoscopy, 831–832

Opioids, and gastrointestinal motility, 759t, 760
Opisthotonos, in heartwater, 629–630, 630
Optic disk, disorders of, 854t, 856
Optic nerve, anatomy of, 852
  disorders of, 854t, 855–856
  myelination of, in llamas, 843, 843
Optimizer. See *Diazinon*.
Oral rehydration solution, 4–5, 5t
  for toxemia of pregnancy, 313
Orbenin, dosage of, 932t
  for keratoconjunctivitis, 835–836
Orbit, anatomy of, in llamas, 843
Orchitis, 795
  in brucellosis, 552, 552
Organoarsenics, in herbicides, toxicity of, 388t, 391
Organophosphates, for external parasitosis, 51, 54t, 55t, 57t
  in anthelmintic therapy, 50
  toxicity of, and miosis, 854t, 855
    in insecticides, 381–382, 382t
Ornithodoros ticks, as vectors, of African swine fever, 486
  of borreliosis, 516
Osteochondrosis, of stifle, 875–876
Osteofluorosis, 399–402, 401
Osteogenesis imperfecta, 94
Osteomyelitis, 881
Osteopetrosis, 94
Ostertagia infestation, 47–50
  in cattle, 743–748, 746t–748t
Otitis media, ocular signs of, 854t
Ova, abnormalities of, and conception failure, 781–782
Ovalocytes, 694t
Ovaries, congenital defects of, 97
  cysts of, in cattle, 774–775
  disorders of, and infertility, 782
  ultrasonography of, 27t, 28–29
Ovine. See *Sheep*.
Ovulation. See also *Estrus*.
  disorders of, and conception failure, 782
  trace minerals in, 294
Oxalate, in urolithiasis, 819
  toxicity of, in sheep, 221
    plant accumulation in, 364–365
    to kidney, 824t
    in neonate, 821
Oxfendazole, dosage of, 932t
  for cestode infestation, 758
  for nematode infestation, in cattle, 748t
Oximes, for organophosphate toxicity, 382
Oxoid CM 161 medium, for *Trichomonas foetus* culture, 610, 610t
Oxygen, arterial, maintenance of, 680
  feed exposed to, 341–343
  in inhalation anesthesia, 68–70, 70
Oxytetracycline (Terramycin), as feed additive, 184, 186, 187t
  dosage of, 933t
  for *Actinobacillus* pleuropneumonia, 550t
  for anaplasmosis, 592–593, 593t, 595
  for anthrax, 566
  for besnoitiosis, 598
  for dermatophilosis, 523
  for ehrlichiosis, 617t
    in petechial fever, 619t, 620
  for eperythrozoonosis, in llamas, 176, 176t
  for ergotism, 336
  for erysipelas, 580
  for heartwater, 631, 632t

Oxytetracycline (Terramycin) *(Continued)*
  for keratoconjunctivitis, in cattle, 835–837
    in sheep, 840
  for mastitis, 767t
  for mycoplasmosis, in cattle, 458
    ocular, in goats, 841
  for pasteurellosis, 557t, 557–560
  for phlegmon, interdigital, 870
  for pleuritis, fibrinous, with pleuropneumonia, 664
  for pneumonia, 658t, 658–659, 659t, 661, 663
    in pasteurellosis, 557, 557t, 558
  for respiratory disease, in sheep, in flock therapy, 672
  for sinusitis, in actinomycosis, 639
  for tick-borne fever, 621, 621t
  for vesiculitis, 794
  nephrotoxicity of, 819
Oxytocin, dosage of, 932t
  for fetal membrane retention, 769, 770
  for lactation failure, 768
  in induction of parturition, 815
  with stripping, for mastitis, 768
Oxytropis species, toxicity of, 348, 357

Palpebral reflex, in ophthalmic examination, 830–831, 853
  blocking of, 834
Panacur. See *Fenbendazole*.
Pancreas, secretions of, drugs affecting, 760t
Pantothenic acid, deficiency of, skin lesions in, 911
  nutritional requirement for, in pigs, 280t, 282
  in pregnancy and lactation, 215
Papilledema, 854t, 856
Papillomas, 916
  digital, 868–869
  in cattle, 430–431
  in goats, 462
  in sheep, 462
  viral, penile, 796
Papovavirus infection, 916
Papular stomatitis, *426*, 426–427, *427*, 898
Parainfluenza-3 virus infection, 443–444
  and pneumonia, 653–654
  serologic test for, 677, 678
  vaccination against, in prevention of pasteurellosis, 558
Parakeratosis, ruminal, 716–717
  zinc deficiency and, 909, 912
Paralysis, congenital defects and, 92–93
  of femoral nerve, 875
  of radial nerve, anesthesia and, 68
Paramphistomum infestation, 755, 756
Paramyxovirus infection, 502–504
Paraquat, toxicity of, 387, 388t
Parasitosis, and blood loss, in anemia, 700
  and bronchitis, treatment of, 678–679, 679t
  cerebellar, 859
  cestode, 757–758
  external, treatment for, 51–58, 52t–57t
  helminthic, treatment for, 47–51
  in goats, 164–165
  in llamas, 175–177, 176t
  in pigs, 170, 171
  in stocker calves, 132
  nematode, cerebrospinal, 863

Parasitosis *(Continued)*
  in cattle, 743–748, 746t–748t
  in goats, 752
  in pigs, 752–754, 754t
  in sheep, 748–752
  ocular, in camelids, 845
    in cattle, 838–839
    in sheep and goats, 841–842
  of respiratory tract, 673–675
  of skin, helminthic, 889–890
    keds in, 887–888
    lice in, 886–887
    maggots in, 888–889
    mites and, 882–886
  protozoal, 584–613, 623–628. See also specific diseases, e.g., *Anaplasmosis.*
  trematode, 755–757, 757t
Parasympathetic nerve, in pupillary light reflex, 830–831
Parasympatholytics, preanesthetic, 60
Paratect (morantel), for nematode infestation, 748t
  in anthelmintic therapy, 50
Parathyroid hormone, in milk fever, 305
  in oxalate poisoning, 364, 365
Paratuberculosis, 533–534
Paravertebral analgesia, 83, *83, 84*
Paregoric, and gastrointestinal motility, 759t, 760
Parelaphostrongylus tenuis infestation, cerebrospinal, 863
  in goats, 165
Paresis, parturient, 304–309, 307t
  dietary management of, 322
  downer syndrome after, 322
Pars esophagea, ulceration of, 735–736
Parsley, skin reactions to, 362–363
Partial thromboplastin time, measurement of, 691, 692t
Parturition, fetal membrane retention after, 769–770
  hemoglobinuria after, 323–326, 325t
  induction of, in cattle, 811, 811t
    in goats, 805, 811t, 814
    in pigs, 815
    in sheep, 805, 811t, 813
  milk fever in, 304–309, 307t
    dietary management of, 268
    downer syndrome after, 322
  uterine infection after, 770–772
Parvaquone, for theileriosis, 628
Parvovirus infection, in cattle, 431–432
  in pigs, and reproductive failure, 484–485
  and vesicular disease, 900
Paspalum grasses, in *Claviceps* toxicity, cerebellar, 860
Pasteurella haemolytica, infection with, parainfluenza-3 virus predisposing to, 443–444
  with mycoplasmosis, in pneumonia, 478
  toxin of, in pneumonia, 635, 637
Pasteurellosis, and keratoconjunctivitis, 837
  in cattle, 555–558, 557t
  in lamb, newborn, 156–158
  in pigs, 559–560
  in pneumonia, 641–643, 655, 662, 663
  serologic tests for, 677
Pasture, grazing on, and nematode infestation, 746, 750–751
  and tetany, hypomagnesemic, 318, 320

Pasture *(Continued)*
  forage resources in, 257, 259t, 285–288, *286*, 287t, *288*, *289*
  management of, 290–291
  nutrient intake from, 289–290, *290*, 293–294
  pneumonia control in, 662–663
  selective, 288–289, *289*
  supplementation of, 291–292
    medicated feed additives in, 300–301
    minerals in, 291–302
Pasture fever, *620*, 620–621, 621t
Patella, luxation of, 874–875
Patellar ligament, medial, trauma to, 874–875
Peas, wild, toxicity of, 345, 350t
Pebulate, toxicity of, 389t, 391
Pediculosis, 886–887
  external parasiticides for, 51–58, 52t–54t, 56t, 57t
  in goats, 165
  in llamas, 176–177
Pelvis, fracture of, 879
Pemphigus foliaceus, 901
  prednisolone for, 912
D-Penicillamine, dosage of, 932t
  for copper toxicosis, 398
Penicillin, dosage of, 932t
  for *Actinobacillus* pleuropneumonia, 550, 550t
  for actinomycosis, 536, 537
  for anthrax, 566
  for bacillary hemoglobinuria, 571
  for blackleg, 570
  for campylobacteriosis, 513, 514
  for clostridial infection, 897
    with malignant edema, 570
  for *Corynebacterium* infection, with caseous lymphadenitis, 538
  for *Corynebacterium pseudotuberculosis* infection, with ulcerative lymphangitis, 539
  for *Corynebacterium renale* infection, with nephritis, 539
    with posthitis, 540
  for cystitis, 827–828
  for dermatitis, digital, 869
  for dermatophilosis, 523, 895
  for endocarditis, 688, 702
  for ergotism, 336
  for erysipelas, 580, 898
  for *Eubacterium suis* infection, 520, 828
  for keratoconjunctivitis, infectious, 835–836
  for listeriosis, 583, 862
  for mastitis, 767t
  for omphalitis, 102t
  for phlegmon, interdigital, 870
  for pneumonia, 658t, 659, 659t
    in pasteurellosis, 557, 557t
  for polyarthritis, 116
  for pyelonephritis, 827, 828
  for respiratory disease, in sheep, in flock therapy, 672
  for staphylococcosis, in exudative epidermitis, 896
  for streptococcosis, 577, 578
  for tetanus, 568
  for uterine infection, 771
    in embryo transfer, 786
Penicillium species, toxins of, 336, 337
Penis, anesthesia of, 84
  congenital defects of, 96

Penis (Continued)
  disorders of, 796–798
  ultrasonography of, 27t, 29
Pennisetum clandestinum, toxicity of, 364
Pentachlorophenol, toxicity of, 410
Pentobarbital, dosage of, 932t
  in anesthesia, 64
  preanesthetic, 63
Pentothal, in anesthesia, 64–65
Pentylenetetrazol, dosage of, 932t
Percussion, in diagnosis, of respiratory diseases, 675–676
Pericardiocentesis, 686, 687
Pericarditis, trauma and, 686–687
  with reticuloperitonitis, 720, 722
Pericardium, ultrasonography of, 27–28
Perilla frutescens, toxicity of, 350t, 352, 368–369
Perineal nerve, block of, in analgesia of udder, 86, 86
Periorchitis, 795
Peritonitis, reticular trauma and, 719–722, 735
Permethrin, for lice, in goats, 165
  for parasitosis, external, 54t–57t
Peroneal nerve, in downer cow syndrome, 322
Peroneus tertius tendon, rupture of, 880
Perosomu elumbis, 94
Persea americana, toxicity of, 351t
Pesticides, in water supply, 376t, 376–377
  toxic, herbicides as, 386–393, 388t–390t
    insecticides as, 380–382, 381t
    rodenticides as, 383–386, 384t, 385t
Petechiae, conjunctival, in heartwater, 629, 630
Petechial fever, 618–620, 619, 619t
Peterson eye block, 87, 87, 834
Petrolatum, liquid, and gastrointestinal motility, 759t, 760
Petroleum, toxicity of, 407–409
Peyronella glomerata, skin infection by, 893
PG600, in estrus management, 165
Phaeohyphomycosis, 893
Phaeosclera dematiodes infection, 893
Phalaris species, toxicity of, and staggers, 860
Pharynx, inflammation of, 639–640
  laceration of, 713–714
  obstruction of, 640
Phenamidine, for babesiosis, 587t
Phenols, toxicity of, 409–411
  in herbicides, 388t, 391
Phenothiazine, for nematode infestation, in cattle, 748t
  in goats, 751, 752
  in sheep, 751–752
  in tranquilizers, preanesthetic, 60
Phenoxy herbicides, toxicity of, 389t, 391
Phenylalanine, dietary, 280t
Phenylarsonic compounds, arsanilic acid in, in prevention of eperythrozoonosis, 616
  ocular toxicity of, 854t, 856
  toxicity of, 395–396
Phenylbutazone, 9t, 10
  dosage of, 930t, 932t
  for bovine ephemeral fever, 449
  for laminitis, aseptic, 868
  for urticaria, 901
Phenylephrine, for hypotension, tranquilizer-induced, 60
Phlebitis, treatment of, 701–702
  umbilical, 101, 102

Phlegmon, interdigital, 869–870
Phoradendron species, toxicity of, 351t
Phorate, toxicity of, 381, 382t
Phormia blowflies, skin infestation by, 888–889
Phosmet, for parasitosis, external, 54t, 57t
Phosphorus, blood level of, 920t
  deficiency of, in hemoglobinuria, postparturient, 324–326, 325t
    in milk fever, 304, 306, 307
  for downer cow syndrome, 323
  in rodenticides, toxicity of, 385t, 386
  in urolithiasis, 819, 820
  nutritional requirement for, 200–203, 202t
    in cattle, 251, 252t
      beef, 122, 123t
        in breeding herd, 253t, 259–260
        in pregnancy and lactation, 206t, 207, 208t, 209
      dairy, 268, 270t, 271t
        in pregnancy and lactation, 211–213, 213t, 214t
    in goats, 273, 274t, 275t, 277, 278
    in pigs, 170, 171, 279, 280t
      in pregnancy and lactation, 214–216
    in sheep, in pregnancy and lactation, 218, 220t
  supplemental, and fluoride toxicosis, 399
  for grazing cattle, 295–296, 298, 299t
Photodermatitis, 904–906, 905t
Photosensitization, plant toxicity and, 354t, 355, 362–363, 363
Phthalamic acids, in herbicides, toxicity of, 389t, 391
Phycomycosis, 524
Phylloerythrin, in photosensitization, 355, 363
Physostigmine, and gastrointestinal motility, 759t, 759t
Phytolacca americana, toxicity of, 351t
Phytonadione. See *Vitamin K_1 (Aquamephyton)*.
Pia mater, anatomy of, 77, 78
Picloram, toxicity of, 390t, 392
Picornavirus infection, in foot-and-mouth disease, 464, 464
  skin lesions in, 899
Pig(s), abortion in, induced, 793, 814
  blood tests in, reference values for, 919t, 920t
  disorders in. See specific disorders, e.g., Cholera, and affected structures, e.g., Lung(s).
  drug residues in, 35
  herd health management in, 167–172
  intubation of, for anesthesia, 72
  nutrition in, 278–285, 280t, 282t
    energy requirement in, 195–196
    in pregnancy and lactation, 214–216
    protein requirement in, 196–197, 197t
  reproduction in, 170, 171
    management of, 776–777, 805–809, 806t, 807t, 808, 810t, 811t, 814–815
    rate of, 787, 788t, 789t
Piglet, anesthesia in, 68, 68
  blood tests in, reference values for, 920t
  diarrhea in, 111–115
  hypoglycemia in, 119–120
  hypothermia in, 119–120
  immunity in, colostrum and, 97–100, 99
  polyarthritis in, 115–116
  weaning of, 170–172

Piglet (Continued)
  in prevention of pneumonia, 667
Pigmentation, disorders of, 913–914
  and photodermatitis, 905t, 906
Pigweed, toxicity of, 350t, 352
  to kidney, 823t, 825t
Pilocarpine, and gastrointestinal motility, 759, 759t
Pimaricin (natamycin), for dermatophytosis, 892
  for fungal infection, 529
  with mastitis, 527
Pine-tar pitch, toxicity of, 410
Pinkeye. See *Conjunctiva, inflammation of.*
Pinus ponderosa, toxicity of, and abortion, 347
Piperazine, dosage of, 932t
  for elaephoriasis, 841
  in anthelmintic therapy, 50
Piperonyl butoxide, for parasitosis, external, 55t
Pirimiphos-methyl, for parasitosis, external, 55t
Pituitary extract, dosage of, 932t
Pituitary gonadotropin, dosage of, 932t
Pityriasis rosea, in pigs, 909–910
Pizzle rot (posthitis), 798
  in *Corynebacterium renale* infection, 540–541
Placenta, inflammation of, and abortion, in listeriosis, 582, 583
  in chlamydiosis, in cattle, 455
  retention of, 769–770
Plants. See also specific types, e.g., *Alfalfa*.
  teratogenic, 359–361
  toxicity of, after herbicide application, 393
  cyanide in, 367–368
  in harvested and prepared feeds, 343–345, 344t
  in United States, in East and Midwest, 349–352, 350t, 351t
    in West, 345–349
  oxalate accumulation in, 364–365
  selenium accumulation in, 347, 366, 366–367, 367, 367t
  to heart, 352t, 352–354, 353t, 371–372
  to liver, 354t, 354–356, 363, 363t
  to nervous system, 352t, 352–353, 356t, 356–358
  to skin, 361–364, 363t, 905t, 906
Plasma, protein in, in dehydration, 2
  transfusion of, 7
    for shock, 682
Plastridge's medium, for *Trichomonas foetus* culture, 610, 610t
Platelets, disorders of, 698
  laboratory count of, 690, 691, 692t
Pleural friction rub, auscultation of, 675–676
Pleuritis, fibrinous, pleuropneumonia with, 664
  vs. pericarditis, traumatic, 686
Pleuropneumonia, actinobacillosis and, 549–551, 550t
  with fibrinous pleuritis, 664
Pneumocytes, alveolar, 634
Pneumonia, 640–643
  actinobacillosis and, 549–551, 550t, 665, 667, 668t, 669
  arthritis-encephalitis virus and, in goats, 473
  ascariasis and, 666, 668t, 674–675

Pneumonia (Continued)
  aspiration, anesthesia and, 59
    in petroleum toxicity, 407–409
  chlamydial, 456, 654
  dimethyl sulfoxide for, 12
  fibrinous, 653–656
    control of, 660–664
    treatment of, 656–660, 657t–659t
  giant cell, in dermatosis vegetans, 909
  in feedlot cattle, 137–140, 660–662
  in feedlot sheep, 161t, 162, 162
  in influenza, 502
  in lamb, 157–158
  in mycoplasmosis, in cattle, 457, 654
    in goats, 478–479
    in pigs, 504–505
    in sheep, 478–479
  in nocardiosis, 521, 522
  in paramyxovirus infection, 503
  in pigs, 664–669, 665t, 668t, 669t
  interstitial, in purple mint toxicosis, 368–369
  pasteurellosis and, 655, 662, 663, 677
    in cattle, 556–558, 557t
    in pigs, 560
  pathologic reactions in, 635, 637
  progressive, in sheep, 470–471
  respiratory syncytial virus and, 447, 653–654, 660, 661, 663
  serologic tests in, 677–678
  with uveitis, in camelids, 846
Pododermatitis, aseptic, 867–868, 868
  infectious, in feedlot cattle, 140
  interdigital, 869–870
Podophyllin, for papillomatosis, 916
Podophyllum peltatum, toxicity of, 351t
Pokeweed, toxicity of, 351t
Polioencephalomalacia, cerebellar, 859–860
  in goats, 861
  in lamb, 157
  in sheep, 861
  ocular signs of, 854t, 854–856
  vs. Haemophilus somnus infection, 548
Polioencephalomyelitis, 490
Polled Hereford cattle, myoclonus in, 859
Poloxalene, dosage of, 933t
Polyacrylate, in prevention of gastric ulcers, 736
Polyarthritis, chlamydial infection and, 456
  in piglet, 115–116
Polybrominated biphenyls, toxicity of, 403t, 403–404, 404t, 904
Polychlorinated biphenyls, toxicity of, 405–407, 904
Polychromasia, in anemia, 693, 694t
Polycystic kidneys, 821
Polycythemia, 695–696
Polyflex. See Ampicillin.
Polymyxin B, dosage of, 930t, 931t
Polyploidy, and conception failure, 781–782
Polyserositis, in mycoplasmosis, 505
Ponderosa pine, toxicity of, and abortion, 347
Pontocaine (tetracaine), dosage of, 932t
  in regional analgesia, 79t
Porphyria, 910
Posthitis, 540–541, 798
Potassium, blood level of, 920t
  in extracellular fluid, 1
  in replacement therapy, 3, 4, 5t

Potassium (Continued)
  in rumen, in hypomagnesemic tetany, 319
  nutritional requirement for, 201–203, 202t
    in cattle, 251, 252t, 260t
    in pregnancy and lactation, 208
    in pigs, 280t
  supplemental, for grazing cattle, 295, 299t
Potassium aluminum sulfate, for dermatophilosis, 895
Potassium chloride, dosage of, 932t
Potassium iodide, for spirochetosis, 897
Potassium permanganate, dosage of, 932t
Pour-On. See Trichlorfon (Neguvon).
Povidone-iodine, for dermatophytosis, 892
Power plants, cooling waters from, toxicants in, 377–378
Poxvirus infection, in cattle, and mammillitis, 423–425, 424, 424t
  in goats, 459, 459–460
  in pigs, 482–483, 483
  in sheep, 459, 459–460
  of skin, 898–899
Pralidoxime, dosage of, 932t
  for organophosphate toxicity, 382
Praziquantel, in anthelmintic therapy, in llamas, 176t
Preanesthetic drugs, 60–63, 61t
Predef (isoflupredone), dosage of, 931t
  for inflammation, 9t, 11, 11t
Prednisolone/prednisone, dosage of, 932t
  for cholecalciferol toxicity, 385
  for endotoxemia, with lactation failure, 769
  for inflammation, 9t, 10–12, 11t
  for leukosis, bovine, enzootic, 704
  for lymphosarcoma, 850
  for pemphigus foliaceus, 912
  for shock, 683
  for spondylitis, 878
  for urticaria, 901
Pregnancy, in cattle, beef, in large herd management, 126, 126, 126t, 127, 129
  nutrition in, 127, 253, 253t, 257
  dairy, in herd health management, 144–145, 145, 145t
  energy requirement in, 192–194, 193t
  heifer, in dairy replacement programs, 151–152, 152t
  in llamas, 173
  in pigs, 170
    nutrition in, 214–216, 284
  in sheep, 155–159
  listeriosis in, 580, 582, 583
  nutrition in, 204–221
  termination of. See Abortion.
  toxemia in, in cattle, 313t, 314–315
    in sheep, 221, 312–314, 313t
    ocular signs of, 854t, 856
    vs. milk fever, 306
  toxoplasmosis in, 623, 625
  ultrasonography of, 27t, 29
Pregnant mare serum gonadotropin, in estrus management, in goats, 165, 777–778, 805, 813
  in pigs, 776, 811t, 814
  in sheep, 158, 777–778, 805, 813
Prepuce, campylobacteriosis of, 510–512
  disorders of, 796–798
  trichomoniasis of, 608–611, 609

Presponse, in vaccination, against pasteurellosis, 558
Prions, in scrapie, 475–477
Privet, toxicity of, 350t
Probiotics, as feed additives, 187
Procaine, in regional analgesia, 79, 79t, 82
Procaine penicillin. See Penicillin.
Progesterone, dosage of, 932t
  imbalance of, and conception failure, 783
  in estrus management, in pigs, 776
    in sheep, 813
  in growth stimulants, 181t
  in ovarian cysts, 774
Progestins, in estrus management, in cattle, 810, 810t, 811t
  in goats, 813
  in pigs, 814
  in sheep, 811t, 812–813
Progestogens, in estrus management, in sheep, 158
Prolactin, in fescue toxicosis, 371
Prolate (phosmet), for parasitosis, external, 54t, 57t
Promazine, dosage of, 932t
  for tetanus, 568
  preanesthetic, 61t
Prometone, toxicity of, 389t, 392
Prometryn, toxicity of, 389t
Propachlor, toxicity of, 387, 388t
Propanil, toxicity of, 387, 388t
Proparacine, dosage of, 932t
Propazine, toxicity of, 390t
Propiopromazine, dosage of, 932t
  preanesthetic, 61t
Propylene glycol, dosage of, 932t
  for acetonemia, 221, 311, 311t
  for toxemia of pregnancy, 313, 313t, 315
  with ronnel, for demodectic mange, 886
Prostaglandins, dosage of, 932t
  for fetal membrane retention, 770–772
  for ovarian cysts, 775
  for uterine infection, 771–772
  in abortion induction, in cattle, 792, 792t
    in goats, 792, 792t, 814
    in pigs, 793
    in sheep, 792, 792t
  in estrus management, in cattle, 144, 146t, 778–779, 809–810, 810t
    in goats, 777, 805, 814
    in pigs, 776, 814
    in sheep, 158, 777, 805, 813
  in inflammation, 8, 8
  in parturition management, in cattle, 812
    in goats, 805, 814
    in pigs, 814
    in sheep, 805
Protamine sulfate, dosage of, 932t
Protein, blood level of, in assessment of colostrum, 148, 149t
  measurement of, 690, 691, 692t
  reference values for, 921t
  deficiency of, and skin lesions, 911
  digestion of, in nonruminants, 225–226, 232–233
    in ruminants, 226–230, 227, 228t, 229, 229t, 233
  in feed, for pigs, 170, 171
    for stocker calves, 131, 132t
    limitation of, for posthitis, 540
  measurement of, 224–225, 233–234
    computer programs for, 245–246

Protein *(Continued)*
    Cornell system for, 240–244, *241, 242,* 243t
    Iowa State system for, 234–236, *235,* 235t–237t
    Wisconsin system for, 236–240, *238,* 240t, 241t
  metabolism of, in stress, 18
  nutritional requirement for, 196–203, 197t, 201t, 202t
    in cattle, 250–251
      beef, 122, 123t
        for weight gain, 244–245
        in breeding herd, 253t, 258t, 259
        in pregnancy and lactation, 206t, 207, 209
      dairy, 264–268, 265t–267t, 270t, 271t
        in pregnancy and lactation, 210–211, 213, 213t
      in lactation, 198–200
    in goats, 273–278, 274t, 275t
    in pigs, 278–280, 280t
      in pregnancy and lactation, 214, 216
    in sheep, 197–198
      in pregnancy and lactation, 217, 220t
  ratio of, to fibrinogen, in inflammation, 697
  structure of, 224, 232, *232*
  supplementation with, for grazing cattle, 292
Prothrombin time, measurement of, 691, 692t
Protoporphyria, 93
Prototheca species, infection with, 525–527
Protozoal diseases, 584–613, 623–628. See also specific diseases, e.g., *Coccidiosis.*
  of skin, 900
  ruminal, assessment of, 710
Prunus laurocerasus, toxicity of, 368
Prunus species, toxicity of, 351t
Prunus virginiana, toxicity of, 347, 368
Pruritus, in pseudorabies, 423
  in scrapie, 476, *476*
Pseudocowpox, 424t, *425,* 425–426, 898
Pseudohermaphroditism, 97
  in goats, 804
Pseudolumpy skin disease, 899
Pseudorabies, 422–423, *423*
  in pigs, 480–481
  respiratory signs of, 668t
  serologic test for, 678
  ocular signs of, 854t
  skin lesions in, 899
Psorergates mites, skin infestation by, 885
Psoriasiform dermatitis, pustular, 909–910
Psoroptes species, infestation by, 48, 882–883
Pteridium aquilinum, toxicity of, 350t
  to eyes, 854t, 856
  to kidney, 823t
Pudendal nerve, anesthetic block of, 84
Puffer sow syndrome, respiratory signs of, 668t
Pulmonary adenomatosis, 477–478, 637
Pulmonary artery, aneurysm of, 647, 648, *649, 651, 652*
  thromboembolism of, 648
Pulmonary edema, acute, 643–647, *644, 645*
  pathology of, 636–637
Pupils, anatomy of, in llamas, 842–843, *843*

Pupils *(Continued)*
  light reflex of, anatomy of, 852–853, *853*
  examination for, 830–831, 853–854
Purple foxglove (*Digitalis purpurea*), toxicity of, 350t, 353
Purple mint, toxicity of, 350t, 352, 368–369
Pustular dermatitis, psoriasiform, 909–910
  viral, 898–899
Pyelonephritis, in cattle, 817t, 826–827
  in pigs, 817t, 828
Pygmy goats, exfoliative dermatitis in, 913
Pylorus, stenosis of, in vagus indigestion, 730, *731*
Pyometra, 772–773
  in trichomoniasis, 608, 609
Pyrantel, for ascariasis, in prevention of pneumonia, 675
  for nematode infestations, 754, 754t
  in anthelmintic therapy, 50–51
Pyrazon, toxicity of, 390t, 392
Pyrethroids, for external parasitosis, 51, 52, 54t–57t
Pyrilamine maleate, for inflammation, 9t
Pyrogallol, in oak poisoning, 822
Pyrogens, in reticuloruminal motility, 707
Pyrrolizidine alkaloids, toxicity of, 343, 344
  to liver, 347, 350t, 354t, 354–356
Pythiosis, 893

Q fever, 622–623
Quadriceps muscle, in femoral nerve paralysis, 875
Quarter cracks, 865
Quercus species, toxicity of, 348, 351t, 372–374, 373t, *374*
  to kidney, 822–826
Quinapyramine, for trypanosomiasis, 607, 607t
Quinidine, for arrhythmia, 702, 702t
  for atrial fibrillation, 689, 702
Quinoline, derivatives of, for babesiosis, 587t
Quinuronium, for babesiosis, 587t

Rabies, fluorescent antibody test for, 414
  ocular signs of, 854t
  vs. hypomagnesemic tetany, 320
Rabon, for parasitosis, external, 54t, 56t
Ractopamine, as growth stimulant, 188, 188t
Radial immunodiffusion test, for passive immunity, 99
Radial nerve, paralysis of, anesthesia and, 68
Radiation therapy, for ocular squamous cell carcinoma, 848
Radiofrequency current hyperthermia, for ocular squamous cell carcinoma, 849
Radiography, of lung, 676–677
Radius, fracture of, 879
Raging cow disease (spongiform encephalopathy), 454–455, 860
Ragwort, toxicity of, 350t, 352
Rain lily, giant, and photosensitization, 363
Ralgro (zeranol), as growth stimulant, 181, 181t, 182, 183t
  dosage of, 934t

Ralgro (zeranol) *(Continued)*
  residue of, in calf, 35
Ram. See also *Sheep.*
  epididymitis in, 796
  examination of, before breeding, 154, 155, 156t
  fertility of, 804
  penile disorders in, 798
Rangeland, grazing on, forage resources in, 257, 259t, 285–288, *286,* 287t, *288,* 289
  management of, 290–291
  nutrient intake from, 289–290, *290,* 293–294
  selective, 288–289, *289*
  supplementation of, 291–292
    medicated feed additives in, 300–301
  minerals in, 291–302
  toxic plants on, 345–349
Ranunculus species, toxicity of, 351t
Rape plant, toxicity of, 350t
Rattlebox, toxicity of, 350t
Rattlepod (*Crotalaria*), toxicity of, 347, 350t, 351t
Rattlesnake bites, 411–412
  antivenin for, 412, 931t
Ravap, for parasitosis, external, 53t
Rayless goldenrod, toxicity of, 348–349
Rebreathing systems, in anesthesia, 68–69, *69*
Re-Covr, dosage of, 933t
  for inflammation, 9t
Rectovaginal constriction, 97
Rectum, atresia of, 742–743
  examination of, in pregnant cow, 144–145, *145,* 145t
  prolapse of, 741–742
    in lamb, 157
  stricture of, 742
  temperature measurement in, in calves, 180
Red blood cells, decreased level of, *693,* 693–695, 694t–696t
  elevated level of, 695–696
  laboratory count of, 690–692, 692t, 919t, 920t
  production of, 692–693
Red clover, in salivary syndrome, 338–339
Red squill, in rodenticides, toxicity of, 385t, 386
Redroot pigweed, toxicity of, 350t, 352
  to kidney, 823t, 825t
Reflexes, neurophthalmic, blocking of, 834
  examination of, 830–831, 853–854
Refractometry, in test for passive immunity, 99
Regumate, for estrus synchronization, 776
Regurgitation, anesthesia and, 59
  with encephalitis and wasting, 492–493
Rehydration solution, 4–5, 5t
  for toxemia of pregnancy, 313
Reovirus infection, in cattle, 434–435
  in goats, 465
  in pigs, 497
  in sheep, 465
Reproductive system. See *Genitalia.*
Resorb oral rehydration solution, 5t
Respiration, in anesthesia, 58–59
  in spinal analgesia, 80–81
Respiratory syncytial virus, 447
  and pneumonia, 653–654, 660, 661, 663
  serologic test for, 677, 678

INDEX 959

Respiratory tract. See also specific
    structures, e.g., *Trachea.*
  clearance mechanisms of, 653
  coronavirus infection of, 498–500
  diseases of, diagnosis of, 675–678
    in cattle, 653–664
      control of, 660–664
      etiology of, 653–654
      fibrinous pleuritis and pleuropneu-
        monia in, 664
      incidence of, 654–655
      on feedlot, 137–140, 140t
      pathology of, 655–656
      signs of, 655
      treatment of, 656–660, 657t–659t
    in heartwater, 629
    in pigs, 667, 668t
    in sheep, 670t, 670–673
    treatment of, 678–680, 679t
  in influenza, 501–502
  infection of. See also *Pneumonia.*
    adenoviruses in, 430
    chlamydial, 456, 654
    Haemophilus somnus in, 547, 548
    in rhinotracheitis, 418
    reoviruses in, 435
    viral, diagnosis of, 416t
  mycoplasmosis of, 457
  parasitosis of, 673–675
  pasteurellosis of, in cattle, 556–558, 557t
  pathologic reactions of, 635–637
  physiology of, 633–635
  upper, bleeding in, and epistaxis, 638–
    639
    inflammation of, 638–640
    obstruction of, 639, 640
Reticulocytes, in anemia, 693–694
  laboratory testing of, reference values
    for, 919t
Reticulopericarditis, traumatic, 686–687
Reticuloperitonitis, traumatic, 719–722,
    735
Reticulum, motility of, 706–709, 707
Retina, anatomy of, in camelids, 843, 843
  diseases of, 839, 841, 854t, 855–856
    in camelids, 845, 846
Retrobulbar space, aspiration from, in
    ocular examination, 833
  ultrasonography of, 27t, 29
Retropharynx, abscess of, traumatic, 713,
    714
  diseases of, 714–718, 715
Revive oral rehydration solution, 5t
Revivon, in capture of ruminants, 63
Rheum raponticum, toxicity of, 351t
Rhinitis, 638
  atrophic, progressive, pasteurellosis
    and, 559–560
  inclusion body, 481–482
Rhinosporidiosis, 525, 638, 639
Rhinotracheitis, infectious, 417–419
  and conjunctivitis, 837
  and keratoconjunctivitis, in goats, 841
  and pneumonia, 653–654, 660–663
  serologic test for, 677
  skin lesions with, 899
  vaccination against, in prevention of
    pasteurellosis, 558
  vs. keratoconjunctivitis, 835
Rhinoviruses, 437
Rhipicephalus ticks. See *Ticks.*
Rhizoctonia species, toxicity of, in salivary
    syndrome, 338, 338–339, 339
Rhododendron, toxicity of, 350t

Rhubarb, toxicity of, 351t
Rib eye, ultrasonography of, 27t, 29
Riboflavin, nutritional requirement for, in
    pigs, 280t, 282
  in pregnancy and lactation, 215
Ribs, fracture of, 879
Ricinus communis, toxicity of, 351t
Rickettsia conjunctivae infection, and
    keratoconjunctivitis, 840–841
Rickettsial diseases, 613–623, 628–632. See
    also specific diseases, e.g.,
    Ehrlichiosis.
Rifamycin, for heartwater, 631
Rift Valley fever, in cattle, 441t, 441–442
  in sheep and goats, 469–470
Rinderpest, 444–446
  skin lesions in, 899
Ringer's solution, for vagus indigestion,
    731
Ripercol. See *Levamisole.*
Rivanol precipitation test, for brucellosis,
    553
Robaxin, dosage of, 932t
Robinia pseudoacacia, toxicity of, 351t
Rodenticides, toxicity of, 383–386, 384t, 385t
Romney Marsh disease, 574
Romney sheep, congenital cataracts in, 93
Rompun. See *Xylazine.*
Ronnel, for demodectic mange, 886
Roridin A, toxicity of, 332, 333
Rose bengal test, for brucellosis, 553, 553
Rotavirus infection, and diarrhea, in
    neonatal ruminants, 104–105
  in piglet, 112–114
  in cattle, 439–440
  in pigs, 497–498
  in sheep, 467–468
Roundworms. See *Nematode infestation.*
Roxarsone (3-nitro-4-hydroxy
    phenylarsonic acid), for
    eperythrozoonosis, 616
  toxicity of, 395–396
RU 38.486, in abortion induction, 793
Rubberweed, toxicity of, 349
Rumatel, for nematode infestation, 748t
  in anthelmintic therapy, 50
Rumen, bloat in, 717–718
  function of, assessment of, 709–710
  in indigestion, 710–711
    vagus, 730
  inflammation of, 716–717
  lactic acidosis in, 714–716, 715
  motility of, 706–709, 707
  protein metabolism in, measurement of,
    in Cornell system, 240–244, 241,
    242
  in Wisconsin system, 236–239
  protein synthesis in, 225
Rumensin. See *Monensin.*
Rumex crispus, toxicity of, to kidney, 824t
Rumex species, toxicity of, 351t, 364
Ruminants. See specific animals, e.g.,
    Cattle.
Rumination, physiology of, 708
Rusterholz ulcer, 866–867
Rye, toxicity of, 351t
Ryegrass, toxicity of, 357, 860

Safe-Guard. See *Fenbendazole.*
Saffan, dosage of, 932t
  in anesthesia, 67

St. Johnswort, and photosensitization,
    350t, 362
Salinomycin, toxicity of, 329–330
Salivation, drugs affecting, 760t
  excessive, mycotoxicosis and, 338, 338–
    339, 339
  in anesthesia, 60
Salmonellosis, 562–565
  and diarrhea, in neonatal ruminants,
    108–109
Salt. See also specific elements, e.g.,
    Sodium.
  in water supply, 375, 375t
Sambucus canadensis, toxicity of, 351t
Samore (trypanosomiasis), 604t, 604–607,
    607t
  of skin, 900
Samorin, for trypanosomiasis, 606–607,
    607t
Saponaria species, toxicity of, 351t
Sarcobatus vermiculatus (greasewood),
    toxicity of, 347, 364
  in sheep, 221
  to kidney, 824t
Sarcocystosis, 625–627, 626, 626t
  of skin, 900
Sarcoptes scabiei infestation, 48, 49, 883–884
Sarsaponin, as feed additive, 187
Satratoxin, 340
Scabies, 48, 49, 883–884
Scarlet drench powder, dosage of, 932t
Schirmer test, 832
  in llama, 843, 844
Schistocytes, 694t
Schistosomia, 96
Sciatic nerve, in downer cow syndrome,
    322
Scilliroside, in rodenticides, toxicity of,
    385t, 386
Scintigraphy, in respiratory disease, 677
Scleroderma, in besnoitiosis, 597, 597, 598
Scorpion stings, 411t, 412
Scours. See *Diarrhea.*
Scrambled eggs plant, toxicity of, 350t
Scrapie, 475–477, 476
  ocular signs of, 841, 854t
  skin lesions in, 900
Screwworm infestation, of skin, 889
  parasiticides for, 51–58, 52t, 53t, 56t, 57t
Scrotum, congenital defects of, 96
  diseases of, 794–796
  ultrasonography of, 27t, 29
Seborrhea, 912–913
  nutritional deficiencies and, 911
Secale cereale, toxicity of, 351t
Sedatives, in capture of ruminants, 62–63
  preanesthetic, 60–62, 61t
Segmental aplasia, of wolffian duct, 96–97
Seizures, strychnine poisoning and, 385–
    386
Selenium, blood level of, in sheep, 154
  deficiency of, in white muscle disease,
    154, 164, 689–690
  skin lesions in, 911
  dietary, for llamas, 175, 175t
  dosage of, 932t, 933t
  for ear necrosis, 903
  in water supply, 376, 376t
  injection of, in pregnant goat, 164
  nutritional requirement for, in cattle,
    251, 252t, 260t
    beef, in pregnancy and lactation,
      208, 208t
    dairy, 268, 270t

Selenium *(Continued)*
   in pigs, 280t, 281
      in pregnancy and lactation, 215
   in sheep, in pregnancy and lactation, 218
   supplemental, for grazing cattle, 296t, 297, 299t
   toxicity of, and fetal malformations, in sheep, 839
      plant accumulation in, 347, 366, 366–367, 367, 367t
      to skin, 904
Semen, artificial instillation of. See *Insemination, artificial*.
Seminal vesicle, inflammation of, 793–794
   in chlamydiosis, 455–456
Senecio species, toxicity of, 343, 344, 347, 350t, 351t, 352
Senna, and gastrointestinal motility, 759, 759t
   toxicity of, 350t
Septicemia, and arthritis, 873–874
   and meningitis, 861
   in actinobacillosis, 535
   in *Escherichia coli* infection, 517, 518
   in *Haemophilus somnus* infection, 547
   in mycoplasmosis, 479
   in nocardiosis, 521
   in pasteurellosis, 555–556
   in salmonellosis, 562–563
Serpula hyodysenteriae infection, in pigs, 560–562, 561t
Serum, constituents of, 920t
   enzyme activity in, 920t
Sesbania species, toxicity of, 350t
Setaria sphacelata, toxicity of, 364, 365
Sevarin, as feed additive, 187
Shaker calves, 92
Shearing, before lambing, 156
Sheep, abortion in, induced, 792, 792t
   blood tests in, normal values for, 919t–921t
   disorders in. See specific disorders, e.g., *Border disease*, and affected structures, e.g., *Foot*.
   herd health management in, 153–159, 154t–156t
   on feedlot, 159t–161t, 159–162, 161, 162
   neonatal. See *Lamb*.
   nutrition in, energy requirement in, 194–195
      in pregnancy and lactation, 216–221, 220
      protein requirement in, 197–198
   reproduction in, management of, 158–159, 777–778, 803–805, 810t, 811t, 812–813
      rate of, 787, 788t, 789t
Sheeppox, 459, 459–460, 898
Shipping fever, antibiotics for, as feed additives, 187t
   in stocker calves, 131, 133–134
Shock, after insect bites, 413
   circulatory, 682t, 682–683, 683t
   drug disposition in, 25
   endotoxic, 7, 7t
   steroids for, 9t, 11, 683
Silage, heat damage to, 341–343
   Listeria contamination of, 580–583, 581, 583t
   mold damage to, 341–343
Silicate, in urolithiasis, 819
Silvex, toxicity of, 391t

Simazine, toxicity of, 390t, 392
Single radial immunodiffusion test, for passive immunity, 99
Sinusitis, 639
Skeleton, congenital defects of, 94
   lupine and, 346
Skin, aplasia of, 909
   appendages of, disorders of, 914–915
   bacterial infection of, 894–898
   besnoitiosis of, 596–598, 597, 598, 900
   congenital defects of, 95, 907–910, 908t
   cysts of, 910, 918
   endocrine disorders of, 912
   farrowing house disorders of, 913
   folliculitis of, eosinophilic, 915
   fungal infection of, 890–894, 891t, 892t
   hypoplasia of, focal, 909
   immune disorders of, 900–901
   in dermatophilosis, 522–524, 894–895
   inflammation of. See *Dermatitis*.
   interdigital fibroma of, 871–872
   lumpy, viral infection and, 427–429, 428, 429, 900
   necrosis of, in pigs, 903
   nodules of, in mammillitis, 420
   nutritional disorders of, 911–912
   parasitosis of, helminths in, 889–890
      keds in, 887–888
      lice in, 886–887
      maggots in, 888–889
      mites and, 882–886
   photodermatitis of, 904–906, 905t
   pigmentation disorders of, 913–914
   plant toxicity in, 361–364, 363t, 905t, 906
      and photosensitization, 354t, 355, 362–363, 363t
   protozoal diseases of, 900
   seborrhea of, 911–913
   staphylococcosis of, 578–579, 895–896
   swine pox of, 482, 483
   toxicosis of, chemical, 904
   trauma to, 901–902
      plants and, 361–362
      thermal, 902–903
   tumors of, 910, 915–918, 916t
   viral infection of, 898–900
      diagnosis of, 416t
   zootoxicoses of, 906
Slaframine (slobber factor), in salivary syndrome, in mycotoxicosis, 338, 338–339, 339
Smallpox, vaccination against, as source of bovine vaccinia, 424
SMEDI syndrome, 493
Snakebite, 411t, 411–412, 906
   antivenin for, 412, 930t
Snakeroot, toxicity of, 349, 350t
Sneezeweed, toxicity of, 349, 350t, 351t, 352
Snout, atrophy of, in pasteurellosis, 559–560
Sodaphos (sodium acid phosphate), for downer cow syndrome, 323
   for hemoglobinuria, postparturient, 325t
Sodium, blood level of, reference values for, 920t
   deficiency of, vs. hypomagnesemic tetany, 320
   for cardiotoxic plant poisoning, 354
   in extracellular fluid, 1
   in replacement therapy, 2–4, 5t
   nutritional requirement for, 200, 202
      in cattle, 251, 252t, 260t, 270t

Sodium *(Continued)*
   beef, in pregnancy and lactation, 207, 208t, 209, 210
   dairy, in pregnancy and lactation, 212, 213, 213t, 214t
   in pigs, 279, 280t
      in pregnancy and lactation, 215
   in sheep, in pregnancy and lactation, 218
   supplemental, for grazing cattle, 295
   toxicity of, 328–329
Sodium acetate phosphate, dosage of, 932t
Sodium acid phosphate, for downer cow syndrome, 323
   for hemoglobinuria, postparturient, 325t
Sodium arsanilate, for dysentery, in pigs, 561t
Sodium bicarbonate (baking soda), and cerebrospinal fluid acidosis, 3
   and esophageal groove closure, 708
   dosage of, 932t
   for acidosis, in listeriosis, 862
      lactic, 716
   for zinc phosphide toxicity, 386
   in replacement therapy, 3, 4, 5t
Sodium cephapirin, dosage of, 931t
Sodium chloride, for hypovolemia, in anemia, 699
   for shock, 683
Sodium formaldehyde sulfoxylate, dosage of, 932t
Sodium hypochlorite, for dermatophytosis, 892
Sodium iodide, for dermatophytosis, 892
Sodium nitrate, dosage of, 932t
Sodium polyacrylate, in prevention of gastric ulcers, 736
Sodium selenite, for ear necrosis, 903
Sodium sulfate, and gastrointestinal motility, 759t, 760
   dosage of, 932t
   for oak toxicity, 374
Sodium sulfite precipitation test, for passive immunity, 99, 99
Sodium thiosulfate, dosage of, 932t
   for arsenic toxicosis, 395
   for cyanide poisoning, 368
Soframycin, dosage of, 932t
Solanum species, toxicity of, 351t
   and cerebellar degeneration, 859
Sole, abscess of, 864–865
   ulcer of, Rusterholz, 866–867
Solenopotes lice, skin infestation by, 887
Solenopsis species, stings of, 412t, 412–413
Solu-Delta-Cortef. See *Prednisolone/ prednisone*.
Somatotropin, 42–46, 43, 44, 188
   in response to estrogen, 181
Sonography, diagnostic, 26–29, 27t, 28
   of heart, 27, 27t, 686
Sorbitol dehydrogenase, blood level of, 920t
Soremouth, vaccination against, in goats, 164
Sorghum, toxicity of, 368
   after herbicide application, 393
Soursob, toxicity of, 364
Sow. See *Pig(s)*.
Soybeans, antitrypsin factors in, 225–226
   nutrients in, in dairy cattle feed, 212, 213t, 214t
   protein in, 196–197, 197t, 245t–247t, 245–246

INDEX □ **961**

Soybeans *(Continued)*
  in dairy cattle feed, 266, 266t, 267t
  metabolism of, 228t, 229t, 235t, 236t, 239, 240, 243, 243t
Spanbolet. See *Sulfamethazine.*
Spanish goats, herd management of, 163–166
Sparine (promazine), dosage of, 933t
  preanesthetic, 61t
Spasticity, congenital defects and, 92–93
Spectinomycin (Spectam), dosage of, 932t
  for pneumonia, in cattle, 658t, 660
Sperm, defects of, and conception failure, 781–783
  in testicular degeneration, 795
Spherocytes, 694t
Spider bites, 411t, 412
Spinal cord, anatomy of, 77–79, *78*, 78t
  congenital defects of, 93
  in analgesia induction, 79–83, *81–84*
  inflammatory disease of, 863
Spine, anatomy of, 77, *78*, 82, *82–84*, 83
  congenital defects of, 94
  inflammation of, 877–878
Spiramycin, dosage of, 932t
Spirochetosis, 897
Spondylitis, 877–878
Spongiform encephalopathy, 454–455, 860
Spot-On Insecticide, for tick-borne fever, 621, 621t
Spotton (fenthion), dosage of, 931t
  for lice, in llamas, 177
  for parasitosis, external, 52, 53t
Spurge, toxicity of, 350t
Squamous cell carcinoma, ocular, 847t, 847–850, 850t
  of skin, 917
Stachybotryotoxicosis, 340–341
  skin lesions in, 906
Stagger grass, toxicity of, 350t
Staggers, in selenium poisoning, 366, 367
  Phalaris species and, 860
  ryegrass ingestion and, 357, 860
Stanchion trauma, ocular, in cattle, 854t, 855
Stanozolol, for anemia, 701
Staphylococcal infection, 578–579
  and mastitis, 763, 765, 765t, 766t
  and polyarthritis, 116
  of skin, 895–896
Starvation, 911
Steer-oid, as growth stimulant, 181t
Stenton's medium, for *Trichomonas foetus* culture, 610, 610t
Stephanofilariasis, of skin, 890
Stephanurus infestation, 49, 50
  in pigs, 752–754, 754t
Sterne strain anthrax vaccine, 566t, 566–567
Steroids. See also specific drugs, e.g., *Dexamethasone.*
  anabolic, for anemia, 701
    in growth stimulation, 181t, 181–183, 184t, 294
  contraindication to, in bronchopneumonia, 419
  effect of, on leukocytes, 697
  for acetonemia, 311, 311t
  for anaphylaxis, 684
  for aspiration pneumonia, in petroleum toxicity, 409
  for *Haemophilus somnus* infection, 548
  for hemoglobinuria, postparturient, 325, 325t

Steroids *(Continued)*
  for inflammation, 9t, 10–12, 11t
  for keratoconjunctivitis, 836
  for laminitis, aseptic, 868
  for pneumonia, 643
  for rhinitis, allergic, 638
  for shock, 9t, 11, 683
  for toxemia of pregnancy, 313, 313t, 315
  for urticaria, 901
  in induced abortion, in cattle, 811, 811t
  in induction of parturition, in cattle, 811, 811t
  in respiratory therapy, 678, 679t, 680
Stibophen, for elaephoriasis, 841
Stifle, injury of, 874–876
Stillbirth, enteroviral infection and, 493
  in pigs, 807t
  leptospirosis and, 543, 544
Stings, 411t, 412t, 412–413
Stirofos, for parasitosis, 53t, 54t, 56t
Stocker calves, management of, 130–134, 132t, *133*, *134*
Stomach, ulceration of, in pigs, 735–736
Stomatitis, in foot-and-mouth disease, 438, *438*
  in goats, 464, *464*
  in pigs, *494*, 494–495
  in sheep, 464, *464*
  papular, *426*, 426–427, *427*
    bovine, 898
  vesicular, viral, 899
    in cattle, 447–448
    in pigs, 504
Strabismus, 854–855
Strawberry foot rot, 522
Streptococcal infection, 575–578
  and mastitis, 763, 765, 765t, 766t
  and meningitis, 861
  and polyarthritis, 115–116
Streptococcus faecium, as feed additives, 187
Streptomycin, dosage of, 932t
  for campylobacteriosis, 512, 513, 785
  for dermatophilosis, 523, 895
  for leptospirosis, 545
  in embryo transfer, 786
Stresnil, preanesthetic, 61t
Stress, and metabolic changes, 16–19
  in calves, nutrition in, 178–180, 179t
    feed additives in, 187–188
  in pigs, respiratory signs of, 668t
  in respiratory disease, in cattle, 654
  in sheep, 671
Strongyloides infestation, 48–50
  in pigs, 752–754, 754t
Struck disease, 574
Strychnine, toxicity of, 384t, 385t, 385–386
Stypandra imbricata, toxicity of, to eyes, 854t, 856
Subarachnoid space, anatomy of, 77, *78*
  injection into, for analgesia, 80–83, *82*
Subconjunctival injection, 834
Subestrus, in cattle, 810–811
Succinylcholine, and hyperthermia, malignant, 74
Sulbactam, for pneumonia, in pasteurellosis, 557t
Sulfabromomethazine, dosage of, 932t
Sulfachlorpyrazine, dosage of, 932t
  for coccidiosis, 602
Sulfachlorpyridazine, dosage of, 932t
Sulfadiazine, for pneumonia, in cattle, 656–657
Sulfadimethoxine (Albon), dosage of, 932t
  for coccidiosis, in llamas, 176, 176t

Sulfadimethoxine (Albon) *(Continued)*
  for pneumonia, 657t
  residues of, tests for, 32t
Sulfadimidine. See *Sulfamethazine.*
Sulfadoxine, for nephritis, in *Corynebacterium renale* infection, 539
  for pneumonia, in pasteurellosis, 557, 557t
Sulfaethoxypyridazine, dosage of, 932t
Sulfaguanidine, for coccidiosis, 602, 603t
Sulfa-Lite, dosage of, 932t
Sulfamethazine, as feed additive, 187t
  dosage of, 932t
  for coccidiosis, 602, 603t
  for keratoconjunctivitis, 836, 837
  for phlegmon, interdigital, 870
  for pneumonia, 657t
    chlamydial, 456
  in prevention of pasteurellosis, 558
  residues of, 32t, 35
Sulfamethoxazole, for *Actinobacillus* pleuropneumonia, in pigs, 550t
Sulfa-on-Site test, 31, 31t, 32t
Sulfaquinoxaline, for coccidiosis, 602, 603t
Sulfathiazole, for phlegmon, interdigital, 870
  residues of, test for, 32t
Sulfisoxazole, dosage of, 932t
Sulfonamides, for coccidiosis, 602, 603t
  for keratoconjunctivitis, 836
  for mastitis, 767t
  for omphalitis, 102t
  for pneumonia, 643
    in cattle, 656–657, 657t
  nephrotoxicity of, 818–819
  residues of, in pigs, 35
  tests for, 31, 31t, 32t
Sulfur, in copper metabolism, 396–397
  nutritional requirement for, in cattle, 251, 252t, 260t
    beef, in pregnancy and lactation, 208, 208t
    dairy, 268, 270t
  in sheep, in pregnancy and lactation, 218
  supplemental, for grazing cattle, 296, 299t
Sunburn, 904
Suramin, for trypanosomiasis, 607, 607t
Surfactants, for gastrointestinal disorders, 761
Surital, dosage of, 932t
  in anesthesia, 64–65
Surra (trypanosomiasis), 604t, 604–607, 607t
  of skin, 900
Swab Test on Premises, 31, 31t
Swainsonine, in salivary syndrome, 338, *338*
  toxicity of, to cerebellum, 860
Swayback, in copper deficiency, 397
Sweet clover, toxicity of, 358–359
Sweet shrub, toxicity of, 350t
Swine. See *Pig(s), Piglet,* and specific disorders, e.g., *Mycoplasmosis.*
Swine fever, African, 486–488, *487*, *488*
  respiratory signs of, 668t
  skin lesions in, 899
Swine pox infection, 482–483, *483*
  of skin, 898
Syncro-Mate B. See *Norgestomet.*
Syndactyly, 94

Synovex, as growth stimulant, 181t, 182, 183t
  dosage of, 932t
Synovial fluid, in septic arthritis, 873–874
Synovitis, of stifle, 876

T-2 toxin, 332–334
T lymphocytes. See *Lymphocytes*.
Tabosa grass, in *Claviceps* toxicity, cerebellar, 860
Taenia species, infestation by, 758
  cerebellar, 859
Tailings, from mines, toxicants in, 377–380, *378*, 378t
Talfan disease, 490
Tannic acid, dosage of, 932t
Tannin, in oak poisoning, 372–374, 822–824
Tapeworm infestations, 757–758
Taractan, dosage of, 932t
  preanesthetic, 61t
Tarsal bones, fracture of, 879
Tarsorrhaphy, 834
Tassels, 910
Taxus species, toxicity of, 350t, 353, 371–372
Tears, deficiency of, and conjunctivitis, 832
  Schirmer test of, in llama, *843*, 844
Teat, analgesia of, 86
  inflammation of. See *Mammillitis* and *Mastitis*.
  ultrasonography of, 27t, 29
Teeth, fluorosis of, 399, 400, *400*
  geothermal water and, 379, *379*
  of llamas, cutting of, 175
Telazol, in anesthesia, 67
  in capture of ruminants, 63
Telmin, in anthelmintic therapy, in llamas, 176t
Telogen, defluxion in, 915
Temperature, and cold exposure, in calves, 116–118
  in goats, 166
  in lambs, 156
  and feed damage, 341–343
  and frostbite, 902–903
  and pneumonia, 666
  and respiratory disorders, in pigs, 668t
  in sheep, 671
  and skin injury, 902–903
  effect of, on fertility, 783
  Fahrenheit to Centigrade conversion of, 934t
  in stocker calves, 131, 133–134
  of scrotum, 794, 795
  rectal, in calves, 180
  regulation of, 116–117
  Weather Safety Index of, 124, 124t
Tendons, trauma to, 880–881
Tenesmus, in vaginitis, 773
Teratogen(s), bluetongue virus as, in cattle, 436
  border disease virus as, 463
  Cache Valley virus as, 474–475, *475*
  in sheep, 839
  lupine as, 346, 360, 361
  plants as, 359–361
Terbufos, toxicity of, 382t
Terminator. See *Diazinon*.
Terramycin. See *Oxytetracycline*.
Teschen disease, 490–491

Testes, disorders of, 794, 795
  hypoplasia of, 96
  ultrasonography of, 27t, 29
Testosterone, for anemia, 701
  in growth stimulants, 181t
  in treatment of posthitis, 540–541
Tetanus, 567–568
  ocular signs of, 854t
  prevention of, in goats, 164
    with dehorning, 861
  in llamas, 174
Tetany, grass diet and, 212
  hypomagnesemia and, 318–321
  transportation and, in lambs, 160
Tetracaine, dosage of, 932t
  in regional analgesia, 79t
Tetrachlorvinphos, for parasitosis, external, 53t, 54t, 56t
Tetracycline. See also *Chlortetracycline* and *Oxytetracycline*.
  dosage of, 932t
  for abortion induction, 791
  for anaplasmosis, 592–593, 593t
  for bacillary hemoglobinuria, 571
  for chlamydiosis, 456, 457
  for clostridial infection, 897
  for dermatitis, digital, 869
  for ehrlichiosis, 617, 617t
  for enteropathy, proliferative, in campylobacteriosis, 514, 515
  for eperythrozoonosis, 616
  for *Eubacterium suis* infection, 520
  for *Haemophilus somnus* infection, 549
  for leptospirosis, 545
  for listeriosis, 862
  for mycoplasmosis, 458
  for petechial fever, 619t, 620
  for polyarthritis, 116
  for tick-borne fever, 621
  for uterine infection, 771
  in prevention of bloat, 718
  nephrotoxicity of, 819
  residues of, test for, 32t
Tetradymia species, toxicity of, 348, 355
Tetrahydropyrimidines, in anthelmintic therapy, 50–51
Thallium, toxicity of, to skin, 904
Thallium sulfate, in rodenticides, toxicity of, 386
Theileriosis, 627–628
  of skin, 900
Thelaziasis, ocular, in camelids, 845
  in cattle, 838–839
Theophylline, for heart failure, 704
Therabloat, dosage of, 932t
Thermal injury, of skin, 902–903
Thiabendazole, dosage of, 932t
  for dermatophytosis, 892
  for nematode infestation, in cattle, 748t
    in goats, 751, 752
    in pigs, 754t
    in sheep, 751–752
  for rumenitis, 717
  in anthelmintic therapy, 49–50
  in llamas, 176t
Thiamine, deficiency of, in lamb, 157
  dosage of, 932t
  for bovine bonkers syndrome, 327
  for polioencephalomalacia, 859–861
  nutritional requirement for, in cattle, 252
  in pigs, 280t
Thiamylal, dosage of, 932t
  in anesthesia, 64–65

Thimble toe, 865–866
Thimet, toxicity of, 381, 382t
Thiobarbiturates, in anesthesia, 64, 64–65
Thiocarbamates, in herbicides, toxicity of, 389t, 391
Thiopental, in anesthesia, 64–65
Thiosulfate, for cyanide toxicity, 368
Thlaspi arvense, toxicity of, 351t
Thomson's gazelle, petechial fever in, 619
Thoracocentesis, for pleural effusion, 678
  in respiratory disease, 676
Thorax, ultrasonography of, 27t, 27–28, *28*
Thorazine (chlorpromazine), and gastrointestinal secretion, 761
  dosage of, 930t
  preanesthetic, 61t
Thornapple, toxicity of, 350t
Thraxol-2 vaccine, against anthrax, 566t, 566–567
Threadworm (*Strongyloides ransomi*) infestation, 49–50, 752–754, 754t
Threonine, dietary, for pigs, 279, 280t
Thrombopathies, 698
Thrombocytopenia, 698
Thrombocytosis, 698
Thromboembolism, pulmonary, with vena caval thrombosis, 648
  with meningoencephalitis, in *Haemophilus somnus* infection, 546–549, *547*
  in pneumonia, 662, 664
  ocular signs of, 838, 854t, 856
Thrombophlebitis, treatment of, 701–702
Thromboplastin time, partial, measurement of, 691, 692t
Thrombosis, vena caval, 647–648, *649*–*652*
Thumps, 674–675
Thyrocalcitonin, in milk fever, 305
Thyroid, enlargement of, hereditary, 910
  hypofunction of, and skin lesions, 912
  hereditary, 910
  in border disease, 463
  iodine deficiency and, in pigs, 280
Thysanosoma species, infestation by, 757–758
Tiamulin, for *Actinobacillus* pleuropneumonia, 550t
  for dysentery, 561t
  for pasteurellosis, 560
  for polyarthritis, 116
Tibia, displacement of, in ligament injury, 875
  fracture of, 879
Tick-borne fever, 620, 620–621, 621t
Ticks, *Amblyomma variegatum*, and immunosuppression, dermatophilosis with, 523, 524
  as vectors, in epizootic bovine abortion, 455
  of African swine fever, 486
  of anaplasmosis, 588, 593–595
  of babesiosis, 584–587
  of borreliosis, 515, 516
  of ehrlichiosis, 616–618
    in tick-borne fever, 620–621
  of heartwater, 628, 629, 632
  of Nairobi sheep disease, 468
  of Q fever, 622
  of theileriosis, 627, 628
  external parasiticides for, 51–58, 52t–57t
  Hyalomma, toxicity of, to skin, 906
  in llamas, 177
Tiguvon (fenthion), dosage of, 932t
  for lice, in llamas, 177
  for parasitosis, external, 53t, 57t

Tiletamine, in anesthesia, 67
    in capture of ruminants, 63
Tilmicosin, for pneumonia, in pasteurellosis, 557, 557t
Timber milkvetch, toxicity of, 348
Timothy, protein in, metabolism of, 243t
Tobacco, as teratogen, 360, 361
    toxicity of, 351t, 358
Togavirus infection, skin lesions in, 899
Tolazoline, as antagonist to xylazine sedation, 62
Toltrazuril, for coccidiosis, 602, 603t
Tomahawk, for parasitosis, external, 55t
Tomanol, for ephemeral fever, 449
Tomato, toxicity of, 350t
Tongue, smooth, congenital, 96
Tonometry, in ocular examination, 832
Tonsils, physiology of, 633
Torovirus infection, 451–452
Toxaphene, in water supply, 376t
Toxemia, engorgement, 714–716, 715
    enteric. See *Enterotoxemia.*
    of pregnancy, in cattle, 313t, 314–315
        in sheep, 221, 312–314, 313t
            ocular signs of, 854t, 856
            vs. milk fever, 306
Toxoplasmosis, 623–625, 624
    ocular signs of, 841–842, 854t
Trachea, aspiration of, diagnostic, 676, 677
    inflammation of, 636, 639–640
    intubation of, for anesthesia, 70–72, 71, 71t, 73, 74
    obstruction of, 640
        prevention of, 679t, 679–680
    physiology of, 633–634
Tramisol. See *Levamisole.*
Tranquilizers, preanesthetic, 60, 61t
Transaminase, glutamic-oxaloacetic, blood level of, 920t
Transfusion, 6–7
    for hypogammaglobulinemia, 13
    for shock, 682
    in anemia, 699–700
Transmissible gastroenteritis virus, in piglets, 112–115
    in pigs, 498–500
Tranvet, dosage of, 932t
    preanesthetic, 61t
Trauma, and coxofemoral luxation, 876–877
    and fractures, 878–880
    and pericarditis, 686–687
    and reticuloperitonitis, 719–722, 735
    cerebellar, 859
    in cattle, on feedlot, 140
    penile, in boar, 797–798
        in bull, 796–797
    stanchion, ocular, in cattle, 854t, 855
    to pharynx, 713–714
    to skin, thermal, 902–903
    to stifle, 874–876
    to tendons, 880–881
Trees, toxins in, 351t
    in oak, 348, 351t, 372–374, 373t, 374
    in yew, 350t, 353, 371–372
Trematode infestations, 755–757, 757t
Trenbolone, as growth stimulant, 181t, 182–183, 184t
    dosage of, 931t
    for acetonemia, 311t
    for toxemia of pregnancy, 313, 313t, 315
Treponema hyodysenteriae infection, 560–562, 561t

Trexel sheep, ocular congenital defects in, 839
Triallate, toxicity of, 389t, 391
Triamcinolone, dosage of, 932t
    for acetonemia, 311t
    for inflammation, 11t
    in induction of parturition, in cattle, 811, 811t
Triazines, in herbicides, toxicity of, 389t–390t, 391–392
Triazoles, in herbicides, toxicity of, 390t, 392
Tribrissen, dosage of, 933t
Tricarboxylic acid cycle, in acetonemia, 310, *310*
Trichloracetate, in herbicides, toxicity of, 387, 388t
Trichlorfon (Neguvon), dosage of, 932t
    for mange, chorioptic, 885
        demodectic, 886
    for parasitosis, external, 54t
2,3,6-Trichlorobenzoic acid, toxicity of, 387, 388t
Trichlorobenzyl chloride, in herbicides, toxicity of, 387, 388t
Trichomoniasis, and infertility, 785, 800
    in cattle, 608, 608–612, 609, 610t, *611*
Trichophyton species, skin infection by, 890–892, 891t, 892t
Trichostrongyliasis, 47–50
    in cattle, 743–748, 746t–748t
    in sheep, 749–752
Trichothecene, toxicity of, 332–334, 340–341
Trichuris suis infestation, 47–50, 752–754, 754t
Triclabendazole, for fluke infestation, 757, 757t
Triclopyr, toxicity of, 390t, 392–393
Triflupromazine, preanesthetic, 61t
Trifluralin, toxicity of, 388t, 391
Trifolium pratense, in salivary syndrome, 338–339
Trifolium species, toxicity of, 351t
Trigeminal nerve, anatomy of, 852
    in palpebral reflex, 830
Triglochon species, cyanide in, 344, 347
Trimethoprim, for *Actinobacillus* pleuropneumonia, 550
    for nephritis, in *Corynebacterium renale* infection, 539
    for pneumonia, 656–657
        in pasteurellosis, 557, 557t
Tripelennamine, dosage of, 933t
    for inflammation, 9t
Triticum aestivum (wheat), protein in, metabolism of, 235t, 243t
    toxicity of, 351t
Trochlear nerve, anatomy of, 852
Trombiculidiasis, 886
Tropicamide, dosage of, 933t
    in ocular examination, in llama, 843–844
Trypamidium, for trypanosomiasis, 606–607, 607t
Trypan blue, for babesiosis, 587t
Trypanosomiasis, 604t, 604–607, 607t
    of skin, 900
Trypsin, in embryo transfer, 787
    inhibition of, in protein digestion, 225–226
Tryptamine alkaloid, toxicity of, and staggers, 860
Tryptophan, dietary, for pigs, 279, 280t
    in pulmonary edema, 643, *644*, 646

Tsetse fly, as vector, of trypanosomiasis, 604, 605, 607
Tuberculosis, in cattle, 531–533, 533t
    in pigs, 529–531
Tumor necrosis factor, metabolic effects of, 18–19
Tumors, cerebellar, 859
    ocular, 846–851, 847t, 850t
        examination of, 833
    of skin, 910, 915–918, 916t
Tunica vaginalis, inflammation of, 795
Turkeys, monensin toxicity in, 330
Twin pregnancy, and toxemia, 312, 313
Tying up syndrome, of horses, vs. lathyrism, 345
Tylosin, as feed additive, 184–186
    dosage of, 933t
    for dysentery, 561, 561t
    for ear necrosis, 903
    for erysipelas, 580
    for mastitis, 767t
    for pneumonia, 658t, 659t, 660
    for polyarthritis, 116
    for staphylococcal infection, in exudative epidermitis, 896
    residues of, test for, 32t
Tympany. See *Bloat.*
Typhlectomy, for cecal necrosis, in volvulus, 740

Udder, analgesia of, 86, *86*
    inflammation of. See *Mastitis.*
    ultrasonography of, 27t, 29
Ulcer(s), abomasal, 708, 735
    gastric, in pigs, 735–736
    in posthitis, in *Corynebacterium renale* infection, 540
    of cornea, in camelids, 844, 845
    in conjunctivitis, 835, 837
    Rusterholz, 866–867
Ulcerative dermatosis, viral, 899
Ulcerative lymphangitis, *Corynebacterium pseudotuberculosis* infection and, 538–539
Ultrasonography, diagnostic, 26–29, 27t, 28
    of heart, 27, 27t, 686
Ultraviolet light, and dermatitis, 904–906, 905t
Umbilical arteries, inflammation of, 101, 102, 821–822
Umbilical hernia, 96, 102
Umbilical vein, inflammation of, 821–822
Umbilicus, inflammation of, 101–103, 102t
Undulant fever, 551
Urachus, inflammation of, 101–103, 821–822
    patent, 821
Uracils, in herbicides, toxicity of, 390t, 392
Uranium, mining of, water pollutants from, 378, 378t
Urea, efflux of, in ruminants, 199
    in herbicides, toxicity of, 390t, 392
    in protein supplementation, 199
        in dairy cattle, 211, 267, 267t
    nitrogen in, blood level of, 920t
    protein synthesis from, 226, 228t, 230, 234, 235t–237t
    toxicity of, 231
Ureaplasma infection, genitourinary, in goats, 479
    in cattle, 457–458

Urethra, hypospadiac, 96, 821
  muscle of, relaxation of, 818
  rupture of, urolithiasis and, 820
Uridine-5-monophosphate synthase, deficiency of, 96
Urinary tract. See also *Bladder* and *Kidney(s)*.
  congenital defects of, 96, 821
  disorders of, in neonate, 821–822
    in pigs, 827–828
  infection of, 817
    Eubacterium suis in, 519–521
  lithiasis of, 817t, 817–820
    in feedlot cattle, 141
    in lambs, 157
    pain in, 735
Urination, induction of, 818
Urticaria, 900–901
Uterine tube, disorders of, and infertility, 782
Uterus, atonic, in fetal membrane retention, 769
  congenital defects of, 97
  examination of, in infertility, in beef cattle, 802
  infection of, in feedlot cattle, 141
  inflammation of, 770–772
    and infertility, 784–785
  infusion into, for abortion induction, 791
  prolapse of, in feedlot cattle, 141
    pudendal nerve block for, 84
  pus in, in cattle, 772–773
    in trichomoniasis, 608, 609
  semen placement in, 780–781
  torsion of, pain in, 735
  tuberculosis of, 532
  ultrasonography of, 27t, 28–29
Uvea, disorders of, in camelids, 845–846
  inflammation of, in cattle, 837–838
    in lambs, 840
    mycoplasmal, in goats, 840, 841

Vaccination, against *Actinobacillus pleuropneumonia*, 551
  against anaplasmosis, 594–596, 595t
  against anthrax, 566t, 566–567
  against babesiosis, 586–587
  against bacillary hemoglobinuria, 571
  against besnoitiosis, 598
  against black disease, 573
  against blackleg, 570
  against border disease, 464
  against botulism, 569
  against bovine ephemeral fever, 449–450
  against bovine respiratory syncytial virus, 447
  against bovine viral diarrhea, 434
  against braxy, 572
  against brucellosis, 555
  against campylobacteriosis, in sheep, 509
  against cholera, 496
  against clostridial enterotoxemia, 575
  against coronavirus infection, 440
  against *Corynebacterium* infection, with lymphadenitis, 538
  against dermatophytosis, 892
  against ecthyma, contagious, 461
  against encephalitis, Japanese, 497

Vaccination (Continued)
  against enteroviral encephalomyelitis, 491
  against *Escherichia coli* infection, 518–519
  against foot rot, 873
  against foot-and-mouth disease, 438–439
  against gastroenteritis virus, transmissible, 499–500
  against *Haemophilus somnus* infection, 548
  against heartwater, 632, 632t
  against keratoconjunctivitis, infectious, 836–837
  against leptospirosis, 545
  against listeriosis, 583
  against papillomatosis, 431, 916
  against parainfluenza-3 virus, 444
  against paratuberculosis, 534
  against pasteurellosis, 556, 558
  against phlegmon, interdigital, 870
  against pneumonia, 643
    in cattle, beef, on feedlot, 660–661
      on pasture, 662
    dairy, 663
  against pox virus infection, 460
  against respiratory diseases, in sheep, 671
  against rhinotracheitis, 419
  against Rift Valley fever, in cattle, 442
    in sheep, 470
  against rinderpest, 446
  against rotavirus infection, in cattle, 440
    in pigs, 498
  against salmonellosis, 564
  against tuberculosis, 533
  against vesicular stomatitis virus, 448
  in prevention of diarrhea, in neonatal ruminant, 104–106, 109
  of calves, feeder, 180
    stocker, 132, 133
  of cattle, beef, calendar for, 123–124
    on feedlot, 141
  of goats, 164
  of llamas, 174
  of pigs, 170, 171
  of sheep, before breeding, 155t
  timing of, and immunoglobulins in colostrum, 98, 100
Vaccinia infection, and mammillitis, 423–425, 424, 424t
  of skin, 898
Vacor, in rodenticides, toxicity of, 385t, 386
Vagina, campylobacterial infection of, 510–513
  congenital defects of, 97
  Eubacterium suis infection of, 519
  infection of, viral, diagnosis of, 416t
  inflammation of, in cattle, 773–774
    in rhinotracheitis, 418
    pudendal nerve block for, 84
  trichomoniasis of, 608–611
Vagus nerve, gastrointestinal innervation by, 706, 706t
  in indigestion, 730–732, 731
  in reticuloperitonitis, traumatic, 720
Valbazen. See *Albendazole*.
Valine, dietary, for pigs, 280t
Valium, dosage of, 933t
  preanesthetic, 61t
Valsyn, dosage of, 931t, 933t
Vanadium, in water supply, 376, 376t

Vapona (dichlorvos), for nematode infestations, 754, 754t
  for parasitosis, external, 53t
  in anthelmintic therapy, 50
Vasopressin, and esophageal groove closure, 708
Veal, drug residues in, 34–35
Vebanol, dosage of, 933t
Vecoxan, for coccidiosis, 602, 603t
Vena cava, thrombosis of, 647–648, 649–652
Venom, toxicity of, 411t, 411–413, 412t
Ventricular septal defects, 96
Veratine, and gastrointestinal motility, 760
Veratrum species, as teratogens, 361, 839
  toxicity of, to heart, 353
    to nervous system, 358
Vermis, cerebellar, absence of, 858
Vernolate, toxicity of, 389t, 391
Verrucae. See *Papillomas*.
Verrucarin A, toxicity of, 332, 333
Verrucose dermatitis, 867
Vertebrae, anatomy of, 77, 78, 83, 83, 84
  congenital defects of, 96
  inflammation of, 877–878
Vertical wall cracks, 865
Vesicles, in ecthyma, 460, 461
  in foot-and-mouth disease, 438, 438
  in pigs, 494, 494–495, 495
Vesicular disease, in pigs, 899
  parvovirus and, 900
  viral, 491–492
Vesicular exanthema, 488–489, 899
Vesicular stomatitis, viral, 899
  in cattle, 447–448
  in pigs, 504
Vesiculitis, 793–794
  in chlamydiosis, 455–456
Vestibular system, disease of, cerebellum in, 860
  ocular signs of, 855
Vestibulocochlear nerve, anatomy of, 852
Vestibulovaginitis, 773
Vetalog. See *Triamcinolone*.
Vetame, dosage of, 933t
  preanesthetic, 61t
Vetch, hairy, toxicity of, to skin, 363–364, 906
Vetisulid, dosage of, 932t
Vetrophin, dosage of, 931t
Vicia villosa (hairy vetch), toxicity of, to skin, 363–364, 906
Vicuñas. See *Camelids*.
Vigilante, for parasitosis, 56t
Villi, intestinal, in diarrhea, in piglet, 113
Vincristine, for lymphosarcoma, 850
Viral infection. See also specific diseases, e.g., *Rabies*.
  control of, embryo transfer in, 786
  diagnosis of, 414–417, 416t
  in cattle, 417–455
  in goats, 459–479
  in pigs, 480–504
  in sheep, 459–479
  nasal, diagnosis of, 676
  of skin, 898–900
Viremia, and hemorrhage, diagnosis of, 416t
Virginiamycin, for dysentery, 561t
Vision, loss of, causes of, 854t, 855, 856
  testing of, 830
Visna, 470–471
Vitamin A, deficiency of, and infertility, 783–784

Vitamin A (Continued)
　　ocular signs of, 854t, 856
　　skin lesions in, 911
　for stocker calves, 132
　nutritional requirement for, 200–203
　　in beef cattle, 122, 123t
　　　in breeding herd, 253t, 259
　　　in pregnancy and lactation, 206t, 208
　　in cattle, 251–252, 252t
　　　dairy, 270t, 271t
　　　　in pregnancy and lactation, 212, 213, 213t, 214t
　　in goats, 274t, 275t, 278
　　in pigs, 280t, 281
　　　in pregnancy and lactation, 215
　　in sheep, in pregnancy and lactation, 219
　supplementation with, for cattle, grazing, 291–292
Vitamin B_1. See Thiamine.
Vitamin B_6, nutritional requirement for, in pigs, 280t, 282
Vitamin B_{12}, for anemia, 701
　nutritional requirement for, in pigs, 280t, 282
　　in pregnancy and lactation, 215, 216
Vitamin C, deficiency of, skin lesions in, 911
　in immunotherapy, 16
Vitamin D, metabolism of, in acidosis, 18
　nutritional requirement for, in cattle, 252, 252t
　　dairy, 268, 270t, 271t
　　in goats, 274t
　　in pigs, 280t, 281
　　in pregnancy and lactation, 215
　toxicity of, to kidney, 825t
Vitamin D_3, in milk fever, 268, 305, 307t, 308
　toxicity of, in rodenticides, 383–385, 384t, 385t
　　to kidney, 825t
Vitamin E, deficiency of, in white muscle disease, 689–690
　　skin lesions in, 911
　dosage of, 933t
　for stocker calves, 131
　nutritional requirement for, for llamas, 175, 175t
　　in cattle, 252, 252t
　　　dairy, 268, 270t
　　in pigs, 280t, 281, 283
　　in pregnancy and lactation, 215
Vitamin K, dosage of, 931t, 933t
　nutritional requirement for, in pigs, 280t, 281
　　in pregnancy and lactation, 215
Vitamin K_1 (Aquamephyton), dosage of, 931t
　for hemorrhage, in mastitis, 768
　for sweet clover poisoning, 359
　in anticoagulant rodenticide poisoning, 383
Vitiligo, 914
Vitreous, examination of, 831
Volvulus, abomasal, 725–730, 727, 729, 730t, 735
　cecocolic, 739–740
　of mesentery, 734, 735
Vomiting, anesthesia and, 59
　with encephalitis and wasting, 492–493
Vomitoxin, 332–334

von Willebrand factor, deficiency of, 698
Vulvovaginitis, in rhinotracheitis, 418
　pustular, 773–774

Wall cracks, horizontal, 865–866
　vertical, 865
Warbex, for parasitosis, external, 53t
Warbles, 888
Warfarin, toxicity of, 383, 384t
Warts. See Papillomas.
Water (fluid), administration of, in anesthesia, 75–76
　geothermal, toxicants in, 377–380, 378, 379
　in mine tailings, toxicants in, 377–380, 378, 378t
　industrial coolant, toxicants in, 377–378
　intake of, in cattle, 252, 252t
　　beef, in breeding herd, 260, 260t
　　range-fed, 292–293
　　in oxalate poisoning, 365
　　in pigs, 282, 282t
　　in sheep, in pregnancy and lactation, 219
　　in sodium toxicosis, 328–329
　loss of, in diarrhea, in neonate, 104
　mineral content of, 292, 295
　quality of, 375t, 375–377, 376t
　replacement therapy with, 1–2
　　in calves, 2t, 2–5, 5t
　　in cattle, 5–6, 7
　total body content of, 1
Water hemlock, toxicity of, 346, 350t
　to central nervous system, 358
Water moccasin bites, 411
Waterbelly, in urolithiasis, 820
　in feedlot cattle, 141
Wattle cysts, 918
Wattles, 910
Weaning, of heifer, in beef herd replacement program, 256–257
　of lamb, 157–158
　　in limited forage conditions, 221
　　in prevention of respiratory disease, 671–672
　of piglet, 170–172
　　in prevention of pneumonia, 667
Weather. See Temperature.
Weaver syndrome, 92
Weight, loss of, in abomasal emptying defect, 736–737
　　with encephalitis and vomiting, 492–493
　pounds to kilograms, conversion of, 934t
Wheat, protein in, metabolism of, 235t, 243t
　toxicity of, 351t
Wheezing, auscultation of, 675
Whipworm infestation, 47–50, 752–754, 754t
White blood cells, disorders of, 696t, 696–698
　laboratory count of, 690–692, 692t, 919t, 920t
　production of, 692–693
White muscle disease, 689–690
　prevention of, in goats, 164
　　in sheep, 154
White snakeroot, toxicity of, 349, 350t
Willebrand factor, deficiency of, 698

Wisconsin system, in feed protein estimation, 236–240, 238, 240t, 241t
Wisteria, toxicity of, 351t
Wolffian duct, defects of, 96–97
Wood shavings, in bedding, and mycobacterial disease, 529, 531
Worms, parasitic, cestode, 757–758
　helminthic, 47–51
　nematode, in cattle, 743–748, 746t–748t
　　in goats, 752
　　in pigs, 752–754, 754t
　　in sheep, 748–752

Xanthine, in urolithiasis, 819
Xanthium species, toxicity of, 350t, 351t, 352
　to kidney, 825t
Xylazine, adverse reactions to, 21
　and hypoxemia, 59
　dosage of, 933t
　for tetanus, 568
　in abscess extirpation, in caseous lymphadenitis, 538
　in anesthesia, with guaifenesin and ketamine, 65–66
　　with Telazol, 67
　in capture of ruminants, 62–63
　in cerebrospinal fluid sampling, 861
　in eye examination, 830
　in induction of parturition, 815
　in reduction of coxofemoral luxation, 877
　in scar removal, in posthitis, 540
　in spinal analgesia, 82–83
　preanesthetic, 60–62, 61t
Xylocaine. See Lidocaine.

Yeasts, as feed additives, 187
　infection with, 524–528
　　cutaneous, 894
Yellow jessamine, toxicity of, 350t
Yellow lamb disease, 573
Yew, toxicity of, 350t, 353, 371–372
Yohimbine, as antagonist to xylazine sedation, 62

Zea mays. See Corn.
Zearalenol, toxicity of, 332, 333
Zearalenone, toxicity of, 332, 333
Zeranol, as growth stimulant, 181, 181t, 182, 183t
　dosage of, 933t
　residue of, in calf, 35
Zinc, deficiency of, hereditary, and parakeratosis, 909
　in keratogenesis imperfecta, 95
　skin lesions in, 912
　in copper metabolism, 397, 398
　in water supply, 376, 376t
　nutritional requirement for, in cattle, 251, 252t, 260t, 270t
　　in pigs, 280, 280t
　　in pregnancy and lactation, 215
　　in sheep, in pregnancy and lactation, 218
　supplemental, for grazing cattle, 296t, 297–298, 299t, 300
　toxicity of, to kidney, 823t

Zinc phosphide, in rodenticides, toxicity of, 384t, 385t, 386
Zinc sulfate, for dermatitis, digital, 869
 for dermatophilosis, 895
 for foot rot, 873
 in precipitation test, for passive immunity, 99
Zolazepam, in anesthesia, 67
 in capture of ruminants, 63
Zona pellucida, in embryo transfer, 785–787, 786
Zootoxins, 411t, 411–413, 412t
Zwoegerziekte, 470–471
Zygadenus species, toxicity of, 346, 351t
Zygomycosis, 524–526, 528
Zygote, abnormalities of, and infertility, 781–782